FIFTH EDITION

WYLLIE'S TREATMENT OF EPILEPSY

PRINCIPLES AND PRACTICE

WYLLIE'S TREATMENT OF EPILEPSY

PRINCIPLES AND PRACTICE

Editor-in-Chief

Elaine Wyllie, MD
Professor of Pediatric Medicine
Cleveland Clinic Lerner College of Medicine
Director of the Center for Pediatric Neurology
Neurological Institute
Cleveland Clinic
Cleveland, Ohio

Associate Editors

**Gregory D. Cascino,
MD, FAAN**
Professor of Neurology
Mayo Clinic College of Medicine
Chair, Division of Epilepsy
Mayo Clinic
Rochester, Minnesota

Barry E. Gidal, PharmD
Professor, School of Pharmacy and
Department of Neurology
Chair, Pharmacy Practice Division
University of Wisconsin
Madison, Wisconsin

Howard P. Goodkin, MD, PhD
The Shure Associate Professor
of Pediatric Neurology
Departments of Neurology and Pediatrics
University of Virginia
Charlottesville, Virginia

Wolters Kluwer | Lippincott Williams & Wilkins
Health

Philadelphia · Baltimore · New York · London
Buenos Aires · Hong Kong · Sydney · Tokyo

Acquisitions Editor: Fran Destefano
Product Manager: Tom Gibbons
Vendor Manager: Alicia Jackson
Senior Manufacturing Manager: Ben Rivera
Marketing Manager: Brian Freiland
Design Coordinator: Steve Druding
Production Service: MPS Limited, a Macmillan Company

5th Edition
© 2011 by Lippincott Williams & Wilkins, a Wolters Kluwer business
Two Commerce Square
2001 Market Street
Philadelphia, PA 19103 USA
LWW.com

Printed in China.

Library of Congress Cataloging-in-Publication Data
Wyllie's treatment of epilepsy : principles and practice. — 5th ed. / editor-in-chief, Elaine Wyllie ; associate editors, Gregory D. Cascino, Barry E. Gidal, Howard P. Goodkin.
    p. ; cm.
  Other title: Treatment of epilepsy
  Rev. ed. of: The treatment of epilepsy. 4th ed. / editor-in-chief, Elaine Wyllie. c2006.
  Includes bibliographical references and index.
  Summary: "In one convenient source, this book provides a broad, detailed, and cohesive overview of seizure disorders and contemporary treatment options. For this Fifth Edition, the editors have replaced or significantly revised approximately 30 to 50 percent of the chapters, and have updated all of them. Dr. Wyllie has invited three new editors: Gregory Cascino, MD, at Mayo Clinic, adult epileptologist with special expertise in neuroimaging; Barry Gidal, PharmD, RPh, at University of Wisconsin, a pharmacologist with phenomenal expertise in antiepileptic medications; and Howard Goodkin, MD, PhD, a pediatric neurologist at the University of Virginia. A fully searchable companion website will include the full text online and supplementary material such as seizure videos, additional EEG tracings, and more color illustrations"—Provided by publisher.
  ISBN-13: 978-1-58255-937-7 (hardback)
  ISBN-10: 1-58255-937-6 (hardback)
  1. Epilepsy. I. Wyllie, Elaine. II. Treatment of epilepsy. III. Title: Treatment of epilepsy.
  [DNLM: 1. Epilepsy—therapy. 2. Epilepsy—diagnosis. WL 385 W983 2011]
  RC372.T68 2011
  616.8'53—dc22

                                        2010024726

To purchase additional copies of this book, call our customer service department at (800) 638-3030 or fax orders to (301) 223-2320. International customers should call (301) 223-2300.

Visit Lippincott Williams & Wilkins on the Internet: at LWW.com. Lippincott Williams & Wilkins customer service representatives are available from 8:30 am to 6 pm, EST.

                                        10 9 8 7 6 5 4 3 2 1

DEDICATION

*To the **Cleveland Clinic,** which brought me on board as a young doctor and provided me career opportunities beyond my wildest imagination*

*To our Chief Executive Officer, **Dr. Delos Cosgrove,** whose visionary leadership has brought the Cleveland Clinic to where we are today, at the forefront of medical care throughout the world*

*And to my husband, **Dr. Robert Wyllie,** Physician-in-Chief of the Cleveland Clinic Children's Hospital, who provides the environment for all of us who care for children to do our best work*

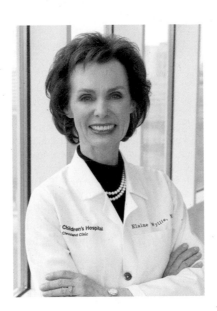

Dr. Elaine Wyllie, on campus at the Cleveland Clinic

CONTRIBUTING AUTHORS

Harry S. Abram, M.D.
Assistant Professor of Pediatrics and Neurology
Mayo Clinic Florida—Nemours Children's Clinic
Director, Neurophysiology Laboratory, Department
of Pediatrics
Wolfson Children's Hospital
Jacksonville, Florida

Andreas V. Alexopoulos, M.D., M.P.H.
Cleveland Clinic Lerner Research Institute
Cleveland Clinic Epilepsy Center
Cleveland Clinic
Cleveland, Ohio

Ulrich Altrup, M.D. (Deceased)
Department of Neurology
Institute for Experimental Epilepsy Research
Muenster, Germany

Frederick Andermann, O.C., M.D., F.R.C.P. (C.)
Professor of Neurology and Pediatrics
McGill University
Director, Epilepsy Service
Montreal Neurological Hospital and Institute
Montreal, Quebec, Canada

Anne Anderson, M.D.
Associate Professor of Pediatrics, Neurology,
and Neuroscience
Baylor College of Medicine
Medical Director, Epilepsy Monitoring Unit
Investigator, Cain Foundation Laboratories
Texas Children's Hospital
Houston, Texas

Gail D. Anderson, Ph.D.
Professor of Pharmacy
University of Washington
Seattle, Washington

Alexis Arzimanoglou, M.D.
Associate Professor
University Hospitals of Lyon and INSERM U821
Head, Institute for Children and Adolescents with Epilepsy
IDEE and Pediatric Neurophysiology
Hopital Femme Mere Enfant (HCL)
Lyon, France

Thomas Bast, M.D.
Head Physician
Epilepsy Clinic for Children and Adolescents
Epilepsy Centre Kork
Kehl, Germany

Jocelyn F. Bautista, M.D.
Assistant Professor of Medicine
Cleveland Clinic Lerner College of Medicine
Cleveland Clinic
Cleveland, Ohio

Selim R. Benbadis, M.D.
Professor of Neurology
University of South Florida
Director of Epilepsy and EEG
Tampa General Hospital
Tampa, Florida

T.A. Benke, M.D., Ph.D.
Associate Professor of Pediatrics, Neurology, and
Pharmacology
University of Colorado Denver, School
of Medicine
Children's Hospital
Aurora, Colorado

Anne T. Berg, Ph.D.
Research Professor of Biology
Northern Illinois University
DeKalb, Illinois
Professor, Epilepsy Center
Northwestern Children's Memorial Hospital
Chicago, Illinois

William E. Bingaman, M.D.
Head, Epilepsy Surgery
Vice Chairman, Neurological Institute
The Richard and Karen Shusterman Family Endowed Chair
in Epilepsy Surgery
Professor in Surgery
Cleveland Clinic Lerner College of Medicine of Case Western
Reserve University
Cleveland Clinic
Cleveland, Ohio

Angela K. Birnbaum, Ph.D.
Associate Professor of Experimental and Clinical
Pharmacology
University of Minnesota
Minneapolis, Minnesota

Jane G. Boggs, M.D.
Associate Professor of Neurology
Wake Forest University
Winston Salem, North Carolina

Blaise F. D. Bourgeois, M.D.
Professor of Neurology
Harvard Medical School
Director, Division of Epilepsy and Clinical Neurophysiology
Children's Hospital
Boston, Massachusetts

Jeffrey W. Britton, M.D.
Assistant Professor of Neurology
Divisions of Clinical Neurophysiology—EEG and Epilepsy
Mayo Clinic
Rochester, Minnesota

Paula M. Brna, M.D., F.R.C.P. (C.)
Assistant Professor of Pediatrics
Dalhousie University
Pediatric Neurologist
IWK Health Centre
Halifax, Nova Scotia, Canada

Martin J. Brodie, M.D.
Professor of Medicine and Clinical Pharmacology
Division of Cardiovascular and Medical Sciences
University of Glasgow
Clinical and Research Director, Epilepsy Unit
Western Infirmary
Glasgow, Scotland

Amy R. Brooks-Kayal, M.D.
Professor of Pediatrics and Neurology
University of Colorado School of Medicine
Chief and Ponzio Family Chair in Pediatric Neurology
Children's Hospital
Aurora, Colorado

Richard C. Burgess, M.D., Ph.D.
Adjunct Professor of Biomedical Engineering
Case Western Reserve University
Director, MEG Laboratory
Cleveland Clinic
Cleveland, Ohio

Richard W. Byrne, M.D.
Professor and Chairman, Department of Neurosurgery
Rush University Medical School
Chicago, Illinois

Carol S. Camfield, M.D.
Professor Emeritus of Child Neurology
Dalhousie University
Halifax, Nova Scotia, Canada

Peter R. Camfield, M.D.
Professor Emeritus of Child Neurology
Dalhousie University
Halifax, Nova Scotia, Canada

Gregory D. Cascino, M.D., F.A.A.N.
Professor of Neurology
Mayo Clinic College of Medicine
Chair, Division of Epilepsy
Mayo Clinic
Rochester, Minnesota

Kevin E. Chapman, M.D.
Department of Pediatric Neurology
Barrow Neurological Institute
St. Joseph's Hospital and Medical Center
Phoenix, Arizona

Jean E. Cibula, M.D.
Assistant Professor of Neurology
University of Florida
Medical Director, EEG Lab
University of Florida Comprehensive Epilepsy Program
Shands Hospital at the University of Florida
Gainesville, Florida

Robert R. Clancy, M.D.
Professor of Neurology and Pediatrics
University of Pennsylvania School of Medicine
Children's Hospital of Philadelphia
Philadelphia, Pennsylvania

J. Helen Cross, M.B., Ch.B., Ph.D., F.R.C.P.C.H., F.R.C.P.
Prince of Wales's Chair of Childhood Epilepsy
UCL Institute of Child Health
Honorary Consultant in Paediatric Neurology
Great Ormond Street Hospital
London, England

Luigi D'Argenzio, M.D.
Epilepsy Fellow, Neuroscience Unit
UCL—Institute of Child Health
London, United Kingdom
Clinical Fellow in Paediatric Neurology
National Centre for Young People with Epilepsy
Lingfield, Surrey, United Kingdom

Stefanie Darnley, B.A.
Research Assistant in Neurology
Johns Hopkins University School of Medicine
Baltimore, Maryland

Rohit R. Das, M.D., M.P.H.
Assistant Professor of Neurology
University of Louisville
Attending Neurologist and Epileptologist
Kosair Children's and University of Louisville Hospitals
Louisville, Kentucky

Anita Datta, M.D., F.R.C.P.C.
Clinical Assistant Professor of Pediatric Neurology
Pediatric Neurologist/Epileptologist
University of Saskatchewan
Royal University Hospital
Saskatoon, Saskatchewan, Canada

Norman Delanty, M.D., F.R.C.P.I.
Honorary Senior Lecturer in Molecular and
Cellular Therapeutics
Royal College of Surgeons in Ireland
Consultant Neurologist, Epilepsy Programme
Beaumont Hospital
Dublin, Ireland

Robert J. DeLorenzo, M.D., Ph.D., M.P.H.
George Bliley Professor of Neurology
Professor of Pharmacology and Toxicology
Professor of Molecular Biophysics and Biochemistry
Virginia Commonwealth University
Virginia Commonwealth University Hospital
Richmond, Virginia

Darryl C. De Vivo, M.D.
Sidney Carter Professor of Neurology and Professor
of Pediatrics
Columbia University College of Physicians and Surgeons
New York Presbyterian Hospital
University Hospital of Columbia and Cornell
New York, New York

Beate Diehl, M.D.
Department of Clinical and Experimental Epilepsy
Institute of Neurology, University College London
Consultant Clinical Neurophysiologist
National Hospital for Neurology and Neurosurgery
London, United Kingdom

Ding Ding, M.D., M.P.H.
Associate Professor of Biostatistics and Epidemiology
Fudan University
Hua Shan Hospital
Shanghai, People's Republic of China

Joseph Drazkowski, M.D.
Associate Professor of Neurology
Mayo Clinic Arizona
Phoenix, Arizona

François Dubeau, M.D.
Assistant Professor of Neurology and Neurosurgery
McGill University
Montreal Neurological Hospital and Institute
Montreal, Quebec, Canada

Michael Duchowny, M.D.
Professor of Neurology and Pediatrics
University of Miami Miller School of Medicine
Director, Comprehensive Epilepsy Center,
Brain Institute
Miami Children's Hospital
Miami, Florida

Stephan Eisenschenk, M.D.
Associate Professor of Neurology
University of Florida
Director, UF/Shands Comprehensive Epilepsy Program
Shands Hospital
Gainesville, Florida

Dana Ekstein, M.D.
Hebrew University School of Medicine
Hadassah University Medical Center
Jerusalem, Israel

Christian E. Elger, M.D., F.R.C.P.
Professor of Epileptology
University of Bonn
Head, Department of Epileptology
University of Bonn Medical Centre
Bonn, Germany

Edward Faught, M.D.
Professor of Neurology
Emory University
Chief, Neurology Service
Emory University Hospital Midtown
Atlanta, Georgia

Jacqueline A. French, M.D.
Professor of Neurology
New York University School of Medicine
Academic Director, Comprehensive
Epilepsy Center
New York University-Langone Medical Center
New York, New York

Neil Friedman, M.D., Ch.B.
Center for Pediatric Neurology
Neurological Institute, Cleveland Clinic
Cleveland, Ohio

William Davis Gaillard, M.D.
Professor of Neurology and Pediatrics
George Washington University and Georgetown University
Chief, Division of Epilepsy, Neurophysiology and Critical
Care Neurology
Children's National Medical Center
Washington, D.C.

Deana M. Gazzola, M.D.
Instructor in Neurology
New York University School of Medicine
New York University-Langone Medical Center
New York, New York

Barry E. Gidal, Pharm.D.
Professor, School of Pharmacy and Department of Neurology
Chair, Pharmacy Practice Division
University of Wisconsin
Madison, Wisconsin

Frank G. Gilliam, M.D., M.P.H.
Director of Neurology
Geisinger Health System
Wilkes-Barre and Danville, Pennsylvania

Robin L. Gilmore, M.D.
Staff Neurologist
Maury Regional Medical Center
Columbia, Tennessee

Tracy A. Glauser, M.D.
Professor of Pediatrics
University of Cincinnati College of Medicine
Director, Comprehensive Epilepsy Center
Cincinnati Children's Hospital Medical Center
Cincinnati, Ohio

Cristina Y. Go, M.D.
Neurologist and Clinical Neurophysiologist
Paediatric Epilepsy Fellowship Training Co-director
The Hospital for Sick Children
Toronto, Ontario, Canada

Jorge A. González-Martínez, M.D., Ph.D.
Staff, Epilepsy Surgery
Epilepsy Center
Cleveland Clinic Neurological Institute
Cleveland, Ohio

Howard P. Goodkin, M.D., Ph.D.
The Shure Associate Professor of Pediatric Neurology
Departments of Neurology and Pediatrics
University of Virginia
Charlottesville, Virginia

L. John Greenfield, Jr., M.D., Ph.D.
Professor and Chairman
Department of Neurology
University of Arkansas for Medical Sciences
Little Rock, Arkansas

Varda Gross-Tsur, M.D.
Associate Professor
Hebrew University—Hadassah Hospital
Director, Child Development Unit
Shaare Zedek Medical Center
Jerusalem, Israel

Carlos A. M. Guerreiro, M.D., Ph.D.
Professor of Neurology
University of Campinas (Unicamp)
Campinas, Sao Paolo, Brazil

Marilisa M. Guerreiro, M.D., Ph.D.
Professor of Pediatric Neurology
Head, Child Neurology Section
University of Campinas (Unicamp)
Campinas, Sao Paolo, Brazil

Renzo Guerrini, M.D.
Professor of Child Neurology and Psychiatry
University of Florence
Director, Pediatric Neurology
Children's Hospital A. Meyer
Florence, Italy

Ajay Gupta, M.D.
Assistant Professor of Pediatric Epilepsy
Cleveland Clinic Lerner College of Medicine
Cleveland Clinic
Cleveland, Ohio

Andreas Hahn, M.D.
Associate Professor of Neuropediatrics
Justus-Liebig-University Giessen
Assistant Medical Director, Neuropediatrics
University Hospital Giessen
Giessen, Germany

Stephen Hantus, M.D.
Associate Staff
Cleveland Clinic Epilepsy Center
Cleveland, Ohio

Cynthia L. Harden, M.D.
Professor of Neurology, Clinical Educator Track
Director, Division of Epilepsy
University of Miami Miller School of Medicine
Attending Neurologist
Jackson Memorial Hospital
University of Miami Hospital
Miami, Florida

W. Allen Hauser, M.D.
Professor of Neurology and Epidemiology
Columbia University
New York, New York

Lara Jehi, M.D.
Assistant Professor of Neurology
Cleveland Clinic Lerner College of Medicine
Epilepsy Center, Cleveland Clinic
Cleveland, Ohio

Stephen E. Jones, M.D., Ph.D.
Imaging Institute
Cleveland Clinic
Cleveland, Ohio

Stephen P. Kalhorn, M.D.
Department of Neurosurgery
New York University Langone Medical Center
New York, New York

Andres M. Kanner, M.D.
Professor of Neurological Sciences and Psychiatry
Rush Medical College at Rush University
Director, Laboratories of Electroencephalography
and Video-EEG Telemetry
Associate Director, Section of Epilepsy and Rush
Epilepsy Center
Rush University Medical Center
Chicago, Illinois

Christoph Kellinghaus, M.D.
Head of Section, Epilepsy/EEG
Klinikum Osnabrück
Osnabrück, Germany

John F. Kerrigan, M.D.
Assistant Professor of Clinical Pediatrics and Neurology
University of Arizona College of Medicine–Phoenix
Director, Pediatric Epilepsy Program
Co-director, Hypothalamic Hamartoma Program
Barrow Neurological Institute
St. Joseph's Hospital and Medical Center
Phoenix, Arizona

Prakash Kotagal, M.D.
Head, Section of Pediatric Epilepsy
Epilepsy Center
Cleveland Clinic
Cleveland, Ohio

Gregory Krauss, M.D.
Professor of Neurology
Johns Hopkins Hospital
Baltimore, Maryland

Ruben Kuzniecky, M.D.
Professor of Neurology
New York University
Co-director, NYU Epilepsy Center
New York University Hospital
New York, New York

Patrick Kwan, M.D.
Division of Neurology
Department of Medicine and Therapeutics
The Chinese University of Hong Kong
Prince of Wales Hospital
Hong Kong

Kay Kyllonen, Pharm.D., F.P.P.A.G.
Clinical Specialist in Pediatrics
Pharmacy Department
Cleveland Clinic
Cleveland, Ohio

Beth A. Leeman, M.D.
Assistant Professor of Neurology
Emory University
Physician, Neurology Service
Atlanta VA Medical Center
Atlanta, Georgia
Assistant in Neuroscience, Department of Neurology
Massachusetts General Hospital
Boston, Massachusetts

Louis Lemieux, B.Sc., M.Sc., Ph.D.
Professor of Physics Applied to Medical Imaging
Department of Clinical and Experimental Epilepsy
UCL Institute of Neurology
London, United Kingdom

Ilo E. Leppik, M.D.
Professor of Pharmacy and Adjunct Professor
of Neurology
Director of Epilepsy Research and Education Program
College of Pharmacy
University of Minnesota
Director of Research
MINCEP Epilepsy Care
Minneapolis, Minnesota

Christine Linehan, Ph.D.
Senior Researcher, Centre for Disability Studies
University College Dublin
Dublin, Ireland

Tobias Loddenkemper, M.D.
Assistant Professor of Neurology
Harvard Medical School
Children's Hospital
Boston, Massachusetts

Hans O. Lüders, M.D., Ph.D.
Professor of Neurology
Case Medical School
Epilepsy Center Director
University Hospitals
Cleveland, Ohio

Susan E. Marino, Ph.D.
Assistant Professor and Director of Experimental
and Clinical Pharmacology
Center for Clinical and Cognitive Neuropharmacology
University of Minnesota
Minneapolis, Minnesota

Robert C. Martinez, M.D.
Instructor in Neurology, Epilepsy Division
University of Miami Miller School of Medicine
Jackson Memorial Hospital, University of Miami Hospital
Miami, Florida

Gary W. Mathern, M.D.
Professor of Neurosurgery and Psychiatry & Behavioral
Sciences
Intellectual and Developmental Disabilities Research Center
Brain Research Institute
David Geffen School of Medicine
University of California, Los Angeles
Neurosurgical Director, Pediatric Epilepsy Surgery Program
and Neurobiology of Epilepsy Research Laboratory
Ronald Reagan Medical Center
Los Angeles, California

Michael J. McLean, M.D., Ph.D.
Associate Professor of Neurology
Vanderbilt University Medical Center
Nashville, Tennessee

Kimford J. Meador, M.D.
Professor of Neurology
Emory University
Director of Epilepsy
Emory University Hospital
Atlanta, Georgia

Mohamad Mikati, M.D.
Wilburt C. Davison Distinguished Professor of Pediatrics
Professor of Neurobiology
Duke University
Chief, Division of Pediatric Neurology
Duke University Medical Center
Durham, North Carolina

Ghayda Mirzaa, M.D.
Fellow, Clinical Genetics
Department of Human Genetics
University of Chicago
Chicago, Illinois

Eli M. Mizrahi, M.D.
Chair of Neurology
Professor of Neurology and Pediatrics
Director, Clinical Neurophysiology Residency Program
Baylor College of Medicine
Chief, Neurophysiology Service
St. Luke's Episcopal Hospital
Houston, Texas

Ahsan N.V. Moosa, M.D.
Epilepsy Center, Neurological Institute
Cleveland Clinic
Cleveland, Ohio

Diego A. Morita, M.D.
Assistant Professor of Pediatrics and Neurology
University of Cincinnati College of Medicine
Director, New Onset Seizure Program
Cincinnati Children's Hospital Medical Center
Cincinnati, Ohio

Bernd A. Neubauer, M.D.
Head, Department of Neuropediatrics
University of Giessen
Giessen, Germany

Katherine C. Nickels, M.D.
Assistant Professor of Neurology
Senior Associate Consultant
Mayo Clinic
Rochester, Minnesota

Soheyl Noachtar, M.D.
Professor of Neurology
Head, Epilepsy Center
University of Munich
Munich, Germany

Douglas R. Nordli, Jr., M.D.
Professor of Pediatrics
Northwestern University Feinberg School of Medicine
Lorna S. and James P. Langdon Chair of
Pediatric Epilepsy
Children's Memorial Hospital
Chicago, Illinois

Christine O'Dell, R.N., M.S.N.
Clinical Nurse Specialist, Neurology
Montefiore Medical Center
New York, New York

Karine Ostrowsky-Coste, M.D.
University Hospitals of France
Institute for Children and Adolescents with Epilepsy—IDEE
and Pediatric Neurophysiology
Hopital Femme Mere Infant (HCL)
Lyon, France

Alison M. Pack, M.D.
Associate Professor of Clinical Neurology
Columbia University
New York Presbyterian Hospital
New York, New York

Sumit Parikh, M.D.
Center for Pediatric Neurology
Neurological Institute
Cleveland Clinic
Cleveland, Ohio

John M. Pellock, M.D.
Professor and Chair of Child Neurology
Virginia Commonwealth University
Richmond, Virginia

Page B. Pennell, M.D.
Associate Professor of Neurology
Harvard Medical School
Director of Research for Division of Epilepsy and Sleep
Brigham and Women's Hospital
Boston, Massachusetts

Andrew Pickens IV, M.D., J.D., M.B.A.
Medical Director, Duke Raleigh Emergency Department,
Quality Improvement
Raleigh, North Carolina

Bernd Pohlmann-Eden, M.D., Ph.D.
Professor of Neurology and Pharmacology
Dalhousie University
Co-director, Epilepsy Program
Queen Elizabeth II Health Science Centre
Halifax, Canada

Richard A. Prayson, M.D.
Professor of Pathology
Cleveland Clinic Lerner College of Medicine
Section Head, Neuropathology
Cleveland Clinic
Cleveland, Ohio

Janet Reid, M.D., F.R.C.P.C.
Section Head of Pediatric Radiology
Children's Hospital Cleveland Clinic
Cleveland, Ohio

James J. Riviello, Jr., M.D.
George Peterkin Endowed Chair in Pediatrics
Professor of Pediatrics and Neurology
Baylor College of Medicine
Chief of Neurophysiology
Texas Children's Hospital
Houston, Texas

Howard C. Rosenberg, M.D., Ph.D.
Professor of Physiology and Pharmacology
University of Toledo College of Medicine
Toledo, Ohio

William E. Rosenfeld, M.D.
Director
Comprehensive Epilepsy Care Center for Children and Adults
Chesterfield, Missouri

Jonathan Roth, M.D.
Pediatric Neurosurgery Fellow
New York University Langone Medical Center
New York, New York

Paul M. Ruggieri, M.D.
Head, Section of Neuroradiology and MRI
Cleveland Clinic
Cleveland, Ohio

Steven C. Schachter, M.D.
Professor of Neurology
Harvard Medical School
Chief Academic Officer
Center for Integration of Medicine and Innovative Technology
Boston, Massachusetts

Stephan Schuele, M.D., M.P.H.
Assistant Professor of Neurology
Northwestern University
Feinberg School of Medicine
Director, Northwestern University Comprehensive
Epilepsy Center
Chicago, Illinois

Raj D. Sheth, M.D.
Professor of Neurology
Mayo Clinic College of Medicine
Nemours Children's Clinic
Jacksonville, Florida

Shlomo Shinnar, M.D., Ph.D.
Professor of Neurology, Pediatrics and Epidemiology and
Population Health
Hyman Climenko Professor of Neuroscience Research
Albert Einstein College of Medicine
Director, Comprehensive Epilepsy Management Center
Montefiore Medical Center
New York, New York

Joseph I. Sirven, M.D.
Professor and Chairman, Neurology
Mayo Clinic
Phoenix, Arizona

Michael C. Smith, M.D.
Professor of Neurological Sciences
Rush University
Director and Senior Attending Neurologist,
Rush Epilepsy Center
Rush University Medical Center
Chicago, Illinois

O. Carter Snead III, M.D.
Professor of Medicine, Paediatrics and Pharmacology
University of Toronto
Head, Division of Neurology (Pediatrics)
Hospital for Sick Children
Toronto, Ontario, Canada

Elson L. So, M.D.
Professor of Neurology
Mayo Clinic
Rochester, Minnesota

Norman K. So, M.B., B.Chir.
Epilepsy Center
Neurological Institute
Cleveland Clinic
Cleveland, Ohio

Erwin-Josef Speckmann, M.D.
Professor Emeritus
Institute of Physiology (Neurophysiology)
University of Münster
Münster, Germany

Martin Staudt, M.D.
Professor of Developmental Neuroplasticity
Eberhard-Karls University
Tübingen, Germany
Vice Director, Clinic for Neuropediatrics and
Neurorehabilitation, Epilepsy Center for Children
and Adolescents
Schön-Klinik Vogtareuth
Vogtareuth, Germany

S. Matthew Stead, M.D., Ph.D.
Assistant Professor of Neurology
Mayo Clinic
Rochester, Minnesota

William O. Tatum IV, D.O.
Professor of Neurology
Mayo Clinic College of Medicine
Director, Epilepsy Monitoring Unit
Mayo Hospital
Jacksonville, Florida

Elizabeth A. Thiele, M.D., Ph.D.
Associate Professor of Neurology
Harvard Medical School
Director, Pediatric Epilepsy Program
Massachusetts General Hospital
Boston, Massachusetts

Elizabeth I. Tietz, M.D.
Professor and Vice-Chair of Physiology and Pharmacology
University of Toledo College of Medicine
Toledo, Ohio

Ingrid Tuxhorn, M.D.
Professor of Medicine
Case Western Reserve University
Cleveland Clinic Lerner Research Center
Neurologic Institute at the Cleveland Clinic Epilepsy Center
Cleveland, Ohio

Basim M. Uthman, M.D., F.A.C.I.P., F.A.A.N.
Professor of Neurology
Director, Neurology Clerkship
Weill Cornell Medical College in Qatar
Qatar Foundation Education City
Doha, Qatar

Fernando L. Vale, M.D.
Professor and Vice-Chair, Department of Neurosurgery
University of South Florida
Tampa General Hospital
Tampa, Florida

Tonicarlo R. Velasco, M.D.
Neurophysiologist
Department of Neurology, Psychiatry and
Behavioral Sciences
University of Sao Paulo
Executive Director, Adult Epilepsy Surgery Program
Hospital das Clinicas de Ribeirao Preto-CIREP
Ribeirao Preto, Sao Paulo, Brazil

Elizabeth Waterhouse, M.D.
Professor of Neurology
Virginia Commonwealth University School of Medicine
Richmond, Virginia

Tim Wehner, M.D.
Department of Neurology
Phillips-University
University Hospital Marburg
Marburg, Germany

Howard L. Weiner, M.D.
Professor of Neurosurgery and Pediatrics
New York University School of Medicine
New York University Langone Medical Center
New York, New York

Timothy E. Welty, Pharm.D., F.C.C.P.
Professor and Chair
Department of Pharmacy Practice
University of Kansas
Lawrence, Kansas
University of Kansas Medical Center
Kansas City, Kansas

James W. Wheless, M.D.
Professor and Chief of Pediatric Oncology
Le Bonheur Chair in Pediatric Neurology
University of Tennessee Health Science Center
Director, Neuroscience Institute
Le Bonheur Comprehensive Epilepsy Program
Le Bonheur Children's Medical Center
Clinical Chief and Director of Pediatric Neurology
St. Jude Children's Research Hospital
Memphis, Tennessee

H. Steve White, Ph.D.
Professor of Pharmacology and Toxicology
College of Pharmacy
University of Utah
Salt Lake City, Utah

L. James Willmore, M.D.
Associate Dean and Professor of Neurology
St. Louis University School of Medicine
St. Louis University Hospital
St. Louis, Missouri

Sara McCrone Winchester, M.D.
Pediatric Neurology Fellow
Department of Pediatrics, Division of Child Neurology
Duke University Medical Center
Durham, North Carolina

S. Parrish Winesett, M.D.
Assistant Professor of Neurosurgery
University of South Florida
Tampa, Florida
Medical Director, Epilepsy Monitoring Unit
All Children Hospital
St. Petersburg, Florida

Elaine Wirrell, B.Sc. (Hon.), M.D., F.R.C.P.(C.)
Professor of Child and Adolescent Neurology and Epilepsy
Director of Pediatric Epilepsy
Mayo Clinic
Rochester, Minnesota

Gregory A. Worrell, M.D., Ph.D.
Assistant Professor of Neurology
Mayo Clinic
Rochester, Minnesota

Elaine Wyllie, M.D.
Professor of Pediatric Medicine
Cleveland Clinic Lerner College of Medicine
Director of the Center for Pediatric Neurology
Neurological Institute
Cleveland Clinic
Cleveland, Ohio

Benjamin G. Zifkin, M.D.C.M., F.R.C.P.C.
Epilepsy Clinic
Montreal Neurological Hospital
Montreal, Quebec, Canada

■ PREFACE

When I started the first edition of this book as a newly minted epileptologist at the Cleveland Clinic, most of our current antiepileptic medications were still on the horizon and epilepsy surgery was in the early stages of development. Each successive edition of the book chronicled sea changes in the field, from the development of powerful neuroimaging techniques, through approval of many new antiepileptic medications, to the emergence of genetics as a force in epilepsy diagnosis. Today, with its own neurodiagnostic procedures and plethora of effective treatment modalities, epileptology is one of the most rewarding and complex fields in medicine. And in society, epilepsy is starting to emerge from the shadows as patients and families band together in support groups and gather information from the internet. Persons with epilepsy are demanding, expecting, state-of-the-art health care at the same time that our field is growing more complex every day.

That's why we need this book now more than ever. Its reason for being is to provide health care professionals with the most up-to-date tools to care for persons with epilepsy, day in and day out. Thanks to the 144 world-renowned experts who shared their knowledge with us, this fifth edition is a ready reference for cutting-edge information about everything from complex drug–drug interactions to age-related EEG manifestations of focal epileptogenic lesions. It's been an honor to craft this work for all of us to use in our clinical practice.

Elaine Wyllie, MD
Professor of Pediatric Medicine
Cleveland Clinic Lerner College of Medicine
Director of the Center for Pediatric Neurology
Neurological Institute
Cleveland Clinic
www.clevelandclinic.org/epilepsy

■ FOREWORD

It is a privilege and honor to be asked to write the foreword of the 5th Edition of *Wyllie's Treatment of Epilepsy*. It is also an easy task since I know the book well. The 4th edition is frequently pulled from my bookshelf when I have a question about a patient with epilepsy, and I am looking forward to replacing it with the 5th. While the first edition, published in 1993, was outstanding, each edition has achieved new heights. Recognizing that it is very difficult to continuously improve a legendary text, the 5th edition will not disappoint.

Advances in the treatment of epilepsy continue to evolve at a rapid rate as there is increasing awareness among both healthcare workers and the public of the enormity of the condition. Epilepsy does not spare age, gender, race, or ethnic group and is one of the most common neurologic disorders encountered. Increased understanding of the etiology, pathophysiology, and genetic underpinnings coupled with advancements in the medical, dietary, and surgical management of patients makes this an ideal time to publish the 5th edition.

Elaine Wyllie, along with her associate editors Gregory Cascino, Barry Gidal, and Howard Goodkin, has recruited an outstanding group of authors who have provided a comprehensive, but not encyclopedic, review of the treatment of epilepsy. Each author is well known for their work in epilepsy.

The book is crafted in a logical and educationally sound manner. Starting with the pathologic substrates and mechanisms of epilepsy, important chapters cover epidemiology, natural history, genetics, and epileptogenesis (Part I). A key tool in the evaluation of patients with epilepsy is the electroencephalogram and Part II of the book covers the basic principles of electroencephalography. A wonderful bonus in this section is a remarkably complete atlas of epileptiform abnormalities.

Epileptic seizures and syndromes are detailed in Part III of the book. The gamut of seizures and syndromes from the neonate to the elderly are covered in considerable detail. Nonepileptic conditions that mimic epileptic seizures are reviewed and there is a heavy emphasis on seizures in special clinical settings, such as seizures in neurometabolic diseases, head trauma, and neurocutaneous disorders.

Antiepileptic medications are reviewed in Part IV and epilepsy surgery in Part V. As the book's title would indicate, these topics are covered in considerable depth, either of which would qualify as a stand-alone monograph. Dr. Wyllie and her colleagues understand that individuals with epilepsy frequently have more issues than just seizures, and have devoted Part VI to psychosocial aspects of epilepsy.

The authors have crafted a highly integrated text, not an easy task when dealing with multiple authors. As such, the book is easy to read and flows from one part to the other rather seamlessly. While few readers will read the book cover to cover, the interested student who wishes to review topics will find the process enjoyable as well as educationally rewarding.

While there are numerous textbooks dealing with epilepsy available, none do as much as Wyllie and colleagues in one volume. Beautifully illustrated and attractively designed, the 5th volume will undoubtedly retain its stature as the best book on epilepsy available. It is highly recommended for everyone interested in epilepsy, from the medical student to the seasoned epileptologist.

Books like *Wyllie's Treatment of Epilepsy* do not happen without a great deal of work from the editors and authors. Kudos to all.

Gregory L. Holmes, MD
Professor of Neurology and Pediatrics
Chair, Department of Neurology
Dartmouth Medical School
Lebanon, New Hampshire

■ ACKNOWLEDGMENTS

The fifth edition's terrific associate editors—Dr. Gregory Cascino, Dr. Barry Gidal, and Dr. Howard Goodkin—each brought their own prodigious expertise, dedication, and good humor to the project. Ms. Jennifer Kowalak provided impeccable editorial assistance, Mr. Arijit Biswas meticulously transformed the manuscript to final printer files, and Mr. Tom Gibbons at Lippincott gracefully shepherded the book through every stage of production. Mr. Dick Blake, master teacher of dance and etiquette, remains a constant inspiration and wellspring of creativity. And I owe everything to Dr. Robert Wyllie, Physician-in-Chief of the Cleveland Clinic Children's Hospital—my husband, dancing partner, and father to our sons, Mr. Robert Wyllie and Mr. James Wyllie, who make us proud.

CONTENTS

PART IV ■ ANTIEPILEPTIC MEDICATIONS

PART V ■ EPILEPSY SURGERY

PART VI ■ PSYCHOSOCIAL ASPECTS OF EPILEPSY

Cover image   Artist's rendition of an axial colorized fiber orientation map from diffusion tensor imaging (DTI) showing displacement of white matter tracts around a grey matter heterotopia in the right posterior quadrant. The original image is shown in Chapter 77.

With thanks to Dr. Beate Diehl and Prof. Louis Lemieux for sharing this case, and to Mr. Jeffrey Loerch for his artistic rendition.

PART I ■ PATHOLOGIC SUBSTRATES AND MECHANISMS OF EPILEPTOGENESIS

CHAPTER 1 ■ EPIDEMIOLOGIC ASPECTS OF EPILEPSY

CHRISTINE LINEHAN AND ANNE T. BERG

An estimated 40 million individuals worldwide have epilepsy. This estimate is based on epidemiological data gathered as part of the Global Burden of Disease (GBD) Study, a study pioneered by the World Health Organisation, the World Bank, and the Harvard School of Public Health (1). Mortality data from GBD, a traditional measure of burden of disease, indicates that 142,000 persons with epilepsy die annually, equating to 0.2% of all deaths worldwide. Mortality statistics, however, mask the burden of disease among those living with epilepsy. Acknowledging the need to define burden beyond mortality, the GBD study introduced a new measure of burden of diseases, injuries, and risk factors, the DALY (disability-adjusted life year). One DALY equates to 1 year of healthy life lost due to disability or poor health. Epilepsy is estimated to contribute 7,854,000 DALYs (0.5%) to the global burden of disease.

A clear pattern emerges from the GBD data whereby over half of all deaths and half of all years of healthy life lost to epilepsy occur in low-income countries. Moreover, almost one in five of all deaths and almost one in four of all years of healthy life lost to epilepsy worldwide occur among children living in these regions. The greater burden of epilepsy observed in these regions is multifaceted but a major contributor is the "treatment gap," that is, the difference between the number of individuals with active epilepsy and the number who are being appropriately treated at a given point in time. Estimates suggest that up to 90% of people with epilepsy in resource-poor countries are inadequately treated (2).

The burden of epilepsy, however, extends beyond physical health status. Stigma and discrimination are common features of the condition worldwide (3). Profound social isolation (4), feeling of shame and discomfort (5), and higher risk of psychiatric disorder (6) are among a host of variables contributing to a compromised quality of life. Poor employment opportunities, lost work productivity, and out of pocket health care expenses contribute to the economic burden of epilepsy not only for the individual with epilepsy but also for the family and the wider community (2,7,8). In combination, these findings leave little doubt regarding the substantial burden of epilepsy.

The first epidemiological study of epilepsy was conducted in 1959 by Leonard T. Kurland and reported population-based data from Rochester, Minnesota, over a 10-year period. Kurland acknowledged that data existed from "numerous reports based on proportionate hospital admission rates and selected case series," but observed that "these data are not necessarily representative of a population from which the patients are drawn" (9). This observation was to profoundly impact not only the future of epidemiological studies in the field but also the prevailing view of epilepsy and its prognosis. What Kurland had observed was that studies based on institutionalized patients suffered an inherent bias whereby those with more severe levels of epilepsy were overrepresented. Those with milder forms of epilepsy were less likely to attend specialist referral centers and were therefore less likely to be identified in these studies. The consequence of failing to include those with milder forms of epilepsy in epidemiological studies was that epilepsy appeared as an unremitting and chronic condition affecting a somewhat smaller proportion of people with epilepsy in the population (10).

Early epidemiological studies that followed from Kurland's work contributed substantially to our current understanding of epilepsy. Additional studies exploring the Rochester longitudinal population-based data sets, for example, illustrated that the occurrence of epilepsy and isolated seizures was relatively common (11). These data sets also revealed that the probability of being in remission, as defined by five consecutive years of seizure freedom, was also more common than previously thought (12), an important consideration for investigators determining prevalence estimates (see Fig. 1.1). These early epidemiological findings provided an evidence base of the occurrence and prognosis of epilepsy

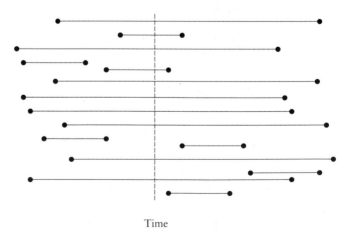

Time

FIGURE 1.1. Prevalence bias. Each horizontal line represents a case with active disease (i.e., a prevalent case). The length of the line represents the time of the active disease, with onset to the left and offset or death to the right. The dashed vertical line represents the day on which prevalence is measured. Long-duration cases are oversampled (8 of 8 are ascertained on the prevalence day) relative to short-duration cases (2 of 7 are ascertained on the prevalence day).

that contributed to advances in the treatment and management of seizures (10).

Epidemiological investigations since these early studies continue to inform and challenge our understanding of epilepsy. This chapter aims to outline current definitions and distinctions in epidemiological research. In addition, findings from more recent studies and the challenges presented to investigators conducting these studies are outlined.

CURRENT DEFINITIONS AND DISTINCTIONS USED IN EPIDEMIOLOGIC EPILEPSY RESEARCH

Epilepsy (recurrent, unprovoked seizures) must be distinguished from many other conditions and situations in which seizures may occur. The following definitions are generally accepted and are in widespread use.

Epileptic Seizure

An epileptic seizure is a "transient occurrence of signs and/or symptoms due to abnormal excessive or synchronous neuronal activity in the brain" (13). Epileptic seizures must be distinguished from nonepileptic seizures and from other conditions that may produce clinical manifestations that are highly similar to those caused by epileptic seizures.

Acute Provoked Seizure

An acute provoked seizure is one that occurs in the context of an acute brain insult or systemic disorder, such as, but not limited to, stroke, head trauma, a toxic or metabolic insult, or an intracranial infection (14).

Unprovoked Seizure

A seizure that occurs in the absence of an acute provoking event is considered unprovoked (14).

Epilepsy

The widely accepted operational definition of epilepsy requires that an individual have at least two unprovoked seizures on separate days, generally 24 hours apart. An individual with a single unprovoked seizure or with two or more unprovoked seizures within a 24-hour period is typically not at that time considered to have met the criteria for labeling him with the diagnosis of epilepsy per se (14). A recent ILAE document attempted to provide a conceptual definition of epilepsy that entailed the notion of an enduring underlying predisposition to unprovoked seizures. The definition was presented, however, as an operational definition and engendered considerable controversy and response (15–17) precisely because there was no way to ensure that it would be consistently and validly applied across different settings by different investigators, a quality that is a prerequisite for

meaningful research. At the same time, we must recognize that a first seizure often is the first identifiable sign of epilepsy and that in some cases, it is possible to recognize the specific underlying disorder (form of epilepsy) at its earliest presentation (18). In the case of Dravet syndrome, the first definitive sign may be a febrile seizure and, with a genetic test, the epilepsy may be diagnosed at that early time (19). Currently in epilepsy, particularly in epidemiological settings, this is the exception rather than the rule.

Etiology

Traditionally and according to ILAE Commission reports of 1989 and 1993, etiology is partitioned into two primary categories. Remote symptomatic refers to epilepsy that occurs in association with an antecedent condition that has been demonstrated to increase the risk of developing epilepsy. Antecedent factors include, but are not limited to, history of stroke, brain malformation, clear neurodevelopmental abnormality such as cerebral palsy, history of bacterial meningitis or viral encephalitis, certain chromosomal and genetic disorders, and tumors. Epilepsy in the context of a progressive condition (e.g., neurodegenerative disease or an aggressive tumor) is often considered a subgroup within the category of remote symptomatic. Idiopathic refers to a group of well-characterized disorders whose initial onset is concentrated during infancy, childhood, and adolescence. The intent of the term is to reflect a presumed genetic etiology in which the primary and often the sole manifestation is seizures. Use of the term idiopathic requires a precise diagnosis of the form of epilepsy. A third term cryptogenic is used and rightfully means that the cause of the epilepsy is unknown; it could be secondary to an insult that has not yet been identified (e.g., a cortical malformation) or it could be a genetic (idiopathic) epilepsy. Both possibilities are realized on a regular basis as new imaging techniques uncover previously unrecognized malformations and genetic investigations identify new genetic syndromes. The International League Against Epilepsy has revised and updated the concepts and terminology to keep them relevant in the context of increasing advances in genomics and neuroimaging and improved understanding of the epilepsies (20).

Gray Areas

Neonatal seizures (i.e., those occurring in an infant <28 days old) are usually differentiated from epilepsy for a variety of reasons; however, several specific forms of epilepsy have been reported in this age group (21). For the epidemiologist, the difficulty is accurate diagnostic information to distinguish well-characterized forms of epilepsy from neonatal seizures that may reflect chronic or transient insults to the developing brain. Febrile seizures are a well-described and recognized seizure disorder that, for historical reasons, has been distinguished (both clinically and in research) from epilepsy. For those involved in detailed genetic investigations, this may be an inappropriate distinction; however, for the epidemiologist who may not always have the necessary clinical and particularly the genetic detail, the distinction is of value. It also has important clinical implications for the treatment of children with such seizures.

Epilepsy Syndromes

Epilepsy syndromes have been alluded to above and are presented in greater detail in subsequent chapters of this book. Epilepsy, like cancer, is not a single disorder, and the efforts to identify specific forms of epilepsy reflect the importance of the diversity within the epilepsies. The epilepsy syndromes represent forms of epilepsy that have different causes, different manifestations, different implications for short- and long-term management and treatment, and different outcomes. Many epidemiological studies do not attempt to identify specific forms of epilepsy; however, in large-scale population- and community-based studies, it is possible to do, provided the investigators have access to the necessary information and the expertise needed to diagnose these syndromes (18,22,23).

EPIDEMIOLOGY

Epidemiological studies have provided valuable insights into the frequency of seizures within the population and have provided the initial impetus for some of the distinctions outlined above. However, as Kurland noted, epidemiologists need to be vigilant to potential sources of bias that threaten the validity of their findings. The ability of diagnosticians to appropriately identify cases and the capabilities of epidemiologists to identify those cases within the population are fundamental issues within the field of epidemiology.

Diagnostic Issues and Considerations in Ascertaining Cases

Seizures and epilepsy present a complex situation because the diagnosis is not based on a single source or type of information. Rather, epilepsy is a clinical diagnosis supported to a greater or lesser extent by a wide range of data obtained from several sources: the medical history, the history (both from the patient and witnesses) of the events believed to be seizures, the circumstances under which the events occur, a neurologic examination, reliable EEG, and increasingly neuroimaging (24). To have a valid diagnosis, one must also be able to rule out many other conditions that mimic seizures. These disorders include, but are not limited to, movement disorders, parasomnias, attention-deficit/hyperactivity disorder, pseudo- or nonepileptic seizures, transient ischemic attacks, and syncope (see Chapters 39 and 40).

Ideally, a diagnosis of epilepsy should be undertaken by medical practitioners with expertise in epilepsy (25). Unfortunately, access to neurologists and epilepsy specialists is generally poor in developing countries and often poor in developed countries as well. Consequently, diagnoses may be made by those with only minimal expertise in the field (26,27). Estimates of misdiagnosis rates suggest that over one fifth of persons with a diagnosis of epilepsy may be misdiagnosed (28,29). Re-evaluation of initial diagnosis of epilepsy in epidemiological studies report rates of 23% (30,31) with diagnostic doubt among patients diagnosed by neurologists and nonspecialists reported at 5.6% and 18.9%, respectively (32).

Epidemiological studies that rely on medical registers for case ascertainment provide valuable insights into levels of misdiagnoses. Christensen et al. (33), for example, randomly selected $n = 200$ patients with an ICD diagnosis of epilepsy from the Danish National Hospital Register, a national register of all discharges and outpatient cases from Danish hospitals. The authors reported that almost one in five (19%) of the patients did not fulfill the ILAE criteria for an epilepsy diagnosis. In fact, approximately 7% of patients were given an epilepsy diagnosis on the basis of one seizure. Christensen et al. (34) also noted that while the validity of epilepsy diagnosis from the register was moderate to high, there was low predictive value for epilepsy syndromes.

Primary care registers, a common source of case ascertainment in epidemiological research, have also been found to include persons incorrectly diagnosed with epilepsy. Gallitto et al. (35) gathered population-based data from general practitioners (GPs) in the Aeolian Islands. All established or suspected cases of epilepsy were evaluated by epileptologists in the local outpatient services with the support of the local GPs or, for those with additional disabilities, within the family home. The evaluations comprised a review of medical notes and where necessary EEG or neuroradiologic investigation. Following the epileptologic evaluation 30% of established and suspected cases were identified as not fulfilling the diagnostic criteria for epilepsy.

While organizations such as the UK-based National Institute for Health and Clinical Excellence have proposed best practice guidelines in diagnosis, currently no agreed criteria exist for what constitutes an adequate diagnostic evaluation including who should perform it. There are also no standards in epidemiological studies for the use of routine diagnostic tests such as EEG and MRI. Unsurprisingly, there has been a call for a gold standard diagnostic criterion to distinguish epileptic seizures from other diagnoses with similar clinical features (28).

In addition to the determination of whether someone has epilepsy, adequate information is needed to identify the specific form of epilepsy and its underlying cause. While this level of detail is frequently absent from traditional epidemiological studies, it must be incorporated in the future if epidemiological studies are to continue to inform scientific and clinical endeavors relevant to epilepsy as it is understood and treated today. Without a meaningful diagnostic evaluation, epidemiological studies can do little more than provide an approximate head count which previous work has shown to be rather error-prone. The lumping together of highly diverse disorders that share the diagnostic label "epilepsy" also limits the ability of epidemiological studies to provide meaningful prognostic information.

Other case ascertainment options have been employed by epidemiologists, each having its own unique challenges. Screening questionnaires, for example, are a common tool used in epidemiologic studies. Methodologies employing screening questionnaires typically comprise two phases. In the first phase, a screen is used to identify positive cases. In the second phase, these positive cases are evaluated clinically to confirm the presence of epilepsy. Noronha et al. (36), for example, used a screening tool developed by Borges et al. (37) in the first phase of their study to determine the prevalence of epilepsy in Brazil. The screening tool reported sensitivity and specificity at 96% and 98%, respectively. Similarly, Melcon et al. (38) used a modified version of a screening tool from the Copiah County study (39) to identify potential cases for inclusion in their prevalence estimate of epilepsy in Argentina. This screening tool also reported acceptable levels of sensitivity and specificity at 95% and 80%, respectively.

Screening tools are also advocated by the World Health Organisation, whose "Global Campaign against Epilepsy" supports those undertaking epidemiological research in resource-poor countries. Demonstration projects managed under this program, in addition to assessments of local knowledge, attitude and health service provision, undertake epidemiological door-to-door studies to determine prevalence estimates. Screening tools developed by WHO (40) have been used in large-scale national epidemiological studies (41). Notwithstanding the successful application of screening tools in many studies, the diagnostic sensitivity and specificity of these tools can, however, be poor and the training of physicians or other health care professionals charged with validating positive screens may be compromised by poor access to such basic diagnostic tools as EEGs.

Other case ascertainment sources used in epidemiological studies include prescription databases recording anti-epilepsy drug usage. By definition, these epidemiological studies estimate "treated epilepsy" and are more common in developed countries where the treatment gap is minimal. Prescription databases have been found to offer a suitable means by which the prevalence of epilepsy can be determined in community samples (42) as the coverage of the databases is typically far broader than medical registers. Purcell et al. (43), for example, examined rates of treated epilepsy in the United Kingdom using the General Practitioner Research Database that provided data on prescription use of over 1.4 million persons.

A potential source of bias in identifying persons with epilepsy from prescription databases is that cases cannot be clinically validated (43,44). This bias is magnified in situations where diagnosis is not recorded on the database and where "estimates" of drug use among people with epilepsy are applied (45,46). While anti-epilepsy drugs have been previously identified as "tracers" of epilepsy due to their chronic and highly specific usage (46) the growing use of anti-epilepsy medication for indications other than epilepsy, such as pain, migraine, bipolar disorders, agitation, hormonal imbalance, and weight reduction must now be considered. In general, reliance on prescription data alone is an inadequate case ascertainment method for epilepsy.

A methodology for case ascertainment that is becoming more frequently used in North American studies is the self-report survey. These studies typically include epilepsy-specific items in large population-based health surveys (47–50). The coverage of these surveys is extensive. The Canadian Health Survey, for example, was completed by over 130,000 persons, all of whom were questioned as to their health status, health care utilization, and determinants of health (47). The California Health Interview Survey 2003 provided similar data on over 41,000 persons (50).

The Behavioral Risk Factor Surveillance System (51) provides an example of the typical type of epilepsy-specific items that can be included in these surveys; "Have you ever been told by a doctor that you have a seizure disorder or epilepsy?" A distinct advantage of this methodology is the opportunity it affords to examine not only the frequency of self-reported epilepsy among very large representative populations but also the impact of epilepsy on their health-related quality of life. Issues such as employment, education, and comorbid conditions can be examined. Where these items are common to both those with and without a self-report of epilepsy, important disparities can be identified. Without doubt, this method

differs from more rigorous epidemiologic studies (49). A selection bias may exist whereby, despite the broad community-dwelling population from which samples are drawn, those who agree to participate in surveys may differ in some fundamental way from those who decline. This method also faces the challenge previously observed among studies examining prescription databases whereby cases are not clinically validated. Whether those who self-disclose epilepsy do in fact have the condition cannot be determined, no more so than those who have epilepsy but chose not to disclose it.

Each of the methods outlined above has its own benefits and challenges. This has led some researchers to propose that the most valid method to identify cases of epilepsy is to access multiple sources of case ascertainment (52). Data linkage studies, for example, provide opportunities simultaneously to examine both population-based and hospital-based registers (53,54). These multicase ascertainment studies make it possible "not only to estimate the number of cases missed by each source but also to indirectly estimate the number of cases missed by the combined dataset" (55). Choice of case ascertainment, however, may not always be at the discretion of the epidemiologist. Resources of appropriately trained personnel, funding, and sophistication of health care services are some of the many factors that influence how the same study might be conducted differently in different jurisdictions.

Variations in methodology can result in highly varying estimates of epilepsy (56,57). A contributing factor is the lack of harmonized definitions employed across studies. Despite the Commission of Epidemiology and Prognosis of the ILAE (14) issuing guidelines for definitions employed in epidemiological studies, specific definitions of what constitutes "epilepsy," "active cases," and "cases in remission" differ markedly among studies. Definition of "active epilepsy," for example, varies in terms of their stated duration since last seizure, with some studies using the ILAE-recommended definition of one seizure or use of anti-epilepsy drugs within the previous 5 years (58) and others truncating this duration to the previous 3 months (49,50). Harmonization of definitions is encouraged as it would permit valuable comparisons of findings across studies.

FREQUENCY MEASURES OF INCIDENCE AND PREVALENCE

Incidence is expressed as the number of new cases of disease in a standard-sized population per unit of time—for example, the number of cases per 100,000 population per year. Prospective studies of incidence are advocated as they permit observation of any changes in the incidence rate (52) and may therefore identify risk factors that play a causal role in the development of epilepsy (33,59). Ongoing surveillance studies of this type however are time-consuming and costly (52,60) and are therefore less common than prevalence studies (52,61) and less likely to be conducted in resource-poor countries (62). Incidence rates for epilepsy are typically between 30 and 80 per 100,000 population per year in developed countries but have been observed to exceed these figures. Table 1.1 presents a selection of studies illustrating this trend.

Worldwide, rates vary across regions, with rates being typically higher in resource-poor countries (59), most especially in Africa and Latin America where figures can exceed 100 per 100,000 population (63–65). Rates also differ by age, but

TABLE 1.1

INCIDENCE AND PREVALENCE OF EPILEPSY AS REPORTED IN SELECTED POPULATION-BASED STUDIES THROUGHOUT THE WORLD

	Studies	Country/region	Methodology	Age group (years)	Incidence/100,000/year	Prevalence/1000
Africa	Mung'ala-Odera et al. (2008) (75)	Kenya	Combined data from two door-to-door studies	Children	187	41 lifetime, 11 active
	Dozie et al. (2006) (77)	Nigeria	Door-to-door survey screening with confirmatory examination of those screening positive for epilepsy	All ages	—	12 active
	Almu et al. (2006) (78)	Ethiopia (Zay Society)	Door-to-door survey screening with confirmatory examination of those screening positive for epilepsy	All ages	—	29.5 active
Latin America	Noronha et al. (2007) (36)	Brazil	Door-to-door survey screening with confirmatory examination of those screening positive for epilepsy	All ages	—	9.2 lifetime, 5.4 active
	Melcon et al. (2007) (38)	Buenos Aires	Door-to-door survey screening with confirmatory examination of those screening positive for epilepsy	All ages	—	6.2 lifetime, 3.8 active
	Medina et al. (2005) (79)	Honduras	Door-to-door survey screening with confirmatory examination of those screening positive for epilepsy	All ages	92.7	23.3 lifetime, 15.4 active
Europe	Dura-Trave et al. (2008) (66)	Spain	Cases referred to neuro-pediatric reference center	Children under 15 years	62.6	—
	Christensen et al. (2007) (33)	Denmark	Data linkage (Civil Registration and Hospital Register Databases)	All ages	68.8	5.7 lifetime
	Olafsson et al. (2005) (80)	Iceland	Cases identified via country wide surveillance system in health care facilities with confirmatory review by neurologists	All ages	56.8 all unprovoked seizures; 23.5 single unprovoked seizures; 33.3 epilepsy	—
North America	Benn et al. (2008) (81)	New York	Cases identified via review of local hospital and nursing home registers with follow up interviews	All ages	41.1[a]	—
	Kobau et al. (2008) (26)	USA	Self-report omnibus health survey	Over 18 years	—	16.5 lifetime, 8.4 active
	Kelvin et al. (2007) (82)	New York	Telephone survey—responses by positive cases reviewed by epileptologists	All ages	—	5.9 lifetime, 5.0 active
Asia	Fong et al. (2008) (83)	Hong Kong	Population-based phone screening followed by neurological validation	All ages	—	8.49 seizure disorders, 3.94 active
	Tran et al. (2006) (84)	Central Lao	Door-to-door survey screening with confirmatory examination of those screening positive for epilepsy	All ages	—	7.7 active
	Mani et al. (1998) (85)	Rural South India	Door-to-door survey screening with confirmatory examination of those screening positive for epilepsy	All ages	49.3	4.19 lifetime, 3.91 active

[a]First unprovoked seizure and newly diagnosed epilepsy.

TABLE 1.2

DISTRIBUTION OF EPILEPSY SYNDROMES IN NEWLY DIAGNOSED PATIENTS FROM EIGHT DIFFERENT COUNTRIES

Syndrome	Connecticut[a] (23) Children <16 years N (%)	France[b] (18) Children <14 years N (%)	France[b] (18) Adults ≥25 years N (%)	The Netherlands (22) Children <16 years N (%)	Italy[c] (86) Children N (%)	Columbia (41) All ages N (%)	Sweden (87) Children <16 years N (%)	Japan (88) Children <16 years N (%)	Iceland (80) All ages N (%)
11 idiopathic focal	61 (10%)	47 (9%)	1 (<1%)	31 (7%)	21 (9%)	2 (2%)	46 (23%)	55 (5%)	16 (6%)
12 symptomatic focal	71 (12%)	34 (7%)	81 (27%)	74 (16%)	92 (38%)	27 (29%)	9 (4%)	345 (29%)	74 (26%)
13 cryptogenic focal	227 (37%)	121 (24%)	107 (35%)	87 (19%)	0 (0)	45 (49%)	49 (24%)	507 (42%)	78 (27%)
21 idiopathic generalized	126 (21)	199 (40%)	15 (5%)	195 (42%)	67 (28%)	9 (9%)	37 (18%)	95 (8%)	30 (10%)
22 cryptogenic/ symptomatic generalized	43 (7%)	39 (8%)	0 (0)	29 (6%)	50 (21%)	2 (2%)	47 (23%)	173 (14%)	6 (2%)
23 symptomatic generalized	9 (1%)	14 (3%)	7 (2%)	41 (9%)	1 (<1%)	0 (0)	0 (0)	0 (0)	1 (<1%)
31 generalized and focal features	5 (1%)	13 (3%)	0 (0)	1 (<1%)	1 (<1%)	0 (0)	0 (0)	0 (0)	8 (3%)
32 unclassified	71 (12%)	34 (7%)	94 (30%)	2 (<1%)	19 (8%)	6 (7%)	17 (8%)	21 (2%)	77 (27%)
Total number of patients	613	501	305	462	251	92[d]	205	1196	290

[a] The cryptogenic and symptomatic localization-related categories were redefined to be consistent with the interpretation of other authors and to facilitate comparisons.
[b] Limited to children <14 years of age.
[c] Pediatric epilepsy center (referral) in Milan—published prior to 1989.
[d] Listed as "special syndrome."

differentially in developed and resource-poor countries. In developed countries, rates are highest among infants and older persons (66–69). Although incidence rates among children have fallen over the last three decades in developed countries, this decrease has been offset by an increase among older persons (70). A different age-related pattern emerges in developing countries, however, where a decrease in incidence is observed with age (59). The larger proportion of children in developing countries is thought to contribute to the higher overall incidence rates when compared with developed countries (34,59).

Prevalence studies measure the total number of persons with epilepsy at a specific moment in time. Prevalence rates are usually expressed as the number of persons with epilepsy per 1000 population. Estimates of active epilepsy are typically the focus of prevalence studies, with those in remission or who are not receiving treatment at the time of case ascertainment being excluded. A *plethora of studies* that consistently report prevalence estimates of active epilepsy in developed countries of between 4 and 10 per 1000 population suggests there is "little justification for further cross-sectional studies of prevalence" (56) in these countries. Recent findings from Norway, however, of 12 per 1000 treated epilepsy and 7 per 1000 active cases in a population that excluded high-risks groups such as older persons have led investigators to suggest that the true prevalence of epilepsy in developed countries may be higher than previously reported (71). Prevalence estimates typically increase with age and are generally higher among males than females (52), although this difference may not always reach statistical significance.

Prevalence estimates in resource-poor countries are generally higher than in developed countries (56). Median prevalence of active epilepsy in Latin America is reported as 12.4 per 1000 population; however, this finding conceals widely varying findings from individual studies ranging from 5.1 to 57 per 1000 population (72). This wide variation in estimates is also observed in Africa where estimates have been reported ranging from 5.2 to 58 per 1000 (73,74). While researchers note that known risk factors, such as environment, contribute to the high-prevalence estimates on the African continent (75), some authors suggest that the true prevalence estimate may actually be higher again as disclosure of the condition is particularly problematic (76). Reviews of studies conducted in Asia, perhaps surprisingly, report findings aligning more closely with those in developed countries. This has led some investigators to speculate whether there is a specific protective factor as yet unknown in Asia or whether the finding reflects specific risk factors in Latin America and Africa (61). Table 1.1 presents findings from some recent studies worldwide (77–85).

Several recent studies have examined the relative frequency, if not absolute incidence, of different forms of epilepsy in well-characterized series of incident patients who were reasonably representative of the populations from which they were drawn (Table 1.2) (86–88). Apart from the obvious difference between adults and children, there is a degree of variation among the studies just of children as well. Whether this represents real differences across populations or methodological difference between studies is not clear. Certainly, patterns of referral to recruitment sources as well as the diagnostic ability of the physicians who evaluate the patients, could create apparent differences between studies where none exist. Such concerns aside, a few generalities can be drawn. Fewer children than adults are likely to have an unclassified form of epilepsy. In children, idiopathic focal epilepsies (largely dominated by Benign Rolandic Epilepsy) comprise about 5% to 10% of childhood-onset epilepsy. The idiopathic generalized epilepsies comprise 20% to 40%. Finally, between 10% and 20% of childhood-onset epilepsy falls into the category of secondary generalized. These are some of the most devastating and intractable forms of epilepsy and include West and Lennox–Gastaut syndrome.

SUMMARY

Epidemiology has been key in demonstrating the relatively high frequency of seizures in the population and in challenging long-held beliefs about the uniformly poor seizure outcomes associated with seizures. Research pursuits within the epidemiology of epilepsy have come a long way from the days of simply counting how many people in a given population had seizures. Some studies are providing estimates of the frequency of specific types of epilepsy with some relatively clear patterns emerging across studies. As diagnostic technology has become more sophisticated, the methods used for ascertaining cases in a population have become appropriately more complex. Representativeness and diagnostic accuracy are increasingly at odds, especially in underdeveloped areas. Once these issues are adequately addressed, cross-regional or cross-national comparisons of similarly conducted studies may help identify forms of epilepsy and causes of epilepsy that are unusually common in certain areas. This may, in turn, lead to insights into prevention. Combining the strengths of epidemiologic methods with the sophistication of new medical diagnostic technology and our growing understanding of epilepsy has the promise of advancing our knowledge of the causes, consequences, and possibly prevention of this common set of disorders.

References

1. World Health Organisation. The global burden of disease: 2004 update. Geneva, World Health Organisation; 2008. Available at: http://www.who.int/healthinfo/global_burden_disease/2004_report_update/en/index.html. Accessed January 28, 2009.
2. Jamison DT, Breman JG, Measham AR, et al. *Disease Control Priorities in Developing Countries.* 2nd ed. New York: Oxford University Press; 2006.
3. Jacoby A, Wang W, Dang V, et al. Meanings of epilepsy in its sociocultural context and implications for stigma: findings from ethnographic studies in local communities in China and Vietnam. *Epilepsy and Behavior.* 2008;12:286–297.
4. Elliot IM, Lach L, Smith ML. I just want to be normal: a qualitative study exploring how children and adolescents view the impact of intractable epilepsy on their quality of life. *Epilepsy and Behavior.* 2005;7:664–678.
5. Scambler G. Sociology, social structure and health-related stigma. *Psychology, Health & Medicine.* 2006;11:288–295.
6. Gaitatzis A, Carroll K, Majeed A, et al. The epidemiology of the comorbidity of epilepsy in the general population. *Epilepsia.* 2004;45:1613–1622.
7. de Boer HM, Mula M, Sander JW. The global burden and stigma of epilepsy. *Epilepsy and Behavior.* 2008;12:540–546.
8. Begley CE, Baker GA, Beghi E, et al. Cross country measures for monitoring Epilepsy Care. *Epilepsia.* 2007;48:990–1001.
9. Kurland LT. The incidence and prevalence of convulsive disorders in a small urban community. *Epilepsia.* 1959;1:143–161.
10. Berg AT, Shinner S. The contribution of epidemiology to the understanding of childhood seizures and epilepsy. *Journal of Child Neurology.* 1994;9:2819–2826.
11. Hauser WA, Kurland LT. The epidemiology of epilepsy in Rochester, Minnesota, 1935 through 1967. *Epilepsia.* 1975;16:1–66.
12. Annegers JF, Hauser WA, Elveback LR. Remission of seizures and relapse in patients with epilepsy. *Epilepsia.* 1979;20:729–737.
13. Fisher RS, Boas WE, Blume W, et al. Epileptic seizures and epilepsy: definitions proposed by the International League against Epilepsy (ILAE) and the International Bureau for Epilepsy (IBE). *Epilepsia.* 2005;46:470.

14. Commission on Epidemiology and Prognosis, International League Against Epilepsy. Guidelines for epidemiologic studies on epilepsy. *Epilepsia.* 1993;34:592–596.

15. Beghi F, Berg A, Carpio A, et al. Comment on epileptic seizure and epilepsy: definitions proposed by the International League against Epilepsy (ILAE) and the International Bureau of Epilepsy (IBE). *Epilepsia.* 2005;46:1698–1699.

16. Gomez-Alonso J, Andrade C, Koukoulis A. Comment on epileptic seizure and epilepsy: definitions proposed by the International League against Epilepsy (ILAE) and the International Bureau of Epilepsy (IBE). *Epilepsia.* 2005;46:1699–1700.

17. Ahmed SN. Comment on epileptic seizure and epilepsy: definitions proposed by the International League against Epilepsy (ILAE) and the International Bureau of Epilepsy (IBE). *Epilepsia.* 2005;46:1700.

18. Jallon P, Loiseau P, Loiseau J. Newly diagnosed unprovoked epileptic seizures: presentation at diagnosis in CAROLE study. *Epilepsia.* 2001;42:464–475.

19. Berkovic SF, Scheffer IE. Febrile seizures: genetics and relationship to other epilepsy. *Current Opinion in Neurology.* 1998;11:129.

20. Berg AT, Berkovic SF, Brodie MJ, et al. Revised terminology and concepts for organization of seizures and epilepsies: Report of the ILAE Commission on Classification and Terminology, 2005–2009. *Epilepsia.* 2010;51:676–685.

21. Plouin P, Raffo E, de Oliveira T. Prognosis of neonatal seizures. In: Jallon P, Berg AT, Dulac O, et al., eds. *Prognosis of Epilepsies.* Montrouge, France: John Libbey Eurotext; 2003:199–209.

22. Callenbach PM, Geerts AT, Arts WF, et al. Familial occurrence of epilepsy in children with newly diagnosed multiple seizures: dutch study of epilepsy in childhood. *Epilepsia.* 1998;39:331–336.

23. Berg AT, Shinnar S, Levy SR, et al. Newly diagnosed epilepsy in children: presentation at diagnosis. *Epilepsia.* 1999;40:445–452.

24. Hirtz D, Ashwal S, Berg AT, et al. Practice parameter: evaluating a first nonfebrile seizure in children. Report of the quality standards committee of the American Academy of Neurology, the Child Neurology Society, and the American Epilepsy Society. *Neurology.* 2000;55:616–623.

25. Stokes T, Shaw EJ, Juarez-Garcia A, et al. *Clinical Guidelines and Evidence Review for the Epilepsies: Diagnosis and Management in Adults and Children in Primary and Secondary Care.* London: Royal College of General Practitioners; 2004.

26. Kobau R, Zahran H, Thurman DJ, et al. Epilepsy Surveillance Among Adults — 19 States, Behavioral Risk Factor Surveillance System, 2005. *Morbidity and Mortality Weekly Report.* 2008;57:SS-6, 1–20.

27. Pal DK, Das T, Sengupta S. Case-control and qualitative study of attrition in a community epilepsy programme in rural India. *Seizure.* 2000;9:119–123.

28. Chowdhury FA, Nashef L Elwes, RDC. Misdiagnosis in epilepsy: a review and recognition of diagnostic uncertainty. *European Journal of Neurology.* 2008;15:1034–1042.

29. Josephson CB, Rahey S, Sadler RM. Neurocardiogenic syncope: frequency and consequences of its misdiagnosis as epilepsy. *Canadian Journal of Neurological Sciences.* 2007;34:221–224.

30. Juarez-Garcia A, Stokes T, Shaw B, et al. The costs of epilepsy misdiagnosis in England and Wales. *Seizure.* 2006;15:598–605.

31. Scheepers B, Clough P, Pickles C. The misdiagnosis of epilepsy: findings of a population study. *Seizure.* 1998;7:403–406.

32. Leach JP, Lauder R, Nicolson A, et al. Epilepsy in the UK: misdiagnosis, mistreatment, and undertreatment? The Wrexham area epilepsy project. *Seizure.* 2005;14:514–520.

33. Christensen J, Vestergaard M, Pedersen MG, et al. Incidence and prevalence of epilepsy in Denmark. *Epilepsy Research.* 2007a;76:60–65.

34. Christensen J, Vestergaard M, Olsen J, et al. Validation of epilepsy diagnoses in the Danish National Hospital Register. *Epilepsy Research.* 2007b;75:162–170.

35. Gallitto G, Serra S, La Spina P, et al. Prevalence and characteristics of epilepsy in the Aeolian Islands. *Epilepsia.* 2005;46:1828–1835.

36. Noronha A, Borges M, Marques L, et al. Prevalence and pattern of epilepsy treatment in different socioeconomic classes in Brazil. *Epilepsia.* 2007;48:880–885.

37. Borges MA, Min LL, Guerreiro CA, et al. Urban prevalence of epilepsy: populational study in Sao Jose do Rio Preto, a medium-sized city in Brazil. *Arquivos de Neuropsiquiatria.* 2004;62:199–204.

38. Melcon M, Kochen S, Vergara R. Prevalence and clinical features of epilepsy in a Argentina — A community-based study. *Neuroepidemiology.* 2007;28:8–15.

39. Anderson DW, Schoenberg BS, Haerer, AF. Racial differentials in the prevalence of major neurological disorders; background and methods of the Copiah County Study. *Neuroepidemiology.* 1982;1:17–30.

40. World Health Organization. *Research Protocol for Measuring the Prevalence of Neurological Disorders in Developing Countries.* Geneva; World Health Organization; 1981.

41. Velez A, Eslava-Cobos, J. Epilepsy in Colombia: epidemiologic profile and classification of epileptic seizures and syndromes. *Epilepsia.* 2006;1: 193–201.

42. Lammers MW, Hekster YA, Keyser A, et al. Use of antiepileptic drugs in a community-dwelling Dutch population. *Neurology.* 1996;46:62–67.

43. Purcell B, Gaitatzis A, Sander JW, et al. Epilepsy prevalence and prescribing patterns in England and Wales. *Office of National Statistics, Health Statistics Quarterly.* 2002;15:23–30.

44. Wallace H, Shorvon S, Tallis R. Age specific incidence and prevalence rates of treated epilepsy in an unselected population of 2,052,922 and age specific fertility rates of women with epilepsy. *Lancet.* 1998;352:1970–1973.

45. Shackleton DP, Westendorp RGJ, Kasteleijn-Nolst Trenite, DGA, et al. Dispensing epilepsy medication: a method of determining the frequency of symptomatic individuals with seizures. *Journal of Clinical Epidemiology.* 1997;50:1061–1068.

46. Banfi R, Borselli G, Marinai C, et al. Epidemiological study of epilepsy by monitoring prescriptions of antiepileptic drugs. *Pharmacy, World and Science.* 1995;17:138–140.

47. Tellez-Zenteno JF, Pondal-Sordo M, Matijevic S, et al. National and regional prevalence of self-reported epilepsy in Canada. *Epilepsia.* 2004;45:1623–1629.

48. Ferguson P, Selassie A, Wannamaker B, et al. Prevalence of epilepsy and health related quality of life and disability among adults with epilepsy – South Carolina 2003–2004. *Morbidity and Mortality Weekly Report MMWR.* 2005;54:1080–1081.

49. Kobau R, Gilliam F, Thurman DJ. Prevalence of self-reported epilepsy or seizure disorder and its associations with self-reported depression and anxiety: results from the 2004 Health Styles Survey. *Epilepsia.* 2006;47:1915–1921.

50. Kobau R, Zahran H, Grant D, et al. Prevalence of active epilepsy and health-related quality of life among adults with self-reported epilepsy in California: California Health Interview Survey, 2003. *Epilepsia.* 2007;48:1904–1913.

51. Centers for Disease Control and Prevention. Behavioural risk factor surveillance system. Available at: http://www.cdc.gov/BRFSS/about.htm. Accessed January 22, 2009.

52. Forsgren L, Beghi E, Oun A, et al. The epidemiology of epilepsy in Europe – a systematic review. *European Journal of Neurology.* 2005;12:245–253.

53. Svendsen T, Lossius M, Nakken KO. Age specific prevalence of epilepsy in Oppland County, Norway. *Acta Neurologica Scandinavica.* 2007;116:307–311.

54. Morgan CL, Kerr MP. Epilepsy and Mortality: a record linkage study in a U.K. population. *Epilepsia.* 2002;43:1251–1255.

55. Koepsell TD, Weiss NS. *Epidemiologic Methods: Studying the Occurrence of Illness.* New York: Oxford University Press; 2003.

56. Sander JW. The epidemiology of epilepsy revisited. *Current Opinion in Neurology.* 2003;16:165–170.

57. Bell GS, Sander JW. The epidemiology of the epilepsies: the size of the problem. *Seizure.* 2001;10:306–314.

58. Õun A, Haldre S, Mägi M. Prevalence of adult epilepsy in Estonia. *Epilepsy Research.* 2003;52:233–242.

59. Kotsopoulos IAW, van Merode T, Kessels FGH, et al. Systematic review and meta-analysis of incidence studies of epilepsy and unprovoked seizures. *Epilepsia.* 2002;43:1402–1409.

60. Sridharan R. Epidemiology of epilepsy. *Current Science.* 2002;82:664–670.

61. Mac T, SiTran D, Quet F, et al. Epidemiology, aetiology and clinical management of epilepsy in Asia: a systematic review. *Lancet Neurology.* 2007;6:533–543.

62. Khatri IA, Iannaccone ST, Ilyas MS, et al. Epidemiology of epilepsy in Pakistan: a review of literature. *Journal of Pakistan Medical Association.* 2003;53:594–596.

63. Lavados J, Germain L, Morales L, et al. A descriptive study of epilepsy in the district of El-Salvador, Chile, 1984–1988. *Acta Neurol Scand.* 1992;85:249–256.

64. Placencia M, Shorvon SD, Paredes V, et al. Epileptic seizures in an Andean region of Ecuador. *Brain.* 1992;115:771–782.

65. Rwiza HT, Kilonzo GP, Haule J, et al. Prevalence and incidence of epilepsy in Ulanga, a rural Tanzanian district: a community-based study. *Epilepsia.* 1992;33:1051–1056.

66. Dura-Trave T, Yoldi-Petri ME, Gallinas-Victoriano F. Incidence of epilepsies and epileptic syndromes among children in Navarre, Spain: 2002 through 2005. *Journal of Child Neurology.* 2008;23:878–882.

67. Hussain SA, Haut SR, Lipton RB, et al. Incidence of epilepsy in a racially diverse, community-dwelling, elderly cohort: results from the Einstein aging study. *Epilepsy Research.* 2006;71:195–205.

68. Forsgren L, Bucht G, Eriksson S, et al. Incidence and clinical characterization of unprovoked seizures in adults: a prospective population-based study. *Epilepsia.* 1996;37:224–229.

69. Hauser WA, Annegers JF, Kurland LT. Incidence of epilepsy and unprovoked seizures in Rochester, Minnesota: 1935–1984. *Epilepsia.* 1993;34:453–468.

70. Duncan JS, Sander JW, Sisodiya SM, et al. Adult epilepsy. *Lancet.* 2006;367:1087–100.

71. Brodtkorb E, Sjaastad O. Epilepsy prevalence by individual interview in a Norwegian community. *Seizure.* 2008;17:646–650.

72. Burneo J, Tellez-Zenteno J, Wiebe S. Understanding the burden of epilepsy in Latin America: a systematic review of its prevalence and incidence. *Epilepsy Research.* 2005;66:63–74.

73. Preux, P-M. *Contribution à la connaissance épidémiologique de l'épilepsie en Afrique subsaharienne.* Thèse; 2000.

74. World Health Organisation. *Epilepsy: A manual for medical and clinical officers in Africa*; 2002 Available at: http://www.who.int/mental_health/media/en/639.pdf. Accessed January 26, 2009.

75. Mung'ala-Odera V, Meehan R, Njuguna P, et al. Prevalence and risk factors of neurological disability and impairment in children living in rural Kenya. *International Journal of Epidemiology.* 2006;35:683–688.

76. Mosser P, Schmutzhard E, Winkler AS. The pattern of epileptic seizures in rural Tanzania. *Journal of the Neurological Sciences.* 2007;258:33–38.

77. Dozie INS, Onwuliri COE, Nwoke BEB, et al. Onchocerciasis and epilepsy in parts of the Imo river basin, Nigeria: a preliminary report. *Public Health.* 2006;120:448–450.

78. Almu S, Tadesse Z, Cooper P, et al. The prevalence of epilepsy in the Zay society, Ethiopia; an area of high prevalence. *Seizure.* 2006;15:211–213.

79. Medina MT, Durón RM, Martínez L, et al. Prevalence, incidence and etiology of epilepsy in rural Honduras; the Salamá Study. *Epilepsia.* 2005;46:124–131.

80. Olafsson E, Ludvigsson P, Gudmundsson G, et al. Incidence of unprovoked seizures and epilepsy in Iceland and assessment of the epilepsy syndrome classification: a prospective study. *Lancet Neurology.* 2005;4:627–634.

81. Benn EKT, Hauser WA, Shih T, et al. Estimating the incidence of first unprovoked seizure and newly diagnosed epilepsy in the low-income urban community of Northern Manhattan, New York City. *Epilepsia.* 2008;49:1431–1439.

82. Kelvin EA, Hesdorffer, DC, Bagiella E, et al. Prevalence of self-reported epilepsy in a multiracial and multiethinic community in New York City. *Epilepsy Research.* 2007;77:141–150.

83. Fong GCY, Kwan P, Hui ACF, et al. An epidemiological study of epilepsy in Hong Kong SAR China. *Seizure.* 2008;17:457–464.

84. Tran D, Odermatt P, Le T, et al. Prevalence of epilepsy in a rural district of central Lao PDR. *Neuroepidemiology.* 2006;26:199–206.

85. Mani KS, Rangan G, Srinivas HV, et al. The Yelandur study: a community-based approach to epilepsy in rural South India – epidemiological aspects. *Seizure.* 1998;7:281–288.

86. Viani F, Beghi E, Atza MG, et al. Classifications of epileptic syndromes: advantages and limitations for evaluation of childhood epileptic syndromes in clinical practice. *Epilepsia.* 1988;29:440–445.

87. Larsson K, Eeg-Olofsson O. A population based study of epilepsy in children from a Swedish county. *European Journal of Paediatric Neurology.* 2006;10:107–113.

88. Oka E, Ohtsuka Y, Yoshinaga H, et al. Prevalence of childhood epilepsy and distribution of epileptic syndromes: a population-based survey in Okayama, Japan. *Epilepsia.* 2006;47:626–630.

CHAPTER 2 ■ THE NATURAL HISTORY OF SEIZURES

D. DING AND W. A. HAUSER

It was not long ago that studies of highly selected populations drawn from tertiary-care centers suggested that epilepsy was predominantly a lifelong condition with a low likelihood of seizure control, much less remission. However, recent retrospective and prospective epidemiologic studies based on community and hospital populations have provided more favorable information regarding the natural history of epilepsy including recurrence after a single seizure, intractability, remission, relapse after drug withdrawal, and mortality. Specific factors that have been studied with respect to the short-term and long-term natural history of seizures and epilepsy include the age of onset, gender, etiology, seizure type, electroencephalogram (EEG) pattern, number of seizures prior to treatment, early response to treatment, medication withdrawal, and epilepsy surgery. For the individual, the outcome of epilepsy strongly reflects the individual's syndromic classification and underlying etiology of the epilepsy (1–3).

RECURRENCE AFTER A SINGLE SEIZURE

A seizure may be the result of an acute precipitant such as a stroke or toxin (i.e., acute symptomatic) or occur in the absence of precipitation factors (i.e., unprovoked). The incidence of acute symptomatic seizures is 29 to 39 per 100,000 per year, and the incidence of single unprovoked seizures is 23 to 61 per 100,000 person-years (4).

Epilepsy is generally defined as a condition in which an individual tends to experience recurrent unprovoked seizures. Overall, the lifetime cumulative risk of developing epilepsy by the age of 80 years ranges from 1.4% to 3.3% (5). Although the person with only one unprovoked seizure does not have epilepsy, their risk that this person will develop epilepsy differs from the general population; and it is estimated that 40% to 50% of incident, single unprovoked seizures will recur (5,6).

The risk of subsequent seizures following a first seizure decreases with time. Prospective studies reported the 2-year recurrence risk ranged from 25% to 66% accounting for 80% of long-term recurrences after the initial seizure (7–17). The heterogeneous nature of clinical epilepsy can influence the reported variation. For example, when several factors were assessed in a single study, recurrence risk at 2 years varied from less than 15% in those with no identified risk factors to 100% in those with a combination of two or more risk factors (7) (Table 2.1).

A prior neurologic insult, such as neurologic deficits from birth (mental retardation and cerebral palsy), is the most powerful and consistent predictor of recurrence after a first seizure (6–8,18,19). Moreover, the risk of a second seizure is increased by partial seizure type (especially in patients with remote symptomatic first seizures, i.e., seizures that occur in the setting of a previous injury to the brain) (6), an abnormal electroencephalogram (e.g., specific epileptiform EEG patterns) (7,8,18–20), prior acute symptomatic seizures including febrile seizures (7,8,16,21), status epilepticus (SE), multiple seizures at the time of the index episode (7,22), and Todd paralysis (7,8).

At 2 years, the pooled estimate of recurrence risk was 32% for patients with idiopathic first seizures and 57% for patients with remote symptomatic first seizures (6). Over a 10-year period, individuals with a first acute symptomatic seizure that occurred in the setting of central nervous system infection, stroke, and traumatic brain injury were 80% less likely to experience a subsequent unprovoked seizure than were individuals with a first unprovoked seizure (23).

The predictive value of specific EEG abnormalities is controversial. Only generalized spike-and-wave discharge was found to be associated with an increased recurrence risk in the idiopathic group (7). The pooled risk of recurrence at 2 years was 27% with a normal EEG, 58% with epileptiform abnormalities, and 37% with non-epileptiform abnormalities (6). EEG findings poorly predict recurrence after a single seizure among neurologically normal children aged 6 to 14 years (15), whereas brain imaging with CT or MRI can predict the risk of seizure recurrence among children and adults (24).

In two randomized clinical trials, use of antiepileptic drugs (AEDs) in doses to maintain serum levels in the therapeutic range was associated with a reduction in the proportion of patients who experienced seizure recurrence after a first seizure (25,26). A prognostic model based on the Medical Research Council's (MRC) "Multi-center trial for Early Epilepsy and Single Seizures (MESS)" data estimated that, for individuals treated immediately following a first seizure, the probabilities of a second seizure by 1, 3, and 5 years were 26%, 35%, and 39% respectively. No significant difference was observed between immediate treatment group and delayed treatment group with respect to being seizure free between 3 and 5 years after randomization, quality of life outcomes, and serious complications (27). In summary, drug initiation after a first seizure decreases early seizure recurrence but does not affect the long-term prognosis of developing epilepsy (28).

TABLE 2.1

SEIZURE RECURRENCE AFTER A FIRST UNPROVOKED SEIZURE: AN EXTENDED FOLLOW-UP

Risk factor	Recurrence in subgroups, % months of follow-up		
	12 months	24 months	36 months
Baseline (N = 78)	7.0	13.0	16.7
Idiopathic or cryptogenic with an affected sibling (N = 10)	20.0	20.0	31.0
Idiopathic or cryptogenic with a generalized spike-and-wave EEG pattern (N = 10)	10.0	55.0	55.0
Idiopathic or cryptogenic with prior acute seizures (all febrile) (N = 7)	0.0	14.0	28.6
Idiopathic or cryptogenic with abnormal neurologic examination (N = 13)	9.3	15.4	20.3
Idiopathic or cryptogenic with abnormal examination and additional feature (N = 23)	14.3	14.3	22.7
Idiopathic or cryptogenic with two or more features and normal examination (N = 5)	40.0	40.0	70.0
Remote symptomatic with no other features (N = 32)	15.9	15.9	24.8
Remote symptomatic with Todd's paresis (N = 4)	0.0	25.0	50.0
Remote symptomatic with prior acute symptomatic seizures (N = 3)	100.0	100.0	100.0
Remote symptomatic with multiple seizures or status epilepticus at presentation (N = 8)	25.0	37.5	37.5
Remote symptomatic with two or more risk factors (N = 12)	41.7	75.0	75.0

EEG, electroencephalogram.
From Hauser WA, Rich SS, Annegers JF, et al. Seizure recurrence after a first unprovoked seizure: an extended follow-up. *Neurology.* 1990;40: 1163–1170, with permission.

REMISSION OF TREATED EPILEPSY

Given that in developed countries antiepileptic medication is usually commenced after two unprovoked seizures, prognostic studies from western countries are essentially those of treated epilepsy. A landmark study of the natural history of treated epilepsy was a community-based project carried out in Rochester, Minnesota, USA. The probability of being in remission for 5 years at 20 years after diagnosis (terminal remission) was 75% (29). The National General Practice Study of Epilepsy (NGPSE) conducted in the United Kingdom is the largest ongoing prospective community-based study of the prognosis of epileptic seizures. When patients with acute symptomatic seizures and those who had only one seizure were excluded, 60% had achieved a 5-year remission by 9 years of follow-up (14,30). Other modern large-scale studies that include only newly diagnosed patients followed for long periods also tend to suggest a remission rate of 60% to 90% (31) (Table 2.2).

Many studies have looked at possible predictors of seizure prognosis, including age of onset, gender, etiology, seizure type, EEG patterns, number of seizures prior to treatment, and early response to treatment (17). When comparing prognosis by etiology, patients with idiopathic generalized epilepsy appear to have a better prognosis than patients with symptomatic or cryptogenic partial epilepsy. In one study 82% of people with idiopathic generalized seizures achieved 1-year seizure freedom compared with only 35% with remote symptomatic partial epilepsy and 45% with cryptogenic partial epilepsy (3). Temporal lobe epilepsy (TLE) is associated

TABLE 2.2

TERMINAL REMISSION DATA FROM SELECTED STUDIES

Reference	Study setting	Special study features	No. of patients	Median follow-up (years)	Years in remission	% in remission at median follow-up
Elwes et al. (32)	Hospital		106	5.5	2	79
Shafer et al. (29)	Community		432	17	5	66
Collaborative Group (33)	Hospital		280	4	1	70
Cockerell et al. (14)	Community	Definite epilepsy	564	7	5	68
Sillanpaa et al. (34)	Hospital	Children only	176	40	1	93
Lindsten et al. (35)	Community	≥1 baseline seizure	107	9	5	64
		≥2 baseline seizures	89	9	5	58

From Kwan P, Sander JW. The natural history of epilepsy: an epidemiological view. *J Neurol Neurosurg Psychiatry.* 2004;75:1376–1381, with permission.

with a poorer prognosis than extra-TLE. The prognosis for mesial TLE or hippocampal sclerosis and another identified pathology (dual pathology) is worse than the prognosis for epilepsy in the setting of other etiologies such as arteriovenous malformation, cerebral infarction, cortical dysplasia, and primary tumor (3,36).

The number of seizures in the first 6 months after onset has been found to be a strong determinant of the probability of subsequent remission, with 95% of those with two seizures in the first 6 months achieving a 5-year remission compared with only 24% of those with more than 10 seizures during this same time period (37). Remote symptomatic epilepsy, the presence of the neurological birth deficit, and learning disability are consistently shown to be associated with a poor prognosis (38).

Seizure type has been an inconsistent prognostic factor with some studies (29,39). People with multiple seizure types, as is typical in the childhood encephalopathies, appear to have a poorer prognosis (33). Children who experience clusters of seizures during treatment are much more likely to have refractory epilepsy than children without clusters and are less likely to achieve 5-year terminal remission (34). Children who continued to have weekly seizures during the first year of treatment had an eightfold increase in the risk of developing intractable epilepsy and a twofold increase in the risk of never achieving 1-year terminal remission (40).

An ongoing long-term study of newly diagnosed patients in Glasgow, Scotland, demonstrated that among the 470 patients who had never previously received AED treatment, 64% entered terminal remission of at least 1 year, including 47% of patients who became and remained seizure-free on the first drug, 13% on the second drug, but only 4% on the third drug or a combination of two drugs. Thus, response to the first AED was the most powerful predictor of prognosis (41).

A meta-analysis of 25 studies concluded that the risk of relapse was 25% at 1 year after discontinuation of antiepileptic medications and 29% at 2 years (42). However, when compared to the MRC's large-scale randomized Antiepileptic Drug Withdrawal Study conducted in the United Kingdom, the rate estimated by the meta-analysis is likely an underestimate. In the MRC study, 25% of patients whose treatment was maintained experienced seizure recurrence, indicating that recurrent seizures following antiepileptic medication withdrawal cannot be attributed solely to medication withdrawal. Even though a substantial proportion of patients in the MRC study remained seizure-free after medication withdrawal, there were no powerful predictors that allowed for the identification of these individuals (43). At a conservative estimate, at least 60% of newly diagnosed patients will enter long-term remission on treatment initiation, and approximately 50% of these patients will remain in remission after antiepileptic medication withdrawal.

SPONTANEOUS REMISSION AND UNTREATED EPILEPSY

Evidence from studies from resource-poor countries where a significant treatment gap exists suggests that many patients may enter spontaneous remission with no AED treatment (44). The similar prevalence rates in resource-poor and developed nations may reflect the occurrence of spontaneous remission of many of the untreated cases. In late 1980s, 49% of 643 patients who lived in northern Ecuador and had never received AED treatment were seizure-free for at least 12 months (44). A recent study from rural Bolivia reported 43.7% of untreated epilepsy cases were seizure-free for more than 5 years when the cohort was revisited after 10 years (45). Besides developing countries, spontaneous remission of epilepsy has also been observed in developed countries. In a Finnish study, it was found that 42% of 33 untreated epilepsy patients entered a 2-year remission within 10 years after onset (46).

PROGNOSIS OF INTRACTABLE EPILEPSY

Only 5% to 10% of all incidence cases of epilepsy ultimately result in truly intractable disease. These cases probably account for half the prevalence cases of epilepsy. Approximately 60% of patients with intractable epilepsy can be expected to suffer from partial seizures. Intractability of epilepsy is difficult to define as it is not simply the converse of seizure freedom. Moreover, the predictors of intractability may differ from those of seizure control or remission, and the definition of drug resistance will vary with the investigator's interest and available procedures (47–50). Etiology, younger age at onset (younger than age 1 year), high initial seizure frequency, and mental retardation are predictors of intractability among children (50,51). The type of syndrome, cryptogenic or symptomatic generalized epilepsies, is a predictor of intractability in multivariate analyses. After adjustment for syndrome, initial seizure frequency, focal EEG slowing, and acute symptomatic or neonatal SE also correlate with an increased risk (48,52).

Studies suggest that failure to control seizures with the first or second AED implies that the probability of subsequent seizure control with further AEDs is only about 4% (31). Recent studies reported that approximately 5% per year of patients with intractable epilepsy are seizure-free for 12 months following medication changes. This finding highlights the fact that, irrespective of the number of previous AEDs, there is still a small possibility of inducing meaningful seizure remission in this population (53,54). One retrospective cohort study of 187 patients with intractable epilepsy who had been followed for a mean of 3.8 years reported a remission rate of 4% per year with 17 of the 20 who went into remission having undergone a medication change just prior to the onset of remission and 3 of the individuals experiencing remission for no obvious reason. Five of these 20 patients subsequently relapsed after 12 months of seizure freedom. No predictors of remission or subsequent relapse were identified (55). However, because the probability of remission in these patients is small, in addition to medication changes in this population, alternative treatments, including surgery, should be considered.

PROGNOSIS AFTER EPILEPSY SURGERY

In a meta-analysis of articles published between 1991 and 2005 that reported on the outcome of ≥20 patients of any age who had undergone resective or nonresective epilepsy surgery with a mean/median follow-up of ≥5 years, 20% (95% confidence interval [95% CI] = 18–23) of patients achieved long-term AED discontinuation, 41% (95% CI = 37–45) were on monotherapy, and 31% (95% CI = 27–35) remained on polytherapy. Of the patients with TLE surgery, 14% (95% CI = 11–17) achieved long-term AED discontinuation, 50% (95% CI = 45–55) achieved monotherapy, and 33% remained on polytherapy (95% CI = 29–38). Children achieved better AED outcomes than adults (56). TLE surgery has also been reported to be four times more likely to render patients seizure-free than medical treatment alone in appropriately selected patients (57).

Recent studies evaluated the long-term efficacy of frontal lobe epilepsy (FLE) surgery and TLE surgery with a large sample size, respectively, of 97 and 434 consecutive adult patients. The likelihood of remaining seizure-free after 2 years of freedom from seizures was 86% for 10 years after FLE surgery and 90% for 16 years after TLE surgery. Etiology has an important role in the prediction of long-term outcome after surgery (58,59). Lesional posterior cortical epilepsy surgery has also proved to be effective in short- and long-term follow-up (60).

MORTALITY OF EPILEPSY

Mortality associated with a specific disease can be an indirect estimator of severity (61). People with epilepsy have a mortality rate (the number of deaths that occur in the defined population divided by the person-years at risk in that population) two to three times higher than that of the general population (62). Mortality rate from epilepsy shows a small peak in early life, which possibly reflects the mortality of those children with severe hypoxic ischemic encephalopathy, brain malformations, and inherited metabolic disorders. The risk then falls to a minimum around the age of 10 years. It rises again in late adolescence and early adulthood before levelling off throughout most of adult life. There is a late peak of epilepsy-related mortality in old age, presumably secondary to cerebrovascular disease (CVD) (63) (Fig. 2.1).

In many countries, death certificates are unreliable with respect to the specific cause of death. The certificates may fail to mention epilepsy as a causative or even a contributory factor. Often, a range of other medical conditions that are irrelevant to the cause of death are listed or the death may be incorrectly attributed to epilepsy (64–66). Thus, the estimates of mortality rate of epilepsy based on death certificates are unlikely to be accurate.

Mortality is best expressed as the standardized mortality ratio (SMR), the ratio of the observed number of deaths in an epilepsy population to that expected based on the age- and sex-specific mortality rates in a reference population, in a given time. The proportional mortality ratio (PMR), the proportion of deaths due to a particular cause in a cohort of patients in a given period, can be used to compare the relative contribution of various causes to the overall mortality in the population. Case fatality rate (CFR), the number of deaths caused by a disease divided by the number of diagnosed cases of the disease, can also be used to describe the severity of mortality (67,68).

The risk of mortality after a single seizure is rarely reported. The SMR in patients following a new diagnosis of unprovoked seizure ranges from 2.5 to 4.1 (4). In the NGPSE,

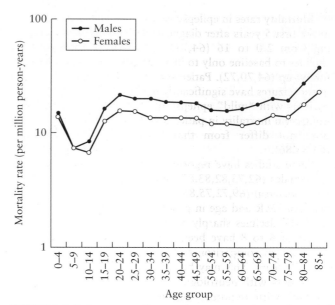

FIGURE 2.1 Epilepsy mortality rates by age group during the period 1950–1994 controlling for the effects of period of death and cohort of birth, in England and Wales. (From O'Callaghan FJK, Osborne JP, Martyn CN. Epilepsy related mortality. *Arch Dis Child.* 2004;89: 705–707, with permission.)

patients with a provoked seizure had an SMR of 3.0 (69,70), whereas a French study reported an SMR of 9.3 as a 1-year mortality in a prospective cohort of 804 patients following a first provoked seizure (71). The high mortality in the French study was due to the inclusion of afebrile, provoked seizures and seizures that were associated with a progressive symptomatic etiology.

Population-based studies provide a more accurate estimate of mortality in the general epilepsy population. In large cohort studies of patients over 15 years, SMRs ranging from 2.1 to 5.1 were reported (70,72–75). The majority of death in people whose seizures start in childhood occur in adulthood (38,76,77). Prospective studies in which children with large sample size were followed for 15 to more than 30 years reported higher SMRs of 8.8 to 13.2 (76,78,79).

There have been only a few mortality-related studies undertaken in the developing world. A recent prospective study of Chinese rural patients with epilepsy reported an SMR of 3.9 (95% CI = 3.8–3.9). This value may be an underestimate as patients with progressive neurological and other chronic medical conditions were not included (80). Two hospital-based studies in Martinique and Ecuador reported SMRs of 4.3 and 6.3. Additionally, a community follow-up study in India reported a higher SMR of 7.8 (81).

Risk factors of mortality in epilepsy include etiology, duration and type of epilepsy, seizure frequency, gender, and age. Idiopathic (and/or cryptogenic) epilepsy has the lowest long-term mortality, with SMRs ranging from 1.5 to 1.8 in population studies (62,64,82). Long-term mortality is greatly increased in remote symptomatic epilepsy, especially in children with gross neurological deficit and/or learning difficulties, with reported SMRs of 2.2 to 49.7 (64,71,73,79,80,83). The SMR for patients with generalized tonic–clonic seizures is 3.5 to 3.9 for the first 5 to 10 years following diagnosis. In contrast, the SMR associated with myoclonic seizures is 4.1 and with partial seizures is 1.5 to 2.1 (64,73,83).

Mortality rates in epilepsy vary over time. The rate is high in the first 5 years after diagnosis with reported SMRs ranging from 2.0 to 16 (64,71,73,75,83,84). The rate then declines to baseline only to increase again in years 9 to 29 of follow-up (64,70,72). Patients with "severe" epilepsy or frequent seizures have significantly higher SMRs compared with patients with "mild" epilepsy or who are seizure-free (62). Long-term mortality in patients with well-controlled seizures does not differ from that of the general population (64,85,86).

Some studies have reported higher SMRs for males than for females (62,73,82,83,87). However, this finding has not been universal (69,72,75,85,88). There is an inverse relation between SMR and age in people under 50 years of age, and the SMR declines sharply after age 60 (64,70,73,74,82,83). SMRs of 6 to 8 have been reported for age groups up to 50 years, in comparison to SMRs of <2 for patients older than 70 years. This may be explained by the high mortality in patients with neurological deficit at birth and in young patients with remote symptomatic epilepsy due to head trauma and brain tumors, as well as the highly increased risk of sudden death in younger adults with epilepsy (62). A study from rural China reported that patients aged 15 to 29 years had higher mortality ratios than did those in other age groups with the SMRs exceeding 23 (80). Epilepsy could pose a potential threat to young people with the disorder especially in resource-poor areas where the high treatment gap exists.

Cause-Specific Mortality

Death in people with epilepsy can be classified into three groups: epilepsy-related deaths, deaths related to the underlying cause of the epilepsy, and deaths that are unrelated to the epilepsy or its underlying etiology (89) (Table 2.3). For patients with epilepsy, population-based studies demonstrate PMRs of 12% to 39% for CVD, 12% to 37% for ischemic heart disease (IHD), 18% to 40% for neoplasia (including brain tumors), 9% to 15% for brain tumors, 8% to 18% for pneumonia, 0% to 7% for suicides, 0% to 12% for accidents, 0% to 4% for SUDEP, 0% to 10% for seizure-related causes (including SE), and 5% to 30% for other causes (64,69,70, 71,72,82,90). A study in rural China illustrated a significantly higher PMR (30%) for accidents, and lower PMR (6%) for myocardial infarction (80).

Deaths directly related to epilepsy include SUDEP, SE, accidents caused by seizures, and suicide (62). The PMRs for epilepsy-related conditions range between 1% and 45% (64,70,72,78,82,91). The wide range of the PMR for epilepsy-related conditions may be explained by differences in patient characteristics and population selection, diagnostic criteria, duration of follow-up, and classification of causes of death (62).

SUDEP is defined as a sudden, unexpected, witnessed or unwitnessed, nontraumatic and nondrowning death in patients with epilepsy, with or without evidence of seizure and excluding documented SE, in which postmortem examination does not reveal a toxicological or anatomical cause of death (92). When an autopsy is not performed, sudden death occurring in benign circumstances with unknown competing cause for death can be categorized as probable or possible SUDEP,

TABLE 2.3

CAUSES OF DEATH IN EPILEPSY

Unrelated deaths
  Neoplasms outside the central nervous system
  Ischemic heart disease
  Pneumonia
  Others

Related to underlying disease
  Brain tumors
  Cerebrovascular disease
  Cerebral infection-abscesses and encephalitis
  Inherited disorders, e.g., Batten's disease

Epilepsy-related deaths
  Suicides
  Treatment-related deaths
  Idiosyncratic drug reactions
  Medication adverse effects
  Seizure-related deaths
  Status epilepticus
  Trauma, burns, drowning
  Asphyxiation, aspiration
  Aspiration pneumonia after a seizure
  Sudden unexpected death in epilepsy

From Nashef L, Shorvon SD. Mortality in epilepsy. *Epilepsia.* 1997;38:1059–1061, with permission.

especially for the purpose of epidemiological studies (93,94). Potential mechanisms for SUDEP include central and obstructive apnea, cardiac arrhythmia, autonomic disturbance, and hypoxia (62,95–98).

The reported incidence of SUDEP has ranged from 0.35 to 9.3 per 1000 person-years depending on the different study population and methodologies employed (99–105). The incidence of death for young adults with intractable epilepsy is many times that of the general population, with a peak between the ages of 20 and 40 years (106). In older age groups the relative increase incidence of SUDEP is difficult to measure since it might be confounded by the co-morbidity such as cardiovascular, respiratory, or CVD. Young age (20 to 45 years old), early onset of epilepsy, acquired epilepsy (primarily from traumatic brain injury or encephalitis/meningitis), primary generalized tonic–clonic seizures, intractable epilepsy, frequent seizures were reported to be the independent risk factors for SUDEP (75,99,100,106–113). A few studies have implicated treatment with carbamazepine as an independent risk factor, even after adjustments for seizure frequency (109,113–115). Frequent drug changes and AED polytherapy, which are conventional markers of severe and unstable epilepsy, may be more common in SUDEP cases than in controls (109).

SE appears to be an important cause of death with an annual incidence of 10 to 60 per 100,000 in the general population (116–120). It accounts for between 0.5% and 10% of all deaths in epilepsy, with an SMR of 2.8 (95% CI 2.1–3.5) (121). The CFR from SE was reported as 7.6% to 22% for short-term mortality (within 30 days of SE) (116,118,119, 122–125) and 43% for long-term mortality (30 days after SE to 10 years) (121). The Higher CFRs were found in patients with acute symptomatic seizures, myoclonic seizures, and people over

65 years (121,124–129). The overtreatment of nonconvulsive SE with benzodiazepines in the elderly may be an additional factor for the increase of CFR (128). With respect to etiology, the highest CFR for adults are reported for hypoxia (secondary to cardiac arrest), cerebral infection, and CVD (116,122,124). Poor compliance, assessed by low AED levels, unprovoked epilepsy, and children with epilepsy were associated with relatively low CFRs (2% to 4%) (116–118, 121–124,130–132). These findings suggest that SE by itself does not alter long-term mortality (124).

People with epilepsy may sustain a fatal accident either during a seizure or as a consequence of a seizure. Accidental deaths related to epilepsy are commonly due to drowning, traffic accidents, trauma, falls, burns, or aspiration. Based on attendance records of four accident and emergency departments, the risk of injury as a result of a seizure was estimated to be 29.5 per 100,000 per year (133). Accident-related deaths in people with epilepsy comprise between 1.2% and 6.5% of all deaths in community-based studies (64,70,76,82) and between 7.3% and 42% in selected population studies with SMRs ranging from 2.4 to 5.6 (62,73,87,88,125,134–137). A study in Iceland reported that the SMR for deaths due to accidents, poisonings, and violence was 7.27 (95% CI = 1.96 to 18.62) for male patients with remote symptomatic epilepsy and 1.76 (95% CI = 0.47 to 4.51) for those with idiopathic/cryptogenic seizures (87). People with epilepsy have an increased risk of drowning with SMR of 5.4 to 96.9 that varied depending on the study population (138). Other accidental deaths related to seizure are reported rarely in the developed countries (139–142).

Studies performed during the 1970 and 1980s demonstrated that people with epilepsy were at an increased risk of suicide (62,73,74,82,87,88,135,137,143). However, this finding has not been replicated, especially in more recent studies (62,64,69,70,125,144). In these studies, the suicide PMRs range between 0% and 20% and the SMRs between 1 and 5.8. Mental illness, drug addiction, TLE, early onset of epilepsy (particularly onset during adolescence), and personality disorder have been associated with increased risk (145–147).

Common nonepileptic causes of death cited in mortality studies include neoplasia, CVD, IHD, and pneumonia. Reports have noted increased SMR for malignant neoplasia of the lung, pancreas, hepatobiliary system, breast, and lymphoid and hematopoietic tissue (116). Cancer accounts for 16% to 29% of deaths with reported SMRs ranging from 3.4 to 5.4 (72,88,134); although in one study, hospitalized patients with epilepsy appeared to be at much higher risk, with a reported SMR of 29.9 (73). The SMR for neoplasia remains at 1.4 to 2.5 even when CNS tumors are excluded (64,70,73,74,88). The SMR for all cancers in an institutional cohort with more severe epilepsy (SMR 1.42; 95% CI = 1.18 to 1.69) was higher than that for the milder cases in a community-based population (SMR = 0.93; 95% CI = 0.84 to 1.03). The SMR for brain and CNS neoplasms was significantly elevated in the group with milder epilepsy (148).

CVD is a significant cause of death in elderly people with epilepsy and accounts for 44% of deaths in patients over 75 years (73). CVD PMR is 14% to 16% in population-based series (64,70,82,87) and in a large hospital-based series (73), and 5% to 6% in referral populations (88,125,134,136,137). The SMR ranged between 1.8 and 5.3, reflecting a mortality

spectrum from epilepsy center cohorts to general population cohorts, with hospital cohorts in the middle (64,70,72,73,88,134). PMRs for IHD are similar to those for CVD. IHD events include angina pectoris, myocardial infarction, and sudden cardiac death (62). Most deaths from IHD were noted in patients over the age of 45 (73,90). Population-based studies have demonstrated a slight increase in mortality from IHD with SMRs ranging between 1.1 and 1.5 (64,70,74,83,88,90).

Especially in institutionalized patients, pneumonia often reflects a terminal event in patients with poorly controlled seizures, poor general condition, and debilitation (70,73,82,88,125,137). PMRs for pneumonia range from 5% to 25% in studies of inpatients in epilepsy institutions and hospitals, as well as patients in the community (4,62,64,73,74,82,88,125,137). SMRs range between 3.5 and 10.3 (64,70,73,88,139). The majority of deaths due to pneumonia occur in elderly patients (69,70,73,82,125), as well as in children with epilepsy, especially those with remote symptomatic seizures (78), infantile spasms, and severe psychomotor retardation (149).

SUMMARY

Epidemiological studies have provided more favorable information of the natural history of seizures. At least 60% of newly diagnosed patients can expect complete seizure control, and approximately 50% of these patients can discontinue medication. Up to one third of premature deaths can be directly or indirectly attributable to epilepsy. Mortality is significantly higher in people with symptomatic epilepsy, in the first 5 to 10 years after diagnosis of epilepsy, and in younger people. Major contributors to death in patients with epilepsy are neoplasia, cerebrovascular disorders, and pneumonia in elderly or institutionalized patients. SUDEP is the most important cause of epilepsy-related deaths, particularly in the young, and people with frequent seizures and/or suboptimal AED treatment. Appropriate postmortem investigations should be conducted in order to accurately classify the cause of death. Management of treatment and care should also be considered to prevent the seizure-related premature death.

References

1. Sander JW. Some aspects of prognosis in the epilepsies: a review. *Epilepsia.* 1993;34:1007–1016.
2. Berg AT, Shinnar S. Do seizures beget seizures? An assessment of the clinical evidence in humans. *J Clin Neurophysiol.* 1997;14:102–110.
3. Semah F, Picot MC, Adam C, et al. Is the underlying caused of epilepsy a major prognostic factor for recurrence? *Neurology.* 1998;51:1256–1262.
4. Hauser WA, Beghi E. First seizure definitions and worldwide incidence and mortality. *Epilepsia.* 2008;49(S1):8–12.
5. Hauser WA, Hesdorffer DC. *Epilepsy: Frequency, Causes, and Consequences.* New York: Demos Publications; 1990.
6. Berg AT, Shinnar S. The risk of seizure recurrence following a first unprovoked seizure: a quantitative review. *Neurology.* 1991;41:965–972.
7. Hauser WA, Rich SS, Annegers JF, Anderson VE. Seizure recurrence after a first unprovoked seizure: an extended follow-up. *Neurology.* 1990;40:1163–1170.
8. Shinnar S, Berg AT, Moshe SL, et al. The risk of seizure recurrence following a first unprovoked seizure in childhood: a prospective study. *Pediatrics.* 1990;85:1076–1085.

9. Lindsten H, Stenlund H, Forsgren L. Seizure recurrence in adults after a newly diagnosed unprovoked epileptic seizure. *Acta Neurol Scand.* 2001; 104:202–207.

10. Hart YM, Sander JW, Johnson AL, et al. National general practice study of epilepsy: recurrence after a first seizure. *Lancet.* 1990;336:1271–1274.

11. Shinnar S, Berg AT, Moshe SL, et al. The risk of seizure recurrence after a first unprovoked afebrile seizure in childhood: an extended follow-up. *Pediatrics.* 1996;98:216–225.

12. Winckler MI, Rotta NT. Clinical and electroencephalographic follow-up after a first unprovoked seizure. *Pediatr Neurol.* 2004;30:201–206.

13. Martinovic Z, Jovic N. Seizure recurrence after a first generalized tonic-clonic seizure, in children, adolescents and young adults. *Seizure.* 1997; 6:461–465.

14. Cockerell OC, Johnson AL, Sander JW, et al. Remission of epilepsy: results from the National General Practice Study of Epilepsy. *Lancet.* 1995; 346:140–144.

15. Arthur TM, deGrauw TJ, Johnson CS, et al. Seizure recurrence risk following a first seizure in neurologically normal children. *Epilepsia.* 2008; 49:1950–1954.

16. Annegers JF, Hauser WA, Shirts SB, et al. Factors prognostic of unprovoked seizures after febrile convulsions. *N Engl J Med.* 1987;316:493–498.

17. Shinnar S, Berg AT, O'dell C, et al. Predictors of multiple seizures in a cohort of children prospectively followed from the time of their first unprovoked seizure. *Ann Neurol.* 2000;48:140–147.

18. Stroink H, Brouwer OF, Arts WF, et al. The first unprovoked, untreated seizure in childhood: a hospital based study of the accuracy of the diagnosis, rate of recurrence, and long term outcome after recurrence. Dutch study of epilepsy in childhood. *J Neurol Neurosurg Psychiatry.* 1998;64: 595–600.

19. Annegers JF, Shirts SB, Hauser WA, et al. Risk of recurrence after an initial unprovoked seizure. *Epilepsia.* 1986;27:43–50.

20. van Donsclaar CA, Gertz AT, Schumsheimer RJ. Idiopathic first seizure in adult life. Who should be treated? *BMJ.* 1991;302:620–623.

21. Nelson KB, Ellenburg JH. Antecedents of seizure disorders in early childhood. *Am Dis Child.* 1986;40:1053–1061.

22. Camfield P, Camfield C. Epilepsy can be diagnosed when the first two seizures occur on the same day. *Epilepsia.* 2000;41:1230–1233.

23. Hesdorffer DC, Benn EK, Cascino GD, et al. Is a first acute asymptomatic seizure epilepsy? Mortality and risk for recurrent seizure. *Epilepsia.* 2009;50:1102–1108.

24. Krumholz A, Wiebe S, Gronseth G, et al. Practice Parameter: evaluating an apparent unprovoked first seizure in adults (an evidence-based review): Report of the Quality Standards Subcommittee of the American Academy of Neurology and the American Epilepsy Society. *Neurology.* 2007;69: 1996–2007.

25. Camfield P, Camfield C, Dooley J, et al. A randomized study of carbamazepine versus no medication after a first unprovoked seizure in childhood. *Neurology.* 1989;39:851–852.

26. Mussico M, First Seizure Trial Group (FIRST Group). Randomized clinical trial on the efficacy of antiepileptic drugs in reducing the risk of relapse after a first unprovoked tonic-clonic seizure. *Neurology.* 1993;43: 478–483.

27. Kim LG, Johnson TL, Marson AG, et al. Prediction of risk of seizure recurrence after a single seizure and early epilepsy: further results from the MESS trial. *Lancet Neurology.* 2006;5:317–322.

28. Shih JJ, Ochoa JG. A systematic review of antiepileptic drug initiation and withdrawal. *Neurologist.* 2009;15:122–131.

29. Shafer SQ, Hauser WA, Annegers JF, et al. EEG and other early predictors of epilepsy remission: a community study. *Epilepsia.* 1988;29:590–600.

30. Cockerell OC, Johnson AL, Sander JW, et al. Prognosis of epilepsy: a review and further analysis of the first nine years of the British National General Practice Study of Epilepsy, a prospective population-based study. *Epilepsia.* 1997;38:31–46.

31. Kwan P, Sander JW. The natural history of epilepsy: an epidemiological view. *J Neurol Neurosurg Psychiatry.* 2004;75:1376–1381.

32. Elwes RD, Johnson AL, Shorvon SD, et al. The prognosis for seizure control in newly diagnosed epilepsy. *N Engl J Med.* 1984;311:944–947.

33. Collaborative group for the Study of Epilepsy. Prognosis of epilepsy in newly referred patients: a multicenter prospective study of the effects of monotherapy on the long-term course of epilepsy. *Epilepsia.* 1992; 33:45–51.

34. Sillanpaa M, Schmidt D. Seizure clustering during drug treatment affects seizure outcome and mortality of childhood-onset epilepsy. *Brain.* 2008;131:938–944.

35. Lindsten H, Stenlund H, Forgren L. Remission of seizures in a population-based adult cohort with a newly diagnosed unprovoked epilepsy seizure. *Epilepsia.* 2001;42:1025–1030.

36. Stephen LJ, Kwan P, Brodie MJ. Does the cause of localisation-related epilepsy influence the response to antiepileptic drug treatment? *Epilepsia.* 2001;42:357–362.

37. MacDonald BK, Johnson AL, Goodridge DM, et al. Factors predicting prognosis of epilepsy after presentation with seizures. *Ann Neurol.* 2000; 48:833–841.

38. Brorson LO, Wranne L. Long-term prognosis in childhood epilepsy: survival and seizure prognosis. *Epilepsia.* 1987;28:324–330.

39. Annegers JF, Hauser WA, Elveback LR. Remission of seizures and relapse in patients with epilepsy. *Epilepsia.* 1979;20:729–737.

40. Sillanpaa M, Schmidt D. Early seizure frequency and aetiology predict long-term medical outcome in childhood-onset epilepsy. *Brain.* 2009; 132(4):989–998.

41. Kwan P, Brodie MJ. Early identification of refractory epilepsy. *N Engl J Med.* 2000;342:314–319.

42. Berg AT, Shinnar S. Relapse following discontinuation of antiepileptic drugs: a meta-analysis. *Neurology.* 1994;44:601–608.

43. Medical Research Council Antiepileptic Drug Withdrawal Study Group. Randomized study of antiepileptic drug withdrawal in patients in remission. *Lancet.* 1991;337:1175–1180.

44. Placencia M, Sander JW, Roman M, et al. The characteristics of epilepsy in a largely untreated population in rural Ecuador. *J Neurol Neurosurg Psychiatry.* 1994;57:320–325.

45. Nicoletti A, Sofia V, Vitale G, et al. Natural history and mortality of chronic epilepsy in an untreated population of rural Bolivia: a follow-up after 10 years. *Epilepsia.* 2009;50:2199–2206.

46. Keranen T, Riekkinen PJ. Remission of seizures in untreated epilepsy. *BMJ.* 1993;307:483.

47. Shinnar S, Berg AT, Moshe SL, et al. Discontinuing antiepileptic drugs in children with epilepsy: a prospective study. *Ann Neurol.* 1994;35:534–545.

48. Berg AT, Shinnar S, Levy SR, et al. Early development of intractable epilepsy in children: a prospective study. *Neurology.* 2001;56:1430–1431.

49. Wakamoto H, Nagao H, Hayashi M, et al. Long-term medical, educational, and social prognoses of childhood-onset epilepsy: a population-based study in a rural district of Japan. *Brain Dev.* 2000;22:246–255.

50. Casetta I, Granieri E, Monetti VC, et al. Early predictors of intractability in childhood epilepsy: a community-based case-control study in Copparo, Italy. *Acta Neurol Scand.* 1999;99:329–333.

51. Berg AT, Novotny EJ, Levy SR, et al. Predictors of intractable epilepsy in children: a case-control study. *Epilepsia.* 1996;37:24–30.

52. Berg AT, Shinnar S, Levy SR, et al. Two-year remission and subsequent relapse in children with newly diagnosed epilepsy. *Epilepsia.* 2001;42: 1553–1562.

53. Luciano AL, Shorvon SD. Results of treatment changes in patients with apparently drug-resistant chronic epilepsy. *Ann Neurol.* 2007;62:375–381.

54. Callaghan BC, Anand K, Hesdorffer D, et al. Likelihood of seizure remission in an adult population with refractory epilepsy. *Ann Neurol.* 2007;62:382–389.

55. Choi H, Heiman G, Pandis D, et al. Seizure remission and relapse in adults with intractable epilepsy: a cohort study. *Epilepsia.* 2008;49:1440–1445.

56. Te'llez-Zenteno JF, Dhar R, Hernandez-Ronquillo L, et al. Long-term outcomes in epilepsy surgery: antiepileptic drugs, mortality, cognitive and psychosocial aspects. *Brain.* 2007;130:334–345.

57. Schmidt D, Stavem K. Long-term seizure outcome of surgery versus no surgery for drug-resistant partial epilepsy: a review of controlled studies. *Epilepsia.* 2009;50:1301–1309.

58. Elsharkawy AE, Alabbashi AH, Pannek H, et al. Outcome of frontal lobe epilepsy surgery in adults. *Epilepsy Res.* 2008;81:97–106.

59. Elsharkawy AE, Alabbashi AH, Pannek H, et al. Long-term outcome after temporal lobe epilepsy surgery in 44 consecutive adult patients. *J Neurosurg.* 2009;110:1135–1146.

60. Elsharkawy AE, El-Ghandour NM, Oppel F, et al. Long-term outcome of lesional posterior cortical epilepsy surgery in adults. *J Neurol Neurosurg Psychiatry.* 2009;80:773–780.

61. Logroscino G, Hesdorffer DC. Methodologic issues in studies of mortality following epilepsy: measures, types of studies, sources of cases, cohort effects, and competing risks. *Epilepsia.* 2005;46:S3–S7.

62. Gaitatzis A, Sander JW. The mortality of epilepsy revisited. *Epileptic Disord.* 2004;6:3–13.

63. O'Callaghan FJK, Osborne JP, Martyn CN. Epilepsy related mortality. *Arch Dis Child.* 2004;89:705–707.

64. Hauser WA, Annegers JF, Elveback LR. Mortality in patients with epilepsy. *Epilepsia.* 1980;21:399–412.

65. Sander JW, Shorvon SD. Incidence and prevalence studies in epilepsy and their methodological problems: a review. *J Neurol Neurosurg Psychiatry.* 1987;50:829–839.

66. Bell GS, Gaitatzis A, Johnson AL, et al. Predictive value of death certification in the case ascertainment of epilepsy. *J Neurol Neurosurg Psychiatry.* 2004;75:1756–1758.

67. Commission on Epidemiology and Prognosis ILAE. Guidelines for epidemiologic studies on epilepsy. *Epilepsia.* 1993;34:592–596.

68. Tomson T. Mortality in epilepsy. *J Neurol.* 2000;247:15–21.

69. Cockerell OC, Johnson AL, Sander JW et al. Mortality from epilepsy: results from a prospective population-based study. *Lancet.* 1994;344: 918–921.

70. Lhatoo SD, Johnson AL, Goodridge DM, et al. Mortality in epilepsy in the first 11 to 14 years after diagnosis: multivariate analysis of a long-term, prospective, population-based cohort. *Ann Neurol.* 2001;49:336–344.

71. Loiseau J, Picot MC, Loiseau P. Short-term mortality after a first epileptic seizure: a population-based study. *Epilepsia.* 1999;40:1388–1392.

72. Lindsten H, Nystrom L, Forsgren L. Mortality risk in an adult cohort with a newly diagnosed unprovoked epileptic seizure: a population-based study. *Epilepsia.* 2000;41:1469–1473.

73. Nilsson L, Tomson T, Farahmand BY, et al. Cause-specific mortality in epilepsy: a cohort study of more than 9,000 patients once hospitalized for epilepsy. *Epilepsia.* 1997;38:1062–1068.
74. Shackleton DP, Westendorp RG, Trenite DG, et al. Mortality in patients with epilepsy: 40 years of follow-up in a Dutch cohort study. *J Neurol Nerosurg Psychiatry.* 1999;66:636–640.
75. Nashef L, Fish DR, Sander JW, et al. Incidence of sudden unexpected death in an adult outpatient cohort with epilepsy at a tertiary referral centre. *J Neurol Nerosurg Psychiatry.* 1995;58:462–464.
76. Sillanpää M, Jalava M, Kaleva O, et al. Long-term prognosis of seizures with onset in childhood. *N Engl J Med.* 1998;338:1715–1722.
77. Kurtz Z, Tookey P, Ross E. Epilepsy in young people: 23 year follow-up of the British national child development study. *BMJ.* 1998;316:339–342.
78. Harvey AS, Nolan T, Carlin JB. Community-based study of mortality in children with epilepsy. *Epilepsia.* 1993;34:597–603.
79. Camfield CS, Camfield PR, Veugelers PJ. Death in children with epilepsy: a population-based study. *Lancet.* 2002;359:1891–1895.
80. Ding D, Wang W, Wu J, et al. Premature mortality in people with epilepsy in rural China: a prospective study. *Lancet Neurol.* 2006;5:823–827.
81. Carpio A, Bharucha NE, Jallon P, et al. Mortality of epilepsy in developing countries. *Epilepsia.* 2005;46:S28–S32.
82. Zielinski JJ. Epilepsy and mortality rate and cause of death. *Epilepsia.* 1974;15:191–201.
83. Olafsson E, Hauser WA, Gudmundsson G. Long-term survival of people with unprovoked seizures: a population-based study. *Epilepsia.* 1998;39:89–92.
84. Cockerell OC. The mortality of epilepsy. *Curr Opin Neurol.* 1996;9:93–96.
85. Sperling MR, Feldman H, Kinman J, et al. Seizure control and mortality in epilepsy. *Ann Neurol.* 1999;46:45–50.
86. Salanova V, Markand O, Worth R. Temporal lobe epilepsy surgery: outcome, complications, and late mortality rate in 215 patients. *Epilepsia.* 2002;43:170–174.
87. Rafnsson V, Olafsson E, Hauser WA, et al. Cause-specific mortality in adults with unprovoked seizures. A population-based incidence cohort study. *Neuroepidemiology.* 2001;20:232–236.
88. White SJ, McLean AE, Howland C. Anticonvulsant drugs and cancer. A cohort study in patients with severe epilepsy. *Lancet.* 1979;2:458–461.
89. Nashef L, Shorvon SD. Mortality in epilepsy. *Epilepsia.* 1997;38:1059–1061.
90. Annegers JF, Hauser WA, Shirts SB. Heart disease mortality and morbidity in patients with epilepsy. *Epilepsia.* 1984;25:699–704.
91. Wannamaker BB. A perspective on death of persons with epilepsy. In: Lathers CM, Schraeder PL, eds. *Epilepsy and Sudden Death.* New York: Dekker; 1990:27–37.
92. Nashef L. Sudden unexplained death in epilepsy: terminology and definitions. *Epilepsia.* 1997;38:S6–S8.
93. Monte CP, Arends JB, Tan IY, et al. Sudden unexpected death in epilepsy patients: risk factors. A systematic review. *Seizure.* 2007;16:1–7.
94. Tellez-zemtemo JF, Ronqiollo LH, Wiebe S. Sudden unexpected death in epilepsy: evidence-based analysis of incidence and risk factors. *Epilepsy Res.* 2005;65:101–115.
95. Nashef L, Walker F, Allen P, et al. Apnoea and bradycardia during epileptic seizures: relation to sudden death in epilepsy. *J Neurol Neurosurg Psychiatry.* 1996;60:297–300.
96. Natelson BH, Suarez RV, Terrence CF, et al. Patients with epilepsy who die suddenly have cardiac disease. *Arch Neurol.* 1998;55:857–860.
97. Hilz MJ, Devinsky O, Doyle W, et al. Decrease of sympathetic cardiovascular modulation after temporal lobe epilepsy surgery. *Brain.* 2002;125:985–995.
98. Lathers CM, Schraeder PL. Clinical pharmacology: drugs as a benefit and/or risk in sudden unexpected death in epilepsy? *J Clin Pharmacol.* 2002;42:123–136.
99. Ficker DM, So EL, Shen WK, et al. Population-based study of the incidence of sudden unexplained death in epilepsy. *Neurology.* 1998;51:1270–1274.
100. Leestma JE, Walczak T, Hughes JR, et al. A prospective study on sudden unexpected death in epilepsy. *Ann Neurol.* 1989;26:195–203.
101. Timmings PL. Sudden unexpected death in epilepsy: a local audit. *Seizure.* 1993;2:287–290.
102. Lip GY, Brodie MJ. Sudden death in epilepsy: an avoidable outcome? *J R Soc Med.* 1992;85:609–611.
103. Nashef L, Fish DR, Garner S, et al. Sudden death in epilepsy: a study of incidence in a young cohort with epilepsy and learning difficulty. *Epilepsia.* 1995;36:1187–1194.
104. Nilson L, Ahlbom A, Farahmand BY, et al. Mortality in a population-based cohort of epilepsy surgery patients. *Epilepsia.* 2003;44:575–581.
105. Dasheiff RM. Sudden unexpected death in epilepsy: a series from an epilepsy surgery program and speculation on the relationship to sudden cardiac death. *J Clin Neurophysiol.* 1991;8:216–222.
106. Hitiris N, Suratman S, Kelly K, et al. Sudden unexpected death epilepsy: a search for risk factors. *Epilepsy & Behavior.* 2007;10:138–141.
107. Langan Y, Nolan N, Hutchinson M. The incidence of sudden unexpected death in epilepsy (SUDEP) in South Dublin and Wicklow. *Seizure.* 1998;7:355–358.
108. Nilsson L, Farahmand BY, Persson PG, et al. Risk factors for sudden unexpected death in epilepsy: a case-control study. *Lancet.* 1999;353:888–893.
109. Nilsson L, Bergman U, Diwan V, et al. Antiepileptic drug therapy and its management in sudden unexpected death in epilepsy: a case-control study. *Epilepsia.* 2001;42:667–673.
110. Ficker DM. Sudden unexplained death and injury in epilepsy. *Epilepsia.* 2000;41:S7–S12.
111. Leestma JE, Kalelkar MB, Teas SS, et al. Sudden unexpected death associated with seizures: analysis of 66 cases. *Epilepsia.* 1984;25:84–88.
112. Lear-Kaul KC, Coughlin L, Dobersen MJ. Sudden unexpected death in epilepsy: a retrospective study. *Am J Forensic Med pathol.* 2005;26:11–17.
113. Langan Y, Nashef L, Sander JW. Case-control study of SUDEP. *Neurology.* 2005;64:1131–1133.
114. Timmings PL. Sudden unexpected death in epilepsy: is carbamazepine implicated? *Seizure.* 1998;7:289–291.
115. Hennessy MJ, Tighe MG, Binnie CD, et al. Sudden withdrawal of carbamazipine increases cardiac sympathetic activity in sleep. *Neurology.* 2001;57:1650–1654.
116. DeLorenzo RJ, Hauser WA, Towne AR, et al. A prospective, population-based epidemiologic study of status epilepticus in Richmond, Virginia. *Neurology.* 1996;46:1029–1235.
117. Hesdorffer DC, Logroscino G, Cascino G, et al. Incidence of status epilepticus in Rochester, Minnesota, 1965–1984. *Neurology.* 1998;50:735–741.
118. Waterhouse EJ, Garnett LK, Towne AR, et al. Prospective population-based study of intermittent and continuous convusive status epilepticus in Richmond, Virginia. *Epilepsia.* 1999;40:752–758.
119. Knake S, Rosenow F, Vescovi M, et al. Incidence of status epilepticus in adults in Germany: a prospective, population-based study. *Epilepsia.* 2001;42:714–718.
120. Vignatelli L, Tonon C, D'Alessandro R. Incidence and short-term prognosis of status epilepticus in adults in Bologna, Italy. *Epilepsia.* 2003;44:964–968.
121. Logroscino G, Hesdorffer DC, Cascino GD, et al. Long-term mortality after a first episode of status epilepticus. *Neurology.* 2002;58:537–541.
122. Logroscino G, Hesdorffer DC, Cascino GD, et al. Short-term mortality after a first episode of status epilepticus. *Epilepsia.* 1997;38:1344–1349.
123. Coeytaux A, Jallon P, Galobardes B, et al. Incidence of status epilepticus in French-speaking Switzerland (EPISTAR). *Neurology.* 2000;55:693–697.
124. Wu YW, Shek DW, Garcia PA, et al. Incidence and mortality of generalized convulsive status epilepticus in California. *Neurology.* 2002;58:1070–1076.
125. Krumholz A, Sung GY, Fisher RS, et al. Complex partial status epilepticus accompanied by serious morbidity and mortality. *Neurology.* 1995;45:1499–1504.
126. Young GB, Jordan KG, Doig GS. An assessment of nonconvulsive seizures in the intensive care unit using continuous EEG monitoring: an investigation of variables associated with mortality. *Neurology.* 1996;47:83–89.
127. Hitiris N, Mohanraj R, Norrie J, et al. Mortality in epilepsy. *Epilepsy & Behavior.* 2007;10:363–376.
128. Litt B, Wityk RJ, Hertz SH, et al. Nonconvulsive status epilepticus in the critically ill elderly. *Epilepsia.* 1998;39:1194–1202.
129. Shneker BF, Fountain NB. Assessment of acute morbidity and mortality in nonconvulsive status epilepticus. *Neurology.* 2003;61:1066–1073.
130. Maytal J, Shinnar S, Moshe SL, et al. Low morbidity and mortality of status epilepticus in children. *Pediatrics.* 1989;83:323–331.
131. Phillips SA, Shanahan RJ. Etiology and mortality of status epilepticus in children. A recent update. *Arch Neurol.* 1989;46:74–76.
132. Towne AR, Pellock JM, Ko D, et al. Determinants of mortality in status epilepticus. *Epilepsia.* 1994;35:27–34.
133. Kirby S, Sadler RM. Injury and death as a result of seizures. *Epilepsia.* 1995;36:25–28.
134. Shackleton DP, Westendorp RG, Kasteleijn-Nolst Trenite DG, et al. Survival of patients with epilepsy: an estimate of the mortality risk. *Epilepsia.* 2002;43:445–450.
135. Hashimoto K, Fukushima Y, Saito F, et al. Mortality and cause of death in patients with epilepsy over 16 years of age. *Jpn J Psychiatry Neurol.* 1989;43:546–547.
136. Henriksen B, Juul-Jensen P, Lund M. The mortality of epilepsy. In: Brackenridge RDC, ed. *Proceedings of the International Congress of Life Assurance Medicine.* London: Pitman; 1970:139–148.
137. Livanainen M, Lehtinen J. Causes of death in institutionalized epileptics. *Epilepsia.* 1979;20:485–491.
138. Bell GS, Gaitatzis A, Bell CL, et al. Drowning in people with epilepsy: how great is the risk? *Neurology.* 2008;71:578–582.
139. Russell-Jones DL, Shorvon SD. The frequency and consequences of head injury in epileptic seizures. *J Neurol Neurosurg Psychiatry.* 1989;52:659–662.
140. Spitz MC. Severe burns as a consequence of seizures in patients with epilepsy. *Epilepsia.* 1992;33:103–107.
141. Buck D, Baker GA, Jacoby A, et al. Patients' experiences of injury as a result of epilepsy. *Epilepsia.* 1997;38:439–444.

142. Spitz MC. Injuries and death as a consequence of seizures in people with epilepsy. *Epilepsia*. 1998;39:904–907.

143. Harris EC, Barraclough B. Suicide as an outcome for mental disorders. A meta-analysis. *Br J Psychiatry*. 1997;170:205–228.

144. Blumer D, Montouris G, Davies K, et al. Suicide in epilepsy: psychopathology, pathogenesis, and prevention. *Epilepsy & Behavior*. 2002; 3:232–341.

145. Barraclough BM. The suicide rate of epilepsy. *Acta Psychiatr Scand*. 1987;76:339–345.

146. Nilsson L, Ahlbom A, Farahmand BY, et al. Risk factors for suicide in epilepsy: a case control study. *Epilepsia*. 2002;43:644–651.

147. Christensen J, Vestergaard M, Mortensen PB, et al. Epilepsy and fisk of suicide: a population-based case-control study. *Lancet Neurol*. 2007;6:693–698.

148. Singh G, Fletcher O, Bell GS, et al. Cancer mortality amongst people with epilepsy: a study of two cohorts with severe and presumed milder epilepsy. *Epilepsy Res*. 2009;83:190–197.

149. Kurokawa T, Fung KC, Hanai T, et al. Mortality and clinical features in cases of death among epileptic children. *Brain Dev*. 1982;4:321–325.

CHAPTER 3 ■ EXPERIMENTAL MODELS OF SEIZURES AND MECHANISMS OF EPILEPTOGENESIS

T. A. BENKE AND A. R. BROOKS-KAYAL

ANIMAL MODELS OF SEIZURES AND EPILEPSY: WHAT IS THE QUESTION?

An editorial (1) began to summarize one of the key issues in experimental models of seizures and epilepsy: how close does your model need to be to the true human condition in order to reach valid translational conclusions? In other words, is the best model for a cat actually a cat, preferably the same cat (2), or will a dog do because it also has fur? To some extent the differences between the cat and dog are irrelevant, as our understanding of the mechanisms of brain processes from development to learning and memory in healthy and diseased states are still in their infancy. The first step, undoubtedly, is to define the pertinent questions. For the pediatric epilepsies, this has been approached in a workshop "Models of Pediatric Epilepsies" sponsored by NIH/NINDS, the American Epilepsy Society and the International League against Epilepsy (3). Those questions were as follows: (i) what are the long-term consequences of seizures? Can these be modified? and (ii) what is the best anticonvulsant therapy? What is the best antiepileptogenic therapy? From these questions, the mechanisms of seizure initiation, prolongation, and termination can be addressed, and their sequelae defined. Further, the mechanisms underlying the development of spontaneous repetitive seizures (SRS) (epileptogenesis) and associated cognitive dysfunction can begin to be addressed. The mechanisms by which modifiers such as genetic background, developmental stage, and other insults (hypoxia, trauma) may also be differentiated. From this, the committee proposed a table listing general strategies for model development (Table 3.1). In brief, models should be clinically relevant, developmentally appropriate, and generalize to a human condition (i.e., have validity).

While entire volumes have been devoted to the subject of this chapter (4,5), we will review the literature involving only a subset of the issues that seem pertinent to a text on clinical epilepsy. Following a review of synaptic transmission mechanisms, we will focus on the methods for invoking status epilepticus (SE) (a "prolonged" single seizure) via chemoconvulsants; single, repetitive, or prolonged seizures via hypoxia, temperature, kindling, or chemoconvulsants; and seizures induced by trauma or genetic alterations. The process by which the initial insult (seizure, SE, or other) may lead to spontaneous SRs (epilepsy) has been the subject of intense study and multiple reviews have been put forth (6,7). Consensus regarding the relationship (cause or effect?) of sclerosis and network reorganization to this process has not been forthcoming. Overall, the field has significantly shifted

TABLE 3.1
STRATEGIES FOR ANIMAL MODEL DEVELOPMENT

1. Address a clinical need for better therapies
2. Address a key question or testable hypothesis
3. Address age specificities of developmental epilepsies and exhibit age-specific manifestations
4. Address normal aspects of development as they relate to models of developmental epilepsies
5. Animal models of seizures and epilepsy should have EEG correlates; spontaneous seizures should be demonstrated in animal models of epilepsy
6. Investigate etiology and natural history of catastrophic/intractable epilepsies
7. Address role(s) of "multihit" mechanisms in epileptogenesis and epilepsies, that is, trauma plus seizure or environment/diet plus genetic susceptibility
8. Address long-term role of seizures and other aspects of epileptic encephalopathies
9. Address model validity to clinical situation by comparisons with pharmacologic response, seizures phenotypes, outcomes, genetics, and so on
10. Allow cross-pollination from related fields: ischemia, sleep, trauma, synaptic plasticity, cancer/cell-signaling, and so on

Modified from Stafstrom CE, Moshe SL, Swann JW, et al. Models of pediatric epilepsies: strategies and opportunities. *Epilepsia.* 2006;47:1407–1414.

from a descriptive to a mechanistic focus involving key receptors, enzymes, and genetic regulation.

GENERAL MECHANISMS OF TRANSMISSION AND NETWORKS

Seizures can be defined as paroxysms of abnormal, rhythmic, synchronized discharges in the brain. Communication in the nervous system is a combination of electrical and chemical signaling with a balance between excitation and inhibition in each, primarily mediated between neurons. Glia modulate both types of communication primarily on a local basis, but frequently with distant consequences. While neurons are largely polarized structures favoring directed communication (an input end and an output end), this is not always the case and how this may change is clearly relevant to seizures. As electrical units, neurons depend on membrane-embedded protein ion channels to maintain their membrane in a polarized state in which, at rest, the inside of the neuron is electronegative compared to the outside. Each ion channel has its own relative ion selectivity and the net directional flux of ions (which depends on both the concentration of ions on either side of the membrane and the membrane polarity or voltage) determines whether this flux will move the neuronal membrane voltage toward, or away from, its resting state. Ionic channels transition between opened and closed states. This gating can be modulated by membrane voltage (voltage-gated channels [VGCs]) and/or the binding of external or internal chemical ligands.

Synaptic transmission is the process by which neurotransmitters (ligands) released from a neighboring neuron diffusively move toward another neuron and bind to receptors on that neuron. Ligand binding to a receptor can result in channel opening within the receptor or lead to the ligand-bound receptor interacting with a separate protein, often another channel, as in the case of G-protein-coupled receptors (GPCRs). Neurotransmitter release involves many tightly linked processes. Only specialized structures and regions are involved in neurotransmitter release. Initiation of release involves either local voltage-gated mediated polarization changes or second messenger systems activated by neurotransmitters themselves. Vesicles, membranous spheres filled with neurotransmitter by pumps within the vesicular membrane, then fuse with presynaptic membranes to release neurotransmitter into the synaptic cleft that separates the presynaptic neuron from the postsynaptic neuron. Less commonly, neurotransmitters may be directly pumped into the cleft. Neurotransmitters are either enzymatically degraded in the cleft or pumped out of the cleft by transporters into the presynaptic terminal, postsynaptic neuron, or surrounding glial support cells. From there it is either enzymatically broken down, recycled and shuttled across membranes, resynthesized or pumped backed into vesicles.

The resulting ionic flux(es) can have several simultaneous consequences. Some ions only affect membrane voltage while certain ions (e.g., calcium) also act as second messengers by activating calcium-dependent enzymes. These enzymes can then exert a cascading effect on ion channels and other enzymes, including those that influence membrane shape and scaffolds that hold and direct protein location (i.e., internal versus external, synaptic versus extrasynaptic), protein translation, protein degradation, and RNA transcription.

Neurons are three-dimensional structures with compartments (dendrite, axon, and soma) and subcompartments in each (e.g., main dendrite, branch, spine; axonal hillock, axon, branch, terminal), and the precise temporal and spatial regulation of neuronal function is mirrored by the segregation of unique, but often similar, ion channels and enzymes to distinct subcompartments. For instance, the molecular diversity of potassium channels, each coded by different genes and often many splice variants, reflects the unique functional needs or duties of each subcompartment where they may be selectively located and regulated. Neurons themselves are also segregated as inhibitory or excitatory, depending on the type of neurotransmitter(s) they may (predominantly) release. Each class of neuron may also express a unique complement of ion channel and receptor subtypes resulting in incredible diversity of neuronal function.

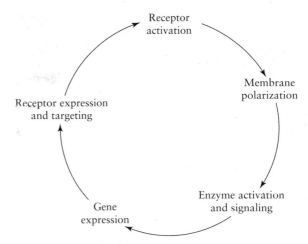

FIGURE 3.1 Proposed cascade of events following a seizure leading to any potential adverse sequelae (status epileptics, epileptogenesis, learning impairment, etc.).

The resulting cascade, beginning with receptor activation, followed by alterations in membrane polarization, potentially loops around to result in alterations of the properties of the initial trigger of receptor activation. Consideration of this simplistic mechanism is important. Such a loop likely underlies normal plasticity associated with processes like learning and memory, but perhaps becomes unstable with seizures and epileptogenesis, leading to aberrant plasticity that could result in both seizures and cognitive dysfunction (Fig. 3.1).

Glutamatergic Ion Channels

At the synaptic level, most excitatory amino acid transmission in the central nervous system (CNS) is mediated by the activation of families of glutamate-activated ligand-gated cation channels classified according to their preferred agonists: kainate, α-amino-3-hydroxy-5-methyl-4-isoxazole propionate (AMPA), or N-methyl-D-aspartate (NMDA) (8). To date, nine subunit subtypes and related isoforms have been cloned with pharmacology in in vitro expression systems similar to the AMPA (GluR1-4) and kainate receptors (GluR5-7, KAR1-2) (9–11). Similarly, five subunit subtypes and related isoforms have been cloned with pharmacology in in vitro expression systems similar to NMDA receptors (NR1, NR2A-D) in vivo (12–16). Some subunit-specific interactions and their role in synaptic transmission have been shown (17–22). Metabotropic glutamate receptors (mGluRs) are GPCRs broadly divided into three classes (Groups I–III) (23). Epileptologists are becoming increasingly interested in ionotropic glutamate receptors as the anticonvulsants topiramate, felbamate, and talampanel likely interact with these receptors. In addition, Group I mGluR agonists or Group II mGluR antagonists are thought to have both anticonvulsant and antiepileptogenic potential (24). Since these modulatory receptors do not directly participate in fast excitatory synaptic transmission, it is hoped that targeting these receptors may be effective with fewer side effects compared to agents that directly modulate GluRs and NRs.

Calcium influx through NRs is thought to mediate the calcium-activated processes involved in long-term potentiation and depression (LTP and LTD) (25–29), neurite outgrowth (30), synaptogenesis (31), and cell death (32–34). LTP and

LTD are thought to be synaptic models of learning and memory (35). "Induction" of LTP/LTD is thought to take place when synaptically activated NRs allow calcium entry and accumulation in the neuron. In order for this to happen, the nearby region of dendrite must be sufficiently depolarized by synaptic activation of GluRs to alleviate the magnesium-dependent block of NRs. "Expression" of LTP/TD is thought to occur when calcium activates a cascade involving protein phosphorylation and dephosphorylation resulting in modifications in synaptic strength (36).

While other possible mechanisms exist (35,37–40), postsynaptic changes in GluR subunit numbers (40–42) or properties (42) are thought to underlie synaptic modification. This has resulted in postulated "subunit rules": (i) for AMPA-type GluRs, synaptic removal of GluR2 subunits drags along GluR1 and GluR3 which underlies LTD, (ii) GluR1 or GluR3 not associated with GluR2 ("homomers") act independently, (iii) insertion and/or modification of GluR1 underlies LTP (43). It is likely that the regulation of GluR subunits and measured properties are exquisitely intertwined (44). Knockout studies of GluR1 (45) and GluR2 (46,47) have shed further light on the relationship of LTP and LTD to behavioral testing of learning and memory such as the Morris Water Maze (MWM). GluR1 knockouts have impaired LTP and LTD with normal MWM testing (48). However, on spatial working memory tasks, they are significantly impaired (48,49).

It has now been shown that AMPA-type glutamate receptors can not only participate in calcium-dependent plasticity, but can also, as a result of plasticity, alter their subunit composition (50,51). Since initial cloning studies, it has been known that GluR2-lacking receptors flux calcium (52), allowing for this to occur. Either downregulation of GluR2 or upregulation of GluR1 would potentially lead to more homomeric, calcium-permeable GluRs. This contributed to the "GluR2 hypothesis" (53,54) whereby preferential removal of GluR2 (with no changes in GluR1) can lead to AMPA-type glutamate receptors that flux calcium.

Kainate receptors have now been proposed to be involved in plasticity at mossy fiber (MFs) synapses independent of NRs (55–57). They share with NRs the cardinal feature of plasticity, namely that they can be highly permeable to the second messenger calcium (58). Kainate receptors at other synapses in the hippocampus and cortex (58–60) may also participate in the induction of plasticity in this fashion.

Glutamate Receptors and Development

Developmentally and regionally specific patterns of expression of the different glutamate receptors and their isoforms have been shown (61–63). NRs appear before GluRs, even prior to the appearance of dendritic spines (64). NR2B-containing receptors appear first with slower kinetic properties, followed by NR2A (after week 1 in the rat) with faster kinetic properties (65,66). In the rat hippocampus, GluR1 and GluR2 primarily exist in a flip isoform prior to adolescence but begin to exist in a flop isoform during adolescence (2–4 weeks of age) (63). These and other related isoforms each have unique kinetic properties (67,68). The mechanisms underlying synaptic plasticity thus vary as the animal ages (69–74) and are partly dependent on anatomic location (72,75–77). LTP remains largely dependent on NRs throughout development.

However, LTD in the hippocampus develops from mostly NR-dependent forms to include NR-independent forms as the animals age (78,79). These NR-dependent and NR-independent forms are differentiated by the effectiveness of different chemical and electrical LTD inducing stimulation paradigms (78–83). Visual development coincides with changes in glutamate receptor composition at thalamo-cortical synapses (84), which has also been shown in the auditory system (85). It appears that calcium permeable or GluR2-lacking receptors are a feature only of early development (84,86–88).

Subsynaptic Machinery Regulating Insertion, Removal, and Maintenance of Glutamate Receptors

The expanding role of the subsynaptic scaffolding that interacts with glutamate receptors has been the subject of intense investigation (89–91). The central organizer appears to be PSD-95 (and related proteins), which contains a sticky tail of PDZ domains. These interactions are thought to regulate the function and targeting of glutamate receptors by tethering them at the synapse and by holding various regulatory kinases and phosphatases in proximity. NRs interact directly with PSD-95 through PDZ domains. GluRs can interact with the PDZ domains of PSD-95 (92) through TARPS (93). Interaction of GluR2 with NSF and GRIP1 seems to hold receptors in the synapse, while interaction with PICK1 removes them to extrasynaptic and subsynaptic or vesicular holding areas (94,95). GluR1 interacts (through a linkage with SAP97, a PSD-95 family member) with AKAP79/150 (96). AKAP79/150 links the complex with PKA (96,97), calcineurin, and the actin cytoskeleton (98). These interactions are thought to bring GluRs to synapses and upregulate them in LTP (99–101) and remove them in LTD (97,101–103). In LTD, the complex dissociates and moves out of dendritic spines (98). These mechanisms may be unique to the CA1 region of hippocampus where AKAP79 is primarily expressed (104).

GABAergic Ion Channels

Gamma-aminobutyric acid (GABA) is the main inhibitory neurotransmitter in the adult brain. Epileptologists have been interested in this system because commonly prescribed anticonvulsant drugs, such as phenobarbital, the benzodiazepines, and to a lesser extent valproate, topiramate, and levitiracetam, reduce seizure activity by augmenting GABA receptor activity. The GABAergic system consists of three main receptor subtypes: $GABA_A$, $GABA_B$, and $GABA_C$. $GABA_A$ receptors (GABARs) are primarily located postsynaptically and mediate most of the fast synaptic inhibition in the brain. They are anion selective and gate primarily chloride, although under certain circumstances they may also gate bicarbonate. $GABA_A$ receptors are heterogeneous complexes composed of multiple protein subunits. Numerous subtypes exist for each subunit ($\alpha1–6$, $\beta1–3$, $\gamma1–3$, δ, ϵ, π, θ, and $\rho1–3$). The most common in vivo GABAR subunit composition is two α, two β, and one γ subunit. There is remarkable receptor heterogeneity, with subtype combinations varying in different brain regions, cell types, and during different times in development (105–108). Different subunit subtypes and the wide variety of combinations confer distinct functional and pharmacological properties to the GABARs (105). The γ subunit, for example, is required for GABA$_A$ receptors to be responsive to benzodiazepine-type drugs, whereas the α subunit subtype determines the type of the benzodiazepine binding site (e.g., type I or II) (109,110). Brain regions that express the highest concentration of the α1 subunit have a correspondingly high number of type I benzodiazepine binding sites and are, in turn, more sensitive to zolpidem-induced augmentation and less sensitive to zinc-induced inhibition (111–113).

GABA$_B$ receptors are G-protein-linked metabotropic receptors that are located both presynaptically and postsynaptically and are responsible for slower, more long-lasting inhibitory currents. Like GABA$_A$ receptors, they are composed of multiple subunits, primarily R1 and R2, which have additional diversity due to splice variation. Also like GABA$_A$, GABA$_B$ receptors are widely distributed in the CNS, particularly in the hippocampus, cerebellum, and thalamus. In contrast, GABA$_C$ receptors are located primarily in the retina and do not appear to play a significant role in epilepsy.

The function of the GABAergic system differs markedly in the mature and immature brain. While GABA$_A$ receptor activation results in neuronal hyperpolarization and an inhibition of cell firing in the mature brain, receptor activation results in membrane depolarization and excitation in the immature brain (114–116). The switch from GABA-mediated excitation to inhibition is related to changes in the chloride gradient that occur during the course of development (117–122). In mature neurons, the intracellular concentration of chloride is low due to the presence of KCC2-extruding transporters. When GABA$_A$ receptors are activated, chloride flows, according to its concentration gradient, into the cell; this causes membrane hyperpolarization and hence an inhibitory postsynaptic response. In contrast, intracellular concentrations of chloride are high in immature brain due to the combined effects of low KCC2 expression and the presence of NKCC1 transporters that actively carry chloride into the neuron. When GABA$_A$ receptors are activated, ion channels open, chloride flows out of the cell, and depolarization occurs. In rodents, KCC2 expression is very low during the first two postnatal weeks. By inference, it is thought that KCC2 expression is low in humans until around the end of gestation (123).

A number of laboratories have shown that depolarizing (e.g., excitatory) GABA currents are critical for the development of calcium-dependent processes, such as neuronal proliferation, migration, targeting, and synaptogenesis (124–128). In addition, there is evidence suggesting that GABAR-mediated currents also play a critical role in the generation of ictal activity in the developing brain. It has been known for some time that synchronous neuronal activity in the hippocampus can be driven by GABA$_A$ receptor activation and inhibited by GABA$_A$ receptor blockade (129). More recent evidence, however, suggests that GABAR-mediated excitation may drive ictal activity in the developing hippocampus as well (130,131).

Plasticity and Trafficking of GABAergic Receptors

During the process of epileptogenesis in animal models there are alterations in the expression and membrane localization of several GABAR subunits (α1, α4, γ2, δ) in hippocampal dentate granule neurons (132–134). These alterations, which are associated with changes in phasic and tonic GABAR-mediated inhibition, and in GABAR modulation by benzodiazepines, neurosteroids, and zinc, begin soon after SE and continue as animals become epileptic (132–135). Several laboratories have documented similar changes in GABAR subunit composition in human temporal lobe epilepsy (TLE) and in animal models of TLE (132,134,136,137). In the pilocarpine model of SE in adult rodents, GABAR α1 subunit mRNA expression decreases, α4 subunit mRNA expression increases in dentate granule cells (DGCs) of the hippocampus, and animals uniformly go on to develop the recurrent spontaneous seizures that define epilepsy (132). The change in subunit expression correlates with a decreased sensitivity to zolpidem augmentation and increased sensitivity to zinc inhibition of GABAR responses (132). Similar functional and subunit expression changes have been observed in DGCs isolated from surgically resected hippocampus from patients with intractable TLE (137). The changes in GABAR subunit expression and function in DGCs of adult epileptic animals precede the development of epilepsy and immature animals exposed to prolonged induced seizures show increased GABAR α1 subunit expression and do not subsequently develop epilepsy (138), suggesting that GABAR changes contribute to the epileptogenic process. Viral gene transfer studies demonstrating that the expression of higher α1 subunit levels inhibits development of epilepsy after SE provide further evidence in support of this (139).

Voltage-Gated Ion Channels

Generically, voltage-gated sodium channels (VGSCs) and voltage-gated calcium channels (VGCCs) are excitatory or depolarizing. VGSCs are somewhat broadly lumped as they each function similarly, with subtypes segregated to unique neuronal populations and subcompartments. However, some VGSCs have unique deactivation characteristics, often prolonged or "reverberant" resulting in unique signaling properties. VGCCs are segregated according to their biophysical properties (T, P/Q, N, and L/HVA-type) and like VGSCs are often segregated to unique neuronal populations and subcompartments. Voltage-gated potassium channels (VGKCs) are typically inhibitory or hyperpolarizing; however, depending on their voltage-dependent gating and subcellular location they can have the opposite influence on membrane potential (e.g., HCN or I$_h$). VGCs often share the same or similar targeting motifs and scaffolds that regulate the expression and targeting ligand-gated ion channels (140).

Neuronal Networks

Neuronal networks refer to the detailed web of connections of inhibitory and excitatory neurons within the different regions of the brain. The activation patterns and activity of different neuronal networks are thought to underlie basic brain function (141). A significant portion of experimental epilepsy research has focused on neuronal networks, specifically within the hippocampus. From a simplistic point of view, information primarily enters the hippocampus in a lamellar fashion via the dentate gyrus, travels from there to the CA3 region, then to CA1, and then out via the entorhinal cortex; however, it is substantially more complicated than this (142,143). The CA3 has an excitatory feedback loop, which participates in normal learning, but can, however, contribute to seizure generation (144). The dentate gyrus is thought to limit CA3 excitation by acting like a filter to incoming inputs (145,146). This is due to the properties of excitatory inputs into the dentate gyrus as well as feedback inhibition within the dentate gyrus (143). Therefore, much research has focused on determining the nature of these mechanisms and how they have been potentially subverted in experimental models to result in epilepsy.

REVIEW OF TECHNIQUES

Experimental models can be divided into whole-animal (in vivo) versus in vitro studies. Whole-animal models of acquired epilepsies typically involve single or multiple treatments to the animal that produce some form of injury or stimulation that results in later development of spontaneous seizures. Examples of these induced injuries include SE (chemoconvulsant and electrical), kindling, hypoxia, and head trauma. In genetic models, a spontaneous or induced genetic mutation or deletion results in seizures that happen spontaneously. Seizure activity must be carefully defined for several reasons. First, the definition of a seizure is often extremely variable, as in the clinical literature. Second, consciousness, routinely used as a modifier in describing clinical seizures, is arbitrarily defined in most animals used. Typically, rhythmic, stereotyped, altered behavior is observed and characterized as seizure activity. As in the clinical literature, EEG has become the gold standard for correlating altered behavior with seizures, but its use is limited due to the time and labor-intensive placement of electrodes, limitations of electrode stability over time, and the fact that electrographic seizures emanating from deeper structures can be missed when recording from the cortical surface.

In Vitro Versus In Vivo Models

In vitro studies involve removal and subsequent manipulations of whole-brain structures, slices of brain structures or isolation, and culture of separated brain cells (neurons and glia). These studies allow detailed manipulations and measurements but are limited in a key way. While it is tempting to designate repetitive electrical discharges as a seizure, seizures defined in the whole animal are associated with a change in behavior or sensation which cannot be appreciated in these in vitro models and thus must be referred to as "seizure-like" events or an ictus to avoid confusion. One researcher's abnormal ictal-induced phenomena may also be interpreted as another researcher's normal activity-dependent changes. In addition, certain seizures, and their sequelae, may involve the interplay of multiple brain structures and are thus difficult if not impossible to recreate in in vitro models. Finally, key processes such as development and epileptogenesis which occur over a prolonged period of time cannot be fully studied in in vitro models as they are limited by the length of time the in vitro preparation is viable (hours to weeks).

There are dozens of in vivo and in vitro models of seizures and epilepsy and as mentioned earlier there is little consensus about which if any are the "optimal model". In reality, each model has its strengths and limitations, and the relative benefits depend on the specific question being asked. Below, we focus on the models that are in common use or emerging.

Pilocarpine and Kainate Models

The pilocarpine and lithium pilocarpine model (147) involves the systemic administration of a muscarinic acetylcholine agonist (pilocarpine) to induce a prolonged electrographic and behavioral seizure that requires cessation by benzodiazepines or barbiturates, typically after 1–2 hours, in order to prevent animal mortality. Clearly, from a clinical standpoint, this is never the cause of SE in humans. Nevertheless, it is widely used because it results in severe SE and eventually develops an epileptic phenotype with features very similar to human TLE resulting in its widespread use for studying both of these conditions.

Kainate, a glutamate analogue that is not metabolized, is either injected systemically or directly into the brain and can result in seizures lasting several hours (148,149). Clinically, kainate originates as a shellfish poison whereby human toxicity during outbreaks results in seizures and in severe cases hippocampal sclerosis (150). While this clinical situation is extremely rare, conditions involving glutamate overload that are known to be associated with seizures such as stroke, hypoxia (151,152), or infection may be mimicked to some degree by kainate administration. Similar to the pilocarpine model, because kainate results in SE, though probably not as severe as pilocarpine, and adult animals eventually develop an epileptic phenotype with features very similar to human TLE, it is widely used for studying both these conditions. In youngest animals, kainate primarily activates the hippocampus while in older animals its effects are widespread (153).

Brief Seizure Models

Pentylenetetrazole and flurothyl are GABAergic antagonists that are administered systemically or inhaled, respectively (154). They both induce relatively short seizures, with flurothyl being very brief and limited nearly to the length of exposure to the vapors. As a result, both agents are used to mimic conditions involving single or multiple brief, generalized seizures (155). The major limitations of these models are that the mechanism of seizure induction does not clearly parallel any human condition, and the animals never develop spontaneous seizures. Both agents are thought to act on all susceptible brain regions, including cortex and hippocampus (154). Electrical kindling, whereby electrodes are implanted in order to stimulate select brain regions, can also be used to study how repeated, brief seizure-like activity can influence outcomes. Depending on the stimulation protocol, eventually kindling can lead to SE. This model, however, is limited by the technicalities of long-term implantation in rodents and the fact that most kindling paradigms do not result in development of spontaneous seizures.

Clinical Models: Fever and Hypoxia/Ischemia

In models where seizures are induced in the setting of increased temperature (fever), hypoxia, and/or ischemia, the ability of these models to generalize to human pathologies is clearly evident. Hypoxia models can involve placing animals in an environment of reduced oxygen content until seizures are observed (156,157). Other methods involve single or multiple cerebral vessel occlusions, often in combination with exposure to an environment with reduced oxygen content. Methods involving vessel occlusion are often time-intensive. These methods are then limited by the elements of hypoxia and ischemia, as these may independently influence outcomes (158). Temperature-induced seizures in developing animals (159,160) involve slowly heating the animal, typically with warmed air, until seizures are initiated. This model is gaining popularity as a model of febrile seizures but may be limited by the fact it is really a model of externally imposed hyperthermia rather than endogenous fever as occurs in the human condition.

Toxin Models

Several models involve direct infusion of toxins, compounds, or even genetic material into specific regions such as the hippocampus. These are each meant to model focal seizures or epileptogenesis, though the result can have distant effects. These include the tetanus-toxin model (161) and more recently the tetrodotoxin model (162), thought to be a model of infantile spasms or West syndrome. Knockdown of GluR2 by injection of antisense probes results in acute seizures (163). Following withdrawal of direct injection of glutamate receptor antagonists, spontaneous seizures are provoked in immature animals, while systemic injection does not cause this to happen (164).

Trauma Models

Experimental models of trauma utilizing either direct impact methods (165) or surgical undercuts (166) have been recently reviewed as models for studying the development of post-traumatic epileptogenesis and epilepsy. As head trauma is a common cause of acquired epilepsy in humans, these models seem very generalizable to human pathology. As a result, these models have been used extensively to study the efficacy of anti-epileptogenic compounds as well as the mechanisms underlying post-traumatic epileptogenesis.

In Vitro Models

In vitro methods involving brain slices or cultures use a variety of methods to induce seizure-like electrical events. These can involve perfusion of compounds that typically enhance or favor membrane excitability alone or in combination with electrical stimulation, akin to kindling. The resulting spontaneous neuronal-mediated discharges can then be recorded from groups of neurons or from individual neurons typically using electrophysiological techniques. Imaging techniques using fluorescent dyes that are able to indicate changes in membrane voltage or secondary changes due to accumulations of specific ions, such as calcium, often complement electrophysiological measurements as they are able to simultaneously record from populations of neurons that may be somewhat distant from each other. The pattern of these discharges is then interpreted either in isolation, in groups or bursts, or when the bursts cluster together as an ictus. The

transitions between these types of discharges are interpreted as indicative of ictal genesis and are thought to generalize to seizure genesis. When the ictus is prolonged, this generalizes to SE. When the ability to generate an ictus becomes more facile, this is thought to generalize to epileptogenesis. Determining how excitation spreads through a slice of brain tissue is generalized to how it may spread in the intact preparation. Thus, application of anticonvulsants to an in vitro preparation has been used to determine their efficacy and precise mechanism(s) of action. In order to circumvent the issues of truly generalizable seizures, SE or epileptogenesis in vitro, brain slices are often prepared at various time points after these phenomenon have developed in vivo. Findings from hippocampal brain slices prepared from animals after experiencing an induced or spontaneous seizure in vivo allow examination of how overall synaptic transmission, plasticity, and seizure thresholds have become altered by these processes (Table 3.2).

MECHANISMS OF SE

Here, there are two basic questions: why did the seizure not stop by itself and why is SE more difficult to stop with anticonvulsants than a single seizure? Was the underlying neuronal network susceptible to this happening or did it become dynamically changed to allow its progression? Given that it has been found that the clinical situation is mimicked by the experiment in which benzodiazepines lose their potency as the seizure progresses (167), much effort has focused on the role of GABAR and inhibitory synaptic transmission (168). These questions have been approached in a variety of ways, using in vitro brain slices or in vivo models employing pilocarpine, kainate, or kindling, sometimes in combination with in vitro brain slices prepared during or after the event. Recent studies suggest that during SE, GABARs at inhibitory synapses onto granule cells of the dentate gyrus are removed from synaptic sites and moved to extrasynaptic sites and internal pools (169) in a subunit-specific manner (170). This likely minimizes their effectiveness in both self-termination of the seizure as well as the loss of effectiveness of benzodiazepines, in part mediated by loss of $\gamma 2$ subunits that modulate benzodiazepine sensitivity. These issues are complicated during development in the CA3 region of the hippocampus, where GABAergic synapses are depolarizing and thus contribute to the development of ictal activity (130,171).

The alterations in GABARs in the dentate gyrus are possibly mediated by NR activation rather than by direct activation of GABARs (170). It has been found that blocking NRs prevents the progression to drug-resistant SE (172). NRs then further contribute to the process as they are progressively recruited to synaptic sites as SE progresses (172). While in vitro studies suggest that NRs and GluRs are involved in epileptogenesis (173–175), it is possible that their contribution to this process may be mediated by their effects on SE. Reductions in GluR2 in CA1 and CA3 (176,177) 6–48 hours after SE, while implicated in cell death after SE, may have also contributed to prolonging SE, perhaps through facilitated GluR function (178). Excess glutamate, which may occur with transporter dysfunction, has been shown to lead to NR activation and seizures (179); however, this may be limited to

TABLE 3.2

ANIMAL MODEL SUMMARY

Model	Questions addressed
Pilocarpine and kainate	• SE: consequences, treatment, role of development • TLE and epileptogenesis: hippocampal networks, mechanisms and therapies • "Multihit" models
Pentylenetetrazole and flurothyl	• Multiple brief seizure models: mechanisms of epileptogenesis • Treatment of brief seizures • Role of development on long-term consequences • "Multihit" models
Temperature	• Febrile seizures in children: mechanisms and therapies • Role of development and long-term consequences • Epileptogenesis • "Multihit" models
HIE	• True "multihit" model • Role of development and long-term consequences • Epileptogenesis: mechanisms and therapies • Focal epilepsy and epileptogenesis: therapies
Toxins: tetrodotoxin and NMDA	• Infantile spasms: mechanisms & therapies • Role of development and long-term consequences • Treatment • Epileptic encephalopathies
Toxins: tetanus toxin	• Focal epilepsy and epileptogenesis: therapies • Role of development and long-term consequences
Trauma	• True "multihit" model • Role of development and long-term consequences • Focal epilepsy and epileptogenesis: mechanisms and therapies
In vitro models	• SE: consequences, treatment, role of development • Role of development • Synaptic and therapeutic mechanisms, especially when coupled with in vivo models
Genetic models	• Catastrophic epilepsies: genesis, therapy, long-term consequences • Linkage of human mutations with synaptic and electrical mechanisms in seizures and epilepsy • "Multihit" models

developing animals in which glial regulation of extracellular glutamate by transporters is immature (180). Indeed, multiple genes, including those involved in transcription, are likely regulated following SE (181).

EPILEPTOGENESIS

Epileptogenesis refers to the process by which a previously "normal" brain becomes capable of producing SRS. Animal models have typically employed prolonged SE to trigger this process; however, models of trauma and injections of toxins have also been used (see Review of Techniques). The nature and mechanisms of this process have each been richly studied. Does this happen gradually, that is, what is the significance of the latent period between trigger and first SRS? This is a critical question as it might represent a window of opportunity for intervention. What is the relationship of the sclerotic pathology, often seen in human TLE and also seen in animal models, to this process? How much of the process is due to network rewiring versus changes in neuronal and/or synaptic function? What are the signaling cascades mediating these processes and how can they be circumvented or reversed?

The appearance of SRS has been taken to indicate the end of the latent period. Enhanced excitability has been shown to gradually develop prior to the appearance of SRS (182), suggesting the end of the latent period is not a stepwise function into SRS and epilepsy. In support of this, an intensive video-EEG monitoring study has challenged the notion of the latent period by showing that the progression into SRS and epilepsy is a sigmoid function of time (183). In other words, after the first SRS, epilepsy continues to progress. Progression clearly represents a worse-case scenario that may not always be present (184). Additional work is needed to determine where and whether there is a window for interventions to prevent this progression. Interestingly, there is a transient period following pilocarpine SE in adult animals when GABAergic inhibition becomes excitatory in some brain regions due to loss of normal chloride regulation (185), suggesting that chloride regulation may be a potential therapeutic target.

Network Reorganization

Network reorganization in the hippocampus has been extensively studied as one of the presumed origins of SRS because of similar findings in human TLE. Primarily this has focused on the output of DGC neurons and has been thoroughly reviewed (143,147,186). Excitotoxic loss of mossy cells (187) in the denate gyrus may lead to sprouting of dentate axons, known as mossy fibers (MFs). The sprouted MFs make aberrant excitatory connections locally in the dentate gyrus and distantly in CA3 creating an abnormal excitatory feedback circuit (188). These abnormal connections are further dysfunctional, with a higher probability of activation, a larger NR component (189,190), and recruitment of kainate receptors (191). These disturbances, coupled with permanent alterations in GABARs (see below), are thought to result in a circuit prone to trigger seizures in other regions, such as CA3 (143). Not without controversy, MFs and SRS have not been proven to be either necessary or sufficient for the development of TLE (7,192). Further aberrant circuits have also been described originating in CA3 (193) and CA1 (194–196). In trauma-induced epilepsy, aberrant connections are formed in the region of injury as well as the hippocampus (6,165,166). In the region of injury, discrete regions of apical dendrites have a selective overabundance of excitatory synaptic inputs and connectivity (197,198), which with alterations in membrane VGC properties (198) may also contribute to the epileptic state.

Excitotoxic cell loss (which may occur following SE or other insults) throughout the hippocampus is thought to be mediated by glutamate toxicity via GluRs (176,199) and NRs (200). Secondary reactive gliosis may also contribute to synaptic dysfunction (201,202). Loss of hilar mossy cells and other neurons mediating inhibition are thought to be critical potential contributors to the hyperexcitable steady state of the epileptic hippocampus. SE also has the paradoxical effect of inducing neurogenesis in the dentate gyrus (203). Some of the newly formed neurons may also participate in MFs or other aberrant circuitry that leads to the epileptic hippocampus (204), although the exact role of newborn neurons in epileptogenesis continues to be studied.

The role of network alterations and other causative phenomena in epileptogenesis appears to be differentially regulated depending on when in development this process is initiated. Kainate-induced SE in adult animals causes, over time, SRS, CA3 cell loss, MFs into CA3 and dentate gyrus, sprouting into CA1 stratum pyramidale and stratum radiatum, and impaired learning in memory tasks (194,205,206). Similar results are found with the pilocarpine model (147,206,207). However if animals younger than 14 days are treated with either kainate or pilocarpine, the animals do not develop spontaneous seizures (see below) (138,208,209). Single or repetitive episodes of SE in infancy caused by pilocarpine are not benign, however, and have been associated with long-term abnormalities of inhibitory neurotransmission (138). Further,

single or multiple episodes of SE induced by pilocarpine at postnatal day 14 or later does result in SRS (210–212) as well as deficits in memory and learning that are inconsistently associated with cell loss and/or MFs (210,212–215). Studies in other models have not provided additional clarity regarding the association of cell loss and MFs to development of epilepsy after early-life seizures. Early-life focal administration of tetanus toxin results in a chronic epileptic state that includes memory impairment without cell loss (161) but does involve MFs (216). In contrast, repetitive flurothyl seizures in early development result in MFs, but they do not apparently result in SRS, only a reduced seizure threshold (217–219). Chronic perforant path kindling is associated with cell loss in the dentate gyrus (220). Similarly, in prolonged temperature-induced seizures, MFs gradually develops; however, reduction in seizure thresholds are seen much earlier and SRS have been reported only infrequently (221–223). Furthermore, MFs appears in a model of early-life stress, apparently unrelated to seizures (224).

Seizure or SE-Induced Alterations in Ion Channels

Early studies of in vitro brain slice models indicated that alterations in NRs with the successive prolongation of seizure-like discharges correlated with epileptogenesis (173–175). The mechanism of non-NR-mediated calcium influx via calcium-permeable GluRs is also thought to underlie cell death in adult models of seizures (176,225–227) and hypoxia (157). GluR1 upregulation has only been found in an adult model of electroconvulsive therapy (228). GluR2 "knockdown" studies have shown that downregulation of GluR2 can lead to seizures and hippocampal injury (163). Clinical evidence from pathological studies might support upregulation of GluR1 (229–231). Seizures or SE in developing animals have found either no change in GluR2 (199,232) or a downregulation of GluR2 (157,233) with no changes in GluR1 (234). Recurrent episodes of kainate-induced SE in developing animals are associated with a decrease in kainate binding (a reflection of GluRs as well as kainate receptors) in CA3 but not CA1 (209). Recurrent flurothyl seizures in developing animals have shown a long-term reduction in NRs and PSD-95 (235). Transient alteration in the properties of synaptically activated GluRs consistent with calcium permeable GluRs following hypoxic seizures in developing animals has been postulated to mediate the cascade resulting in later-life alterations in this model (236). Seizures induced by kainate in infant rats results in altered LTP, LTD, kindling and learning associated with enhanced inhibition in the dentate gyrus (237) and mechanistically linked to reduced NR2A, altered trafficking of GluR1 and increased PSD-95 (232).

In adult, epileptic animals following pilocarpine SE, GABAergic signaling is altered by specific reduction of $GABA_A$ receptor $\alpha1$ subunits and an increase in $\alpha4$ subunits in the dentate gyrus, resulting in a reduction in benzodiazepine sensitivity and enhanced inhibition by zinc (132). (This contrasts markedly to the developing hippocampus where pilocarpine SE does not result in epilepsy but results in an upregulation of $\alpha1$, overall receptor numbers and enhanced benzodiazepine sensitivity [138].) Altered function of VGSCs (238,239), T-type calcium channels (240,241), and potassium channels (242) have been described in epileptic animals and are thought to contribute to the epileptic state. In the hyperthermia model of febrile seizures, a single prolonged seizure results in permanent susceptibility to convulsants, enhanced in vitro kindling, mechanistically linked to enhancement of the voltage-gated potassium channel HCN (222,243,244).

The signaling pathways that regulate the plasticity in ion channel expression during epileptogenesis are just beginning to be elucidated. For example, recent studies have demonstrated that the mechanisms that regulate differential expression of GABAR α-subunits in hippocampus after SE include the CREB/ICER, JAK/STAT, BDNF, and Egr3 signaling pathways (245). Targeting signaling pathways that alter the expression of genes involved in epileptogenesis may provide novel therapeutic approaches for preventing or inhibiting the development of epilepsy after a precipitating insult.

SEQUELAE BEYOND EPILEPTOGENESIS

In adult models of epileptogenesis associated with cell loss and/or MFs, uniformly there is learning and memory impairment when assessed with the MWM, a behavior test used to assess spatial, long-term memory formation (246). Altered emotionality is also noted with fear conditioning (247). Mechanistically, this impairment is thought to be mediated by the anatomical damage, as similar deficits are observed in hippocampal lesion studies not associated with seizures or epileptogenesis (248). Similarly, in immature animals, abnormalities in the MWM are associated with histological changes following repetitive SE (213–215), repetitive flurothyl seizures (219,249), tetanus toxin (161), hypoxia/ischemia (250), and hyperthermia (222,243,244)-induced seizures. In models where immature animals develop SRS, there is altered emotionality (211). Furthermore, kainate insult in infancy and again later in adulthood results in more prominent memory impairment than a single insult at either time (251). In immature animals following a kainate-induced seizure, there have not been any detectable problems with the MWM or histological changes (206,252), including an absence of MFs; similar findings have been reported for repeated episodes of kainate-induced SE in immature animals (209). As adults, these animals have only subtle abnormalities in the MWM (253) and in more difficult mazes these animals have abnormalities most consistent with defective working memory (232,237,253,254); emotionality may be unaffected (253,254). Thus, permanent impairments in learning and memory are more severe in animal models when associated with significant histological abnormalities. However, significant impairments can also exist without histological abnormalities, which possibly reflect pathology limited to abnormal synaptic function isolated to the hippocampus.

GENETIC SUSCEPTIBILITY

Advances in genetics have allowed for several human epilepsy syndromes associated with single gene defects to be further characterized (255). Following determination of the analogous gene in mice, similar defects can be introduced through cloning techniques in order to better understand how epilepsy develops in these syndromes as well as determine which treatments might be more efficacious. Often, the nature of the genetic defect, whether it represents a gain or loss of function, is not clear until the altered resulting protein is expressed in an intact, cloned animal model. In the animal model of Dravet syndrome, genetic knock-in of human mutations in VGSCs (NaV1.1) results in a phenotype very similar to that seen in humans (256,257). Importantly, these studies have highlighted how the balance between excitation and inhibition is a critical modifier in this disorder (258). Similarly, genetic knock-in of human mutations in KCNQ2 and KCNQ3 has many similarities to the human phenotype of benign familial neonatal convulsions (259). Enhanced function of T-type calcium channels in thalamocortical circuits has been postulated to mediate childhood absence epilepsy. While specific mutations in T-type calcium channels have not been determined in the human condition; specific genetic targeting of enhanced expression of T-type calcium channels in this circuit have been found to mimic the human condition (260). However, genetic knock-in of human mutations in GABA receptors associated with generalized epilepsy syndromes has not resulted in phenotypes similar to the human conditions (261,262). Similarly, knock-in of human mutations in nicotinic acetylcholine receptors seen in autosomal-dominant nocturnal frontal lobe epilepsy also does not reproduce features similar to the human syndromes (263). These negative results suggest not only the complexities of genetic technologies, but also likely reflect basic underlying differences in rodent and human physiology, especially susceptibility to seizures and epilepsy.

SUMMARY

Animal models, despite their limitations, have advanced our understanding of the mechanisms of seizures and epileptogenesis. Specifically, substantial gains have been made in understanding the ability of the hippocampus and cortex to rewire themselves following insults to result in circuits capable of spontaneous seizures. Developmental models have shown how significant physiological and behavioral alterations can result without obvious histological changes. Important questions remain to be answered in further understanding the signaling pathways, genetic programs, and subsequent synaptic modifications that underlie epileptogenesis as well as the behavioral consequences of seizures. These discoveries are crucial to determine safe and effective pharmacological targets for stopping seizures and curing epilepsy and its consequences.

References

1. Mazarati A. The best model for a cat is the same cat...Or is it? *Epilepsy Curr.* 2007;7:112–114.
2. Rosenblueth A, Wiener, N. The role of models in science. *Philos Sci.* 1945;12:316–321.
3. Stafstrom CE, Moshe SL, Swann JW, et al. Models of pediatric epilepsies: strategies and opportunities. *Epilepsia.* 2006;47:1407–1414.
4. *Recent Advances in Epilepsy Research.* 548 vol. New York, NY: Kluwer, 2004.
5. *Models of Seizures and Epilepsy.* Amsterdam: Elsevier, 2006.
6. Pitkanen A, Kharatishvili I, Karhunen H, et al. Epileptogenesis in experimental models. *Epilepsia.* 2007;48(suppl 2):13–20.

7. Williams PA, Hellier JL, White AM, et al. Development of spontaneous seizures after experimental status epilepticus: implications for understanding epileptogenesis. *Epilepsia.* 2007;48(suppl 5):157–163.
8. Dingledine R, Borges K, Bowie D, et al. The glutamate receptor ion channel. *Pharmacol Rev.* 1999;51(1):7–61.
9. Hollman M, O'Shea-Greenfield A, Rogers SW, et al. Cloning by functional expression of a member of the glutamate receptor familly. *Nature.* 1989;342:643–648.
10. Egebjerg J, Bettler B, Hermans-Borgmeyer I, et al. Cloning of a cDNA for a glutamate receptor subunit activated by kainate but not AMPA. *Nature.* 1991;351:745–748.
11. Keinänen K, Wisden W, Sommer B, et al. A Family of AMPA-Selective Glutamate Receptors. *Science.* 1990;249:556–560.
12. Moriyoshi K, Masu M, Ishii T, et al. Molecular cloning and characterization of the rat NMDA receptor. *Nature.* 1991;354:31–37.
13. Monyer H, Sprengel R, Schoepfer R, et al. Heteromeric NMDA receptors: molecular and functional distinction of subtypes. *Science.* 1992;256: 1217–1221.
14. Meguro H, Mori H, Araki K, et al. Functional characterization of a heteromeric NMDA receptor channel expressed from cloned cDNAs. *Nature.* 1992;357:70–74.
15. Kutsuwada T, Kashiwabuchi N, Mori H, et al. Molecular diversity of the NMDA receptor channel. *Nature.* 1992;358:36–41.
16. Sugihara H, Moriyoshi K, Ishii T, et al. Structures and properties of seven isoforms of the NMDA receptor generated by alternative splicing. *Biochem Biophys Res Commun.* 1992;185:826–832.
17. Nishimune A, Isaac JTR, Molnar E, et al. NSF binding to GluR2 regulates synaptic transmission. *Neuron.* 1998;21:87–97.
18. Osten R, Srivastava S, Inman GJ, et al. The AMPA receptor GluR2 C terminus can mediate a reversible, ATP-dependent interaction with NSF and a- and b-SNAPs. *Neuron.* 1998;21:99–110.
19. Noel J, Ralph GS, Pickard L, et al. Surface expression of AMPA receptors in hippocampal neurons is regulated by an NSF-dependent mechanism. *Neuron.* 1999;23:365–376.
20. Luthi A, Chittajallu R, Duprat F, et al. Hippocampal LTD expression involves a pool of AMPARs regulated by the NSF-GluR2 interaction. *Neuron.* 1999;24:389–399.
21. Luscher C, Xia H, Beattie EC, et al. Role of AMPA receptor cycling in synaptic transmission and plasticity. *Neuron.* 1999;24:649–658.
22. Derkach V, Barria A, Soderling TR. Ca2+/calmodulin-kinase II enhances channel conductance of alpha-amino-3-hydroxy-5-methyl-4-isoxazolepropionate type glutamate receptors. *Proc Natl Acad Sci USA.* 1999; 96(6):3269–3274.
23. Alexander GM, Godwin DW. Metabotropic glutamate receptors as a strategic target for the treatment of epilepsy. *Epilepsy Res.* 2006;71:1–22.
24. Ure J, Baudry M, Perassolo M. Metabotropic glutamate receptors and epilepsy. *J Neurol Sci.* 2006;247:1–9.
25. Collingridge GL, Kehl SJ, McLennan H. Excitatory amino acids in synaptic transmission in the Schaffer-collateral commissural pathway of the rat hippocampus. *J Physiol.* 1983;334:33–46.
26. Lynch G, Larson J, Kelso S, et al. Intracellular injections of EGTA block induction of hippocampal long-term potentiation. *Nature.* 1983;305: 719–721.
27. Malenka RC, Kauer JA, Zucker RS, et al. Postsynaptic calcium is sufficient for potentiation of hippocampal synaptic transmission. *Science.* 1988;242:81–84.
28. Cummings JA, Mulkey RM, Nicoll RA, et al. Ca²⁺ signaling requirements for long-term depression in the hippocampus. *Neuron.* 1996;16:825–833.
29. Malenka RC, Bear MF. LTP and LTD: an embarrassment of riches. *Neuron.* 2004;44:5–21.
30. Mattson MP, Dou P, Kater SB. Outgrowth-regulating actions of glutamate in isolated hippocampal pyramidal neurons. *J Neurosci.* 1988;8: 2087–2100.
31. Rabacchi S, Bailly Y, Delhaye-Bouchaud N, et al. Involvement of the N-methyl D-aspartate (NMDA) receptor in synapse elimination during cerebellar development. *Science.* 1992;256:1823–1825.
32. Simon RP, Swan JH, Griffiths T, et al. Blockade of N-methyl-D-aspartate receptors may protect against ischemic damage in the brain. *Science.* 1984;226:850–852.
33. Choi DW. Calcium-mediated neurotoxicity: relationship to specific channel types and role in ischemic damage. *Trends Neurosci.* 1988;11:465–469.
34. McNamara D, Dingledine R. Dual effect of glycine on NMDA-induced neurotoxicity in rat cortical cultures. *J Neurosci.* 1990;10:3970–3976.
35. Bliss TVP, Collingridge GL. A synaptic model of memory: long-term potentiation in the hippocampus. *Nature.* 1993;361:31–39.
36. Ben-Ari Y, Aniksztejn L, Bregestovski P. Protein Kinase-C Modulation of NMDA Currents – An Important Link for LTP Induction. *Trends Neurosci.* 1992;15:333–339.
37. Bekkers JM, Stevens CF. Presynaptic mechanism for long-term potentiation in the hippocampus. *Nature.* 1990;346:724–729.
38. Lisman JE, Harris KM. Quantal analysis and synaptic anatomy—Integrating two views of hippocampal plasticity. *Trends Neurosci.* 1993;16:141–147.
39. Sorra KE, Harris KM. Stability in synapse number and size at 2 hr after long-term potentiation in hippocampal area CA1. *J Neurosci.* 1998;18(2): 658–671.
40. Kullmann DM, Nicoll RA. Long-term potentiation is associated with increases in quantal content and quantal amplitude. *Nature.* 1992;357: 240–244.
41. Davies SN, Lester RAJ, Reymann KG, et al. Temporally distinct pre- and post-synaptic mechanisms maintain long-term potentiation. *Nature.* 1989;338:500–503.
42. Benke TA, Luthi A, Isaac JTR, et al. Modulation of AMPA receptor unitary conductance by synaptic activity. *Nature.* 1998;395:793–797.
43. Lee SH, Simonetta A, Sheng, M. Subunit rules governing the sorting of internalized AMPA receptors in hippocampal neurons. *Neuron.* 2004;43: 221–236.
44. Oh MC, Derkach VA. Dominant role of the GluR2 subunit in regulation of AMPA receptors by CAMKII. *Nat Neurosci.* 2005;8(7):853–854.
45. Jensen V, Kaiser KMM, Borchardt T, et al. A juvenile form of postsynaptic hippocampal long-term potentiation in mice deficient for the AMPA receptor subunit GluR-A. *J Physiol.* 2003;553(3):843–856.
46. Jia ZP, Agopyan N, Miu P, et al. Enhanced LTP in mice deficient in the AMPA receptor GluR2. *Neuron.* 1996;17:945–956.
47. Feldmeyer D, Kask K, Brusa R, et al. Neurological dysfunctions in mice expressing different levels of the Q/R site-unedited AMPAR subunit GluR-B. *Nat Neurosci.* 1999;2:57–64.
48. Reisel D, Bannerman DM, Schmitt WB, et al. Spatial memory dissociations in mice lacking GluR1. *Nat Neurosci.* 2002;5(9):868–873.
49. Schmitt WB, Sprengel R, Mack V, et al. Restoration of spatial working memory by genetic rescue of GluR-A-deficient mice. *Nat Neurosci.* 2005;8(3):270–272.
50. Liu S-QJ, Cull-Candy SG. Synaptic activity at calcium permeable AMPA receptors induces a switch in receptor subtype. *Nature.* 2000;405: 454–457.
51. Liu SJ, Cull-Candy SG. Subunit interaction with PICK and GRIP controls Ca2+ permeability of AMPARs at cerebellar synapses. *Nat Neurosci.* 2005;8(6):768–775.
52. Spencer HJ, Tominez G, Halpern B. Mass spectrograhic analysis of stimulated release of endogenous amino acids from rat hippocampal slices. *Brain Res.* 1981;212:194–197.
53. Pellegrini-Giampietro DE, Gorter JA, Bennett MVL, et al. The GluR2 (GluR-B) hypothesis: Ca(2+)-permeable AMPA receptors in neurological disorders. *Trends Neurosci.* 1997;20:464–470.
54. Pellegrinigiampietro DE, Bennett MVL, Zukin RS. Are Ca²⁺ Permeable Kainate/Ampa Receptors More Abundant in Immature Brain. *Neurosci Lett.* 1992;144:65–69.
55. Contractor A, Swanson G, Heinemann SF. Kainate receptors are involved in short- and long-term plasticity at mossy fiber synapses in the hippocampus. *Neuron.* 2001;29:209–216.
56. Bortolotto ZA, Clarke VRJ, Delany CM, et al. Kainate receptors are involved in synaptic plasticity. *Nature.* 1999;402:297–301.
57. Bortolotto ZA, Lauri S, Isaac JTR, et al. Kainate receptors and the induction of mossy fibre long-term potentiation. *Proc R Soc Lond B Biol Sci.* 2003;358:657–666.
58. Vissel B, Royle GA, Christie BR, et al. The role of RNA editing of kainate receptors in synaptic plasticity and seizures. *Neuron.* 2001;29: 217–227.
59. Vignes M, Clarke VRJ, Parry MJ, et al. The GluR5 subtype of kainate receptor regulates excitatory synaptic transmission in areas CA1 and CA3 of the rat hippocampus. *Neuropharmacology.* 1998;37:1269–1277.
60. Kidd FL, Isaac JT. Developmental and activity-dependent regulation of kainate receptors at thalamocortical synapses. *Nature.* 1999;400: 569–573.
61. Watanabe M, Inoue Y, Sakimura K, et al. Developmental changes in distribution of NMDA receptor channel subunit messenger RNAs. *NeuroReport.* 1992;3:1138–1140.
62. Monyer H, Burnashev N, Laurie DJ, et al. Developmental and regional expression in the rat brain and functional properties of four NMDA receptors. *Neuron.* 1994;12:529–540.
63. Monyer H, Seeburg PH, Wisden W. Glutamate-operated channels: developmentally early and mature forms arise by alternative splicing. *Neuron.* 1991;6:799–810.
64. Durand GM, Kovalchuk Y, Konnerth A. Long-term potentiation and functional synapse induction in developing hippocampus. *Nature.* 1996; 381:71–75.
65. Hestrin S. Developmental regulation of NMDA receptor-mediated synaptic currents at a central synapse. *Nature.* 1992;357:686–689.
66. Burgard EC, Hablitz JJ. Developmental changes in NMDA and non-NMDA receptor mediated synaptic potentials in rat neocortex. *J Neurophysiol.* 1993;69:230–240.
67. Lomeli H, Mosbacher J, Melcher T, et al. Control of kinetic properties of AMPA receptor channels by nuclear RNA editing. *Science.* 1994;266: 1709–1713.
68. Mosbacher J, Schoepfer R, Monyer H, et al. A molecular determinant for submillisecond desensitization in glutamate receptors. *Science.* 1994;266: 1059–1062.
69. Harris KM, Teyler TJ. Developmental onset of long-term potentiation in area CA1 of the rat hippocampus. *J Physiol.* 1984;346:27–48.
70. Dudek SM, Bear MF. Bidirectional long-term modification of synaptic effectiveness in the adult and immature hippocampus. *J Neurosci.* 1993; 13:2910–2918.

71. Izumi Y, Zorumski CF. Developmental changes in the effects of metabotropic glutamate receptor antagonists on CA1 long-term potentiation in rat hippocampal slices. *Neurosci Lett.* 1994;176:89–92.

72. Isaac JTR, Crair MC, Nicoll RA, et al. Silent synapses during development of thalamocortical inputs. *Neuron.* 1997;18:269–280.

73. Bolshakov VY, Siegelbaum SA. Regulation of hippocampal transmitter release during development and long-term potentiation. *Science.* 1995; 269:1730–1734.

74. Palmer MJ, Isaac JTR, Collinridge GL. Multiple, developmentally regulated expression mechanisms of long-term potentiation at CA1 synapses. *J Neurosci.* 2004;24(21):4903–4911.

75. Isaac JTR, Nicoll RA, Malenka RC. Evidence for silent synapses: implications for the expression of LTP. *Neuron.* 1995;15:427–434.

76. Teyler TJ, Perkins AT, Harris KM. The development of long-term potentiation in hippocampus and neocortex. *Neuropsychologia.* 1989;27:31–39.

77. Kirkwood A, Bear MF. Homosynaptic long-term depression in the visual cortex. *J Neurosci.* 1994;14:3404–3412.

78. Kemp N, Bashir ZI. Induction of LTD in the adult hippocampus by the synaptic activation of AMPA/kainate and metabotropic glutamate receptors. *Neuropharmacology.* 1999;38:495–504.

79. Kemp N, Bashir ZI. NMDA receptor-dependent and -independent long-term depression in the CA1 region of the adult rat hippocampus in vitro. *Neuropharmacology.* 1997;36:397–399.

80. Kamal A, Ramakers GM, Urban IJ, et al. Chemical LTD in the CA1 field of the hippocampus from young and mature rats. *Eur J Neurosci.* 1999; 11(10):3512–3516.

81. Kemp N, McQueen J, Faulkes S, et al. Different forms of LTD in the CA1 region of the hippocampus: role of age and stimulus protocol. *Eur J Neurosci.* 2000;12(1):360–366.

82. Berretta N, Cherubini, E. A novel form of long-term depression in the CA1 area of the adult rat hippocampus independent of glutamate receptors activation. *Eur J Neurosci.* 1998;10(9):2957–2963.

83. Otani S, Connor JA. Requirement of rapid Ca²⁺ entry and synaptic activation of metabotropic glutamate receptors for the induction of long-term depression in the adult rat hippocampus. *J Physiol.* 1998;511:761–770.

84. Bannister NJ, Benke TA, Mellor J, et al. Developmental changes in AMPA and kainate receptor mediated quantal transmission at thalamocortical synapses in the barrel cortex. *J Neurosci.* 2005;25(21):5259–5271.

85. Eybalin M, Caicedo A, Renard N, et al. Transient Ca²⁺-permeable AMPA receptors in postnatal rat primary auditory neurons. *Eur J Neurosci.* 2004;20:2981–2989.

86. Yin HZ, Sensi SL, Carriedo SG, et al. Dendritic localization of Ca²⁺ permeable AMPA/kainate channels in hippocampal pyramidal neurons. *J Comp Neurol.* 1999;409:250–260.

87. Yuste R, Majewska A, Cash SS, et al. Mechanisms of calcium influx into hippocampal spines: heterogeneity among spines, coincidence detection by NMDA receptors, and optical quantal analysis. *J Neurosci.* 1999; 19(6):1976–1987.

88. Ogoshi F, Weiss JH. Heterogeneity of Ca²⁺ permeable AMPA/kainate channel expression in hippocampal pyramidal neurons: fluorescence imaging and immunocytochemical assessment. *J Neurosci.* 2003;23(33): 10521–10530.

89. Collingridge GL, Isaac JTR, Wang YT. Receptor trafficking and synaptic plasticity. *Nat Rev Neurosci.* 2004;5:952–962.

90. Smith KE, Gorski JA, Dell'Acqua ML. Modulation of AMPA receptor activity by associated proteins. *CellScience Reviews.* 2005.

91. Kim E, Sheng, M. PDZ domain proteins of synapses. *Nat Rev Neurosci.* 2004;5:771–781.

92. El-Husseini AED, Schnell E, Chetkovich DM, et al. PSD-95 involvement in maturation of excitatory synapses. *Science.* 2000;290:1364–1368.

93. Tomita S, Fukata M, Nicoll RA, et al. Dynamic Interaction of stargazin-like TARPs with cycling AMPA receptors at synapses. *Science.* 2004;303: 1508–1511.

94. Iwakura Y, Nagano T, Kawamura M, et al. N-methyl-D-aspartate-induced α-amino-3-hydroxy-5-methyl-4-isoxazolepropionic acid (AMPA) receptor down-regulation involves interaction of the carboxy terminus of GluR2/3 with Pick1. *J Biol Chem.* 2001;276:40025–40032.

95. Terashima A, Cotton L, Dev KK. Regulation of synaptic strength and AMPA receptor subunit composition by PICK1. *J Neurosci.* 2004; 24(23):5381–5390.

96. Colledge M, Dean RA, Scott GK, et al. Targeting of PKA to glutamate receptors through a MAGUK-AKAP complex. *Neuron.* 2000;27:107–119.

97. Cho K, Brown MW, Bashir ZI. Mechanisms and physiological role of enhancement of mGluR5 receptor function by group II mGlu receptor activation in rat perirhinal cortex. *J Physiol.* 2002;540.3:895–906.

98. Gomez LL, Alam S, Smith KE, et al. Regulation of A-kinase anchoring protein79/150-cAMP-dependent protein kinase postsynaptic targeting by NMDA receptor activation of calcineurin and remodeling of dendritic actin. *J Neurosci.* 2002;22(16):7027–7044.

99. Genin A, French P, Doyere V, et al. LTP but not seizure is associated with up-regulation of AKAP-150. *Eur J Neurosci.* 2003;17:331–340.

100. Hayashi Y, Shi S-H, Esteban JA, et al. Driving AMPA receptors into synapses by LTP and CaMKII: Requirement for GluR1 and PDZ domain interaction. *Science.* 2000;287:2262–2267.

101. Ehlers MD. Reinsertion or degradation of AMPA receptors determined by activity-dependent endocytic sorting. *Neuron.* 2000;28:511–525.

102. Snyder EM, Colledge M, Crozier RA, et al. Role of A kinase-anchoring proteins (AKAPs) in glutamate receptor trafficking and long term synaptic depression. *J Biol Chem.* 2005;280(17):16962–16968.

103. Tan S-E, Liang K-C. Spatial learning alters hippocampal calcium calmodulin-dependent protein kinase II activity in rats. *Brain Res.* 1996;711: 234–240.

104. Sik A, Gulacsi A, Lai Y, et al. Localization of the A kinase anchoring protein AKAP79 in the human hippocampus. *Eur J Neurosci.* 2000;12:1155–1164.

105. Vicini S. Pharmacologic significance of the structural heterogeneity of the GABAA receptor-chloride ion channel complex. *Neuropsychopharmacology.* 1991;4:9–15.

106. Laurie DJ, Wisden W, Seeburg PH. The distribution of thirteen GABAA receptor subunit mRNAs in the rat brain. III. Embryonic and postnatal development. *J Neurosci.* 1992;12:4151–4172.

107. Wisden W, Laurie DJ, Monyer H, et al. The distribution of 13 GABAA receptor subunits in the rat brain. I. Telencephalon, diencephalon, mesencephalon. *J Neurosci.* 1992;12:1040–1062.

108. MacDonald RL, Olsen RW. GABAA receptor channels. *Annu Rev Neurosci.* 1994;17:569–602.

109. Klepner CA, Lippa AS, Benson DI, et al. Resolution of two biochemically and pharmacologically distinct benzodiazepine receptors. *Pharmacol Biochem Behav.* 1979;11:457–462.

110. Pritchett DB, Sontheimer H, Shivers BD, et al. Importance of a novel GABAA receptor subunit for benzodiazepine pharmacology. *Nature.* 1989;338:582–585.

111. Niddam R, Dubois A, Scatton B, et al. Autoradiographic localization of [3H]zolpidem binding sites in the rat CNS:comparison with the distribution of [3H]flunitrazepam binding sites. *J Neurochem.* 1987;49: 890–899.

112. Sieghart W. Multiplicity of GABAA-benzodiazepine receptors. *Trends Pharmac Sci.* 1989;10:407–411.

113. Brooks-Kayal AR, Shumate MD, Jin H, et al. Gamma-Aminobutyric acid(A) receptor subunit expression predicts functional changes in hippocampal dentate granule cells during postnatal development. *J Neurochem.* 2001;77:1266–1278.

114. Mueller AL, Taube JS, Schwartzkroin PA. Development of hyperpolarizing inhibitory postsynaptic potentials and hyperpolarizing response to gamma-aminobutyric acid in rabbit hippocampus studied in vitro. *J Neurosci.* 1984;4:860–867.

115. Ben Ari Y, Rovira C, Gaiarsa JL, et al. GABAergic mechanisms in the CA3 hippocampal region during early postnatal life. *Prog Brain Res.* 1990;83: 313–321.

116. Cherubini E, Rovira C, Gaiarsa JL, et al. GABA mediated excitation in immature rat CA3 hippocampal neurons. *Int J Dev Neurosci.* 1990;8: 481–490.

117. Rivera C, Voipio J, Payne JA, et al. The K+/Cl- co-transporter KCC2 renders GABA hyperpolarizing during neuronal maturation. *Nature.* 1999; 397:251–255.

118. Plotkin MD, Snyder EY, Hebert SC, et al. Expression of the Na-K-2Cl cotransporter is developmentally regulated in postnatal rat brains: a possible mechanism underlying GABA's excitatory role in immature brain. *J Neurobiol.* 1997;33:781–795.

119. Clayton GH, Owens GC, Wolff JS, et al. Ontogeny of cation-Cl- cotransporter expression in rat neocortex. *Brain Res Dev Brain Res.* 1998;109: 281–292.

120. Lu J, Karadsheh M, Delpire E. Developmental regulation of the neuronal-specific isoform of K-Cl cotransporter KCC2 in postnatal rat brains. *J Neurobiol.* 1999;39:558–568.

121. Ganguly K, Schinder AF, Wong ST, et al. GABA itself promotes the developmental switch of neuronal GABAergic responses from excitation to inhibition. *Cell.* 2001;105:521–532.

122. Payne JA, Rivera C, Voipio J, et al. Cation-chloride co-transporters in neuronal communication, development and trauma. *Trends Neurosci.* 2003;26:199–206.

123. Romijn HJ, Hofman MA, Gramsbergen A. At what age is the developing cerebral cortex of the rat comparable to that of the full-term newborn human baby? *Early Hum Dev.* 1991;26:61–67.

124. Barbin G, Pollard H, Gaiarsa JL, et al. Involvement of GABAA receptors in the outgrowth of cultured hippocampal neurons. *Neurosci Lett.* 1993; 152:150–154.

125. LoTurco JJ, Owens DF, Heath MJ, et al. GABA and glutamate depolarize cortical progenitor cells and inhibit DNA synthesis. *Neuron.* 1995;15: 1287–1298.

126. Leinekugel X, Khalilov I, McLean H, et al. GABA is the principal fast-acting excitatory transmitter in the neonatal brain. *Adv Neurol.* 1999;79: 189–201.

127. Owens DF, Boyce LH, Davis MBE, et al. Excitatory GABA responses in embryonic and neonatal cortical slices demonstrated by gramicidin perforated-patch recordings and calcium imaging. *J Neurosci.* 1996;16: 6414–6423.

128. Ben Ari Y, Khazipov R, Leinekugel X, et al. GABAA, NMDA and AMPA receptors: a developmentally regulated 'menage a trois'. *Trends Neurosci.* 1997;20:523–529.

129. Ben-Ari Y, Cherubini E, Corradetti R, et al. Giant synaptic potentials in immature rat CA3 hippocampal neurones. *J Physiol (Lond).* 1989;416: 303–325.

130. Dzhala VI, Staley KS. Excitatory action of endogenously released GABA contribute to initiation of ictal epileptiform activity in the developing hippocampus. *J Neurosci.* 2003;23(5):1840–1846.

131. Khalilov I, Holmes GL, Ben-Ari, Y. In vitro formation of a secondary epileptogenic mirror focus by interhippocampal propagation of seizures. *Nat Neurosci.* 2003;6(10):1079–1085.

132. Brooks-Kayal AR, Shumate MD, Jin H, et al. Selective changes in single cell GABA(A) receptor subunit expression and function in temporal lobe epilepsy. *Nat Med.* 1998;4:1166–1172.

133. Peng Z, Huang CS, Stell BM, et al. Altered expression of the delta subunit of the GABAA receptor in a mouse model of temporal lobe epilepsy. *J Neurosci.* 2004;24:8629–8639.

134. Zhang N, Wei W, Mody I, et al. Altered localization of GABA(A) receptor subunits on dentate granule cell dendrites influences tonic and phasic inhibition in a mouse model of epilepsy. *J Neurosci.* 2007;27:7520–7531.

135. Cohen AS, Lin DD, Quirk GL, et al. Dentate granule cell GABA(A) receptors in epileptic hippocampus: enhanced synaptic efficacy and altered pharmacology. *Eur J Neurosci.* 2003;17:1607–1616.

136. Houser CR, Esclapez M. Downregulation of the alpha5 subunit of the GABA(A) receptor in the pilocarpine model of temporal lobe epilepsy. *Hippocampus.* 2003;13:633–645.

137. Brooks-Kayal AR, Shumate MD, Jin H, et al. Human neuronal gamma-aminobutyric acid(A) receptors: coordinated subunit mRNA expression and functional correlates in individual dentate granule cells. *J Neurosci.* 1999;19:8312–8318.

138. Zhang G, Raol YH, Hsu FC, et al. Effects of status epilepticus on hippocampal GABA$_A$ receptors are age-dependent. *Neuroscience.* 2004; 125:299–303.

139. Raol YH, Lund IV, Bandyopadhyay S, et al. Enhancing GABA(A) receptor alpha 1 subunit levels in hippocampal dentate gyrus inhibits epilepsy development in an animal model of temporal lobe epilepsy. *J Neurosci.* 2006;26:11342–11346.

140. Kornau HC, Seeburg PH, Kennedy MB. Interaction of ion channels and receptors with PDZ domain proteins. *Curr Opin Neurobiol.* 1997;7: 368–373.

141. Hasselmo ME. Neuromodulation and cortical function: Modeling the physiological basis of behavior. *Behav Brain Res.* 1995;67:1–27.

142. Amaral DG, Witter MP. The three-dimensional organization of the hippocampal formation: A review of anatomical data. *Neuroscience.* 1989; 31:571–591.

143. Scharfman HE. The CA3 "backprojection" to the dentate gyrus. *Prog Brain Res.* 2007;163:627–637.

144. Dzhala VI, Staley KJ. Transition from interictal to ictal activity in limbic networks in vitro. *J Neurosci.* 2003;23(21):7873–7880.

145. Heinemann U, Beck H, Dreier JP, et al. The dentate gyrus as a regulated gate for the propagation of epileptiform activity. *Epilepsy Res Suppl.* 1992;7:273–280.

146. Feng L, Molnar P, Nadler JV. Short-term frequency-dependent plasticity at recurrent mossy fiber synapses of the epileptic brain. *J Neurosci.* 2003; 23(12):5381–5390.

147. Curia G, Longo D, Biagini G, et al. The pilocarpine model of temporal lobe epilepsy. *J Neurosci Methods.* 2008;172:143–157.

148. Ben-Ari Y, Cossart, R. Kainate, a double-agent that generates seizures: two decades of progress. *Trends Neurosci.* 2000;23(11):580–587.

149. Holmes GL. Effects of seizures on brain development: lesssons from the laboratory. *Pediatr Neurol.* 2005;33:1–11.

150. Peng YG, Taylor TB, Finch RE, et al. Neuroexcitatory and neurotoxic actions of the amnesic shellfish poison, domoic acid. *NeuroReport.* 1994; 5:981–985.

151. Yager JY, Armstrong EA, Miyashita H, et al. Prolonged neonatal seizures exacerbate hypoxic-ischemic brain damage: correlation wiht cerebral energy metabolism and excitatory amino acid release. *Dev Neurosci.* 2002;24:367–381.

152. Wirrell EC, Armstrong EA, Osman LD, et al. Prolonged seizures exacerbate perinatal hypoxic-ischemic brain damage. *Pediatr Res.* 2001;50(4): 445–454.

153. Tremblay E, Nitecka L, Berger ML, et al. Maturation of kainic acid seizure-brain damage syndrome in the rat. I. Clinical, electrographic and metabolic observations. *Neuroscience.* 1984;13:1051–1072.

154. Velisek L, Veliskova J, Ptachewich Y, et al. Age-dependent effects of gamma-aminobutyric acid agents of flurothyl seizures. *Epilepsia.* 1995; 36(7):636–643.

155. Holmes GL. The long-term effects of seizures on the developing brain: clinical and laboratory issues. *Brain Dev.* 1991;13:393–409.

156. Jensen FE, Holmes GL, Lombroso CT, et al. Age-dependent changes in long-term seizure susceptibility and behavior after hypoxia in rats. *Epilepsia.* 1992;33:971–980.

157. Jensen FE. The role of glutamate receptor maturation in perinatal seizures and brain injury. *Int J Dev Neurosci.* 2002;20:339–347.

158. Zhang K, Peng BW, Sanchez RM. Decreased IH in hippocampal area CA1 pyramidal neurons after perinatal seizure-inducing hypoxia. *Epilepsia.* 2006;47:1023–1028.

159. Bender RA, Baram TZ. Epileptogenesis in the developing brain: what can we learn from animal models? *Epilepsia.* 2007;48(suppl 5):2–6.

160. Dube CM, Brewster AL, Baram TZ. Febrile seizures: mechanisms and relationship to epilepsy. *Brain Dev.* 2009;31:366–371.

161. Benke TA, Swann J. The Tetanus Toxin Model of Chronic Epilepsy. In: Binder DK, Sharfman HE, eds. *Recent Advances in Epilepsy Research.* 16th ed. New York: Kluwer Academic, 2003.

162. Lee CL, Frost JD, Jr., Swann JW, et al. A new animal model of infantile spasms with unprovoked persistent seizures. *Epilepsia.* 2008;49:298–307.

163. Friedman LK, Koudinov AR. Unilateral GluR2(B) hippocampal knockdown: a novel partial seizure model in the developing rat. *J Neurosci.* 1999;19:9412–9425.

164. Tandon P, Liu Z, Stafstrom CE, et al. Long-term effects of excitatory amino acid antagonists NBQX and MK-801 on the developing brain. *Brain Res Dev Brain Res.* 1996;95:256–262.

165. Pitkanen A, Immonen RJ, Grohn OH, et al. From traumatic brain injury to posttraumatic epilepsy: what animal models tell us about the process and treatment options. *Epilepsia.* 2009;50(suppl 2):21–29.

166. Prince DA, Parada I, Scalise K, et al. Epilepsy following cortical injury: cellular and molecular mechanisms as targets for potential prophylaxis. *Epilepsia.* 2009;50(suppl 2):30–40.

167. Goodkin HP, Kapur J. Responsiveness of status epilepticus to treatment with diazepan decreases rapidly as seizure duration increases. *Epilepsy Curr.* 2003;3:11–12.

168. Wasterlain CG, Chen JW. Mechanistic and pharmacologic aspects of status epilepticus and its treatment with new antiepileptic drugs. *Epilepsia.* 2008;49(suppl 9):63–73.

169. Naylor DE, Liu H, Wasterlain CG. Trafficking of GABAA receptors, loss of inhibition, and a mechanism for pharmacoresistance in status epilepticus. *J Neurosci.* 2005;25:7724–7733.

170. Goodkin HP, Joshi S, Mtchedlishvili Z, et al. Subunit-specific trafficking of GABA(A) receptors during status epilepticus. *J Neurosci.* 2008;28: 2527–2538.

171. Khazipov R, Holmes GL. Synchronization of kainate-induced epileptic activity via GABAergic inhibition in the superfused rat hippocampus in vivo. *J Neurosci.* 2003;23(12):5337–5341.

172. Mazarati AM, Wasterlain CG. N-methyl-D-asparate receptor antagonists abolish the maintenance phase of self-sustaining status epilepticus in rat. *Neurosci Lett.* 1999;265:187–190.

173. Croucher MJ, Collins JF, Meldrum BS. Anticonvulsant action of excitatory amino acid antagonists. *Science.* 1982;21:899–901.

174. Baudry M, Oliver M, Creager R, et al. Increase in glutamate receptors following repetitive electrical stimulation in hippocampal slices. *Life Sci.* 1980;27:325–330.

175. Stasheff SF, Anderson WW, Clark S, et al. NMDA antagonists differentiate epileptogenesis from seizure expression in an in vitro model. *Science.* 1989;245:648–651.

176. Grooms SY, Opitz T, Bennett MVL, et al. Status epilepticus decreases glutamate receptor 2 mRNA and protein expression in hippocampal pyramidal cels before neuronal death. *Proc Natl Acad Sci USA.* 2000;97: 3631–3636.

177. Sommer C, Roth SU, Kiessling M. Kainate-induced epilepsy alters protein expression of AMPA receptor subunits GluR1, GluR2 and AMPA receptor binding protein in the rat hippocampus. *Acta Neuropathologica.* 2001;101:460–468.

178. Standley S, Baudry M. Rapid effects of kainate administration on a-amino-3-hydroxy-5-methyl-4-isoxazole propionic acid (AMPA) receptor properties in rat hippocampus. *Exp Neurol.* 1998;152:208–213.

179. Demarque M, Villeneuve N, Manent JB, et al. Glutamate transporters prevent the generation of seizures in the developing rat neocortex. *J Neurosci.* 2004;24(13):3289–3294.

180. Fellin T, Gomez-Gonzalo M, Gobbo S, et al. Astrocytic glutamate is not necessary for the generation of epileptiform neuronal activity in hippocampal slices. *J Neurosci.* 2006;26:9312–9322.

181. Hunsberger JG, Bennett AH, Selvanayagam E, et al. Gene profiling the response to kainic acid induced seizures. *Mol Brain Res.* 2005;141: 95–112.

182. El Hassar L, Esclapez M, Bernard C. Hyperexcitability of the CA1 hippocampal region during epileptogenesis. *Epilepsia.* 2007;48(suppl 5): 131–139.

183. Williams PA, White AM, Clark S, et al. Development of spontaneous recurrent seizures after kainate-induced status epilepticus. *J Neurosci.* 2009;29:2103–2112.

184. Sutula TP. Mechanisms of epilepsy progression: current theories and perspectives from neuroplasticity in adulthood and development. *Epilepsy Res.* 2004;60:161–171.

185. Pathak HR, Weissinger F, Terunuma M, et al. Disrupted dentate granule cell chloride regulation enhances synaptic excitability during development of temporal lobe epilepsy. *J Neurosci.* 2007;27:14012–14022.

186. Nadler JV. The recurrent mossy fiber pathway of the epileptic brain. *Neurochem Res.* 2003;28:1649–1658.

187. Andre V, Marescaux C, Nehlig A, et al. Alterations of hippocampal GABAergic system contribute to development of spontaneous recurrent seizures in the rat lithium-pilocarpine model of temporal lobe epilepsy. *Hippocampus.* 2001;11:452–468.

188. Buckmaster PS, Zhang GF, Yamawaki R. Axon sprouting in a model of temporal lobe epilepsy creates a predominantly excitatory feedback circuit. *J Neurosci.* 2002;22(15):6650–6658.

189. Okazaki MM, Molnar P, Nadler JV. Recurrent mossy fiber pathway in rat dentate gyrus: synaptic currents evoked in presence and absence of seizure-induced growth. *J Neurophysiol.* 1999;81:1645–1660.

190. Okazaki MM, Nadler JV. Glutamate receptor involvement in dentate granule cell epileptiform activity evoked by mossy fiber stimulation. *Brain Res.* 2001;915:58–69.

191. Epsztein J, Represa A, Jorquera I, et al. Recurrent mossy fibers establish aberrant kainate receptor-operated synapses on granule cells from epileptic rats. *J Neurosci.* 2005;25:8229–8239.

192. Lombroso CT. Neonatal seizures: gaps between the laboratory and the clinic. *Epilepsia.* 2007;48(suppl 2):83–106.

193. Siddiqui AH, Joseph SA. CA3 axonal sprouting in kainate-induced chronic epilepsy. *Brain Res.* 2005;1066:129–146.

194. Esclapez M, Hirsch JC, Ben-Ari Y, et al. Newly formed excitatory pathways provide a substrate for hyperexcitability in experimental temporal lobe epilepsy. *J Comp Neurol.* 1999;498:449–460.

195. Cossart R, Dinocourt C, Hirsch JC, et al. Dendritic but not somatic GABAergic inhibition is decreased in experimental epilepsy. *Nat Neurosci.* 2001;4:52–62.

196. Cavazos JE, Jones SM, Cross DJ. Sprouting and synaptic reorganization in the subiculum and CA1 region of the hippocampus in acute and chronic models of partial-onset epilepsy. *Neuroscience.* 2004;126:677–688.

197. Jin X, Prince DA, Huguenard JR. Enhanced excitatory synaptic connectivity in layer v pyramidal neurons of chronically injured epileptogenic neocortex in rats. *J Neurosci.* 2006;26:4891–4900.

198. Avramescu S, Timofeev I. Synaptic strength modulation after cortical trauma: a role in epileptogenesis. *J Neurosci.* 2008;28:6760–6772.

199. Friedman LK, Pellegrini-Giampietro DE, Sperber EF, et al. Kainate-induced status epilepticus alters glutamate and GABA_A receptor gene expression in adult rat hippocampus: an insitu hybridization study. *J Neurosci.* 1994;14:2697–2707.

200. Rice AC, Floyd CL, Lyeth BG, et al. Status epilepticus causes long-term NMDA receptor-dependent behavioral changes and cognitive deficits. *Epilepsia.* 1998;39:1148–1157.

201. Oberheim NA, Tian GF, Han X, et al. Loss of astrocytic domain organization in the epileptic brain. *J Neurosci.* 2008;28:3264–3276.

202. Tian GF, Azmi H, Takano T, et al. An astrocytic basis of epilepsy. *Nat Med.* 2005;11:973–981.

203. Parent JM, Elliott RC, Pleasure SJ, et al. Aberrant seizure-induced neurogenesis in experimental temporal lobe epilepsy. *Ann Neurol.* 2006;59:81–91.

204. Parent JM, Murphy GG. Mechanisms and functional significance of aberrant seizure-induced hippocampal neurogenesis. *Epilepsia.* 2008;49(suppl 5):19–25.

205. Stafstrom CE, Thompson JL, Holmes GL. Kaininc acid seizures in the developing brain: status epilepticus and spontaneous recurrent seizures. *Brain Res Dev Brain Res.* 1992;21:227–236.

206. Yang Y, Tandon P, Liu Z, et al. Synaptic reorganization following kainic acid-induced seizures during development. *Dev Brain Res.* 1998;107:169–177.

207. Cilio MR, Sogawa Y, Cha B, et al. Long-term effects of status epilepticus in the immature brain are specific for age and model. *Epilepsia.* 2003;44(4):518–528.

208. Sarkisian MR, Tandon P, Liu Z, et al. Multiple kainic acid seizures in the immature and adult brain: ictal manifestations and long-term effects on learning and memory. *Epilepsia.* 1997;38:1157–1166.

209. Tandon P, Yang Y, Stafstrom CE, et al. Downregulation of kainate receptors in the hippocampus following repeated seizures in immature rats. *Dev Brain Res.* 2002;136:145–150.

210. Raol YSH, Budreck EC, Brooks-Kayal AR. Epilepsy after early-life seizures can be independent of hippocampal injury. *Ann of Neurol.* 2003;53:503–511.

211. Kubova H, Mares P, Suchomelova L, et al. Status epilepticus in immature rats leads to behavioral and cognitive impairment and epileptogenesis. *Eur J Neurosci.* 2004;19:3255–3265.

212. Sankar R, Shin DH, Liu H, et al. Patterns of status epilepticus-induced neuronal injury during development and long-term consequences. *J Neurosci.* 1998;18:8382–8393.

213. Priel MR, dos Santos NF, Cavalheiro E. A. Developmental aspects of the pilocarpine model of epilepsy. *Epilepsy Res.* 1996;26:115–121.

214. dos Santos NF, Arida RM, Filho EM, et al. Epileptogenesis in immature rats following recurrent status epilepticus. *Brain Res Rev.* 2000;32: 269–276.

215. Santos NF, Marques RH, Correia L, et al. Multiple pilocarpine-induced status epilepticus in developing rats: a long-term behavioral and electrophysiological study. *Epilepsia.* 2000;41(suppl 6):S57–S63.

216. Anderson AE, Hrachovy RA, Antalffy BA, et al. A chronic focal epilepsy with mossy fiber sprouting follows recurrent seizures induced by intrahippocampal tetanus toxin injection in infant rats. *Neuroscience.* 1999;92(1):73–82.

217. Sogawa Y, Monokoshi M, Silveira DC, et al. Timing of cognitive deficits following neonatal seizures: relationship to histological changes in the hippocampus. *Dev Brain Res.* 2001;131:73–83.

218. de Rogalski Landrot I, Minokoshi M, Silveria DC, et al. Recurrent neonatal seizures: relationship of pathology to the electroencephalogram and cognition. *Dev Brain Res.* 2001;129:27–38.

219. Holmes GL, Gairsa J-L, Chevassus-Au-Louis N, et al. Consequences of neonatal seizures in the rat: morphological and behavioral effects. *Ann Neurol.* 1998;44:845–857.

220. Thompson K, Holm AM, Schousboe A, et al. Hippocampal stimulation produces neuronal death in the immature brain. *Neuroscience.* 1998;82:337–348.

221. Bender RA, Dube C, Gonzalez-Vega R, et al. Mossy fiber plasticity and enhanced hippocampal excitability, without hippocampal cell loss or altered neurogenesis, in an animal model of prolonged febrile seizures. *Hippocampus.* 2003;13:399–412.

222. Dube C, Chen K, Eghbal-Ahmadi M, et al. Prolonged febrile seizures in the immature rat model enhance hippocampal excitability long term. *Ann Neurol.* 2000;47:336–344.

223. Dube C, Richichi C, Bender RA, et al. Temporal lobe epilepsy after experimental prolonged febrile seizures: prospective analysis. *Brain.* 2006;129: 911–922.

224. Brunson KL, Kramar E, Lin B, et al. Mechanisms of late-onset cognitive decline after early-life stress. *J Neurosci.* 2005;25(14):9328–9338.

225. Hu RQ, Cortez MA, Man HY, et al. Alteration of GluR2 expression in the rat brain following absence seizures induced by g-hydroxybutyric acid. *Epilepsy Res.* 2001;44:41–51.

226. Koh S, Tibayan FD, Simpson JN, et al. NBQX or topiramate treatment after perinatal hypoxia-induced seizures prevents later increases in seizure-induced neuronal injury. *Epilepsia.* 2004;45:569–575.

227. Prince HC, Tzingounis AV, Levey AI, et al. Functional downregulation of GluR2 in piriform cortex of kindled animals. *Synapse.* 2000;38: 489–498.

228. Naylor P, Stewart CA, Wright SR, et al. Repeated ECS induces GluR1 mRNA bunt NMDAR1A-G mRNA in the rat hippocampus. *Brain Res.* 1996;35:349–353.

229. Ying Z, Babb TL, Comair YG, et al. Increased densities of AMPA GluR1 subunit proteins and presynaptic mossy fiber sprouting in the rascia dentata of human hippocampal epilepsy. *Brain Res.* 1998;798: 239–246.

230. Ying Z, Babb TL, Hilbig A, et al. Hippocampal chemical anatomy in pediatric and adolescent patients with hippocampal or extrahippocampal epilepsy. *Dev Neurosci.* 1999;21:236–247.

231. Eid T, Kovacs I, Spencer DD, et al. Novel expression of AMPA-receptor subunit GluR1 on mossy cells and CA3 pyramidal neuons in the human epileptogenic hippocampus. *Eur J Neurosci.* 2002;15:517–527.

232. Cornejo BJ, Mesches MH, Coultrap S, et al. A single episode of neonatal seizures permanently alters glutamatergic synapses. *Ann Neurol.* 2007;61:411–426.

233. Sanchez RM, Koh S, Rio C, et al. Decreased glutamate receptor 2 expression and enhanced epileptogenesis in immature rat hippocampus after perinatal hypoxia-induced seizures. *J Neurosci.* 2001;21: 8154–8163.

234. Zhang G, Raol YSH, Hsu F-C, et al. Long-term alterations in glutamate receptor and transporter expression following early-life seizures are associated with increased seizure susceptibility. *J Neurochem.* 2004;88:91–101.

235. Swann JW, Le JT, Lee CL. Recurrent seizures and the molecular maturation of hippocampal and neocortical glutamatergic synapses. *Dev Neurosci.* 2007;29:168–178.

236. Rakhade SN, Zhou C, Aujla PK, et al. Early alterations of AMPA receptors mediate synaptic potentiation induced by neonatal seizures. *J Neurosci.* 2008;28:7979–7990.

237. Lynch M, Sayin U, Bownds J, et al. Long-term consequences of early postnatal seizures on hippocampal learning and plasticity. *Eur J Neurosci.* 2000;12:2252–2264.

238. Ellerkmann RK, Remy S, Chen J, et al. Molecular and functional changes in voltage-dependent Na(+) channels following pilocarpine-induced status epilepticus in rat dentate granule cells. *Neuroscience.* 2003;119:323–333.

239. Blumenfeld H, Lampert A, Klein JP, et al. Role of hippocampal sodium channel Nav1.6 in kindling epileptogenesis. *Epilepsia.* 2009;50:44–55.

240. Yaari Y, Yue C, Su H. Recruitment of apical dendritic T-type Ca^{2+} channels by back propagating spikes underlies de novo intrinsic bursting in hippocampal epileptogenesis. *J Physiol.* 2007;580:435–450.

241. Su H, Sochivko D, Becker A, et al. Up regulation of a T-type Ca^{2+} channel causes a long-lasting modification of neuronal firing mode after status epilepticus. *J Neurosci.* 2002;22:3645–3655.

242. Bernard C, Anderson A, Becker A, et al. Acquired dendritic channelopathy in temporal lobe epilepsy. *Science.* 2004;305:532–535.

243. Chen K, Baram TZ, Soltesz, I. Febrile seizures in the developing brain result in persistent modification of neuronal excitability in limbic circuits. *Nat Med.* 1999;5:888–894.

244. Chan K, Aradi I, Thon N, et al. Persistently modified h-channels after complex febrile seizures convert the seizure-induced enhancement of inhibition to hyperexcitability. *Nat Med.* 2001;7:331–337.

245. Lund IV, Hu Y, Raol YH, et al. BDNF selectively regulates GABAA receptor transcription by activation of the JAK/STAT pathway. *Sci Signal.* 2008;1:ra9.

246. Morris RGM, Frey, U. Hippocampal synaptic plasticity: role in spatial learning or the automatic recording of attended experience. *Philos Trans R Soc Lond B Biol Sci.* 1997;352(1360):1489–1503.

247. Kemppainen EJS, Nissinen J, Pitkänen, A. Fear conditioning is impaired in systemic kainic acid and amygdala-stimulation models of epilepsy. *Epilepsia.* 2006;47:820–829.

248. de Hoz L, Moser EI, Morris RG. Spatial learning with unilateral and bilateral hippocampal networks. *Eur J Neurosci.* 2005;22:745–754.

249. Huang L, Cilio MR, Silveira DC, et al. Long-term effects of neonatal seizures: a behavioral, electrophysiological and histological study. *Brain Res Dev Brain Res.* 1999;118:99–107.

250. Mikati MA, Zeinieh MP, Kurdi RM, et al. Long-term effects of acute and of chronic hypoxia on behavior and on hippocampal histology in the developing brain. *Brain Res Dev Brain Res.* 2005;157:98–102.

251. Koh S, Storey TW, Santos TC, et al. Early-life seizures in rats increase susceptibility to seizure-induced brain injury in adulthood. *Neurology.* 1999;53(5):915–921.

252. Stafstrom CE. Assessing the behavioral and cognitive effects of seizures on the developing brain. *Prog Brain Res.* 2002;135:377–390.

253. Cornejo BJ, Mesches MH, Benke TA. A single early-life seizure impairs short-term memory but does not alter spatial learning, recognition memory, or anxiety. *Epilepsy Behav.* 2008;

254. Sayin U, Sutula TP, Stafstrom CE. Seizures in the developing brain cause adverse long-term effects on spatial learning and anxiety. *Epilepsia.* 2004;45(12):1539–1548.

255. Avanzini G, Franceschetti S, Mantegazza M. Epileptogenic channelopathies: experimental models of human pathologies. *Epilepsia.* 2007; 48(suppl 2):51–64.

256. Oakley JC, Kalume F, Yu FH, et al. Temperature- and age-dependent seizures in a mouse model of severe myoclonic epilepsy in infancy. *Proc Natl Acad Sci U S A.* 2009;106:3994–3999.

257. Kalume F, Yu FH, Westenbroek RE, et al. Reduced sodium current in Purkinje neurons from Nav1.1 mutant mice: implications for ataxia in severe myoclonic epilepsy in infancy. *J Neurosci.* 2007;27: 11065–11074.

258. Catterall WA, Dib-Hajj S, Meisler MH, et al. Inherited neuronal ion channelopathies: new windows on complex neurological diseases. *J Neurosci.* 2008;28:11768–11777.

259. Singh NA, Otto JF, Dahle EJ, et al. Mouse models of human KCNQ2 and KCNQ3 mutations for benign familial neonatal convulsions show seizures and neuronal plasticity without synaptic reorganization. *J Physiol.* 2008;586:3405–3423.

260. Ernst WL, Zhang Y, Yoo JW, et al. Genetic enhancement of thalamocortical network activity by elevating alpha 1g-mediated low-voltage-activated calcium current induces pure absence epilepsy. *J Neurosci.* 2009;29: 1615–1625.

261. MacDonald RL, Gallagher MJ, Feng HJ, et al. GABA(A) receptor epilepsy mutations. *Biochem Pharmacol.* 2004;68:1497–1506.

262. Kang JQ, Shen W, MacDonald RL. The GABRG2 mutation, Q351X, associated with generalized epilepsy with febrile seizures plus, has both loss of function and dominant-negative suppression. *J Neurosci.* 2009;29: 2845–2856.

263. Marini C, Guerrini R. The role of the nicotinic acetylcholine receptors in sleep-related epilepsy. *Biochem Pharmacol.* 2007;74:1308–1314.

CHAPTER 4 ■ GENETICS OF THE EPILEPSIES

JOCELYN BAUTISTA AND ANNE ANDERSON

The importance of genetics is becoming increasingly recognized in epilepsy syndromes, as in nearly all human disease. Genetics plays a role not only in causation or susceptibility to disease, but also in responsiveness to medications and adverse effects. This chapter will provide an overview of the genetic contribution to human epilepsy in general, the genetics of specific idiopathic epilepsy syndromes, and genetic testing principles in the epilepsies.

GENETIC CONTRIBUTION TO EPILEPSY

Although suspected for centuries, the genetic contribution to epilepsy was difficult to establish historically due to difficulties defining epilepsy, misdiagnosis of seizures, inaccurate family histories due to insufficient medical information, embarrassment and concealment of seizures among family members, as well as the presence of multiple causative factors, aside from genetic risk. Epidemiological studies eventually confirmed the importance of genetics by demonstrating an increased risk of epilepsy in family members of persons with epilepsy, compared to the general population (1). Offspring of individuals with focal epilepsy were found to be just as likely to have epilepsy as offspring of individuals with generalized epilepsy, and both were three times more likely than the general population (2). These population-based studies were further supported by twin studies, which showed higher concordance among monozygotic compared to dizygotic twins (3,4), as well as heritability studies (5), segregation analyses (6,7), and linkage studies (8,9). Animal genetic models of epilepsy have lent further support, but the strongest evidence has come from the finding of specific mutations in human epilepsy syndromes. Genetics appears to play a disease-causing role in the symptomatic epilepsies such as the progressive myoclonic epilepsies (Chapter 21), as well as those associated with malformations of cortical development (Chapter 27), neurocutaneous syndromes (Chapter 31), inherited metabolic and mitochondrial disorders (Chapter 32), and chromosomal disorders. Aside from disease genes, there also appear to be genes that mediate responsiveness to antiepileptic medications (Chapter 49). Disease genes identified in idiopathic epilepsy syndromes will be the focus of this present chapter.

GENETICS OF IDIOPATHIC EPILEPSY SYNDROMES

The majority of the currently known genetic mutations associated with idiopathic epilepsy syndromes involve genes encoding ion channels or the regulatory molecules associated with them. More recently, mutations in several additional non-ion channel genes have been linked to idiopathic epilepsy syndromes. Of note however is that while the first gene mutation associated with idiopathic epilepsy was described in 1995 and a number of other genes have been identified since then, the genetic cause of the majority of idiopathic epilepsy syndromes remains to be elucidated. In the sections that follow we present an overview of the major mutations identified to date and the functional consequences.

Ion channels are critical determinants of neuronal membrane excitability. While there are specific differences in the structure and function of the various ion channels for which mutations have been described, in general these channels are composed of primary pore-forming subunit proteins that flux ions and a number of associated proteins that serve regulatory functions. Mutations in the genes encoding any one of these proteins may disrupt channel function. The expression of ion channels in the pre- and postsynaptic membranes is highly regulated and is a dynamic, activity-dependent process. Mutations in the proteins encoding these channels can affect the biophysical properties of the channels as well as their trafficking to and from the surface membrane. Thus, mutations in ion channel proteins can have dramatic effects on the intrinsic membrane properties of a neuron. Depending on the type of neurons affected, there may be marked alterations in neuronal firing patterns and the network properties of the system, which may lead to seizures or a predisposition to them.

Ion Channel Gene Mutations

Mutations in both nicotinic acetylcholine receptors (nAChRs) and γ-aminobutyric acid (GABA) receptors, and in voltage-dependent sodium, potassium, calcium, and chloride channels have been identified in some idiopathic epilepsy syndromes. While these receptors and ion channels are functionally and molecularly distinct, they flux ions in response to binding of a ligand to the extracellular domains of the pore-forming regions of the channels or in response to a change membrane potential.

Nicotinic Acetylcholine Receptors

Background. Neuronal nAChRs are ionotropic receptors formed by a pentamer of subunits that are arranged in the lipid bilayer of the surface membrane creating a pore that fluxes cations in response to ligand (acetylcholine) binding. There have been 17 different genes identified that encode for ACh receptor subunits, which include α1–10, β1–4, δ, ε, and γ (10). In the forebrain, α and β subunits are the most abundant, and mutations in both these subgroups have been identified in epilepsy. Under physiological conditions, binding of the endogenous agonist acetylcholine to the receptor induces permeability of the pore region to Na^+, Ca^{2+}, and K^+ ions

(Na^+ and Ca^{2+} moving inward and K^+ outward). Nicotine is an exogenous agonist of the channel as the name implies. A preponderance of evidence indicates that the receptors are primarily localized to presynaptic membranes where they function to modulate neurotransmitter release in both inhibitory and excitatory neurons (GABA and glutaminergic, respectively). Nicotinic AChRs are critical to a number of physiological processes of the central nervous system (CNS) including arousal and sleep as well as cognitive functions. At a cellular level, these receptors regulate neurotransmitter release and neuronal excitability and integration (11).

Epilepsy Genetics. Aberrations in the nAChRs at a protein level have been identified in a number of diseases involving the CNS, including schizophrenia and Alzheimer disease. The only known gene mutations in AChRs subunits associated with a neurological disorder are those associated with autosomal dominant nocturnal frontal lobe epilepsy (ADNFLE). In 1995, a mutation in *CHRNA4*, the gene encoding the α-4 nicotinic acetylcholine receptor subunit was described in ADNFLE. This was the first gene mutation identified in association with an epilepsy syndrome. Subsequently, additional mutations have been described in *CHRNA4*; in the genes encoding the nicotinic acetylcholine receptor α-2 and β-2 subunits, *CHRNA2* and *CHRNB2*, respectively; and in genes encoding other ion channels. The majority of the mutations described so far involve the pore-forming region of the channel (12). At the molecular level, a number of effects have been described for the various mutations identified (13). One common effect appears to be an overall increased sensitivity of the receptor to acetylcholine. Although several models have been proposed, exactly how the aberrant channel function leads to the clinical syndrome is unclear.

Epilepsy Syndrome. ADNFLE is characterized by seizures consisting of hyperkinetic limb movements or tonic posturing of the extremities, with onset in late childhood or early adolescence. These can occur multiple times during periods of non-rapid eye movement (NREM) sleep and may be confused with nocturnal parasomnias. The incidence is unknown but ADNFLE is thought to be under-recognized and easily misdiagnosed. In some cases, there are rare daytime seizures as well, including generalized tonic–clonic (GTC), generalized atonic, and complex partial seizures (CPS) (14). The ictal electroencephalogram (EEG) may demonstrate bifrontal slowing and epileptiform activity, but it also may be normal. ADNFLE has been associated with mutations in *CHRNA4*, *CHRNB2*, and *CHRNA2*. Penetrance is incomplete, approximately 70% (approximately 30% of individuals who carry the mutation will never show clinical disease). Of over 100 ADNFLE families reported in the literature, *CHRNA4* and *CHRNB2* mutations have been identified in about 10%. The majority of cases of ADNFLE have seizures that respond well to antiepileptic medications. Several cases of sporadic nocturnal frontal lobe epilepsy have also been associated with mutations in *CHRNA4*; these cases tend to be more refractory (15,16). Neuropsychological assessment of patients with ADNFLE and mutations in the nAChr receptor revealed impairments in cognitive function involving executive tasks and memory (17).

GABA_A Receptors

Background. GABA_A receptors are ionotropic receptors that flux chloride (Cl^-) in response to ligand binding. GABA_A receptors underlie fast inhibition and regulate neuronal activity at a cellular and network level. The balance of inhibitory and excitatory neurotransmission is critical to physiologic functions of the CNS. There are 18 genes encoding a number of different GABA_A receptor subunits (α1–6, β1–3, γ1–3, δ, ε1–3, θ, π). Various combinations of these subunits associate to compose the pentameric pore-forming functional GABA_A channels in the CNS. Pentamers of two α, two β, and one γ or one δ subunit compose most GABA_A receptors (18). The heterogeneity in the subunit composition of the receptor contributes to the pharmacological profile and localization at a subcellular and regional level in the brain. These receptors are activated through ligand binding to the extracellular domains of the receptor. The endogenous ligand is GABA; however, the channels are well-known targets for a number of exogenous drugs, including benzodiazepines, barbiturates, and other sedative agents such as alcohol, which enhance inhibitory neurotransmission (19). Importantly, the pharmacology of these channels has been critical to the medical management of a number of neurological disorders including epilepsy. Application of an antagonist of these receptors can evoke seizures, which is a phenomenon that has been exploited in basic science epilepsy laboratories.

Epilepsy Genetics. GABA_A receptors composed of α1β2γ2 subunits are the most common form of the receptor found in brain. Mutations in *GABRG2* and *GABRA1* have been described in epilepsy; these are the genes encoding the γ2 and α1 subunits, respectively. The first *GABRG2* mutations were identified by two independent groups in families with generalized epilepsy with febrile seizures plus (GEFS+) and childhood absence epilepsy (CAE). Shortly thereafter additional mutations in *GABRG2* were described in families with GEFS+, severe myoclonic epilepsy of infancy (SMEI) or Dravet syndrome, CAE, and febrile seizures (FS). A separate mutation in *GABRG2* has been described in isolated FS. Mutations in the *GABRA1* subunit have been described in familial juvenile myoclonic epilepsy (JME) and a sporadic case of CAE. These mutations have been characterized in a number of laboratories, and a variety of functional effects have been identified including alterations in GABA sensitivity, reduced surface expression, and alterations in the biophysical properties of the receptor. The net result of these alterations is a reduction in GABA-activated Cl^- currents and thereby alterations in inhibitory neurotransmission (12). Mutations in *GABRD*, the gene encoding the δ subunit, have been suggested as susceptibility alleles in GEFS+ and JME. The δ subunit is found in GABA_A receptors localized exclusively to the extra- or perisynaptic regions, while those containing γ subunits are found both in the synaptic and extrasynaptic regions. These channels contribute to the tonic inhibitory current, and studies have shown that the mutations described in epilepsy reduce this current and the surface expression of the channels (12).

Epilepsy Syndromes. GEFS+ is a familial epilepsy syndrome, with at least two affected family members, encompassing a wide range of phenotypes from simple FS to FS persisting beyond 6 years of age (FS+), to afebrile GTC seizures, absence, myoclonic, or atonic seizures, and even focal seizures. While many patients have seizures that remit spontaneously, others may develop refractory epilepsy, including SMEI or Dravet syndrome. Mutations in *GABRG2* have been described in GEFS+ and Dravet syndrome. A mutation in *GABRG2* has also been identified in a family with CAE and FS (20). In another family, two siblings and their father had isolated FS with onset between 13 and 18 months of age, resolving by 5 years of age; all three affected individuals had a mutation in *GABRG2* (21). The last two families are arguably still within the spectrum of the GEFS+ phenotype. Mutations in *GABRA1* have been described in familial JME, in one family with 14 affected individuals over four generations, all with a similar phenotype of myoclonic and GTC seizures and generalized spike–wave complexes on EEG (22). Mutations in *GABRA1* have also been described in a sporadic case of CAE. Out of 98 individuals with idiopathic generalized epilepsy (IGE), one individual with clusters of daily absence seizures from 3 to 5 years of age was identified as having a heterozygous mutation in *GABRA1*; there was no history of FS and no family history of seizures (23). *GABRD* is thought to be a susceptibility locus for IGE, and a mutation has been identified in one small family with GEFS+ (24). Clinical descriptions of IGE syndromes of childhood and adolescence, such as CAE and JME, can be found in Chapter 20. Clinical features of affected individuals in the families described above do not differ significantly from nonfamilial forms of IGE.

Sodium Channels

Background. Voltage-gated sodium channels (Na_v) are composed of a complex formed by a large α subunit and smaller auxiliary β subunits. The Na_v α subunit consists of four internally repeated domains that each have six transmembrane spanning regions and a pore loop, which together form the ion-conducting pore that fluxes Na^+ ions. The β subunits associate with the α subunit complex and modify the channel biophysical properties and interact with the cytoskeleton. Four of the nine genes encoding the α subunit of Na_v channels are expressed in the mammalian CNS. These are *SCN1A*, *SCN2A*, *SCN3A*, and *SCN8A*, which encode $Na_v1.1$, $Na_v1.2$, $Na_v1.3$, and $Na_v1.6$, respectively. The Na_v1 channels are responsible for action potential initiation and propagation in neurons. The subcellular localization varies depending upon the subunit composition (25,26). These channels are critical to physiological functions of the CNS, and the aberrant regulation or genetic mutation of these channels has been associated with neuropathology, including epilepsy. Furthermore, these channels have been the target of therapeutics in epilepsy. The mechanism of action of some anticonvulsant drugs such as phenytoin is thought to be in part through modulation of these channels.

Epilepsy Genetics. Mutations in *SCN1A*, *SCN2A*, and *SCN1B* have been described in epilepsy. The first sodium channel mutation in epilepsy was described in 2000 in *SCN1A* (27). Subsequently, over 100 mutations have been described in this channel subunit. *SCN1A* mutations have been described in GEFS+ and in SMEI or Dravet syndrome. The mutations associated with GEFS+ are missense mutations in *SCN1A*, while those associated with Dravet are missense and nonsense mutations with protein truncation. Deletions of entire exons or multiple exons have also been described in association with a Dravet phenotype. There is phenotypic variability and complex inheritance, suggesting a role for modifier genes. *SCN2A* missense mutation has been described in benign neonatal–infantile familial seizures, and a nonsense or trunca-

tion mutation has been described in Dravet syndrome. The mutations in *SCN1A* and *SCN2A* that led to more dramatic alteration in the protein product were associated with the more severe phenotype (Dravet syndrome). *SCN1B* mutations have been described in GEFS+, FS, early onset absence epilepsy, and temporal lobe epilepsy (TLE) (12).

Epilepsy Syndrome. As mentioned above, GEFS+ is a familial epilepsy syndrome with a highly variable phenotype, typically involving FS persisting beyond 6 years of age, followed by afebrile seizures. At the more severe end of the GEFS+ spectrum is SMEI or Dravet syndrome. Mutations in *SCN1A*, *SCN2A*, and *SCN1B* have been described in GEFS+. While approximately 10% of GEFS+ families will have *SCN1A* mutations (typically missense), over 70% of Dravet patients will have *SCN1A* mutations (both missense and truncation). Most of the *SCN1A* mutations that occur in Dravet syndrome (60% to 85%) appear to be de novo mutations. The afebrile seizures that follow FS can be either generalized or focal, including mesial TLE. Affected family members can have isolated FS, afebrile seizures, or both. De novo mutations in *SCN1A* have also been identified in cases of alleged pertussis vaccine-induced encephalopathy which can resemble SMEI clinically (28).

Potassium Channels

Background. Potassium channels are major determinants of the intrinsic membrane excitability of neurons and thus alterations in these channels will have profound effects on network behavior within the CNS. These channels are critical to physiological functions of the CNS including development, plasticity, learning and memory, and many other functions. Mutations or aberrant regulation of a number of the K^+ channels expressed within the CNS have been described in neurological disorders, including epilepsy. These channels are extremely diverse and there are many different subunits described. The functional channel complexes flux K^+ ions outward. There are three major classes of K^+ channels that are defined by the number of transmembrane domains within each α subunit. Mutations in channels falling into two of these classes have been described in epilepsy. These include the voltage-dependent potassium (K_v) channel α subunits that are characterized by six transmembrane domains and the inward-rectifier K^+ (K_{ir}) channels that are characterized by two transmembrane domains. Each of these groups is characterized by subfamilies encoded by numerous genes. The functional channel is formed by multimerization of the α subunits and a host of associated or auxiliary subunits that influence the channel properties and trafficking (12,26).

Epilepsy Genetics. *KCNQ2* and *KCNQ3* from the K_v family, which encode K_v7 α subunits, have been clearly linked to epilepsy. Channels composed of these subunits underlie the M-current, named so due to the observation that stimulation of muscarinic cholinergic receptors suppresses the current. M-channels contribute to a portion of the afterhyperpolarization (AHP), known as the medium AHP (mAHP). These channels are expressed early during development in the human brain. Interestingly, a number of mutations have been identified in *KCNQ2* in families with benign familial neonatal convulsions (BFNC). A few de novo mutations have also been identified in association with benign neonatal convulsions. Relatively fewer mutations in *KCNQ3* have been identified in families with this syndrome (29). The described mutations are predicted to result in truncation of the channel protein and others are missense mutations. Evidence suggests that the net effect of these mutations is a loss of function. The decreased level of functional M-channels is predicted to lead to increased excitability within the CNS, particularly during the neonatal period. Indeed, under physiological conditions these likely play an important inhibitory role early postnatally when GABA neurotransmission is depolarizing and thereby excitatory. The remission in the epilepsy in the affected individuals is thought to be due to the developmental switch in GABA when it changes to become inhibitory (12).

KCNA1 encodes $K_v1.1$ α subunits. The K_v1 subfamily of K^+ channels is found throughout the brain and is localized to axonal regions. Kv1.1 α subunits heteromultimerize with other K_v1 subunits, and the channels may be dramatically altered in their properties by inclusion of the $K_v\beta1.1$ auxiliary subunit in the supramolecular channel complex (26). These channels function to repolarize the postsynaptic membrane and play a role in shaping the action potential. Mutations in *KCNA1* underlie autosomal dominant episodic ataxia type 1 (EA1), and some families with this disorder have epilepsy. The effect of this mutation on channel function is an overall loss of function with altered channel assembly, trafficking, and kinetics (12).

KCNMA1 encodes the α subunit of the large-conductance voltage- and Ca^{2+}-activated K^+ channel, also called the BK channel (KCa1.1). The BK channel is distinct from other K^+ channels in that it can be activated by both intracellular Ca^{2+} and membrane depolarization. BK channels are highly conserved throughout evolution and are widely expressed in multiple mammalian cells including smooth muscle, inner ear hair cells, and neurons throughout the brain. The channels consist of a pore-forming α subunit (*KCNMA1*), which has at least nine splice variants in the human brain (30), and a regulatory β subunit, of which there are four isoforms (*KCNMB1-4*). A mutation in *KCNMA1* has been identified in a family with generalized epilepsy and paroxysmal dyskinesia (GEPD) (31). The mutation increases the sensitivity of the channel to calcium, compared to the wild-type channel. This gain of function appears to cause more rapid action potential repolarization. The end result is that neurons fire at a higher sustained rate, likely due to a reduction of action potential width (32).

A mutation in *KCND2*, the gene encoding the $K_v4.2$ α subunit, has been described in an individual with medically intractable TLE. This same mutation was present in the father, suggesting that this gene may be considered a susceptibility locus (33). Missense variations in the gene encoding the $K_{ir}4.1$ potassium channel (*KCNJ10*) have been associated with susceptibility to IGE syndromes of absence epilepsy and JME (34).

Epilepsy Syndromes. BFNC associated with *KCNQ2* and *KCNQ3* mutations have onset at several days of life in an otherwise normal neonate. The seizures are characterized by clonic limb movements and apnea. A small percentage of these individuals go on to have seizures later in life. Myokymia later in life has been described in one family with *KCNQ2* mutation and BFNC (35). *KCNA1* mutations have been described in families with episodic ataxia (type 1), which is a rare disorder that is characterized by intermittent episodes of ataxia and myokymia as well as partial seizure in a few kindreds. Because not all families with this gene defect exhibit epilepsy as part of the phenotype, this gene locus is considered a susceptibility gene or risk factor for epilepsy. A *KCNMA1* mutation has been identified in a family with coexistent GEPD (31). Sixteen affected individuals developed epileptic seizures ($n = 4$), paroxysmal nonkinesigenic dyskinesia ($n = 7$), or both ($n = 5$).

Calcium Channels

Background. Voltage-dependent calcium (Ca_v) channels flux calcium intracellularly in response to depolarization and thereby mediate a number of physiological processes in the CNS including the activation of signaling pathways, gene transcription, and neurotransmitter release. Similar to the Na_v channel α subunit, Ca_v channels are characterized by a large α (or $\alpha1$) subunit composed of four internally repeated domains that associate to compose a pore-forming region. There are associated auxiliary subunits that contribute to the regulation and diversity of these channels. The α and auxiliary subunits for Ca_v channels are classified in three major families for each. There are Ca_v1 (L-type), Ca_v2 (P/Q-, N-, and R-type), and Ca_v3 (T-type) α subunits and $\alpha2\delta$, β, and γ auxiliary subunits. Ca_v1 channels are typically localized postsynaptically in the somatodendritic regions and contribute to calcium signaling in response to action potential backpropagation, synaptic activity, and activity-dependent gene regulation. Ca_v2 channels are localized both pre- and postsynaptically with both axonal and somatodendritic expression. An important function for these channels is the regulation of presynaptic neurotransmitter release. Ca_v3 channels underlie a transient calcium current that activates at subthreshold potentials and is critical for the regulation of calcium flux at near resting membrane potential and also during action potentials. These channel subfamily members are fairly broadly distributed within the CNS (26). A number of the antiepileptic drugs mediate an anticonvulsant effect through altering the function of these channels (see Chapter 50).

Epilepsy Genetics. Mutations in the genes encoding Ca_v channels and their auxiliary subunits were first described in mice with naturally occurring mutations in these channels that were associated with generalized spike and wave activity (36). Subsequently, mutations in Ca_v channels associated with idiopathic epilepsy in humans have been described. The most common mutations in Ca_v channels associated with epilepsy involve *CACNA1H*, which encodes the $Ca_v3.2$ channels, also known as T-type calcium channels. $Ca_v3.2$ channels are localized primarily in dendritic regions where they modulate neuronal excitability through supporting burst firing and boosting synaptic inputs. These channels contribute to the thalamocortical circuitry with expression both in neurons in cortical layer V and in reticular thalamic nuclei, and over 30 mutations have been described in the families with IGE and CAE. Interestingly, aberrant oscillations in the thalamocortical circuitry are thought to contribute to the generalized spike and slow wave activity characteristic of IGE. A variety of different mutations have been described for *CACNA1H* in epilepsy. Some are associated with a gain of function but others have effects on channel kinetics, trafficking, or decrease the underlying current. In addition, a number of sites for alternative splicing of $Ca_v3.2$ are present and some of the identified mutations occur in these regions (12). Thus, additional work is warranted to understand the mechanisms involved.

The *CACNA1A* gene encodes the Ca$_v$2.1 α subunit, which underlies the P/Q-type calcium current and is widely expressed in the CNS both in regions of the forebrain such as cortex and hippocampus and in the cerebellum (26). Subcellularly, these channels are localized presynaptically where they play a critical role in initiating neurotransmitter release. The channels are also localized in the somatodendritic regions where they modulate excitability of the postsynaptic membrane in neurons (26). Mutations in *CACNA1A* have a strong link with familial hemiplegic migraine (FHM), episodic ataxia type 2, and spinocerebellar ataxia type 6 (37). Some kindreds with mutations in this gene express a phenotype that also includes epilepsy. There are different mutations described and functional characterization of some of them suggests that channel function is impaired in the mutant channel.

The *CACNB4* gene encodes the Ca$_v$ auxiliary β$_4$ subunit. Mutation in the mouse ortholog resulting in a neurological phenotype associated with epilepsy was first described in 1997 (38). Subsequently, mutations in *CACNB4* were described in humans with IGE/JME and episodic ataxia (39). Recent evidence suggests that the mutation in *CACNB4* may be a genetic modifier in individuals with *SCNA1* mutations and SMEI or Dravet syndrome (40).

Epilepsy Syndromes. Susceptibility to IGE/CAE is associated with variants in the *CACNA1H* gene. In one study, missense mutations were identified in 12% of children of Chinese descent with CAE, with each child inheriting the missense mutation from one of his or her unaffected parents; there was no difference in clinical CAE phenotypes between individuals with mutations and those without (41). Two possible explanations for the presence of missense mutations in unaffected parents are: (i) the parents might have had CAE early in life that was undetected and (ii) the missense mutations only increase susceptibility to CAE but alone are not sufficient to cause CAE. Variants in *CACNA1H* were also identified among 240 Caucasian individuals in Australia, from 167 unrelated IGE and GEFS+ families, with a wide variety of individual epilepsy syndromes including CAE, juvenile absence epilepsy (JAE), JME, myoclonic astatic epilepsy, GEFS+, FS, and TLE (42). All variants were also observed in some unaffected individuals, suggesting the variants are susceptibility alleles. The types of variants identified in the studies above are population specific and present at low frequencies. Mutations in the *CACNA1A* gene have also been found to be associated with epilepsy. In one Swedish family of three mutation carriers, all had FHM and ataxia, and two had CPS (43). In a second family, five members had absence epilepsy with 3 Hz spike and wave activity and cerebellar ataxia (44). Finally, coding variants in the *CACNB4* gene were identified in two families with IGE and one family with episodic ataxia (39).

Chloride Channels

Background. This section is focused on voltage-gated chloride channels (ClCs), which contrasts an earlier section in this chapter covering ligand-gated chloride (GABA$_A$) receptors. There are a number of mammalian genes encoding ClCs. These channels flux chloride and serve a number of important functions throughout the organism. This discussion will focus on CLC-2 channels, which are encoded by *CLCN2*. Mutations in this gene have been reported in JME. CLC-2 channels are homodimers, and each subunit composing the dimer has a pore region that fluxes Cl$^-$. Channel opening to flux Cl$^-$ out of the cell occurs in response to hyperpolarization and acidic extracellular pH (45). The channel is expressed in the CNS and has a critical role in GABA inhibition through maintaining a low intracellular concentration gradient (46,47).

Epilepsy Genetics and Syndromes. Three mutations in the *CLCN2* gene were identified in three of 46 unrelated families with IGE (48). Of the three families, one family had four members with JME and one member with epilepsy with grand mal seizures upon awakening (EGMA), another family had several members with EGMA and one member with CAE, and the third family had JAE. All three families had different mutations in the *CLCN2* gene. These mutations result in a premature stop codon, an atypical splicing, and a single amino acid substitution. All three mutations result in altered channel function, either a loss of function or altered gating voltage-dependent gating. In another study of 112 patients with familial generalized and focal epilepsies, three additional mutations were identified (49,50).

Non-Ion Channel Gene Mutations

Leucine-Rich Gene, Glioma-Inactivated-1 (*LGI1*) Gene

Background. Most genes mutated in idiopathic epilepsy syndromes encode ion channel subunits. There are several notable exceptions including *LGI1* and the *MASS1* gene, which is mutated in the Frings mouse model of audiogenic epilepsy. Each contains a novel domain consisting of seven repeats, each consisting of a 44-residue EAR (epilepsy-associated repeat) domain. The encoded protein contains three leucine-rich repeats (LRRs) in the N-terminal domain, surrounded by cysteine-rich clusters. Other LRR-containing proteins are involved in signal transduction, cell growth regulation, adhesion, and migration.

Epilepsy Genetics. The *LGI1* gene product enhances AMPA receptor-mediated synaptic transmission in hippocampal slices. Mutations in *LGI1* have been identified in individuals with autosomal dominant partial epilepsy with auditory features (ADPEAF) (51). There is evidence for allelic heterogeneity, as 10 different mutations have been described in various families with ADPEAF.

Epilepsy Syndrome. ADPEAF is characterized by focal seizures with auditory auras ranging from unformed sounds, such as humming or ringing, to distortions and volume changes, to more organized sounds such as singing and music. Some affected individuals have seizures provoked by auditory stimuli. Age of onset can vary from 4 to 50 years, with mean age of onset in the late teens. Interictal EEG is often normal, as is magnetic resonance imaging (MRI). ADPEAF exhibits decreased penetrance, approximately 70%, regardless of the specific *LGI1* mutation. *LGI1* mutations have been described in approximately 50% of the families tested, with no clear clinical distinction between those families with mutations and those without. A subset of affected individuals with *LGI1* mutations has IGE. An *LGI1* mutation also has been identified in a woman with sporadic lateral TLE with telephone-induced seizures. Focal seizures were characterized by distortion or attenuation of sound and were triggered almost exclusively by answering the telephone, although other auditory stimuli could also evoke seizures. She was found to have a de novo mutation in the *LGI1* gene (52).

Na+,K+-ATPase Pump Gene (*ATP1A2*)

Background. The Na+,K+-ATPase catalyzes the ATP-driven exchange of three intracellular Na+ ions for two extracellular K+ ions across the plasma membrane. The enzyme plays a crucial role in maintaining the transmembrane cation gradients that are dissipated in the propagation of action potentials. The α-2 isoform of the major subunit of the Na+,K+-ATPase is predominantly found in neural and muscle tissues. The *ATP1A2* protein is thought to play a role in calcium signaling during cardiac muscle contraction. In the CNS, *ATP1A2* is expressed in neurons throughout the brain in the neonatal period, becoming more abundant in glia in adulthood. In the CNS, the α-2 isoform is thought to play a critical role in calcium signaling, although the exact mechanism of its pathogenesis is still unclear.

Epilepsy Genetics and Syndromes. In a five-generation Dutch-Canadian family with FHM and benign familial infantile convulsions (BFIC), a mutation was identified in the *ATP1A2* gene, regardless of whether the affected family member had FHM, BFIC, or both (53). In a case-control study of 152 German individuals with nonfamilial IGE and 111 healthy German controls, no significant association was found with seven polymorphisms of the *ATP1A2* gene and IGE compared to controls, suggesting *ATP1A2* was not a major susceptibility gene in their epilepsy population (54). The *ATP1A2* gene appears to play a more significant role in FHM. Clinical features of BFIC are described in Chapter 19, Idiopathic and Benign Partial Epilepsies of Childhood.

Myoclonin1/EFHC1 Gene

Background. *Myoclonin1/EFHC1* encodes a 640-amino acid protein that consists of three DM10 domains of unknown function and a C-terminal region with calcium-binding EF hand motifs. Mutations in *Myoclonin1/ EFHC1* occur in JME. In functional characterization of the *EFHC1* mutation studies have shown that Ca$_v$2.3 currents (R-type calcium currents) are increased in the presence of cotransfection with *Myoclonin1/EFHC1* constructs in HEK cells. In hippocampal neurons, *EFHC1* appears to be involved in apoptosis through modulation of R-type calcium currents. Additional studies have suggested that *EFHC1* is a ciliary component.

Epilepsy Genetics and Syndrome. Notably, while JME is also seen in mutations of the *GABRA1* or the *CLCN2* genes (see relevant sections above), a recent study suggests that *Myoclonin1/EFHC1* mutations may be more common in association with JME (55). The characterization of some of the initially defined *Myoclonin1/EFHC1* mutations in JME revealed that R-type calcium current–mediated apoptosis was attenuated with mutant *EFHC1* (56). Additional mutations in *Myoclonin1/EFHC1* in JME have subsequently been identified, which remain to be characterized. Furthermore, the effect of *EFHC1* mutations identified in JME on ciliary function has not been characterized to our knowledge. Thus, the mechanism whereby mutations in *EFHC1* lead to the development of JME has not been fully elucidated.

GENETIC TESTING

Genetic testing is available for a number of the idiopathic epilepsy syndromes described above, as highlighted in Table 4.1 (for more information on currently available genetic tests, check www.genetests.org). It is important to differentiate genetic testing to establish a diagnosis in a patient with epilepsy or suspected epilepsy (diagnostic testing) from genetic testing in asymptomatic individuals to identify future risk of developing epilepsy (screening or predictive testing). It is also important to differentiate genetic testing in monogenic disorders (caused by a single "major" gene) versus genetic testing in complex genetic disorders, which may be caused by multiple genes and/or environmental factors. The ethical implications of genetic testing are complex and need to be addressed before testing is ordered, ideally with a geneticist or genetic counselor. Genetic testing has implications for the entire family, and yet each individual family member has the right to decide whether to participate in testing. The testing can involve the analysis of DNA, RNA, chromosomes, proteins, or metabolites. Genetic testing of symptomatic individuals (diagnostic testing) is most helpful when the test has high sensitivity and specificity, when the results will influence clinical management, when the disease is preventable or treatable, or when the results provide important information for other family members. Even without effective treatment, genetic testing can be valuable by establishing the diagnosis and excluding other possibilities, thus limiting further testing.

Complicating genetic testing in the idiopathic epilepsies is incomplete penetrance and genetic heterogeneity. Many of the mutations identified to date have less than 100% penetrance; some individuals who carry the disease mutation will never have clinical disease. Most idiopathic epilepsy syndromes also display genetic heterogeneity in that they can be caused by more than one mutation in more than one gene; this clearly complicates the interpretation of a "negative" test of a single gene. Consider the case of a child diagnosed clinically with SMEI. Approximately 60% to 85% of patients with SMEI will have *SCN1A* mutations, with the vast majority occurring de novo. Mutations in *GABRG2* have also been identified in SMEI patients, and *SCN1A* mutations have also been identified in patients with GEFS+, a typically more benign phenotype. The child's parents request genetic testing to determine the risk to future offspring. If an *SCN1A* mutation is identified in the affected child, and not in the parents, the mutation is likely to have occurred de novo, and the risk to future offspring is low. However, it is difficult to exclude the possibility of gonadal mosaicism (the presence of the mutation in a subset of the gametes of one parent), in which case there would be a risk to future offspring. If an *SCN1A* mutation is not identified in the affected child, one cannot rule out the possibility of a gene mutation in another gene, such as *GABRG2*. If an *SCN1A* mutation is identified in both the affected child and one parent, there is a 50% chance of transmitting that *SCN1A* mutation to future offspring, but the clinical phenotype would be difficult to predict, as *SCN1A* mutations have been identified in a wide range of phenotypes, from benign FS to severe intractable epilepsy.

As another example, consider the case of a 28-year-old woman with intractable nocturnal frontal lobe epilepsy. Her brother, father, paternal uncle, and paternal grandfather all

TABLE 4.1

SELECTED INHERITED IDIOPATHIC HUMAN EPILEPSIES

Epilepsy syndrome	Seizure types/clinical features	Chromosomal segment	Gene
Idiopathic focal			
Benign focal epilepsy of childhood, benign rolandic epilepsy	Focal and secondarily GTC, nocturnal	15q14	Unknown
Benign familial infantile convulsions (BFIC)	Focal and secondarily GTC	19q (BFIC1)	Unknown
		16p12-q12 (BFIC2)	Unknown
		2q23-q24 (BFIC3)	SCN2A
		1p36-p35 (BFIC4)	Unknown
Benign familial neonatal–infantile convulsions (BFNIC)	Focal and secondarily GTC	2q24	SCN2A
Benign familial neonatal convulsions (BFNC)	Tonic, neonatal	20q13.3 (EBN1)	KCNQ2[a]
		8q24 (EBN2)	KCNQ3
		pericentric inversion, chr 5 (EBN3)	Unknown
Autosomal dominant nocturnal frontal lobe epilepsy (ADNFLE)	Focal and secondarily GTC, nocturnal	20q13.2-q13.3 (ENFL1)	CHRNA4[a]
		15q24 (ENFL2)	Unknown
		1q21(ENFL3)	CHRNB2[a]
		8p21 (ENFL4)	CHRNA2
Autosomal dominant partial epilepsy with auditory features (ADPEAF)	Focal, often with auditory auras	10q24 (ETL1)	LGI1
Familial partial epilepsy with variable foci (FPEVF)	Focal, arising from different foci within the same family	22q11	Unknown
Familial occipitotemporal lobe epilepsy and migraine with visual aura	Visual, cognitive, and autonomic auras; focal motor seizures, CPS, secondarily GTC; migraine with aura	9q21-q22 (ETL4)	Unknown
Familial temporal lobe epilepsy	FS with childhood afebrile seizures, GTC	12q22-q23 (ETL2)	Unknown
	Déjà vu aura, CPS, rare secondarily GTC, relatively benign course, normal MRI	4q13-q21 (ETL3)	Unknown
Idiopathic generalized			
Childhood absence epilepsy (CAE)	Typical absence, GTC	8q24 (ECA1)	Unknown
		5q31.1 (ECA2)	GABRG2[a]
		3q26 (ECA3)	CLCN2
		5q34 (ECA4)	GABRA1
		15q11-q12 (ECA5)	GABRB3
Juvenile myoclonic epilepsy (JME)[b]	Myoclonic, absence, and GTC	6p12-p11 (EJM1)	EFHC1[a]
		15q14 (EJM2)	Unknown
		6p21 (EJM3)	Unknown
		5q12-q14 (EJM4)	Unknown
		2q22-q23 (EMJ5)	CACNB4
		5q34-q35	GABRA1
		3q26	CLCN2
Idiopathic generalized epilepsy (IGE) comprising CAE, JAE, JME, and epilepsy with grand mal seizures on awakening (EGMA)[b]	Absence, myoclonic, GTC	8q24 (IGE1/EIG1)	Unknown
		14q23 (IGE2/EIG2)	Unknown
		9q32-q33 (IGE3/EIG3)	Unknown
		10q25-q26 (IGE4/EIG4)	Unknown
		10p11 (EIG5)	Unknown
		16p13 (EIG6)	CACNA1H
		15q13 (EIG7)	Unknown
		3q26	CLCN2
		2q22-q23	CACNB4

TABLE 4.1 *(Continued)*

Epilepsy syndrome	Seizure types/clinical features	Chromosomal segment	Gene
Generalized epilepsy with febrile seizures plus (GEFS+)	Febrile seizures often beyond 6 years of age, followed by GTC, absence, myoclonic, atonic	19q13	*SCN1B*[a]
		2q24	*SCN1A*[a]
		5q31	*GABRG2*[a]
		2q24	*SCN2A*
		1p36	*GABRD*
Familial adult myoclonic epilepsy	GTC, myoclonus	8q24	Unknown
		2p11-q12	Unknown
Idiopathic autosomal recessive infantile myoclonic epilepsy; familial infantile myoclonic epilepsy (FIME)	Myoclonic, febrile seizures, GTC	16p13	Unknown
Other syndromes			
Familial febrile seizures	GTC with fever	8q13-q21 (FEB1)	Unknown
		19p (FEB2)	Unknown
		2q23-q24 (FEB3)	*SCN1A*[a]
		5q14-q15 (FEB4)	*GPR98*
		6q22-q24 (FEB5)	Unknown
		18p11.2 (FEB6)	Unknown
		21q22 (FEB7)	Unknown
		5q31-q33 (FEB8)	*GABRG2*[a]
		3p24-p23 (FEB9)	Unknown
		3q26 (FEB10)	Unknown

[a]Clinical genetic testing available.
[b]There are other potential susceptibility alleles that have been reported in the literature that are not listed here. We have attempted to list the epilepsy genes that have the strongest evidence for disease association.

have similar seizures at night. She plans to have children, and she wants to know the risk of epilepsy in her offspring. Based on her family history, her diagnosis is most likely ADNFLE, which has been associated with mutations in *CHRNA4*, *CHRNB2*, and *CHRNA2*. Mutations in *CHRNA4* and *CHRNB2* account for only a small percentage of all patients with ADNFLE, implying that other genes are involved. As with many autosomal dominant epilepsies, there is incomplete penetrance, estimated at 50% to 70%. If a *CHRNA4* mutation is identified in this patient, there is a 50% chance of transmitting the mutation, and a 25% to 35% chance of transmitting nocturnal frontal lobe epilepsy to her offspring. If a *CHRNA4* mutation is not identified in this patient, she may still have a mutation in another gene, with a similar risk of transmitting the disease. In a patient with a clinical diagnosis of nocturnal frontal lobe epilepsy and a family history consistent with autosomal dominant inheritance, genetic testing would not necessarily change treatment or genetic counseling.

CONCLUSION

Genetics plays a role in virtually all epilepsy syndromes, through a diversity of mechanisms. The identification of specific mutations in ion channel subunits has contributed significantly to our knowledge of underlying pathogenic pathways leading to seizures and epilepsy. Further work in the identification of gene defects and their functional characterization will continue to advance our understanding of basic mechanisms. Work toward better phenotype–genotype correlations and the functional significance of both common and rare polymorphisms in "epilepsy genes" will allow us to make better use of genetic testing in epilepsy.

The eventual hope is that knowledge of the role of genetics in human epilepsy will improve recognition, diagnosis, and treatment. In the search for new strategies to reduce the burden of disease, the discovery of epilepsy genetic risk factors offers a novel opportunity to identify individuals susceptible to epilepsy before it develops, and to treat and prevent seizures in those individuals at risk.

References

1. Annegers JF, Hauser WA, Anderson VE, et al. The risks of seizure disorders among relatives of patients with childhood onset epilepsy. *Neurology.* 1982;32:174–179.
2. Ottman R, Annegers JF, Hauser WA, et al. Seizure risk in offspring of parents with generalized versus partial epilepsy. *Epilepsia.* 1989;30:157–161.
3. Sillanpaa M, Koskenvuo M, Romanov K, et al. Genetic factors in epileptic seizures: Evidence from a large twin population. *Acta Neurol Scand.* 1991;84:523–526.
4. Berkovic SF, Howell RA, Hay DA, et al. Epilepsies in twins: genetics of the major epilepsy syndromes. *Ann Neurol.* 1998;43:435–445.
5. Kjeldsen MJ, Kyvik KO, Christensen K, et al. Genetic and environmental factors in epilepsy: a population-based study of 11900 danish twin pairs. *Epilepsy Res.* 2001;44:167–178.
6. Greenberg DA, Delgado-Escueta AV, Maldonado HM, et al. Segregation analysis of juvenile myoclonic epilepsy. *Genet Epidemiol.* 1988;5:81–94.

7. Ottman R, Hauser WA, Barker-Cummings C, et al. Segregation analysis of cryptogenic epilepsy and an empirical test of the validity of the results. *Am J Hum Genet.* 1997;60:667–675.

8. Durner M, Keddache MA, Tomasini L, et al. Genome scan of idiopathic generalized epilepsy: evidence for major susceptibility gene and modifying genes influencing the seizure type. *Ann Neurol.* 2001;49:328–335.

9. Sander T, Schulz H, Saar K, et al. Genome search for susceptibility loci of common idiopathic generalised epilepsies. *Hum Mol Genet.* 2000;9:1465–1472.

10. Kalamida D, Poulas K, Avramopoulou V, et al. Muscle and neuronal nicotinic acetylcholine receptors. Structure, function and pathogenicity. *FEBS J.* 2007;274:3799–3845.

11. Gotti C, Zoli M, Clementi F. Brain nicotinic acetylcholine receptors: native subtypes and their relevance. *Trends Pharmacol Sci.* 2006;27:482–491.

12. Reid CA, Berkovic SF, Petrou S. Mechanisms of human inherited epilepsies. *Prog Neurobiol.* 2009;87:41–57.

13. McLellan A, Phillips HA, Rittey C, et al. Phenotypic comparison of two scottish families with mutations in different genes causing autosomal dominant nocturnal frontal lobe epilepsy. *Epilepsia.* 2003;44:613–617.

14. Oldani A, Zucconi M, Asselta R, et al. Autosomal dominant nocturnal frontal lobe epilepsy. A video-polysomnographic and genetic appraisal of 40 patients and delineation of the epileptic syndrome. *Brain.* 1998;121(Pt 2):205–223.

15. Chen Y, Wu L, Fang Y, et al. A novel mutation of the nicotinic acetylcholine receptor gene CHRNA4 in sporadic nocturnal frontal lobe epilepsy. *Epilepsy Res.* 2009;83:152–156.

16. Phillips HA, Marini C, Scheffer IE, et al. A de novo mutation in sporadic nocturnal frontal lobe epilepsy. *Ann Neurol.* 2000;48:264–267.

17. Picard F, Pegna AJ, Arntsberg V, et al. Neuropsychological disturbances in frontal lobe epilepsy due to mutated nicotinic receptors. *Epilepsy Behav.* 2009;14:354–359.

18. Jacob TC, Moss SJ, Jurd R. GABA(A) receptor trafficking and its role in the dynamic modulation of neuronal inhibition. *Nat Rev Neurosci.* 2008;9:331–343.

19. Olsen RW, Sieghart W. GABA A receptors: subtypes provide diversity of function and pharmacology. *Neuropharmacology.* 2009;56:141–148.

20. Wallace RH, Marini C, Petrou S, et al. Mutant GABA(A) receptor gamma2-subunit in childhood absence epilepsy and febrile seizures. *Nat Genet.* 2001;28:49–52.

21. Audenaert D, Schwartz E, Claeys KG, et al. A novel GABRG2 mutation associated with febrile seizures. *Neurology.* 2006;67:687–690.

22. Cossette P, Liu L, Brisebois K, et al. Mutation of GABRA1 in an autosomal dominant form of juvenile myoclonic epilepsy. *Nat Genet.* 2002;31:184–189.

23. Maljevic S, Krampfl K, Cobilanschi J, et al. A mutation in the GABA(A) receptor alpha(1)-subunit is associated with absence epilepsy. *Ann Neurol.* 2006;59:983–987.

24. Dibbens LM, Feng HJ, Richards MC, et al. GABRD encoding a protein for extra- or peri-synaptic GABAA receptors is a susceptibility locus for generalized epilepsies. *Hum Mol Genet.* 2004;13:1315–1319.

25. Catterall WA, Dib-Hajj S, Meisler MH, et al. Inherited neuronal ion channelopathies: new windows on complex neurological diseases. *J Neurosci.* 2008;28:11768–11777.

26. Vacher H, Mohapatra DP, Trimmer JS. Localization and targeting of voltage-dependent ion channels in mammalian central neurons. *Physiol Rev.* 2008;88:1407–1447.

27. Escayg A, MacDonald BT, Meisler MH, et al. Mutations of SCN1A, encoding a neuronal sodium channel, in two families with GEFS+2. *Nat Genet.* 2000;24:343–345.

28. Berkovic SF, Harkin L, McMahon JM, et al. De-novo mutations of the sodium channel gene SCN1A in alleged vaccine encephalopathy: a retrospective study. *Lancet Neurol.* 2006;5:488–492.

29. Turnbull J, Lohi H, Kearney JA, et al. Sacred disease secrets revealed: the genetics of human epilepsy. *Hum Mol Genet.* 2005;14(Spec No. 2):2491–2500.

30. Tseng-Crank J, Foster CD, Krause JD, et al. Cloning, expression, and distribution of functionally distinct Ca(2+)-activated K+ channel isoforms from human brain. *Neuron.* 1994;13:1315–1330.

31. Du W, Bautista JF, Yang H, et al. Calcium-sensitive potassium channelopathy in human epilepsy and paroxysmal movement disorder. *Nat Genet.* 2005;37:733–738.

32. Diez-Sampedro A, Silverman WR, Bautista JF, et al. Mechanism of increased open probability by a mutation of the BK channel. *J Neurophysiol.* 2006;96:1507–1516.

33. Singh B, Ogiwara I, Kaneda M, et al. A Kv4.2 truncation mutation in a patient with temporal lobe epilepsy. *Neurobiol Dis.* 2006;24:245–253.

34. Lenzen KP, Heils A, Lorenz S, et al. Supportive evidence for an allelic association of the human KCNJ10 potassium channel gene with idiopathic generalized epilepsy. *Epilepsy Res.* 2005;63:113–118.

35. Scheffer IE, Berkovic SF. The genetics of human epilepsy. *Trends Pharmacol Sci.* 2003;24:428–433.

36. Burgess DL, Noebels JL. Voltage-dependent calcium channel mutations in neurological disease. *Ann N Y Acad Sci.* 1999;868:199–212.

37. Ophoff RA, Terwindt GM, Vergouwe MN, et al. Familial hemiplegic migraine and episodic ataxia type-2 are caused by mutations in the Ca^{2+} channel gene CACNL1A4. *Cell.* 1996;87:543–552.

38. Burgess DL, Jones JM, Meisler MH, et al. Mutation of the Ca^{2+} channel beta subunit gene Cchb4 is associated with ataxia and seizures in the lethargic (lh) mouse. *Cell.* 1997;88:385–392.

39. Escayg A, De Waard M, Lee DD, et al. Coding and noncoding variation of the human calcium-channel beta4-subunit gene CACNB4 in patients with idiopathic generalized epilepsy and episodic ataxia. *Am J Hum Genet.* 2000;66:1531–1539.

40. Ohmori I, Ouchida M, Miki T, et al. A CACNB4 mutation shows that altered Ca(v)2.1 function may be a genetic modifier of severe myoclonic epilepsy in infancy. *Neurobiol Dis.* 2008;32:349–354.

41. Chen Y, Lu J, Pan H, et al. Association between genetic variation of CACNA1H and childhood absence epilepsy. *Ann Neurol.* 2003;54:239–243.

42. Heron SE, Khosravani H, Varela D, et al. Extended spectrum of idiopathic generalized epilepsies associated with CACNA1H functional variants. *Ann Neurol.* 2007;62:560–568.

43. Kors EE, Melberg A, Vanmolkot KR, et al. Childhood epilepsy, familial hemiplegic migraine, cerebellar ataxia, and a new CACNA1A mutation. *Neurology.* 2004;63:1136–1137.

44. Imbrici P, Jaffe SL, Eunson LH, et al. Dysfunction of the brain calcium channel CaV2.1 in absence epilepsy and episodic ataxia. *Brain.* 2004;127:2682–2692.

45. Verkman AS, Galietta LJ. Chloride channels as drug targets. *Nat Rev Drug Discov.* 2009;8:153–171.

46. Staley K. The role of an inwardly rectifying chloride conductance in postsynaptic inhibition. *J Neurophysiol.* 1994;72:273–284.

47. Staley K, Smith R, Schaack J, et al. Alteration of GABAA receptor function following gene transfer of the CLC-2 chloride channel. *Neuron.* 1996;17:543–551.

48. Haug K, Warnstedt M, Alekov AK, et al. Mutations in CLCN2 encoding a voltage-gated chloride channel are associated with idiopathic generalized epilepsies. *Nat Genet.* 2003;33:527–532.

49. D'Agostino D, Bertelli M, Gallo S, et al. Mutations and polymorphisms of the CLCN2 gene in idiopathic epilepsy. *Neurology.* 2004;63:1500–1502.

50. Stogmann E, Lichtner P, Baumgartner C, et al. Mutations in the CLCN2 gene are a rare cause of idiopathic generalized epilepsy syndromes. *Neurogenetics.* 2006;7:265–268.

51. Kalachikov S, Evgrafov O, Ross B, et al. Mutations in LGI1 cause autosomal-dominant partial epilepsy with auditory features. *Nat Genet.* 2002;30:335–341.

52. Michelucci R, Mecarelli O, Bovo G, et al. A de novo LGI1 mutation causing idiopathic partial epilepsy with telephone-induced seizures. *Neurology.* 2007;68:2150–2151.

53. Vanmolkot KR, Kors EE, Hottenga JJ, et al. Novel mutations in the Na$^+$, K$^+$-ATPase pump gene ATP1A2 associated with familial hemiplegic migraine and benign familial infantile convulsions. *Ann Neurol.* 2003;54:360–366.

54. Lohoff FW, Ferraro TN, Sander T, et al. No association between common variations in the human alpha 2 subunit gene (ATP1A2) of the sodium-potassium-transporting ATPase and idiopathic generalized epilepsy. *Neurosci Lett.* 2005;382:33–38.

55. Medina MT, Suzuki T, Alonso ME, et al. Novel mutations in Myoclonin1/EFHC1 in sporadic and familial juvenile myoclonic epilepsy. *Neurology.* 2008;70:2137–2144.

56. Suzuki T, Delgado-Escueta AV, Aguan K, et al. Mutations in EFHC1 cause juvenile myoclonic epilepsy. *Nat Genet.* 2004;36:842–849.

CHAPTER 5 ■ PICTORIAL ATLAS OF EPILEPSY SUBSTRATES

AJAY GUPTA, MD, RICHARD A. PRAYSON, MD, AND JANET REID, MD

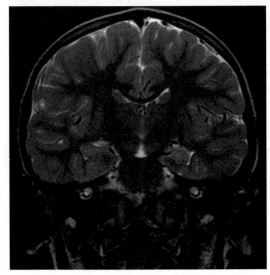

FIGURE 5.1 **Mesiotemporal sclerosis.** Coronal T2-weighted image from MRI without gadolinium in a 7-year-old male with temporal lobe epilepsy shows increased signal intensity and decreased size of the left hippocampal formation (*arrow*) and mesiotemporal lobe (*arrows*).

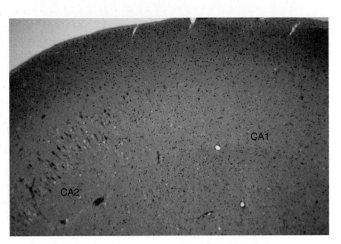

FIGURE 5.3 Higher magnification appearance of the hippocampus in **hippocampal sclerosis** at the interface between CA2 and CA1 regions. There is a marked loss of neurons in the CA1 region with gliosis.

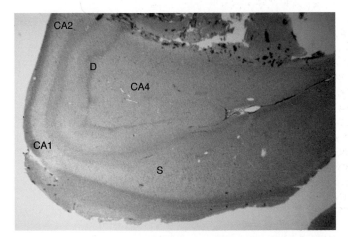

FIGURE 5.2 Low magnification appearance of hippocampus in **hippocampal sclerosis (HS)**. An adult patient who underwent anterior temporal lobectomy for treatment of intractable temporal lobe epilepsy. HS is the most common cause of intractable partial epilepsy in adults. HS is generally marked by preferential loss of neurons in the dentate (D), CA4 region, CA1 region, and subiculum (S). A lesser degree of neuronal loss may be observed in the CA3 and CA2 regions. Loss of neurons is accompanied by gliosis and in severe cases, grossly evident atrophy.

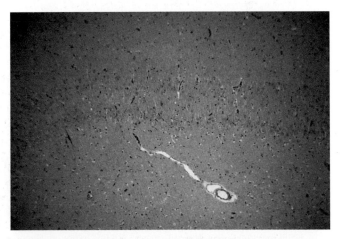

FIGURE 5.4 Histologic appearance of **double dentate** marked by two bands of neurons in the hippocampus. This represents a form of a hippocampal dysplasia. Hippocampal dysplasia is an infrequent cause of temporal lobe epilepsy, and may be seen as a dysmorphic hippocampal formation on a high-definition three-dimensional volume acquisition sequence on brain MRI.

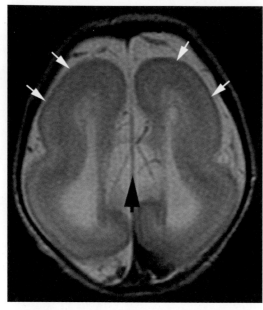

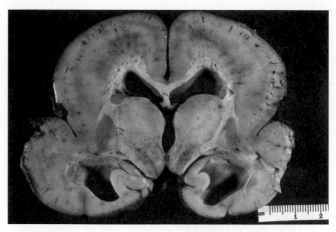

FIGURE 5.7 The gross appearance of **lissencephaly (agyria)** characterized by a lack of gyral formation and a decreased number of sulci. Note enlargement of ventricles suggesting parenchymal volume loss. The cortex is usually thickened on cross section. Microscopically, there is abnormally layered cortex, typically three to five layers.

FIGURE 5.5 **Lissencephaly**. Axial T2-weighted image from MRI without gadolinium in a newborn shows lack of normal sulcation (*white arrows*), parallel lateral ventricles, and absence of the corpus callosum (*black arrow*). Children with lissencephaly usually present with epileptic spasms, severe global developmental delay, microcephaly, and marked hypotonia during early infancy.

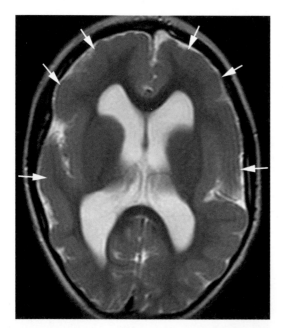

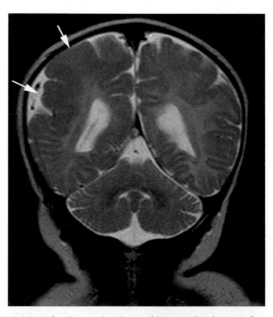

FIGURE 5.6 **Pachygyria**. Axial T2-weighted image from MRI without gadolinium in a 4 year old with spastic quadriplegia and generalized seizures shows a paucity of sulcal markings and thickened cortex bilaterally (*arrows*).

FIGURE 5.8 **Polymicrogyria**. Coronal T2-weighted image from MRI without gadolinium in a newborn with motor seizures shows generalized thickening of the cortex of the right parietal lobe characterized by multiple small gyri (*arrows*). Polymicrogyria are usually epileptogenic lesions, sporadic or familial in occurrence, and various brain MRI patterns have been recognized that help in making an accurate diagnosis.

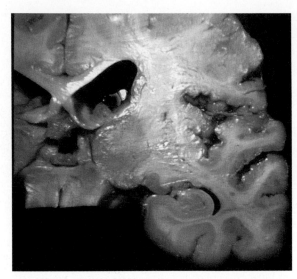

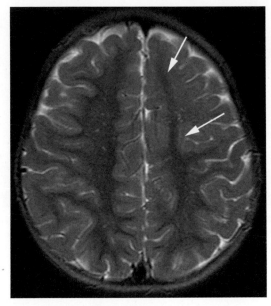

FIGURE 5.9 Gross appearance of **perisylvian polymicrogyria (micropolygyria)** marked by the focal presence of small, irregular gyri separated by shallow sulci. The cortex is often thinned and microscopically comprises two- to four-layered cortex. The leptomeninges overlying polymicrogyria may be abnormally hypervascular due to persistence of fetal leptomeningeal vascularization. (Photograph courtesy of Dr. Bette Kleinschmidt-DeMasters.). Congenital bilateral perisylvian polymicrogyria (CBPP) usually presents with seizures during childhood. Other clinical findings in the patients with CBPP include pseudobulbar paresis, dysarthria, swallowing difficulties, and tongue paresis with inability to protrude tongue and perform lateral tongue movements.

FIGURE 5.11 Lobar cortical dysplasia. Axial T2-weighted image from MRI without gadolinium in a 3 year old with infantile spasms shows generalized blurring of the gray/white interface with lack of normal white matter arborization in the left frontal lobe (*arrows*).

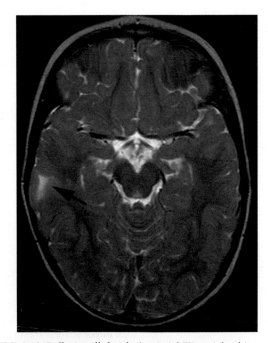

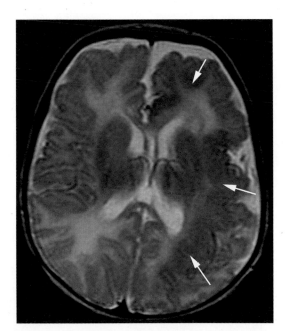

FIGURE 5.10 Balloon cell dysplasia. Axial T2-weighted image from MRI without gadolinium in an 18-month-old male with intractable seizures shows high signal in the right parietal subcortical white matter subtending a broad-based gyrus (*arrow*). Most focal cortical dysplasias are sporadic congenital malformations, and as a group are one of the most important causes of intractable epilepsy that is surgically remediable.

FIGURE 5.12 Hemispheric malformation of cortical development. Axial T2-weighted image from MRI without gadolinium in a 4-year-old boy with intractable infantile spasms since birth shows diffuse left hemispheric cortical thickening with lack of normal arborization of white matter (*arrows*).

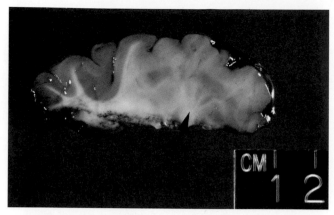

FIGURE 5.13 Gross appearance of **cortical dysplasia** marked by an indistinct gray/white interface (right portion of cross section—*arrow*) with evidence of gray matter tissue abnormally placed in white matter (**nodular heterotopia**).

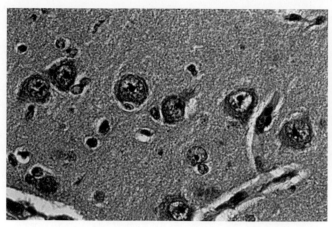

FIGURE 5.15 High magnification appearance of neurons in cortical layer II of the parietal lobe in a patient with **cortical dysplasia**. The neurons are abnormally enlarged in size (**neuronal cytomegaly**) without any other evidence of dysmorphic features.

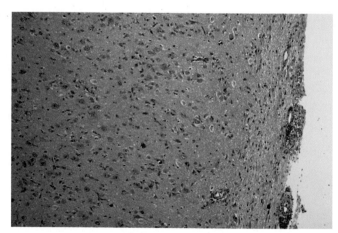

FIGURE 5.14 Histologic appearance of **cortical dysplasia** marked by a loss of normal cortical lamination, increased cellularity, and malpositioning of neurons within the cortex. Neurons normally have their apical dendrites oriented perpendicular with respect to the surface of the brain.

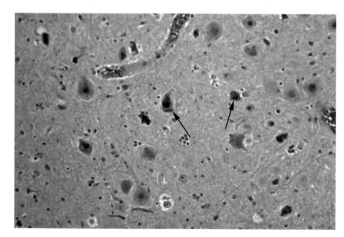

FIGURE 5.16 Histologic appearance of neurons in cortical layer III of the temporal lobe in a patient with **cortical dysplasia**. The neurons are marked by abnormal cytologic appearance (**dysmorphic neurons**) (*arrows*) including abnormal nuclear morphology and atypical distribution of Nissl substance. In addition, neurons are haphazardly arranged within the cortex.

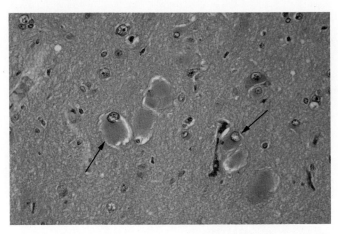

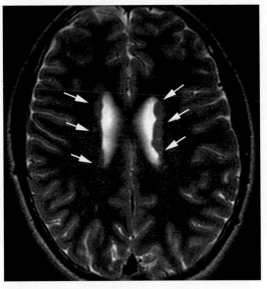

FIGURE 5.17 Histologic appearance of **balloon cells** (*arrows*) in the setting of **cortical dysplasia**. Balloon cells are marked histologically by the presence of abundant eosinophilic cytoplasm and eccentrically placed nuclei. Multinucleation may be observed. The derivation of these cells is still debated. A subset of balloon cells stain with markers of both glial differentiation (glial fibrillary acidic protein) and neural differentiation (neuron-specific enolase).

FIGURE 5.18 Subependymal (periventricular) heterotopia. Axial T2 weighted image from MRI without gadolinium in a 14-year-old female with history of ptosis and tremors shows gray matter nodularity lining the lateral ventricles bilaterally (*arrows*). Bilateral periventricular nodular heterotopia could be an X-linked dominant condition due to Filamin-A gene mutations.

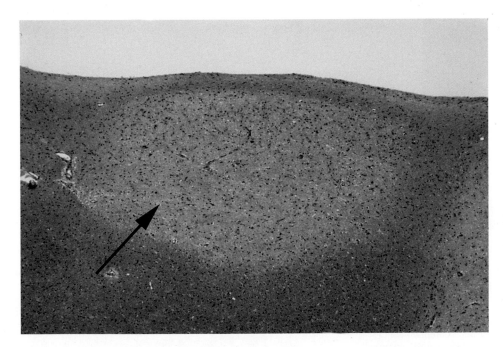

FIGURE 5.19 Microscopic appearance of a **subependymal (periventricular) nodular heterotopia** of gray matter (*arrow*). The nodule microscopically is marked by a mixture of neural and glial cells arranged in a disorganized fashion. Heterotopias are collections of mostly normal appearing neurons in abnormal location presumably due to a disturbance in migration.

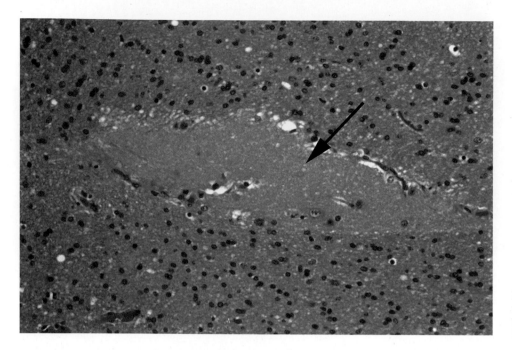

FIGURE 5.20 Small focus of **heterotopic gray matter** situated in the deep white matter of the frontal lobe region (*arrow*).

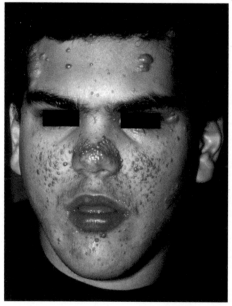

FIGURE 5.21 A patient with facial adenoma sebaceum, a diagnostic finding in tuberous sclerosis (TS). TS is an autosomal dominant condition that involves multiple organs and systems besides central nervous system. Clinical spectrum is highly variable and the diagnosis is usually made by looking for other findings like hypomelanotic skin patches, fibromatous skin plaques, dental pits, ungual fibromas, retinal hamartomas, cardiac rhabdomyomata, and renal cysts. TS is caused by mutations in the TSC 1 (Hamartin) and 2 (Tuberin) genes located on the chromosomes 9 and 16, respectively. The phenotype due to TSC 1 and 2 mutations is generally difficult to distinguish clinically.

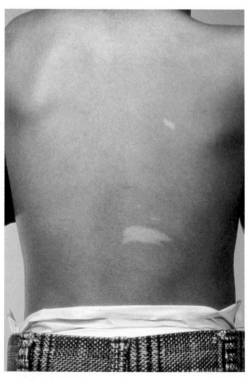

FIGURE 5.22 "Ash leaf macule" in a patient with tuberous sclerosis. Hypopigmented macules may only be visible under ultraviolet light in patients with fair skin color.

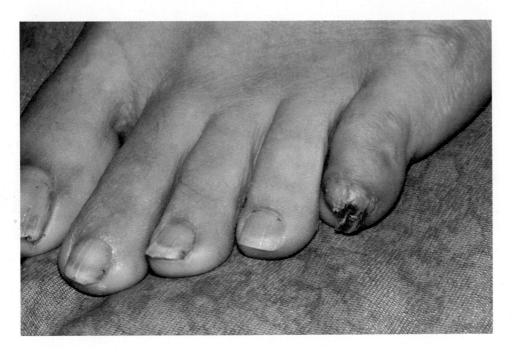

FIGURE 5.23 Ungual fibroma involving the little toe.

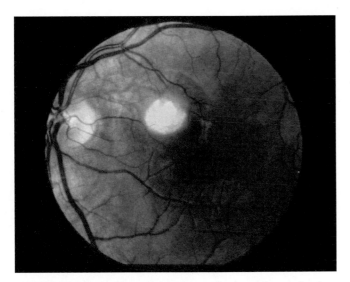

FIGURE 5.24 Retinal hamartoma seen on fundoscopic examination.

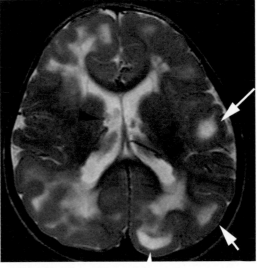

FIGURE 5.25 **Tuberous sclerosis.** Axial T2-weighted image from MRI without gadolinium in a 9-year-old male with over 20 seizures per day shows multiple subependymal low signal intensity nodules (*black arrows*) and multiple bilateral malformations of cortical development characterized by gyral broadening and subcortical white matter hyperintensity (*white arrows*).

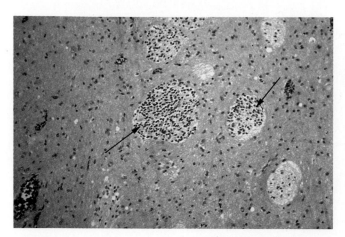

FIGURE 5.26 Histologic appearance of **hamartia** (*arrows*) characterized by an aggregation of small, immature appearing neurons. This lesion most likely represents a form of cortical dysplasia and is seen in patients with tuberous sclerosis.

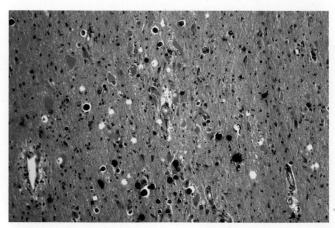

FIGURE 5.28 Histologic appearance of parenchyma from a **cortical tuber** of tuberous sclerosis. The histologic findings are generally that of a cortical dysplasia and are marked by abnormal cortical lamination, a malorientation of neurons within the cortex and dysmorphic neurons frequently accompanied by ballooned cells. Microcalcifications are also prominently noted in this particular microscopic field.

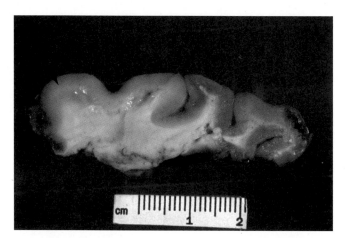

FIGURE 5.27 Gross appearance of a **cortical tuber** marked by obliteration of the gray/white interface (left most gyrus—*arrow*). Cortical tubers often have a firm, consistency related to gliosis and microcalcifications. Other pathological findings in the brain of tuberous sclerosis patients include subependymal nodules and giant cell astrocytomas typically located at the foramen of Monro leading to obstructive hydrocephalus in some patients.

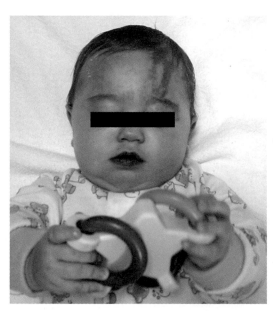

FIGURE 5.29 A child with Sturge–Weber syndrome. The presence of nevus flameus in the distribution of the first division (ophthalmic) of the trigeminal nerve high correlates with the central nervous system involvement.

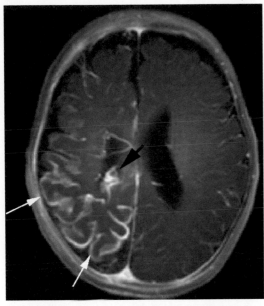

FIGURE 5.30 Sturge–Weber syndrome. Axial MPRAGE image from MRI with gadolinium in a 12-month-old girl with left tonic–clonic seizures shows diffuse gyriform enhancement (*white arrows*) with enlargement of the glomus of the right choroid plexus (*black arrow*).

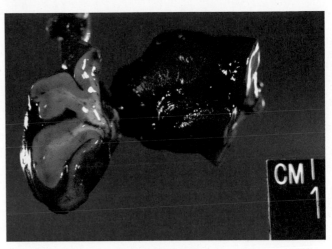

FIGURE 5.32 Cross-sectional (left) and external (right) views from a resection in a patient with **Sturge–Weber disease.** The leptomeninges appear hemorrhagic due to proliferation of vessels.

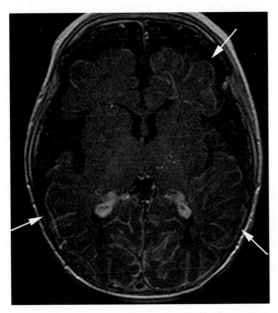

FIGURE 5.31 Sturge–Weber syndrome. Axial T1-weighted image from MRI with gadolinium in a 4-month-old girl with bilateral facial port wine stains shows left frontal and bilateral parieto-occipital gyriform enhancement (*white arrows*) with bilateral enlargement of the glomus of the choroid plexus (*black arrows*).

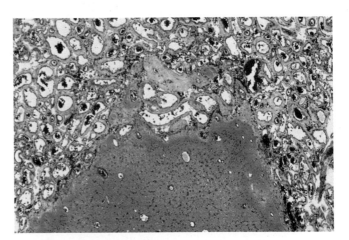

FIGURE 5.33 Histologic appearance of the leptomeninges in the setting of **Sturge–Weber** disease. The leptomeninges are marked by a proliferation of venous and capillary vessels arranged in a hemangiomatous configuration. There is no malignant potential to the lesion. The underlying cortex often demonstrates gliosis with prominent microcalcifications.

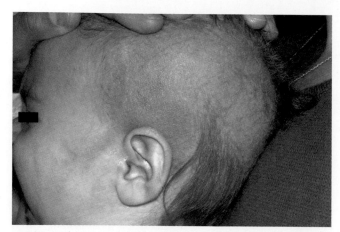

FIGURE 5.34 A child with a nevus on the cheek and left temple extending on to the scalp with loss of hair. She presented with partial seizures. Her brain MRI showed an extensive malformation of cortical development in the left temporo-parieto-occipital region. The constellations of findings suggest epidermal nevus syndrome, which is a sporadic condition. Epidermal nevus syndromes may be associated with hemimegalencephaly ipsilateral to the facial cutaneous findings.

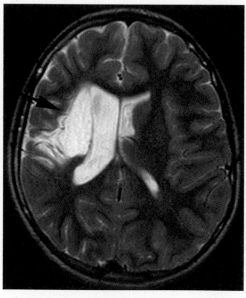

FIGURE 5.36 **Remote infarction.** Axial T2-weighted image from MRI without gadolinium in a 9-year-old boy with a history of post-traumatic occlusion of the right internal carotid artery as an infant shows cystic encephalomalacia in the right MCA territory (*arrow*).

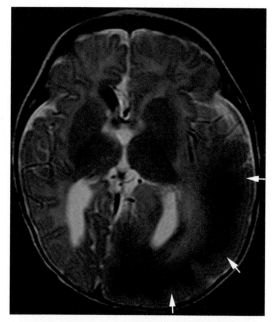

FIGURE 5.35 **Epidermal nevus syndrome with hemimegalocephaly.** Axial T2-weighted image from MRI without gadolinium in a 6-month-old child with facial linear shows generalized enlargement of the left hemisphere with gyral thickening, decreased cortical signal, and blurring of the gray/white interface (*arrows*).

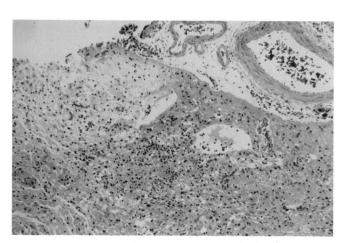

FIGURE 5.37 Histologic appearance of a **remote infarct** resulting in chronic epilepsy. The parenchyma is marked by cystic degeneration accompanied by macrophages and gliosis. Note the relative sparing of the molecular layer that is more commonly observed with infarcts versus contusion.

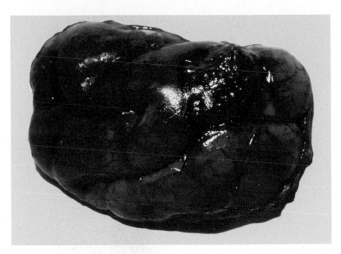

FIGURE 5.38 Gross appearance of a circumscribed hemorrhagic appearing lesion situated in the temporal lobe corresponding to a **cavernous angioma** (*arrow*).

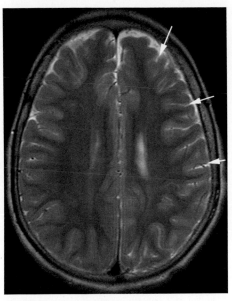

FIGURE 5.40 Rasmussen encephalitis. Axial T2-weighted image from MRI without gadolinium in a 3-year-old boy with a 1-year history of right tonic–clonic seizures progressive hemiparesis shows widening of the left frontal sulcal markings consistent with mild volume loss (*arrows*). Rasmussen encephalitis typically presents with intractable partial seizures (usually focal motor seizures and epilepsia partialis continua), progressive hemiparesis, cognitive decline, and unilateral cerebral atrophy with early and prominent involvement of the insular region.

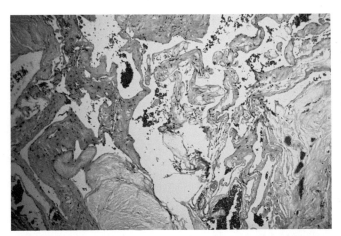

FIGURE 5.39 Microscopic appearance of the **cavernous angioma** in Fig. 5.24. Cavernous angiomas are marked by a proliferation of dilated venous vessels, typically arranged in back-to-back fashion, without intervening neural parenchyma. Thickening of venous vessel walls may be observed. The lesions are often accompanied by adjacent gliosis and hemosiderin deposition.

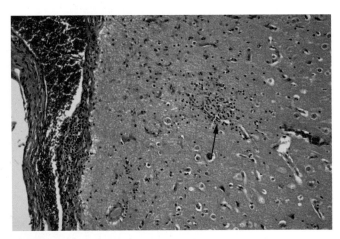

FIGURE 5.41 The histopathologic findings of **Rasmussen encephalitis** often resemble those of viral encephalitis. These findings that are illustrated here include leptomeningeal chronic inflammation, perivascular parenchymal inflammation with microglial nodule formation (*arrow*), and gliosis.

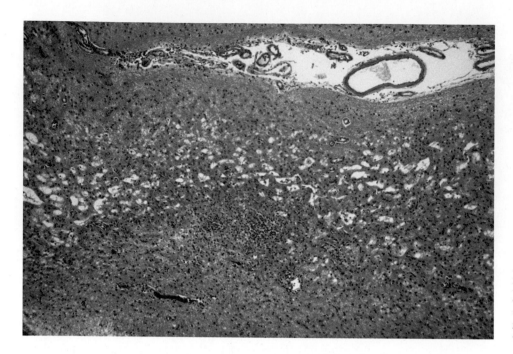

FIGURE 5.42 Many patients with **Rasmussen encephalitis** demonstrate cortical atrophy that microscopically is seen here and is marked by prominent gliosis, inflammation, and vacuolar degenerative changes in the cortex.

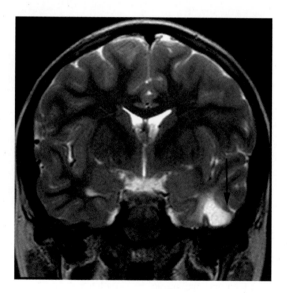

FIGURE 5.43 **Ganglioglioma.** Coronal T2-weighted image from MRI without gadolinium in a 9-year-old boy with a 6-year history of seizures consisting of staring spells shows a cystic cortical lesion of the left inferior temporal gyrus (*arrow*).

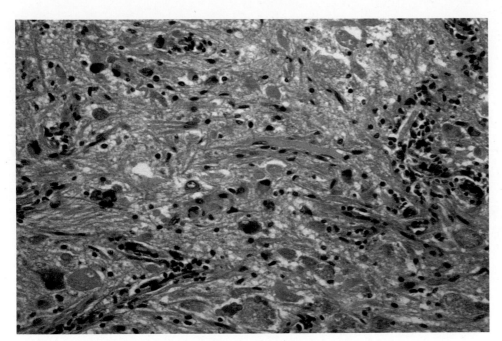

FIGURE 5.44 Histologic appearance of a **ganglioglioma**. The tumor represents a low-grade neoplasm (WHO grade I) tumor. It is marked by a proliferation of atypical ganglion cells intermixed with an atypical gliomatous component, most commonly resembling low-grade astrocytoma. Gangliogliomas most commonly arise in the temporal lobe, often in childhood, and are associated with cortical dysplasia. Perivascular chronic inflammation and eosinophilic granular bodies are also common features of this tumor type. This photomicrograph shows rare atypical large neuronal cells intermixed with a more spindle cell glioma component.

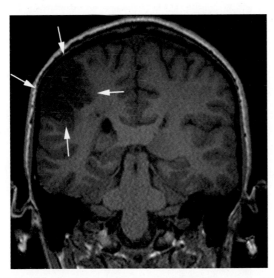

FIGURE 5.45 Dysembryoplastic neuroepithelial tumor. Coronal MPRAGE image from MRI without gadolinium in a 13-year-old girl with a 1-year history of left arm somatosensory progressing to dialeptic seizures shows a cortical lesion involving the right inferior parietal lobule characterized by multiple cystic structures, gyral broadening, and mild inner table scalloping (*arrows*).

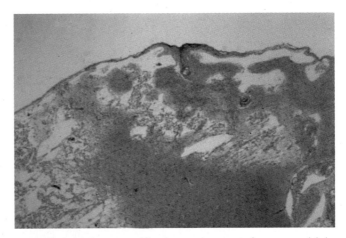

FIGURE 5.46 Low magnification appearance of a temporal lobe dysembryoplastic neuroepithelial tumor. These WHO grade I lesions most commonly arise in the temporal lobe and are predominantly cortical based. Typically, they have multinodular architectural pattern and a microcystic appearance as seen in this photomicrograph.

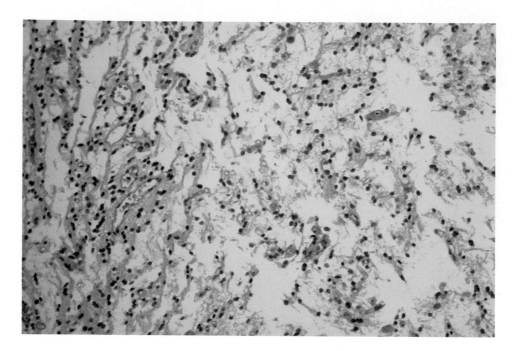

FIGURE 5.47 Higher magnification appearance of a **dysembryoplastic neuroepithelial tumor** showing a proliferation of predominantly oligodendroglial-like rounded cells arranged against a mucoid background. Intermixed with these cells are smaller numbers of major appearing neuronal cells and astrocytic cells. Dysembryoplastic neuroepithelial tumors are also frequently accompanied by adjacent cortical dysplasia.

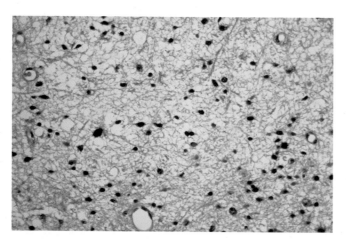

FIGURE 5.48 Histologic appearance of a **low-grade diffuse fibrillary astrocytoma** (WHO grade II). The tumor is marked by a mildly hypercellular parenchyma and cytologic atypia, as evidenced by nuclear enlargement and hyperchromasia and angularity to the nuclear contours. Areas of ganglioglioma may resemble low-grade astrocytoma, underscoring the importance of tissue sampling in order to identify the atypical ganglion cell component that helps define ganglioglioma. This tumor has the potential of degenerating into a higher-grade lesion over time (glioblastoma multiforme).

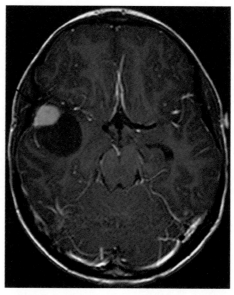

FIGURE 5.49 **Pleomorphic xanthoastrocytoma.** Axial T1-weighted image from MRI with gadolinium in a 10-year-old boy with a 1-year history of headache shows a lesion involving the cortex and subcortical white matter of the right temporal pole characterized by a large cyst with an enhancing mural nodule (*arrow*) without significant surrounding edema.

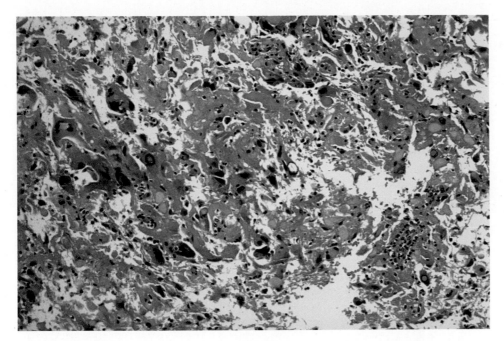

FIGURE 5.50 **Pleomorphic xanthoastrocytomas** are generally low-grade astrocytic tumors (WHO grade II) marked by prominent hypercellularity and nuclear pleomorphism, lipidized astrocytic cells, perivascular lymphocytes, and increased reticulin staining between individual tumors cells. In contrast to high-grade astrocytic tumors, most pleomorphic xanthoastrocytomas lack appreciable mitotic activity or necrosis. Most of these tumors arise either in the temporal or parietal lobe region in younger patients.

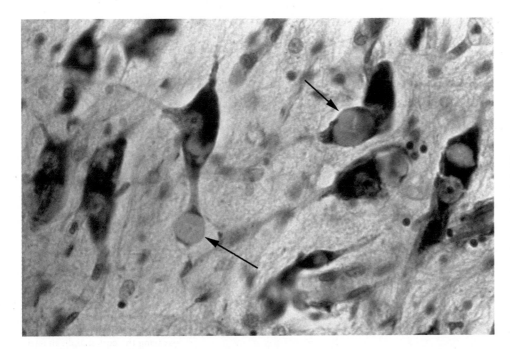

FIGURE 5.51 **Lafora bodies** (*arrows*) are intracytoplasmic neuronal polyglucosan structures that are seen in Lafora disease, which is an inherited progressive myoclonic epilepsy syndrome. It is an autosomal-recessive disorder with onset in late childhood and adolescence. Characteristic seizures include myoclonic and occipital lobe seizures with visual hallucinations, scotomata, and photoconvulsions. The disease leads to an inexorable decline in the cognitive and neurologic functions resulting in dementia and death usually within 10 years of onset.

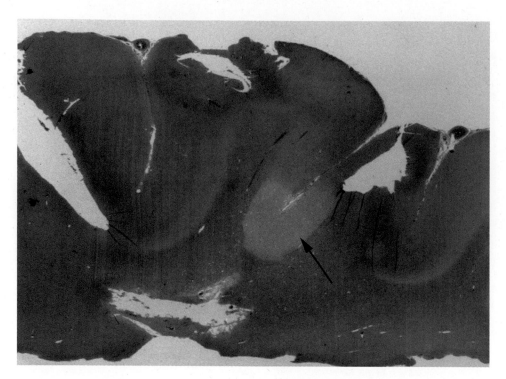

FIGURE 5.52 Invasive seizure monitoring with depth electrodes may occasionally result in infarcts associated with disruption of vessels. This low magnification photomicrograph shows a pale zone of cortex (*arrow*) representing acute infarct due to placement of electrodes (**electrode-related infarct**).

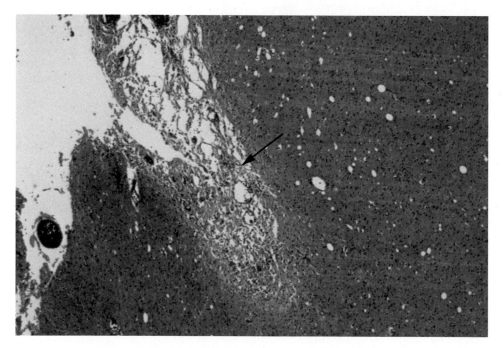

FIGURE 5.53 The tract along which a depth electrode was placed is observed. Evidence of **infarct/contusion along the electrode tract** as marked by vacuolated changes, surrounding gliosis, and a macrophage infiltrate (*arrow*).

PART II ■ BASIC PRINCIPLES OF ELECTROENCEPHALOGRAPHY

CHAPTER 6 ■ NEUROPHYSIOLOGIC BASIS OF THE ELECTROENCEPHALOGRAM

ERWIN-JOSEF SPECKMANN, CHRISTIAN E. ELGER, AND ULRICH ALTRUP

Field potentials appear and are detectable in the space surrounding cellular elements of the nervous system. They comprise rapid waves and baseline shifts; the former correspond to the conventional electroencephalogram (EEG), and both phenomena are included in the so-called direct current (DC) potential. Field potentials are essential in the diagnosis and classification of epileptic seizures as well as in the control of antiepileptic therapy. This chapter describes the elementary mechanisms underlying the generation of field potentials and the special functional situations leading to "epileptic" field potentials.

BIOELECTRICAL ACTIVITY OF NEURONAL AND GLIAL CELLS

The cells of the nervous system are generally differentiated into neurons and glial cells, whose processes intermingle and form a dense, highly complex matrix (Fig. 6.1). Because the

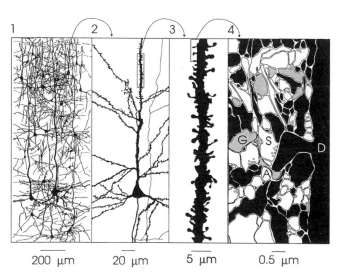

FIGURE 6.1 Morphology and histology of neuronal and glial elements in the neocortex. *Rectangles* and *arrows* indicate extended sections. In section 1, only a minor portion of the neurons is stained. *A*, axon; *D*, dendrite; *G*, glial cell; *S*, synapse. (Modified from Gaze RM. *The Formation of Nerve Connections.* New York: Academic Press; 1970. Purpura DP. Dendritic differentiation in human cerebral cortex: normal and aberrant developmental patterns. In: Kreutzberg GW, ed. *Advances in Neurology.* Vol 12. New York: Raven Press; 1975:91–116; Valverde F. The organization of area 18 in the monkey: a golgi study. *Anat Embryol.* 1978;154:305–334; and Westrum LE, Blackstad TW. An electromicroscopic study of the stratum radiatum of the rat hippocampus (regio superior, CA1) with particular emphasis on synaptology. *J Comp Neurol.* 1962;113:281–293, with permission.)

actual interactions of these cellular elements are barely recognizable in spatiotemporal dimensions, principles of their structure and function inevitably are taken into account.

Neurons

A typical neuron consists of a soma (body, perikaryon) and fibers (dendrites and axons). In functional terms, with respect to information input, the relatively short and highly arborized dendrites can be considered extensions of the soma, as reflected in their being covered by thousands of synaptic endings. Axons are relatively long and, especially in their terminal regions, branch into collaterals. These neuronal output structures carry information into the terminal regions. Information is transferred to other neurons by way of synaptic endings (1–9).

Neuronal function is closely correlated with bioelectrical activity, which can be studied with intracellular microelectrode recordings. When a neuron is impaled by a microelectrode, a membrane potential of approximately 70 mV with negative polarity in the intracellular space becomes apparent. This resting membrane potential, existing in the soma and all its fibers, is based mainly on a potassium-outward current through leakage channels. If the resting membrane potential is critically diminished, that is, if a threshold is surpassed, an action potential (AP) is triggered, which is based on sodium-inward and potassium-outward currents through voltage-dependent membrane channels. APs are conducted along the axons to the terminations, where they lead to a release of transmitter substances. These transmitters open another class of membrane channels in the postsynaptic neuron. Dependent on the ionic composition of the currents flowing through the transmitter (ligand)-operated channels, two types of membrane potential changes, commonly called postsynaptic potentials (PSPs), are induced in the postsynaptic neuron. When a sodium-inward current prevails, depolarization of the postsynaptic neuron occurs. This synaptic depolarization is called an excitatory postsynaptic potential (EPSP) because it increases the probability that an AP will be triggered. When a potassium-outward current or a chloride-inward current prevails, hyperpolarization of the postsynaptic neuron occurs. Because hyperpolarization increases the distance between membrane potential and threshold, the synaptic hyperpolarization is called an inhibitory postsynaptic potential (IPSP) (10–12).

The EPSPs and IPSPs can interact with each other (Fig. 6.2). Electrical stimulation of an axon (ST1 in Fig. 6.2A) forming an excitatory synapse on a postsynaptic neuron can induce an AP at the site of stimulation. Conducted along the axon, the AP

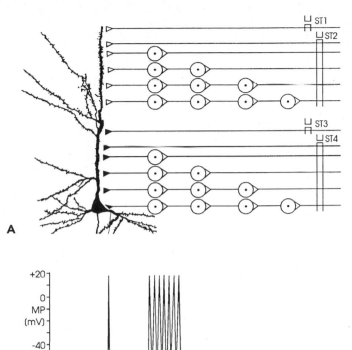

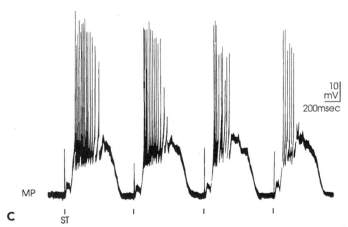

FIGURE 6.2 Bioelectrical activity of neuronal elements: membrane potential (MP), action potential (AP), excitatory postsynaptic potential (EPSP), and inhibitory postsynaptic potential (IPSP). **A:** Indicated are stimulation sites and the pyramidal neuron from which the recording was made. Open symbols represent excitatory synapses and filled symbols inhibitory synapses. Up to four interneurons are schematically drawn between stimulation sites (ST1 to ST4) and the neuron. **B:** Intracellular recording from the pyramidal neuron in **A** is shown. Single electrical stimuli applied at ST1 and ST3 evoked monosynaptic EPSP and IPSP, respectively. Paired stimulation at ST1 and ST3 led to a summation of the corresponding monosynaptic responses. After stimulation at ST2 and ST4, polysynaptic EPSP and IPSP, respectively, were elicited. **C:** Original tracing of synaptically mediated neuronal depolarizations in a spinal motoneuron of the cat is shown. Stimulation (ST) of pathways oligosynaptically and polysynaptically linked to the neuron led to early (oligosynaptic) and late (polysynaptic) potentials. (**A** and **B** adapted from Speckmann E-J. *Experimentelle Epilepsieforschung.* Darmstadt, Germany: Wissenschaftliche Buchgesellschaft; 1986:13, with permission.)

finally induces an EPSP in the postsynaptic neuron (ST1 in Fig. 6.2B). When only one synapse separates the site of stimulation from the site of EPSP generation, a monosynaptic EPSP appears. One way in which a summation of EPSP takes place is when the stimulation is repeated with an interstimulus interval shorter than the duration of the EPSP. With this temporal summation, the second EPSP can surpass the threshold and induce an AP (ST1 in Fig. 6.2B). A summation of EPSPs also can occur when monosynaptic EPSPs are evoked simultaneously at several locations on the postsynaptic neuron (spatial summation). Temporal and spatial summations are often combined with each other and are essential for information processing in the central nervous system, as when the AP reaches the target neuron by different ways. With stimulation at ST2 in Figure 6.2A, the triggered APs pass through varying numbers of relays before reaching their target. As APs are delayed with each synaptic transmission, they appear with temporal dispersion at the postsynaptic neuron and induce a long-lasting depolarization (ST2 in Fig. 6.2B). Because many synapses are involved, such a depolarization is called a polysynaptic EPSP. When a polysynaptic network is activated repeatedly, EPSPs of considerable amplitude and duration can appear, as demonstrated by the original recording in Figure 6.2C. As with EPSPs, IPSPs can be induced both monosynaptically and polysynaptically and also are subject to temporal and spatial summation (ST3 and ST4 in Figs. 6.2A and B) (5,11,12).

In complex neuronal systems, EPSPs and IPSPs are often superimposed and induce long-lasting sequences of fluctuations of the membrane potential. These kinds of postsynaptic responses play a prominent role in the generation of extracellular potential fields, such as the EEG.

Glial Cells

Consisting of a soma and fibers, glial cells intermingle with the neuronal structures. Glial cell fibers are electrically coupled, building up an extended functional network (3,8,13).

Glial cells also show a membrane potential (Fig. 6.3A). Unlike neurons, glial cells do not generate APs and PSPs. Because their resting membrane potential is based exclusively on potassium-outward current through leakage channels, its value is close to the potassium equilibrium potential. With an increase and a subsequent decrease in extracellular potassium concentration, glial cells depolarize and repolarize, respectively (Fig. 6.3A). Changes in the extracellular concentration of other cations have only small effects on the membrane potential of glial cells (14,15).

Glial cells and neurons are functionally linked by way of the extracellular potassium concentration (Figs. 6.3B and C). As mentioned, neuronal APs are associated with an outflow of potassium ions (Fig. 6.3B). Thus, with an increase in the repetition rate of neuronal APs, the extracellular potassium concentration increases, resulting in depolarization of glial cells adjacent to the active neurons (Fig. 6.3C) (11,14–16).

PRINCIPLES OF FIELD POTENTIAL GENERATION

Changes in membrane potential of neurons and glial cells are the basis of changes in extracellular field potential. The mechanisms involved can be described as follows: (i) primary

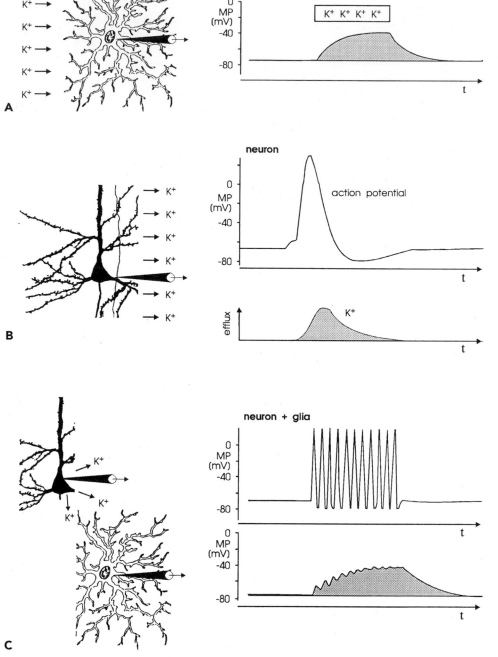

FIGURE 6.3 Changes in membrane potential (MP) of a glial cell induced by an increase in extracellular potassium concentration (**A**) and functional linkage between neuronal and glial activity (**B**) and (**C**). **A:** The increased extracellular concentration of K⁺ led to a sustained depolarization of the glial cell. **B:** During a neuronal action potential, an efflux of K⁺ occurred. **C:** The K⁺ concentration in the extracellular space close to the glial cell was raised during the repetitive firing of a neuron. This led to sustained depolarization of the neighboring glial cell. (**A** and **C** adapted from Zenker W. Feinstruktur des Nervengewebes. In: Zenker W, ed. *Makroskopische und Mikroskopische Anatomie des Menschen.* Vol 3. Munich, Germany: Urban & Schwarzenberg; 1985:3–55, and **B** and **C** adapted from Valverde F. The organization of area 18 in the monkey: a golgi study. *Anat Embryol.* 1978;154:305–334, with permission.)

transmembranous ion fluxes at a restricted membrane area of cells and consequent localized membrane potential changes; (ii) development of potential gradients between sites of primary events and the remaining areas of the membrane; and (iii) secondary ion currents because of the potential gradient along the cell membrane in the intracellular and extracellular spaces. The secondary current flowing through the extracellular space is directly responsible for the generation of field potentials (9,17). Because EPSPs and IPSPs are important in the generation of the EEG findings, the processes are explained in greater detail using the examples of an excitatory synaptic input (2,12,18,19).

A vertically oriented neuronal element, shown schematically in Figure 6.4, is impinged on by a single excitatory synapse whose afferent fiber can be stimulated. The resulting net influx of cations leads to depolarization of the membrane, that is, to an EPSP. Consequently, a potential gradient exists along the neuronal membrane and evokes an intracellular and extracellular current flow. As a result of the intracellular current, the EPSP spreads electrotonically; the extracellular current induces field potentials. The polarity depends on the site of recording. The electrode near the synapse "sees" the inflow of cations (a negativity), whereas the electrode distant from the synapse "sees" the outflow of cations (a positivity).

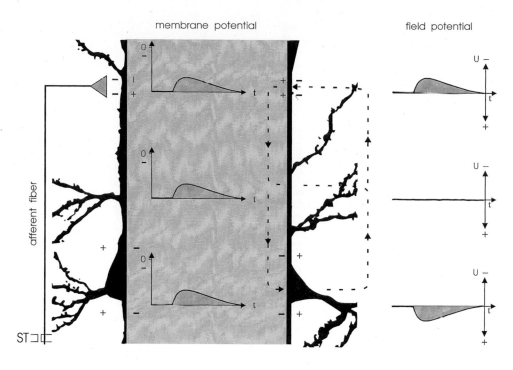

membrane potential   field potential

FIGURE 6.4 Principles of field potential generation in the neocortex. A perpendicular pyramidal neuron with an extended intracellular space (*hatched area*) is shown. An afferent fiber (**left**) formed an excitatory synaptic contact at the superficial aspect of the apical dendrite. Changes in membrane potential and in corresponding field potential are given in the intracellular and extracellular spaces, respectively. After stimulation of the afferent fiber (ST), an excitatory postsynaptic potential developed in the upper part of the dendrite and spread electrotonically to the lower parts. The local excitation (+ and −) led to tangential current flows (*broken lines*) and to the field potential changes in the extracellular space.

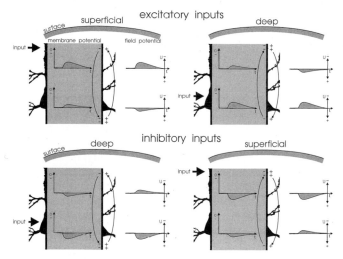

FIGURE 6.5 Generation of field potential in the neocortex by excitatory and inhibitory synaptic inputs reaching the superficial and deep parts of perpendicular pyramidal neurons. The intracellular space is extended (*hatched areas*). Changes in membrane potential and in the corresponding field potential are given in the intracellular and extracellular spaces, respectively. Locations of active inputs are indicated (*heavy arrows*). EPSP and IPSP, excitatory and inhibitory postsynaptic potentials, respectively. Excitatory inputs: With superficial excitation, an inward current generated an EPSP in upper and lower regions. Because of the direction of the extracellular current flow (*light arrows*), the field potential had negative polarity at the surface and positive polarity in the deep recording (*cf.* Fig. 6.4). With deep excitation, the current flow—and the field potentials—had inverse direction to that elicited by superficial excitation. Inhibitory inputs: With deep inhibition, an outward current generated an IPSP in lower and upper regions. Because of the direction of the extracellular current flow (*arrows*), the field potential had positive polarity in the deep recording and negative polarity at the surface. With superficial inhibition, the direction of current flow was inverse to that seen with deep inhibition; the field potentials were inverted as well. Differences in the shape of the various potentials were caused by the electrical properties of the tissue.

Between the two electrodes is the reversal point of the field potentials (12,20).

Corresponding effects occur with the generation of IPSPs. Activation of an inhibitory synapse induces an outflow of cations or an inflow of anions at the synaptic site. In this way, the membrane potential is increased at the synaptic site, and a potential gradient develops along the cell membrane, similar to that described for EPSPs. The potential gradient evokes a current flow from the synaptic site to the surrounding regions of the membrane. Compared with EPSPs, the extracellular current flow is inverted, as is the polarity of field potentials. Thus, the electrode near the synapse "sees" a positivity and the electrode distant from the synapse a negativity.

Field potentials are generated by extracellular currents, and their polarity depends on the direction of the current as well as on the positions of the extracellular electrodes. Figure 6.5 illustrates the generation and polarity of field potentials, as elicited by excitatory and inhibitory inputs to superficial and deep regions of vertical neuronal elements. Negative field potentials at the cortical surface may be based on superficial EPSPs as well as on deep IPSPs, and positive field potentials at the surface may be based on superficial IPSPs as well as on deep EPSPs (Fig. 6.6) (12,19,20).

POTENTIAL FIELDS IN NEURONAL NETWORKS

Many neuronal elements contribute to the extracellular currents that generate field potentials recorded at the surface of central nervous system structures. The spatial arrangement of the neuronal elements and the positions of the recording electrodes play an essential role in establishing and detecting extracellular potential fields (2,12,21).

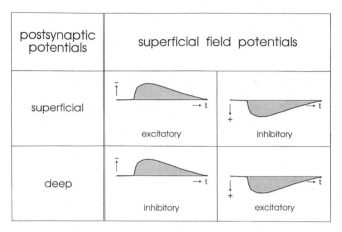

FIGURE 6.6 Synopsis of the synaptic processes underlying the generation of superficial field potentials in the cerebral cortex. Different mechanisms may lead to uniform superficial field potentials.

Two principal types of neuronal arrangements can be identified (Fig. 6.7). In the parallel type, the somata are in one layer and the dendrites are in opposite layers (Fig. 6.7A). In the other type, the somata are in the center of a pool and the dendrites extend to its periphery (Fig. 6.7B). The first arrangement is realized in the cortex and the second in brainstem nuclei.

The two neuronal arrangements build up the so-called open and closed fields. In open fields, one electrode (E2 in Fig. 6.7A) largely integrates the potentials of the population (i.e., it is near the zero potential line), and the other electrode (E1 in Fig. 6.7A) sees only the positive or negative field, permitting the recording of a field potential. In closed fields, external electrodes do not see significant potential differences because the current flows within the pool compensate for each other (Fig. 6.7B) (2,21).

TYPES OF FIELD POTENTIAL CHANGES

With respect to the time course, two types of field potentials can be differentiated, depending on the time constant of the amplifying recording device. The conventional EEG is

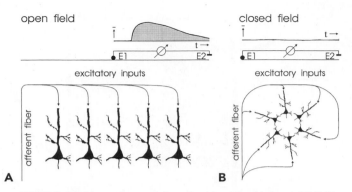

FIGURE 6.7 Neurons arranged to give open (**A**) and closed (**B**) fields. Field potentials are present (**A**) or missing (**B**) during excitatory inputs by way of afferent fibers. E1 and E2 indicate different and reference electrodes.

recorded with a time constant of 1 second or less. Amplification with an infinite time constant, that is, by a DC amplifier, permits additional recording of baseline shifts and wavelike potentials (EEG/DC) (22–24).

Wave Generation (Conventional Electroencephalogram)

The generation of wavelike potentials is described in Figure 6.8, a representation of a column of neocortex. In its upper dendritic region, the neuron is activated by an afferent fiber by way of an excitatory synapse. The superficial EEG and the membrane potentials of the dendrite and afferent fiber are recorded. The afferent fiber shows grouped, followed by regular, discharges. With grouped discharges prominent, summated EPSPs occur in the dendrite; with sustained regular activity, a depolarizing shift of the membrane potential appears. The changes in membrane potential in the upper dendrite lead to field potentials. When amplifiers with a finite time constant are used, only fluctuations in field potential are recorded, corresponding to findings on conventional EEG. The shift of the membrane potential is not reflected (21,25).

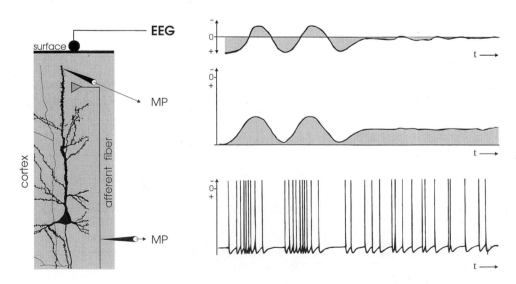

FIGURE 6.8 Wave generation in the electroencephalogram (EEG) at the surface of the cerebral cortex. A perpendicular pyramidal neuron is shown. An afferent fiber formed an excitatory synaptic contact at the superficial part of the apical dendrite. Simultaneous recordings of the membrane potentials (MPs) of the afferent fiber and the dendritic element, as well as of the EEG, are displayed. Groups of action potentials in the afferent fiber generate wavelike excitatory postsynaptic potentials (EPSPs) in the dendritic region and corresponding waves in the EEG recording. Tonic activity in the afferent fiber results in long-lasting EPSP with only small fluctuations. The long-lasting depolarization is not reflected on the conventional EEG recording.

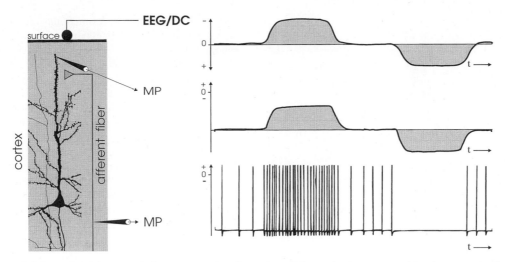

FIGURE 6.9 Sustained shifts in the electroencephalogram (EEG) at the surface of the cerebral cortex resulting from sustained neuronal activities. If recordings are performed with a direct current (DC) amplifier (EEG/DC), sustained potentials can also be recorded at the surface. In the perpendicular pyramidal neuron depicted, an afferent fiber formed an excitatory synaptic contact at the superficial part of the apical dendrite. The membrane potentials (MPs) of the afferent fiber and the dendritic element were recorded simultaneously, as was the EEG/DC. Increased and decreased sustained activity in the afferent fiber generated sustained depolarizations and hyperpolarizations of the dendritic region and corresponding negative and positive shifts of the EEG/DC recording.

Baseline Shifts (Electroencephalogram/ Direct Current)

The generation of baseline shifts is described in Figures 6.9 and 6.10. In a column of the neocortex (Fig. 6.9), a neuron is activated in its upper dendritic region by an afferent fiber by way of an excitatory synapse. In this case, the afferent fiber displays three levels of sustained activity. Medium regular activity is interrupted by periods of high repetition and silence. Consequently, owing to facilitation, the upper dendrite is depolarized during the high discharge in the afferent fiber and is hyperpolarized in the silent period because of disfacilitation. This results in corresponding field potential shifts. When amplifiers with an infinite time constant are used, these baseline shifts, which reflect sustained values of the membrane potential of neuronal elements, are recorded. With a sufficiently high upper-frequency limit, the DC recording comprises conventional EEG waves as well as slow potential deviations (26–32).

Glial cells also are involved in the generation of baseline shifts (Figs. 6.10 and 6.11). As noted, a functional coupling between neurons and glial cells exists (see Fig. 6.3). Figure 6.10 shows a neuron in deep cortical layers and a network of electrically coupled glial cells extending to the surface. The superficial EEG/DC and the membrane potentials of a glial cell and the neuron are recorded. With increased discharge frequency of the neuron, extracellular potassium concentration rises, evoking a depolarization of the adjacent glial cell. The potassium-induced depolarization is conducted electrotonically

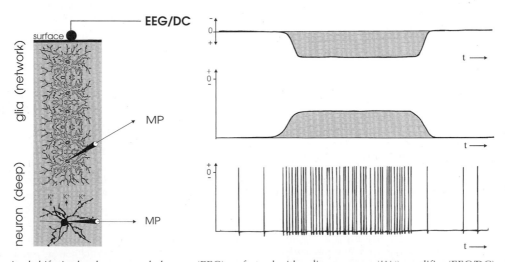

FIGURE 6.10 Sustained shifts in the electroencephalogram (EEG) performed with a direct current (DC) amplifier (EEG/DC) at the surface of the cerebral cortex generated by neuronal activity and mediated by a glial network. If recordings are performed with a DC amplifier, sustained potentials can also be recorded. A deep neuron functionally coupled to a perpendicularly oriented glial network is shown. The membrane potentials (MPs) of the deep neuron and of a glial cell as well as the EEG/DC were recorded simultaneously. Sustained increased activity of the deep neuron induced an increase in extracellular K+ concentration and a corresponding depolarization of the glial cells. Because of the electrotonically coupled network of glial cells, a sustained positive potential was induced in the surface EEG/DC recording.

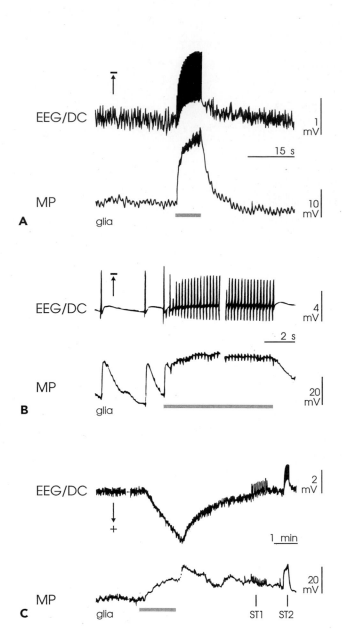

FIGURE 6.11 Simultaneous recordings of the electroencephalogram (EEG) potential performed with a direct current (DC) amplifier (EEG/DC) at the surface of the cerebral cortex and of the membrane potential (MP) of glial cells in an anesthetized and artificially ventilated rat. **A:** High-frequency electrical stimulation of the cortical surface (*horizontal bar*) is indicated. **B:** Focal epileptic activity induced by penicillin is indicated. Repetitive cortical stimulation (*horizontal bar*) increased the frequency of epileptic discharges (interruption, approximately 5 seconds). **C:** Increase of the local partial pressure of carbon dioxide (PCO_2) during apnea (*horizontal bar*) is shown. ST1 and ST2, low- and high-frequency electrical stimulation of the cerebral cortex, respectively. Depolarization of glial cells can be associated with both a positive (**C**) and a negative (**A** and **B**) shift in the EEG/DC. (**A** adapted from Caspers H, Speckmann E-J, Lehmenkühler A. DC potentials of the cerebral cortex. Seizure activity and changes in gas pressures. *Rev Physiol Biochem Pharmacol.* 1987;106:127–178; **B** adapted from Speckmann E-J. *Experimentelle Epilepsieforschung.* Darmstadt, Germany: Wissenschaftliche Buchgesellschaft; 1986; and **C** adapted from Caspers H, Speckmann E-J, Lehmenkühler A. Electrogenesis of slow potentials of the brain. In: Elbert T, Rockstroh B, Lutzenberger W, et al., eds. *Self-regulation of the Brain and Behavior.* New York: Springer; 1984:26–41, with permission.)

within the glial network. A functional situation is present similar to that in a perpendicular neuron with a deep excitatory synaptic input (see Figs. 6.5 and 6.6). The superficial EEG/DC electrode sees a long-lasting positivity because of an outflow of cations from the glial cells in the upper layers. In other respects, this corresponds to the well-known spatial buffering of potassium. In principle, the aforementioned mechanism can make visible the activity of closed fields (Fig. 6.7B) in baseline shifts of field potentials (31,33,34).

Glial cells contribute to the generation of field potentials, although this mechanism is not dominant. Thus, the original recordings of cortical EEG/DC and membrane potentials of cortical glial cells demonstrate that glial depolarization occurs parallel to negative (Figs. 6.11A and B) and positive (Fig. 6.11C) baseline shifts of field potentials. On the whole, field potential changes can be thought to be generated primarily by neuronal structures (16,31).

BASICS OF EPILEPTIC FIELD POTENTIALS

As described, field potentials recorded during epileptic activity are based on changes in neuronal membrane potential. The amplitudes of field potentials exceed those of nonepileptic potentials because the underlying neuronal activity is highly synchronized. As a result of the synchronization, the activity of a single element represents that of the entire epileptic population. On that basis, changes in field potentials and neuronal membrane potential can clearly be related to one another (12,35–39).

Figure 6.10 shows typical recordings of epicortical EEG and of the membrane potential of a neuron in upper cortical layers. During the development of epileptic activity, flat depolarizations superimposed by APs appear first. These membrane potential changes evolve into typical paroxysmal depolarizations that consist of a steep depolarization triggering a burst of APs, a plateau-like diminution of the membrane potential, and a steep repolarization followed by an afterhyperpolarization or an afterdepolarization. With the appearance of the epileptic neuronal depolarizations, negative fluctuations of the local field potential develop. As Figure 6.12 shows, a close temporal relationship exists between development of the intracellularly recorded membrane potential and the extracellularly generated field potentials. Later the duration and amplitude of the neuronal depolarizations and of the negative field potentials increase and reach a final level. The transition from epileptic to normal activity is also associated with a parallelism between field potentials and membrane potential changes. Thus, the epileptic negative field potentials represent the activity of an epileptic neuronal network (35–37,39).

Epileptic foci can induce evoked potentials (EP) in nonepileptic areas (Fig. 6.13). In Figure 6.13A, two cortical columns generate epileptic activity, as indicated by the neuronal paroxysmal depolarizations and the concomitant negative spikes in the EEG. The epileptic activities at both sites are not necessarily synchronous. In Figure 6.13B, only one column is epileptically active. The epileptic discharges elicit synaptic potentials in the neighboring nonepileptic area. The synchronized burst discharges induced in the nonepileptic column then give rise to "epileptic evoked potentials."

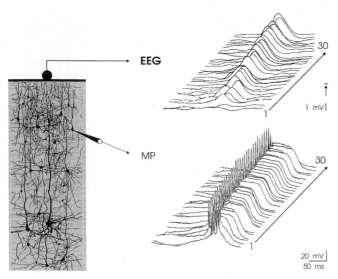

FIGURE 6.12 Simultaneous establishment of paroxysmal depolarizations of a neuron in superficial cortical layers and of sharp waves in the electroencephalogram at the cortical surface during development of an epileptic focus. Focal epileptic activity was induced by local penicillin application. MP, membrane potential. Graphic superposition of 30 successive potentials with the commencement of focal epileptic activity is shown. (Adapted from Elger CE, Speckmann E-J. Vertical inhibition in motor cortical epileptic foci and its consequences for descending neuronal activity to the spinal cord. In: Speckmann E-J, Elger CE, eds. *Epilepsy and Motor System.* Baltimore, MD: Urban & Schwarzenberg; 1983: 152–160, with permission.)

FIELD POTENTIALS WITH FOCAL EPILEPTIC ACTIVITY

For practical reasons, the description of field potential generation with focal epileptic activity takes into account the functional significance of an epileptic focus, especially motor phenomena (12,35,38,40,41).

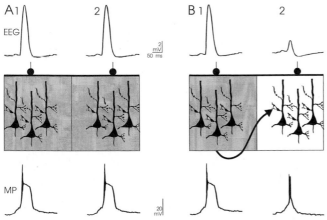

FIGURE 6.13 Electroencephalographic waves at the cortical surface representing locally generated (**A1** and **A2** and **B1**) and synaptically transmitted (**B2**) epileptiform neuronal discharges. Cortical columns with (*hatched areas*) and without (*open area*) locally generated epileptic activity are shown. Both **A1** and **A2** potentials represent directly epileptiform neuronal depolarizations. The potential in **B1** represents directly epileptiform neuronal discharges, and that in **B2** represents indirectly epileptiform discharges in the primary nonepileptic neighboring column, that is, a potential synaptically evoked by the epileptically active neurons (*arrow*). MP, membrane potential.

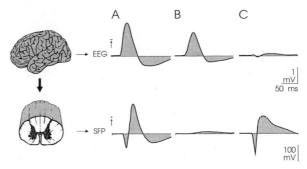

FIGURE 6.14 Dissociation in occurrence of epileptiform potentials on the surface electroencephalogram and of spinal field potentials (SFPs). Focal epileptiform activity was restricted to motor cortical layers. **A:** Simultaneous appearance of cortical and spinal activity is indicated. **B:** Presence of cortical activity and failure of spinal activity are shown. **C:** Failure of cortical activity and presence of spinal activity are shown. (Adapted from Elger CE, Speckmann E-J, Prohaska O, et al. Pattern of intracortical potential distribution during focal interictal epileptiform discharges (FIED) and its relation to spinal field potentials in the rat. *Electroencephalogr Clin Neurophysiol.* 1981;51: 393–402, with permission.)

The relationship between epileptic field potentials in motor cortical areas and their output to the spinal cord is detailed in Figure 6.14. In Figure 6.14A, the epicortical EEG spike is associated with a defined high-amplitude spinal field potential, indicating synchronized descending neuronal activity. These events result finally in muscular clonus. Superficial EEG potentials and spinal output are not always closely related, however. Each of these motor phenomena may be present without the other (Fig. 6.14B and C) (42–47).

The aforementioned discrepancies between superficial EEG potentials and cortical output can be clarified by recording field potentials from within the cortex. In Figure 6.15, the superficial EEG was recorded simultaneously with intracortical field potentials at three depths, including layer V, and with spinal field potentials. With positive field potentials in layer V, spinal field potentials are missing (Fig. 6.15A and B). Synchronized motor output appears only when the typical epileptic negative spike occurs in layer V (Fig. 6.15C). In all these cases, the EEG spikes at the cortical surface are identical (42–44,46,47).

The situations presented in Figure 6.15A and C are shown at the level of intracellular recordings in Figure 6.16. The positive field potentials in layer V parallel long-lasting and highly effective neuronal inhibitions, and the negative field potentials at the same site are based on typical neuronal paroxysmal depolarization shifts. Thus, the synchronized excitation of pyramidal neurons in layer V is a prerequisite for epileptic motor output. This excitation is not necessarily reflected in the superficial EEG, however (Fig. 6.14C). Epileptic motor reactions based on a cortical focus may occur without appropriate signs on such a recording (43,44,46–48).

The difference between bioelectrical activity at the cortical surface and in deeper cortical layers becomes very clear when voltage-sensitive dyes are used instead of field potential recordings (49–51). With this technique, neuronal activity can be seen, although the requirements for the generation of field potentials are not fulfilled (*cf.* Fig. 6.7).

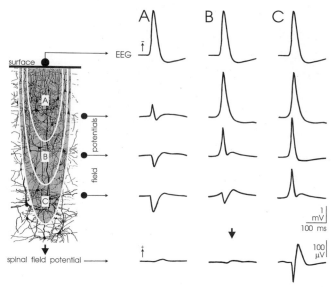

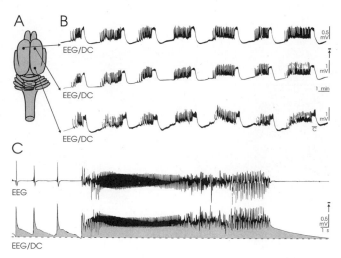

FIGURE 6.15 Epicortical (electroencephalogram), intracortical, and spinal field potentials during focal epileptiform activity. The actual vertical extension of the focus is indicated on the left and related to the tracings by letters. The occurrence of synchronized spinal field potentials is linked to the appearance of negative field potentials in lamina V (**A–C**). (Adapted from Elger CE, Speckmann E-J, Caspers H, et al. Focal interictal epileptiform discharges in the cortex of the rat: laminar restriction and its consequences for activity descending to the spinal cord. In: Klee MR, Lux HD, Speckmann E-J, eds. *Physiology and Pharmacology of Epileptogenic Phenomena.* New York: Raven Press; 1982:13–20, with permission.)

FIGURE 6.17 Experimental animal model of generalized tonic–clonic seizures elicited by repeated systemic administration of pentylenetetrazol. **A:** The recording arrangement is shown. **B:** Simultaneous recordings of the epicortical direct current (DC) potential from the motor regions of both hemispheres and from an occipital area are presented. **C:** Part C in **B** is displayed as a conventional electroencephalogram (EEG) and EEG/DC potential with an extended timescale. (Adapted from Speckmann E-J. *Experimentelle Epilepsieforschung.* Darmstadt, Germany: Wissenschaftliche Buchgesellschaft; 1986:69, with permission.)

FIELD POTENTIALS WITH GENERALIZED TONIC–CLONIC ACTIVITY

Observations made during tonic–clonic seizures in experimental animal studies are used to explain the generation of field potentials during generalized seizures. After repeated injec-

tions of pentylenetetrazol, typical tonic–clonic seizures appear (Fig. 6.17) accompanied by field potential changes consisting of baseline shifts and superimposed rapid waves. The latter allow the differentiation between tonic and clonic phases (Fig. 6.17C) (12,35–38,41).

Baseline Shifts (Electroencephalogram/ Direct Current)

Figure 6.18 shows the relationship between baseline shifts of field potentials, from both surface and deep recordings, and membrane potential changes of pyramidal neurons in layer V.

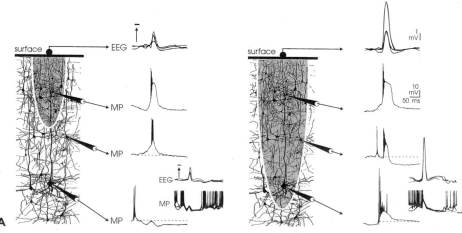

FIGURE 6.16 Membrane potential (MP) changes of single neurons in layers of the motor cortex during focal epileptic activity with different vertical extensions. Epileptic activity was recorded 5 (**A**) and 15 (**B**) minutes after local application of penicillin to the cortical surface. The drawings indicate vertical extension of the focus. The MP changes were recorded simultaneously with the electroencephalographic changes, which are superimposed to show the relationship of the curves to each other. *Insets:* Shown are three superimposed superficial electroencephalographic and deep MP recordings. (Adapted from Speckmann E-J. *Experimentelle Epilepsieforschung.* Darmstadt, Germany: Wissenschaftliche Buchgesellschaft; 1986: 122, with permission.)

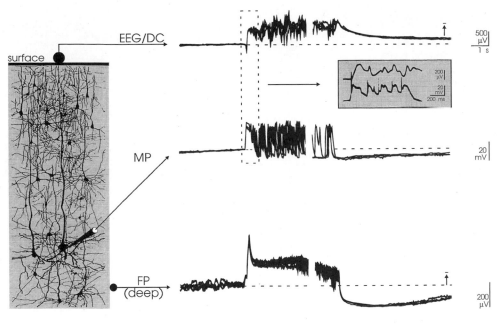

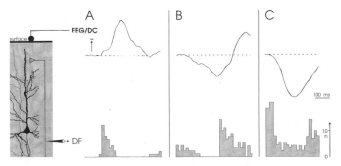

FIGURE 6.18 Relationship between shifts of the epicortical (electroencephalogram [EEG] performed with a direct current [DC] amplifier [EEG/DC]) and laminar field potentials (FPs) and changes in the membrane potential (MP) of a pyramidal tract cell during tonic–clonic seizures (inkwriter recordings with graphic superpositions). Epileptic activity was elicited by repeated systemic administrations of pentylenetetrazol. Interruptions were 30 to 60 seconds. *Inset:* Shown are parts of the EEG/DC and MP recordings displayed on an oscilloscope with an extended timescale.

During tonic–clonic seizures, a series of paroxysmal depolarizations occurs in pyramidal tract neurons. This means that neuronal depolarization parallels a negative shift of the baseline of field potentials on superficial and deep recordings. The close temporal relationship can be discerned also on recordings with an extended timescale. Although the bioelectrical events are similar, discrepancies exist in the commencement of seizures and in the postictal phase. With seizure onset, a monophasic negative shift always occurs on deep recordings of field potentials. In contrast, the superficial EEG/DC findings can start with a monophasic negative or positive as well as a biphasic negative–positive fluctuation. In the postictal period, deep recordings always show a positive displacement of the baseline of field potentials and superficial recordings a negative displacement. Comparison of the different simultaneous recordings of field potentials and membrane potential reveals the following findings. The initial negative fluctuation and the postictal positive displacement of the field potential in deeper layers correspond, respectively, to the initial highly synchronized depolarization and to the postictal hyperpolarization of pyramidal tract neurons. This close correspondence is missing when superficially recorded EEG/DC shifts and neuronal membrane potential changes are compared. Thus, the mean neuronal activity is well represented in the baseline shift of deep field potentials. As far as the superficial field potentials are concerned, additional generators, for example, glial networks, must be taken into account (14–16,18,52–54).

Waves (Conventional Electroencephalogram)

The rapid waves superimposed on the baseline shifts of the EEG/DC can best be interpreted when the afferent impulse inflow to the upper cortical layers is evaluated. Figure 6.19 represents a cortical column with a perpendicularly oriented neuron. An afferent fiber forms an excitatory synapse in upper dendritic regions. The discharge frequency of the afferent fiber was recorded simultaneously with the surface EEG/DC. For further description, three types of waves were selected: monophasic negative (Fig. 6.19A), monophasic positive (Fig. 6.15C), and biphasic positive–negative (Fig. 6.19B) waves. With the commencement of negative waves, the discharge rate increased from a low initial level (Fig. 6.15A and B); during positive waves, the discharge rate decreased from a high level (Fig. 6.19C). Thus, the generation of superficial waves can be explained as resulting from facilitation (negative waves) and disfacilitation (positive waves) of neuronal structures in upper cortical layers (20,22–24,40,46,47).

FIGURE 6.19 Relationship between different patterns of fluctuations of the epicortical field potential (electroencephalogram [EEG] performed with direct current [DC] amplifier [EEG/DC]) and changes in discharge frequency (DF) of neuronal elements in superficial cortical layers during tonic–clonic seizures. Epileptic activity was elicited by repeated systemic administrations of pentylenetetrazol. Up to 16 single events were averaged: monophasic negative (A) and positive (C), as well as biphasic positive–negative (B), fluctuations of EEG/DC. N, number of action potentials. (Adapted from Speckmann E-J. *Experimentelle Epilepsieforschung.* Darmstadt, Germany: Wissenschaftliche Buchgesellschaft; 1986:143, with permission.)

CORRELATIONS OF MEMBRANE POTENTIAL CHANGES IN A NEURONAL POPULATION AND OF EEG SIGNALS

In addition to electroencephalography, there is a variety of other methods for detecting brain activity. Among these, single photon emission tomography (SPECT), positron emission tomography (PET), functional magnetic resonance imaging (fMRI), and intrinsic optical imaging (IOI) are based on metabolic changes associated with increases of local neuronal activity. Besides the latter "very indirect" methods EEG including EP and magnetoencephalography (MEG) represent "more direct ones" since they measure the field effects of the proper neuronal activity and therewith of the information processing brain activity. For the analysis of neuronal network functions, the immediate and simultaneous recording of membrane potentials of all neurons in a population by application of voltage-sensitive dyes is the "only direct" method available yet (55–60). Without doubt, all these methods have advantages and disadvantages. Thus, the functional imaging using voltage-sensitive dyes cannot be applied in patients for several reasons, for example, prerequisite of direct access to the brain structure to be investigated, photo toxicity and pharmacological side effects of the dyes. But, this method is helpful to analyze the functional meaning of field potentials in living human brain slices in vitro, especially with spontaneously occurring epileptic discharges.

Principle and schematic example of recording neuronal membrane potentials using voltage-sensitive dyes are displayed in Figures 6.14–6.20. The living brain slices are stained with fluorescence (or absorption) dyes (A1 in Fig. 6.20). With depolarization and hyperpolarization the fluorescence is decreased and increased, respectively (A2 and A3 in Fig. 6.20). The changes in fluorescence are measured via a microscope by an array of detectors and therewith the actual membrane potentials of the neurons are observed (B1 and B2 in Fig. 6.20).

The method of simultaneous measurement of neuronal membrane potentials of all neurons in a population is successfully applied in living human brain slices (0.5 mm thick) in vitro obtained from neurosurgical interventions (tumor and epilepsy surgery) (57–59,61).

A comparison of the field potentials, that is, the local EEG, and of the neuronal membrane potentials detected by the aid of voltage-sensitive dyes is given in Figure 6.21. The tissue is a slice preparation from the temporal neocortex resected from a patient suffering from pharmacoresistant complex partial seizures. Most of these living human brain slices show spontaneous epileptic EEG potentials, that is, epileptic discharges not induced by experimental procedures. One can derive from the recordings:

(1) During epileptic discharges only a certain portion of the neurons in the population is active simultaneously, that is, a complete synchronization is missing (Fig. 6.21, numbers 2 through 4).

(2) Similar epileptic potentials in the EEG (Fig. 6.21, numbers 2 and 3) are associated with different extents of neuronal depolarizations and similar extents of neuronal

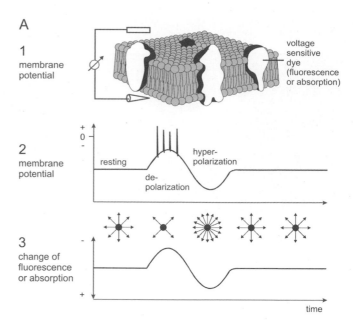

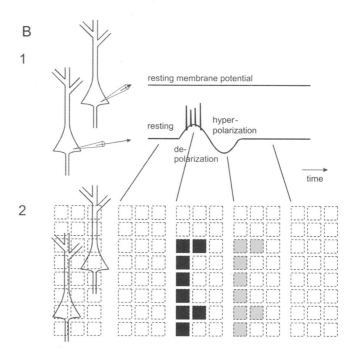

FIGURE 6.20 Recording of neuronal membrane potentials using voltage-sensitive dyes, principles and schematic example of application. **A:** (1) A dye is incorporated into the double lipid membrane of nerve cells and illuminated by light with dye-specific wavelength; simultaneously the membrane potential is recorded with an intracellular microelectrode against a reference electrode in the extracellular space. (2) Changes of the membrane potential (MP) starting from the resting level passing a decrease (depolarization) with action potentials superimposed and a subsequent Increase (hyperpolarization) and eventually returning to resting level. (3) In correspondence to the different MP levels fluorescence and absorption of the dye changes. With fluorescent dyes a depolarization is associated with decrease and a hyperpolarization with an increase of fluorescence (*symbols*). **B:** (1) Two neurons in a population; one stays in the resting state, the other changes its MP as in A (2). (2) By the aid of a microscope and a connected array of diodes (*squares*) the different MP changes of both neurons can be detected via the different optical behaviors (62).

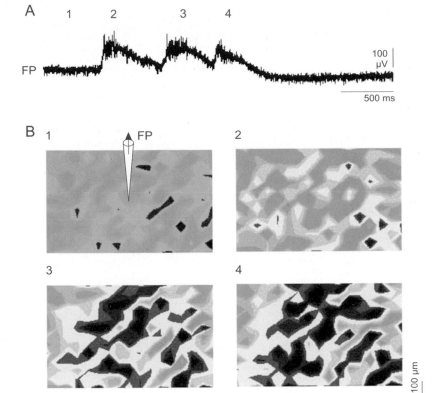

FIGURE 6.21 Simultaneous detection of membrane potentials (MP) of all neurons in a population (voltage-sensitive dye) and conventional recording of the local field potential (FP) at the same time. Living brain tissue (0.5 mm thick) from the temporal lobe of a patient who underwent epilepsy surgery. **A:** Recording of the local FP ("local EEG"). (1) Resting state, (2–4) epileptic discharges of different intensities. Epileptic discharges appeared spontaneously, i.e. they were not induced experimentally. **B:** MP changes indicated by the intensity of fluorescence of the dye (black = decrease of the MP, depolarization). Similar epileptic potentials in the FP (2 and 3) are associated with different extents of neuronal depolarizations and similar extents of neuronal depolarizations with different epileptic potentials in the FP (3 and 4) (62).

depolarizations with different epileptic potentials in the EEG (numbers 3 and 4).

CONCLUSION

Changes of neuronal activity associated with net current flows in the extracellular space produce field potentials. In clinical practice, a synchronization of the activity of neuronal elements is needed to recognize signals. As seen in superficial and deep potential fields, field potentials are generated in functionally different structures and may be based on different elementary mechanisms. Field potentials at the cortical surface, for example, can be interpreted in a variety of ways because they are not constantly related to neuronal activity in deep cortex.

References

1. Gaze RM. *The Formation of Nerve Connections.* New York: Academic Press; 1970.
2. Hubbard JI, Llinas R, Quastel DMJ. *Electrophysiological Analysis of Synaptic Transmission.* London: Edward Arnold; 1969.
3. Palay SL, Chan-Palay V. General morphology of neurons and neuroglia. In: Kandel ER, ed. *Handbook of Physiology, the Nervous System.* Vol 1. Bethesda, MD: American Physiological Society; 1977:5–37.
4. Purpura DP. Dendritic differentiation in human cerebral cortex: normal and aberrant developmental patterns. In: Kreutzberg GW, ed. *Advances in Neurology* Vol 12. New York: Raven Press; 1975:91–116.
5. Shepherd GM. *The Synaptic Organization of the Brain.* London: Oxford University Press; 1974.
6. Valverde F. The organization of area 18 in the monkey: a golgi study. *Anat Embryol.* 1978;154:305–334.
7. Westrum LE, Blackstad TW. An electromicroscopic study of the stratum radiatum of the rat hippocampus (regio superior, CA1) with particular emphasis on synaptology. *J Comp Neurol.* 1962;113:281–293.
8. Zenker W. Feinstruktur des Nervengewebes. In: Zenker W, ed. *Makroskopische und Mikroskopische Anatomie des Menschen.* Vol 3. Munich, Germany: Urban & Schwarzenberg; 1985:3–55.
9. Zschocke ST. *Klinische Elektroenzephalographie.* Berlin: Springer; 1995.
10. Eccles JC. *The Physiology of Synapses.* Berlin: Springer; 1964.
11. Rall W. Core conductor theory and cable properties of neurons. In: Kandel ER, ed. *Handbook of Physiology. The Nervous System.* Vol 1. Bethesda, MD: American Physiological Society; 1977:39–97.
12. Speckmann E-J. *Experimentelle Epilepsieforschung.* Darmstadt, Germany: Wissenschaftliche Buchgesellschaft; 1986.
13. De Robertis EDP, Carrea R, eds. *Biology of Neuroglia.* New York: Elsevier; 1965:15.
14. Kuffler SW, Nicholls JG. The physiology of neuroglial cells. *Erg Physiol.* 1966;57:1–90.
15. Kuffler SW, Nicholls JG, Orkand RK. Physiological properties of glial cells in the central nervous system of amphibia. *J Neurophysiol.* 1966;29:768–780.
16. Somjen GG, Trachtenberg M. Neuroglia as generator of extracellular current. In: Speckmann E-J, Caspers H, eds. *Origin of Cerebral Field Potentials.* Stuttgart, Germany: Thieme; 1979:21–32.
17. Speckmann E-J, Bingmann D. Komplexe Hirnfunktionen im Spiegel des EEG. In: Deetjen P, Speckmann E-J, eds. *Physiologie.* Vol 5.1. Munich, Germany: Urban & Fischer; 1999:225–232.
18. Speckmann E-J, Caspers H, Janzen RWC. Laminar distribution of cortical field potentials in relation to neuronal activities during seizure discharges. In: Brazier MAB, Petsche H, eds. *Architectonics of the Cerebral Cortex.* Vol 3. New York: Raven Press; 1978:191–209.
19. Speckmann E-J, Walden J. Mechanisms underlying the generation of cortical field potentials. *Acta Otolaryngol Suppl.* 1991;491:17–24.
20. Speckmann E-J, Caspers H, Elger CE. Neuronal mechanisms underlying the generation of field potentials. In: Elbert T, Rockstroh B, Liitzenberger W, et al., eds. *Self-regulation of the Brain and Behavior.* New York: Springer; 1984:9–25.
21. Creutzfeldt O, Houchin J. Neuronal basis of EEG waves. In: Remond A, ed. *Handbook of Electroencephalography and Clinical Neurophysiology.* Vol 2. Amsterdam: Elsevier; 1974:71–79.
22. Speckmann E-J, Caspers H. The effect of O_2- and CO_2-tensions in the nervous tissue on neuronal activity and DC potentials. In: Remond A, ed. *Handbook of Electroencephalography and Clinical Neurophysiology.* Vol 2. Amsterdam: Elsevier; 1974:71–89.
23. Speckmann E-J, Caspers H. Cortical field potentials in relation to neuronal activities in seizure conditions. In: Speckmann E-J, Caspers H, eds. *Origin of Cerebral Field Potentials.* Stuttgart, Germany: Thieme; 1979:205–213.

24. Speckmann E-J, Caspers H, eds. *Origin of Cerebral Field Potentials.* Stuttgart, Germany: Thieme; 1979.

25. Andersen P, Andersson SA. *Physiological Basis of the Alpha Rhythm.* New York, NY: Meredith Corp.; 1968.

26. Caspers H. Relations of steady potential shifts in the cortex to the wakefulness-sleep spectrum. In: Brazier MAB, ed. *Brain Function.* Berkeley: University of California Press; 1963:177–200.

27. Caspers H. DC potentials recorded directly from the cortex. In: Remond A, ed. *Handbook of Electroencephalography and Clinical Neurophysiology.* Vol 10. Amsterdam: Elsevier; 1974:3.

28. Caspers H, Speckmann E-J. DC potential shifts in paroxysmal states. In: Jasper HH, Ward AA Jr, Pope A, eds. *Basic Mechanisms of the Epilepsies.* Boston: Little, Brown; 1969:375–395.

29. Caspers H, Speckmann E-J. Cortical DC shifts associated with changes of gas tensions in blood and tissue. In: Remond A, ed. *Handbook of Electroencephalography and Clinical Neurophysiology.* Vol 10. Amsterdam: Elsevier; 1974:41–65.

30. Caspers H, Speckmann E-J, Lehmenkühler A. Effects of CO_2 on cortical field potentials in relation to neuronal activity. In: Speckmann E-J, Caspers H, eds. *Origin of Cerebral Field Potentials.* Stuttgart, Germany: Thieme; 1979:151–163.

31. Caspers H, Speckmann E-J, Lehmenkühler A. DC potentials of the cerebral cortex. Seizure activity and changes in gas pressures. *Rev Physiol Biochem Pharmacol.* 1987;106:127–178.

32. Goldring S. DC shifts released by direct and afferent stimulation. In: Remond A, ed. *Handbook of Electroencephalography and Clinical Neurophysiology.* Vol 10. Amsterdam: Elsevier; 1974:12–24.

33. Caspers H, Speckmann E-J, Lehmenkühler A. Electrogenesis of cortical DC potentials. In: Kornhuber HH, Deecke L, eds. *Motivation, Motor and Sensory Processes of the Brain: Electrical Potentials, Behaviour and Clinical Use.* Vol 54. New York: Elsevier; 1980:3–15.

34. Caspers H, Speckmann E-J, Lehmenkühler A. Electrogenesis of slow potentials of the brain. In: Elbert T, Rockstroh B, Lutzenberger W, et al., eds. *Self-regulation of the Brain and Behavior.* New York: Springer; 1984:26–41.

35. Jasper HH, Ward AA, Pope A, eds. *Basic Mechanisms of the Epilepsies.* Boston: Little, Brown; 1969.

36. Klee MR, Lux HD, Speckmann E-J, eds. *Physiology and Pharmacology of Epileptogenic Phenomena.* New York: Raven Press; 1982.

37. Klee MR, Lux HD, Speckmann E-J, eds. *Physiology, Pharmacology and Development of Epileptogenic Phenomena.* Berlin: Springer; 1991:20.

38. Purpura DP, Penry JK, Tower DE, et al., eds. *Experimental Models of Epilepsy.* New York: Raven Press; 1972.

39. Speckmann E-J, Elger CE. The neurophysiological basis of epileptic activity: a condensed review. In: Degen R, Niedermeyer E, eds. *Epilepsy, Sleep and Sleep Deprivation.* Amsterdam: Elsevier; 1984:23–34.

40. Speckmann E-J, Elger CE, eds. *Epilepsy and Motor System.* Baltimore, MD: Urban & Schwarzenberg; 1983.

41. Wieser HG. *Electroclinical Features of the Psychomotor Seizure. A Stereoencephalographic Study of Ictal Symptoms and Chronotopographical Seizure Patterns Including Clinical Effects of Intracerebral Stimulation.* New York: Gustav Fischer; 1983.

42. Elger CE, Speckmann E-J. Focal interictal epileptiform discharges (FIED) in the epicortical EEG and their relations to spinal field potentials in the rat. *Electroencephalogr Clin Neurophysiol.* 1980;48:447–460.

43. Elger CE, Speckmann E-J. Vertical inhibition in motor cortical epileptic foci and its consequences for descending neuronal activity to the spinal cord. In: Speckmann E-J, Elger CE, eds. *Epilepsy and Motor System.* Baltimore, MD: Urban & Schwarzenberg; 1983:152–160.

44. Elger CE, Speckmann E-J, Caspers H, et al. Focal interictal epileptiform discharges in the cortex of the rat: laminar restriction and its consequences for activity descending to the spinal cord. In: Klee MR, Lux HD, Speckmann E-J, eds. *Physiology and Pharmacology of Epileptogenic Phenomena.* New York: Raven Press; 1982:13–20.

45. Elger CE, Speckmann E-J, Prohaska O, et al. Pattern of intracortical potential distribution during focal interictal epileptiform discharges (FIED) and its relation to spinal field potentials in the rat. *Electroencephalogr Clin Neurophysiol.* 1981;51:393–402.

46. Petsche H, Müller-Paschinger IB, Pockberger H, et al. Depth profiles of electrocortical activities and cortical architectonics. In: Brazier MAB, Petsche H, eds. *Architectonics of the Cerebral Cortex.* Vol 3. New York: Raven Press; 1978:257–280.

47. Petsche H, Pockberger H, Rappelsberger P. Current source density studies of epileptic phenomena and the morphology of the rabbit's striate cortex. In: Klee MR, Lux HD, Speckmann E-J, eds. *Physiology and Pharmacology of Epileptogenic Phenomena.* New York: Raven Press; 1981:53–63.

48. Elger CE, Speckmann E-J. Penicillin-induced epileptic foci in the motor cortex: vertical inhibition. *Electroencephalogr Clin Neurophysiol.* 1983;56:604–622.

49. Köhling R, Höhling J-M, Straub H, et al. Optical monitoring of neuronal activity during spontaneous sharp waves in chronically epileptic human neocortical tissue. *J Neurophysiol.* 2000;84:2161–2165.

50. Köhling R, Reindel J, Vahrenhold J, et al. Spatio-temporal patterns of neuronal activity: analysis of optical imaging data using geometric shape matching. *J Neurosci Meth.* 2002;114:17–23.

51. Straub H, Kuhnt U, Höhling J-M, et al. Stimulus induced patterns of bioelectric activity in human neocortical tissue recorded by a voltage sensitive dye. *Neuroscience.* 2003;121:587–604.

52. Gumnit RJ, Matsumoto H, Vasconetto C. DC activity in the depth of an experimental epileptic focus. *Electroencephalogr Clin Neurophysiol.* 1970;28:333–339.

53. Gumnit RJ. DC shifts accompanying seizure activity. In: Remond A, ed. *Handbook of Electroencephalography and Clinical Neurophysiology.* Vol 10. Amsterdam: Elsevier; 1974:66–77.

54. Speckmann E-J, Caspers H, Janzen RWC. Relations between cortical DC shifts and membrane potential changes of cortical neurons associated with seizure activity. In: Petsche H, Brazier MAB, eds. *Synchronization of EEG Activity in Epilepsies.* New York: Springer; 1972:93–111.

55. Cohen LB, Salzberg BM. Optical measurement of membrane potential. *Rev Physiol Biochem Pharmacol.* 1978;83:35–83.

56. Ebner TJ, Chen G. Use of voltage-sensitive dyes and optical recordings in the central nervous system. *Prog Neurobiol.* 1985;46:463–506.

57. Köhling R, Höhling J-M, Straub H, et al. Optical monitoring of neuronal activity during spontaneous sharp waves in chronically epileptic human neocortical tissue. *J Neurophysiol.* 2000;84:2161–2165.

58. Köhling R, Reinel J, Vahrenhold J, et al. Spatio-temporal patterns of neuronal activity: analysis of optical imaging data using geometric shape matching. *J Neurosci Meth.* 2002;114:17–23.

59. Straub H, Kuhnt U, Höhling J-M, et al. Stimulus induced patterns of bioelectric activity in human neocortical tissue recorded by a voltage sensitive dye. *Neurosci.* 2003;121:587–604.

60. Grinvald A, Hildesheim R. VSDI: A new era in functional imaging of cortical dynamics. *Nat Rev Neurosci.* 2004;5:874–885.

61. Gorji A, Straub H, Speckmann E-J. Epilepsy surgery: perioperative investigations of intractable epilepsy. *Anat Embryol* (Berlin). 2005;210:525–537.

62. Speckmann, E.-J. The brain of my art. *Creativity and Self-Conscious Brain.* Münster;2008:232.

CHAPTER 7 ■ LOCALIZATION AND FIELD DETERMINATION IN ELECTROENCEPHALOGRAPHY

RICHARD C. BURGESS

LOCALIZATION AND MAPPING

The word "electroencephalogram" (EEG) is derived from Greek roots to create a term meaning an electrical picture of the brain. While interpreting an EEG, electroencephalographers maintain a three-dimensional picture of the brain/head in their minds. In principle, there are an infinite number of different source configurations of an electrical event within the head that may give rise to the same electrical field distribution at the scalp. Despite this theoretical constraint, one of the key functions of the electroencephalographer is to conceptualize the generators in relationship to this vision and to build an increasingly clear mental image of the foci of these generators. Methods for localization and field determination are tools to help the electroencephalographer infer the location, strength, and orientation of generator sources within the cortex, based on their manifestation at 21 or more EEG recording sites.

Scalp electrical activity arises from both physiological and pathological brain generators. Localization of epileptiform potentials from scalp EEG is critically important to pinpoint the epileptic focus and identify the region of brain pathology (1). Many electroencephalographers have taken a simplistic approach, assuming that the generator source must be close to the point where the maximum voltage is recorded. Attempts to systematize the localization of specific EEG activity date back to the early years of electroencephalography. In the mid-1930s, Adrian and Matthews (2) as well as Adrian and Yamagiwa (3) employed phase reversal techniques to localize normal rhythms, and Walter (4) used phase reversals for localization of abnormal EEG activity, as did Gibbs and Gibbs (5) in 1941 in their classic atlas. More recently, a variety of reviews have outlined general principles for the use of polarity, montages, and localization (5–11). It should be emphasized that phase reversals are not inherently an indicator of abnormality. Phase reversals occur as a result of both normal and abnormal activities. Phase reversals are most obvious for sharply contoured transient activity and therefore in the case of epileptiform abnormalities provide a dramatic visual clue.

Despite the critical importance of accuracy in localization, there has been an absence in the literature of descriptions of systematic methods for accomplishing this localization in a simple, manual fashion (12,13). Most textbooks emphasize the distribution that would occur as a result of an assumed generator (i.e., the "forward" problem). With the evolution of digital EEG (14) a variety of methods for computerized source localization have become available (15,16) at the push of a button within the EEG machine itself or as stand-alone software (17,18). These techniques are model-based and have significant limitations; they have generally not been employed in routine clinical practice. A practical guide for the step-by-step identification of the origin of epileptiform activity has been developed at the Cleveland Clinic Foundation (19) and is covered in some detail here.

The principles of source localization apply to any type of brain electrical activity; however this review will concentrate primarily on defining the electrophysiologic origin of epileptiform activity. While epileptologists generally rely heavily on the location of interictal discharges in the workup of patients leading up to epilepsy surgery (20,21), the relationship of the irritative zone (as manifest by interictal spikes) to the epileptogenic zone (identification of which is obviously crucial for surgical success) has been the subject of much debate (22,23). Nevertheless, the majority of the points covered in this review will be illustrated using interictal spikes.

There are two steps in the interpretation of epileptiform discharges: *surface field determination* and *source localization*. Proper determination of the electrical field results from knowledge of the electrode positions and head shape, and has only one answer. Accurate field determination is essential not only for accurate source localization but also for discrimination of epileptic activity from other nonepileptic transients. For source localization on the other hand, no single unique solution exists. In order to arrive at a plausible solution for the source location, several assumptions are useful. In this chapter, practical neurophysiological concepts that relate the generator to the surface electrical fields will be described in the first section. Then, the next three sections describe important conventions used in visual interpretation of EEG regarding instrumentations, the field determination, and the source localization. Lastly, the application of computer-based techniques that aim to assist in the localization problem will be briefly discussed.

PRACTICAL CONCEPTS OF ELECTRICAL FIELDS APPLIED TO BRAIN GENERATORS

Sources

The electrical sources seen at the scalp arise from intracranial focal dipoles or sheets of dipoles. These dipoles represent the postsynaptic potentials originating from vertically oriented neurons. A unit current dipole is created by the intercellular laminar currents in the apical dendrites arising from the pyramidal cells in the outer layer of the cerebral cortex. Specifically, superficial excitatory postsynaptic potentials and deep inhibitory postsynaptic potentials generate almost all spontaneous EEG activities (24), particularly the epileptogenic abnormalities. When populations of neurons are more or less synchronously activated for relatively long durations, the activity can be macroscopically recorded from a certain distance as a linear summation of the unit dipoles (25–27). This summated activity may also be represented as a dipole or sheet of dipoles along the cortex. Thus the generator of epileptic activity can be explained by a single or multiple equivalent current dipoles (8,13,28,29). The surface potential can be thought of as a two-dimensional projection or shadow of a complex three-dimensional electrical object residing inside the head.

Fundamental to scalp localization is the concept of the "inverse" problem, which entails an estimate, based on surface data, of the magnitude, location, and distribution of electrical fields throughout the brain. Whereas the forward problem is solvable with unique solutions, the inverse problem is not. The mathematical representation of the biophysics underlying volume conduction is covered by Nunez (9).

The forward problem can be stated as follows: Given known charge distributions and volume conductor geometries and properties, predict the resulting surface potential distribution. The solution involves applying numerical or analytical methods for any known set of geometries and boundary conditions (9,30) to solve Poisson's equation:

$$\nabla^2 \Phi = -\frac{\rho}{\varepsilon}$$

where ∇^2 is the second spatial gradient operator, Φ is the scalar potential in volts, ρ is the free charge density, and ε is the permittivity of the mass of tissue. Multiple sources can be shown to combine linearly, so that a combination of sources results in the arithmetic sum of the potential distributions that each would produce individually.

The corresponding inverse problem can be stated as follows: Given a surface potential distribution and the volume conductor geometries and properties, determine the underlying charge distribution. Unfortunately, a given surface map can be produced by any of an infinite number of possible source distributions. EEG records at a distance from the sources, and employs only a limited number of sensors—typically 20 to 30 in a routine scalp EEG. Therefore, this problem generally has no unique solution (31). Nevertheless, simplifying assumptions are usually made: (i) The source dipole is near the surface; (ii) the source dipole is perpendicular to the surface; (iii) the head is a uniform, homogeneous volume conductor; (iv) at least one recording electrode is essentially over the source; and (v) the reference is not contained in the active region.

On the basis of these assumptions, one generally looks for a single predominating potential maximum on the surface, with the source lying directly below it; however, a variety of nondipolar source configurations could produce the same observation. For example, a simple monopolar charge buildup, a curved dipole sheet, or a finite-thickness dipole "pancake" would all produce a single well-defined maximum. In addition, signals originating from confined but deep-seated generators will be broadly distributed when recorded from the surface (32,33), and these cannot be reliably distinguished from more superficial but widespread epileptic regions.

In addition to these "equivalent" source possibilities, others are physiologically similar but generate very different surface maps. Through variations in orientation and shape, dipole sheets can produce charge reorientation and cancellation. The resultant range of possible scalp distributions serves as a reminder that observed scalp maxima do not necessarily lie directly above maximal brain activity. Jayakar et al. (34) have pointed out the difficulties in localizing epileptic foci on the basis of simple models, owing to effects from dipolar orientation, anatomic variations, and inhomogeneities, among other factors.

Volume Conduction

In a volume conductor, the electrical field spreads instantaneously over an infinite number of pathways between the positive and negative ends of the dipole. Outside the neuron, the circuit is completed by the current flowing through the extracellular fluid in a direction opposite to the intracellular current. Through the process of volume conduction, electrical activity originates from a generator and spreads through a conductive medium to be picked up by a distant recording electrode. Volume conduction is passive—that is, it does not involve active regeneration of the signal by intervening neurons or synaptic relays—and occurs as easily through saline as through brain parenchyma. Potentials recorded by way of volume conduction are picked up synchronously and at the speed of light at all recording electrodes. Although attenuated with distance by the medium, volume-conducted components preserve their original polarity and morphology.

The attenuation factor is defined by the inverse square law: That is, the recorded electrical potential falls off in direct proportion to the square of the distance from the generator (35,36). For example, a 100 microvolt potential seen at the electrode directly overlying a cortical generator (assume a distance of 1 cm away) will be reflected as a 4 microvolt potential at an electrode that is 5 cm away and as only a 1 microvolt potential at 10 cm away. The rapidity of this falloff is a function of the depth of the generator, with more superficial generators falling off much more rapidly. Distant generators have a "flat" falloff, one of the hallmarks of a "far-field" potential (Fig. 7.1).

The medium through which current travels to reach the recording electrode is not homogeneous but rather exhibits a variety of conductivities (37). As the current attempts to complete its circuit by following the path of least resistance, these differences in conductivities, especially differences among cerebrospinal fluid (CSF), skull, and scalp, and their associated boundaries affect the electrical potential recorded on the scalp. The signal is not only altered in amplitude but also undergoes an apparent low-pass-filtering during its passage to the surface because of the spatial summation and shunting effects of the intervening layers. In the skull, the conductivity in a tangential direction is higher than in a direction perpendicular to the surface. This produces a "smearing effect" on the surface potential distribution (38). Although the current tends to flow along the path of least resistance, there is still some flow throughout the volume conductor, thereby permitting recording of the electrical potential at all sites on the

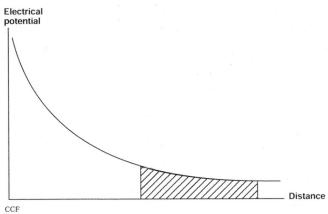

FIGURE 7.1 The electrical potential recorded by an electrode decreases in a parabolic fashion the farther away from the source it is. The difference recorded between two electrodes close to the source (near-field potentials) will be greater than the differential recordings from the tail of the curve. These far-field potentials (in the shaded region) are also lower in absolute amplitude.

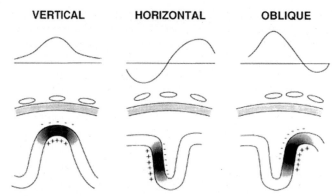

FIGURE 7.2 There are unusual sources wherein both the negative and the positive poles are recorded on the surface. The bottom row of figures shows a patch of cortex containing gyri and sulci. The darker areas represent the cortical mantle that is activated by an epileptic discharge, with negative and positive poles highlighted. In the middle row of illustrations, the positions of the electrodes on the scalp, relative to the discharging cortex are shown. The top row illustrates the voltage that would be recorded on the EEG as a function of the distance along the scalp right below it.

volume conductor, albeit with the amplitude inversely related to the square of the distance from the source (see Fig. 7.1).

The head also contains normal or abnormal openings that present low-resistance paths to conducted currents. The current tends to flow toward skull defects, whether physiologic (such as foramina) or acquired through trauma or surgery, and around cavities (such as the ventricles), markedly distorting the field in the region of the defect. The resistivity of scalp or brain tissue is many times smaller than that of bone (39–41). As a result, surface potentials near these openings will be unusually high and the largest potentials can be seen at the location of the defect even when the source is several centimeters away from the defect (38,42,43).

Surface Electrical Manifestations

A variety of real-world considerations complicate the interpretation of surface recordings. Because the dipoles measured at the scalp ordinarily are oriented radially, scalp electrodes see primarily the positive or the negative pole. Although generators located at the apex of a gyrus lie perpendicular to the scalp (i.e., vertical dipoles), any generator within a cortical fissure will present a dipole at an angle to the scalp. Nearly 70% of the cortical surface lies within the sulcal depths (44). In addition, many brain areas—most notably the mesial frontal, parietal, occipital, and basal temporal cortex—are diversely oriented and lie at varying distances from surface electrodes. Hence, it is not sufficient to assume that the generator must be close to the point where the maximum potential is recorded (7). Finally, the choice of reference affects the form of the EEG measurements.

When a generator dipole is oblique or parallel to the scalp, the resulting surface potentials can lead to false localization of the potential maximum. The typical bell-shaped distribution of the electrical field is replaced by one shaped like a sideways "S." Because both the positive and the negative ends of the dipole may be recorded at the scalp, the surface potential can exhibit two "maxima" of opposite polarity. Between the two ends will be a zero isopotential boundary where the generator will not be picked up at all (Fig. 7.2).

It is important to distinguish true horizontal dipoles, such as those arising at a sulcus or the interhemispheric fissure, from field distributions resulting from widely separated activity but giving rise to distinct negative and positive maxima. For example, bisynchronous temporal spikes differing slightly in phase, such that the negative component on the left aligns with the positive component on the right, may appear to represent huge transverse dipoles (34); however, careful evaluation with an alternative reference (or the demonstration that the spikes also occur asynchronously) can prove that the fields represent not the source and sink of a single dipole but rather two generators (45) linked by corticocortical propagation.

When a source lies deeper in the brain, two changes occur: The surface potential becomes smaller and the field becomes more widespread relative to the surface maximum (32,33,46). Although the shape of the electrical field gradient can indicate the type of field and the distance of the generator, identifying the source on the basis of the potential difference between any scalp electrodes becomes increasingly difficult. When the potential field gradient is relatively flat, as is the case in the far-field potential from a deep-seated source, a bipolar montage will display the waveform at relatively smaller amplitude (see Fig. 7.1). Diffuse discharges may be better appreciated on referential montages, assuming that the reference is not involved. An adequate "vantage point" may be impossible with surface electrodes when the focus is deep. It may be impossible to find a scalp electrode reference that is not electrically involved in the active region, and some cases can only be resolved by invasive electrode placements that can monitor more limited areas (see Chapter 82) (30,47–50).

The combination of multiple sources can produce a variety of results. A superficial source can overshadow a deep one, distorting or even hiding it. Because the amplitude of a measured potential is inversely proportional to the square of the distance from the recording electrode, nearby sources can appear significantly higher at the recording electrodes. A given electrode thus has a "view" of the nearby generators, such that dipoles that combine to reinforce each other will have a large net effect, whereas those that cancel will produce a smaller or null potential (51).

Complicating this problem is the fact that the equivalent dipole is an abstraction. In reality, only sources that extend over multiple layers of several square centimeters of cortical tissue have sufficient energy to generate detectable scalp discharges (46,52). An epileptogenic zone almost always consists of a continuum of dipoles, resulting in a sheet or "patch" (53) dipole. Such a source may cover an extended brain region, with the constituent areas lying at various depths and orientations. Again, both reinforcement and cancellation are possible to produce a variety of surface potential distributions. Overall, the conduction phenomena leading to surface potentials follow the "solid-angle" rule (54), that is, the net surface potential is proportional to the solid angle subtended by the recording electrode. Unless a dipole sheet parallels the surface, the maximum surface potential may be elsewhere than directly over the affected area, as illustrated in Figure 7.3. The solid angle theorem helps to explain the results of multiple synchronously discharging pyramidal neurons arrayed over a cortical region containing both sulci and gyri.

In the same way that opposing dipoles can cancel each other relative to a distant electrode, a sheet of nonparallel dipoles can produce a "closed" field (55) whose potential contributions will cancel, resulting in a negligible potential at the surface (56). These generators, usually not visible on scalp EEG, are observed primarily on invasive recordings (51). Even when not a completely closed field, multipolar source–sink configurations tend to produce more cancellation than dipolar generators and to attenuate more quickly as a function of distance (9). This irregular structure is particularly likely in the basal and mesial areas of the temporal cortex and the hippocampus, where cortical infolding is so prevalent (57).

The head consists of a series of roughly concentric layers that separate the brain from the scalp surface. Each of these layers—CSF, meninges, bone, and skin— presents different electrical characteristics to the currents that conduct the EEG to the surface. These layers occasion considerable current spreading, which causes the potential from localized foci to appear in a much broader scalp area (9,58). Spreading in itself would not be an insurmountable problem, because it is theoretically possible to recover deep dipole sources based on observed surface potentials, using appropriate mathematical transformations. Such recovery, however, is guaranteed only in a perfectly spherical concentric conductor, onto which electrodes can be placed in any location. The head is not a perfect globe, however, and significant constraints disqualify the face or neck, which may be preferred for certain sources, as electrode sites.

Electrode Placement as Spatial Sampling

Placement of scalp electrodes should be considered an exercise in spatial sampling. Electrode density must be generous enough to capture the available information but not so closely spaced as to overwhelm with redundant data. Inability to precisely locate a cortical generator may be the result of spatial undersampling ("aliasing"). The assumption that a potential will decrease monotonically as distance increases from the involved electrode is based not only on an uncomplicated electrical field, that is, a monopole, but also on an electrode placement sufficiently dense to accurately represent the spatial contours of the field. Cooper et al. (52) suggested that at least 6 cm^2 of cortex discharging simultaneously is required to reflect a visible potential on the scalp surface, and more recently it has been suggested that the required area for surface detectability is even larger, based on simultaneous intracranial and scalp EEG recordings (22,59). Because most epileptogenic potentials seen on the scalp are visible at multiple electrodes, a considerably larger cortical area must be synchronously discharging to produce these potentials.

Especially controversial is the detectability of spikes generated in the mesial temporal lobe. Some authors believe that scalp EEG recording of deep sources is possible (121), while others have found it impossible to record spikes from the mesial temporal structures (60,61). Sphenoidal electrodes provide a significantly better view of the mesial area, as shown in Figure 7.4, and are frequently employed in epilepsy monitoring units.

The widely accepted International 10–20 Electrode Placement System (62), although relatively easy to apply reproducibly, has some inherent limitations in terms of the accuracy of localization (63). When more precise localization is indicated to avoid spatial aliasing, scalp electrodes should be placed at least once every 2.5 cm (64). The maximum spacing can be determined theoretically (65) as well as experimentally, and as many as 128 electrodes (spaced approximately 2 cm apart) may sometimes be necessary (66).

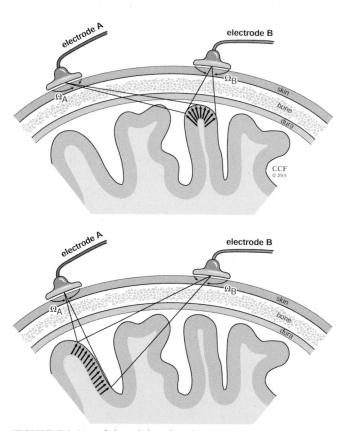

FIGURE 7.3 Use of the solid-angle rule to ascertain the signal measured on the scalp surface relative to the orientation of the dipole. **Top:** Surface electrode B sees a large electrical potential because of the orientation and proximity of the dipole layer, as borne out by the solid angle Ω_B. **Bottom:** In this case, the potential seen by electrode A is actually lower than that measured by the more distant electrode B because of the arrangement of the dipoles in the discharging region. The smaller solid angle, Ω_A, is proportional to the voltage measured on the scalp.

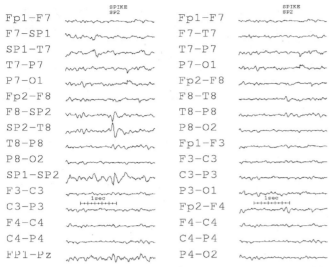

FIGURE 7.4 This EEG shows an example of a spike that is highly focal in the right sphenoidal electrode. Note that in the conventional double-banana longitudinal montage without the sphenoidals, this discharge is almost invisible.

Boundary Problems

Regardless of the fineness of the scalp electrode grid, boundary effects will occur at the edges of the array. The maximum potential must be well within the scope of the recording electrodes to ascertain that a physiologic gradient exists away from the electrode. For example, epileptic sharp waves arising from mesial temporal structures are frequently localized outside the area covered by the 10–20 placement (67–70). It is impossible to determine the complete extent of the maximum fields unless the area is surrounded by regions of lesser activity. Recordings in which the activity is large all the way to the boundary of the region defined by the montage must be "remontaged" to include, if possible, all the relevant electrodes, or further recording must be carried out with additional electrodes. This may be especially complicated when it is difficult to position electrodes inferior to the customary borders of scalp coverage.

A significant portion of the head cannot be practically surveyed and important brain areas such as the basomesial temporal cortex and other deep sources are only indirectly accessible with standard scalp electrodes. Additional electrodes inferior to the 10–20 System (62) must be employed to provide a better view. In certain circumstances, the information obtained from a combination of closely spaced scalp electrodes such as the International 10–10 System (71–73) and sphenoidal electrodes can obviate the need for more invasive recordings (74).

EEG INSTRUMENTATION CONSIDERATIONS RELATED TO LOCALIZATION

Differential Amplifiers

Amplifiers used in clinical neurophysiology measure the difference between two potentials at the inputs to the amplifier and provide an amplified version of this difference at the

output. These devices, called differential amplifiers, eliminate unwanted signals that are identical at both inputs, called common-mode signals. The two terminals at the input to a differential amplifier are sometimes labeled G1 and G2, recalling when a screened "grid" within the vacuum tube amplifier controlled the flow of electrons from cathode to plate. Modern opamp-based differential amplifiers employ complex integrated circuits, and the terms "input 1" and "input 2" are used throughout this chapter.

The amplifier itself has no concept of polarity; it simply does the subtraction and the gain multiplication and then provides an output voltage that is a linear function of the input voltages, according to the following equation:

$$V_{\text{output}}(t) = G \times [V_{\text{input1}}(t) - V_{\text{input2}}(t)]$$

where $V_{\text{output}}(t)$ and $V_{\text{input}N}(t)$ are the output and input voltages and G is the gain of the amplifier. Only during interpretation of the EEG waveform in the context of the underlying generators does the concept of polarity have any meaning. Inexperienced electroencephalographers often mistakenly ascribe a polarity at the input to a specific pen deviation at the output (12). It should be remembered that there are no positive deflections and no negative deflections. There are only upward and downward deflections (12). Figure 7.5 illustrates four different input conditions that give rise to exactly the same deflection.

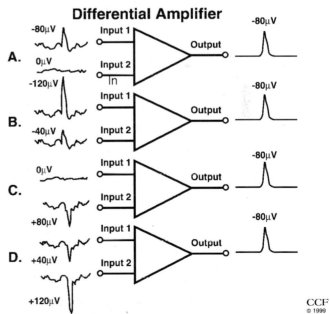

FIGURE 7.5 A and B illustrate a surface-negative spike. Input 1 is more negative than input 2. Because a differential amplifier responds only to the difference between the two inputs (input 1 − input 2), the spikes illustrated will yield identical output voltages; (−80) − (0) is the same as (−120) − (−40). The background electroencephalogram activity, because it is more widespread than the spikes and therefore almost the same at both inputs, is largely canceled out. In C and D, the spike is surface positive, that is, input 2 is more positive than input 1. The calculations (0) − (+80) and (+40) − (+120) both result in an answer of −80, and the background is still canceled out. All four circumstances yield identical outputs despite the differing amplitudes and polarities.

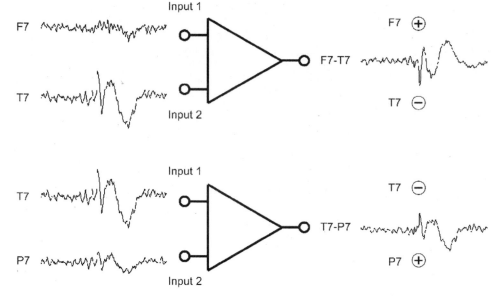

Differential amplifiers and polarity convention

FIGURE 7.6 Differential amplifier and polarity conventions. The differential amplifier is designed to amplify only the difference between the signals at the two inputs. An upward deflection appearing at the output is caused by input 1 being more negative than input 2. A downward deflection results from input 1 being more positive than input 2. This convention is common to all clinical EEG machines. When the name of the electrode (i.e., its "derivation") connected to input 1 is written above the waveform and that connected to input 2 is written below as in this figure, the deflection always points to the electrode of higher "relative" negativity.

Polarity Conventions

Deflection refers to the direction on the page or display screen in which the waveform component under study appears to go, and it is a function only of the display instrumentation. By EEG convention, upward deflections are caused by input 1 being more negative than input 2. Downward deflections are caused by input 1 being more positive than input 2 (75). These relationships imply nothing about the underlying polarity of the signals at inputs 1 and 2—only the polarity of their *differences*. When the name of electrode connected to input 1 is written above the deflection and the name of input 2 below, the deflection will point to the electrode with the "relative" negativity as has been done in Figure 7.6.

If the difference between the two signals at the input is zero, no deflection will occur. When two electrodes (no matter how close to the source of the sharp wave or spike) that lie along the same isopotential line (typically at the same distance from the generator) are input to a differential amplifier, the output will reflect no activity, even though both electrodes may be measuring high amplitudes in an absolute sense. Some amplifiers used in basic neurophysiology research and in clinical evoked potentials employ another convention, designed to display positive input 1 as an upward deflection.

Derivations and Montages

A derivation describes the connections of the electrodes to the amplifier inputs. A montage is a combination of derivations arranged down the EEG page to display many amplifier channels simultaneously in a way that aids in the identification and localization of abnormalities (76). Each amplifier could be connected to any pair of electrodes available. Likewise, these amplifier outputs could be arranged in any fashion on the screen; the arrangement in *chains* assists our visual localization capabilities.

The arrangement of derivations into a montage determines whether it is called bipolar or referential. Derivations in bipolar montages are established between neighboring electrodes to emphasize focal activity. They take advantage of the subtractive nature of differential amplifiers to effect a high degree of cancellation. Any montage can be analyzed to locate the maximum of a sharp wave or spike, provided that the montage has a logical order (6,77,78). It is convenient to link the electrodes in a systematic "chain" of bipolar derivations. Because input 1 of each succeeding channel in the montage is the same as input 2 of the preceding channel, the electrodes are all electrically linked in a structured way, and—more importantly—mathematically.

Bipolar montages are of maximum advantage when attempting to pick out localized potentials, as they help to cancel out more widespread activity. Bipolar montages are most logically arranged in a longitudinal or transverse direction. In a referential montage, the same electrode is connected to input 2 of every channel, while each channel has a different electrode connected to input 1. In contrast to bipolar montages, referential montages do a better job of picking up activity that has a more widespread distribution.

ELECTRICAL FIELD DETERMINATION ON THE SCALP

Identification of Peaks; Measurement of the Amplitude

Interictal epileptiform abnormalities are recognized by their morphology—an impression of "standing out" from the background—and by their electrical field distribution, which must demonstrate a realistic relationship between the electrical potentials at topographically associated electrode positions. In choosing an abnormality to localize, the peak selected must be representative of the patient's population of spikes, and the sample must be as clean as possible.

It is assumed that an activity starts from "zero" and reaches its maximum after a certain time. The amplitude of the activity is measured between the zero and the maximum peak. However, it is often difficult to identify the level of the "zero" in each EEG channel correctly, because the activity is superimposed on the background, arises from the noise level, or continues from the preceding activity. Sometimes sharp activity can be separated from a slower background, if the frequency of the epileptic activity is clearly different, by using filtering.

Practically, the amplitude is measured as peak-to-peak or baseline-to-peak. Identification of the baseline and peak may be particularly troublesome in the case of polyphasic discharges, in which each phase is brief and difficult to line up temporally. When analyzing a peak, the maximum value in each EEG channel should be identified at exactly the same time point. During visual analysis of a waveform, the montage selected will influence identification of the peak, resulting in different, or sometimes erroneous, field determinations. Multiple peaks or phase reversals with small time shifts reflect sequential change in the location of the maximum. In the EEG tracings shown in Figure 7.7, note that the peaks of several of the channels were reached on different phases of the waveform, giving the erroneous appearance of a phase reversal. Computerized source localization techniques are especially sensitive to the selection of the appropriate time frame. Errors in identifying the peaks that are to be mapped can cause extraordinary displacements in the apparent localization of the sources (79,80).

The peak of the sharp wave (i.e., the negative extrema) generally has the highest amplitude at the electrode closest to the involved cortical epileptogenic neurons (7). The main component of an epileptic discharge may be preceded by a smaller deflection of the opposite polarity. Early components show a more localized field than later ones (81,82), and they are more synchronous than the slow wave that frequently follows a spike. Thus, the initial deflection probably contains more localizing information (34), and employing the lower-frequency waves for localization may not always represent the epileptogenic region.

Mapping the Electrical Field

The two-dimensional display of the scalp regions involved in epileptiform or other activity is called mapping. Isopotential lines are drawn on a representation of the scalp to specify the topography of equivalent electrical potentials, similar to the isocontour lines drawn by a surveyor on a land map. From the area where the activity is maximum, succeeding regions that are further away will show a lower amplitude and can be divided into convenient isopotential contours. Because EEG amplitude is always measured with respect to a reference, the absolute amplitude will be dependent on the reference. But as shown in Figure 7.8, the *shape* of the contour distribution does not change with the reference.

The potential fields of spikes and sharp waves can be mapped even without electronic assistance by tracking the relationships of the electrical potential level between electrodes. As the initial step, a longitudinal or transverse chain of the electrodes is used to map the one-dimensional relationship of voltage level to electrode position, as illustrated in Figure 7.9, top. Then, two chains are connected to each other through a common electrode to obtain the two-dimensional relationship. To create an isopotential contour map, a 100% value is assigned to the maximum and a 0% value is assigned to the minimum. However, as discussed later, the polarity of the maximum depends on an assumption about the generator. The "maximum" may be the highest negative point or the

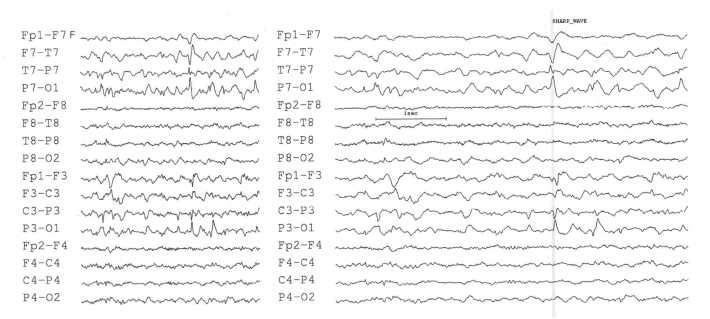

FIGURE 7.7 Phase reversals—choosing the same component. Be certain to select the proper phase of the discharge. The EEG on the left appears to show a confusing distribution, at first glance, with phase reversals at multiple sites. On the right, the timescale of the same epoch has been doubled. The vertical marker reveals that the discharge actually consists of three phases, with each peak at a slightly different time. The phase revereal at T_7–P_7 occurs prior to the phase reversal at P_3.

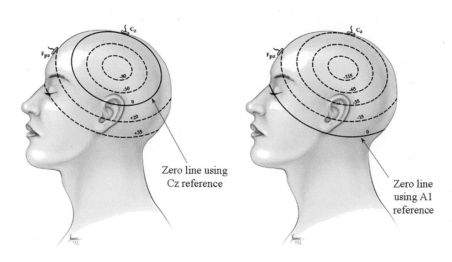

Zero line using
Cz reference

Zero line
using A1
reference

FIGURE 7.8 Topographical distribution of electrical potentials (in microvolts). EEG amplitudes are always measured *relative* to another reference. Note that the specific choice of reference electrode does not affect the *shape* of the isocontours of this left temporal discharge.

highest positive point. Similarly, the "minimum" may be negative or positive, or may have a mid-curve value when two maxima of opposite polarity are assumed, for example, a horizontal dipole generator. Depending on the polarity of the maximum, that is the point given a 100% value, at least two different isocontour maps can be obtained, as shown in Figure 7.10. To make the correct choice, some assumptions must be introduced, as described later.

The ideal situation in referential recording occurs when the reference electrode is totally inactive or picks up activity of negligible amplitude. In this situation, those channels showing some activity will deflect in one direction only, as illustrated in Figure 7.9, bottom. The electrode closest to the generator will show the largest pen deflection, and the amplitude of the deflection in all the other channels will be directly proportional to the magnitude of the activity recorded from each of those electrodes. This situation makes it especially easy to find the maximum and to assess the extent of the field distribution (see Fig. 7.9). To achieve this ideal situation, an alert technologist will recognize a contaminated reference and construct a "distribution montage," typically with a reference electrode from the other hemisphere (Fig. 7.11).

In mapping potentials measured from a bipolar recording, the bipolar measurements first must be converted to voltages relative to a selected "reference" electrode. The wisest choice usually is to select the least involved electrode at the beginning

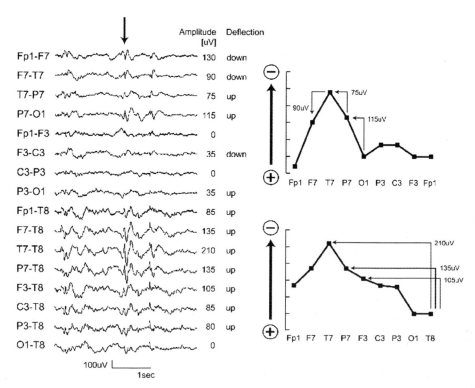

Voltage / Electrode map

FIGURE 7.9 Voltage/electrode map. The EEG shows the same activity in two different montages: a bipolar montage in the top eight traces and a referential montage in the bottom eight. Two voltage/electrode maps for the spike indicated by the *arrow* are reconstructed manually from the two montages, respectively. In the bipolar montage, the difference of the potential level (amplitude) and relative polarity (deflection) between neighboring electrodes is sequentially tracked along the "chain" of the montage. Here, the potential mapping was started from a common electrode O_1 with a value of 0 μV assumed. Employing the algebraic relationships between the electrode derivations, the calculated amplitudes at each individual electrode are graphed. The resulting voltage level at Fp_1 differed slightly between the two bipolar chains, owing to minor differences in manual measurement of the amplitudes. For the referential montage, the measured amplitudes are written down directly, as no calculations are necessary. If all the deflections are in the same direction and the referential electrode (input 2) is located at the minimum, as seen in this example, then the amplitude of the deflection simply reflects the voltage level of the electrode. No matter which montage is used, the field determination should be same in terms of location of the maximum. The voltage/electrode maps may differ in detail, however, reflecting a varying degree of visibility of the spike between montages.

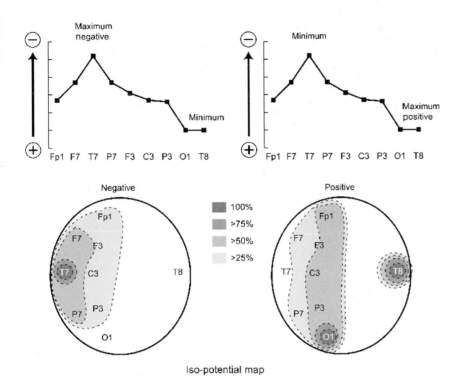

FIGURE 7.10 Isopotential map. As in Figure 7.1, the vertical axis of the top figures represents electrical potential, and the horizontal axis shows electrode location. A 100% value is assigned to the maximum and a 0% value is assigned to the minimum. Depending on the polarity of the maximum, at least two different maps can be obtained, illustrated on the bottom row. In the map on the left side the maximum is assumed to be negative, and the falloff of potential with distance is physiological. On the right, the opposite assumption was made, that is, the maximum is a positive potential, resulting in a very unphysiological distribution. Thus, it was deduced that this spike has maximum negativity from the left temporal area.

or end of the chains, taking advantage of the fact that certain electrodes are common to more than one chain. For instance, in the "double-banana" longitudinal montage, the frontal polar and occipital electrodes occur in both ipsilateral chains. These common electrodes provide an electrical connection between chains and allow an algebraic determination of the potential gradient of the electrical field over the entire area covered by the two chains. Because all the electrodes in both chains are related to each other by a sequence of subtractions, one can determine the relative amplitude at any electrode to the reference electrode. Of course, the exact amplitude (in absolute terms) at any scalp electrode is unknown. However, electrodes relatively distant from the site of maximum activity "see" a negligible potential, hence the assumption that the potential of the particular transient under study at these uninvolved electrodes is zero. The fact that the potential at this

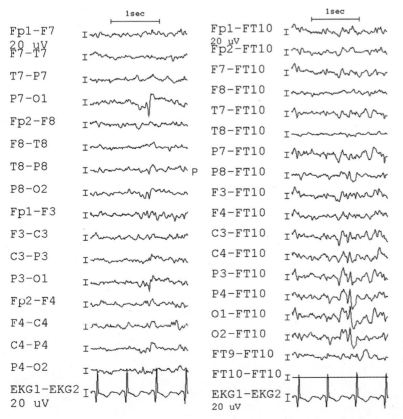

FIGURE 7.11 On the left, a bipolar montage with no phase reversal suggests that the activity is either at the beginning or the end of the chain. The same time period is shown on the right, and the distribution montage to an uninvolved contralateral electrode confirms the left posterior maximum of this surface-negative discharge.

uninvolved electrode may not be exactly zero is unimportant because the relative differences between electrodes will be appropriately preserved.

Although it is possible to localize a spike or sharp wave from a single montage if electrical connections between the chains (or appropriate assumptions) exist, recording from multiple montages, especially "crisscrossing" montages, will help to confirm the topography of the discharge and can better define the topographic distribution. When the amplitudes of the potential distribution do not match exactly between chains or montages, the discrepancies most likely arise from errors in visual measurement, erroneous assumptions of zero potential, or difficulty recognizing the same waveform in different montages. Generally, referential montages with uninvolved references will be better able to map the distribution of the activity.

The procedure for mapping the potential field, illustrated in Figures 7.9 and 7.10, can be summarized as follows:

1. Measure the amplitude of the component of interest in each channel.
2. Select an electrode that appears to be uninvolved. Assume a value of zero for that electrode.
3. Calculate the amplitude of all the electrodes relative to the selected electrode, based on the algebraic relationship established by the montage.
4. Follow this procedure for all the chains connected by common electrodes.
5. Assume another zero electrode to calculate the distribution in chains not connected by a common electrode.
6. If the resulting distribution has potentials both above and below zero, start with another "zero" electrode.
7. Draw isopotential contours around the resulting distribution.
8. If the topographic distribution is unphysiologic, assume the opposite polarity for the waveform.

These principles can be applied most profitably when electrode montages are simple and systematic, as recommended by the American Clinical Neurophysiology Society (76).

Rules for Field Identification

A practical set of rules for identification of the electrical fields seen on the EEG is outlined in Table 7.1.

TABLE 7.1

RULES FOR POTENTIAL DISTRIBUTION

Montage type	Phase reversal	Conclusion
Bipolar	No	Maximum or minimum is located at the end of the chain
Bipolar	Yes	Maximum or minimum is located at the electrode of the phase reversal
Referential	No	Referential electrode is either maximum or minimum
Referential	Yes	Referential electrode is neither maximum nor minimum

The following sections provide more detailed instructions for the application of these rules.

Bipolar Montage

Derivations in a bipolar montage are customarily arranged in chains (6,76,77); that is, the electrode connected to input 2 of one channel is also connected to input 1 of the next channel. Electrode chains are usually parallel, along transverse or sagittal axes, and contain no single electrode common to all channels.

When the deflections of two channels move simultaneously in opposite directions, this defines a "phase reversal." The presence or absence of phase reversals provides useful and immediate clues to localize maxima and minima. Whether the montage is bipolar or referential radically alters the meaning of the phase reversal (Table 7.1). In bipolar montages, there are two types of phase reversals: negative phase reversals (wherein the deflections point toward each other), and positive phase reversals (wherein they point away from each other).

If there is a phase reversal, the electrode where it occurs is either the minimum or the maximum of the electrical field. (The term "maximum" denotes absolute value, not necessarily maximum negativity.) The location of the maximum depends on the assumed polarity of the generator. Phase reversals involving surface-negative activity generate a negative phase reversal, in which the deflections "point" toward each other. However, the same picture theoretically could result from a positive electrical field that is minimum at the site of the phase reversal and larger at the ends of the chain. Conversely, a positive potential maximum at an electrode in the middle of a bipolar chain will cause the deflections to point away from each other, that is, a positive phase reversal.

If there is no phase reversal, then the electrical field maximum must be located under either the first or the last electrode of the chain (Fig. 7.12). The potential field minimum must then be at the opposite end of the chain. Because the potential gradient for each pair of electrodes in the chain is in the same direction, the potential decreases progressively from the electrode with the highest potential to the one with the lowest potential.

In a bipolar montage, the amplitude may be misleading because it indicates differences in electrical potential and not the electrode of maximal involvement (Fig. 7.13). Because the gradients tend to be steeper in regions of highest activity, the electroencephalographer may habitually but unwisely determine the maximum on the basis of amplitude. Inexperienced electroencephalographers will often (erroneously) localize by a cursory impression of the "maximum field." It is very important, however, to keep in mind that recordings made between a pair of electrodes (a derivation) are actually measuring the electrical gradient.

Referential Montage

All derivations in a referential montage connect the same electrode (or electrode combination) to input 2. If some derivations within a given montage use one reference electrode (e.g., the left ear) whereas others use a different reference (e.g., the right ear), only those sets of channels with a common reference should be analyzed together.

If there is no phase reversal (as shown in Fig. 7.14), the reference electrode (i.e., the one connected to input 2) is either

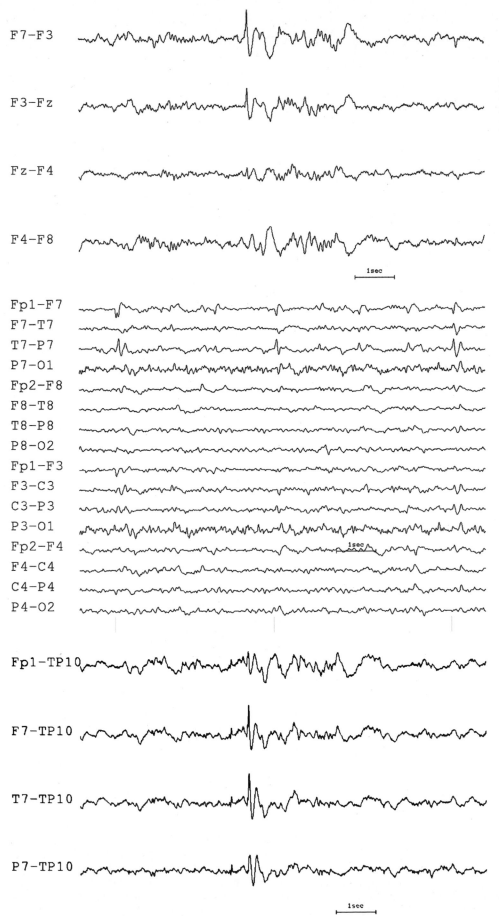

F7–F3

F3–Fz

Fz–F4

F4–F8

1sec

Fp1–F7
F7–T7
T7–P7
P7–O1
Fp2–F8
F8–T8
T8–P8
P8–O2
Fp1–F3
F3–C3
C3–P3
P3–O1
Fp2–F4
F4–C4
C4–P4
P4–O2

1sec

Fp1–TP10

F7–TP10

T7–TP10

P7–TP10

1sec

FIGURE 7.12 Bipolar montage with no phase reversal. Electroencephalographers are used to looking for phase reversals in a bipolar montage. In this tracing there is no phase reversal; therefore, the discharge must be coming from either the beginning or the end of the chain. If the sharp wave is negative, implying that the activity is at the beginning of the chain (F_7), the distribution has a much more realistic falloff (i.e., it has a single peak with a monotonic decline). If the sharp wave is assumed to be positive, then the maximum would have to be at the end of the chain (F_8) with an oddly flat distribution on the right and a rapid falloff on the left.

FIGURE 7.13 Bipolar montage with phase reversal. The amplitudes of the differences between the voltages at input 1 and input 2 do not indicate the maximum of the electrical field. In this circumstance, the amplitude of the sharp wave is actually maximum at F_7 and T_7, but approximately equal in those two adjacent eletrodes, so the discharge is localized to both electrodes.

FIGURE 7.14 Referential montage with no phase reversal. This montage, which employs a contralateral reference chosen because it appeared to be uninvolved in the discharge, helps to clarify the location of a spike widely distributed across the left temporal region.

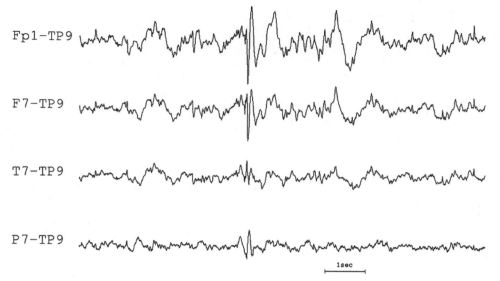

Fp1-TP9

F7-TP9

T7-TP9

P7-TP9

1sec

FIGURE 7.15 Referential montage with phase reversal. Since there is a phase reversal between channels 2 and 3, the reference is neither minimum nor maximum, that is, it must be "involved." This tracing is actually of the same discharge as shown in Figure 7.14, employing a less wisely chosen reference.

the minimum or the maximum of the electrical field. If the reference electrode is the minimum of the electrical field, the maximum will be at the electrode with the largest amplitude. This situation is the easiest to analyze, because the amplitude of the deflection in each channel directly reflects the level of activity in input 1 of the channel.

If the reference is maximum, the electrode at input 1 of the largest-amplitude channel is at the minimum of the electrical field. If the reference is maximum and some channels show no deflection, the electrodes connected to input 1 of those channels are also maximum.

If there is a phase reversal, then the reference electrode is neither the minimum nor the maximum of the electrical field (Fig. 7.15). Hence, the reference is "involved," that is, at some intermediate potential. This indicates that some electrodes connected to input 1 have a greater potential and some a lower potential than the reference. If, for instance, the polarity of the discharge is negative, those electrodes connected to input 1 that have a higher potential than the reference will point upward, whereas those less negative than the reference will point downward. The channels that show no activity (isopotential with the reference) measure a negativity at input 1 equal to that at the reference. If the recorded potential has two maxima of opposite polarity, such as seen in tangential dipole sources, then referential montages will show phase reversals even if the reference is the minimum.

Choice of a Reference

In a referential montage, any electrode may be the reference, but ordinarily it is the one uninvolved in the electrical field. The voltage difference between any pair of electrodes is entirely unrelated to the choice of reference (83,84); subtracting the voltage measured referentially at electrode B from that measured referentially at electrode A will produce exactly the voltage measured bipolarly from the A-B derivation, regardless of the reference chosen. This is true for a single electrode or a mathematically calculated one such as the

average reference (85–87) and is the principle of computer-aided montage reformatting.

The amplifiers in a reference montage perform their differential function exactly as in a bipolar montage. Referential recordings measure not the absolute potential under the various scalp electrodes but the potential difference, as do bipolar recordings. Specifically, however, they measure the difference between each electrode and a chosen common reference. Instead of chains of electrodes, with each succeeding amplifier sharing one input from the previous amplifier, all the amplifiers share a common input 2. What the amplifier "sees" depends on the electrical relationship between the reference and the field of the waveform. The reference may be completely uninvolved in the field (a minimum), may be in an area that picks up a higher value of the waveform than any of the other electrodes (a maximum), or may lie somewhere in between (neither a maximum nor a minimum).

When mapping the distribution of a particular wave, the choice of reference electrode will affect the appearance of the traces as well as the electroencephalographer's ability to localize. For evaluating epileptic foci, the reference is normally chosen to be completely uninvolved in the electrical field distribution of the spike or sharp wave (all deflections should point in the same direction). Typically, the electrode most distant from the activity of interest will be the least involved reference. "Standard" referential montages occasionally include the reference in the field distribution (some deflections pointing upward, some downward). An electrode at the vertex (C_z) is an excellent reference for displaying temporal spikes but may be a poor choice during sleep when it is very active. In the linked-ears reference (88) (frequently used to decrease electrocardiographic artifact), the reference electrode (A_1 connected to A_2) connects the two brain regions. This electrical shunt changes the field generated (89), decreasing, for example, asymmetries between the temporal regions (9) and producing other distortions (90). The "weighting" applied to activity from each side will depend entirely on the electrode impedances, with the ear having the lower impedance predominating. When temporal lobe epileptiform activity spreads to the ipsilateral ear, the linked-ear reference will inappropriately reveal spikes in both hemispheres.

A common average reference has been advocated (86) to avoid the problem of an "active reference." Using passive summing networks, active amplifier configurations, or combinatorial software, it is possible to devise a reference that combines all the electrodes applied to the head, the so-called common average reference (85,86). The disadvantages of this system are threefold: (i) The common average reference is, by definition, contaminated because the abnormal potential will influence all of the channels (91); (ii) depending on the number of electrodes included in the average, the potential under study will be reduced by a small proportion; and (iii) large-amplitude focal pathologic activities will be reflected proportionally in all the inactive channels as well, albeit with apparently opposite polarity.

A variety of calculated references and transformations are available, but these must be used with caution. The "source derivation" provides useful "deblurring" by arithmetically estimating the cortical sources that generate a scalp distribution; however, this method gives increasing weight to distant electrodes and can produce erroneous results when these sites are active (34,36,92,93). Because there is no ideal reference for all cases, it is usually best to distribute the electrical field potentials by manual selection of an uninvolved and quiet electrode as a reference.

SOURCE LOCALIZATION

Assumptions

After determination of the electrical field, the sources responsible for the production of the field can be localized with the aid of a number of simplifications. The procedure for determining the polarity and location of the generator is based on the following four specific assumptions:

1. Epileptogenic sources are simple dipoles or sheets of dipoles obeying a simple principle of superposition (46).
2. Dipoles are fundamentally oriented perpendicularly, with only one pole generally detectable on the scalp (75), and therefore can be treated as if they were monopoles. When both the positive and the negative poles are recorded from the surface, the localization system outlined below will not apply.
3. Epileptiform discharges are chiefly surface-negative phenomena. In the absence of a skull defect, a transverse-lying dipole (as in benign focal epileptiform discharges of childhood), or other evidence of an unusual discharge, the assumption of surface negativity will usually result in the proper distribution.
4. The head is essentially a uniform, homogeneous volume conductor.

Choosing Between Two Possibilities

The application of the rules above will yield two possible hypotheses in each case. In a bipolar chain, for example, a

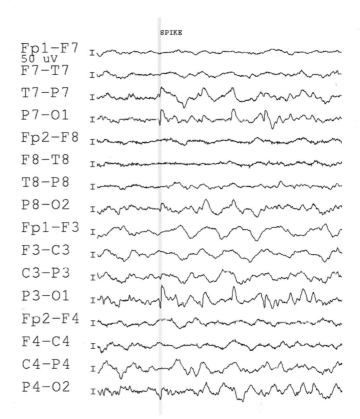

FIGURE 7.16 Bipolar montage with maximum negativity at the end of the chain. The marker brackets the downgoing negative component.

downward deflection with no phase reversals may be generated by either a negativity maximum at the last electrode of the chain (Fig. 7.16) or a positivity maximum at the first electrode of the chain. To choose between the two possibilities in any given case, one must guess about the polarity of the source generator or the relative likelihood of one of the two electrodes being the more active.

Because the localization of a transient will depend on a correct assumption about its polarity, all possible clues must be used to make an educated guess about polarity. For example, if the transient appears to be epileptiform, it is most likely to be surface negative, whereas if morphology and location suggest a positive occipital sharp transient (POST), it can be expected to be surface positive (Fig. 7.17). The best strategy is to see if the distribution based on the assumed polarity makes physiologic sense; if not, the opposite polarity will have to be tried. In Figure 7.10, the isopotential map based on an assumption that the polarity of the maximum is negative displays a more logical potential falloff for focal activity than the opposite assumption. Therefore, it is most likely that this activity has negative polarity with a maximum at electrode T_7.

Determination of the electrical field of a discharge may help to differentiate artifacts or extracortical physiologic activity from abnormal brain activity (Fig. 7.18). Because the electrical gradient is steepest at the electrodes closest to the source, the electrical potential difference between inputs 1 and 2 becomes

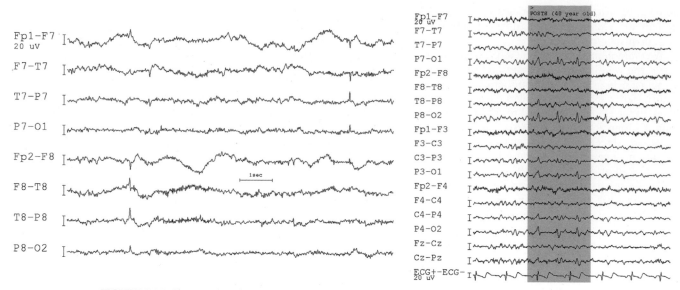

FIGURE 7.17 Clues to identifying the origin of sharply contoured waveforms. **Left:** Although these discharges stand out dramatically from the background, their presence during sleep and their very brief duration suggest that the transients here are "benign epileptiform transients of sleep (BETS)." BETS are often multiphasic, but the predominant component is negative, as in this example. **Right:** The electrical field distribution of these sharply contoured waves is consistent with POSTS (positive occipital sharp transients), that is, a positivity at the end of the chain. If the electroencephalographer assumed instead that they were negative, suggesting epileptiform discharges, their distribution across the entire head would have been more difficult to explain physiologically.

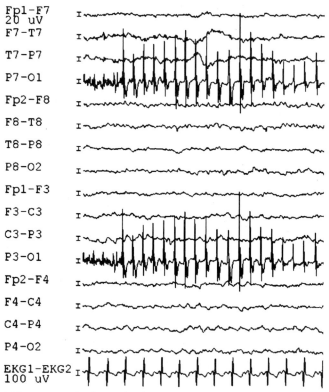

FIGURE 7.18 Artifacts. The sharply contoured discharges emanating from the left posterior region cannot be dismissed as artifacts on the basis of morphology alone, nor do they match up with the EKG artifact. However, since they appear only in channels 4 and 12, they must be arising solely from electrode O_1. If these large-amplitude occipital "spikes" were epileptogenic, electrical field theory would dictate a much more gradual falloff. Because the field shows a precipitous, and therefore impossible, distribution, these discharges must be artifacts.

smaller as one moves farther away from the generator source (94). For this reason, the steepest potential gradient, and the largest deflection, will most often appear in the channels nearest the source.

When dealing with an invariant spike, seen in various chains and montages, analyses based on any of the multiple electrode chains or montages should all reach the same conclusion (see Figs. 7.9 and 7.19). Corroborating a potential localized on a longitudinal montage by using a transverse montage (i.e., montages that are at right angles to each other), for example, can be helpful. If different conclusions result from the analysis of different montages, the assumptions about polarity or location were probably incorrect on one of the montages. Nevertheless, consistent conclusions across montages do not prove that the assumptions were correct, as the same error about polarity or location may have been made throughout the analysis.

Localization Rules: Cautions and Limitations

The simple rules and procedures for manual localization of electrical activity on the basis of bipolar or referential montages, outlined above, are valid only for single sources; that is, they presuppose a single monopolar generator. Regional abnormalities such as those encountered in focal epilepsy quite frequently satisfy this assumption as an approximation. Some EEG patterns, however, are produced by two or more generators of the same or different polarity acting simultaneously. When multiple sources or horizontal dipoles are involved, even highly sophisticated mathematical source localization

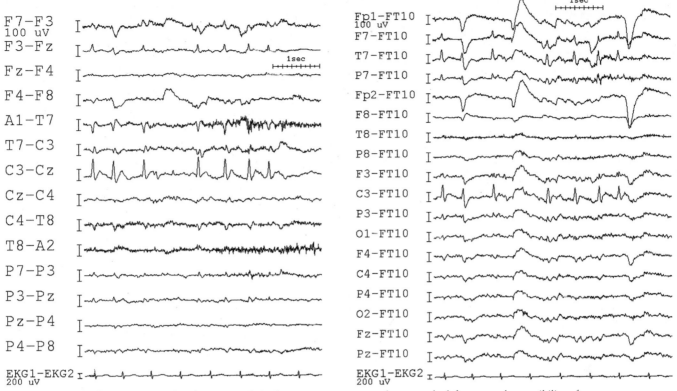

FIGURE 7.19 The phase reversals in the transverse montage shown on the left suggest the possibility of benign rolandic spikes. On the right, an ad hoc distribution montage employing a contralateral electrode clearly shows a typical centro-temporal distribution. It is also easier to distiguish the eye movement artifacts from the sharp waves in this montage.

techniques may not enable us to identify the exact composition of such generators.

Although both poles of the dipolar generator must be present by definition, one of them is oriented deep within the head, allowing assumption of a monopole. On occasion, however, both poles may be represented on the scalp surface, precluding the use of these rules. This occurs, for example, in the case of an epileptogenic focus originating from the superior mesial portion of the motor strip (95). Cortical regions involving the interhemispheric fissure, such as the foot area or the calcarine cortex, are especially likely to produce these horizontal dipoles. Specifically, the end of the dipole traditionally at the surface will be buried within the fissure with its maximum seen on the contralateral scalp, and the ordinarily deep end of the dipole may be close to the scalp surface on the ipsilateral side. Because of their location, horizontal dipoles also can be seen in benign focal epileptiform discharges of childhood (96).

The electrical fields resulting from these transverse dipoles are characterized by a simultaneous surface-negative and surface-positive potential seen at different electrodes on the scalp or by a double-phase reversal (13,97). Note that when double-phase reversals or other factors indicate, for example, a huge anteroposterior dipole or a transverse dipole extending from one hemisphere to the other (45), the physiologic meaning of such an unusual field must be questioned. A horizontal dipole should not be the first thought when the electroencephalographer confronts deflections pointing in opposite directions. An involved reference, the most common cause for this phenomenon, must be excluded.

As noted, in a bipolar montage, the channels of highest amplitude must not be confused with the area of greatest activity. This mistake is most likely to occur when the chain has no phase reversals, indicating that the maximum of the discharge originates from either the beginning or the end of the chain or when the maximum is broadly distributed across several channels (Fig. 7.20). A greater amplitude seen in one or more channels is solely a manifestation of a greater potential *difference*.

Obviously, determining whether a phase reversal is present is a key aspect of the localization procedure. Multiple fast components may be confusingly mixed when viewed from a bipolar montage and are more accurately represented in a referential montage to identify the individual components that are phase reversing across channels. A discharge with an extremely broad field can result in rather tiny differences between adjacent electrodes.

Because the brain, skull, and scalp do not have homogeneous conductivity, current pathways from active epileptogenic areas can vary dramatically among the recording sites. This variability may lead to a site of maximal scalp activity considerably distant from the fundamental generator (98).

Although general physiologic and physical principles can explain the phenomena involved, clinical interpretation of a particular set of measurements often will have to be based on experience and information that is not easily derivable from first principles. Nevertheless, by remaining aware of alternative possibilities, the electroencephalographer can avoid misinterpreting unusual recordings.

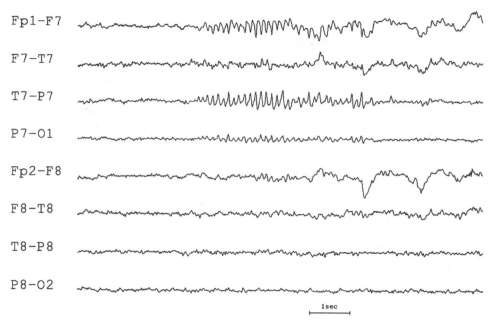

Fp1-F7

F7-T7

T7-P7

P7-O1

Fp2-F8

F8-T8

T8-P8

P8-O2

1sec

FIGURE 7.20 Bipolar montage with phase reversal. Phase reversals need not always occur in adjacent channels. This EEG shows the phenomonon for some normal activity rather than the abnormal discharges seen in Figure 7.13. The phase reversal of this arciform activity spans the isoelectric channels, consistent with the broad distribution of a wicket rhythm.

COMPUTER-AIDED METHODOLOGY FOR LOCATING EEG SOURCES

Topographic Mapping of Voltage and Other Parameters

Topographic EEG mapping is the generation of a pictorial representation based on measurements obtained from multi-channel EEG analysis—usually simultaneous, instantaneous, amplitudes of some parameter. Computer-aided mapping can accurately summarize the field distribution and may help to highlight locally originating activity (99). Computed topographic maps can be used (i) to describe an already known localization (perhaps for communication with non-neurophysiologists), (ii) to confirm a conventionally determined localization, (iii) to identify changes not detected in the original interpretation, and (iv) to display statistical differences between patient populations (so-called Z scores) (100). These maps should always be used in conjunction with the raw EEG data (101,102).

Automated mapping may be used to represent the topographic distribution of any variable, whether derived from complex calculations or simply displaying electrical field distributions as shown in Figure 7.21, depending on the application. In the evaluation of epileptic patients, the topographic distribution of sharp waves may present a valuable display, once their characteristics have been reduced to a metric (103). It is important to remember that a computerized system is unlikely to perform the measurement in every case as it would have been done manually, so that visual inspection of the waveform is essential for each map (101).

When used to map the amplitude of the EEG or evoked potential at a specific point in time, interpolation between the voltages measured at the electrodes must be carried out to

present a smooth contour on the map. The most practical interpolation method is the one based on spherical splines (104). Unlike magnetic resonance imaging and computed tomography, in which the intensity of every pixel is based on a measurement, topographic maps are derived from measurements at

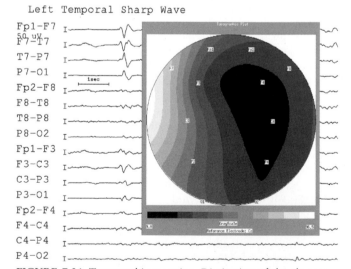

Left Temporal Sharp Wave

Fp1-F7
50 uV
F7-T7
T7-P7
P7-O1
Fp2-F8
F8-T8
T8-P8
P8-O2
Fp1-F3
F3-C3
C3-P3
P3-O1
Fp2-F4
F4-C4
C4-P4
P4-O2

1sec

FIGURE 7.21 Topographic mapping. Digtization of the electroencephalogram offers the opportunity for interactive postprocessing that may help to convey location in an easy to understand way. In this figure, the electrical field of the sharp wave seen phase reversing at T_7 in the EEG has been automatically mapped onto a top view of a spherical model of the head. Using baseline-to-peak amplitude measurements from a C_z reference, interpolating the amplitudes at every scalp location between electrodes, dividing into 10 isocontours, the amplitude map has been plotted as a gray-scale intensity. Koszer et al. (110) have demonstrated relatively good congruence between the manual process carried out by electroencephalographers described in the text and computerized topographic mapping methods.

only 16 to 32 points, with the balance obtained via interpolation, creating the illusion of a higher resolution than actually exists.

Once the computer has associated the amplitude information with its topographic location, mathematical techniques even more powerful than electrical field mapping can be brought to bear. As a result of volume conduction, potentials generated within a small brain region will be seen over a wide area of scalp. The spreading of the field to the scalp can be mathematically reduced by current source derivation methods (99,105). These spatial deblurring techniques such as the Laplacian operator (106) can narrow the apparent distribution of the electrical field, thereby emphasizing discrete foci (91). The Laplacian operator supplies information about the locally occurring activity in a "reference-free" manner (78), taking into account the direction of the field along the scalp to define the differences between adjacent electrodes.

Commercial instrumentation for topographic mapping is relatively easy to use. Although much attention has been paid to the algorithms for generating and presenting these displays, there is a danger that the relatively complex calculations that go into generating these maps will lead to gross misinterpretation as a result of the wide range of variables (98,102,107,108). There are a number of pitfalls and caveats associated with topographic mapping (108,109) that have prevented widespread acceptance of this technique for most clinical applications (98). Jayakar et al. (34) have described several limitations of these methods.

Computer-aided topographic mapping actually is not well suited to display epileptiform EEG elements owing to their rapid time course. Because not all the channels may be at their peak simultaneously, the maps may show an unexpected result, that is, the maps may demonstrate spike progression but will not necessarily reflect the manually determined localization (110). Moreover, computer topographic mapping of the amplitude of the EEG signal (or of evoked potentials, spectral measurements, or statistical analysis) provides no new information and cannot be used to make classifications not apparent in the raw data. Topographic mapping techniques, even with sophisticated enhancements such as the Laplacian operator or spatial deblurring, do not provide any conclusive three-dimensional information about the source of scalp-recorded signals (111). Nevertheless, they can make it easier to grasp the special relationships existing between electrodes in various neighborhoods of the scalp or to chart the progress of an epileptic discharge across the scalp as shown in Figure 22 in color plate section. To decrease errors, several restrictions imposed by the interpolation methods and the boundary value problem dictate the use of more electrodes than are conventionally placed. Indeed, adding closely spaced electrodes alone may reveal new information.

Dipole Modeling and Source Localization

Visual inspection, aided by simple enhancements such as distribution montages and the rules outlined above, is the time-honored method to identify the location from which epileptic EEG activity arises. There are, however, difficulties in identifying the source of a scalp potential that derive, in part, from the fact that the amplitude seen on the scalp is a function of not only its distance from the generator but also the orientation of the dipolar generator. Not only do the generators of the EEG dipoles possess an orientation, but they are complex sheets of dipoles arranged on a convoluted surface, following the contours of the cortex. The other problem that distorts the relationship between scalp potentials and the underlying cortical generators is the nonhomogeneity of the cerebral tissue, scalp, and skull.

There are computerized methods for EEG source localization that attempt to address some of these difficulties. These packages (such as BESA) (15) were initially developed in the realm of research, and they provide myriad tools to calculate and extract quantities from electrophysiological data (112–116). Computerized source analysis is an attempt to identify the origin of electrical potentials seen on the scalp by solving the "inverse problem." Source analysis is carried out by postulating a single or multiple spatiotemporal dipole models chosen to account for the surface signals and their timing relationships (117–119). Although the sources of electrical activity recorded by the EEG are actually folded sheets of dipolar pyramidal neurons, the traditional computer model typically uses only a single dipole with no spatial extent. In order to explain a widespread scalp distribution, the computer model tends to locate these dipoles deep to the actual cortical location. Solutions to the inverse problem involve simplifications and approximations and, even when well-defined dipoles using implanted sources in the human brain are employed, often produce errors of a few centimeters (120,121). Although it is not possible to uniquely identify the positions of the electrical sources in the brain from the scalp electrodes (122), appropriate assumptions can yield useful information in some cases (16,123). An illustration of the practical use of the equivalent current source dipole method to localize an epileptic discharge is shown in Figure 7.23 (in color plate section).

Localization using dipole source analysis has been the subject of many validation (124) and comparison studies (125). In recent years, purveyors of these packages have enhanced their offerings to be of more use in clinical medicine. Several journals have dedicated special issues to the various aspects of this methodology (126). Although computerized "source analysis" was applied beginning in the mid-1980s to identify single or multiple foci (117,118), and has been continuously developed for more than 20 years, the extra time and effort required have discouraged use of these techniques on a routine basis. This software methodology is sometimes limited, because in clinical use only the simplest of models of the source (e.g., equivalent current dipole) and the head (e.g., concentric spheres) are employed. The temporal dynamics of the source and the intracranial anatomic pathology associated with epilepsy often make these models inexact, and the results may be misleading (127). The modeling required for source localization of magneto-encephalography (MEG) signals—which arise from the same neuronal activity that generates EEG signals—is much simpler, providing a generally more accurate computerized solution to this sophisticated inverse problem. The volume conductor model that represents the physical properties of the medium between the sources and the sensors is especially complex for the electroencephalography of patients with highly distorted head anatomy. MEG, on the other hand, is unaffected by the tissue variations inherent in scalp, skull, CSF, dura, and brain parenchyma. The use of MEG for evaluation of epileptic patients is covered in detail in Chapter 77.

While new imaging techniques have decreased the importance of EEG for many neurological disorders, EEG is still the sine qua non for the diagnosis of epilepsy. If the seizure semiology, ictal scalp EEG features, and the neuroimaging fail to produce a consensus regarding the focus localization, then further studies—usually including even more EEG from intracranial recordings—will be required in order to outline a target for surgical resection.

References

1. Engel J., Jr., ed. Approaches to localization of the epileptogenic lesion. *Surgical Treatment of the Epilepsies.* New York, NY: Raven Press; 1987:75–95.
2. Adrian ED, Matthews BHC. The Berger rhythm: potential changes from the occipital lobes in man. *Brain.* 1934;57:355–385.
3. Adrian ED, Yamagiwa K. The origin of the Berger rhythm. *Brain.* 1935; 58(323):351.
4. Walter WG. The localization of cerebral tumours by electroencephalography. *Lancet.* 1936;2:305–308.
5. Gibbs FA, Gibbs EL. *Atlas of Electroencephalography.* Reading, MA: Addison-Wesley Publishing; 1941.
6. Gloor P. Application of volume conduction principles to montage design. *Am J EEG Technol.* 1977;17:520.
7. Gloor P. Neuronal generators and the problem of localization in electroencephalography: application of volume conductor theory to electroencephalography. *J Clin Neurophysiol.* 1985;2(4):327–354.
8. Magnus O. On the technique of location by electroencephalography. *Electroencephalogr Clin Neurophysiol.* 1961;19(suppl):135.
9. Nunez PL. *Electrical Fields of the Brain.* New York, NY: Oxford University Press; 1981.
10. Osselton JW. Bipolar, unipolar and average reference recording methods, I: mainly theoretical considerations. *Am J EEG Technol.* 1966;5:53–64.
11. Osselton JW. Bipolar, unipolar and average reference recording methods, II: mainly practical considerations. *Am J EEG Technol.* 1969;9: 117–133.
12. Knott JR. Further thoughts on polarity, montages, and localization. *J Clin Neurophysiol.* 1985;2(1):63–75.
13. Lesser RP, Luders H, Dinner DS, et al. An introduction to the basic concepts of polarity and localization. *J Clin Neurophysiol.* 1985;2(1): 45–61.
14. Burgess RC. Design and evolution of a system for long-term electroencephalographic and video monitoring of epilepsy patients. *Methods.* 2001;25(2):231–248.
15. Scherg M, Ebersole JS. Models of brain sources. *Brain Topogr.* 1993; 5(4):419–423.
16. Scherg M, Ebersole JS. Brain source imaging of focal and multifocal epileptiform EEG activity. *Neurophysiol Clin.* 1994;24(1):51–60.
17. Lantz G, Holub M, Ryding E, et al. Simultaneous intracranial and extracranial recording of interictal epileptiform activity in patients with drug resistant partial epilepsy: patterns of conduction and results from dipole reconstructions. *Electroencephalogr Clin Neurophysiol.* 1996; 99(1):69–78.
18. Santiago-Rodriguez E, Harmony T, Fernandez-Bouzas A, et al. EEG source localization of interictal epileptiform activity in patients with partial complex epilepsy: comparison between dipole modeling and brain distributed source models. *Clin Electroencephalogr.* 2002;33(1):42–47.
19. Hamer HM, Luders H. Electrode montages and localization of potentials in clinical electroencephalography. In: Levin KH, Luders H, eds. *Comprehensive Clinical Neurophysiology.* Philadelphia, PA: Lippincott, Williams and Wilkins; 2000:358–387.
20. Blume WT, Borghesi JL, Lemieux JF. Interictal indices of temporal seizure origin. *Ann Neurol.* 1993;34(5):703–709.
21. Blume WT, Holloway GM, Wiebe S. Temporal epileptogenesis: localizing value of scalp and subdural interictal and ictal EEG data. *Epilepsia.* 2001;42(4):508–514.
22. Ebersole JS. Defining epileptogenic foci: past, present, future. *J Clin Neurophysiol.* 1997;14(6):470–483.
23. Janszky J, Fogarasi A, Jokeit H, et al. Spatiotemporal relationship between seizure activity and interictal spikes in temporal lobe epilepsy. *Epilepsy Res.* 2001;47(3):179–188.
24. Okada Y. Neurogenesis of evoked magnetic fields. In: Williamson RJ, Romani GL, Kaurman L, eds. *Biomagnetism, An Interdisciplinary Approach.* New York, NY: Plenum Press; 1983:399–408.
25. Creutzfeldt OD, Watanabe S, Lux HD. Relations between EEG phenomena and potentials of single cortical cells. I. Evoked responses after thalamic and erpicortical stimulation. *Electroencephalogr Clin Neurophysiol.* 1966;20(1):1–18.
26. Creutzfeldt OD, Watanabe S, Lux HD. Relations between EEG phenomena and potentials of single cortical cells. II. Spontaneous and convulsoid activity. *Electroencephalogr Clin Neurophysiol.* 1966;20(1):19–37.
27. Elul R. The genesis of the EEG. *Int Rev Neurobiol.* 1971;15:227–272.
28. Brazier MAB. A study of the electrical fields at the surface of the head. *Electroencephalogr Clin Neurophysiol.* 1951;2:38–52.
29. Shaw JC, Roth M. Potential distribution analysis. I and II. *Electroencephalogr Clin Neurophysiol.* 1955;7:273–292.
30. Plonsey R. *Bioelectric Phenomena.* New York, NY: McGraw-Hill; 1969.
31. Helmholtz HLF. Ueber einige Gesetze der Vertheilung elektrischer Strome in korperlichen Leitern mit Anwendung. *Ann Physik und Chemie.* 1853;9: 211–377.
32. Ludwig BI, Marsan CA. Clinical ictal patterns in epileptic patients with occipital electroencephalographic foci. *Neurology.* 1975;25(5): 463–471.
33. Olivier A, Gloor P, Andermann F, et al. Occipitotemporal epilepsy studied with stereotaxically implanted depth electrodes and successfully treated by temporal resection. *Ann Neurol.* 1982;11(4):428–432.
34. Jayakar P, Duchowny M, Resnick TJ, et al. Localization of seizure foci: pitfalls and caveats. *J Clin Neurophysiol.* 1991;8(4):414–431.
35. Brazier MA. The electrical fields at the surface of the head during sleep. *Electroencephalogr Clin Neurophysiol.* 1949;1:195–204.
36. Nunez PL, Pilgreen KL. The spline-Laplacian in clinical neurophysiology: a method to improve EEG spatial resolution. *J Clin Neurophysiol.* 1991; 8(4):397–413.
37. Nicholson PW. Specific impedance of cerebral white matter. *Exp Neurol.* 1965;13(4):386–401.
38. van den Broek SP, Reinders F, Donderwinkel M, et al. Volume conduction effects in EEG and MEG. *Electroencephalogr Clin Neurophysiol.* 1998;106(6):522–534.
39. Nunez PL, ed. An overview of electromyogenic theory. *Electrical Fields of the Brain.* New York, NY: Oxford University Press; 1981:42–74.
40. Goncalves SI, de Munck JC, Verbunt JP, et al. In vivo measurement of the brain and skull resistivities using an EIT-based method and realistic models for the head. *IEEE Trans Biomed Eng.* 2003;50(6):754–767.
41. Hoekema R, Wieneke GH, Leijten FS, et al. Measurement of the conductivity of skull, temporarily removed during epilepsy surgery. *Brain Topogr.* 2003;16(1):29–38.
42. Haueisen J, Ramon C, Eiselt M, et al. Influence of tissue resistivities on neuromagnetic fields and electric potentials studied with a finite element model of the head. *IEEE Trans Biomed Eng.* 1997;44(8):727–735.
43. Heasman BC, Valentin A, Alarcon G, et al. A hole in the skull distorts substantially the distribution of extracranial electrical fields in an in vitro model. *J Clin Neurophysiol.* 2002;19(2):163–171.
44. Carpenter MB. *Core Text of Neuroanatomy,* 4th Edition. Philadelphia, PA: Lippincott, Williams & Wilkins; 1991:210.
45. Ebersole JS, Wade PB. Intracranial EEG validation of single versus dual dipolar sources for temporal spikes in presurgical candidates. *Epilepsia.* 1990;31:621.
46. Lutzenberger W, Elbert T, Rockstroh B. A brief tutorial on the implications of volume conduction for the interpretation of the EEG. *J Psychophysiol.* 1987;1:81–89.
47. Awad IA, Luders H, Burgess RC. Epidural pegs and foramen ovale electrodes: a new class of electrodes of intermediate invasiveness for the mapping of seizure foci. *J Clin Neurophysiol.* 1989;6:338.
48. Erenberg G. Localization of epileptogenic spike foci: comparative study of closely spaced scalp electrodes, nasopharyngeal, sphenoidal, subdural, and depth electrodes. In: Akimoto H, Kazamatsuri H, Seino M, eds. *Advances in Epileptology: XIIIth International Symposium.* New York, NY: Raven Press; 1982:185–189.
49. Friedman L, Skipper G, Wyllie E. Commentary: chronic intracranial recording and stimulation with subdural electrodes. In: Engel J,Jr (ed.) *Surgical Treatment of the Epilepsies.* New York, NY: Raven Press; 1987:297–321.
50. Wyllie E, Luders H, Morris HH, III, et al. Subdural electrodes in the evaluation for epilepsy surgery in children and adults. *Neuropediatrics.* 1988;19(2):80–86.
51. Gregory DL, Wong PKH. Clinical and EEG features of "tripole" spike discharges in children. *Epilepsia.* 1986;27:605.
52. Cooper R, Winter AL, CROW HJ, et al. Comparison of subcortical, cortical and scalp activity using chronically indwelling electrodes in man. *Electroencephalogr Clin Neurophysiol.* 1965;18:217–228.
53. Ebersole JS, Hanes-Ebersole S. EEG dipole patch: a realistic extended source model for spikes and seizures. *Muscle and Nerve.* 2003;12(suppl):S-37.
54. Woodbury JW. Potentials in volume conductor. In: Ruch TC, Fulton JF, eds. *Medical Physiology and Biophysics.* Philadelphia, PA: Saunders; 1960:83–91.
55. Klee M, Rall W. Computed potentials of cortically arranged populations of neurons. *J Neurophysiol.* 1977;40(3):647–666.
56. Lorente De No R. Correlation of nerve activity with polarization phenomona. *Harvey Lect.* 1947;42:43–105.

57. Gloor P, Vera CL, Sporti L. Electrophysiological studies of hippocampal neurons. I. Configuration and laminar analysis of the "resting" potential gradient, of the main transient response to perforant path, fimbrial and mossy fiber volleys and of "spontaneous" activity. *Electroencephalogr Clin Neurophysiol.* 1963;15:353–378.

58. Neshige R, Luders H, Shibasaki H. Recording of movement-related potentials from scalp and cortex in man. *Brain.* 1988;111(Pt 3):719–736.

59. Tao JX, Baldwin M, Hawes-Ebersole S, et al. Cortical substrates of scalp EEG epileptiform discharges. *J Clin Neurophysiol.* 2007;24(2):96–100.

60. Marks DA, Kratz A, Booke J, et al. Comparison and correlation of surface and sphenoidal electrodes with simultaneous intracranial recording: an interictal study. *Electroencephalogr Clin Neurophysiol.* 1992;82:23–29.

61. Fernandez Torre JL, Alarcon G, Binnie CD, et al. Generation of scalp discharges in temporal lobe epilepsy as suggested by intraoperative electrocorticographic recordings. *J Neurol Neurosurg Psychiatry.* 1999;67:51–58.

62. Jasper HH. The ten twenty electrode system of the international federation. *Electroencephalogr Clin Neurophysiol.* 1958; 10:371–375.

63. Myslobodsky MS, Coppola R, Bar-Ziv J, et al. Adequacy of the international 10–20 electrode system for computed neurophysiologic topography. *J Clin Neurophysiol.* 1990;7(4):507–518.

64. Gevins AS. Analysis of the electromagnetic signals of the human brain: milestones, obstacles, and goals. *IEEE Trans Biomed Eng.* 1984;31(12): 833–850.

65. Lopes da Silava FH, van Rotterdam A. Biophysical aspects of EEG and magnetoencephalogram generation. In: Niedermeyer E, ed. *EEG Basic Principles, Clinical Applications and Related Fields.* Baltimore, MD: Lippincott, Williams and Wilkins; 1999:93–109.

66. Gevins AS, Bressler SL. Functional topography of the human brain. In: Pfurtscheller G, ed. *Functional Brain Imaging.* Toronto, Canada: Hans Huber Publishers; 1988:99–116.

67. Gibbs EL, Gibbs FA, Fuster B. Psychomotor epilepsy. *Arch Neurol Psychiatry.* 1948;60:331–339.

68. Luders H, Hahn J, Lesser RP, et al. Basal temporal subdural electrodes in the evaluation of patients with intractable epilepsy. *Epilepsia.* 1989;30(2):131–142.

69. Rovit RL, Gloor P, Henderson LR. Temporal lobe epilepsy—a study using multiple basal electrodes, I: description of method. *Neurochirurgia.* 1960;3:634.

70. Sperling MR, Engel J, Jr. Electroencephalographic recording from the temporal lobes: a comparison of ear, anterior temporal, and nasopharyngeal electrodes. *Ann Neurol.* 1985;17(5):510–513.

71. Chatrian GE, Lettich E, Nelson PL. Ten percent electrode system for topographic studies of spontaneous and evoked EEG activities. *Am J Electroencephalogr Clin Neurophysiol.* 1985;25:83–92.

72. Morris HH, III, Luders H, Lesser RP, et al. The value of closely spaced scalp electrodes in the localization of epileptiform foci: a study of 26 patients with complex partial seizures. *Electroencephalogr Clin Neurophysiol.* 1986;63(2):107–111.

73. Nuwer MR. Recording electrode site nomenclature. *J Clin Neurophysiol.* 1987;4(2):121–133.

74. Morris HH, III, Kanner A, Luders H, et al. Can sharp waves localized at the sphenoidal electrode accurately identify a mesio-temporal epileptogenic focus? *Epilepsia.* 1989;30(5):532–539.

75. Niedermeyer E. The EEG signal: polarity and field determination. In: Niedermeyer E, Lopes da Silva F, eds. *Electroencephalography—Basic Principles, Clinical Applications, Associated Fields.* 4th ed. Baltimore, MD: Lippincott, William and Wilkins; 1999:143–148.

76. Klass DW, Bickford RG, Ellingson RJ. A proposal for standard EEG montages to be used in clinical electroencephalography. *Guidelines in EEG.* Atlanta, GA: American Electroencephalography Society; 1980.

77. MacGillivray BB, Binnie CD, Osselton JW. Traditional methods of examination in clinical EEG. Derivations and montages. In: Delucchi MR, ed. *Handbook of Electroencephalography and Clinical Neurophysiology, III.* Amsterdam, Netherlands: Elsevier Scientific Publishing Co.; 1974: C22–C57.

78. Sharbrough FW. The mathematical logic for the design of montages. *Am J EEG Technol.* 1977;17:73–83.

79. Merlet I, Paetau R, Garcia-Larrea L, et al. Apparent asynchrony between interictal electric and magnetic spikes. *Neuroreport.* 1997;8(5):1071–1076.

80. Minami T, Gondo K, Yamamoto T, et al. Magnetoencephalographic analysis of rolandic discharges in benign childhood epilepsy. *Ann Neurol.* 1996;39(3):326–334.

81. Takahashi H, Yasue M, Ishijima B. Dynamic EEG topography and analysis of epileptic spikes and evoked potentials following thalamic stimulation. *Appl Neurophysiol.* 1985;48(1–6):418–422.

82. Thickbroom GW, Davies HD, Carroll WM, et al. Averaging, spatio-temporal mapping and dipole modelling of focal epileptic spikes. *Electroencephalogr Clin Neurophysiol.* 1986;64(3):274–277.

83. Lehmann D, Skrandies W. Reference-free identification of components of checkerboard-evoked multichannel potential fields. *Electroencephalogr Clin Neurophysiol.* 1980;48(6):609–621.

84. Walter DO, Etevenon P, Pidoux B, et al. Computerized topo-EEG spectral maps: difficulties and perspectives. *Neuropsychobiology.* 1984;11(4): 264–272.

85. Goldman D. The clinical use of the "average" electrode in monopolar recording. *Electroencephalogr Clin Neurophysiol.* 1950;2:211–214.

86. Lehmann D, Michel CM. Intracerebral dipole sources of EEG FFT power maps. *Brain Topogr.* 1989;2(1–2):155–164.

87. Osselton JW. Acquisition of EEG data by bipolar, unipolar and average reference methods: a theoretical comparison. *Electroencephalogr Clin Neurophysiol.* 1965;19(5):527–528.

88. John ER, Prichep LS, Fridman J, et al. Neurometrics: computer-assisted differential diagnosis of brain dysfunctions. *Science.* 1988;239(4836): 162–169.

89. Katznelson RD. EEG recording, electrode placement, and aspects of generator localization. In: Nunez PL, Katznelson RD, eds. *Electric Fields of the Brain: The Neurophysics of EEG.* London, UK: Oxford University Press; 1981:176–213.

90. Fisch BJ, Pedley TA. The role of quantitative topographic mapping or "neurometrics" in the diagnosis of psychiatric and neurological disorders: the cons. *Electroencephalogr Clin Neurophysiol.* 1989;73(1):5–9.

91. Lopes da Silava FH. A critical review of clinical applications of topographic mapping of brain potentials. *J Clin Neurophysiol.* 1990;7: 535–551.

92. Burgess RC. Editorial: localization of neural generators. *J Clin Neurophysiol.* 1991;8:369.

93. van Oosterom A. History and evolution of methods for solving the inverse problem. *J Clin Neurophysiol.* 1991;8(4):371–380.

94. Morris HH, III, Luders H. Electrodes. *Electroencephalogr Clin Neurophysiol Suppl.* 1985;37:3–26.

95. Lueders H, Dinner DS, Lesser RP, et al. Origin of far-field subcortical evoked potentials to posterior tibial and median nerve stimulation. A comparative study. *Arch Neurol.* 1983;40(2):93–97.

96. Luders H, Lesser RP, Dinner DS. Benign focal epilepsy of childhood. In: Luders H, Lesser RP, eds. *Epilepsy: Electroclinical Syndromes.* Berlin, Germany: Springer-Verlag; 1987:303–346.

97. Adelman S, Lueders H, Dinner DS, et al. Paradoxical lateralization of parasagittal sharp waves in a patient with epilepsia partialis continua. *Epilepsia.* 1982;23(3):291–295.

98. Perrin F, Bertrand O, Giard MH, et al. Precautions in topographic mapping and in evoked potential map reading. *J Clin Neurophysiol.* 1990;7(4): 498–506.

99. Hjorth B. Principles for transformation of scalp EEG from potential field into source distribution. *J Clin Neurophysiol.* 1991;8(4):391–396.

100. Duffy FH, Bartels PH, Burchfiel JL. Significance probability mapping: an aid in the topographic analysis of brain electrical activity. *Electroencephalogr Clin Neurophysiol.* 1981;51(5):455–462.

101. American Electroencephalography Society. Statement on the clinical use of quantitative EEG. *J Clin Neurophysiol.* 1987;4:197.

102. Nuwer MR. Frequency analysis and topographic mapping of EEG and evoked potentials in epilepsy. *Electroencephalogr Clin Neurophysiol.* 1988;69(2):118–126.

103. Burgess RC. Neurophysiological mapping systems (editorial). *J Clin Neurophysiol.* 1990;7(4):552.

104. Perrin F, Pernier J, Bertrand O, et al. Spherical splines for scalp potential and current density mapping. *Electroencephalogr Clin Neurophysiol.* 1989;72(2):184–187.

105. Rodin E, Cornellier D. Source derivation recordings of generalized spike-wave complexes. *Electroencephalogr Clin Neurophysiol.* 1989;73(1): 20–29.

106. Babiloni F, Babiloni C, Carducci F, et al. High resolution EEG: a new model-dependent spatial deblurring method using a realistically-shaped MR-constructed subject's head model. *Electroencephalogr Clin Neurophysiol.* 1997;102(2):69–80.

107. Herrman WM, Kubicki ST, Kunkel H. Empfehlungen der Deutschen EEG-Gesellschaft fur das Mapping von EEG-Parametern. *Z EEG-EMG.* 1989; 20:125–132.

108. Kahn EM, Weiner RD, Brenner RP, et al. Topographic maps of brain electrical activity—pitfalls and precautions. *Biol Psychiatry.* 1988;23(6): 628–636.

109. Duffy FH. Brain electrical activity mapping: issues and answers. *Topographic Mapping of Brain Electrical Activity.* Boston, MA: Butterworths; 1986:401–418.

110. Koszer S, Moshe SL, Legatt AD, et al. Surface mapping of spike potential fields: experienced EEGers vs. computerized analysis. *Electroencephalogr Clin Neurophysiol.* 1996;98(3):199–205.

111. Gevins A, Le J, Leong H, et al. Deblurring. *J Clin Neurophysiol.* 1999;16(3):204–213.

112. Wood CC. Application of dipole localization methods to identification of human evoked potentials. *Ann N Y Acad Sci.* 1982;388:139–155.

113. Scherg M, Von Cramon D, Two bilateral sources of late AFP as indentified by a spatio-temporal dipole model. *Electroencephalogr Clin Neurophysiol.* 1985;62:32–44.

114. Fender DH. Source localization of brain electrical activity. In: Gevins AS, Redmond A, eds. *Methods of Analysis of Brain Electrical and Magnetic Signals.* Amsterdam: Elsevier; 1987:355–403.

115. Synder AZ. Dipole source localization in the study of EP generators: a critique. *Electroencephalogr Clin Neurophysiol.* 1991;80:321–325.

116. Mosher JC, Lewis PS, Leahy RM. Multiple dipole modeling and localization from spatio-temporal MEG data. *IEEE Trans Biomed Eng.* 1992; 39(6):541–557.

117. Scherg M, Von Cramon D. Evoked dipole source potentials of the human auditory cortex. *Electroencephalogr Clin Neurophysiol.* 1986;65(5): 344–360.

118. Scherg M. Fundamentals of dipole source potential analysis. In: Gradori F, Hoke M, Romani GL, eds. *Auditory Evoked Magnetic Fields and Electric Potentials.* Basel, Switzerland: Karger; 1990:40–69.

119. Scherg M, Bast T, Berg P. Multiple source analysis of interictal spikes: goals, requirements, and clinical value. *J Clin Neurophysiol.* 1999;16(3):214–224.

120. Cuffin BN, Cohen D, Yunokuchi K, et al. Tests of EEG localization accuracy using implanted sources in the human brain. *Ann Neurol.* 1991; 29(2):132–138.

121. Smith DB, Sidman RD, Flanigin H, et al. A reliable method for localizing deep intracranial sources of the EEG. *Neurology.* 1985;35(12):1702–1707.

122. Regan D. *Human Brain Electrophysiology: Evoked Potentials and Evoked Magnetic Fields in Science and Medicine.* New York, NY: Elsevier Science Publishing Co.; 2003.

123. Scherg M. Functional imaging and localization of electromagnetic brain activity. *Brain Topogr.* 1992;5(2):103–111.

124. Cohen D, Cuffin BN, Yunokuchi K, et al. MEG versus EEG localization test using implanted sources in the human brain. *Ann Neurol.* 1990; 28(6):811–817.

125. Sutherling WW, Levesque MF, Crandall PH, et al. Localization of partial epilepsy using magnetic and electric measurements. *Epilepsia.* 1991; 32(suppl 5):S29–S40.

126. He B, Sekihara K. Functional source imaging (editorial). *IEEE Trans BME.* 2006;53(9): 1729–1731.

127. Kobayahsi K, Yoshinaga H, Ohtsuka Y, et al. Diple modeling of epileptic spikes can be accurate or misleading. *Epilepsia.* 2005;46(3):397–408.

CHAPTER 8 ■ APPLICATION OF ELECTROENCEPHALOGRAPHY IN THE DIAGNOSIS OF EPILEPSY

KATHERINE C. NICKELS AND GREGORY D. CASCINO

The electroencephalogram (EEG) is the most frequently performed neurodiagnostic study in patients with seizure disorders and, despite its introduction more than 60 years ago, still has important clinical and research applications (1). Due to the paroxysmal nature of epilepsy, an EEG is usually obtained between seizure episodes (1,2). The interictal EEG may be useful in confirming the diagnosis of epilepsy, in addition to monitoring and predicting response to treatment (1,3–7). Correlation of the ictal and interictal EEG changes with ictal semiology underlies the current classification of seizures (1,8). Furthermore, localized electrographic alterations such as continuous focal slowing and certain epileptiform discharges may even "suggest" the presence of underlying pathology (9,10).

This chapter discusses the relationship between extracranial EEG studies and epilepsy and the clinical applications of interictal and ictal EEG recordings.

HISTORICAL PERSPECTIVE

In 1933, Berger (11) published his observations of EEG changes in patients during "convulsions" but failed to recognize the tremendous potential of these studies in epilepsy. In 1935, Gibbs and colleagues (12) documented the association of specific interictal and ictal EEG alterations in patients with seizures. They also indicated that interictal EEG findings may localize the epileptogenic zone (13). Various interictal EEG patterns in patients with partial and generalized epilepsy were subsequently recognized, and attempts were made to classify seizures according to electroclinical correlations (12). Penfield and Jasper later revealed the importance of electrocorticography in recording interictal EEG abnormalities during focal cortical resective surgery for intractable partial epilepsy (14).

CLINICAL APPLICATIONS

Rationale

Despite impressive technical advances, the purpose of the EEG has not changed since the days of Gibbs and Gibbs (13). The EEG identifies specific interictal or ictal abnormalities that are associated with an increased epileptogenic potential and correlate with a seizure disorder (8). This is important in determining whether a patient's recurrent spells represent seizures.

However, the specificity and sensitivity of the EEG is variable and EEG findings must be correlated with the clinical history. A persistently normal EEG recording does not exclude the diagnosis of epilepsy, and false interpretation of nonspecific changes with hyperventilation or drowsiness may lead to an error in diagnosis and treatment (2). Furthermore, epileptiform alterations may occur without a history of seizures, although this is rare (15).

For patients with a known seizure disorder, the EEG is helpful in classification of seizure disorder, determination of seizure type and frequency, and seizure localization (2). Seizure classification may be difficult to determine by ictal semiology alone. The appropriate classification affects subsequent diagnostic evaluation and therapy, and may have prognostic importance. Therefore, the EEG is essential in determining the appropriate treatment for patients with epilepsy.

The EEG has fundamental value in evaluating surgical candidacy and determining operative strategy in selected patients with intractable partial epilepsy (16). In these individuals, interictal epileptiform alterations identified on EEG provide only limited information about lateralization and localization of the epileptic brain tissue, as the diagnostic yield depends on the site of seizure onset. Identification of ictal EEG patterns, performed in an inpatient unit with concomitant video recordings, is necessary to localize the epileptogenic zone preoperatively (2,9).

Methods

Recordings should be performed according to the methodology established by the American Clinical Neurophysiology Society (formerly the American Electroencephalography Society) (17). Standard activation procedures such as hyperventilation and photic stimulation should be included. The recording of drowsiness and nonrapid eye movement (NREM) sleep, facilitated by sleep deprivation, may increase the sensitivity of the EEG to demonstrate interictal epileptiform alterations, especially in patients with partial epilepsy. Adequate levels of sleep may be attained after administration of chloral hydrate. Benzodiazepines should not be used as sedatives because of their associated increase in β activity and the possible masking of epileptiform alterations. During the recording, the EEG technologist should obtain information about seizure manifestations, time of the latest seizure, current medications and antiepileptic drug levels, and precipitating events.

Interictal Recording

The recording of interictal epileptiform activity depends on the seizure type, localization of the epileptogenic zone, recording methodology, age at seizure onset, and frequency of seizure activity (1,4,18). The diagnostic yield of the interictal EEG can be increased by performing multiple EEG recordings, increasing the duration of the EEG, and timing a study shortly after a seizure, because interictal epileptiform discharges may be potentiated following an attack (18).

Ictal Recording

When routine interictal EEG recordings prove diagnostically inadequate, long-term EEG studies may be used to improve the yield of EEG abnormalities (9). Ictal EEGs are used to determine whether recurrent spells represent seizures, to classify seizure type, and to localize the epileptogenic zone (9,19). This is typically accomplished with inpatient prolonged video-EEG monitoring. However, in patients with very frequent paroxysmal events, short-duration video EEG may be effective in characterizing the events (20). Furthermore, ambulatory EEG is also useful in spell classification, as well as seizure quantification, classification, and localization, especially in children (21).

Recognition of ictal EEG patterns is indicated in patients with medically refractory partial epilepsy being considered for surgical treatment. The effectiveness of scalp-recorded ictal EEG for identifying the seizure onset zone may be enhanced by altering the recording technique (2,8–10,22,23). Closely spaced scalp electrodes increase the diagnostic accuracy of such monitoring. With application of the standard extension of the 10–20 Electrode Placement System, as outlined in the American Clinical Neurophysiology Society guidelines, inferolateral temporal electrode positions, namely, F_9, F_{10}, T_9, and T_{10}, may be used to record epileptiform activity of anterior temporal lobe origin (22). Special extracranial electrodes also may improve diagnostic effectiveness. Sphenoidal electrodes may reveal the topography of interictal and ictal epileptiform discharges in patients with temporal lobe seizures and indicate the mesial temporal localization of the epileptogenic region (9). Supraorbital electrodes, which record from the orbitofrontal region, may be useful in patients with partial epilepsy of frontal lobe origin (2). Digital EEG acquisition and storage in a format suitable for subsequent remontaging and filtering have improved the speed with which interpretable ictal recordings may be obtained over paper recordings.

Limitations of Extracranial Recordings

There are limitations of scalp-recorded, or extracranial, EEG, which may affect the interpretation of these studies (24). Potentially epileptogenic activity may be attenuated by dura, bone, and scalp, or degraded by muscle artifacts (1). Therefore, epileptiform activity generated in cortex remote from the surface electrodes, such as amygdala and hippocampus, may not be associated with interictal extracranial EEG alterations (24). Approximately 20% to 70% of cortical spikes are recorded on the scalp EEG and patients with seizure disorders may have repetitively normal interictal EEG studies (1,18,24).

Extracranial EEG recordings may also inaccurately localize the epileptogenic zone. For example, interictal scalp EEG may fail to detect specific alterations arising from the amygdala only to reveal distant, more widespread cortical excitability (24). Furthermore, the interictal and ictal EEG patterns may have discordant localization of the epileptogenic zone (25).

Pitfalls in Interpretation

Differentiating artifact from electrical activity of cerebral origin represents a challenge for both the EEG technologist and the electroencephalographer (1). Artifacts can mimic interictal and ictal epileptiform patterns. Artifacts can be related to *extrinsic* factors (such as the electrical interference generated by power cables and fluorescent lights), *biological* factors (e.g., myogenic and eye movement artifacts), and *technological* factors (such as poor electrical impedance causing an electrode "pop"). Changes during drowsiness, hyperventilation, photic stimulation, and arousal from sleep can be particularly confounding in pediatric patients. Thus, knowledge of the normal EEG background for age is critical to appropriate interpretation.

Some EEG patterns—such as small sharp spikes (see Fig. 9.4), 14- and 6-Hz positive bursts (see Fig. 9.5), 6-Hz spike and wave (see Fig. 9.6), wicket waves, rhythmic temporal θ activity of drowsiness, psychomotor variant pattern, and subclinical rhythmic epileptiform discharges of adults—are not associated with increased epileptogenic potential (5).

SPECIFIC INTERICTAL EPILEPTIFORM PATTERNS IN PARTIAL EPILEPSIES

EEG abnormalities in patients with seizure disorders may be categorized as *specific* or *nonspecific*. Specific patterns, including the spike, sharp wave, spike–wave complex, temporal intermittent rhythmic delta activity (TIRDA), and periodic lateralized epileptiform discharges (PLEDs), are potentially epileptogenic and provide diagnostically useful information (24). Nonspecific changes, such as generalized or focal slow-wave activity and amplitude asymmetries, are not unique to epilepsy and do not indicate an increased epileptogenic potential (24). Potentially epileptogenic EEG alterations identified in patients with seizure disorders are rarely detected in nonepileptic patients (15). Interictal epileptiform alterations identify the irritative zone that may mark the epileptic brain tissue (26). Patients with seizures beginning in childhood typically display a higher incidence of EEG abnormalities than do those with adult-onset epilepsy (18).

Spikes and Sharp Waves

The main types of epileptiform discharges are spikes and sharp waves, occurring either as single potentials or with an after-following slow wave, known as a spike-wave complex. Spike-wave complexes may occur in isolation or in a repetitive fashion. Spike-wave discharges are predominantly negative transients easily recognized by their characteristic steep ascending and descending limbs and duration of 20 to 70 msec. Sharp-wave discharges are broader potentials with a pointed

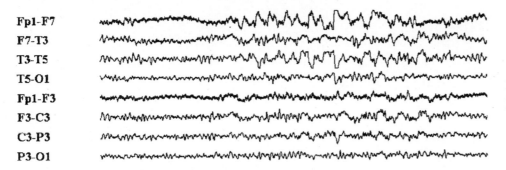

FIGURE 8.1 Temporal intermittent rhythmic delta activity (TIRDA) appears to increase in amplitude, slow in frequency, and spread slightly in distribution (note the late development of rhythmic slowing over the frontocentral region) over 3 to 4 seconds.

peak that lasts between 70 and 200 msec (27). These abnormalities should have a physiologic potential field and should involve more than one electrode to exclude electrode artifact.

Temporal Intermittent Rhythmic Delta Activity (TIRDA)

The interictal potentially epileptogenic pattern TIRDA (Fig. 8.1) has been identified in patients with partial epilepsy of temporal lobe origin and has the same epileptogenic significance as temporal lobe spike or sharp-wave discharges (5). This pattern, most prominent during drowsiness and NREM sleep, consists of rhythmic trains of low- to moderate-amplitude δ frequency slow waves over the temporal region, unilaterally or bilaterally, without apparent clinical accompaniment (5). This should be differentiated from persistent polymorphic δ frequency activity over the temporal region due to a focal structural brain lesion.

Periodic Epileptiform Discharges

The focal or lateralized sharp-wave discharges called PLEDs may have a wide field of distribution and occur in a periodic or quasiperiodic fashion (Fig. 8.2) (28). Typically occurring at 0.5 to 2.0 Hz, they vary in amplitude and duration (100 to 200 msec) and most commonly appear as broad diphasic or triphasic waves (5), although complexes of repetitive discharges also may be seen (29). This EEG pattern is not specific for any one pathologic lesion and is often the result of an acute or subacute insult, including infarct, tumor, or infection. PLEDs are usually transient, but persistent PLEDs have been reported (5).

Typical, uniform PLEDs are known as PLEDs-proper. In addition, the discharges may also be associated with low amplitude rhythmic discharges, known as PLEDs-plus. The risk of acute seizures is much greater if the EEG demonstrates PLEDs-plus. Up to 74% of the patients with PLEDs-plus monitored have been reported to have seizures, whereas only 6% of those with PLEDs-proper developed seizures during acute illness (30).

Occasionally, asynchronous PLEDs can be seen in both hemispheres, known as BiPLEDs. This most commonly occurs in patients with encephalitis, meningitis, seizure disorders, or hypoxic encephalopathy (30,31). PLEDs can also involve multiple independent sites, or multifocal PLEDs. Up to 89% of patients with multifocal PLEDs have developed clinical seizures (31). Rarely, the periodic complexes can be more diffuse, referred to as generalized epileptiform discharges (GPEDs). A study of patients with GPEDs found 89.2% of the patients experienced seizures within 48 hours and 32.4% of these patients were in status epilepticus (32).

CLINICAL USE OF THE ELECTROENCEPHALOGRAPH IN THE PARTIAL EPILEPSIES

Ictal Patterns in Partial Epilepsies

Partial, or localization-related, epilepsy implies seizure activity of focal onset (1,7,24). The electrographic onset of a seizure is characterized by a sudden change of frequency and the appearance of a new rhythm. An aura preceding impairment of consciousness may be without obvious electrographic accompaniment, and the new EEG rhythm may be intermittent at first but may evolve into more distinct patterns. Focal onset of the electrographic seizure may evolve through several phases: (i) focal desynchronization or attenuation of EEG activity; (ii) focal, rhythmic, low-voltage, fast-activity discharge; and (iii) progressive increase in amplitude with slowing that spreads to a regional anatomic distribution. Focal epileptiform discharges, such as repetitive spikes or fast activity recorded at

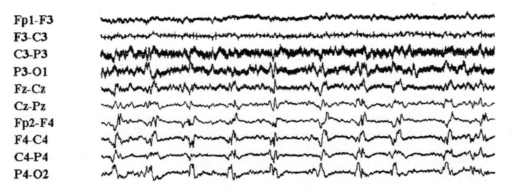

FIGURE 8.2 Periodic lateralizing epileptiform discharges (PLEDs), maximum over the right centroparietal region, with some spread to the left posterior head regions.

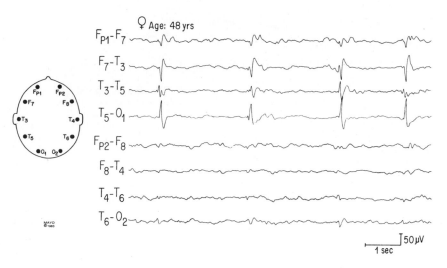

MAYO
©1983

FIGURE 8.3 Left temporal spikes. Characteristic interictal left temporal spike discharges. (Courtesy of B.F. Westmoreland, Mayo Clinic, Rochester, MN.)

a single electrode, are a relatively rare but important first change localizing the epileptogenic zone, provided an electrode artifact is ruled out (33).

Various areas of the brain differ significantly in their susceptibility to epilepsy. The temporal lobe has the lowest threshold for seizures, followed by the rolandic motor strip area and portions of the frontal lobe. The parietal and occipital lobes have the lowest degree of epileptogenicity. Focal epileptiform discharges may occur over any location on the scalp and depend on the age of the individual and the site of the pathologic lesion. This is particularly important in newborns and infants, whose brain maturation is incomplete or abnormal. Epileptiform discharges may appear to be generalized or multiregional (hypsarrhythmia) even in the presence of a focal brain lesion on magnetic resonance imaging (see Chapter 74).

Furthermore, extracranial EEG monitoring may be unremarkable in most patients experiencing simple partial seizures (34). A localized epileptiform abnormality on interictal scalp EEG may aid in the diagnostic classification of simple partial seizures, but those associated with transient psychic or visual experiential phenomena rarely occur with a precise, focal, epileptiform discharge on extracranial EEG. Therefore, the lack of EEG changes alone should not be used to establish the diagnosis of nonepileptic clinical behavior.

Temporal Lobe Epilepsy

Temporal spikes are highly epileptogenic and represent the most common interictal EEG alteration in adults with partial epilepsy (Fig. 8.3). The spike discharge amplitude is maximal over the anterior temporal region (in contrast to the centrotemporal spike) and may prominently involve the ear leads. Sleep markedly potentiates the presence of temporal spikes; approximately 90% of patients with temporal lobe seizures show spikes during sleep (5).

The ictal extracranial EEG during an anterior temporal lobe seizure typically demonstrates lobar seizure onset (Fig. 8.4). A

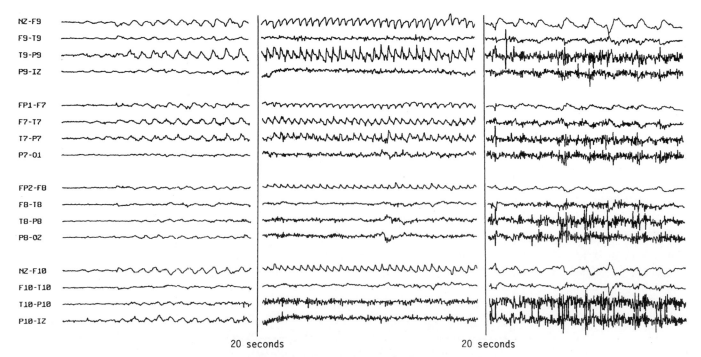

FIGURE 8.4 Scalp-recorded left temporal lobe seizure showing θ-, α-, and δ-frequency activity during consecutive phases.

lateralized moderate- to high-amplitude rhythmic paroxysm of activity is most prominent in the temporal scalp electrodes and may progress to generalized rhythmic slowing maximal on the side of seizure onset. Focal temporal lobe or generalized arrhythmic slow-wave activity may occur postictally. Interictal temporal lobe spiking may increase at the termination of the seizure (35).

In patients with partial seizures of temporal lobe origin, the localizing value of scalp EEG has ranged from approximately 40% to 90% (2,36). This variability may depend on whether the predominant apparent ictal EEG change occurs with the initial epileptiform discharges or with subsequent focal rhythmic abnormalities. Sphenoidal and inferolateral temporal scalp (T_1, T_2, F_9, F_{10}) electrodes, as well as closely placed scalp electrodes, can be useful in delineating the topography of the interictal activity (2,4,22,23,33). Sphenoidal electrodes record epileptiform activity emanating from the mediobasal limbic region and help to localize the epileptogenic zone prior to an anterior temporal lobectomy (2). In patients with temporal lobe epilepsy, the sensitivity of sphenoidal electrodes compared with scalp electrodes is unclear (4). Sphenoidal electrodes are artifact prone and poorly tolerated (which may interfere with a sleep recording) and have not demonstrated more sensitivity or specificity than lateral inferior scalp electrodes (4).

Patients with complex partial seizures of anterior temporal lobe origin may demonstrate localized, lateralized, or generalized ictal scalp EEG patterns (8,10). Most patients with independent bilateral and bisynchronous temporal spikes are ultimately found to have unilateral temporal lobe seizures (2). Prior to the seizure, an increase in interictal temporal lobe (or bitemporal) spiking may be evident. However, robust interictal spike discharges must be distinguished from electrographic seizure activity (10).

Frontal Lobe Epilepsy

The second most common site of seizure onset in partial epilepsy is the frontal lobe (8). This region presents difficult challenges in attempts to localize the epileptogenic zone with interictal scalp EEG recordings (2,33). The interictal EEG is not as sensitive and specific in frontal lobe epilepsy as it is in temporal lobe epilepsy (2). Epileptogenic zones in the frontal lobe remote from scalp electrodes (orbitofrontal and mesiofrontal regions) may not be associated with interictal activity despite multiple or prolonged EEG recordings. Supraorbital surface electrodes may increase the sensitivity and specificity of EEG scalp recordings in patients with frontal lobe epilepsy associated with seizures originating from the orbitofrontal region (2). These electrodes are preferred for nocturnal recordings because of the artifact generated by eye movement and blinking (2).

In frontal lobe epilepsy, seizures may begin in the dorsolateral frontal cortex, orbitofrontal region, cingulate gyrus, supplementary cortex, or frontal pole (7). Interictal frontal lobe epileptogenic discharges may be associated with simple partial, complex partial, atonic, or secondarily generalized tonic–clonic seizures (5,12). Ictal behavior in frontal lobe epilepsy is highly variable, and establishing the diagnosis based on ictal semiology alone may be difficult (7). Frontal lobe seizures, especially those arising from the supplementary sensorimotor region, may be confused with nonepileptic behavioral events (7).

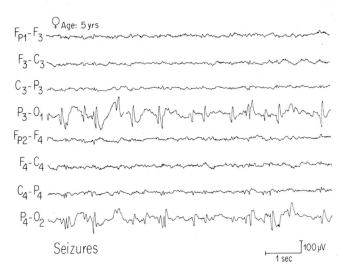

FIGURE 8.5 Occipital spikes. Bilateral occipital lobe interictal spiking in a child with a seizure disorder. (Courtesy of B.F. Westmoreland, Mayo Clinic, Rochester, MN.)

Occipital Lobe Epilepsy

Occipital spike-wave activity occurs less frequently than does epileptiform activity from the temporal or frontal regions (Fig. 8.5). Interictal occipital epileptiform activity is most common in children and indicates only moderate epileptogenicity. Approximately 40% to 50% of patients with occipital spikes have seizures (5). As described by Gastaut in 1982, occipital spike-waves also may occur in patients with idiopathic age-related occipital epilepsy, a less common variant of benign rolandic epilepsy (37). The seizures begin with a visual phenomenon and may be followed by generalized tonic–clonic episodes. Headache may occur during or after the seizures. The typical interictal occipital spikes attenuate with eye opening (37). Patients with this "benign partial" disorder have an excellent prognosis, and the seizures usually do not persist into adulthood (3,5,37).

Occipital "needle-sharp spikes" may also occur in congenitally blind individuals (usually children) who do not have epilepsy (38). Interictal occipital spike-waves may be unilateral or bilateral and may be associated with simple or complex partial seizures (3,5).

Perirolandic Epilepsy

The most common cause of perirolandic epilepsy is benign childhood epilepsy with centrotemporal spikes, or "rolandic epilepsy." The interictal EEG pattern in benign focal epilepsy of childhood is a high-voltage diphasic or polyphasic spike followed by a slow wave with the duration of 200 to 300 msec (Fig. 8.6) (1,3,5). Scalp EEG spike-wave activity appears to be maximal over the lower rolandic and midtemporal regions. The central midtemporal spike-wave may exhibit a surrounding region of positivity, suggesting a tangential dipole source (3,5). The discharges may be unilateral or bilateral, shift from side to side, and may not correspond to the hemisphere associated with ictal symptoms (5). Spiking is usually more abundant during drowsiness and sleep and is not a good predictor of the severity of seizure activity. Central spikes-waves have a moderate degree of epileptogenicity, with approximately 40% to 60% of patients having clinical seizures (5).

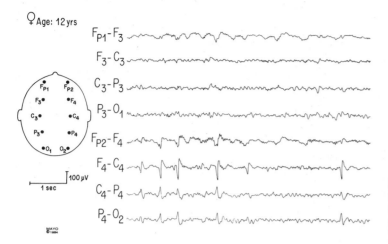

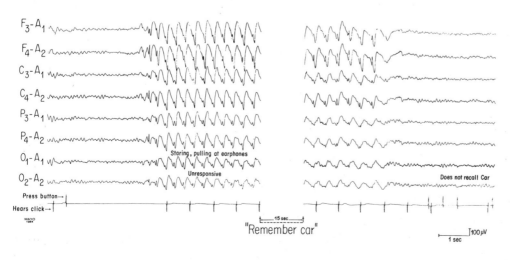

FIGURE 8.6 Right central spikes. Bipolar electroencephalogram (EEG) tracing shows interictal spiking in the right central region in a patient with benign rolandic epilepsy. Note normal background EEG activity. (Courtesy of B.F. Westmoreland, Mayo Clinic, Rochester, MN.)

Benign childhood epilepsy with centrotemporal spikes is a common and distinct seizure disorder. Seizure onset is typically between 2 and 12 years of age, and seizures disappear between 15 and 18 years of age (39). Antiepileptic drug therapy can usually be deferred, although the seizures typically respond well if treatment is elected. The ictal behavior includes focal motor or sensory seizures with frequent secondary generalization, excessive salivation and drooling, and motor speech arrest (40).

ELECTROENCEPHALOGRAPHY IN THE PRIMARY GENERALIZED EPILEPSIES

The specific interictal patterns associated with generalized epilepsies are easily distinguishable from normal background activity and include 3-Hz generalized spike and wave, slow spike and wave, atypical generalized spike and wave, and generalized paroxysmal fast activity. Generalized epilepsies are classified further as symptomatic or idiopathic, depending on etiology, seizure activity, and EEG alterations (40). Seizure types include absence, generalized tonic–clonic, atonic, myoclonic, tonic, clonic–tonic–clonic, and atypical absence (40).

SPECIFIC PATTERNS

3-Hz Spike and Wave

This morphologic pattern of the spike-wave complexes is similar in both interictal and ictal recordings. The EEG alteration consists of generalized, often anterior predominant, repetitive, bisynchronous, symmetric spike- and slow-wave discharges occurring at approximately 3 Hz (Fig. 8.7) (1,3,5,24,41). The typical pattern often varies, however. The frequency may be faster than 4.0 Hz at the beginning of the discharge and slower than 2.5 Hz at the end (42). Shifting minor asymmetries may occur over homologous head regions. Double spikes may be associated with an aftercoming slow wave (41). Hyperventilation, hypoglycemia, drowsiness, and eye closure may potentiate the generalized spike-wave discharge (41). During sleep, the morphology of the interictal abnormality may appear as fragmented or asymmetric spike-wave bursts (41). Background activities are usually normal. However, some intermittent, rhythmic, bisynchronous slow waves may be present over the posterior head regions (41).

This highly epileptogenic pattern occurs typically in children 3 to 15 years old with idiopathic generalized epilepsy and absence seizures (41). Absence seizures are more frequent in

FIGURE 8.7 Absence seizure (hyperventilation: 80 seconds). Electrographic correlate of a typical absence seizure precipitated by hyperventilation. Response testing during the seizure shows that the patient stopped pressing the button when a clicking sound was made in his ear. (Courtesy of J.D. Grabow, Mayo Clinic, Rochester, MN.)

girls and display a strong genetic predisposition. They usually occur frequently (multiple daily) as brief absences that typically last less than 30 seconds. Clinical seizures characterized by staring, automatisms, rapid eye blinking, and myoclonic movements of the extremities are closely correlated to the EEG recording and may occur when EEG changes persist for more than 3 to 4 seconds (8).

Multiple Spike and Wave

The multiple spike-and-wave pattern (also called atypical spike and wave and fast spike and wave) consists of a generalized mixture of intermittent brief spike and polyspike complexes associated with slow waves of variable frequency (3.5 to 6 Hz), morphology, and spatial distribution (Fig. 8.8) (43). The typical 1- to 3-second bursts are usually subclinical. The background between bursts may be normal or contain focal or generalized slow irregularities.

This pattern is associated with generalized tonic–clonic, clonic, atonic, myoclonic, and atypical absence seizures (24). In a generalized tonic–clonic seizure, the ictal EEG alterations at onset are bilateral, symmetric, and synchronous. The tonic phase begins with generalized, low-voltage, fast activity (the "epileptic recruiting rhythm") that progresses to a generalized spike and polyspike burst (Fig. 8.9) (8). The spike discharges gradually slow in frequency as they increase in amplitude. The clonic phase is associated with muscular relaxation and generalized EEG suppression with intermixed generalized spike and polyspike discharges. Postictally, at the termination of the seizure, prominent generalized background slowing gradually returns to baseline.

Slow Spike and Wave

The slow spike-and-wave pattern (see Fig. 9.24) consists of generalized, repetitive, bisynchronous, sharp-wave or spike discharges occurring at 1.5 to 2.5 Hz and is electrographically and clinically distinct from the 3-Hz pattern

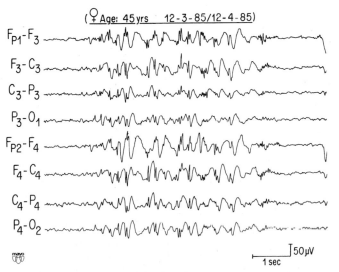

FIGURE 8.8 Generalized atypical spike and wave in an adult patient with a mixed seizure disorder that includes atypical absence seizures. (Courtesy of F.W. Sharbrough, Mayo Clinic, Rochester, MN.)

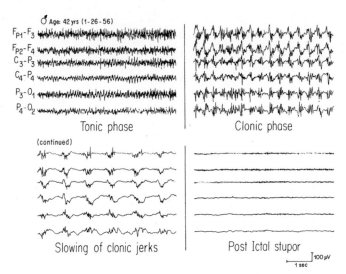

FIGURE 8.9 Multiple scalp-recorded electroencephalogram phases of a generalized tonic–clonic seizure. (From Westmoreland BF. The electroencephalogram in patients with epilepsy. In: Aminoff MJ, ed. *Neurology Clinics.* Philadelphia: WB Saunders, 1985:599–613, by permission of Mayo Foundation for Medical Education and Research.)

(1,3,24,37,43). The interictal and ictal EEG alterations are widely distributed, may occur asymmetrically with a shifting focal emphasis (44), and may be prolonged. Often, no clinical manifestations are apparent, although appropriate testing may disclose some alteration in psychomotor performance. Focal spikes and focal or generalized background slowing between the spike-wave bursts may also be present (44). Slow spike-and-wave discharges are less likely than the 3-Hz discharge to be activated by hyperventilation and hypoglycemia (43). Sleep recordings may show generalized spikes and multiple spike-wave discharges (43). The unusual similarity of the ictal and interictal EEG patterns may complicate the assessment of epilepsy in a child with severe cognitive impairment and reported frequent staring.

Seizures in these patients can vary but usually consist of tonic–clonic, tonic, atonic, atypical absences, and myoclonic types. Compared with the 3-Hz spike and wave, which rarely is present before the child is 4 years of age, the slow discharge may begin as early as age 6 months (45). The slow spike-and-wave pattern is most common in children with symptomatic generalized epilepsies, and may persist into adulthood (43–45).

The EEG may be helpful in classifying seizure syndromes. The two most common syndromes associated with the slow spike-and-wave pattern are Lennox–Gastaut syndrome and myoclonic-astatic epilepsy of Doose (Doose syndrome). Lennox–Gastaut syndrome typically presents in the preschool years in children who usually have a prior history of neurological disease. Children are usually delayed and the interictal EEG shows background slowing with frontally predominant, slow spike-wave, usually less than 2 Hz. In comparison, myoclonic-astatic epilepsy of Doose also affects preschoolers. However, children are neurologically normal prior to presentation. The interictal EEG also shows slow spike-wave, but it is usually 2 to 3 Hz, with theta rhythms in the parietal regions (46).

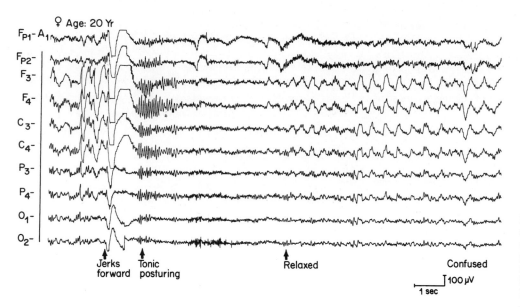

FIGURE 8.10 High-amplitude generalized sharp wave followed by desynchronization and generalized paroxysmal fast activity during a tonic seizure. (Courtesy of F.W. Sharbrough, Mayo Clinic, Rochester, MN.)

Paroxysmal or Rhythmic Fast Activity

This pattern of repetitive spike discharges with a frequency of 8 to 20 Hz often occurs at the onset of generalized tonic–clonic seizures, in association with tonic seizures, and during sleep recordings in patients with generalized seizures. The ictal scalp EEG reveals a generalized, synchronous, symmetric alteration, usually in the form of low-voltage fast-frequency (approximately 20 to 25 Hz) activity that progressively increases in amplitude (Fig. 8.10).

Electrodecremental Response

This ictal EEG pattern, seen mostly with tonic and atonic seizures and with infantile spasms, consists of an abrupt generalized "flattening" or desynchronization of activity, usually arising from an abnormal background (Fig. 8.11). The EEG desynchronization may last longer than the clinical seizure. The degree of EEG suppression may depend on the duration of the seizure and the alteration in mentation. Muscle artifact may make identification difficult when the seizure is brief (8).

Photoparoxysmal Response

This abnormal cerebral response to photic stimulation consists of generalized multiple spike-wave complexes and is likely a variant of the atypical spike and wave (47). It is best seen at flash frequencies between 10 and 20 Hz, and the resulting seizure discharge may outlast the stimulus by a few seconds. The response may be accompanied by brief body jerks or impaired consciousness (48). Photoparoxysmal responses may be seen at any age, as a familial trait or an acquired phenomenon (47,48), but maximal expression is between ages 8 and 20 years. Acquired photoparoxysmal responses may be seen following withdrawal from various medications and alcohol and in metabolic derangements (48).

The photoparoxysmal response must be contrasted with the noncerebral, nonepileptogenic, photomyogenic response to photic stimulation. Brief muscle spikes and eye movement artifacts are time-locked to the photic flashes that cease when the stimulus is discontinued (49). Again, this response is best seen at flash frequencies of 8 to 15 Hz. The EEG artifacts may become more prominent as the stimulus continues, and may be attenuated with eye opening. Myoclonic or oscillatory

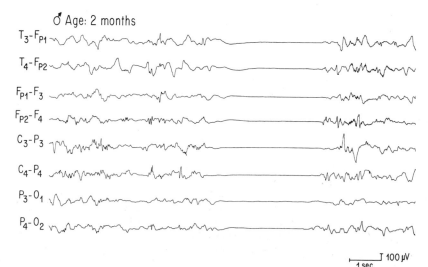

FIGURE 8.11 Electrodecremental episode associated with infantile spasms (onset 3 weeks, cause unknown). (Courtesy of D.W. Klass, Mayo Clinic, Rochester, MN.)

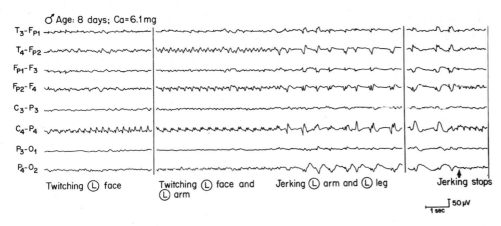

FIGURE 8.12 Scalp-recorded right hemisphere seizure in a neonate with hypocalcemia. (Courtesy of B.F. Westmoreland, Mayo Clinic, Rochester, MN.)

movements of the eyes may accompany the photomyogenic response, which is seen mainly in adults and is related to nervousness, as well as to drug and alcohol withdrawal (49).

SPECIAL ELECTROENCEPHALO-GRAPHIC PATTERNS IN NEWBORNS AND INFANTS

Neonatal Recording

Ictal EEG seizure discharges in neonates may vary in frequency, amplitude, morphology, and duration. These paroxysms of rhythmic sharp-wave discharges or rhythmic activity in the θ-, α-, or β-frequency ranges may occur in a focal or multifocal distribution (Fig. 8.12). The seizure discharges may shift from one location to another. The epileptiform activity may be associated with clinical seizures. However, subclinical EEG phenomena without an observed clinical accompaniment are common. The interictal background activity is prognostically important in this population. Neonatal seizures associated with symptomatic neurologic disease such as anoxic encephalopathy may feature a low-voltage background abnormality or a burst-suppression pattern indicative of a poor prognosis.

Due to the association of neonatal seizures with neurodevelopmental abnormalities, early and accurate detection is important (50). Over the past two decades, amplitude-integrated electroencephalography (aEEG) has been used with increasing frequency as a cerebral function monitor (50). This monitor typically uses one EEG channel placed over the biparietal head region, which is close to the "watershed" regions of the neonatal brain (51). This information is then filtered and compressed to show the upper and lower amplitudes of the EEG signal. While this technology allows monitoring without the need of experienced EEG technicians and electroencephalographers, the sensitivity of aEEG has been questioned. Depending on the expertise of the interpreting neonatologist, the sensitivity may range from 12% to 55% (50).

Hypsarrhythmia

Hypsarrhythmia is a chaotic mixture of high-amplitude (exceeding 300 mV), generalized, continuous, arrhythmic slow-wave activity intermixed with spike and multifocal spike discharges (Fig. 8.13) (44,52). Nearly continuous during

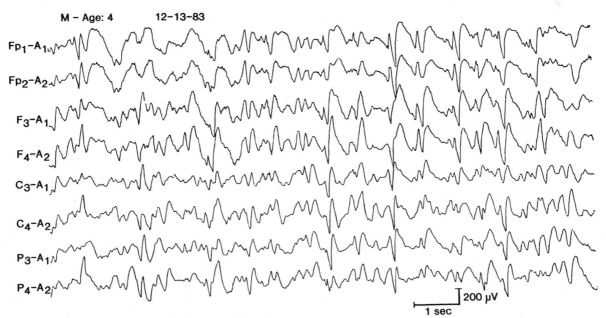

FIGURE 8.13 Interictal EEG reveals high-amplitude generalized background activity intermixed with multifocal spike discharges (hypsarrhythmia) in a child with infantile spasms. (Courtesy of B.F. Westmoreland, Mayo Clinic, Rochester, MN.)

wakefulness, it becomes more discontinuous during NREM sleep, with high-voltage spikes and sharp waves alternating with lower-voltage irregular slow-wave activity (52). Epileptiform activity decreases during rapid eye movement sleep. Hypsarrhythmia occurs most commonly from 4 months to 5 years of age in children with infantile spasms (West syndrome). Nevertheless, not all patients with infantile spasms have this EEG alteration, and not all patients with hypsarrhythmia have infantile spasms. Infantile spasms may be symptomatic (cause can be determined) or cryptogenic (cause is unknown). However, the EEG cannot distinguish one etiology from another (52). The hypsarrhythmic pattern likely represents a response of the immature brain to a variety of disturbances in cerebral function.

References

1. Daly DD. Epilepsy and syncope. In: Pedley TA, Daly DD, eds. *Current Practice of Clinical Electroencephalography.* New York: Raven Press; 1990:269–334.
2. Quesney LF. Extracranial EEG evaluation. In: Engel J Jr, ed. *Surgical Treatment of the Epilepsies.* New York: Raven Press; 1987:129–166.
3. Niedermeyer E, da Silva FL. Abnormal EEG patterns (epileptic and paroxysmal). In: *Electroencephalography: Basic Principles, Clinical Applications, and Related Fields.* 2nd ed. Baltimore, MD: Urban & Schwarzenberg; 1987:183–207.
4. Sharbrough FW. Commentary: extracranial EEG monitoring. In: Engel J Jr, ed. *Surgical Treatment of the Epilepsies.* New York: Raven Press; 1987: 167–171.
5. Westmoreland BF. The electroencephalogram in patients with epilepsy. In: Aminoff MJ, ed. *Neurology Clinics.* Philadelphia: WB Saunders; 1985: 599–613.
6. Williamson PD, Spencer DD, Spencer SS. Complex partial seizures of frontal lobe origin. *Ann Neurol.* 1985;18:497–504.
7. Williamson PD, Weiser H-G, Delgado-Escueta AV. Clinical characteristics of partial seizures. In: Engel J Jr, ed. *Surgical Treatment of the Epilepsies.* New York: Raven Press; 1987:101–120.
8. Engel J Jr. Epileptic seizures. In: Engel J Jr, ed. *Seizures and Epilepsy.* Philadelphia: FA Davis; 1989:137–178.
9. Risinger MW, Engel J Jr, Van Ness PC, et al. Ictal localization of temporal lobe seizures with scalp-sphenoidal recordings. *Neurology.* 1989;39: 1288–1293.
10. Sharbrough FW. Complex partial seizures. In: Lüders H, Lesser RP, eds. *Epilepsy: Electroclinical Syndromes.* Berlin: Springer-Verlag; 1987: 279–302.
11. Berger H. Uber das Elektrenkephalogram des menschen. *Arch Psychiatry.* 1933;100:301–320.
12. Gibbs FA, Davis H, Lennox WG. The electroencephalogram in epilepsy and in conditions of impaired consciousness. *Arch Neurol Psychiatry.* 1935;34:1133–1148.
13. Gibbs EL, Gibbs FA. Diagnostic and localizing value of electroencephalographic studies in sleep. *Res Publ Assoc Res Nerv Ment Dis.* 1947;23: 366–376.
14. Penfield W, Jasper H, eds. *Epilepsy and the Functional Anatomy of the Brain.* Boston: Little, Brown; 1954.
15. Zivin L, Ajmone-Marsan C. Incidence and prognostic significance of epileptiform activity in the EEG of nonepileptic subjects. *Brain.* 1969; 91:751–778.
16. Andermann FA. Identification of candidates for surgical treatment of epilepsy. In: Engel J Jr, ed. *Surgical Treatment of the Epilepsies.* New York: Raven Press; 1987:51–70.
17. Guidelines in electroencephalography, evoked potentials and polysomnography. *J Clin Neurophysiol.* 1994;11(1):1–147.
18. Ajmone-Marsan C, Zivin LS. Factors related to the occurrence of typical paroxysmal abnormalities in the EEG records of epileptic patients. *Epilepsia.* 1970;11:361–381.
19. Cascino GD. Clinical indications and diagnostic yield of video-electroencephalographic monitoring in patients with seizures and spells. *Mayo Clinic Proceedings.* 2002;77:1111–1120.
20. Watemberg N, Tziperman B, Dabby R, et al. Adding video recording increases the diagnostic yield of routine electroencephalograms in children with frequent paroxysmal events. *Epilepsia.* 2005;46(5):716–719.
21. Wirrell E, Kozlik S, Tellez J, et al. Ambulatory electroencephalography (EEG) in children: diagnostic yield and tolerability. *J Child Neurol.* 2008;23(6):655–662.
22. Sharbrough FW. Electrical fields and recording techniques. In: Daly D, Pedley TA, eds. *Current Practice of Clinical Electroencephalography.* New York: Raven Press; 1990:29–49.
23. Sperling MR, Engel J Jr. Comparison of nasopharyngeal with scalp electrodes including ear and true temporal electrodes in the detection of spikes. *Electroencephalogr Clin Neurophysiol.* 1984;58:39.
24. Pedley TA. Interictal epileptiform discharges: discriminating characteristics and clinical correlations. *Am J EEG Technol.* 1980;20:101–119.
25. Ojemann GA, Engel J Jr. Acute and chronic intracranial recording and stimulation. In: Engel J Jr, ed. *Surgical Treatment of the Epilepsies.* New York: Raven Press; 1987:263–288.
26. Schwartzkroin PA, Wyler AR. Mechanisms underlying epileptiform burst discharges. *Ann Neurol.* 1980;7:95–107.
27. International Federation of Society for Electroencephalography and Clinical Neurophysiology. *Electroencephalography and Clinical Neurophysiology.* New York: Elsevier; 1974.
28. de la Paz D, Brenner RP. Bilateral independent periodic epileptiform discharges. *Arch Neurol.* 1981;38:713–715.
29. Reiher J, Rivest J, Grand'Maison F, et al. Periodic lateralized epileptiform discharges with transitional rhythmic discharges: association with seizures. *Electroencephalogr Clin Neurophysiol.* 1991;78:12–17.
30. Yemisci M, Gurer G, Saygi S, et al. Generalised periodic epileptiform discharges: clinical features, neuroradiological evaluation and prognosis in 37 adult patients. *Seizure.* 2003;12(7):465–472.
31. Brenner R. Is it status? *Epilepsia.* 2002;43(Suppl 3):103–113.
32. Jirsch J, Hirsch LJ. Nonconvulsive seizures: developing a rational approach to the diagnosis and management in the critically ill population. *Clin Neurophysiol.* 2007;118(8):1660–1670.
33. Quesney LF, Constain M, Fish DR, et al. Frontal lobe epilepsy: a field of recent emphasis. *Am J EEG Technol.* 1990;30:177–193.
34. Devinsky O, Sato S, Kufta CV, et al. Electroencephalographic studies of simple partial seizures with subdural electrode recordings. *Neurology.* 1989;39:527–533.
35. Gotman J, Marciani MG. Electroencephalographic spiking activity, drug levels, and seizure occurrence in epileptic patients. *Ann Neurol.* 1985;17:597–603.
36. Wyllie E, Lüders H, Morris HH, et al. Clinical outcome after complete or partial resection for intractable partial epilepsy. *Neurology.* 1987;33: 1634–1641.
37. Gastaut H. A new type of epilepsy: benign partial epilepsy of childhood with occipital spike-waves. *Clin Electroencephalogr.* 1982;13:13–22.
38. Gibbs FA, Gibbs EL. *Atlas of Electroencephalography, IV.* Reading, MA: Addison-Wesley; 1978.
39. Kellaway P. The incidence, significance and natural history of spike foci in children. In: Henry CE, ed. *Current Clinical Neurophysiology. Update of EEG and Evoked Potentials.* New York: Elsevier; 1980: 151–175.
40. Gastaut H. Clinical and electroencephalographic classification of epileptic seizures. *Epilepsia.* 1970;11:102–113.
41. Dalby MA. Epilepsy and 3 per second spike and wave rhythms. *Acta Neurol Scand.* 1969;45(Suppl 40):1–180.
42. Gibbs FA, Gibbs EL. *Atlas of Electroencephalography, III.* 2nd ed. Reading, MA: Addison-Wesley Publishing; 1964.
43. Blume WT, David RB, Gomez MR. Generalized sharp and slow wave complexes—associated clinical features and long-term follow-up. *Brain.* 1973;289:306.
44. Gastaut H, Roger J, Soulayrol R, et al. Childhood epileptic encephalography with diffuse slow spike-waves (otherwise known as "petit mal variant") or Lennox syndrome. *Epilepsia.* 1966;7:139–179.
45. Markand O. Slow spike and wave activity in EEG and associated clinical features: often called "Lennox-Gastaut" syndrome. *Neurology.* 1977; 25:463–471.
46. Roger J, Bureau M, Dravet C, et al., eds. *Epileptic Syndromes of Infancy, Childhood, and Adolescence.* 2nd ed. London: John Libbey; 1992.
47. Newmark ME, Penry KJ. *Photosensitivity and Epilepsy. A Review.* New York: Raven Press; 1979.
48. Fisch BJ, Hauser WA, Brust JCM, et al. The EEG response to diffuse and patterned photic stimulation during acute untreated alcohol withdrawal. *Neurology.* 1989;39:434–436.
49. Meier-Ewert K, Broughton RJ. Photomyoclonic response of epileptic and nonepileptic subjects during wakefulness, sleep, and arousal. *Electroencephalogr Clin Neurophysiol.* 1976;23:301–304.
50. Shellhaas RA, Soaita AI, Clancy RR. Sensitivity of amplitude-integrated electroencephalography for neonatal seizure detection. *Pediatrics.* 2007; 120(4):770–777.
51. Shah DK, Mackay MT, Lavery S, et al. Accuracy of bedside electroencephalographic monitoring in comparison with simultaneous continuous conventional electroencephalography for seizure detection in term infants. *Pediatrics.* 2008;121(6):1146–1154.
52. Hrachovy RA, Frost JD Jr, Kellaway P. Hypsarrhythmia: variations on a theme. *Epilepsia.* 1984;35:317–325.

CHAPTER 9 ■ ELECTROENCEPHALOGRAPHIC ATLAS OF EPILEPTIFORM ABNORMALITIES

SOHEYL NOACHTAR AND ELAINE WYLLIE

Electroencephalography (EEG) is generally considered the single most important laboratory tool in the evaluation of patients with epilepsy. This atlas of material from patients seen at the Cleveland Clinic Foundation and the University of Munich illustrates some of the EEG findings discussed throughout this book. Additional EEG atlases and textbooks are listed in the bibliography at the end of this chapter.

METHODS

These tracings were made following American Electroencephalographic Society guidelines (1), with electrodes placed according to the International 10-20 Electrode Placement System (2). Additional closely spaced electrodes according to the 10-10 system (Fig. 9.1) were used in some cases to better define a focal epileptogenic zone. The combinatorial electrode nomenclature used here is that recently proposed by the American Electroencephalographic Society (3) and the International Federation of Clinical Neurophysiology (2). The EEG terminology used in this chapter follows the recommendation of the International Federation of Clinical Neurophysiology (4).

For consistency and ease of interpretation, we displayed most tracings with the same longitudinal bipolar montage (Fig. 9.2). Occasionally, the activity was best shown with a transverse bipolar montage (Fig. 9.3), a longitudinal bipolar montage with anterior temporal or sphenoidal electrodes (Fig. 9.2), or a referential montage.

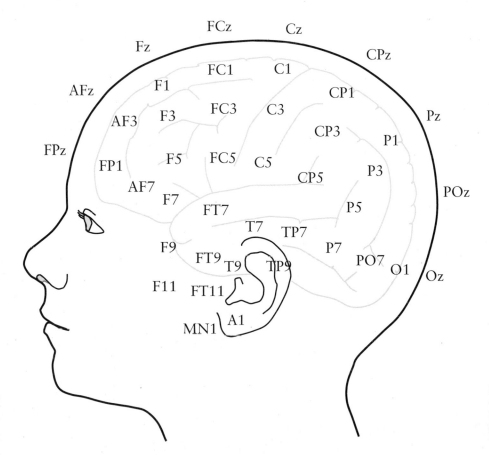

FIGURE 9.1 Electrode positions and nomenclature of the combinatorial 10-10 system proposed by the American Electroencephalographic Society (1) and the International Federation of Clinical Neurophysiology (2).

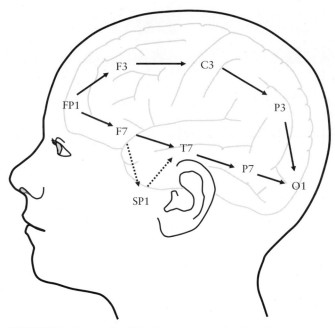

FIGURE 9.2 Longitudinal bipolar montage, left-sided electrodes. The "double-banana" montage used for almost all the tracings in this atlas includes the channels shown with *filled arrows*, ordered as follows: left temporal chain, right temporal chain, left parasagittal chain, and right parasagittal chain. The "anterior temporal" montage used in some of the tracings is modified to include the channels shown with *broken arrows* to reflect anterior, basal, or mesial temporal discharges with anterior temporal (FT9, FT10) or sphenoidal (SP1, SP2) electrodes.

PART I: NORMAL ELECTROENCEPHALOGRAPHIC PATTERNS AND VARIANTS SOMETIMES CONFUSED WITH EPILEPTIFORM ACTIVITY

For epileptologists to fulfill the basic obligation to "do no harm," they must avoid "overreading" normal variants on EEG (5,6). This section includes several normal patterns that may be easily mistaken for epileptiform discharges, resulting

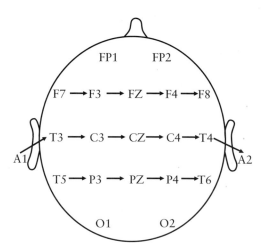

FIGURE 9.3 Transverse bipolar montage, vertex view. Channels are arrayed in order, as follows: frontal chain, temporocentral chain, and parietal chain.

in an incorrect diagnosis of epilepsy and inappropriate recommendations for antiepileptic medication.

Small sharp spike	Figure 9.4
14- and 6-Hz positive spikes	Figure 9.5
6-Hz "phantom" spike and wave	Figure 9.6
Wicket spikes	Figure 9.7
Subclinical rhythmical electrographic discharges of adults	Figure 9.8
Rhythmic temporal theta bursts of drowsiness	Figure 9.9
Hypnagogic hypersynchrony	Figure 9.10
V-waves and positive occipital sharp transients (POSTS)	Figure 9.11
Sleep spindle	Figure 9.12
Hyperventilation effect	Figure 9.13
Photic driving	Figure 9.14
Breach rhythm	Figure 9.15

PART II: ELECTROENCEPHALO-GRAPHIC ABNORMALITIES OF THE GENERALIZED EPILEPSIES

Childhood Absence Epilepsy

Absence seizure	Figure 9.16
Absence status epilepticus	Figures 9.17 and 9.18

Juvenile Myoclonic Epilepsy

Myoclonic jerk with photic stimulation	Figure 9.19
Cluster of myoclonic jerks	Figure 9.20

Infantile Spasms

Hypsarrhythmia	Figure 9.21
Seizure	Figure 9.22

Lennox–Gastaut Syndrome

Generalized sharp- and slow-wave complexes	Figure 9.23
Generalized paroxysmal fast and polyspikes in sleep	Figure 9.24
Atonic seizures	Figure 9.25

Intractable Epilepsy with Multifocal Spikes

Intractable epilepsy with multifocal spikes	Figure 9.26

Stimulation-Related Epilepsy

Reading-induced spike-and-wave complexes	Figure 9.27

PART III: ELECTROENCEPHALO-GRAPHIC ABNORMALITIES OF THE FOCAL EPILEPSIES

Localization-related (partial, focal, or local) epilepsies (15) involve seizures arising from a cortical region within one hemisphere. The first several illustrations are from children who had benign epileptiform discharges of childhood on EEG, with or without clinical seizures. The rest of the figures are from patients with symptomatic epilepsy and focal seizures arising from specific cortical regions, grouped by location of the epileptogenic zone. For most of the titles and legends, we use terminology from the most recent seizure and epilepsy classification systems of the International League Against Epilepsy (16). Some additional terms are also used here, such as "aura" instead of "simple partial seizure with special sensory symptoms" and "focal clonic seizure" instead of "simple partial seizure with focal motor signs." Some newer terms were also included (17); these are discussed further in Chapter 10.

Benign Focal Epileptiform Discharges of Childhood

Centrotemporal sharp waves	Figure 9.28
Dipole potential	Figure 9.29
Occipital sharp waves	Figure 9.30
Left and right central sharp waves	Figure 9.31

Temporal Lobe Epilepsy

Temporal sharp wave	Figure 9.32
Complex partial ("hypomotor") seizure	Figure 9.33
Bitemporal sharp waves	Figures 9.34 and 9.35
Temporal lobectomy: positive left temporal spike waves	Figures 9.36
Complex partial seizure with automatisms	Figures 9.37 and 9.38
Lateral (neocortical) temporal lobe epilepsy: temporo-parietal polyspikes	Figures 9.39

Frontal Lobe Epilepsy

Frontal sharp waves	Figure 9.40
Secondary bilateral synchrony	Figure 9.41
Subclinical EEG seizure	Figures 9.42 and 9.43

Occipital Lobe Epilepsy

Visual aura and focal clonic seizure	Figures 9.44 and 9.45

Supplementary Motor Area Epilepsy

Sharp waves at vertex	Figure 9.46
Tonic seizure	Figure 9.47

Paracentral Epilepsy

Focal clonic seizure	Figures 9.48 and 9.49
Right frontocentral sharp waves	Figure 9.50
Left arm tonic seizure	Figure 9.51
Epilepsia partialis continua	Figure 9.52

PART IV: ELECTROENCEPHALO-GRAPHIC FINDINGS IN NONEPILEPTIC PAROXYSMAL DISORDERS

The differential diagnosis of epilepsy includes a wide variety of paroxysmal disorders (see Chapter 43). During a clinical episode, the EEG recording may be crucial to clarifying the exact nature of the spells. In most of these disorders, the ictal electroencephalogram is normal. Three nonepileptic paroxysmal disorders with abnormal EEG findings are syncope, breath-holding spells, and sleep attacks caused by narcolepsy.

Pallid infantile syncope	Figures 9.53 and 9.54
Cyanotic breath-holding spell	Figures 9.55 and 9.56
Narcolepsy	Figure 9.57

SMALL SHARP SPIKE

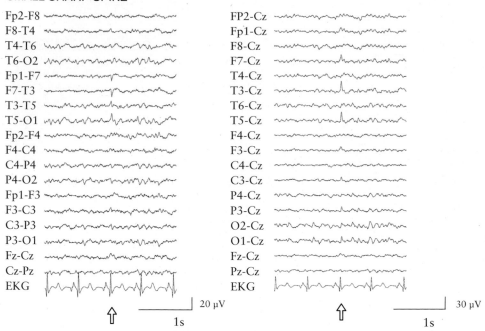

FIGURE 9.4 Twenty-five-year-old man, otherwise normal, with chronic tension headache. Note the low-amplitude monophasic sharp transient *(arrow)* followed by a minimal slow wave, maximum negativity in the left temporal region, undisturbed background rhythms, during light sleep. Small, sharp spikes have also been called benign epileptiform transients of sleep (7).

14-HZ AND 6-HZ POSITIVE SPIKES

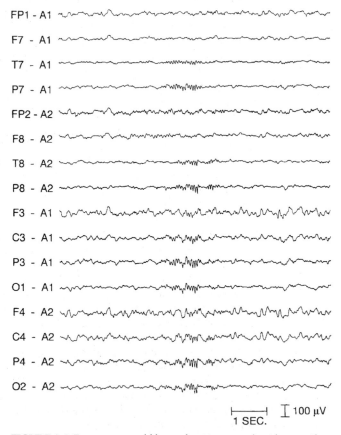

FIGURE 9.5 Fourteen-year-old boy, otherwise normal, with nonepileptic episodes of dizziness. Note the burst of sharply contoured 14-Hz activity with maximum positivity posteriorly, occurring in light sleep (8). Elsewhere in the recording were similar bursts with predominantly 6-Hz frequency. Positive spikes of 14- and 6-Hz have also been called ctenoids.

6-HZ "PHANTOM" SPIKE AND WAVE

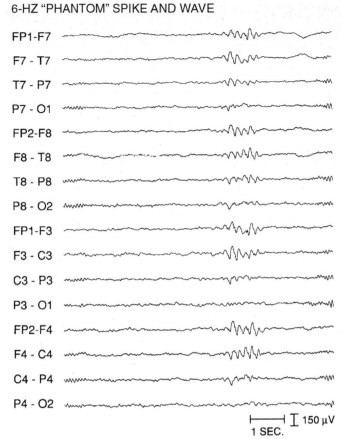

FIGURE 9.6 Fourteen-year-old boy with muscle contraction headaches, dizziness, and syncope. Note the generalized burst of 6-Hz low-amplitude spikes with prominent slow waves occurring during drowsiness (6).

WICKET SPIKES

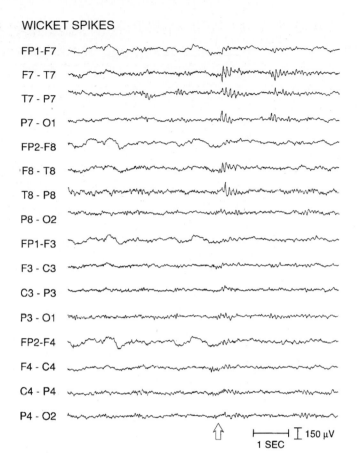

FIGURE 9.7 Seventy-five-year-old woman with gait disturbance and no seizures. Note the 9-Hz, rhythmic, sharply contoured waves with maximum negativity in midtemporal regions, occurrence during drowsiness, and undisturbed background rhythms. The typical frequency of wicket spikes is 6- to 11-Hz (9).

SUBCLINICAL RHYTHMICAL ELECTROGRAPHIC DISCHARGES OF ADULTS

RHYTHMICAL TEMPORAL THETA BURSTS OF DROWSINESS

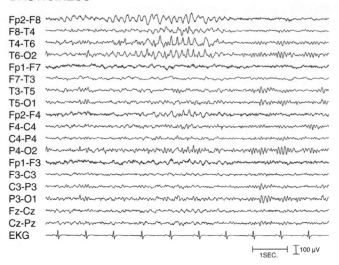

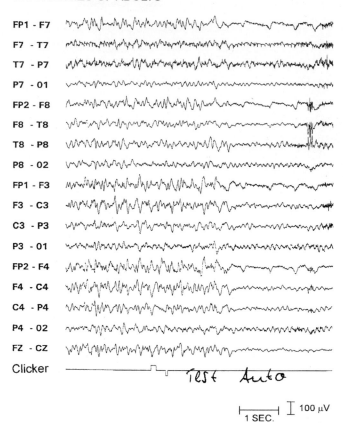

FIGURE 9.9 Forty-eight-year-old woman with benign paroxysmal vertigo. This rhythmic theta activity during drowsiness, with sharply contoured waves maximal in the left midtemporal region, has also been called psychomotor variant (6,11). Note that the patterns cease as soon as the patient alerts, which is associated with occipital alpha activity.

FIGURE 9.8 Sixty-one-year-old woman with depression. Note the diffuse frontal-maximum, rhythmic, sharply contoured theta and delta activity (10) that ended after 34 seconds and was immediately followed by a normal posterior-dominant alpha rhythm. During the rhythmic activity, the patient responded appropriately to an auditory stimulus (clicker). In the last channel, the upward deflection was from the technician's sound stimulus, and the subsequent downward deflection was from the button pressed by the patient in response. The patient remained awake and responsive throughout the recording and afterward recalled the test word ("auto").

HYPNAGOGIC HYPERSYNCHRONY

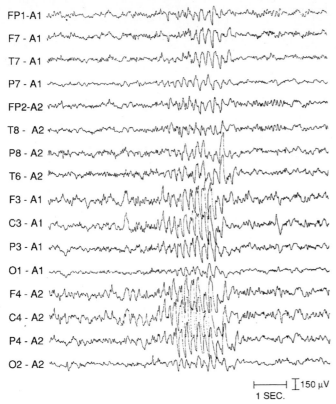

FIGURE 9.10 One-and-a-half-year-old normal boy. Note the generalized, rhythmic, high-amplitude theta activity with intermixed sharp transients during drowsiness.

V-WAVES AND POSITIVE OCCIPITAL SHARP TRANSIENTS

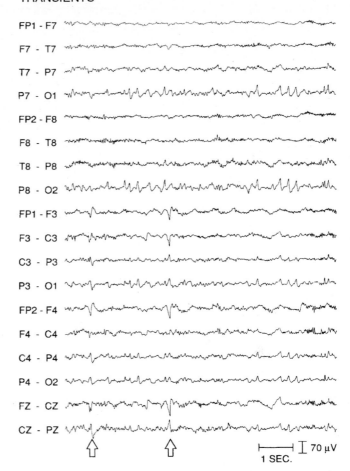

FIGURE 9.11 Sixteen-year-old girl with vasovagal syncope. Note the central vertex waves (*arrows*) and runs of positive occipital sharp transients of sleep (POSTS) (channels 4 and 8), both normal features of stage I or II non-rapid eye movement (non-REM) sleep.

SLEEP SPINDLE

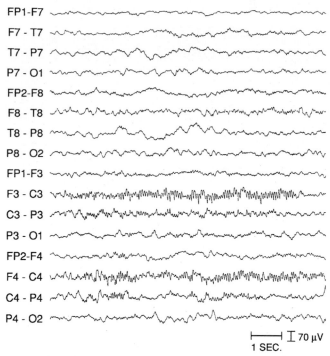

FIGURE 9.12 Two-month-old normal infant. Prolonged spindles with 12-Hz μ-like waveforms are common in infants during stage II non-REM sleep and may be asynchronous over the right and left hemispheres.

HYPERVENTILATION EFFECT

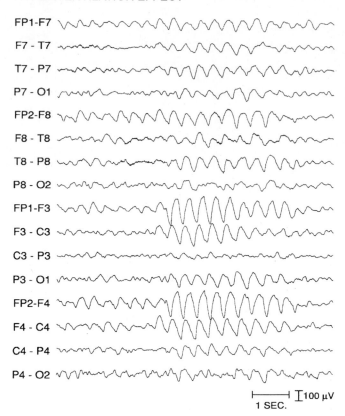

FIGURE 9.13 Eight-year-old girl with school problems. She was misdiagnosed as having absence epilepsy because of hyperventilation-induced high-amplitude rhythmic slowing. The girl was alert and responsive during this tracing, which was obtained after 2 minutes of hyperventilation.

PHOTIC DRIVING

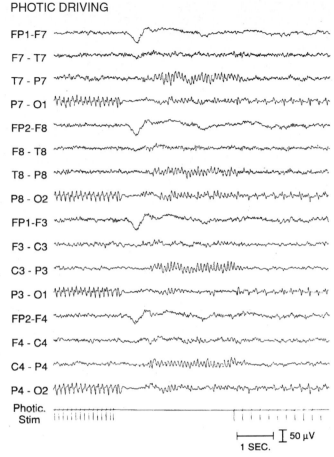

FIGURE 9.14 Twelve-year-old boy with childhood absence epilepsy since 4 years of age, seizure free on medication for the last 1.5 years. Note the time-locked, unsustained, bioccipital response to 8- and 4-Hz photic stimulation, separated by normal posterior background activity. Photic driving represents a normal response to photic stimulation and is not related to the epilepsy of the patient.

BREACH RHYTHM

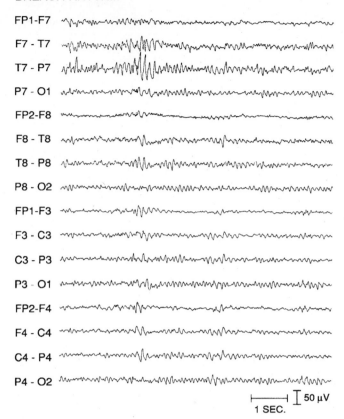

FIGURE 9.15 Twenty-one-year-old woman with trigeminal neuralgia, status after left parietotemporal craniotomy for vascular decompression. Note the asymmetry of background rhythms owing to the skull defect (12), maximum at the left temporal (T7) electrode.

CHILDHOOD ABSENCE EPILEPSY: ABSENCE SEIZURE

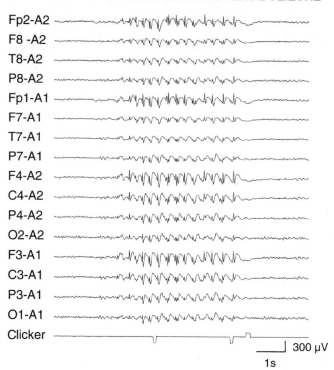

FIGURE 9.16 Twelve-year-old boy, otherwise normal, with recent onset of absence seizures. These generalized 3-Hz spike-and-wave complexes were precipitated by hyperventilation and lasted for 4 seconds, with staring and unresponsiveness. Note that the patient failed to press a button as a response to an auditory stimulus given to him during the SWC but he responded to a second stimulus at the end of the discharge.

ABSENCE STATUS EPILEPTICUS: GENERALIZED POLYSPIKE-AND-WAVE COMPLEXES

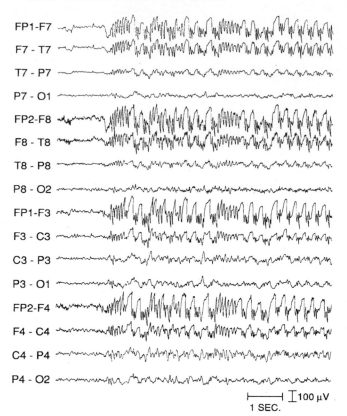

FIGURE 9.17 Forty-three-year-old woman with absence seizures during childhood. She was seizure free throughout adulthood until absence status epilepticus began during chemotherapy for breast cancer. During this episode, with generalized polyspike-and-wave complexes, she had unresponsiveness and eyelid fluttering. Electroencephalographic findings and behavior returned to normal after intravenous injection of diazepam.

ABSENCE STATUS EPILEPTICUS: GENERALIZED SHARP AND SLOW WAVE COMPLEXES

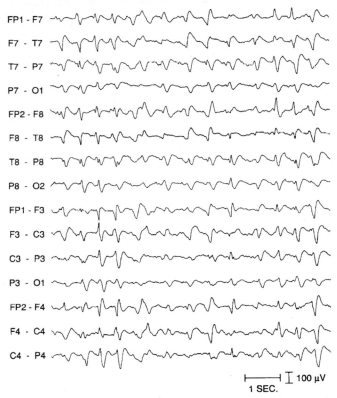

FIGURE 9.18 Fifty-eight-year-old woman with a 3-day history of confusion and agitation prior to this electroencephalogram (EEG). She had no previous history of seizures, and this was her first manifestation of generalized absence epilepsy. EEG findings and behavior returned to normal after intravenous injection of diazepam.

JUVENILE MYOCLONIC EPILEPSY: MYOCLONIC JERK WITH PHOTIC STIMULATION

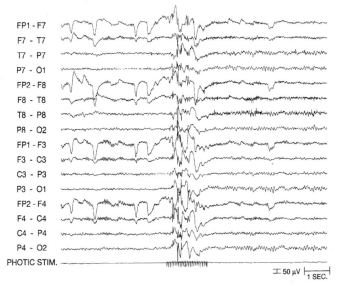

FIGURE 9.19 Fifteen-year-old boy with an 8-month history of myoclonic jerks of the upper extremities in the morning after awakening. A generalized tonic–clonic seizure occurred in the morning 2 weeks before this electroencephalogram. Note the polyspike component of the spike-and-wave complexes during the myoclonic jerk precipitated by photic stimulation.

JUVENILE MYOCLONIC EPILEPSY: CLUSTER OF MYOCLONIC JERKS

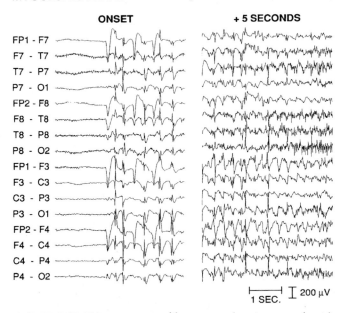

FIGURE 9.20 Thirty-two-year-old woman, otherwise normal, with myoclonic and generalized tonic–clonic seizures on awakening since adolescence. This episode began with repeated myoclonic jerks of the arms and upper body synchronous with the generalized spike-and-wave complexes. This flurry evolved after 20 seconds into a generalized tonic–clonic convulsion ("clonic–tonic–clonic seizure").

INFANTILE SPASMS: HYPSARRHYTHMIA

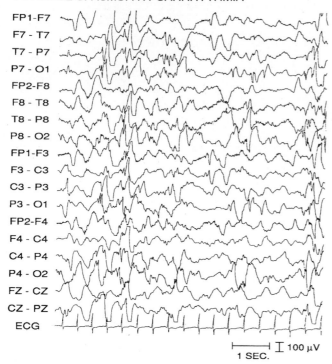

FIGURE 9.21 Eight-month-old boy with infantile spasms and developmental delay. Awake electroencephalographic record showed disorganized background rhythms dominated by multifocal spikes and high-amplitude slowing.

INFANTILE SPASMS: SEIZURE

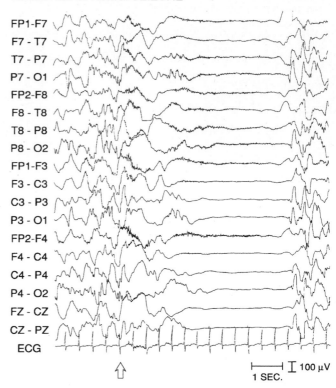

FIGURE 9.22 EEG during a spasm (*arrow*), from the same infant as in Figure 9.21. Note the generalized high-amplitude slow transient followed by a generalized electrodecremental pattern for 3 seconds. The spasm involved tonic abduction and extension of both arms with flexion of the trunk and neck.

LENNOX-GASTAUT SYNDROME: GENERALIZED SHARP- AND SLOW-WAVE COMPLEX

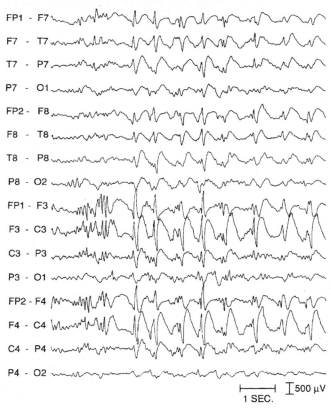

LENNOX-GASTAUT SYNDROME: GENERALIZED PAROXYSMAL FAST AND POLYSPIKES IN SLEEP

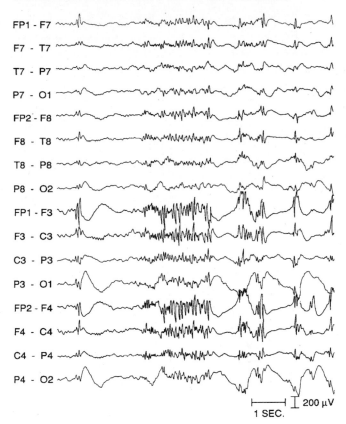

FIGURE 9.23 Six-year-old girl with developmental delay and intractable generalized tonic, tonic–clonic, and atypical absence seizures since age 3 years. Note the bifrontal polyspikes preceding the generalized sharp- and slow-wave complexes (5), also called slow spike-and-wave complexes.

FIGURE 9.24 Eleven-year-old boy with moderately severe mental retardation and intractable generalized tonic, atonic, myoclonic, and atypical absence seizures since age 4 years. Awake EEG showed generalized sharp- and slow-wave complexes.

LENNOX-GASTAUT SYNDROME: ATONIC SEIZURES

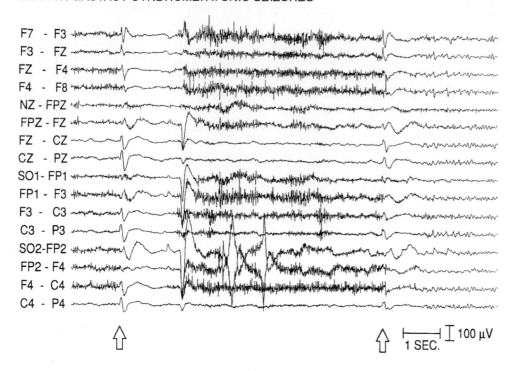

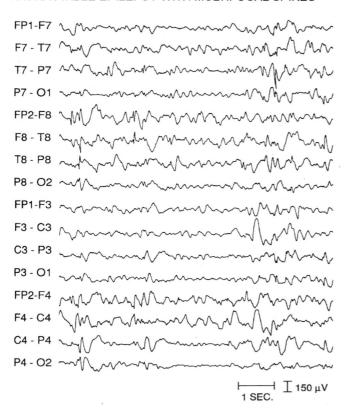

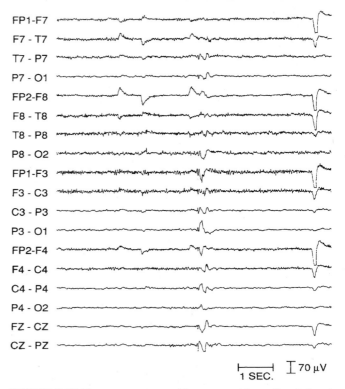

FIGURE 9.25 Forty-one-year-old man with borderline intelligence and intractable generalized tonic, atonic, generalized tonic–clonic, and atypical absence seizures since age 3 years. Interictal electroencephalogram showed generalized sharp- and slow-wave complexes. Two seizures are recorded here, with limp head nodding plus tonic stiffening and elevation of both arms. Each seizure began with a generalized sharp wave (*arrows*) followed by attenuation of electroencephalograph activity and cessation of muscle artifact.

INTRACTABLE EPILEPSY WITH MULTIFOCAL SPIKES

FIGURE 9.26 Three-year-old boy with developmental delay and intractable clusters of generalized tonic, myoclonic, and atypical absence seizures. This electroencephalographic pattern is not uncommon in children with clinical features similar to those of Lennox–Gastaut syndrome (13).

STIMULATION-RELATED EPILEPSY: READING-INDUCED SPIKE-AND-WAVE COMPLEXES

FIGURE 9.27 Twenty-seven-year-old woman with reading-induced brief myoclonic or (rarely) generalized tonic–clonic seizures since age 12 years (14). During this electroencephalography, the patient was reading; note the horizontal eye movement artifact. She consistently reported a feeling of "jerking" in her body and eyelids and "loss of function" in her arms whenever the electroencephalograph recorded an isolated spike-and-wave discharge, as shown here.

BENIGN FOCAL EPILEPTIFORM DISCHARGES OF
CHILDHOOD: CENTROTEMPORAL SHARP WAVES

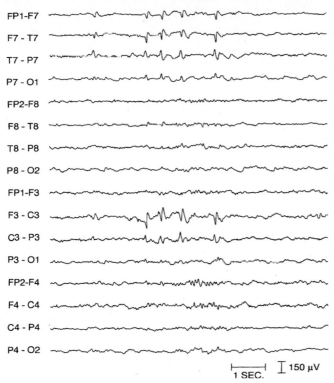

FIGURE 9.28 Eight-year-old boy with attention deficit hyperactivity disorder and no history of seizures. Awake electroencephalogram showed normal findings, but recording during drowsiness and light sleep showed left centrotemporal sharp waves (benign focal epileptiform discharges of childhood) (18). Many children with benign focal epileptiform discharges of childhood do not have seizures (19), and the finding may be incidental.

BENIGN FOCAL EPILEPTIFORM DISCHARGES OF
CHILDHOOD: DIPOLE POTENTIALS

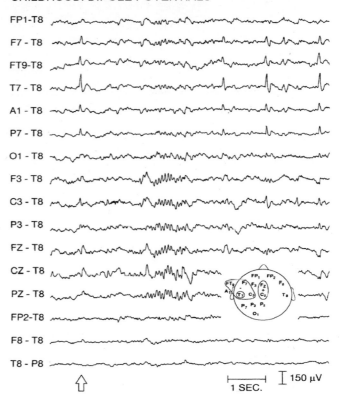

FIGURE 9.29 This referential electroencephalogram was from the patient described in Figure 9.28. Note that the sharp waves were reflected at the scalp as dipoles, with maximum negativity over the left centrotemporal region and maximum positivity over the vertex. Dipole potentials are typical of benign focal epileptiform discharges of childhood, possibly as a result of horizontal orientation along banks of the sylvian or rolandic fissures (18).

BENIGN FOCAL EPILEPTIFORM DISCHARGES OF CHILDHOOD: OCCIPITAL SHARP WAVES

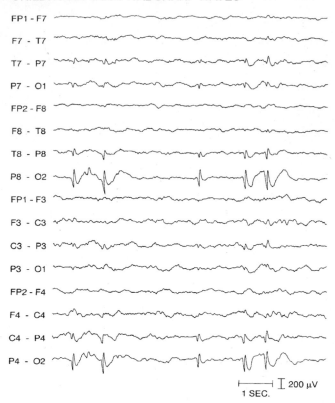

FIGURE 9.30 Eight-year-old boy with mild language delay and no history of seizures. The right occipital sharp waves with typical morphology of benign focal epileptiform discharges of childhood (18) were abundant in light sleep but rare during wakefulness.

BENIGN FOCAL EPILEPTIFORM DISCHARGES OF CHILDHOOD: LEFT AND RIGHT CENTRAL SHARP WAVES

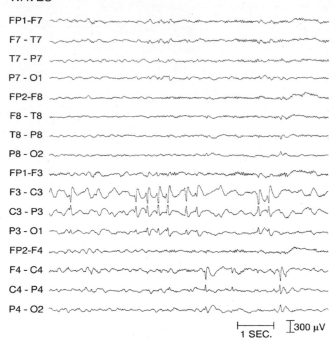

FIGURE 9.31 Eight-year-old boy, otherwise normal, with rare nocturnal generalized tonic–clonic convulsions since age 4 years. Benign focal epileptiform discharges of childhood are commonly bifocal or multifocal, often from homologous areas of both hemispheres (18).

TEMPORAL LOBE EPILEPSY: TEMPORAL SHARP WAVE

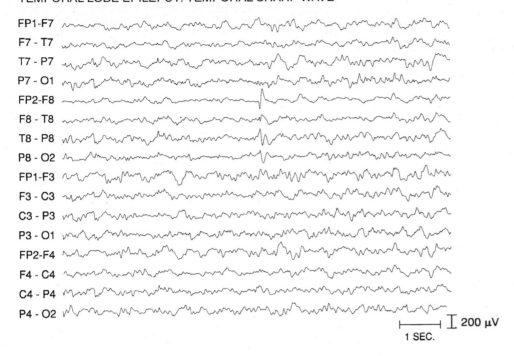

FIGURE 9.32 Twenty-three-year-old woman with complex partial seizures with automatisms since age 15 years. Interictal electroencephalogram showed sharp waves from the right anterior temporal region, with maximum amplitude at electrode F8.

TEMPORAL LOBE EPILEPSY: COMPLEX PARTIAL ("HYPOMOTOR") SEIZURE

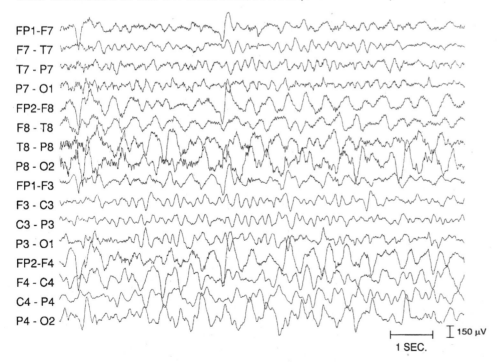

FIGURE 9.33 Sixteen-month-old girl with complex partial seizures since age 6 years. Episodes involved a subtle change of facial expression and decreased responsiveness with minimal or no automatisms ("hypomotor" symptomatology, as discussed in Chapter 14). Magnetic resonance imaging disclosed a large cystic ganglioglioma in the right temporal lobe. Ictal electroencephalogram showed paroxysmal delta activity in the right hemisphere.

TEMPORAL LOBE EPILEPSY: BITEMPORAL SHARP WAVES

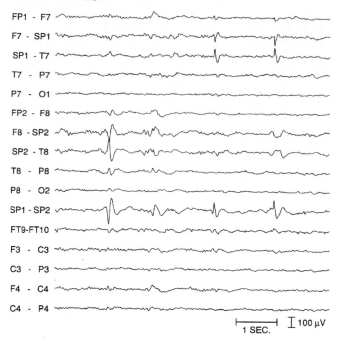

FP1 - F7
F7 - SP1
SP1 - T7
T7 - P7
P7 - O1
FP2 - F8
F8 - SP2
SP2 - T8
T8 - P8
P8 - O2
SP1 - SP2
FT9-FT10
F3 - C3
C3 - P3
F4 - C4
C4 - P4

1 SEC.   100 µV

FIGURE 9.34 Thirty-seven-year-old man with adult-onset complex partial seizures with automatisms. Interictal sharp waves were left or right temporal, maximal at sphenoidal electrodes. All recorded seizures were from the right temporal lobe.

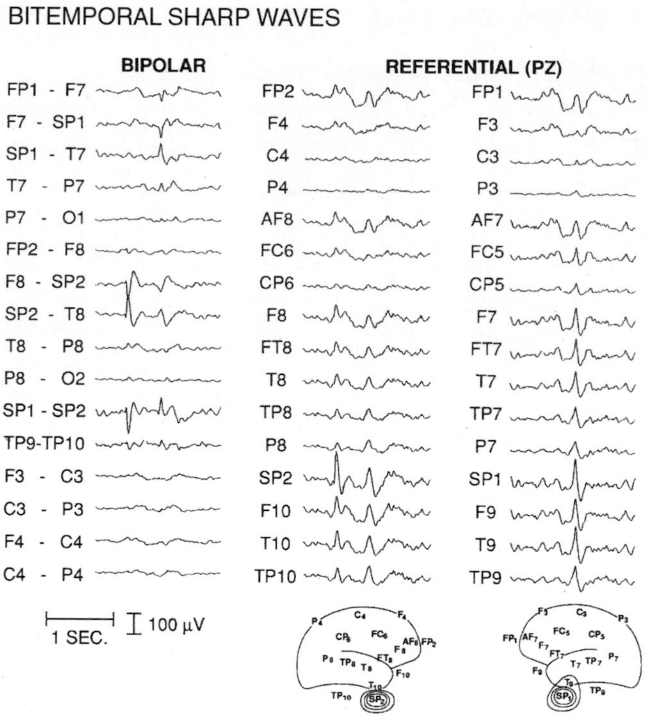

BITEMPORAL SHARP WAVES

BIPOLAR

FP1 - F7
F7 - SP1
SP1 - T7
T7 - P7
P7 - O1
FP2 - F8
F8 - SP2
SP2 - T8
T8 - P8
P8 - O2
SP1 - SP2
TP9-TP10
F3 - C3
C3 - P3
F4 - C4
C4 - P4

1 SEC.   100 µV

REFERENTIAL (PZ)

FP2   FP1
F4   F3
C4   C3
P4   P3
AF8   AF7
FC6   FC5
CP6   CP5
F8   F7
FT8   FT7
T8   T7
TP8   TP7
P8   P7
SP2   SP1
F10   F9
T10   T9
TP10   TP9

FIGURE 9.35 Two-second sample of electroencephalogram from the patient in Figure 9.34, showing the distribution of the left and right temporal sharp waves.

TEMPORAL LOBE EPILEPSY: POSITIVE POLARITY SPIKES AFTER RESECTION

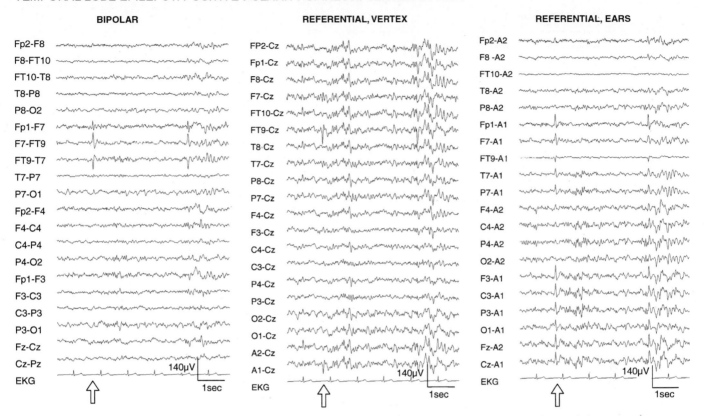

FIGURE 9.36 Bipolar and referential montages of the same spike (*arrow*) of a patient who underwent left anterior temporal lobe resection for medically intractable temporal lobe epilepsy. Note that the left anterior spike (electrode FT9) has a positive polarity. This a rare finding in patients following temporal resections. The downward deflection in the vertex reference (Cz) in the electrodes FT9 and A1 reflects the positivity. The ear reference montage shows that the electrode FT9 shows the maximum positivity (downward deflection) whereas the other left sided electrodes are relatively negative with regard to left ear electrode (A1) and, therefore, point upward. This may give rise to the false impression of a negative spike in the left frontal region in the ipsilateral ear reference montage.

TEMPORAL LOBE EPILEPSY: COMPLEX PARTIAL SEIZURE WITH AUTOMATISMS

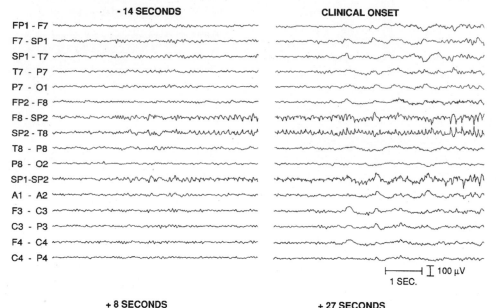

FIGURE 9.37 Thirty-one-year-old woman with complex partial seizures with automatisms since age 5 years. Fourteen seconds before clinical onset, an electroencephalographic seizure pattern was maximal at the right sphenoidal electrode.

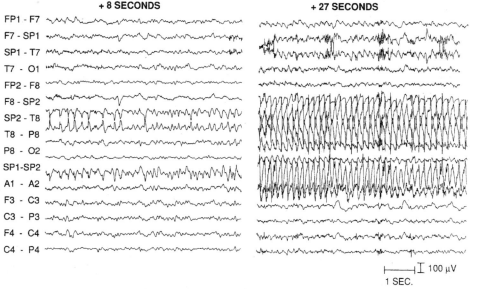

FIGURE 9.38 Continuation of the seizure shown in Figure 9.37. Clinical features included staring, unresponsiveness, and oral automatisms.

NEOCORTICAL TEMPORAL LOBE EPILEPSY: POLYSPIKES

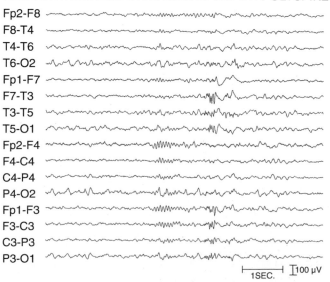

FIGURE 9.39 Thirty-year-old man with lateral neocortical temporal lobe epilepsy due to left lateral temporal focal cortical dysplasia (20). A sleep spindle precedes the left temporo-parietal polyspike. The patient is seizure free following resection of the focal cortical dysplasia sparing the left temporal speech area.

FRONTAL LOBE EPILEPSY: FRONTAL SHARP WAVES

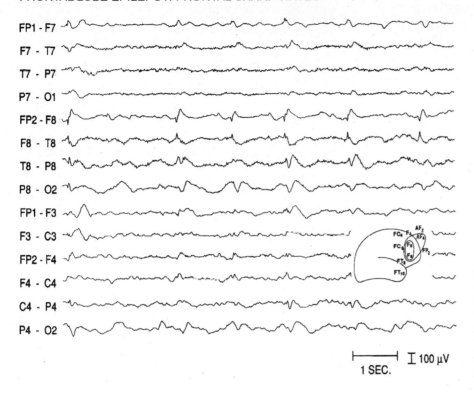

FIGURE 9.40 Twenty-one-month-old boy with intractable daily focal clonic seizures involving the left side of the body. Interictal electroencephalogram showed nearly continuous periodic sharp waves from the right frontal lobe, with the distribution shown in the inset. MRI disclosed an area of increased signal in the same area, and histologic examination of resected tissue showed cortical dysplasia.

FRONTAL LOBE EPILEPSY: FRONTAL SHARP WAVES WITH SECONDARY BILATERAL SYNCHRONY

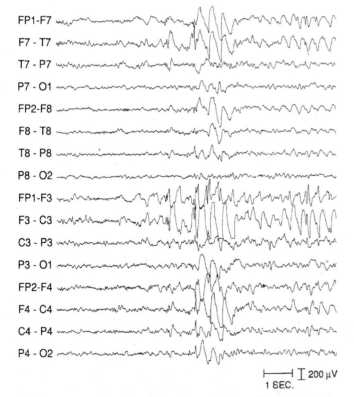

FIGURE 9.41 Seventeen-year-old boy with intractable complex partial and generalized tonic–clonic seizures and extensive encephalomalacia of the left frontal lobe as a result of head trauma at age 13 years. Interictal sharp waves were maximum in the left frontal region but frequently showed secondary bilateral synchrony with generalization.

FRONTAL LOBE EPILEPSY: SUBCLINICAL ELECTROENCEPHALOGRAPHIC SEIZURE, ONSET

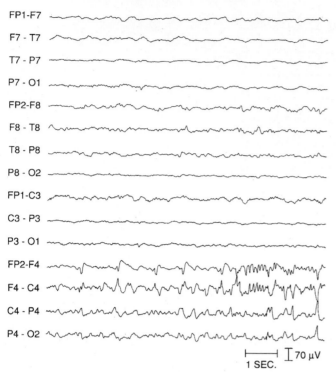

FRONTAL LOBE EPILEPSY: SUBCLINICAL EEG SEIZURE, +50 SECONDS

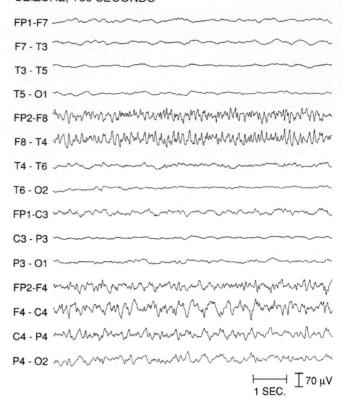

FIGURE 9.42 Fifty-year-old man with focal clonic seizures involving the left face and arm. Seizures began after right frontotemporal craniotomy and evacuation of right frontal intracerebral hemorrhage. The electroencephalographic seizure pattern begins in the region of the F4 electrode.

FIGURE 9.43 Evolution of the subclinical seizure in Figure 9.42. The seizure pattern has spread to involve more widespread frontal and central regions of the right hemisphere.

OCCIPITAL LOBE EPILEPSY: VISUAL AURA AND FOCAL
CLONIC SEIZURE, -10 SECONDS

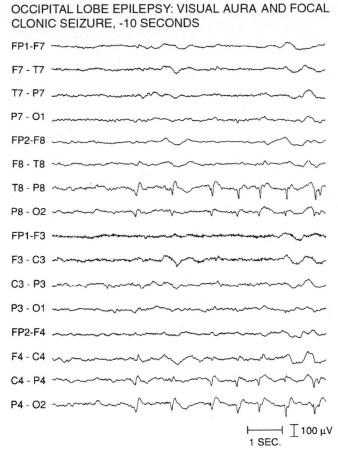

OCCIPITAL LOBE EPILEPSY: VISUAL AURA AND FOCAL
CLONIC SEIZURE, CLINICAL ONSET

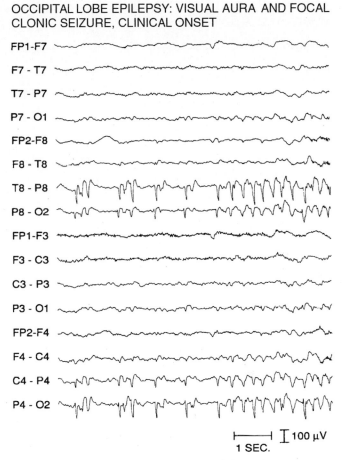

FIGURE 9.44 Sixty-year-old woman with recent onset of visual aura of flashing lights followed by version of eyes to the left and clonic jerking of the left face and arm. Ictal electroencephalogram showed repetitive sharp waves in the right occipitoparietal area.

FIGURE 9.45 Evolution of the electroencephalographic seizure pattern in Figure 9.44.

SUPPLEMENTARY MOTOR AREA EPILEPSY: SHARP WAVES AT VERTEX

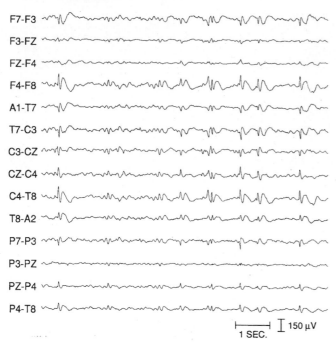

FIGURE 9.46 Seventeen-year-old woman with a low-grade astrocytoma in the left mesial frontal lobe (paracentral lobule). Intractable seizures involved brief tonic abduction of both arms, version of head and eyes to the right, and falling backward without loss of consciousness.

SUPPLEMENTARY MOTOR AREA EPILEPSY: TONIC SEIZURE

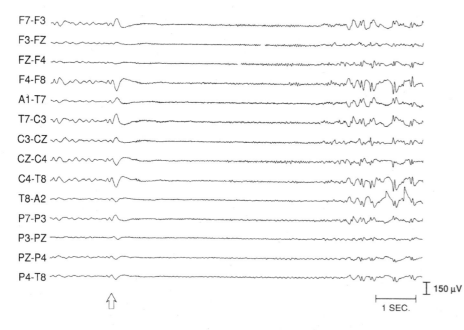

FIGURE 9.47 Electroencephalogram during a typical seizure from the patient described in Figure 9.46. At clinical onset (*arrow*), a vertex slow transient and then a generalized electrodecremental pattern with paroxysmal fast activity were recorded, followed by paroxysmal vertex sharp waves.

PERIROLANDIC EPILEPSY: FOCAL CLONIC SEIZURE, CLINICAL ONSET

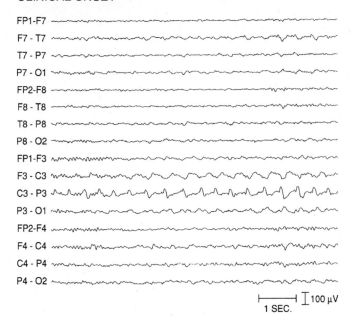

PERIROLANDIC EPILEPSY: FOCAL CLONIC SEIZURE, +10 SECONDS

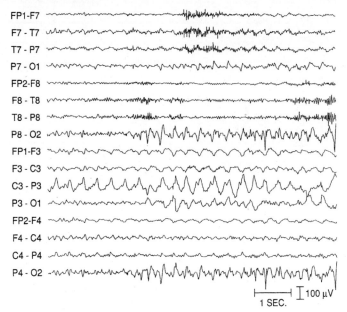

FIGURE 9.48 Four-year-old girl with frequent nocturnal focal clonic seizures with jacksonian spread. Seizures began with twitching of the right shoulder and thoracic wall, followed by version of the head to the right and clonic jerking of the right arm and leg without loss of consciousness. Seizure pattern on electroencephalogram was maximum at the left central region.

FIGURE 9.49 Evolution of the seizure in Figure 9.48, with spread of the ictal discharge into left parietal and occipital regions.

PERIROLANDIC EPILEPSY: RIGHT FRONTOCENTRAL SHARP WAVES

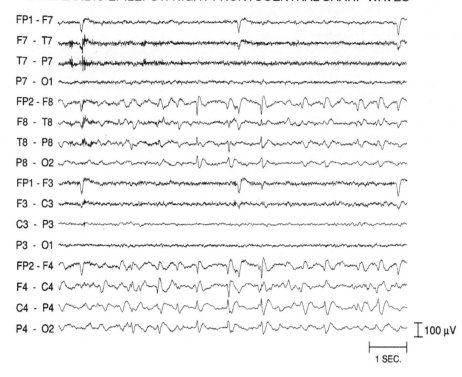

FIGURE 9.50 Eight-year-old boy with left hemiparesis and posttraumatic encephalomalacia in the right frontocentral white matter as a result of a motor vehicle accident at age 3 months. Interictal electroencephalogram showed right hemisphere slowing with sharp waves over the right frontocentral region (maximum at the C4 electrode).

PERIROLANDIC EPILEPSY: LEFT ARM TONIC SEIZURE

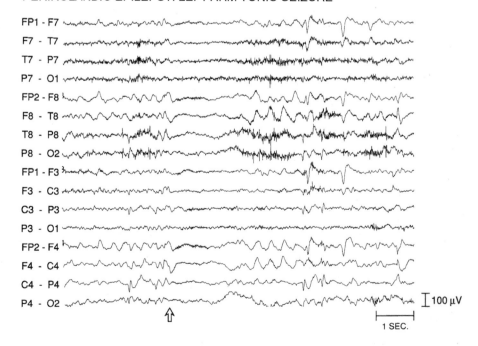

FIGURE 9.51 Same patient as in Figure 9.50. Electroencephalography showed diffuse electrodecrement during brief tonic seizures with stiffening and extension of the left arm and leg. Seizures ceased after right frontocentral resection.

PERIROLANDIC EPILEPSY: EPILEPSIA PARTIALIS CONTINUA

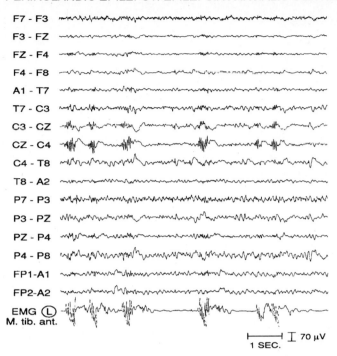

FIGURE 9.52 Sixty-nine-year-old man with continual jerking of the left foot and leg for 6 weeks, without loss of consciousness. Electromyography from the left tibialis anterior muscle showed that jerks occurred synchronously with each burst of polyspikes on electroencephalogram. Polyspikes were maximum at left vertex electrodes, presumably as a result of paradoxical lateralization of the discharge from the right interhemispheric region (21).

PALLID INFANTILE SYNCOPE: OCULAR COMPRESSION TEST

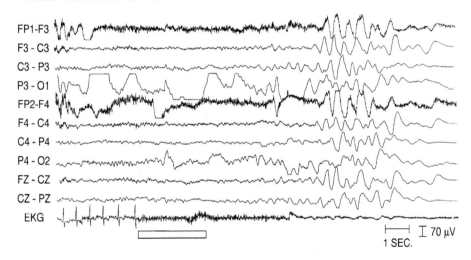

FIGURE 9.53 Two-year-old boy with pallid infantile syncope. Ocular compression (22,23) (*bar*), a controversial provocative maneuver, resulted in syncope with cardiac asystole for 12.5 seconds. Electroencephalography showed diffuse high-amplitude slowing followed by cerebral suppression as a result of global cerebral ischemia.

PALLID INFANTILE SYNCOPE: OCULAR COMPRESSION TEST, CONTINUED

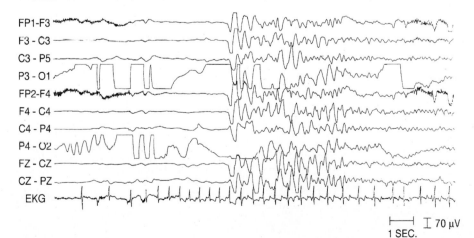

FIGURE 9.54 With recovery of the patient shown in Figure 9.53, electroencephalogram showed high-amplitude slowing followed by normal rhythms. Asystole with ocular compression may be caused by activation of the oculocardiac reflex (trigeminal afferent, vagal efferent pathways) (22,23).

CYANOTIC BREATH-HOLDING SPELL

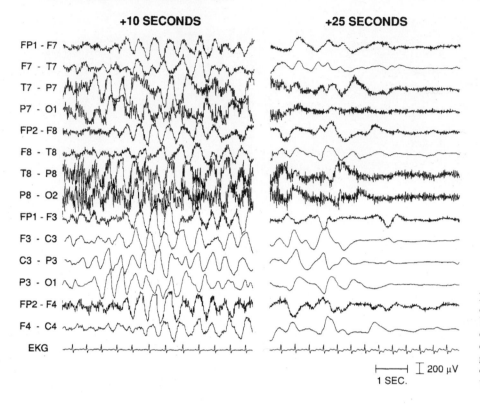

FIGURE 9.55 Two-year-old boy with cyanotic breath-holding spells sometimes followed by generalized tonic–clonic seizures. This episode occurred during crying and involved cessation of respiration for 40 seconds, oxygen desaturation to 73%, cyanosis, loss of consciousness, opisthotonic posturing, and urinary incontinence.

CYANOTIC BREATH-HOLDING SPELL

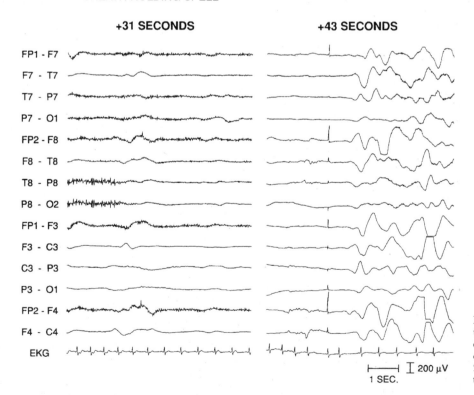

FIGURE 9.56 As the episode continued in the patient shown in Figure 9.55, electroencephalographic activity was similar to that during the syncopal attack in Figures 9.53 and 9.54, but the electroencephalogram showed tachycardia instead of asystole.

NARCOLEPSY

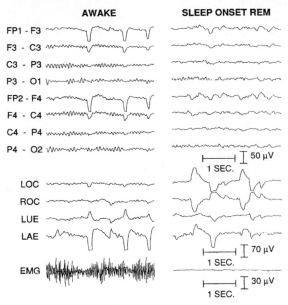

FIGURE 9.57 Fifty-six-year-old man with episodes of loss of consciousness (sleep attacks) and automatic behavior (minisleeps). Multiple sleep latency test gave evidence of narcolepsy with short sleep latency (2 minutes) and sleep-onset rapid eye movement periods (REM latency, 1 minute). Typical features during rapid eye movement sleep included rapid eye movements, absent muscle artifact, and drowsy electroencephalographic pattern. LOC and ROC, left and right outer canthus; LUE and RUE, left and right under eye. Ocular electrodes were referential to A1/A2.

ACKNOWLEDGMENTS

Most EEG tracings in this atlas were prepared by Diana Roth, R EEGT, and Jim Reed.

References

1. American Electroencephalographic Society. Guidelines in EEG, 1–7 (revised 1985). *J Clin Neurophysiol.* 1986;3:133–168.
2. Klem GH, Lüders HO, Jasper HH, et al. The ten-twenty electrodes system of the International Federation. *Electroenceph Clin Neurophysiol Suppl.* 1999;52:3–6.
3. Sharbrough F, Chatrian GE, Lesser RP, et al. American EEG Society: guidelines for standard electrode position nomenclature. *J Clin Neurophysiol.* 1991;8:200–202.
4. Noachtar S, Binnie C, Ebersole J, et al. A glossary of terms most commonly used by clinical electroencephalographers and proposal for the report form for the EEG findings. *Electroenceph Clin Neurophysiol Suppl.* 1999; 52:21–41.
5. Daly DD. Epilepsy and syncope. In: Daly DD, Pedley TA, eds. *Current Practice of Clinical Electroencephalography.* 2nd ed. New York: Raven Press; 1990:306–310.
6. Klass DW, Westmoreland BF. Nonepileptogenic epileptiform electroencephalographic activity. *Ann Neurol.* 1985;18:627–635.
7. White JC, Langston JW, Pedley TA. Benign epileptiform transients of sleep. *Neurology.* 1977;27:1061–1068.
8. Lombroso CT, Schwartz IH, Clark DM, et al. Ctenoids in healthy youths. Controlled study of 14- and 6-per-second positive spiking. *Neurology.* 1966;16:1152–1158.
9. Reiher J, Lebel M. Wicket spikes: clinical correlations of a previously undescribed EEG pattern. *Can J Neurol Sci.* 1977;4:39–47.
10. Westmoreland BF, Klass DW. A distinctive rhythmic EEG discharge of adults. *Electroencephalogr Clin Neurophysiol.* 1981;51:186–191.
11. Gibbs FA, Rich CL, Gibbs EL. Psychomotor variant type of seizure discharge. *Neurology.* 1963;13:991–998.
12. Cobb WA, Guiloff RF, Cast J. Breach rhythm: the EEG related to skull defects. *Electroencephalogr Clin Neurophysiol.* 1979;47:251–271.
13. Kotagal P. Multifocal independent spike syndrome: relationship to hypsarrhythmia and the slow spike-wave (Lennox-Gastaut) syndrome. *Clin Electroencephalogr.* 1995;26:23–29.
14. Bickford RG, Whelan JL, Klass DW, et al. Reading epilepsy: clinical and electroencephalographic studies of a new syndrome. *Trans Am Neurol Assoc.* 1956;81:100–102.
15. Commission on Classification and Terminology of the International League against Epilepsy. Proposal for revised clinical and electroencephalographic classification of epileptic seizures. *Epilepsia.* 1981;22:489–501.
16. Commission on Classification and Terminology of the International League against Epilepsy. Proposal for revised classification of epilepsies and epileptic syndromes. *Epilepsia.* 1989;30:389–399.
17. Luders H, Acharya J, Baumgartner C, et al. Semiological seizure classification. *Epilepsia.* 1998;39:1006–1013.
18. Lüders H, Lesser RP, Dinner DS, et al. Benign focal epilepsy of childhood. In: Lüders H, Lesser RP, eds. *Epilepsy: Electroclinical Syndromes.* London: Springer-Verlag; 1987:303–346.
19. Eeg-Olofsson O. The development of the electroencephalogram in normal children from age 1 through 15 years: 14- and 6-Hz positive spike phenomena. *Neuropaediatrie.* 1971;2:405–427.
20. Noachtar S, Bilgin O, Remi J, et al. Interictal regional polyspikes in noninvasive EEG suggest cortical dysplasia as etiology of focal epilepsies. *Epilepsia.* 2008;49:1011–1017.
21. Adelman S, Lüders H, Dinner DSD, et al. Paradoxical lateralization of parasagittal sharp waves in a patient with epilepsia partialis continua. *Epilepsia.* 1982;23:291–295.
22. Lombroso CT, Lerman P. Breath-holding spells (cyanotic and pallid infantile syncope). *Pediatrics.* 1967;39:563–581.
23. Stephenson JBP. Two types of febrile seizures: anoxic (syncopal) and epileptic mechanisms differentiated by oculocardiac reflex. *Br Med J.* 1978;2:726–729.

Bibliography

Blume WT, Kaibara M. *Atlas of Adult Electroencephalography.* New York: Raven Press; 1995.

Blume WT, Kaibara M. *Atlas of Pediatric Electroencephalography.* 2nd ed. Philadelphia: Lippincott-Raven; 1999.

Ebersole JS, Pedley TA, eds. *Current Practice of Clinical Electroencephalography.* 3rd ed. Philadelphia: Lippincott Williams & Wilkins; 2003.

Gubermann A, Couture M. *Atlas of Electroencephalography.* Boston: Little Brown; 1989.

Lüders H, Noachtar S. *Atlas and Classification of Electroencephalography.* Philadelphia: WB Saunders; 2000.

Niedermeyer E, Lopez da Silva FH, eds. *Electroencephalography: Basic Principles, Clinical Applications and Related Fields.* 3rd ed. Baltimore, MD: Urban & Schwarzenberg; 1993.

Osselton R, Cooper JW, Shaw JC. *EEG Technology.* 3rd ed. London: Butterworths; 1980.

Spehlmann E. *EEG Primer.* 2nd ed. Amsterdam: Elsevier; 1991.

Stockard-Pope JE, Werner SS, Bickford RG. *Atlas of Neonatal Electroencephalography.* 2nd ed. New York: Raven Press; 1992.

Tyner FS, Knott JR, Mayer WB Jr. *Fundamentals of EEG Technology, Vol 1. Basic Concepts and Methods.* New York: Raven Press; 1983.

PART III ■ EPILEPTIC SEIZURES AND SYNDROMES

CHAPTER 10 ■ CLASSIFICATION OF SEIZURES

CHRISTOPH KELLINGHAUS AND HANS O. LÜDERS

Efforts to categorize epileptic seizures and syndromes date to classic medical literature (1). Various classifications were developed for different purposes (2–11), so that by the middle of the twentieth century, a large number of classifications were in active use. As more diagnostic and treatment modalities became available, the resulting confusion pointed to the need for a widely accepted system.

The classification system currently used most extensively is the International Classification of Epileptic Seizures (ICES). This classification was developed by the Commission on Classification and Terminology of the International League Against Epilepsy (ILAE) in 1964 (12), and the system was revised in 1981 (13). The current ICES is used worldwide and is reproduced in its entirety as an appendix immediately following this chapter. In light of still unresolved issues and controversies, however, the Commission is further revising this seizure classification system (14).

EVOLUTION OF THE CURRENT SYSTEM

Early observers of epileptic seizures noted that seizure symptomatology could shed some insight into the underlying epileptic process, with focal seizures usually occurring in patients with focal lesions and bilateral or generalized seizures occurring in patients with more generalized pathologies. These observations suggested a strong correlation between the clinical characteristics of seizures and the underlying epileptic process. With the advent of electroencephalography (EEG) in the 1930s, however, it became clear that similar semiological seizure types could be present in patients with either generalized or focal EEG abnormalities. For example, episodes of staring and loss of consciousness could occur in patients with either generalized 3-Hz spike–wave complexes or anterior temporal sharp waves.

Continued research identified various electroclinical syndromes whose correct identification was considered essential for the correct diagnosis and management of a patient with epilepsy. This philosophy dominated during the development of the 1964 ICES, which used terms derived from descriptions of symptomatology to characterize electroclinical syndromes. The 1981 ICES added new terminology that divided seizures into focal or generalized types on the basis of electroclinical features (i.e., its clinical semiology and EEG characteristics). For example, seizures characterized by staring and impaired consciousness are called "absences" if the patient's EEG showed generalized epileptiform discharges and "complex partial seizures" if the epileptiform discharges are focal. This

approach reflected the assumption that a strict one-to-one relationship exists between the electroclinical syndromes and the corresponding epilepsy syndromes.

LIMITATIONS OF THE ELECTROCLINICAL APPROACH TO SEIZURE CLASSIFICATION

Although EEG features are an integral part of the 1981 ICES, they are not always available in clinical practice. Routine interictal EEG frequently may not show epileptiform discharges, and only a small minority of patients with epilepsy undergo prolonged video-EEG recording. In these cases, assumptions are often based on other lines of evidence. In a patient with no interictal epileptiform discharges on the EEG, for example, episodes of loss of consciousness are assumed to be complex partial seizures if magnetic resonance imaging (MRI) shows a temporal lobe tumor. If neither test is revealing, or before any test has been performed (as may be the case at a patient's initial visit), the focal or generalized nature of the epilepsy may not be apparent solely from a description of the seizures. In this situation, precise use of the 1981 ICES is not possible.

Moreover, the 1981 ICES does not allow for easy expression of many potentially important seizure signs and symptoms. By focusing heavily on the presence or absence of altered consciousness as the key distinction between complex and simple types of focal seizures, the 1981 ICES de-emphasizes much of the rich symptomatology that may carry localizing or lateralizing significance. Consciousness during a seizure may be difficult to determine and offers little localizing information because seizures with or without loss of consciousness may arise from any region of the brain. Other seizure signs or symptoms may greatly enhance epileptogenic localization, but they are not easily expressed in the 1981 ICES. For example, a seizure characterized as "simple partial seizure with focal motor signs" using the 1981 ICES system would be more easily expressed as a "left arm clonic seizure" in the semiological classification system described in the next subsection. A classification system encompassing a broad range of seizure symptomatology would be especially valuable to neurologists evaluating patients for epilepsy surgery because convergence of data from different lines of testing is key to localization of the epileptogenic zone.

Recently, it has become clear that a strict one-to-one relationship between electroclinical syndromes and the corresponding epilepsy syndromes does not exist. Modern neuroimaging has allowed neurologists to identify important etiologies in vivo, such as cortical dysplasia and hippocampal sclerosis, that were previously often found only on histopathologic analysis. Correlation of neuroimaging and video-EEG results demonstrates the variable relationship between an electroclinical syndrome and the underlying epileptogenic process (15), especially among infants (16) in whom interrater agreement for seizure classification according to the 1981 ICES proved to be poor (17). Whereas focal epilepsy in children, adolescents, and adults tend to present with features commonly associated with focal epilepsies—for example, auras and clonic jerking of one extremity—infants with focal epilepsy frequently only exhibit subtle focal motor signs or symmetric tonic movements commonly thought to be associated with generalized epileptogenicity (18,19). For example, it is now generally accepted that epileptic spasms and hypsarrhythmia, traditionally thought to occur only in infants with generalized epilepsy, not infrequently may be due to a focal brain lesion identified on MRI or positron-emission topography (PET) studies (20–22). In other words, the assumption of a one-to-one relationship between semiological seizure type and epilepsy (as assumed in the 1981 ICES) leads to confusion between the classification of epileptic seizures and epilepsy syndromes.

ADVANTAGES OF A SEIZURE CLASSIFICATION SYSTEM BASED SOLELY ON SYMPTOMATOLOGY

In an effort to avoid these limitations, Lüders and colleagues (16,23–28) have proposed a seizure classification system based solely on the main signs and symptoms of the seizures identified by a patient or by a direct observer, or by analysis of ictal videotapes. This system, which has been used at selected epilepsy centers for more than 10 years, and has been slightly modified since its first publication in 1998, has several advantages.

"Unbundling" the signs and symptoms of seizures from EEG, neuroimaging, and other clinical information allows neurologists to contribute independently to the diagnosis of patients with epilepsy. The decision if the epilepsy is generalized or focal is thus deferred until the entire clinical picture—available results from family history, a patient's past and present history, neurologic and physical examination, seizure symptomatology, EEG, neuroimaging, and genetic testing—becomes available. This system recognizes that seizure symptomatology alone provides limited information about the best choice of antiepileptic drugs, prognosis, and other therapeutic considerations. Management of seizures, prognosis, and so on will require additional information (EEG, MRI, etc.) to properly classify the epilepsy itself.

Classifying seizure symptomatology separately from other clinical and laboratory features eliminates the current confusion between seizures (electroclinical complexes in the ICES) and epilepsies, and at the same time emphasizes the importance of seizure semiology in the diagnosis of epilepsies.

THE SEMIOLOGICAL SEIZURE CLASSIFICATION (SSC)

The seizure classification system proposed by Lüders and colleagues subdivides ictal signs and symptoms into one of four domains: sensation, cognitive function, autonomic function, or motor function (Table 10.1).

TABLE 10.1

SEMIOLOGICAL SEIZURE CLASSIFICATION

Epileptic seizure	Complex motor seizure
Aura	Automotor seizure
Somatosensory aura	Hypermotor seizure
Auditory aura	Gelastic seizure
Olfactory aura	
Visual aura	Dyscognitive seizure
Autonomic aura	Dialeptic seizure
Psychic aura	Typical dialeptic seizure
Gustatory aura	Delirious seizure
Motor seizure	Autonomic seizure
Simple motor seizure	Special seizure
Tonic seizure	Atonic seizure
Clonic seizure	Hypomotor seizure
Myoclonic seizure	Astatic seizure
Versive seizure	Aphasic seizure
Tonic–clonic seizure	Akinetic seizure
Epileptic spasm	Negative myoclonic seizure

Seizures characterized by sensory or psychic disturbances without loss of consciousness or other features are called auras; seizures in which the most prominent feature is an alteration or loss of cognitive functions (e.g., perception, attention, emotion, consciousness) are referred to as dyscognitive seizures; seizures with predominantly autonomic (i.e., involuntary) features are considered autonomic seizures; and seizures characterized by abnormal movements, with or without loss of consciousness, are known as motor seizures.

Motor seizures are subdivided into simple and complex types. In simple motor seizures, unnatural and apparently involuntary motor movements are similar to those elicited by electrical stimulation of the primary motor areas. Simple motor seizures may be further subdivided into clonic, tonic, tonic–clonic, myoclonic, and versive seizures, and epileptic spasms. In complex motor seizures, relatively complicated movements simulate natural movements but are inappropriate for the situation ("automatisms"). The term "complex" here does not mean that the patient loses awareness during the seizures, although impaired consciousness is common. Complex motor seizures may be further subdivided into (1) automotor seizures with repetitive oral or gestural automatisms (often seen in temporal lobe epilepsy); (2) hypermotor seizures with violent proximal movements (frequently seen in seizures arising from mesial or orbitofrontal regions); and (3) gelastic seizures with inappropriate laughter, typically seen with hypothalamic hamartoma.

Dyscognitive seizures are subdivided into dialeptic seizures (predominant loss of consciousness) and delirious seizures (predominant confusion or emotional alteration, disordered thinking). The term "dyscognitive seizures" was not part of the original publication of the SSC, but has been chosen in accordance with the Glossary of Descriptive Terminology for Ictal Semiology developed by the ILAE (29). Knowledge of the focal or generalized nature of the epilepsy is not required for this classification. For example, dialeptic seizures characterized by quiet unconsciousness without significant motor activity may be seen in childhood absence epilepsy, as well as in some cases of frontal or temporal lobe epilepsy. The neutral but unfamiliar term "dialeptic" was proposed to avoid confusion with the traditional use of "absence" as an electroclinical syndrome.

Seizures that do not fit into any of the four categories mentioned above are classified as special seizures. This includes many seizures with "negative" or "inhibitory" features. Aphasic seizures are seizures with predominant dysphasia or aphasia and preserved consciousness. Atonic seizures involve loss of postural tone, resulting in head drops or limp falling. Astatic seizures consist of epileptic falls. Videopolygraphic studies show that these may be caused by pure atonia, atonia following a myoclonic jerk, or pure tonic stiffening, but in clinical practice, the exact pathogenesis is often unclear. Hypomotor seizures are characterized by decreased or absent behavioral motor activity without the emergence of new motor manifestations; this descriptive term is only needed for infants or severely mentally impaired individuals, in whom it is not possible to test consciousness directly (16,30). Akinetic seizures are characterized by the inability to perform voluntary movements despite preserved consciousness, as may occur with activation of the negative motor areas in the mesial frontal and inferior frontal gyri. Negative myoclonic seizures consist of a brief (50 to 200 msec) interruption of tonic muscle activity caused by an epileptiform discharge; the resulting brief, sudden movement is caused by loss of muscle tone.

Modifiers may be added to classify the somatotopic distribution of ictal signs and symptoms, as, for example, "left-hand clonic seizure" or "generalized clonic seizure." These modifiers refer to the part(s) of the body involved in the seizure, not to the side or lobe of the brain generating the ictal discharge. To express the evolution of symptoms that occurs as the seizure discharge spreads to new cortical areas, the components can be listed in order of appearance and linked by arrows (see examples below).

Precise definitions of the state of consciousness is necessary only for some specific seizure types, such as dialeptic seizures, in which loss of consciousness is the predominant symptom, and auras, in which consciousness is always preserved. However, the state of consciousness is always an important semiological variable. The semiological seizure classification allows for the specification at which point in the sequence of symptoms the patient lost consciousness by inserting the expression "loss of consciousness" (LOC) after the seizure component during which consciousness was lost (see example below).

There are several semiological features of the ictal or postictal state that are not necessarily the main element of a seizure component, but have been established as reliably lateralizing the hemisphere of seizure onset—for example, dystonic posturing (31), ictal speech (32), or postictal weakness (33). These lateralizing signs can be listed following the seizure sequence (see example below).

Examples:

- left visual aura → left versive seizure (LOC) → generalized tonic–clonic seizure
- abdominal aura → automotor seizure; lateralizing sign: left arm dystonic posturing

This system permits classification of seizures with different degrees of precision to match the available information. If information is limited, as in the absence of a witness or a complete or accurate history, a less detailed classification may be appropriate (e.g., "motor seizure"). Progressively greater amounts of information may permit further categorization of the seizure as "simple motor seizure," "right arm motor seizure," or "right arm clonic seizure."

The semiological seizure classification has also been adapted successfully to characterize the semiology of status epilepticus (28). Like the SSC, the semiological classification of status epilepticus (SCSE) focuses on the main clinical manifestations and evolution of the episode. It allows for classification of complex evolutions that defy classification based on the current ILAE classification. Thus, important information may be preserved and misclassification (or no classification at all) may be prevented.

The 1981 ICES, which defines epileptic syndromes on the basis of electroclinical syndromes, has provided a common language for the advancement of patient care and research. However, the authors of the 1981 ICES revision expected (and actually hoped for) further revisions of the classification, as they were aware that increasing knowledge would lead to modification of their approaches and concepts (13). Recent advances in neuroimaging and molecular biology have revolutionized the definition of epileptic syndromes, providing insights beyond those obtained from EEG alone and demonstrating that a strict one-to-one relationship between electroclinical syndromes and the underlying epileptic processes does not exist. In addition, an alternative seizure classification system based solely on symptomatology has been proposed by Lüders and colleagues (25,26). As a result of those developments, the Commission on Classification and Terminology of the ILAE is revising the classification (14).

A few years ago, a proposal for a five-axis diagnostic scheme was put forth by the ILAE Task Force on Classification and Terminology (34). This proposal uses the strictly descriptive terminology of the semiological seizure classification, but categorizes it as a glossary (29). The second axis contains the epileptic seizure types "that present diagnostic entities with physiologic, therapeutic, and/or prognostic implications" (34). In this axis, the ICES dichotomy of focal and generalized seizures remains essentially unchanged, complemented by some semiological details, as well as by status epilepticus types and reflex seizure types. This approach, with its imminent redundancy of information as well as the whole proposal of the diagnostic scheme, has been hotly debated (35–39) and remains controversial (see also Chapter 18). On the other hand, the semiological seizure classification has been used successfully in the clinical management of patients, as well as in the scientific investigation of epilepsy in various settings and age-groups (18,40–42). In addition, some studies (43–45) have compared the semiological seizure classification with the current ILAE seizure classification and have found it to be more useful particularly in localized epilepsies. However, health professionals who are not yet acquainted with the SSC should undergo a training program with video samples (46).

Regardless of the seizure classification system that is used, one must bear in mind that in every case, the seizure classification must be complemented by an epilepsy classification that specifies the etiology of the epilepsy, the location of the epileptogenic zone, and other important medical or neurological conditions the patient has.

References

1. Wolf P. *Epileptic Seizures and Syndromes: Terms and Concepts.* London: Libbey; 1994.
2. Gastaut H. Classification of the epilepsies. Proposal for an international classification. *Epilepsia.* 1969;10(suppl):13–21.
3. Gastaut H. Clinical and electroencephalographic classification of epileptic seizures. *Epilepsia.* 1969;10(suppl 2):13–21.
4. Gastaut H. Clinical and electroencephalographical classification of epileptic seizures. *Epilepsia.* 1970;11:102–113.
5. Gastaut H. *Dictionary of Epilepsy.* Geneva: World Health Organization; 1973.
6. Masland RL. Classification of the epilepsies. *Epilepsia.* 1959;1:512–520.
7. Masland RL. Comments on the classification of epilepsy. *Epilepsia.* 1969;10(suppl):8.
8. Masland RL. The classification of the epilepsies. A historical review. In: Vinken PJ, Bruzn GW, ed. *The Classification of the Epilepsies. A Historical Review* ed. Amsterdam: Elsevier; 1974;1–29.
9. McNaughton FL. The classification of the epilepsies. *Epilepsia.* 1952;1:7–16.
10. Merlis JK. Proposal for an international classification of the epilepsies. *Epilepsia.* 1970;11:114–119.
11. Merlis JK. Treatment in relation to classification of the epilepsies. *Acta Neurol Latinoam.* 1972;18:42–51.
12. Commission on Classification and Terminology of the International League Against Epilepsy. A proposed international classification of epileptic seizures. *Epilepsia.* 1964;5:297–306.
13. Commission on Classification and Terminology of the International League Against Epilepsy. Proposal for revised clinical and electroencephalographic classification of epileptic seizures. *Epilepsia.* 1981;22:489–501.
14. Engel J, Jr. Classifications of the International League Against Epilepsy: time for reappraisal. *Epilepsia.* 1998;39:1014–1017.
15. Manford M, Fish DR, Shorvon SD. An analysis of clinical seizure patterns and their localizing value in frontal and temporal lobe epilepsies. *Brain.* 1996;119(pt 1):17–40.
16. Acharya JN, Wyllie E, Lüders HO, et al. Seizure symptomatology in infants with localization-related epilepsy. *Neurology.* 1997;48:189–196.
17. Nordli DR, Jr., Bazil CW, Scheuer ML, et al. Recognition and classification of seizures in infants. *Epilepsia.* 1997;38:553–560.
18. Hamer HM, Wyllie E, Luders HO, et al. Symptomatology of epileptic seizures in the first three years of life. *Epilepsia.* 1999;40:837–844.
19. Nordli DR, Jr., Kuroda MM, Hirsch LJ. The ontogeny of partial seizures in infants and young children. *Epilepsia.* 2001;42:986–990.
20. Chugani HT, Shields WD, Shewmon DA, et al. Infantile spasms: I. PET identifies focal cortical dysgenesis in cryptogenic cases for surgical treatment. *Ann Neurol.* 1990;27:406–413.
21. Chugani HT, Shewmon DA, Shields WD, et al. Surgery for intractable infantile spasms: neuroimaging perspectives. *Epilepsia.* 1993;34:764–771.
22. Wyllie E, Comair YG, Kotagal P, et al. Epilepsy surgery in infants. *Epilepsia.* 1996;37:625–637.
23. Bautista JF, Lüders HO. Semiological seizure classification: relevance to pediatric epilepsy. *Epileptic Disord.* 2000;2:65–72.
24. Lüders HO, Noachtar S. *Atlas und Video epileptischer Anfälle und Syndrome.* Wehr, Germany: Ciba-Geigy Verlag; 1995.
25. Lüders HO, Acharya J, Baumgartner C, et al. Semiological seizure classification. *Epilepsia.* 1998;39:1006–1013.
26. Lüders HO, Acharya J, Baumgartner C, et al. A new epileptic seizure classification based exclusively on ictal semiology. *Acta Neurol Scand.* 1999;99:137–141.
27. Lüders HO, Rosenow F, Arnold S, et al. A semiological classification of status epilepticus. *Epileptic Disord.* 2005;7:149–150.
28. Rona S, Rosenow F, Arnold S, et al. A semiological classification of status epilepticus. *Epileptic Disord.* 2005;7:5–12.
29. Blume WT, Lüders HO, Mizrahi E, et al. Glossary of descriptive terminology for ictal semiology: report of the ILAE Task Force on Classification and Terminology. *Epilepsia.* 2001;42:1212–1218.
30. Kallen K, Wyllie E, Lüders HO, et al. Hypomotor seizures in infants and children. *Epilepsia.* 2002;43:882–888.
31. Bleasel A, Kotagal P, Kankirawatana P, et al. Lateralizing value and semiology of ictal limb posturing and version in temporal lobe and extratemporal epilepsy. *Epilepsia.* 1997;38:168–174.
32. Marks WJ, Jr., Laxer KD. Semiology of temporal lobe seizures: value in lateralizing the seizure focus. *Epilepsia.* 1998;39:721–726.
33. Kellinghaus C, Kotagal P. Lateralizing value of Todd's palsy in patients with epilepsy. *Neurology.* 2004;62:289–291.
34. Engel J, Jr. A proposed diagnostic scheme for people with epileptic seizures and with epilepsy: report of the ILAE Task Force on Classification and Terminology. *Epilepsia.* 2001;42:796–803.
35. Avanzini G. Of cabbages and kings: do we really need a systematic classification of epilepsies? *Epilepsia.* 2003;44:12–13.
36. Berg AT, Blackstone NW. Of cabbages and kings: perspectives on classification from the field of systematics. *Epilepsia.* 2003;44:8–11.
37. Engel J. Reply to "Of cabbages and kings: some considerations on classifications, diagnostic schemes, semiology, and concepts". *Epilepsia.* 2003;44:4–5.
38. Lüders HO, Najm I, Wyllie E. Reply to "Of cabbages and kings: some considerations on classifications, diagnostic schemes, semiology, and concepts". *Epilepsia.* 2003;44:6–7.
39. Wolf P. Of cabbages and kings: some considerations on classifications, diagnostic schemes, semiology, and concepts. *Epilepsia.* 2003;44:1–3.
40. Henkel A, Noachtar S, Pfander M, et al. The localizing value of the abdominal aura and its evolution: a study in focal epilepsies. *Neurology.* 2002;58:271–276.
41. Hirfanoglu T, Serdaroglu A, Cansu A, et al. Semiological seizure classification: before and after video-EEG monitoring of seizures. *Pediatr Neurol.* 2007;36:231–235.
42. Werhahn KJ, Noachtar S, Arnold S, et al. Tonic seizures: their significance for lateralization and frequency in different focal epileptic syndromes. *Epilepsia.* 2000;41:1153–1161.
43. Baykan B, Ertas NK, Ertas M, et al. Comparison of classifications of seizures: a preliminary study with 28 participants and 48 seizures. *Epilepsy Behav.* 2005;6:607–612.
44. Benbadis SR, Thomas P, Pontone G. A prospective comparison between two seizure classifications. *Seizure.* 2001;10:247–249.
45. Parra J, Augustijn PB, Geerts Y, et al. Classification of epileptic seizures: a comparison of two systems. *Epilepsia.* 2001;42:476–482.
46. Isler A, Basbakkal Z, Serdaroglu G, et al. Semiologic seizure classification: the effectiveness of a modular education program for health professionals in pediatrics. *Epilepsy Behav.* 2008;13:387–390.

APPENDIX 10.A ■ PROPOSAL FOR REVISED CLINICAL AND ELECTROGRAPHIC CLASSIFICATION OF EPILEPTIC SEIZURES[1]

Commission on Classification and Terminology of the International League Against Epilepsy (1981)

PART I: PARTIAL (FOCAL, LOCAL) SEIZURES

Partial seizures are those in which, in general, the first clinical and electroencephalographic changes indicate initial activation of a system of neurons limited to part of one cerebral hemisphere. A partial seizure is classified primarily on the basis of whether or not consciousness is impaired during the attack (Table 10.A1). When consciousness is not impaired, the seizure

is classified as a simple partial seizure. When consciousness is impaired, the seizure is classified as a complex partial seizure. Impairment of consciousness may be the first clinical sign, or simple partial seizures may evolve into complex partial seizures. In patients with impaired consciousness, aberrations of behavior (automatisms) may occur. A partial seizure may not terminate, but instead progress to a generalized motor seizure. Impaired consciousness is defined as the inability to respond

---

[1]From Commission on Classification and Terminology of the International League Against Epilepsy. Proposal for revised clinical and electroencephalographic classification of epileptic seizures. *Epilepsia.* 1981;22:489–501, with permission.

TABLE 10.A1

CLASSIFICATION OF PARTIAL SEIZURES

Clinical seizure type	EEG seizure type	EEG interictal expression
A. *Simple partial seizures* (consciousness not impaired) 　1. With minor signs 　　(a) Focal motor without march 　　(b) Focal motor with march (jacksonian) 　　(c) Versive 　　(d) Postural 　　(e) Phonatory (vocalization or arrest of speech) 　2. With somatosensory or special-sensory symptoms (simple hallucinations, e.g., tingling, light flashes, buzzing) 　　(a) Somatosensory 　　(b) Visual 　　(c) Auditory 　　(d) Olfactory 　　(e) Gustatory 　　(f) Vertiginous 　3. With autonomic symptoms or signs (including epigastric sensation, pallor, sweating, flushing, piloerection, and pupillary dilation) 　4. With psychic symptoms (disturbance of higher cerebral function); these symptoms rarely occur without impairment of consciousness and are much more commonly experienced as complex partial seizures 　　(a) Dysphasic 　　(b) Dynamic (e.g., déjà vu) 　　(c) Cognitive (e.g., dreamy states, distortions of time sense) 　　(d) Affective (fear, anger, etc.) 　　(e) Illusions (e.g., macropsia) 　　(f) Structured hallucinations (e.g., music, scenes)	Local contralateral discharge starting over the corresponding area of cortical representation (not always recorded on the scalp)	Local contralateral discharge
B. Complex *partial seizures* (with impairment of consciousness; may sometimes begin with simple symptomatology) 　1. Simple partial onset followed by impairment of consciousness 　　(a) With simple partial features (A.1–A.4.) followed by impaired consciousness 　　(b) With automatisms 　2. With impairment of consciousness at onset 　　(a) With impairment of consciousness only 　　(b) With automatisms	Unilateral or, frequently, bilateral discharge, diffuse or focal in temporal or frontotemporal regions	Unilateral or bilateral generally asynchronous focus; usually in temporal or frontal regions
C. *Partial seizures evolving to secondarily generalized seizures* (may be generalized tonic–clonic, tonic, or clonic) 　1. Simple partial seizures (A) evolving to generalized seizures 　2. Complex partial seizures (B) evolving to generalized seizures 　3. Simple partial seizures evolving to complex partial seizures evolving to generalized seizures	Above discharges become secondarily and rapidly generalized	

normally to exogenous stimuli by virtue of altered awareness and/or responsiveness (see "Definition of Terms").

There is considerable evidence that simple partial seizures usually have unilateral hemispheric involvement and only rarely have bilateral hemispheric involvement; complex partial seizures, however, frequently have bilateral hemispheric involvement.

Partial seizures can be classified into one of the following three fundamental groups:

A. Simple partial seizures
B. Complex partial seizures

1. With impairment of consciousness at onset
2. Simple partial onset, followed by impairment of consciousness

C. Partial seizures evolving to generalized tonic–clonic convulsions (GTCs)

1. Simple evolving to GTC
2. Complex evolving to GTC (including those with simple partial onset)

PART II: GENERALIZED SEIZURES (CONVULSIVE OR NONCONVULSIVE)

Generalized seizures are those in which the first clinical changes indicate initial involvement of both hemispheres (Table 10.A2). Consciousness may be impaired and this impairment may be the initial manifestation. Motor manifestations are bilateral. The ictal electroencephalographic patterns initially are bilateral, and presumably reflect neuronal discharge, which is widespread in both hemispheres.

PART III: UNCLASSIFIED EPILEPTIC SEIZURES

Includes all seizures that cannot be classified because of inadequate or incomplete data and some that defy classification in hitherto described categories. This includes some neonatal seizures, for example, rhythmic eye movements, chewing, and swimming movements.

PART IV: ADDENDUM

Repeated epileptic seizures occur under a variety of circumstances: (1) as fortuitous attacks, coming unexpectedly and without any apparent provocation; (2) as cyclic attacks, at more or less regular intervals (e.g., in relation to the menstrual cycle or the sleep-waking cycle); and (3) as attacks provoked by: (a) nonsensory factors (fatigue, alcohol, emotion, etc.) or (b) sensory factors, sometimes referred to as reflex seizures.

Prolonged or repetitive seizures (status epilepticus). The term "status epilepticus" is used whenever a seizure persists for a sufficient length of time or is repeated frequently enough that recovery between attacks does not occur. Status epilepticus may be divided into partial (e.g., jacksonian) or generalized (e.g., absence status or tonic–clonic status). When very localized motor status occurs, it is referred to as epilepsia partialis continua.

PART V: DEFINITION OF TERMS

Each seizure type will be described so that the criteria used will not be in doubt.

Partial Seizures

The fundamental distinction between simple partial seizures and complex partial seizures is the presence or the impairment of the fully conscious state.

Consciousness has been defined as "that integrating activity by which Man grasps the totality of his phenomenal field" (21) and incorporates it into his experience. It corresponds to *Bewusstsein* and is thus much more than "vigilance," for were it only vigilance (which is a degree of clarity) then only confusional states would be representative of disordered consciousness.

Operationally in the context of this classification, *consciousness* refers to the degree of awareness and/or responsiveness of the patient to externally applied stimuli. *Responsiveness* refers to the ability of the patient to carry out simple commands of willed movement; *awareness* refers to the patient's contact with events during the period in question and its recall. A person aware and unresponsive will be able to recount the events that occurred during an attack and his or her inability to respond by movement or speech. In this context, unresponsiveness is other than the result of paralysis, aphasia, or apraxia.

With Motor Signs

Any portion of the body may be involved in focal seizure activity depending on the site of origin of the attack in the motor strip. Focal motor seizures may remain strictly focal or they may spread to contiguous cortical areas producing a sequential involvement of body parts in an epileptic "march." The seizure is then known as a jacksonian seizure. Consciousness is usually preserved; however, the discharge may spread to those structures whose participation is likely to result in loss of consciousness and generalized convulsive movements. Other focal motor attacks may be versive with head turning to one side, usually contraversive to the discharge. If speech is involved, this is either in the form of speech arrest or, occasionally, vocalization. Occasionally, a partial dysphasia is seen in the form of epileptic palilalia with involuntary repetition of a syllable or phrase.

Following focal seizure activity, there may be a localized paralysis in the previously involved region. This is known as Todd paralysis and may last from minutes to hours.

When focal motor seizure activity is continuous, it is known as epilepsia partialis continua.

With Autonomic Symptoms

Vomiting, pallor, flushing, sweating, piloerection, pupil dilation, borborygmi, and incontinence may occur in case of simple partial seizures.

TABLE 10.A2

CLASSIFICATION OF GENERALIZED SEIZURES

Clinical seizure type	EEG seizure type	EEG interictal expression

A. 1. *Absence seizures*
  (a) Impairment of consciousness only
  (b) With mild clonic components
  (c) With atonic components
  (d) With tonic components
  (e) With automatism
  (f) With autonomic components
    (*b* through *f* may be used alone or in combination)
	Usually regular and symmetrical 3 Hz but may be 2- to 4-Hz spike-and-slow-wave complexes and may have multiple spike-and-slow-wave complexes; abnormalities are bilateral	Background activity usually normal, although paroxysmal activity (such as spikes or spike-and-slow-wave complexes) may occur; this activity is usually regular and symmetric

2. *Atypical absence*
May have:
  (a) Changes in tone that are more pronounced than in A.1
  (b) Onset and/or cessation that is not abrupt
	EEG more heterogeneous: may include irregular spike-and-slow-wave complexes, fast activity, or other paroxysmal activity, abnormalities are bilateral but often irregular and asymmetric	Background usually abnormal; paroxysmal activity (such as spikes or spike-and-slow-wave complexes) frequently irregular and asymmetric

B. *Myoclonic seizures* Myoclonic jerks (single or multiple)	Polyspike and wave, or sometimes spike and wave or sharp and slow waves	Same as ictal
C. *Clonic seizures* Myoclonic jerks (single or multiple)	Fast activity (10 Hz or more) and slow waves: occasional spike-and-wave patterns	Spike-and-wave or polyspike-and-wave discharges
D. *Clonic seizures*	Low voltage, fast activity or a fast rhythm of 9–10 Hz or more, decreasing in frequency and increasing in amplitude	More or less rhythmic discharges of sharp and slow waves, sometimes asymmetric, background often abnormal for age
E. *Tonic–clonic seizures*	Rhythm at 10 Hz or more, decreasing in frequency and increasing in amplitude during tonic phase, interrupted by slow waves during clonic phase	Polyspikes and waves or spike and wave or, sometimes, sharp and slow-wave discharge
F. *Atonic seizures* (astatic) Combinations of the above may occur, for example, B and F, B and D	Polyspikes and wave or flattening or low-voltage fast activity	Polyspikes and slow wave

With Somatosensory or Special Sensory Symptoms

Somatosensory seizures arise from those areas of cortex subserving sensory function, and they are usually described as pins-and-needles or a feeling of numbness. Occasionally, a disorder of proprioception or spatial perception occurs. Like motor seizures, somatosensory seizures also may march and spread at any time to become complex partial or generalized tonic–clonic seizures as in A.1. Special sensory seizures include visual seizures varying in elaborateness and depending on whether the primary or association areas are involved, from flashing lights to structured visual hallucinatory phenomena, including persons, scenes, and so on. Like visual seizures, auditory seizures may also run the gamut from crude auditory sensations to such highly integrated functions as music.

Olfactory sensations, usually in the form of unpleasant odors, may occur.

Gustatory sensations may be pleasant or odious taste hallucinations. They vary in elaboration from crude (salty, sour, sweet, bitter) to sophisticated. They are frequently described as "metallic."

Vertiginous symptoms include sensations of falling in space and floating, as well as rotatory vertigo in a horizontal or vertical plane.

With Psychic Symptoms (Disturbance of Higher Cerebral Function)

These usually occur with impairment of consciousness (i.e., complex partial seizures).

Dysphasia

This was referred to earlier.

Dysmnesic Symptoms

A distorted memory experience such as distortion of the time sense, a dreamy state, a flashback, or a sensation as if a naïve experience had been experienced before, known as déjà vu, or as if a previously experienced sensation had not been experienced, known as jamais-vu, may occur. When this refers to auditory experience, these are known as déjà-entendu or jamais-entendu. Occasionally, as a form of forced thinking, the patient may experience a rapid recollection of episodes from his or her past life, known as panoramic vision.

Cognitive Disturbances

These include dreamy states; distortions of the time sense; and sensations of unreality, detachment, or depersonalization.

With Affective Symptomatology

Sensation of extreme pleasure or displeasure as well as fear and intense depression with feelings of unworthiness and rejection may be experienced during seizures. Unlike those of psychiatrically induced depression, these symptoms tend to come in attacks lasting for a few minutes. Anger or rage is occasionally experienced, but unlike temper tantrums, epileptic anger is apparently unprovoked and abates rapidly. Fear or terror is the most frequent symptom; it is sudden in onset, usually unprovoked, and may lead to running away. Associated with the terror, there are frequently objective signs of autonomic activity, including pupil dilatation, pallor, flushing, piloerection, palpitation, and hypertension.

Epileptic or gelastic seizure laughter should not, strictly speaking, be classed as an affective symptom because the laughter is usually without affect and hollow. Like other forms of pathologic laughter, it is often unassociated with true mirth.

Illusions

These take the form of distorted perceptions in which objects may appear deformed. Polyoptic illusions such as monocular diplopia and distortions of size (macropsia or micropsia) or of distance may occur. Similarly, distortions of sound, including microacusia and macroacusia, may be experienced. Depersonalization, as if the person were outside his or her body, may occur. Altered perception of size or weight of a limb may be noted.

Structured Hallucinations

Hallucinations may occur as manifestations or perceptions without a corresponding external stimulus and may affect somatosensory, visual, auditory, olfactory, or gustatory senses. If the seizure arises from the primary receptive area, the hallucination would tend to be rather primitive. In the case of vision, flashing lights may be seen; in the case of auditory perception, rushing noises may occur. With more elaborate seizures involving visual or auditory association areas with participation of mobilized memory traces, formed hallucinations occur, and these may take the form of scenery, persons, spoken sentences, or music. The character of these perceptions may be normal or distorted.

Seizures with Complex Symptomatology

Automatisms

(These may occur in both partial and generalized seizures. They are described in detail here for convenience.) In the *Dictionary of Epilepsy* (5), automatisms are described as "more or less coordinated adapted (eupractic or dyspractic) involuntary motor activity occurring during the state of clouding of consciousness either in the course of, or after, an epileptic seizure, and usually followed by amnesia for the event. The automatism may be simply a continuation of an activity that was going on when the seizure occurred, or, conversely, a new activity developed in association with the ictal impairment of consciousness. Usually, the activity is commonplace in nature, often provoked by the subject's environment, or by his sensations during the seizure; exceptionally, fragmentary, primitive, infantile, or antisocial behavior is seen. From a symptomatological point of view, the following are distinguished: (a) eating automatisms (chewing, swallowing); (b) automatisms of mimicry, expressing the subject's emotional state (usually of fear) during the seizure; (c) gestural automatisms, crude or elaborate, directed toward either the subject or his environment; (d) ambulatory automatisms; and (e) verbal automatisms."

Ictal epileptic automatisms usually represent the release of automatic behavior under the influence of clouding of consciousness that accompanies a generalized or partial epileptic seizure (confusional automatisms). They may occur in complex partial seizures as well as in absence seizures. Postictal epileptic automatisms may follow any severe epileptic seizure, especially a tonic–clonic one, and are usually associated with confusion.

While some regard masticatory or oropharyngeal automatisms as arising from the amygdala or insular and opercular regions, these movements are occasionally seen in the generalized epilepsies, particularly absence seizures, and are not of localizing help. The same is true of mimicry and gestural automatisms. In the latter, fumbling of clothes, scratching, and other complex motor activity may occur in both complex partial and absence seizures. Ictal speech automatisms are occasionally encountered. Ambulatory seizures again may occur either as prolonged automatisms of absence, particularly prolonged absence continuing, or of complex partial seizures. In the latter, a patient may occasionally continue to drive a car, although may contravene traffic light regulations.

There seems to be little doubt that automatisms are a common feature of different types of epilepsy. While they do not lend themselves to simple anatomic interpretation, they appear to have in common a discharge involving various areas of the limbic system. Crude and elaborate automatisms do occur in patients with absence, as well as complex partial seizures. Of greater significance is the precise descriptive history of the seizures; the age of the patient; and the presence or absence of an aura and of postictal behavior, including the presence or absence of confusion. The EEG (electroencephalogram) is of cardinal localizational importance here.

Drowsiness or Somnolence

Drowsiness or somnolence implies a sleep state from which the patient can be aroused to make appropriate motor and verbal responses. In stupor, the patient may make some spontaneous movement and, by painful or other vigorously applied stimuli, can be aroused to make avoidance movements. The patient in confusion makes inappropriate responses to his or her environment and is disoriented with regard to place, time, or person.

Aura

A frequently used term in the description of epileptic seizures is aura. According to the *Dictionary of Epilepsy*, this term was introduced by Galen to describe the sensation of a breath of air felt by some subjects prior to the onset of a seizure. Others have referred to the aura as the portion of a seizure experienced before loss of consciousness occurs. This loss of consciousness may be the result of secondary generalization of the seizure discharge or of alteration of consciousness imparted by the development of a complex partial seizure.

The aura is that portion of the seizure that occurs before consciousness is lost and for which memory is retained afterward. It may be that, as in simple partial seizures, the aura is the whole seizure. Where consciousness is subsequently lost, the aura is, in fact, the signal symptom of a complex partial seizure.

An aura is a retrospective term that is described after the seizure has ended.

Generalized Seizures: Absence Seizures

The hallmark of the absence attack is a sudden onset, interruption of ongoing activities, a blank stare, possibly a brief upward rotation of the eyes. If the patient is speaking, speech is slowed or interrupted; if walking, he or she stands transfixed; if eating, he or she will stop the food on the way to the mouth. Usually the patient will be unresponsive when spoken to. In some, attacks are aborted when the patient is spoken to. The attack lasts from a few seconds to half a minute and evaporates as rapidly as it commenced.

Absence with Impairment of Consciousness Only

The above description fits the description of absence simple in which no other activities take place during the attack.

Absence with Mild Clonic Components

Here, the onset of the attack is indistinguishable from the above, but clonic movements may occur in the eyelids, at the corner of the mouth, or in other muscle groups, which may vary in severity from almost imperceptible movements to generalized myoclonic jerks. Objects held in the hand may be dropped.

Absence with Atonic Components

Here, there may be a diminution in tone of muscles subserving posture, as well as in the limbs, leading to drooping of the head, occasionally slumping of the trunk, dropping of the arms, and relaxation of the grip. Rarely, tone is sufficiently diminished to cause one to fall.

Absence with Tonic Components

Here, during the attack, tonic muscular contraction may occur, leading to an increase in muscle tone, which may affect the extensor muscles or the flexor muscles symmetrically or asymmetrically. If the patient is standing, the head may be drawn backward and the trunk may arch. This may lead to retropulsion. The head may tonically draw to one or another side.

Absence with Automatisms

Purposeful or quasipurposeful movements occurring in the absence of awareness during an absence attack are frequent and may range from lip licking and swallowing to clothes fumbling or aimless walking. If spoken to, the patient may grunt or turn to the spoken voice, and when touched or tickled, may rub the site. Automatisms are quite elaborate and may include combinations of the above-described movements or may be so simple as to be missed by casual observation. Mixed forms of absence frequently occur.

Tonic–Clonic Seizures

The most frequently encountered of the generalized seizures are the generalized tonic–clonic seizures, often known as grand mal. Some patients experience a vague ill-described warning, but the majority lose consciousness without any premonitory symptoms. There is a sudden, sharp tonic contraction of muscles, and when this involves the respiratory muscles, there is stridor, a cry or moan, and the patient falls to the ground in the tonic state, occasionally injuring himself or herself. The patient lies rigid, and during this stage, tonic contraction inhibits respiration and cyanosis may occur. The tongue may be bitten and urine may be passed involuntarily. This tonic stage then gives way to clonic convulsive movements lasting for a variable period of time. During this stage, small gusts of grunting respiration may occur between the convulsive movements, but usually the patient remains cyanotic and saliva may froth from the mouth. At the end of this stage, deep respiration occurs and all the muscles relax, after which the patient remains unconscious for a variable period of time and often awakes feeling stiff and sore all over. He or she then frequently goes into a deep sleep and when awakened feels quite well apart from soreness and, frequently, headache. GTCs may occur in childhood and in adult life; they are not as frequent as absence seizures, but vary from one a day to one every 3 months and occasionally to one every few years. Very short attacks without postictal drowsiness may occur on occasion.

Myoclonic Seizures

Myoclonic jerks (single or multiple) are sudden, brief shock-like contractions that may be generalized or confined to the face and trunk or to one or more extremities or even to individual muscles or groups of muscles. Myoclonic jerks may be rapidly repetitive or relatively isolated. They may occur predominantly around the hours of going to sleep or awakening from sleep. They may be exacerbated by volitional movement (action myoclonus). At times, they may be regularly repetitive.

Many instances of myoclonic jerks and action myoclonus are not classified as epileptic seizures. The myoclonic jerks of myoclonus due to spinal cord disease, dyssynergia cerebellaris myoclonica, subcortical segmental myoclonus, paramyoclonus multiplex, and opsoclonus–myoclonus syndrome must be distinguished from epileptic seizures.

Clonic Seizures

Generalized convulsive seizures occasionally lack a tonic component and are characterized by repetitive clonic jerks. As the frequency diminishes, the amplitude of the jerks do not. The postictal phase is usually short. Some generalized convulsive seizures commence with a clonic phase passing into a tonic phase, as described below, leading to a "clonic–tonic–clonic" seizure.

Tonic Seizures

To quote Gowers, a tonic seizure is "a rigid, violent muscular contraction, fixing the limbs in some strained position. There is usually deviation of the eyes and of the head toward one side, and this may amount to rotation involving the whole body (sometimes actually causing the patient to turn around, even two or three times). The features are distorted; the color of the face, unchanged at first, rapidly becomes pale and then flushed and ultimately livid as the fixation of the chest by the spasms stops the movements of respiration. The eyes are open or closed; the conjunctiva is insensitive; the pupils dilate widely as cyanosis comes on. As the spasm continues, it commonly changes in its relative intensity in different parts, causing slight alterations in the position of the limbs." Tonic axial seizures with extension of head, neck, and trunk may also occur.

ATONIC SEIZURES

A sudden diminution in muscle tone occurs, which may be fragmentary, leading to a head drop with slackening of the jaw, the dropping of a limb or a loss of all muscle tone leading to a slumping to the ground. When these attacks are extremely brief, they are known as "drop attacks." If consciousness is lost, this loss is extremely brief. The sudden loss of postural tone in the head and trunk may lead to injury by projecting objects. The face is particularly subject to injury. In the case of more prolonged atonic attacks, the slumping may be progressive in a rhythmic, successive relaxation manner.

(So-called drop attacks may be seen in conditions other than epilepsy, such as brainstem ischemia and narcolepsy cataplexy syndrome.)

Unclassified Epileptic Seizures

This category includes all seizures that cannot be classified because of inadequate or incomplete data and includes some seizures that, by their natures, defy classification in the previously defined broad categories. Many seizures occurring in the infant (e.g., rhythmic eye movements, chewing, swimming movements, jittering, and apnea) will be classified here until such time as further experience with videotape confirmation and electroencephalographic characterization entitles them to subtyping in the extant classification.

Epilepsia Partialis Continua

Under this name have been described cases of simple partial seizures with focal motor signs without a march, usually consisting of clonic spasms, which remain confined to the part of the body in which they originate, but which persist with little or no intermission for hours or days at a stretch. Consciousness is usually preserved, but postictal weakness is frequently evident.

POSTICTAL PARALYSIS (TODD PARALYSIS)

This category refers to the transient paralysis that may occur following some partial epileptic seizures with focal motor components or with somatosensory symptoms. Postictal paralysis has been ascribed to neuronal exhaustion due to the increased metabolic activity of the discharging focus, but it may also be attributable to increased inhibition in the region of the focus, which may account for its appearance in nonmotor somatosensory seizures.

CHAPTER 11 ■ EPILEPTIC AURAS

NORMAN K. SO

The word "aura" (from Greek for air, Latin for breeze) was first applied to epilepsy by Galen's teacher, Pelops (1), who interpreted reports of altered sensations ascending to the head from an extremity as support for a humoral mechanism in which a vapor passed up the blood vessels. For many centuries, Galen's followers believed that somatosensory auras starting in the extremities indicated a peripheral origin of epileptic seizures.

The aura, of course, is the start, not the cause, of a seizure, as Erastus pointed out around 1580. Jackson's systematic study of auras ushered in a new era when he correlated the sensations with functional localization in the brain (2). The 1981 International Classification of Epileptic Seizures (3) defined the aura as "that portion of the seizure which occurs before consciousness is lost and for which memory is retained afterwards." An aura in isolation thus corresponds to a simple partial sensory seizure. Conventional usage further limits the word to the initial sensations of a seizure, without observable signs, that the patient is aware of and recollects. This definition specifically separates an aura from a focal motor seizure and is used in this chapter. Whether autonomic phenomena in seizures should be considered auras is debatable. To the extent that patients can clearly recollect such symptoms as shivering with piloerection at seizure onset, autonomic phenomena can be experienced as an aura. However when flushing or pupillary dilatation are reported by others without the patient's awareness, the term aura would not be appropriate.

PRODROMES AND PREMONITIONS

The aura usually lasts seconds to minutes and immediately precedes the signs of an attack. On occasion, auras can be long-lasting, continuous, or recurrent with short intervening breaks. Intracranial electroencephalographic (EEG) studies have shown that prolonged auras (aura continua) can represent continuous or recurrent seizures, a form of focal status epilepticus (4).

More frequently, for hours to days before attacks, patients may experience prodromal symptoms of nervousness, anxiety, dizziness, and headache that should not be regarded as auras. The prodrome may be evident on awakening and signals a seizure that will occur later in the day. Sometimes the patient may not be conscious of anything untoward, but family members or friends may describe irritability or "a mean streak." Such prodromal symptoms resemble those recounted by patients with migraine. Gowers' speculation (1) that the prodrome is "indicative of slight disturbance of the nerve centers" has not been improved on.

Less commonly, some patients with generalized epilepsy can experience stereotyped sensations before a generalized seizure. Like an aura, these premonitory symptoms immediately precede the seizure and can be varied but lack the character that suggests activation of a circumscribed area of the cortex. Sensations include dizziness, warmth, cold, generalized tingling, anxiety, and a "spaced-out" or confused feeling. On occasions, ill-formed visual imagery and abdominal sensations have been reported before generalized tonic–clonic seizures. Some of the sensations likely correspond to a buildup of absence (dizziness, lightheadedness, and confusion) or myoclonic seizures (anxiety, restlessness, jumpiness, and jerking) before loss of consciousness or convulsive activity.

AURA COMBINATIONS AND MARCH

Although an aura reflects activation of functional cortex by a circumscribed seizure discharge, the seizure discharge frequently spreads. When the seizure discharge spreads along a single functional area such as the postcentral gyrus, the sensory equivalent of focal motor Jacksonian march is seen. An aura can also spread across different functional regions. A seizure that starts in the primary visual area of the occipital lobe and spreads to the temporal limbic structures may present with initial transient blindness followed by other sensations referable to the temporal lobe (5).

Multiple sensations can occur even when seizure activity is relatively confined to one region, as at the start of temporal lobe seizures. In some cases, the multiple auras can be dissected out along a sequence, implying spread of the seizure discharge. Anxiety, epigastric, and "indescribable" sensations commonly precede the more complex phenomena of deja vu and other illusions of vision or sound (6), although the sequence is not always stable in different attacks. In other cases, a time series cannot be discerned, and the multiple sensations seem to occur simultaneously. An alternative explanation for multiple auras could be that they are secondary to activation of a system with access to more than one functional region. The temporal limbic system, with extensive connections to the septum, hypothalamus, temporal neocortex, insula, and parieto-occipital association cortex, is an example (7). In support of this hypothesis, electrical stimulation of temporal limbic structures by depth electrodes can produce different sets of sensations at different times, despite stimulation of the same contact (8).

PRESENCE AND ABSENCE OF AURAS

The incidence of auras in large populations is imprecise. In the 32-year epidemiologic study from Rochester, Minnesota (9), epilepsy with focal sensory seizures was seen in 3.7% of all patients. A further 26.4% were classified to have temporal lobe epilepsy, but the incidence of aura in this group was not separately reported. In the two large series of clinic- and office-based epileptic patients studied by Gowers (1) and by Lennox and Cobb (10) (Table 11.1), an aura was present in 56% of patients. Although notable discrepancies exist between the two series in relative frequencies of unilateral somatosensory auras, bilateral general sensations, and visual auras, other categories are remarkably consistent. Differences are most likely explained on the basis of definitions of aura type.

The figures in other series were more variable. In patients with complex partial seizures or temporal lobe epilepsy, the incidence of auras ranged between 22.5% and 83% (6,11–15). During long-term scalp and sphenoidal or intracranial EEG monitoring of seizures, 46% to 70% of patients reported auras, either independent of or as part of their habitual seizures (16–18).

Some patients who do not describe auras may have had them early in the illness. Anecdotal experience suggests that auras may disappear as the disease progresses and seizures cause increasingly profound loss of awareness and postictal confusion. As Lennox and Cobb (10) stated, "It is more accurate to speak of the recollection of aura[s] rather than of their presence." Young children may lack the verbal capacity to describe the sensations that herald a seizure, even though their actions indicate some awareness of the impending event. Similarly, adults who deny any warning, nevertheless, may press the seizure alarm button during video-EEG monitoring but have no recollection of having done so. The seizure either induces an amnesia so immediate that there is no memory of a warning or causes retrograde amnesia. This is supported by a study that showed that amnesia for auras depended on the severity of the seizure (19). An isolated aura is nearly always recollected and associated with either no or a unilateral EEG ictal discharge. The aura is more likely to be forgotten if the seizure becomes secondarily generalized and involves bilateral EEG ictal discharge.

The complete cessation of all seizures, the desired goal of successful epilepsy surgery, cannot always be achieved. Auras can persist as isolated phenomena after epilepsy surgery, when complex partial or secondarily generalized seizures no longer occur, even after discontinuation of antiepileptic drugs. Isolated postoperative auras are often ignored and classified among the "seizure-free" outcomes. In a few studies, isolated postoperative auras occurred in 20% (20,21) to 35% (22) of patients after surgery for temporal lobe epilepsy and in 22% of a series after focal resective surgery unselected for location (23). Residual auras seem particularly common after temporal lobe surgery and may relate to incomplete removal of the mesial temporal structures comprising the amygdala, hippocampus, and parahippocampal gyrus. The persistence of epigastric auras after functional hemispherectomy, in which the insula is the only cortical structure still functionally connected on the side of surgery, suggests that continuing seizure activity in that structure may be another mechanism. Postoperative auras commonly recurred within the first 6 months of operation and tended to persist (22). Although isolated postoperative auras are widely regarded as of little significance, they may accompany an increased risk of recurrence of complex partial seizure (22) and reduced quality of life on self-assessment (23).

A small number of patients may lose their aura after temporal lobectomy even as they continue to have postoperative complex partial seizures; others may experience a different aura. These alterations occurred in 55% of patients who had residual postoperative seizures (20).

INDIVIDUAL DETERMINANTS

A long duration of epilepsy has been correlated with an increase in the incidence of auras, which Lennox and Cobb (10) thought was "presumably due to the greater total number of seizures and the greater likelihood of experiencing aura." An early onset of epilepsy, lower intelligence quotient, male gender, and right temporal lobe focus have been associated with a higher incidence of "simple primitive" auras, whereas complex "intellectual" auras with illusions or hallucinations accompanied male gender and a verbal intelligence quotient of greater than 100 (24).

Aura content may be related to the patient's psychological makeup. Stimulation of various mesial limbic structures elicited auras with features that were intimately related to ongoing psychopathologic processes (25). Emotional responses and hallucinations produced by electrical stimulation were reported to depend on the background affective

TABLE 11.1

INCIDENCE OF AURA IN TWO SERIES OF CLINIC- AND OFFICE-BASED EPILEPTIC PATIENTS

Aura	Gowers (1) %[a] (n = 2013)	Lennox and Cobb (10) % (n = 1359)
Present	1145 (57%)	764 (56%)
Somatosensory[b]	18.0	8.5
Bilateral sensations	4.5	38.0
Visceral/epigastric	18.0	14.5
Vertiginous	19.0	12.0
Cephalic	8.0	5.5
Psychical	8.0	11.0
Visual[c]	16.0	6.5
Auditory	6.0	2.0
Olfactory	1.0	1.0
Gustatory	1.5	0.1

[a]Percentages apply to patients with aura.
[b]Includes motor phenomena at onset.
[c]Includes illusions and hallucinations.
From Gowers WR. *Epilepsy and Other Chronic Convulsive Diseases: Their Causes, Symptoms & Treatment.* 2nd ed. London, UK: J & A Churchill; 1901 and Lennox WG, Cobb S. Aura in epilepsy: a statistical review of 1,359 cases. *Arch Neurol Psychiatry.* 1933;30:374–387, with permission.

state (26,27). Similarly, patients who experienced anxiety or fear during temporal lobe electrical stimulation scored higher on the "psychasthenia" scale of the Minnesota Multiphasic Personality Inventory, whereas those experiencing dreamlike or memorylike hallucinations scored higher on the "schizophrenia" scale (8). The aura phenomena shown to be sensitive to personality factors are precisely those that make up an individual's personality. Thus, the memory flashback that may be recalled in an aura is not a generic item but an experience specific to the patient.

CLINICAL LOCALIZATION

An aura provides evidence of focal seizure onset. The nature of the symptoms may localize the epileptogenic zone. Not all sensations near the onset of seizures are necessarily auras, however. It is important to differentiate auras from prodromes and from nonspecific premonitions before generalized seizures. Auras may vary in the same patient or occur in combination but should show a certain stereotypy and consistency. It may be particularly difficult to classify a first seizure based on the report of a preceding sensation. One study (28) noted poor interobserver agreement about the nature of such preceding sensations. In the same study, the incidence of generalized versus focal epileptiform EEG abnormalities and of structural abnormalities on computed tomography was similar in the 67 patients with and the 82 patients without sensations preceding a generalized convulsion. At 1-year follow-up, seizures had recurred in 22 of the 67 patients with preceding sensations, but only 11 of these had clinical indications that the recurrences were of focal onset. Thus, self-report of a preceding sensation in an isolated first convulsion may not be a reliable indicator of focal epilepsy.

The sensation before an ictal event can be misleading in another situation. Sometimes, though rarely, patients have pseudoseizures starting with an epileptic aura (29). Often, the epileptic seizures are well controlled except for auras. Whether the pseudoseizure that follows the aura represents a learned response or occurs from other psychogenic mechanisms cannot be determined.

Current concepts of the localizing value of auras rely heavily on the pioneering studies of Penfield and Jasper (14) who correlated sensations and signs obtained through electrical stimulation of the awake patient with those of the patient's spontaneous seizures. Subsequent studies with long-term intracranial electrodes for the recording of spontaneous seizures and extraoperative electrical brain stimulation have extended early observations (30–34).

Although an aura may help to localize the epileptogenic zone, an important point must be kept in mind. The initial sensation of an aura is related to the first functional brain area activated by the seizure that has access to consciousness, but this may not be the site of seizure origin. A seizure starting in the posterior parietal region may be initially asymptomatic until ictal activity spreads to adjacent functional areas. Spread to the postcentral gyrus may elicit a somatosensory sensation as the first warning; propagation to parieto-occipital association cortex may give rise to initial visual illusions or hallucinations. Furthermore, it remains unclear whether experience of an aura is contingent on direct ictal involvement of the cortical areas subserving those functions or whether an aura sensation

may also be evoked by excitation at a distance, provided a pathway of projection or facilitation exists between the site of excitation and an eloquent cortical structure. Both mechanisms are probably operative in human epilepsy. A sensory Jacksonian march cannot be explained by other than ictal spread along the somatosensory cortex. The indistinguishable auras found in patients with hippocampal sclerosis and temporal neocortical pathology underlie the distributed network that functionally links the limbic and neocortical structures in the temporal lobe. Cortical stimulation in extratemporal epilepsy also showed that sites at which an aura is reproduced can extend well beyond the expected functional map for those sensations (33).

The localizing value of auras has been studied in a number of ways. Penfield and Kristiansen (35) recorded the initial seizure phenomenon in 222 patients with focal epilepsy and commented on the likely localization of different auras. Auras reported in patients with well-defined epileptogenic foci in different brain regions can be compared from different series (Table 11.2) or, better yet, prospectively (36) (Table 11.3). Data from patients (37,38) who become seizure free after localized brain resections are particularly important because their surgical outcome is absolute proof of the correct localization of the epileptogenic zone. Making comparisons from different series in the literature is hampered by several problems: Definitions of aura type are not uniform, data on different auras are often grouped in dissimilar ways, and classification rules may differ when multiple sensations occur in the same aura. In spite of the different approaches, however, retrospective and prospective series yielded a remarkably similar conclusion: Auras have localizing significance. Patients with temporal lobe epilepsy have the highest incidence of epigastric, emotional, and psychic auras (36,37). Frontal lobe epilepsy is distinguished by frequent reports of no aura (36,38). When an aura is present in frontal lobe epilepsy, cephalic and general body sensations predominate (36). Perirolandic epilepsy with centroparietal foci is most likely to involve somatosensory aura (39). Not surprisingly, occipital lobe epilepsy has the highest incidence of visual aura (36,40). No single aura sensation is necessarily restricted to a single lobe, however.

Except for unilateral somatosensory and visual auras contralateral to the site of seizure onset, the nature of an aura provides no reliable lateralizing information. Penfield and colleagues (14,41) reported that psychic illusions were lateralized mainly to the nondominant temporal lobe. Subsequently, these findings have been confirmed by some researchers (42) but refuted by others (6,12,16).

EEG LOCALIZATION

The EEG signature of auras depends on the recording technique. An isolated aura is a focal seizure of restricted extent with an intensity between that of a subclinical EEG seizure and a complex partial seizure. Because the success of an ictal EEG recording is determined by the proximity of the electrode(s) to the epileptogenic trigger zone, scalp EEGs frequently fail to detect any changes during an isolated aura and during the aura component of a complex partial seizure. In one study (43) of depth electrode-recorded temporal lobe seizures, only 19% of auras had surface ictal EEG changes.

TABLE 11.2

RELATIVE INCIDENCE OF AURAS IN FOCAL EPILEPSIES (%)

	Temporal[a] Rasmussen (37) (n = 147)	Frontal[a] Rasmussen (38) (n = 140)	Centroparietal Ajmone-Marsan and Goldhammer (39) (n = 40)	Occipital Ludwig and Ajmone-Marsan (40) (n = 18)
Somatosensory	5	17.5	52[b]	0
Epigastric/emotional	52[b]	12.5	22	6
Cephalic	5	12.5	7	6
General body	8	12.5	7	6
Psychical	15	7.5	10	17
Visual	11	5.0	25	56[b]
Auditory	11	—	25	—
Olfactory	11	—	25	11
Gustatory	11	—	25	11
Vertiginous	11	2.5	—	—
None	15	42.5[b]	22	6

[a]Seizure free after surgery.
[b]Indicates highest incidence for location.
From Rasmussen T. Localizational aspects of epileptic seizure phenomena. In: Thompson RA, Green JR, eds. *New Perspectives in Cerebral Localization*. New York: Raven Press; 1982:177–203; Rasmussen T. Characteristics of a pure culture of frontal lobe epilepsy. *Epilepsia*. 1983;24:482–493; Ajmone-Marsan C, Goldhammer L. Clinical ictal patterns and electrographic data in cases of partial seizures of frontal-central-parietal origin. In: Brazier MAB, ed. *Epilepsy: Its Phenomena in Man*. New York: Academic Press; 1973:235–259; Ludwig BI, Ajmone-Marsan C. Clinical ictal patterns in epileptic patients with occipital electroencephalographic foci. *Neurology*. 1975;25:463–471, with permission.

TABLE 11.3

FREQUENCY OF AURAS IN FOCAL EPILEPSIES

	n	Retrospective series			Prospective series		
		Temporal	Frontal	Postero-occipital	Temporal	Frontal	Postero-occipital
Somatosensory	32	1	8	15	0	1	7
Epigastric	47	20	3	3	20	0	1
Cephalic	22	5	13	1	3	0	0
Diffuse warm sensation	10	1	9	0	0	0	0
Psychic	51	27	2	2	19	0	1
Elementary visual	13	1	0	12	0	0	0
Elementary auditory	3	3	0	0	0	0	0
Vertiginous	7	0	1	2	1	1	2
Conscious confusion	11	4	3	1	2	1	0
Total	196	62	39	36	42	3	11

Adapted from Palmini A., Gloor P. The localizing value of auras in partial seizures: a prospective and retrospective study. *Neurology*. 1992;42:801–808, with permission.

In the same study, 10% of subclinical EEG seizures and 86% of clinical (psychomotor) seizures were accompanied by surface changes. An EEG that incorporates sphenoidal electrodes may have a better chance (28%) of detecting an electrographic change during auras (17). The surface EEG ictal pattern is often incomplete and subtle compared with that of a complex partial seizure and may appear as low-frequency rhythmic sharp waves, sudden attenuation of the ongoing background, or abrupt cessation of ongoing interictal spikes sometimes followed by rhythmic slow waves.

Depth electrodes targeted directly at mesial limbic structures (where the majority of temporal lobe seizures originate) have been more successful in demonstrating EEG ictal activity in temporal lobe auras than were simultaneous recordings from subdural electrodes over the lateral temporal convexity (44,45). Nevertheless, even in patients with seizure onset in one temporal lobe, localized by depth electrode recording, only about half the isolated auras showed an ictal EEG correlate (18,46). In neurophysiologic terms, these observations support the belief that only a very small portion of the brain must be activated to produce aura sensations. On the basis of firing patterns of limbic neurons recorded by microelectrode techniques in patients with temporal lobe epilepsy, only 14% of neurons at the epileptogenic trigger zone are estimated to increase their firing rate in an aura. The corresponding estimate for a subclinical seizure is 7% and for a clinical complex partial seizure 36% (47). In the same patient, some auras may be associated with ictal EEG changes, whereas others show no change (46). This suggests that seizures may arise dynamically from different discrete areas within a larger epileptic zone. That identical auras may arise from sites remote from those where they were successfully recorded is unlikely. These patients had electrodes implanted into homologous regions of the opposite hemisphere and often became seizure free after temporal lobectomy.

SOMATOSENSORY AURAS

Tingling, numbness, and an electrical feeling are common, whereas absence of sensation or a sensation of movement is less. A sensation that starts focally or shows a sensory march, such as an ascent up the arm from the hand in the course of seconds, points to a seizure discharge in the primary somatosensory area of the contralateral postcentral gyrus. A primary somatosensory aura can be interrupted by clonic jerking, usually of the part with the abnormal sensation, which presumably reflects spread from the postcentral to the precentral gyrus. Occasionally, a seizure starting in the primary motor area of the precentral gyrus also causes a somatosensory aura, which is usually followed rapidly or simultaneously accompanied by clonic motor phenomena. A clinically identical seizure may have started more posteriorly in "silent" parietal cortex and caused symptoms only after it spread to the postcentral gyrus.

Somatic sensations with a wide segmental or bilateral distribution indicate seizure activity outside the primary somatosensory area. Seizures arising from or involving the second sensory area, situated in the superior bank of the sylvian fissure anterior to the precentral gyrus (14,48), evoke somatic sensations of the contralateral or ipsilateral sides of the body or both. The sensation is often rudimentary, as in primary somatosensory auras; however, second sensory auras include pain, coldness, and a desire for movement (49). The sensation occasionally is followed by inability to move or control the affected part, an example of a "sensory inhibitory seizure."

Seizures arising from the supplementary motor area were preceded by an aura in nearly half the patients in one study (50). Penfield and Jasper (14) elicited somatic sensations from the supplementary sensory area, a part of the mesial cortex in the interhemispheric fissure, posterior to the supplementary motor area. Recently, extraoperative stimulation using chronically implanted subdural electrodes not only confirmed the existence of supplementary sensory areas but also showed that they intermingle and overlap with the supplementary motor area, so that the two regions can best be regarded as a single functional entity (51,52). Auras from the supplementary motor and sensory areas include nonspecific tingling, desire for or sensation of movement, and feelings of stiffness, pulling, pulsation, and heaviness. These sensations usually involve extensive areas of a contralateral extremity or side of the body or bilateral body parts. They may be perceived as a generalized body sensation as well. Penfield and Jasper (14)

also elicited epigastric sensations on stimulation of the supplementary motor area.

Chronic recordings and stimulation studies of depth electrodes implanted into the posterior insular cortex revealed another brain region that can give rise to contralateral somatosensory sensations (34,53). The sensations include those of tingling, electrical shock, heat, and sometimes pain. They can involve more localized or more extensive regions on the contralateral side of the body.

As an aura, a general body sensation, including diffuse warm and cold thermal sensations, has little value in cortical localization, having been reported as seizure aura from all regions of the brain. Besides the supplementary motor area, the mesial temporal structures (54) have responded to stimulation with such diffuse sensations.

Ictal pain as aura can be classified according to the affected parts: cephalic, abdominal, and somesthetic. Ictal headache will be discussed with other cephalic auras, and abdominal pain with epigastric aura. Painful body sensations may represent the initial aura or occur as a component of an aura or seizure. The pain may be sharp, burning, electric, cold, or cramplike and may be focally to diffusely distributed. Pain as an isolated symptom is much less common than as an association of paresthesias and other somatic sensations (55,56). Some patients experience cramplike pain with tonic muscle spasm of an affected part. Well-localized and unilateral ictal pain generally occurs contralateral to an epileptic focus in the postcentral gyrus or neighboring parietal lobe (55–59). Electrical stimulation of the postcentral gyrus can elicit contralateral pain (57,60). Resection of the parietal cortex with the epileptic focus has successfully abolished painful seizures (56,57). Other areas reported to produce painful somesthetic auras are the second sensory area (14,48) and insular cortex (53). The localization of heat, cold, warmth, and flushing is variable or poorly understood. When these sensations are focal and unilateral, the same cortical regions described above are likely responsible. When they are felt over wide segmental areas, on both sides of the body or in a generalized distribution, they lack reliable localizing value. Pharyngeal dysesthesias of tingling and burning are uncommon auras, sometimes reported in patients with temporal lobe epilepsy or seizures arising from the insula (53).

VISUAL AURAS

Spots, stars, blobs, bars, or circles of light, monochromatic or variously colored, implicate seizure activity in the visual areas of the occipital lobes (14). These stationary or moving images may be lateralized to the visual field contralateral to the involved lobe but also may appear directly ahead. When they are lateralized and move across the field of vision, the patient's head may turn to follow them. Some patients describe darkness proceeding to blindness, which can also occur as a postictal phenomenon in those with visual auras. An occipital seizure may propagate to the temporal lobe or the parietal cortex. In the former instance, a visual aura may be followed by psychic experiences, epigastric aura, or emotional feelings, whereas a somatosensory aura may follow in the latter case. Auras with formed visual hallucinations are discussed under psychic auras, as are visual illusions such as macropsia and micropsia.

AUDITORY AURAS

The auditory area lies in the transverse gyrus of Heschl. Electrical stimulation there and in the adjacent superior temporal gyrus produces simple sounds variously described as ringing, booming, buzzing, chirping, or machinelike (14). A lateralized sound is usually contralateral to the side of stimulation. At other times, partial deafness may occur. Auras with such unformed auditory hallucinations suggest seizure activity in the superior temporal neocortex and temporal operculum (14,61). Because seizures can spread to other portions of the temporal lobe, auditory auras are frequently accompanied by other temporal lobe phenomena. Other auditory illusions and hallucinations are discussed later on in this chapter.

VERTIGINOUS AURAS

Stimulation of the superior temporal gyrus can elicit feelings of displacement or movement, including rotatory sensations (14). True vertiginous auras are probably uncommon but may be localized to the posterior part of the superior temporal neocortex (61). More frequently, patients report dizziness, which, on questioning, may be clarified into a cephalic aura, blurring of vision, or knowledge of impending loss of awareness. Early reports of patients with so-called vertiginous seizures probably included a large number with nonspecific dizziness (62,63). Vertiginous auras usually form only one element of the sensations experienced before a seizure.

OLFACTORY AURAS

Jackson and Beevor (64) reported a "case of tumor of the right temporosphenoidal lobe bearing on the localization of the sense of smell and on the interpretation of a particular variety of epilepsy." The patient experienced a "very horrible smell which she could not describe." The term "uncinate fits" has been used to describe seizures with this aura because pathologic lesions are frequently found in the medial temporal lobe. The smell of an olfactory aura is often unpleasant or disagreeable (14,65). Odors akin to burning rubber, sulfur, or organic solvents have been reported. However the smell can be neutral or even pleasant (66). The incidence of olfactory aura is generally about 1% (see Table 11.1). Whether patients with this symptom are disproportionately likely to have temporal lobe tumor is open to debate (65,67), as non-neoplastic lesions such as mesial temporal sclerosis can also be found responsible (66,68).

Other than the medial temporal lobe, the olfactory bulb is the only structure that can produce an olfactory sensation on electrical stimulation. It remains to be seen whether seizure activity starting in the orbitofrontal region will cause an olfactory aura. Olfactory aura rarely occurs in isolation; gustatory or other sensations referable to the temporal lobe may also be experienced.

GUSTATORY AURAS

Usually disagreeable, the taste experienced may be described as sharp, bitter, acid, or sickly sweet. The incidence is low (see Table 11.1). Penfield and Jasper (14) ascribed the representation of taste deep in the sylvian fissure adjacent to and above the insular cortex. Hausser-Hauw and Bancaud (69) localized gustatory hallucinations to the parietal or rolandic operculum. They also recorded spontaneous and electrically induced seizures from the temporal limbic structures that were associated with gustatory phenomena, but believed that the aura resulted from seizure propagation to the opercular region. Temporal lobectomies failed to abolish the gustatory hallucinations in three of their patients. The course of seizures with gustatory aura depends on the site of the epileptogenic zone (69). Suprasylvian seizures are likely to involve salivation, second sensory area sensations, and clonic facial contractions. Seizures of temporal origin may have epigastric aura and develop into typical psychomotor attacks.

EPIGASTRIC OR ABDOMINAL AURAS

Under this heading are various sensations localized to the abdomen or lower chest that may move to the throat and head but rarely descend in the opposite direction. "Visceral" and "viscerosensory" are other terms to describe this aura. Commonly characterized as a feeling of nausea, epigastric aura may also be like butterflies in the stomach, emptiness, "going over a hill," tightness, and churning; occasionally, it may be painful (58,70). This aura is frequently associated with or preceded or followed by other sensory, psychic, emotional, or autonomic phenomena (71). The sensation cannot be considered secondary to altered gastroesophageal function, as direct intraesophageal and intragastric pressure recording showed its occurrence with and without peristalsis (71,72). Although epigastric aura is most common in temporal lobe epilepsy, it has been associated with epilepsies from all lobes (see Tables 11.2 and 11.3). Epigastric sensations can be elicited in epileptic and nonepileptic individuals by electrical stimulation of the amygdala, hippocampus, anteromedial temporal region, sylvian fissure, insula, supplementary motor area, pallidum, and centrum medianum of the thalamus (14,49,71).

CEPHALIC AURAS AND ICTAL HEADACHES

Cephalic aura includes ill-defined sensations felt within the head, such as dizziness, electrical shock, tingling, fullness, or pressure. For this reason, it cannot be confused with a somatosensory aura arising from the primary sensory area. Moreover, electrical stimulation studies have provided no clear localization, and cephalic sensations have been reported as auras in focal seizures arising from all brain regions (see Tables 11.2 and 11.3).

The relationship of headache to seizures is complex and is still the subject of considerable scrutiny (73). Patients often experience a diffuse postictal headache that is generally related to the intensity of the seizure (74). Headaches also may occur as an epileptic prodrome. Some patients with migraines and epilepsy may note that their seizures seem to be triggered by their headaches. Other headaches of abrupt onset signal the beginning of a seizure and can be considered an aura or an ictal headache. An ictal headache can be pounding like a migraine but also sharp and steady. The pain may build gradually, but several patients studied with scalp or intracranial recording showed abrupt pain onset and offset synchronous with EEG seizure activity (75,76).

Ictal headache is not well localized to any specific region and has been described in generalized epilepsy (75). A lateralized headache is likely to be ipsilateral to the side of the epileptogenic focus (56,75). Many well-studied patients had temporal lobe epilepsy, probably reflecting the increased likelihood of intensive presurgical EEG monitoring in this group. Patients with occipital lobe epilepsy represent the other major population with ictal headache. In classic migraine, the occipital cortex seems to be a primary site of dysfunction, as evidenced by early migrainous aura with visual phenomena and spreading oligemia that starts from the occipital pole (77). Ictal or postictal headache is often a striking symptom in benign epilepsy of childhood with occipital paroxysms (78) and in occipital seizures of patients with Lafora disease (79) and other progressive myoclonus epilepsies. The physiologic mechanism of ictal headaches remains unclear. It is possible that ictal headaches are often not auras at all in the ordinary sense of the term, but that many of them result "from an alteration in intracranial circulation either preceding the attack or coincidental with its onset" (14).

EMOTIONAL AURAS

Fear ranges from mild anxiety to intense terror and is "unnatural," out of proportion to, and separable from the understandable apprehension that accompanies the beginning of a seizure. In some patients, the fear resembles a real-life experience, such as suddenly finding a stranger standing close behind, and also may be associated with an unpleasant psychic hallucination of past events. Others seemingly localize the sensation to the chest or stomach, and fear is frequently associated with epigastric aura (80). Ictal fear may be accompanied by symptoms and signs of autonomic activation such as mydriasis, piloerection, tachycardia, and hyperventilation. On the basis of lesions in epileptic patients, an aura of fear has been linked to temporal lobe epilepsy (80,81). Fear also has been elicited on stimulation of the temporal lobe, particularly the mesial structures (31,82). An aura of fear must be distinguished from a panic attack, and correct identification as an epileptic aura is helped by subsequent ictal phenomena;

however, the distinction may be difficult if an aura of fear occurs in isolation, as at the onset of epilepsy.

Elation and pleasure are infrequent auras. The preictal happiness and ecstasy reported by Dostoyevski have often been cited as examples. Pleasurable sensations have not been elicited by electrical stimulation in the vicinity of epileptogenic lesions (8,14,31) and are not held to be of localizing value.

Depression as an aura or ictal phenomenon is rare. In the largest series, reported by Williams (80), many of the patients had depression that lasted for hours to days, making it likely that this state constituted a prodromal mood change rather than an aura. No consistent cortical localization has been demonstrated.

PSYCHIC AURAS

In 1880, Hughlings Jackson (2) described "certain psychical states during the onset of epileptic seizures" that included "intellectual aurae . . . reminiscence . . . dreamy feelings . . . dreams mixing up with present thoughts . . . double consciousness . . . 'as if I went back to all that occurred in my childhood'. These are all voluminous mental states and yet of different kinds . . ." Admittedly, the range of experiences encompassed by the term "psychical auras" is imprecise. Both Gowers (1) and Penfield and Jasper (14) included emotional auras under this heading. Such states have also been called "experiential" phenomena, particularly those related to psychic hallucinations (31,82).

An illusion results from faulty interpretation of present experience in relation to the environment. Aware of the error in perception, the patient has "mental diplopia" in the Jacksonian sense. A hallucination is a sensory lifelike experience unrelated to present environment and reality. Psychic hallucinations usually consist of dreamlike events or memory flashbacks that are complex and "formed," in contrast to the elementary "unformed" hallucinations that characterize excitation of the primary sensory areas. Nevertheless, epileptic patients invariably sense that the hallucinations are not real.

The nature of psychic auras is as varied as their complexity. Many attempts at classification have been made (Table 11.4), but it may be fruitless to adhere to an overly rigid categorization of these rich phenomena that offer glimpses into the workings of human consciousness. For example, deja vu can be

TABLE 11.4

PSYCHIC AURAS

	Illusion	Hallucination
Memory	Deja vu, jamais vu, deja entendu, jamais entendu, strangeness	Memory flashbacks, dreams of past
Vision	Macropsia, micropsia, objects nearer or farther, clearer or blurred	Objects, faces, scenes
Sound	Advancing or receding, louder or softer, clearer or fainter	Voices, music
Self-image	Mental diplopia, depersonalization, derealization, remoteness	Autoscopy
Time	Standstill, rushing, or slowing	—
Others	Increased awareness, decreased awareness	—

considered an illusion of familiar memory; the converse, when what should have been a familiar visual experience becomes unfamiliar, is called jamais vu. The corresponding auditory illusions are deja entendu and jamais entendu. Autoscopy, a hallucination of self-image, is seeing oneself in external space, as a "double," or as an external entity observed from a distance after the mind is felt to have left the body (83).

Despite reports that psychic auras can occur with focal seizures from elsewhere in the brain, the consensus ascribes them to epileptic activation of the temporal lobe. Penfield and Jasper's assertion (14) that "a psychical hallucination or dream is produced only by discharge in the temporal cortex" remains valid, based on the vast experience with intracranial electrical stimulation that has since accumulated. Penfield and Perot (41) found that the sites eliciting psychic phenomena were nearly all in the lateral temporal neocortex, particularly along its superior border, and only occasionally from basal or mesial temporal regions. In contrast, later studies from the same institution (31), identified the mesial temporal limbic structures, especially the amygdala, as the sites most frequently producing psychic phenomena, even in the absence of an electrical afterdischarge. Gloor (84) pointed to methodologic differences to account for the discrepant results: Penfield and colleagues (14,41) stimulated mainly the lateral neocortical surface intraoperatively, whereas Gloor et al. (31) based their observations on extraoperative stimulation in patients with chronically implanted depth electrodes to explore the temporal lobes. To reconcile these differences, Gloor (84) proposed a hypothesis based on the model of a neuronal network with reciprocal connections—in this case, between the limbic structures and the temporal isocortex. Psychic phenomena arising "from the activation of matrices in distributed neuronal networks" could presumably be elicited from different locations within the temporal lobe, including temporal isocortex and various limbic structures.

Forced thinking refers to an awareness of intrusive stereotyped thoughts, fixation on, or crowding of thoughts. Penfield and Jasper (14) separated it from psychic auras and localized it to the frontal lobe.

AUTONOMIC AURAS

There is no consensus on the range of phenomena to be included in this category. Epigastric sensations are considered an autonomic aura by some, although there is insufficient evidence for implication of autonomic afferent or efferent pathway activation. To be discussed are sensations that are clearly experienced by the patient.

One of the commonest sensation is that of palpitations. This can usually be verified by accompanying tachycardia on the electrocardiogram. It is usually associated with auras of fear, anxiety, or epigastric sensation. These are auras frequent in temporal lobe epilepsy. Tachycardia of course occurs not just with the aura, but even more frequently in complex partial or generalized seizures.

Respiratory symptoms experienced as an aura include such sensations as not being able to breathe, a need to breathe more deeply, and of a breath filling the chest that would not expire. Alterations in respiratory rhythms have been reported on stimulation of temporal limbic structures and in seizures of insular origin (53).

Cold shivering and associated piloerection as auras are usually experienced over diffuse or extended areas, but can be localized. There are usually other associated auras. It is probably not localized to a single cortical area, but seems most common in temporal lobe epilepsy (85,86). It has been reported to show a left hemispheric predominance in lateralization.

Urinary urgency has been reported both at seizure onset or afterwards. The same can be said of the rectal sensation to defecate. The localization of these sensations is not clear.

SEXUAL AURAS

These uncommon erotic feelings may or may not be accompanied by genital sensations or symptoms or signs of sexual arousal. They are distinguished from the sometimes unpleasant superficial genital sensations without sexual content that arise from stimulation of the primary somatosensory area at the parasagittal convexity or interhemispheric fissure and possibly the perisylvian region. Sexual auras seem to arise most frequently from the temporal lobe (87) with other cases reported from the parasagittal area implicating the sensory cortex. The cases reported thus far have shown a female preponderance. Of those patients whose sexual aura resulted in orgasm, a right hemisphere lateralization has been found in one review (88).

References

1. Gowers WR. *Epilepsy and Other Chronic Convulsive Diseases: Their Causes, Symptoms & Treatment.* 2nd ed. London, UK: J & A Churchill; 1901.
2. Jackson JH. On right or leftsided spasm at the onset of epileptic paroxysms, and on crude sensation warnings, and elaborate states. *Brain.* 1880/1881;3:192–206.
3. Commission on Classification and Terminology of the International League against Epilepsy. Proposal for revised clinical and electroencephalographic classification of epileptic seizures. *Epilepsia.* 1981;22:489–501.
4. Wieser HG, Hailemariam S, Regard M, et al. Unilateral limbic epileptic status activity: stereo EEG, behavioral, and cognitive data. *Epilepsia.* 1985;26:19–29.
5. Olivier A, Gloor P, Andermann F, et al. Occipitotemporal epilepsy studied with stereotaxically implanted depth electrodes and successfully treated by temporal resection. *Ann Neurol.* 1982;11:428–432.
6. Kanemoto K, Janz D. The temporal sequence of aura-sensations in patients with complex focal seizures with particular attention to ictal aphasia. *J Neurol Neurosurg Psychiatry.* 1989;52:52–56.
7. Gloor P. Physiology of the limbic system. In: Penry JK, Daly DD, eds. *Complex Partial Seizures and Their Treatment. Advances in Neurology.* New York, NY: Raven Press; 1975;11:27–53.
8. Halgren E, Walter RD, Cherlow D, et al. Mental phenomena evoked by electrical stimulation of the human hippocampal formation and amygdala. *Brain.* 1978;101:83–117.
9. Hauser EA, Kurland LT. The epidemiology of epilepsy in Rochester, Minnesota, 1935 through 1967. *Epilepsia.* 1975;16:1–66.
10. Lennox WG, Cobb S. Aura in epilepsy: a statistical review of 1,359 cases. *Arch Neurol Psychiatry.* 1933;30:374–387.
11. Gibbs FA, Gibbs EL. *Atlas of Electroencephalography, II. Epilepsy.* 2nd ed. Cambridge, MA: Addison-Wesley Press; 1952.
12. Janati A, Nowack WJ, Dorsey S, et al. Correlative study of interictal electroencephalogram and aura in complex partial seizures. *Epilepsia.* 1990;31:41–46.
13. King DW, Ajmone-Marsan C. Clinical features and ictal patterns in epileptic patients with EEG temporal lobe foci. *Ann Neurol.* 1977;2:7.
14. Penfield W, Jasper H. *Epilepsy and the Functional Anatomy of the Human Brain.* Boston, MA: Little, Brown & Co; 1954.
15. Theodore WH, Porter RJ, Penry JK. Complex partial seizures: clinical characteristics and differential diagnosis. *Neurology.* 1983;33:1115–1121.
16. Marks WJ Jr, Laxer KD. Semiology of temporal lobe seizures: value in lateralizing the seizure focus. *Epilepsia.* 1998;39:721–726.
17. Sirven JI, Sperling MR, French JA, et al. Significance of simple partial seizures in temporal lobe epilepsy. *Epilepsia.* 1996;37:450–454.
18. Sperling MR, O'Connor MJ. Auras and subclinical seizures: characteristics and prognostic significance. *Ann Neurol.* 1990;28:320–329.

19. Schulz R, Lüders HO, Noachtar S, et al. Amnesia of the epileptic aura. *Neurology.* 1995;45:231–235.
20. Blume WT, Girvin JP. Altered seizure patterns after temporal lobectomy. *Epilepsia.* 1997;38:1183–1187.
21. Lund JS, Spencer SS. An examination or persistent auras in surgically treated epilepsy. *Epilepsia.* 1992;33(suppl 3):95.
22. Tuxhorn I, So N, Van Ness P, et al. Natural history and prognostic significance of auras after temporal lobectomy. *Epilepsia.* 1992;33(suppl 3):95.
23. Vickrey BG, Hays RD, Engel J Jr, et al. Outcome assessment for epilepsy surgery: the impact of measuring health-related quality of life. *Ann Neurol.* 1995;37:158–166.
24. Taylor DC, Lochery M. Temporal lobe epilepsy: origin and significance of simple and complex auras. *J Neurol Neurosurg Psychiatry.* 1987;50:673–681.
25. Ferguson SM, Rayport M. Psychosis in epilepsy. In: Blumer D, ed. *Psychiatric Aspects of Epilepsy.* Washington, DC: American Psychiatric Press; 1984:229–270.
26. Mahl GF, Rothenberg A, Delgado JMR, et al. Psychological response in humans to intracerebral stimulation. *Psychosom Med.* 1964;26:337–368.
27. Rayport M, Ferguson SM. Qualitative modification of sensory responses to amygdaloid stimulation in man by interview content and context. *Electroencephalogr Clin Neurophysiol.* 1974;34:714. Abstract.
28. Van Donselaar CA, Geerts AT, Schimsheimer RJ. Usefulness of an aura for classification of a first generalized seizure. *Epilepsia.* 1990;31:529–535.
29. Kapur J, Pillai A, Henry TR. Psychogenic elaboration of simple partial seizures. *Epilepsia.* 1995;36:1126–1130.
30. Bancaud J, Talairach J, Bonis A, et al. *La Stéréo-Électro-Encéphalographie dans l'Épilepsie.* Paris: Masson & Co; 1965.
31. Gloor P, Olivier A, Quesney LF, et al. The role of the limbic system in experiential phenomena of temporal lobe epilepsy. *Ann Neurol.* 1982;12:129–144.
32. Lüders H, Lesser R, Dinner DS, et al. Commentary: chronic intracranial recording and stimulation with subdural electrodes. In: Engel J Jr, ed. *Surgical Treatment of the Epilepsies.* New York: Raven Press; 1987:297–321.
33. Schulz R, Lüders HO, Tuxhorn H, et al. Localization of epileptic auras induced on stimulation by subdural electrodes. *Epilepsia.* 1997;38:1321–1329.
34. Ostrowsky K, Isnard J, Guénot M, et al. Functional mapping of the insular cortex: clinical implication in temporal lobe epilepsy. *Epilepsia.* 2000;41:681–686.
35. Penfield W, Kristiansen K. *Epileptic Seizure Patterns.* Springfield, IL: Charles C Thomas; 1951.
36. Palmini A, Gloor P. The localizing value of auras in partial seizures: a prospective and retrospective study. *Neurology.* 1992;42:801–808.
37. Rasmussen T. Localizational aspects of epileptic seizure phenomena. In: Thompson RA, Green JR, eds. *New Perspectives in Cerebral Localization.* New York: Raven Press; 1982:177–203.
38. Rasmussen T. Characteristics of a pure culture of frontal lobe epilepsy. *Epilepsia.* 1983;24:482–493.
39. Ajmone-Marsan C, Goldhammer L. Clinical ictal patterns and electrographic data in cases of partial seizures of frontal-central-parietal origin. In: Brazier MAB, ed. *Epilepsy: Its Phenomena in Man.* New York: Academic Press; 1973:235–259.
40. Ludwig BI, Ajmone-Marsan C. Clinical ictal patterns in epileptic patients with occipital electroencephalographic foci. *Neurology.* 1975;25:463–471.
41. Penfield W, Perot P. The brain's record of auditory and visual experience. A final summary and discussion. *Brain.* 1963;86:595–694.
42. Gupta K, Jeavons PM, Hughes RC, et al. Aura in temporal lobe epilepsy: clinical and electroencephalographic correlation. *J Neurol Neurosurg Psychiatry.* 1983;46:1079–1083.
43. Lieb JP, Walsh GO, Babb TL, et al. A comparison of EEG seizure patterns recorded with surface and depth electrodes in patients with temporal lobe epilepsy. *Epilepsia.* 1976;17:137–160.
44. Spencer SS, Spencer DS, Williamson PD, et al. Combined depth and subdural electrode investigation in uncontrolled epilepsy. *Neurology.* 1990;40:74–79.
45. Sperling MR, O'Connor MJ. Comparison of depth and subdural electrodes in recording temporal lobe seizures. *Neurology.* 1989;39:1497–1504.
46. Sperling MR, Lieb JP, Engel J Jr, et al. Prognostic significance of independent auras in temporal lobe epilepsy. *Epilepsia.* 1989;30:322–331.
47. Babb TL, Wilson CL, Isokawa-Akesson M. Firing patterns of human limbic neurons during stereoencephalography (SEEG) and clinical temporal lobe seizures. *Electroencephalogr Clin Neurophysiol.* 1987;66:467–482.
48. Woolsey CN, Erickson TC, Gilson WE. Localization in somatic sensory and motor areas of human cerebral cortex as determined by direct recording of evoked potentials and electrical stimulation. *J Neurosurg.* 1979;51:476–506.
49. Penfield W, Rasmussen T. *The Cerebral Cortex of Man.* New York: Macmillan; 1950.
50. Morris HH, Dinner DS, Lüders H, et al. Supplementary motor seizures: clinical and electroencephalographic findings. *Neurology.* 1988;38:1075–1082.
51. Fried I, Katz A, Sass J, et al. Functional organization of supplementary motor cortex: evidence from electrical stimulation. *Epilepsia.* 1989;30:725. Abstract.
52. Lim SH, Dinner DS, Pillay PK, et al. Functional anatomy of the human supplementary sensorimotor area: results of extraoperative electrical stimulation. *Electroencephalogr Clin Neurophysiol.* 1994;91:179–193.
53. Isnard J, Guénot M, Ostrowsky K, et al. The role of the insular cortex in temporal lobe epilepsy. *Ann Neurol.* 2000;48:614–623.
54. Weingarten SM, Cherlow DG, Halgren E. Relationship of hallucinations to the depth structures of the temporal lobe. In: Sweet WR, Obrador S, Martin-Rodriguez JG, eds. *Neurosurgical Treatment in Psychiatry, Pain and Epilepsy.* Baltimore, MD: University Park Press; 1976:553–568.
55. Mauguiere F, Courjon J. Somatosensory epilepsy. *Brain.* 1978;101:307–332.
56. Young GB, Blume WT. Painful epileptic seizures. *Brain.* 1983;106:537–554.
57. Lewin W, Phillips CG. Observations on partial removal of the postcentral gyrus for pain. *J Neurol Neurosurg Psychiatry.* 1952;15:143–147.
58. Siegel AM, Williamson PD, Roberts DW, et al. Localized pain associated with seizures originating in the parietal lobe. *Epilepsia.* 1999;40:845–855.
59. Wilkinson HA. Epileptic pain. An uncommon manifestation with localizing value. *Neurology.* 1973;23:518–520.
60. Hamby WB. Reversible central pain. *Arch Neurol.* 1961;5:82–86.
61. Wieser HG. *Electroclinical Features of the Psychomotor Seizure.* London, UK: Butterworths; 1983.
62. Berman S. Vestibular epilepsy. *Brain.* 1955;78:471–486.
63. Smith BH. Vestibular disturbances in epilepsy. *Neurology.* 1960;10:465–469.
64. Jackson JH, Beevor CE. Case of tumour of the right temporosphenoidal lobe bearing on the localization of the sense of smell and on the interpretation of a particular variety of epilepsy. *Brain.* 1889;12:346–357.
65. Daly DD. Uncinate fits. *Neurology.* 1958;8:250–260.
66. Acharya V, Acharya J, Lüders H. Olfactory epileptic auras. *Neurology.* 1998;51:56–61.
67. Howe JG, Gibson JD. Uncinate seizures and tumors, a myth reexamined. *Ann Neurol.* 1982;12:227. Letter.
68. Fried I, Spencer DD, Spencer SS. The anatomy of epileptic auras: focal pathology and surgical outcome. *J Neurosurg.* 1995;83:60–66.
69. Hausser-Hauw C, Bancaud J. Gustatory hallucinations in epileptic seizures. Electrophysiological, clinical and anatomical correlates. *Brain.* 1987;110:339–359.
70. Nair DR, Najm I, Bulacio J, et al. Painful auras in focal epilepsy. *Neurology.* 2001;57:700–702.
71. Van Buren JM. The abdominal aura: a study of abdominal sensations occurring in epilepsy produced by depth stimulation. *Electroencephalogr Clin Neurophysiol.* 1963;15:1–19.
72. Van Buren JM, Ajmone-Marsan C. A correlation of autonomic and EEG components in temporal lobe epilepsy. *Arch Neurol.* 1960;3:683–693.
73. Andermann F, Lugaresi E, eds. *Migraine and Epilepsy.* Boston, MA: Butterworths; 1987.
74. Schon F, Blau JN. Postepileptic headache and migraine. *J Neurol Neurosurg Psychiatry.* 1987;50:1148–1152.
75. Isler H, Wieser HG, Egli M. Hemicrania epileptica: synchronous ipsilateral ictal headache with migraine features. In: Andermannn F, Lugaresi E, eds. *Migraine and Epilepsy.* Boston, MA: Butterworths; 1987:249–264.
76. Laplante P, Saint-Hilaire JM, Bouvier G. Headache as an epileptic manifestation. *Neurology.* 1983;33:1493–1495.
77. Olesen J, Larsen B, Lauritzen M. Focal hyperemia followed by spreading oligemia and impaired activation of RCBF in classic migraine. *Ann Neurol.* 1981;9:344–352.
78. Gastaut H. A new type of epilepsy: benign partial epilepsy of childhood with occipital spike-waves. *Clin Electroencephalogr.* 1982;13:13–22.
79. Kobayashi K, Iyoda K, Ohtsuka Y, et al. Longitudinal clinicoelectrophysiologic study of a case of Lafora disease proven by skin biopsy. *Epilepsia.* 1990;31:194–201.
80. Williams D. The structure of emotions reflected in epileptic experiences. *Brain.* 1956;79:29–67.
81. Macrae D. Isolated fear. A temporal lobe aura. *Neurology.* 1954;4:479–505.
82. Mullan S, Penfield W. Illusions of comparative interpretation and emotion. *Arch Neurol Psychiatry.* 1959;81:269–284.
83. Devinsky O, Feldmann E, Burrowes K, et al. Autoscopic phenomena with seizures. *Arch Neurol.* 1989;46:1080–1088.
84. Gloor P. Experiential phenomena of temporal lobe epilepsy. Facts and hypotheses. *Brain.* 1990;113:1673–1694.
85. Green JB. Pilomotor seizures. *Neurology.* 1984;34:837–839.
86. Stefan H, Pauli E, Kerling F, et al. Autonomic auras: left hemispheric predominance of epileptic generators of cold shivers and goose bumps? *Epilepsia.* 2002;43:41–45.
87. Remillard GM, Andermann F, Testa GF, et al. Sexual ictal manifestations predominate in women with temporal lobe epilepsy: a finding suggesting sexual dimorphism in the human brain. *Neurology.* 1983;33:323–330.
88. Jansky J, Szücs A, Halász P, et al. Orgasmic aura originates from the right hemisphere. *Neurology.* 2002;58:302–304.

CHAPTER 12 ■ FOCAL SEIZURES WITH IMPAIRED CONSCIOUSNESS

LARA JEHI AND PRAKASH KOTAGAL

Awareness and responsiveness are the two sides of the coin characterizing a clinically applicable definition of consciousness as proposed by the International Classification of Epileptic Seizures (ICES) (1). These two concepts are intimately related, but it is important to recognize that they are essentially distinct: while consciousness as a whole is clearly impaired in epilepsy patients who are completely unresponsive during their spells, and are later amnestic of their events, the question is a bit more controversial in other cases. For example, we know now that up to 10% of patients with right temporal lobe epilepsies may be fully responsive and interactive during focal seizures associated with automatisms, and yet not be able postictally to recall any of the events that occurred during the seizure (2). Conversely, some patients may not obey any commands during a seizure, but do recall when interviewed postictally all the commands and instructions given during the ictus. This may be seen with several possible scenarios including ictal aphasia, inability to perform voluntary movements secondary to stimulation of negative motor areas, or diversion of attention by a hallucinated experience (3). These examples illustrate the conceptual complexity of assessing consciousness in relation to epileptic seizures and highlight the practical importance of a thorough seizure and postseizure interview while patients are being evaluated in epilepsy clinics and video-EEG monitoring units. Recently, some epilepsy centers have even proposed the use of a standardized "Consciousness Inventory" to assess the level and content of ictal consciousness (4,5). For the purposes of this chapter, we will use the term "focal epilepsy with impaired consciousness" to refer to focal epilepsies where either responsiveness or awareness/recall is disturbed during the ictal period.

Another issue that needs to be spelled out prior to proceeding with this discussion of epilepsy and consciousness would be a clear definition and distinction of the following terms: "complex partial seizure," "dialeptic seizure," and "automotor seizure." The ICES defines as "complex partial" any seizure consisting of a lapse of consciousness and minimum motor activity *IF* the ictal EEG shows focal epileptiform activity. A seizure with exactly the same symptomatology or "semiology" would be classified as an "absence seizure" *IF* the ictal EEG shows generalized spike–wave complexes. The terms complex partial and absence refer therefore to electroclinical complexes where both clinical semiology *AND* knowledge of the ictal EEG patterns—information that is not necessarily always available in an initial outpatient evaluation—are required for an accurate definition. Furthermore, the broad umbrella of "complex partial" seizures encompasses various seizure types that have little in common except a focal onset.

For example, partial seizures arising from the perirolandic region or supplementary motor area may involve impairment of consciousness but are very different from complex partial seizures arising from the mesial temporal lobe with an aura of deja vu, staring, unresponsiveness, and stereotyped oroalimentary and hand automatisms. These issues lead to the proposition of a five-tier classification system that distinguishes the *seizure* characteristics (including semiological features and frequency) of a given patient from the *epilepsy* characteristics (including etiology, associated neurological deficits, and location of the epilepsy, as determined through various diagnostic modalities including EEG, imaging, etc.) (6). In this semiological classification, a seizure is defined solely based on its clinical characteristics. A "dialeptic" (from the Greek word dialeptin meaning "to stand still," "to interrupt," or "to pass out") seizure is one with impairment of consciousness as the predominant feature. An "automotor" seizure would be one with predominant automatisms regardless of whether consciousness was impaired or not. In this chapter, we will use the general term of complex partial seizures, as well as the more specific terms of dialeptic and automotor seizures when a distinction between the two is needed.

In the following sections, we will first provide a brief historical overview and briefly discuss features that allow differentiation of focal from generalized seizures causing an impairment of awareness. Then, we will focus on characterizing the localizing value of focal seizures with impaired consciousness, and discuss lateralizing features that may help in further defining the epileptogenic focus. We then describe typical electroencephalographic findings and conclude with a section on the proposed mechanisms of impaired consciousness in partial epilepsy.

HISTORICAL BACKGROUND

Although descriptions of seizures with loss of consciousness and automatisms suggesting focal origin date to the days of Hippocrates, Galen, and Areatus, Hughlings Jackson first suggested their origin in the temporal lobe and called them "uncinate fits" (7). The introduction of the EEG in 1929 made it possible to identify the characteristic interictal and ictal features of these seizures. In 1937, Gibbs and Lennox proposed the term "psychomotor epilepsy" to describe a characteristic EEG pattern of temporal lobe seizures accompanied by mental, emotional, motor, and autonomic phenomena (8). Gibbs, Gibbs, and Lennox also noted interictal sharp waves in the temporal regions in patients with this seizure type. Penfield and Kristiansen (9) and Penfield and Jasper (10) observed that some patients with seizures and loss of consciousness had extratemporal sharp waves. Jasper and colleagues first pointed out that the localization of the EEG ictal discharge was more important than its actual pattern, and that this pattern originated from "deep within the temporal lobes, near the midline" (11).

The early work of investigators at the Montreal Neurological Institute in Canada, and in Paris, France, contributed immensely to our understanding of various types of epilepsy, including temporal and extratemporal, and used information from multiple techniques: scalp recordings, invasive recordings from depth electrodes and intraoperative corticography, and cortical stimulation studies (9,10,12,13). Ajmone-Marsan and colleagues (14,15) used chemical activation with pentylenetetrazol to study partial seizures from various locations. The Paris group (16) published a number of papers on frontal lobe epilepsy. Tharp (17) was the first to identify seizures with loss of consciousness arising from the orbitofrontal regions.

Early work on the symptomatology of focal seizures with impaired consciousness was based on eyewitness descriptions by family members, nurses, or physicians (12,15). Some studies employed cine film and analyzed photographs taken at three per second (18). The introduction of videotape technology provided an inexpensive and effective way to easily record and play back seizures as often as needed, resulting in a better grasp of phenomenology. The observations of Delgado-Escueta, Theodore, Williamson, Quesney, Bancaud, and others vastly improved our understanding of focal seizures with impaired consciousness (19–24). Crucial insights were provided by Gastaut, who proposed the first ICES in 1970 (25).

In his 1983 monograph, *Electroclinical Features of the Psychomotor Seizure*, Wieser (26) described the order of symptom onsets and symptom clusters, and attempted to correlate these clusters with electrographic activity recorded with depth electrodes. Maldonado et al. (27) also examined the sequences of symptoms in hippocampal-amygdalar–onset seizures. Using methods similar to those of Wieser, Kotagal examined temporal lobe psychomotor seizures in patients who were seizure-free after temporal lobectomy (28). Similar methods also have been used to study frontal lobe seizures (29,30).

FOCAL VERSUS GENERALIZED SEIZURES WITH IMPAIRMENT OF CONSCIOUSNESS

Focal seizures with impairment of consciousness can present with or without an aura. The auras last from a few seconds to as long as 1 to 2 minutes before consciousness is actually lost. Impairment of consciousness is maximal initially. Partial recovery later in the seizure may allow the patient to look at an observer walking into the room or interact in some other way with the environment (28). Most of these seizures with automatisms last longer than 30 seconds—up to 1 to 2 minutes (sometimes as long as 10 minutes). Very few are briefer than 10 seconds, which helps to distinguish them clinically from typical absence seizures characterized by 3-Hz spike-wave complexes (23).

Conversely, blinking has been described more often in generalized absence as opposed to focal seizures with impaired

consciousness. Automotor activity is not restricted to focal seizures and subtle automatisms may be seen in typical absence (generalized) epilepsy (1). So, a clear distinction between dialeptic seizures seen in the setting of frontal or temporal lobe epilepsy from those in absence epilepsy may not be possible without obtaining an electrophysiological confirmation and recording an ictal EEG (1).

LOCALIZING VALUE OF FOCAL SEIZURES WITH IMPAIRMENT OF CONSCIOUSNESS

Research during the past two decades has advanced our understanding of the symptomatology of focal seizures with impairment of consciousness arising from various locations (22,28). Most such seizures arise in the temporal lobe; however, in at least 10% to 30% of patients evaluated in epilepsy surgery programs, the origin is extratemporal, most commonly the frontal lobe (1).

Escueta and colleagues described three types of complex partial seizures (23). Type I (24–30% of mesial temporal lobe seizures) begins with a motionless stare or behavioral arrest (phase 1) quickly followed by a period of unresponsiveness and stereotyped automatisms (phase 2) evolving to a final phase of a "clouded state" and semipurposeful reactive automatisms. Type II events are uncommon and similar to Type I events except that phase I is absent. Type III complex partial seizures, previously called temporal lobe syncope, begin with a drop attack, followed by confusion, amnesia, and gradual return of composure (23). The localizing value of the motionless stare was believed to indicate mesial temporal lobe epilepsy (23). However, behavioral arrest is also seen in 20% of patients with frontal lobe epilepsy (31). Types II and III are thought to be of extratemporal origin (32).

Different components of consciousness may be impaired depending on the location of the ictal seizure pattern. Frontal lobe seizures are more likely to manifest with loss of orientation behavior and expressive speech; left temporal lobe seizures lead to impairments of memory and expressive and receptive speech; and right temporal lobe seizures rarely involve impairment of consciousness (33).

Seizures of Frontal Lobe Origin

Seizures arising from the frontal lobes occur in up to 30% of patients with focal epilepsy, and represent the second most common focal type after temporal lobe seizures (20). In 50% of patients with frontal lobe epilepsy, seizures are accompanied by loss of consciousness. Seizures with loss of consciousness can arise from various locations within the frontal lobe (except from the rolandic strip) (17,29,30,34). Semiologic features include occurrence in clusters, occurrence many times a day, occurrence for brief duration (lasting about 30 seconds with a sudden onset), and minimal postictal confusion. Bizarre attacks with prominent motor automatisms involving the lower extremities (pedaling or bicycling movements), sexual automatisms, and prominent vocalizations are common, and the seizures are remarkably stereotyped for each patient (29,30,32). Identification of seizure onset within the frontal lobe by semiology alone and differentiation of mesial temporal lobe epilepsy and frontal lobe epilepsy may be misleading and difficult; however, analysis of the earliest signs and symptoms, as well as their order of appearance, may allow this distinction in onset (29). Clonic seizures frequently arise from the frontal convexity, tonic seizures from the supplementary motor area, and automotor seizures from the orbitofrontal region (35). Seizures with "motor agitation" and hypermotor features are more likely to arise from the orbitofrontal and frontopolar regions, as opposed to seizures with oroalimentary automatisms, gesturing, fumbling, and looking around, which are more suggestive of a temporal lobe focus (29). Up to 50% of patients develop complex partial status epilepticus (35).

The unique symptomatology of supplementary motor seizures includes an onset with abrupt tonic extension of the limbs that is often bilateral but may be asymmetric and is accompanied by nonpurposeful movements of uninvolved limbs and vocalizations. Typically, these occur out of sleep and recur many times a night. Because of their bizarre symptomatology, they are sometimes mistaken for nonepileptic seizures. Consciousness is often preserved in supplementary motor area seizures, and postictally baseline mentation returns quickly.

Cingulate gyrus seizures may also vary in semiology. Seizures arising from the anterior portion of the cingulate present with predominantly motor manifestations such as bilateral asymmetric tonic seizures, hypermotor seizures, and complex motor seizures, while posterior cingulate cortex epilepsies tend to predominantly have alterations of consciousness (dialeptic seizures) and automatisms of the distal portions of the limbs (automotor seizures) as the main clinical manifestations.

Orbitofrontal seizures manifest prominent autonomic phenomena, with flushing, mydriasis, vocalizations, and automatisms. The vocalizations may consist of unintelligible screaming or loud expletives of words or short sentences. Patients also may get up and run around the room.

Quesney and associates (24) reported that seizures of the anterolateral dorsal convexity may manifest with auras such as dizziness, epigastric sensation, or fear in 50% of patients; behavioral arrest in 20%; and speech arrest in 30%. One third of the patients exhibited sniffing, chewing or swallowing, laughing, crying, hand automatisms, or kicking. A tendency to partial motor activity in the form of tonic or clonic movements contralateral to the side of the focus was also noted. Bancaud and colleagues described speech arrest, visual hallucinations, illusions, and forced thinking in some patients during seizures of dorsolateral frontal origin. These patients may also show contralateral tonic eye and head deviation or asymmetric tonic posturing of the limbs before contralateral clonic activity or secondary generalization. Other patients may have autonomic symptoms such as pallor, flushing, tachycardia, mydriasis, or apnea (20).

Seizures of Temporal Lobe Origin

Approximately 40% to 80% of patients with temporal lobe epilepsy have seizures with stereotyped automatisms. In fact, seizures with predominantly oral and manual automatisms in addition to few other motor manifestations (excluding focal clonic activity and version) are highly suggestive of a temporal lobe origin (22–24,28). Secondary generalization occurs

in approximately 60% of temporal lobe seizures (28). Postictally, gradual recovery follows several minutes of confusion; however, patients may carry out automatic behavior, such as getting up, walking about, or running, of which they have no memory. Attempts to restrain them may only aggravate matters. Violence, invariably nondirected, may be seen during this period. The patient is usually amnestic for the seizure but may be able to recall the aura. A few patients may exhibit retrograde amnesia for several minutes before the seizure.

In young children, partial seizures of temporal lobe onset are characterized predominantly by behavioral arrest with unresponsiveness (36); automatisms are usually oroalimentary, whereas discrete manual and gestural automatisms tend to occur in children older than age 5 or 6 years. In younger children, symmetric motor phenomena of the limbs, postures similar to frontal lobe seizures in adults, and head nodding as in infantile spasms were typical (37). Because it is impossible to test for consciousness in infants, focal seizures with impairment of consciousness may manifest as hypomotor seizures, a bland form of complex partial seizure with none or only few automatisms. In very young infants, these may also occasionally be accompanied by central apnea (38).

Seizures of Parietal Lobe Origin

Like seizures of occipital lobe onset, partial seizures from the parietal lobe may manifest loss of consciousness and automatisms when they spread to involve the temporal lobe. Initial sensorimotor phenomena may point to onset in the parietal lobe, as do vestibular hallucinations such as vertigo, described in seizures beginning near the angular gyrus. Language dysfunction may occur in seizures arising from the dominant hemisphere. Also described in parietal lobe complex partial seizures have been auras including epigastric sensations, formed visual hallucinations, behavioral arrest, and panic attacks (39). In a study of 40 patients with parietal lobe epilepsy as established by standard presurgical evaluation, including MRI, fluorodeoxyglucose–positron emission tomography (FDG-PET), ictal single-photon emission tomography (SPECT), and scalp video-EEG monitoring, with additional intracranial EEG monitoring in selected cases, 27 patients experienced at least one type of aura. The most common auras were somatosensory (13 patients), followed by affective, vertiginous, and visual auras. Seizures had diverse manifestations. Eighteen patients showed simple motor seizure, followed by automotor seizure and dialeptic seizure (39).

A limiting factor in many studies of seizure symptomatology is that relatively few reported patients with extratemporal complex partial seizures become seizure-free after cortical resection, casting some doubt on the localization of the epileptic focus.

Seizures of Occipital Lobe Origin

The following features suggest the occipital lobe as the origin of a complex partial seizure: (i) Visual auras, usually of elementary sensations such as white or colored flashing lights, are often in the part of the visual field corresponding to the focus; the visual phenomena may remain stationary or move across the visual field. (ii) Ictal blindness in the form of a whiteout or blackout may be reported. (iii) Version of the eyes and head to the opposite side is common and is a reliable lateralizing sign; patients may report a sensation of eye pulling to the opposite side even in the absence of eye deviation. (iv) Rapid, forced blinking and oculoclonic activity also may be seen (40–42). Other symptoms may result from spread to the temporal or parietal lobes (42). Suprasylvian spread to the mesial or parietal cortex produces symptomatology similar to that in supplementary motor seizures, whereas spread to the lateral parietal convexity gives rise to sensorimotor phenomena. Spread to the lateral temporal cortex followed by involvement of the mesial structures may produce formed visual hallucinations, followed by automatisms and loss of consciousness. Direct spread to the mesial temporal cortex may mimic mesial temporal epilepsy. The visual auras may be the only clue to recognizing the occipital lobe onset of these seizures; however, the patient may not recall them because of retrograde amnesia, if the aura was fleeting or if the seizure is no longer preceded by the aura as it was in the past (40).

In a study of 42 patients with occipital lobe epilepsy, 73% experienced visual auras frequently followed by loss of consciousness possibly as a consequence of ictal spread into the frontotemporal region. Vomiting is more common in benign than in symptomatic occipital lobe seizures, and may also represent ictal spread to the temporal lobes (43).

LATERALIZING FEATURES ASSOCIATED WITH FOCAL SEIZURES WITH IMPAIRED CONSCIOUSNESS

The complex partial seizures with automatisms—or automotor seizures—are the commonest type of seizures observed in video-EEG monitoring units. The number of clinical symptoms per seizure and the duration of the seizures are usually higher than in other motor seizures, especially when observed in relation to temporal lobe epilepsy, allowing for a rich spectrum of lateralizing semiological findings (44). The following section will review some of the most salient lateralizing signs potentially seen in this context.

Dystonic Limb Posturing

Unilateral dystonic posturing defined as forced, unnatural, unilateral (or predomiantly unilateral) posturing of an arm or leg—either in flexion or extension, proximal or distal, or usually with a rotatory component—is probably the most reliable lateralizing sign in temporal lobe automotor seizures (44–46). It could be easily distinguished from tonic posturing, in which there is only extension or flexion without accompanying rotation or assumption of unnatural postures. It occurs contralateral to the epileptogenic zone in about 90% of temporal and extratemporal seizures. When occurring in conjunction with unilateral automatisms of the opposite limb and head turning, it also has an excellent localizing value suggesting a mesial temporal lobe onset (44). It likely reflects direct or indirect basal ganglia activation, in addition to widespread subcortical and cortical involvement of different neural networks, as

suggested by associated PET and SPECT changes and invasive EEG recordings (44–47).

Head Version

Classically, a versive head movement is defined as a tonic, unnatural, and forced lateral gyratory head movement, as opposed to head turning or deviation where more natural and unforced head gyratory movements occur. While the lateralizing value of simple head turning or deviation is questionable at best, classical head version strongly lateralizes the seizure onset to the contralateral side in >90% of the cases, especially when it occurs with conjugate eye version and shortly precedes secondary generalization (within less than 10 seconds) (44,46,48). It occurs in both temporal (about 35% of cases) and extratemporal (20–60%) seizures, and may be caused by seizure spread to the premotor areas (Broadman's areas 6 and 8) (44).

A careful evaluation of the ictal head movements is also important in determining the lateralizing value of "whole body" versive activity, or gyratory seizures (GSs) defined as a rotation around the body axis during a seizure for at least 180°. In a recent video-EEG series (49), this occurred more often in FLE (4/47 patients) versus TLE (8/169 patients). The direction of rotation lateralized seizure onset depending on the seizure evolution: (i) GSs starting with a forced version of the head ensuing into a body rotation lateralized seizure onset zone contralateral to the direction of rotation. (ii) In GSs without a preceding gyratory forced head version; the direction of rotation was toward the side of seizure onset.

Postictal Todd's Palsy

Although the occurrence of postictal hemiparesis (Todd's palsy) is a very rare occurrence (less than 1% of seizures), it is a very reliable lateralizing sign suggesting an epileptogenic focus in the contralateral hemisphere. It has, however, also been described in generalized epilepsies, and after seizures without focal motor features or secondary generalization (50).

Automatisms

The broad term of "automatisms" refers to stereotyped complex behavior seen during seizures. Gastaut and Broughton (51) listed five subclasses of automatisms: alimentary, mimetic, gestural, ambulatory, and verbal. This list does not include stereotyped bicycling or pedaling movements or sexual automatisms.

Oroalimentary automatisms such as lip smacking, chewing, swallowing, and other tongue movements tend to occur early in the seizure, often with hand automatisms, and may be elicited by electrical stimulation of the amygdala (20). They may occur without loss of consciousness in temporal lobe seizures when the ictal discharge is confined to the amygdala and anterior hippocampus (2). A complex automatism such as singing has been described (52). As such, oroalimentary automatisms have no lateralizing value. Preserved responsiveness during automatisms does, however, lateralize to the

TABLE 12.1

FREQUENCY AND RELIABILITY OF VARIOUS LATERALIZING SIGNS SEEN IN FOCAL SEIZURES WITH IMPAIRED CONSCIOUSNESS

Sign	Frequency	Lateralizing value
Postictal palsy (50)	Less than 1% of patients	Contralateral in 100% of patients
Unilateral dystonic limb posturing (45,47,53)	15–70% of FLE or TLE patients	Contralateral in >90% of cases
Head version (29,48)	35% of TLE patients, 20–60% of FLE patients	Contralateral in >90% of the cases
Unilateral tonic posturing (46)	15–20% of TLE patients, 50% of FLE patients	Contralateral in 40–90% of the cases
Unilateral immobile limb (46)	5–28% of TLE patients	Contralateral in most cases
Unilateral eye blinking (54)	0.8–1.5% of patients	Ipsilateral in 80% of patients
Postictal nosewiping (55)	50–85% of mesial TLE patients, 10–33% of FLE patients	Ipsilateral in 70–90% of TLE patients, nonlateralizing in FLE patients

nondominant hemisphere: while most automatisms are usually accompanied by impaired consciousness and subsequent amnesia, Ebner and coworkers (2) found that 10% of patients with right temporal lobe epilepsy had automatisms with preservation of consciousness; this was never observed in those with left temporal lobe epilepsy. Other researchers have made similar observations (44).

Hand automatisms, also referred to as simple discrete movements by Maldonado and colleagues (27) or bimanual automatisms, are rapid, repetitive, pill-rolling movements of the fingers or fumbling, grasping movements in which the patient may pull at sheets and manipulate any object within reach. Searching movements may also be seen. Some authors believed that unilateral automatisms had a lateralizing value (44). In our experience, they did not, unless accompanied by tonic/dystonic posturing in the opposite limb. In these patients, the seizures may begin with bilateral hand automatisms that are interrupted by dystonic posturing on one side while the automatisms continue on the other side (ipsilateral to the ictal discharge) (45) (Table 12.1).

Like oroalimentary automatisms, the hand automatisms suggest onset from the mesial temporal region. In extratemporal seizures with unilateral tonic posturing, thrashing to-and-fro movements, which are more proximal and not discrete, are sometimes seen in the opposite limb.

Eye blinking or fluttering may be observed. Although usually symmetric, unilateral blinking has been reported ipsilateral to the seizure focus (54). A mechanism similar to unilateral hand automatisms may be operative, but this has not been documented. Rapid, forced eye blinking when the seizure begins is thought to indicate occipital lobe onset (54). Seizures arising from the occipital region may produce version of the eyes to the opposite side (44).

Truncal or body movements may be seen, usually in the middle or late third of the seizure, when the patient attempts to sit up, turn over, or get out of bed (28).

Bicycling or pedaling movements of the legs are more commonly observed in complex partial seizures arising from the mesial frontal and orbitofrontal regions (24) than in temporal lobe seizures. They are sometimes seen in temporal lobe seizures but probably reflect spread of the ictal discharge to the mesial frontal cortex.

Mimetic automatisms, with changes in facial expression, grimacing, smiling, or pouting, are common in complex partial seizures (44). Crying has been noted in complex partial seizures arising from the nondominant temporal lobe (44).

Sexual or genital automatisms such as pelvic or truncal thrusting, masturbatory activity, or grabbing or fondling of the genitals are relatively uncommon during complex partial seizures. However, they have been reported in complex partial seizures of frontal lobe origin, as well as in those arising from the temporal lobes (44). Leutmezqwer and colleagues (56) postulate that discrete genital automatisms such as fondling or grabbing the genitals are seen in temporal lobe seizures, whereas hypermotoric sexual automatisms such as pelvic or truncal thrusting usually occur in frontal lobe seizures.

So, in summary, although various types of automatisms may have a useful localizing value, it is mainly unilateral distal limb automatisms with contralateral dystonia that is useful as a lateralizing sign.

Postictal Nose Wiping

Nosewiping or rubbing that occurs within 60 seconds of the seizure end has good localizing and lateralizing value: it occurs in 50% to 85% of TLE patients, but in only 10% to 33% of extratemporal epilepsy patients. It is performed with the hand ipsilateral to the epileptogenic focus in 75% to 90% of the cases when seen in the context of a temporal lobe automotor seizure, but has no lateralizing value when seen with an extratemporal seizure. Postulated mechanisms leading to its occurrence include ictal activation of the amygdala with subsequent olfactory hallucinations or increased nasal secretions, and postictal contralateral hand movement abnormalities or neglect (44,55).

ELECTROENCEPHALOGRAPHIC FINDINGS

Interictal Electroencephalography

Most complex partial seizures with automatisms arise from the anterior temporal regions of one side or the other. Temporal intermittent rhythmic delta activity (TIRDA) is found in up to 28% of patients evaluated for temporal lobe

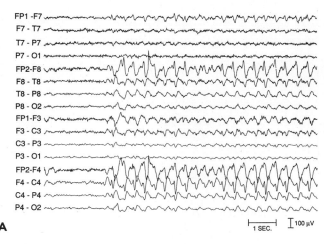

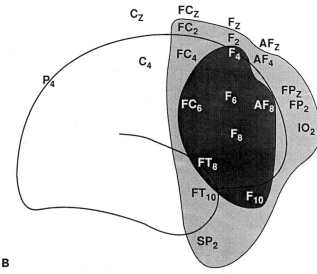

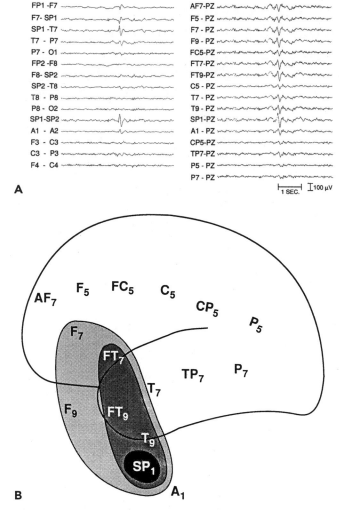

FIGURE 12.1 Left mesial temporal lobe. Interictal sharp wave focus (**left**). A and B: Distribution of the field of an interictal spike from a patient with temporal lobe epilepsy. The spike amplitude is maximal at SP_1 (measured on referential recordings), greater than 90% at T_9, FT_9, and FT_7 electrodes, and greater than 70% at F_7 and F_9.

FIGURE 12.2 Run of focal spike-and-wave discharge in right frontal lobe with no clinical signs (**left**) and right frontal lobe, interictal spikes (**right**). A and B: Distribution of the field of interictal spikes occurring in runs from a patient with frontal lobe complex partial seizures. The field is widespread, involving most of the right frontal convexity.

epilepsy as opposed to only 0.3% of the general population, and is therefore felt to be significantly predictive of TLE. Bitemporal sharp-wave foci are noted in 25% to 33% of patients and may be independent or synchronous. Mesial temporal spikes may not be well seen at the surface, and intermittent rhythmic slowing may be the only clue to deep-seated spikes (57). On a single routine EEG recording, 30% to 40% of patients may have normal interictal findings; activating techniques can reduce this to approximately 10% (58).

At the scalp, the field of mesial temporal spikes is often maximal at the anterior temporal electrodes (T_1 or T_2, FT_9 or FT_{10}). When nasopharyngeal or sphenoidal electrodes are used (especially in prolonged monitoring), the amplitude of the spike is usually maximal at these electrodes, consistent with their origin in the amygdalar–hippocampal region (Fig. 12.1).

Less frequently, sharp-wave foci are seen in the midtemporal or posterior temporal region. Interictal foci may be mapped according to amplitude, and the relative frequency of various sharp-wave foci may be taken into account during

monitoring of epilepsy surgery candidates. A fair degree of correlation is present between the predominant spike focus and side of ictal onset (63% in Wieser and coworkers' series of 133 patients (59)). Hyperventilation may activate focal temporal slowing or spikes and may provoke a clinical seizure.

In 10% to 30% of patients with complex partial seizures, an extratemporal focus is seen, usually in the frontal lobes (Fig. 12.2). In some patients with mesial frontal foci, the interictal discharge may take the form of a bifrontal spike-and-wave discharge.

Care should be taken to exclude nonepileptiform sharp transients such as benign epileptiform transients of sleep or small sharp spikes, wicket spikes, complex partial variant, and 14- and 6-Hz spikes. Evidence suggests that when benign epileptiform transients of sleep occur in epileptic individuals, they do so frequently and in runs (60). Transients resembling benign epileptiform transients of sleep sometimes are found to be maximal at the sphenoidal electrode; such discharges should be interpreted cautiously.

Ictal Electroencephalography

Although interictal EEGs may show normal findings in some patients with complex partial seizures, ictal changes are seen in 95% of patients (except during isolated auras) (61). In frontal lobe seizures from the mesial frontal or orbitofrontal cortex, ictal and interictal activities may not be reflected at the surface or are often masked by electromyographic and movement artifacts (Fig. 12.3).

An electrodecremental pattern is seen at the onset of a complex partial seizure in about two thirds of patients. It is usually quite diffuse (perhaps owing to an associated arousal); if focal or accompanied by low-voltage fast activity, it has lateralizing significance. The low-voltage fast activity, best seen with depth electrodes, may appear only as flattening at the surface. Alternatively, diffuse bitemporal slowing, higher on one side, may occur (61,62).

Approximately 50% to 70% of patients with temporal lobe epilepsy exhibit a so-called prototype pattern (62) consisting of a 5- to 7-Hz rhythmic θ discharge in the temporal regions, maximum at the sphenoidal electrode (Fig. 12.4). This pattern may appear as the first visible EEG change or follow diffuse or lateralized slowing in the δ range (often within 30 seconds of clinical onset). Depth electrode studies have shown this pattern to have 80% accuracy in localizing the onset to the ipsilateral mesial temporal structures (63). Postictal slowing is also helpful in lateralization. In patients with unitemporal interictal spikes, the lateralizing value of the ictal data was excellent (61). Seizure rhythms at ictal onset confined to the sphenoidal electrode are often seen in patients

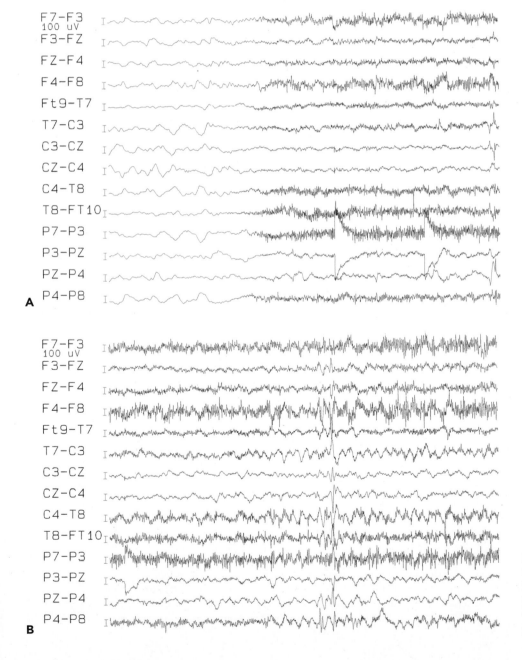

FIGURE 12.3 A and B: Ictal onset of a frontal lobe complex partial seizure arising out of sleep, beginning with low-amplitude fast rhythms, followed by rhythmic slowing near the vertex. The electroencephalographic seizure pattern cannot be lateralized.

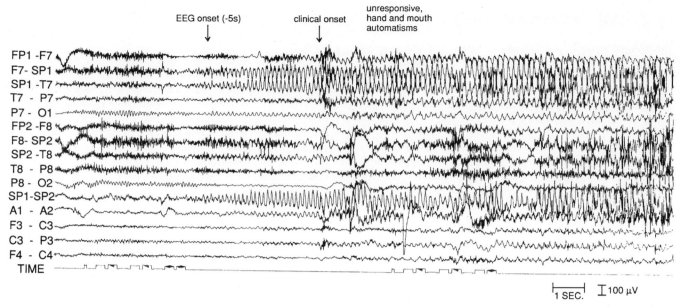

FIGURE 12.4 Ictal onset of a complex partial seizure (same patient as in Fig. 12.1). A brief electrodecremental response in the left temporal region is followed by the buildup of a rhythmic 5- and 6-Hz theta pattern, maximal at the left sphenoidal electrode. The electroencephalographic changes preceded the clinical onset by 5 seconds.

with mesial temporal lobe epilepsy as opposed to those with non–temporal lobe epilepsy. Use of coronal transverse montages incorporating the sphenoidal electrodes may permit earlier identification of seizure onset (61).

Although previous reports described false lateralization on the basis of scalp EEG, subsequent systematic studies have shown this to be infrequent except in the presence of a structural lesion that may mask or attenuate the amplitude of the ictal discharge on that side (61). Although lateralization from scalp EEG is usually satisfactory, localization within a lobe is sometimes incorrect, because seizures from an extratemporal site may spread to the temporal lobe and produce similar EEG patterns. The ictal discharge may then propagate to the rest of the hemisphere, or it may propagate bilaterally. Spread to the opposite temporal lobe is common. With some frontal lobe seizures, scalp ictal changes are difficult to appreciate because of electromyographic and movement artifacts. Occasionally, a generalized spike-and-wave discharge with a mesial frontal focus is seen (61).

PATHOPHYSIOLOGY OF IMPAIRED CONSCIOUSNESS IN FOCAL SEIZURES

Gloor believed in 1986 that while a "satisfactory explanation of consciousness . . . may never be possible . . . there are, however, aspects of conscious experience such as perception, cognition, memory, affect, and voluntary motility that are open to neurobiological research" (3). Since that time, and because of multiple "neurobiological research" attempts, significant advances have been made in the understanding of altered consciousness in the setting of focal seizures, and various mechanisms have been proposed.

Epileptic Activation of Subcortical Structures, Mainly the Thalamus and Upper Brainstem

Close connections exist between the prefrontal cortex and the nonspecific thalamic nucleus and the midline region of the intralaminar thalamic complex. Since epileptiform discharges arising from various regions within the frontal lobe—including the intermediate frontal region, orbitofrontal region, and cingulate gyrus—may elicit dialeptic seizures, and generalized discharges can be seen with epileptic activation of the mesial frontal lobe (secondary bilateral synchrony), it has been proposed that rapid epileptic spread from all of those frontal regions to the reticular formation is actually responsible for the impaired consciousness observed in FLE (1).

In TLE, a similar mechanism with additional spread to the upper brainstem structures has been suggested based on ictal SPECT perfusion studies (64).

Epileptic Activation of the Limbic System

Invasive EEG recordings have shown that ictal discharges in the mesial temporal lobes may be associated with the dialeptic symptomatology (1). In a recent study of 134 patients with complex partial seizures, Heo et al. found that interictal epileptiform discharges (IEDs) localized primarily to the temporal region and were more frequently detected in patients who were unaware of their seizures (94%) than in those who were aware (55%). Bilateral independent IEDs were found more frequently in the unawareness group than in the awareness group (48% vs. 13%). The bilateral presence of lesions was also more frequent in the unawareness group than the awareness group (16.1% vs. 4.9%). The authors conclude that complete loss of consciousness was caused by rapid spread of ictal discharges to the contralateral hemisphere in association with bilateral independent IEDs and bilateral presence of lesions (65).

Epileptic Disturbance of the Normal Balance between Excitation and Inhibition of Various Cortical/Subcortical Networks

Some authors suggest that arrest of activity during a seizure may either be the result of interference with the normal activity of the primary motor cortex, or epileptic activation of the negative motor areas during frontal lobe involvement, or both (1). Abnormal increased activity in frontoparietal association cortex and related subcortical structures is associated with loss of consciousness in generalized seizures. Abnormal decreased activity in these same networks may cause loss of consciousness in complex partial seizures. Thus, abnormally increased or decreased activity in the same networks can cause loss of consciousness. Information flow during normal conscious processing may require a dynamic balance between these two extremes of excitation and inhibition (66).

References

1. Noachtar S. Dialeptic seizures: localizing and lateralizing value. In: Lüders HO, ed. *Textbook of Epilepsy Surgery.* United Kingdom: Informa Healthcare; 2008:479–487.
2. Ebner A, Dinner DS, Noachtar S, et al. Automatisms with preserved responsiveness: a lateralizing sign in psychomotor seizures. *Neurology.* 1995;45(1):61–64.
3. Gloor P. Consciousness as a neurological concept in epileptology: a critical review. *Epilepsia.* 1986;27(suppl 2):S14–S26.
4. Cavanna AE, Mula M, Servo S, et al. Measuring the level and content of consciousness during epileptic seizures: the Ictal Consciousness Inventory. *Epilepsy Behav.* 2008;13(1):184–188.
5. Johanson M, Valli K, Revonsuo A, et al. Alterations in the contents of consciousness in partial epileptic seizures. *Epilepsy Behav.* 2008;13(2):366–371.
6. Lüders HO. *Textbook of Epilepsy Surgery.* United Kingdom: Informa Healthcare; 2008.
7. Temkin O. *The Falling Sickness: A History of Epilepsy from the Greeks to the beginning of Modern Neurology.* Baltimore, MD: Johns Hopkins; 1971.
8. Gibbs FA, Gibbs EL, Lennox WG. Epilepsy: a paroxysmal cerebral dysrhythmia. *Epilepsy Behav.* 2002;3(4):395–401.
9. Penfield W, Kristiansen K. *Epileptic Seizure Pattern.* Springfield, IL: Charles C. Thomas; 1951.
10. Penfield W, Jasper H. *Epilepsy and the Functional Anatomy of the Human Brain.* Boston: Little, Brown and Company; 1954.
11. Tudor M, Tudor L, Tudor KI. Hans Berger (1873–1941)—the history of electroencephalography. *Acta Med Croatica.* 2005;59(4):307–313.
12. Daly D. Uncinate fits. *Neurology.* 1958;8(4):250–260.
13. Feindel W, Penfield W. Localization of discharge in temporal lobe automatism. *AMA Arch Neurol Psychiatry.* 1954;72(5):603–630.
14. Ajmone Marsan C, Stoll Jr J. Subcortical connections of the temporal pole in relation to temporal lobe seizures. *AMA Arch Neurol Psychiatry.* 1951;66(6):669–686.
15. Ludwig BI, Marsan CA. Clinical ictal patterns in epileptic patients with occipital electroencephalographic foci. *Neurology.* 1975;25(5):463–471.
16. Geier S, Bancaud J, Talairach J, et al. Automatisms during frontal lobe epileptic seizures. *Brain.* 1976;99(3):447–458.
17. Tharp BR. Orbital frontal seizures. A unique electroencephalographic and clinical syndrome. *Epilepsia.* 1972;13(5):627–642.
18. Ajmone-Marsan J, Ralston B. *The Epileptic Seizure. Its Functional Morphology and Diagnostic Significance.* Springfield, IL: Charles C. Thomas; 1957.
19. Bancaud J. Clinical symptomatology of epileptic seizures of temporal origin. *Rev Neurol.* (Paris) 1987;143(5):392–400.
20. Bancaud J, Talairach J. Clinical semiology of frontal lobe seizures. *Adv Neurol.* 1992;57:3–58.
21. Delgado-Escueta AV, Walsh GO. Type I complex partial seizures of hippocampal origin: excellent results of anterior temporal lobectomy. *Neurology.* 1985;35(2):143–154.
22. Escueta AV, Bacsal FE, Treiman DM. Complex partial seizures on closed-circuit television and EEG: a study of 691 attacks in 79 patients. *Ann Neurol.* 1982;11(3):292–300.
23. Escueta AV, Kunze U, Waddell G, et al. Lapse of consciousness and automatisms in temporal lobe epilepsy: a videotape analysis. *Neurology.* 1977;27(2):144–155.
24. Quesney LF, Constain M, Fish DR, et al. The clinical differentiation of seizures arising in the parasagittal and anterolaterodorsal frontal convexities. *Arch Neurol.* 1990;47(6):677–679.
25. Merlis JK. Proposal for an international classification of the epilepsies. *Epilepsia.* 1970;11(1):114–119.
26. Wieser HG. *Electroclinical Features of the Psychomotor Seizure.* London: Butterworths; 1983.
27. Maldonado HM, Delgado-Escueta AV, Walsh GO, et al. Complex partial seizures of hippocampal and amygdalar origin. *Epilepsia.* 1988;29(4):420–433.
28. Kotagal P, Luders HO, Williams G, et al. Psychomotor seizures of temporal lobe onset: analysis of symptom clusters and sequences. *Epilepsy Res.* 1995;20(1):49–67.
29. Kotagal P, Arunkumar G, hammel J, et al. Complex partial seizures of frontal lobe onset statistical analysis of ictal semiology. *Seizure.* 2003;12(5):268–281.
30. Salanova V, Morris HH, Van Ness P, et al. Frontal lobe seizures: electroclinical syndromes. *Epilepsia.* 1995;36(1):16–24.
31. Kellinghaus C, Luders HO. Frontal lobe epilepsy. *Epileptic Disord.* 2004;6(4):223–239.
32. Walsh GO, Delgado-Escueta AV. Type II complex partial seizures: poor results of anterior temporal lobectomy. *Neurology.* 1984;34(1):1–13.
33. Lux S, Kurthen M, Helmstaedter C, et al. The localizing value of ictal consciousness and its constituent functions: a video-EEG study in patients with focal epilepsy. *Brain.* 2002;125(Pt 12):2691–2698.
34. Inoue Y, Mihara T. Awareness and responsiveness during partial seizures. *Epilepsia.* 1998;39(suppl 5):7–10.
35. Jobst BC, Siegel AM, Thadani VM, et al. Intractable seizures of frontal lobe origin: clinical characteristics, localizing signs, and results of surgery. *Epilepsia.* 2000;41(9):1139–1152.
36. Acharya JN, Wyllie E, Luders HO, et al. Seizure symptomatology in infants with localization-related epilepsy. *Neurology.* 1997;48(1):189–196.
37. Wyllie E. Developmental aspects of seizure semiology: problems in identifying localized-onset seizures in infants and children. *Epilepsia.* 1995;36(12):1170–1172.
38. Kallen K, Wyllie E, Luders HO, et al. Hypomotor seizures in infants and children. *Epilepsia.* 2002;43(8):882–888.
39. Kim DW, Lee SK, Yun CH, et al. Parietal lobe epilepsy: the semiology, yield of diagnostic workup, and surgical outcome. *Epilepsia.* 2004;45(6):641–649.
40. Williamson PD, Thadani VM, Darcey TM, et al. Occipital lobe epilepsy: clinical characteristics, seizure spread patterns, and results of surgery. *Ann Neurol.* 1992;31(1):3–13.
41. Aykut-Bingol C, Spencer SS. Nontumoral occipitotemporal epilepsy: localizing findings and surgical outcome. *Ann Neurol.* 1999;46(6):894–900.
42. Blume WT, Wiebe S, Tapsell LM. Occipital epilepsy: lateral versus mesial. *Brain.* 2005;128(Pt 5):1209–1225.
43. Salanova V, Andermann F, Olivier A, et al. Occipital lobe epilepsy: electroclinical manifestations, electrocorticography, cortical stimulation and outcome in 42 patients treated between 1930 and 1991. Surgery of occipital lobe epilepsy. *Brain.* 1992;115(Pt 6):1655–1680.
44. Bianchin MM, Sakamoto AC. Complex motor seizures: localizing and lateralizing value. In: Lüders HO, ed. *Textbook of Epilepsy Surgery.* United Kingdom: Informa Healthcare; 2008:462–478.
45. Kotagal P, Luders H, Morris HH, et al. Dystonic posturing in complex partial seizures of temporal lobe onset: a new lateralizing sign. *Neurology.* 1989;39(2 Pt 1):196–201.
46. Bleasel A, Kotagal P, Kankirawatana P, et al. Lateralizing value and semiology of ictal limb posturing and version in temporal lobe and extratemporal epilepsy. *Epilepsia.* 1997;38(2):168–174.
47. Rusu V, Chassoux F, Landre E, et al. Dystonic posturing in seizures of mesial temporal origin: electroclinical and metabolic patterns. *Neurology.* 2005;65(10):1612–1619.
48. Wyllie E, Luders H, Morris HH, et al. Ipsilateral forced head and eye turning at the end of the generalized tonic–clonic phase of versive seizures. *Neurology.* 1986;36(9):1212–1217.
49. Dobesberger J, Walser G, Embacher N, et al. Gyratory seizures revisited: a video-EEG study. *Neurology.* 2005;64(11):1884–1887.
50. Kellinghaus C, Kotagal P. Lateralizing value of Todd's palsy in patients with epilepsy. *Neurology.* 2004;62(2):289–291.
51. Gastaut H, Broughton R. *Epileptic Seizures: Clinical and Electrographic Features, Diagnosis and Treatment.* Springfield, IL: Charles C. Thomas; 1972.
52. Doherty MJ, Wilensky AJ, Holmes MD, et al. Singing seizures. *Neurology.* 2002;59(9):1435–1438.

53. Marks Jr WJ, Laxer KD. Semiology of temporal lobe seizures: value in lateralizing the seizure focus. *Epilepsia*. 1998;39(7):721–726.

54. Benbadis SR, Kotagal P, Klem GH. Unilateral blinking: a lateralizing sign in partial seizures. *Neurology*. 1996;46(1):45–48.

55. Geyer JD, Payne TA, Faught E, et al. Postictal nose-rubbing in the diagnosis, lateralization, and localization of seizures. *Neurology*. 1999;52(4): 743–745.

56. Leutmezer F, Serles W, Bacher J, et al. Genital automatisms in complex partial seizures. *Neurology*. 1999;52(6):1188–1191.

57. Marks DA, Katz A, Booke J, et al. Comparison and correlation of surface and sphenoidal electrodes with simultaneous intracranial recording: an interictal study. *Electroencephalogr Clin Neurophysiol*. 1992;82(1):23–29.

58. Dinner DS, Luders H, Rothner AD, et al. Complex partial seizures of childhood onset: a clinical and encephalographic study. *Cleve Clin Q*. 1984; 51(2):287–291.

59. Wieser HG, Bancaud J, Talairach J, et al. Comparative value of spontaneous and chemically and electrically induced seizures in establishing the lateralization of temporal lobe seizures. *Epilepsia*. 1979;20(1):47–59.

60. Molaie M, Santana HB, Otero C, et al. Effect of epilepsy and sleep deprivation on the rate of benign epileptiform transients of sleep. *Epilepsia*. 1991;32(1):44–50.

61. Foldvary-Schaeffer N. Non-invasive electroencephalography in the evaluation of the ictal onset zone. In: Lüders HO, ed. *Textbook of Epilepsy Surgery*. United Kingdom: Informa Healthcare; 2008:603–613.

62. Blume WT, Young GB, Lemieux JF. EEG morphology of partial epileptic seizures. *Electroencephalogr Clin Neurophysiol*. 1984;57(4):295–302.

63. Risinger MW, Engel Jr J, Van Ness PC, et al. Ictal localization of temporal lobe seizures with scalp/sphenoidal recordings. *Neurology*. 1989;39(10): 1288–1293.

64. Lee KH, Meador KJ, Park YD, et al. Pathophysiology of altered consciousness during seizures: subtraction SPECT study. *Neurology*. 2002;59(6): 841–846.

65. Heo K, Han SD, Lim SR, et al. Patient awareness of complex partial seizures. *Epilepsia*. 2006;47(11):1931–1935.

66. Blumenfeld H, Taylor J. Why do seizures cause loss of consciousness? *Neuroscientist*. 2003;9(5):301–310.

CHAPTER 13 ■ FOCAL MOTOR SEIZURES, EPILEPSIA PARTIALIS CONTINUA, AND SUPPLEMENTARY SENSORIMOTOR SEIZURES

ANDREAS V. ALEXOPOULOS AND STEPHEN E. JONES

In memoriam: Dudley S. Dinner, MD (1947–2007)
"One who is the giver of knowledge is the giver of life"

HISTORY

Focal motor seizures have been recognized since the time of Hippocrates, who first observed seizures affecting the body contralateral to the side of head injury (1). Hughlings Jackson was the first to theorize that focal seizures are caused by "*a sudden and excessive discharge of gray matter in some part of the brain*" and that the clinical manifestations of the seizure depend on the "*seat of the discharging lesion*" (2,3).

During the second half of the 19th century, Fritsch and Hitzig pioneered stimulation of the brain in animals (4). They discovered that electrical stimulation of the exposed cerebral cortex produced contralateral motor responses in dogs (5,6). Experimental faradic stimulation of the human cerebral cortex was first performed by Bartholow in 1874 (7). In 1909, Cushing reported that faradic stimulation of the postcentral gyrus could be used to determine the anatomic relationship of the sensory strip to an adjacent tumor (8). Motor responses elicited by electrical stimulation in humans were first described by Krause in the beginning of the 20th century (9), and by Foerster more than 70 years ago (2). These early observations led to the fundamental work of Penfield and Brodley, who used electrical stimulation to elucidate the motor and sensory representation of the human cerebral cortex and pioneered the techniques for the functional localization of the sensorimotor cortex during surgery (10).

FUNCTIONAL ANATOMY OF THE MOTOR CORTEX

Strictly speaking, the motor cortex (Fig. 13.1) consists of three motor areas: the primary motor area (PMA or M1) in the precentral gyrus, which houses a complete representation of body movements; the supplementary sensorimotor area (SSMA or SMA) on the mesial surface rostral to the PMA, also containing a complete motor representation (hence the term *supplementary*); and a more loosely defined premotor cortex (PreMC) on the lateral convexity (11).

The prefrontal and orbitofrontal cortices, as well as the dorsolateral and mesial frontal cortices anterior to the SSMA, are not considered part of the motor cortex. The term *prefrontal cortex* is used to define the extensive part of the frontal lobe

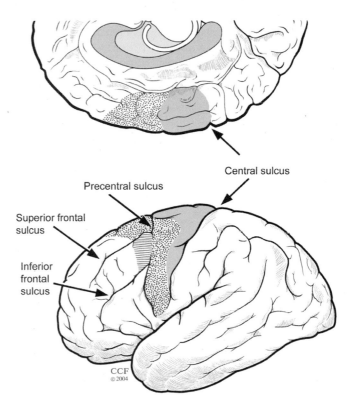

FIGURE 13.1 Mesial and lateral aspects of the left hemisphere: schematic representation of the three motor areas and their approximate relationship to the surface hemispheric anatomy. The *shaded area* corresponds to the primary motor cortex (Brodmann area 4). The *stippled area* illustrates the supplementary sensorimotor cortex on the mesial aspect. On the lateral view, the *stippled area* represents the premotor cortex. Also note the approximate location of the frontal eye field (*hatched area*).

that lies anterior to the motor and premotor zones (12). Modern anatomic and physiologic studies in humans and primates challenge the traditional division of motor areas (13). For example, part of the cingulate cortex, which was previously linked to the limbic system, is now considered as a fourth main motor area, the so-called cingulate motor area (CMA) (14,15).

Activation studies using positron emission tomography (PET) or functional magnetic resonance imaging (fMRI) allude to the complex organization of the motor system. The breadth of cortical and subcortical areas activated with even the simplest movements attests to the wide distribution and extent of interconnected neural networks underlying motor control (14). Observed movements presuppose a series of parallel or sequential processes involving the selection, planning, preparation, and initiation of action (14,16).

Efferent and Afferent Connections

The familiar hierarchical model of motor control is based on the four levels of spinal cord, brainstem, PMA, and PreMC SSMA. This concept has influenced our understanding of the various motor manifestations of seizures (17). Motor commands are organized hierarchically from the most automatic (e.g., deep tendon reflexes) to the least (e.g., skilled and precise voluntary movements). Each level of motor control retains a somatotopic organization and receives peripheral sensory information that is used to modify the motor output at that level (18). The cerebral cortex exerts its motor control by way of the corticospinal and corticobulbar pathways. The cortex also modulates the action of motor neurons in the brainstem and spinal cord indirectly through its influence on the brain's various descending systems.

To this day, limited direct information exists about specific neuronal connections between functional brain regions of the human cortex (19). Our knowledge of detailed connectivities is derived from invasive tracer studies in primates. Recent imaging advances are now permitting noninvasive studies of neuronal connections in humans, using the techniques of diffusion tensor imaging (DTI) and functional connectivity MRI (fcMRI)—the latter technique aims to identify highly correlative BOLD signal changes present in different regions of the cortex during the resting state or during specific tasks (20). Importantly, cortical regions identified by fcMRI may reside at a considerable distance from each other.

Brainstem Motor Efferents

The brainstem gives rise to several descending motor pathways, which are divided into ventromedial and dorsolateral groups (21,22). The ventromedial system sends fibers through the ventral columns of the spinal cord and terminates predominantly in the medial part of the ventral horn, which contains the motor nuclei controlling proximal limb and axial muscle groups. In contrast, the dorsolateral system descends in the lateral part of the spinal cord and terminates on the lateral motor cell complex, which innervates more distal limb muscles (23). Thus, *the dorsolateral motor system places its emphasis on muscles devoted to fine motor control.*

Motor Cortex Efferents

The *axons that project from layer V of the cortex* to the spinal cord run together in the corticospinal tract (a massive bundle of fibers containing approximately 1 million axons). About one-third of corticospinal and corticobulbar fibers arise from the PMA. Another third originate from the SSMA and PreMC, and the rest have their origin in the parietal lobe (arising mainly from the somatosensory cortex of the postcentral gyrus) (24). The *corticospinal fibers together with the corticobulbar fibers run through the posterior limb of the internal capsule* to reach the ventral portion of the brainstem and send collaterals to the striatum, thalamus, red nucleus, and other brainstem nuclei (25). Many of these relationships can now be visualized noninvasively using combined fMRI and DTI techniques (Fig. 13.2). In the brainstem, *the corticobulbar fibers terminate bilaterally in cranial nerve motor*

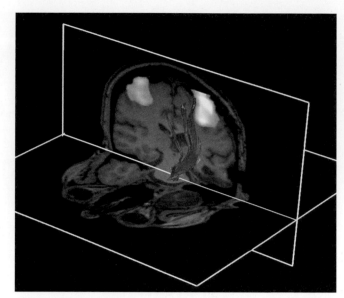

FIGURE 13.2 Combination of DTI, fMRI, and anatomic imaging demonstrating relationship of the left corticospinal tract to the motor regions using a finger-tapping paradigm. The fMRI and anatomic images are displayed as cut-planes, with 3D superimposition of a surface representation of DTI tracks. A seed region for deterministic tracking is placed in the central pons—from this structure the tracks ascend superiorly through the internal capsule, and corona radiata to terminate in peri-central cortex. Note the expected close approximation of central tracks to the hand area.

nuclei (either directly via a monosynaptic route or indirectly), with the exception of motor neurons innervating the lower face, which receive mostly contralateral corticobulbar input. About *three-fourths of the corticospinal fibers cross the midline* in the pyramidal decussation at the junction of the medulla and spinal cord and descend in the spinal cord as the lateral corticospinal tract (19). Uncrossed fibers descend as the ventral corticospinal tract. The lateral and ventral divisions of the corticospinal tract terminate in approximately the same regions of spinal gray matter along with corresponding brainstem-originating pathways. *The majority of corticospinal tract terminals project on spinal interneurons.* An estimated 5% of the fibers synapse directly on (both alpha and gamma) motor neurons (26).

These anatomic arrangements of descending tracts underlie the contralateral and/or bilateral motor manifestations of focal seizures arising from the motor cortex (17).

Motor Cortex Afferents

The major cortical inputs to the motor areas of cortex are from the prefrontal and parietal association areas (18). These are focused mainly on the PreMC and the SSMA, whereas the PMA receives a large input from the primary somatosensory cortex (27). In addition, the PMA receives direct and indirect inputs from the PreMC and the SSMA. In particular, *the SSMA projects bilaterally to the primary motor cortex in a somatotopically organized manner.* Other corticocortical inputs arrive from the opposite hemisphere through the corpus callosum (Fig. 13.3), which interconnects heterotopic as well as homologous areas of the two hemispheres (28,29). The major subcortical input to the motor cortical areas comes from the thalamus, where separate nuclei convey modulating inputs from the basal ganglia and the cerebellum (27).

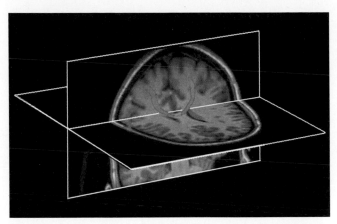

FIGURE 13.3 Example of corticocortical connectivity using probabilistic tractography from high-resolution DTI images. One seed region is placed in one motor area and the target region is placed in the contralateral motor area. Computed tracts course across the corpus callosum as expected. The tracts are displayed as a red 3D overlay on black and white anatomic cut-planes.

Stimulation Studies

In clinical practice, insights into the functional anatomy of the motor cortex and other eloquent brain cortical areas are afforded by direct cortical stimulation. At the same time, electrical stimulation of the human cortex provides an experimental model that can be used to reproduce the effects of cortical activation after an ictal discharge (30). Several groups use cortical stimulation to trigger habitual auras and/or seizures in an attempt to better delineate the ictal onset zone before epilepsy surgery.

In general, the observed clinical response is assumed to arise from cortex below the stimulated electrode or from the region between two closely spaced electrodes, given that the current density drops off rapidly with increasing distance from the tissue underlying the stimulated electrode (31,32). Electrical stimulation can elicit "positive" responses (such as localized movements resulting from activation of the PMA or SSMA cortex) or "negative" responses (such as inhibition of motor activity). The latter becomes apparent only if the patient engages in specific tasks during stimulation. In areas such as the supplementary motor cortex, both positive responses in the form of bilateral motor movements and negative responses such as speech arrest can be demonstrated. The area of stimulation gives rise to distinctive patterns of motor activation of the PMA, SSMA, or premotor regions. Overlapping clinical manifestations are commonly observed as a result of the highly developed interconnectivity between these regions (33).

Negative motor responses interfere with a person's ability to perform a voluntary movement or sustain a voluntary contraction when cortical stimulation is applied (34). *The patient is unaware of the effects of stimulation unless asked to perform the specific function* integrated by the stimulated cortical region. In a systematic review of 42 patients who had subdural electrodes over the perirolandic area, the Cleveland Clinic group observed *negative motor responses over both hemispheres,* when stimulating the agranular cortex immediately in front of the primary and supplementary face areas (34). To distinguish the two negative motor areas, investigators proposed the terms *primary negative motor area* (PNMA,

in regard to the region of the inferior frontal gyrus immediately in front of the face PMA) and *supplementary negative motor area* (SNMA, in reference to the mesial portion of the superior frontal gyrus immediately in front of the face SSMA). Other investigators have been able to confirm and extend these observations using similar techniques of direct cortical stimulation with subdural electrodes, and have concluded that negative motor areas are in fact widely distributed throughout the perirolandic region and within the PreMC (35). These areas are considered a part of the cortical inhibitory motor system, the epileptic activation of which may give rise to *focal inhibitory motor seizures* (also referred to by some authors as "*akinetic*" seizures). Such seizures can be easily overlooked because patients may remain unaware of their weakness and/or inability to execute specific movements, unless they are carefully examined.

The effects of functional localization and effects of electrical stimulation in the three broad motor areas are briefly discussed below:

Primary Motor Area

The PMA resides in the anterior wall of the central sulcus (see Fig. 13.1) and corresponds to Brodmann's area 4. On the basis of cytoarchitectonic criteria, area 4 is recognized primarily by the presence of Betz cells (giant pyramidal cells) in cortical layer V and the absence of a granular layer IV (36). The central sulcus marks the border between the agranular motor cortex and the granular somatosensory cortex (37).

Radiographically, the central sulcus appears as a prominent, almost always continuous, sulcus, which extends from the mesial aspect (near the brain's apex) along an oblique coronal trajectory towards (and near to) the sylvian fissure. The superior and inferior aspects of the central sulcus are terminated by the paracentral lobule and subcentral gyrus, respectively, which effectively appear as a joining of the pre- and postcentral gyri. *The radiographic identification of the central sulcus is often critical to interpretation of imaging studies and planning surgical procedures,* as it provides a central landmark from which other topology can be located. There are several characteristic features identifying the central sulcus, three of which are shown in the cartoon of Figure 13.4 and on the T1-weighted MRI images of Figure 13.5. Most easily identified is the so-called "hand knob," which assumes the form of an upside-down omega ("Ω") *on axial images* (38). Formed by a relative gyral hypertrophy corresponding to the PMA of the hand, the "hand knob" appears to project posteriorly from the precentral gyrus into the contour of the central sulcus. Due to anatomic variation, this feature sometimes assumes the shape of a horizontal epsilon ("ε"), rather than the inverted omega (38). Another confirmatory feature of the "hand knob" *on the sagittal plane* is that it appears as if forming a backwards "hook" (see Fig. 13.5), but this appearance is less reliable than the characteristic axial morphology. A second helpful landmark is the topology of the superior central gyrus, which is easily seen running along an anterior–posterior direction along the medial frontal lobe, and whose posterior margin is the precentral gyrus. Identification of the precentral gyrus is further aided by demarcation of the pre- and postcentral sulci. Lastly, axial images nicely portray *the pars marginalis,* which is the

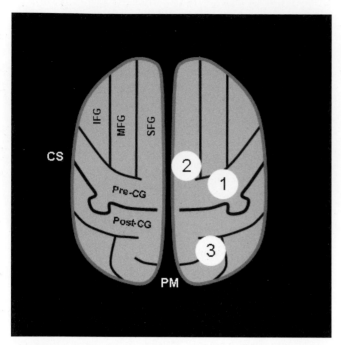

FIGURE 13.4 Key features for identifying the sensorimotor cortex. The essential step is identification of the central sulcus (CS), which separates the precentral gyrus anteriorly (motor cortex) from the postcentral gyrus posteriorly (sensory cortex). This schematic of an axial section illustrates three classic features that aid in the identification of the CS. (1) the "hand knob" is a posterior protuberance of the precentral gyrus, which corresponds to relative "hypertrophy" of the primary hand motor area. The shape of the sulcus in this area is often described as that of an upside-down omega ("Ω"). (2) The anterior–posterior orientation of the superior frontal gyrus is often easily identified, as it aligns along a paramedian plane. While the anterior margin of the SFG extends to the frontal poles, the posterior margin merges with the precentral gyrus, such that the most posterior margin often appears as the central sulcus. (3) Posterior to the medial aspect of the central sulcus is the pars marginalis, which often has a slight concavity—when pairing together the left and right pars marginalis assume the characteristic appearance that resembles a "smile" or "bracket," which can be seen on multiple axial sections, making identification easy. IFG, inferior frontal gyrus; MFG, middle frontal gyrus; SFG, superior frontal gyrus; Pre-CS, precentral gyrus; post-CD, postcentral gyrus; CS, central sulcus; PM, pars marginalis.

ascending ramus arising from the posterior cingulate sulcus. The left and right ascending rami appear on axial images as bilaterally paired paramedian features that together form the shape of a "bracket" or "smile" (39). This characteristic appearance is often preserved over multiple axial slices and can be used to identify the central sulcus, and differentiate it from the adjacent postcentral sulcus.

The somatotopic organization of the PMA was elucidated by the pioneering work of Krause (9), Penfield, Jasper, and Rasmussen (40,41), and others (Fig. 13.6). In this region of the PMA, *simple movements were elicited with the lowest intensity of electrical stimulation* (42). The resulting motor maps show an orderly arrangement with the tongue and lips near the sylvian fissure and the thumb, digits, arm, and trunk represented successively along the central sulcus, ending with the leg, foot, and toes on the mesial surface. The somatotopic organization of the motor cortex is not fixed and can be altered during motor learning or after injury (43). The layout of the motor homunculus is topographically similar to that of

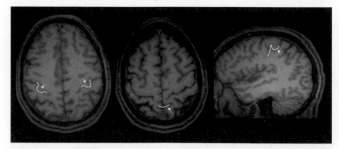

FIGURE 13.5 MRI examples of the landmark features described in Figure 13.4, which help locate the central sulcus. Shown as overlaid white line segments are the "omega" of the hand knob (left image) and the pars marginalis "smile" (middle image). The middle image also demonstrates the architecture of the superior frontal gyrus terminating posteriorly in the precentral gyrus. The right image displays the backwards "hook" as described in the text—this feature is appreciated on sagittal images passing through the hand knob.

the somatosensory homunculus, which resides immediately behind the PMA. Contemporary noninvasive methods, such as BOLD imaging fMRI, nicely confirm and recapitulate the classic homunculus (see Fig. 13.6). Output of the PMA is directed to the corticospinal and corticobulbar tracts, as well as to the SSMA and homologous areas in the opposite hemisphere via the corpus callosum (44).

Stimulation Studies

In the PMA, single stimuli typically elicit single clonic movements of the contralateral somatic muscles represented by the area of the motor homunculus being stimulated. High-frequency (50 to 60 Hz) stimulus series result in slower, tonic contralateral motor responses (45). Intraoperative application of electrical stimulation mapping under local or general anesthesia provides the most direct and easy way to localize the perirolandic cortex in most adults (46). When local anesthesia is used, motor responses are usually evoked with currents of 2 to 4 mA. Sensory responses are elicited with stimulation of the postcentral gyrus, often at slightly lower thresholds (47). *The threshold for eliciting a motor response in humans is lowest in the PMA.* Electrical cortical stimulation studies uncover the individual variability in the topographic organization of sensorimotor maps in humans with structurally normal anatomy (48). The importance of direct cortical stimulation studies in patients with lesions and/or epileptogenic foci encroaching on the sensorimotor cortex cannot be overemphasized (49).

Supplementary Sensorimotor Area

The SSMA is a distinct anatomic region located on the mesial surface of the superior frontal gyrus and its adjacent dorsal convexity (50). The cerebral cortex of the SSMA corresponds to the mesial portion of area 6 of Brodmann's cytoarchitectonic map of the brain (40,51) (see Fig. 13.1). Phylogenetically, the SSMA may be viewed as older motor cortex derived from the anterior cingulate periarchicortical limbic system (52). Similar to the primary motor cortex, the SSMA is referred to as agranular cortex, because the internal granular layer (layer IV) is not prominent. In contrast to area 4, area 6 does not contain Betz cells (51). The medial precentral sulcus defines the border between the PMA for the foot and the posterior limit of the

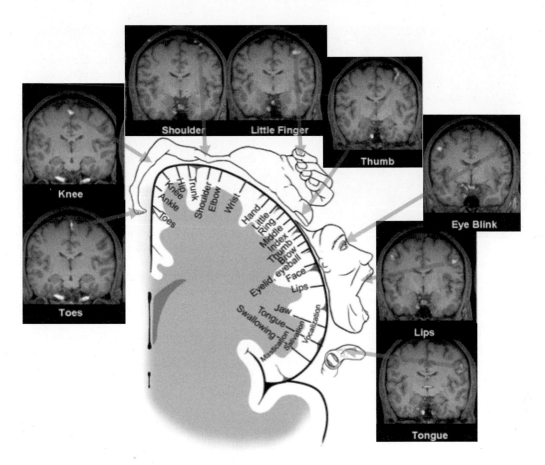

FIGURE 13.6 The motor homunculus after Penfield and Rasmussen depicting the somatotopic arrangement of the primary motor cortex (PMA) (with the tongue and lips near the sylvian fissure and the thumb, fingers, arm, and trunk represented successively along the precentral gyrus ending with the leg, foot, and toes on the mesial surface) occupies the center of this figure. Muscle groups involved in fine movements feature a disproportionately large representation. (Adapted from Penfield W, Rasmussen T. *The Cerebral Cortex of Man—A Clinical Study of Localization of Function.* New York: The MacMillan Company; 1950, with permission.) Surrounding this schematic representation of the motor homunculus are corresponding images of fMRI activation of the primary motor cortex obtained with eight different motor tasks—the fMRI images nicely recapitulate the classic—motor homunculus. Images are provided in coronal oblique reformatted planes that are roughly parallel to the motor strip. Significant activity is shown as color overlay. The toe, knee, shoulder, and finger tasks employed flexion/extension or tapping at a rate of about 2 per second, using the right-sided limb only. The eye blink, lip (pursing), and tongue (pressing against palate) tasks were bilateral motions performed at a similar rate. Right lower extremity movements are clearly localized along the left superior-medial cortical surfaces, with right upper extremity movements localized along left superior-lateral cortical surfaces. Note bilateral motions from eyes, lips, and tongue show corresponding bilateral activation.

SSMA (13,53). No clear cytoarchitectonic or anatomic boundary separates the SSMA from the adjacent PreMC (54).

The macaque and human mesial area 6 (SSMA) is further subdivided into pre-SSMA (rostrally) and SSMA proper (caudally) on the basis of comparable cytoarchitectonic and transmitter receptor studies (37). Studies in primates suggest that the pre-SSMA holds a hierarchically higher role in motor control. The functional properties of the SSMA subdivisions have not been detailed in humans (55). The border between the pre-SSMA and SSMA proper corresponds to the VAC line (i.e. the vertical line passing through the anterior commissure and perpendicular to the AC-PC line, which connects the anterior and posterior commissures) (Fig. 13.7). The border between SSMA proper and PMA corresponds approximately to the VPC line (i.e. the vertical line that traverses the posterior commissure and is perpendicular to the AC-PC line) (56).

Stimulation Studies

More than 70 years ago, Foerster was the first to describe motor responses in humans elicited by electrical stimulation of the mesial aspect of the superior frontal gyrus anterior to the primary motor representation of the lower extremity (2). Systematic study of this region with electrical stimulation was carried out at the Montreal Neurological Institute (MNI) during the intraoperative evaluation of patients with intractable focal epilepsy preceding surgical resection (57).

This was the first group to use the term *supplementary motor area* (SMA). Direct intraoperative electrical stimulation of the SMA produced vocalization, speech arrest, postural movements of all extremities, inhibition of voluntary movements, paresthesias, and autonomic changes. The rich repertoire of combined or postural movements included the so-called *"fencing posture,"* a term coined by the MNI group to

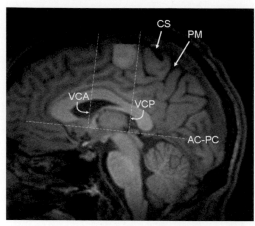

FIGURE 13.7 Functional MRI using a finger-tapping paradigm (paramedian sagittal plane) shows activation of the supplementary sensorimotor area (SSMA), which lies within the paracentral lobule, and is located anteriorly to medial margin of the central sulcus. In addition cerebellar activation is also present. Note the anatomical relationships of the SSMA to the AC-PC line, as described on page 167. The border between the pre-SSMA anteriorly and SSMA proper corresponds to the VAC line, and the border between SSMA proper and PMA posteriorly corresponds approximately to the VPC line. AC-PC refers to the line that connects the anterior and posterior commissures; VAC (or VCA as depicted above) refers to the vertical line passing through the anterior commissure and perpendicular to the AC-PC line; VPC (or VCP as depicted above) refers to the vertical line that traverses the posterior commissure and is perpendicular to the AC-PC line; CS, central sulcus; PM, pars marginalis.

describe the classical stimulation-induced postural response that consists of elevation of the contralateral arm with the head and eyes turned toward the raised hand (40). The Montreal studies demonstrated that both positive (such as bilateral motor movements) and negative responses (such as speech arrest) could be elicited by stimulating this region. The intra-operative study of the mesial interhemispheric surface carries significant limitations, because of the tedious and potentially dangerous surgical approach (in proximity to the superior sagittal sinus and its cerebral bridging veins), the restricted amount of time, and the relative difficulty in recognizing the specific gyral landmarks during surgery in this region.

With the advent of subdural electrodes, the Cleveland Clinic series of extraoperative stimulation studies showed that positive motor responses were not restricted to the mesial aspect of the superior frontal gyrus, but could also be elicited from its dorsal convexity, the lower half of the paracentral lobule, and the precuneus (58). The same group confirmed the presence of sensory symptoms that were elicited along with the positive motor responses after stimulation of the SMA and coined the term *supplementary sensorimotor area* (SSMA) instead of SMA.

Using depth electrodes, Talairach and Bancaud were the first to describe a somatotopic organization within the SSMA (59). The Yale group confirmed the presence of somatotopic distribution in the SSMA, where the face, upper extremity, and lower extremity responses are oriented in a rostrocaudal direction, with the lower extremities represented posteriorly, head and face most anteriorly, and the upper extremities between these two regions (60). Likewise, studies of movement-related potentials (MRPs) using subdural electrodes implanted over the SSMA region demonstrated that MRPs for different types of movements (finger, foot, tongue, vocalization, etc.) also have a somatotopic distribution within the SSMA, which is consistent with the

organization defined by electrical stimulation (61–63). Notably, fMRI studies using motor activation paradigms, such as finger tapping for example, demonstrate strong activations of the SSMA in addition to the primary motor cortex (see Fig. 13.7).

Premotor Cortex

Fulton coined the term *premotor cortex* (PreMC) in 1935 to describe the third major component of motor cortex (64). This area encompasses the more loosely defined agranular cortex of the lateral frontal convexity rostral to the PMA (11,22), which corresponds to the lateral portion of Brodmann's area 6 (see Fig. 13.1). It is difficult to define the anterior border of the agranular PreMC in humans, where a broad zone of progressive transition exists between area 6 and the granular cortex of Brodmann's frontal area 9 (65). In the macaque, the PreMC is further subdivided into a dorsal portion on the dorsolateral convexity and a ventral portion on the ventrolateral convexity (11). Despite the lack of direct correlation between microstructure and function in humans, the two subdivsions of the premotor area are considered to have homologous counterparts in the human brain. The motor and premotor cortices, as well as the frontal eye fields (FEFs) and the anterior cingulate cortex of area 24, have reciprocal connections with the SSMA (51). Anatomic labeling experiments in the macaque have demonstrated that the more anterior dorsal PreMC projects to the spinal cord, challenging the notion that the PreMC, unlike the PMA and SSMA, lacks prominent corticospinal connections (22,66,67).

According to the classic schema, the PreMC is responsible for the preparation and organization of movements (54). Several recent studies show that the PreMC also plays a central role in nonmotor attentional and receptive domains. Therefore, our current understanding suggests a dual PreMC function pertaining to motor and cognitive behaviors (68).

Stimulation Studies

On the basis of early electrical stimulation studies of the monkey brain (69), the agranular lateral PreMC (area 6) has been subdivided into a rostral section (6aβ or 6r) and a caudal section (6aα or 6c). Recent quantitative architectonic and neurotransmitter studies have corroborated the presence of similar topographic boundaries in the human brain (37,65). The rostral subdivision covers the anterior part of the precentral gyrus, and its caudal counterpart resides in the posterior part of the superior and middle frontal gyri, in front of the precentral sulcus (70).

Eye movements can be electrically induced from a large area of the human dorsolateral frontal cortex and the precentral gyrus. These stimulation-elicited responses have been attributed to electrical interference with the human homolog of the monkey FEF (71). Electrical stimulation studies in humans have confirmed the functional location of the eye movement sites anterior to the motor representation of arm and face (71,72). However, some ambiguity exists as regards the exact location of the human FEF within this rather extensive oculomotor region. The divergence is largely caused by the methodological differences of neuroimaging and electrical cortical stimulation studies.

The electrically defined human FEF is located in the posterior end of the middle frontal gyrus (see Fig. 13.1) immediately anterior to the precentral sulcus (and in proximity to the superior frontal sulcus). Electrical cortical stimulation of this area produces constant oculomotor responses characterized by low stimulation thresholds (71). Conversely, neuroimaging studies of cerebral blood flow (CBF) changes suggest that the homologous region in humans lies posterior to the electrically defined FEF. Indeed, the CBF-defined FEF is located between the central and precentral sulci in front of the primary hand representation, suggesting that the eye movement field lies in Brodmann area 6 (i.e., in a PreMC region homologous to the ventral PreMC) (73,74).

FOCAL MOTOR SEIZURES

Focal seizure is the term proposed by the Task Force of the International League Against Epilepsy (ILAE) to describe seizures in which the initial activation involves a limited number of neurons in part of one hemisphere (75). The terms *localization-related* or *partial* seizures have been used to describe the same seizure type. However, the more recently proposed diagnostic scheme of the ILAE Task Force prefers the less ambiguous term *focal* to partial or localization-related seizures (76).

Motor phenomena constitute the main clinical manifestations of motor seizures. As a rule, consciousness is retained in the majority of seizures arising from discrete motor regions. It is possible, however, for an ictal discharge to remain localized and still produce alteration of consciousness. Furthermore, certain motor manifestations and a patient's anxious reaction to the seizure symptoms may prevent the patient from responding appropriately during seizures. It may, therefore, be difficult to ascertain the level of consciousness in several patients with focal motor seizures. In the past, the presence or absence of altered awareness was used to dichotomize seizures of focal onset into "simple partial" and "complex partial." It is now proposed to move away from this dichotomy, which seems to have "*lost its meaningful precision*" (76).

The established International Classification of Epileptic Seizures (75) divides focal motor seizures into those with or without a march, versive, postural, and phonatory seizures. The diagnostic scheme proposed in 2001 is based on the use of a system of five axes (levels) intended to provide a standardized description of individual patients (76). Axis 2 now defines the epileptic seizure type or types experienced by the patient. Hence, focal motor seizures may present with *elementary clonic motor signs*, with *asymmetric tonic motor seizures* (a term commonly used to describe seizures arising from the SSMA), *typical automatisms* (a term that refers to seizures arising from the temporal lobe), with *hyperkinetic automatisms*, with *focal negative myoclonus*, and, finally, with *inhibitory motor seizures*. The addition of axis 1 allows for the systematic description of ictal semiology observed during seizures utilizing a standardized glossary of descriptive terminology (77). Ictal motor phenomena may be subdivided into **elementary motor manifestations** (such as tonic, clonic, dystonic, versive) and **automatisms**. Automatisms consist of a more or less co-ordinated, repetitive motor activity (such as oroalimentary, manual or pedal, vocal or verbal, hyperkinetic or hypokinetic) (77). Somatotopic modifiers may be added to describe the body part producing motor activity during seizures.

Another recent seizure classification is based on the clinical symptomatology and is independent of electroencephalographic (EEG), neuroimaging, and historical information (78). This classification uses terms such as *focal clonic, focal tonic,* or *versive,* and evolution during the seizure is indicated by arrows. For example: left hand somatosensory aura → left arm clonic seizure → left versive seizure.

Clinical Semiology

This section reviews the elementary motor phenomena resulting from a variety of focal motor seizures. These seizures typically present with clonic or tonic manifestations. Hyperkinetic manifestations are usually attributed to seizures arising from (or spreading to) the frontal lobe. Other motor automatisms seen with focal seizures (such as oroalimentary, mimetic, or gestural automatisms) are reviewed elsewhere.

In a population-based study conducted in Denmark of 1054 patients with epilepsy who were between the age of 16 and 66 years, 18% had "simple partial" seizures (79). Mauguiere and Courjon examined the presenting seizure type in a large series of 8938 patients with seizures admitted to a single hospital over a 10-year period. They found that 1158 patients (12.9%) had focal tonic or clonic seizures without march (the most common presentation of focal seizures in this series); 582 patients (6.5%) presented with hemitonic or clonic seizures; 461 (5.2%) had adversive seizures; and only 199 (2.2%) had Jacksonian seizures (80). Perirolandic epileptogenic lesions often involve both the precentral and postcentral gyri, giving rise to both motor and sensory phenomena. In one video-EEG study of 14 patients with a total of 87 "simple partial" seizures, sensory phenomena were observed in approximately one-third of patients exhibiting focal motor seizures (81).

Postictally, patients may experience a transient functional deficit, such as localized paresis (Todd paralysis), which may last for minutes or hours (up to 48 hours or longer). This interesting clinical phenomenon of "postepileptic paresis" is the signature of a focal seizure and bears the name of Dr. Bentley Todd, who first described it in the mid-19th century (82). Todd paralysis is believed to result from persistent focal dysfunction of the involved epileptogenic region. Postictal Todd paralysis is a clinical sign of substantial value in lateralizing the hemisphere of seizure onset (83).

Clonic Seizures

Clonic seizures consist of repeated, short contractions of various muscle groups characterized by rhythmic jerking or twitching movements (84). These movements recur at regular intervals of less than 1 to 2 seconds. Most clonic seizures are brief and last for less than 1 or 2 minutes. During this period, clonic movements may remain restricted to one region or spread in a Jacksonian manner. The majority of focal motor seizures tend to involve the hand and face, although any body part may potentially be affected (85). Such predilection is attributed to the large cortical representation of the hand and face area. The typical manifestation of a localized discharge within the precentral gyrus is clonic twitching of specific contralateral muscle groups, as determined by their proportionate somatotopic representation.

The clonic movements are usually limited to the corresponding area of the body, but may spread during the attack. Such spread (e.g., from the muscles of the face to the ipsilateral hand or arm) is known as the "*Jacksonian march.*" During these "*Jacksonian attacks,*" motor symptoms travel slowly from one territory to another, typically following the order of the corresponding somatotopic representation. The term *Jacksonian seizures* was proposed by Charcot in 1887 to describe the characteristic march seen with this particular subtype of clonic seizures (86). The continued use of the term serves to remind us of Hughlings Jackson's astute clinical observations, which provided the basis for his revolutionary principles of functional localization long before the era of EEG and neuroimaging correlations (87). In his own words:

> "*The part of the body where the convulsion begins indicates the part of the brain where the discharge begins and where the discharging lesion is situated. But from the focus discharging primarily the discharge spreads laterally to the adjacent "healthy" foci. One focus after the other is seized by the radiating waves of impulses. The march of the attack, the order in which the different parts of the body become involved, reveals the arrangement of the corresponding foci in the precentral convulsion*" (2)

The march usually starts from a distal body region (such as the thumb, fingers, great toe, mouth, or eyelids) and spreads toward a more proximal part. Jackson astutely described three variants: (i) "*fits starting in the hand (most often in the thumb or both),*" (ii) "*fits starting in one side of the face (most often near the mouth),*" and (iii) "*fits starting in the foot (nearly always in the great toe)*" (3). Typically, consciousness remains intact and secondary generalization of Jacksonian seizures is uncommon. At times, the march may skip some areas, a phenomenon that may be related to different seizure thresholds within the symptomatogenic region. Holowach and associates reviewed 60 *Jacksonian seizures* in children and found that the majority (25 out of 60) began in the face (eight in the periocular and five in the perioral region), 17 in the hand, seven in the arm, two in the shoulder, and nine in the leg and foot (88).

Lastly, the term *hemiconvulsions* refers to unilateral clonic seizures (i.e., clonic activity affecting one side of the body). Prolonged unilateral convulsions followed by the onset of hemiparesis are described in the childhood syndrome of hemiconvulsion-hemiplegia-epilepsy.

Myoclonus and Myoclonic Seizures

Many types of myoclonic phenomena (e.g., myoclonus caused by spinal cord disease or essential myoclonus) do not have an epileptic origin and need to be differentiated from (focal) myoclonic seizures. Typically, *myoclonic jerks* are arrhythmic compared with clonic motor activity. Notable exceptions discussed under *the broad definition of myoclonus* include the more rhythmic motoric manifestations of *epilepsia partialis continua* (see below, pages 161–162) and the nonepileptic *segmental myoclonus* or *palatal myoclonus* (also called palatal tremor) (89).

Epileptic myoclonus is typically accompanied by an EEG correlate of spike or multispike–wave complexes (90,91). Polygraphic recordings combining EEG with electromyography (EMG) of affected muscles may be necessary to unmask the relationship or the epileptic EEG activity to the myoclonic jerk. Video recordings can be helpful, but cannot replace polygraphy in ambiguous cases. The term *myoclonic seizure* is reserved for epileptic seizures, whose main components are single or repeated epileptic myoclonias (92). Gastaut distinguished epileptic myoclonic events into generalized, segmental, and focal, according to whether the seizures affected the entire body, one or more limbs, ipsilateral body parts/segments, or only one part of a single limb, respectively (93).

Although an accurate distinction may oftentimes prove difficult, some authors do not consider epileptic myoclonus as part of focal motor seizures (91). Others view focal cortical myoclonus as one manifestation of focal motor seizures, given that myoclonus in this instance results from a hypersynchronous discharge arising from a distinct population of cortical cells within the PMA and/or premotor areas (94). Focal cortical myoclonus has been described in patients with focal lesions involving the motor cortex, such as tumors, trauma, cortical dysplasia, or vascular lesions (Fig. 13.8). In a report of four children with perirolandic cortical dysplasia presenting with focal cortical myoclonus, the authors observed that

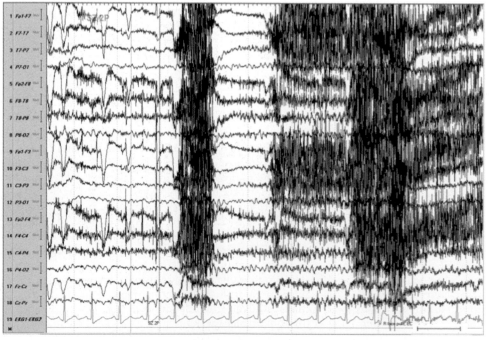

A

FIGURE 13.8 Consecutive scalp electroencephalogram tracings (A to C, longitudinal bipolar montage) during a typical stereotyped event do not disclose a definite evolving ictal pattern, in a 39-year-old patient with exquisitely focal motor seizures since childhood. In the last 3 years, she has been experiencing daily very brief seizures involving the muscles of the lower face on the right side without alteration of awareness. There is no history of Jacksonian march or secondarily generalized tonic–clonic seizures. Interictal EEG is normal. Although EEG activity is predominantly obscured by the presence of high voltage myogenic artifact, the sequence of motor manifestations can be discerned from the appearance of this same artifact. **A:** Clinical onset in the middle of this 10-second page punctuated by tonic contraction of the right facial musculature with involuntary right eye closure and deviation of the jaw towards the right, associated with voluntary reactive tensing of the entire face, as evidenced by the widespread and asymmetric "tonic muscle artifact."

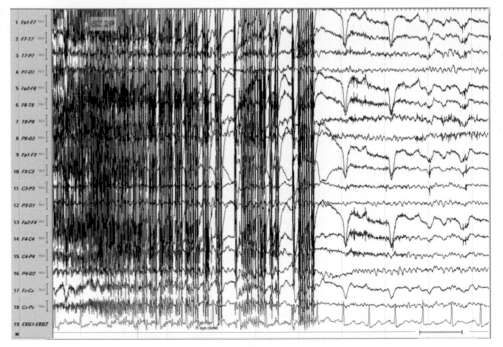

B

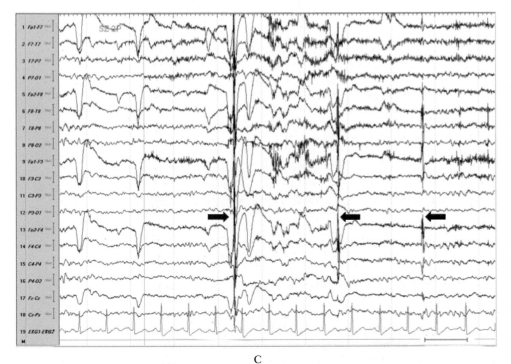

C

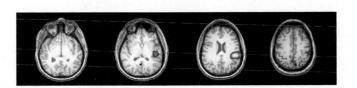

D

FIGURE 13.8 (*continued*) **B:** Clinical evolution with a brief cluster of repetitive focal myoclonic seizures involving the right side of the lower face, as evidenced by the corresponding repetitive, nonrhythmic and almost instantaneous, muscle artifact. Because of its very high voltage, the artifact appears widespread on this printed page. Digital reformatting confirms that the myogenic artifact is in fact picked up predominantly by the right-sided EEG electrodes, which are adjacent and susceptible to the contracting ipsilateral facial muscles. **C:** After the end of this motor sequence, the patient experiences three isolated, less intense, but otherwise identical muscle jerks in the span of 5 seconds, which are associated with myogenic artifact of relatively lower voltage (*arrows*) interrupting the otherwise normal awake EEG recording. Note that in this instance, the terminal muscle jerk is indeed associated with myogenic artifact primarily involving the right-sided derivations. **D:** Subtraction ictal SPECT (single photon emission computed tomography) study co-registered to the patient's MRI, as depicted in these selected axial images, revealed a small, discrete, and isolated area of hyperperfusion in the left precentral region, ventral to the expected location of the hand motor area. The patient's MRI was normal except for a small, questionable, but concordant (based on clinical semiology, EEG and ictal SPECT findings) area of faint signal increase in the depth of the left precentral sulcus at the level of the middle frontal gyrus. Surgical pathology revealed a balloon-cell cortical dysplasia. The location of the lesion (in the depth of the sulcus) and the exquisitely focal nature of the patient's habitual seizures likely account for the lack of interictal and ictal EEG abnormalities in this case.

localization of the recorded epileptiform discharges correlated with the body part affected by the myoclonus (C3 electrode in two patients whose myoclonus involved predominantly the right upper extremity, C3-T7 electrodes in one patient with myoclonus affecting the face, and Cz electrode in the other patient with focal myoclonus of the left leg) (95).

Finally, the paradoxical term *negative myoclonus* is reserved for cases of sudden, brief relaxations in tonic muscle contraction (89). Negative myoclonus (which also encompasses the phenomenon of *asterixis* typically seen in toxic-metabolic encephalopathies) is a nonspecific manifestation and can be associated with a variety of neurological disorders. Epileptic negative myoclonus can be either unilateral or bilateral and can be seen in relationship with a number of heterogeneous epilepsies ranging from the benign idiopathic epilepsies to severe epileptic encephalopathies (96).

Tonic Seizures

Tonic seizures consist of sustained muscle contractions that usually last for more than 5 to 10 seconds and result in posturing of the limbs or whole body (97). From the standpoint of clinical semiology, tonic seizures can be described according to the distribution and symmetry of tonic contractions with involvement of the axial (neck, trunk, and pelvis) and limb musculature. Generalized tonic seizures involve axial and limb muscles in a symmetric and synchronous fashion. Unequal or asynchronous contraction of muscle groups involving both sides of the body results in bilateral asymmetric tonic seizures. Contraction restricted to a portion of the body on one side only gives rise to focal tonic seizures (98).

In contrast to focal clonic seizures, which represent epileptic activation of a restricted region of the precentral gyrus, tonic motor seizures may implicate a wider area of motor cortex including the SSMA and the PreMC (17,99). Even though focal tonic seizures are attributed to activation of Brodmann area 6 (and the mesial frontal region in particular), some overlap in symptomatology occurs, with ictal involvement of the premotor and/or PMAs (100).

In a video-EEG study of 481 consecutive patients with focal epilepsy—evaluated at two tertiary epilepsy centers over a period of 4 years—a total of 123 patients were observed to have tonic seizure manifestations during at least one of their video-EEG recorded seizures. The vast majority of these patients had extratemporal epilepsy. Tonic seizures more frequently involved both sides of the body (76% bilateral vs. 24% unilateral). Importantly, when seen at the beginning of the seizure evolution, tonic seizures were more frequently associated with frontal lobe epilepsy as compared to epilepsy arising from the posterior neocortex. Furthermore, auras were more likely to precede tonic seizures originating from the parieto-occipital regions, and were less frequently reported in frontal lobe epilepsy (101).

Stimulation of the SSMA elicits bilateral, asymmetric tonic contractions affecting primarily the more proximal muscles. Less frequently, focal tonic contractions may be seen. The symptomatogenic zone is less clear in cases of symmetric, bilateral tonic seizures. However, these seizures are believed to be generated by simultaneous bilateral activation of Brodmann area 6, rostral to the precentral region, in both hemispheres (30). It is also possible that generalized tonic seizures result from direct activation of brainstem

reticular-activating systems (102,103). The fact that slow-wave and Rapid Eye Movement (REM) sleep, as well as decreased levels of vigilance, appear to facilitate some tonic seizures, for example in patients with Lennox-Gastaut syndrome, further implicates the brainstem in the generation of these phenomena (104). It becomes evident that different types of tonic seizures utilize different neuroanatomical pathways, which is hardly surprising given that tonic seizures may be a common clinical manifestation resulting from a variety of different pathophysiologies underlying symptomatic and less frequently idiopathic epilepsies.

Nonepileptic focal tonic symptoms can result from subcortical pathology (e.g., spinal cord or brainstem dysfunction in the case of compression or multiple sclerosis). In addition, paroxysmal tonic phenomena may be seen as part of certain movement disorders (such as paroxysmal choreoathetosis or spasmodic torticollis) or other nonepileptic paroxysmal disorders (e.g., in the setting of convulsive syncope) (98).

Oculocephalic Deviation and Versive Seizures

Foerster and Penfield first described versive seizures in 1930. The seizures consist of a sustained, unnatural turning of the eyes and head to one side, as a result of a predominantly tonic contraction of head and eye muscles (105). Although consciousness is often lost by the time a patient experiences version, occasionally patients may be aware of the forced, involuntary head and eye deviation (44,106).

As discussed, cortical stimulation studies have confirmed the functional location of eye movement sites in proximity to the primary motor representation of the arm and face (72). On stimulating this region, Rasmussen and Penfield observed that the more anterior points were responsible for contralateral rotation (107). Stimulation of more posterior points (closer to the central sulcus) elicited contralateral, ipsilateral, or upward eye movements. Head rotation was usually seen in conjunction with contralateral eye rotation.

The lateralizing significance of oculocephalic deviation has met with controversy. Indeed a number of authors use the terms *head turning* and *head version* interchangeably (108–110). This lexical ambiguity prompted Wyllie and colleagues to restrict the term *version* to "*unquestionably forced, involuntary head and eye deviation to one side resulting in sustained unnatural positioning of the head and eyes*" (105). In this important study, the authors reviewed retrospectively all lateral head and eye movements observed during 74 seizures in 37 patients and classified as "nonversive" any mild, unsustained, wandering, or seemingly voluntary head and eye movements. Visual analysis of video recordings was performed without prior knowledge of EEG findings. By adhering to the strict definition of "version," the authors showed that the presence of a contralateral versive head and eye movement provides reliable lateralizing information (especially when this movement precedes secondary generalization) (105). On the other hand, one should be cautious about interpreting the direction of eye and head turning, if the seizure does not become secondarily generalized (111,112).

Version may result from seizures originating from various locations and spreading to the PreMC. A noteworthy clinical observation is that extratemporal seizures give rise to version earlier in the seizure (within 18 seconds from seizure onset), compared with seizures of temporal lobe origin (in which version is usually seen after 18 seconds or later) (111).

Seizures Manifested by Vocalization or Arrest of Vocalization

Several types of utterances can occur during epileptic seizures. A prolonged continuous or interrupted vocalization may occur in seizures involving the SSMA or lower PMA on either hemisphere (59). Vocalization, when it occurs as part of SSMA seizures, tends to be more sustained (113). Penfield and Jasper produced such phonatory phenomena in humans by stimulating the SSMA or the PMA below the lip or tongue area (40). Finally, the so-called epileptic cry is frequently seen at the onset of generalized tonic–clonic seizures.

Speech arrest, defined as inability to speak during a seizure despite conscious attempts by the patient (44), may result from involvement of the PMA (114) or SSMA in either the dominant or the nondominant hemisphere. Electrical cortical stimulation studies suggest that the speech arrest observed in cases of

SSMA stimulation represents a negative motor response (resulting from inhibition of tongue movement) (115).

EEG Findings

The ability of scalp electroencephalography to detect interictal activity depends on the extent of the irritative zone and the orientation of the dipole. Special techniques may be required to demonstrate epileptiform activity in patients with focal seizures. Sleep recordings, for example, have been reported to increase the yield of interictal epileptiform abnormalities (116–118). Special electrodes (such as sphenoidal, anterior temporal, or ear electrodes) and closely spaced additional scalp electrodes (Fig. 13.9A) may help to distinguish temporal from frontal foci and determine whether the electrical field of a midline sharp wave is higher over the left or right hemisphere (119–121).

Small epileptogenic foci may be entirely missed with interictal (and even ictal) surface EEG recordings (see Fig. 13.8). On the other hand, interictal epileptiform abnormalities may

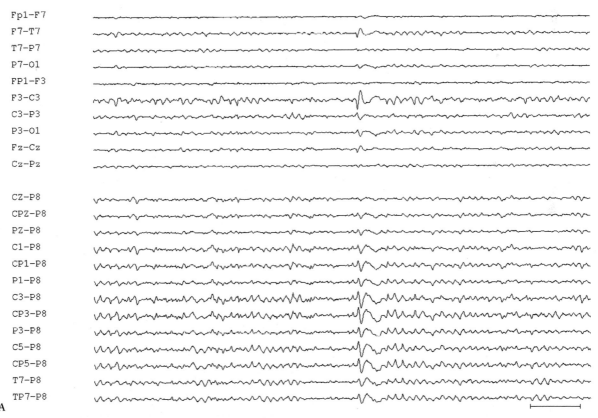

FIGURE 13.9 Scalp EEG tracings (**A, B,** and **C**) from a 41-year-old patient with intractable left perirolandic epilepsy of unknown etiology since age 11 years. He presented with daily focal motor seizures involving the right leg and shoulder sometimes preceded by a somatosensory aura (tingling sensation in the right foot) and rare secondarily generalized tonic–clonic seizures. **A:** Interictal left centroparietal sharp wave as seen on a longitudinal bipolar (*upper part*) and referential montage (*lower part*). The P8 reference derivation of the sharp wave shows maximum negativity at electrode CP3. The addition of closely spaced surface electrodes (placed according to the 10–10 Electrode Placement System) provides for a more accurate distribution map. In this instance, the potential amplitude at electrode C5 is 85% and at electrodes C3 and CP3 is 83% of the amplitude recorded at the maximally involved electrode CP3.

(continued)

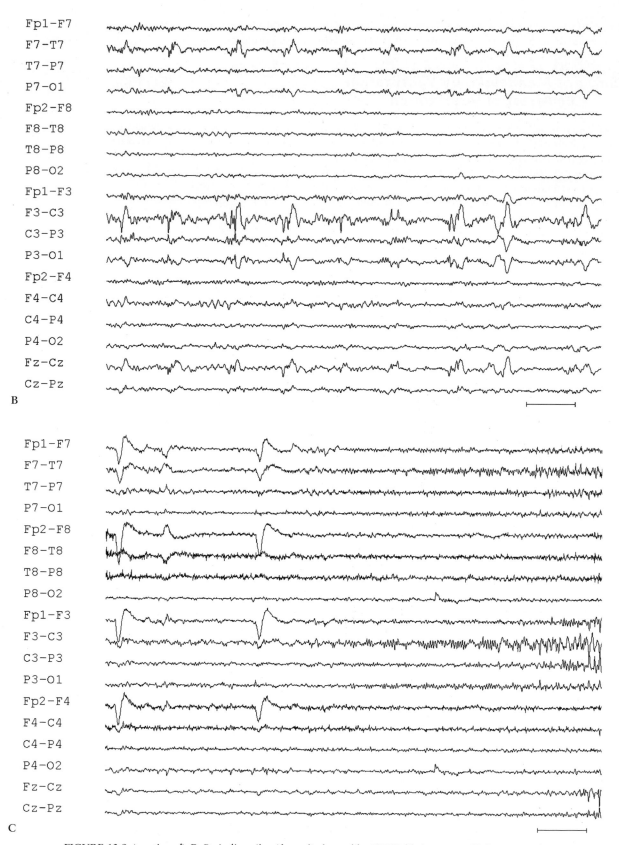

FIGURE 13.9 (*continued*) **B:** Periodic epileptiform discharge-like (PLED-like) pattern of left centroparietal sharp waves and polyspikes. This interictal finding was present during the first 24 hours of admission for acute exacerbation of his habitual focal motor seizures. **C:** The ictal onset is punctuated by the appearance of evolving low- to high-amplitude paroxysmal fast activity arising from the left centroparietal region.

have a misleadingly widespread appearance because of the large distance and intervening cortical area that separates the epileptogenic zone from the scalp EEG electrodes (122).

Random EEG tracings in patients with focal epilepsy may not show evidence of focal epileptiform activity. In a case series of 19 patients with refractory frontal lobe epilepsy, Salanova and associates reported absence of interictal sharp waves in 7 of 19 (37%) patients (123). Secondary bilaterally synchronous discharges may be seen in up to two-thirds of patients with frontal lobe epilepsy (124). EEG interpretation should take into account the possibility of "secondary bilateral synchrony," a term introduced by Tükel and Jasper to describe the bilateral discharges seen in patients with parasagittal epileptogenic lesions (125).

Ictal recordings may show regional seizure patterns (Fig. 13.9C) or may have limited localizing or lateralizing value. As a rule, the patterns are more widespread and more difficult to lateralize compared with those seen with seizures of temporal lobe origin. Studies show that ictal electroencephalography may be nonlocalizing in more than half of patients with frontal lobe epilepsy (123,126). False localization may occur with an erroneous temporal ictal pattern on surface EEG as a result of underlying frontolimbic connections (122).

Particular EEG patterns may sometimes be seen in relationship to the corresponding seizure type: generalized tonic seizures, for example, may be associated with ictal EEG activity, which consists of repetitive rhythmic spiking of variable frequency (8–25 Hz, or faster) and amplitude (127). More recently, investigators have been able to ascertain the presence of gamma rhythms in the frequency range of 50 to 100 Hz associated with generalized tonic seizures during scalp EEG recordings in patients with Lennox-Gastaut syndrome (128).

Invasive recordings using subdural electrodes in frontal lobe epilepsies may only show evidence for a focal onset in a relatively small number of patients; often, a more diffuse "regional" pattern may be seen (123,129). This, of course, depends on the nature, location, extent, and connectivity of the underlying epileptogenic substrate and its relationship to the recording electrodes. In a careful invasive study of patients presenting with circumscribed focal clonic seizures, investigators observed that these seizures were always associated with a localized polyspike and wave *intracranial ictal EEG* pattern involving the subdural electrodes overlying the PMA, while neighboring subdural electrodes not overlying the precentral gyrus showed various other ictal patterns (130). Such ictal patterns associated with focal clonic seizures may occasionally be discernible by scalp EEG recordings.

EPILEPSIA PARTIALIS CONTINUA

The *epileptic seizure types*, which constitute axis 2 of the recently proposed ILAE diagnostic scheme (76), have been divided into self-limited and continuous. The term "*continuous seizure types*" encompasses the diverse presentations of status epilepticus.

Status epilepticus can be broadly divided into status epilepticus with motor or without motor phenomena (131). Subcategories of motor status epilepticus include generalized and secondarily generalized status, as well as *focal motor*

status epilepticus. The latter is characterized by repetitive typical somatomotor seizures with or without Jacksonian march originating from the perirolandic region. This condition may occur at the onset or during the course of epilepsies manifesting with focal motor seizures. Consciousness is usually preserved, and cerebral function of the uninvolved cortex remains intact. A variety of motor phenomena may be observed in the context of focal motor status ranging from overt to more subtle motor manifestations, such as epileptic nystagmus for example, which may be seen in patients with oculoclonic status epilepticus (132,133).

Epilepsia partialis continua of Kojevnikov (EPC or partial continuous epilepsy) constitutes one form of focal motor status epilepticus, characterized by localized unremitting myoclonus. The condition was first described by Kojevnikov in 1895 as a disorder of persistent localized motor seizures (134). In published literature, EPC has been referred to as "Kojevnikov," "Kojewnikow," or "Kozhevnikov" syndrome.

Clinical Semiology

EPC has been regarded by some as "the semiological epitome of a focal seizure" (135), as it usually involves a restricted area of the motor cortex of one hemisphere and presents with clinically localized motor manifestations. EPC is defined by the occurrence of almost continuous and rhythmic or semirhythmic muscular contractions (*myoclonic jerks*) that remain localized to a limited area on one side of the body and persist for hours, days, or even years (136,137). The definition has undergone several revisions in the past, reflecting differences of opinion among various authors. In 1989, the ILAE Commission defined EPC as a specific form of continuous somatomotor seizures involving the Rolandic cortex (138). Any muscle group may be involved, but *distal musculature is more commonly affected*. The myoclonic jerks may appear isolated or in clusters, with a regular or irregular occurrence at a frequency of 1 to 2 per second. In general, unilateral involvement with synchronous activation of agonists and antagonists is observed. The jerks are predominantly seen involving the muscles of the upper half of the body. In a study of 151 patients presenting with EPC, the authors observed that during its course the disease involved the head in 16% of patients, the head and upper limb in 14%, the upper limb only in 40%, the trunk in 5%, the lower extremity in 14%, and the whole side of the body in 11% (139).

By definition, the jerks are spontaneous, although they may be aggravated by physical activity, psychic exertion, and/or sensory stimuli (140). In most cases, the jerks may be reduced in amplitude but persist during sleep (141,142). Other seizure types (such as Jacksonian or generalized seizures) and a variety of neurologic deficits may be seen in these patients depending on the underlying etiology.

The pathophysiology of EPC is not well understood. It has been postulated that the absence of seizure propagation is associated with the specific anatomical location of the epileptic focus within a neocortical area of sufficiently preserved inhibition. Virtually all authors today agree that involvement of the PMA is indispensable for the generation and sustainment of EPC (143). Bancaud and coworkers divided EPC into two broad categories based on the presence (type 2) or absence (type 1) of a progressive brain lesion (136): Type 1 was associated with a regional nonprogressive lesion in the sensorimotor cortex, whereas type 2 was typically seen in the setting of Rasmussen syndrome.

EPC may develop at any age. The usual etiology of EPC is a focal lesion involving the cortex (principally the sensorimotor cortex) that results from stroke, trauma, infection, metastasis, or primary tumor. A hypoxic, metabolic, or septic encephalopathy may predispose patients with a pre-existing focal lesion to develop EPC. All patients presenting with EPC should be carefully evaluated for an underlying lesion that may be amenable to curative resective surgery. EPC is, of course, a common manifestation of Rasmussen syndrome (seen in almost 50% of cases) (144). Despite its focal expression, EPC in Rasmussen syndrome may be associated with MRI and EEG evidence of more diffuse hemispheric abnormalities. In the U.K. series of 36 patients from ages 1 to 84 years, who presented with EPC over the period of one year the commonest isolated etiology was Rasmussen syndrome in seven (19%; five were children), followed by stroke in five (14%). In seven patients, the cause of their presentation remained undetermined (137). EPC and its variants have also been reported in the setting of multiple sclerosis (145), human immunodeficiency virus infection (146,147), Creutzfeldt-Jakob disease (148), and other neurodegenerative diseases such as mitochondrial disorders (149,150) or Alpers syndrome (151).

Focal motor seizures or EPC, or both, may be the presenting feature of *nonketotic hyperglycemia* or may occur as a later complication, especially in the presence of an underlying focal cerebral lesion (152). Hyperglycemia, hyponatremia, mild hyperosmolarity, and lack of ketoacidosis were found to contribute to the development of EPC predominantly in areas of pre-existing focal cerebral damage in 21 patients with evidence of nonketotic hyperglycemia (153). One should note, however, that EPC has also been reported in the setting of *ketotic hyperglycemia* (137,154). Depending on the etiology, EPC may be an early or late feature in the course of the underlying disease and may be seen either in isolation or in association with other seizure types (155). Similar to EPC, focal somatomotor status may reflect an underlying focal brain lesion (secondary to a vascular, neoplastic, traumatic, or infectious etiology) or may present in the context of toxic-metabolic abnormalities. In patients without pre-existing epilepsy, the onset of focal motor status may signify underlying "asymptomatic" ischemia or interterritorial cerebral infarction (infarction in watershed territories).

Subcortical or spinal myoclonus and certain forms of tremor and other extrapyramidal movement disorders should be considered in the differential diagnosis of EPC. Clinical differentiation is often challenging, and special neurophysiologic examinations may be necessary (155,156).

EEG Findings

The conventional scalp EEG may be unrevealing or misleadingly normal. There may be very few or no paroxysmal abnormalities; and the background rhythm may be normal. In some cases, time-locked EEG events preceding the EPC-associated myoclonic jerks can be detected by back-averaging. In addition, special stereoencephalographic or electrocorticographic recordings may prove helpful in resolving the underlying spike focus.

In other cases, irregular 0.5- to 3-Hz slowing may be seen in the frontocentral region along with reduction of the beta activity in the same area (44), but there are no characteristic EEG findings to aid in the diagnosis of EPC. In a study of 32 cases, the most common EEG finding was regional spiking (141). Other abnormalities included bursts of sharp waves or spike-and-wave discharges and unilateral or bilateral runs of abnormal rhythms. In a study of 21 adults presenting with EPC, the authors found EEGs to be abnormal in all but one patient. Each patient underwent at least two EEGs in the course of the disease; consequently more than one pattern was seen in some patients. The most common EEG finding was the presence of unilateral lateralized and/or localized spike or sharp-wave discharges in 10 patients (48%). Other lateralized abnormalities ranged from periodic lateralized epileptiform discharges (PLEDs) in three, paroxysmal slow-wave activity in two, and lateralized continuous slow activity in four patients. Four patients exhibited diffuse, continuous slow activity, one showed paroxysmal generalized slow-wave activity, and one patient had periodic generalized epileptiform discharges (157). In this study, only seven patients (33%) were found to have epileptiform discharges during EPC that correlated to the myoclonic jerks.

On rare occasions, PLEDs and PLED-like patterns that are time locked to the jerks are observed in the course of EPC (158). PLEDs are commonly viewed as a transient interictal pattern (see Fig. 13.9B), which usually disappears within a few days, but may last as long as 3 months or longer (159). PLEDs can occur in a variety of structural and metabolic disorders usually of acute or subacute nature (160,161). It is important to note that depending on the clinical scenario there are occasions when PLEDs in fact represent an ictal EEG pattern (162). Furthermore, one should not overlook the common occurrence of seizures in association to the presence of PLEDs on EEG recordings—seizures have been reported to occur with a frequency ranging from 58% to 100% in some studies (160). The most common seizure type seen in the presence of PLEDs is focal motor seizures affecting the contralateral body (163), often presenting as status epilepticus or as repetitive focal motor seizures (160,163,164).

In Rasmussen encephalitis, it is important to identify and document MRI evidence of progressive atrophy, which usually involves only one hemisphere. An abnormal EEG with progressive regional or lateralized slowing and ipsilateral regional or multiregional spiking is the rule. In a case report of an 11-year-old girl with Rasmussen syndrome, and a 5-month history of EPC, fluorodeoxyglucose–positron emission tomography (FDG-PET) studies demonstrated an area of hypermetabolism in the right central cortex and ipsilateral thalamus. A congruent sharp-wave focus was present in the same region on scalp EEG recordings. Using simultaneously recorded EMG of the left tibialis anterior muscle, the authors demonstrated regular jerks, time locked with the right central sharp waves (165). With time, the EEG abnormalities of Rasmussen encephalitis may become bilateral or more widespread, multiregional, or synchronous suggesting progression of a more diffuse process than indicated by the clinical manifestation of EPC.

SUPPLEMENTARY SENSORIMOTOR SEIZURES

Clinical Semiology

Seizures arising from the SSMA are of brief duration, usually lasting only 10 to 40 seconds. Rapid onset of asymmetric tonic posturing involving one or more extremities is characteristically observed (50,166). While it is common for both sides of the body to be affected simultaneously, unilateral tonic motor activity may occur (167). The typical seizure is frequently referred to as a *bilateral asymmetric tonic seizure.*

Speech arrest and vocalization are common. Somatosensory symptoms, such as numbness, tingling, or pressure sensation may precede the phase of tonic posturing (40); these body sensations are not well localized in contradistinction to somatosensory symptoms that result from epileptic activation of the postcentral gyrus (168). Common descriptions include a feeling of tension, pulling, or heaviness in an extremity or a sense that the extremity is "about to move" (169). In addition, the sensation of either an urge to perform a movement or an anticipation that some movement is about to occur has been reported in response to electrical stimulation (60). Although consciousness is usually preserved, patients may not be able to respond verbally during the tonic phase. Toward the end of the seizure, a few rhythmic clonic movements of the extremities may be observed (169). Postictal confusion is absent in the majority of SSMA seizures.

Asymmetric involvement of the upper extremities usually manifests with abduction at the shoulders, flexion of one elbow, and extension of the other upper extremity. As a rule, the lower extremities are also involved in the tonic posturing, with abduction at the hips and flexion or extension at the knees (50). Even patients, in whom tonic posturing appears to be unilateral, have bilaterally increased (or decreased) tone (33).

In their original report and illustrations of "somatic sensory seizures" arising from the SSMA, Penfield and Jasper described head turning to the side of the flexed upper extremity (40). They observed that the head and eyes appear as if looking toward the flexed and raised arm with the patient adopting the so-called *"fencing posture"*—a motor response reminiscent of the asymmetric tonic neck reflex (33). Ajmone Marsan and Ralston subsequently coined the term *"M2e"* to describe the abduction and elevation of the contralateral arm with external rotation at the shoulder and slight flexion at the elbow (170). The patient's head and eyes deviate as if looking at the raised arm, while both lower extremities remain extended or slightly flexed at the hips and knees.

In contrast to these early reports, further analysis of SSMA seizures showed that assumption of the classic *"fencing"* or *"M2e"* posture is not common (100,171). Among the less common motor manifestations, coarse movements of the tonic postured extremities may be observed (172). If present, vocalization may be prominent during the tonic phase reflecting the tonic involvement of the diaphragm and laryngeal muscles, which contract against semiclosed vocal cords (169).

Ictal activity may spread to involve the PMA of the face on the dorsolateral convexity, resulting in unilateral clonic movements or contralateral head version. Secondary generalization may lead to a generalized tonic–clonic seizure. Clonic movements can be seen toward the end of the tonic seizure (169). Unusual hyperkinetic automatisms (involving the ipsilateral upper extremity) have been described with seizures involving the SSMA (173). Finally, writhing movements may be seen as some patients attempt to move around or sit up during the tonic seizure.

SSMA seizures may be frequent (up to 5 to 10 per day) and can occur in clusters. They tend to occur predominantly during sleep (168,174). In a systematic review of their relationship with sleep, almost two-thirds of a total of 322 SSMA seizures in 24 patients occurred during sleep, almost exclusively during nonrapid eye movement (NREM) sleep stages I and II—as demonstrated by video-EEG recordings (175).

It should be emphasized that only a minority of patients with seizures displaying the clinical features of SSMA activation (*"SSMA seizures"*) actually have *"SSMA epilepsy"* (176). In most cases, the SSMA functions as the symptomatogenic zone: the observed seizures reflect the expression of ictal discharges originating from clinically silent regions that have anatomical or functional proximity to the SSMA, such as the basal frontal regions, the dorsolateral convexity of the frontal lobe, and the mesial parietal regions (50). This important point is illustrated by a recent stereo-EEG study of 14 patients with intractable focal epilepsy presenting with SSMA seizure semiology. Invasive EEG recordings showed evidence of seizure origin within the SSMA region in only six (43%) patients. The eight remaining patients were found to have diffuse unilateral or bilateral seizure onset. The authors concluded that SSMA semiology is suggestive of early involvement of this region, but is *by no means a reliable indicator that the SSMA itself contains the seizure focus* (177). Consequently, the SSMA itself may not need to be sacrificed in patients presenting with intractable SSMA seizures. Moreover, unless the location of the epileptogenic focus/generator has been carefully defined, resection of the SSMA may not be associated with a favorable postoperative outcome (178). Lastly, the clinical picture of SSMA seizures with involvement of all four extremities and simultaneous preservation of awareness may be misleading, and it is not unusual for patients with this type of paroxysmal activity to be misdiagnosed as having psychogenic nonepileptic seizures (113).

EEG Findings

Interictal sharp waves, when present, are usually found at the midline, maximum at the vertex, or just adjacent to the midline in the frontocentral region (Fig. 13.10A). Only 50% of 16 patients with supplementary sensorimotor seizures, who underwent evaluation with subdural electrodes, had shown scalp EEG evidence of midline frontocentral interictal epileptiform activity (179).

It is important to distinguish midline interictal epileptiform discharges from vertex sharp transients of sleep. This distinction may not be possible, when sharp waves are seen only during sleep. The presence of prominent after-going slow waves, occurrence of polyspikes, and/or consistently asymmetric distribution of the electrical field may raise the suspicion of epileptiform activity (179,180). In general, normal sleep-related transients display a symmetric field pattern, whereas midline sharp waves may be asymmetric. *Appearance of the same midline sharp waves or spikes during wakefulness* (see Fig. 13.10A) will lead to the correct diagnosis of underlying epilepsy.

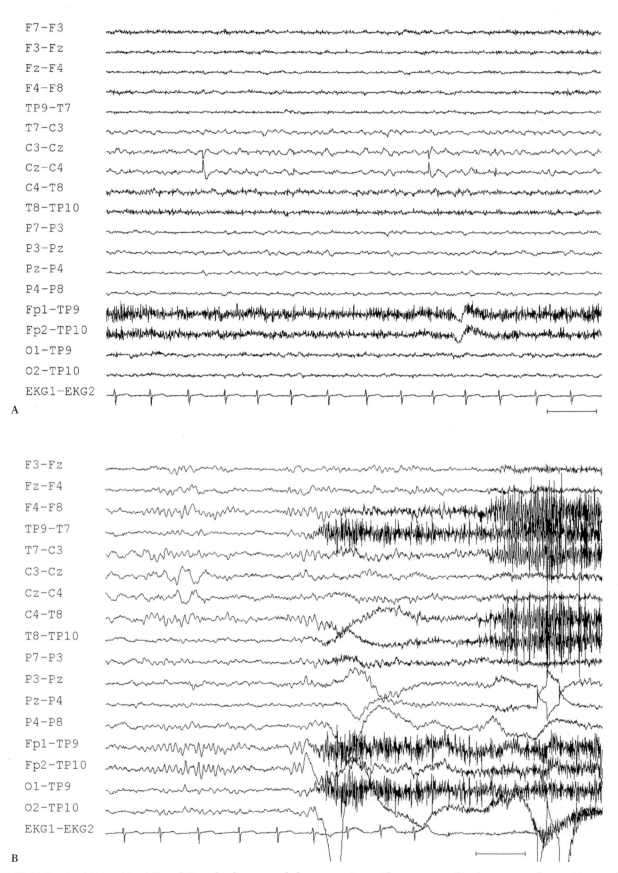

FIGURE 13.10 Interictal (**A**) and ictal (**B** and **C**) scalp electroencephalogram tracings with a transverse bipolar montage from a 12-year-old girl with left SSMA epilepsy. Bilateral asymmetric tonic seizures arising from sleep and wakefulness were captured during video-electroencephalograph evaluation. **A:** This awake recording shows sharp waves at the vertex (virtually confined to the Cz electrode). Note that the potential amplitude is slightly higher on the left (C3) than on the right (C4) central electrode. **B:** Clinical onset of typical seizure occurring out of sleep coincides with the appearance of bilateral myogenic artifact. Scalp EEG does not reveal a clear ictal pattern at the time of clinical onset.

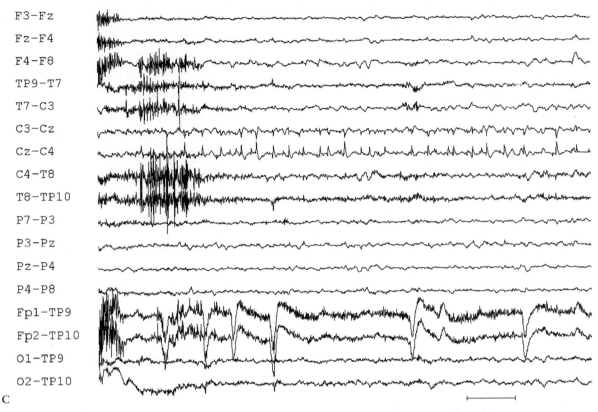

FIGURE 13.10 (*continued*) C: Rhythmic, repetitive sharp waves are present at the vertex within 15 seconds of clinical onset.

During seizures originating from the SSMA (Fig. 13.10B), the EEG is frequently obscured by prominent EMG artifact owing to the associated tonic activity and the midline location of the ictal EEG discharges. However, careful review of the vertex region with the appropriate (usually transverse bipolar) montage and use of closely spaced parasagittal scalp electrodes may reveal the ictal EEG pattern despite considerable EMG artifact. Frequently, an initial high-amplitude slow transient or sharp wave may be seen at the vertex followed by midline low-amplitude fast activity or an electrodecremental pattern (169,180). These early changes are often followed by the development of high-amplitude rhythmic slowing distributed bilaterally in the frontocentral regions. Ictal activity may remain restricted to the vertex (Fig. 13.10C) or have a more widespread distribution. In general, the lateralizing value of such ictal EEG changes is rather limited. Moreover, paradoxical, erroneous scalp EEG lateralization is possible, when the generator of sharp waves is situated in the interhemispheric fissure producing a transverse or oblique dipole orientation (181). Lastly, a small percentage of patients with SSMA seizures will have no identifiable scalp EEG change during the ictus.

DIFFERENTIAL DIAGNOSIS

The differential diagnosis of focal motor seizures includes nonepileptic myoclonus (182) or tonic spasms (183,184), psychogenic nonepileptic seizures, complex motor sterotypies/tics (185), and other paroxysmal movement disorders such as paroxysmal choreoathetosis (186) and tremor (187).

As mentioned, the absence of abnormalities on outpatient EEGs does not exclude the possibility of focal motor seizures. When available, home videotape recordings can provide valuable diagnostic information by capturing the episodes in question. Otherwise, prolonged inpatient video-EEG monitoring may be necessary. Patients who present with infrequent attacks of unclear etiology pose considerable diagnostic challenges, given the low diagnostic yield of prolonged EEG recordings. Ambulatory EEGs are not particularly helpful in this setting, especially if no ictal EEG patterns are seen during the paroxysmal behavior.

Seizures arising from the frontal lobe can be bizarre (such as seizures characterized by prominent thrashing movements and preserved consciousness) and may be misdiagnosed as nonepileptic seizures of psychogenic origin. The reverse can also be true. Saygi and coworkers compared the ictal manifestations of 63 frontal lobe seizures in 11 patients with the clinical features of 29 psychogenic seizures in 12 patients (188). The authors did not find any single clinical criterion that would sufficiently differentiate these two groups. Seizure characteristics favoring an epileptic diagnosis included younger age at onset, stereotyped patterns of movements, turning to a prone position during seizures, shorter duration of seizures, nocturnal occurrence, and the presence of MRI and EEG abnormalities. In another study, which only compared the clinical features of SSMA and nonepileptic seizures, the duration of SSMA seizures was much shorter than that of psychogenic events (113). None of the SSMA seizures lasted longer than 38 seconds, whereas psychogenic seizures had a mean duration of 173 seconds. In addition, SSMA seizures occurred predominantly out of sleep, whereas psychogenic seizures usually occurred from the waking state.

Epileptic motor seizures may manifest themselves at any time of the day or night. However, a number of epilepsy syndromes (including SSMA epilepsy, frontal lobe epilepsy, benign focal epilepsy of childhood, generalized epilepsy, and autosomal dominant nocturnal frontal lobe epilepsy [ADNFLE]) tend to manifest with seizures occurring predominantly during sleep. In addition, sleep-related paroxysmal motor phenomena can be seen with various sleep disorders (including NREM arousal disorders, REM behavior disorder of sleep, and sleep–wake transition disorder). The differential diagnosis of such nocturnal paroxysmal events is broad and often challenging, given the frequently poor clinical description and overlap of clinical manifestations (189).

It is not understood why certain seizure types occur preferentially during sleep (190). In a study of patients with intractable focal epilepsy, continuous video-electroencephalography and polysomnography were used to compare sleeping–waking distribution of seizures and quality of sleep organization in 15 patients with frontal lobe epilepsy and 15 patients with temporal lobe epilepsy (191). The authors demonstrated that seizures of frontal lobe origin occurred more frequently during the night compared with seizures arising from the temporal lobe in this group of patients with pharmacoresistant epilepsy.

More recently, ADNFLE has been identified as a distinctive clinical syndrome (192,193). The disorder is characterized by clusters of brief nocturnal motor seizures with hyperkinetic or tonic manifestations. Stereotyped attacks are frequently seen in individual family members despite the significant intrafamilial variation. Interictal EEGs are frequently normal, and the diagnosis is established on a clinical basis. Seizures usually begin in childhood and may persist throughout life, although the overall seizure frequency tends to decrease over time (192). A strong linkage with the neuronal nicotinic acetylcholine receptor has been established in the years following initial description of this syndrome (194,195).

Several case reports highlight the unusual occurrence of repetitive involuntary movements in the setting of transient cerebral ischemia (the so-called limb-shaking transient ischemic attacks or "*limb-shaking TIAs*") that may be mistaken for focal motor seizures (196–198). These episodic attacks are often precipitated by standing up or walking and seem to involve only the limbs (hand-arm alone or hand-arm and ipsilateral leg) without spreading to the facial or truncal musculature (196,199). The need to recognize these paroxysmal positive motor manifestations as a sign of severe contralateral carotid occlusive disease is emphasized (196,197).

References

1. Souques A. *Étapes de la Neurologie dans l'Antiquité Grecque*. Paris: Masson et Cie; 1936.
2. Foerster O. The motor cortex in man in the light of Hughlings Jackson's doctrines. *Brain*. 1936;59(2):135–139.
3. Taylor J. *Selected Writings of John Hughlings Jackson*. London: Hodder and Stoughton; 1931.
4. Fritsch G, Hitzig E. Über die elektrische Erregbarkeit des Grosshirns. *Arch Anat Physiol Wiss Med*. 1870;37:300–332.
5. Wieser HG. Historical review of cortical electrical stimulation. In: Lüders HO, Noachtar S, eds. *Epileptic Seizures—Pathophysiology and Clinical Semiology*. Philadelphia: Churchill Livingstone; 2000:141–152.
6. Uematsu S, Lesser RP, Gordon B. Localization of sensorimotor cortex: the influence of Sherrington and Cushing on the modern concept. *Neurosurgery*. 1992;30(6):904–912.
7. Bartholow R. Experimental investigations into functions of the human brain. *Am J Med Sci*. 1874;67:305–313.
8. Cushing H. A note upon the faradic stimulation of the psotcentral gyrus in conscious patients. *Brain*. 1909;32(1):44–53.
9. Zimmermann M. Electrical stimulation of the human brain. *Hum Neurobiol*. 1982;1(4):227–229.
10. Penfield W, Brodley E. Somatic motor and sensory representation in the cerebral cortex of man as studied by electrical stimulation. *Brain*. 1937;60(4):389–443.
11. Geyer S, Matelli M, Luppino G, et al. Functional neuroanatomy of the primate isocortical motor system. *AnatEmbryol(Berl)*. 2000;202(6):443–474.
12. Petrides M. Mapping prefrontal cortical systems for the control of cognition. In: Toga A, Mazziotta J, eds. *Brain Mapping: The Systems*. San Diego: Academic Press; 2000:159–176.
13. Roland PE, Zilles K. Functions and structures of the motor cortices in humans. *Curr Opin Neurobiol*. 1996;6(6):773–781.
14. Fink GR, Frackowiak RS, Pietrzyk U, et al. Multiple nonprimary motor areas in the human cortex. *J Neurophysiol*. 1997;77(4):2164–2174.
15. Mayer AR, Zimbelman JL, Watanabe Y, et al. Somatotopic organization of the medial wall of the cerebral hemispheres: a 3 Tesla fMRI study. *Neuroreport*. 2001;12(17):3811–3814.
16. Grafton ST, Hari R, Salenius S. The human motor system. In: Toga AW, Mazziotta JC, eds. *Brain Mapping: The Systems*. San Diego: Academic Press; 2000:331–363.
17. Blume W. Focal motor seizures and epilepsia partialis continua. In: Wyllie E, ed. *The Treatment of Epilepsy: Principles and Practice*, 3rd ed. Philadelphia: Lippincott Williams & Wilkins; 2001:329–343.
18. Ghez C, Krakauer J. The organization of movement. In: Kandel ER, Schwartz JH, Jessell TM, eds. *Principles of Neural Science*. New York: McGraw-Hill; 2000:653–673.
19. Crick F, Jones E. Backwardness of human neuroanatomy. *Nature*. 1993;361(6408):109–110.
20. Guye M, Bartolomei F, Ranjeva JP. Imaging structural and functional connectivity: towards a unified definition of human brain organization? *Curr Opin Neurol*. 2008;21(4):393–403.
21. Kuypers H. Anatomy of the descending pathways. In: Brookhart JM, Mountcastle VB, Brooks VB, Geiger SR, eds. *The Nervous System, II Motor Control*. Bethesda: American Physiological Society; 1981: 597–666.
22. Blume WT. Motor cortex: anatomy, physiology and epileptogenesis. In: Wyllie E, ed. *The Treatment of Epilepsy: Principles and Practice*. 1st ed. Philadelphia: Lea & Febiger; 1993:16–25.
23. Carpenter MB. Tracts of the spinal cord. In: Carpenter MB, ed. *Human Neuroanatomy*. 7th ed. Baltimore, MD: Williams & Wilkins; 1976:238–284.
24. Galea MP, Darian-Smith I. Multiple corticospinal neuron populations in the macaque monkey are specified by their unique cortical origins, spinal terminations, and connections. *Cereb Cortex*. 1994;4(2):166–194.
25. Arslan O. Motor neurons. *Neuroanatomical Basis of Clinical Neurology*. New York: The Parthenon Publishing Group; 2001:361–385.
26. Nauta WJ, Feirtag M. Descending paths; the motor system. *Fundamental Neuroanatomy*. New York, NY: WH Freeman; 1986:91–107.
27. Passingham R. Lateral premotor cortex (area 6). *The Frontal Lobes and Voluntary Action*. Oxford: Oxford University Press; 1993:38–68.
28. Goldman-Rakic PS. Anatomical and functional circuits in prefrontal cortex of nonhuman primates—relevance to epilepsy. *Adv Neurol*. 1995;66:51–65.
29. Terada K, Usui N, Umeoka S, et al. Interhemispheric connection of motor areas in humans. *J Clin Neurophysiol*. 2008;25(6):351–356.
30. Lüders HO. Symptomatogenic areas and electrical stimulation. In: Lüders HO, Noachtar S, eds. *Epileptic Seizures—Pathophysiology and Clinical Semiology*. Philadelphia: Churchill Livingstone; 2000:131–140.
31. Lesser RP, Gordon B. Methodologic considerations in cortical electrical stimulation in adults. In: Lüders HO, Noachtar S, eds. *Epileptic Seizures—Pathophysiology and Clinical Semiology*. Philadelphia: Churchill Livingstone; 2000:153–165.
32. Nathan SS, Sinha SR, Gordon B, et al. Determination of current density distributions generated by electrical stimulation of the human cerebral cortex. *Electroencephalogr Clin Neurophysiol*. 1993;86(3):183–192.
33. Arzimanoglou A, Guerrini R, Aicardi J. *Aicardi's pilepsy in Children*. Philadelphia: Lippincott Williams & Wilkins; 2004.
34. Lüders HO, Dinner DS, Morris HH, et al. Cortical electrical stimulation in humans. The negative motor areas. *Adv Neurol*. 1995;67:115–129.
35. Mikuni N, Ohara S, Ikeda A, et al. Evidence for a wide distribution of negative motor areas in the perirolandic cortex. *Clin Neurophysiol*. 2006;117(1):33–40.
36. White LE, Andrews TJ, Hulette C, et al. Structure of the human sensorimotor system. I: Morphology and cytoarchitecture of the central sulcus. *Cereb Cortex*. 1997;7(1):18–30.
37. Zilles K, Schlaug G, Matelli M, et al. Mapping of human and macaque sensorimotor areas by integrating architectonic, transmitter receptor, MRI and PET data. *J Anat*. 1995;187(Pt 3):515–537.
38. Yousry TA, Schmid UD, Alkadhi H, et al. Localization of the motor hand area to a knob on the precentral gyrus. A new landmark. *Brain*. 1997;120(Pt 1):141–157.

39. Naidich TP, Brightbill TC. The pars marginalis. I. A "bracket" sign for the central sulcus in axial plane CT and MRI. *Int J Neuroradiol.* 1996;2:3–19.

40. Penfield W, Jasper H. *Epilepsy and the Functional Anatomy of the Human Brain.* Boston: Little, Brown & Company; 1954.

41. Penfield W, Rasmussen T. *The Cerebral Cortex of Man—A Clinical Study of Localization of Function.* New York: The MacMillan Company; 1950.

42. Krakauer J, Ghez C. Voluntary movement. In: Kandel ER, Schwartz JH, Jessell TM, eds. *Principles of Neural Science.* New York: McGraw-Hill; 2000:756–781.

43. Donoghue JP. Plasticity of adult sensorimotor representations. *Curr Opin Neurobiol.* 1995;5(6):749–754.

44. Kotagal P, Lüders HO. Simple motor seizures. In: Engel J, Pedley TA, edis. *Epilepsy: The Comprehensive CD-Rom.* Philadelphia: Lippincott Williams & Wilkins; 1999.

45. Neuloh G, Schramm J. Intraoperative neurophysiological mapping and monitoring. In: Deletis V, Shils JL, eds. *Neurophysiology in Neurosurgery—A Modern Intraoperative Approach.* San Diego: Academic Press; 2002: 339–401.

46. Wood CC, Spencer DD, Allison T, et al. Localization of human sensori-motor cortex during surgery by cortical surface recording of somatosen-sory evoked potentials. *J Neurosurg.* 1988;68(1):99–111.

47. Toga AW, Ojemann GA, Ojemann JG, et al. Intraoperative brain map-ping. In: Toga AW, Mazziotta JC, Frackowiak RSJ, eds. *Brain Mapping: The Disorders.* San Diego: Academic Press; 2000:77–105.

48. Nii Y, Uematsu S, Lesser RP, et al. Does the central sulcus divide motor and sensory functions? Cortical mapping of human hand areas as revealed by electrical stimulation through subdural grid electrodes. *Neurology.* 1996;46(2):360–367.

49. Lado FA, Legatt AD, LaSala PA, et al. Alteration of the cortical motor map in a patient with intractable focal seizures. *J Neurol Neurosurg Psychiatry.* 2002;72(6):812–815.

50. Dinner DS. Supplementary sensorimotor area epilepsy. In: Bazil CW, Malow BA, Sammaritano MR, eds. *Sleep and Epilepsy: The Clinical Spectrum.* Amsterdam: Elsevier; 2002:223–236.

51. Wiesendanger M. Recent developments in studies of the supplementary motor area of primates. *Rev Physiol Biochem Pharmacol.* 1986;103:1–59.

52. Sanides F. Functional architecture of motor and sensory cortices in pri-mates in the light of a new concept of neocortex evolution. In: Noback R, Montagna W, eds. *The Primate Brain.* New York, NY: Appleton; 1970:137–208.

53. Zilles K, Schlaug G, Geyer S, et al. Anatomy and transmitter receptors of the supplementary motor areas in the human and nonhuman primate brain. *Adv Neurol.* 1996;70:29–43.

54. Wise SP. The primate premotor cortex: past, present, and preparatory. *Annu Rev Neurosci.* 1985;8:1–19.

55. Tanji J. New concepts of the supplementary motor area. *Curr Opin Neurobiol.* 1996;6(6):782–787.

56. Vorobiev V, Govoni P, Rizzolatti G, et al. Parcellation of human mesial area 6: cytoarchitectonic evidence for three separate areas. *Eur J Neurosci.* 1998;10(6):2199–2203.

57. Penfield W, Welch K. The supplementary motor area in the cerebral cortex of man. *Trans Am Neurol Assoc.* 1949;74:179–184.

58. Lim SH, Dinner DS, Pillay PK, et al. Functional anatomy of the human supplementary sensorimotor area: results of extraoperative electrical stim-ulation. *Electroencephalogr Clin Neurophysiol.* 1994;91(3):179–193.

59. Talairach J, Bancaud J. The supplementary motor area in man (anatomo-functional findings by stereo-encephalography in epilepsy). *Int J Neurol.* 1966;5:330–347.

60. Fried I, Katz A, McCarthy G, et al. Functional organization of human supplementary motor cortex studied by electrical stimulation. *J Neurosci.* 1991;11(11):3656–3666.

61. Ikeda A, Luders HO, Burgess RC, et al. Movement-related potentials recorded from supplementary motor area and primary motor area: role of supplementary motor area in voluntary movements. *Brain.* 1992;115(Pt 4): 1017–1043.

62. Ikeda A, Luders HO, Burgess RC, et al. Movement-related potentials associated with single and repetitive movements recorded from human supplementary motor area. *Electroencephalogr Clin Neurophysiol.* 1993;89(4):269–277.

63. Ikeda A, Luders HO, Shibasaki H, et al. Movement-related potentials associated with bilateral simultaneous and unilateral movements recorded from human supplementary motor area. *Electroencephalogr Clin Neurophysiol.* 1995;95(5):323–334.

64. Fulton JF. A note on the definition of the "motor" and "premotor" areas. *Brain.* 1935;58:311–316.

65. Baleydier C, Achache P, Froment JC. Neurofilament architecture of supe-rior and mesial premotor cortex in the human brain. *Neuroreport.* 1997;8(7):1691–1696.

66. Dum RP, Strick PL. The origin of corticospinal projections from the pre-motor areas in the frontal lobe. *J Neurosci.* 1991;11(3):667–689.

67. Schluter ND, Rushworth MF, Mills KR, et al. Signal-, set-, and move-ment-related activity in the human premotor cortex. *Neuropsychologia.* 1999;37(2):233–243.

68. Schubotz RI, von Cramon DY. Functional-anatomical concepts of human premotor cortex: evidence from fMRI and PET studies. *Neuroimage.* 2003;20(Suppl 1):S120–S31.

69. Vogt C, Vogt OJ. Allgemeine Ergebnisse unserer Hirnforschung. *J Psychol Neurol.* 1919;25(Suppl 1):273–462.

70. Duffau H, Capelle L, Denvil D, et al. The role of dominant premotor cor-tex in language: a study using intraoperative functional mapping in awake patients. *Neuroimage.* 2003;20(4):1903–1914.

71. Blanke O, Spinelli L, Thut G, et al. Location of the human frontal eye field as defined by electrical cortical stimulation: anatomical, functional and electrophysiological characteristics. *Neuroreport.* 2000;11(9): 1907–1913.

72. Godoy J, Lüders H, Dinner DS, et al. Versive eye movements elicited by cortical stimulation of the human brain. *Neurology.* 1990;40(2): 296–299.

73. Luna B, Thulborn KR, Strojwas MH, et al. Dorsal cortical regions sub-serving visually guided saccades in humans: an fMRI study. *Cereb Cortex.* 1998;8(1):40–47.

74. Paus T. Location and function of the human frontal eye-field: a selective review. *Neuropsychologia.* 1996;34(6):475–483.

75. ILAE. Proposal for revised clinical and electroencephalographic classifica-tion of epileptic seizures. From the Commission on Classification and Terminology of the International League Against Epilepsy. *Epilepsia.* 1981;22:489–501.

76. Engel Jr J. A proposed diagnostic scheme for people with epileptic seizures and with epilepsy: report of the ILAE task force on classification and ter-minology. *Epilepsia.* 2001;42(6):796–803.

77. Blume WT, Lüders HO, Mizrahi E, et al. Glossary of descriptive terminol-ogy for ictal semiology: report of the ILAE task force on classification and terminology. *Epilepsia.* 2001;42(9):1212–1218.

78. Lüders HO, Burgess R, Noachtar S. Expanding the international classifi-cation of seizures to provide localization information. *Neurology.* 1993;43(9):1650–1655.

79. Wagner AL. A clinical and epidemiological study of adult patients with epilepsy. *Acta Neurol Scand Suppl.* 1983;94:63–72.

80. Mauguiere F, Courjon J. Somatosensory epilepsy: a review of 127 cases. *Brain.* 1978;101(2):307–332.

81. Devinsky O, Kelley K, Porter RJ, et al. Clinical and electroencephalographic features of simple partial seizures. *Neurology.* 1988;38(9):1347–1352.

82. Todd RB. *Clinical Lectures on Paralysis, Certain Diseases of the Brain, and Other Affections of the Nervous System.* 2nd ed. London: John Churchill; 1856.

83. Kellinghaus C, Kotagal P. Lateralizing value of Todd's palsy in patients with epilepsy. *Neurology.* 2004;62(2):289–291.

84. Noachtar S, Arnold S. Clonic seizures. In: Lüders HO, Noachtar S, eds. *Epileptic Seizures: Pathophysiology and Clinical Semiology.* Philadelphia: Churchill Livingstone; 2000:412–424.

85. Matsuo F. Partial epileptic seizures beginning in the truncal muscles. *Acta Neurol Scand.* 1984;69(5):264–269.

86. Holmes G. Local epilepsy. *Lancet.* 1927(1):957–962.

87. Sengoku A. The contribution of J. H. Jackson to present-day epileptology. *Epilepsia.* 2002;43(Suppl 9):6–8.

88. Holowach J, Thurston DL, O'Leary J. Jacksonian seizures in infancy and childhood. *J Pediatr.* 1958;52(6):670–686.

89. Faught E. Clinical presentations and phenomenology of myoclonus. *Epilepsia.* 2003;44(Suppl 11):7–12.

90. Hallett M. Myoclonus: relation to epilepsy. *Epilepsia.* 1985;26(Suppl 1): S67–S77.

91. Leppik IE. Classification of the myoclonic epilepsies. *Epilepsia.* 2003;44(Suppl 11):2–6.

92. Serratosa JM. Myoclonic seizures. In: Wyllie E, edr. *The Treatment of Epilepsy, Principles and Practice.* 3rd ed. Philadelphia: Lippincott Williams and Wilkins; 2001:395–404.

93. Gastaut H. Semeiology of myoclonus and analytic nosology of myoclonic syndromes. *Rev Neurol (Paris).* 1968;119(1):1–30.

94. Noachtar S, Peters AS. Semiology of epileptic seizures: a critical review. *Epilepsy Behav.* 2009;15(1):2–9.

95. Kuzniecky R, Berkovic S, Andermann F, et al. Focal cortical myoclonus and rolandic cortical dysplasia: clarification by magnetic resonance imag-ing. *Ann Neurol.* 1988;23(4):317–325.

96. Tassinari CA, Rubboli G, Parmeggiani L, et al. Epileptic negative myoclonus. *Adv Neurol.* 1995;67:181–197.

97. Lüders HO, Noachtar S, Burgess RC. Semiologic classification of epileptic seizures. In: Lüders HO, Noachtar S, eds. *Epileptic Seizures—Pathophysiology and Clinical Semiology.* Philadelphia: Churchill Livingstone; 2000:263–285.

98. Bleasel AF, Lüders HO. Tonic seizures. In: Lüders HO, Noachtar S, eds. *Epileptic Seizures—Pathophysiology and Clinical Semiology.* Philadelphia: Churchill Livingstone; 2000:389–411.

99. Geier S, Bancaud J, Talairach J, et al. The seizures of frontal lobe epilepsy: a study of clinical manifestations. *Neurology.* 1977;27(10):951–958.

100. Chauvel P, Trottier S, Vignal JP, et al. Somatomotor seizures of frontal lobe origin. *Adv Neurol.* 1992;57:185–232.

101. Werhahn KJ, Noachtar S, Arnold S, et al. Tonic seizures: their significance for lateralization and frequency in different focal epileptic syndromes. *Epilepsia.* 2000;41(9):1153–1161.

102. Egli M, Mothersill I, O'Kane M, et al. The axial spasm—the predominant type of drop seizure in patients with secondary generalized epilepsy. *Epilepsia.* 1985;26(5):401–415.

103. Fromm GH. The brain-stem and seizures: summary and synthesis. In: Fromm GH, Feingold CL, Browning RA, eds. *Epilepsy and the Reticular Formation: The Role of the Reticular Core in Convulsive Seizures.* New York: Alan R Liss; 1987.

104. Horita H, Kumagai K, Maekawa K. Overnight polygraphic study of Lennox-Gastaut syndrome. *Brain Dev.* 1987;9(6):627–635.

105. Wyllie E, Luders H, Morris HH, et al. The lateralizing significance of versive head and eye movements during epileptic seizures. *Neurology.* 1986;36(5):606–611.

106. McLachlan RS. The significance of head and eye turning in seizures. *Neurology.* 1987;37(10):1617–1619.

107. Rasmussen T, Penfield W. Movement of head and eyes from stimulation of the human frontal cortex. *Res Pub Assoc Res Nerv Mental Dis.* 1947;27:346–361.

108. Ochs R, Gloor P, Quesney F, et al. Does head-turning during a seizure have lateralizing or localizing significance? *Neurology.* 1984;34(7):884–890.

109. Quesney LF. Clinical and EEG features of complex partial seizures of temporal lobe origin. *Epilepsia.* 1986;27(Suppl 2):S27–S45.

110. Robillard A, Saint-Hilaire JM, Mercier M, et al. The lateralizing and localizing value of adversion in epileptic seizures. *Neurology.* 1983;33(9):1241–1242.

111. Chee MW, Kotagal P, Van Ness PC, et al. Lateralizing signs in intractable partial epilepsy: blinded multiple-observer analysis. *Neurology.* 1993;43(12):2519–2525.

112. Kotagal P, Arunkumar GS. Lateral frontal lobe seizures. *Epilepsia.* 1998;39(Suppl 4):S62–S68.

113. Kanner AM, Morris HH, Luders H, et al. Supplementary motor seizures mimicking pseudoseizures: some clinical differences. *Neurology.* 1990;40(9):1404–1407.

114. Gabor AJ. *Physiological Basis of Electrical Activity of Cerebral Origin.* Quincy, MA: Grass Instrument Co.; 1978.

115. Dinner DS, Lüders HO, Shih-Hui L, et al. Electrical stimulation of the supplementary sensorimotor area. In: Lüders HO, Noachtar S, eds. *Epileptic Seizures—Pathophysiology and Clinical Semiology.* Philadelphia: Churchill Livingstone; 2000:192–198.

116. Gibbs EL, Gibbs FA. Diagnostic and localizing value of electroencephalographic studies in sleep. *Proc Assoc Res Nerv Ment Dis.* 2004;26:366–376.

117. Martins dS, Aarts JH, Binnie CD, et al. The circadian distribution of interictal epileptiform EEG activity. *Electroencephalogr Clin Neurophysiol.* 1984;58(1):1–13.

118. Rossi GF, Colicchio G, Pola P. Interictal epileptic activity during sleep: a stereo-EEG study in patients with partial epilepsy. *Electroencephalogr Clin Neurophysiol.* 1984;58(2):97–106.

119. Kanner AM, Jones JC. When do sphenoidal electrodes yield additional data to that obtained with antero-temporal electrodes? *Electroencephalogr Clin Neurophysiol.* 1997;102(1):12–19.

120. Morris HH, III, Luders H, Lesser RP, et al. The value of closely spaced scalp electrodes in the localization of epileptiform foci: a study of 26 patients with complex partial seizures. *Electroencephalogr Clin Neurophysiol.* 1986;63(2):107–111.

121. Sperling MR, Engel Jr J. Electroencephalographic recording from the temporal lobes: a comparison of ear, anterior temporal, and nasopharyngeal electrodes. *Ann Neurol.* 1985;17(5):510–513.

122. Pedley TA, Mendiratta A, Walczak TS. Seizures and epilepsy. In: Ebersole JS, Pedley TA, eds. *Current Practice of Clinical Electroencephalography.* Philadelphia: Lippincott Williams & Wilkins; 2003:506–587.

123. Salanova V, Morris HH, III, Van Ness PC, et al. Comparison of scalp electroencephalogram with subdural electrocorticogram recordings and functional mapping in frontal lobe epilepsy. *Arch Neurol.* 1993;50(3):294–299.

124. Rasmussen T. Characteristics of a pure culture of frontal lobe epilepsy. *Epilepsia.* 1983;24(4):482–493.

125. Tükel K, Jasper H. The electroencephalogram in parasagittal regions. *Electroencephalogr Clin Neurophysiol.* 1952;4:481–494.

126. Lee SK, Kim JY, Hong KS, et al. The clinical usefulness of ictal surface EEG in neocortical epilepsy. *Epilepsia.* 2000;41(11):1450–1455.

127. Miyakoshi M, Yagi K, Osawa T, et al. Correlative study on symptomatology of epileptic seizures—behavioral manifestation and electroencephalographic modalities. *Folia Psychiatr Neurol Jpn.* 1977;31(3):451–461.

128. Kobayashi K, Inoue T, Watanabe Y, et al. Spectral analysis of EEG gamma rhythms associated with tonic seizures in Lennox-Gastaut syndrome. *Epilepsy Res.* 2009;86(1):15–22.

129. Quesney LF, Constain M, Rasmussen T, et al. Presurgical EEG investigation in frontal lobe epilepsy. In: Theodore W, ed. *Surgical Treatment of Epilepsy.* Amsterdam: Elsevier; 1992:55–69.

130. Hamer HM, Luders HO, Knake S, et al. Electrophysiology of focal clonic seizures in humans: a study using subdural and depth electrodes. *Brain.* 2003;126(Pt 3):547–555.

131. Logroscino G, Hesdorffer DC, Cascino G, et al. Time trends in incidence, mortality, and case-fatality after first episode of status epilepticus. *Epilepsia.* 2001;42(8):1031–1035.

132. Gastaut H, Roger A. Une forme inhabituelle de l'épilepsie: le nystagmus épileptique. *Rev Neurol.* 1954;90:(130):132.

133. Kanazawa O, Sengoku A, Kawai I. Oculoclonic status epilepticus. *Epilepsia.* 1989;30(1):121–123.

134. Kojewnikoff AY. Eine besondere form von corticaler epilepsie. *Neurologie Zentralblatt.* 1895;14:47–48.

135. Engel J. Can we replace the terms "focal" and "generalized"? In: Hirsch E, Andermann F, Chauvel P, Engel J, Lopes da Silva F, Lüders H, eds. *Generalized Seizures: From Clinical Phenomology to Underlying Systems and Networks.* Montrouge, France: John Libbey Eurotext; 2006: 263–285.

136. Bancaud J, Bonis A, Trottier S, et al. L'epilepsie partielle continue: syndrome et maladie. *Rev Neurol (Paris).* 1982;138(11):803–814.

137. Cockerell OC, Rothwell J, Thompson PD, et al. Clinical and physiological features of epilepsia partialis continua. Cases ascertained in the UK. *Brain.* 1996;119(Pt 2):393–407.

138. ILAE. Proposal for revised classification of epilepsies and epileptic syndromes. Commission on classification and terminology of the International League Against Epilepsy. *Epilepsia.* 1989;30(4): 389–399.

139. Lohler J, Peters UH. Epilepsia partialis continua (Kozevnikov epilepsy). *Fortschr Neurol Psychiatr Grenzgeb.* 1974;42(4):165–212.

140. Obeso JA, Rothwell JC, Marsden CD. The spectrum of cortical myoclonus. From focal reflex jerks to spontaneous motor epilepsy. *Brain.* 1985;108(Pt 1):193–224.

141. Thomas JE, Reagan TJ, Klass DW. Epilepsia partialis continua: a review of 32 cases. *Arch Neurol.* 1977;34(5):266–275.

142. Wieser HG, Graf HP, Bernoulli C, et al. Quantitative analysis of intracerebral recordings in epilepsia partialis continua. *Electroencephalogr Clin Neurophysiol.* 1978;44(1):14–22.

143. Bien CG, Elger CE. Epilepsia partialis continua: semiology and differential diagnoses. *Epileptic Disord.* 2008;10(1):3–7.

144. Panayiotopoulos CP. Kozhevnikov-Rasmussen syndrome and the new proposal on classification. *Epilepsia.* 2002;43(8):948–949.

145. Hess DC, Sethi KD. Epilepsia partialis continua in multiple sclerosis. *Int J Neurosci.* 1990;50(1–2):109–111.

146. Bartolomei F, Gavaret M, Dhiver C, et al. Isolated, chronic, epilepsia partialis continua in an HIV-infected patient. *Arch Neurol.* 1999;56(1): 111–114.

147. Ferrari S, Monaco S, Morbin M, et al. HIV-associated PML presenting as epilepsia partialis continua. *J Neurol Sci.* 1998;161(2):180–184.

148. Lee K, Haight E, Olejniczak P. Epilepsia partialis continua in Creutzfeldt-Jakob disease. *Acta Neurol Scand.* 2000;102(6):398–402.

149. Antozzi C, Franceschetti S, Filippini G, et al. Epilepsia partialis continua associated with NADH-coenzyme Q reductase deficiency. *J Neurol Sci.* 1995;129(2):152–161.

150. Veggiotti P, Colamaria V, Dalla BB, et al. Epilepsia partialis continua in a case of MELAS: clinical and neurophysiological study. *Neurophysiol Clin.* 1995;25(3):158–166.

151. Wilson DC, McGibben D, Hicks EM, et al. Progressive neuronal degeneration of childhood (Alpers syndrome) with hepatic cirrhosis. *Eur J Pediatr.* 1993;152(3):260–262.

152. Schomer DL. Focal status epilepticus and epilepsia partialis continua in adults and children. *Epilepsia.* 1993;34(Suppl 1):S29–S36.

153. Singh BM, Strobos RJ. Epilepsia partialis continua associated with nonketotic hyperglycemia: clinical and biochemical profile of 21 patients. *Ann Neurol.* 1980;8(2):155–160.

154. Placidi F, Floris R, Bozzao A, et al. Ketotic hyperglycemia and epilepsia partialis continua. *Neurology.* 2001;57(3):534–537.

155. Cock HR, Shorvon SD. The spectrum of epilepsy and movement disorders in EPC. In: Guerrini R, Aicardi J, Andermann F, Hallett M, eds. *Epilepsy and Movement Disorders.* Cambridge, U.K.: Cambridge University Press; 2002:211–226.

156. Shorvon S. Clinical forms of status epilepticus. *Status Epilepticus: Its Clinical Features and Treatment in Children and Adults.* Cambridge: Cambridge University Press; 1994:84–98.

157. Gurer G, Saygi S, Ciger A. Epilepsia partialis continua: clinical and electrophysiological features of adult patients. *Clin Electroencephalogr.* 2001;32(1):1–9.

158. PeBenito R, Cracco JB. Periodic lateralized epileptiform discharges in infants and children. *Ann Neurol.* 1979;6(1):47–50.

159. Westmoreland BF, Klass DW, Sharbrough FW. Chronic periodic lateralized epileptiform discharges. *Arch Neurol.* 1986;43(5):494–496.

160. Pohlmann-Eden B, Hoch DB, Cochius JI, et al. Periodic lateralized epileptiform discharges—a critical review. *J Clin Neurophysiol.* 1996;13(6): 519–530.

161. Lüders HO, Noachtar S. *Atlas and Classification of Electroencephalography.* Philadelphia: WB Saunders; 2000.

162. Garzon E, Fernandes RM, Sakamoto AC. Serial EEG during human status epilepticus: evidence for PLED as an ictal pattern. *Neurology.* 2001;57(7):1175–1183.

163. Garcia-Morales I, Garcia MT, Galan-Davila L, et al. Periodic lateralized epileptiform discharges: etiology, clinical aspects, seizures, and evolution in 130 patients. *J Clin Neurophysiol.* 2002;19(2):172–177.

164. Snodgrass SM, Tsuburaya K, Ajmone-Marsan C. Clinical significance of periodic lateralized epileptiform discharges: relationship with status epilepticus. *J Clin Neurophysiol.* 1989;6(2):159–172.

165. Hajek M, Antonini A, Leenders KL, et al. Epilepsia partialis continua studied by PET. *Epilepsy Res.* 1991;9(1):44–48.

166. Laich E, Kuzniecky R, Mountz J, et al. Supplementary sensorimotor area epilepsy: seizure localization, cortical propagation and subcortical activation pathways using ictal SPECT. *Brain.* 1997;120(Pt 5):855–864.

167. Morris HH, III. Supplementary motor seizures. In: Wyllie E, ed. *The Treatment of Epilepsy: Principles and Practice.* 1st ed. Philadelphia: Lea & Febiger; 1993:541–546.
168. Lim SH, Dinner DS, Luders HO. Cortical stimulation of the supplementary sensorimotor area. *Adv Neurol.* 1996;70:187–197.
169. Morris HH, III, Dinner DS, Luders H, et al. Supplementary motor seizures: clinical and electroencephalographic findings. *Neurology.* 1988;38(7):1075–1082.
170. Ajmone-Marsan C, Ralston BL. The epileptic seizure: its functional morphology and diagnostic significance. *A Clinical-Electroencephalographic Anslysis of Metrazole-Induced Attacks.* Springfield, IL: Charles C. Thomas; 1957.
171. Quesney LF, Constain M, Fish DR, et al. The clinical differentiation of seizures arising in the parasagittal and anterolaterodorsal frontal convexities. *Arch Neurol.* 1990;47(6):677–679.
172. So NK. Mesial frontal epilepsy. *Epilepsia.* 1998;39(Suppl 4):S49–S61.
173. Barba C, Doglietto F, Policicchio D, et al. Unusual ipsilateral hyperkinetic automatisms in SMA seizures. *Seizure.* 2005;14(5):354–361.
174. Bass N, Wyllie E, Comair Y, et al. Supplementary sensorimotor area seizures in children and adolescents. *J Pediatr.* 1995;126(4):537–544.
175. Anand I, Dinner DS. Relationship of supplementary motor area epilepsy and sleep. *Epilepsia.* 1997;38(S8):48–49.
176. Lüders HO. The supplementary sensorimotor area: an overview. *Adv Neurol.* 1996;70:1–16.
177. Aghakhani Y, Rosati A, Olivier A, et al. The predictive localizing value of tonic limb posturing in supplementary sensorimotor seizures. *Neurology.* 2004;62(12):2256–2261.
178. Ikeda A, Sato T, Ohara S, et al. "Supplementary motor area (SMA) seizure" rather than "SMA epilepsy" in optimal surgical candidates: a document of subdural mapping. *J Neurol Sci.* 2002;202(1–2):43–52.
179. Bleasel AF, Morris HH, III. Supplementary sensorimotor area epilepsy in adults. *Adv Neurol.* 1996;70:271–284.
180. Pedley TA, Tharp BR, Herman K. Clinical and electroencephalographic characteristics of midline parasagittal foci. *Ann Neurol.* 1981;9(2):142–149.
181. Adelman S, Lueders H, Dinner DS, et al. Paradoxical lateralization of parasagittal sharp waves in a patient with epilepsia partialis continua. *Epilepsia.* 1982;23(3):291–295.
182. Krauss GL, Mathews GC. Similarities in mechanisms and treatments for epileptic and nonepileptic myoclonus. *Epilepsy Curr.* 2003;3(1):19–21.
183. Plant G. Spinal meningioma presenting as focal epilepsy. *Br Med J (Clin Res Ed).* 1981;282(6280):1974–1975.
184. Waubant E, Alize P, Tourbah A, et al. Paroxysmal dystonia (tonic spasm) in multiple sclerosis. *Neurology.* 2001;57(12):2320–2321.
185. Mahone EM, Bridges D, Prahme C, et al. Repetitive arm and hand movements (complex motor stereotypies) in children. *J Pediatr.* 2004;145(3):391–395.
186. Plant G. Focal paroxysmal kinesigenic choreoathetosis. *J Neurol Neurosurg Psychiatry.* 1983;46(4):345–348.
187. Vanasse M, Bedard P, Andermann F. Shuddering attacks in children: an early clinical manifestation of essential tremor. *Neurology.* 1976;26(11):1027–1030.
188. Saygi S, Katz A, Marks DA, et al. Frontal lobe partial seizures and psychogenic seizures: comparison of clinical and ictal characteristics. *Neurology.* 1992;42(7):1274–1277.
189. Vaughn BV. Differential diagnosis of paroxysmal nocturnal events in adults. In: Bazil CW, Malow BA, Sammaritano MR, eds. *Sleep and Epilepsy: The Clinical Spectrum.* 1st ed. Amsterdam: Elsevier Science B.V.; 2002:325–338.
190. Sammaritano MR. Focal epilepsy and sleep. In: Dinner DS, Lüders HO, eds. *Epilepsy and Sleep: Physiologic and Clinical Relationships.* San Diego: Academic Press; 2001:85–100.
191. Crespel A, Baldy-Moulinier M, Coubes P. The relationship between sleep and epilepsy in frontal and temporal lobe epilepsies: practical and physiopathologic considerations. *Epilepsia.* 1998;39(2):150–157.
192. Scheffer IE, Bhatia KP, Lopes-Cendes I, et al. Autosomal dominant nocturnal frontal lobe epilepsy: a distinctive clinical disorder. *Brain.* 1995;118(Pt 1):61–73.
193. Scheffer IE, Bhatia KP, Lopes-Cendes I, et al. Autosomal dominant frontal epilepsy misdiagnosed as sleep disorder. *Lancet.* 1994;343(8896):515–517.
194. Anderson E, Berkovic S, Dulac O, et al. ILAE genetics commission conference report: molecular analysis of complex genetic epilepsies. *Epilepsia.* 2002;43(10):1262–1267.
195. Bertrand D, Picard F, Le Hellard S, et al. How mutations in the nAChRs can cause ADNFLE epilepsy. *Epilepsia.* 2002;43(Suppl 5):112–122.
196. Baquis GD, Pessin MS, Scott RM. Limb shaking—a carotid TIA. *Stroke.* 1985;16(3):444–448.
197. Schulz UG, Rothwell PM. Transient ischaemic attacks mimicking focal motor seizures. *Postgrad Med J.* 2002;78(918):246–247.
198. Yanagihara T, Piepgras DG, Klass DW. Repetitive involuntary movement associated with episodic cerebral ischemia. *Ann Neurol.* 1985;18(2):244–250.
199. Baumgartner RW, Baumgartner I. Vasomotor reactivity is exhausted in transient ischaemic attacks with limb shaking. *J Neurol Neurosurg Psychiatry.* 1998;65(4):561–564.

CHAPTER 14 ■ GENERALIZED TONIC–CLONIC SEIZURES

TIM WEHNER

Generalized tonic–clonic seizures (GTCSs) are among the most commonly encountered seizures in both children and adults. More than half of all patients with epilepsy may experience a GTCS in the course of their illness (1). A GTCS may have a generalized onset (primarily GTCS), or it may begin focally, followed by secondary generalization (secondarily GTCS) (2). "Generalized" or "generalization" is commonly defined as the simultaneous, symmetrical, and synchronous involvement of both cerebral hemispheres. The limitations of this definition are discussed later in this chapter.

The glossary of descriptive terminology for ictal semiology provided by the International League Against Epilepsy (ILAE) task force describes a tonic–clonic seizure as "a sequence consisting of a tonic followed by a clonic phase. Variants such as clonic–tonic–clonic may be seen" (3).

GTCSs occur in a variety of both generalized and focal epilepsy syndromes as well as both idiopathic and symptomatic epilepsies. Examples of generalized epilepsy syndromes that may manifest with GTCSs are childhood absence epilepsy, juvenile myoclonic epilepsy, myoclonic-astatic epilepsy, and generalized epilepsy with febrile seizures plus. Idiopathic focal epilepsy syndromes that may manifest with GTCSs include benign focal epilepsy of childhood and autosomal dominant nocturnal frontal lobe epilepsy. Symptomatic epilepsies that may comprise GTCS include progressive myoclonic epilepsies (such as Unverricht–Lundborg disease), epilepsy seen in the setting of neuronal ceroid lipofuscinosis, as well as epilepsy complicating diffuse brain disorders or lesions such as Alzheimer disease, hypoxic–ischemic encephalopathy, multiple sclerosis, or meningoencephalitis. All epilepsies related to circumscribed structural brain lesions such as ischemic stroke, intracranial hemorrhage, brain tumors, vascular malformations, infections, or brain development disorders may include GTCSs as well. For this reason, the presence or absence of GTCSs does not help in the diagnosis of a specific epilepsy syndrome.

CLINICAL MANIFESTATIONS

Gastaut and Broughton provided a detailed description of the semiology and pathophysiology of GTCSs (4). They stressed the stereotypical nature of GTCSs and divided them into the following phases:

1. Preictal manifestations
2. Ictal manifestations (with loss of consciousness)
   a. the tonic phase (including an "intermediate vibratory period")
   b. the clonic phase
   c. (concurrent) autonomic changes
3. Immediate postictal features
4. Late postictal features

Video 14.1 illustrates phases 1–3 of a GTCS in a 27-year-old woman with idiopathic generalized epilepsy.

Preictal manifestations of GTCSs, according to Gastaut and Broughton, are brief bilateral myoclonic contractions immediately preceding the onset of the tonic phase. Others define this phase more broadly and include a variety of nonspecific symptoms that may precede a GTCS by hours, sometimes even days. These include anxiety, behavioral withdrawal, changes in appetite, dizziness, headache, irritability, lethargy, lightheadedness, mood changes, and sleep disturbances (5). These symptoms most likely reflect physiologic changes that lower the seizure threshold; they do not represent an epileptic aura.

The tonic phase is typically initiated by a brief phase of flexion that begins in the muscles of the body axis and subsequently spreads to the limb girdles. In the upper limbs, the combination of shoulder and arm elevation and elbow semiflexion results in a "hands-up" gesture, as illustrated in Video 14.1. The lower limbs somewhat less consistently demonstrate a combination of flexion, abduction, and external rotation in the hips. At this moment, the body assumes an emprosthotonic position. The muscular contractions in this stage are most intense in the limb girdle region and decrease towards the periphery.

This tonic flexion is followed by tonic extension that again starts in the axial muscles. Tonic contraction of the thoracoabdominal muscles causes prolonged expiration across the spasmodic glottis, producing the tonic epileptic cry that may last 2 to 12 seconds. The arms become extended with forearm pronation, wrist flexion, and finger extension (as seen in Video 14.1) or wrist extension and fist clenching. The legs move into forced extension in the hip, knee, ankle and toe joints, combined with adduction and external rotation in the hips. Thus, the body assumes an opisthotonic position.

These sustained tetanic muscular contractions then resolve into a tremor of decreasing frequency and increasing amplitude, caused by recurrent decreases in muscle tone. This constitutes the so-called "intermediate vibratory period" that affects the peripheral limb muscles first and subsequently spreads to the limb girdle and axial muscles.

The clonic phase follows when the recurrent contractions of the intermediate vibratory period become prolonged and intense enough to completely interrupt the tonic contraction, thereby producing repetitive myoclonic jerks of progressively decreasing frequency. This phase typically lasts about 30 seconds.

Concurrent autonomic changes include an increase in heart rate and blood pressure, either mediated directly through ictal activation of structures of the central autonomic network (insular cortex, amygdala, hypothalamus, periaqueductal gray matter, parabrachial complex, nucleus of the tractus solitarius, and ventrolateral medulla) (6) or reflecting the high metabolic demand of the tonic and clonic phase. Involvement of the diaphragm and thoracoabdominal muscles during the tonic phase results in insufficient air exchange, which in turn may lead to alveolar hypoventilation causing decrease in blood oxygen saturation and cyanosis (7). Tonic contraction of thoracoabdominal and urinary sphincter muscles also results in up to sixfold increased bladder pressure.

The pupils are markedly dilated; the skin may show piloerection and diffuse perspiration. Hypersecretion of salivary and tracheobronchial glands results in excessive oral secretions, which contribute to the risk of postictal aspiration.

The immediate postictal phase is characterized by a few seconds of muscular flaccidity, during which the loss of bladder sphincter tone can result in urinary incontinence. Following this short period of relaxation, muscle tone increases again, in particular in facial and masticatory muscles. Regular, though often labored, respirations return, as the airway is partially blocked by orotracheal secretions and the closed jaw. Nausea, retching, and vomiting may occur and can result in aspiration if the reflexes protecting the airway are still suppressed.

A longer, late postictal phase follows, during which muscle tone, heart, and respiration rate as well as pupils normalize. The patient gradually awakens, though it may take many minutes to hours until the patient has fully recovered consciousness (8). Tiredness, headache, and diffuse muscle soreness are common. Some patients are belligerent and combative postictally.

Video-EEG studies have demonstrated a marked variability in the semiology of GTCSs. In a study of 120 secondarily GTCSs in 47 patients, only 27% of seizures contained the motor manifestations (myoclonic jerks—tonic phase—intermediate vibratory period—clonic phase) as described by Gastaut. There was marked variability in the duration of the individual phases, even in seizures occurring in the same patient (9).

Asymmetries of the tonic phase were observed in the majority of 35 secondarily GTCSs in 29 patients with pharmacoresistant temporal lobe epilepsy (TLE) studied by Jobst et al. The semiology of individual GTCSs differed in half of the patients who had more than one GTCS, suggesting that the evolution of GTCSs may utilize different pathways in the brain (10).

In two studies of patients with pharmacoresistant temporal lobe epilepsy, the clonic phase of secondarily GTCSs ended asymmetrically in 68% of patients, with the last beat occurring on the side ipsilateral to the electrographical seizure onset in 79% of patients (11,12).

In contrast to the description provided by Gastaut, the mouth was found to be open or partially open during all 64 secondarily GTCSs observed in a study of 13 children. In addition, "jerking" motor activity was observed in the first minute of the postictal phase with little or no EEG correlate in 10 of the 13 children (13).

Asymmetries in the motor manifestations of secondarily GTCSs may provide information about the hemisphere of seizure origin and therefore serve as lateralizing signs. Forced and sustained head version at the onset of a GTCS, with the chin pointing upward, lateralizes the seizure to the contralateral hemisphere with 90% to 100% specificity. Unilateral or asymmetrical tonic limb posture ("figure of four") likewise lateralizes the seizure origin to the hemisphere contralateral to the extended arm with a specificity of more than 90% (14).

Patients with idiopathic generalized epilepsy are infrequently evaluated by video-EEG. Nonetheless, focal features or lateralizing signs have been reported during GTCSs occurring in this patient population as well (15). Head version is described most frequently; it may occur to either site in different GTCSs in the same patient (16).

In a study of 10 GTCSs in patients with idiopathic generalized epilepsy, adversive head turn occurred in six, and asymmetry or asynchrony during the clonic phase was seen in three (17). Another study of GTCSs in 20 patients with idiopathic generalized epilepsy (IGE) found the "figure of four" sign in three patients; tonic unilateral posturing in two; and version, postictal hemiparesis, and unilateral mouth deviation in one patient each (18). Of 26 patients with juvenile myoclonic epilepsy (JME), five patients had lateralizing signs (version to the left or "figure of four") immediately preceding or during a GTCS (19).

Video 14.2 and Fig. 14.2 provide an example of a GTCS with focal semiological features. Here, the initial phase of the seizure is characterized by staring and nonresponsiveness for approximately 30 seconds. At the onset of the convulsive phase, the patient turns her head to the right, this is followed by extension of the left arm and flexion of the right arm in the elbow, combining for a "figure of four" sign. Although the head turn to the right suggests ictal activation of the left hemisphere, it is not forced and sustained enough to qualify as a "lateralizing" version (20). On the other hand, the left arm extension suggests seizure origin in the right hemisphere (21). Note also that there are a few clonic beats at the onset of the convulsive phase, followed by tonic stiffening of the entire body that ultimately progresses into clonic contractions of decreasing frequency, similar to those observed in Video 14.1.

Primarily GTCSs on average are shorter (on average 60 seconds) than secondarily GTCSs (73–93 seconds), in particular if the latter arise from the temporal lobe (9). Observers tend to overestimate the duration of GTCSs or they may include the postictal phase. Video-EEG studies have demonstrated that GTCSs rarely last longer than 3 minutes. If a seizure does not terminate within 3 minutes, it may lead to status epilepticus, and benzodiazepines (rectal diazepam, 0.5 mg/kg in children age 2–5 years, 0.3 mg/kg in children age 6–11 years, 0.2 mg/kg in children older than 12 years) or intravenous lorazepam (0.05–0.1 mg/kg) should be administered. It is not necessary to administer benzodiazepines after a single GTCS has terminated; in fact this may hamper the patient's ability to control his airway and necessitate endotracheal intubation.

GTCSs with the above sequence of events or variations are not seen in infants younger than 6 months and rarely, if ever, in the first three years of life. In two video-EEG studies combining 397 seizures in 145 patients aged 1 to 35 months, not a single GTCS was found (22,23). This is presumably due to immaturity of cortical neurons as well as incomplete myelination of major nerve fiber tracts that mediate the rapid spread of the seizure activity.

Immediately following a GTCS, marked acidosis with arterial pH < 7.0 may be recorded; the acid–base equilibrium is restored within 60 minutes (24). Serum glucose levels may increase transiently, usually less than 200 mg/dL. A minor pleocytosis may be found in the cerebrospinal fluid following a single GTCS (25). Transient elevations in plasma levels of adrenocorticotropic hormone (ACTH), beta endorphin, beta lipotropin, prolactin, and vasopressin, and a later increase in plasma cortisol have been observed following a GTCS, presumably reflecting ictal activation of the hypothalamus (26). Of these, serum prolactin levels may help differentiating generalized seizures from nonepileptic events. The American Academy of Neurology (AAN) has addressed the value of serum prolactin measurements in a guideline published in 2005 (27). Pooled statistical analysis of nine class II and one class I study for the differentiation of GTCSs from nonepileptic seizures revealed a sensitivity of 60% and a specificity of 96%. Thus, the AAN recommends that measurements within 10 to 20 minutes after the event is a useful adjunct for the differentiation of GTCSs or complex-partial seizures from psychogenic nonepileptic seizures in adults and older children. Elevated serum prolactin levels have been demonstrated following syncope as well (28), therefore they cannot be used to differentiate between seizure and syncope.

Postictal serum elevation of creatine kinase is a highly specific though not very sensitive marker for GTCSs (29).

Complications of GTCSs include tongue or oral lacerations, head trauma, posterior dislocation of the shoulder, bone fractures, in particular of the thoracic vertebrae, as well as aspiration pneumonia and pulmonary edema (5). To prevent these complications, it is recommended that observers remove hazardous items from the scene and place the patient in a lateral decubitus position. If the patient needs to be moved, this should be done at the trunk to avoid joint luxations. No attempt should be made to place items between the jaws as this may result in dental injury. In epilepsy monitoring units, oxygen should be administered via a face mask, and oral secretions should be suctioned in the postictal phase.

ELECTROENCEPHALOGRAPHIC MANIFESTATIONS

Interictal Findings

The EEG in patients with idiopathic GTCSs typically contains normal background activity, although rhythmic slowing in the delta or theta range is more common in patients with idiopathic GTCSs as well as their family members compared to the general population. In patients with secondarily GTCSs, nonspecific EEG abnormalities such as background slowing, asymmetries, and generalized or regional slowing are common indirect clues to the symptomatic nature of the epilepsy.

Epileptiform activity is observed in about half of all patients with GTCSs on their first EEG. Interictal generalized epileptiform activity is an incidental finding in only about 1% of healthy humans; therefore, it is a highly specific marker for epilepsy (30). About one third of patients with GTCSs have interictal epileptiform abnormalities on every serial EEG. Four main interictal epileptiform patterns have been described in patients with idiopathic GTCSs:

1. Typical 3-Hz spike-and-wave complexes
2. Spike-and-wave complexes that are irregular in frequency and amplitude; these may be seen in patients with idiopathic or symptomatic epilepsy
3. Four- to 5- Hz spike-and-wave complexes
4. Polyspike complexes of short duration

These patterns may occur in combination in one patient, even in the same recording. Asymmetrical fragments of these patterns are observed in patients with primarily and secondarily GTCSs; asymmetry of a generalized epileptiform discharge therefore by itself does not imply that the patient's epilepsy is focal or symptomatic. In a longitudinal study of a rigorously selected cohort of patients with idiopathic generalized epilepsy and GTCSs, 65% of patients had persistent focal abnormalities (slowing or epileptiform discharges) over a median time frame of 16 years (31). In patients with secondarily GTCSs, focal abnormalities may be observed, reflecting the extent of the irritative zone.

In some patients with focal epilepsy, a focal epileptiform discharge may spread so rapidly throughout the brain that its distribution on scalp EEG resembles that of a "genuine" generalized discharge. This phenomenon is called secondary bilateral synchrony. It may occur as a generalized interictal discharge or at the onset of a generalized EEG seizure. Although generalized epileptiform discharges are not always perfectly symmetrical or synchronous, subtle asymmetries should not be interpreted as secondary bilateral synchrony unless focal epileptiform activity occurs persistently in one area, and precedes and initiates consistently most or all bursts of generalized epileptiform discharges (32,33).

Ictal Findings

The ictal EEG at the onset of a GTCS is ideally recorded simultaneously from the onset over the entire scalp.

The clinical seizure onset may be preceded by preictal generalized bursts of polyspikes, spike-and-wave complexes, or a mixture of both (Fig. 14.1). Tonic contractions of facial and masticatory muscles at the onset of the tonic phase create diffuse muscle artifacts that obscure the ictal EEG, relatively sparing the vertex derivations. The underlying EEG activity may be a brief period (1–3 seconds) of diffuse flattening or low voltage activity of approximately 20 Hz. During the tonic phase, a surface negative rhythm of about 10 Hz evolves with rapidly increasing amplitude, for which Gastaut and Fischer-Williams proposed the term epileptic recruiting rhythm (4). After about 10 seconds, this rhythm is gradually replaced by a slower rhythm that increases in amplitude and decreases in frequency. When the slow activity reaches a frequency of about 4 Hz, polyspike-and-wave-complexes of progressively decreasing frequency become discernible, which are associated with the myoclonic jerks of the clonic phase.

After the final ictal polyspike-and-wave complex, the EEG may become isoelectric for a few seconds before diffuse slow activity in the delta range appears. During the postictal phase, this activity gradually increases in frequency until a normal alpha rhythm returns. This "recovery" of the EEG correlates with the postictal recovery of mental function. Mild degrees of slowing may be observed for more than 24 hours after a single uncomplicated GTCS (5). The EEG corresponding to the seizure in Video 14.1 (Fig. 14.1) illustrates the typical electroencephalographic evolution of a GTCS.

The electroencephalographic patterns of primarily and secondarily GTCSs are virtually indistinguishable once the tonic phase has been established. Rarely, marked asymmetry in the slowing of the postictal phase may provide a lateralizing or even localizing clue in a GTCS that otherwise lacks focal clinical or electrographic features.

Detailed analysis of synchrony using magnetencephalography revealed variations in the extent of synchrony preceding and during different types of seizures. In general, synchrony was higher in generalized absence seizures compared to GTCSs, and in the latter, synchrony was higher locally than globally, and fluctuations in synchrony were observed between specific cortical areas in different seizures in the same patient (34).

Lhatoo and Lüders analyzed nine secondarily GTCSs in nine patients who underwent invasive electrocorticography for medically refractory focal epilepsy. They found asynchronous ictal rhythms occurring in the two hemispheres or even within one hemisphere. These findings suggest that synchronization of brain regions does not appear to be necessary during secondarily GTCSs (35).

Thus, the distinction between GTCSs of generalized and focal onset (primarily and secondarily GTCS) is not always straightforward. Frontal lobe seizures in particular may be characterized by rapid generalization, and neither seizure semiology nor surface EEG may provide clues to the focal onset.

TREATMENT

A monotherapeutic anticonvulsant trial should be the initial approach in any patient presenting with epilepsy. The discussion in this chapter focuses on the initial anticonvulsant treatment of patients with a presenting complaint of new-onset GTCS. Medications that are indicated in rare epilepsy syndromes only as well as epilepsy surgery and stimulation therapies such as vagus nerve stimulation are discussed in detail elsewhere in this book.

Although a considerable number of randomized controlled trials are available comparing individual anticonvulsants with each other or placebos, few if any studies meet the rigorous criteria imposed by expert review committees to determine "best evidence" (36,37). Thus, the ILAE treatment guideline in 2006 stated that GTCSs in children and adults had "no anticonvulsant with level A or B efficacy and effectiveness evidence as initial monotherapy" (38). The practice parameter of the subcommittee of the AAN and the American Epilepsy Society on the newer anticonvulsants (in 2004) found that "lamotrigine, tiagabine, topiramate, and oxcarbazepine are effective in a mixed population of newly diagnosed partial and generalized tonic–clonic seizures. Insufficient data exist to make a recommendation for the syndromes individually" (39). Keeping these limitations in mind, the findings of some key studies on anticonvulsant monotherapy are summarized later in this paragraph.

Studies on anticonvulsants in epilepsy tend to categorize patients according to their epilepsy syndrome rather than seizure types. As discussed above, GTCSs occur in generalized and focal epilepsy syndromes. In clinical practice, the physician may have to choose an anticonvulsant even though description of clinical semiology, interictal EEG findings, and neuroimaging studies may not yield precise information about the patient's epilepsy syndrome. In this situation, a "broad spectrum" anticonvulsant should be used. This group includes lamotrigine (LTG), levetiracetam (LEV), phenobarbital (PB), primidone (PRM), topiramate (TPM), and valproic acid (VPA). Of these, LEV, PB, and VPA can be given intravenously.

If the patient's semiology or EEG clearly indicates a focal epilepsy, carbamazepine (CBZ), gabapentin (GBP), oxcarbazepine (OXC), or phenytoin (PHT, intravenous formulations available) may be used in addition to the above. These anticonvulsants may exacerbate seizures or induce status epilepticus in patients with idiopathic generalized epilepsies (40–42). Thus, they should not be used as initial monotherapy in these patients.

In the Veterans Affairs cooperative study that compared CBZ, PB, PHT, and PRM, no difference was found in control of GTCSs. Patients taking PRM experienced significantly more adverse effects that lead to therapy failure. PHT was associated with dysmorphic effects and hypersensitivity (43). In a follow-up study, VPA was as effective as CBZ for the control of GTCSs; however CBZ was better in a composite score that combined seizure control and side effects (44). No difference was found in terms of efficacy for CBZ, PB, PHT, and VPA in a study conducted in the United Kingdom. More patients discontinued PB and CBZ than PHT and VPA, though the numbers were too small to reach statistical significance (45).

More recently, standard and new antiepileptic drugs were compared in the SANAD study that was undertaken in the United Kingdom. Patients were randomized to anticonvulsants in an unblinded fashion, and both time to one year remission and treatment failure (defined as inadequate seizure control or intolerable side effects) were analyzed as primary outcomes. One part addressed patients with generalized and unclassifiable epilepsies. For these two groups together, VPA was as effective but better tolerated than TPM, whereas no difference was found between VPA and LTG in both measures. In the subgroup of patients with generalized epilepsy, fewer patients failed VPA compared to TPM and LTG. VPA was more effective in controlling seizures compared to LTG, but there was no difference compared to TPM. The authors concluded that in patients with generalized and unclassifiable epilepsies, VPA is better tolerated than TPM and more efficacious than LTG (46). Due to the well-known teratogenic effects of VPA, these results may not apply to women with childbearing potential.

The other part of SANAD addressed patients with focal epilepsies. Fewer patients failed LTG compared to CBZ, GBP, TPM; and LTG had a nonsignificant advantage compared to OXC. CBZ was more efficacious than GBP and had a nonsignificant advantage compared to LTG, OXC, and TPM. The authors concluded that LTG is clinically better than CBZ for time to treatment failure outcomes (47).

Interestingly, these results could not be replicated in a study comparing LTG and sustained-release CBZ in patients age 65 and above with newly diagnosed epilepsy. Whereas LTG had a nonsignificant advantage in terms of tolerability, CBZ had a nonsignificant advantage in terms of efficacy (48).

LEV, which was not evaluated in the SANAD studies, has subsequently been compared with controlled-release (CR) CBZ (49,50), extended-release (ER) VPA (50), or LTG (51) in three recent European studies as a monotherapy option in adults with new-onset epilepsy. To this point, the results of the second (50) and third (51) studies have only been published in abstract form. In the first study (49), LEV and CR-CBZ were equally effective and time to discontinuation was equal for LEV and CR-CBZ. In the second study (50), time to first seizure was slightly longer in subjects randomized to CR-CBZ or ER-VPA. In both of these studies, fewer patients discontinued LEV due to adverse events, though this finding did not

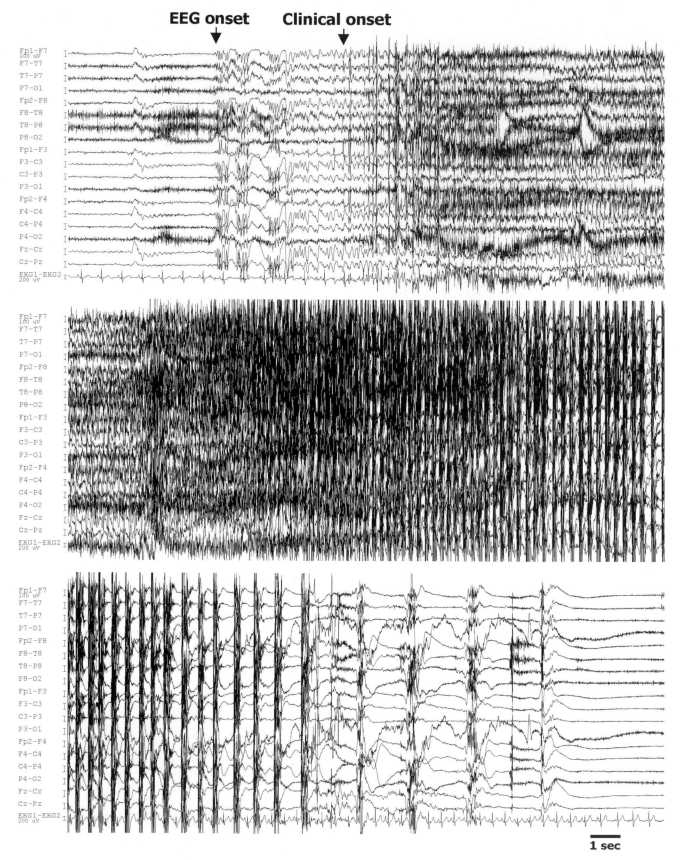

FIGURE 14.1. EEG corresponding to Video 14.1, subsequent 20-second pages. At seizure onset, the EEG is characterized by generalized 5-Hz polyspike-and-wave complexes, subsequently it becomes obscured by muscle artifacts, with relative sparing of the vertex channels (Fz-Cz and Cz-Pz). Towards the seizure end, the frequency of the spike-and-wave complexes decreases to 2 Hz. Note the postictal flattening of the EEG. Scalebar 1 second.

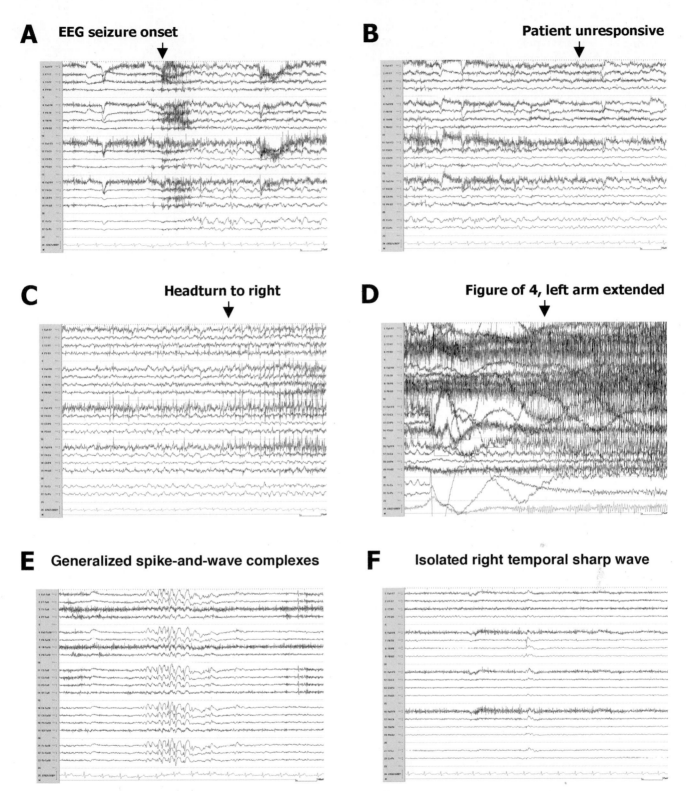

A   EEG seizure onset

B   Patient unresponsive

C   Headturn to right

D   Figure of 4, left arm extended

E Generalized spike-and-wave complexes

F   Isolated right temporal sharp wave

FIGURE 14.2. EEG findings in the patient whose seizure is shown in Video 14.2, 10-second pages.
A: EEG onset of the seizure is characterized by rhythmic slowing. Generalized spike-and-wave complexes
are seen a few seconds later, less prominent compared to the seizure in Figure 14.1. The patient initially
seems to be engaged in the conversation with her roommate. A few seconds later, she does not respond to
the monitoring assistant (**B**). At the beginning of the convulsive phase, marked by the head turn to the
right (**C**, 38 seconds after the EEG onset), the frequency of the ictal rhythm increases from 3 to 4.5 Hz.
The potentially lateralizing semiological features occur while the EEG continues to show a generalized
distribution (**C, D**). Note that pages **A** and **B** are continuous, whereas 10-second epochs were omitted
between pages (**B** and **C**) and (**C** and **D**). Interictally, this patient manifested both generalized spike-and-
wave complexes SWC (**E**) and isolated right temporal sharp waves (**F**). Her high-resolution brain MRI
did not reveal any abnormalities, and an ictal SPECT did not provide a clear metabolic correlate of focal
seizure origin. Therefore, it remains unclear whether this patient has idiopathic generalized epilepsy or
focal epilepsy with rapid secondarily GTCSs, or both.

reach statistical significance (49,50). In the third study (51) comparing LEV and LTG, time to first seizure occurrence was equal for both drugs, with nonsignificant trends favoring LEV in terms of efficacy and LTG in terms of tolerability. Interestingly, there was also no difference in terms of seizure control at 6 weeks, although patients in the LTG arm had not reached their target dose yet (51).

To date, there are no controlled studies on pregabalin (PGB) or zonisamide (ZNS) monotherapy in patients with either generalized or focal epilepsy.

Again, it should be emphasized that in none of the studies evaluating the newer anticonvulsants results were stratified according to seizure type. In fact, the proportion of patients with GTCSs was as low as 20% (49). The available data show that a variety of anticonvulsants can be chosen as the initial treatment of patients with generalized and focal epilepsy. Since many patients require life-long therapy, an individual drug should be chosen based on efficacy, tolerability, potential interactions with other drugs, potential long-term side effects or toxicity, and cost.

The studies cited above also demonstrated that the majority of patients with epilepsy respond well to their first anticonvulsant. Complete seizure cessation with the use of anticonvulsants can be achieved in more than half of patients with GTCSs (5). Those who continue to experience disabling seizures despite adequate trials of two anticonvulsants should be referred to an epilepsy center.

CONCLUSION

In summary, the semiology of GTCSs may vary and differ from the classic description by Gastaut. Primarily and secondarily GTCSs may represent a spectrum where clinical and electrographic synchrony and symmetry are seen more often in primarily GTCSs, whereas secondarily GTCSs more likely feature asymmetry and asynchrony, both in their clinical and electrographic manifestations (35). The majority of patients with GTCSs can expect complete seizure cessation with monotherapy of an appropriate anticonvulsant.

References

1. Hauser WA, Kurland LT. The epidemiology of epilepsy in Rochester, Minnesota, 1935 through 1967. *Epilepsia.* 1975;16:1–66.
2. Kotagal P. Generalized tonic-clonic seizures. In: Lüders HO, Noachtar S, eds. *Epileptic Seizures: Pathophysiology and Clinical Semiology.* Philadelphia: Churchill Livingstone; 2000:425–432.
3. Blume WT, Luders HO, Mizrahi E, et al. Glossary of descriptive terminology for ictal semiology: report of the ILAE task force on classification and terminology. *Epilepsia.* 2001;42:1212–1218.
4. Gastaut H, Broughton R. *Epileptic Seizures: Clinical and Electrographic Features, Diagnosis and Treatment.* Springfield, IL: Charles C. Thomas; 1972:25–90.
5. Fisch BJ, Olejniczak PW. Generalized tonic-clonic seizures. In: Wyllie E, ed. *The Treatment of Epilepsy. Principles and Practice.* 4th ed. Philadelphia: Lippincott, Williams & Wilkins; 2006:279–304.
6. Benarroch EE. The central autonomic network: functional organization, dysfunction, and perspective. *Mayo Clin Proc.* 1993;68:988–1001.
7. Bateman LM, Li CS, Seyal M. Ictal hypoxemia in localization-related epilepsy: analysis of incidence, severity and risk factors. *Brain.* 2008;131: 3239–3245.
8. Helmstaedter C, Elger CE, Lendt M. Postictal courses of cognitive deficits in focal epilepsies. *Epilepsia.* 1994;35:1073–1078.
9. Theodore WH, Porter RJ, Albert P, et al. The secondarily generalized tonic-clonic seizure: a videotape analysis. *Neurology.* 1994;44:1403–1407.
10. Jobst BC, Williamson PD, Neuschwander TB, et al. Secondarily generalized seizures in mesial temporal epilepsy: clinical characteristics, lateralizing signs, and association with sleep-wake cycle. *Epilepsia.* 2001;42:1279–1287.
11. Leutmezer F, Woginger S, Antoni E, et al. Asymmetric ending of secondarily generalized seizures: a lateralizing sign in TLE. *Neurology.* 2002;59: 1252–1254.
12. Trinka E, Walser G, Unterberger I, et al. Asymmetric termination of secondarily generalized tonic-clonic seizures in temporal lobe epilepsy. *Neurology.* 2002;59:1254–1256.
13. Kirton A, Darwish H, Wirrell E. Unique clinical phenomenology can help distinguish primary from secondary generalized seizures in children. *J Child Neurol.* 2004;19:265–270.
14. Loddenkemper T, Kotagal P. Lateralizing signs during seizures in focal epilepsy. *Epilepsy Behav.* 2005;7:1–17.
15. Casaubon L, Pohlmann-Eden B, Khosravani H, et al. Video-EEG evidence of lateralized clinical features in primary generalized epilepsy with tonic-clonic seizures. *Epileptic Disord.* 2003;5:149–156.
16. Chin PS, Miller JW. Ictal head version in generalized epilepsy. *Neurology.* 2004;63:370–372.
17. Niaz FE, Abou-Khalil B, Fakhoury T. The generalized tonic-clonic seizure in partial versus generalized epilepsy: semiologic differences. *Epilepsia.* 1999;40:1664–1666.
18. Leutmezer F, Lurger S, Baumgartner C. Focal features in patients with idiopathic generalized epilepsy. *Epilepsy Res.* 2002;50:293–300.
19. Usui N, Kotagal P, Matsumoto R, et al. Focal semiologic and electroencephalographic features in patients with juvenile myoclonic epilepsy. *Epilepsia.* 2005;46:1668–1676.
20. Wyllie E, Luders H, Morris HH, et al. The lateralizing significance of versive head and eye movements during epileptic seizures. *Neurology.* 1986;36:606–611.
21. Kotagal P, Bleasel A, Geller E, et al. Lateralizing value of asymmetric tonic limb posturing observed in secondarily generalized tonic-clonic seizures. *Epilepsia.* 2000;41:457–462.
22. Hamer HM, Wyllie E, Luders HO, et al. Symptomatology of epileptic seizures in the first three years of life. *Epilepsia.* 1999;40:837–844.
23. Korff C, Nordli DR, Jr. Do generalized tonic-clonic seizures in infancy exist? *Neurology.* 2005;65:1750–1753.
24. Orringer CE, Eustace JC, Wunsch CD, et al. Natural history of lactic acidosis after grand-mal seizures: a model for the study of an anion-gap acidosis not associated with hyperkalemia. *N Engl J Med.* 1977;297:796–799.
25. Edwards R, Schmidley JW, Simon RP. How often does a CSF pleocytosis follow generalized convulsions? *Ann Neurol.* 1983;13:460–462.
26. Aminoff MJ, Simon RP, Wiedemann E. The hormonal responses to generalized tonic-clonic seizures. *Brain.* 1984;107(Pt 2):569–578.
27. Chen DK, So YT, Fisher RS, et al. Use of serum prolactin in diagnosing epileptic seizures: report of the therapeutics and technology assessment subcommittee of the American Academy of Neurology. *Neurology.* 2005;65:668–675.
28. Oribe E, Amini R, Nissenbaum E, et al. Serum prolactin concentrations are elevated after syncope. *Neurology.* 1996;47:60–62.
29. Wyllie E, Lueders H, Pippenger C, et al. Postictal serum creatine kinase in the diagnosis of seizure disorders. *Arch Neurol.* 1985;42:123–126.
30. Zivin L, Marsan CA. Incidence and prognostic significance of "epileptiform" activity in the EEG of non-epileptic subjects. *Brain.* 1968;91:751–778.
31. Lombroso CT. Consistent EEG focalities detected in subjects with primary generalized epilepsies monitored for two decades. *Epilepsia.* 1997;38: 797–812.
32. Pedley TA, Mendiratta A, Walczak TS. Seizures and epilepsy. In: Ebersole JS, Pedley TA, eds. *Current Practice of Electroencephalography.* 3rd ed. Philadelphia: Lippincott Williams & Wilkins; 2003:506–587.
33. Gotman J. Interhemispheric relations during bilateral spike-and-wave activity. *Epilepsia.* 1981;22:453–466.
34. Garcia Dominguez L, Wennberg RA, Gaetz W, et al. Enhanced synchrony in epileptiform activity? Local versus distant phase synchronization in generalized seizures. *J Neurosci.* 2005;25:8077–8084.
35. Lhatoo SD, Lüders HO. Secondary generalized tonic-clonic seizures. In: Lüders HO, ed. *Textbook of Epilepsy Surgery.* 1st ed. London, UK: Informa Healthcare; 2008:492–500.
36. French JA. Can evidence-based guidelines and clinical trials tell us how to treat patients? *Epilepsia.* 2007;48:1264–1267.
37. Panayiotopoulos CP. Evidence-based epileptology, randomized controlled trials, and SANAD: a critical clinical view. *Epilepsia.* 2007;48:1268–1274.
38. Glauser T, Ben-Menachem E, Bourgeois B, et al. ILAE treatment guidelines: evidence-based analysis of antiepileptic drug efficacy and effectiveness as initial monotherapy for epileptic seizures and syndromes. *Epilepsia.* 2006;47:1094–1120.
39. French JA, Kanner AM, Bautista J, et al. Efficacy and tolerability of the new antiepileptic drugs, I: treatment of new-onset epilepsy: report of the TTA and QSS subcommittees of the American Academy of Neurology and the American Epilepsy Society. *Epilepsia.* 2004;45:401–409.
40. Perucca E, Gram L, Avanzini G, et al. Antiepileptic drugs as a cause of worsening seizures. *Epilepsia.* 1998;39:5–17.

41. Gelisse P, Genton P, Kuate C, et al. Worsening of seizures by oxcarbazepine in juvenile idiopathic generalized epilepsies. *Epilepsia*. 2004;45: 1282–1286.

42. Thomas P, Valton L, Genton P. Absence and myoclonic status epilepticus precipitated by antiepileptic drugs in idiopathic generalized epilepsy. *Brain*. 2006;129:1281–1292.

43. Mattson RH, Cramer JA, Collins JF, et al. Comparison of carbamazepine, phenobarbital, phenytoin, and primidone in partial and secondarily generalized tonic-clonic seizures. *N Engl J Med*. 1985;313:145–151.

44. Mattson RH, Cramer JA, Collins JF. A comparison of valproate with carbamazepine for the treatment of complex partial seizures and secondarily generalized tonic-clonic seizures in adults. The department of veterans affairs epilepsy cooperative study no. 264 group. *N Engl J Med*. 1992;327: 765–771.

45. Heller AJ, Chesterman P, Elwes RD, et al. Phenobarbitone, phenytoin, carbamazepine, or sodium valproate for newly diagnosed adult epilepsy: a randomised comparative monotherapy trial. *J Neurol Neurosurg Psychiatry*. 1995;58:44–50.

46. Marson AG, Al-Kharusi AM, Alwaidh M, et al. The SANAD study of effectiveness of valproate, lamotrigine, or topiramate for generalised and unclassifiable epilepsy: an unblinded randomised controlled trial. *Lancet*. 2007;369:1016–1026.

47. Marson AG, Al-Kharusi AM, Alwaidh M, et al. The SANAD study of effectiveness of carbamazepine, gabapentin, lamotrigine, oxcarbazepine, or topiramate for treatment of partial epilepsy: an unblinded randomised controlled trial. *Lancet*. 2007;369:1000–1015.

48. Saetre E, Perucca E, Isojarvi J, et al. An international multicenter randomized double-blind controlled trial of lamotrigine and sustained-release carbamazepine in the treatment of newly diagnosed epilepsy in the elderly. *Epilepsia*. 2007;48:1292–1302.

49. Brodie MJ, Perucca E, Ryvlin P, et al. Comparison of levetiracetam and controlled-release carbamazepine in newly diagnosed epilepsy. *Neurology*. 2007;68:402–408.

50. Pohlmann-Eden B, Van Paesschen W, Hallström Y, et al. The KOMET study: an open-label, randomized, parallel-group trial comparing the efficacy and safety of levetiracetam with sodium valproate and carbamazepine as monotherapy in subjects with newly diagnosed epilepsy. Abstract no 3.242, presented at 62nd Annual Meeting of the American Epilepsy Society, Seattle, WA, December 5–9, 2008. Available at: http://www.aesnet.org/go/publications/aes-abstracts/abstract-search/. Accessed March 23, 2009.

51. Rosenow F, Bauer S, Reif P, et al. Lamotrigine versus levetiracetam in the initial monotherapy of epilepsy—results of the LaLiMo study—an open randomized controlled head to head phase 3b trial including 410 patients. Abstract no 1.242, presented at 62nd Annual Meeting of the American Epilepsy Society, Seattle, WA, December 5–9, 2008. Available at: http://www.aesnet.org/go/publications/aes-abstracts/abstract-search/. Accessed March 23, 2009.

CHAPTER 15 ■ ABSENCE SEIZURES

ALEXIS ARZIMANOGLOU AND KARINE OSTROWSKY-COSTE

Although the first clinical description of absence seizures was provided by Poupart in 1705 (1,2), it was not until 1824 that Calmiel introduced the term "absence seizures" to describe these brief episodes reminiscent of *the spirit fleeing from the eyes* (*absence seizures d'espirit*) (3).

The association of clinical absence seizures with generalized spike and wave discharges was recognized soon after the advent of the electroencephalography, first by Berger in 1933 (4) followed by Gibbs and colleagues in 1935 (5). The combination of a relatively stereotyped clinical manifestation and an easily recognizable and consistent electroencephalographic (EEG) pattern has made absence seizures the paradigm for detailed electroclinical correlations (4,6–10).

Under the 1981 International League Against Epilepsy (ILAE) revision of epileptic seizures, absence seizures are recognized as either typical or atypical (11) according to specific clinical characteristics and generalized spike and wave EEG discharges (12–14). As discussed in Chapter 10, the terms "absence seizures" and "dialeptic seizures" have been proposed in a semiologic classification based on signs and symptoms only, regardless of whether EEG findings are generalized or focal. In contrast to the purely symptomatologic approach, this chapter discusses absence seizures as defined by the International Classification of Epileptic Seizures.

CLINICAL FEATURES

Absence seizures were categorized into various subtypes by the ILAE (11), based on clinical features (Table 15.1).

Typical Absence Seizures

A typical absence seizure is defined by the ILAE (11) as a generalized epileptic seizure that is clinically characterized by impairment of consciousness alone (simple typical absence seizures) or in combination with mild clonic, atonic, or atonic movements, autonomic components, or automatisms (complex typical absence seizure) (15,16). Of the two types, complex typical absence seizures are the more common (17,18).

Typical absence seizures most frequently commence during childhood. Most often they remit spontaneously, but they may persist into adulthood (19,20) or even start in adulthood (21).

TABLE 15.1

SUMMARY OF CLINICAL CHARACTERISTICS OF DIALEPTIC SEIZURES

	Typical absence seizures	Atypical absence seizures	Myoclonic absence seizures	Focal seizure
Syndrome	IGEs, CAE, JAE, JME	Generalized symptomatic epilepsies, LGS, MAE, CSWSS	Cryptogenic/symptomatic generalized epilepsies, EMA	Idiopathic/cryptogenic/ symptomatic partial epilepsies
Onset/offset	Obvious	Subtle	Obvious	Variable
Electroencephalography	3 Hz regular spike and wave complexes	Irregular slow spike and wave complexes <2.5 Hz	3 Hz regular spike and wave complexes	Variable, from minor rhythm modification (diffuse or focal) to clear focal discharge
Mean duration	5–20 seconds	5–30 seconds	10–60 seconds	From seconds to minutes
Automatism	Simple	Elaborate	No	Possibly
Motor symptoms	No or mild	No or mild	Severe myoclonic jerks at 3 Hz	Possibly
Aura	Never	Rare	Never	Possibly
Postictal confusion	No	Possibly	Possibly	Possibly
Mental state	Normal	Impaired	Impaired	Variable
Inducibility	Yes	No	No	Sometimes
Prognosis	Good	Poor	Poor	Variable

IGE, idiopathic generalized epilepsy; CAE, childhood absence epilepsy; JAE, juvenile absence epilepsy; JME, juvenile myoclonic epilepsy; LGS, Lennox–Gastaut syndrome; MAE, myoclonic astatic epilepsy; CSWSS, continuous spike and wave during slow sleep; EMA, epilepsy with myoclonic absence.

Typical absence seizures often occur at times of boredom or tiredness. They may be avoided by focusing on a particular task, especially if enjoyable (22–24). There have been reports of typical absence seizures triggered by arithmetic and other spatial tasks (25,26). An important characteristic of typical absence seizures is susceptibility to induction by hyperventilation in virtually all untreated patients. Absence seizures may also be precipitated by photic stimulation or watching television in approximately 15% of patients, especially adolescents and adults (27–30). The level of hypocapnia required to induce typical absence seizures appears to vary among individuals (31). Interestingly, overbreathing during physical exercise can decrease the frequency (32).

Typical absence seizures are almost exclusively observed in idiopathic generalized epilepsies (IGEs), that is, childhood absence seizures epilepsy (CAE), juvenile absence seizures epilepsy (JAE), and juvenile myoclonic epilepsy (JME).

Simple Typical Absence Seizures

The majority of simple typical absence seizures last between 5 and 20 seconds (24). Seizure onset is sudden and the child becomes motionless with a vacant stare. The eyes may drift upwards. Often, there is a slight beating of the eyelids at a rhythm of 3 Hz. The seizure ends abruptly, sometimes with the presence of a smile. The patient may rarely be in a dazed state for 2 to 3 seconds, suggestive of a very brief postictal phase (4).

During the seizure, there is impairment of consciousness, although there may not be complete abolition of awareness, responsiveness, or memory. Often, the patient is aware of the time that has elapsed during the seizure, but only rarely has a confused memory of the events that occurred during the time of the seizure.

Simple typical absence seizures are frequently repeated many times per day with reports of as many as a hundred or more per day (33). However, the occurrence of extremely brief "micro-absence seizures," during which the state of consciousness may be almost impossible to assess, makes any precise evaluation of the number of attacks difficult.

Complex Typical Absence Seizures

Complex typical absence seizures are differentiated from the simple typical absence seizures due to the presence of mild motor components, autonomic components, or commonly automatisms (8,27). However, as with simple typical absence seizures, these seizures are brief and impairment of consciousness is the predominant feature.

Of the motor components, the mild clonic movements are common and involve the eyelids, corners of the mouth, and sometimes the deltoid muscles. Atonic components involve a sudden loss of tone causing the head or trunk to slump forward. There may be a slight myoclonic jerk but rarely does this jerk result in a fall. Mild tonic components may result in a slight retropulsion of the head and trunk or a resultant gaze deviation and head rotation to one side (versive absence seizures) (34).

The autonomic phenomena include changes in respiratory rhythms or apnea, pallor, heart rate modification, and mydriasis (24). Urination has been reported to occur in 5% to 17% of patients (29,34,35).

The automatisms are typically oral (e.g., licking, lip-smacking, and swallowing) but can also involve simple leg or arm gestures. The automatisms may evolve in a craniocaudal fashion

with elevation of the eyelids, licking and swallowing, and, finally, fiddling and scratching movements of the hands (9,10). Automatisms generally occur in more prolonged absence seizures when the loss of consciousness is more severe (8), analogous to complex partial seizures. However, in contrast to the automatisms associated with complex partial seizures, the automatisms of complex typical absence seizures stop abruptly, coincident with the termination of the ictal EEG discharge, and do not progressively merge with the postictal automatisms and confusion.

Like simple typical absence seizures, these events may occur frequently throughout the day.

Atypical Absence Seizures

Atypical absence seizures generally last between 5 and 30 seconds (4,36), which is slightly longer than the typical absence seizures. In some cases loss of consciousness is incomplete, allowing the child to partially continue an ongoing activity. The decreased consciousness is often associated with some loss of muscle tone, erratic myoclonic movements, sialorrhea, or mild hypertonia of the neck and spinal muscles. Unlike typical absence seizures, atypical absence seizures are not susceptible to induction by hyperventilation or photic stimulation (36,37).

Atypical absence seizures most commonly occur in children with mental retardation who also exhibit multiple other seizure types such as concomitant tonic, atonic, or myoclonic seizures and who can be classified as having one of the symptomatic or cryptogenic generalized epilepsies (see Chapter 22). In the case of Lennox–Gastaut syndrome, atypical absence seizures represent the second most common seizure type for these children (38–40).

Myoclonic Absence Seizures

Absence seizures with a pronounced clonic or myoclonic jerk, in which the motor component dominates the clinical picture, were initially reported in 1966 (41) and later defined by Tassinari and colleagues as a specific seizure type (42).

Myoclonic absence seizures usually last for 10 to 60 seconds. The myoclonic jerk typically involves the upper extremities but may also occur in the lower limbs (proximal limb musculature) resulting in a loss of posture (43,44). Rhythmic jerks may occur at a frequency of approximately three times per second and are more violent than those that occur during typical absence seizures with twitches of eyelid or facial muscles (45,46). Frequently, an associated tonic contraction is predominant in the proximal appendicular and axial muscle that causes the head to be tilted backwards and the arms to be raised (46). Autonomic manifestations such as arrest of breathing and urinary incontinence may also occur (45,46). These seizures may be precipitated by photic stimulation, hyperventilation, or watching television (43).

Although myoclonic absence seizures are not specifically identified by the ILAE seizure classification, these seizures are listed as a component of the syndrome of epilepsy with myoclonic absence seizures (44,46), which is a cryptogenic or symptomatic epilepsy according to the 1989 ILAE epilepsy syndrome classification (47). The typical age of onset of this syndrome is 7 years. The children often have prior mental impairment (19,43,48). These seizures are often resistant to therapy and the prognosis is poor.

ELECTROENCEPHALOGRAPHIC FEATURES

Typical Absence Seizures

For either simple or complex typical absence seizures, the ictal EEG discharge is concurrent with clinical symptoms, essentially consisting of generalized symmetric, synchronous complexes that feature a negative slow wave preceded by one (occasionally two or more) negative spike or sharp wave, repeating at a rhythm of about 3 Hz in regularly organized bursts. The spike corresponds to positive (excitatory) phenomena, particularly the mild myoclonic jerks of eyelids or limbs, whereas the slow wave appears to be inhibitory in nature (49).

The basic frequency of 3 Hz does not tend to vary, although it may be slightly faster and more irregular in the first few seconds, progressively slowing to 2.5 Hz (29,50). In addition, toward the end of the discharge, the spikes may become less apparent and drop out.

Although there is a strong relationship between changes in awareness and the occurrence of ictal 3 Hz discharges, the extent of unconsciousness does not appear to correlate with EEG characteristics such as amplitude or diffusion of the ictal pattern (24,51).

Interictally, the background activity is normal; with the exception of intermittent rhythmic posterior delta activity seen in some children (52,53).

In addition, brief generalized 3 Hz spike and wave discharges may occur without obvious clinical change. It is debatable whether these bursts are ictal or interictal (54,55). The distinction likely depends on the sophistication of the testing. A generally accepted observation is that discharges lasting longer than 3 seconds can be noticed in everyday life by an attentive observer. However, continuous response tasks have demonstrated decreased performance during even briefer discharges and sometimes even slightly before the discharge.

These interictal discharges are characteristically bilateral and symmetric; however, in some cases, unilateral or asymmetric discharges that change from side to side occur. Exceptionally, persistently unilateral discharges may occur. Such asymmetries should not lead to an erroneous diagnosis of partial seizures (56,57). These localized or focal interictal paroxysms are not common (14,58,59) and have been associated with late onset (27).

During light sleep, the interictal paroxysms may become fragmented and irregular, and may develop into multiple spike and wave discharges (Fig. 15.1). In stages III and IV of sleep, the number of spikes increases and the waves become longer and more distorted. The basic morphology during rapid eye movement sleep is similar to that during resting wakefulness. Polyspikes during sleep appear to be associated with a less favorable prognosis (60).

Atypical Absence Seizures

Although the ictal bursts of atypical absence seizures have a similar distribution to those of typical absence seizures, the generalized slow spike and wave discharges that accompany an atypical absence seizure are lower in amplitude, broader and blunter (Fig. 15.2), and more irregular (e.g., less perfectly monomorphic), and the frequency is approximately 1.5 Hz (<2.5 Hz). Asymmetries may correlate with focal neurologic signs or radiologic deficits on the affected side.

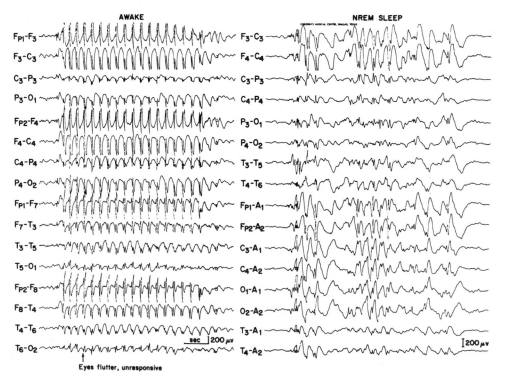

FIGURE 15.1 Typical absence seizures recorded in a 7-year-old girl. The awake record shows a classic generalized 3-Hz spike and wave discharge. In nonrapid eye movement sleep, the discharges are more irregular, and the one-to-one relationship between spikes and waves is lost. (From Daly DD. Epilepsy and syncope. In: Daly DD, Pedley TA, eds. *Current Practice of Clinical Electroencephalography.* New York: Raven Press; 1990: 269–334, with permission.)

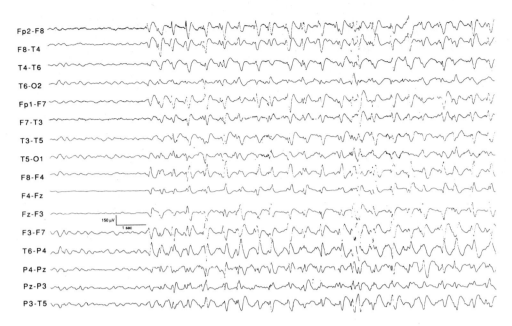

Fp2-F8
F8-T4
T4-T6
T6-O2
Fp1-F7
F7-T3
T3-T5
T5-O1
F8-F4
F4-Fz
Fz-F3
F3-F7
T6-P4
P4-Pz
Pz-P3
P3-T5

150 µV
1 sec

FIGURE 15.2 Slow spike and wave discharge (2 Hz) in an 18-year-old boy with atypical absence seizures as a consequence of Lennox–Gastaut syndrome.

Interictally, there are brief bursts of slow spike and wave discharges and focal or multifocal spikes superimposed on a diffusely slow background. The discharges are activated in sleep and interspersed with brief runs of generalized rapid spikes, with or without clinical tonic seizures (4,6,14,61–63). This combination of findings is characteristic of symptomatic or cryptogenic generalized epilepsies (see Chapter 22).

Myoclonic Absence Seizures

Myoclonic absence seizures share the EEG signature of typical absence seizures (20,25): a bilateral, synchronous and symmetric discharges of 3 Hz spike and wave; however, the myoclonic absence seizures are easily differentiated from absence seizures based on their obvious clinical features.

The background activity is usually slowed but may be normal. In addition to generalized spikes, focal or multifocal spike and waves may be present (45).

Other Electroencephalographic Patterns

A number of other EEG patterns are associated with staring spells, although their clinical significance is controversial.

Generalized Rhythmic Delta Activity

Lee and Kirby (64) described seven children who experienced brief periods of loss of awareness associated with generalized high-amplitude rhythmic delta activity, without a spike component. Nearly all electroclinical observations were made during hyperventilation. The authors characterized these events as absence seizures because of the consistent electroclinical features and the response to antiabsence medications. However, their interpretation is not universally accepted (37,65,66).

Low-Voltage Fast Rhythms

Gastaut and Broughton (4) described patterns of diffuse flattening, low-voltage fast activity at about 20 Hz, and rhythmic 10-Hz sharp waves associated with atypical absence seizures, in addition to the classic slow spike and wave discharges. These patterns also typically accompany tonic seizures in patients with Lennox–Gastaut syndrome. It is therefore arguable whether the staring spells associated with the faster rhythms and often with increased axial tone should be regarded as atypical absence seizures or as tonic seizures (4,67). Similarly, staring spells with generalized fast rhythms or diffuse EEG flattening are occasionally observed without tonic seizures or Lennox–Gastaut syndrome (68,69). Some episodes may represent partial seizures from occult frontal lobe foci, whereas others remain unclassified (58,70,71). Generalized fast activity has also been described during clinically typical absence seizures (72).

Mixed Patterns

Exceptional patients with staring spells show mixed slow and diffused fast rhythms during attacks (Fig. 15.3), whose nosologic position is uncertain. The fast rhythms are likely caused by a neurophysiologic mechanism different from that of spike and wave discharges. Until the neurobiologic differences of these discharges are better understood, the value of classification remains dubious.

DIAGNOSIS

Typical Absence Seizures

Establishing the diagnosis of typical absence seizures in children is usually not difficult. Children are usually referred for frequent, repeated episodes of staring of very short duration. Such episodes are often so subtle that parents report the episodes are almost exclusively present at lunchtime or dinner,

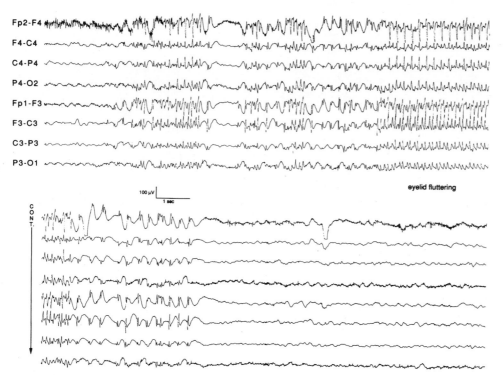

FIGURE 15.3 Staring spell associated with eyelid fluttering in a 45-year-old man with refractory generalized epilepsy since adolescence. Other family members had well-controlled generalized epilepsy. The clinical attack was associated with a complex generalized EEG abnormality comprising periods of 9- to 13-Hz spikes, intermingled with 2- to 4-Hz spike and wave discharges and periods of generalized flattening.

when the family is sitting face-to-face (e.g., "he suddenly stares and drops his spoon and then takes it back again as if nothing happened"). It is the repetitive and stereotyped pattern of such episodes in an otherwise normal child that suggests the diagnosis.

In adolescents and adults, typical absence seizures may be mild and inconspicuous, occurring infrequently with only incomplete loss of awareness.

The provocation of an attack by hyperventilation while the patient is being watched is a highly useful test when an attack is produced. The diagnosis of typical absence seizures can be confirmed by a single electroencephalogram recording. Provided that hyperventilation is well performed, the lack of spike and wave discharges should cast serious doubt on the diagnosis of typical absence seizures. If 3 minutes of hyperventilation is ineffective, an extension to 5 minutes may be valuable.

Hyperventilation can also induce other types of clinical attacks including brief complex partial seizures or psychogenic events including "pseudo-absence seizures" (20,66). Although clinically distinguishing these from typical absence seizures is not difficult, there are rare occasions when it can be difficult to differentiate a more prolonged absence seizures with automatisms from a brief focal-onset seizure. In general, however, focal seizures of temporal origin are associated with an aura that lasts longer than 30 seconds, involve complex automatisms or postictal confusion, and are usually infrequent and clustered rather than frequent and related to the time of day or fatigue (15,70,73,74). Video–EEG monitoring (74) is occasionally required to make the distinction—a crucial one, because of the greatly different prognostic and therapeutic implications.

In rare cases, focal-onset seizures of frontal lobe origin can mimic typical absence seizures. Clinical, EEG, or radiologic features of a frontal focus usually lead to the correct diagnosis (70,75–78). However, an occult frontal focus, especially on the mesial surface of one hemisphere, can occasionally cause brief seizures with generalized discharges (i.e., "secondary bilateral synchrony") (71,79–81). Clues from the electroencephalography include irregular epileptiform discharges with a maximum field in or just adjacent to the midline rather than the characteristic bilateral maximum field at F7/F8 and occasional focal discharges (82,83).

One common error is confusing simple daydreaming and inattentiveness at school or in front of the television for a typical absence seizure. Many children are occasionally inattentive. The family or teacher reports brief episodes of staring and unresponsiveness with no significant motor manifestations. Is the child having absence seizures or nonepileptic staring spells? Based on a questionnaire given to parents, several features were identified that can help distinguish the two scenarios in an otherwise normal child (84). Three features suggest nonepileptic events: (a) the events do not interrupt play; (b) the events were first noticed by a professional (e.g., schoolteacher or speech therapist) rather than a parent; and (c) the staring child is responsive to touch or "interruptible" by other external stimuli. Each of these features has approximately 80% specificity for suggesting nonepileptic staring episodes. Several factors are associated with an epileptic etiology including twitches of the arms or legs, loss of urine, or upward eye movement. Other features suggestive of nonepileptic or behavioral rather than epileptic etiology include lower age and lower frequency of episodes (85). Similarly, sustained inattention is more often associated with attention-deficit hyperactivity disorder than with absence seizures (86).

Tics or other stereotyped movements (e.g., head thrusts observed with oculomotor apraxia) also are mistaken for typical absence seizures surprisingly often. Careful questioning about the abruptness of onset, the circumstances of occurrence, repetition, the appearance of the eyes, and the movements of the eyelids usually permits easy differentiation.

Atypical Absence Seizures

Atypical absence seizures rarely exist alone. They often signal a more serious disorder associated with mental retardation and multiple other seizure types, particularly tonic and atonic attacks (62,87).

Associated Brain Anomalies

We do not typically obtain brain imaging in a child in whom a diagnosis of typical absence seizures is made. As the term idiopathic (IGE) suggests, the brain of patients with an IGE is expected to be anatomically normal, based on magnetic resonance imaging (MRI) or routine histologic examination. However, brain abnormalities may be present in patients with typical absence seizures, although determination of their exact significance may not always be straightforward. Bamberger and Matthes (88) identified some forms of brain lesion in 39% of patients with typical absence seizures, and brain damage was also reported in a similar percentage of patients by Dalby (27). Minor morphologic changes (i.e., microdysgenesis) have been noted in some patients with IGE (89), but this remains controversial (90).

TREATMENT

The treatment of typical absence seizures is generally of great benefit and seizure control may be rapidly obtained in most patients. The disappearance of the rhythmic ictal spike and wave bursts in response to hyperventilation confirms the effectiveness of the therapy (91). A monotherapy approach is preferred at onset and for subsequent maintenance.

The first effective drugs to treat typical absence seizures were diones (e.g., trimethadione and paramethadione), but these have since been superseded by other less toxic drugs. Frontline drugs for absence seizures include valproic acid, which is reported to result in complete control of typical absence seizures in 80% of children (91,92), and ethosuximide, which may be moderately less efficacious (93). In cases where neither drug is efficacious, the combination of both may prove to be of benefit (94). This combination is reported to be particularly effective against myoclonic absence seizures and other syndromes with myoclonias (48).

Lamotrigine is useful in the treatment of typical absence seizures when valproate or ethosuximide have failed (95,96). A combination of lamotrigine and valproate may also be effective when neither drug is efficacious alone (97,98). Recent data suggest that levetiracetam may be effective in the treatment of typical absence seizures and therefore may be tried in pharmacoresistant cases (99).

Clonazepam, nitrazepam (91), and clobazam are effective in controlling absence seizure attacks, but their associated side effects do not make these drugs an obvious choice. Tolerance is usually achieved after a few months, but sometimes as long as a year (100,101). Other antiepileptic drugs generally are not effective. Indeed, some agents, especially those that interfere with GABA turnover and influence GABAergic mechanisms, such as vigabatrin (60), tiagabine (102), and carbamazepine (103), may aggravate absence seizures.

For atypical absence seizures, treatment is more challenging and depends on the associated syndrome. For Lennox–Gastaut syndrome, the treatment options are poor and limited success has been reported using lamotrigine, topiramate, and rufinamide (39). Drugs that may exacerbate atypical seizures across the different syndromes include carbamazepine, vigabatrin, phenobarbital, tiagabin and possibly phenytoin and oxcarbazepine.

COURSE AND PROGNOSIS

Discrepant views have been expressed regarding the outcome of patients with typical absence seizures (15). These discrepancies have resulted from the differing diagnostic criteria used by various investigators, the differences in origin and composition of the patients in the series, the variable duration of follow-up, and the heterogeneity of the epilepsies featuring typical absence seizures. All of these factors have resulted in differences in the definition of what constitutes typical absence seizures epilepsy.

With respect to course and prognosis, it is best to note that although descriptively interesting, the distinctions among multiple subtypes of typical absence seizures likely has no clinical or neurobiologic significance (104). The important and practical diagnosis is that of IGE with absence seizures (105) for the typical absence seizures, and for atypical absence seizures and its variants a diagnosis of a symptomatic or cryptogenic generalized epilepsy of the Lennox–Gastaut type. It is the syndromic diagnosis, not the identification of the seizure type, which is most useful for management (106) and for predicting course and outcome. The reader is referred to the excellent discussion of these topics in Chapters 20 and 22.

PATHOPHYSIOLOGY

Functional Anatomy

Generation of absence seizures is dependent on an intact thalamocortical network, and the generalized spike and wave discharges associated with absence seizures are believed to reflect a widespread phase-locked oscillation between excitation (spike) and inhibition (wave) in mutually connected thalamocortical networks (107). However, the site of initiation is not known.

Penfield, Jasper, and colleagues (108–111) initially proposed the centrencephalic theory in which a subcortical neuronal system centered on the midline structures of the upper brainstem and diencephalon (centrocephalic system) gave rise to discharges that synchronously entrain cortical regions in both hemispheres. Although this hypothesis is intuitively appealing, it is not universally accepted (112) and, as elegantly reviewed by Meeren and colleagues (113), other theories have been proposed that posit the thalamus or cortex as the site of origin of the absence seizures. Although an impressive body of data from human studies (71,79,81,114) point to the cerebral cortex as the site of the primary abnormality, recent functional MRI studies suggest thalamic onset (115–117).

Although the finding that the antiabsence drug ethosuximide specifically affects low threshold calcium currents in thalamic neurons (118,119) also suggests the primacy of the thalamus in generating the seizures (120), a defect of the

T-type calcium channels responsible for this current are unlikely to be the primary cause of absence seizures. Rather, the thalamocortical system must be viewed as an oscillating network that generates a variety of physiologic and pathologic rhythms (121). Thus, interference at many points in the network can precipitate or interrupt absence seizures.

GABA-mediated Inhibition

GABA-mediated inhibition plays a critical role in the synchronization and desynchronization of thalamocortical circuits (122–124). In experimental models of absence seizures, GABA-mediated inhibition potentiates spike and wave discharges (50). Furthermore, absence seizures are aggravated in patients who receive either vigabatrin (60) or tiagabine (102), both of which influence GABA turnover.

GABA$_A$ receptors are ligand-gated ion channels that mediate fast inhibitory synaptic transmission within the central nervous system. GABA$_A$ receptors are deemed benzodiazepine-sensitive or benzodiazepine-insensitive based on the receptor's subunit compositions. Within the thalamus, benzodiazepine-sensitive GABA$_A$ receptors are expressed by the neurons within the nucleus reticularis of the thalamus (nRT), whereas benzodiazepine-insensitive receptors are expressed by the glutamatergic thalamocortical relay neurons. The oscillatory firing of thalamocortical circuitry is dependent on the ability of the nRT to entrain the thalamocortical relay neurons. It is the differential expression of GABA$_A$ receptors that underlies the therapeutic role of benzodiazepines in the treatment of absence seizures as the net effect of benzodiazepine administration is the selective inhibition of the nRT (124,125).

GABA$_B$ receptors are G-protein–coupled receptors that regulate neuronal excitability by modulation of postsynaptic potassium-dependent hyperpolarization and release of neurotransmitter at the presynaptic terminals. These receptors are capable of mediating the long-lasting thalamic inhibitory postsynaptic potentials that are critical to the generation of normal thalamocortical rhythms. GABA$_B$ receptor antagonists block absence seizures in experimental models (50,126) and the somatosensory cortex of epileptic rats exhibits alteration in GABA$_B$ receptor subunit expression and localization (127), which has been proposed to contribute to neocortical hyperexcitability (128).

Glutamate–Glutamine Cycling

Curiously, there are differences of cerebral glucose utilization between the rodent strain GAERS (genetic absence seizures epilepsy rat from Strasbourg), which exhibits a propensity for absence seizures, and non-epileptic rodents. In the GAERS strain, glucose utilization is increased (129) as are metabolic enzyme activities (29,130,131). It is proposed that the increased cycling of glutamate and glutamine between astrocytes and glutamatergic neurons, combined with decreased GABAergic function in the cortex of GAERS, may be the underlying cause of absence seizures (132). However, in children there are conflicting reports with regards to any associations between fluctuations of cerebral glucose metabolism and absence seizures and further research is required.

Genetic Factors

The importance of genetic factors in the pathogenesis of typical absence seizures has been long recognized. Strong genetic evidence was provided by monozygotic twin studies demonstrating 70% concordance of absence seizures and 84% concordance of the 3 Hz spike and wave trait (24). The incidence of seizures or EEG paroxysmal abnormalities in first-degree relatives is estimated to lie between 15% and 44% (44,53,133–135).

In patients with IGE, genes that encode for subunits of receptors involved in GABAergic mediated-inhibition and deactivation of calcium currents have been identified; both of which are essential for the maintenance of thalamic oscillations.

Mutations in the GABA$_A$ γ_2 receptor subunit gene, *GABRG2*, have been identified in patients with CAE (136,137) as well as in families with a spectrum of epilepsy syndromes consistent with generalized epilepsy with febrile seizures *plus* (138–140). For patients with JME, mutations have also been identified in the GABA$_A$ receptor α_1 subunit gene *GABRA1* (141) as well as other susceptibility alleles (142).

Mutations in the *CLCN2* gene that encodes the voltage-gated chloride channel subunit was identified in a cohort of common IGE syndromes (CAE, JAE, and JME) (143,144). *CLCN2* is expressed in neurons that are sensitive to GABA and is believed to play a role in maintaining the low intracellular chloride concentration that is necessary for an inhibitory GABA response.

In patients with typical absence seizures, mutations have been identified in genes that encode for two low-voltage–gated T-type calcium channels, *CACNA1G* (Cav3.1) and *CACNA1H* (Cav3.2). In 2003, Chen and colleagues (145) initially identified mutations in *CACNA1H* in patients with CAE. Although subsequently confirmed (140,146), mutations were not identified in all studies (147). Mutations in *CACNA1G* have been identified in patients with IGEs (148). In addition to low-voltage–gated T-type calcium channels, mutations have also been identified in the calcium subunit gene *CACNA1A*, which encodes the α_{1A} subunit of neuronal P/Q-type (Cav2.1) (147,149,150) and the calcium-channel β_4 subunit gene *CACNB4* (151) in patients with IGE phenotypes.

In recent years, knockout studies in mice have demonstrated the importance of calcium channels in the etiology of absence seizures. In mice lacking the Cav2.3, R-type calcium channel, an altered thalamocortical rhythmicity was identified (152). In the "stargazer" mouse with mutation in the calcium channel γ_2 subunit (stargazin), several neurologic disorders including spontaneous absence seizure, cerebellar ataxia, and head tossing were observed (153); this mutation was also associated with aberrant GABA$_A$ receptor expression in the dentate gyrus (154).

Linkage experiments in IGE patients have identified other chromosomal loci; however, the genetic significance of these sites is unknown (144,155–158). In one identified locus, 6p11-12 (159), mutations were further identified in the *EFHC1* gene (160), whose function is so far unclear.

However, it is important to note that these mutations have only been identified in a subset of patients and are not common to different syndromes, underlying the polygenic nature of seizures. Moreover, rodent models with single gene defects present major neurologic defects (161) and are not appropriate for the study of absence seizures, whereas polygenic models (GAERS or WAG/Rij rats) appear to better resemble human idiopathic absence seizures epilepsies (162), consistent with the current view that typical absence seizures, as well as associated seizure types, are predominantly polygenic in nature.

References

1. Adie W. Pyknolepsy: a form of epilepsy occuring in children with a good prognosis. *Brain*. 1924;47:96–102.
2. Drury I, Dreifuss FE. Pyknoleptic petit mal. *Acta Neurol Scand*. 1985;72:353–362.
3. Dreifuss FE. Historical Aspects. In: Duncan J, Panayiotopoulos C, eds. *Typical Absences and Related Epileptic Syndromes*. London: Churchill Communications; 1995:1–7.
4. Gastaut H, Broughton R. *Epileptic Seizures: Clinical and Electroencephalographic Features, Diagnosis and Treatment*. Springfield: Charles C. Thomas; 1972.
5. Gibbs F, Davis H, Lennox WG. The electroencephalogram in epilepsy and conditions of impaired consciousness. *Arch Neurol Psychiatry*. 1935;34:1133–1148.
6. Gastaut H. Clinical and electroencephalographic correlates of generalized spike and wave bursts occurring spontaneously in man. *Epilepsia*. 1968;9:179–184.
7. Panayiotopoulos CP, Obeid T, Waheed G. Differentiation of typical absence seizures in epileptic syndromes. A video EEG study of 224 seizures in 20 patients. *Brain*. 1989;112:1039–1056.
8. Penry JK, Porter RJ, Dreifuss FE. Simultaneous recording of absence seizures with video tape and electroencephalography. A study of 374 seizures in 48 patients. *Brain*. 1975;98:427–440.
9. Stefan H. *Epileptische Absencen*. Stuttgart, Germany: Thieme; 1982.
10. Stefan H, Burr W, Hildenbrand K, et al. Basic temporal structure of absence symptoms. In: Akimoto H, Kazamatsuri H, Seino M, et al., eds. *Advances in Epileptology: XIIIth Epilepsy International Symposium*. New York: Raven Press; 1982;55–60.
11. Proposal for revised clinical and electroencephalographic classification of epileptic seizures. From the Commission on Classification and Terminology of the International League Against Epilepsy. *Epilepsia*. 1981;22:489–501.
12. Gibbs F, Lennox WG, Gibbs E. The electroencephalogram in diagnosis and in localization of epileptic seizures. *Arch Neurol Psychiatry*. 1936;36:1225–1235.
13. Gibbs F, Gibbs E, Lennox WG. The influence of blood sugar level on the wave and spike formation in petit mal epilepsy. *Arch Neurol Psychiatry*. 1939;41:1111–1116.
14. Gibbs F, Gibbs E. *Atlas of Electroencephalography*. Vol II. Cambridge: Addison-Wesley; 1952.
15. Arzimanoglou A, Guerrini R, Aicardi J. *Aicardi's Epilepsy in Children*. 3rd ed. Philadelphia: Lippincott Williams & Wilkins; 2004.
16. Dreifuss FE. Absence epilepsies. In: Dam M, Gram L, eds. *Comprehensive Epileptology*. New York: Raven Press; 1991:1–14, 145–153.
17. Penry JK. Perspectives in complex partial seizures. *Adv Neurol*. 1975;11:1–14.
18. Porter RJ. Current medical therapy of epilepsy. *Acta Neurol Scand Suppl*. 1992;140:59–64.
19. Gastaut H, Zifkin BG, Mariani E, et al. The long-term course of primary generalized epilepsy with persisting absences. *Neurology*. 1986;36:1021–1028.
20. Panayiotopoulos C. The clinical spectrum of typical absence seizures and absence epilepsies. In: Malafosse A, Genton P, Hirsch E, et al., eds. *Idiopathic Generalized Epilepsies: Clinical, Experimental and Genetic Aspects*. London: John Libbey; 1974:75–85.
21. Thomas P, Beaumanoir A, Genton P, et al. 'De novo' absence status of late onset: report of 11 cases. *Neurology*. 1992;42:104–10.
22. Guey J, Bureau M, Dravet C, et al. A study of the rhythm of petit mal absences in children in relation to prevailing situations. The use of EEG telemetry during psychological examinations, school exercises and periods of inactivity. *Epilepsia*. 1969;10:441–451.
23. Guey J, Tassinari CA, Charles C, et al. Variations in the efficiency level in relation to paroxysmal epileptic discharges. *Rev Neurol (Paris)*. 1965;112:311–317.
24. Lennox WG, Lennox MA. *Epilepsy and Related Disorders*. Boston: Little, Brown, and Company; 1960.
25. Goossens LA, Andermann F, Andermann E, et al. Reflex seizures induced by calculation, card or board games, and spatial tasks: a review of 25 patients and delineation of the epileptic syndrome. *Neurology*. 1990;40:1171–1176.
26. Senanayake N. Epilepsia arithmetices revisited. *Epilepsy Res*. 1989;3:167–173.
27. Dalby MA. Epilepsy and 3 per second spike and wave rhythms. A clinical, electroencephalographic and prognostic analysis of 346 patients. *Acta Neurol Scand*. 1969;(suppl 40):3+.
28. Harding GFA, Jeavons PM. *Photosensitive Epilepsy*. 2nd ed. London: MacKeith Press, 1994.
29. Loiseau P, Cohadon F. *Le Petit Mal et Ses Frontieres*. Paris: Masson; 1970.
30. Roger J, Genton P. Definitions and ictal manifestations of typical. In: Duncan J, Panayiotopoulos CP, eds. *Typical Absences and Related Syndromes*. London: Churchill Communication; 1995:145–151.
31. Wirrell EC, Camfield PR, Gordon KE, et al. Will a critical level of hyperventilation-induced hypocapnia always induce an absence seizure? *Epilepsia*. 1996;37:459–462.
32. Esquivel E, Chaussain M, Plouin P, et al. Physical exercise and voluntary hyperventilation in childhood absence epilepsy. *Electroencephalogr Clin Neurophysiol*. 1991;79:127–132.
33. Browne TR, Dreifuss FE, Penry JK, et al. Clinical and EEG estimates of absence seizure frequency. *Arch Neurol*. 1983;40:469–472.
34. Janz D. *Spezielle Pathologie und Therapie*. Stuttgart: Thieme; 1969.
35. Holowach J, Thurston DL, O'Leary JL. Petit mal epilepsy. *Pediatrics*. 1962;30:893–901.
36. Holmes,GL, McKeever M, Adamson M. Absence seizures in children: clinical and electroencephalographic features. Ann Neurol. 1987;21:268–273.
37. Epstein MA, Duchowny M, Jayakar P, et al. Altered responsiveness during hyperventilation-induced EEG slowing: a non-epileptic phenomenon in normal children. *Epilepsia*. 1994;35:1204–1207.
38. Aicardi J, Gomes A. Clinical and EEG symptomatology of the "genuine" Lennox-Gastaut syndrome and its differentiation from other forms of epilepsy in early childhood. In: Degen R, ed., *The Benign Localized and Generalized Epilepsies of Early Childhood*. Amsterdam: Elsevier; 1992:185–193.
39. Arzimanoglou A., French J, Blume WT, et al. Lennox-Gastaut syndrome: a consensus approach on diagnosis, assessment, management, and trial methodology. *Lancet Neurol*. 2009;8:82–93.
40. Gastaut H, Dravet C, Loubier D. Evolution clinique et pronostic du syndrome de Lennox-Gastaut. In: Lugaresi E, Pazzaglia P, Tassinari C, eds. *Evolution and Prognosis of Epilepsies*. Bologna: Aulo Gaggi; 1973:133–154.
41. Gibberd FB. The prognosis of petit mal. *Brain*. 1966;89:531–238.
42. Tassinari CA, Lyagoubi S, Santos V, et al. Study on spike and wave discharges in man. II. Clinical and electroencephalographic aspects of myoclonic absences. *Rev Neurol (Paris)*. 1969;121:379–383.
43. Lugaresi EP, Pazzaglia P, Roger J, et al. Evolution and prognosis of petit mal. In: Harris P, Mawdsley C, eds. *Epilepsy: Proceedings of the Hans Berger Centenary Symposium*. Edinburgh: Churchill Livingstone; 1974:151–153.
44. Lugaresi EP, Pazzaglia P, Franck L. Evolution and prognosis of primary generalized epilepsies of the petit mal absence type. In: Lugaresi E, Ed., *Evolution and Prognosis of Epilepsy*. Bologna: Aulo Gaggi; 1973:3–22.
45. Tassinari C, Burea M. Epilepsy with myoclonic absences. In: Roger J, Dravet C, Bureau M, eds. *Epileptic Syndromes in Infancy, Childhood and Adolescence*. London: John Libbey; 1985:121–129.
46. Tassinari C, Bureau M, Homas P. Epilepsy with myoclonic absences. In: Roger J, Dravet C, Bureau M, eds. *Epileptic Syndromes in Infancy, Childhood and Adolescence*. London: John Libbey; 1992:151–160.
47. Proposal for revised classification of epilepsies and epileptic syndromes. Commission on Classification and Terminology of the International League Against Epilepsy. *Epilepsia*. 1989;30:389–399.
48. Tassinari CA, Michelucci R, Rubboli G, et al. Myoclonic absence epilepsy. In: Duncan JS, Panayiotopoulos CP, eds. *Typical Absences and Related Syndromes*. London: Churchill Communications; 1995:187–195.
49. Tassinari CA, Lyagoubi S, Gambarelli S, et al. Relationships between EEG discharge and neuromuscular phenomena. *Electroencephalogr Clin Neurophysiol*. 1971;31:171–182.
50. Snead OC III . Basic mechanisms of generalized absence seizures. *Ann Neurol*. 1995;37:146–157.
51. Aarts JH, Binnie CD, Smit AM, et al. Selective cognitive impairment during focal and generalized epileptiform EEG activity. *Brain*. 1984;107: 293–308.
52. Riviello JJ, Foley CM. The epileptiform significance of intermittent rhythmic delta activity in childhood. *J Child Neurol*. 1992;7:56–60.
53. Sato S, Dreifuss FE, Penry JK. Prognostic factors in absence seizures. *Neurology*. 1976;26:788–796.
54. Browne TR, Mirsky AF. Absence (petit mal) seizures. In: Browne TR, Feldman RG, eds. *Epilepsy: Diagnosis and Management*. Boston: Little, Brown and Company; 1983:61–74.
55. Browne TR, Penry JK, Proter RJ, et al. Responsiveness before, during, and after spike-wave paroxysms. *Neurology*. 1974;24:659–665.
56. Benbadis SR. Observations on the misdiagnosis of generalized epilepsy as partial epilepsy: causes and consequences. *Seizure*. 1999;8:140–145.
57. Panayiotopoulos CP. Diagnosis in epilepsies: still a central problem. *Eur J Neurol*. 1996;3(suppl 3):3–8.
58. Niedermeyer E. *The Generalized Epilepsies*. Springfield, IL: Charles C. Thomas Publishers; 1972.

59. Ricci GB, Vizzioli R. Bilateral spike and wave complexes and cortical focus. *Electroencephalogr Clin Neurophysiol.* 1964;6:534.
60. Parker AP, Agathonikou A, Robinson RO, et al. Inappropriate use of carbamazepine and vigabatrin in typical absence seizures. *Dev Med Child Neurol.* 1998;40:517–519.
61. Gastaut H. The Lennox-Gastaut syndrome: comments on the syndrome's terminology and nosological position amongst the secondary generalized epilepsies of childhood. *Electroencephalogr Clin Neurophysiol Suppl.* 1982;35:71–84.
62. Gastaut H, Roger J, Soulayrol R, et al. Epileptic encephalopathy of children with diffuse slow spikes and waves (alias "petit mal variant") or Lennox syndrome. *Ann Pediatr (Paris).* 1966;13:489–499.
63. Lennox WG, Davis JP. Clinical correlates of the fast and the slow spike-wave electroencephalogram. *Pediatrics.* 1950;5:626–644.
64. Lee SI, Kirby D. Absence seizure with generalized rhythmic delta activity. *Epilepsia.* 1988;29:262–267.
65. Lafleur J, Reiher J. Pseudo-absences. *Electroencephalogr Clin Neurophysiol.* 1977;43:279–280.
66. North KN, Ouvrier, RA, Nugent M. Pseudoseizures caused by hyperventilation resembling absence epilepsy. *J Child Neurol.* 1990;5:288–294.
67. Erba G, Browne TR. Atypical absence, myoclonic, atonic and tonic seizures, and the "Lennox-Gastaut syndrome". In: Browne TR, Feldman RG, eds. *Epilepsy: Diagnosis and Management.* Boston: Little, Brown and Company; 1983:75–94.
68. Blume WT. *Atlas of Pediatric Electroencephalography.* New York: Raven Press; 1982.
69. Delgado-Escueta AV, Treiman DM, Walsh GO. The treatable epilepsies. *N Engl J Med.* 1983;308:1508–1514.
70. Berkovic SF, Andermann F, Andermann E, et al. Concepts of absence epilepsies: discrete syndromes or biological continuum? *Neurology.* 1987;37:993–1000.
71. Niedermeyer E, Laws Jr ER, Walker EA. Depth EEG findings in epileptics with generalized spike-wave complexes. *Arch Neurol.* 1969;21:51–58.
72. Fakhoury T, Abou-Khalil B. Generalized absence seizures with 10–15 Hz fast discharges. *Clin Neurophysiol.* 1999;110:1029–1035.
73. Aicardi J. *Epilepsy in Children.* 2nd ed. New York: Raven Press; 1994.
74. So EL, King DW, Murvin AJ. Misdiagnosis of complex absence seizures. *Arch Neurol.* 1984;41:640–641.
75. Geier S, Bancaud J, Talairach J, et al. Automatisms during frontal lobe epileptic seizures. *Brain.* 1976;99:447–458.
76. Rasmussen T. Characteristics of a pure culture of frontal lobe epilepsy. *Epilepsia.* 1983;24:482–493.
77. Tukel K, Jasper H. Electroencephalogram in parasagittal lesions. *Electroencephalogr Clin Neurophysiol.* 1952;4:481–494.
78. Williamson PD. Complex partial seizures of frontal lobe origin. *Ann Neurol.* 1985;18:497–504.
79. Bancaud J, Talairach J, Morel P, et al. "Generalized" epileptic seizures elicited by electrical stimulation of the frontal lobe in man. *Electroencephalogr Clin Neurophysiol.* 1974;37:275–282.
80. Ferrie CD, Robinson RO, Knott C, et al. Symptomatic typical absence seizures. In: Duncan JS, Panayiotopoulos CP, eds. *Typical Absences and Related Epileptic Syndromes.* London: Churchill Communications; 1995:241–252.
81. Gloor P, Rasmussen T, Altuzarra A, et al. Role of the intracarotid amobarbital-pentylenetetrazol EEG test in the diagnosis and surgical treatment of patients with complex seizure problems. *Epilepsia.* 1976;17:15–31.
82. Blume WT, Pillay N. Electrographic and clinical correlates of secondary bilateral synchrony. *Epilepsia.* 1985;26:636–641.
83. Daly DD. Epilepsy and syncope. In: Daly DD, Pedley TA, eds. *Current Practice of Clinical Electroencephalography.* New York: Raven Press; 1990:269–334.
84. Rosenow F, Wyllie E, Kotagal P, et al. Staring spells in children: descriptive features distinguishing epileptic and nonepileptic events. *J Pediatr.* 1998;133:660–663.
85. Carmant L, Kramer U, Holmes GL, et al. Differential diagnosis of staring spells in children: a video-EEG study. *Pediatr Neurol.* 1996;14:199–202.
86. Williams J, Sharp GB, DelosReyes E, et al. Symptom differences in children with absence seizures versus inattention. *Epilepsy Behav.* 2002;3:245–248.
87. Chevrie JJ, Aicardi J. Childhood epileptic encephalopathy with slow spike-wave. A statistical study of 80 cases. *Epilepsia.* 1972;13:259–271.
88. Bamberger P, Matthes A. *Anfalle im Kindesalter.* Basel: Karger; 1959.
89. Meencke HJ, Janz D. Neuropathological findings in primary generalized epilepsy: a study of eight cases. *Epilepsia.* 1984;25:8–21.
90. Opeskin K, Kalnins RM, Halliday G, et al. Idiopathic generalized epilepsy: lack of significant microdysgenesis. *Neurology.* 2000;55:1101–1106.
91. Sherwin AL. Absence seizures. In: Morselli PL, Pippenger CE, Penry JK, eds. *Antiepileptic Drug Therapy in Pediatrics.* 1983:153–161. New York: Rave Press;
92. Covanis A, Gupta AK, Jeavons PM. Sodium valproate: monotherapy and polytherapy. *Epilepsia.* 1982;23:693–720.
93. Sato S, White BG, Penry JK, et al. Valproic acid versus ethosuximide in the treatment of absence seizures. *Neurology.* 1982;32:157–163.
94. Rowan AJ, Meijer JW, de Beer-Pawlikowski N, et al. Valproate-ethosuximide combination therapy for refractory absence seizures. *Arch Neurol.* 1983;40:797–802.
95. Frank LM, Enlow T, Holmes GL, et al. Lamictal (lamotrigine) monotherapy for typical absence seizures in children. *Epilepsia.* 1999;40:973–939.
96. Holmes GL, Frank LM, Sheth RD, et al. Lamotrigine monotherapy for newly diagnosed typical absence seizures in children. *Epilepsy Res.* 2008;82:124–132.
97. Arzimanoglou A, Kulak I, Bidaut-Mazel C, et al. Optimal use of lamotrigine in clinical practice: results of an open multicenter trial in refractory epilepsy. *Rev Neurol (Paris).* 2001;157:525–536.
98. Panayiotopoulos CP, Ferrie CD, Knott C, et al. Interaction of lamotrigine with sodium valproate. *Lancet.* 1993;341:445.
99. Verrotti A, Cerminara C, Domizio S, et al. Levetiracetam in absence epilepsy. *Dev Med Child Neurol.* 2008;50:850–853.
100. Allen JW, Oxley J, Robertson MM, et al. Clobazam as adjunctive treatment in refractory epilepsy. *Br Med J (Clin Res Ed).* 1983;286:1246–1247.
101. Schmidt D. Benzodiazepines-an update. In: Pedley TA, Meldrum BS, eds. *Recent Advances in Epilepsy.* Edinburgh: Churchill Livingstone; 1985:125–135.
102. Knake S, Hamer HM, Schomburg U, et al. Tiagabine-induced absence status in idiopathic generalized epilepsy. *Seizure.* 1999;8:314–317.
103. Snead OC III. Hosey LC. Exacerbation of seizures in children by carbamazepine. *N Engl J Med.* 1985;313:916–921.
104. Reutens DC, Berkovic SF. Idiopathic generalized epilepsy of adolescence: are the syndromes clinically distinct? *Neurology.* 1995;45:1469–1476.
105. Benbadis SR, Tatum WO, Gieron M. Idiopathic generalized epilepsy and choice of antiepileptic drugs. *Neurology.* 2003;61:1793–1795.
106. Benbadis SR, Luders HO. Epileptic syndromes: an underutilized concept. *Epilepsia.* 1996;37:1029–1034.
107. Gloor P, Avoli PM, Kostopoulos G. Thalamocortical relationships in generalized epilepsy with bilaterally synchronous spike-and-wave discharge. In: Avoli M, Gloor P, Kostopoulos G, eds. *Generalized Epilepsy: Neurobiological Approaches.* Boston: Birkhauser; 1990:190–212.
108. Jasper HH, Kershman J. Electroencephalographic classification of the epilepsies. *Arch Neurol Psychiatry.* 1941;45:903–943.
109. Jasper HH, Droogleever-Fortuyn J. Experimental studies on the functional anatomy of petit mal epilepsy. *Res Publ Assoc Res Nerv Ment Dis.* 1947;26:272–298.
110. Penfield W, Jasper HH. Highest level of seizures. *Res Publ Assoc Res Nerv Ment Dis.* 1947;26:252–271.
111. Penfield W, Jasper HH. *Epilepsy and the Functional Anatomy of the Human Brain.* Boston: Little, Brown and Company; 1954.
112. Jasper HH. Current evaluation of the concepts of centrencephalic and cortico-reticular seizures. *Electroencephalogr Clin Neurophysiol.* 1991;78:2–11.
113. Meeren H, van Luijtelaar G, Lopes da Silva F, et al. Evolving concepts on the pathophysiology of absence seizures: the cortical focus theory. *Arch Neurol.* 2005;62:371–376.
114. Holmes, MD, Brown M, Tucker DM. Are "generalized" seizures truly generalized? Evidence of localized mesial frontal and frontopolar discharges in absence. *Epilepsia.* 2004;45:1568–1579.
115. Hamandi K, Salek-Haddadi A, Laufs H, et al. EEG-fMRI of idiopathic and secondarily generalized epilepsies. *Neuroimage.* 2006;31:1700–1710.
116. Moeller F, Siebner HR, Wolff S, et al. Simultaneous EEG-fMRI in drug-naive children with newly diagnosed absence epilepsy. *Epilepsia.* 2008;49:1510–1519.
117. Labate A, Briellmann RS, Abbott DF, et al. Typical childhood absence seizures are associated with thalamic activation. *Epileptic Disord.* 2005;7:373–377.
118. Coulter DA, Huguenard JR, Prince DA. Differential effects of petit mal anticonvulsants and convulsants on thalamic neurones: calcium current reduction. *Br J Pharmacol.* 1990;100:800–806.
119. Drinkenburg WH, Coenen AM, Vossen JM, et al. Spike-wave discharges and sleep-wake states in rats with absence epilepsy. *Epilepsy Res.* 1991;9:218–224.
120. Coulter DA, Huguenard JR, Prince DA. Characterization of ethosuximide reduction of low-threshold calcium current in thalamic neurons. *Ann Neurol.* 1989;25:582–593.
121. Steriade M, McCormick DA, Sejnowski TJ. Thalamocortical oscillations in the sleeping and aroused brain. *Science.* 1993;262:679–685.
122. Gibbs JW III, Zhang YF, Kao CQ, et al. Characterization of GABA$_A$ receptor function in human temporal cortical neurons. *J Neurophysiol.* 1996;75:1458–1471.
123. Hosford DA, Lin FH, Wang Y, et al. Studies of the lethargic (lh/lh) mouse model of absence seizures: regulatory mechanisms and identification of the lh gene. *Adv Neurol.* 1999;79:239–252.
124. Wong CG, Snead OC III. The GABA$_A$ receptor: Subunit-Dependent Functions and Absence Seizures. *Epilepsy Curr.* 2001;1:1–5.
125. Huguenard JR, Prince DA. Intrathalamic rhythmicity studied in vitro: nominal T-current modulation causes robust antioscillatory effects. *J Neurosci.* 1994;14:5485–5502.
126. Hosford DA, Clark S, Cao Z, et al. The role of GABA$_B$ receptor activation in absence seizures of lethargic (lh/lh) mice. *Science.* 1992;257:398–401.

127. Merlo D, Mollinari C, Inaba Y, et al. Reduced GABA$_B$ receptor subunit expression and paired-pulse depression in a genetic model of absence seizures. *Neurobiol Dis.* 2007;25:631–641.

128. Inaba Y, D'Antuono M, Bertazzoni G, et al. Diminished presynaptic GABA$_B$ receptor function in the neocortex of a genetic model of absence epilepsy. *Neurosignals.* 2009;17:121–131.

129. Nehlig A, Vergnes M, Marescaux C, et al. Local cerebral glucose utilization in rats with petit mal-like seizures. *Ann Neurol.* 1991;29:72–77.

130. Dufour F, Koning E, Nehlig A. Basal levels of metabolic activity are elevated in Genetic Absence Epilepsy Rats from Strasbourg (GAERS): measurement of regional activity of cytochrome oxidase and lactate dehydrogenase by histochemistry. *Exp Neurol.* 2003;182:346–352.

131. Dutuit M, Didier-Bazès M, Vergnes M, et al. Specific alteration in the expression of glial fibrillary acidic protein, glutamate dehydrogenase, and glutamine synthetase in rats with genetic absence epilepsy. *Glia.* 2000; 32:15–24.

132. Melø TM, Sonnewald U, Touret M, et al. Cortical glutamate metabolism is enhanced in a genetic model of absence epilepsy. *J Cereb Blood Flow Metab.* 2006;26:1496–1506.

133. Currier RD, Kooi KA, Saidman LJ. Prognosis of "Pure" Petit Mal; a follow-up study. *Neurology.* 1963;13:959–967.

134. Degen R, Degen HE, Roth C. Some genetic aspects of idiopathic and symptomatic absence seizures: waking and sleep EEGs in siblings. *Epilepsia.* 1990;31:784–794.

135. Rocca WA, Sharbrough FW, Hauser WA, et al. Risk factors for absence seizures: a population-based case-control study in Rochester, Minnesota. *Neurology.* 1987;37:1309–1314.

136. Kananura C, Haug K, Sander T, et al. A splice-site mutation in GABRG2 associated with childhood absence epilepsy and febrile convulsions. *Arch Neurol.* 2002;59:1137–1141.

137. Wallace RH, Scheffer IE, Barnett S, et al. Neuronal sodium-channel α1-subunit mutations in generalized epilepsy with febrile seizures plus. *Am J Hum Genet.* 2001;68:859–865.

138. Baulac S, Huberfeld G, Gourfinkel-An I, et al. First genetic evidence of GABA$_A$ receptor dysfunction in epilepsy: a mutation in the γ2-subunit gene. *Nat Genet.* 2001;28:46–48.

139. Harkin LA, Bowser DN, Dibbens LM, et al. Truncation of the GABA$_A$-receptor γ2 subunit in a family with generalized epilepsy with febrile seizures plus. *Am J Hum Genet.* 2002;70:530–536.

140. Lü JJ, Zhang YH, Chen YC, et al. T-type calcium channel gene-CACNA1I is a susceptibility gene to childhood absence epilepsy. *Zhonghua Er Ke Za Zhi.* 2005;43:133–136.

141. Cossette P, Liu L, Brisebois K, et al. Mutation of GABRA1 in an autosomal dominant form of juvenile myoclonic epilepsy. *Nat Genet.* 2002;31:184–189.

142. Delgado-Escueta AV. Advances in genetics of juvenile myoclonic epilepsies. *Epilepsy Curr.* 2007;7:61–67.

143. Haug K, Warnstedt M, Alekov AK, et al. Mutations in CLCN2 encoding a voltage-gated chloride channel are associated with idiopathic generalized epilepsies. *Nat Genet.* 2003;33:527–532.

144. Sander T, Schulz H, Saar K, et al. Genome search for susceptibility loci of common idiopathic generalised epilepsies. *Hum Mol Genet.* 2000;9:1465–1472.

145. Chen Y, Lu J, Pan H, et al. Association between genetic variation of CACNA1H and childhood absence epilepsy. *Ann Neurol.* 2003;54:239–243.

146. Liang J, Zhang Y, Chen Y, et al. Common polymorphisms in the CACNA1H gene associated with childhood absence epilepsy in Chinese Han population. *Ann Hum Genet.* 2007;71:325–335.

147. Chioza B, Wilkie H, Nashef L, et al. Association between the α$_{1a}$ calcium channel gene CACNA1A and idiopathic generalized epilepsy. *Neurology.* 2001;56:1245–1246.

148. Singh B, Monteil A, Bidaud I, et al. Mutational analysis of CACNA1G in idiopathic generalized epilepsy. Mutation in brief #962. Online. *Hum Mutat.* 2007;28:524–525.

149. Chioza B, Osei-Lah A, Nashef L, et al. Haplotype and linkage disequilibrium analysis to characterise a region in the calcium channel gene CACNA1A associated with idiopathic generalised epilepsy. *Eur J Hum Genet.* 2002;10:857–864.

150. Imbrici P, Jaffe SL, Eunson LH, et al. Dysfunction of the brain calcium channel CaV2.1 in absence epilepsy and episodic ataxia. *Brain.* 2004;127:2682–2692.

151. Escayg A, De Waard M, Lee DD, et al. Coding and noncoding variation of the human calcium-channel beta4-subunit gene CACNB4 in patients with idiopathic generalized epilepsy and episodic ataxia. *Am J Hum Genet.* 2000;66:1531–1539.

152. Weiergraber M, Henry M, Ho MS, et al. Altered thalamocortical rhythmicity in Ca(v)2.3-deficient mice. *Mol Cell Neurosci.* 2008;39:605–618.

153. Ryu MJ, Lee C, Kim J, et al. Proteomic analysis of stargazer mutant mouse neuronal proteins involved in absence seizure. *J Neurochem.* 2008;104:1260–1270.

154. Payne HL, Donoghue PS, Connelly WM, et al. Aberrant GABA$_A$ receptor expression in the dentate gyrus of the epileptic mutant mouse stargazer. *J Neurosci.* 2006;26:8600–8608.

155. Elmslie FV, Rees M, Williamson MP, et al. Genetic mapping of a major susceptibility locus for juvenile myoclonic epilepsy on chromosome 15q. *Hum Mol Genet.* 1997;6:1329–1334.

156. Izzi C, Barbon A, Kretz R, et al. Sequencing of the GRIK1 gene in patients with juvenile absence epilepsy does not reveal mutations affecting receptor structure. *Am J Med Genet.* 2002;114:354–359.

157. Sander T, Hildmann T, Kretz R, et al. Allelic association of juvenile absence epilepsy with a GluR5 kainate receptor gene (GRIK1) polymorphism. *Am J Med Genet.* 1997;74:416–421.

158. Zara F, Bianchi A, Avanzini G, et al. Mapping of genes predisposing to idiopathic generalized epilepsy. *Hum Mol Genet.* 1995;4:1201–1207.

159. Suzuki T, Morita R, Sugimoto Y, et al. Identification and mutational analysis of candidate genes for juvenile myoclonic epilepsy on 6p12: LRRC1, GCLC, KIAA0057 and CLIC5. *Epilepsy Res.* 2002;50:265–275.

160. Suzuki T, Delgado-Escueta AV, Aguan K, et al. Mutations in EFHC1 cause juvenile myoclonic epilepsy. *Nat Genet.* 2004;36:842–849.

161. Steinlein OK, Noebels JL. Ion channels and epilepsy in man and mouse. *Curr Opin Genet Dev.* 2000;10:286–291.

162. Rudolf G, Thérèse Bihoreau M, Godfrey F, et al. Polygenic control of idiopathic generalized epilepsy phenotypes in the genetic absence rats from Strasbourg (GAERS). *Epilepsia.* 2004;45:301–308.

CHAPTER 16 ■ ATYPICAL ABSENCE SEIZURES, MYOCLONIC, TONIC, AND ATONIC SEIZURES

WILLIAM O. TATUM IV

Atypical absence seizures, myoclonic, tonic, and atonic seizures are types of generalized seizures that occur when an initial electroclinical onset arises simultaneously from both hemispheres. These seizure types typically reflect the symptom of an underlying condition or disease process (1–3) that affects the cerebral cortex in patients with an encephalopathic generalized epilepsy (EGE) and Lennox–Gastaut Syndrome (LGS) (see Chapter 22) unlike those patients with an idiopathic generalized epilepsy (IGE) where a genetic substrate is suspect (4). Despite the apparent homogeneous classification of seizure semiology, various underlying pathophysiologic mechanisms occur. Additionally, a heterogeneous combination of several seizure types may also coexist; yet they may share a single epileptogenic symptomatic substrate (2,3). Atypical absence seizures, myoclonic, tonic, and atonic seizures frequently coexist with mental retardation, an abnormal electroencephalogram (EEG), and a poor response to therapy in patients with EGE. Still, some seizures defy classification due to their multiple handicaps that limit both subjective reporting as well as objective behavioral description. Furthermore, seizures may appear to possess a generalized semiology even though they are the manifestation of focal epilepsy (5,6). Video-EEG monitoring has improved our recognition, identification, and classification of patients with atypical absence seizures, myoclonic, tonic, and atonic seizures with revision of former classifications (7) and semiologic-based classifications that assist with diagnosis and treatment (8).

SEIZURE TYPES

Atypical Absence Seizures

Semiology

Absence seizures are generalized seizures that have long been subdivided into *typical* and *atypical* forms (9). *Petit mal* is the colloquialism used to describe typical absence seizures. Petit mal variant is an older term that was used to reflect conditions of a childhood epileptic encephalopathy with diffuse slow spike wave (aka LGS) (10). The semiology of atypical absence seizures may have *simple* or *complex* behavioral features that are usually associated with multiple seizure types, mental retardation, and neurological disabilities of varying severity, as well as characteristic EEG features (11,12). Atypical absence seizures may occur at any age, but they rarely begin before 2 years of age or after the teenage years (11). Behaviorally, atypical absence seizures may appear as brief or prolonged staring with variable degrees of impaired consciousness. They have a high incidence of associated motor signs, particularly changes in muscle tone including tonic posturing, clonic jerks, or atonia resulting in falls (Video 16.1) (11,12). Atypical absence seizures begin and evolve gradually, with less abrupt onsets and termination than typical absence seizures. Automatisms or autonomic features may also occur. Seizure duration unlike typical absence seizures may last longer than 5 to 20 seconds, possibly even minutes (11,12). Consciousness is variably impaired, and postictal confusion may occur though briefly (11). Atypical absence seizures are most likely to occur during states of drowsiness and less frequently with concentration, and do not activate with hyperventilation and photic stimulation. Atypical absence seizures may be combined with tonic seizures and slow spike wave (SSW) especially in patients with LGS. When more than a single seizure manifestation occurs with absence seizures, the semiology is identified by the primary component (i.e., myoclonic absence seizures). Counting behavioral seizures is challenging since isolated clinical observation omits subclinical SSW discharges that could alter cognitive abilities.

Electrophysiology

Atypical absence seizures have a characteristic pattern on EEG (11), with interictal generalized SSW discharges that are often irregular, asymmetrical, and lower in amplitude, with spikes (or sharp waves) that occur at <3 Hz and usually between 1.5 and 2.5 Hz. This is in contrast to the regular 3-Hz generalized spike wave (GSW) pattern that occurs at onset of a burst that is classically associated with typical absence seizures (Fig. 16.1). In atypical absence seizures, the EEG background typically manifests diffuse slowing with focal or multifocal independent epileptiform discharges and generalized polyspike-and-waves. The individual SSW discharges may occur as single complexes or in bursts that are usually longer in duration than typical absence seizures with a 3-Hz GSW pattern, and are more blunted in morphology (Fig. 16.2) (11,12). The SSW pattern on EEG is typically a malignant pattern and may not always be associated with a discernible change in clinical behavior. Identifying bursts of SSW alone ignores the differences in the impact of clinical versus subclinical discharges, and counting seizures with video-EEG (i.e., in antiepileptic drug [AED] clinical trials of LGS) is reliable only when clinical semiologies are used to determine whether the discharge is clinical or subclinical. Patients with cryptogenic EGE and SSW are more likely to show bilaterally symmetrical SSW, while those with concomitant structural lesions may show asymmetrically higher-amplitude discharges over the unaffected hemisphere (13).

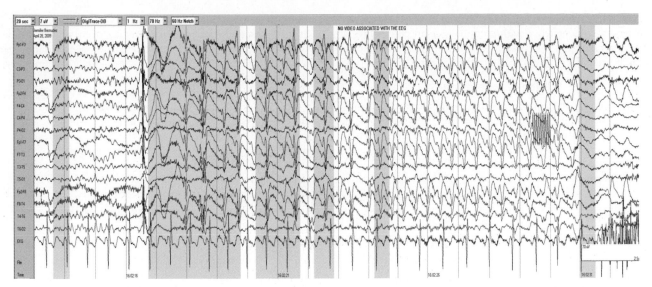

FIGURE 16.1 Slow spike waves that evolve to faster frequencies in a patient with atypical absence seizures. Note this is the reverse of 3 Hz spike waves in typical absence seizures that slow to <3 Hz at the termination of a burst.

The ictal EEG associated with atypical absence seizures typically demonstrates diffuse, irregular SSW discharges with or without lateralization; however, irregular diffuse fast activity at 10 to 13 Hz or a combination of fast spike wave or sharp waves of increasing amplitude may also be seen (16). Patients with absence seizures that are "intermediate" between typical absence seizures associated with IGE and atypical absence seizures associated with EGE have been described, with cognitive impairment, social and learning handicaps, intractability to AEDs, and a poorer prognosis than patients with typical absence seizures (14). Depth electrode recording from the centromedian thalamic nuclei during atypical absence seizures has shown simultaneous 1- to 2-Hz SSW discharges (15). Quantitative EEG may show interhemispheric asynchrony and

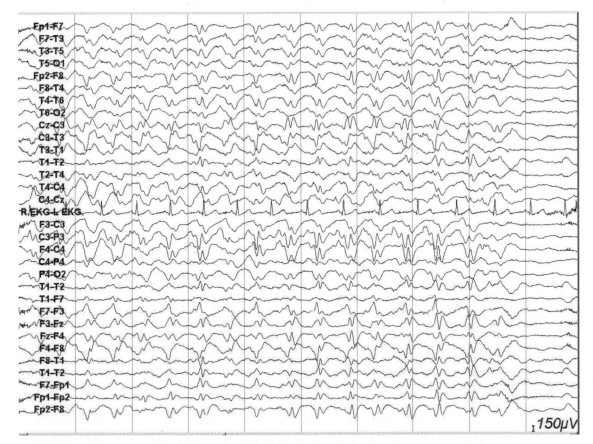

FIGURE 16.2 A burst of slow spike wave discharges in a 10-year-old girl with EGE and atypical absence seizures. Note the blunted appearance of the sharp waves and 2 Hz repetition frequency. With permission from Tatum WO, Husain A, Benbadis S, Kaplan P. *Handbook of EEG Interpretation*. New York: Demos Medical Publishing; 2008:93.

morphologic asymmetries of the SSW discharges to help distinguish frontal lobe epilepsy with secondary bilateral synchrony (16). Antiepileptic drugs may also modify the atypical spike wave pattern underlying atypical absence seizures (17).

Clinical Correlation

The spectrum of clinical and electroencephalographic manifestations of atypical absence seizures has been furthered by video-EEG monitoring (18). The differential diagnosis of atypical absence seizures broadly encompasses staring spells as well as behavioral semiologies of SSW during EEG. The principle differential diagnosis of atypical absence seizures lies in the potential to miss or dismiss their occurrence (19). When staring is noticed, separating nonepileptic behavior from atypical absence seizures is an important diagnostic distinction for the purposes of treatment (20). In one study, episodes of staring were found to be epileptic in origin in only 27% of patients with video-EEG monitoring (18) emphasizing the importance of considering nonepileptic staring despite a diagnosis of EGE. Distinguishing atypical absence seizures from complex typical absence seizures may be challenging electrographically, though the clinical course, additional seizure types, semiology with a relative paucity of automa-

tisms, presence of changes in muscle tone, and longer seizure duration usually helps distinguish patients with atypical absence seizures (21). Secondary bilateral synchronous spike wave discharges on EEG may occur with focal epilepsy of frontal lobe origin (22) that appears as SSW (Fig. 16.3). Conversely, atypical absence seizures may exist if the characteristic generalized clinical and electrographic abnormalities are noted despite the presence of a focal pathological process (23,24). They may overlap with spike wave complexes during slow sleep and occur with the Landau–Kleffner syndrome and the syndrome of continuous spike wave during slow sleep (25). Atypical semiologies have been reported with the benign partial epilepsies with a disconnection between the electrographic and clinical features mimicking atypical absence seizures (26).

Myoclonic Seizures

Semiology

Myoclonic seizures or jerks are generalized epileptic seizures (6) that may occur either as part of an IGE syndrome or as a feature of EGE. *Myoclonus* is a brief, sudden, involuntary,

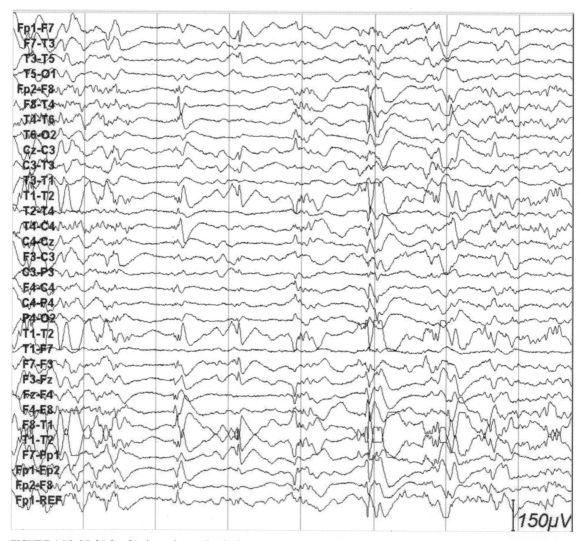

FIGURE 16.3 Multi-focal independent spike discharges in a patient with EGE and atypical absence seizures. With permission from Tatum WO, Husain A, Benbadis S, Kaplan P. *Handbook of EEG Interpretation.* New York: Demos Medical Publishing; 2008:86.

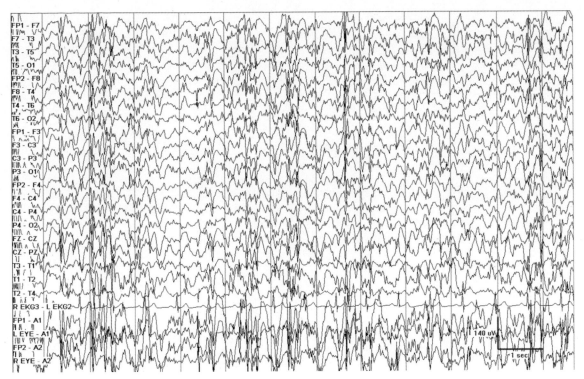

FIGURE 16.4 Myoclonic seizures were occurring continuously with concomitant polyspike- and polysharp-and-slow-wave discharges on EEG (see in seconds 1, 2, 5–7, 11) in a patient with LaFora Body Disease.

shock-like muscular contraction of the body that results in a movement that may be either epileptic or nonepileptic. Myoclonic seizures imply a generalized onset in patients with epilepsy. *Cortical reflex myoclonus* is a term that reflects a motor movement resulting from focal epilepsy and reflects the segment of the brain responsible for motor activation. *Reticular reflex myoclonus*, on the other hand, may occur with generalized epilepsy but originates in the subcortical structures and brainstem.

Myoclonic seizures are characterized by brief, sudden, involuntary muscle contractions involving different combinations of the head, trunk, and limbs (Video 16.2). They usually occur without detectable loss of consciousness and may be generalized, regional (involving two adjacent areas), or focal (confined to one area). They may be regular or irregular, symmetrical or asymmetrical, and synchronous or asynchronous. Myoclonic jerks may occur as a positive or negative motor movement manifesting extra movement or a sudden loss of movement and postural tone (27). Myoclonic seizures are often bilateral jerks that vary from subtle restricted twitches of the periocular or facial muscles to massive movements involving generalized jerks of the arms and legs that may be accompanied by retropulsion and falls. *Massive* epileptic myoclonus implies that a bilateral jerk is large enough to create a fall, and semiologic difficulty may arise when massive myoclonic seizures result in a fall similar to tonic and atonic seizures (drop attacks). Partial seizures with tonic posturing may occasionally mimic myoclonic seizures, though the presence of a relative asymmetry or sustained increase in motor tone should help distinguish this semiology. Additionally, other nonepileptic conditions including psychogenic nonepileptic seizures may masquerade as myoclonic seizures (28). Some patients may have combined seizure types (i.e., epilepsy

with myoclonic absence seizures) with both absence seizures and myoclonic semiologies and carry a guarded prognosis despite the presence of a regular 3-Hz GSW pattern on the EEG that usually denotes a favorable prognosis. Brief myoclonic seizures may occur singly or serially in clusters associated with impaired cognition when they are frequent and repetitive. Myoclonic status epilepticus typically occurs in patients with EGE (29), and occurs less frequently during sleep (Fig. 16.4).

Electrophysiology

In general, myoclonic jerks have a high-amplitude, bisynchronous, diffuse spike wave or polyspike-and-wave discharge as their electrophysiological correlate (Fig. 16.5). A very brief latency between short bursts of synchronized electromyographic potentials in both agonist and antagonist muscles and that of the corresponding spikes occur. The spikes are time-locked events that are coupled with the myoclonic jerks that follow. By using back-averaging techniques, latencies are found to occur between 21 and 80 msec (30,31). When a myoclonic jerk is generated by subcortical structures, a generalized epileptiform discharge follows the first electromyographic sign of myoclonus; however, in this situation a primary epileptogenic mechanism has been disputed by some (31). Negative myoclonus, if due to a lapse of tone, can be seen only during antigravity posture and is coupled with either the slow-wave or the second positive component of a polyspike-and-wave discharge (31). Myoclonic seizures have semiologies with an electromyographic pattern, demonstrating a brief synchronous potential of <50 msec that is seen simultaneously in the involved muscle groups (27). During the myoclonic jerks, medium- to high-amplitude repetitive 16-Hz spikes are seen on the surface of the scalp EEG (32).

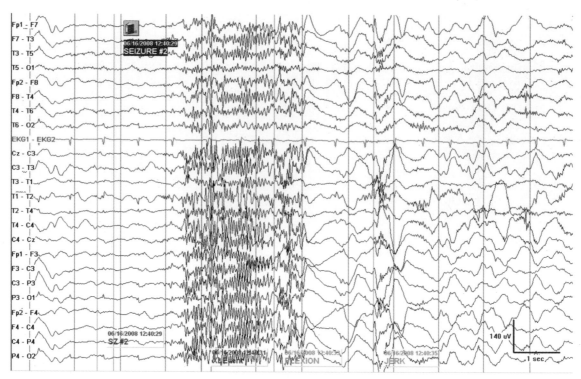

FIGURE 16.5 EEG with GPFA (generalized paroxysmal fast activity) and a brief tonic (flexion) seizure followed by a single myoclonic jerk in second 6 associated with a polyspike-and-wave discharge.

Recordings from thalamic nuclei during myoclonic seizures demonstrate subcortical slow polyspike-and-wave discharges that lead the seizures recorded on the scalp surface in patients with LGS (15,33). A unique EEG pattern is seen in early myoclonic encephalopathy and neonatal myoclonic seizures with burst-suppression or multiple paroxysmal abnormalities with asynchronous attenuations (see Chapter 21) (21). Giant visual evoked potentials appearing as occipital high-amplitude polyphasic spikes may be observed during intermittent photic stimulation at low repetition rates of <3 Hz in patients with EGE due to neuronal ceroid lipofuscinosis of late infancy, where myoclonic (as well as atypical absence seizures and atonic) seizures are commonly encountered (34).

Focal myoclonias are suspected to be derived from a hyperexcitable cortex responsible for motor activation. Electrographic secondary bilateral synchrony in patients with myoclonic jerks and focal epilepsy has been noted with generalized epileptiform discharges that show a slight delay in interhemispheric propagation as a function of coherence and phase analysis suggesting a frontal lobe onset (35).

Clinical Correlation

Myoclonic seizures are clinically heterogeneous and represent a group of disorders that may occur in many different types of epilepsies and epilepsy syndromes from early infancy into adulthood. Causes of myoclonic seizures vary greatly from acquired etiologies to familial epilepsies with varied inheritance patterns (36–39) where it is the associated features that are present as opposed to the semiology of the myoclonus that helps to define the epilepsy syndrome. Epilepsies that possess a myoclonic component may include combined myoclonic seizure types (Chapter 10), myoclonic seizures associated with IGE syndromes (Chapter 20), myoclonic seizures associated with EGE syndromes (Chapters 21 and 22), and infantile spasms (Chapter 17). Epilepsy with myoclonic absence seizures is an epilepsy syndrome that is intermediate between IGE and EGE with prolonged and prominent rhythmic generalized myoclonic jerks involving both shoulders, arms, and legs associated with absence seizures. The myoclonic jerks in this syndrome may repeat at 3 Hz during activation techniques helping to distinguish myoclonic absence seizures from simple absence seizures (25). Epilepsy with myoclonic–astatic seizures is also a syndrome intermediate between IGE and EGE with febrile seizures and subsequent myoclonic jerks during childhood that involve mainly the axial muscles, more than the face, upper trunk, and arms with jerks strong enough to cause patients to fall (i.e., astatic seizures) (40,41). Furthermore, there are less commonly patients with IGE due to a presumed genetic etiology that manifest refractory myoclonic seizures and developmental delay to mimic an EGE (31). Myoclonic–astatic epilepsy and severe myoclonic epilepsy in infancy (Dravet syndrome) represent more severe phenotypes of *generalized epilepsy with febrile seizures plus (GEFS+)*, which mimic patients with EGE, but do not possess a discernible etiology and have a genetic foundation for expression (39). A symptomatic or cryptogenic etiology is often found when myoclonic seizures begin before the age of 4 years (39), and myoclonic seizures associated with EGE represent an important but challenging treatment group for the clinician. Early myoclonic encephalopathy manifests during the neonatal period with onset of irregular myoclonic jerks (36). Severe myoclonic epilepsy of infancy (Dravet syndrome) occurs with myoclonic seizures following febrile seizures during the first year of life (39,42). Myoclonic seizures are common but least characteristic in patients with LGS, although a myoclonic variant of LGS that has a better prognosis for cognitive development has been reported to occur (43). The progressive myoclonic epilepsies (see Chapter 21) are a rare but extremely debilitating and progressive heterogeneous subgroup of EGE with myoclonic seizures as the hallmark of the conditions serving as the clinical marker (44). The presence of mental retardation and abnormal neurologic examination does not absolutely preclude an independent IGE, though it should always raise suspicion of EGE (45). Severe myoclonic epilepsy of infancy, early myoclonic encephalopathy, LGS, the progressive myoclonus epilepsies, and the mitochondrial encephalopathies are strongly associated with myoclonic seizures and portend an unfavorable prognosis for response to treatment as well as for longevity. Lastly, myoclonic seizures must be differentiated from infantile spasms. Infantile spasms may have a shock-like appearance with lightning like quickness, although they have dissimilar EEG semiologies manifesting a hypsarrhythmia pattern when compared to myoclonic seizures with polyspikes.

Tonic Seizures

Semiology

Tonic seizures are generalized *convulsive* seizures (7,46), even though they may be very brief and appear nonconvulsive. In an effort to distinguish between different forms of tonic seizures that may appear, the taxonomy has included (i) *tonic axial seizures* with abrupt tonic muscular contraction and rigidity of the neck, facial, and masticatory muscles; (ii) *global tonic seizures* involving widespread contraction of the axial and appendicular musculature (Video 16.3); and (iii) *tonic axorhizomelic seizures* as an intermediate form with contraction of the upper limb muscles and deltoid muscles that lead to elevation of the shoulders. Partial seizures with asymmetrical tonic posturing are referred to as *tonic postural seizures*. Short tonic seizures have high-amplitude, rapid muscular contractions that involve mainly the axis of the body and trunk, maximal in the neck and shoulder girdle, and last only 500 to 800 msec with forward positioning that resembles infantile spasms (47). When tonic posturing is observed in patients with infantile spasms and West syndrome, the term *tonic spasms* describes the seizure type and is often refractory to treatment (48,49). Myoclonic jerks may appear to represent brief tonic seizures but are actually single muscular contractions that last <200 msec, while tonic seizures are more intense and sustained lasting for seconds (50), although they may be associated with a myoclonic (or atonic) component (15). *Prolonged tonic seizures* may occur with a vibratory component that resembles a generalized tonic–clonic seizure (51), although tonic seizures are much briefer, averaging 10 to 15 seconds (50).

Tonic seizures may vary from a short, upward deviation of the eyeballs with or without nystagmoid eye movements to more intense generalized symmetrical or asymmetrical tonic stiffening, loss of consciousness, falls, and repeated injury (10,16). Falls from tonic seizures may be forward or backward depending on whether the axial and lower limb musculature is fixed in flexion or (less frequently) in extension. Tonic seizures are associated with falls less consistently than atonic seizures because the leg muscles are often not involved or have an increased extensor tone to maintain an upright posture (11). While both tonic and atonic seizures are referred to as *drop attacks*, the semiology of tonic seizures consists of a rigid muscular extension (like a falling tree), whereas atonic seizures manifest as an abrupt loss of muscle tone (like a shot

duck) (personal communication Dr. Jackie French, 1991). Scars from old injuries on the forehead and occipital regions may reflect injury patterns associated with propulsive or retropulsive seizures. Contraction of the respiratory and abdominal muscles may create a high-pitched cry or a period of hypopnea. Seizure intensities may vary among patients and individuals, and combined seizure types may also occur (52). The duration of tonic seizures is several seconds to a minute, although most last for 5 to 20 seconds. Tonic seizures are most frequent during stages I and II of nonrapid eye movement (NREM) sleep (6). Autonomic features may include respiratory, heart rate, or blood pressure increases; pupillary dilation; and facial flushing. Postictal features demonstrate a variable degree of cognitive and motor recovery (Video 16.4) (53), with the depth of the postictal state usually proportional to the seizure intensity (6). In patients with LGS, tonic seizures have been reported to occur in large numbers during NREM sleep and may be "subclinical" depending on the method of measurement used during EEG and clinical testing performed (54). Tonic status epilepticus is not uncommon and may occur in 54% to 97% of patients with an insidious or brief initial tonic component (50).

Electrophysiology

The interictal EEG characteristics seen with tonic seizures are dependent on the specific epileptic syndrome. In most patients with tonic seizures associated with EGE, a diffusely slow background with multifocal spikes and sharp waves is noted on the EEG that is typically the reflection of a diffuse structural injury of the brain (50). In patients with LGS beginning before the age of 5 years, the generalized SSW complexes may not appear until the onset of epilepsy is well established (9,10,20,55).

The ictal EEG manifestations of tonic seizures associated with EGE reveal a generalized frontally predominant initial attenuation of background activity that is associated with desynchronization that precedes the bilateral 10- to 25-Hz spikes with the amplitude ranging from flattened scalp EEG to >100 µV (Fig. 16.6) (56). Generalized paroxysmal fast activity (GPFA) often appears as the electrographic counterpart of tonic seizures during slow-wave sleep and consists of diffuse, repetitive, medium- to high-amplitude spike discharges that usually have malignant albeit variable clinical semiologies with increased muscular tone (Fig. 16.7) (56,57). Mixtures of clinical and EEG patterns may also be seen with tonic absence seizures that occur with a tonic component and staring that is associated with GPFA followed by SSW on the EEG (52). Fast ictal spike discharges have been noted in the centromedian nuclei of the thalamus bilaterally with invasive electrodes that correlate with the onset of tonic seizures and concomitant diffuse scalp EEG changes in patients with LGS (15). Rhythmic ictal theta and delta patterns that differ from the background activity have been described in patients with tonic status epilepticus and LGS (58).

Tonic postural seizures associated with focal epilepsy often have interictal midline spikes when interictal epileptiform discharges are observed (59). However interictal epileptiform discharges are often notably absent with scalp recording due to inadequate scalp representation of the midline cortical generators. Because the ictal discharges in patients with tonic postural seizures may arise from "deep" in the mesial frontal cortex, scalp EEG even during the seizure may be unrevealing,

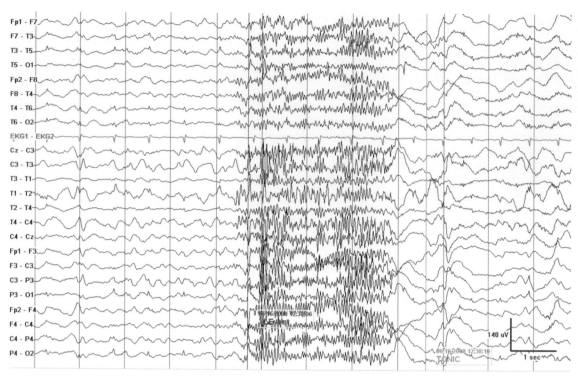

FIGURE 16.6 A tonic seizure in a patient with LGS associated with GPFA. Note the intermixed myogenic artifact and subsequent post-ictal slowing that occurs.

resulting from a low-amplitude, regional, high-frequency ictal discharge (60) or from diffuse attenuation of background in patients with tonic seizures of focal origin (61).

Clinical Correlation

Tonic seizures may present as either the initial or the primary manifestation of EGE (50). Tonic seizures are the most common cause of a sudden fall in children with LGS (61) and a major cause of morbidity and mortality, often necessitating the use of a protective helmet (50,62). The prevalence of tonic seizures is inadequately represented given the discrepancy between observed clinical seizure incidence and subclinical seizures noted electrographically during video-EEG monitoring (11). Mental retardation is less common when tonic seizures begin later in childhood or in adulthood, and is associated with a poor prognosis for seizure control and normal development with seizure onset before the age of 2 years (50).

Nonepileptic tonic or opisthotonic posturing should also be considered when painful tonic spasms or posturing occur, even though treatment may include AEDs (63). Nonepileptic tonic posturing is readily differentiated from epileptic tonic seizures by normal interictal and ictal EEG (64). Identifying tonic seizures is based on the clinical history and disease course (64–66) in patients with EGE and represents one of the cardinal seizure types in LGS (2). Although tonic seizures are characteristic of LGS and affect between 74% and 90% of patients (50), they may be notably absent in other "secondary" generalized epilepsies as well as atypical benign partial epilepsy of childhood (pseudo-Lennox syndrome) (67). When seizures are present during neonatal development, tonic seizures represent one of the earliest clinically identifiable forms (68). Although infantile spasms may appear to be clinically similar to tonic seizures, spasms are more rapid in onset (lasting for 1 to 2 seconds), peak more slowly than a myoclonic jerk, occur in

clusters, and have unique EEG characteristics (47–49). Secondarily generalized seizures with asymmetrical tonic abduction and elevation of the arms may occur in patients with focal epilepsy and may mimic tonic seizures seen in patients with LGS, although they are differentiated by the presence of associated simple partial and complex partial seizures as well as the absence seizures of associated electrographic changes seen in EGE (59,69–71). When tonic postural seizures occur, they are often frequent, nocturnal, and associated with episodes of recurrent status epilepticus given their predisposition to emanate from the frontal cortex (69,72).

Atonic Seizures

Semiology

Epilepsy received early recognition as "the falling sickness" due to the falls associated with recurrent seizures (73). Atonic seizures are generalized seizures associated with a sudden loss of postural tone that predisposes an individual to epileptic falls (51,61). Atonic seizures are frequently and incorrectly used synonymously with the term *drop attacks* (7), though seizures that result in falls are not synonymous with atonic seizures and may also occur with tonic, myoclonic, as well as partial seizures. Unfortunately, limited uniformity of taxonomy exists with respect to atonic seizures and attempts to categorize them as drop attacks, astatic, akinetic, static drops, apoplectic, and inhibitory seizures by applying descriptive terminology that only serves to worsen the difficulty with classification (51). Atonic seizures may occur as brief seizures (drop attacks) lasting second, or prolonged seizures with more protracted loss of muscular control and lasting 1 to several minutes (akinetic seizures) (51). Atonic seizures begin suddenly and without warning with a

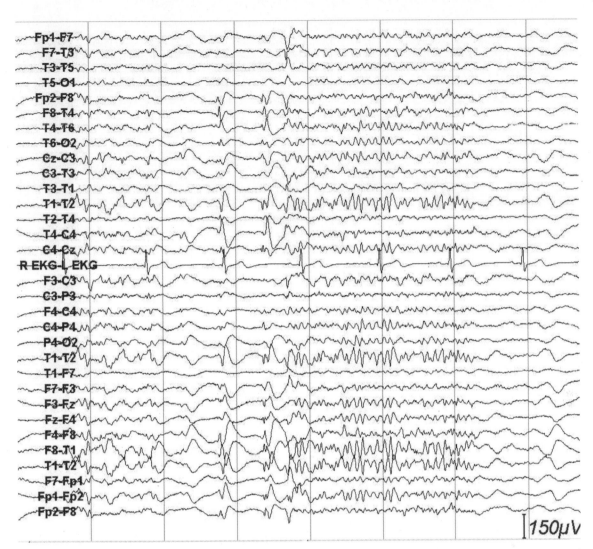

FIGURE 16.7 An asymptomatic burst of GPFA in sleep beginning at the end of second 4 through second 6. Interictal epileptiform discharges are noted bilaterally before the onset.

sudden loss of postural tone in the flexor and extensor muscles of the limbs, trunk, or neck (Video 16.5). They range in severity, from a brief head nod to a sudden intense loss of tone in the extensor and flexor postural muscles that leads to an abrupt fall. Brief atonic seizures can result in a fall within 1 to 2 seconds (11,50). An initial head drop lasting approximately 250 msec is followed by truncal and leg collapse that occurs within 800 msec (51,74). Video-EEG analysis of drop attacks with the patient in the standing position demonstrates the first manifestations to be flexion at the waist and knees, followed by additional knee buckling leading to a fall straight downward, such that the individual lands on his or her buttocks (75). In contrast, tonic seizures may occur with either tonic flexion at the hips and propulsive or retropulsive falls (51). While consciousness is impaired during the fall, postictal confusion is rare and recovery may vary depending on the duration of the attack. Return of consciousness occurs immediately with the patient capable of returning to the standing position within a few seconds (51,61). Pure atonia is unusual and seizures often appear along with other motor components such as a myoclonic jerk (11,76). The atonic seizure component (such as in patients with myoclonic–astatic epilepsy) may have late motor features too, with

transient changes in facial expression or twitching of the extremities that follows the initial atonia challenging classification of the clinical semiology (75).

Electrophysiology

In most patients with atonic seizures, a diffusely slow posterior dominant rhythm with bursts of SSW or polyspike-and-wave complexes is seen on the interictal EEG (11). Generalized SSW discharges occur most often in the first 5 years of life, waning with increasing age and rarely seen in patients >40 years (50). Common epileptiform abnormalities associated with EGE including focal, lateralized, multifocal independent spike discharges, or diffuse irregular epileptiform discharges may also occur (Fig. 16.8). Activation of SSW by intermittent photic stimulation is not typically noted.

During atonic seizures, scalp EEG characteristically reveals polyspike-and-wave discharges or more infrequently, generalized irregular SSW discharges. The discharges are followed immediately by diffuse, generalized slow waves, maximal in the vertex and central regions that correlate with the generalized atonia (Fig. 16.9) (74). During a prolonged atonic seizure, the diffuse, bilateral slow waves often mask an underlying discharge of bilateral, synchronous, symmetrical sharp waves

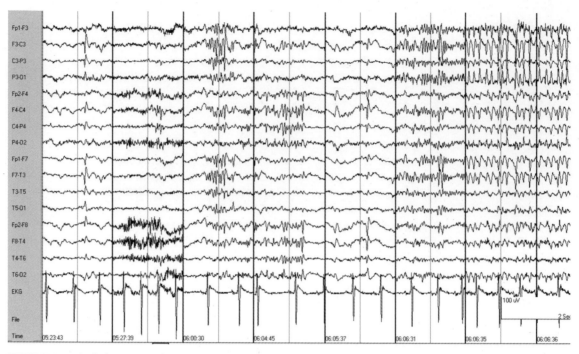

FIGURE 16.8 Ambulatory EEG demonstrating 2 second epochs of left (second 1) and right (second 5) hemispheric spikes, left (second 3) and right (second 4) hemispheric polyspikes, and generalized polysharps (second 7) during a single recording in a patient with EGE.

recurring at approximately 10 Hz (51,76), with the morphology of the initial discharge characterized by positive-negative-deep-positive waveforms followed by a larger surface-negative aftergoing slow wave. A correlation between the intensity of the atonia and the depth of the positive components of the spike-and-wave complex has been reported (40).

Patients with extratemporal localization-related epilepsy may manifest brief focal atonias lasting from 100 to 150 msec

corresponding to low-voltage fast activity or repetitive spikes in the contralateral frontocentral cortex (77), though the relationship between EEG amplitude and intensity of focal atonia is not consistent (78). Intraoperative EEG during corpus callosotomy has been performed in patients with atonic–tonic seizures demonstrating a transformation of generalized to lateralized epileptiform discharges, although this did not always correlate with the degree of clinical seizure reduction (79).

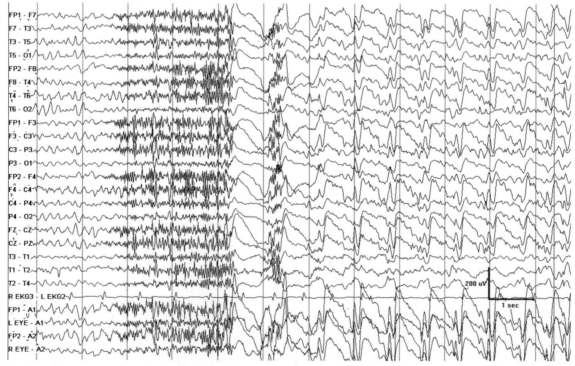

FIGURE 16.9 EEG demonstrating a burst of polyspikes at the onset that precedes a burst of generalized slow spike waves in a patient with EGE and atonic seizures.

Clinical Correlation

Atonic seizures associated with an abrupt loss of brief postural tone are commonly observed in patients with EGE but they may also occur with atypical absence seizures that have a prominent postural component (71). Video-EEG monitoring may be necessary in order to classify the individual seizure type (Video 16.6). Because of the risk for falls and seizure-related injury, atonic seizures are one of the most common and disabling seizure types (51). Atonic seizures often occur as a combination of different seizure types (16). Myoclonic and atonic seizures often coexist during a single event or individually in the same patient (i.e., myoclonic–astatic epilepsy) (71).

Partial seizures resulting in a fall may mimic the atonic seizures of EGE, although this is relatively uncommon, though drop attacks and focal atonic seizures may occur. In addition, the ictal paresis, when it occurs, may range from the less severe epileptic negative myoclonus to the more severe transient unsteadiness or episodes of falling to the ground. When atonic seizures are observed in patients with focal epilepsy, they are similar to asymmetrical tonic postural seizures and usually arise from the mesial frontal or parietal lobe (80). This category of partial atonic seizures represents an important distinction for patients with atonic seizures due to the implications of surgical therapy when AEDs are ineffective.

PATHOPHYSIOLOGY

The pathophysiologic basis for atypical absence seizures, myoclonic, tonic, and atonic seizures is poorly understood (81,82). Some neural connections have been elucidated with brain stimulation and with epilepsy surgery in patients with refractory seizures, and the genetic basis for many of the individuals that possess these seizure types is unfolding (2,31,83). A heterogenous group of structural pathologies may also underlie similar ictal behavior associated with these seizure types despite the vast differences in anatomic substrates (84,85).

In atypical absence seizures, frontal lobe connections appear to play a role in the expression of the spike wave pattern on EEG and may, thus, be operational with the precise events that herald the transition from the interictal to ictal state yet to be fully identified (86). Genetic causes are infrequently associated with atypical absence seizures, although underlying developmental abnormalities associated with a disordered cerebral cortex may be influenced by inherited patterns (85,87) and are probably underestimated (88). The neurochemical mechanism of atypical absence seizures seizures is incompletely delineated. However, increased γ-aminobutyric acid (GABA) antagonism potentiates spike wave discharges and may therefore involve a central role (89), although the lack of an appropriate model has limited investigation (81).

Myoclonic seizures are hypothesized to be produced by both cortical and subcortical generators that involve the thalamocortical and reticular projections (30,31). Because of the wide variety of mechanisms associated with the clinical expression of myoclonic seizures, no single pathology has been identified (27). In patients with EGE, a wide range of pathologic substrates may exist, although frontal lobe abnormalities may favor a predisposition (35,90). A genetic propensity or the existence of a structural lesion underscores the best-described pathophysiological mechanisms for myoclonic seizures with various modes of inheritance observed (91,37,92). For example, the progressive myoclonus epilepsy syndromes have isolated gene loci involved in the majority of the disorders (44). Myoclonic seizures associated with X-linked inheritance (92), chromosomal abnormalities (93), mutant mitochondrial DNA (94), ion channelopathies (95), and defects of neurotransmitter systems (96) form part of the wide variety of the genetic influences that have been reported.

Tonic seizures often have a cryptogenic etiology, although congenital brain malformation, hypoxic-ischemic encephalopathy, and central nervous system infections are the symptomatic causes most often found. Tonic seizures and LGS involve subcortical structures (47), whereas tonic postural (focal) seizures usually arise from the contralateral mesial frontal or parietal cortex (70) from a structural basis (97) or less frequently through genetic means (i.e., autosomal dominant frontal lobe epilepsy) (98). During AED development, the maximal electroshock model produces generalized tonic extensor rigidity during electrical stimulation to mimic human partial seizures (99). Other animal models have shown that an intact brainstem is a requirement to produce atonic seizure and that it is not entirely dependent on intact frontal cortex (100). The reticular formation within the upper mid-brainstem is probably involved, given that electrical stimulation will reproduce similar behaviors and lesioning that area will suppress them (101). Blocking extra pyramidal motor inhibition with tonic spasms occurring as a release phenomenon has also been postulated (47). The GABA–chloride ionophore complex appears to play a role in the development of tonic seizures (81). Neuroimaging with magnetic resonance imaging (MRI) has demonstrated altered anatomic architecture near the red nucleus of the brainstem in patients with LGS and tonic seizures, providing further support for brainstem involvement (23), although neuronal migration disorders and cortical malformations may also coexist (101).

Atonic seizures also have subcortical brainstem structures implicated in their pathophysiology (51). The reticular formation within the brainstem has efferent neuronal synaptic connections with the medial medulla reported to be involved in atonia during REM sleep, and is suspected to play a central role in the atonia via motor inactivation, disturbed integration, or activation of inhibitory neural connections (102,103). When the fast-conducting corticoreticulospinal pathways are activated by subcortical brainstem inhibitory centers, bilateral atonia of axial postural muscles may occur (104). The motor cortex probably participates in production of some atonic seizures, with negative motor features (i.e., "inhibitory seizures") (103,105–107). Inhibition of bilateral motor cortices in conjunction with bilateral spike wave complexes on EEG has been noted (107); a subcortical–cortical polysynaptic connection seems plausible given the clinical observation that corpus callosotomy has a beneficial effect in patients with atonic seizures (108).

TREATMENT

The treatment of patients with atypical absence seizures, myoclonic, tonic, and atonic seizures is predicated upon appropriate recognition and classification of the specific type of seizure, type of epilepsy, and epilepsy syndrome (17,109,110). Atypical absence seizures, myoclonic, tonic, and atonic seizures are grouped together due to their common clinical coexistence in patients with EGE. Evidence-based medical and surgical outcomes for these individual seizure types are limited (111,108). However, treatment is often ineffective and unrewarding with AED resistance commonly encountered in clinical practice (112).

Atypical absence seizures seizures are best approached with the use of divalproex sodium, lamotrigine, and ethosuximide either alone or in combination, and these are often used as first-line therapies (113). While valproate is commonly recommended as a first-line therapy, rare cases of seizure aggravation have been reported in patients with myoclonic absence seizures (114). A synergistic combination has been noted using valproate plus ethosuximide or valproate plus lamotrigine (113,115,116). Lamotrigine is effective for the treatment of absence seizures but may have an inconsistent effect on myoclonic jerks with exacerbation reported in rare cases (117,118). Polytherapy using benzodiazepines such as clonazepam may also be useful, especially if absence seizures are combined with a myoclonic component (119). Other AEDs not commonly available may be effective as well (120).

Myoclonic seizures are usually treated with valproate due to the broad spectrum of efficacy in patients with LGS, with myoclonic seizures responding in the majority of cases (121,122). Valproate resistance (122) or unusual presentations of medical illness with myoclonic seizures (123) may occur with seizures of frontal lobe origin. Lamotrigine has been used as an initial treatment approach in patients with LGS and in those with myoclonic–astatic epilepsy (124), although caution is advised because of the possibility of aggravating myoclonic seizures (117). Topiramate has been useful in patients with the most severe myoclonic seizure types as well (125). Benzodiazepines, valproate, lamotrigine, topiramate, zonisamide, and levetiracetam may all be effective AEDs in patients with myoclonic seizures (113), whereas phenytoin, carbamazepine, gabapentin, and vigabatrin may aggravate these seizure types (126–129). Rufinamide is a recently approved AED that has shown a primary benefit in drop attacks and severe disabling seizures that may be useful for patients with LGS and atypical absence seizures, myoclonic, tonic, and atonic seizures (130). Other less commonly used agents include acetazolamide, piracetam, and stiripentol (131–133). The ketogenic diet should be considered if AEDs are ineffective for myoclonic seizures (134), although exacerbation of behavioral problems has been noted following successful treatment (135). Vagus nerve stimulation (VNS) may also be useful in patients with myoclonic seizures, and may be beneficial in some cases of progressive myoclonic epilepsy (136).

Tonic seizures are a clinical marker for medical intractability in patients with epilepsy, and AED resistance is the rule rather than the exception (11,66,124). Phenytoin is an effective treatment for patients with tonic seizures and tonic status epilepticus (137). Valproate is a useful alternative, with an intravenous preparation available for rapid loading (138). Patients with LGS who have tonic seizures may respond to carbamazepine; however, it can aggravate atypical absence seizures in patients with EGE and mixed seizure types and should be used with caution (139). Lamotrigine, topiramate, zonisamide, levetiracetam, and rufinamide are AEDs that are evolving in the treatment of patients with mixed seizure types including tonic seizures. Rufinamide has recently become available for patients with generalized seizures associated with LGS, noting a >40% median percent reduction in tonic–atonic seizures (drop attack), seizure frequency, improvement in seizure severity, and >50% responder rate for total seizures with adjunctive use when compared to placebo (130). Benzodiazepines may also be beneficial; however, tolerance limits long-term efficacy, and tonic seizures have occurred paradoxically from IV benzodiazepine administration (140). Resective surgery may be an effective option for patients with tonic seizures in whom a focal structural lesion is responsible for the seizures (141–144), although it is rarely efficacious when mixed seizure types associated with EGE exist (145,146). Corpus callosal section is an effective palliative treatment for most patients with drop attacks due to tonic or atonic seizures (108). Vagus nerve stimulation is a less invasive adjunctive treatment that may be useful (147). Responsive neurostimulation systems and stimulation of the anterior nucleus of the thalamus may be promising for patients with tonic seizures (148). The modified Atkins diet that is high in fat and low in carbohydrates may prove to be beneficial for adult patients with intractable epilepsy and tonic seizures given the nearly 50% responder rate in 30 patients that has been recently described (149).

The treatment of atonic seizures is usually disappointing and unsatisfying due to the pharmacoresistance observed with AEDs. Valproate is often recommended as the initial treatment for patients with atonic seizures (50) when a generalized origin is encountered, though other effective broad-spectrum AEDs include felbamate, lamotrigine, topiramate (111) in addition to promising efficacy with rufinamide (130) and benzodiazepines. Felbamate was the first new AED with class 1 evidence of efficacy as add-on therapy in patients with LGS, demonstrating the best response in patients with atonic seizures (150). Patients with atonic and absence seizures respond most favorably to lamotrigine therapy (151). Topiramate reduces the number of drop attacks in patients with LGS and also improves seizure severity (152). Combinations of valproate with lamotrigine or benzodiazepines may also be helpful (119). Steroids and adrenocorticotropic hormone (ACTH) may have a dramatic response but these are usually followed by relapse. Atonic seizures were noted to decrease rapidly in children with LGS after fasting prior to introduction of the ketogenic diet (153). Children with atonic seizures may respond quite favorably to vagal nerve stimulation (154–156), and this procedure has been recommended prior to corpus callosotomy by some (147). Tolerance does not appear to develop with VNS (157) and drug reduction is possible (158), although children with swallowing problems should be monitored for potential aspiration (155). Corpus callosotomy is the surgical procedure of choice when resection is not feasible, though it renders few patients seizure-free (144,147). Atonic seizures, followed by tonic, generalized tonic–clonic, and atypical absence seizures are often improved with up to 80% reduction whereas myoclonic seizures and partial seizures are not (108). A palliative benefit is noted in most patients (159), and an improved response to AED therapy may follow sectioning (160). Radiosurgical corpus callosotomy may ultimately prove to be a promising alternative (161).

SUMMARY

Atypical absence seizures, myoclonic, tonic, and atonic seizures in patients with EGE or LGS are among the most difficult seizure types to diagnose and treat successfully (162). Seizure identification directs not only the evaluation for the underlying condition or disease process, but also aids in classifying the most appropriate treatments (5). The clinical and EEG manifestations of these seizure types are often syndrome-related, with genetic influences, associated developmental disorders, and multiple handicaps. When it appears, the SSW pattern on EEG is typically an unfavorable one that is not specific for a single seizure type but occurs in patients with atypical absence seizures, myoclonic, tonic, and atonic seizures and may also occur in patients with partial seizures (163). The long-term prognosis for patients with atypical absence seizures, myoclonic, tonic, and atonic seizures seen in conjunction with EGE and LGS is typically poor. The prognosis is often associated with uncontrolled seizures, cognitive, psychosocial, and physical deterioration, and the consequences of recurrent seizure-related injuries include greater morbidity and mortality (164). Over time, the clinical course of an individual patient may change. Loss of the initial electroclinical features may occur with evolution into different seizure semologies or even different epilepsy syndrome classifications such as patients with EGE that evolve to manifest predominately partial seizures. Newer AEDs, pharmacogenomics, dietary manipulation, palliative surgical techniques, and neurostimulation offer hope (165,166) to patients and the families of patients (167) with EGE and LGS (see Chapter 22) associated with refractory atypical absence seizures, myoclonic, tonic, and atonic seizures given the attendant risks for injury (168) and the impaired quality of the lives involved with their care.

References

1. Blume WT, Luders HO, Mizrhai E, et al. Glossary of descriptive terminology for ictal semiology: report of the ILAE task force on classification and terminology. *Epilepsia.* 2001;42:1212–1218.
2. Pedley TA. Overview: diseases associated with epilepsy. In: Engel J Jr, Pedley TA, eds. *Epilepsy: A Comprehensive Textbook.* Philadelphia: Lippincott-Raven Publishers; 1997:2515–2516.
3. Jallon P, Loiseau P, Loiseau J. Newly diagnosed unprovoked epileptic seizures: presentation at diagnosis in CAROLE study. Coordination Active du Reseau Observatoire Longitudinal de l'Epilepsie. *Epilepsia.* 2001;42:464–475.
4. Mattson RH. Overview: idiopathic generalized epilepsies. *Epilepsia.* 2003;44(suppl 2):2–6.
5. Hamer HM, Wyllie E, Luders HO, et al. Symptomatology of epileptic seizures in the first three years of life. *Epilepsia.* 1999;40:837–844.
6. Niaz FE, Abou-Khalil B, Fakhoury T. The generalized tonic-clonic seizure in partial versus generalized epilepsy: semiologic differences. *Epilepsia.* 1999;40:1664–1666.
7. Engel J Jr. A proposed diagnostic scheme for people with epileptic seizures and with epilepsy: report of the ILAE Task Force on Classification and Terminology. *Epilepsia.* 2001;42:796–803.
8. Luders H, Acharya J, Baumgartner C, et al. Semiological seizure classification. *Epilepsia.* 1998;39:1006–1013.
9. Lennox WG, Davis JP. Clinical correlates of the fast and slow spike-wave electroencephalogram. *Pediatrics.* 1950;5:626–644.
10. Gastaut H, Roger J, Soulayrol R, et al. Childhood epileptic encephalopathy with diffuse slow spike-waves (otherwise known as "petit mal variant") or Lennox syndrome. *Epilepsia.* 1966;7:139–179.
11. Yaqub BA. Electroclinical seizures in Lennox-Gastaut syndrome. *Epilepsia.* 1993;34:120–127.
12. Stefan H, Snead III OC. Absence seizures. In: Engel J Jr, Pedley TA, eds. *Epilepsy: A Comprehensive Textbook.* Philadelphia: Lippincott-Raven Publishers; 1997:579–590.
13. Velasco AL, Boleaga B, Santos N, et al. Electroencephalographic and magnetic resonance correlations in children with intractable seizures of Lennox-Gastaut syndrome and epilepsia partialis continua. *Epilepsia.* 1993;34:262–270.
14. Guye M, Bartolomei F, Gastaut JL, et al. Absence epilepsy with fast rhythmic discharges during sleep: an intermediary form of generalized epilepsy? *Epilepsia.* 2001;42:351–356.
15. Velasco M, Velasco F, Alcala H, et al. Epileptiform EEG activity of the centromedian thalamic nuclei in children with intractable generalized seizures of the Lennox-Gastaut syndrome. *Epilepsia.* 1991;32:310–321.
16. Matsuzaka T, Ono K, Baba H, et al. Quantitative EEG analyses and surgical outcome after corpus callosotomy. *Epilepsia.* 1999;40:1269–1278.
17. Marciani MG, Spanedda F, Placidi F, et al. Changes of the EEG paroxysmal pattern during felbamate therapy in Lennox-Gastaut syndrome: a case report. *Int J Neurosci.* 1998;95:247–253.
18. Bare MA, Glauser TA, Strawsburg RH. Need for electroencephalogram video confirmation of atypical absence seizures in children with Lennox-Gastaut syndrome. *J Child Neurol.* 1998;13:498–500.
19. Carmant L, Kramer U, Holmes GL, et al. Differential diagnosis of staring spells in children: a video-EEG study. *Pediatr Neurol.* 1996;14:199–202.
20. Gloor P. Generalized epilepsy with spike-and-wave discharge: a reinterpretation of its electrographic and clinical manifestations. *Epilepsia.* 1979;20:571–588.
21. Chaix Y, Daquin G, Monteiro F, et al. Absence epilepsy with onset before age three years: a heterogeneous and often severe condition. *Epilepsia.* 2003;44:944–949.
22. Rasmussen T. Characteristics of a pure culture of frontal lobe epilepsy. *Epilepsia.* 1983;24:482–493.
23. Goldsmith IL, Zupanc ML, Buchalter JR. Long-term seizure outcome in 74 patients with Lennox-Gastaut syndrome: effects of incorporating MRI head imaging in defining the cryptogenic subgroup. *Epilepsia.* 2000;41:395–399.
24. Barkovich AJ, Kuzniecky RI. Gray matter heterotopia. *Neurology.* 2000;55:1603–1608.
25. Tatum WO IV, Genton P, Bureau M, et al. Less common epilepsy syndromes. In: Wyllie E, ed. *The Treatment of Epilepsy: Principles & Practice.* 3rd ed. Philadelphia: Lippincott Williams and Wilkins; 2001:551–575.
26. Aicardi J. Atypical semiology of rolandic epilepsy in some related syndromes. *Epileptic Disord.* 2000;2(suppl 1):S5–S9.
27. Hallet M. Myoclonus: relation to epilepsy. *Epilepsia.* 1985;26(suppl 1):S67–S77.
28. Bauer J, Elger CE. Psychogenic seizures mimicking juvenile myoclonic epilepsy: case reports. *Seizure.* 2001;10:208–211.
29. Tatum WO IV, French JA, Benbadis SR, et al. The etiology and diagnosis of status epilepticus. *Epilepsy Behav.* 2001;2:311–317.
30. Oguni H, Mukahira K, Uehara T, et al. Electrophysiological study of myoclonic seizures in children. *Brain Dev.* 1997;19:279–284.
31. Dulac O, Plouin P, Shewmon A. Myoclonus and epilepsy in childhood: 1996 Royaumont meeting. *Epilepsy Res.* 1998;30:91–106.
32. Renganathan R, Delanty N. Juvenile myoclonic epilepsy: under-appreciated and under-diagnosed. *Postgrad Med J.* 2003;79:78–80.
33. Spiegel EA, Wycis HT. Thalamic recordings in man: special reference to seizure discharges. *Electroencephalogr Clin Neurophysiol.* 1950;2:23–27.
34. Rapin I. Myoclonus in neuronal storage and Lafora diseases. In: Fahn S, Marsden CD, Van Woert MH, eds. *Myoclonus. Advances in Neurology.* Vol 43. New York: Raven Press; 1986:65–85.
35. Kobayashi K, Maniwa S, Ogino T, et al. Myoclonic seizures combined with partial seizures and probable pathophysiology of secondary bilateral synchrony. *Clin Neurophysiol.* 2000;111:1813–1816.
36. Aicardi J. Early myoclonic encephalopathy. In: Roger J, Bureau M, Dravet C, et al, eds. *Epileptic Syndromes in Infancy, Childhood and Adolescence.* 2nd ed. London: John Libbey; 1992;13–23.
37. Zara F, Gennaro E, Stabile M, et al. Mapping of a locus for a familial autosomal recessive idiopathic myoclonic epilepsy of infancy to chromosome 16p13. *Am J Hum Genet.* 2000;66:1552–1557.
38. Plaster NM, Uyama E, Uchino M, et al. Genetic localization of the familial adult myoclonic epilepsy (FAME) gene to chromosome 8q24. *Neurology.* 1999;53:1180–1183.
39. Scheffer IE, Wallace R, Mulley JC, et al. Clinical and molecular genetics of myoclonic-astatic epilepsy and severe myoclonic epilepsy in infancy (Dravet syndrome). *Brain Dev.* 2001;23:732–735.
40. Oguni H, Fukuyama Y, Tanaka T, et al. Myoclonic astatic epilepsy of early childhood—clinical and EEG analysis of myoclonic-astatic seizures, and discussions on the nosology of the syndrome. *Brain Dev.* 2001;23:757–764.
41. Doose H. Myoclonic astatic epilepsy of early childhood. In: Roger J, Bureau M, Dravet C, et al., eds. *Epileptic Syndromes in Infancy, Childhood and Adolescence.* 2nd ed. London: John Libbey; 1992:103–114.
42. Gennaro E, Veggiotti P, Malacarne M, et al. Familial severe myoclonic epilepsy of infancy: truncation of Nav1.1 and genetic heterogeneity. *Epileptic Disord.* 2003;5:21–25.
43. Aicardi J, Chevrie JJ. Myoclonic epilepsies of childhood. *Neuropadiatrie.* 1971;3:177–190.
44. Conry JA. Progressive myoclonic epilepsies. *J Child Neurol.* 2002;17(suppl 1):S80–S84.
45. Gelisse P, Genton P, Raybaud C, et al. Is it juvenile myoclonic epilepsy? *Epileptic Disord.* 2000;2:27–32.
46. Commission on Classification and Terminology of the International League Against Epilepsy. Proposal for revised classification of epilepsies and epileptic syndromes. *Epilepsia.* 1989;30:389–399.
47. Egli M, Mothersill I, O'Kane M, et al. The axial spasm—the predominant type of drop seizure in patients with secondary generalized epilepsy. *Epilepsia.* 1985;26:401–415.
48. Fusco L, Vigevano F. Ictal clinical electroencephalographic findings of spasms in West syndrome. *Epilepsia.* 1993;34:671–678.
49. Pachatz C, Fusco L, Vigevano F. Epileptic spasms and partial seizures as a single ictal event. *Epilepsia.* 2003;44:693–700.

50. Farrell K, Tatum WO. Encephalopathic generalized epilepsy and Lennox-Gastaut syndrome. In Wyllie E, ed. *The Treatment of Epilepsy; Practice and Principals.* 4th ed. Chapter 33. Baltimore: Lippincott, Williams and Williams; 2006:429–440.

51. Tassinari CA, Michelucci R, Shigematsu H, et al. Atonic and falling seizures. In: Engel J Jr, Pedley TA, eds. *Epilepsy: A Comprehensive Textbook.* Philadelphia: Lippincott-Raven Publishers; 1997:605–616.

52. Shih TT, Hirsch LJ. Tonic-absence seizures: an underrecognized seizure type. *Epilepsia.* 2003;44:461–465.

53. Ishida S, Kato M, Oonuma T, et al. Tonic-automatism complex: cases with violent gestural automatisms following a brief tonic seizure. *Jpn J Psychiatry Neurol.* 1993;47:271–272.

54. Froscher W. Sleep and prolonged epileptic activity (status epilepticus). *Epilepsy Res Suppl.* 1991;2:165–176.

55. Chevrie JJ, Aicardi J. Childhood epileptic encephalopathy with slow spike-wave. A statistical study of 80 cases. *Epilepsia.* 1972;13:259–271.

56. Niedermeyer E. Lennox-Gastaut syndrome. Clinical description and diagnosis. *Adv Exp Med Biol.* 2002;497:61–75.

57. Halasz P. Runs of rapid spikes in sleep: a characteristic EEG expression of generalized malignant epileptic encephalopathies. A conceptual review with new pharmacological data. *Epilepsy Res Suppl.* 1991;2:49–71.

58. Hoffmann-Riem M, Diener W, Benninger C, et al. Nonconvulsive status epilepticus—a possible cause of mental retardation in patients with Lennox-Gastaut syndrome. *Neuropediatrics.* 2000;31:169–174.

59. Kutluay E, Passaro EA, Gomez-Hassan D, et al. Seizure semiology and neuroimaging findings in patients with midline spikes. *Epilepsia.* 2001;42:1563–1568.

60. Ikeda A, Yazawa S, Kunieda T, et al. Scalp-recorded, ictal focal DC shift in a patient with tonic seizure. *Epilepsia.* 1997;38:1350–1354.

61. Arroyo S, Lesser RP, Fisher RS, et al. Clinical and electroencephalographic evidence for sites of origin of seizures with diffuse electrodecremental pattern. *Epilepsia.* 1994;35:974–987.

62. Besag FM. Lesson of the week: tonic seizures are a particular risk factor for drowning in people with epilepsy. *Br Med J.* 2001;322:975–976.

63. Solaro P, Tanganelli P. Tiagabine for treating painful tonic spasms in multiple sclerosis: A pilot study. *J Neurol Neurosurg Psychiatry.* 2004;75:341–343.

64. Vigevano F, Lispi ML. Tonic reflex seizures of early infancy: an age-related non-epileptic paroxysmal disorder. *Epileptic Disord.* 2001;3:133–136.

65. Libenson MH, Stafstrom CE, Rosman NP. Tonic "seizures" in a patient with brainstem demyelination: MRI study of brain and spinal cord. *Pediatr Neurol.* 1994;11:258–262.

66. Ko TS, Holmes GL. EEG and clinical predictors of medically intractable childhood epilepsy. *Clin Neurophysiol.* 1999;110:1245–1251.

67. Hahn A, Pistohl J, Neubauer BA, et al. Atypical "benign" partial epilepsy or pseudo-Lennox syndrome. Part 1: symptomatology and long-term prognosis. *Neuropediatrics.* 2001;32:1–8.

68. Scher MS, Aso K, Beggarly ME, et al. Electrographic seizures in preterm and full-term neonates: clinical correlates, associated brain lesions, and risk for neurologic sequelae. *Pediatrics.* 1993;91:128–134.

69. Vigevano F, Fusco L. Hypnic tonic postural seizures in healthy children provide evidence for a partial epileptic syndrome of frontal lobe origin. *Epilepsia.* 1993;34:110–119.

70. Ikeda A, Matsumoto R, Ohara S, et al. Asymmetric tonic seizures with bilateral parietal lesions resembling frontal lobe epilepsy. *Epileptic Disord.* 2001;3:17–22.

71. Werhahn KJ, Noachtar S, Arnold S, et al. Tonic seizures: their significance for lateralization and frequency in different focal epileptic syndromes. *Epilepsia.* 2000;41:1153–1161.

72. Salanova V, Morris HH, Van Ness P, et al. Frontal lobe seizures: electroclinical syndromes. *Epilepsia.* 1995;36:16–24.

73. Tempkin O. *The Falling Sickness.* Baltimore: The Johns Hopkins Press; 1945.

74. Gastaut H, Tassinari CA, Bureau-Paillas M. Polygraphic and clinical study of "epileptic atonic collapses." *Riv Neurol (Paris).* 1966;36:5–21. [French]

75. Oguni J, Uehara T, Imai K, et al. Atonic epileptic drop attacks associated with generalized spike-and-slow wave complexes: video-polygraphic study in two patients. *Epilepsia.* 1997;38:813–818.

76. Meletti S, Tinuper P, Bisulli F, et al. Epileptic negative myoclonus and brief asymmetric tonic seizures. A supplementary sensorimotor area involvement both for negative and positive motor phenomena. *Epileptic Disord.* 2000;2:163–168.

77. Satow T, Ikeda A, Yamamoto J, et al. Partial epilepsy manifesting atonic seizure: report of two cases. *Epilepsia.* 2002;43:1425–1431.

78. Oguni H, Sato F, Hayashi K, et al. A study of unilateral brief focal atonia in childhood partial epilepsy. *Epilepsia.* 1992;33:75–83.

79. Fiol ME, Gates JR, Mireles R, et al. Value of intraoperative EEG changes during corpus callosotomy in predicting surgical results. *Epilepsia.* 1993;34:74–78.

80. Tinuper P, Cerullo A, Marini C, et al. Epileptic drop attacks in partial epilepsy: clinical features, evolution, and prognosis. *J Neurol Neurosurg Psychiatry.* 1998;64:231–237.

81. Vergnes M, Marescaux C. Pathophysiological mechanism underlying genetic absence epilepsy in rats. In: Malafosse A, Genton P, Mirsch E, et al., eds. *Idiopathic Generalized Epilepsies: Clinical, Experimental, and Genetic Aspects.* London: John Libbey; 1994:151–168.

82. Gastaut H. The Lennox-Gastaut syndrome: comments on the syndrome's terminology and nosological position amongst the secondary generalized epilepsies of childhood. *Electroencephalogr Clin Neurophysiol Suppl.* 1982;35:71–84.

83. Capovilla G, Rubboli G, Beccaria F, et al. A clinical spectrum of the myoclonic manifestations associated with typical absences in childhood absence epilepsy. A video-polygraphic study. *Epileptic Disord.* 2001;3:57–62.

84. Meencke HJ, Janz D. The significance of microdysgenesis in primary generalized epilepsy: an answer to the considerations of Lyon and Gastaut. *Epilepsia.* 1985;26:368–371.

85. Kuznicky R. Familial diffuse cortical dysplasia. *Arch Neurol.* 1994;51:307–310.

86. Pavone A, Niedermeyer E. Absence seizures and the frontal lobe. *Clin Electroencephalogr.* 2000;31:153–156.

87. Blume WT. Pathogenesis of Lennox-Gastaut syndrome: considerations and hypothesis. *Epileptic Disord.* 2001;3:183–196.

88. Berkovic SF, Howell RA, Hay DA, et al. Epilepsies in twins. In: Wolf P, ed. *Epileptic Seizures and Syndromes.* London: John Libbey; 1994:157–164.

89. Snead OC III. Basic mechanisms of generalized absence seizures. *Ann Neurol.* 1995;37:146–157.

90. Devinsky O, Gershengorn J, Brown E, et al. Frontal functions in juvenile myoclonic epilepsy. *Neuropsychiatry Neuropsychol Behav Neurol.* 1997;10:243–246.

91. Sano A, Mikami M, Nakamura M, et al. Positional candidate approach for the gene responsible for benign adult familial myoclonic epilepsy. *Epilepsia.* 2002;43(suppl 9):26–31.

92. Scheffer IE, Wallace RH, Phillips FL, et al. X-linked myoclonic epilepsy with spasticity and intellectual disability: mutation in the homeobox gene ARX. *Neurology.* 2002;59:348–356.

93. Elia M, Guerrini R, Musumeci SA, et al. Myoclonic absence-like seizures and chromosome abnormality syndromes. *Epilepsia.* 1998;39:660–663.

94. Fang W, Huang CC, Chu NS, et al. Myoclonic epilepsy with ragged-red fibers (MERRF) syndrome: report of a Chinese family with mitochondrial DNA point mutation in tRNA (Lys) gene. *Muscle Nerve.* 1994;17:52–57.

95. Claes L, Del-Favero J, Ceulemans B, et al. De novo mutations in the sodium-channel gene SCN1A cause severe myoclonic epilepsy of infancy. *Am J Hum Genet.* 2001;68:1327–1332.

96. Cossette P, Liu L, Brisebois K, et al. Mutation of GABRA1 in an autosomal dominant form of juvenile myoclonic epilepsy. *Nat Genet.* 2002;31:184–189.

97. So NK. Mesial frontal epilepsy. *Epilepsia.* 1998;39(suppl 4):S49–S61.

98. Ito M, Kobayashi K, Fuji T, et al. Electroclinical picture of autosomal dominant frontal lobe epilepsy in a Japanese family. *Epilepsia.* 2000;41:52–58.

99. Gale K. Animal models of generalized convulsive seizures: some neuroanatomical differentiations of seizure types. In: Avoli M, Gloor P, Kostopoulos G, et al., eds. *Generalized Epilepsy. Neurobiological Approaches.* Boston: Birkhauser; 1990:329–343.

100. Browning RA, Nelson DK. Modification of electroshock and pentylenetetrazol seizure patterns in rats after precollicular transections. *Exp Neurol.* 1986;93:546–556.

101. Ricci S, Cusmai R, Fariello G, et al. Double cortex. A neuronal migration anomaly as a possible cause of Lennox-Gastaut syndrome. *Arch Neurol.* 1992;49:61–64.

102. Guerrini R, Genton P, Bureau M, et al. Multilobar polymicrogyria, intractable drop attack seizures, and sleep-related electrical status epilepticus. *Neurology.* 1998;51:504–512.

103. So NK. Atonic phenomena and partial seizures: a reappraisal. In: Fahn S, Hallett M, Luders H, et al., eds. *Negative Motor Phenomena. Advances in Neurology.* Vol 67. Philadelphia: Lippincott-Raven; 1995:29–39.

104. Siegel JM, Nienhuis R, Fahringer HM, et al. Neuronal activity in narcolepsy: identification of cataplexy-related cells in the medial medulla. *Science.* 1991;252:1315–1318.

105. Luders HO, Dinner DS, Morris HH, et al. Cortical electrical stimulation in humans. The negative motor areas. *Adv Neurol.* 1995;67:115–129.

106. Andermann F, Tenembaum S. Negative motor phenomena in generalized epilepsies. A study of atonic seizures. *Adv Neurol.* 1995;67:9–28.

107. Ikeda A, Ohara S, Matsumoto R, et al. Role of primary sensorimotor cortices in generating inhibitory motor response in human. *Brain.* 2000;123:1710–1721.

108. Cendes F, Ragazzo PC, da Costa V, et al. Corpus callosotomy in treatment of medically resistant epilepsy: preliminary results in a pediatric population. *Epilepsia.* 1993;34:910–917.

109. Chabolla DR. Characteristics of the epilepsies. *Mayo Clin Proc.* 2002;77:981–990.

110. Tatum WO IV. Long-term EEG monitoring: a clinical approach to electrophysiology. *J Clin Neurophysiol.* 2001;18:442–455.

111. Bergin AM. Pharmacotherapy of paediatric epilepsy. *Expert Opin Pharmacother.* 2003;4:421–431.

112. Sisodiya SM. Mechanisms of antiepileptic drug resistance. *Curr Opin Neurol.* 2003;16:197–201.

113. Panayiotopoulos CP. Treatment of typical absence seizures and related epileptic syndromes. *Paediatr Drugs.* 2001;3:379–403.

114. Lerman-Sagie T, Watemberg N, Kramer U, et al. Absence seizures aggravated by valproic acid. *Epilepsia.* 2001;42:941–943.

115. Alvarez N, Besag F, Iivanainen M. Use of antiepileptic drugs in the treatment of epilepsy in people with intellectual disability. *J Intellect Disabil Res.* 1998;42(suppl 1):1–15.

116. Arzimanoglou A, French J, Blume WT et al. Lennox-Gastaut syndrome: a consensus approach on diagnosis, assessment, management, and trial methodology. *Lancet Neurology.* 2009;8:82–93.

117. Guerrini R, Dravet C, Genton P, et al. Lamotrigine and seizure aggravation in severe myoclonic epilepsy. *Epilepsia.* 1998;39:508–512.

118. Carrazana EJ, Wheeler SD. Exacerbation of juvenile myoclonic epilepsy with lamotrigine. *Neurology.* 2001;56:1424–1425.

119. Czuczwar SJ, Borowicz KK. Polytherapy in epilepsy: the experimental evidence. *Epilepsy Res.* 2002;52:15–23.

120. Farwell JR, Anderson GD, Kerr BM, et al. Stiripentol in atypical absence seizures in children: an open trial. *Epilepsia.* 1993;34:305–311.

121. Kanazawa O. Refractory grand mal seizures with onset during infancy including severe myoclonic epilepsy in infancy. *Brain Dev.* 2001;23:749–756.

122. Fernando-Dongas MC, Radtke RA, VanLandingham KE, et al. Characteristics of valproic acid resistant juvenile myoclonic epilepsy. *Seizure.* 2000;9:385–388.

123. Bassan H, Bloch AM, Mesterman R, et al. Myoclonic seizures as a main manifestation of Epstein-Barr virus infection. *J Child Neurol.* 2002;17:446–447.

124. Dulac O, Kaminska A. Use of lamotrigine in Lennox-Gastaut and related epilepsy syndromes. *J Child Neurol.* 1997;12(suppl 1):S23–S28.

125. Nieto-Barrera M, Candau R, Nieto-Jimenez M, et al. Topiramate in the treatment of severe myoclonic epilepsy in infancy. *Seizure.* 2000;9:590–594.

126. Perucca E, Gram L, Avanzini G, et al. Antiepileptic drugs as a cause of worsening seizures. *Epilepsia.* 1998;39:5–17.

127. Berkovic SF. Aggravation of generalized epilepsies. *Epilepsia.* 1998;39(suppl 3):S11–S14.

128. Asconape J, Diedrich A, DellaBadia J. Myoclonus associated with the use of gabapentin. *Epilepsia.* 2000;41:479–481.

129. Appleton RE. Vigabatrin in the management of generalized seizures in children. *Seizure.* 1995;4:45–48.

130. Glauser T, Kluger G, Sachdeo R, et al. Rufinamide for generalized seizures associated with Lennox-Gastaut syndrome. *Neurology.* 2008;70(21):1950–1958.

131. Resor SR Jr, Resor LD. Chronic acetazolamide monotherapy in the treatment of juvenile myoclonic epilepsy. *Neurology.* 1990;40:1677–1681.

132. Koskiniemi M, Van Vleymen B, Hakamies L, et al. Piracetam relieves symptoms in progressive myoclonus epilepsy: a multicentre, randomised, double-blind, crossover study comparing the efficacy and safety of three dosages of oral piracetam with placebo. *J Neurol Neurosurg Psychiatry.* 1998;64:344–348.

133. Chiron C, Marchand MC, Tran A, et al. Stiripentol in severe myoclonic epilepsy in infancy: a randomised placebo-controlled syndrome-dedicated trial. STICLO study group. *Lancet.* 2000;356:1638–1642.

134. Prasad AN, Stafstrom CE, Holmes GL. Alternative epilepsy therapies: the ketogenic diet, immunoglobulins, and steroids. *Epilepsia.* 1996;37(suppl 1):S81–S95.

135. Yamamoto T, Pipo JR, Akaboshi S, et al. Forced normalization induced by ethosuximide therapy in a patient with intractable myoclonic epilepsy. *Brain Dev.* 2001;23:62–64.

136. Smith B, Shatz R, Elisevich K, et al. Effects of vagus nerve stimulation on progressive myoclonus epilepsy of Unverricht-Lundborg type. *Epilepsia.* 2000;21:1046–1048.

137. Vigevano F, Fusco L, Kazuichi Y, et al. Tonic seizures. In: Engel J Jr, Pedley TA, eds. *Epilepsy: A Comprehensive Textbook.* Philadelphia: Lippincott-Raven; 1997:617–625.

138. Tatum WO IV, Galvez R, Benbadis S, et al. New antiepileptic drugs: into the new millennium. *Arch Fam Med.* 2000;9:1135–1141.

139. Genton P. When antiepileptic drugs aggravate epilepsy. *Brain Dev.* 2000;22:75–80.

140. DiMario FJ Jr, Clancy RR. Paradoxical precipitation of tonic seizures by lorazepam in a child with atypical absence seizures. *Pediatr Neurol.* 1988;4:249–251.

141. Jobst BC, Siegel AM, Thadani VM, et al. Intractable seizures of frontal lobe origin: clinical characteristics, localizing signs, and results of surgery. *Epilepsia.* 2000;41:1139–1152.

142. Lee SA, Ryu JY, Lee SK, et al. Generalized tonic seizures associated with ganglioglioma: successful treatment with surgical resection. *Eur Neurol.* 2001;46:225–226.

143. Wiebe S, Blume WT, Girvin JP, et al. A randomized, controlled trial of surgery for temporal-lobe epilepsy. *N Engl J Med.* 2001;345:311–318.

144. Bourgeois M, Sainte-Rose C, Lellouch-Tubiana A, et al. Surgery of epilepsy associated with focal lesions in childhood. *J Neurosurg.* 1999;90:833–842.

145. Holmes GL. Overtreatment in children with epilepsy. *Epilepsy Res.* 2002;52:35–42.

146. Wheless JW. The ketogenic diet: an effective medical therapy with side effects. *J Child Neurol.* 2001;16:633–635.

147. Benbadis SR, Tatum WO, Vale FL. When drugs don't work: an algorithmic approach to medically intractable epilepsy. *Neurology.* 2000;55:1780–1784.

148. Cascino GD. When drugs and surgery don't work. *Epilepsia.* 2008;49(suppl 9):79–84.

149. Kossof EH, Rowley H, Sinha SR, et al. A prospective study of the modified Atkins diet for intractable epilepsy in adults. *Epilepsia.* 2008;49:316–319.

150. Felbamate Study Group in Lennox-Gastaut Syndrome. Efficacy of felbamate in childhood epileptic encephalopathy (Lennox-Gastaut syndrome). *N Engl J Med.* 1993;328:29–33.

151. Donaldson JA, Glauser TA, Olberding LS. Lamotrigine adjunctive therapy in childhood epileptic encephalopathy (the Lennox-Gastaut syndrome). *Epilepsia.* 1997;38:68–73.

152. Sachdeo RC, Glauser TA, Ritter F, et al. A double-blind, randomized trial of topiramate in Lennox-Gastaut syndrome. Topiramate YL Study Group. *Neurology.* 1999;52:1882–1887.

153. Freeman JM, Kossoff EH, Hartman AL. The ketogenic diet: one decade later. *Pediatrics.* 2007;119(3):535–543.

154. Patwardhan RV, Stong B, Bebin EM, et al. Efficacy of vagal nerve stimulation in children with medically refractory epilepsy. *Neurosurgery.* 2000;47:1353–1357.

155. Frost M, Gates J, Helmers SL, et al. Vagus nerve stimulation in children with refractory seizures associated with Lennox-Gastaut syndrome. *Epilepsia.* 2001;42:1148–1152.

156. Hosain S, Nikalov B, Harden C, et al. Vagus nerve stimulation treatment for Lennox Gastaut syndrome. *J Child Neurol.* 2000;15:509–512.

157. Morris GL III, Mueller WM. Long-term treatment with vagus nerve stimulation in patients with refractory epilepsy. The Vagus Nerve Stimulation Study Group E01–E05. *Neurology.* 1999;53:1731–1735.

158. Tatum WO, Johnson KD, Goff S, et al. Vagus nerve stimulation and drug reduction. *Neurology.* 2001;56:561–563.

159. Maehara T, Shimizu H. Surgical outcome of corpus callosotomy in patients with drop attacks. *Epilepsia.* 2001;42:67–71.

160. Vossler DG, Lee JK, Ko TS. Treatment of seizures in subcortical laminar heterotopia with corpus callosotomy and lamotrigine. *J Child Neurol.* 1999;14:282–288.

161. Pendl G, Eder HG, Schroettner O, et al. Corpus callosotomy with radiosurgery. *Neurosurgery.* 1999;45:303–307.

162. Dulac O, N'Guyen T. The Lennox-Gastaut syndrome. *Epilepsia.* 1993;34(suppl 7):S7–S17.

163. Martinez-Menendez B, Sempere AP, Mayor PP, et al. Generalized spike-and-wave patterns in children: clinical correlates. *Pediatr Neurol.* 2000;22:23–28.

164. Hauser WA. The natural history of drug resistant epilepsy: epidemiologic considerations. *Epilepsy Res Suppl.* 1992;5:25–28.

165. Ogawa K, Kanemoto K, Ishii Y, et al. Long-term follow-up study of Lennox-Gastaut syndrome in patients with severe motor and intellectual disabilities: with special reference to the problem of dysphagia. *Seizure.* 2001;10:197–202.

166. Ohtahara S, Ohtsuka Y, Kobayashi K. Lennox-Gastaut syndrome: a new vista. *Psychiatry Clin Neurosci.* 1995;49:S179–S183.

167. Thompson PJ, Upton D. The impact of chronic epilepsy on the family. *Seizure.* 1992;1:43–48.

168. Nakken KO, Lossius R. Seizure-related injuries in multihandicapped patients with therapy-resistant epilepsy. *Epilepsia.* 1993;34:836–840.

CHAPTER 17 ■ EPILEPTIC SPASMS

INGRID TUXHORN

Infantile spasms (IS) were first described in 1841 by James West in a letter to the *Lancet* titled "On a particular form of infantile convulsions" after he had observed these events in his own son (1). He described a "peculiar seizure disorder," which was later named West syndrome in his honor, that manifested with axial spasms in clusters and failure of normal development. With the clinical application of electroencephalography (EEG) approximately 100 years later by the Gibbs in the 1950s, the triad of West syndrome as an epileptic encephalopathy of infancy manifesting with spasms, psychomotor retardation, and hypsarrhythmia as a specific electroencephalographic signature was completely described (2).

Epileptic spasms (ES) are either brief myoclonic or tonic seizures and are a pervasive seizure type in a number of epilepsy syndromes of infancy and childhood such as the West syndrome, Ohtahara syndrome or early epileptic encephalopathy with burst suppression, and Lennox–Gastaut syndrome (LGS). However, older children and even adults may have seizures that are semiologically similar to IS such that the general term *epileptic spasms* may be more encompassing and appropriate (3). Although ES are a common seizure type in infancy making up about half of all seizure types, not all exhibit hypsarrhythmia. Similarly, the etiologies are quite varied, and although the prognosis is frequently guarded and often grave, a small proportion of children may show complete recovery without sequelae.

ES manifesting in infancy were considered to be a generalized seizure type in the past classification framework of the International League Against Epilepsy (ILAE), when IS were placed among the generalized seizure disorders in the first 1970 classification schema. In the 1981 revision schema, IS were not featured, while in the 1989 epilepsy classification update, IS were reintroduced as an age-related generalized seizure type and epilepsy. In the 2001 and 2006 ILAE task force reports on epileptic syndromes, the concept of epileptic encephalopathies was introduced for the first time and specific age-related features further characterized. Of the eight epileptic encephalopathies featured, early myoclonic encephalopathy, Ohtahara syndrome, and West syndrome are invariably associated with IS or ES as a leading seizure type, while Dravet syndrome and LGS only variably so (4). With the recent extensive use of video-EEG monitoring, it has become more obvious that ES, particularly in infancy, may be a feature of generalized as well as focal epilepsy due to varied etiologies and pathologies that may include metabolic and structural brain disease. IS and ES are, therefore, not a diagnosis but an age-related seizure type seen in a number of epilepsy syndromes. This is an important consideration for appropriate medical or surgical management that significantly impacts on the short- and long-term prognosis.

EPIDEMIOLOGY

Epidemiologic studies from various countries show an incidence of ES of approximately 2 to 5 per 10,000 live births worldwide (5–9), with an estimated lifetime prevalence by age 10 years of 1.5 to 2 per 10,000 children (6,10). The lower prevalence rates most likely are a result of the associated mortality, evolution of ES into other seizure types, and incomplete determination in population-based studies of older children (11). A genetic predisposition may exist as IS have been reported in both monozygotic and dizygotic twins (12,13). Boys appear to be affected in 60% of cases, but in some studies sex differences are inconsistent (5,8,14).

CLINICAL SEMIOLOGY OF IS AND ES

IS are seizures usually associated with a severe developmental epilepsy syndrome with onset in the first year of life, peaking between 3 and 10 months of age (15).

IS or ES are brief axial movements that frequently appear in clusters. The seizure starts with a phasic contraction that lasts for less than 2 seconds, followed by an ensuing tonic contraction for 2 to 10 seconds, although only the phasic contraction may be present (16). Sometimes called tonic spasms, prolonged muscle or tonic contractions are seen in intractable cases (17). The three types of spasms—flexion, extension, and mixed—are classified by the type of contraction. In flexion spasms, the trunk, arms, legs, and head flex. In extension spasms, the back arches and arms and legs extend, while mixed spasms combine extension of the legs and flexion of the neck, trunk, and arms. Mixed spasms are the commonest type, accounting for 42% of all ES. Flexion spasms account for 35% and extensor spasms comprise only 23% of all ES (16). Many children have more than one type, even in the same cluster, often influenced by position (17). If the trunk remains vertical, the resemblance is to a flexion spasm; if the patient is horizontal, what looks like an extension spasm is seen (18). The contractions themselves also may vary in intensity, and ES can range from only a subtle head drop or shoulder shrug, which usually occur at the beginning of an episode, building up to more marked muscle contractions (17,19). Videotelemetry with electromyography (EMG) of ES has shown that the first activated muscle can vary in the same patient between different clusters or even from spasm to spasm within the same cluster, while the EEG shows no variation of the patterns. Even if the same muscle were initially activated with every spasm, the ensuing sequence or pattern of muscle involvement may differ within the same cluster (20).

At the onset of seizures, the spasms are usually mild before they become more characteristic and full-blown, as described above, which may produce a delay in diagnosis.

Complex rotation of the eyes, deviation, or nystagmoid movements may occur in two thirds of all IS (16). Eye movements may be independent of the spasm or may precede its development by weeks, which may result in delayed diagnosis of the epileptic nature, or occur as part of the motor features associated with the spasm (19). In addition, abnormal eye movements may suggest altered consciousness but decreased responsiveness may follow ES or occur independently as a second seizure type. Between spasms, most children cry, although this is probably not an ictal phenomenon but may be a result of surprise or pain (16). Up to 60% of all patients have respiratory pauses, while pulse changes occur less often. Some spasms are induced by sound or touch, rarely by photic stimulation (21).

Rarely, one arm or leg is more extended or the head deviates to one side. Spasms are usually asymmetric on the side contralateral to a unilateral lesion such as hemimegalencephaly. Symmetric spasms and a symptomatic etiology usually indicate diffuse lesions such as in Down syndrome or neurofibromatosis (22); however, some children with focal or unilateral lesions may have only symmetric spasms (21,22). Recently, videotelemetry has allowed more frequent detection of asymmetric spasms. These patients may either have consistently asymmetric spasms or alternate between asymmetric or symmetric spasms.

Spasms may be intermixed with other seizure types in one third to one half of patients (23–25). The muscle contraction in spasms is faster than that in tonic seizures but slower than that in myoclonic seizures (26,27). Tonic seizures can occur simultaneously with or precede spasms and may be difficult to differentiate, requiring videotelemetry to define the seizure type. Tonic seizures last longer than spasms and lack the initial phasic component. Both may be generated by a similar mechanism or have a similar origin such as the brainstem (16).

Asymmetry of eye movements, head, neck, and limb jerks during the spasms is often documented by video-EEG recording implying a focal component. Partial seizures may occur before, during, or after a spasm and frequently precede a cluster of spasms (18).

There is frequently a diurnal variation of spasm frequency. Most spasms occur on awakening or after feeding, less often during sleep, and the typical clustering lasting less than 1 to 5 seconds have been documented (16). Clusters typically consist of 3 to 20 spasms that occur several times a day although single spasms may also occur (11). The spasms decrease in intensity at the end of longer clusters; however, the number and type of spasms may vary markedly from week to week with less day-to-day variation (16,28).

Partial seizures suggest a symptomatic cortical lesion, and a prenatal etiology is likely if the partial seizure precedes the spasms (29). Partial seizures may precede the spasms or appear to induce the appearance of spasms that are usually asymmetric spasms with the predominant side conforming to that of the preceding partial seizure.

The effects of brain maturation on seizure semiology have been recently studied in children with well-defined "pure cultures" of temporal and extratemporal lobe focal epilepsy (30). It has been shown that axial or bilateral motor components comprising brief myoclonic IS or ES (depending on the patient's age) frequently appear in an age-dependent fashion in young children with well-localized temporal lobe seizure onset (30). The more typical behavioral, psychomotor type semiology only invariably manifests after 4 years of age while there is an inverse linear correlation of the motor ES components with age, and very young children may only manifest with ES. Only later does the semiology transition from the IS seizure type to the more adult type behavioral complex partial seizure. The semiology of temporal lobe epilepsy may, therefore, mimic generalized epilepsy with ES in the very young child or infant. Animal studies in immature rats, investigating the ontogenetic expression of drug-induced limbic seizures, have shown a similar age-dependent phenomenology in addition to high after-discharge thresholds that suggest a relative resistance of the immature limbic system to synchronization, so that extratemporal and possibly subcortical neuronal networks primarily contribute to the seizure semiology and not to the limbic system (31).

ASSOCIATED NEUROLOGIC FINDINGS

Psychomotor development may be normal or abnormal prior to onset of ES and reflects the etiology and presence of an underlying brain injury.

Abnormal neurologic findings on presentation of ES are quite frequent and may include motor impairments including tetraparesis, diplegia, hemiplegia, ataxia, athetosis as well as blindness, deafness, and microcephaly. These findings have been described in 30% to 89% of patients and may be considered a prognostic factor for underlying brain injury as 85% to 90% of this group will eventually have developmental delay (14,28,32,33). Other studies have documented mental retardation in 75% and cerebral palsy in 50% of patients (10,24,25,34–36). Children with cryptogenic ES are frequently neurologically normal prior to the onset of ES. Deterioration and loss of acquired milestones including head control, reaching for objects, and visual tracking may be affected. Loss of visual tracking may reflect the degree of epileptic encephalopathy present and appears to be a neurologic risk factor for poor prognosis of psychomotor development (37).

ETIOLOGY

A variety of disorders can cause infantile and epileptic spasms that drive management, prognosis, and overall outcome. Pre-existing brain damage has been demonstrated in 60% to 90% of cases reflecting pre-, peri-, or postnatal brain injury that may usually be determined by history and clinical neurologic examination. Symptomatic patients account for 70% to 80% of all cases, and generally have a poorer prognosis than cryptogenic children (8,25,38–40). Symptomatic patients usually have more focality on neurologic examination, a history of partial seizures evolving into spasms, or lateralization on EEG (41). Prenatal causes include congenital malformation, congenital infections, neurocutaneous disorders, chromosomal abnormalities, metabolic disorders, and congenital syndromes. Prenatal etiologies account for 30% to 45%, perhaps as many as 50%, of all cases (23,36,42,43). Tuberous sclerosis may be found as a cause in 10% to 30% of patients whose spasms are the result of a prenatal etiology (24,42,43). There is some radiologic evidence that a larger tuber burden is more likely to produce spasms rather than partial seizures, but this may also reflect an age-specific seizure manifestion (44). Although partial seizures are most common with focal cortical dysplasia (FCD), ES can occur (45); positron emission tomography (PET) scans may help to identify these patients (46). Occipital lesions are associated with earlier onset of ES than are frontal lesions (47). Neurofibromatosis type I can also cause spasms, but these usually have a better prognosis than other symptomatic causes (48). Chromosomal abnormalities, most commonly Down syndrome (43,49), represent approximately 13% of prenatal etiologies; these children usually do not have a poor prognosis compared to other symptomatic cases (50).

Perinatal causes account for 14% to 25% of spasms but may be decreasing in frequency (51), perhaps because of a lowered incidence of neonatal hypoglycemia (52). Perinatal causes include hypoxic–ischemic encephalopathy and hypoglycemia. The difference may be relative, however, and reflect an increased survival in low-birth-weight infants rather than a true decrease in perinatal causes. Hypoxic–ischemic encephalopathy often involves severe neonatal electroencephalographic findings such as markedly or maximally depressed backgrounds in the first week of life (53). In children with cerebral palsy, deep white-matter injuries are not associated with West syndrome; therefore, spasms are less likely in premature infants (52). Spasms associated with periventricular leukomalacia are typically hypsarrhythmic and located more posteriorly than anteriorly (27,54).

Postnatal causes include meningoencephalitis and other types of infections, stroke and trauma, hypoxic–ischemic insult such as near drowning and cardiac arrest, and tumors.

Besides the above-mentioned acquired brain injuries, cerebral malformations may account for up to 30% of cases and may include the various neurocutaneous syndromes, Aicardi syndrome, polymicrogyria, lissencephaly, hemimegalencephaly, schizencephaly, and FCD.

In addition, rare inborn errors of metabolism may manifest with infantile seizures and encephalopathy resembling IS. These conditions include Menkes disease, phenylketonuria and tetrahydrobiopterin deficiency, and mitochondrial diseases.

When the underlying cause cannot be identified, spasms are classified as cryptogenic; in the past, this category accounted for up to 50% of cases. However, since the advent of magnetic resonance imaging (MRI) and further technical developments in resolution and newer sequences, only 10% to 15% of cases are still cryptogenic (28,55–57). In fact, some imaging studies that were normal early in life may later demonstrate lesions on MRI after normal myelination has progressed (58). This time window in the first and second year of life may require serial imaging to detect the underlying pathology that will usually turn out to be type 1 FCD. ^{18}FDG-PET may also increase the likelihood for picking up a malformation of cortical development not visualized with MRI scan in some cryptogenic patients. Cryptogenic patients often are products of a normal pregnancy and birth, with normal development prior to the onset of spasms and normal findings on physical examination. The spasms begin abruptly without a background of previous partial seizures. Results of neuroimaging and laboratory evaluations are frequently normal. Cryptogenic patients have been shown to have higher levels of

CSF corticotropin, serum progesterone, CSF GABA, and CSF nerve growth factor (59), which may reflect brain damage from the spasms or that stress hormones may play a role in the pathogenesis of spasms.

Although most children with spasms have no family history, 7% to 17% may have a positive history of febrile seizures, which may reach an incidence of up to 40% in cryptogenic cases (24). Autosomal dominant inheritance is found in patients with tuberous sclerosis complex (TSC) and neurofibromatosis type I presenting as IS. Sex-linked dominant inheritance may be seen in incontinentia pigmenti, double cortex syndrome, and lissencephaly. Some families have been reported with an X-linked transmission that has been mapped to regions Xp11.4-Xpter and Xp21.3-Xp22.1 and that also is associated with mental retardation (60). One of these loci is implicated in neuroaxonal processing (radixin, RDXP2) (61). Chromosomal translocations may be implicated in Wilson's syndrome and Down syndrome presenting with ES.

CURRENT MODELS AND THEORIES OF THE PATHOPHYSIOLOGY OF ES

Several promising animal models to study the pathophysiology of IS and ES have recently emerged. However, an ideal model that recapitulates every aspect of human IS and ES does not exist and may not be expected. Some of the issues are interspecies differences in brain development and the lack of comparative developmental biomarkers across the species for variable seizure phenotypes and EEG signatures. However, each model will hopefully add another piece to the puzzle to give a clearer picture that will potentially translate experimental findings into clinically useful therapies. Six different models have been recently reviewed: (i) the corticotrophin-releasing hormone model examining the role of stress and response to adrenocorticotropic hormone (ACTH) in the developing brain; (ii) the N-methyl-D-aspartic acid (NMDA) model examining cryptogenic IS; (iii) the tetrodotoxin (TTX) model examining hyperexcitability provoked decrease of neuronal activity; (iv) the multiple hit model examining cortical and subcortical lesions mimicking symptomatic IS; (v) the aristaless gene (ARX) mutation model, a genetic knock out model that recapitulates human mutations of ARX with an IS and MR phenotype and may prove the hypothesis that a deficiency of cortical interneuronal GABAergic inhibition (interneuonopathy) underlies developmental epileptic encephalopathies; and lastly (vi) the Down syndrome model, Ts65Dn Mouse model, that suggests that $GABA_B$ receptor alterations (agonists) may be a prospasm mechanism (62).

From a recent human tissue study of four infants with FCD and IS treated with surgical resection, $GABA_A$ receptor abnormalities have been described using a novel technique of electrophysiologic recording after oocyte membrane injection from cortical brain tissue of these infants. Characterization of the cortical $GABA_A$ receptor properties demonstrated unaltered intrinsic physiology but altered neuromodulation to neurosteroids and zinc, which parallels the response of IS to ACTH (63).

Current theories on the generation of IS are that they represent a nonspecific age-dependent reaction of the immature brain to injury involving subcortical structures that acts diffusely on the cortex, leading to the hypsarrhythmic electroencephalogram pattern and the generalized spasms (11). Individual case reports have described abnormalities in the pons and involvement of the serotonergic, noradrenergic, or cholinergic neurons in the brainstem nuclei to support this assumption (64–66). Brainstem origin has also been postulated on the basis of abnormalities in brainstem auditory evoked responses in patients with spasms and disruptions of rapid eye movement (REM) sleep (67–69). Because hypsarrhythmia occurs mainly during sleep and the brainstem controls sleep cycles, this sleep association again suggests that the brainstem plays a role in the manifestations of IS and possibly ES (69,70).

The frequent intermixture of partial seizures with generalized or asymmetric spasms suggests a cortical–subcortical interaction, a hypothesis supported by the effectiveness of cortical resection in controlling generalized IS (18). In other words, the cortical lesion interacts with developing brainstem pathways, causing motor spasms that are similar to startle or cortical reflex myoclonus (71,72).

Further supporting the brainstem hypothesis are results of PET scans in patients with ES showing hypermetabolism of the lenticular nuclei (73). That serotonergic ([11C]-methyl-L-tryptophan) and α-aminobutyric acid (GABA)-ergic ([11C]-flumazenil) tracers may be more effective than FDG-PET in defining a focus in patients with ES also suggests brainstem involvement, because the raphe-cortical or striatal projections use serotonin as a neurotransmitter and these pathways cause the diffuse hypsarrhythmic patterns on EEG (40). On ictal single-photon-emission computed tomography studies, both subcortical and cortical structures were activated (74).

The response to corticotropin suggests involvement of the hypothalamus and pituitary–adrenal axis. Baram has proposed that a nonspecific stressor releases the proconvulsant corticotropin-releasing hormone (CRH), which may be the final common pathway for the multitude of etiologies of IS (75). CRH causes severe seizures and death in neurons associated with learning and memory, and its effects are especially important in infants because CRH receptors are most abundant during the early developmental period (76). To support the hypothesis that corticotropin inhibits the release and production of CRH through a negative feedback mechanism, Nagamitsu and colleagues (77) measured CSF levels of β-endorphin (also derived from a common precursor of corticotropin), corticotropin, and CRH (which releases both corticotropin and β-endorphin) in 20 patients with spasms. The CSF levels of β-endorphin and corticotropin were lower than in controls, as was the CRH level, although not significantly. Riikonen observed that CSF corticotropin levels were higher in infants with cryptogenic than symptomatic spasms (59).

Because IS typically begin at the time when the first immunizations are administered, the question has been whether the association is causative or coincidental. Numerous anecdotal reports have noted the appearance of IS within a few hours to a few days after a diphtheria, pertussis, tetanus (DPT) vaccination, although all controlled studies to date have failed to demonstrate any association (78–80). Some proposed immunologic mechanisms have been based on antibodies to brain tissue in blood samples from patients with IS (81,82), or increased numbers of activated B and T cells in the blood (83), or increased levels of HLA-DRw52 antigen (33). Finally, calcium-mediated models have been postulated, but further studies are needed to substantiate this (84).

INTERICTAL AND ICTAL EEG

IS and ES are commonly associated with the characteristic interictal EEG pattern termed hypsarrhythmia that literally translates from the Greek as high-amplitude irregular waves. This pathognomonic electrographic pattern consists of random high-voltage slow waves and spikes that may vary from moment to moment in localization, amplitude, and duration (19). As early as 1952, Gibbs and Gibbs noted that the abnormality was almost continuous and represents a highly abnormal, chaotically disorganized EEG pattern signaling the grave prognosis of a severe epileptic encephalopathy. The spike discharges are usually multifocal, independently arising from multiple regions of the brain. Rarely, the spike discharges may generalize, but it is not common to have rhythmic, repetitive, and synchronously organized runs of spike discharge patterns that resemble the petit mal variant or slow spike-wave EEG phenotype. Synchrony may significantly increase with age, while increasing asynchrony may occur with advancing sleep stages. On serial EEG recordings, fluctuation and a waxing and waning of the basic pattern may be seen (85–87). The interictal pattern may vary with some aspects being determined by the underlying pathology, some by the type of epilepsy syndrome, but also by age, sleep stages, and a variable combination of these (Figs. 17.1–17.6).

Rarely the interictal EEG may be normal early in the onset of IS and should, therefore, be repeated serially at close intervals if there is a high index of suspicion for the diagnosis of ES (16). By the same token, IS caused by a localized cortical pathology involving a single lobe or hemisphere may not be associated with hypsarrhythmia, and focal slow-wave activity or a persistently interictal spike focus localizing to one brain region even in the presence of multifocal spikes may point to focal epileptiform pathology such as cortical dysplasia, porencephaly, or a developmental tumor.

The background activity never approaches normal frequencies or amplitudes and is characteristically of high voltage (500 to 1000 mV), disorganized, and asynchronous with a waxing and waning quality (2).

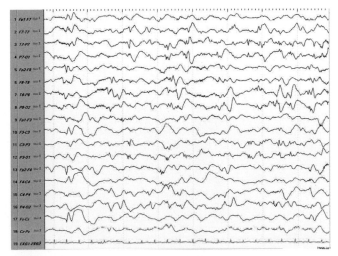

FIGURE 17.1 EEG showing classic hypsarrhythmia consisting of high-amplitude polymorphic delta waves and multiregional spike waves.

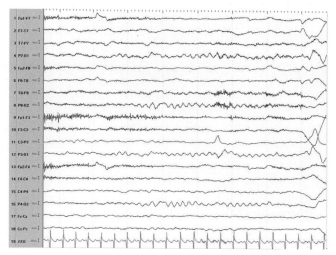

FIGURE 17.2 EEG of patient in Figure 17.1 shows normal background and resolution of hypsarrythmia within 4 weeks on ACTH.

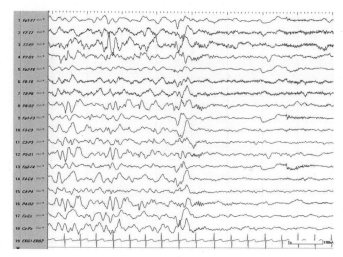

FIGURE 17.5 EEG showing an ictal change associated with an epileptic spasm in the form of a generalized wave followed by an electrodecremental pattern.

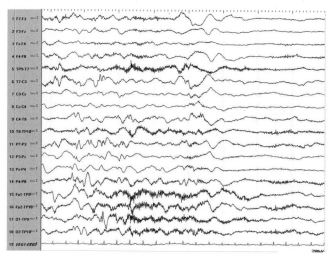

FIGURE 17.3 Electrodecremental pattern associated with an IS preceded by a broad central slow wave.

The sleep–wake cycle has a significant effect on the manifestation of the pattern of hypsarrhythmia. During non-REM sleep, there may be fragmentation of the hypsarrhythmic pattern, while by the end of REM sleep or during arousal from sleep, near-normal activity may occur; this "pseudonormalization" may also immediately precede a cluster of spasms (88,89). Long-term monitoring has disclosed variable patterns throughout the day, with more hypsarrhythmia noted in slow-wave sleep and less in REM sleep (21). Fast-wave bursts were seen during REM sleep in 35% of patients with spasms, sometimes occurring periodically until clinical spasms appeared and the patient awakens (20). Spasms may start subclinically in REM sleep (90).

Any variation in the characteristic hypsarrhythmic pattern as described above has been termed modified hypsarrhythmia and includes background synchronization, very focal features, voltage asymmetries, generalized background burst suppression, and slow waves without spikes (16). In an analysis of

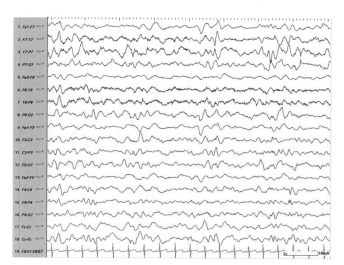

FIGURE 17.4 EEG showing a modified hypsarrhythmia pattern consisting of more lateralized high-amplitude multifocal spikes over the left hemisphere suggesting a structural lesion.

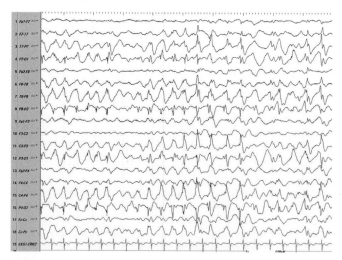

FIGURE 17.6 Modified hypsarrhythmia in an older child with more synchronized posterior hypersynchronous activity.

precorticotropin electroencephalograms, the modified pattern occurred in up to 36 (69%) of 53 patients with spasms; cortical dysplasia was associated with hemihypsarrhythmia or burst suppression (91).

Regarding the role of the EEG as a prognostic tool, a burst-suppression pattern, as seen in children with Ohtahara syndrome, suggests a poor prognosis; a lower-voltage EEG may indicate a better outcome (90), as may preservation of hypsarrhythmia between spasms (27,50), faster background activity, and absence of electrodecremental responses. However, less-typical features of hypsarrhythmia such as disorganization, slowing, high amplitude, spike and electrodecremental response, absent normal sleep architecture, relative normalization, burst suppression, hemihypsarrhythmia, occipital hypsarrhythmia, interhemispheric asymmetry, and interhemispheric synchronization may predict a better prognosis (91). This view is controversial, however, as modified hypsarrhythmia has been linked to a poorer prognosis than typical hypsarrhythmia; and in late-onset ES, a more organized electroencephalographic background predicts better development while persistent hypsarrhythmia and a disorganized background may be a risk factor for poorer prognosis (92).

The most common ictal discharge that has been described consists of an initial multiphasic, high-amplitude slow wave sometimes of positive polarity or less frequently a de novo low-amplitude, brief, fast frequency discharge (18,27). The generalized positive slow waves are followed by attenuation or an electrodecremental response, observed mainly at PZ (parietal midline), FZ/PZ, or FZ (frontal midline) with some variable degree of laterality (16,22). Because the decremental activity follows the slow wave and clinical spasm, it most likely is a postictal phenomenon (18,27) and the slow wave corresponds to the actual epileptic spasm. An electrodecremental response can also be seen in the absence of a clinical seizure (11). Slow-sharp and slow-wave complexes, although less frequent with spasms, differ from the elongated appearance of those in myoclonic seizures (27). Diffuse attenuation, generalized spike wave, paroxysmal fast activity or fast frequencies, and slow wave are also associated with IS. There is no correlation between the semiology of the spasms and the different ictal patterns. The ictal pattern usually is brief, only lasting for approximatley 1 second, while longer patterns are usually also associated with behavioral arrest (21). EMG shows that the axial muscles contract earlier than the limb muscles and the head earlier than the arms (22). A review of the EEG and behavioral changes before and between the spasms suggests that a cluster of spasms may represent a single sustained ictal event rather than brief, repetitive seizures (93). Pseudonormalization and high-amplitude slowing may precede the spasms and are associated with decreased activity and interaction (90), while subclinical discharges without clinical manifestations are also possible at the end of a spasm cluster; however, surface EMG may confirm subclinical contractions without actual perceptible movement on video-EEG during the subclinical discharges (27,50).

Fast activity is often associated with tonic spasms with sustained tonic muscle contraction and may be more common in asymmetric spasms, suggesting a cortical onset for spasms (90,94–97). Fast activity can also fade during repeated spasms or in partial seizures that occur with spasms (72).

DIFFERENTIAL DIAGNOSIS AND EVALUATION

The true epileptic nature of spasms may be easily missed in the beginning and considered to be colic, gastroesophageal reflux, or paroxysmal crying (15). Other paroxysmal disorders that may mimic ES include *benign myoclonus of infancy* in which the interictal and ictal EEGs are normal including in sleep; *hyperekplexia* in which the jerks may be triggered by touching the nose; *Sandifer syndrome* due to *gastroesophageal reflux*, *paroxysmal tonic upward gaze*, *jactatio capitis*, *spasmus nutans*, *breath holding spells*, and *infantile gratification behavior* (15).

West syndrome is the classic epileptic encephalopathy of infancy associated with IS and is characterized by a triad of ES, hypsarrhythmia, and developmental failure or regression. Over the years, salaam seizures, jack-knife seizures, axial spasms, periodic spasms, and serial spasms have been used to describe events that are not ES (22).

The age of onset is typically between 4 and 8 months (16), but ES can occur as early as 2 weeks or as late as 18 months of age (11,98) and, rarely, can begin in adulthood. In some studies (98), late-onset spasms may be cryptogenic or associated with cortical dysplasia, hypoxic–ischemic encephalopathy, or genetic anomalies, and were refractory to medications (16). Late-onset spasms may be intermixed with atonic, tonic, partial, myoclonic, or generalized tonic–clonic seizures or atypical absences. The characteristic spasms generally resolve spontaneously or evolve into LGS or intractable partial seizures but may persist in 15% to 23% of patients beyond 3 to 7 years of age (34,35).

Watanabe has suggested that a subset of the cryptogenic group may be truly an "idiopathic" form of West syndrome (51). These patients have normal development, and the spasms usually remit after a short period. Developmental regression and focal interictal EEG abnormalities are usually not present; hypsarrhythmia disappears between each spasm, which is symmetric; and a family history of seizures is common. This group may represent from approximately half to 80% of the cryptogenic cases (24,75).

IS and West syndrome eventually evolve into the *LGS* in many children. Tonic seizures usually coexist with and are more marked during this stage of the syndrome. Seizure clustering is seen more frequently in West syndrome, but less frequently in LGS (22). Clusters of ES will usually become single spasms in LGS in parallel, with the changed interictal pattern from hypsarrhythmia to a generalized slow spike-and-wave pattern at 1 to 2.5 Hz (71). This evolution has been reported in patients with tuberous sclerosis who present with IS and develop the LGS (71).

IS, due to an epileptic encephalopathy such as West syndrome, need to be differentiated from more benign epilepsy syndromes, particularly *benign familial infantile convulsions* (BFIC) and *benign myoclonic epilepsy of infancy* (BMEI) (99–101). A firm diagnosis is necessary before initiation of therapy because many common medications (specifically corticotropin and vigabatrin) carry a higher risk of morbidity or mortality than most commonly used anticonvulsants. Like IS, BFIC and BMEI present in the first year of life. The seizures of BFIC are usually partial, but the EEG may be normal (100). Myoclonic seizures in BMEI can occur in clusters. The EEG may be normal or show generalized spike-and-wave discharges but not the hypsarrhythmia or multifocal independent spike discharges typically seen in IS. Because patients with IS may not display the distinguishing EEG abnormalities early in the disease, a normal or mildly abnormal record does not rule out IS in the early disease stage and follow-up EEG studies are essential for clarification. A pattern of normal development prior to seizure onset and continued normal development after seizures start is highly suggestive of benign epilepsy syndromes and not an epileptic encephalopathy with IS. In contrast, children with IS may or may not be normal at seizure onset, but will invariably demonstrate either developmental regression or failure to achieve developmental milestones in a timely fashion.

As with all forms of epilepsy, the evaluation begins with the history and physical/neurologic examination. The skin should be examined for evidence of neurocutaneous disorders and the fundi for a cherry-red macula suggestive of a storage or mitochondrial disorder or for chorioretinitis indicating possible transplacental infection. Nearly half of all of the etiologic diagnoses are established or suspected by the historical and physical data. Many diagnoses, however, require confirmatory MRI, and once imaging is complete, approximately 70% of patients will have a confirmed etiologic diagnosis (102). In many cases, expensive and time-consuming laboratory studies can be avoided. In the remaining 30% of cases, an etiology will be established for no more than one third, leaving about 10% of cases in which a diagnosis is determined by results of lumbar puncture or metabolic or genetic testing.

Neuroimaging

Much of the decrease in cryptogenic cases is a result of the advances in MRI techniques of the past 10 to 15 years. Comparing etiologic categories of IS, Riikonen noted that identification of brain malformations increased from 10%

between 1960 and 1977 to nearly 35% between 1977 and 1991 (102). Imaging should be considered essential to the evaluation. MRI is preferred to computed tomography (CT) scanning because of the greater sensitivity for brain malformations. CT, however, can show subtle calcifications caused by transplacental infections. In a study of 86 patients with IS, MRI assigned 91% to a symptomatic etiology, most commonly hypoxic–ischemic encephalopathy (30%) (103) characterized by diffuse atrophy and thinning of the corpus callosum. Delayed myelination in 27% of patients did not appear to be associated with any specific etiology (Table 17.1).

Some MRI abnormalities suggest specific etiologies, many genetically based, that may require further evaluation. Genetic etiologies including Rett syndrome due to various mutations in the MeCP2 gene, atypical Rett syndrome due to CDKL5 mutations, and X-linked ARX homeobox gene mutations need to also be considered in the etiologic diagnosis and diagnosed with chromosomal microarrays and specific mutational studies. Additional genetic and metabolic etiologies are continuing to be added to this list as our understanding of the genetic contributions to IS advances (104).

Metabolic Studies

Metabolic studies are indicated to identify more than 50 disorders associated with infantile seizures (105–107). A trial of folinic acid is warranted (108), as is a 100-mg intravenous pyridoxine bolus to rule out pyridoxine-dependent seizures. Complete blood count, electrolytes (looking for an anion gap), and glucose determinations are appropriate. Measurements of uric acid, transaminases, lactate, pyruvate, ammonia, urine organic acids, and serum amino acids will identify the vast majority of inborn errors of metabolism linked to IS. In the past, phenylketonuria was a relatively common inborn error

---

TABLE 17.1

MAGNETIC RESONANCE IMAGING FINDINGS IMPLYING A GENETIC ETIOLOGY

Abnormality	Possible genetic association
Lissencephaly	
■ Posterior predominant lissencephaly or Miller–Dieker syndrome	LIS1 gene on chromosome 17
■ Anterior predominant lissencephaly or band heterotopia	XLIS gene on X chromosome
■ Lissencephaly with cerebellar hypoplasia	Reelin gene
Cortical tubers, periventricular nodules	Tuberous sclerosis; TSC1 or TSC2 mutations; 75% to 85% are spontaneous mutations; parents should be evaluated
Perisylvian polymicrogyria	Some are familial; multiple associations
	X-linked recessive
	X-linked dominant
	Autosomal recessive
	22q11.2 deletions
Cerebral calcifications	Transplacental infections
Loss of cerebral white matter	Pyruvate carboxylase deficiency
Hypoplasia of corpus callosum	Nonketotic hyperglycemia

TABLE 17.2

ETIOLOGIES OF SYMPTOMATIC INFANTILE SPASMS THAT MAY RESPOND TO
SPECIFIC THERAPIES

Symptomatic IS	Therapy
Pyridoxine-dependent seizures	Pyridoxine[a]
Phenylketonuria	Diet[a]
Maple-syrup urine disease	Diet[a]
Glucose transporter defect	Ketogenic diet
Tumor	Surgery to remove tumor[b]
Arteriovenous malformation	Surgery to treat the malformation[b]
Sturge–Weber syndrome	Surgery if medications fail[a]
Tuberous sclerosis	Vigabatrin, possible surgery if medications fail[a]
Biotinidase deficiency	Biotin[a]
Menkes disease	Copper histidinate[a]
Hyperammonemia disorders	Possible diet, depending on the disorder[a]
Nonketotic hyperglycinuria	Benzoate[a]
Cortical dysplasias	Possible cortical resection if medications fail[b]
Focal cortical dysplasia	
Hemimegalencephaly	

[a]Symptomatic with a specific therapy and a genetic etiology.
[b]Symptomatic with a specific therapy without an identified genetic etiology.

identified by testing that has been nearly eliminated by neonatal screening. Nevertheless, such screening is not routine in all countries, and measurement of urine amino acid levels will detect phenylketonuria and maple-syrup urine disease, as well as other, rarer, metabolic diseases. Zellweger syndrome and neonatal adrenoleukodystrophy are other rare causes of hypsarrhythmia that can be diagnosed with the serum very-long-chain fatty acid test (Table 17.2).

Lumbar Puncture

A few very rare disorders, such as nonketotic hyperglycinemia, may be detected only by study of the CSF (109). In addition to routine evaluations for glucose, protein, and cells, the CSF should be assessed for amino acids plus lactate and pyruvate to detect possible mitochondrial disorders.

PHARMACOLOGIC TREATMENT

Recovery is only considered to have occurred when both the ES and the EEG abnormality of hypsarrhythmia have responded to treatment and ceased. More than 100 years after James West's initial description of IS, the effectiveness of steroids was first recognized and to date only two medications have class 1 evidence of efficacy: corticotropin and vigabatrin (110,111). Corticotropin and, as of 2009, vigabatrin are approved by the Food and Drug Administration for use in the United States. In addition, some patients respond to valproic acid, lamotrigine, high-dose pyridoxine, topiramate, and zonisamide, while most conventional antiepileptic drugs are ineffective. Some drugs such as carbamazepine or oxcarbazepine may even worsen the seizures which should be considered when IS are associated with focal features.

Corticotropin and Steroids

The effectiveness of corticotrophin and steroids underscores how IS differ from all other epilepsy syndromes. In 1958, Sorel and colleagues administered 4 to 10 IU/day of corticotropin to seven patients, four of whom responded within a few days while therapy failed in only one patient (110). In the 45 years since that report, efficacy has been repeatedly confirmed, but agreement is still lacking on the most appropriate dose and duration of treatment. Dosing is complicated by the existence of natural and synthetic forms of corticotropin. Studies of the synthetic product generally used much lower doses than studies of the natural product. It is estimated that 1 IU of synthetic corticotropin is equivalent to 40 IU of natural corticotropin. The synthetic version is used primarily in Japan where a low dose is 0.2 IU/kg/day and a high dose is 1 IU/kg/day. Even with the low dose, 75% of patients responded in one study (112). In contrast, natural corticotropin at doses up to 150 IU/m^2 body surface area/day succeeded in 14 of 15 patients; five later had relapses for a long-term response rate of 60% (109). A review of seven studies did not confirm a better response with 150 IU/day with 40 IU/day being a common dose (35). The overall long-term response rate ranged from 53% to 91%. When treating IS, I initially begin treatment with 40 IU/day for 1 to 2 weeks and increase to 60 IU/day or even to 80 IU/day if the response is incomplete. If spasms are controlled and hypsarrhythmia disappears, I taper the dose over 1 to 4 months, while failed responders are rapidly tapered and the drug discontinued from a risk–benefit perspective.

Despite its effectiveness for IS, no medication carries a higher potential for significant side effects. Most children develop a Cushing syndrome with obesity, plethora, hypertension, and intense irritability. All patients are at-risk for arterial hypertension, electrolyte imbalance, gastric ulcer, growth retardation, cardiomyopathy, or immunosuppression with increased risk of infection. In one study, the risk of serious side effects was 43% with 160 IU/day; the incidence was lower with lower doses (113). Death from infection and cardiomyopathy has ranged from 2% to 5% in some series. Sepsis, tuberculosis, meningoencephalitis, and protracted cytomegalovirus infection are major infections that have been reported. Corticotropin exacerbates the seizures in a few infants, and treatment for more than a few weeks leads to steroid insufficiency if the drug is stopped abruptly (114). Parents must be fully informed of the associated morbidity and mortality risks (reported at approximately 2% to 5%) before the therapy begins, and these must be balanced against the virtual certainty of mental retardation if the spasms are not rapidly controlled. Careful follow-up with regular measurements of blood pressure, electrolytes, and urinalysis is mandatory. The current risk-to-benefit assessment favors corticotropin, but if another, less hazardous medication proves to be as effective, it would be the drug of choice.

There are few comparative trials of the efficacy of steroids and ACTH but one double-blind trial showed that a 2-week trial of high-dose ACTH was superior to 2 weeks of prednisone, while another found no difference with either compound (115). In addition, some patients may respond to one drug but not the other. Following response to steroids or corticotrophin, the relapse rate is high and variably reported between 33% and 56% (34). Relapses usually occur within the first 2 months following the end of treatment, but a second course may give a remission and response in up to 75% of patients (35). Recovery of mental function has been reported between 14% and 58%, particularly in patients with a cryptogenic etiology (116).

Vigabatrin (VGB)

This drug has been reported to be highly effective in the treatment of IS of all etiologies, and in patients with tuberous sclerosis it was superior to steroids (117). Particularly in new onset cases under 3 months of age, VGB monotherapy has a higher efficacy, reported up to 90%, than in older patients.

In 1991, 29 of 68 patients with medically refractory IS achieved complete resolution with VGB as add-on therapy, as did 12 of 14 patients who had tuberous sclerosis (118). VGB also might be effective in Down syndrome (119).

Since 1997, four controlled trials have been reported. Vigevano and Cilio (120) administered either corticotropin 10 IU/day or VGB 100 to 150 mg/kg/day to children with newly diagnosed IS. Eleven of 23 VGB patients responded (one late relapse) compared with 14 of 19 corticotropin patients (six late relapses). Vigabatrin was more effective in patients with tuberous sclerosis or cerebral malformations; corticotropin was more effective in patients with perinatal hypoxic–ischemic encephalopathy. There was no difference in cryptogenic cases. Appleton and colleagues (121) used VGB or placebo for 5 days, followed by open-label VGB. Seven of 20 patients in the VGB group were seizure-free at the end of 5 days, as were two of 20 in the placebo group. For 14 days, Elterman and associates (122) treated 75 patients with 18 to 36 mg/kg/day (low dose) and 67 patients with 100 to 148 mg/kg/day (high dose) of VGB. Eight low-dose patients and 24 high-dose patients achieved complete control. In a study involving

underlying tuberous sclerosis, all 11 patients treated with VGB responded, compared with only 5 of 11 patients treated with hydrocortisone (123).

VGB appears to be well tolerated. The reports of hypotonia, somnolence, or insomnia (124) are expected in a drug that enhances GABA activity. Constriction of peripheral visual fields, which substantially limits the drug's use, was not reported until 1997 (125) and now affects from 15% to 50% of patients. In one report (126), constriction occurred in more than 90% of patients who had been taking VGB for a mean of 8.5 years. Foveal function also may be impaired (127). Most studies have suggested that the constriction is not reversible; however, eight of 12 patients who underwent full withdrawal improved significantly; none of the 12 who continued taking the drug did so (125). The problem is mild enough that most patients are unaware of the disturbance, which becomes apparent only on perimetric studies.

Unfortunately, visual fields are virtually impossible to evaluate in these very young children, many with cortical visual impairment and visual inattention unrelated to VGB therapy. Given the catastrophic nature of IS, visual-field constriction may be an acceptable price for seizure control and improved opportunity for normal development (126).

Valproic Acid

Before the availability of VGB around the world, single reports of seizure response to valproic acid were reported with tolerable side effects. In a 1981 report, valproic acid produced an "excellent" response in four of 18 patients treated with 20 mg/kg/day (128). A year later, seven of 19 patients achieved good control (11 had also been treated with corticotropin) (129). Seizures were controlled in 11 of 22 patients treated with up to 100 mg/kg/day for 4 weeks (130). Other patients later responded but also received dexamethasone or carbamazepine, so the effect of valproic acid was less clear. Prospective randomized studies of efficacy against IS are lacking. Because liver failure is a risk in children younger than 2 years of age (131), although none of the reported patients were affected, valproic acid should be used cautiously and probably not as a first line of therapy for IS particularly if metabolic etiologies have not been excluded (132).

Pyridoxine

A trial of 100 mg of pyridoxine intravenously is appropriate for patients with an unclear etiologic diagnosis because pyridoxine (vitamin B_6) dependence can be a rare but highly treatable cause of IS (133). Seizures caused by pyridoxine-dependent epilepsy cease immediately following intravenous administration of vitamin B_6. As early as 1968, however, it has been known that long-term oral administration of high doses of pyridoxine has been effective against nonpyridoxine-dependent seizures (134). In 1993, five of 17 patients treated with 100 to 300 mg/kg/day responded within 4 weeks—most within 1 week (135). In Japan, high-dose vitamin B_6 has been the drug of choice (135,136), with reported response rates of 10% to 30%. Loss of appetite, irritability, and vomiting are modest compared with the side effects of corticotropin or VGB, but there may be a high risk of gastric hemorrhage.

Pyridoxine is not used as frequently outside of Japan but given its relatively low-risk profile, a 1- to 2-week trial of 100 to 400 mg may be reasonable before or in addition to other therapies.

Nitrazepam

One of the earliest nonsteroid treatments for IS, the benzodiazepines succeed only occasionally but may be useful if more effective therapies have failed (137–139). Nitrazepam administered to 24 children controlled IS in 11 but hypotonia was reported as a significant side effect (140). A multicenter, randomized comparison of corticotropin and nitrazepam demonstrated no statistical difference between the two medications in significantly reducing spasms (141). Side effects with corticotropin were more severe, leading to discontinuation in six patients. Many reports noted an increase in oral secretions and a higher incidence of aspiration and pneumonia with nitrazepam. Several deaths occurred in one series (142). The incidence of mortality was 3.98 deaths per 100 patient-years when young epilepsy patients were taking nitrazepam and 0.26 deaths per 100 patient-years if the medication had been discontinued (143).

Other Antiepileptic Drugs

None of the new anticonvulsants have enough evidence of efficacy to permit a recommendation. The Japanese experience suggests that zonisamide may be effective in about one third of patients (144), but controlled and comparison trials are lacking. Five of 25 patients had a complete clinical and electrographic response to doses ranging from 8 to 32 mg/kg/day; most responses occurred in 1 to 2 weeks (145). Zonisamide was well tolerated, but 20% of the patients in one study experienced anorexia and one patient lost weight (146). If the more than 30% efficacy figures hold up in controlled studies, zonisamide could become a first-line therapy.

Topiramate up to 25 mg/kg/day was effective in four of 11 patients with intractable IS (147). Seizures decreased in 43% of 14 patients, but worsened in 29%; no patient became seizure-free (148).

Before reports of aplastic anemia, three of four patients with medically intractable IS responded to felbamate as add-on therapy (149). Because aplastic anemia has not been noted in prepubertal patients, felbamate may be as safe as some other drugs and could be recommended if other medications have failed.

Anecdotal evidence, but no prospective controlled trials, supports the efficacy of lamotrigine. One report noted that 25 of 30 patients became seizure-free (150). The usual dose is 6 to 10 mg/kg/day; however, three patients in whom VGB and corticotropin had failed responded to less than 1 mg/kg/day (150). Use of a low dose is important because rash, the major side effect, depends to some extent on how rapidly the dose is increased. The usual recommendation is a slow rise over 2 months to the minimum expected therapeutic dose. Given the need to control IS as soon as possible, this 2-month requirement decreases the therapeutic value of lamotrigine. If the very low dose is effective, however, lamotrigine becomes a fallback drug (151).

KETOGENIC DIET

The ketogenic diet is a decades-old therapy enjoying a resurgence of interest and wide spread application. Two retrospective reports of 40 children suggest control of spasms in 20% to 35% of patients with otherwise intractable disease (152,153). Children younger than 1 year of age can achieve ketosis and may benefit from the diet. Despite generally good tolerability, renal stones, gastritis, hyperlipidemia, and gastroesophageal reflux may occur.

INTRAVENOUS IMMUNOGLOBULIN

High-dose intravenous immunoglobulin (IVIG) is another effective nonantiepileptic drug therapy that may be effective in a variety of seizure disorders, especially when associated with an epileptic encephalopathy. All six children with cryptogenic IS, but only one of five symptomatic patients, achieved complete remission (154). IVIG may also improve juvenile spasms (155). Doses range from 100 to 200 mg/kg administered every 2 to 3 weeks to 400 mg/kg/day for 5 consecutive days. Actual efficacy is unclear, however, and the most appropriate doses and duration have not been determined.

SURGICAL MANAGEMENT

Removal of an epileptogenic cortical lesion may be highly effective in treating IS and hypsarrythmia. Patients with single lesions including tumors, FCD porencephaly, hemimegalencephaly, and catastrophic epilepsy are ideal surgical candidates that should be selected early for surgery as there is compelling evidence that earlier surgery and shorter duration of epilepsy predict improved cognitive outcome (156).

A history of partial seizures that preceded or accompanied IS, cortical disturbances on MRI, or localized EEG abnormalities that suggest a cortical defect should prompt referral to a pediatric epilepsy surgery center (157).

COURSE AND PROGNOSIS

Prognostic features are overall difficult to assess. Signs of brain injury usually preclude complete recovery even in cases where seizure remission is achieved. In cryptogenic cases without evidence of brain lesions the best outcome appears to be predictable in patients who do not lose visual eye contact (37). Although IS are self-limited and approximately 6% to 15% will recover spontaneously after a few weeks or months, control of epilepsy is difficult to predict in the individual case.

However, IS are a seizure type that are generally associated with a severe epileptic encephalopathy and carry a grave prognosis associated with significant morbidity and also mortality. Intractable epilepsy, mental retardation, and autism are possible consequences of IS. Mortality is increased in the acute short term due to treatment complications and neurologic morbidity underlying various etiologies. In addition, the long-term mortality may be high: a 25- to 35-year follow-up of 214 patients demonstrated that 31% died, many in the first 3 years of life (35,158). Eight of the 24 deaths by age 3 years were a consequence of complications of corticotropin therapy. The most common cause of death overall was infection. Of the 147 survivors, 25 (17%) had an intelligence quotient (IQ) of 85 or higher; 11 others (7%) were in the dull-normal range with IQs of 68 to 84; and 45% were retarded. Overall outcome is driven by the underlying etiology and seizure control. While some etiologies, such as severe hypoxic–ischemic encephalopathy and lissencephaly, will lead to death or mental retardation regardless of whether IS develop children with cryptogenic spasms or spasms caused by FCD may have a normal or near-normal developmental outcome if the second factor, seizure control, is achieved. Accurate diagnosis and appropriate medical or surgical management need to be the gold standard in these cases to reduce the severe cognitive sequelae of this epileptic encephalopathy.

References

1. West W. On a particular form of infantile convulsions. *Lancet.* 1841;1: 724–725.
2. Gibbs F, Gibbs E. Atlas of electroencephalography. In: Gibbs F, Gibbs E, eds. *Epilepsy.* Reading, MA: Addison-Wesley; 1952.
3. Cerullo A, Marini C, Carcangiu R, et al. Clinical and video-polygraphic features of epileptic spasms in adults with cortical migration disorder. *Epileptic Disord.* 1999;1:27–33.
4. Tuxhorn I, Kotagal P. Classification. *Semin Neurol.* 2008;28:277–288.
5. Riikonen R, Donner M. Incidence and aetiology of infantile spasms from 1960 to 1976: a population study in Finland. *Dev Med Child Neurol.* 1979;21:333–343.
6. Cowan LD, Hudson LS. The epidemiology and natural history of infantile spasms. *J Child Neurol.* 1991;6:355–364.
7. Ludvigsson P, Olafsson E, Sigurthardottir S, et al. Epidemiologic features of infantile spasms in Iceland. *Epilepsia.* 1994;35:802–805.
8. Sidenvall R, Eeg-Olofsson O. Epidemiology of infantile spasms in Sweden. *Epilepsia.* 1995;36:572–574.
9. van den Berg B, Yerushalmy J. Studies on convulsive disorders in young children, I: incidence of febrile and nonfebrile convulsions by age and other factors. *Pediatr Res.* 1969;3:298–304.
10. Trevathan E, Murphy C, Yeargin-Allsopp M. The descriptive epidemiology of infantile spasms among Atlanta children. *Epilepsia.* 1999;40: 748–751.
11. Wong M, Trevathan E. Infantile spasms. *Pediatr Neurol.* 2001;24:89–98.
12. Pavone L, Mollica F, Incorpa G, et al. Infantile spasms syndrome in monozygotic twins. *Arch Dis Child.* 1980;55:870–872.
13. Senga P, Mayanda H, Yidika M. Spasmes infantiles chez deux jumeaux monozygotiques: une novelle observation. *Presse Med.* 1986;15:485.
14. Lacy J, Penry J. Infantile spasms. In: Lacy J, Penry J, eds. *Infantile Spasms.* New York: Raven Press; 1976.
15. Dulac O, Tuxhorn I. Infantile spasms and West Syndrome. In: Roger J, Bureau M, Dravet C, et al., eds. *Epileptic Syndromes in Infancy, Childhood and Adolescence.* 3rd ed. London: John Libbey; 2002;47–63.
16. Hrachovy R. West's syndrome (infantile spasm). Clinical description and diagnosis. *Adv Exp Med Biol.* 2002;497:33–50.
17. Fusco L, Vigevano F. Tonic spasm seizures: a particular and previously unreported type of seizure. *Epilepsia.* 1994;35(Suppl 7):87.
18. Vigevano F, Fusco L, Pachatz C. Neurophysiology of spasms. *Brain Dev.* 2001;23:467–472.
19. Donat J, Wright F. Seizures in series: similarities between seizures of the West and Lennox-Gastaut syndromes. *Epilepsia.* 1991;32:504–509.
20. Bisulli F, Volpi L, Meletti S, et al. Ictal pattern of EEG and muscular activation in symptomatic infantile spasms: a videopolygraphic and computer analysis. *Epilepsia.* 2002;43:1559–1563.
21. Ohtahara S, Yamatogi Y. Severe encephalopathic epilepsy in infants: West syndrome. In: Pellock J, Dodson W, Bourgeois B, eds. *Pediatric Epilepsy: Diagnosis and Therapy.* New York: Demos Medical; 2001:177–192.
22. Watanabe K, Negoro T, Okumura A. Symptomatology of infantile spasms. *Brain Dev.* 2001;23:453–466.
23. Lombroso C. A prospective study of infantile spasms: clinical and therapeutic correlations. *Epilepsia* 1983;24:135–158.
24. Matsumoto A, Watanabe K, Negoro T, et al. Infantile spasms: etiologic factors, clinical aspects and long term prognosis in 200 cases. *Eur J Pediatr.* 1981;135:239–244.
25. Koo B, Hwang P, Logan W. Infantile spasms: outcome and prognostic factors of cryptogenic and symptomatic groups. *Neurology.* 1993;43: 2322–2327.
26. Holmes G, Vigevano F. Infantile spasms. In: Engel J Jr, Pedley T, eds. *Epilepsy: A Comprehensive Textbook.* Philadelphia: Lippincott Williams & Wilkins; 1998:627–660.
27. Vigevano F, Fusco L, Cusmai R, et al. The idiopathic form of West syndrome. *Epilepsia.* 1993;34:743–746.
28. Hrachovy R, Frost J Jr. Intensive monitoring of infantile spasms. In: Schmidt D, Morselli P, eds. *Intractable Epilepsy: Experimental and Clinical Aspects.* New York: Raven Press; 1986:87–97.
29. Dulac O. Infantile spasms and West syndrome. In: Engel J Jr, Pedley T, eds. *Epilepsy: A Comprehensive Textbook.* Philadelphia: Lippincott-Raven; 1997:2277–2283.
30. Fogarasi, A, Tuxhorn I, Jansky J, et al. Age-dependent seizure semiology in temporal lobe epilepsy. *Epilepsia.* 2007;48(9):1697–1702.
31. Moshe S. The effects of age on kindling phenomenon. *Dev Psychobiol.* 1981;14:75–81.
32. Kellaway P. Neurologic status of patients with hypsarrhythmia. In: Gibbs F, ed. *Molecules and Mental Health.* Philadelphia, PA: JB Lippincott; 1959:134–149.
33. Hrachovy R, Frost JD Jr, Pollack MS, et al. Serologic HLA typing in infantile spasms. *Epilepsia.* 1988;29:817–819.
34. Jeavons P, Bower B, Dimitrakoudi M. Long-term prognosis of 150 cases of West syndrome. *Epilepsia.* 1973;14:153–164.
35. Riikonen R. A long-term follow-up study of 214 children with syndrome of infantile spasms. *Neuropediatrics.* 1982;13:14–23.
36. Kurokawa T, Goya N, Fukuyama Y, et al. West syndrome and Lennox-Gastaut syndrome: a survey of natural history. *Pediatrics.* 1980;65:81–88.
37. Jambaque I, Chiron C, Dulac O, et al. Visual inattention in West Syndrome: a neuropsychological and neurofunctional imaging study. *Epilepsia.* 1993;34:692–700.
38. Rantala H, Putkonen T. Occurrence, outcome and prognostic factors of infantile spasms and Lennox-Gastaut syndrome. *Epilepsia.* 1999;40: 287–289.
39. Carmant L. Infantile spasms: West syndrome. *Arch Neurol.* 2002;59: 317–318.
40. Juhasz C, Chugani HT, Muzik O, et al. Neuroradiological assessment of brain structure and function and its implication in the pathogenesis of West syndrome. *Brain Dev.* 2001;23:488–495.
41. Carranza E, Lombroso CT, Mikati M, et al. Facilitation of infantile spasms by partial seizures. *Epilepsia.* 1993;34:94–109.
42. Watanabe K. Recent advance and some problems in the delineation of epileptic syndromes in children. *Brain Dev.* 1996;18:423–437.
43. Ohtahara S, Ohtsuka Y, Yamatogi Y, et al. Prenatal etiologies of West syndrome. *Epilepsia.* 1993;34:716–722.
44. Shephard C, Houser O, Gomez M. MR findings in tuberous sclerosis complex and correlation with seizure development and mental impairment. *Am J Neuroradiol.* 1995;16:149–155.
45. Dulac O, Pinard J, Plouin P. Infantile spasms associated with cortical dysplasia and tuberous sclerosis. In: Guerrini R, ed. *Dysplasias of Cerebral Cortex and Epilepsy.* Philadelphia: Lippincott-Raven; 1996:217–225.
46. Koo B, Hwang P. Localization of focal cortical lesions influences age of onset of infantile spasms. *Epilepsia.* 1996;37:1068–1071.
47. Chugani H, Shewmon DA, Shields WD, et al. Surgery for intractable infantile spasms: neuroimaging perspectives. *Epilepsia.* 1993;34:764–771.
48. Motte J, Billard C, Fejerman N, et al. Neurofibromatosis type one and West syndrome: a relatively benign association. *Epilepsia.* 1993;34: 723–726.
49. Mizukawa M, Ohtsuka Y, Murashima I, et al. West syndrome associated with chromosome abnormalities: clinicoelectrical study. *Jpn J Psychiatr Neurol.* 1992;46:435–436.
50. Silva M, Cieuta C, Guerrini R, et al. Early clinical and EEG features of infantile spasms in Down syndrome. *Epilepsia.* 1996;37:977–982.
51. Watanabe K. West syndrome: etiological and prognostic aspects. *Brain Dev.* 1998;20:1–8.
52. Riikonen R. Decreasing perinatal mortality: unchanged infantile spasm morbidity. *Dev Med Child Neurol.* 1995;37:232–238.
53. Yamamoto N, Watanabe K, Negoro T, et al. Long-term prognosis of tuberous sclerosis with epilepsy in children. *Brain Dev.* 1987;9:292–295.
54. Okumura A, Hayakawa F, Kuno K, et al. Periventricular leucomalacia and West syndrome. *Dev Med Child Neurol.* 1996;38:13–18.
55. Hrachovy RA, Frost JD Jr, Kellaway P, et al. A controlled study of prednisone therapy in infantile spasms. *Epilepsia.* 1979;20:403–407.
56. Hrachovy R, Frost JD Jr, Kellaway P, et al. A controlled study of ACTH therapy in infantile spasms. *Epilepsia.* 1980;21:631–636.
57. Hrachovy R, Frost JD Jr, Kellaway P, et al. Double-blind study of ACTH vs prednisone therapy in infantile spasms. *J Pediatr.* 1983; 103:641–645.
58. Sankar R, Curran JG, Kevill JW, et al. Microscopic cortical dysplasia in infantile spasms: evolution of white matter abnormalities. *Am J Neuroradiol.* 1995;16:1265–1272.
59. Riikonen R. How do cryptogenic and symptomatic infantile spasms differ? Review of biochemical studies in Finnish patients. *J Child Neurol.* 1996;11:383–388.
60. Claes S, Devriendt K, Lagae L, et al. The X-linked infantile spasms syndrome (MIM 308350) maps to Xp11.4-Xpter in two pedigrees. *Ann Neurol.* 1997;42:360–364.

61. Brueyere H, Lewis S, Wood S, et al. Confirmation of linkage in X-linked infantile spasms (West syndrome) and refinement of the disease locus to Xp21.3-Xp22.1. *Clin Genet.* 1999;55:173–181.

62. Stafstrom C. Infantile spasms: a critical review of emerging animal models. Current review in basic science. *Epilepsy Curr.* 2009;9:75–81.

63. Jansen L, Peugh L, Ojemann. GABA$_A$ receptor properties in catastrophic infantile epilepsy. *Epilepsy Res.* 2008;81:188–197.

64. Morimatsu Y, Murofuchi K, Handa T. Pathology in severe physical and mental disabilities in children—with special reference to four cases of nodding spasms. *Adv Neurol Sci.* 1972;20:465–470.

65. Satho J, Mizutani T, Morimatsu Y. Neuropathology of the brainstem in age dependent epileptic encephalopathy—especially in cases of infantile spasms. *Brain Dev.* 1986;8:443–449.

66. Pranzatelli M. Putative neurotransmitter abnormalities in infantile spasms: cerebrospinal fluid neurochemistry and drug effects. *J Child Neurol.* 1994;9:119–129.

67. Kaga K, Mark R, Fukuyama Y. Auditory brainstem responses in infantile spasms. *J Pediatr Otorhinolaryngol.* 1982;4:57–67.

68. Fukuyama Y, Shionaga A, Idia Y. Polygraphic study during night sleep in infantile spasms. *Eur Neurol.* 1979;18:302–311.

69. Hrachovy R, Frost J Jr, Kellaway P. Sleep characteristics in infantile spasms. *Neurology.* 1981;31:688–694.

70. Hrachovy R, Frost J Jr. Infantile spasms: a disorder of the developing nervous system. In: Kellaway P, Noebels J, eds. *Problems and Concepts in Developmental Neurophysiology.* Baltimore, MD: Johns Hopkins University Press; 1989:131–147.

71. Ohtsuka Y, Ohmori I, Oka E. Long-term follow-up of childhood epilepsy associated with tuberous sclerosis. *Epilepsia.* 1998;39:1158–1163.

72. Panzica F, Franceschetti S, Binelli S, et al. Spectral properties of EEG fast activity ictal discharges associated with infantile spasms. *Clin Neurophysiol.* 1999;110:593–603.

73. Shields WD, Shewmon DA, Chugani HT, et al. Treatment of infantile spasms: medical or surgical? *Epilepsia.* 1992;33(Suppl 4):S26–S31.

74. Haginoya K, Munakata M, Yokoyama H, et al. Mechanism of tonic spasms in West syndrome viewed from ictal SPECT findings. *Brain Dev.* 2001;23:496–501.

75. Baram T. Pathophysiology of massive infantile spasms: perspective on the putative role of brain adrenal axis. *Ann Neurol.* 1993;33:231–236.

76. Brunson K, Eghbal-Ahmadi M, Baram T. How do the many etiologies of West syndrome lead to excitability and seizures? The corticotropin releasing hormone excess hypothesis. *Brain Dev.* 2001;23:533–538.

77. Nagamitsu S, Matsuishi T, Yamashita Y, et al. Decreased cerebrospinal fluid levels of beta-endorphin and ACTH in children with infantile spasms. *J Neural Transm.* 2001;108:363–371.

78. Bellman MH, Ross EM, Miller DL. Infantile spasms and pertussis immunisation. *Lancet.* 1983;1:1031–1034.

79. Fukuyama Y, Tomori N, Sugitate M. Critical evaluation of the role of immunization as an etiological factor of infantile spasms. *Neuropadiatrie.* 1977;8:224–237.

80. Melchior J. Infantile spasms and early immunization against whooping cough. Danish survey from 1970 to 1975. *Arch Dis Child.* 1977;52:134–137.

81. Reinskov T. Demonstration of precipitating antibody to extract of brain tissue in patients with hypsarrhythmia. *Acta Paediatr Scand.* 1963;(suppl):140–173.

82. Mota N, Rezkallah-Iwasse MT, Peracoli MT, et al. Demonstration of antibody and cellular immune response to brain extract in West and Lennox-Gastaut syndromes. *Arq Neuropsiquiatr.* 1984;42:126–131.

83. Hrachovy R, Frost J Jr, Shearer W. Immunological evaluation of patients with infantile spasms. *Ann Neurol.* 1985;18:414.

84. Carmant L, Goodyear E, Sauerwein C. The use of calcium channel blockers in the treatment of West syndrome [abstract]. *Neurology.* 2000;54(Suppl 3):A295.

85. Friedman E, Pampiglione G. Prognostic implications of electroencephalographic findings of hypsarrhythmia in first year of life. *Br Med J.* 1971;4:323–325.

86. Watanabe K, Iwase K, Hara K. The evolution of EEG features in infantile spasms: a prospective study. *Dev Med Child Neurol.* 1973;15:584–596.

87. Kotagal P. Multifocal independent spike syndrome: relationship to hypsarrhythmia and the slow spike-wave (Lennox-Gastaut) syndrome. *Clin Electroencephalogr.* 1995;26:23–29.

88. Hrachovy R, Frost J Jr, Kellaway P. Hypsarrhythmia: variation on a theme. *Epilepsia.* 1984;25:317–325.

90. Kellaway P, Hrachovy RA, Frost JD Jr, et al. Precise characterization and quantification of infantile spasms. *Ann Neurol.* 1979;6:214–218.

91. Kramer U, Sue W, Mikati M. Hypsarrhythmia: frequency of variant patterns and correlation with etiology and outcome. *Neurology.* 1997;48:197–203.

92. Foley C, Bowens P, Riviello J. Low voltage EEG predicts the prognosis of infantile spasm. *Epilepsy.* 1989;30:654.

93. Shewmon D. Ictal aspects with emphasis on unusual variants. In: Dulac O, Chugani H, Dalla Bernardina B, eds. *Infantile Spasms and West Syndrome.* London: WB Saunders; 1994:36–51.

94. Foley C, Bowens P, Riviello J. *Epilepsia.* 1989;30:654.

95. Aicardi J. Infantile spasms and related syndromes. In: Aicardi J, ed. *Epilepsy in Children.* New York: Raven Press; 1994:18–43.

96. Dulac O, Plouin P, Jambaque I, et al. Benign infantile spasms [French]. *Rev Electroencephalogr Neurophysiol Clin.* 1986;16:371–382.

97. Gailey EK, Shewmon DA, Chugani HT, et al. Asymmetric and asynchronous infantile spasms. *Epilepsia.* 1995;36:873–882.

98. Bednarek N, Motte J, Soufflet C, et al. Evidence of late-onset infantile spasms. *Epilepsia.* 1998;39:55–60.

99. Vigevano F, Fusco L, Di Capua M, et al. Benign infantile familial convulsions. *Eur J Pediatr.* 1992;151:608–612.

100. Caraballo RH, Cersosimo RO, Amartino H, et al. Benign familial infantile seizures: further delineation of the syndrome. *J Child Neurol.* 2002;17:696–699.

101. Dravet C, Giraud N, Bureau M, et al. Benign myoclonus of early infancy or benign non-epileptic infantile spasms. *Neuropediatrics.* 1986;17:33–38.

102. Riikonen R. Epidemiological data of West syndrome in Finland. *Brain Dev.* 2001;23:539–541.

103. Saltik S, Kocer N, Dervent A. Magnetic resonance imaging findings in infantile spasms: etiologic and pathophysiologic aspects. *J Child Neurol.* 2003;18:241–246.

104. Parikh S, Cohen B, Gupta A, et al. Metabolic testing in the pediatric epilepsy unit. *Pediatr Neurol.* 2008;38(3):191–195.

105. Nordli DR Jr, De Vivo DC. Classification of infantile seizures: implications for identification and treatment of inborn errors of metabolism. *J Child Neurol.* 2002;17(suppl 3):3S3–3S7; discussion 3S8.

106. Trasmonte JV, Barron TF. Infantile spasms: a proposal for a staged evaluation. *Pediatr Neurol.* 1998;19:368–371.

107. Saudubray JM, Nassogne MC, de Lonlay P, et al. Clinical approach to inherited metabolic disorders in neonates: an overview. *Semin Neonatol.* 2002;7:3–15.

108. Torres OA, Miller VS, Buist NM, et al. Folinic acid-responsive neonatal seizures. *J Child Neurol.* 1999;14:529–532.

109. Dalla Bernardina B, Aicardi J, Goutieres F, et al. Glycine encephalopathy. *Neuropadiatrie.* 1979;10:209–225.

110. Sorel L, Dusaucy-Bauloye A. A propos de 21 cas d'hyparrthmie de Gibbes. Son traitement spectaculaire par l'ACTH. *Acta Neurol Belg.* 1958;58:130–141.

111. Mackay M, Weiss S, Snead OC III. Treatment of infantile spasms: an evidence-based approach. *Int Rev Neurobiol.* 2002;49:157–184.

112. Yanagaki S, Ogoni H, Hayashi K, et al. A comparative study of high-dose and low-dose ACTH therapy for West syndrome. *Brain Dev.* 1999;21:461–467.

113. Riikonen R, Donner M. ACTH therapy in infantile spasms: side effects. *Arch Dis Child.* 1980;55(9):664–672.

114. Perheentupa J, Riikonen R, Dunkel L, et al. Adrenocortical hyporesponsiveness after treatment with ACTH of infantile spasms. *Arch Dis Child.* 1986;61:750–753.

115. Baram TZ, Mitchell W, Tournay A et al. High-dose corticotrophin (ACTH) versus prednisone for infantile spasms: a prospective, randomized, blinded study. *Pediatrics.* 1996;95:375–379.

116. Snead OC III, Benton JW Jr, Hosey LC, et al. Treatment of infantile spasms with high-dose ACTH: efficacy and plasma levels of ACTH and cortisol. *Neurology.* 1989;39:1027–1031.

117. Chiron C, Dulac O, Beaumont D, et al. Therapeutic trial of vigabatrin in refractory infantile spasms. *J Child Neurol.* 1991;Suppl 2:S52–9.

118. Jambaque I, Chiron C, Dumas C, et al. Mental and behavioural outcome of infantile epilepsy treated by vigabatrin in tuberous sclerosis patients. *Epilepsy Res.* 2000;38:151–160.

119. Nabbout R, Melki I, Gerbaka B, et al. Infantile spasms in Down syndrome: good response to a short course of vigabatrin. *Epilepsia.* 2001;42:1580–1583.

120. Vigevano F, Cilio MR. Vigabatrin versus ACTH as first line treatment for infantile spasms: a randomized, prospective study. *Epilepsia.* 1997;38:1270–1274.

121. Appleton RE, Peters AC, Mumford JP, et al. Randomised, placebo-controlled study of vigabatrin as first-line treatment of infantile spasms. *Epilepsia.* 1999;40:1627–1633.

122. Elterman RD, Shields WD, Mansfield KA, et al. Randomized trial of vigabatrin in patients with infantile spasms. *Neurology.* 2001;57:1416–1421.

123. Chiron C, Dumas C, Jambaque I, et al. Randomized trial comparing vigabatrin and hydrocortisone in infantile spasms due to tuberous sclerosis. *Epilepsy Res.* 1997;26:389–395.

124. Eke T, Talbot JF, Lawden MC. Severe persistent visual field constriction associated with vigabatrin. *Br Med J.* 1997;314:180–181.

125. Fledelius HC. Vigabatrin-associated visual field constriction in a longitudinal series. Reversibility suggested after drug withdrawal. *Acta Ophthalmol Scand.* 2003;81:41–46.

126. Banin E, Shelev RS, Obolensky A, et al. Retinal function abnormalities in patients treated with vigabatrin. *Arch Ophthalmol.* 2003;121:811–816.

127. Shields WD, Sankar R. Vigabatrin. *Semin Pediatr Neurol.* 1997;4:43–50.

128. Pavone L, Incorpora G, La Rosa M, et al. Treatment of infantile spasms with sodium dipropylacetic acid. *Dev Med Child Neurol.* 1981;23: 454–461.

129. Bachman DS. Use of valproic acid in treatment of infantile spasms. *Arch Neurol.* 1982;39:49–52.

130. Siemes H, Spohr HL, Michael T, et al. Therapy of infantile spasms with valproate: results of a prospective study. *Epilepsia.* 1988;29:553–560.

131. Bryant AE III, Dreifuss FE. Valproic acid hepatic fatalities. III. U.S. experience since 1986. *Neurology.* 1996;46:465–469.

132. Baxter P. Epidemiology of pyridoxine dependent and pyridoxine responsive seizures in the UK. *Arch Dis Child.* 1999;81:431–433.

133. Hansson O, Hagberg B. Effect of pyridoxine treatment in children with epilepsy. *Acta Soc Med Ups.* 1968;73:35–43.

134. Pietz J, Benninger C, Schafer H, et al. Treatment of infantile spasms with high-dosage vitamin B_6. *Epilepsia.* 1993;34:757–763.

135. Ohtsuka Y, Matsuda M, Ogino T, et al. Treatment of the West syndrome with high-dose pyridoxal phosphate. *Brain Dev.* 1987;9:418–421.

136. Watanabe K. Medical treatment of West syndrome in Japan. *J Child Neurol.* 1995;10:143–147.

137. Hanson RA, Menkes JH. A new anticonvulsant in the management of minor motor seizures. *Neurology.* 1970;20:379–380.

138. Jan JE, Riegl JA, Crichton JU, et al. Nitrazepam in the treatment of epilepsy in childhood. *Can Med Assoc J.* 1971;104:571–575.

139. Gibbs FA, Anderson EM. Treatment of hypsarrhythmia and infantile spasms with a Librium analogue. *Neurology.* 1965;15:1173–1176.

140. Volzke E, Doose H, Stephan E. The treatment of infantile spasms and hypsarrhythmia with Mogadon. *Epilepsia.* 1967;8:64–70.

141. Dreifuss F, Farwell J, Holmes G, et al. Infantile spasms. Comparative trial of nitrazepam and corticotropin. *Arch Neurol.* 1986;43:1107–1110.

142. Murphy JV, Sawasky F, Marquardt KM, et al. Deaths in young children receiving nitrazepam. *J Pediatr.* 1987;111:145–147.

143. Rintahaka PJ, Nakagawa JA, Shewmon DA, et al. Incidence of death in patients with intractable epilepsy during nitrazepam treatment. *Epilepsia.* 1999;40:492–496.

144. Glauser TA, Pellock JM. Zonisamide in pediatric epilepsy: review of the Japanese experience. *J Child Neurol.* 2002;17:87–96.

145. Suzuki Y. Zonisamide in West syndrome. *Brain Dev.* 2001;23:658–661.

146. Lotze TE, Wilfong AA. Zonisamide treatment for symptomatic infantile spasms. *Neurology.* 2004;62:296–298.

147. Glauser TA, Clark PO, McGee K. Long-term response to topiramate in patients with West syndrome. *Epilepsia.* 2000;41(suppl 1):S91–S94.

148. Mikaeloff Y, de Saint-Martin A, Mancini J, et al. Topiramate: efficacy and tolerability in children according to epilepsy syndromes. *Epilepsy Res.* 2003;53:225–232.

149. Hurst DL, Rolan TD. The use of felbamate to treat infantile spasms. *J Child Neurol.* 1995;10:134–136.

150. Veggiotti P, Cieuta C, Rex E, et al. Treatment of infantile spasms with lamotrigine. *Lancet.* 1994;344:1375–1376.

151. Cianchetti C, Pruna D, Coppola G, et al. Low-dose lamotrigine in West syndrome. *Epilepsy Res.* 2002;51:199–200.

152. Kossoff EH, Pyzik PL, McGregan JR, et al. Efficacy of the ketogenic diet for infantile spasms. *Pediatrics.* 2002;109:780–783.

153. Nordli DR Jr, Kureda MM, Carroll J, et al. Experience with the ketogenic diet in infants. *Pediatrics.* 2001;108:129–133.

154. Bingel U, Pinter JD, Sotero de Menezes M, et al. Intravenous immunoglobulin as adjunctive therapy for juvenile spasms. *J Child Neurol.* 2003; 18:379–382.

155. Ariizumi M, Baba K, Hibio S, et al. Immunoglobulin therapy in the West syndrome. *Brain Dev.* 1987;9:422–425.

156. Freitag H, Tuxhorn I. Cognitive function in preschool children after epilepsy surgery: rationale for early intervention. *Epilepsia.* 2005;46(4): 561–567.

157. Chugani HT, Shewmon DA, Sankar R, et al. Infantile spasms: II. Lenticular nuclei and brain stem activation on positron emission tomography. *Ann Neurol.* 1992;31:212–219.

158. Riikonen R. ACTH therapy of West syndrome: Finnish views. *Brain Dev.* 2001;23:642–646.

CHAPTER 18 ■ CLASSIFICATION OF THE EPILEPSIES

TOBIAS LODDENKEMPER

The most widely used system for classification of epilepsies was proposed in 1989 by the Commission on Classification and Terminology of the International League Against Epilepsy (ILAE) (1). This epilepsy classification remains in place despite ongoing discussion and is appended to this chapter. ILAE's 1981 seizure classification (2) and its 1985 and 1989 classifications of the epilepsies (1,3) have given physicians around the world a common language. These ILAE classifications were derived from earlier classification approaches in 1969 and 1970 (4,5) and were mainly based on two features: (a) distinction between generalized and focal seizure types and (b) etiologic considerations. This classification, like all other classification systems, is not without its shortcomings, and new approaches have been proposed.

TERMINOLOGY AND DEFINITIONS

Concepts and terminology of epilepsy have been changing throughout the centuries (6). It is important to differentiate between epilepsy, epilepsy syndrome, and seizure types as different entities. Seizure types are discussed separately in chapter 10.

The term epilepsy initially characterized both the disease and its attacks (6). An operational definition has been provided previously by the ILAE: "A condition characterized by recurrent (two or more) epileptic seizures, unprovoked by any immediate identified cause. Multiple seizures occurring in a 24-h period are considered a single event. An episode of status epilepticus is considered a single event. Individuals who have had only febrile seizures or only neonatal seizures as herein defined are excluded from this category" (7). The ILAE also provided the following conceptual definition: "epilepsy is a disorder of the brain characterized by an enduring predisposition to generate epileptic seizures and by the neurobiologic, cognitive, psychological, and social consequences of this condition. The definition of epilepsy requires the occurrence of at least one epileptic seizure. Elements in the definition of epilepsy include history of at least one seizure, enduring alteration in the brain that increases the likelihood of future seizures, and associated neurobiologic, cognitive, psychological, and social disturbances" (8).

The concept of epilepsy syndromes was introduced relatively recently (6), and epilepsy syndromes were only introduced in 1985 into the classification (3). An epilepsy syndrome is defined as "a complex of signs and symptoms that define a unique epileptic condition. This must involve more than just a seizure type: thus frontal lobe seizures per se, for instance, do not constitute a syndrome" (9). The ILAE furthermore distinguishes epileptic diseases which are defined as "a pathologic condition with a single, specific, well-defined etiology. Thus progressive myoclonic epilepsy is a syndrome, but Unverricht–Lundborg is a disease" (9).

THE 1989 ILAE CLASSIFICATION

The 1989 ILAE epilepsy classification is used worldwide and is reproduced in the appendix to this chapter. It was revised from proposals made in 1970 (4,5) and 1985 (3) and, like the 1981 ILAE seizure classification (2), is based primarily on the definition of electroclinical syndromes. In 1969, Henri Gastaut proposed the first classification of epilepsies (4), which was used as the basis of the first ILAE epilepsy classification system that was proposed 1 year later (5). This classification provided the major division between "partial" (focal) and generalized epilepsies. Each seizure type was grouped according to this dichotomy and associated with interictal and ictal electroencephalographic (EEG) findings, etiology and pathologic findings, and age of manifestation.

About 15 years later, a revision introduced the concept of epilepsy syndromes "defined as an epileptic disorder characterized by a cluster of signs and symptoms customarily occurring together. The signs and symptoms may be clinical (e.g., case history, seizure type, modes of seizure recurrence, and neurological and psychological findings) or as a result of findings detected by ancillary studies (e.g., EEG, X-ray, CT [computed tomography], and NMR [nuclear magnetic resonance])" (3). This revision divided many specific epilepsy syndromes under the major dichotomy of generalized and "localization-related" (focal) epilepsies and associated them with clinical and EEG findings, etiologies, and disease severity.

The primary dichotomy of these classification systems was set between localization-related (focal) epilepsies, "in which seizure semiology or findings at investigation disclose a localized origin of the seizures" (1), and generalized epilepsies, characterized by "seizures in which the first clinical changes indicate initial involvement of both hemispheres . . . [and] the ictal encephalographic patterns initially are bilateral" (1). EEG findings are the laboratory results that carry the most weight for defining a focal epilepsy syndrome.

In addition to localizing information, previous epilepsy classifications also contained etiologic information. The 1970 epilepsy classification[5] further divided the generalized epilepsies into *primary*—those occurring in the setting of normal neurologic status, with seizures that begin in childhood or adolescence and lack any clear cause—and *secondary*—those involving abnormal neurologic or psychological findings and diffuse or multifocal brain lesions. Because the term *secondary generalized epilepsy* was sometimes confused with the different concept of "secondary" or "secondarily" generalized tonic-clonic seizures, it was abandoned in the 1985 (3) and 1989 (1) revisions. Primary and secondary were replaced with *idiopathic* and *symptomatic*. The 1970 classification[5] applied the etiologic dichotomy only to generalized epilepsies because all focal epilepsies were assumed to be associated with some type of brain lesion. This neglected the idiopathic syndrome of benign epilepsy of childhood with centrotemporal spikes, and therefore the 1985 (3) and 1989 (1) revisions applied idiopathic and symptomatic to the focal epilepsies as well. The term *cryptogenic* was added in the 1989 (1) classification to describe epilepsy syndromes that are presumed to be symptomatic but are of unknown cause in specific patients.

Discussion of the 1989 Proposal

Despite its widespread use, the 1989 proposal has been criticized because of its stiff separation between "partial" and "generalized" epilepsies neglecting multiregional epilepsies and other conditions on the borderline between generalized and focal epilepsies. Furthermore the terms "idiopathic," "cryptogenic," and "symptomatic" have frequently been misunderstood and were thought to be imprecise. Additionally, this system did not accommodate the rapidly growing knowledge in the field and did not differentiate between "well-accepted" and "controversial" syndromes (9,10). Additionally, the system accommodated didactic grouping purposes but was not helpful in clinical practice: a working diagnosis is usually assigned first and subsequently etiologies are explored. A final diagnosis and classification was frequently not possible before workup was completed. Additionally, the system did not provide sufficient description of seizure semiology, and mingled seizure semiology and epilepsy type or syndrome and only allowed a strict one-to-one relationship between seizure type and epilepsy.

2001 ILAE PROPOSAL: A SYNDROME-ORIENTED CLASSIFICATION

To resolve these existing controversies, the ILAE's Commission on Classification and Terminology published a common terminology for ictal semiology (11) and a revised five-axis classification scheme of epilepsies (9). This proposal (9) was again based on epilepsy syndromes that appeared in previous classifications. The authors defined an epileptic syndrome as "[a] complex of signs and symptoms that define a unique epilepsy condition" (9). However, after discussion and debate this proposal was again revised 5 years later and another progress report was issued 5 years later (12).

Axes of the 2001 ILAE Proposal

The different axes in the 2001 ILAE proposal included seizure description (axis 1), seizure type (axis 2), epilepsy syndrome (axis 3), etiology (axis 4), and impairment (axis 5).

Axis 1 described ictal seizure semiology through a standardized glossary of descriptive ictal terminology (11). This terminology was independent of pathophysiological mechanisms, epilepsy focus, or seizure etiology.

Axis 2 was based on a list of accepted epileptic seizure types constructed by the task force. These seizure types were closely related to diagnostic epilepsy entities or indicated underlying mechanisms, pathophysiology, or etiology, or implicated related prognosis and therapy.

Axis 3 identified the epilepsy syndrome diagnosis and separated epilepsy syndromes from entities with epileptic seizures. Epilepsy syndromes were divided into "syndromes in development" and fully characterized syndromes (10).

Axis 4 delineated the etiology of epilepsies, which included pathologic and genetic causes as well as diseases frequently associated with epilepsy and this list was a work in progress at the time of publication.

Axis 5 was incomplete at the time of publication and was intended to include an optional classification of the degree of disability and impairment caused by the epilepsy.

Discussion of the 2001 ILAE Proposal

Compared with the 1989 version of epilepsy classification, the diagnostic scheme of the 2001 proposal overcame several shortcomings and confusion among EEG features, clinical seizure semiology, and syndromatic classification efforts. By dividing the seizure classification into several axes, the ILAE responded to the criticism that a strict one-to-one relationship is lacking between epilepsy syndromes and seizure types. The introduction of a multiaxial diagnostic scheme reflected the recognition of epilepsy as a clinical symptom that can manifest with different semiologic seizure types and be intertwined with different etiologies. It also responded to criticism that seizure semiology was not sufficiently emphasized in previous classifications. Furthermore, it addressed the more and more confluent borders between generalized and focal epilepsies. The term partial was replaced by focal. Additionally, it modeled epilepsy syndromes more flexibly by defining "accepted syndromes" versus "syndromes in development."

However, the 2001 proposal also attracted criticism for its incomplete presentation, lack of inclusion criteria for "accepted" syndromes, redundancy among classification axes, lack of information on age of onset, and inability to use this classification in all patients (13–16).

Limitations for applicability of the proposed ILAE epilepsy syndromes in clinical practice were demonstrated in several studies (15–17). In a general family practice, only 5% of all patients could be classified according to the ILAE syndromes (18). In a general neurology practice, 11% of all epilepsy patients could be classified according to the ILAE syndromes (19), and epileptologists could sort only 12 to 25% of all patients into ILAE epilepsy syndrome categories (15,20). These studies indicate that more patients can be classified as further information becomes available in each case and the more skilled the classifying physician is. Nevertheless, up to 75% of all patients were not classifiable according to the ILAE syndrome-oriented classification even by fully trained epileptologists, indicating that the majority of epilepsy patients do not fit any syndromic category. To address these limitations, the ILAE core group on classification revised this approach and provided an update on attempts to establish a new classification (12).

THE 2006 REPORT OF THE ILAE CLASSIFICATION CORE GROUP

In this proposal, it was attempted to outline "scientifically rigorous criteria for identification of specific epileptic seizure types and specific epilepsy syndromes as unique diagnostic entities" (12). Criteria included epileptic seizure types, age of onset, progressive nature, interictal EEG, associated interictal signs and symptoms, pathophysiological mechanisms, anatomical substrate, and etiological categories, as well as genetic basis. Subsequently, the group scored epilepsy syndromes listed in the 2001 proposal on a scale from 1 to 3, with 3 being the most clearly and reproducibly defined. The proposal mentioned that this was a very preliminary method and intended to ignite further research and category suggestions or possible cluster analysis of signs and symptoms (12). Based on this proposal epilepsy syndromes could be assigned in up to 70% of cases in a first comparison (17). However, ongoing inter- and intra-axial discordance was noted.

THE 2010 REVISED TERMINOLOGY AND CONCEPTS FOR ORGANIZATION OF SEIZURES AND EPILEPSIES

This additional update is an "interim organization" and tries to address ongoing criticisms to concepts and terminology (21). Classification is not treated as a rigid doctrine but a guide to summarize our current understanding about seizures and epilepsies in a useful manner. This revision resurrects the concept of electroclinical accepted syndromes and leaves the suggested syndrome list from 2006 unchanged (21). It also tries to address the variable degrees of precision of diagnosis and attempts to include the natural evolution. Epilepsies are now organized by specificity into three major divisions of electroclinical syndromes, nonsyndromic epilepsies with structural-metabolic causes, and epilepsies of unknown cause. This organization allows further description within divisions by dimensions as previously suggested in a five-dimensional epilepsy classification (13) that are only loosely defined. These may include cause, seizure types, age at onset, and others. Furthermore, it emphasizes the descriptive seizure terminology from 2001 (11) within these dimensions, at least for focal epilepsies. Seizures are now recognized as "occurring in and rapidly engaging bilaterally distributed networks (generalized) and within networks limited to one hemisphere and either discretely localized or more widely distributed (focal)" and terms such as complex-partial and simple partial have been abandoned. It also rekindles the terminology "focal" and differentiates from "generalized" seizures, while recognizing that generalized epileptic seizures do not necessarily include the entire cortex. Suggested etiologic concepts within the causal dimension include genetic, structural-metabolic, and unknown replacing idiopathic, symptomatic, and cryptogenic. Changes in terminology and classification remain work in progress.

While the ILAE continues to improve this epilepsy classification, alternative approaches have been proposed. One is a patient-oriented five-dimensional epilepsy classification that has been shown to be useful for everyday use and particularly in epilepsy surgery patients (6,13,16).

FIVE-DIMENSIONAL PATIENT-ORIENTED EPILEPSY CLASSIFICATION PROPOSAL

An potential application of this new revised approach to epilepsies is the patient-oriented epilepsy classification (13). This uses five dimensions to capture the critical features in patients with epilepsy.

Dimensions of the Patient-Oriented Classification

Dimension 1: The Epileptogenic Zone

The first dimension characterizes the localization of the epileptogenic zone, as determined by all available clinical information (e.g., history, examination, electroencephalography, MRI). Classification is recognized as an ongoing interactive process with an increasing degree of precision as additional clinical data become available. If it is uncertain whether the patient has epilepsy or nonepileptic seizures, the term *paroxysmal event* is used. If these results indicate that the patient has nonepileptic seizures, other classification systems can further characterize the event (22).

As further information becomes available (e.g., an electroencephalogram demonstrating left mesial temporal sharp waves, left temporal EEG seizures, and an MRI showing left hippocampal atrophy), the classification becomes more precise (left mesial temporal lobe epilepsy). If the patient has epilepsy but the epileptogenic zone cannot be determined further, the expression *unclassified epileptogenic zone* is used. If additional localizing evidence is available, a subcategory such as focal, multifocal, multilobar, generalized, or other is used. The categories focal, multilobar, and multifocal allow for further specification (Table 18.1) (23). Multifocal indicates more than one epileptogenic zone in different lobes. The term *generalized* is used if the cortex is diffusely epileptogenic without a localizable epileptogenic zone. Further characterization of the localization of the epileptogenic zone is possible by the addition of "left" or "right." The traditional ILAE epilepsy syndrome (if applicable) can be added in parentheses after the epileptogenic zone (e.g., Rasmussen encephalitis) to provide clinicians with traditionally used key words. Single seizures and situation-related seizures (e.g., febrile seizures and seizures induced by electrolyte or metabolic disturbances) can also be classified within certain limits by this system.

Dimension 2: Seizure Classification

The clinical signs and symptoms are the most important pieces of information for localizing a lesion in the central nervous system. Seizures and seizure semiology are the clinical manifestation of epilepsy. A seizure classification based solely on this clinical presentation of the epilepsy has been used successfully at several centers (24–31) and is outlined in detail in chapter 10.

This seizure classification uses only the clinical semiology and does not require any additional diagnostic techniques other than analysis of an observed or videotaped seizure. Information from MRI, EEG, or positron emission tomography (PET) is unnecessary. The semiologic seizure classification distinguishes among auras, autonomic seizures, dialeptic

TABLE 18.1

CLASSIFICATION OF THE EPILEPTOGENIC ZONE
(FIVE-DIMENSIONAL EPILEPSY CLASSIFICATION)

Unclassified epileptogenic zone

Focal—if the epileptogenic zone can be localized to a single area within one lobe of the brain on the basis of findings from the history, semiology, electroencephalogram, and imaging, the category focal or the more specific characterizations, frontal, temporal, parietal, occipital, or perirolandic (central), are used

    Frontal

    Perirolandic (central)[a]

    Temporal

      • Neocortical temporal

      • Mesial temporal

    Parietal

    Occipital

    Other[b]

Multilobar—one extensive epileptogenic zone within two or more adjacent lobes of the same hemisphere

    Frontotemporal

    Temporoparietal

    Frontoparietal

    Temporoparietooccipital

    Other

Hemispheric—the epileptogenic zone involves the whole hemisphere; a distinction of noninvolved area is not possible

Multifocal—multiple separate zones of epileptogenicity from distinct brain regions

    Bitemporal

    Other

    Other[c]

    Generalized

---

[a]The perirolandic (or central) area is defined as the precentral gyrus and the postcentral gyrus containing the primary motor and sensory areas. Anterior border to the frontal lobe is the precentral sulcus; inferior border to the temporal lobe is the sylvian fissure (14).
[b]Other locations, such as subcortical regions (e.g., hypothalamus), are suspected to be capable of generating seizures and can be included in this category.
[c]Other multifocal epileptogenic zones can include multiple combinations of epilepsy locations, such as "left frontal and right parietooccipital" or "right and left parieto-occipital."

seizures (characterized primarily by loss of awareness), motor seizures, and special seizures such as atonic, hypomotor, and negative myoclonic seizures (27–30).

Seizures frequently consist of more than one clinical component and follow a certain time sequence (e.g., an aura of nausea and uprising epigastric discomfort can be followed by distal picking hand movements; this can evolve into generalized stiffening and generalized rhythmic jerking of the body). This sequential evolution is considered in the semiologic seizure classification through linkage of separate seizure phases by arrows in the order of occurrence (e.g., abdominal aura → automotor seizure → generalized tonic-clonic seizure). To avoid excessive semiologic detail, up to four seizure phases can be separately classified. This restriction is arbitrary but usually sufficient to classify all the important seizure components based on clinical experience with this system in the past two decades.

Dimension 3: Etiology

Seizures are caused by the co-occurrence of multiple triggering factors. On the basis of investigational methods used to determine the cause of the epilepsy (e.g., histopathology, metabolic testing, MRI imaging, genetic testing), factors responsible for the generation of seizures can be found simultaneously at different diagnostic levels. To account for multiple coexisting etiologic factors, the etiology dimension permits the classification of several factors in one patient. A list of 12 etiologic categories has been proposed (Table 18.2) with the expectation that scientific progress, especially in genetics, will lead to addition of coexisting causes.

Dimension 4: Seizure Frequency

Severity of the epilepsy, as quantified by combined frequency of all seizure types, indicates the acuity of the disease. Categories include "daily," "persistent," "rare or none," "undefined," and "unknown" (Table 18.3). More specific information may also be added (e.g., '1 per day' or '4 per week').

Dimension 5: Related Medical Information

This dimension provides additional information in free text on associated medical conditions acquired in the history and examination or in previous diagnostic procedures. Samples include "history of febrile convulsions at age 1 year," "developmental delay," "right hemianopia," or "generalized slow spike-and-wave complexes on routine EEG."

A 3-year-old patient with daily myoclonic seizures followed by astatic seizures frequently triggered by light and photic stimulation would be classified by the above methods as follows:

    Epileptogenic zone: generalized (epilepsy with myoclonic-astatic seizures/Doose syndrome)
    Semiology: myoclonic seizure → astatic seizure
    Etiology: unknown
    Seizure frequency: daily (20/day)
    Related medical information: seizures triggered by photic stimulation

Advantages of the Five-Dimensional Patient-Oriented Classification

Independence of Dimensions

Except for dimension 1 (epileptogenic zone), which summarizes all dimensions, the other four dimensions are independent and separate entities without overlap or duplication of information.

Classification of all Patients is Possible

The classification process is independent of the amount of available diagnostic information (medical history, electroencephalography, MRI, PET, single-photon-emission CT), so it allows for categorization of every patient at different stages in the diagnostic process. The more information is available, the more specific the classification becomes.

Essential Characterization of Patients

The five-dimensional classification conveys the information necessary for a brief assessment of each case. A syndromic term can be added when the case represents a typical syndromic manifestation and use of the syndromic name can convey more information with fewer words. Important variations in clinical presentation can be encoded and accounted for in the classification.

TABLE 18.2

ETIOLOGIES (FIVE-DIMENSIONAL EPILEPSY CLASSIFICATION)

Hippocampal sclerosis
Tumor
- Glioma
- Dysembryoplastic neuroepithelial tumor
- Ganglioglioma
- Other

Malformation of cortical development
- Focal malformation of cortical development
- Hemimegalencephaly
- Malformation of cortical development with epidermal nevi (epidermal nevus syndrome)
- Heterotopic grey matter
- Hypothalamic hamartoma
- Hypomelanosis of Ito
- Other

Malformation of vascular development
- Cavernous angioma
- Arteriovenous malformation
- Sturge–Weber syndrome
- Other

CNS infection
- Meningitis
- Encephalitis
- Abscess
- Other

(Immune-mediated) CNS inflammation
- Rasmussen encephalitis
- Vasculitis
- Other

Hypoxic–ischemic brain injury
- Focal ischemic infarction
- Diffuse hypoxic–ischemic injury
- Periventricular leukomalacia
- Hemorrhagic infarction
- Venous sinus thrombosis
- Other

Head trauma
- Head trauma with intracranial hemorrhage
- Penetrating head injury
- Closed head injury

Inheritable conditions
- Tuberous sclerosis
- Progressive myoclonic epilepsy
- Metabolic syndrome
- Channelopathy
- Mitochondrial disorder
- Chromosomal aberration
- Presumed genetic cause
- Other

Structural brain abnormality of unknown cause
Other
Unknown—unclear etiology based on the current information

CNS, central nervous system.

TABLE 18.3

SEIZURE FREQUENCY (FIVE-DIMENSIONAL EPILEPSY CLASSIFICATION)

Daily
One or more seizures per day
Rare or none
Fewer than one seizure per 6 months; these patients are required to have had more than two documented seizures, with the last seizure occurring more than 6 months ago
Persistent
Fewer than one seizure per day but at least one seizure within the past 6 months. A persistent pattern must be recognizable in the period before the past 6 months. Single seizures, recent onset of epilepsy, breakthrough seizures in an otherwise well-controlled patient, and patients with fewer than 6 months of follow-up are classified as undefined (see below)
Undefined
Impossible to predict seizure frequency because of unknown frequency, recent onset of epilepsy, breakthrough seizures in an otherwise well-controlled patient caused by medication change/reduction or other provoking factors (sleep deprivation, alcohol, hypoxia, chemotherapy, etc.), and patients with fewer than 6 months follow-up after epilepsy surgery

Independence of Investigational Techniques

Many recent electroclinical syndromes are tightly locked to investigational devices, such as the electroencephalograph or the MRI. Sooner or later, additional techniques for localizing the epileptogenic zone will become available. The five-dimensional patient-oriented classification can be performed solely on the basis of observation and history taking and is flexible enough to incorporate future localizing tools and techniques.

Applicability to Research

The five-dimensional classification allows for reproducible and objective encoding and decoding of information in research (16). Whereas a syndrome-based classification of patients encodes a variety of heterogeneous patients into one category (e.g., Lennox–Gastaut syndrome), the five-dimensional classification sorts these patients by well-delineated homogenous criteria, with high inter-rater reliability (16). Therefore, the five-dimensional classification also opens new perspectives for research trials to recognize groups of seizures, etiologies, and epileptogenic zones that may represent clinically or scientifically important entities. Data can be analyzed in a multidimensional fashion by grouping patients according to each dimension.

Close Relationship to General Neurologic Localization Principles

The patient-oriented epilepsy classification follows general neurologic localization principles of symptom description, localization of the brain lesion, and search for etiology. On the basis of a presenting symptom (seizure), a working hypothesis on the localization of the lesion is generated (epileptogenic zone), and further information is gathered to determine the cause of the lesion (etiology). This process includes a continuous refinement of the seizure semiology, epileptogenic zone, and etiology as more information (e.g., from video-electroencephalography, MRI) becomes available and as the patient is referred and evaluated by a more experienced physician (e.g., from general practitioner to neurologist to epileptologist).

Seizures Listed as Independent Neurologic Symptoms

Repeated epileptic seizures are the presenting symptoms of localized or widespread cortical lesions caused by multiple etiologic factors. There is no one-to-one relationship between seizure semiology and etiologies as frequently suggested by epilepsy syndromes. This multifaceted approach pictures the epileptic seizure as an independent neurologic symptom due to multiple etiologies at various cortical locations occurring at different frequencies and in conjunction with other clinical findings.

Limitations of the Patient-Oriented Classification

Orientation Toward Focal Epilepsy and Epilepsy Surgery Candidates

The five-dimensional classification places more emphasis on focal epilepsies and is designed to provide the epileptologist with a brief outline of important presurgical information. It is therefore more surgically oriented and neglects subtypes of generalized epilepsies at first sight.

Concept of the Epileptogenic Zone

Although the concept of the epileptogenic zone is congenial to the multifactorial approach to epilepsy, it always remains a hypothetical construct, "the best possible guess," and its accuracy may be influenced by the extent of the observers' training and the available tests. However, these arguments apply also to a syndromatic approach and any kind of classification that requires decision making.

Inconsistencies in Etiological Dimension

Despite attempts to base the etiologic dimension on an isolated modality such as genetics, pathology, pathophysiology, or anatomy, we were not able to describe epilepsy etiology at only one level. This makes the etiologic dimension itself a multifaceted approach with different layers. Frequently, it is difficult to name a single etiology, as in a patient with a malformation of cortical development, a related neurotransmitter imbalance in the region of the malformation, and an underlying genetic mutation accounting for the malformation.

CONCLUSION

The classification of epilepsies is currently controversial, with various proposals under discussion. The terminology of the 1989 ILAE proposal (1) is in widespread use and is reproduced here as an Appendix. Newer approaches (12,13) are an attempt to improve its limitations, with the ultimate goal of improving diagnosis, treatment, and patient care.

References

1. Commission on Classification and Terminology of the International League Against Epilepsy. Proposal for revised classification of epilepsies and epileptic syndromes. *Epilepsia.* 1989;30(4):389–399.
2. From the Commission on Classification and Terminology of the International League Against Epilepsy. Proposal for revised clinical and electroencephalographic classification of epileptic seizures. *Epilepsia.* 1981;22(4):489–501.
3. Commission on Classification and Terminology of the International League Against Epilepsy. Proposal for classification of epilepsies and epileptic syndromes. *Epilepsia.* 1985;26(3):268–278.
4. Gastaut H. Classification of the epilepsies: proposal for an international classification. *Epilepsia.* 1969;10(Suppl):14–21.
5. Merlis JK. Proposal for an international classification of the epilepsies. *Epilepsia.* 1970;11(1):114–119.
6. Loddenkemper T, Lüders HO. History of epilepsy and seizure classification. In: Lüders HO, ed. *Textbook of Epilepsy Surgery.* London: Informa Healthcare; 2008:160–173.
7. Commission on Epidemiology and Prognosis, International League Against Epilepsy. Guidelines for epidemiologic studies on epilepsy. *Epilepsia.* 1993;34(4):592–596.
8. Fisher RS, van Emde BW, Blume W, et al. Epileptic seizures and epilepsy: definitions proposed by the International League Against Epilepsy (ILAE) and the International Bureau for Epilepsy (IBE). *Epilepsia.* 2005;46(4): 470–472.
9. Engel J, Jr. A proposed diagnostic scheme for people with epileptic seizures and with epilepsy: report of the ILAE Task Force on Classification and Terminology. *Epilepsia.* 2001;42(6):796–803.
10. Engel J, Jr. Classifications of the International League Against Epilepsy: time for reappraisal. *Epilepsia.* 1998;39(9):1014–1017.
11. Blume WT, Luders HO, Mizrahi E, et al. Glossary of descriptive terminology for ictal semiology: report of the ILAE task force on classification and terminology. *Epilepsia.* 2001;42(9):1212–1218.
12. Engel J, Jr. Report of the ILAE classification core group. *Epilepsia.* 2006; 47(9):1558–1568.
13. Loddenkemper T, Kellinghaus C, Wyllie E, et al. A proposal for a five-dimensional patient-oriented epilepsy classification. *Epileptic Disord.* 2005;7(4):308–320.
14. Luders H, Najm I, Wyllie E. Reply to "Of Cabbages and kings: some considerations on classifications, diagnostic schemes, semiology, and concepts". *Epilepsia.* 2003;44(1):6–7.
15. Akiyama T, Kobayashi K, Ogino T, et al. A population-based survey of childhood epilepsy in Okayama Prefecture, Japan: reclassification by a newly proposed diagnostic scheme of epilepsies in 2001. *Epilepsy Res.* 2006;70(Suppl 1):S34–S40.
16. Kellinghaus C, Loddenkemper T, Najm IM, et al. Specific epileptic syndromes are rare even in tertiary epilepsy centers: a patient-oriented approach to epilepsy classification. *Epilepsia.* 2004;45(3):268–275.
17. Kinoshita M, Takahashi R, Ikeda A. Application of the 2001 diagnostic scheme and the 2006 ILAE report of seizure and epilepsy: a feedback from the clinical practice of adult epilepsy. *Epileptic Disord.* 2008;10(3): 206–212.
18. Manford M, Hart YM, Sander JW, et al. The National General Practice Study of Epilepsy. The syndromic classification of the International League Against Epilepsy applied to epilepsy in a general population. *Arch Neurol.* 1992;49(8):801–808.
19. Murthy JM, Yangala R, Srinivas M. The syndromic classification of the International League Against Epilepsy: a hospital-based study from South India. *Epilepsia.* 1998;39(1):48–54.
20. Osservatorio Regionale per L'Epilessia (OREp). ILAE classification of epilepsies: its applicability and practical value of different diagnostic categories. Lombardy. *Epilepsia.* 1996;37(11):1051–1059.
21. Berg AT, Berkovic SF, Brodie MJ, et al. Revised terminology and concepts for organization of seizures and epilepsies: report of the ILAE Commission on Classification and Terminology, 2005–2009. *Epilepsia.* 2010;51:676–685.
22. Gates JR. Epidemiology and classification of non-epileptic events. In: Gates JR, Rowan AJ, eds. *Non-Epileptic Seizures.* Boston: Butterworth Heinemann; 2000:3–14.
23. Kuzniecky R, Morawetz R, Faught E, et al. Frontal and central lobe focal dysplasia: clinical, EEG and imaging features. *Dev Med Child Neurol.* 1995;37(2):159–166.
24. Baykan B, Ertas NK, Ertas M, et al. Comparison of classifications of seizures: a preliminary study with 28 participants and 48 seizures. *Epilepsy Behav.* 2005;6(4):607–612.
25. Hirfanoglu T, Serdaroglu A, Cansu A, et al. Semiological seizure classification: before and after video-EEG monitoring of seizures. *Pediatr Neurol.* 2007;36(4):231–235.
26. Kim KJ, Lee R, Chae JH, et al. Application of semiological seizure classification to epileptic seizures in children. *Seizure.* 2002;11(5):281–284.
27. Luders H, Acharya J, Baumgartner C, et al. Semiological seizure classification. *Epilepsia.* 1998;39(9):1006–1013.
28. Luders H, Acharya J, Baumgartner C, et al. A new epileptic seizure classification based exclusively on ictal semiology. *Acta Neurol Scand.* 1999; 99(3):137–141.
29. Luders H, Noachtar S. *Epileptic Seizures: Pathophysiology and Clinical Semiology.* Philadelphia: W.B.Saunders; 2000.
30. Luders HO, Burgess R, Noachtar S. Expanding the international classification of seizures to provide localization information. *Neurology.* 1993;43(9):1650–1655.
31. Rona S, Rosenow F, Arnold S, et al. A semiological classification of status epilepticus. *Epileptic Disord.* 2005;7(1):5–12.

APPENDIX 18.A ■ PROPOSAL FOR REVISED CLASSIFICATION OF EPILEPSIES AND EPILEPTIC SYNDROMES[1]

Commission on Classification and Terminology of the International League Against Epilepsy (1989)

PART I: INTERNATIONAL CLASSIFICATION OF EPILEPSIES AND EPILEPTIC SYNDROMES

1. Localization-related (focal, local, partial) epilepsies and syndromes
   1.1 Idiopathic (with age-related onset)
   At present, the following syndromes are established, but more may be identified in the future:
   ■ Benign childhood epilepsy with centrotemporal spike
   ■ Childhood epilepsy with occipital paroxysms
   ■ Primary reading epilepsy

   1.2 Symptomatic (Part III)
   ■ Chronic progressive epilepsia partialis continua of childhood (Kojewnikow syndrome)
   ■ Syndromes characterized by seizures with specific modes of precipitation (see Part IV)

Apart from these rare conditions, the symptomatic category comprises syndromes of great individual variability which are based mainly on seizure types and other clinical features, as well as anatomic localization and etiology—as far as these are known.

The seizure types refer to the International Classification of Epileptic Seizures. Inferences regarding anatomic localization must be drawn carefully. The scalp EEG (both interictal and ictal) may be misleading, and even local morphological findings detected by neuroimaging techniques are not necessarily identical with an epileptogenic lesion. Seizure symptomatology and, sometimes, additional clinical features often provide important clues. The first sign or symptom of a seizure is often the most important indicator of the site of origin of seizure discharge, whereas the following sequence of ictal events can reflect its further propagation through the brain. This sequence, however, can still be of high localizing importance. One must bear in mind that a seizure may start in a clinically silent region, so that the first clinical event occurs only after spread to a site more or less distant from the locus of initial discharge. The following tentative descriptions of syndromes related to anatomic localizations are based on data which include findings in studies with depth electrodes.

Temporal Lobe Epilepsies

Temporal lobe syndromes are characterized by simple partial seizures, complex partial seizures, and secondarily generalized seizures, or combinations of these. Frequently, there is a history of febrile seizures, and a family history of seizures is common. Memory deficits may occur. On metabolic imaging studies, hypometabolism is frequently observed (e.g., PET). Unilateral or bilateral temporal lobe spikes are common on EEG. Onset is frequently in childhood or young adulthood. Seizures occur in clusters at intervals or randomly.

General Characteristics

Features strongly suggestive of the diagnosis when present include the following:

1. Simple partial seizures typically characterized by autonomic and/or psychic symptoms and certain sensory phenomena such as olfactory and auditory (including illusions). Most common is an epigastric, often rising, sensation.
2. Complex partial seizures often but not always beginning with motor arrest typically followed by oroalimentary automatism. Other automatisms frequently follow. The duration is typically >1 min. Postictal confusion usually occurs. The attacks are followed by amnesia. Recovery is gradual.

Electroencephalographic Characteristics

In temporal lobe epilepsies the interictal scalp EEG may show the following:

1. No abnormality.
2. Slight or marked asymmetry of the background activity.
3. Temporal spikes, sharp waves and/or slow waves, unilateral or bilateral, synchronous but also asynchronous. These findings are not always confined to the temporal region.
4. In addition to scalp EEG findings, intracranial recordings may allow better definition of the intracranial distribution of the interictal abnormalities.

In temporal lobe epilepsies various EEG patterns may accompany the initial clinical ictal symptomatology, including (a) a unilateral or bilateral interruption of background activity and (b) temporal or multilobar low-amplitude fast activity, rhythmic spikes, or rhythmic slow waves. The onset of the EEG may not correlate with the clinical onset depending on methodology. Intracranial recordings may provide additional information regarding the chronologic and spatial evolution of the discharges.

Amygdalo-Hippocampal (Mesiobasal Limbic or Rhinencephalic) Seizures

Hippocampal seizures are the most common form; the symptoms are those described in the previous paragraphs except that auditory symptoms may not occur. The interictal scalp EEG may be normal, may show interictal unilateral temporal sharp or slow waves, and may show bilateral sharp or slow waves, synchronous or asynchronous. The intracranial interictal EEG may show mesial anterior temporal spikes or sharp waves. Seizures are characterized by rising epigastric discomfort, nausea, marked autonomic signs, and other symptoms,

---

[1]Reproduced, with permission, from Commission on Classification and Terminology of the International League Against Epilepsy. Proposal for revised classification of epilepsies and epileptic syndromes. *Epilepsia.* 1989;30(4):389–399.

including borborygmi, belching, pallor, fullness of the face, flushing of the face, arrest of respiration, pupillary dilatation, fear, panic, and olfactory-gustatory hallucinations.

Lateral Temporal Seizures

Simple seizures characterized by auditory hallucinations or illusions or dreamy states, visual misperceptions, or language disorders in case of language-dominant hemisphere focus. These may progress to complex partial seizures if propagation to mesial temporal or extratemporal structures occurs. The scalp EEG shows unilateral or bilateral midtemporal or posterior temporal spikes which are most prominent in the lateral derivations.

Frontal Lobe Epilepsies

Frontal lobe epilepsies are characterized by simple partial, complex partial, secondarily generalized seizures, or combinations of these. Seizures often occur several times a day and frequently occur during sleep. Frontal lobe partial seizures are sometimes mistaken for psychogenic seizures. Status epilepticus is a frequent complication.

General Characteristics

Features strongly suggestive of the diagnosis include the following:

1. Generally short seizures.
2. Complex partial seizures arising from the frontal lobe, often with minimal or no postictal confusion.
3. Rapid secondary generalization (more common in seizures of frontal than of temporal lobe epilepsy).
4. Prominent motor manifestations that are tonic or postural.
5. Complex gestural automatisms frequent at onset.
6. Frequent falling when the discharge is bilateral.

A number of seizure types are described below; however, multiple frontal areas may be involved rapidly and specific seizure types may not be discernible.

Supplementary Motor Seizures

In supplementary motor seizures, the seizure patterns are postural, focal tonic, with vocalization, speech arrest, and fencing postures.

Cingulate

Cingulate seizure patterns are complex partial with complex motor gestural automatisms at onset. Autonomic signs are common, as are changes in mood and affect.

Anterior Frontopolar Region

Anterior frontopolar seizure patterns include forced thinking or initial loss of contact and adversive movements of head and eyes, with possible evolution including contraversive movements and axial clonic jerks and falls and autonomic signs.

Orbitofrontal

The orbitofrontal seizure pattern is one of complex partial seizures with initial motor and gestural automatisms, olfactory hallucinations and illusions, and autonomic signs.

Dorsolateral

Dorsolateral seizure patterns may be tonic or, less commonly, clonic with versive eye and head movements and speech arrest.

Opercular

Opercular seizure characteristics include mastication, salivation, swallowing, laryngeal symptoms, speech arrest, epigastric aura, fear, and autonomic phenomena. Simple partial seizures, particularly partial clonic facial seizures, are common and may be ipsilateral. If secondary sensory changes occur, numbness may be a symptom, particularly in the hands. Gustatory hallucinations are particularly common in this area.

Motor Cortex

Motor cortex epilepsies are mainly characterized by simple partial seizures, and their localization depends on the side and topography of the area involved. In cases of the lower pre-rolandic area, there may be speech arrest, vocalization or dysphasia, tonic-clonic movements of the face on the contralateral side, or swallowing. Generalization of the seizure frequently occurs. In the rolandic area, partial motor seizures without march or Jacksonian seizures occur, particularly beginning in the contralateral upper extremities. In the case of seizures involving the paracentral lobule, tonic movements of the ipsilateral foot may occur, as well as the expected contralateral leg movements. Postictal or Todd paralysis is frequent.

Kojewnikow's Syndrome

Two types of Kojewnikow syndrome are recognized, one of which is also known as Rasmussen syndrome and is included among the epileptic syndromes of childhood noted under symptomatic seizures. The other type represents a particular form of rolandic partial epilepsy in both adults and children and is related to a variable lesion of the motor cortex. Its principal features are (a) motor partial seizures, always well localized; (b) often late appearance of myoclonus in the same site where somatomotor seizures occur; (c) an EEG with normal background activity and a focal paroxysmal abnormality (spikes and slow waves); (d) occurrence at any age in childhood and adulthood; (e) frequently demonstrable etiology (tumor, vascular); and (f) no progressive evolution of the syndrome (clinical, electroencephalographic or psychological, except in relation to the evolution of the causal lesion). This condition may result from mitochondrial encephalopathy (MELAS). NOTE: Anatomical origins of some epilepsies are difficult to assign to specific lobes. Such epilepsies include those with pre- and postcentral symptomatology (perirolandic seizures). Such overlap to adjacent anatomic regions also occurs in opercular epilepsy.

In frontal lobe epilepsies, the interictal scalp recordings may show (a) no abnormality; (b) sometimes background asymmetry, frontal spikes, or sharp waves; or (c) sharp waves or slow waves (either unilateral or frequently bilateral or unilateral multilobar). Intracranial recordings can sometimes distinguish unilateral from bilateral involvement.

In frontal lobe seizures, various EEG patterns can accompany the initial clinical symptomatology. Uncommonly, the EEG abnormality precedes the seizure onset and then provides important localizing information, such as (a) frontal or multilobar, often bilateral, low-amplitude fast activity, mixed spikes, rhythmic spikes, rhythmic spike-waves, or rhythmic slow waves; or (b) bilateral high-amplitude single sharp waves followed by diffuse flattening.

Depending on the methodology, intracranial recordings may provide additional information regarding the chronologic and spatial evolution of the discharges; localization may be difficult.

Parietal Lobe Epilepsies

Parietal lobe epilepsy syndromes are usually characterized by simple partial and secondarily generalized seizures. Most seizures arising in the parietal lobe remain as simple partial seizures, but complex partial seizures may arise out of simple partial seizures and occur with spread beyond the parietal lobe. Seizures arising from the parietal lobe have the following features: Seizures are predominantly sensory with many characteristics. Positive phenomena consist of tingling and a feeling of electricity, which may be confined or may spread in a Jacksonian manner. There may be a desire to move a body part or a sensation as if a part were being moved. Muscle tone may be lost. The parts most frequently involved are those with the largest cortical representation (e.g., the hand, arm, and face). There may be tongue sensations of crawling, stiffness, or coldness, and facial sensory phenomena may occur bilaterally. Occasionally an intra-abdominal sensation of sinking, choking, or nausea may occur, particularly in cases of inferior and lateral parietal lobe involvement. Rarely, there may be pain, which may take the form of a superficial burning dysesthesia or a vague, very severe, painful sensation. Parietal lobe visual phenomena may occur as hallucinations of a formed variety. Metamorphopsia with distortions, foreshortenings, and elongations may occur and are more frequently observed in cases of nondominant hemisphere discharges. Negative phenomena include numbness, a feeling that a body part is absent, and a loss of awareness of a part or a half of the body, known as asomatognosia. This is particularly the case with nondominant hemisphere involvement. Severe vertigo or disorientation in space may be indicative of inferior parietal lobe seizures. Seizures in the dominant parietal lobe result in a variety of receptive or conductive language disturbances. Some well-lateralized genital sensations may occur with paracentral involvement. Some rotatory or postural motor phenomena may occur. Seizures of the paracentral lobule have a tendency to become secondarily generalized.

Occipital Lobe Epilepsies

Occipital lobe epilepsy syndromes are usually characterized by simple partial and secondarily generalized seizures. Complex partial seizures may occur with spread beyond the occipital lobe. The frequent association of occipital lobe seizures and migraine is complicated and controversial. The clinical seizure manifestations usually, but not always, include visual manifestations. Elementary visual seizures are characterized by fleeting visual manifestations that may be either negative (scotoma, hemianopsia, amaurosis) or, more commonly, positive (sparks or flashes, phosphenes). Such sensations appear in the visual field contralateral to the discharge in the specific visual cortex but can spread to the entire visual field. Perceptive illusions, in which the objects appear to be distorted, may occur. The following varieties can be distinguished: a change in size (macropsia or micropsia) or a change in distance, an inclination of objects in a given plane of space, and distortion of objects or a sudden change of shape (metamorphopsia). Visual hallucinatory seizures are occasionally characterized by complex visual perceptions (e.g., colorful scenes of varying complexity). In some cases, the scene is distorted or made smaller, and in rare instances, the subject sees his own image (heutoscopy). Such illusional and hallucinatory visual seizures involve epileptic discharge in the temporoparieto-occipital junction. The initial signs may also include tonic and/or clonic contraversion of eyes and head or eyes only (oculoclonic or oculogyric deviation), palpebral jerks, and forced closure of eyelids. Sensation of ocular oscillation or of the whole body may occur. The discharge may spread to the temporal lobe, producing seizure manifestations of either lateral posterior temporal or hippocampoamygdala seizures. When the primary focus is located in the supracalcarine area, the discharge can spread forward to the suprasylvian convexity or the mesial surface, mimicking those of parietal or frontal lobe seizures. Spread to contralateral occipital lobe may be rapid. Occasionally the seizure tends to become secondarily generalized.

1.3 Cryptogenic

Cryptogenic epilepsies are presumed to be symptomatic and the etiology is unknown. Thus, this category differs from the previous one by the lack of etiologic evidence (see definitions).

2. Generalized epilepsies and syndromes
    2.1 Idiopathic (with age-related onset—listed in order of age)
    - Benign neonatal familial convulsions
    - Benign neonatal convulsions
    - Benign myoclonic epilepsy in infancy
    - Childhood absence epilepsy (pyknolepsy)
    - Juvenile absence epilepsy
    - Juvenile myoclonic epilepsy (impulsive petit mal)
    - Epilepsy with grand mal (GTCS) seizures on awakening
    - Other generalized idiopathic epilepsies not defined above
    - Epilepsies with seizures precipitated by specific modes of activation (see Appendix II)
    2.2 Cryptogenic or symptomatic (in order of age)
    - West syndrome (infantile spasms, Blitz–Nick–Salaam Krämpfe)
    - Lennox–Gastaut syndrome
    - Epilepsy with myoclonic-astatic seizures
    - Epilepsy with myoclonic absences
    2.3 Symptomatic
        2.3.1 Nonspecific etiology
        - Early myoclonic encephalopathy
        - Early infantile epileptic encephalopathy with suppression burst
        - Other symptomatic generalized epilepsies not defined above
        2.3.2 Specific syndromes
        - Epileptic seizures may complicate many disease states. Under this heading are included diseases in which seizures are a presenting or predominant feature.
3. Epilepsies and syndromes undetermined whether focal or generalized
    3.1 With both generalized and focal seizures
    - Neonatal seizures
    - Severe myoclonic epilepsy in infancy
    - Epilepsy with continuous spike-waves during slow wave sleep
    - Acquired epileptic aphasia (Landau–Kleffner syndrome)
    - Other undetermined epilepsies not defined above

3.2 Without unequivocal generalized or focal features. All cases with generalized tonic-clonic seizures in which clinical and EEG findings do not permit classification as clearly generalized or localization related, such as in many cases of sleep-grand mal (GTCS), are considered not to have unequivocal generalized or focal features.

4. Special syndromes
4.1 Situation-related seizures (Gelegenheitsanfälle)
- Febrile convulsions
- Isolated seizures or isolated status epilepticus
- Seizures occurring only when there is an acute metabolic or toxic event due to factors such as alcohol, drugs, eclampsia, and nonketotic hyperglycemia.

PART II: DEFINITIONS

Localization-Related (Focal, Local, Partial) Epilepsies and Syndromes

Localization-related epilepsies and syndromes are epileptic disorders in which seizure semiology or findings at investigation disclose a localized origin of the seizures. This includes not only patients with small circumscribed constant epileptogenic lesions (anatomic or functional), that is, true focal epilepsies, but also patients with less well-defined lesions, whose seizures may originate from variable loci. In most symptomatic localization-related epilepsies, the epileptogenic lesions can be traced to one part of one cerebral hemisphere, but in idiopathic age-related epilepsies with focal seizures, corresponding regions of both hemispheres may be functionally involved.

Generalized Epilepsies and Syndromes

According to the International Classification of Epilepsies and Epileptic Syndromes, generalized epilepsies and syndromes are epileptic disorders with generalized seizures, that is, "seizures in which the first clinical changes indicate initial involvement of both hemispheres. The ictal encephalographic patterns initially are bilateral."

Epilepsies and Syndromes Undetermined as to Whether They Are Focal or Generalized

There may be two reasons why a determination of whether seizures are focal or generalized cannot be made: (a) the patient has both focal and generalized seizures together or in succession (e.g., partial seizures plus absences), and has both focal and generalized EEG seizure discharges (e.g., temporal spike focus plus independent bilateral spike-wave discharges); and (b) there are no positive signs of either focal or generalized seizure onset. The most common reasons for this are the seizures occur during sleep, the patient recalls no aura, and ancillary investigations, including EEG, are not revealing.

Idiopathic Localization-Related Epilepsies

Idiopathic localization-related epilepsies are childhood epilepsies with partial seizures and focal EEG abnormalities. They are age-related, without demonstrable anatomic lesions, and are subject to spontaneous remission. Clinically, patients have neither neurologic and intellectual deficit nor a history of antecedent illness, but frequently have a family history of benign epilepsy. The seizures are usually brief and rare, but may be frequent early in the course of the disorder. The seizure patterns may vary from case to case, but usually remain constant in the same child. The EEG is characterized by normal background activity and localized high-voltage repetitive spikes, which are sometimes independently multifocal. Brief bursts of generalized spike-waves can occur. Focal abnormalities are increased by sleep and are without change in morphology.

Benign Childhood Epilepsy with Centrotemporal Spikes

Benign childhood epilepsy with centrotemporal spikes is a syndrome of brief, simple, partial, hemifacial motor seizures, frequently having associated somatosensory symptoms that have a tendency to evolve into GTCS. Both seizure types are often related to sleep. Onset occurs between the ages of 3 and 13 years (peak, 9–10 years), and recovery occurs before the age of 15–16 years. Genetic predisposition is frequent, and there is male predominance. The EEG has blunt high-voltage centrotemporal spikes, often followed by slow waves that are activated by sleep and tend to spread or shift from side to side.

Childhood Epilepsy with Occipital Paroxysms

The syndrome of childhood epilepsy with occipital paroxysms is, in general respects, similar to that of benign childhood epilepsy with centrotemporal spikes. The seizures start with visual symptoms (amaurosis, phosphenes, illusions, or hallucinations) and are often followed by a hemiclonic seizure or automatisms. In 25% of cases, the seizures are immediately followed by migrainous headache. The EEG has paroxysms of high-amplitude spike-waves or sharp waves recurring rhythmically on the occipital and posterior temporal areas of one or both hemispheres, but only when the eyes are closed. During seizures, the occipital discharge may spread to the central or temporal region. At present, no definite statement on prognosis is possible.

Idiopathic Generalized Epilepsies (Age-Related)

Idiopathic generalized epilepsies are forms of generalized epilepsies in which all seizures are initially generalized, with an EEG expression that is a generalized, bilateral, synchronous, symmetrical discharge (such as is described in the seizure classification of the corresponding type). The patient usually has a normal interictal state, without neurologic or neuroradiologic signs. In general, interictal EEGs show normal background activity and generalized discharges, such as spikes, polyspike, spike-wave, and polyspike-waves ≥3 Hz. The discharges are increased by slow sleep. The various syndromes of idiopathic generalized epilepsies differ mainly in age of onset.

Benign Neonatal Familial Convulsions

Benign neonatal familial convulsions are rare, dominantly inherited disorders manifesting mostly on the second and third days of life, with clonic or apneic seizures and no specific EEG criteria. History and investigations reveal no etiologic factors. About 14% of these patients later develop epilepsy.

Benign Neonatal Convulsions

Benign neonatal convulsions are very frequently repeated clonic or apneic seizures occurring at about the fifth day of life, without known etiology or concomitant metabolic disturbance. Interictal EEG often shows alternating sharp theta waves. There is no recurrence of seizures, and the psychomotor development is not affected.

Benign Myoclonic Epilepsy in Infancy

Benign myoclonic epilepsy in infancy is characterized by brief bursts of generalized myoclonus that occur during the first or second year of life in otherwise normal children who often have a family history of convulsions or epilepsy. EEG recording shows generalized spike-waves occurring in brief bursts during the early stages of sleep. These attacks are easily controlled by appropriate treatment. They are not accompanied by any other type of seizure, although GTCS may occur during adolescence. The epilepsy may be accompanied by a relative delay of intellectual development and minor personality disorders.

Childhood Absence Epilepsy (Pyknolepsy)

Pyknolepsy occurs in children of school age (peak manifestation, ages 6–7 years), with a strong genetic predisposition in otherwise normal children. It appears more frequently in girls than in boys. It is characterized by very frequent (several to many per day) absences. The EEG reveals bilateral, synchronous symmetrical spike-waves, usually 3 Hz, on a normal background activity. During adolescence, GTCS often develop. Otherwise, absences may remit or, more rarely, persist as the only seizure type.

Juvenile Absence Epilepsy

The absences of juvenile absence epilepsy are the same as in pyknolepsy, but absences with retropulsive movements are less common. Manifestation occurs around puberty. Seizure frequency is lower than in pyknolepsy, with absences occurring less frequently than every day, mostly sporadically. Association with GTCS is frequent, and GTCS precede the absence manifestations more often than in childhood absence epilepsy, often occurring on awakening. Not infrequently, the patients also have myoclonic seizures. Sex distribution is equal. The spike-waves are often >3 Hz. Response to therapy is excellent.

Juvenile Myoclonic Epilepsy (Impulsive Petit Mal)

Impulsive petit mal appears around puberty and is characterized by seizures with bilateral, single or repetitive, arrhythmic, irregular myoclonic jerks, predominantly in the arms. Jerks may cause some patients to fall suddenly. No disturbance of consciousness is noticeable. The disorder may be inherited, and sex distribution is equal. Often, there are GTCS and, less often, infrequent absences. The seizures usually occur shortly after awakening and are often precipitated by sleep deprivation.

Interictal and ictal EEG have rapid, generalized, often irregular spike-waves and polyspike-waves; there is no close phase correlation between EEG spikes and jerks. Frequently, the patients are photosensitive. Response to appropriate drugs is good.

Epilepsy with GTCS on Awakening

Epilepsy with GTCS on awakening is a syndrome with onset occurring mostly in the second decade of life. The GTCS occur exclusively or predominantly (>90% of the time) shortly after awakening regardless of the time of day or in a second seizure peak in the evening period of relaxation. If other seizures occur, they are mostly absence or myoclonic, as in juvenile myoclonic epilepsy. Seizures may be precipitated by sleep deprivation and other external factors. Genetic predisposition is relatively frequent. The EEG shows one of the patterns of idiopathic generalized epilepsy. There is a significant correlation with photosensitivity.

Generalized Cryptogenic or Symptomatic Epilepsies (Age-Related)

West Syndrome (Infantile Spasms, Blitz–Nick–Salaam Krämpfe)

Usually, West syndrome consists of a characteristic triad: infantile spasms, arrest of psychomotor development, and hypsarrhythmia although one element may be missing. Spasms may be flexor, extensor, lightning, or nods, but most commonly they are mixed. Onset peaks between the ages of 4 and 7 months and always occurs before the age of 1 year. Boys are more commonly affected. The prognosis is generally poor. West syndrome may be separated into two groups. The symptomatic group is characterized by previous existence of brain damage signs (psychomotor retardation, neurologic signs, radiologic signs, or other types of seizures) or by a known etiology. The smaller, cryptogenic group is characterized by a lack of previous signs of brain damage and of known etiology. The prognosis appears to be partly based on early therapy with adrenocorticotropic hormone (ACTH) or oral steroids.

Lennox–Gastaut Syndrome

Lennox–Gastaut syndrome manifests itself in children ages 1–8 years, but appears mainly in preschool-age children. The most common seizure types are tonic-axial, atonic, and absence seizures, but other types such as myoclonic, GTCS, or partial are frequently associated with this syndrome. Seizure frequency is high, and status epilepticus is frequent (stuporous states with myoclonias, tonic, and atonic seizures). The EEG usually has abnormal background activity, slow spike-waves <3 Hz and, often, multifocal abnormalities. During sleep, bursts of fast rhythms (~10 Hz) appear. In general, there is mental retardation. Seizures are difficult to control, and the development is mostly unfavorable. In 60% of cases, the syndrome occurs in children suffering from a previous encephalopathy but is primary in other cases.

Epilepsy with Myoclonic-Astatic Seizures

Manifestations of myoclonic-astatic seizures begin between the ages of 7 months and 6 years (mostly between the ages of 2 and 5 years), with (except if seizures begin in the first year) twice as many boys affected. There is frequently hereditary predisposition and usually a normal developmental background. The seizures are myoclonic, astatic, myoclonic-astatic, absence with clonic and tonic components, and tonic-clonic. Status frequently occurs. Tonic seizures develop late in the course of unfavorable cases. The EEG, initially often normal except for 4–7 Hz rhythms, may have irregular fast spike-wave or polyspike-wave. Course and outcome are variable.

Epilepsy with Myoclonic Absences

The syndrome of epilepsy with myoclonic absences is clinically characterized by absences accompanied by severe bilateral rhythmical clonic jerks, often associated with a tonic contraction. On the EEG, these clinical features are always accompanied by bilateral, synchronous, and symmetrical discharge of rhythmical spike-waves at 3 Hz, similar to childhood absence. Seizures occur many times a day. Awareness of the jerks may be maintained. Associated seizures are rare. Age of onset is ~7 years, and there is a male preponderance. Prognosis is less favorable than in pyknolepsy owing to resistance to therapy of the seizures, mental deterioration, and possible evolution to other types of epilepsy such as Lennox–Gastaut syndrome.

Symptomatic Generalized Epilepsies and Syndromes

Symptomatic generalized epilepsies, most often occurring in infancy and childhood, are characterized by generalized seizures with clinical and EEG features different from those of idiopathic generalized epilepsies. There may be only one type, but more often there are several types, including myoclonic jerks, tonic seizures, atonic seizures, and atypical absences. EEG expression is bilateral but less rhythmical than in idiopathic generalized epilepsies and is more or less asymmetrical. Interictal EEG abnormalities differ from idiopathic generalized epilepsies, appearing as suppression bursts, hypsarrhythmia, slow spike-waves, or generalized fast rhythms. Focal abnormalities may be associated with any of the above. There are clinical, neuropsychologic, and neuroradiologic signs of a usually diffuse, specific, or nonspecific encephalopathy.

Generalized Symptomatic Epilepsies of Nonspecific Etiology (Age-Related)

Early Myoclonic Encephalopathy

The principal features of early myoclonic encephalopathy are onset occurring before age 3 months, initially fragmentary myoclonus, and then erratic partial seizures, massive myoclonias, or tonic spasms. The EEG is characterized by suppression-burst activity, which may evolve into hypsarrhythmia. The course is severe, psychomotor development is arrested, and death may occur in the first year. Familial cases are frequent and suggest the influence of one or several congenital metabolic errors, but there is no constant genetic pattern.

Early Infantile Epileptic Encephalopathy with Suppression Burst

This syndrome is defined by very early onset, within the first few months of life, frequent tonic spasms, and suppression-burst EEG pattern in both waking and sleeping states. Partial seizures may occur. Myoclonic seizures are rare. Etiology and underlying pathology are obscure. The prognosis is serious with severe psychomotor retardation and seizure intractability; often there is evolution to the West syndrome at age 4–6 months.

Epilepsies and Syndromes Undetermined as to Whether They Are Focal or Generalized

Neonatal Seizures

Neonatal seizures differ from those of older children and adults. The most frequent neonatal seizures are described as subtle because the clinical manifestations are frequently overlooked. These include tonic, horizontal deviation of the eyes with or without jerking, eyelid blinking or fluttering, sucking, smacking, or other buccal-lingual oral movements, swimming or pedaling movements and, occasionally, apneic spells. Other neonatal seizures occur as tonic extension of the limbs, mimicking decerebrate or decorticate posturing. These occur particularly in premature infants. Multifocal clonic seizures characterized by clonic movements of a limb, which may migrate to other body parts or other limbs, or focal clonic seizures, which are much more localized, may occur. In the latter, the infant is usually not unconscious. Rarely, myoclonic seizures may occur, and the EEG pattern is frequently that of suppression-burst activity. The tonic seizures have a poor prognosis, because they frequently accompany intraventricular hemorrhage. The myoclonic seizures also have a poor prognosis, because they are frequently a part of the early myoclonic encephalopathy syndrome.

Severe Myoclonic Epilepsy in Infancy

Severe myoclonic epilepsy in infancy is a recently defined syndrome. The characteristics include a family history of epilepsy or febrile convulsions, normal development before onset, seizures beginning during the first year of life in the form of generalized or unilateral febrile clonic seizures, secondary appearance of myoclonic jerks, and often partial seizures. EEGs show generalized spike-waves and polyspike-waves, early photosensitivity, and focal abnormalities. Psychomotor development is retarded from the second year of life on, and ataxia, pyramidal signs, and interictal myoclonus appear. This type of epilepsy is very resistant to all forms of treatment.

Epilepsy with Continuous Spike-Waves During Slow-Wave Sleep

Epilepsy with continuous spike-waves during slow-wave sleep results from the association of various seizure types, partial or generalized, occurring during sleep, and atypical absences when awake. Tonic seizures do not occur. The characteristic EEG pattern consists of continuous diffuse spike-waves during slow wave sleep, which is noted after onset of seizures. Duration varies from months to years. Despite the usually benign evolution of seizures, prognosis is guarded because of the appearance of neuropsychologic disorders.

Acquired Epileptic Aphasia (Landau–Kleffner Syndrome)

The Landau–Kleffner syndrome is a childhood disorder in which an acquired aphasia, multifocal spike, and spike-and-wave discharges are associated. Epileptic seizures and behavioral and psychomotor disturbances occur in two thirds of the patients. There is verbal auditory agnosia and rapid reduction of spontaneous speech. The seizures, usually GTCS or partial motor, are rare and remit before the age of 15 years, as do the EEG abnormalities.

Special Syndromes

Febrile Convulsions

Febrile convulsions are an age-related disorder almost always characterized by generalized seizures occurring during an acute febrile illness. Most febrile convulsions are brief and uncomplicated, but some may be more prolonged and followed by transient or permanent neurological sequelae, such as the hemiplegia–hemiatrophy–epilepsy (HHE) syndrome. Febrile convulsions tend to recur in about one third of affected patients. Controversy about the risks of developing epilepsy later has largely been resolved by some recent large studies; the overall risk is probably not more than 4%. The indications for prolonged drug prophylaxis against recurrence of febrile convulsions are now more clearly defined, and most individuals do not require prophylaxis. Essentially, this condition is a relatively benign disorder of early childhood.

PART III: SYMPTOMATIC GENERALIZED EPILEPSIES OF SPECIFIC ETIOLOGIES

Only diseases in which epileptic seizures are the presenting or a prominent feature are classified. These diseases often have epileptic pictures that resemble symptomatic generalized epilepsies without specific etiology, appearing at similar ages.

Malformations

Aicardi syndrome occurs in females and is noted for retinal lacunae and absence of the corpus callosum; infantile spasms with early onset; and often asymmetric, diffuse EEG abnormalities generally asynchronous with suppression burst and/or atypical hypsarrhythmia.

Lissencephaly–pachygyria is characterized by facial abnormalities and specific CT scan features, axial hypotonia, and infantile spasms. The EEG shows fast activity of high-voltage "alpha-like" patterns without change during wakefulness and sleep.

The individual phacomatoses have no typical electroclinical pattern. We emphasize that West syndrome is frequent in tuberous sclerosis and that generalized and partial seizures may follow the otherwise typical course of infantile spasms. Sturge–Weber syndrome is a frequent cause of simple partial seizures followed by hemiparesis.

Hypothalamic hamartomas may present with gelastic seizures, precocious puberty, and retardation.

Proven or Suspected Inborn Errors of Metabolism

Neonate

Metabolism errors in the neonate include nonketotic hyperglycinemia and D-glyceric acidemia, showing early myoclonic encephalopathy with erratic myoclonus, partial seizures, and suppression-burst EEG patterns.

Infant

The classical phenylketonuria can express itself as a West syndrome. A variant of phenylketonuria with biopterin deficiency causes seizures starting in the second 6 months of life in infants who have been hypotonic since birth. The seizures are generalized motor seizures associated with erratic myoclonic jerks and oculogyric seizures.

Tay–Sachs and Sandhoff disease present with acoustic startle or myoclonus in the first months of life, without EEG manifestations. In the second year, myoclonic jerks and erratic partial seizures occur, along with marked slowing of the background rhythms.

Another type of metabolic error is early infantile type of ceroid-lipofuscinosis (Santavuori–Haltia–Hagberg disease). Massive myoclonus begins between the ages of 5 and 18 months, with a highly suggestive EEG pattern of vanishing EEG.

Pyridoxine dependency is manifested by seizures that have no suggestive characteristics, but this condition must always be suspected since therapeutic intervention is possible.

Child

Late infantile ceroid-lipofuscinosis (Jansky–Bielschowsky disease) is characterized by onset between the ages of 2 and 4 years of massive myoclonic jerks, atonic, or astatic seizures. The EEG shows slow background rhythms, multifocal spikes, and a characteristic response to intermittent photic stimulation at a slow rate.

An infantile type of Huntington disease appears after age 3 years, with a slowing of mental development, followed by dystonia, GTCS, atypical absence seizures, and myoclonic seizures. The EEG shows discharges of generalized spike-waves and polyspike-waves, with the usual photic stimulation rate.

Child and Adolescent

A juvenile form of Gaucher disease is marked by onset at approximately 6–8 years of age, with epileptic seizures of various types, most commonly GTCS or partial motor. The EEG shows progressive deterioration of background activity, abnormal photic response, diffuse paroxysmal abnormalities, and multifocal abnormalities with a clear posterior predominance.

The juvenile form of ceroid-lipofuscinosis (Spielmeyer–Vogt–Sjögren disease) is characterized by onset between the ages of 6 and 8 years, a decrease in visual acuity, slowing of psychomotor development, and appearance of cerebellar and extrapyramidal signs. After 1 to 4 years, GTCS and fragmentary, segmental, and massive myoclonus occur. The EEG shows bursts of slow waves and slow spikes and waves.

Onset of Lafora disease occurs between the ages of 6 and 19 years (mean 11.5 years) and is characterized by generalized clonic, GTCS, with a frequent association of partial seizures with visual symptomatology, constant myoclonic jerks (fragmentary, segmental, and massive myoclonus), and rapidly progressive mental deterioration. The EEG shows discharges of fast spike-waves and polyspike-waves, photosensitivity, deterioration of background activity, and the appearance of multifocal abnormalities, particularly posteriorly. On the average, death occurs 5.5 years after onset.

The so-called degenerative progressive myoclonic epilepsy (Lundborg type) also falls into this category. The only significant well-individualized group is the Finnish type, described by Koskiniemi et al. Onset occurs between the ages of 8 and 13 years, with myoclonus (segmental, fragmentary, and massive) and GTCS, associated cerebellar ataxia, and slowly progressive although generally mild mental deterioration. The EEG shows slow abnormalities (theta rhythms and later, delta rhythms), with generalized spike-waves predominantly in the frontal area and photosensitivity. Patients survive ≥15 years.

Dyssynergia cerebellaris myoclonia (DCM) with epilepsy (Ramsay–Hunt syndrome) appears between the ages of 6 and 20 years (mean 11 years) with myoclonias or GTCS. Above all, the myoclonic syndrome is characterized by action and intention myoclonus. The GTCS are rare and sensitive to therapy. Mental deterioration, when present, is slow. Most of the neurologic manifestations are limited to cerebellar signs. In the EEG, the background activity remains normal, with generalized paroxysmal abnormalities (spikes, spike-waves, and polyspike-waves) and photosensitivity. During REM sleep, rapid polyspikes appear, localized in the central and vertex regions.

The clinical picture for the cherry red spot myoclonus syndrome (sialidosis with isolated deficit in neuraminidase) is very similar to that of the Ramsay–Hunt syndrome, with myoclonus, photosensitivity, and cerebellar syndrome. Other characteristics include the nearly constant existence of amblyopia and presence of a cherry red spot on funduscopic examination. The EEG is similar to that of DCM with the following specific features: the polyspike-wave discharges always correspond to a massive myoclonus and there is no photosensitivity.

A Ramsay–Hunt-like syndrome can also be associated with a mitochondrial myopathy, with abnormalities of lactate and pyruvate metabolism (7).

Adult

Kuf disease (adult ceroid-lipofuscinosis) is a relatively slow, progressive storage disease with frequent generalized seizures that may be very intractable. Unlike juvenile storage disease, the optic fundi may be normal. The main characteristic is an extreme photic sensitivity on slow photic stimulation.

A large number of epilepsy-related diseases in childhood, adulthood, and old age are not enumerated here because the seizures are not distinctively different from other seizure types and are not critical for diagnosis.

PART IV

Precipitated seizures are those in which environmental or internal factors consistently precede the attacks and are differentiated from spontaneous epileptic attacks in which precipitating factors cannot be identified. Certain nonspecific factors (e.g., sleeplessness, alcohol or drug withdrawal, or hyperventilation) are common precipitators and are not *specific* modes of seizure precipitation. In certain epileptic syndromes, the seizures clearly may be somewhat more susceptible to nonspecific factors, but this is only occasionally useful in classifying epileptic syndromes. An epilepsy characterized by specific modes of seizure precipitation, however, is one in which a consistent relationship can be recognized between the occurrence of one or more definable nonictal events and subsequent occurrence of a specific stereotyped seizure. Some epilepsies have seizures precipitated by specific sensation or perception (the reflex epilepsies) in which seizures occur in response to discrete or specific stimuli. These stimuli are usually limited in individual patients to a single specific stimulus or a limited number of closely related stimuli. Although the epilepsies that result are usually generalized and of idiopathic nature, certain partial seizures may also occur following acquired lesions, usually involving tactile or proprioceptive stimuli.

Epileptic seizures may also be precipitated by sudden arousal (startle epilepsy); the stimulus is unexpected in nature. The seizures are usually generalized tonic but may be partial and are usually symptomatic.

Seizures precipitated by integration of higher cerebral function such as memory or pattern recognition are most often associated with complex partial epilepsies but are occasionally observed in generalized epilepsies (such as reading epilepsy). Seizures also occur spontaneously in most such patients.

Primary Reading Epilepsy

All or almost all seizures in this syndrome are precipitated by reading (especially aloud) and are independent of the content of the text. They are simple partial motor-involving masticatory muscles, or visual, and if the stimulus is not interrupted, GTCS may occur. The syndrome may be inherited. Onset is typically in late puberty and the course is benign with little tendency to spontaneous seizures. Physical examination and imaging studies are normal, but EEG shows spikes or spike-waves in the dominant parieto-temporal region. Generalized spike and wave may also occur.

CHAPTER 19 ■ IDIOPATHIC AND BENIGN PARTIAL EPILEPSIES OF CHILDHOOD

ELAINE C. WIRRELL, CAROL S. CAMFIELD, AND PETER R. CAMFIELD

The idiopathic partial epilepsies (IPEs) of childhood account for one fifth of all epilepsies in children and adolescents and differ in two ways from other focal epilepsy syndromes. First, IPEs are genetically determined focal disturbances of cerebral activity without any apparent structural abnormality detectable on magnetic resonance imaging (MRI), whereas most focal epilepsies are "lesional," resulting from a localized area of cortical damage or dysgenesis. Second, most IPEs remit by adolescence, unlike lesional focal epilepsies, which are often refractory.

In a survey of seizure disorders in the southwest of France, the annual incidence of IPEs in children 0 to 15 years of age was 8.63 per 100,000 (1), representing half of all partial seizures in this age group. Identification of these syndromes is paramount to providing these children and their families a favorable prognosis and appropriate management. Although controversy surrounds their exact clinical boundaries, IPEs of childhood include (2,3):

- Age-dependent occurrence, with specific peak ages for each subtype
- Absence of significant anatomic lesions on neuroimaging
- Normal neurologic status, with most children intellectually intact and without prior neurologic insult
- Favorable long-term outcome, with remission occurring prior to adolescence in most children, even those whose seizures were initially frequent or difficult to control
- Strong genetic predisposition: Other family members with benign forms of epilepsy that resolved in adolescence
- Specific semiology: Most seizures are simple partial motor or sensory, although complex partial and secondarily generalized seizures also may be seen; nocturnal occurrence is common and frequency is usually low
- Rapid response to antiepileptic medication in most cases
- Specific electroencephalographic (EEG) features: Spikes of distinctive morphology and variable location superimposed on a normal background, with occasional multifocal sharp waves or brief bursts of generalized spike wave; epileptiform discharges are often activated by sleep

The International League Against Epilepsy (ILAE) currently recognizes two types of IPE in childhood (4): benign epilepsy of childhood with centrotemporal spikes (BECTS, also known as benign rolandic epilepsy) and benign occipital epilepsy (BOE). BOE has been further subdivided into early-onset (Panayiotopoulos) and late-onset (Gastaut) types. Other proposed but less well-studied syndromes include benign epilepsy in infancy (BPEI) (5,6), benign partial epilepsy with affective symptoms (BPEAS) (7–10), benign partial epilepsy with extreme somatosensory-evoked potentials (BPE-ESEP) (11–13), benign frontal epilepsy (BFE) (14), and benign partial epilepsy of adolescence (BPEA) (15,16). Table 19.1 summarizes the core/classic features of these syndromes.

BENIGN PARTIAL EPILEPSY SYNDROMES RECOGNIZED BY THE ILAE

Benign Epilepsy of Childhood with Centrotemporal Spikes

First described in 1597 (17), the specific electrographic and clinical features of BECTS have been recognized only during the past 55 years. Rolandic spikes were noted to be unrelated to focal pathology in 1952 (18) and could be observed without clinical seizures (19). In 1958, Nayrac and Beaussart (20) described the clinical symptoms of BECTS, and its excellent prognosis was apparent in the early literature (21,22). Although BECTS is easily recognized in its "pure" form, atypical features are common and may make a confident diagnosis difficult.

Epidemiology

With an incidence of 6.2 to 21 per 100,000 children 15 years and younger (23–25), BECTS accounts for 13% to 23% of all childhood epilepsies (23,26) and approximately two thirds of all IPEs (27–30). Onset is between 3 and 13 years, with a peak at 7 to 8 years, and BECTS always resolves by age 16 (26). Boys are more commonly affected (31–33).

Genetics

An autosomal dominant inheritance of centrotemporal spikes with an age-specific expression has been suggested (34,35), and a recent report documents that the centrotemporal sharp wave trait maps to Elongator Protein Complex 4, which has roles in transcription and tRNA modification (36). Depletion of this protein results in downregulation of genes implicated in the actin cytoskeleton, which may impact neuronal migration during development. Rare cases of BECTS may be associated with KCNQ2 and KCNQ3 mutations (37), and these mutation should be suspected in cases with prior benign neonatal convulsions. The development of actual epilepsy is likely dependent on several other modifying genes and/or environmental

TABLE 19.1

BENIGN PARTIAL EPILEPSY SYNDROMES

Syndrome	Age of presentation	Clinical features	Interictal EEG features	Prognosis
Well-defined syndromes accepted in 1989 ILAE classification				
Benign epilepsy of childhood with centrotemporal spikes	Range, 3–13 years Peak, 7–8 years	Diurnal or nocturnal simple partial seizures affecting the lower face with numbness, clonic activity, drooling, and/or dysarthria; nocturnal generalized seizure	High-voltage centro-temporal spikes with horizontal dipole, activated with sleep; normal background	Remission by adolescence
Early-onset benign occipital epilepsy (Panayiotopoulos type)	Range, 2–8 years Peak, 5 years	Nocturnal seizure with tonic eye deviation, nausea, and vomiting; often prolonged	High-amplitude, repetitive, occipital, centrotemporal or parietal spike and wave, with fixation-off sensitivity EEG may be normal or nonspecific	Remission by 1–2 years after onset
Late-onset benign occipital epilepsy (Gastaut type)	Range, 3–16 years Peak, 8 years	Brief diurnal seizures with elementary visual hallucinations, often with migraine-like, postictal headache	As above	5% suffer recurrent seizures in adulthood
Less common syndromes				
Benign partial epilepsy in infancy	Range, 3–10 months Peak, 4–6 months	Motion arrest, decreased responsiveness, staring, simple automatisms, mild convulsive movements with possible secondary generalization	Normal- or low-voltage rolandic or vertex spikes in sleep	Remission by age 2 years
Benign partial epilepsy in adolescence	Range, adolescence Peak, 13–14 years	Motor or sensory symptoms, often with jacksonian march; auditory, olfactory, or gustatory symptoms never seen	Normal or nonspecific epileptiform discharge	Infrequent seizures that usually abate soon
Benign frontal epilepsy	Range, 4–8 years	Head version +/− trunk turning; fencing posture, sometimes followed by truncal, bipedal, or pelvic movements	Unilateral or bilateral frontal or posterior-frontal foci	May persist into adulthood
Benign partial epilepsy in infancy with midline spikes and waves during sleep	Range 4 months to 2 years	Cyanosis and motion arrest, at times with stiffening	Low-voltage, fast spike followed by higher bell-shaped slow wave over midline region in sleep	Remission by age 2–3 years
Benign partial epilepsy with extreme somatosensory-evoked potentials	Range, 4–6 years	Diurnal partial motor seizures with head and body version	High-voltage spikes in parietal and parasagittal regions evoked by tapping of feet	Resolution by adolescence
Benign partial epilepsy with affective symptoms	Range, 2–9 years	Brief episodes with sudden fear, screaming, autonomic disturbance, automatisms, and altered awareness	Rolandic-like spikes in frontotemporal and parietotemporal regions in wakefulness and sleep	Remission within 1–2 years

factors. Vadlamudi, in a search of four twin registries, found 18 twin pairs, where one twin had classic BECTS, and all 18 were discordant, suggesting noninherited factors are important in development of epilepsy (38).

Two familial syndromes of BECTS have been reported with other neurological features: (i) autosomal dominant rolandic epilepsy with oromotor and speech dyspraxia which

worsens in subsequent generations (39) and (ii) rolandic epilepsy with paroxysmal exercise-induced dystonia and writers cramp which has been linked to the chromosome 16p12-11.2 region (40).

Families with coexistence of BECTS and continuous spike wave in sleep have also been reported, suggesting a common genetic basis for both syndromes (41).

Pathophysiology

Seizures in BECTS involve the lower portion of the perirolandic region in the upper sylvian bank. BECTS most likely represents a "hereditary impairment in brain maturation" (42–44) favoring excitation. The number of axonal branches and synaptic connections is greater early in development and "pruning" of these connections may limit the expression of epilepsy in older individuals. Developmental regulation of voltage-dependent channels may also explain decreased cortical excitability with age.

Clinical Manifestations

Seizures frequently occur either shortly after falling asleep or before awakening; however, 15% have seizures both in sleep and wakefulness, and 20% to 30% in the waking state alone (31,32). The classic semiology consists (i) unilateral numbness or parasthesias of the tongue, lips, gum, and cheek; (ii) unilateral clonic or tonic activity involving the face, lips, and tongue; the tongue may have bilateral movements (iii) dysarthria or anarthria; and (iv) drooling (21). Stiffness of the jaw or tongue and a choking sensation are common. During sleep, seizures may secondarily generalize (32). Postictal confusion and amnesia are rare (45). Very young children with BECTS commonly present with hemiconvulsions instead of the typical facial seizure (32). Rarely, partial motor seizures may change sides without becoming generalized (32). Unusual parasthesias or jerking of a single arm or leg, abdominal pain, blindness, or vertigo may be seen and likely reflect seizure foci outside the centrotemporal region.

Single seizures are seen in 13% to 21% (46,47). Only 6% have frequent events, and this occurrence is most common with onset before 3 years of age (47). Seizures often occur in clusters, followed by long seizure-free intervals. There is no known correlation between severity of the EEG abnormality, seizure frequency, and final outcome (32).

Postictal Todd paresis occurs in 7% to 16% of cases and may suggest focal onset in patients who present with a generalized seizure (48,49).

Seizure duration is typically brief, lasting seconds to several minutes; however, status epilepticus has been described (48,49). Temporary oromotor and speech disturbances with intermittent facial twitching may suggest anterior opercular syndrome and correlates with very frequent or continuous spike discharge in the perisylvian region (50–54). This opercular status epilepticus may persist for weeks to months and may not respond well to antiepileptic medication. Steroids, however, have proven beneficial (50). Eventually, all children recover over 6 months to 8 years but may be left with mild speech dysfluency or minor slowing of tongue or jaw movements. Positron emission tomography demonstrated a bilateral increase of glucose metabolism in the opercular regions in one patient with this type of nonconvulsive status (55).

BECTS can rarely evolve to Landau–Kleffner syndrome, with progressive language deterioration and auditory agnosia or CSWS with a variety of cognitive problems.

Rarely, evolution to "atypical benign partial epilepsy" or "pseudo-Lennox" syndrome has been reported (56–60). In addition to partial motor seizures, frequent atonic, atypical absence and myoclonic seizures, often with nonconvulsive

status epilepticus, as well as cognitive and behavioral disturbances are seen. Sleep EEGs show nearly continuous, bilaterally synchronous anterior spike-and-wave activity. Although these children ultimately have remission of their epilepsy, many are left with varying degrees of mental handicap.

The medical history is usually uneventful, although 6% to 10% experience neonatal difficulties (including 3% with neonatal seizures), 4% to 5% have preceding mild head injuries, and up to 16% have antecedent febrile seizures (32). While prior studies reported an increased incidence of migraine in BECTS compared to controls or children with other types of epilepsy (61,62), these were limited by lack of uniformity in migraine diagnosis. A more recent case control study documented equivalent rates of migraine in BECTS and symptomatic partial epilepsy, but these rates were higher than for normal controls without seizures (63).

EEG Manifestations

The characteristic EEG findings are high-amplitude diphasic spikes or sharp waves with prominent aftercoming slow waves (Fig. 19.1). Spikes have a characteristic horizontal dipole, with maximal negativity in centrotemporal (inferior rolandic) and positivity in frontal regions (64,65). They frequently cluster and are markedly activated in drowsiness and non–rapid-eye-movement sleep (Fig. 19.2); approximately 30% of patients show spikes only during sleep (66). At times, a continuous spike-and-wave in slow sleep pattern is seen. The focus is unilateral in 60% of cases, bilateral in 40%, and may be synchronous or asynchronous (32). While the location is usually centrotemporal, atypical locations are frequent, and spikes may shift location on subsequent EEG recordings. Two electroclinical subgroups of BECTS are a high-central group, with maximum electronegativity at C_3/C_4 and seizures with frequent hand involvement, and a low-central group, with maximum electronegativity at C_5/C_6, ictal drooling, and oromotor involvement are described (67). Atypical spike location is not uncommon. On 24-hour EEGs, 21% of children with typical BECTS had a single focus outside the centrotemporal area and half lacked a horizontal dipole (68). Follow-up recordings showed shifts in foci both toward and away from the centrotemporal area. Usually the background is normal, although mild slowing has been observed (48). Cases with both generalized spike-and-wave discharge and centrotemporal spikes in the same EEG have been reported; however, not all children had a clinical history suggestive of BECTS, indicating that BECTS is an electroclinical syndrome—spikes alone do not make the diagnosis (69). With remission, spikes disappear first from the waking record and later from the sleep recording (32). Few reports of recorded rolandic seizures exist (Fig. 19.3), but two unique features are noted (32,70–74). Ictal spike-and-wave discharges may show dipole reversal, with electropositivity in the centrotemporal region and negativity in the frontal area; postictal slowing is not seen.

Typical rolandic discharges are seen in 0.7% of awake recordings of normal children without a history of seizures (75); if recordings had included sleep, the actual number likely would have been higher. The percentage of children with rolandic sharp waves who develop clinically apparent seizures is unclear. The risk is probably less than 10%, on the basis of reported incidences of BECTS and of rolandic EEG discharge

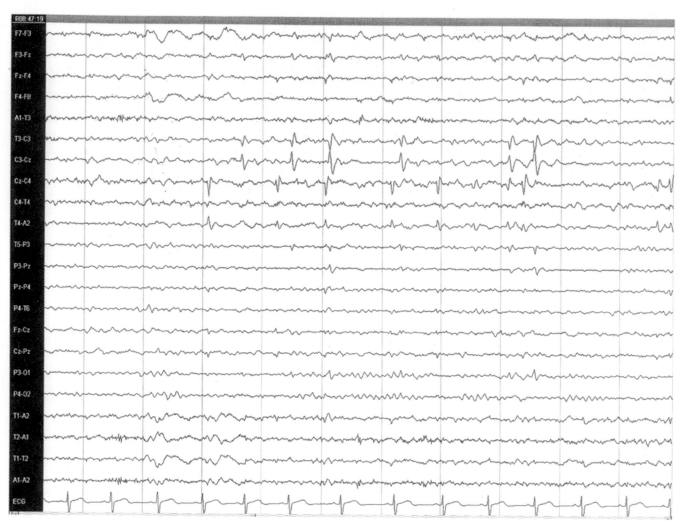

FIGURE 19.1 Typical rolandic spikes at C_3 and C_4-T_4.

in normal children. Therefore, rolandic discharges should be considered most likely an incidental finding in children with seizures or spells whose semiology is not suggestive of BECTS. Rolandic spikes have also been reported in children with brain tumors, cortical dysplasia, Fragile X syndrome, and Rett syndrome.

Neuropsychological Aspects

While early studies noted frequent behavior problems, hyperactivity, inattention, and learning disorders in BECTS, these were attributed to the social stigma of epilepsy or to side effects of antiepileptic medication (33,46,76). However, a recent systemic review of 14 studies evaluating impairments in attention in children with BECTS showed impairment in the alerting, orienting, and executive networks of attention in children with active centrotemporal spikes, which resolve upon EEG remission (77).

Specific neuropsychological deficits have been demonstrated in one quarter to one half of children with BECTS during the period of active epilepsy (78–80). Reading disability and speech sound disorder occur more commonly both in children with BECTS and their siblings (81). Neurocognitive deficits appear to correlate with the amount and location of interictal spike discharge. In a test of short-term memory, four of seven children with BECTS showed a significantly increased error rate during trials with epileptiform discharge compared to those without discharge, and all of these children had behavioral or learning problems (82). A recent study of 28 children showed that several EEG factors were predictive of educational impairment in BECTS: (i) an intermittent slow-wave focus during wakefulness, (ii) a high number of spikes in the first hour of sleep, and (iii) multiple asynchronous bilateral spike-wave foci in the first hour of sleep (83).

Several studies have suggested that the laterality of the EEG discharge predicts the nature of the neurocognitive deficit and that patients with bilateral discharges have the greatest difficulties. D'Alessandro studied attention and visuomotor skills in 44 right-handed children with BECTS (84). Those with bilateral discharge scored the lowest overall; those with only right-sided discharge performed best. After at least 4 years without seizures and EEG abnormalities, resolution of the neuropsychological abnormalities was seen, indicating that they are also "benign" and resolve around the time of puberty.

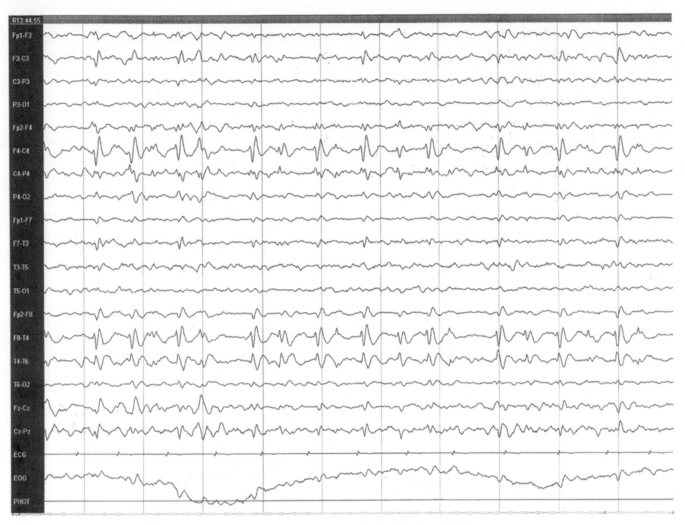

FIGURE 19.2 Marked activation of rolandic spikes with sleep.

In a study assessing language lateralization in 22 right-handed children with BECTS and unilateral EEG discharge, the expected left lateralization of language was seen in all patients with right centrotemporal discharge (85). However, those with left centrotemporal discharge demonstrated bihemispheric representation of language, raising the possibility that focal epileptic activity may alter cerebral mechanisms that underlie cognitive functioning.

Similarly, in a study of attention and processing of visuomotor information, a right hemispheric task, in 43 right-handed children with BECTS, those with bilateral or right centrotemporal discharge scored significantly lower than either controls or those with left centrotemporal discharge, suggesting that focal epileptic discharge in the right hemisphere may interfere with visuomotor processing (86). By contrast, Laub and coworkers (87) found no correlation between neuropsychological test results, EEG focus, and single-photon emission computed tomography findings in nine children with BECTS.

Higher spike frequency on EEG appears to correlate with poorer neuropsychological outcome. Weglage studied 40 right-handed children with rolandic spikes (20 with and 20 without seizures) (88). Neuropsychological deficits were not related to presence or absence of seizures, seizure frequency, lateraliza-

tion of the rolandic focus, or time since diagnosis, but higher spike frequency correlated with greater deficits. Younger age at seizure onset also appears predictive of cognitive difficulties. In a study of academic performance in 20 children with rolandic epilepsy, Piccinelli found greater cognitive difficulties in those with seizure onset before age 8 years and those with greater activation of epileptiform discharge during sleep (89).

Prospective studies (80,90,91) have shown that, like the seizures and epileptiform discharges, the cognitive difficulties also appear to resolve with time.

In summary, neurocognitive deficits are seen in a significant proportion of children with BECTS. Because they appear to correlate with the amount and side of interictal spike discharge, these discharges may cause "transient cognitive impairment." The neurocognitive deficits also resolve as seizures and epileptiform discharges abate with age.

Investigations

If the clinical history and EEG suggest BECTS and the child is neurologically and developmentally intact, no further investigations are required. An MRI scan should be considered if

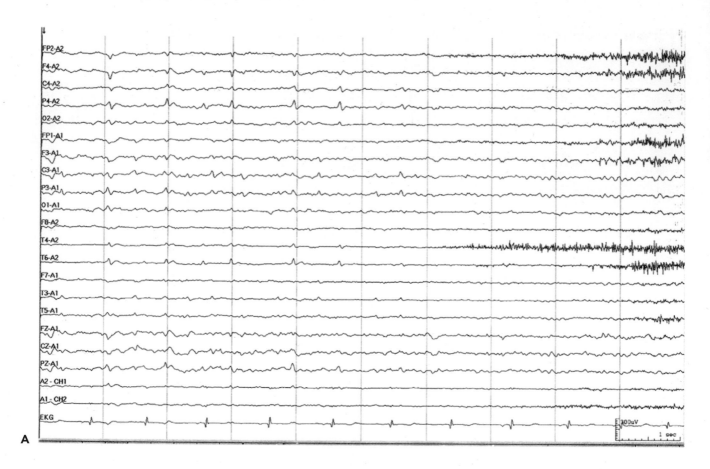

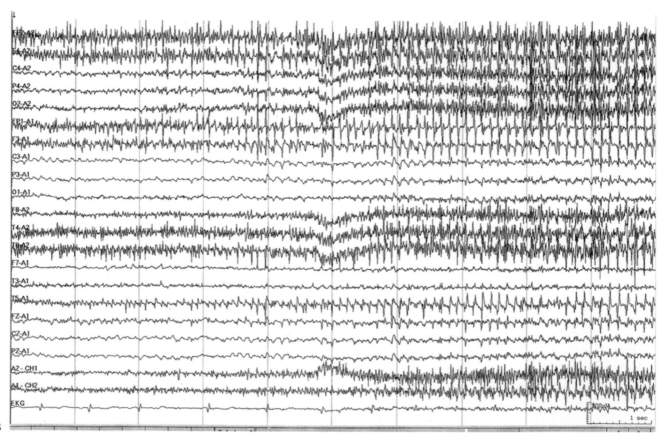

FIGURE 19.3 A–C Recorded rolandic seizure. **A:** Start of seizure. **B:** Ten seconds later.

(continued)

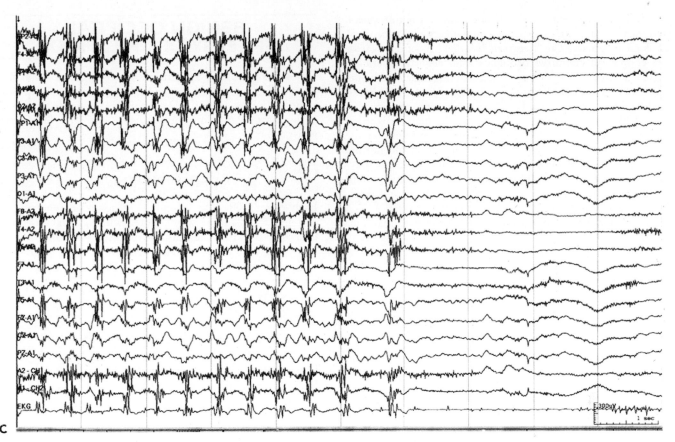

FIGURE 19.3 (*continued*) C: End of seizure. (Courtesy of Mary Connolly, Children's Hospital and University of British Columbia.)

atypical clinical or EEG features are present. EEG recordings of age-appropriate siblings may help support the diagnosis of highly atypical cases. BECTS has been reported in children with other central nervous system pathologic findings, yet the prognosis appears to be as favorable in brain-injured patients as in normal children (33,68,92).

A small study of MRI findings in typical BECTS found hippocampal asymmetries in 28% and white-matter abnormalities in 17% (93). The latter finding may indicate maturational delay with defective myelination, but the hippocampal changes were unexplained. In a larger study of 71 children, neuroimaging abnormalities were found in 14.8%, including ventricular enlargement, white-matter hyperintensities, hippocampal atrophy, cortical dysplasia, and agenesis of the corpus callosum and cavum septum pellucidum (94), suggesting that these brain lesions may lower the epileptogenic threshold and transform a "genetic predisposition" into a clinical condition. However, their presence did not alter the benign course of BECTS; and, a recent unmatched case control study of MRI findings in BECTS suggests that although MRI abnormalities are common in BECTS, they may be no more common than controls (95).

Treatment

Children with BECTS achieve remission regardless of antiepileptic drug therapy. We are unaware of any peer-reviewed reports of children with BECTS dying of sudden unexpected death in epilepsy (SUDEP) or sustaining brain injury from a seizure. A no-medication strategy is reasonable for the majority of children who have infrequent, nocturnal, partial seizures. If recurrent generalized or diurnal seizures occur, or if the seizures are sufficiently disturbing to the child or the family, treatment is generally started. However, treatment does not necessarily relieve parental anxiety or monitoring (96). Short intervals between the initial seizures and younger age at onset predict higher seizure frequency. In a child who presents with status as their first manifestation of rolandic epilepsy, abortive therapy with benzodiazepines is a reasonable therapeutic option.

Only sulthiame and gabapentin have been studied in randomized trials. On the basis of case series and a recent meta-analysis of 794 children (97), the usual antiepileptic drugs prescribed for partial seizures—phenytoin, phenobarbital, valproate, carbamazepine, clobazam, and clonazepam—have equivalent efficacy, and 50% to 65% of patients will have no further seizures once medication is started (26,31,33). Gabapentin was shown to be probably more effective than placebo in a study of 220 children although the results did not reach statistical significance (98). Sulthiame significantly improves the EEG and decreases clinical seizures. In a randomized, double-blind trial comparing sulthiame to placebo in 66 children, 81% taking sulthiame completed 6 months of therapy with no further seizures or adverse events, compared with only 29% taking placebo ($P < 0.00002$) (99). Of 25 children remaining on sulthiame at 6 months, 10 (40%) had a normal EEG, compared with only 1 of 10 (10%) in the placebo group.

The ideal treatment for BECTS should relieve both seizures and interictal discharges, especially in patients with neuropsychological deficits. The literature is largely silent as regards the child with cognitive problems and frequent interictal spikes. Sulthiame does decrease interictal discharge, and while it is tempting to think that it may improve neuropsychological dysfunction, one small study suggests the opposite might be true (100). Hence, while treatment with sulthiame might be warranted in atypical cases of BECTS with nearly continuous spike wave and cognitive decline, it probably should not be used in more typical cases. Rarely, antiepileptic drugs may aggravate BECTS, markedly increasing EEG discharge, often with continuous spike and wave during slow sleep, and causing neuropsychological deterioration. This deterioration has been reported with carbamazepine (101–103), phenobarbital (101), and lamotrigine (104).

Seizures may initially appear refractory in a small number of children (105). Deonna (53) reported that one third of 38 children with BECTS had persistent seizures despite treatment, and 24% had severe seizures. Beaussart (31) noted that 14% of 221 children had occurrence of seizures that lasted longer than 1 year despite medication or that recurred after 1 to many years.

Prognosis

The long-term prognosis of BECTS is excellent, even in those with initially frequent, troublesome seizures, with all patients achieving remission by mid-adolescence (31,46,105,106). In a meta-analysis, 50% of patients were in remission at age 6 years, 92% at age 12 years, and 99.8% at age 18 years (Fig. 19.4) (97). Remission occurs sooner in children older at onset and in those with sporadic seizures or seizure clusters (46). Although learning and behavior problems may be seen in the acute phase, long-term psychosocial outcome is excellent (107), with no increase in psychiatric problems or personality problems, and excellent occupational status.

BENIGN OCCIPITAL EPILEPSY OF CHILDHOOD

Gibbs and Gibbs were the first to recognize that some children with occipital epilepsy had a benign course (108). BOE is now divided into two syndromes: the more common, early-onset (Panayiotopoulos) type and the later-onset (Gastaut) type.

Epidemiology

Early-onset BOE, the second most common type of IPE, accounts for 6% to 13% of children with localization-related epilepsy (109,110). The peak age of onset is 5 years (range, 2 to 8 years) with a female preponderance.

Late-onset BOE begins in mid- to late-childhood, with a peak age of 8 years (range, 3 to 16 years); both sexes are equally affected (110).

Genetics

Reporting a large kindred with BOE, Kuzniecky and Rosenblatt (111) suggested that, as in BECTS, the EEG abnormality was inherited in an autosomal dominant pattern, with age-dependent expression and variable penetrance of the disorder. Other investigators (112,113) have found that most affected children lack a family history of similar disorders. In a study of 16 probands with benign occipital epilepsy, including seven twins, Taylor found that monozygotic twin pairs did not show a higher concordance rate than dizygotic twin pairs, suggesting that this condition was not purely a genetic disorder and that nonconventional genetic influences or environmental factors play a major role (114).

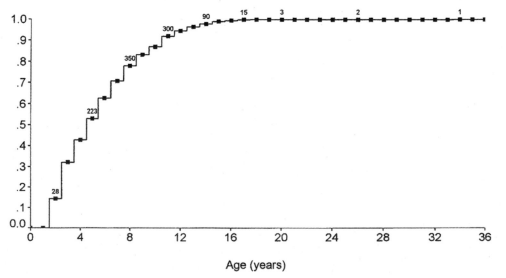

Proportion remission

FIGURE 19.4 Remission of BECTS by age. Numbers in the figure represent the number of patients in the analysis. (From Bouma PAD, Bovenkerk AC, Westendorp RGJ, et al. The course of benign partial epilepsy of childhood with centrotemporal spikes: a meta-analysis. *Neurology.* 1997;48:430–437, with permission.)

Pathophysiology

Koutroumanidis proposed that early-onset BOE is the result of a combination of multifocal cortical hyperexcitability and an unstable autonomic nervous system (115). If the cortical region exceeds a critical epileptogenic level, the autonomic nervous system is first activated, as it is of lower threshold. The autonomic network may then become involved in cortical/subcortical self-sustaining oscillations. These oscillations may eventually synchronize abnormal cortical activity in a critical neuron number with resultant focal cortical symptoms.

Clinical

Early-Onset BOE

Autonomic symptoms especially nausea, retching, and vomiting are the most characteristic symptoms (116). Other autonomic symptoms may include pallor, urinary or fecal incontinence, hypersalivation, mydriasis, miosis, coughing and respiratory or cardiac irregularities. Syncopal-like symptoms may also occur. Tonic eye deviation is common but other ictal visual symptoms such as visual hallucinations are rare, affecting less than 10% of patients (116). The majority of seizures are nocturnal (112,117).

Consciousness may be impaired, and seizures evolve to hemiconvulsions or become secondarily generalized in a significant minority. Seizures are often long, and one third develop partial status epilepticus (116,117). Seizure frequency varies but one third have only a single event (112,116–118). A history of febrile seizures is found in approximately 17% of children (116). Rarely, early-onset BOE may evolve atypically, with appearance of many seizure types, including absences and atonic seizures, and intellectual deterioration (119).

Late-Onset BOE

Late-onset syndrome is rare and manifests as diurnal, brief, visual seizures consisting of visual hallucinations or brief amaurosis, which may result in brief, but total blindness (110,120). Visual hallucinations are most commonly elementary and consist of multicolored, circular patterns which move and multiply during the seizure. More complex visual hallucinations such as faces or figures, or visual illusions such as micropsia or palinopsia are rare. Other occipital symptoms, such as sensory illusions of ocular movements or pain, tonic eye and head deviation, or eyelid closure, may coexist. Consciousness is typically intact unless the seizure progresses or becomes secondarily generalized. Seizure frequency is greater than in early-onset BOE—isolated seizures are rare and seizures may occur daily. There is a complex relationship with migraine. Postictal headache, indistinguishable from migraine, is seen in 25–50% of cases, and headache may precede the seizure or occur at the same time (121). Several features may help distinguish migraine with visual aura from late-onset benign occipital epilepsy. The visual aura of migraine evolves more slowly (over 10–20 minutes rather than 1–3 minutes) and tends to be achromatic and linear rather than multicolored and circular (122).

Rarely, late-onset BOE may have a stormy onset. Verrotti and coworkers (123) described six children presenting with loss of consciousness lasting 6 to 14 hours that was preceded by visual symptoms. Only two of these patients had further seizures, and all did well at follow-up.

The diagnosis of late-onset BOE should be made cautiously, as the semiology may also be seen with symptomatic occipital epilepsy. In Gastaut's series, prognosis was not always benign, and many patients had ongoing seizures (27).

EEG Manifestations

Despite its name, the interictal EEG changes in early-onset BOE are quite variable and do not always involve the occipital regions—an equal number of cases show centrotemporal/parietal foci, and discharges are frequently multifocal, with a marked increase in sleep (115,116). Discharges often shift in foci on subsequent EEGs and some children show irregular, generalized spike-wave discharge (124). Similar to rolandic spikes, they are high-voltage and frequent. Rarely, wake recordings can be normal, with the discharges seen only when sleep is obtained. Some cases show the typical high-amplitude, often bilateral, runs of repetitive occipital spikes and sharp waves similar to what is seen in late-onset BOE (Fig. 19.5). Magnetoencephalography shows dipole clusters along the parieto-occipital, calcarine and rolandic fissures (125).

Extraoccipital spikes are much less common in Gastaut-type BOE (27). The spikes are said to show "fixation-off sensitivity," that is, they attenuate with eye opening and are induced by elimination of central vision such as eye closure, darkness, or vision through +10 spherical lenses (Fig. 19.6) (110). Suppression of epileptiform discharges with eye opening is not specific for BOE, however, and may be seen in symptomatic epilepsies with poorer prognoses (126,127). A superficial rather than a deep dipole source location of the occipital spikes suggests a benign disorder rather than symptomatic occipital epilepsy (128).

The ictal EEG in early-onset BOE shows rhythmic theta or delta activity with intermixed spikes that usually starts posteriorly, although anterior onset has been reported (28,129–131). In late-onset BOE, the discharge is more localized, with fast rhythms appearing in the occipital lobe at the onset of visual symptoms (129).

Neuropsychology

One study (132) examined neuropsychological functioning in 21 children with BOE and in normal controls, matched for age, sex, and socioeconomic status. Compared to controls, the patients had lower scores in attention, memory, and intellectual functioning and performed significantly more poorly on all verbal and visual tests combined. This study, however, included both early- and late-onset cases and recruited the entire control group from a single private school that may have represented a higher-than-usual educational standard. In addition, neuroimaging was not performed to rule out symptomatic occipital epilepsies. No comment was made about whether the observed differences resolved with remission of epilepsy and no distinction between early- and late-onset cases were made. Some studies have suggested that in rare cases BOE may evolve to continuous spike wave in slow-wave sleep (133,134).

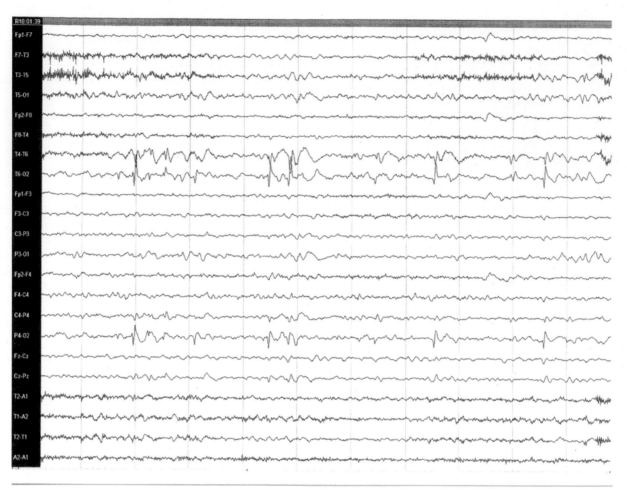

FIGURE 19.5 Posterior temporal-occipital spikes in a 4-year-old girl who presented with a 65-min seizure consisting of focal eye deviation and retching.

Investigations

Imaging is probably not required in a neurologically and developmentally normal child with a typical clinical history of early-onset BOE and an EEG showing occipital paroxysms with fixation-off sensitivity. Nevertheless, MRI is usually performed to rule out a symptomatic etiology, particularly if the typical EEG is not present or the clinical picture is atypical. Because lesional occipital lobe epilepsy due to such etiologies as cortical dysplasia, mitochondrial disease, Lafora disease or celiac disease may mimic the semiologic and EEG features of Gastaut-type BOE, MRI should always be obtained.

Treatment

Most children with early-onset BOE have infrequent seizures and do not need antiepileptic drug treatment. Intermittent use of benzodiazepines could be considered for the child with rare but prolonged events. No particular antiepileptic drug has been shown to be superior (112), although carbamazepine is most frequently prescribed. Spikes may persist for several years after clinical remission.

In contrast, most cases of late-onset BOE require treatment, as seizures are more frequent. Although Panayiotopoulos

reported a favorable response to carbamazepine (27,135), only 60% of 63 patients reported by Gastaut achieved complete seizure control (136).

Prognosis

In Panayiotopoulos syndrome, remission of active epilepsy occurs 1 to 2 years from onset, although up to 15% of patients have concurrent symptoms of rolandic epilepsy or later develop BECTS (118). As in BECTS, even those with many seizures usually achieve long-term remission.

The prognosis is less clear in Gastaut syndrome, although Gastaut reported that 5% of his 63 cases had recurrent seizures into adulthood (136).

PROPOSED BENIGN PARTIAL EPILEPSY SYNDROMES NOT YET RECOGNIZED BY THE ILAE

Five syndromes have been proposed as possible subtypes of idiopathic and benign focal epilepsy, but not all may be confirmed as diagnostically discrete. The diagnosis is usually made after initiation of treatment and observation of the clinical course.

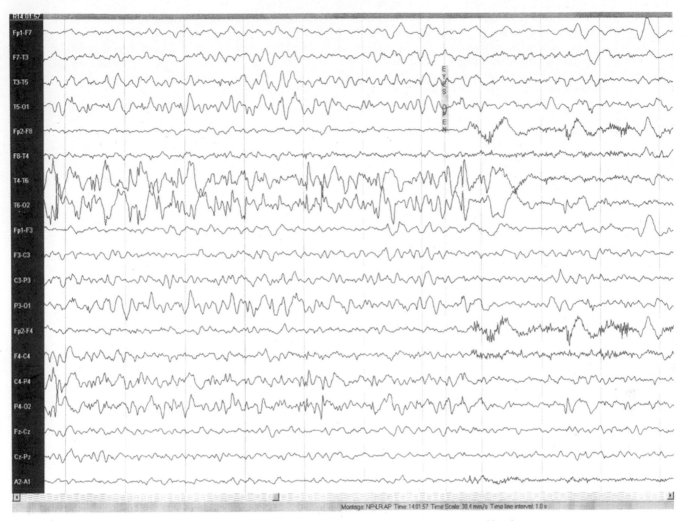

FIGURE 19.6 Prominent fixation-off sensitivity in the same 4-year-old girl.

Benign Partial Epilepsy in Infancy

Watanabe proposed this disorder in 1987, and described two forms: one with partial complex seizures alone (5) and another with partial complex and secondarily generalized seizures (6).

BPEI represents approximately 6.6% to 29% of all epilepsies in the first 2 years of life and may be somewhat more common in Japan. Okumura and colleagues (137) noted that 22 of 75 (29%) infants under 2 years of age presenting with epilepsy met the criteria for BPEI, while Nelson and coworkers (138) made this diagnosis in only 22 of 331 (6.6%) in their population. Both reports noted that the form with secondarily generalized seizures was slightly more common, accounting for 64% to 73% of all BPEI cases. Peak age at onset is 4 to 6 months, with a range of 3 to 10 months.

Seizures occur in 50% of developmentally normal infants whose family histories reveal benign forms of infantile seizures (5,6). Motion arrest, decreased responsiveness, staring, simple automatisms, and mild convulsive movements are usual, with possible secondary generalization. Seizures frequently cluster. Neuroimaging is normal, and seizures are easily controlled with antiepileptic drugs. Remission occurs in 91% within 4 months (138) and in all children by age 2 years.

To determine how confidently BPEI can be recognized in infancy, Okumura and coworkers followed-up 39 children who were believed to have the syndrome (139). At 5 years, 33 had achieved remission, no longer received antiepileptic drugs, and were developmentally normal. In retrospect, six were thought to not have BPEI, as they had recurrent seizures after 2 years or showed developmental delay. Clearly, this diagnosis is not always easy to make prospectively, with the experts being incorrect in 15% of cases.

The interictal EEG is said to be normal, but some infants show low-voltage rolandic and vertex spikes in sleep (140). Ictal recordings demonstrate spikes that are maximal in the temporal and occipital regions, in infants with partial complex seizures alone, or in the central with involvement of parietal, or occipital regions, in those with secondarily generalized seizures.

Benign Partial Epilepsy of Adolescence

Difficult to recognize with any certainty at presentation, BPEA was initially described by Loiseau and Orgogozo in 1978 (15) and accounts for approximately one quarter of all partial epilepsies with onset in the teen years (16,141). Seizures are typically diurnal and occur in neurologically normal adolescents, mainly boys (16,142) with a peak age of 13–14 years. A family history of epilepsy is exceptional (only 3% of Loiseau's cohort) (16). Either motor or sensory manifestations may be present and a jacksonian-type march is frequently described. Auditory, olfactory, or gustatory symptoms are never reported. Seizures may be partial simple, partial complex, or secondarily generalized and are usually infrequent (16). In Loiseau's series, approximately 80% had an isolated seizure only, while most of the remainder had a cluster of two to five attacks within 36 hours with no recurrences (16). Imaging is normal, and the interictal EEG is either normal or may show bilateral posterior slowing, of diffuse slow waves if done shortly after a seizure. Although no interictal epileptiform discharges were noted in the Loiseau cohort (15), 63% of the King group showed epileptiform abnormalities, but these lacked distinctive morphology or distribution (141). Definitive diagnosis usually requires neuroimaging and long-term follow-up to confirm the benign course.

Benign Frontal Epilepsy (BFE)

In 1983, Beaumanoir and Nahory (14) described 11 cases of frontal lobe epilepsy with normal neurologic status and benign course that involved head deviation, sometimes with trunk turning. All patients had a frontal spike focus on EEG but both seizures and EEG discharge resolved within 5 years of follow-up. Four, however, had rare generalized or partial seizures that reappeared years later. Vigevano and Fusco (143) described 10 children with tonic partial seizures in sleep, all of whom had a benign course, many with a positive family history. These cases may represent the early presentation of autosomal dominant frontal lobe epilepsy (144).

Benign Focal Epilepsy in Infancy With Midline Spikes and Waves During Sleep

Capovilla and Beccaria described this entity initially in 2000 (145) and provided details of a larger cohort of these cases in 2006 (146). This syndrome begins in neurologically and developmentally normal children between 4 months and 2 years of age with sporadic seizures, which cluster in 31% of cases. Seizures semiology consists of cyanosis and motion arrest, and stiffening is reported in nearly half of cases. Automatisms or lateralizing signs are rare and secondary generalization has not been reported. Seizures are brief, lasting 1–5 minutes and occur during wakefulness, as well as during sleep in some cases. A family history of epilepsy is present in 47% of cases. The EEG shows a low-voltage, fast spike followed by a higher bell-shaped slow wave over the midline region during sleep only, which spreads to the central or less commonly the temporal region. Outcome is excellent—seizures resolve by 2–3 years of age, and many cases did not require antiepileptic drug treatment.

Benign Partial Epilepsy with Extreme Somatosensory-Evoked Potentials

BPE-ESEP was initially described in 1981 (12). De Marco noted that approximately 1% of children showed high-voltage

spikes in parietal and parasagittal regions (extreme SSEPs) evoked by tapping of their feet during routine EEG (11). This pattern was seen at a peak age of 4 to 6 years, occurred in neurologically normal children without any lesions on imaging, and was more common in males. An increased risk of febrile seizures was noted.

Of the 155 patients in De Marco's group, 46 (30%) either had (N=30) or went on to develop (N=16) epilepsy (13). In another report, 91 (24%) of 385 children with this pattern had afebrile seizures (147). Diurnal partial motor seizures with head and body version were most frequent; however, BECTS and BOE have also been reported with this EEG picture. Seizure frequency is usually low, but more frequent events are possible and focal motor status epilepticus has also been reported. In all cases, seizures resolved by 9 years, with slower resolution of EEG changes and extreme SSEPs.

Benign Partial Epilepsy with Affective Symptoms (BPEAS)

BPEAS, or benign psychomotor epilepsy, was proposed as a distinct entity in 1980 (7–9), with 26 documented cases (10). Over one third have a family history of epilepsy. Onset is between 2 and 9 years of age but 19% have had prior febrile seizures. Seizures are brief, usually lasting 1–2 minutes and occur in either wakefulness or sleep. They begin with sudden fear, with screaming, autonomic disturbance (pallor, sweating, abdominal pain), automatisms such as chewing or swallowing, and altered awareness. Seizures may be followed by brief postictal confusion and fatigue but not unilateral deficits. Secondary generalization does not occur. Although seizures may occur up to several times per day shortly after onset, they respond promptly to antiepileptic drugs.

The EEG background is normal, but rolandic-like spikes are seen in frontotemporal and parietotemporal regions both in wakefulness and sleep. Remission occurs within 1 to 2 years, and long-term intellectual and social outcome is excellent.

SUMMARY

The IPEs of childhood account for a significant proportion of seizure disorders in the pediatric group. In its classic form, BECTS is easily recognizable, occurring in neurologically normal children and having a distinct semiology and EEG pattern. Early-onset BOE, with characteristic ictal semiology also lends itself to a confident diagnosis. Such is not the case for the other IPEs or for BECTS or early-onset BOE with atypical clinical or electrographic features. These diagnoses may be made definitively only in retrospect.

Minor cognitive changes during the active period of epilepsy occur in some children with IPE, but also appear to remit with time. In these cases, treatment to ameliorate the EEG changes as well as the clinical seizures may be beneficial. Many children with IPEs, however, will not require antiepileptic drugs, as most have infrequent seizures. Recognition of these benign epilepsy syndromes is important for appropriate counseling of the child and family.

References

1. Loiseau J, Loiseau P, Guyot M, et al. Survey of seizure disorders in the French Southwest, I: incidence of epileptic syndromes. *Epilepsia.* 1990;31:391–396.

2. Dalla Bernardina B, Sgrò V, Fontana E, et al. Idiopathic partial epilepsies in children. In: Roger J, Dravet C, Bureau M, et al., eds. *Epileptic Syndromes in Infancy, Childhood and Adolescence.* 2nd ed. London: John Libbey; 1992:173–188.

3. Holmes G. Benign focal epilepsies of childhood. *Epilepsia.* 1993;(suppl 3):S49–S61.

4. Commission on Classification and Terminology of the International League Against Epilepsy. Proposal for revised classification of epilepsies and epileptic syndromes. *Epilepsia.* 1989;30:389–399.

5. Watanabe K, Yamamoto N, Negoro T, et al. Benign complex partial epilepsies in infancy. *Pediatr Neurol.* 1987;3:208–211.

6. Watanabe K, Negoro T, Aso K. Benign partial epilepsy with secondarily generalized seizures in infancy. *Epilepsia.* 1993;34:635–638.

7. Dalla Bernardina B, Bureau M, Dravet C, et al. Affective symptoms during attacks of epilepsy in children. *Rev Electroencephalogr Neurophysio Clin.* 1980;10:8–18. French.

8. Plouin P, Lerique A, Dulac O. Etude électroclinique et évolution dans 7 observations de crises partielles complexes dominées par un comportement de terreur chez l'enfant. *Boll Lega Ital Epil.* 1980;29/30:139–143.

9. Dulac O, Arthuis M. Epilepsie psychomotrice bénigne de l'enfant. In: *Journées Parisiennes de Pédiatrie.* Paris: Flammarion; 1980:211–220.

10. Dalla Bernardina B, Colamaria V, Chiamenti C, et al. Benign partial epilepsy with affective symptoms (benign psychomotor epilepsy). In: Roger J, Dravet C, Bureau M, et al., eds. *Epileptic Syndromes in Infancy, Childhood and Adolescence.* 2nd ed. London: John Libbey; 1992:219–223.

11. De Marco P. Possibilities of a temporal relationship between the morphology and frequency of a parietal somatosensory evoked spike and the occurrence of epileptic manifestations. *Clin Electroencephalogr.* 1980;11:132–135.

12. De Marco P, Tassinari CA. Extreme somatosensory evoked potentials (ESEP): an EEG sign forecasting the possible occurrence of seizures in children. *Epilepsia.* 1981;22:569–585.

13. Tassinari CA, De Marco P. Benign partial epilepsy with extreme somatosensory evoked potentials. In: Roger J, Dravet C, Bureau M, et al., eds. *Epileptic Syndromes in Infancy, Childhood and Adolescence.* 2nd ed. London: John Libbey; 1992:225–229.

14. Beaumanoir A, Nahory A. Benign partial epilepsies: 11 cases of frontal partial epilepsy with favorable prognosis. *Rev Electroencephalogr Neurophysiol Clin.* 1983;13:207–211. French.

15. Loiseau P, Orgogozo JM. An unrecognized syndrome of benign focal epileptic seizures in teenagers. *Lancet.* 1978;2:1070–1071.

16. Loiseau P, Louiset P. Benign partial seizures of adolescence. In: Roger J, Dravet C, Bureau M, et al., eds. *Epileptic Syndromes in Infancy, Childhood and Adolescence.* 2nd ed. London: John Libbey; 1992:343–345.

17. van Huffelen AC. A tribute to Martinus Rulandus: a 16th-century description of benign focal epilepsy of childhood. *Arch Neurol.* 1989;46:445–447.

18. Gastaut Y. Un element deroutant de la sémeiologie electroencephalographique: les pointes prerolandiques sans signification focale. *Rev Neurol (Paris).* 1952;87:488–490.

19. Gibbs EL, Gillen HW, Gibbs PA. Disappearance and migration of epileptic foci in children. *Am J Dis Child.* 1954;88:596–603.

20. Nayrac P, Beaussart M. Pre-rolandic spike-waves: a very peculiar EEG reading; electroclinical study of 21 cases. *Rev Neurol (Paris).* 1958;99:201–206. French.

21. Lombroso CT. Sylvian seizures and midtemporal spike foci in children. *Arch Neurol.* 1967;17:52–59.

22. Gibbs FA, Gibbs EL. Good prognosis of midtemporal epilepsy. *Epilepsia.* 1960;1:448–453.

23. Cavazzuti GB. Epidemiology of different types of epilepsy in school age children of Modena, Italy. *Epilepsia.* 1980;21:57–62.

24. Astradsson A, Olafsson E, Ludvigsson P, et al. Rolandic epilepsy: an incidence study in Iceland. *Epilepsia.* 1998;39:884–886.

25. Heijbel J, Blom S, Bergfors PG. Benign epilepsy of children with centrotemporal EEG foci: a study of incidence rate in outpatient care. *Epilepsia.* 1975;16:657–664.

26. Kriz M, Gadzik M. Epilepsy with centrotemporal (rolandic) spikes. A peculiar seizure disorder of childhood. *Neurol Neurochir Pol.* 1978;12:413–419.

27. Panayiotopoulos CP. *Benign Childhood Partial Seizures and Related Epileptic Syndromes.* London: John Libbey; 1999.

28. Oguni H, Hayashi K, Imai K, et al. Study on the early-onset variant of benign childhood epilepsy with occipital paroxysms, otherwise described as early-onset benign occipital seizure susceptibility syndrome. *Epilepsia.* 1999;40:1020–1030.

29. Carabello R, Cersósimo R, Fejerman N. Idiopathic partial epilepsies with rolandic and occipital spikes appearing in the same children. *J Epilepsy.* 1998;11:261–264.

30. Guerrini R, Belmonte A, Veggiotti P, et al. Delayed appearance of interictal EEG abnormalities in early onset childhood epilepsy with occipital paroxysms. *Brain Dev.* 1997;19:343–346.

31. Beaussart M. Benign epilepsy of children with rolandic (centro-temporal) paroxysmal foci: a clinical entity. Study of 221 cases. *Epilepsia.* 1972;13:795–811.

32. Lerman P. Benign partial epilepsy with centrotemporal spikes. In: Roger J, Bureau M, Dravet C, et al., eds. *Epileptic Syndromes in Infancy, Childhood and Adolescence.* London: John Libbey; 1992:189–200.

33. Lerman P, Kivity S. Benign focal epilepsy of childhood: a follow-up study of 100 recovered patients. *Arch Neurol.* 1975;32:261–264.

34. Bray PF, Wiser WC. Evidence for a genetic etiology of temporal-central abnormalities in focal epilepsy. *N Engl J Med.* 1964;271:926–933.

35. Bali B, Kull LL, Strug LJ, et al. Autosomal dominant inheritance of centrotemporal sharp waves in rolandic epilepsy families. *Epilepsia.* 2007;48:2266–2272.

36. Strug LJ, Clarke T, Chiang T, et al. Centrotemporal sharp wave EEG trait in Rolandic epilepsy maps to Elongator Protein Complex 4. *Eur J Hum Genet.* 2009;17:1171–1181.

37. Neubauer BA, Waldegger S, Heinzinger J, et al. KCNQ2 and KCNQ3 mutations contribute to different idiopathic epilepsy syndromes. *Neurology.* 2008;71:177–183.

38. Vadlamudi L, Kjeldsen MJ, Corey LA, et al. Analyzing the etiology of benign rolandic epilepsy: a multicenter twin collaboration. *Epilepsia.* 2006;47:550–555.

39. Scheffer IE, Jones L, Pozzebon M, et al. Autosomal dominant rolandic epilepsy and speech dyspraxia: a new syndrome with anticipation. *Ann Neurol.* 1995;38:633–642.

40. Guerrini R, Bonanni P, Nardocci N, et al. Autosomal recessive rolandic epilepsy with paroxysmal exercise-induced dystonia and writers cramp: delineation of the syndrome and mapping to chromosome 16p12-11.2. *Ann Neurol.* 1999;45:344–352.

41. De Tiege X, Goldman S, Verheulpen D, et al. Coexistence of idiopathic rolandic epilepsy and CSWS is two families. *Epilepsia.* 2006;47:1723–1727.

42. Doose H, Baier WK. Benign partial epilepsy and related conditions: multifactorial pathogenesis with hereditary impairment of brain maturation. *Eur J Pediatr.* 1989;149:152–158.

43. Doose H, Neubauer B, Carlsson G. Children with benign focal sharp waves in the EEG—developmental disorders and epilepsy. *Neuropediatrics.* 1996;27:227–241.

44. Doose H, Neubauer BA, Peterson B. The concept of hereditary impairment of brain maturation. *Epileptic Disord.* 2000;2(suppl 1):S45–S46.

45. Holmes GL. Rolandic epilepsy: clinical and electroencephalographic features. *Epilepsy Res Suppl.* 1992;6:29–43.

46. Loiseau P, Duche B, Cordova S, et al. Prognosis of benign childhood epilepsy with centrotemporal spikes: a follow-up study of 168 patients. *Epilepsia.* 1988;29:229–235.

47. Kramer U, Zelnick N, Lerman-Sagie T, et al. Benign childhood epilepsy with centrotemporal spikes: clinical characteristics and identification of patients at risk for multiple seizures. *J Child Neurol.* 2002;17:17–19.

48. Wirrell EC, Camfield PR, Gordon KE, et al. Benign rolandic epilepsy: atypical features are very common. *J Child Neurol.* 1995;10:455–458.

49. Deonna T, Ziegler AL, Despland PA, et al. Partial epilepsy in neurologically normal children: clinical syndromes and prognosis. *Epilepsia.* 1986;27:241–247.

50. Fejerman N, Di Blasi AM. Status epilepticus of benign partial epilepsies in children: report of two cases. *Epilepsia.* 1987;28:351–355.

51. Colamaria V, Sgro V, Caraballo R, et al. Status epilepticus in benign rolandic epilepsy manifesting as anterior operculum syndrome. *Epilepsia.* 1991;32:329–334.

52. Boulloche J, Le Luyer B, Husson A, et al. Dysphagie et troubles du langage: manifestations d'un état de mal épileptique à pointes temporales. In: *Proceedings IVeme Congres de la Société Européenne de Neurologie Pédiatrique.* Barcelona, November 1989,131.

53. Deonna TW, Roulet E, Fontan D, et al. Speech and oromotor deficits of epileptic origin in benign partial epilepsy of childhood with rolandic spikes (BPERS): relationship to the acquired aphasia-epilepsy syndrome. *Neuropediatrics.* 1993;24:83–87.

54. Roulet E, Deonna T, Despland PA. Prolonged intermittent drooling and oromotor dyspraxia in benign childhood epilepsy with centrotemporal spikes. *Epilepsia.* 1989;30:564–568.

55. de Saint-Martin A, Petiau C, Massa R, et al. Idiopathic rolandic epilepsy with "interictal" facial myoclonia and oromotor deficit: a longitudinal EEG and PET study. *Epilepsia.* 1999;40:614–620.

56. Aicardi J, Chevrie JJ. Atypical benign partial epilepsy of childhood. *Dev Med Child Neurol.* 1982;24:281–292.

57. Fejerman N, Caraballo R, Tenembaum SN. Atypical evolutions of benign partial epilepsy of infancy with centro-temporal spikes. *Rev Neurol.* 2000;31:389–396. Spanish.

58. Hahn A, Pistohl J, Neubauer BA, et al. Atypical "benign" partial epilepsy or pseudo-Lennox syndrome. Part 1: symptomatology and long-term prognosis. *Neuropediatrics.* 2001;32:1–8.

59. Dalla Bernardina B, Tassinari CA, Dravet C, et al. Benign focal epilepsy and "electrical status epilepticus" during sleep. *Rev Electroencephalogr Neurophysiol Clin.* 1978;8:350–353.

60. Deonna T, Ziegler AL, Despland PA. Combined myoclonic-astatic and "benign" focal epilepsy of childhood ("atypical benign partial epilepsy of childhood"). A separate syndrome? *Neuropediatrics.* 1986;17:144–151.
61. Giroud M, Couillault G, Arnould S, et al. Centro-temporal epilepsy and migraine. A controlled study. Evidence for a non-fortuitous association. *Pediatrie.* 1989;44:659–664.
62. Bladin PF. The association of benign rolandic epilepsy with migraine. In: Andermann F, Lugaresi E, eds. *Migraine and Epilepsy.* Boston: Butterworths; 1987:145–152.
63. Wirrell EC, Hamiwka LD. Do children with benign rolandic epilepsy have a higher prevalence of migraine than those with other partial epilepsies or nonepilepsy controls? *Epilepsia.* 2006;47:1674–1681.
64. Gregory DL, Wong PK. Topographic analysis of the centrotemporal discharges in benign rolandic epilepsy of childhood. *Epilepsia.* 1984;25:705–711.
65. Gregory DL, Wong PK. Clinical relevance of a dipole field in rolandic spikes. *Epilepsia.* 1992;33:36–44.
66. Blom S, Heijbel J. Benign epilepsy of children with centro-temporal EEG foci. Discharge rate during sleep. *Epilepsia.* 1975;16:133–140.
67. Legarda S, Jayakar P, Duchowny M, et al. Benign rolandic epilepsy: high central and low central subgroups. *Epilepsia.* 1994;35:1125–1129.
68. Drury I, Beydoun A. Benign partial epilepsy of childhood with monomorphic sharp waves in centrotemporal and other locations. *Epilepsia.* 1991;32:662–667.
69. Ramelli GP, Donati F, Moser H, et al. Concomitance of childhood absence and rolandic epilepsy. *Clin Electroencephalogr.* 1998;29:177–180.
70. Dalla Bernardina BD, Tassinari CA. EEG of a nocturnal seizure in a patient with "benign epilepsy of childhood with rolandic spikes." *Epilepsia.* 1975;16:497–501.
71. Wirrell EC. Benign epilepsy of childhood with centrotemporal spikes. *Epilepsia.* 1998;39(suppl 4):S32–S41.
72. Gutierrez AR, Brick JF, Bodensteiner J. Dipole reversal: an ictal feature of benign partial epilepsy with centrotemporal spikes. *Epilepsia.* 1990;31:544–548.
73. Silva DF, Lima MM, Anghinah R, et al. Dipole reversal: an ictal feature in a patient with benign partial epilepsy of childhood with centro-temporal spike. *Arq Neuropsiquiatr.* 1995;53:270–273.
74. Clemens B. Ictal electroencephalography in a case of benign centrotemporal epilepsy. *J Child Neurol.* 2002;17:297–300.
75. Cavazzuti GB, Cappella L, Nalin A. Longitudinal study of epileptiform EEG patterns in normal children. *Epilepsia.* 1980;12:43–55.
76. Heijbel J, Bohman M. Benign epilepsy of children with centrotemporal EEG foci: intelligence, behavior and school adjustment. *Epilepsia.* 1975;16:679–687.
77. Kavros PM, Clarke T, Strug LJ, et al. Attention impairment in rolandic epilepsy: systemic review. *Epilepsia.* 2008;49:1570–1580.
78. Croona C, Kihlgren M, Lundberg S, et al. Neuropsychological findings in children with benign childhood epilepsy with centrotemporal spikes. *Dev Med Child Neurol.* 1999;41:813–818.
79. Gunduz E, Demirbilek V, Korkmaz B. Benign rolandic epilepsy: neuropsychological findings. *Seizure.* 1999;8:246–249.
80. Baglietto MG, Battaglia FM, Nobili L, et al. Neuropsychological disorders related to interictal epileptic discharges during sleep in benign epilepsy of childhood with centrotemporal or rolandic spikes. *Dev Med Child Neurol.* 2001;43:407–412.
81. Clarke T, Strug LJ, Murphy PL, et al. High risk fo reading disability and speech sound disorder in rolandic epilepsy families: case-control study. *Epilepsia.* 2007;48:2258–2265.
82. Binnie CD, Marston D. Cognitive correlates of interictal discharges. *Epilepsia.* 1992;33(suppl 6):S11–S17.
83. Nicolai J, van der Linden I, Arends JB, et al. EEG characteristics related to educational impairments in children with benign childhood epilepsy with centrotemporal spikes. *Epilepsia.* 2007;48:2093–2100.
84. D'Alessandro P, Piccirilli M, Tiacci C, et al. Neuropsychological features of benign partial epilepsy in children. *Ital J Neurol Sci.* 1990;11:265–269.
85. Piccirilli M, D'Alessandro P, Tiacci C, et al. Language lateralization in children with benign partial epilepsy. *Epilepsia.* 1988;29:19–25.
86. Piccirilli M, D'Alessandro P, Sciarma T, et al. Attention problems in epilepsy: possible significance of the epileptogenic focus. *Epilepsia.* 1994;35:1091–1096.
87. Laub MC, Funke R, Kirsch CM, et al. BECTS: comparison of cerebral blood flow imaging, neuropsychological testing and long-term EEG findings. *Epilepsy Res Suppl.* 1992;6:95–98.
88. Weglage J, Demsky A, Pietsch M, et al. Neuropsychological, intellectual, and behavioral findings in patients with centrotemporal spikes with and without seizures. *Dev Med Child Neurol.* 1997;39:646–651.
89. Piccinelli P, Borgatti R, Aldini A, et al. Academic performance in children with rolandic epilepsy. *Dev Med Child Neurol.* 2008;50:353–356.
90. Deonna T, Zesiger P, Davidoff V, et al. Benign partial epilepsy of childhood: a longitudinal neuropsychological and EEG study of cognitive function. *Dev Med Child Neurol.* 2000;42:595–603.
91. Metz-Lutz MN, Kleitz C, de Saint-Martin A, et al. Cognitive development in benign focal epilepsies of childhood. *Dev Neurosci.* 1999;21:182–190.
92. Santanelli P, Bureau M, Magaudda A, et al. Benign partial epilepsy with centrotemporal (or rolandic) spikes and brain lesion. *Epilepsia.* 1989;30:182–188.
93. Lundberg S, Eeg-Olofsson O, Raininko R, et al. Hippocampal asymmetries and white matter abnormalities on MRI in benign childhood epilepsy with centrotemporal spikes. *Epilepsia.* 1999;40:1808–1815.
94. Gelisse P, Corda D, Raybaud C, et al. Abnormal neuroimaging in patients with benign epilepsy with centrotemporal spikes. *Epilepsia.* 2003;44:372–378.
95. Boxerman JL, Hawash K, Bali B, et al. Is rolandic epilepsy associated with abnormal findings on cranial MRI? *Epilepsy Res.* 2007;75(2–3):180–185.
96. Peters JM, Camfield CS, Camfield PR. Population study of benign rolandic epilepsy: is treatment needed? *Neurology.* 2001;57:537–539.
97. Bouma PAD, Bovenkerk AC, Westendorp RGJ, et al. The course of benign partial epilepsy of childhood with centrotemporal spikes: a meta-analysis. *Neurology.* 1997;48:430–437.
98. Bourgeois BF, Brown LW, Pellock JM, et al. Gabapentin (Neurontin) monotherapy in children with benign childhood epilepsy with centrotemporal spikes (BECTS): a 36 week, double-blind, placebo-controlled study. *Epilepsia.* 1998;39(suppl 6):163.
99. Rating D, Wolf C, Bast T. Sulthiame as monotherapy in children with benign childhood epilepsy with centrotemporal spikes: a 6-month randomized, double-blind, placebo-controlled study. *Epilepsia.* 2000;41:1284–1288.
100. Wirrell E, Sherman EM, Vanmastrigt R, et al. Deterioration in cognitive function in children with benign epilepsy of childhood with central temporal spikes treated with sulthiame. *J Child Neurol.* 2008;23:14–21.
101. Corda D, Gelisse P, Genton P, et al. Incidence of drug-induced aggravation in benign epilepsy with centrotemporal spikes. *Epilepsia.* 2001;42:754–759.
102. Prats JM, Garaizar C, Garcia-Nieto ML, et al. Antiepileptic drugs and atypical evolution of idiopathic partial epilepsy. *Pediatr Neurol.* 1998;18:402–406.
103. Nanba Y, Maegaki Y. Epileptic negative myoclonus induced by carbamazepine in a child with BECTS. Benign childhood epilepsy with centrotemporal spikes. *Pediatr Neurol.* 1999;21:664–667.
104. Catania S, Cross H, de Sousa C, et al. Paradoxic reaction to lamotrigine in a child with benign focal epilepsy of childhood with centrotemporal spikes. *Epilepsia.* 1999;40:1657–1660.
105. Blom S, Heijbel J. Benign epilepsy of children with centrotemporal EEG foci: a follow-up in adulthood of patients initially studied as children. *Epilepsia.* 1982;23:629–631.
106. De Romanis F, Feliciani M, Ruggieri S. Rolandic paroxysmal epilepsy: a long term study in 150 children. *Ital J Neurol Sci.* 1986;7:77–80.
107. Loiseau P, Pestre M, Dartigues JF, et al. Long-term prognosis in two forms of childhood epilepsy: typical absence seizures and epilepsy with rolandic (centrotemporal) EEG foci. *Ann Neurol.* 1983;13:642–648.
108. Gibbs F, Gibbs E. *Atlas of Electroencephalography, Epilepsy, II.* Cambridge: Addison-Wesley Press; 1952:222–224.
109. Panayiotopoulos CP. Benign childhood epilepsy with occipital paroxysms: A 15-year prospective study. *Ann Neurol.* 1989;26:51–56.
110. Panayiotopoulos CP. Benign childhood epileptic syndromes with occipital spikes: new classification proposed by the International League Against Epilepsy. *J Child Neurol.* 2000;15:548–552.
111. Kuzniecky R, Rosenblatt B. Benign occipital epilepsy: a family study. *Epilepsia.* 1987;28:346–350.
112. Ferrie CD, Beaumanoir A, Guerrini R, et al. Early onset benign occipital seizure susceptibility syndrome. *Epilepsia.* 1997;38:285–932.
113. Lada C, Skiadas K, Theodorou V, et al. A study of 43 patients with Panayiotopoulos syndrome, a common and benign childhood seizure susceptibility. *Epilepsia.* 2003;44:81–88.
114. Koutroumanidis M. Panayiotopoulos syndrome: an important electroclinical example of benign childhood system epilepsy. *Epilepsia.* 2007;48:1044–1053.
115. Panayiotopoulos CP. *Panayiotopoulos Syndrome: A Common and Benign Childhood Epileptic Syndrome.* London: John Libbey; 2002.
116. Caraballo R, Cersosimo R, Medina C, et al. Panayiotopoulos-type benign childhood occipital epilepsy: a prospective study. *Neurology.* 2000;55:1096–1100.
117. Panayiotopoulos CP. Early onset benign childhood occipital seizure susceptibility syndrome: a syndrome to recognize. *Epilepsia.* 1999;40:621–630.
118. Ferrie CD, Koutroumanidis M, Rowlinson S, et al. Atypical evolution of Panayiotopoulos syndrome: a case report. *Epileptic Disord.* 2002;4:35–42.
119. Taylor I, Berkovic SF, Kivity S, et al. Benign occipital epilepsies of childhood: clinical features and genetics. *Brain.* 2008;131:2287–2294.
120. Gastaut H. Benign spike-wave occipital epilepsy in children. *Rev Electroencephalogr Neurophysiol Clin.* 1982;12:179–201.
121. Caraballo RH, Cersósimo RO, Fejerman N. Childhood occipital epilepsy of Gastaut: a study of 33 patients. *Epilepsia.* 2008;49:288–297.
122. Panayiotopoulos CP, Michael M, Sanders S, et al. Benign childhood focal epilepsies: assessment of established and newly recognized syndromes. *Brain.* 2008;131:2264–2286.
123. Verrotti A, Domizio S, Melchionda D, et al. Stormy onset of benign childhood epilepsy with occipital paroxysmal discharges. *Childs Nerv Syst.* 2000;16:35–39.

124. Ohtsu M, Oguni H, Hayashi K, et al. EEG in children with early-onset benign occipital seizure susceptibility syndrome: Panayiotopoulos syndrome. *Epilepsia.* 2003;44:435–442.

125. Kanazawa O, Tohyama J, Akasaka N, et al. A magnetoencephalographic study of patients with Panayiotopoulos syndrome. *Epilepsia.* 2005;46:1106–1113.

126. Maher J, Ronen GM, Ogunyemi AO, et al. Occipital paroxysmal discharges suppressed by eye opening: variability in clinical and seizure manifestations in childhood. *Epilepsia.* 1995;36:52–57.

127. Cooper GW, Lee SI. Reactive occipital epileptiform activity: is it benign? *Epilepsia.* 1991;32:63–68.

128. Van der Meij W, Van der Dussen D, Van Huffelen AC, et al. Dipole source analysis may differentiate benign focal epilepsy of childhood with occipital paroxysms from symptomatic occipital lobe epilepsy. *Brain Topogr.* 1997;10:115–120.

129. Beaumanoir A. Semiology of occipital seizures in infants and children. In: Andermann F, Beaumanoir A, Mira L, et al., eds. *Occipital Seizures and Epilepsies in Children.* London: John Libbey; 1993:71–86.

130. Vigevano F, Lispi ML, Ricci S. Early onset benign occipital susceptibility syndrome: video-EEG documentation of an illustrative case. *Clin Neurophysiol.* 2000;111(suppl 2):S81–S86.

131. Vigevano F, Ricci S. Benign occipital epilepsy of childhood with prolonged seizures and autonomic symptoms. In: Andermann F, Beaumanoir A, Mira L, et al., eds. *Occipital Seizures and Epilepsies in Children.* London: John Libbey; 1993:133–140.

132. Gulgonen S, Demirbilik V, Korkmaz B, et al. Neuropsychological functions in idiopathic occipital lobe epilepsy. *Epilepsia.* 2000;41:405–411.

133. Tenembaum SN, Deonna TW, Fejerman N, et al. Continuous spike-waves and dementia in childhood epilepsy with occipital paroxysms. *J Epilepsy.* 1997;10:139–145.

134. Nass R, Gross A, Devinsky O. Autism and autistic epileptiform regression with occipital spikes. *Dev Med Child Neurol.* 1998;40:453–458.

135. Panayiotopoulos CP. Elementary visual hallucinations, blindness and headache in idiopathic occipital epilepsy: differentiation from migraine. *J Neurol Neurosurg Psychiatry.* 1999;66:536–540.

136. Gastaut H. Benign epilepsy of childhood with occipital paroxysms. In: Roger J, Dravet C, Bureau M, et al., eds. *Epilepsy Syndromes in Infancy, Childhood and Adolescence.* London: John Libbey; 1985:159–170.

137. Okumura A, Hayakawa F, Kuno K, et al. Benign partial epilepsy in infancy. *Arch Dis Child.* 1996;74:19–21.

138. Nelson GB, Olson DM, Hahn JS. Short duration of benign partial epilepsy in infancy. *J Child Neurol.* 2002;17:440–445.

139. Okumura A, Watanabe K, Negoro T, et al. Long-term follow-up of patients with benign partial epilepsy in infancy. *Epilepsia.* 2006;47:181–185.

140. Bureau M, Cokar O, Maton B, et al. Sleep-related, low voltage rolandic and vertex spikes: an EEG marker of benignity in infancy-onset focal epilepsies. *Epileptic Disord.* 2002;4:15–22.

141. King MA, Newton MR, Berkovic SF. Benign partial seizures of adolescence. *Epilepsia.* 1999;40:1244–1247.

142. Capovilla G, Gambardella A, Romeo A, et al. Benign partial epilepsies of adolescence: a report of 37 new cases. *Epilepsia.* 2001;42:1549–1552.

143. Vigevano F, Fusco L. Hypnic tonic postural seizures in healthy children provide evidence for a partial epileptic syndrome of frontal lobe origin. *Epilepsia.* 1993;34:110–119.

144. Scheffer IE, Bhatia KP, Lopes-Cendes I, et al. Autosomal dominant nocturnal frontal lobe epilepsy: a distinctive clinical disorder. *Brain.* 1995;118(pt 1):61–73.

145. Capovilla G, Beccaria F. Benign partial epilepsy in infancy and early childhood with vertex spikes and waves during sleep: a new epileptic form. *Brain Dev.* 2000;22:93–99.

146. Capovilla G, Beccaria F, Montagnini A. "Benign focal epilepsy in infancy with vertex spikes and waves during sleep". Delineation of the syndrome and recalling as "benign infantile focal epilepsy with midline spikes and waves during sleep" (BIMSE). *Brain Dev.* 2006;28:85–91.

147. Fonseca LC, Tedrus GM. Somatosensory evoked spikes and epileptic seizures: a study of 385 cases. *Clin Electroencephalogr.* 2000;31:71–75.

CHAPTER 20 ■ IDIOPATHIC GENERALIZED EPILEPSY SYNDROMES OF CHILDHOOD AND ADOLESCENCE

STEPHEN HANTUS

Idiopathic generalized epilepsy (IGE) represents 20% of all epilepsies. It occurs mostly in young people, and with proper diagnosis and management are controlled with medications in 80% of cases. Diagnosis is important as certain medications can aggravate these epilepsies and lead to increased seizures, absence status, and pseudointractability. Proper medication management is often able to allow patients to live an otherwise unaffected life, although persistent social and psychological problems are reported in some studies (1,2).

IGEs are defined by the International League Against Epilepsy (ILAE) as an epilepsy that arises spontaneously, with no associated structural lesion or neurologic sign or symptom, and is of presumed genetic origin (3,4). IGE is a group of epilepsies that give rise to three types of seizures that occur in various combinations depending on the syndrome.

TYPICAL ABSENCE SEIZURES

These seizures are clinically characterized by unresponsiveness of short duration (5 to 15 seconds) with abrupt onset and termination. Patients are unresponsive during the seizures and have no memory of these brief events. Occassionally, there is associated eye fluttering or automatisms. There is little or no postictal confusion or disorientation associated with this seizure type. Electroencephalogram (EEG) demonstrates the typical 3 Hz spike-and-wave complexes that is often most prominent during hyperventilation.

MYOCLONIC SEIZURES

This is a seizure type characterized by brief jerks (1 second or less) that occur sporadically and often involve the upper extremities bilaterally as well as the trunk. They are often described as "shock-like" muscle contractions and occur most frequently in the morning. Patients typically deny any alteration in conciousness during these jerks and have no associated postictal confusion or disorientation, and most often drop objects or spill drinks when these occur. EEG demonstrates a generalized polyspike discharge prior to the muscle jerk of the myoclonic seizure.

GENERALIZED TONIC–CLONIC SEIZURES

These seizures typically last 1 to 3 minutes, and are associated with loss of conciousness and a muscular convulsion. The tonic phase lasts for 10 to 45 seconds and may involve bilateral arm stiffening and often a vocalization. This is followed by a clonic phase with rhythmic jerking of various muscle groups. There is often an extensive postictal period of confusion and disorientation that may last from 5 minutes to several hours. EEG during these seizures shows generalized spike-and-wave discharges that evolve in frequency and amplitude.

IDIOPATHIC GENERALIZED EPILEPSY SYNDROMES

IGE syndromes are best viewed as a spectrum of disorders with these three seizure types expressed in variable amounts as different clinical phenotypes. These syndromes often have overlapping genetic etiologies as well. It is most important to distiguish the focal/localization-related epilepsies from the generalized epilepsies because the treatment and prognosis are very different. The risk of intractability is much higher in focal epilepsies, and the drugs that treat focal epilepsy can exacerbate IGE. The following will describe the diagnostic criteria of the IGE syndromes and what is known about their etiology and prognosis.

CHILDHOOD ABSENCE EPILEPSY

Childhood absence epilepsy (CAE) is a widely recognized syndrome with absence seizures as the only manifestation in many patients, while generalized tonic–clonic (GTC) seizures can also occur in up to 40%, although GTC seizures are more common in the juvenile form (5,6). Recent studies have questioned the concept of generalized epilepsy and have focused on specific cortical networks thought to be involved (6).

Epidemiology

CAE has been estimated to comprise 2% to 8% of epilepsy in the total population, but appears to be heavily age-dependent. Studies of childhood cohorts (0 to 15 age group) estimate 13% to 18%, with 3% to 6% in patients in the older than

15 age group. Large epidemiologic studies in Europe and the United States have shown an incidence of 6 to 8 per 100,000 in the 0 to 15 age group (7). There has been a female predominance noted in several studies (5,8).

Clinical Features

CAE characteristically begins between the ages of 4 and 8 years with absence seizures, but the age of onset can vary between ages 2 to 10 years (9). The absence seizures are often able to be demonstrated by having the patient hyperventilate in the office, effective in up to 98% of patients. A smaller amount of patients (16% noted in one study) are found to be photosensitive (10). In addition to the typical abrupt loss of consciousness and quick recovery of a typical absence, automatisms, transient loss of tone, fluttering of the eyelids, and brief myoclonic jerks are also common. Seizures typically last from 9 to 12 seconds and without medications may occur hundreds of times per day. Patients with CAE have been noted to have cognitive, linguistic, and psychiatric comorbidities (11). In the study by Caplan et al., one fourth of patients had subtle cognitive difficulties, almost half had linguistic deficits, and approximately 67% had a psychiatric diagnosis with attention deficit hyperactivity disorder (ADHD) and anxiety being most common (11). There is some indication that treatment with medications can improve some neurocognitive skills (e.g., visual memory), and the results are dependent on seizure control (12). Although it is a defining characteristic that patients with CAE (and IGEs in general) have normal intelligence, recent studies have emphasized that untreated behavioral and psychiatric problems are common (11,13).

IGEs are also by definition not related to a structural or anatomic cause, and normal imaging with magnetic resonance imaging (MRI) is the most common clinical finding. However, there are some volumetric studies that suggest that the anterior half to the thalamus is larger in patients with absence epilepsy, suggesting a possible structural correlate (14). This finding was not present in patients with other seizure types (GTC seizures).

EEG

The EEG in CAE shows monomorphic high voltage generalized spike-and-slow-wave complexes at 3 Hz (2.5 to 4.0 Hz). These spike-and-wave complexes may occur interictally or as an ictal pattern depending on the duration and responsiveness of the patient. The typical length of an ictal event is 9 to 12 seconds and may begin with 3.0 to 3.5 Hz spike-and-wave complexes that may slow to 2.5 to 3.0 Hz discharges. The background EEG is typically normal. In up to 50% of patients, bursts of rhythmic slowing lasting 2 to 4 seconds can be seen in the occipital leads. A small study suggested that occipital intermittent rhythmic delta activity (ORIDA) indicated a good prognosis for response to medication in typical absence epilepsy (15).

Generalized epilepsies have been considered to arise from the bilateral, global neocortex by definition, but have been noted to have a frontal predominance on EEG. The use of dense array EEG (256 channels) and software to superimpose the electrical signals over the patients MRI have suggested that there are discrete areas that are activated during an absence seizure (16,17). Dense array EEG would suggest a corticothalamic circuit involving the medial frontal and orbitofrontal cortex is maximally involved.

Genetics

Classic family studies have suggested that one third of patients with CAE have a family history of epilepsy and siblings of affected individuals have an approximately 10% chance of suffering seizures (18). The essential genetic nature of IGE is demonstrated in twin studies that show an 81% concordance among monozygotic twins, while dizygotic twins are only 26% concordant for epilepsy (19). The genetics of CAE is a complex pattern with most patients having multiple genetic factors likely contributing to their epilepsy and rare cases with a monogenetic etiology reported (20). Most of the genes that have been identified are subunits of ion channels, with some exceptions. Identified mutations have been shown in the γ-aminobutyric acid receptor γ2 (GABRG2), chloride channel receptor 2 (CLCN2), γ-aminobutyric acid receptor α1 (GABRA1), and the calcium channel voltage-dependent, T-type α1H subunit (CACNA1H) genes (21). A study that examined gene expression in monozygotic twins that were discordant for epilepsy identified altered expression of early growth response 1 (EGR 1) and reticulocalbin 2 (RCN 2) suggesting a role for these proteins in CAE (22).

Treatment

Medical treatment has been shown to suppress absence seizures in more than 80% of patients. Studies that have compared ethosuximide, valproate, and lamotrigine were not able to establish a difference in efficacy and are all considered first-line medications (23). Ethosuximide does not protect against GTC seizures, and has neurotoxic and gastrointestinal side effects that limit its use. Valproate is effective as a broad spectrum agent treating absence, GTC seizures, and myoclonic seizures. Valproate use is limited due to side effects of weight gain and potential tetratogenicity. Lamotrigine is effective in treating absence, has fewer cognitive side effects, and is the preferred medication for females due to the lower rate of tetratogenicity as compared to valproate (23). Levetiracetam and zonisamide have been shown to decrease absence seizures by 50% to 60% in small studies and are considered second-line medications (24,25). Refractory absence epilepsy occurs in 5% to 20% of cases (5). Treatment with an inappropriate antiepileptic drug (AED) is a frequent cause of "pseudointractability," as some drugs have been shown to exacerbate absences (26,27). Carbamazepine is the most frequent cause of worsening seizures and has been associated with absence status epilepticus (26). Phenytoin, tiagabine, vigabatrin, and oxcarbazepine have also been shown to cause a paradoxical increase in seizures in patients with absence epilepsy. Combinations of medications, particularly with valproate, have been shown to be more effective than single medications alone (27).

The decision to stop therapy is often difficult. A minimum seizure-free interval of 2 years is usually recommended before withdrawal of medication. However, each case must be evaluated individually in terms of the attitude of the patient and the family, participation in sports, occupation, and driving an automobile. The EEG findings may help guide the decision, but the presence of occasional brief epileptiform discharges should not preclude drug withdrawal in the seizure-free patient (28).

Prognosis

CAE is one the relatively benign childhood epilepsies, but not all patients become seizure-free. Approximately 50% of patients with CAE will have a spontaneous remission by the age of 10 to 12 years, with a range of 21% to 89% remission (29). In patients with absence seizures only, the seizure-free rate is approximately 80%, while patients with GTC seizures and absence were only 30% seizure-free (29). Early institution of effective therapy is believed to improve prognosis in terms of the later development of tonic–clonic seizures and relapse of absences. A Dutch study with long-term follow up (12 to 17 years) indicated that seizure freedom in the first 6 months of treatment predicted outcome, while EEG and baseline characteristics did not impact outcome (30).

JUVENILE ABSENCE EPILEPSY

Juvenile absence epilepsy (JAE) has a number of features that are clinically distinct from those of the other absence epilepsies and has been recognized as a separate syndrome (3,4). It is often diagnosed retrospectively after a GTC seizure occurs or other associated features are noted.

Epidemiology

There are no definitive epidemiologic studies for JAE, but large studies of absence epilepsy have shown a peak at age 6 to 7 years (consistent with the peak ages of the onset of CAE) and another around age 12 (7). Several cohort studies have estimated that JAE comprises 0.2% to 3.0% of childhood epilepsies and has a prevalence of 0.1 per 100,000 persons in the general population, which is much less common than CAE (7,31).

Clinical Features

Most cases begin on or near puberty, with a range of 10 to 17 years and an average onset at age 12 (7,31). The absences are less frequent that those of CAE, and occur once per day or several per week (as compared to the 100 per day often seen in CAE). The absences of JAE have been described in various clinical reports as resulting in less severe loss of consciousness, having a retropulsive component (backward motion of the eyes), and lasting longer than CAE at approximately 10 to 60 seconds (8,32). GTC seizures have been reported in 47% to 80% of patients with JAE, and frequently occur upon awakening (8,31). Myoclonic jerks are less frequent and occur in 10% to 15% of patients, and illustrate the clinical overlap with some features of juvenile myoclonic epilepsy (8).

EEG

JAE is associated with generalized spike-and-wave discharges that occur typically at 3 to 4 Hz, which is slightly faster than CAE. They have also been reported to be slightly less rhythmic and less organized than the spike-and-wave complexes seen in CAE. Photosensitivity is rare, but appears to be more common in females and in the juvenile form (33,34). The interictal background activity is normal.

Genetics

The genetic origin of JAE is largely undiscovered at this point. It is known from twin studies that genetics play a large role in JAE (35) and that patients with JAE have a family history of epilepsy in 29% to 35% of cases (8,31). Sander et al. reported that the kainate-selective glutamate receptor gene (*GRIK1*) is a susceptibility gene for developing JAE (36). The chloride channel ClCN2 that has also been implicated in CAE and JME is also thought to play a role in JAE (37).

Treatment

Valproate has been the historically most effective treatment choice. It treats the absences and also treats the possible associated GTC seizures and/or myoclonic jerks. However, due to the side effects of weight gain and tetratogenicity, it is generally used with caution in young females. Lamotrigine has also been shown to be an effective choice, treating absence seizures as well as GTC seizures. If myoclonus is present, then treatment with levetiracetam may be an alternative to valproate. Due to the frequent occurrence of GTC seizures with JAE, ethosuximide is not recommended as first-line medication. Education about avoiding sleep deprivation and alcohol consumption is also important in adolescent patients.

Prognosis

The response of JAE to pharmacologic therapy is typically very good. Valproate alone has been shown to treat over 80% of cases. However the seizure-free rates tend to be less than in patients with CAE (8). Patients with GTC seizures tended to have a worse prognosis (8).

JUVENILE MYOCLONIC EPILEPSY

Juvenile myoclonic epilepsy (JME) is a well-known IGE syndrome that involves adolescents. JME often goes undiagnosed until a GTC seizure occurs, because myoclonic jerks are often ignored or attributed to morning clumsiness. Increased awareness by clinicians and the availability of video-EEG has helped make this diagnosis more expedient.

Epidemiology

The incidence of JME has been estimated to be 1 per 100,000 persons, with a prevalence of 0.1 to 0.2 per 100,000. The frequency of JME in large cohorts has been estimated to be

5% to 10% of all epilepsies, and 18% of IGEs (7). Certain populations or family groups have been reported to have a higher incidence of JME such as Saudi Arabia and sections of India (38,39).

Clinical Features

The age of onset for JME is typically 12 to 18 years, with a peak onset at age 15, but can manifest in all age groups (40). The clinical presentation of JME is typically a GTC seizure that occurs in the morning after a night of sleep deprivation and/or alcohol consumption in an otherwise healthy individual. A detailed history will often reveal whole body jerks that occur mostly in the morning and result in spilling drinks and dropping objects and/or brief spells of unresponsiveness that have occurred for several months prior to the GTC seizure. Patients with JME will most frequently have myoclonic seizures (100%), with 87% to 95% having GTC seizures and 10% to 33% having absence seizures (41,42).

Myoclonic seizures are brief jerks that affect the neck, shoulders, arms, or legs. The jerks are more frequent in the upper than lower extremities and are typically bilateral and symmetric, but on occasion may be unilateral (43). Asymmetric myoclonic seizures may delay the diagnosis of JME and video-EEG should be used to make the definitive diagnosis (43). Myoclonic jerks of the upper extremities can often cause patients to drop objects and can interfere with morning activities such as eating breakfast, brushing teeth, or applying cosmetics. The jerks can be single or repetitive and often involve extensor muscles. Falling to the floor is uncommon, but falls may occur when patients are in an awkward position and are surprised by the jerk. The amplitude of the jerk is variable, but is typically not forceful or massive and recovery is immediate with no loss of consciousness. Some patients report electric shock type feelings only, with no physical signs of the myoclonic seizure. The relatively mild myoclonic seizures in JME are in contrast to the myoclonic seizures in Lennox–Gastaut syndrome and some progressive myoclonic epilepsies, which are massive and propel patients to the ground with great force.

GTC seizures in JME are often described as clonic–tonic–clonic due to the several repetitive myoclonic jerks that often precede a GTC seizure. The patient has no loss of awareness during the myoclonic jerks, and this serves as a warning to some patients to get to a safe place seconds prior to a GTC seizure (41). Consciousness is abruptly lost with the onset of the GTC seizure, with tonic extension of the head, face, neck, trunk, and extremities. The tonic phase lasts for 10 to 30 seconds and leads to the final phase of clonic trunk and limb jerks. Patients often emit a high-pitched "ictal cry" during the initial tonic phase. Due to the forceful contraction of many agonist and antagonist muscles simultaneously, patients are often very sore and tired after the seizure. Tongue and/or lip biting and loss of urinary or bowel continence is common. After the seizure, confusion and disorientation typically take 5 to 30 minutes to resolve. Patients typically have no memory of the event.

Absence seizures in JME are less common, occurring in 10% to 33% of patients and tend to be relatively infrequent, of short duration, and not associated with automatisms. In a prospective video-EEG study of JME patients, 16 of 42 (31.9%) were found to have absence seizures (44). When the seizures occurred prior to the age of 10, the patient would stop activities, not answer questions, and stare without postictal symptoms and without memory of the event. When the seizures occurred after the age of 10, the manifestations were usually less severe and consisted of subjective instant loss of contact and concentration or of brief impairment of concentration revealed by testing only (44).

Precipitating factors are commonly reported in patients with JME. Myoclonic and GTC seizures occur most often in the morning or upon awakening (42). Studies of cortical excitability with transcranial magnetic stimulation suggest an increase in cortical excitability/loss of intracortical inhibition in the early morning hours with drug naïve JME patients (45). Sleep deprivation, fatigue, alcohol use, photic stimulation (video games, strobe lights), and menstruation have also been shown to precipitate seizures in patients with JME (41,46). Patients should be counseled to maintain good sleep hygiene and to avoid excessive alcohol consumption since these precipitants can contribute to poor seizure control despite good AED management.

The neurologic exam in JME patients is generally normal, although some neuropsychological tests have suggested cognitive dysfunction with deficits in executive function and expressive language consistent with frontal lobe dysfunction (47,48). The neuroimaging studies in patients with JME typically do not reveal the etiology for the epilepsy, but may show nonspecific abnormalities or subtle changes in cortical volumes (49). A quantitative voxel-based MRI study has shown increased cortical gray matter in the medial frontal lobes in 40% of patients with JME (50). FDG-PET and proton MRS studies have also shown metabolic frontal lobe dysfunction in JME patients (51,52). However, not all studies have been able to duplicate the frontal dysfunction in JME patients, demonstrating the pathophysiological diversity of this condition (53).

EEG

The interictal EEG in JME is abnormal in 50% to 85% of untreated patients, while only 5% to 10% of patients treated with AEDs will have an abnormal EEG (42,54). The characteristic EEG pattern of JME consists of discharges of diffuse bilateral, symmetric, and synchronous 4 to 6 Hz polyspike-and-wave complexes (Fig. 20.1). These discharges may be accentuated over the frontocentral regions. The interictal complexes usually have two or more higher voltage (150 to 300 μV) surface negative spikes that are maximum in the anterior head regions. Focal abnormalities have been reported in up to 30% of cases (42). Response to photic stimulation with myoclonic seizures or epileptiform discharges after 12 to 16 Hz stimulation is common, and occurs in 30% to 50% of cases of JME (42,34). Dense array EEG studies have contested the "generalized" nature of the interictal discharges in JME and have suggested that they are localized to a thalamocortical network that involves the medial orbitofrontal cortex and anterior basal–medial temporal lobes maximally (55).

Genetics

The genetic nature of JME has been well established, and is likely complex and polygenic in most patients, though some rare monogenic forms are being identified. About 40% of

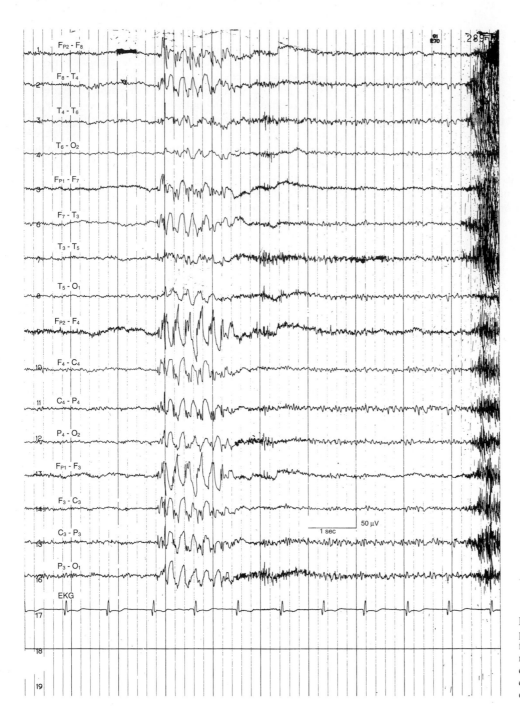

FIGURE 20.1 Interictal 4 to 6 Hz polyspike-and-wave discharge of frontocentral predominance in juvenile myoclonic epilepsy. No clinical changes were seen, and the patient could recall a word given during the discharge.

patients with JME report a positive family history for epilepsy (56). Genetics studies to date suggest that JME is a heterogeneous condition with multiple different mutations and susceptibility loci that have different modes of inheritance and possible mechanisms of action (21). Autosomal recessive, autosomal dominant, and complex polygenic models have been proposed in different family pedigrees (21). Analysis of JME families has identified linkages to multiple chromosomal loci that may contain genes that are causative or increase the susceptibility for developing JME. Chromosomal locations that demonstrate increased susceptibility in JME families include 6p12-p11 (EFHC1), 6p21 (BRD2/RING3), 15q13-14 (Cx-36), 5q34 (GABRA1), 2q22-23 (CACNB4), 8q24, 5q12-q14, 6q24, 16p13, 7q32, and 10q25-26 (20,21,57–59).

Several studies have also identified mutations that are rare, but appear to be causative in selected families. Mutations have been identified in EFHC1/Myoclonin1, CLCN2, GABRA1, and CACNB4 (57). In addition, single nucleotide polymorphism susceptibility alleles have been identified in the bromodomain-containing protein 2 (BRD2) and connexin 36 (Cx-36) (60–62).

EFHC1/Myoclonin1

Studies of multiple families of JME have implicated the 6p12-p11 region as a susceptibility focus, and the potential gene was referred to as EJM1. Mutational analysis was able to narrow this locus to the candidate gene EFHC1, which encodes for the protein Myoclonin1 (63). Proposed mechanisms of action for EFHC1/Myoclonin1 include promoting apoptosis, regulating R-Type calcium currents, cell cycle regulation, and neuronal migration (63–65). Animal studies have shown that mice deficient in EFHC1 have spontaneous myoclonus and increased seizure susceptibility (66). Mutations of EFHC1/Myoclonin1 have been reported in 9% of JME patients in Mexico and Honduras, and 3% of JME patients in Japan, which is more frequent than any other identified mutations in JME thus far (65).

CLCN2

Mutations of the CLCN2 chloride channels were found in three families of JME patients (37). The proposed mechanism was a reduction in chloride channel activity and increased neuronal excitability. The mutations were detected in patients with JME and also some apparently unaffected family members as well, but not in a control population (67). The authors concluded that CLCN2 mutations may act as susceptibility factors for epilepsy among other unknown genetic alterations (67).

GABRA1

Studies of a large French–Canadian family with JME led to the discovery of a mutation in the α1 subunit of the γ-aminobutyric acid receptor subtype A (GABRA1). Studies in vitro suggested a loss of gamma aminobutyric acid (GABA)-activated currents in receptors containing the mutant subunit (68). Expression of the mutant protein revealed a misfolded protein with impaired insertion into the plasma membrane (69). The proposed mechanism of action is a loss of inhibitory signals due to the defective GABA receptors and subsequent increased cortical excitability (68).

CACNB4

A single patient diagnosed with JME was found to have a mutation in the calcium channel β_4 subunit (CACNB4) and her daughter with the same mutation had epilepsy with 3 Hz spike-and-wave complexes (70). This mutation is thought to impair the channel function by shifting the voltage dependence of activation and inactivation. Additional mutations of the same subunit were associated with epilepsy and episodic ataxia (70).

It should be noted that although progress in identifying a few of the genes involved in JME is beginning to emerge, the vast majority of genes and combinations of genes that are involved are yet to be discovered (20,21). While the clinical presentation in JME is fairly homogenous, the pathogenesis appears to be complex and diverse (41).

Treatment

Appropriate management of a patient with JME requires consideration of multiple factors including AED selection, avoiding precipitating factors and anticipating special considerations that might impact their care (pregnancy, driving, behavioral issues). Response to medical therapy is generally good, with 60% to 80% seizure-free rate on medications. However, noncompliance and lifestyle choices that involve sleep deprivation, alcohol use, and other precipitants often lead to ongoing seizures. AED selection is also critical as some AEDs can exacerbate JME and lead to a pseudointractable state (26,32). Quality of life dramatically improves if a patient is able to reach seizure freedom, which can lead to driving employment

and a higher likelihood of social success. In addition to an appropriate AED choice, patients should be counseled to obtain adequate sleep, avoid alcohol, and wear polarized sunglasses if their seizures are sensitive to photic stimulation.

Valproate

Valproic acid is the treatment of choice for JME as it effectively treats absence, myoclonic, and GTC seizures in 86% to 90% of patients (71,72). A recent large, unblinded, randomized, controlled study of patients with IGE treated with Standard and New Antiepileptic Drugs (SANAD) suggested that valproate was preferred to lamotrigine due to better control of seizures, and preferred over topiramate due to lower rates of discontinuation due to side effects (73). Valproate is associated with a number of side effects that can sometimes limit its use or warrant reconsideration, including weight gain, hair loss, tremor, and tetratogenicity. Weight gain is a frequent reason for discontinuing valproate, with 50% to 70% of patients gaining greater than 4 kg (74). The standard dosing of valproate is 20 to 30 mg/kg/day, but patients with JME often respond to low doses, such as 500 mg/day (75). Valproate at low doses (below 1000 mg/day) and with extended release preparations has significantly less side effects and is often well tolerated.

Lamotrigine

Lamotrigine is a useful alternative for patients with JME, especially when valproate alone is not effective or not well tolerated. In a retrospective cohort study, no difference in seizure control was found between valproate monotherapy and lamotrigine monotherapy, and the authors concluded that lamotrigine was an acceptable alternative to valproate (76). When compared in a randomized, controlled trial (SANAD), valproate had better efficacy in terms of seizure control than lamotrigine (73). There have also been some reports of exacerbation of myoclonic seizures with lamotrigine (77). In a study using lamotrigine as an add-on agent in treatment-resistant generalized epilepsy, 80% of patients had a greater than 50% reduction in seizure frequency and 25% became seizure-free (74). In an open-label study of lamotrigine monotherapy in patients who had failed valproate, there was no significant change in their underlying seizures, but 67% of patients reported improvement in their global clinical status on lamotrigine and 76% of patients rated lamotrigine as better tolerated than valproate (78). The major side effect of lamotrigine reported was a rash, which in some patients can be severe. An allergic skin reaction occurs in approximately 10% of patients with severe rash (such as Steven–Johnson syndrome) occurring in 0.3% of adults and 1% of children (79). The lamotrigine-associated rash may be more severe when combined with valproic acid (79). Lamotrigine is well tolerated and effective as an adjunctive therapy for JME, but concerns over decreased seizure control compared to valproate and exacerbation of myoclonic seizures in some limit its use as a monotherapy.

Topiramate

Topiramate is another possible adjunctive or alternative therapy to valproate, but has limited data in treating JME. In double blind, placebo-controlled studies of topiramate, 73% of patients in the JME subgroup had a greater than 50% reduction in primary GTC seizures and 16% became seizure-free (80). In a randomized open-label comparison, topiramate and valproate had similar rates of seizure freedom (67% and 57%, respectively) and both treatment groups had 11% of patients stop the medication due to adverse effects (81). In the SANAD study, topirimate had similar efficacy to valproate, but was associated with more side effects (73). Typical side effects with topiramate include cognitive dysfunction, anomia, weight loss, and nephrolithiasis.

Levetiracetam

A number of studies have shown the efficacy of levetiracetam as an adjunctive therapy for IGE, and its features of no known drug interactions and overall good tolerability have made this drug a useful asset. Using a retrospective design, Kumar reported on 25 patients with IGE treated with levetiracetam and found 68% of patients had some improvement in their seizures and 16% became seizure-free (82). In an open-label study, Kraus et al. studied 55 patients with GTC, myoclonic, and absence seizures and found that 76% had a greater than 50% reduction in seizures and 40% became seizure-free (83). They also found that 15% of the patients discontinued levetiracetam due to adverse events (sedation being the most common). In a multicenter, double blind, placebo-controlled study, Bervokic et al. examined 164 patients with IGE. They reported that 72.2% of patients had a greater than 50% reduction in seizures, with 34% of patients seizure-free from GTC seizures and 24% seizure-free from all seizure types (84). Levetiracetam was well tolerated in this study with only 1.3% of patients discontinuing therapy for adverse events. A randomized, double blind, placebo-controlled, multicenter trial by Noachtar et al. addressed the effects of levetiracetam on myoclonic seizures (85). They examined 120 patients and found 58.3% had a greater than 50% reduction in days/week with myoclonic seizures. The rate of myoclonic seizure freedom was 25% and seizure freedom from all seizure types was seen in 21%. Levetiracetam has been shown to be efficacious in JME for all seizure types including myoclonic seizures as an adjunctive therapy. Adverse events of somnolence, headache, and irritability are relatively rare in 1% to 15% of patients.

Zonisamide

There have been relatively few studies on the efficacy of zonisamide in IGE and JME, but initial data have shown efficacy as an adjunctive agent for multiple seizure types, including JME. Zonisamide has been available in Japan since 1989 and much of the data are from the Japanese experience. In a prospective postmarketing survey, Yamauchi et al. reported that 78% of patients with IGE and 50% of patients with myoclonic seizures had a greater than 50% reduction in their seizures with zonisamide (86). Yagi reported on the pooled efficacy data of 1008 patients collected from controlled and uncontrolled phase II and phase III studies, and found 59% of GTC seizures, 62% of absence seizures, and 43% of myoclonic seizures were reduced by greater than 50% with zonisamide (87). In a small open-label retrospective study, Kothare et al. reported 80% of patients with JME had a greater than 50% reduction in seizures on zonisamide monotherapy (88). They also reported seizure freedom in 69% of GTC seizures, 62% of myoclonic seizures, and 38% of absence seizures. Preliminary data suggest that zonisamide is efficacious as an adjunctive medication for JME, but further data with randomized, controlled trials will help delineate this. The advantages of zonisamide are once daily dosing. Common side effects include weight loss, cognitive problems, and nephrolithiasis.

A number of medications have been reported to exacerbate JME, especially the myoclonic seizures (26). The most common medications causing seizure aggravation are carbamazepine and oxcarbazepine. Phenytoin, gabapentin, and vigabatrin may also exacerbate seizures in JME or do not have efficacy.

Special Considerations of Treating JME in Pregnancy

Child-bearing-age females represent 25% of the population being treated for epilepsy, and the possibility of pregnancy often influences AED selection (89). While all of the AEDs have some risk of tetratogenicity, valproate has the highest risk, especially when given in doses greater than 1000 mg/day (6% to 11% chance of birth defects) (90). This is balanced by the evidence that valproate is the most clinically effective medication to prevent seizures based on the SANAD study (73). Lamotrigine has been the best studied of the newer medications in pregnancy, has been followed in multiple pregnancy registries, and has a reported 2.7% risk of major congenital malformations (91,92). However, the actual risk of birth defects with lamotrigine is unclear since pregnancy induces the clearance of this drug by up to 94%, and this decrease in drug levels is not accounted for in the pregnancy registries (93). There has also been noted increased seizure frequency in mothers taking lamotrigine during pregnancy (93). There has been some indication of a dose responsive risk of birth defects with lamotrigine with an increased malformation rate in patients taking more than 200 mg/day, reported in the UK pregnancy registry, but not in the International Lamotrigine Pregnancy registry (91,92). There is little information of the other medications generally considered useful in JME such as topiramate, zonisamide, and levetiracetam. Monotherapy in general had less risk of malformations (3.7%) than polytherapy (6.0%) regardless of AEDs involved (92). There is some evidence that exposure to AEDs during pregnancy can affect the cognitive development of the fetus, with valproate associated with the worse cognitive outcome (90,94). In the Neurodevelopmental Effects of Antiepileptic Drugs (NEAD) study, children exposed to valproate had a lower intelligence quotient (IQ) on average by 9 points compared to patients exposed to lamotrigine (94). The effect of valproate was dose-dependent and was not observed at dosages below 800 mg/day.

A cautious and informed approach is needed in treating women patients in their child-bearing years. Valproate is generally considered the most efficacious drug at suppressing the seizures in JME and is a reasonable choice if levels of less than 800 to 1000 mg/day can be used. Lamotrigine has shown fewer incidences of birth defects and potential cognitive problems, but has fewer efficacies in preventing maternal seizures and increased seizure frequency has been reported (93). Young women with JME should not be discouraged from having children in general, as greater than 90% of women have normal pregnancies. However, placement on monotherapy and preconceptual planning should be encouraged to reduce the risk of fetal malformations and potential cognitive delays.

Prognosis

The prognosis for JME is generally considered excellent as the majority of patients are able to be treated successfully with AEDs. Seizure-free rates of 60% to 90% have been reported. It has been noted that while response to medication is good, patients do tend to have breakthrough seizures due to noncompliance, sleep deprivation, alcohol use, or other precipitants. Achieving seizure freedom often involves lifestyle modifications as well as compliance with AEDs. Multiple studies in the past have suggested that JME is a lifelong condition and the medications were not to be discontinued (95). Delgado-Escueta and Enrile-Bacsal have reported a 90% relapse rate with withdrawal of medications. A recent study followed patients with JME for 25 years and found that 48% had voluntarily stopped their medications, 17% were without seizures on no medication, and 13% had myoclonus only, also without medication (1). It should also be noted that 36% of patients followed in the study had an episode of convulsive status epilepticus and 13% had medically intractable seizures. While a small percentage of patients with JME could likely come off medications at some time interval as suggested in the study, determining who will remain seizure-free and who will continue to have seizures is less clear.

EPILEPSY WITH GENERALIZED TONIC–CLONIC SEIZURES ONLY

Epilepsy with GTC seizures only has recently been described by the ILAE in their most recent proposed diagnostic scheme for people with epileptic seizures and epilepsy as a separate syndrome (3). It includes "Epilepsy with GTC seizures on awakening," which was previously described as a separate syndrome. The diagnosis of this syndrome can be challenging as many IGEs as well as focal epilepsies have some component of GTC seizures.

Epidemiology

There is limited information on the epidemiology of patients presenting with GTC seizures only. In a population-based study, epilepsy with Grand mal upon awakening was reported as 23% of generalized epilepsies (96). A population-based study in France reported an incidence of 1.8 per 100,000 people (96).

Clinical Features

The peak age of onset is at 15 with an age range between 5 and 50 years (7). Neurological exam and imaging is normal, and other tests except for the EEG do not reveal any other neurological abnormalities.

The predominant seizure type is GTC. Dialeptic seizures and myoclonic seizures are seen less frequently. Seizures are mainly provoked by alcohol and sleep deprivation, and can also be brought out by photic stimulation. Seizures tend to worsen with age. Wolf reported GTC seizures on awakening in 17% to 53%, during wakefulness in 23% to 36%, during sleep in 27% to 44%, and not related to pattern in 13% to

26% of patients (97). In the subcategory of GTC seizures on awakening, GTC seizures occur in more than 90% upon 1 to 2 hours after awakening or at the end of the day (during relaxation), with only rare myoclonic or dialeptic seizures. Unterberger et al. compared epilepsy with GTC seizures on awakening and randomly occurring GTC seizures and found that patients with early morning seizures had a longer duration of epilepsy, a higher relapse rate, and a stronger relationship to seizure provoking factors (98).

EEG

Interictal features on EEG consist of generalized epileptiform discharges presenting either as generalized 4 to 5 Hz spike and wave complexes or as generalized polyspikes. Discharges can be seen bilaterally with occasional asynchrony or asymmetry of bursts.

Ictal EEG is characterized by generalized fast rhythmic spiking, with a bifrontal maximum during the tonic phase of a GTC seizure. EEG activity is frequently obscured by tonic or clonic muscle artifact. Spiking can be asymmetric and asynchronous. This activity slows down and evolves into discontinuous repetitive generalized bursts of generalized (poly) spikes and waves intermingled with rhythmic slow waves. Clonic jerks start approximately at a spike frequency of 4 Hz. Postictally, electrical activity is reduced and can occasionally appear silent (less than 10 µV) for a brief period and is usually followed by irregular diffuse slowing.

Genetics

Patients with epilepsy with GTC seizures only frequently have a positive family history of epilepsy. Most recently, different mutations in unrelated families of the chloride channel-2 gene (CLCN2) on chromosome 3q26-qter have been found to be associated with GTC seizures on awakening (37). Interestingly, CAE, JAE, and JME were also found in families with this mutation (37).

Treatment

Monotherapy with lamotrigine or valproate is recommended, with valproate having higher efficacy and lamotrigine fewer side effects (73). Other options include topiramate, levetiracetam, and zonisamide. If the maximum tolerated dose does not reduce seizure frequency, an alternative medication should be tried. In case of monotherapy failure, combination therapy of lamotrigine and valproate may be effective (99). Gabapentin is not helpful, and tiagabine and vigabatrine may exacerbate seizures in some cases, (26). Additionally, the prevention of precipitating factors of seizures such as sleep deprivation and alcohol intake drug treatment is beneficial.

Prognosis

The prognosis of patients with GTC seizures only is very good and usually better than in patients with focal epilepsy and secondary generalized seizures (100). Up to 95% of patients with

GTC seizures of unknown origin will have a continuous 5-year seizure-free period within 20 years after epilepsy onset (100). Twenty-one percent of patients who have been seizure-free for 5 years or longer relapse within a 20-year observation period (100). Frequency of GTC seizure at the time of diagnosis predicts outcome and remission (101). Failure to remit within 2 years of diagnosis reduces the chance or remission in the following years (102).

GENERALIZED EPILEPSY WITH FEBRILE SEIZURES PLUS (GEFS+)

Generalized epilepsy with febrile seizures plus (GEFS+) is a heterogeneous disorder with some features of an IGE. Generalized epilepsy seizure types as well as febrile seizures, focal seizures, and progressive epilepsy syndromes such as Dravet syndrome have been described (103–104). There is an underlying genetic basis for this disorder with four genes identified thus far, but the clinical features of GEFS+ are divergent from typical IGE in some patients. GEFS+ illustrates the complexity of epilepsy syndromes with multiple different phenotypes arising from the same mutation and different mutations giving rise to clinically similar phenotypes, all-in-one syndrome.

Epidemiology

The epidemiology of GEFS+ has not been studied in a large epidemiologic study and the incidence/prevalence is unknown. It has been speculated that GEFS+ is a common childhood syndrome, and detailing this will be a challenge given the clinical heterogeneity that has been attributed to this syndrome thus far (105).

Clinical Features

Most patients with GEFS+ present with febrile seizures in the typical ages between 3 months and 6 years, then continue to either have additional febrile seizures outside of this age range or begin having afebrile seizures as well (103,104). Seizures can persist into late adolescence or longer, and may remit in the early teenage years. A history of febrile seizures in other family members is crucial to the diagnosis.

Febrile seizures begin approximately at the age of 1 year, slightly earlier than in the average infant with febrile seizures. Onset of afebrile seizures may overlap with febrile seizures or may occur after a seizure-free interval between febrile and afebrile seizures.

Neurological exam is normal in the majority of patients described, but may also show cognitive impairment and developmental abnormalities (103,105,106).

Clinical seizures consist of febrile seizures in association with afebrile seizures presenting as GTC seizures or dialeptic seizures (absences). Other seizure types of myoclonic-astatic, atonic, tonic and complex partial seizures have also been described (103,105,106). Seizures usually persist beyond 6 years of age until adolescence or longer.

EEG

The syndrome lacks a clear electroclinical pattern and interictal EEG can be normal. However, interictal epileptiform discharges frequently consist of irregular generalized spike and waves or polyspikes with infrequent 2 to 3 Hz generalized spike-and-wave complexes (103). Due to variable clinical presentations, interictal EEG may also present with focal epileptiform discharges, for example, in the frontal, temporal, and occipital regions (107).

Genetics

Mode of inheritance has been described as autosomal dominant with incomplete penetrance in a number of family pedigrees (103–106).

Five genes have been associated with GEFS+ thus far, three genes encode for a sodium channel subunit and two encode for $GABA_A$ receptor subunit. SCN1A encodes the α1 subunit of the neuronal voltage-gated sodium channel and was implicated in GEFS+ by identified mutations (108). It is suspected to increase excitability by decreasing the inactivation of the channel. SCN1B, which encodes the β1 subunit of the neuronal voltage-gated sodium channel, has also been found to be mutated in families with GEFS+ (109). This mutation is suspected to interfere with the modulation of the gating of the sodium channel leading to neuronal hyperexcitability. SCN2A has also been implicated by a missense mutation in a patient with GEFS+ (110). The γ-2 subunit of the $GABA_A$ receptor (GABRG2) has also been shown to be mutated in patients with the clinical phenotype of GEFS+ at that benzodiazepine-binding site (111). The mutation is predicted to reduce the flow through the channel, decreasing its inhibitory effect.

Treatment

The decision to treat pharmacologically should be made based on seizure frequency and severity of afebrile seizures. Clinical presentation and individual seizure types should determine the treatment approach and selection of AED if applicable. Due to paucity of reported cases, only little information on the efficacy of specific pharmacological treatments is available. Gerard et al. report pharmacological treatment in six out of 15 affected individuals "with success and seizure control in most" after analysis of a multigeneration pedigree of GEFS+ patients in France (112). Interestingly, in one family with a mutation in the GABRG2 gene (GEFS+ Type 3), decreased benzodiazepine sensitivity has been reported (113).

Prognosis

The prognosis is usually very good, but is dependent on the variable clinical phenotypes associated with GEFS+. Spontaneous remission occurs frequently in the early teenage years (10 to 12 years) (111). However, seizures can persist, and several other epilepsy syndromes can develop (CAE, JME, myoclonic–astatic epilepsy, focal epilepsy) (111,114).

IDIOPATHIC GENERALIZED EPILEPSY SYNDROMES AS PART OF THE GENERALIZED EPILEPSY SPECTRUM

Overall, there are many similarities among the above-described types of IGE syndromes. According to Janz (2), 4.6% of cases of CAE evolve into JME when patients reach the usual age of JME onset. A population-based study of 81 children with CAE found that 15% had progressed to JME 9 to 25 years after seizure onset (115). In this study, the development of GTC or myoclonic seizures in a patient with CAE receiving AEDs made the progression to JME very likely (115). Syndromes manifest with the same seizure types, have similar EEG changes, may evolve into one another, and have overlapping genetic origins. Neurologic exams as well as imaging studies are typically normal. Therefore, IGEs may be viewed as a continuous spectrum of conditions, representing common clinical presentations, and overlapping and complex genetic etiologies.

References

1. Camfield CS, Camfield PR. Juvenile myoclonic epilepsy 25 years after seizure onset: a population-based study. *Neurology.* 2009;73(13):1041–1045.
2. Janz D. Juvenile myoclonic epilepsy. epilepsy with impulsive petit mal. *Cleve Clin J Med.* 1989;56(suppl Pt 1):S23–S33; discussion S40–S42.
3. Engel J Jr. A proposed diagnostic scheme for people with epileptic seizures and with epilepsy: report of the ILAE task force on classification and terminology. *Epilepsia.* 2001;42(6):796–803.
4. Engel J Jr. Report of the ILAE classification core group. *Epilepsia.* 2006;47(9):1558–1568.
5. Loiseau P, Duche B, Pedespan JM. Absence epilepsies. *Epilepsia.* 1995;36(12):1182–1186.
6. Hughes JR. Absence seizures: a review of recent reports with new concepts. *Epilepsy Behav.* 2009;15(4):404–412.
7. Jallon P, Latour P. Epidemiology of idiopathic generalized epilepsies. *Epilepsia.* 2005;46(suppl 9):10–14.
8. Tovia E, Goldberg-Stern H, Shahar E, et al. Outcome of children with juvenile absence epilepsy. *J Child Neurol.* 2006;21(9):766–768.
9. Durón RM, Medina MT, Martínez-Juárez IE, et al. Seizures of idiopathic generalized epilepsies. *Epilepsia.* 2005;46(suppl 9):34–47.
10. Dura Trave T, Yoldi Petri ME. Typical absence seizure: epidemiological and clinical characteristics and outcome. *An Pediatr (Barc).* 2006;64(1):28–33.
11. Caplan R, Siddarth P, Stahl L, et al. Childhood absence epilepsy: behavioral, cognitive, and linguistic comorbidities. *Epilepsia.* 2008;49(11):1838–1846.
12. Sirén A, Kylliäinen A, Tenhunen M, et al. Beneficial effects of antiepileptic medication on absence seizures and cognitive functioning in children. *Epilepsy Behav.* 2007;11(1):85–91.
13. Bhise VV, Burack GD, Mandelbaum DE. Baseline cognition, behavior, and motor skills in children with new-onset, idiopathic epilepsy. *Dev Med Child Neurol.* 2009.
14. Betting LE, Mory SB, Lopes-Cendes Í, et al. MRI volumetry shows increased anterior thalamic volumes in patients with absence seizures. *Epilepsy Behav.* 2006;8(3):575–580.
15. Guilhoto LM, Manreza ML, Yacubian EM. Occipital intermittent rhythmic delta activity in absence epilepsy. *Arq Neuropsiquiatr.* 2006;64(2A):193–197.
16. Holmes MD, Brown M, Tucker DM. Are "generalized" seizures truly generalized? Evidence of localized mesial frontal and frontopolar discharges in absence. *Epilepsia.* 2004;45(12):1568–1579.
17. Holmes MD. Dense array EEG: methodology and new hypothesis on epilepsy syndromes. *Epilepsia.* 2008;49(suppl 3):3–14.
18. Metrakos K, Metrakos JD. Genetics of convulsive disorders. II. Genetic and electroencephalographic studies in centrencephalic epilepsy. *Neurology.* 1961;11:474–483.
19. Berkovic SF, Mulley JC, Scheffer IE, et al. Human epilepsies: interaction of genetic and acquired factors. *Trends Neurosci.* 2006;29(7):391–397.
20. Gardiner M. Genetics of idiopathic generalized epilepsies. *Epilepsia.* 2005;46(suppl 9):15–20.
21. Lu Y, Wang X. Genes associated with idiopathic epilepsies: a current overview. *Neurol Res.* 2009;31(2):135–143.
22. Helbig I, Matigian NA, Vadlamudi L, et al. Gene expression analysis in absence epilepsy using a monozygotic twin design. *Epilepsia.* 2008;49(9):1546–1554.
23. Posner EB, Mohamed K, Marson AG. Ethosuximide, sodium valproate or lamotrigine for absence seizures in children and adolescents. *Cochrane Database Syst Rev.* 2005;(4):CD003032.
24. Striano P, Sofia V, Capovilla G, et al. A pilot trial of levetiracetam in eyelid myoclonia with absences (jeavons syndrome). *Epilepsia.* 2008;49(3):425–430.
25. Kim HL, Aldridge J, Rho JM. Clinical experience with zonisamide monotherapy and adjunctive therapy in children with epilepsy at a tertiary care referral center. *J Child Neurol.* 2005;20(3):212–219.
26. Somerville ER. Some treatments cause seizure aggravation in idiopathic epilepsies (especially absence epilepsy). *Epilepsia.* 2009;50(suppl 8):31–36.
27. Perucca E. The management of refractory idiopathic epilepsies. *Epilepsia.* 2001;42(suppl 3):31–35.
28. Appleton RE, Beirne M. Absence epilepsy in children: the role of EEG in monitoring response to treatment. *Seizure.* 1996;5(2):147–148.
29. Bouma PA, Westendorp RG, van Dijk JG, et al. The outcome of absence epilepsy: a meta-analysis. *Neurology.* 1996;47(3):802–808.
30. Callenbach PMC, Bouma PAD, Geerts AT, et al. Long-term outcome of childhood absence epilepsy: Dutch study of epilepsy in childhood. *Epilepsy Res.* 2009;83(2–3):249–256.
31. Obeid T. Clinical and genetic aspects of juvenile absence epilepsy. *J Neurol.* 1994;241(8):487–491.
32. Benbadis SR. Practical management issues for idiopathic generalized epilepsies. *Epilepsia.* 2005;46(suppl 9):125–132.
33. Baykan B, Matur Z, Gurses C, et al. Typical absence seizures triggered by photosensitivity. *Epilepsia.* 2005;46(1):159–163.
34. Lu Y, Waltz S, Stenzel K, Muhle H, et al. Photosensitivity in epileptic syndromes of childhood and adolescence. *Epileptic Disord.* 2008;10(2):136–143.
35. Beck-Mannagetta G, Janz D. Syndrome-related genetics in generalized epilepsy. *Epilepsy Res Suppl.* 1991;4:105–111.
36. Sander T, Hildmann T, Kretz R, et al. Allelic association of juvenile absence epilepsy with a GluR5 kainate receptor gene (GRIK1) polymorphism. *Am J Med Genet.* 1997;74(4):416–421.
37. Haug K, Warnstedt M, Alekov AK, et al. Mutations in CLCN2 encoding a voltage-gated chloride channel are associated with idiopathic generalized epilepsies. *Nat Genet.* 2003;33(4):527–532.
38. Obeid T, Panayiotopoulos CP. Juvenile myoclonic epilepsy: a study in Saudi Arabia. *Epilepsia.* 1988;29(3):280–282.
39. Nair RR, Thomas SV. Genetic liability to epilepsy in Kerala state, India. *Epilepsy Res.* 2004;62(2–3):163–170.
40. Gram L, Alving J, Sagild JC, et al. Juvenile myoclonic epilepsy in unexpected age groups. *Epilepsy Res.* 1988;2(2):137–140.
41. Welty TE. Juvenile myoclonic epilepsy: epidemiology, pathophysiology, and management. *Paediatr Drugs.* 2006;8(5):303–310.
42. Panayiotopoulos CP, Obeid T, Tahan AR. Juvenile myoclonic epilepsy: a 5-year prospective study. *Epilepsia.* 1994;35(2):285–296.
43. Lancman ME, Asconape JJ, Penry JK. Clinical and EEG asymmetries in juvenile myoclonic epilepsy. *Epilepsia.* 1994;35(2):302–306.
44. Panayiotopoulos CP, Obeid T, Waheed G. Absences in juvenile myoclonic epilepsy: a clinical and video-electroencephalographic study. *Ann Neurol.* 1989;25(4):391–397.
45. Badawy RAB, Macdonell RAL, Jackson GD, et al. Why do seizures in generalized epilepsy often occur in the morning? *Neurology.* 2009;73(3):218–222.
46. Badawy RAB, Curatolo JM, Newton M, et al. Sleep deprivation increases cortical excitability in epilepsy: syndrome-specific effects. *Neurology.* 2006;67(6):1018–1022.
47. Pascalicchio TF, de Araujo Filho GM, da Silva Noffs MH, et al. Neuropsychological profile of patients with juvenile myoclonic epilepsy: a controlled study of 50 patients. *Epilepsy Behav.* 2007;10(2):263–267.
48. Iqbal N, Caswell HL, Hare DJ, et al. Neuropsychological profiles of patients with juvenile myoclonic epilepsy and their siblings: a preliminary controlled experimental video-EEG case series. *Epilepsy Behav.* 2009;14(3):516–521.
49. Betting LE, Mory SB, Lopes-Cendes I, et al. MRI reveals structural abnormalities in patients with idiopathic generalized epilepsy. *Neurology.* 2006;67(5):848–852.
50. Woermann FG, Free SL, Koepp MJ, et al. Abnormal cerebral structure in juvenile myoclonic epilepsy demonstrated with voxel-based analysis of MRI. *Brain.* 1999;122(11):2101–2108.
51. Swartz BE, Simpkins F, Halgren E, et al. Visual working memory in primary generalized epilepsy: an 18FDG-PET study. *Neurology.* 1996;47(5):1203–1212.
52. de Araujo Filho GM, Lin K, Lin J, et al. Are personality traits of juvenile myoclonic epilepsy related to frontal lobe dysfunctions? A proton MRS study. *Epilepsia.* 2009;50(5):1201–1209.
53. Roebling R, Scheerer N, Uttner I, et al. Evaluation of cognition, structural, and functional MRI in juvenile myoclonic epilepsy. *Epilepsia.* 2009;50(11):2456–2465.
54. Aslan K, Bozdemir H, Yapar Z, et al. The effect of electrophysiological and neuroimaging findings on the prognosis of juvenile myoclonic epilepsy proband. *Neurol Res.* 2009, PMID: 19660236.

55. Holmes MD, Quiring J, Tucker DM. Evidence that juvenile myoclonic epilepsy is a disorder of frontotemporal corticothalamic networks. *Neuroimage.* 2010;49(1):80–93.

56. Liu AW, Delgado-Escueta AV, Gee MN, et al. Juvenile myoclonic epilepsy in chromosome 6p12-p11: locus heterogeneity and recombinations. *Am J Med Genet.* 1996;63(3):438–446.

57. Andrade DM. Genetic basis in epilepsies caused by malformations of cortical development and in those with structurally normal brain. *Hum Genet.* 2009;126(1):173–193.

58. Marini C, King MA, Archer JS, et al. Idiopathic generalized epilepsy of adult onset: clinical syndromes and genetics. *J Neurol Neurosurg Psychiatry.* 2003;74(2):192–196.

59. Mulley JC, Scheffer IE, Petrou S, et al. Channelopathies as a genetic cause of epilepsy. *Curr Opin Neurol.* 2003;16(2):171–176.

60. Delgado-Escueta A. Advances in genetics of juvenile myoclonic epilepsies. *Epilepsy Curr.* 2007;7(3):61–67.

61. Pal DK, Evgrafov OV, Tabares P, et al. BRD2 (RING3) is a probable major susceptibility gene for common juvenile myoclonic epilepsy. *Am J Hum Gen.* 2003;73(2):261–270.

62. Hempelmann A, Heils A, Sander T. Confirmatory evidence for an association of the connexin-36 gene with juvenile myoclonic epilepsy. *Epilepsy Res.* 2006;71(2–3):223–228.

63. Suzuki T, Delgado-Escueta AV, Aguan K, et al. Mutations in EFHC1 cause juvenile myoclonic epilepsy. *Nat Genet.* 2004;36(8):842–849.

64. de Nijs L, Leon C, Nguyen L, et al. EFHC1 interacts with microtubules to regulate cell division and cortical development. *Nat Neurosci.* 2009;12(10):1266–1274.

65. Medina MT, Suzuki T, Alonso ME, et al. Novel mutations in Myoclonin1/EFHC1 in sporadic and familial juvenile myoclonic epilepsy. *Neurology.* 2008;70(22 Part 2):2137–2144.

66. Suzuki T, Miyamoto H, Nakahari T, et al. Efhc1 deficiency causes spontaneous myoclonus and increased seizure susceptibility. *Hum Mol Genet.* 2009;18(6):1099–1109.

67. Kleefuss-Lie A, Friedl W, Cichon S, et al. CLCN2 variants in idiopathic generalized epilepsy. *Nat Genet.* 2009;41(9):954–955.

68. Cossette P, Liu L, Brisebois K, et al. Mutation of GABRA1 in an autosomal dominant form of juvenile myoclonic epilepsy. *Nat Genet.* 2002;31(2):184–189.

69. Gallagher MJ, Ding L, Maheshwari A, et al. The GABAA receptor α1 subunit epilepsy mutation A322D inhibits transmembrane helix formation and causes proteasomal degradation. *Proc Natl Acad Sci USA.* 2007;104(32):12999–13004.

70. Escayg A, De Waard M, Lee DD, et al. Coding and noncoding variation of the human calcium-channel β4-subunit gene CACNB4 in patients with idiopathic generalized epilepsy and episodic ataxia. *Am J Hum Genet.* 2000;66(5):1531–1539.

71. Penry JK, Dean JC, Riela AR. Juvenile myoclonic epilepsy: long-term response to therapy. *Epilepsia.* 1989;30(suppl 4):S19–S23; discussion S24–S27.

72. Delgado-Escueta AV, Treiman DM, Walsh GO. The treatable epilepsies. *N Engl J Med.* 1983;308(25):1508–1514.

73. Marson AG, Al-Kharusi AM, Alwaidh M, et al. The SANAD study of effectiveness of valproate, lamotrigine, or topiramate for generalised and unclassifiable epilepsy: an unblinded randomised controlled trial. *Lancet.* 2007;369(9566):1016–1026.

74. Corman CL, Leung NM, Guberman AH. Weight gain in epileptic patients during treatment with valproic acid: a retrospective study. *Can J Neurol Sci.* 1997;24(3):240–244.

75. Karlovassitou-Koniari A, Alexiou D, Angelopoulos P, et al. Low dose sodium valproate in the treatment of juvenile myoclonic epilepsy. *J Neurol.* 2002;249(4):396–399.

76. Prasad A, Kuzniecky RI, Knowlton RC, et al. Evolving antiepileptic drug treatment in juvenile myoclonic epilepsy. *Arch Neurol.* 2003;60(8):1100–1105.

77. Crespel A, Genton P, Berramdane M, et al. Lamotrigine associated with exacerbation or de novo myoclonus in idiopathic generalized epilepsies. *Neurology.* 2005;65(5):762–764.

78. Morris GL, Hammer AE, Kustra RP, et al. Lamotrigine for patients with juvenile myoclonic epilepsy following prior treatment with valproate: results of an open-label study. *Epilepsy Behav.* 2004;5(4):509–512.

79. Guberman AH, Besag FM, Brodie MJ, et al. Lamotrigine-associated rash: risk/benefit considerations in adults and children. *Epilepsia.* 1999;40(7):985–991.

80. Wheless JW. Use of topiramate in childhood generalized seizure disorders. *J Child Neurol.* 2000;15(suppl 1):S7–S13.

81. Levisohn PM, Holland KD. Topiramate or valproate in patients with juvenile myoclonic epilepsy: a randomized open-label comparison. *Epilepsy Behav.* 2007;10(4):547–552.

82. Kumar SP, Smith PE. Levetiracetam as add-on therapy in generalised epilepsies. *Seizure.* 2004;13(7):475–477.

83. Krauss GL, Betts T, Abou-Khalil B, et al. Levetiracetam treatment of idiopathic generalised epilepsy. *Seizure.* 2003;12(8):617–620.

84. Berkovic SF, Knowlton RC, Leroy RF, et al. On behalf of the Levetiracetam N01057 Study Group. Placebo-controlled study of levetiracetam in idiopathic generalized epilepsy. *Neurology.* 2007;69(18):1751–1760.

85. Noachtar S, Andermann E, Meyvisch P, et al. Levetiracetam for the treatment of idiopathic generalized epilepsy with myoclonic seizures. *Neurology.* 2008;70(8):607–616.

86. Yamauchi T, Aikawa H. Efficacy of zonisamide: our experience. *Seizure.* 2004;13(suppl 1):S41–S48.

87. Yagi K. Overview of japanese experience—controlled and uncontrolled trials. *Seizure.* 2004;13(suppl 1):S11–S15.

88. Kothare SV, Valencia I, Khurana DS, et al. Efficacy and tolerability of zonisamide in juvenile myoclonic epilepsy. *Epileptic Disord.* 2004;6(4):267–270.

89. Craig JJ, Hunt SJ. Treating women with juvenile myoclonic epilepsy. *Pract Neurol.* 2009;9(5):268–277.

90. Eriksson K, Viinikainen K, Mönkkönen A, et al. Children exposed to valproate in utero: population based evaluation of risks and confounding factors for long-term neurocognitive development. *Epilepsy Res.* 2005;65(3):189–200.

91. Cunnington M, Ferber S, Quartey G, International Lamotrigine Pregnancy Registry Scientific Advisory Committee. Effect of dose on the frequency of major birth defects following fetal exposure to lamotrigine monotherapy in an international observational study. *Epilepsia.* 2007;48(6):1207–1210.

92. Morrow J, Russell A, Guthrie E, et al. Malformation risks of antiepileptic drugs in pregnancy: a prospective study from the UK epilepsy and pregnancy register. *J Neurol Neurosurg Psychiatry.* 2006;77(2):193–198.

93. Pennell PB, Peng L, Newport DJ, et al. Lamotrigine in pregnancy: clearance, therapeutic drug monitoring, and seizure frequency. *Neurology.* 2008;70(22 Part 2):2130–2136.

94. Meador KJ, Baker GA, Browning N, et al. Cognitive function at 3 years of age after fetal exposure to antiepileptic drugs. *N Engl J Med.* 2009;360(16):1597–1605.

95. Delgado-Escueta AV, Enrile-Bacsal F. Juvenile myoclonic epilepsy of janz. *Neurology.* 1984;34(3):285–294.

96. Zarrelli MM, Beghi E, Rocca WA, et al. Incidence of epileptic syndromes in Rochester, Minnesota: 1980–1984. *Epilepsia.* 1999;40(12):1708–1714.

97. Wolf P. Epilepsy with grand mal on awakening. In: Roger J, Bureau M, Dravet C, eds. *Epilepsy with Grand Mal on Awakening.* London: John Libbey & Company; 1992:329–341.

98. Unterberger I, Trinka E, Luef G, et al. Idiopathic generalized epilepsies with pure grand mal: clinical data and genetics. *Epilepsy Res.* 2001;44(1):19–25.

99. Panayiotopoulos CP. Idiopathic generalized epilepsies: a review and modern approach. *Epilepsia.* 2005;46(suppl 9):1–6.

100. Annegers JF, Hauser WA, Elveback LR. Remission of seizures and relapse in patients with epilepsy. *Epilepsia.* 1979;20(6):729–737.

101. Emerson R, D'Souza BJ, Vining EP, et al. Stopping medication in children with epilepsy: predictors of outcome. *N Engl J Med.* 1981;304(19):1125–1129.

102. Elwes RD, Johnson AL, Shorvon SD, et al. The prognosis for seizure control in newly diagnosed epilepsy. *N Engl J Med.* 1984;311(15):944–947.

103. Scheffer IE, Berkovic SF. Generalized epilepsy with febrile seizures plus. A genetic disorder with heterogeneous clinical phenotypes. *Brain.* 1997;120 (Pt 3):479–490.

104. Scheffer IE, Harkin LA, Dibbens LM, et al. Neonatal epilepsy syndromes and generalized epilepsy with febrile seizures plus (GEFS+). *Epilepsia.* 2005;46(suppl 10):41–47.

105. Singh R, Scheffer IE, Crossland K, et al. Generalized epilepsy with febrile seizures plus: a common childhood-onset genetic epilepsy syndrome. *Ann Neurol.* 1999;45(1):75–81.

106. Scheffer IE, Wallace R, Mulley JC, et al. Clinical and molecular genetics of myoclonic–astatic epilepsy and severe myoclonic epilepsy in infancy (dravet syndrome). *Brain Dev.* 2001;23(7):732–735.

107. Deng YH, Berkovic SF, Scheffer IE. GEFS+ where focal seizures evolve from generalized spike wave: video-EEG study of two children. *Epileptic Disord.* 2007;9(3):307–314.

108. Escayg A, MacDonald BT, Meisler MH, et al. Mutations of SCN1A, encoding a neuronal sodium channel, in two families with GEFS+2. *Nat Genet.* 2000;24(4):343–345.

109. Wallace RH, Wang DW, Singh R, et al. Febrile seizures and generalized epilepsy associated with a mutation in the Na+-channel beta1 subunit gene SCN1B. *Nat Genet.* 1998;19(4):366–370.

110. Sugawara T, Tsurubuchi Y, Agarwala KL, et al. A missense mutation of the Na+ channel alpha II subunit gene na(v)1.2 in a patient with febrile and afebrile seizures causes channel dysfunction. *Proc Natl Acad Sci USA.* 2001;98(11):6384–6389.

111. Baulac S, Huberfeld G, Gourfinkel-An I, et al. First genetic evidence of GABA(A) receptor dysfunction in epilepsy: a mutation in the γ2-subunit gene. *Nat Genet.* 2001;28(1):46–48.

112. Gerard F, Pereira S, Robaglia-Schlupp A, et al. Clinical and genetic analysis of a new multigenerational pedigree with GEFS+ (generalized epilepsy with febrile seizures plus). *Epilepsia.* 2002;43(6):581–586.

113. Wallace RH, Scheffer IE, Barnett S, et al. Neuronal sodium-channel alpha1-subunit mutations in generalized epilepsy with febrile seizures plus. *Am J Hum Genet.* 2001;68(4):859–865.

114. Marini C, Harkin LA, Wallace RH, et al. Childhood absence epilepsy and febrile seizures: a family with a GABA(A) receptor mutation. *Brain.* 2003;126(Pt 1):230–240.

115. Wirrell EC, Camfield CS, Camfield PR, et al. Long-term prognosis of typical childhood absence epilepsy: remission or progression to juvenile myoclonic epilepsy. *Neurology.* 1996;47(4):912–918.

CHAPTER 21 ■ PROGRESSIVE AND INFANTILE MYOCLONIC EPILEPSIES

BERND A. NEUBAUER, ANDREAS HAHN, AND INGRID TUXHORN

Myoclonus is defined as a sudden, brief (<100 msec) involuntary contraction of one muscle or muscle groups. Topography can be variable. Typically, agonistic and antagonistic muscles are involved simultaneously. Epileptic myoclonus is characterized by electromyographic (EMG) discharges of 10–100 ms duration. This EMG burst may be preceded by discharge (spikes or polyspikes in general) that may be easily visible on surface electroencephalography (EEG) (Fig. 21.1) or that may only be detectable when jerk-locked back-averaging or other sophisticated techniques are applied. Epileptic negative myoclonus is defined as an interruption of tonic muscular activity for <500 msec without evidence of antecedent myoclonia (Fig. 21.2). The term clonic means the rhythmic repetition of a myoclonic jerk, mainly at a rate of 2–3 sec. Myoclonic seizures predominantly affect limb, axial, neck, and shoulder muscles, and less frequently facial and extraocular muscles. Rarely, myoclonic seizures occur in series and evolve into a myoclonic status epilepticus, with or without complete loss of consciousness. In most epilepsy syndromes with myoclonic seizures as the cardinal feature additional seizure types occur at lesser frequency. Mostly, these other seizure types include generalized tonic–clonic seizures (GCTS), generalized clonic seizures, atonic seizures, absence seizures, and atypical absences (1).

ETIOLOGY

Myoclonic epilepsies are predominantly genetic in origin. In terms of classification they may be grouped as idiopathic epilepsies (e.g., benign myoclonic epilepsy in infancy [BMEI]), epileptic encephalopathies (e.g., Dravet syndrome), or progressive myoclonic epilepsies (e.g., Unverricht–Lundborg disease).

BMEI usually presents in normally developed children, and in the majority of cases anitepileptic treatment may be weaned after some years of active epilepsy. Behavioral and cognitive prognosis is good in the majority of cases. Familial cases are extremely rare, with the exception of one case identified in the context of a generalized epilepsy with febrile seizures plus (GEFS+) family (2) and a family with three affected children (3). However, a positive family history for febrile seizures or idiopathic epilepsies was repeatedly reported (4). Altogether, classification as an idiopathic generalized epilepsy syndrome seems unequivocal. The etiology is most likely oligogenic or complex (several genes and possibly environmental factors involved).

Myoclonic astatic epilepsy (MAE) or Doose syndrome, initially described by Doose and coworkers, was reported to be an idiopathic generalized epilepsy syndrome (5). The separation of this syndrome from a group of epilepsies that were formerly classified as symptomatic (many of them as Lennox–Gastaut syndrome) was only reluctantly accepted. This is mirrored by the fact that MAE was classified among the "cryptogenic or symptomatic generalized epilepsies and syndromes" for many years. Now it is recognized that the initial description of Doose et al. included cases that from today's point of view might also be diagnosed as benign myoclonic and severe myoclonic epilepsies, but the current classification scheme now accepts Doose syndrome as an idiopathic generalized epilepsy syndrome (6). As with BMEI, familial cases are exceptional, but retrospective studies demonstrated positive family histories for febrile seizures and idiopathic epilepsy syndromes at a clearly elevated rate (7). Although in single cases genetic defects in the genes (mostly *SCN1A*) known to be involved in GEFS+ families were reported, the majority of patients do not carry an identifiable defect in these genes (8).

Severe myoclonic epilepsy of infancy (SMEI) or Dravet syndrome from one point of view may be classified as an idiopathic genetic disorder, since children are healthy and normally developed until onset of the epilepsy, and there is a clear genetic cause (usually a *SCN1A* defect) in the majority of cases. The syndrome may even be observed in GEFS+ families (9). However, Dravet syndrome is a devastating disorder with an extremely severe course in most patients, hence it was declared an epileptic encephalopathy (6).

Progressive myoclonus epilepsies (PMEs) are defined as neurometabolic or neurodegenerative diseases with myoclonias and myoclonic seizures as dominating clinical features.

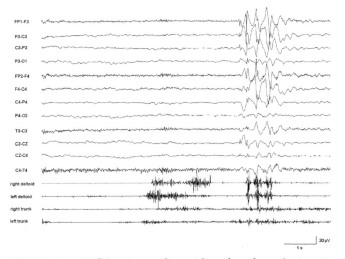

FIGURE 21.1 EEG-EMG recording with surface electrodes in a 3-year-old boy with myoclonic astatic epilepsy (Doose syndrome). Three brief and symmetric myoclonic jerks each time-locked to single generalized single spike wave discharges are recorded from both deltoid muscles.

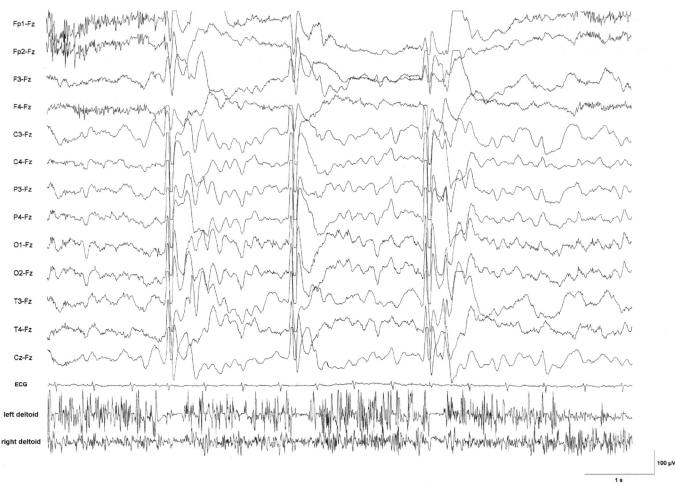

FIGURE 21.2 EEG-EMG recording with surface electrodes in a 6-year-old boy with epileptic negative myoclonus due to lesion-related epilepsy. Silent periods in the EMG from the deltoid muscles lasting between 100 and 150 msec are time-locked to a generalized sharp slow wave complex. Clinically, each brief EMG pause was associated with nodding of the head and sinking of the arms during sustained muscle contraction.

Frequently myoclonic seizures represent the initial clinical symptom. These disorders are in general progressive, however, course varies from moderately mild (e.g., Unverricht–Lundborg) to rapidly progressive and fatal (e.g. NCL type 2). PMEs follow a monogenic, mostly autosomal recessive mode of inheritance (10). Some diseases such as Rett-like syndrome (CDKL-5 defects) are usually not regarded as "classic" PME, but may at certain stages and in individual patients show the typical symptomatology and course of a PME. These disorders, which frequently manifest during infancy or early childhood, may be summarized as progressive encephalopathies with myoclonic seizures (Table 21.1).

BENIGN MYOCLONIC EPILEPSY IN INFANCY (BMEI)

Definition and Epidemiology

BMEI is a rare epilepsy syndrome. Its classic description was done by Dravet and Bureau (11). Altogether about 110 cases have been reported and it is estimated that BMEI accounts for less than 1% of childhood epilepsies (12). BMEI is mainly recognized in Europe (France, Italy), and it may be suspected that in cases with rare myoclonic seizures or seizures that respond quickly to therapy, correct classification may not be applied, thereby underestimating its real prevalence. Some cases may overlap with MAE (Doose syndrome). Boys are affected twice as much (4).

Symptomatology

Onset is mostly between 4 months and 3 years, but may extend up to the 5 years. Febrile seizures antecedent to myoclonic seizures are reported in about 30% of cases. In the beginning, myoclonic seizures are often rare and brief, involving predominantly the upper limbs. But intensity and frequency of the seizures increase often early during course. In the largest series reported, polygraphic video EEG recordings revealed that myoclonic seizures consisted of axial jerks with head drop, elevation and extension of both arms, flexion of the legs, and upward gaze. Myoclonic seizures may vary in intensity ranging from simple head nods to severe falls, when generalized. Seizures may occur repetitively, but usually only in short trains lasting 1–3 sec. Usually they are symmetrical, but rarely may be unilateral. In about a third of patients they are triggered by stimuli like noise, startle, or photic stimulation. Drowsiness is also known to provoke myoclonic seizures (4).

TABLE 21.1

PROGRESSIVE MYOCLONIC EPILEPSIES AND PROGRESSIVE ENCEPHALOPATHIES WITH MYOCLONIC SEIZURES

- *With manifestation during neonatal period/early infancy*
  - Vitamin B6-dependent epilepsy/pyridoxal-phosphate-dependent epilepsy
  - Folinic acid-responsive seizures
  - Nonketotic hyperglycinemia
  - Sulphite oxidase deficiency/molybdenum cofactor deficit
  - X-linked cyclin-dependent kinase-like 5 (*CDKL5*) encephalopathy
  - X-linked myoclonic epilepsy with spasticity and intellectual disability associated with mutations in the *ARX* gene
  - Urea cycle deficits
  - Zellweger syndrome/other peroxisomal disorders
  - GABA-transaminase deficiency
  - Others (e.g., aminoacidopathies, organic acidurias, deficits of β-oxidation of fatty acids, CDG-syndrome variants)
- *With manifestation during late infancy/early childhood*
  - Glucose transporter (GLUT-1) deficiency (De Vivo disease)
  - Early infantile neuronal ceroid lipofuscinosis (*CLN 1*)
  - Late infantile neuronal ceroid lipofuscinosis (*CLN 2*)
  - Mitochondrial cytopathies (e.g., Alpers–Huttenlocher disease, Leigh syndrome)
  - Menkes disease
  - GM2 gangliosidosis
  - Holocarboxlase synthetase deficiency/biotinidase deficiency
  - Hereditary anomalies in serine synthesis
  - Succinic semialdehyde dehydrogenase deficiency
  - Others (e.g., glutathione peroxidase deficiency, methylenetetrahydrofolate reductase deficiency)
- *With manifestation during late childhood/adolescence*
  - Juvenile neuronal ceroid lipofuscinosis (*CLN3*)
  - Adult neuronal ceroid lipofuscinosis (*CNL 4*)
  - Neuronal ceroid lipofuscinosis variants (*CLN 3, CLN 5, CLN 6*)
  - Myoclonic epilepsy with ragged red fibers (MERRF)
  - Unverricht–Lundborg disease
  - Lafora disease
  - Sialidosis types I and II
  - Galactosialidosis
  - Neuroserpinosis
  - Dentato-rubro-pallido-luysian atrophy
  - Juvenile form of Huntington disease
  - Gaucher disease (type III)
  - Action myoclonus-renal failure syndrome
  - Leukoencephalopathy with vanishing white matter
  - Others

EEG

Background activity is normal. Myoclonic jerks are associated with generalized spike waves and polyspike waves. Ictal spikes last for 1–3 sec. Most, if not all, myoclonic seizures are associated with discharges on the surface EEG. EEG discharges are generalized with a fronto-central accentuation. After the myoclonia there may be a short atonia that may result in a drop, that is, a myoclonic astatic seizure. Focal abnormalities, usually spike waves in sleep recordings, were reported in some patients (4). Its significance is unknown.

Treatment and Prognosis

Valproic acid is the drug of first choice and is usually the only drug needed to control the seizures in the majority of cases. Some authors recommend high plasma levels at the start of treatment (up to 100 mg/L) (13). Ethosuximide, benzodiazepines, and phenobarbitale were also effective in the few cases reported who did not receive valproic acid. Altogether there seems to be no specific difference in treatment compared to MAE. Untreated cases continue with pure myoclonic seizures even if the epilepsy lasts for years. Developmental delay and behavioral disturbances are reported in a substantial number of patients. Precise numbers vary substantially between different series, ranging from 0 to 86% (14). A rate of 20–30% seems acceptable. This renders the term "benign" questionable and makes it difficult to differentiate cases with frequent generalized myoclonic seizures and evolving developmental delay from patients with MAE. Bureau and Dravet are convinced that mental prognosis depends on early diagnosis and successful treatment (4). However, there are no controlled studies with antiepileptic drugs (AED) on record and there are no good data on required treatment duration. By definition, myoclonic seizures will disappear eventually in all cases. Most reported children older than 6 years were already weaned off medication without seizure relapse. But in some patients, generalized tonic–clonic seizures (GTCS) occurred when valproate treatment was stopped. While a subgroup with overt reflex seizures appears to be very easily controlled by AED, cases with marked photosensitivity may be more difficult to control (4).

MYOCLONIC ASTATIC EPILEPSY (MAE)/DOOSE SYNDROME

Definition and Epidemiology

The prominent genetic etiology together with the characteristic seizure symptomatology dominated by myoclonic and myoclonic astatic seizures led Doose and coworkers to delineate MAE as an idiopathic generalized epilepsy syndrome of its own right (5). MAE, as a rule, occurs in children with an uneventful history. The epilepsy starts in 94% during the first 5 years of age and accounts for 1–2% of all childhood epilepsies (15). Doose and coworkers reported that in about 20% the seizures have their onset during the first year of life (7,16). Today, many authors feel that onset before the second year of life is exceptional. The age of peak presentation is 3 years (17). Like most other myoclonic epilepsies of early childhood, it affects more boys than girls. The sex ratio is about 2.7/1 (16). If the inclusion criteria include all children older than 1 year, this ratio might even reach 3/1 (17).

Symptomatology

In about 60% of cases, the epilepsy starts with febrile or afebrile GTCS. Alternating grand mal (i.e., hemi-grand mal, unilateral seizures) is a possible presentation. Some days or short weeks later, myoclonic and/or myoclonic-astatic seizures set in in abundance, frequently in combination with brief absences. At first, this occurs predominantly after awakening. Tonic axial seizures may manifest during long-term course, frequently occurring during sleep. Myoclonic seizures consist of symmetric, mostly generalized jerks, accentuated in the arms and the shoulders, and are frequently associated with a simultaneous flexion of the head. The intensity of these seizures is variable and ranges from violent myoclonic jerks with sudden falls to abortive forms merely presenting as short irregular twitches of the face. Myoclonic-astatic seizures are characterized by a loss of muscle tone preceded by a (short) myoclonia. In polygraphic recordings, the loss of muscle tone corresponds to a silent period in the EMG that is paralleled by the slow wave in the EEG following the spikes or polyspikes of the myoclonus. Myoclonic seizures with and without discernable myotonia frequently occur together. The initial myoclonia and the subsequent myotonia equally contribute to the characteristic myoclonic astatic seizure (18–20). Absences are seen in more than half of the children with MAE. Myoclonic and astatic seizures, when they come in series, are frequently accompanied by absences often combined with myoclonic jerks. A unique type of nonconvulsive-status epilepticus ("status of minor seizures") is a rather specific finding observed in 36% (5,7,18) to 95% (17) of MAE patients. The characteristic clinical picture is a somnolent, stuporous child with subtle myoclonic seizures, frequently involving the face and the extremities. The child is unresponsive, drools, has a slurred speech, or is even aphasic. This status may continue for days if not interrupted by adequate means.

EEG

Background activity is of special interest in MAE. In cases starting with GTCS, the EEG may stay entirely normal for weeks. However, almost in all instances a rhythmic, parietally accentuated 4- to 7-Hz activity develops early in the course. This rhythmic slowing of background activity was frequently questioned and falsely attributed to drowsiness. In patients with MAE (and other idiopathic generalized epilepsies of early childhood with myoclonic seizures) it represents a constant trait that is not related to the state of vigilance (Fig. 21.3). This has been documented by EEG recordings of children who were kept attentive by displaying cartoons and so on (20). During the early stages, spikes, irregular spikes, and polyspikes may well be absent and appear only after some delay starting during sleep. If myoclonic seizures dominate the course at a given time, the EEG shows short paroxysms of irregular spikes and polyspikes. In children with astatic and myoclonic astatic seizures, 2- to 3-Hz spikes and waves appear. As the epilepsy progresses, typical absence patterns may appear. During a status of myoclonic-astatic seizures, the EEG displays continuous spike waves with interposed slow waves. Especially in younger children, an irregular polymorphous hypersynchronous activity, sometimes resembling

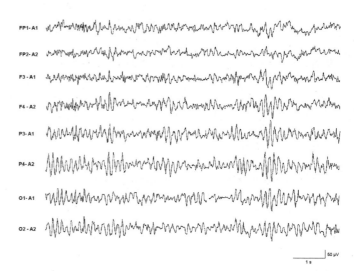

FIGURE 21.3 EEG recording in a 10-year-old boy with Doose syndrome and favorable course of epilepsy, showing a persistent fast theta activity several years after his last seizure. (With permission from Doose H. *EEG in Childhood Epilepsy—Initial Presentation and Long-Term Follow-Up.* First ed. Montrouge: John Libbey; 2003.)

hypsarrhythmia may be recorded. During nocturnal tonic seizures typical 10- to 15-Hz spike series can be observed. In distinction to the tonic seizures observed in Lennox–Gastaut syndrome the EEG onset is generalized in MAE.

Therapy and Prognosis

Revised treatment standards over the last years have significantly improved outcome and prognosis (21). Valproic acid is still the drug of first choice. If efforts fail to achieve complete remission the decision which drug to use next depends on the predominating seizure type. If absences prevail, ethosuximide should be commenced as the next step. If GTCS represent the leading semiology, bromide is frequently the most effective drug, even superior to phenobarbital or primidone (22). Lamotrigine may be effective, but is also known to provoke myoclonic seizures in generalized myoclonic epilepsies. It therefore may represent a valuable option, but has to be used with caution (23). Basing on the broad mechanism of action, topiramate is an additional possibility. However, no data on its effectiveness in MAE are yet available. Carbamazepine, phenytoin, and vigabatrin should be avoided, for they frequently provoke seizure exacerbation (17,24,25). In cases with refractory nonconvulsive status epilepticus adrenocorticotrophic hormone (ACTH) or high-dose steroid-pulse therapy may be alternatives to be considered (24). Zonisamide is effective in myoclonic epilepsies of different etiology (26). Levetiracetam may be used successfully in myoclonic epilepsies; however, it may also aggravate seizures (27). Ketogenic diet is a further possibility that was reported as effective (28).

Already from the early descriptions of the disorder it becomes clear that outcome is highly variable. The spectrum ranges from complete remission (frequently obtained within the first 3 years) and totally normal intellectual development to therapy resistant epilepsy with severe cognitive disability (5,21,24,29). Over the years, however, therapeutic possibilities constantly improved and the danger of seizure and epilepsy aggravation by carbamazepine and phenytoin was more and more recognized. In a series of 81 patients with MAE, 68% became eventually seizure-free. In this retrospective Japanese series, ACTH, ethosuximide, and ketogenic diet proved especially effective (21). Repetitive nonconvulsive status epilepticus ("status of minor seizures") and nocturnal tonic seizures were frequently associated with an unfavorable prognosis (16,21). This is however not unequivocal (17).

SEVERE MYOCLONIC EPILEPSY OF INFANCY (SMEI)/DRAVET SYNDROME

Definition and Epidemiology

This electro-clinical syndrome was delineated by Dravet in 1978 and soon was labeled SMEI (30). Later it was recognized that in a substantial number of cases myoclonic seizures and single other features may be lacking, and still the epilepsy will take the same course. This led to the proposal to rename the epilepsy to Dravet syndrome, which is now recognized as an epileptic encephalopathy (6). In order to include cases that seemed to belong to the same entity but lacked single features of classic SMEI recently the term "borderline SMEI" (SMEB) was introduced. Different variants of what is now called SMEB were earlier recognized independently by different authors, such as "intractable childhood epilepsy with GCTS," "severe idiopathic epilepsy of infancy with generalized tonic–clonic convulsions," "severe polymorphic epilepsy of infants," and even a few others (cited in 8).

The rate of cases with Dravet syndrome seems to augment constantly as the syndrome may be diagnosed increasingly frequently by *SCN1A* (alpha subunit of the neuronal type I sodium channel) gene analysis (31,32). This unique opportunity has sharpened the diagnostic view of the medical community. After one has succeeded in diagnosing a few cases, it frequently becomes an experience of pattern recognition. Therefore, the formerly calculated incidence of 1/40,000 may be an underestimate (33). It is of note that many epileptic vaccine encephalopathies in which an immunization-provoked fever triggered the epilepsy were retrospectively identified as having a *SCN1A* mutation (34).

Symptomatology

The disease most frequently starts with febrile seizures within the first year of life, in an up to then healthy child. These seizures may initially be indiscernible from regular febrile seizures, but frequently become prolonged. Fever, infections without fever, vaccinations, hot baths, or even only hot weather may trigger recurrent seizures. These may occur generalized or unilateral affecting different sides of the body on different occasions (i.e., alternating hemi-grand mal, unilateral seizures, hemi-clonic convulsions). The tendency to suffer temperature-sensitive seizures seems to persist over many years. In the series of Dravet and coworkers, short, single myoclonias were noted by some parents before onset of febrile seizures (33). Even though approximately 70% of cases begin with generalized or unilateral febrile seizures, focal seizures may occur already early in the course, but this is not the rule. Febrile seizures typically occur repeatedly within the first year of life and are frequently the dominating manifestation of the epilepsy in the first 9 months of age. Later, afebrile generalized seizures add to the febrile seizures and are soon followed by myoclonic seizures and atypical absences (33).

Dravet and coworkers define "steady-state seizures" as those that prevail in many cases throughout the course (33). The authors recognize 10 different seizure types:

1. "GCTS" basically identical to those encountered in idiopathic generalized epilepsy syndromes.
2. "Hemi-clonic convulsions" are frequent in the first 3 years of life, then they become rare. Postictal hemiparesis is a frequent feature. If they—by chance—reoccur on a specific side of the body, they may falsely be taken for focal seizures.
3. "Falsely generalized seizures" clinically appear like GCTS. On polygraphic recordings this seizure can be resolved as bilateral asymmetric tonic contractions of different muscle groups.
4. "Unstable seizures" are clinically related to "falsely generalized seizures" with concomitant focal EEG discharges that change their origin between and during seizures.
5. Myoclonic seizures predominantly affect the axial muscles and may range from mild to severe, from simple head nodding to violent thrashes involving the entire body. Severe myoclonic seizures may result in falls and injuries. Repeated twitching of the head is a third observed type. These seizures may precede generalized tonic–clonic convulsions. Interictal myoclonias (without concomitant epileptic discharges on surface EEG) are a frequent feature, mainly observed in periods with high seizure frequency (roughly 70% of cases). Myoclonic seizures may abate over time.
6. Atypical absences may appear at any age during course; however, mostly after the first year of life. In our view absences are not always "atypical" because regular 3-Hz spike slow wave absences may be recorded. Absences may range from pure impairment of consciousness to absences with intermixed myoclonic seizures. Duration varies between 3 and 10 sec in most cases.
7. Simple and complex focal seizures, frequently associated with strong autonomic reactions such as pallor, cyanosis, and sweating, are detectable in about two third of cases. They may start already within the first year of life, but usually begin later. Adversive seizures and clonic seizures frequently in combination are typical manifestations.
8. Tonic seizures are rare in this syndrome. They seem to resemble those seen in Lennox–Gastaut syndrome, often with a myoclonic component.
9. Obtundation states are episodes of reduced attention (drowsy states). They occur in more than one third of children. Usually, they are associated with erratic myoclonias involving the limbs or the face. These drowsy states may continue for hours or even days. In the EEG dysrhythmic slow waves intermingled with spikes and sharp waves are characteristic. This state may evolve from an overt seizure or end in one.

10. A status of generalized tonic–clonic convulsions may occur without warning. Frequently fever, infection, or even photic stimulation may act provocative. If the status is then falsely treated by phenytoin (a sodium channel blocker) it may have an unfavorable outcome.

Besides intractable epilepsy, a variable degree of developmental delay (usually severe) characterizes the course. Children frequently develop an ill defined moderately severe ataxia (60–70%) and mild pyramidal signs. Usually, ataxia is not disabling, will not prevent from walking, and will attenuate over the years. Besides fever, infection and hot weather conditions, seizures may also be triggered by (hot) water immersion, joyful mood (e.g., birthday party), or physical exercise. Hyperkinetic behavior, especially at times of high seizure frequency, and autistic features are frequent findings. In general, the more severe the epilepsy, the more marked will be the developmental and behavioral problems. Death is reported in about 10% of larger historic series. Causes were mixed, ranging from status epilepticus to drowning, sudden unexplained death in epilepsy, and accidents (33).

EEG

In the first 1 or 2 years of life, the interictal EEG is frequently normal. Photosensitivity may be found in about 40% of cases. Over time, the background activity deteriorates. As reported by Doose, a rhythmic theta activity with accentuation over the central channels and independent of vigilance develops (20). Generalized regular and irregular spike waves as well as multifocal spikes and sharp waves may evolve during the course. In unilateral seizures, lateralized spike wave or slow spike wave activity with intermittent irregular spike wave is observed. In "falsely generalized seizures" an initial amplitude reduction and spike wave and slow spike wave activity with changing asymmetry is observed. In unstable seizures, the epileptic EEG activity is similar, but migrates from one brain region to another during the same seizure. In myoclonic seizures spike wave and polyspike wave discharges occur simultaneously with the myoclonias. Absences are accompanied by irregular 2.5–3.5 generalized spike wave discharges lasting mostly 3–10 sec. Obtundation states (nonconvulsive status epilepticus) are characterized by generalized spike wave and slow spike wave discharges with intermixed fast and slow activities (30).

Treatment and Prognosis

Maybe the most important therapy option is to avoid provocative AED. In most cases of Dravet syndrome, *SCN1A*, the major sodium channel of inhibitory interneurons is reduced in activity or function to as low as 50% of normal. Application of sodium channel blockers (e.g., carbamazepine, oxcarbazepine, phenytoin, lamotrigine) may further aggravate this defect, resulting in seizure provocation up to status epilepticus. Head-to-head studies are impossible to conduct; however, retrospective analyses and clinical observation show that several agents are effective. Frequently, in the first 2 years of life, valproic acid is commenced. The next step would be to add either clobazam or topiramate, or successively both (35). If generalized tonic–clonic (especially fever or infection trig-

gered) seizures and status still prevail bromides (potassium bromide) may be of great help (22). From our point of view bromides are possibly the most powerful drugs available for children with Dravet syndrome. Its potency in this syndrome should not be underestimated, but however, bromides predominantly control only GCTS. Children already treated with valproate and clobazam had a 70% seizure reduction under added stiripentol. The reduction of clonic and tonic–clonic seizures was most marked (36). Other drugs used with partial success are zonisamide, phenobarbital, and chloral hydrate. In addition the ketogenic diet was reported to be successful by several authors (37,38). In children with a severe course implantation of a permanent i.v. line (e.g., Port-a-Cath) is helpful to prevent or shorten repeated status epilepticus by rapidly administering phenobarbital and benzodiazepines.

Prognosis is dismal in basically all patients who bear the diagnosis Dravet syndrome by right. Developmental delay usually becomes evident during the second or third year of life. Complete seizure freedom is not a realistic option. However, in some cases reasonable results may be obtained by antiepileptic (combination) therapy. There are cases in the borderland (SMEB) who come closer to the clinical spectrum of GEFS+ and who may respond better to therapy.

Genetics and Molecular Diagnostics

Family history was formerly reported to be frequently positive for febrile convulsions and idiopathic epilepsy syndromes. However, a recent study could not reproduce these findings (39). By far the most cases of Dravet syndrome are caused by defects in the *SCN1A* gene. In cases diagnosed by applying strict inclusion criteria (SMEI) heterozygous *SCN1A* mutations may be detected in up to 80% of cases (40). Other genes like *SCN1B*, *SCN2A*, and *GABRG2* were detected in single patients or families with Dravet syndrome, but quantitatively do not play a significant role. About 95% of *SCN1A* mutations detected in Dravet syndrome patients appear de novo. The remaining 5% that are inherited are usually connected with milder epilepsy phenotypes resembling the GEFS+ spectrum. This is consistent with a mostly negative family history. *SCN1A* mutations are distributed over the entire gene. Truncating mutations are found in about 50% of SMEI patients. The remaining are mostly missense mutations loosely clustering at the ion pore positions of the channel protein. Splice site mutations and heterozygous deletions ranging from single exons to the entire gene are rare. Borderland patients (SMEB) also frequently show *SCN1A* mutations, but at a lesser degree (60–70%).

The spectrum of epilepsies associated with the *SCN1A* gene, however, is broader than Dravet syndrome (SMEI and SMEB), and GEFS+. It also covers some less well-defined infantile epileptic encephalopathies. All of them start within the first year of life and are therapy resistant. These are denoted "cryptogenic generalized epilepsy," "cryptogenic focal epilepsy," and "severe infantile multifocal epilepsy" (40).

Selection criteria to maximize chances of a *SCN1A* mutation detection are given in Table 21.2 (31). If four or more criteria are fulfilled detection chances are about 70% or higher, using a combination of DNA sequencing and exon quantification assay (MLPA).

TABLE 21.2

COMMON FEATURES RECOGNIZED IN CHILDREN WITH *SCN1A* MUTATIONS THAT MAY BE USED AS A GUIDANCE IN ORDER TO ESTIMATE CHANCES OF DETECTION IN MUTATIONAL ANALYSIS

1. Normal development prior to start of epilepsy (~99% of reported cases)
2. Onset of febrile or afebrile GTCS within the first year of life (~96% of reported cases)
3. Unilateral motor seizures (~73% of reported cases)
4. Myoclonic seizures (~75% of reported cases)
5. Temperature sensitivity (~74% of reported cases)
6. Therapy resistance, continuous seizures to adulthood (~89% of reported cases)
7. Development of mostly mild to moderate ataxia (~70% of reported cases)
8. Mental decline (~92% of reported cases)

With permission from: Ebach K, Joos H, Doose H, et al. SCN1A mutation analysis in myoclonic astatic epilepsy and severe idiopathic generalized epilepsy of infancy with generalized tonic–clonic seizures. *Neuropediatrics.* 2005;36(3):210–213.

PROGRESSIVE MYOCLONUS EPILEPSIES (PMEs)

Unverricht–Lundborg disease, Lafora disease, myoclonic epilepsy with ragged red fibers (MERRF), neuronal ceroid lipofuscinoses (NCL), sialidosis, and dentato-rubro-pallido-luysian atrophy (DRPLA) are the archetypes of this albeit rare disease group. Other disorders with variable phenotypes may—in some of the affected—take the course of a PME (see Table 21.1). PME are rare and comprise less than 1% of epilepsies. In their early course, some of them may be difficult to differentiate from idiopathic generalized epilepsies. Precise personal and family history and a thorough clinical and neurological examination are pertinent to obtain diagnostic clues at an early stage (41). Extremely enlarged somatosensory evoked (Fig. 21.4) or visually evoked potentials induced by flashlight, an enhanced long-latency reflex in response to electric stimuli referred to as C-reflex (Fig. 21.5), and an abnormal reaction to paired pulse transcranial magnetic stimulation (Fig. 21.6), all reflecting increased cortical excitation or decreased cortical inhibition, may be diagnostically helpful neurophysiological findings.

Unverricht–Lundborg Disease

This disease clusters in Finland and in Mediterranean countries, where the prevalence reaches up to 1/20,000. The age of onset ranges from 6 to 18 years. The disorder is characterized by a stimulus-sensitive myoclonus, elicited by passive joint movement, startle, and light. Myoclonus becomes more and more severe, until finally patients are wheelchair-dependent. Ataxia, intention tremor, and dysarthria develop. Generalized tonic–clonic convulsions are the presenting sign in 50% of cases. Absences are also observed. Epilepsy is usually easy to control. Mental decline occurs late and is frequently mild. In

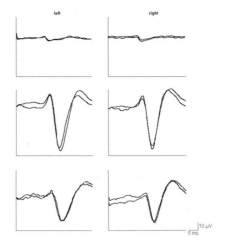

FIGURE 21.4 Somato-sensory-evoked potentials (SEPs) in a 13-year-old boy with progressive myoclonus epilepsy (PME) and in a healthy male of same age (*top*). Giant SEPs are recorded in the patient with PME reflecting extreme cortical hyperexcitability to sensory stimuli (*middle*). Notice the substantial reduction of the SEP amplitude during treatment with levetiracetam (*bottom*).

the beginning, the EEG is indiscernible from idiopathic generalized epilepsy. Over time, background activity deteriorates, and frequent spikes and polyspikes are seen. Photosensitivity is a constant feature. Reduced cortical inhibition results in giant somatosensory potentials. The disease stabilizes over time and the affected survive to old age (42).

Recessive mutations in cystatin B (*CSTB, EPM1*), a protease inhibitor, are causative for the disease. The disease mechanism is still to be elucidated, but it is believed that the defective gene deregulates apoptosis. The by far most common mutation is an expanded dodocamer repeat in the untranslated 5´ promotor region. Point mutations within the gene are much rarer (41,42).

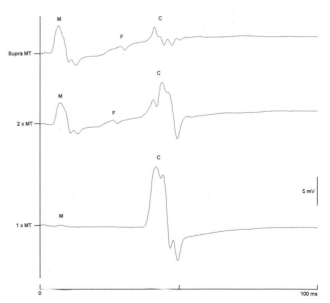

FIGURE 21.5 Positive C-reflex demonstrating decreased cortical inhibition in a 10-year-old girl affected by myoclonic epilepsy with ragged red fibers (MERRF). M, motor response; F, F-wave; C, C-reflex; MT, motor threshold.

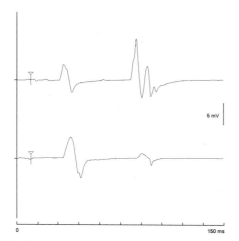

FIGURE 21.6 Motor-evoked potentials elicited by paired pulse transcranial magnetic stimulation at an interstimulus interval of 50 msec in a 10-year-old girl with MERRF (*top*) and a healthy control of same age (*bottom*). Note extreme enhancement of cortical excitability in the patient.

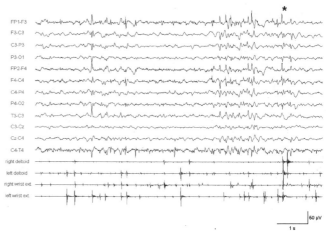

FIGURE 21.7 EEG-EMG recording in a 14-year-old girl affected by Lafora body disease. Numerous predominantly multifocal and asynchronous positive myoclonic jerks of short duration (50–100 msec) and varying intensity are recorded from different muscles. Note that only one myoclonic jerk is associated with a spike wave discharge in the EEG (*).

Valproate and add on clobazam are effective to control seizures and ameliorate myoclonus. Myoclonus responds to piracetam and possibly to levetiracetam. Other agents and vagus nerve stimulation have been used with success in some patients. Phenytoin is strictly to be avoided, for it aggravates the disease (42).

Lafora Disease

Lafora body disease is an autosomal recessively inherited generalized polyglucosan storage disorder that takes a rapidly progressive course. It is characterized by epilepsy, stimulus-sensitive myoclonus, blindness, and mental deterioration. Mutations in the *EPM2A* gene (laforin) cause about 60% of cases, and mutations in *EPM2B* gene (malin) are found in about 35% of patients. Polyglucosan inclusion bodies may be detected in (e.g., axillary) sweat glands by biopsy. How polyglucosan inclusion bodies accumulate is still not entirely understood. The disorder is most prevalent in the Mediterranean countries. Amazingly, it can also be observed in inbred dogs (43).

The disease starts with seizures in normally developed children between 6 and 19 years. Febrile seizures may precede, and initially the epilepsy may be difficult to be held apart from juvenile myoclonic epilepsy. Visual seizures, absences, GCTS, and astatic seizures are characteristic. Myoclonus is usually mild at the beginning but becomes disabling over time. Patients usually die within one decade after onset of the symptoms, frequently in status epilepticus. The EEG is normal at the beginning, but later background activity deteriorates with interposed generalized spikes, polyspikes, and occipital sharp slow waves (Fig. 21.7). Therapy of epilepsy and myoclonus is unspecific (41,43).

Myoclonic Epilepsy with Ragged Red Fibers (MERRF)

MERRF is one of the more common forms of PME (44). It may be sporadic or familial. Some cases show a clear maternal mode of inheritance, and frequently point mutations in the

mitochondrial tRNALys can be detected. Other cases are sporadic or autosomal inherited. In approximately 90% of cases three point mutations of the tRNALys gene may be revealed (8344A>G, 8356T>C, and 8363G>A). In older children ragged red fibers may be found in muscle biopsy representing aggregates of abnormal mitochondria. In adults, ragged red fibers are detectable in 90% of cases. In children these numbers are much smaller. Cytochrome C oxidase-negative fibers in muscle biopsy may also be a characteristic finding. The syndrome is clinically variable as patients may carry different proportions of defective mitochondria in single tissues ("heteroplasmia"). Typical manifestations include generalized epilepsy, myoclonus, and ataxia. The onset may range from childhood to young adulthood with remarkable intrafamilial variation. The disease may present insidiously or set in as a metabolic crisis. Optional additional features are cognitive impairment, spasticity, myopathy, deafness, failure to thrive, lipomas, neuropathy, optic atrophy, cardiomyopathy, external ophthalmoplegia, and diabetes. MERRF may clinically overlap with MELAS (mitochondrial encephalopathy, lactic acidosis, and stroke like episodes). Background EEG activity slows with progression of the disease. Generalized spike waves and focal sharp waves may be observed. In full-blown cases, the EEG is grossly abnormal, but unspecific. It may show background slowing with rhythmic delta activity, bilateral synchronous spike waves, irregular spike waves, and occipital spikes and sharp waves. Many patients are photosensitive and also show a photomyoclonic response. In MRI, signal intensity changes may be seen in the basal ganglia (low signal of the globus pallidus in T2-weighted images). In CT basal ganglia calcifications may be detected. Cortical atrophy may be present early or will ensue over time. There are no approved therapies. Valproate may result in metabolic crisis and hepatic failure, probably because it reduces the cellular uptake of carnitine. However, many patients who were erroneously treated did well with valproate for many years. L-carnitine supplementation may be indicated, but its effectiveness is unproven (41,44).

Neuronal Ceroid Lipofuscinoses (NCL)

NCL constitute the most frequent neurodegenerative disorder in children. Abnormal amounts of lipopigments are stored in lysosomes. Several subtypes, mostly following an autosomal recessive mode of inheritance, are distinguished. Five of them are recognized as PME. MRI reveals cerebral and cerebellar atrophy with signal hypertensities observed in the white matter on T2-weighted images. The cerebral cortex is progressively thinning. Muscle, skin, conjunctival, rectal, or brain biopsies show inclusions of different shapes, depending of the specific type of NCL. The most relevant form in childhood is the "late infantile variant" (NCL type 2, Jansky–Bielschowsky disease). The disease starts at 2–4 years. Generalized tonic–clonic convulsions, astatic seizures, and atypical absences are characteristic. Developmental regression is recognized shortly after onset of the epilepsy while spasticity and ataxia follow early on. Loss of vision occurs at 4–6 years and patients die about 5 years after onset of first symptoms. EEG frequently shows massive background slowing from the beginning of the epilepsy. Slowing is pronounced over the occipital regions. Generalized irregular spike waves are present. The characteristic EEG response to low frequency photic stimulation (1–3 Hz) may not be present at the beginning of the seizures but will follow shortly thereafter. Visual evoked potentials lack cortical inhibition and have a greatly increased amplitude ("giant visual potentials"). Curvilinear bodies may be detected by skin biopsy or buffy coat. The causative enzyme is tripeptidyl peptidase 1 (TPP1). A multitude of mutations have been detected in this gene. Enzyme activity can be measured even from dried blood samples ("Guthrie cards") (41,45).

There are several other, extremely rare variants of the late infantile type, which are mostly restricted to certain ethnic groups. Among those are the "late infantile finish variant" (NCL type 5), the "late infantile variant" (NCL type 6), and the "Turkish variant late infantile form" (NCL type 7) (41).

Juvenile NCL (NCL type 3, Batten disease, Spielmeyer–Vogt–Sjögren disease), the most common variant, presents with loss of vision before the onset of epilepsy. Generalized tonic–clonic convulsions are frequent. Myoclonus remains subtle. Disease onset is at 4–7 years of age. Behavioral problems and psychotic symptoms are prevalent. Later, dementia and extrapyramidal signs will develop. The course is relentless. Death occurs within 5–10 years after onset. The causative gene is identified, but its function remains unknown. Multiple gene defects are on record. The most common one is a deletion of exons 7 and 8. In skin biopsy a "fingerprint" pattern is detectable, and lymphocytes may show vacuoles reflecting enlarged lysosomes. Some rare patients show defects in the CLN1 gene (41). EEG findings are similar to NCL 1 except that there is no photosensitivity.

The adult type (NCL type 4 or Kuf's disease) is a rare autosomal dominant disorder that may begin in adolescence or adulthood. Dementia, ataxia, and later myoclonus and seizures will develop. Vision remains intact. Most patients die within 10 years. EEG shows background slowing and generalized spike wave discharges. Photosensitivity at low frequencies (1–3 Hz) may be present. Visual evoked potentials remain normal while somatosensory potentials are enlarged. There is no known gene (45).

Sialidoses

Sialidosis type 1 (cherry red spot myoclonus syndrome) is an autosomal recessive disorder caused by a deficiency of neuraminidase A (46). Sialidated oligosaccharides are detectable in urine. Multiple gene defects of the gene Neu1 are on record. Truncating mutations are most common. Action and intention tremor, and generalized tonic–clonic convulsions start in adolescence or early adulthood. Visual impairment is mild or even absent, and cognitive decline occurs during course. Spasticity, ataxia, and a painful sensory peripheral neuropathy may be observed. There is no hepatomegaly or skeletal dysplasia. Vacuolated Kupffer cells are hallmarks in histology. EEG shows few epileptic discharges and a low-amplitude fast background activity. Myoclonic attacks are paralleled by central 10–20 Hz activity. Somatosensory potentials are enlarged and visual evoked potentials are reduced in amplitude. Enzyme replacement therapy may become a therapeutic possibility in the near future (41,46).

Sialidosis type II is also caused by neuraminidase deficiency but runs a more severe course than type I. Affected patients show dysostosis multiplex, hepatosplenomegaly, mental deterioration, corneal clouding, and a Hurler-like phenotype. Onset ranges from the neonatal period to adolescence. EEG features are similar to sialidosis type 1 (41).

Dentato-Rubro-Pallido-Luysian Atrophy (DRPLA)

DRPLA is a rare autosomal-dominant repeat extension disorder with the highest prevalence in Japan. The disease is variable with three different main phenotypes recognized. General symptoms include epilepsy, extrapyramidal symptomatology, myoclonus, and dementia (47). One form presents as a PME, one as a pseudo-Huntington disease, and one as the ataxo-choreoathetoid form. The PME form has its onset before 20 years of age. Seizures, myoclonus, and mental deterioration are characteristic. EEG shows a normal background activity, spike waves, and frequently photosensitivity (41,47).

Other Rare Types of Progressive Myoclonus Epilepsies

Gaucher disease is caused by a deficiency of the lysosomal enzyme glucocerebrosidase which cleaves glucose from cerebroside. The subacute neuronopathic form of the disease (type III) may manifest as a typical PME. Hepatomegaly, splenomegaly, thrombopenia, anemia, and osseus symptoms such as osteopenia, pain, and deformations are systemic signs of the disease. Myoclonus, myoclonic seizures, and GCTS may occur in adolescents and young adults. Typically, the EEG shows generalized spike waves and marked photosensitivity. Beneath a mild mental decline, supranuclear horizontal ophthalmoplegia, ataxia, dystonia, and spasticity are additional, but inconstant neurological symptoms. Enzyme replacement therapy is available for Gaucher disease and has been shown to prevent or reverse systemic signs, but its value in improving the neurological manifestations of the disease has not yet been shown (48).

Huntington disease may manifest as early as during the first decade of life. Such children may suffer from severe dystonia and rapidly progressive myclonus epilepsy. Since the disorder is caused by an autosomal-dominant CAG repeat expansion in the so-called Huntingtin gene, careful anamnesis should identify at least one other near relative with Huntington disease.

The clinical and electroencephalographic findings in patients with *Galactosialidosis* are similar to those observed in subjects affected by sialidosis type II. But in divergence from sialidosis type I and II, there is a combined deficiency of sialidase and β-galactosidase due to a primary defect in protective protein/cathepsin A. Three subtypes are recognized: the early infantile type, the late infantile type, and the juvenile/adult type (49).

The list of neurometabolic disorders which, in single cases, may present as a PME is even longer, and some authors still mention *neuroaxonal dystrophy, Hallervorden Spatz disease (neurodegeneration with brain iron accumulation)*, and *GM2 gangliosidosis*. In virtually all cases, other clinical symptoms, besides myoclonic seizures, will aid diagnostic efforts.

PROGRESSIVE ENCEPHALOPATHIES WITH MYOCLONIC SEIZURES

Vitamin B6 (pyridoxine) is present in various dietary products. The phosphorylated active form pyridoxal-phosphate is required as a cofactor to glutamic acid decarboxylase that catalyzes the conversion of glutamate to the inhibitory neurotransmitter GABA (γ-amino-butyric acid).

Pyridoxine-dependent epilepsy is a rare autosomal recessive disorder with a prevalence of 1 in 400,000–700,000 births (50). Typically, first seizures occur within hours after birth and are not sufficiently controlled by conventional antiepileptic medication, but resolve promptly after intravenous administration of high doses of pyridoxine. Affected infants show hyperexitability with marked agitation, irritability, hypervigilance, and startle responses to touch and sounds. Usually, various seizure types are observed including myoclonic, partial clonic, and generalized clonic seizures. After administration of 50–100 mg pyridoxine, seizures may cease within minutes and the EEG normalizes within hours. Life-long pyridoxine-medication is necessary, but even in early treated subjects, mental retardation seems to be the rule. Besides this neonatal type, an increasing number of patients has been reported with therapy-resistant myoclonic, focal clonic, partial motor, generalized tonic–clonic, and complex-partial seizures, beginning beyond the neonatal period and resolving partly (pyridoxine-responsive) or completely (pyridoxine-dependent) after administration of pyridoxine. Moreover, recent reports have been published describing patients with intractable epilepsy that would not or only partially respond to vitamin B6 but resolved completely after the administration of pyridoxal-phosphate (*pyridoxal-phosphate-dependent epilepsy*) (50).

Based on the biochemical function of pyridoxal-phosphate, it had been hypothesized that abnormalities of the genes encoding the two isoforms of glutamic acid decarboxylase underlie pyrdoxine-dependent seizures, but mutations of these genes have been definitely ruled out. Plecko and coworkers reported about increased levels of pipecolic acid in urine, plasma, and CSF of patients that can be used as a diagnostic marker (51). Linkage for several families with pyridoxine-dependent seizures from North Africa and North America had been established at chromosome 5q31, but no obvious candidate gene had initially emerged (52). Recently, Mills et al. deducted from observations of a child with hyperprolinemia type II that accumulation of Δ^1-piperidine-6-carboxylate that reacts with pyridoxal-phosphate should lead to inactivation of the latter. This led to the identification of ALHD7A1 encoding for antiquitin, which is the α-aminoadipic acid semialdehyde dehydrogenase in the pipecolic acid pathway of lysine catabolism, as a candidate gene. Indeed, the authors found homozygous and compound-heterozygous mutations in 13 patients from eight families with a classical neonatal onset of seizures (53).

Because of CSF abnormalities indicating a reduction of intracellular pyridoxal phosphate in patients in whom pyridoxal phosphate stopped the seizures where pyridoxine had failed, Mills and coworkers sequenced the pyridox(am)ine 5′-phosphate oxidase (PNPO) gene. The authors found homozygous missense, splice site, and stop codon mutations in five affected infants (53). Except for one, all patients died within the neonatal period. Whether mutations of the PNPO-gene also contribute to less severe forms of pyridoxal-phosphate-dependent seizures remains to be elucidated.

Several patients with otherwise intractable *neonatal seizures responding to treatment with folinic acid* have been described. Most patients presented with myoclonic or clonic seizures, apneas, and irritability within the first 5 days of life. An autosomal-recessively inherited abnormality of folate metabolism has been postulated, but no specific defect could be identified. Nevertheless, it has been recommended to treat neonates with folinic acid for 24–48 h in case of intractable seizures not responding to a trial with vitamin B6 (54). However, recent research revealed that folinic acid-responsive seizures are identical to pyridoxine-dependent epilepsy (55). Their experience of cases treated with folinic acid, pyridoxine, or both prompted the authors to recommend treatment with pyridoxine, folinic acid, and a low lysine diet for all patients diagnosed with alpha-aminoadipic semialdehyde dehydrogenase deficiency (55).

Biotin is a water-soluble vitamin that is an indispensable coenzyme for four important carboxylases. There are two autosomal-recessive defects of biotin metabolism, *holocarboxylase synthetase deficiency and biotinidase deficiency*, which result in multiple carboxylase deficiency and which can be effectively treated with pharmacological doses of biotin (56). While the very rare holocarboxylase synthetase deficiency manifests during the neonatal period, the first signs of biotinidase deficiency emerge by 3 to 6 months or even later. Frequently, therapy-resistant myoclonic or tonic seizures are the initial symptoms. Erythematous or seborrheic skin lesions beginning around the mouth, conjunctivitis, and alopecia are important diagnostics that are present in about 70% of cases. Without biotin treatment, irreversible neurological damage including psychomotor retardation, ataxia, optic atrophy, and deafness can occur (54).

In addition to the above-mentioned disorders, myoclonic seizures may represent a prominent symptom in a variety of other metabolic encephalopathies presenting during infancy or early childhood (see Table 21.1).

RECENTLY RECOGNIZED TYPES OF PROGRESSIVE MYOCLONUS EPILEPSIES (PMEs) AND PROGRESSIVE MYOCLONIC ENCEPHALOPATHIES

Leukoencephalopathy with vanishing white matter is caused by mutations in genes encoding for the subunits of the eukaryotic subscription factor 2B (eIF2B). Although epileptic seizures are frequent in affected infants and children, the disease is usually not linked to PMEs. But recently, Jansen and colleagues reported on a young adult showing symptoms that justified the diagnosis of PME and who was found to have a homozygous mutation in the EIF2B5 gene after other causes underlying PME had been ruled out (57).

Action myoclonus-renal failure syndrome is a rare autosomal-recessive disorder first reported in the French-Canadian population (58). Recently, it has been shown that the disease is caused by mutations in the SCARB2/LIMP2 gene encoding for the lysosomal membrane protein SCARB2 (59). Severe focal glomerulosclerosis and PME associated with accumulation of storage material in the brain are the clinico-pathological hallmarks of the disease. An increasingly disabling action myoclonus and cerebellar features emerge during the second or third decade of life. Proteinuria progressing to renal failure may occur before or after the onset of neurological symptoms.

Familial encephalopathy with neuroserpin inclusion bodies is a very rare disease that has been recently identified as a cause of PME (60). The disorder may manifest as early as during the second or third decade and may take a rapidly progressive course. It is transmitted in an autosomal-dominant mode and caused by heterozygous point mutations in the *SERPIN1* gene. Neuroserpin belongs to the superfamily of SERPIN (serine proteinase inhibitor), but its exact function in the CNS is still not clear. Mutated neuroserpin accumulates in neuronal inclusions (Collins bodies) throughout the gray matter of the cerebral cortex and in certain subcortical nuclei (60,61) but is not detected in muscle, skin, and rectal biopsies (61).

GLUT-1 deficiency which was first described by de Vivo in 1991 is caused by a defect in the facilitative glucose transporter GLUT1. Impaired glucose transport across brain tissue barriers is reflected by hypoglycorrhachia and results in an epileptic encephalopathy with developmental delay and motor disorders (62). Usually, patients present with seizures during infancy. Among other seizure types, myoclonic seizures, myoclonias, and prolonged absence seizures with myoclonias can be observed. In some subjects, seizure frequency is increased and the EEG is more abnormal during fasting than shortly after a meal. In most patients, motor and mental developments are substantially delayed, and microcephaly evolves in a substantial number. Typically, liquor glucose levels are less than 0.33 g/L and glucose liquor/blood ratios are lower than 0.35. But the diagnosis may be missed if lumbar puncture is not performed after a sufficient period of fasting. EEG findings are variable and compromise mutlifocal or generalized paroxysmal abnormalities and slowing of background activity. Epileptic seizures do not respond well to anticonvulsants, but usually cease when commencing a ketogenic diet.

X-linked cyclin-dependent kinase-like 5 encephalopathy is another recently recognized epileptic entity caused by mutations in the CDKL5 gene (63). The phenotype is reminiscent of the Hanefeld variant of Rett syndrome. As in girls with Rett syndrome, patients are severely mentally retarded, have autistic features, no purposeful hand use, and demonstrate the characteristic stereotypic hand movements. While Classic Rett syndrome is caused by mutations in the gene encoding for methyl-CpG-binding protein 2 (MECP2), the product of the CDKL5 gene has been shown to be involved in the activation of MECP2 (64). About 40 girls with CDKL5 gene mutations have been reported and the electro-clinical picture of the disease has been recently defined (65). In all patients, frequent brief tonic and tonic–clonic seizures start within the first 3 months of life. From 6 months to 3 years, infantile spasms intermixed with short tonic seizures are the dominating seizure types, while profound psychomotor retardation and severe muscular hypotonia become evident. In some subjects, seizures may respond to anticonvulsant therapy, whereas in others the occurrence of myoclonias and myoclonic seizures heralds the terminal stage of epilepsy.

Mutations of the human Aristaless-related homeobox (ARX) gene are associated with a variety of pathological conditions including X-linked syndromic and nonsyndromic mental retardation, dystonia, and X-linked lissencephaly with abnormal genitalia. Polyamine tract expansions of the ARX gene are the commonly observed genetic defect in subjects with X-linked infantile spasms, whereas longer expansions have been detected in two males with early infantile epileptic encephalopathy with suppression-burst pattern (Ohtahara syndrome) (66). In addition, Scheffer and colleagues described a family with six affected boys over two generations who had a missense mutation in the ARX gene. Since all boys had myoclonic seizures as the dominating seizure type, spasticity, and profound mental retardation, the authors termed the disorder *X-linked myoclonic epilepsy with spasticity and intellectual disability* (67).

MANAGEMENT OF PROGRESSIVE MYOCLONIC EPILEPSIES

Therapy is mainly symptomatic. Seizures and myoclonus may be treated with valproic acid, benzodiazepines, levetiracetam, zonisamide, and phenobarbital. Myoclonus may respond well to a high dose of piracetam. Phenytoin, carbamazepine, oxcarbazepine, gabapentin, tiagabine, and vigabatrin may aggravate myoclonus. In Unverricht–Lundborg disease phenytoin is strictly contraindicated. Acetylcysteine has been shown to be effective in a mouse model of Unverricht–Lundborg disease. Lamotrigine may aggravate or attenuate myoclonus. Therefore, it should be tested with caution. In mitochondrial disorders (MERRF, MELAS) valproic acid should be avoided. Vagus nerve stimulation may offer help when other therapeutic options are lacking (10,41).

References

1. Guerrini R, Bonanni P, Rothwell J, et al. Myoclonus and epilepsy. In: Guerrini R, Aicardi J, Andermann F, et al., eds. *Epilepsy and Movement Disorders*. Cambridge, UK: Cambridge University Press; 2002:165–210.
2. Bonanni P, Malcarne M, Moro F, et al. Generalized epilepsy with febrile seizures plus (GEFS+): clinical spectrum in seven Italian families unrelated to SCN1A, SCN1B, and GABRG2 gene mutations. *Epilepsia.* 2004;45(2): 149–158.

3. Galletti F, Brinciotti M, Emanuelli O, et al. Familial occurrence of benign myoclonus of early infancy. *Epilepsia*. 1989;30(5):579–581.
4. Dravet C, Bureau M. Benign myoclonic epilepsy in infancy. In: Roger J, Bureau M, Dravet C, et al., eds. *Epileptic Syndromes in Infancy, Childhood and Adolescence*. 3rd ed. London: John Libbey; 2002:69–79.
5. Doose H, Gerken H, Leonhardt R. et al. Centrencephalic myoclonic-astatic petit mal. Clinical and genetic investigations. *Neuropaediatrie*. 1970;2:59–78.
6. Engel J Jr, International League Against Epilepsy (ILAE). A proposed diagnostic scheme for people with epileptic seizures and with epilepsy: report of the ILAE Task Force on Classification and Terminology. *Epilepsia*. 2001;42(6):796–803.
7. Doose H, Baier WK. Epilepsy with primarily generalized myoclonic-astatic seizures: a genetically determined disease. *Eur J Pediatr*. 1987;146:550–554.
8. Ebach K, Joos H, Doose H, et al. SCN1A mutation analysis in myoclonic astatic epilepsy and severe idiopathic generalized epilepsy of infancy with generalized tonic-clonic seizures. *Neuropediatrics*. 2005;36(3):210–213.
9. Singh R, Andermann E, Whitehouse WP, et al. Severe myoclonic epilepsy of infancy: extended spectrum of GEFS+? *Epilepsia*. 2001;42(7):837–844.
10. Rho JM. Basic science behind the catastrophic epilepsies. *Epilepsia*. 2004;45(Suppl 5):5–11.
11. Dravet C, Bureau M. The benign myoclonic epilepsy of infancy. *Rev Electroencephalogr Neurophysiol Clin*. 1981;11:438–444.
12. Loiseau P, Duché B, Loiseau J. Classification of epilepsies and epileptic syndromes in two different samples of patients. *Epilepsia*. 1991;32(3):303–309.
13. Lin Y, Itomi K, Takada H, et al. Benign myoclonic epilepsy in infants: video-EEG features and long-term follow-up. *Neuropediatrics*. 1998;29(5):268–271.
14. Mangano S, Fontana A, Cusumano L, et al. Benign myoclonic epilepsy in infancy: neuropsychological and behavioural outcome. *Brain Dev*. 2005;27(3):218–223.
15. Doose H, Sitepu B. Childhood epilepsy in a German city. *Neuropediatrics*. 1983;14(4):220–224.
16. Doose H. Myoclonic-astatic epilepsy. *Epilepsy Res Suppl*. 1992;6:163–168.
17. Kaminska A, Ickowicz A, Plouin P, et al. Delineation of cryptogenic Lennox-Gastaut syndrome and myoclonic astatic epilepsy using multiple correspondence analysis. *Epilepsy Res*. 1999;36:15–29.
18. Oguni H, Fukuyama Y, Imaizumi Y, et al. Video-EEG analysis of drop seizures in myoclonic astatic epilepsy of early childhood (Doose syndrome). *Epilepsia*. 1992;33(5):805–813.
19. Oguni H, Uehara T, Imai, et al. Atonic epileptic drop attacks associated with generalized spike-and-slow wave complexes: video-polygraphic study in two patients. *Epilepsia*. 1997;38(7):813–818.
20. Doose H. *EEG in Childhood Epilepsy—Initial Presentation and Long-Term Follow Up*. 1st ed. Montrouge: John Libbey Eurotext; 2003.
21. Oguni H, Tanaka T, Hayashi K, et al. Treatment and long-term prognosis of myoclonic-astatic epilepsy of early childhood. *Neuropediatrics*. 2002;33(3):122–132.
22. Ernst JP, Doose H, Baier WK. Bromides were effective in intractable epilepsy with generalized tonic-clonic seizures and onset in early childhood. *Brain Dev*. 1988;10(6):385–388.
23. Guerrini R, Dravet C, Genton P, et al. Lamotrigine and seizure aggravation in severe myoclonic epilepsy. *Epilepsia*. 1998;39(5):508–512.
24. Doose H. Myoclonic astatic epilepsy of early childhood. In: Roger J, Bureau M, Dravet C, Dreifuss FE, Perret A, Wolf P, eds. *Epileptic Syndromes in Infancy, Childhood and Adolescence*. 2nd ed. London: John Libbey; 1992:103–114.
25. Lortie A, Chiron C, Mumford J, et al. The potential for increasing seizure frequency, relapse, and appearance of new seizure types with vigabatrin. *Neurology*. 1993;43(11 Suppl 5):S24–S27.
26. Ohtahara S. Zonisamide in the management of epilepsy-Japanese experience. *Epilepsy Res*. 2006;68(Suppl 2):S25–S33.
27. Kröll-Seger J, Mothersill IW, Novak S, et al. Levetiracetam-induced myoclonic status epilepticus in myoclonic-astatic epilepsy: a case report. *Epileptic Disord*. 2006;8(3):213–218.
28. Caraballo RH, Cersósimo RO, Sakr D, et al. Ketogenic diet in patients with myoclonic-astatic epilepsy. *Epileptic Disord*. 2006;8(2):151–155.
29. Dulac O. Epileptic encephalopathy. *Epilepsia*. 2001;42(Suppl 3):23–26.
30. Dravet C. Les epilepsies graves de le enfant. *Vie Med*. 1978;8:543–548.
31. Yamakawa K. Molecular basis of severe myoclonic epilepsy in infancy. *Brain Dev*. 2009, Feb 7. [Epub ahead of print]
32. Mulley JC, Scheffer IE, Petrou S, et al. SCN1A mutations and epilepsy. *Hum Mutat*. 2005;25(6):535–542.
33. Dravet C, Bureau M, Oguni H, et al. Severe myoclonic epilepsy in infancy (Dravet syndrome). In: Roger J, Bureau M, Dravet C, et al., eds. *Epileptic Syndromes in Infancy, Childhood and Adolescence*. 3rd ed. London: John Libbey; 2002:81–103.
34. Berkovic SF, Harkin L, McMahon JM, et al. De-novo mutations of the sodium channel gene SCN1A in alleged vaccine encephalopathy: a retrospective study. *Lancet Neurol*. 2006;5(6):488–492.
35. Kröll-Seger J, Portilla P, Dulac O. Topiramate in the treatment of highly refractory patients with Dravet syndrome. *Neuropediatrics*. 2006;37(6):325–329.
36. Chiron C, Marchand MC, Tran A, et al. Stiripentol in severe myoclonic epilepsy in infancy: a randomised placebo-controlled syndrome-dedicated trial. STICLO study group. *Lancet*. 2000;356:1638–1642.
37. Oguni H, Hayashi K, Awaya Y, et al. Severe myoclonic epilepsy in infants—a review based on the Tokyo Women's Medical University series of 84 cases. *Brain Dev*. 2001;23(7):736–748.
38. Caraballo RH, Cersósimo RO, Sakr D, et al. Ketogenic diet in patients with Dravet syndrome. *Epilepsia*. 2005;46(9):1539–1544.
39. Mancardi MM, Striano P, Gennaro E, et al. Familial occurrence of febrile seizures and epilepsy in severe myoclonic epilepsy of infancy (SMEI) patients with SCN1A mutations. *Epilepsia*. 2006;47(10):1629–1635. [Erratum in: *Epilepsia*. 2007;48(2):409.]
40. Harkin LA, McMahon JM, Iona X, et al. The spectrum of SCN1A-related infantile epileptic encephalopathies. *Brain*. 2007;130(Pt 3):843–852.
41. Shahwan A, Farrell M, Delanty N. Progressive myoclonic epilepsies: a review of genetic and therapeutic aspects. *Lancet Neurol*. 2005;4(4):239–248.
42. Kälviäinen R, Khyuppenen J, Koskenkorva P, et al. Clinical picture of EPM1-Unverricht-Lundborg disease. *Epilepsia*. 2008;49(4):549–556.
43. Delgado-Escueta AV. Advances in lafora progressive myoclonus epilepsy. *Curr Neurol Neurosci Rep*. 2007;7(5):428–433.
44. DiMauro S. Mitochondrial diseases. *Biochim Biophys Acta*. 2004;1658(1–2):80–88.
45. Jalanko A, Braulke T. Neuronal ceroid lipofuscinoses. *Biochim Biophys Acta*. 2008, Nov 24. [Epub ahead of print]
46. Federico A, Battistini S, Ciacci G, et al. Cherry-red spot myoclonus syndrome (type I sialidosis). *Dev Neurosci*. 1991;13(4–5):320–326.
47. Oyanagi S. Hereditary dentatorubral-pallidoluysian atrophy. *Neuropathology*. 2000;20(Suppl):S42–S46.
48. Sedel F, Gourfinkel-An I, Lyon-Caen O. et al. Epilepsy and inborn errors of metabolism in adults: a diagnostic approach. *J Inherit Metab Dis*. 2007;30(6):846–854.
49. Matsumoto N, Gondo K, Kukita J, et al. A case of galactosialidosis with a homozygous Q49R point mutation. *Brain Dev*. 2008;30(9):595–598.
50. Gospe SM. Pyridoxine-dependent seizures: new genetic and biochemical clues to help with diagnosis and treatment. *Curr Opin Neurol*. 2006;19:148–153.
51. Plecko B, Hikel C, Korenke GC. et al. Pipecolic acid as a diagnostic marker of pyridoxine-dependent epilepsy. *Neuropediatrics*. 2005;36:200–205.
52. Bennet CL, Huynh HM, Chance PF. et al. Genetic heterogeneity for autosomal recessive pyridoxine dependent seizures. *Neurogenetics*. 2005;6:143–149.
53. Mills PB, Struys E, Jakobs C. et al. Mutations in antiquitin in individuals with pyridoxine-dependent seizures. *Nat Med*. 2006;12:307–309.
54. Livet M-O, Aicardi J, Plouin P, et al. Epilepsies in inborn errors of metabolism. In: Roger J, Bureau M, Dravet C, Genton P, Tassinari CA, Wolf P, eds. *Epileptic Syndromes in Infancy, Childhood and Adolescence*. 3rd ed. London: John Libbey & Company Ltd; 2002:p81–p103.
55. Gallagher RC, Van Hove JL, Scharer G, et al. Folinic acid-responsive seizures are identical to pyridoxine-dependent epilepsy. Ann Neurol, 2009. [Epub ahead of print]
56. Hymes J, Stanley CM, Wolf B. Mutations in BTD causing biotinidase deficiency. *Hum Mutat*. 2001;18(5):375–381.
57. Jansen AC, Andermann E, Niel F. et al. Leucoencephalopathy with vanishing white matter may cause progressive myoclonus epilepsy. *Epilepsia*. 2008;49(5):910–913.
58. Andermann E, Andermann F, Carpenter S. et al. Action myoclonus-renal failure syndrome: a previously unrecognized neurological disorder unmasked by advances in nephrology. *Adv Neurol*. 1986;43:87–103.
59. Berkovic SF, Dibbens LM, Oshlack A, et al. Array-based gene discovery with three unrelated subjects shows SCARB2/LIMP-2 deficiency causes myoclonus epilepsy and glomerulosclerosis. *Am J Hum Genet*. 2008;82(3):673–684.
60. Davis RL, Shrimpton AE, Holohan PD, et al. Familial dementia caused by polymerization of mutant neuroserpin. *Nature*. 1999;401(6751):376–379.
61. Gourfinkel-An I, Duyckaerts C, Camuzat A, et al. Clinical and neuropathologic study of a French family with a mutation in the neuroserpin gene. *Neurology*. 2007;69(1):79–83.
62. Klepper J, Willemsen M, Verrips A, et al. Autosomal dominant transmission of GLUT1 deficiency. *Hum Mol Genet*. 2001;10(1):63–68.
63. Weaving LS, Christodoulou J, Williamson SL, et al. Mutations of CDKL5 cause a severe neurodevelopmental disorder with infantile spasm and mental retardation. *Am J Hum Genet*. 2004;75:1079–1093.
64. Tao J, van Esch H, Hagedorn-Greiwe M, et al. Mutations in the X-linked cyclin-dependent kinase-like 5 (CDKL5/STK9) gene are associated with severe neurodevelopmental retardation. *Am J Hum Genet*. 2004;75:1149–1154.
65. Bahi-Buisson N, Nectoux J, Rosas-Vargas H, et al. Key clinical features to identify girls with CDKL5 mutations. *Brain*. 2008;131(Pt 10):2647–2661.
66. Kato M, Saitoh S, Kamei A, et al. A longer polyalanine expansion mutation in the ARX gene causes early infantile epileptic encephalopathy with suppression-burst pattern (Ohtahara syndrome). *Am J Hum Genet*. 2007;81(2):361–366.
67. Scheffer IE, Wallace RH, Phillips FL, et al. X-linked myoclonic epilepsy with spasticity and intellectual disability: mutation in the homeobox gene ARX. *Neurology*. 2002;59(3):348–356.

CHAPTER 22 ■ ENCEPHALOPATHIC GENERALIZED EPILEPSY AND LENNOX–GASTAUT SYNDROME

S. PARRISH WINESETT AND WILLIAM O. TATUM IV

Encephalopathic generalized epilepsy (EGE) constitutes a heterogeneous group of conditions that involve the brain and are associated with epileptiform abnormalities that contribute to cerebral dysfunction. Patients with EGE routinely often occupy a disproportionate amount of effort in clinical practice due to the care necessary for the accompanying frequent, refractory, multiple seizure types, in addition to the care required for the underlying condition that creates the encephalopathy that is often severe. The Lennox–Gastaut syndrome (LGS) is the prototypic EGE that reflects a common group of patients with epilepsy. Patients with LGS possess a unique electro-clinical profile that becomes apparent in infancy or early childhood. This electro-clinical profile is characterized by frequent uncontrolled seizures, mental retardation (MR), and the presence of slow-spike-and-wave (SSW) on the interictal electroencephalogram (EEG). The EEG was initially used to help classify the epileptic encephalopathies in 1939 when Gibbs noted a "petit mal variant" with SSW that differed from the findings in patients with "true petit mal seizures" and a 3-Hz generalized spike-and-wave (GSW) pattern (1). In 1945, William Lennox noted that unlike those patients with the 3-Hz GSW, the "petit mal variant" with SSW often occurred in brain injured patients with no clinical accompaniment during the discharge and a poor prognosis (2). Under the direction of Henri Gastaut, Charlotte Dravet documented the clinical profile including cognitive impairment, multiple seizure types, and emphasized the interictal features of SSW in the awake state as well as paroxysmal fast activity during sleep (3). The Lennox syndrome was later expanded by Lennox's daughter to bear the name LGS in an effort to recognize the clinical contribution of Gastaut and his colleagues in France (4). Subsequently, Doose noted a lack of homogeneity in patients with SSW including a group of patients with a clinical picture dominated by myoclonic and atonic seizures with a variable and sometimes more favorable prognosis to which he attached the label myoclonic astatic epilepsy (MAE) (5). Furthermore, in 1982, atypical benign partial epilepsy of childhood was described with continuous SSW in sleep termed "pseudo-Lennox–Gastaut" due to the electroclinical features that included multiple seizure types with falls (6).

EGE may begin at different times in life and may be due to a variety of etiologies. For example, early in life, severe myoclonic epilepsy in infancy (Dravet syndrome) can manifest as an EGE that is associated with a channelopathy (7). EGE may manifest as a refractory epilepsy with multiple seizure types, arrested psychomotor development, and behavioral disorders but occur without SSW. Patients with epilepsy and multiple independent spike foci (MISF) may be clinically similar to LGS but manifest a nonprogressive course but SSW is absent (8). Conversely, other patients with encephalopathy may have SSW and a predominance of focal seizures due to secondary bilateral synchrony mimicking EGE and LGS (9). This chapter looks at the spectrum of etiologies and manifestations that are critical for diagnosis and treatment in patients with EGE and LGS.

DEMOGRAPHICS

Population-based studies demonstrate that EGE is not uncommon, representing approximately 11.6% of all the childhood epilepsies in one study (10). In one group of patients with EGE, LGS was the final diagnosis in 20%, while 16% had West Syndrome (WS), 11% had myoclonic-astatic (Doose) syndrome, and 3% had Dravet syndrome (10). However, more than 40% were unable to be classified into a recognizable syndrome (10). In a southeastern metropolitan city of the United States, the incidence of LGS at age 10 was 0.26 per thousand children or approximating 4% of all childhood epilepsy (11), very similar to an annual incidence obtained from a retrospective community report from Finland. (12,13). The actual prevalence may be lower when rigorous criteria for the diagnosis of LGS are used. Epidemiologic studies from industrialized nations have shown that the proportion of patients with LGS is consistent over different westernized countries similar to the US. Among those children with profound MR, 17% have the LGS (11). LGS has an enormous detrimental effect upon the patient's physical and developmental health and also takes its toll on the patient's family well-being and often may warrant institutionalization (14). Males are more often affected than females among patients with the LGS, and no ethnic predisposition is encountered.

PATHOPHYSIOLOGY

There is no single pathophysiology underlying EGE and the LGS. Instead, a variety of pathophysiologies have been implicated (4,15). EGE and the LGS are usually subdivided into symptomatic and cryptogenic forms. The majority of patients with LGS have a demonstrable etiology (4,15). Symptomatic LGS accounts for approximately 70% of cases (15–17). Most symptomatic causes are present in the first year of life even though the syndrome may present later in life. The various etiologies include hypoxic–ischemic encephalopathy, cerebrovascular injury, perinatal meningoencephalitis, structural abnormalities of the brain, and malformations of cortical development (17). Cortical malformations include focal cortical dysplasia, diffuse subcortical laminar heterotopia, frontal lobe tumors, bilateral perisylvian dysplasia, and Sturge–Weber syndrome (4,15). The relationship of infantile spasms (IS) with WS and LGS has been evaluated across multiple studies as a common parallel and preceding epileptic encephalopathy (12,13,17–19). Approximately 28 to 60% (10–13,18) of children diagnosed with LGS had preceding IS; and this group appears to have a particularly poor prognosis relative to seizure control (12). Cryptogenic cases have normal development prior to the onset of LGS and no identifiable etiology by history, physical, or with neuroimaging. Cryptogenic LGS in a cohort from Atlanta, Georgia, represented 44% of patients. (11). Conversely 39% of the children with LGS had preceding IS (12). There is a low incidence of hereditary predisposition in symptomatic LGS with a family history present in <10% (4,15,19). Conversely, a genetic influence and a family history of epilepsy or febrile seizures has been noted in nearly 50% of patients with cryptogenic LGS (20) and a family history of seizures in 40% of patients with MAE (5). Classification may be challenging and unreliable in patients with EGE and LGS. Therefore the genetic influences described with cryptogenic LGS may overlap with patients possessing MAE or frontal lobe epilepsy with SSW from secondary bilateral synchrony. Earlier studies might demonstrate a less significant family history of epilepsy if reclassified today. The lack of a biological marker for EGE and LGS with similar clinical features complicates the ability to differentiate different syndromes when coupled with the heterogeneity of etiology and clinical manifestations. Even taxonomy may be challenging with authors who consider LGS and MAE to be a continuum with an intermediate form of LGS that overlap with MAE when "myoclonic variants" are described (20,21). As neuroimaging improves, many patients previously placed in the cryptogenic group have been found to have neuronal migrational disorders and have subsequently been moved to the symptomatic group. Recent molecular studies have led to the identification of the responsible gene defects for several of the epilepsy syndromes with onset in the first part of life (22). Inheritance patterns may be complex, associated with environmental factors, or monogenetic with recent identification of causative genes for a number of early-onset epilepsies creating the possibility of genetic testing (22).

LENNOX–GASTAUT SYNDROME

The LGS is the prototypic EGE and represents a devastating pediatric epilepsy syndrome accounting for approximately 1% to 4% of all childhood epilepsies (11,14). It is an epilepsy syndrome that is characteristically refractory to antiepileptic drugs (AEDs). LGS has been used loosely and misidentified as any severe epilepsy syndrome of childhood with MR that includes different types of seizures with drop attacks or injury and refractory to AED treatment (4). Additionally, LGS may be applied incorrectly to any severe childhood epilepsy that is associated with SSW on the EEG (23).

The clinical triad of LGS includes:

1. Multiple mixed seizure types including tonic, atonic, and atypical absence with a high seizure frequency, often with a history of status epilepticus.
2. Impaired intellectual function or behavior disturbance.

3. Interictal EEG demonstrating an abnormal background with SSW while awake. There are frequently MISF and frequent bursts of paroxysmal fast activity during sleep.

When all the components are present, the diagnosis is clear. Unfortunately, all of the features of LGS may not be present at the time of presentation. Thus far, the minimum criteria for a diagnosis of LGS have not been determined (23). Many authors do not insist on the EEG finding of generalized paroxysmal fast activity (GPFA) during sleep. Epidemiology studies recently performed do not include the paroxysmal fast activity as criteria (10,11), though some insist that it is an integral component (3,4,15).

Clinical Course

The clinical presentation depends on whether the etiology is symptomatic or cryptogenic (23). In symptomatic cases, the syndrome is often diagnosed after the patient has evolved from another type of epilepsy such as WS. There does appear to be a window of susceptibility for the development of LGS in infancy since most known causes are present in the first year of life (4). In cryptogenic cases, the initial symptom in very young children is usually atonic seizures manifesting as head drops (23). In older children, drop attacks or behavioral disturbances are more common (23). Cognitive deterioration may precede the seizures (3). There are reports of developing the clinical triad of LGS during adolescence (19).

Evolution of EGE and LGS usually involves progressive intellectual deterioration, increasing frequencies of seizures and episodes of status epilepticus. There can be periods of remission, but they are short. Seizures persist in the majority with less than 10% having seizure remission (10,11). In a population-based study, 94% of patients with LGS continued to have intractable epilepsy at the end of over 20 years of follow-up (10). Intellectual outcome is poor with the majority being mentally retarded. Cryptogenic cases may have a slightly better prognosis, but in one group of cryptogenic LGS, only 4 of 23 had resolution of seizures and 3 of 23 had normal intelligence (19). Patients with earlier onset, higher frequency of tonic seizures, repeated episodes of nonconvulsive status epilepticus, and constantly slow interictal background do worse (19) whereas patients with onset >4 years and prominent myoclonus tend to do better (15).

Individual Seizure Types

The characteristic seizure types that define LGS are tonic, atonic, and atypical absence (see Chapter 16), though myoclonic, clonic, partial, and generalized tonic–clonic (GTC) seizures may also occur and be the initial seizure type, particularly in symptomatic LGS. GTC seizures are reported in 15% of patients and partial seizures occur in approximately 7% of patients (3).

Tonic

Tonic seizures are the most characteristic seizure in LGS and help to distinguish LGS from the other epileptic encephalopathies. Tonic seizures can manifest as an increase in muscle tone that may be quite subtle and often "subclinical" (4,15,19). Polygraphic recording with video demonstrates tonic seizures in over 75% of patients (19). They can be manifested as brief episodes of eye or neck movement or appear more prominent with bilateral elevation and extension of the limbs. Tonic seizures are commonly associated with autonomic symptoms such as loss of bladder control, apnea, tachypnea, tachycardia, flushing, or papillary dilation (4). The ictal EEG of tonic seizures may reflect low-voltage 15- to 25-Hz fast activity, voltage attenuation, or rhythmic 10- to 15-Hz activity with high amplitude at the start of the seizure. (4). The 10- to 15-Hz EEG pattern is commonly seen during sleep in LGS. Although tonic seizures may appear to be subclinical in sleep, careful polygraphic recordings will often show subtle clinical changes in muscle tone which can be identified with electromyographic, respiratory, or cardiovascular monitoring (19).

Atonic Seizures

Atonic seizures are generalized seizures associated with a loss of postural tone that occur suddenly, without warning, and may result in falling. They can be subtle with the manifestation of a simple head nod or result in a fall. They are not synonymous with drop attack as this collective terminology reflects many different seizure types that represent seizures that may cause episodes of falls and injury through a variety of different mechanisms including tonic, atonic, and myoclonic seizures. Atonic seizures are a common seizure type that occurs in patients with LGS; however, the majority of epileptic falls including LGS occur due to tonic seizures (24,25) with sudden forceful flexion or extension at the hips that results in a loss of balance and fall. The ictal EEG correlate for atonic seizures is most often a burst of generalized spike- or polyspike-and-wave discharge.

Atypical Absence Seizures

Atypical absence seizures may be seen in more than 75% of LGS patients (19). Atypical absences are characterized by a transitory loss of consciousness. Seizures are often delayed up to 1 second after the onset is noted on EEG and usually last less than 30 sec. Patients may continue purposeful activity during atypical absences and the seizure may be difficult to recognize with the accompanying cognitive impairment. Associated clinical signs during atypical absence seizures include drooling, changes in postural tone, and irregular periocular or perioral movements. Unlike typical absence, these seizures are not precipitated by hyperventilation or intermittent photic stimulation.

The EEG correlate of atypical absence seizures is generalized SSW with a repetition rate of 1.5 to 2.5 Hz that is similar to the interictal SSW pattern, but usually more regular and of higher amplitude (26). The clinical impairment that accompanies atypical absence seizures starts and recovers gradually unlike typical absence seizures with a dramatic onset and termination. Generalized fast paroxysmal activity or voltage attenuation may also be seen (27).

Myoclonic Seizures

Myoclonic seizures are not specific for LGS and may occur with idiopathic (e.g. juvenile myoclonic epilepsy) as well as with EGE. They are seen in approximately 30% of patients diagnosed with LGS (19). Myoclonic seizures are brief, shock-like muscle contractions that may be single or in repetitive clusters that last for a few seconds to hours. Myoclonus may be subtle or massive with generalized lightening-like jerks that

result in a fall through abduction of both extremities and flexion of the axial muscle. Infrequently, patients with LGS may demonstrate myoclonic jerks that are generated focally in one hemisphere with rapid secondary generalization (28). When patients demonstrate prominent myoclonus with additional mixed seizure types, a myoclonic variant of LGS has been described that may possess a better prognosis (15). Ictal EEG demonstrates bursts of polyspike-and-waves during the episodes of myoclonus (4).

Status Epilepticus

At least half of LGS patients will experience episodes of nonconvulsive status epilepticus though any type of status can occur (29). There is concern that many of these are precipitated by overtreatment from hypnotic/sedative AEDs including the benzodiazepines (30,31). Tonic status and atypical absence status epilepticus are most common, although any seizure type may result in status epilepticus. Tonic status can be life threatening because of accompanying autonomic symptoms such as apnea and bronchial hypersecretion (15). The autonomic symptoms may continue even when the tonic seizures are not grossly evident. Commonly, an episode of status may have features of both tonic seizures and atypical absence seizures that last several days (4). Atypical absence seizures that result in nonconvulsive status epilepticus as well as tonic seizure that result in convulsive status epilepticus can occur and be refractory to treatment (29). Even atypical absence status can be difficult to recognize in LGS patients who are often cognitively delayed (29) and are characterized by incomplete clouding of consciousness that may appear as confusion, lethargy, or behavioral changes with increased irritability. They may demonstrate a preserved ability to complete tasks, though they do it in a slower and less complete fashion than they otherwise would be able to do at a baseline. The EEG during status epilepticus may not appear to be distinctly different than the interictal EEG with SSW. Often, the SSW may be more persistent or regular (29).

COGNITIVE ASPECTS OF EGE

MR is a component of EGE and one criteria of the classic triad seen in patients with LGS. However, MR is not inevitable with up to 10% of patients remaining in the normal IQ range although most still demonstrate slowed mental processing (16). Symptomatic patients generally are delayed prior to the onset of LGS and they have particularly marked cognitive delay. Symptomatic cases of LGS had a 72% risk of having severe MR, while cryptogenic cases had only a 22% risk (19). Furthermore, patients with LGS accounted for 17% of all the profoundly MR children in one US metropolitan area (11). Cryptogenic LGS patients do not have developmental delay at the onset, and it is unclear due to the lack of protracted longitudinal study whether progressive cognitive deterioration does occur as it appears to occur clinically (23). To further complicate the difficulty with identifying deterioration from the underlying encephalopathy, effects may result from prolonged episodes of status epilepticus or from AED treatment. Overmedication in this syndrome merits particular caution to avoid sedation and improve alertness, as well as to prevent an iatrogenic increase in seizure frequency and status epilepticus (4,15).

Morbidity and Mortality

A high incidence of injuries is associated with drop attacks (predominantly tonic and atonic seizures) (see chapter 2). Tonic seizures are the most common cause of falls in children with LGS and a major cause of morbidity with repeated injury often encountered (32). The location of scars seen over the forehead or the occiput may impart the means of injury through forward or backward falls, depending upon whether the axial and lower limbs are fixed in flexion or extension. Seizures that result in drop attacks are what often necessitate a protective helmet to protect the head from injury during the course of a fall. Other facial and dental injuries are also not uncommon (33). Beyond the frequent injuries from breakthrough seizures, behavior and cognitive problems often lead to overtreatment with medication that can compromise balance and gait and lead to an iatrogenic component of morbidity. Mortality is often associated with accidental injury and is estimated up to 10% over a 10-year follow-up period (32).

EEG

LGS is characterized by the presence of interictal SSW during the awake state and GPFA during non-REM sleep. Interictal SSW during the awake state is one of the cardinal features of LGS (Fig. 22.1). There is controversy about including GPFA as criteria for the diagnosis of LGS (4,15). The SSW pattern of LGS consists of a spike (70 msec) or more commonly a sharp wave (70 to 200 msec) that is followed by an aftergoing electronegative slow wave of 350 to 400 msec in duration. The field of distribution in 90% of patients is maximal in the frontal regions but can be posterior-predominant in 10% (27). The SSW discharges are not always symmetrical and may be lateralized to one hemisphere. Photic stimulation, hyperventilation, and sleep do not activate the SSW. Occasionally the frequency of SSW can approximate 3 Hz though usually a frequency of 1.5 to 2.5 Hz is seen. When the SSW is present only during sleep, then atypical benign partial epilepsy with

continuous spike and wave of sleep should be considered. In addition, Landau–Kleffner syndrome (with electrical status epilepticus in sleep) and continuous spike waves of slow sleep syndrome also manifests SSW on EEG during sleep, though distinct clinical differences readily distinguish the electroclinical features from LGS.

The finding of SSW on the EEG is an ominous finding. Medically intractable generalized epilepsy is present in most patients with SSW (16,27). In one unselected group of patients with SSW on EEG, a greater than 95% likelihood of manifesting seizures was predicted with a >60% chance of having multiple seizure types, and a 70% chance of having difficult to control seizures (27).

The cause of this constellation of SSW and GPFA with multiple seizure types and MR is unclear. It has been noted that children with interictal SSW discharges had underlying diffuse structural brain injury and a poor prognosis (27). Antecedent conditions associated with LGS almost always involve the cerebral cortex (34). Bilateral frontal lesions and diffuse dysplastic lesions of the cortex are commonly implicated. Interesting, patients with Aicardi syndrome do not have LGS suggesting spread through the corpus callosum is important (15). Lissencephaly is rarely associated with LGS (15). It has been suggested that this is due to an impediment of cortical discharges preventing propagation due to myelinated bundles separating the deep cortical layer into columns (34). There also appears to be an association of SSW with GPFA (34,35).

GPFA and tonic seizures are important because they serve to separate LGS from other epileptic encephalopathies which may have a better prognosis. The electrographic pattern of GPFA is a 10-Hz burst of bilateral fast activity that occurs during NREM sleep (Fig. 22.2). These bursts are generally brief and may appear frequently during sleep and disappear during REM sleep (15). They are identical to the discharges seen with tonic seizures but may have minimal clinical signs such as brief apnea or mild axial contraction that is best illustrated on electromyography. GPFA is not pathognomic for LGS since it may also occur in focal lesional epilepsy but is suggestive of LGS especially when it is bilateral. In patients with EGE, when tonic seizures are the predominant seizure

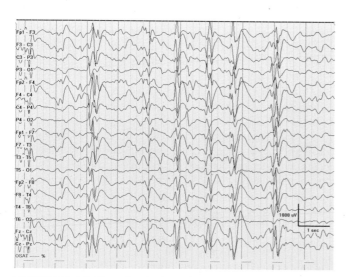

FIGURE 22.1 Diffuse slow spike-and-wave complexes on interictal EEG in a 7-year old with LGS.

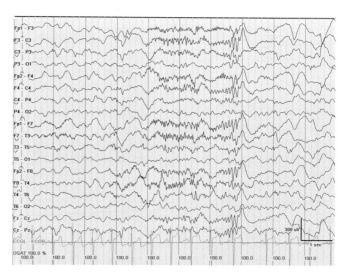

FIGURE 22.2 GPFA in a 4-year old with EGE and mixed seizures. Tonic seizures were noted in sleep with eye opening, mild axial stiffening, and apnea (EEG courtesy of Joseph Casadonte MD).

type as opposed to predominately atypical absence, myoclonic or atonic seizures, the patients with GPFA and tonic seizures had a uniformly poor prognosis (36).

In animal models, the pathogenesis of the SSW and GPFA components results from a heightened cortical excitability (34). Inhibitory systems involved in the interaction of cortical and thalamic reticular neurons and the thalamo-cortical radiations appear to underlie the generation of SSW complexes (34). The heightened cortical excitability is proposed to underlie the SSW complexes as compared to typical 3 Hz GSW (34).

DIFFERENTIAL DIAGNOSIS

Most of the epileptic encephalopathies evolve over the first few years after the clinical presentation. Certain epileptic encephalopathies, such as severe myoclonic epilepsy of infancy (Dravet syndrome) and epilepsy with MISF, rarely have SSW at presentation (7,8). In contrast, LGS almost always has SSW. If the SSW is intermixed with 3-Hz or greater fast spike-and-wave discharges, then idiopathic generalized epilepsy (IGE) such as one of the myoclonic epilepsies should be strongly considered. If there is predominantly SSW during sleep, and focal IEDs while awake, then atypical benign partial epilepsy with continuous SSW of sleep and localization-related epilepsy with secondary bilateral synchrony should be considered. The presence of focal abnormalities on neuroimaging, the EEG, clinical semiology, or the physical examination may suggest focal epilepsy with secondary bilateral synchrony. This is particularly important because resective surgery in localization-related epilepsy may be a curative treatment option. The most difficult differential diagnostic distinction is between MAE and LGS. Some authors considered these two entities a spectrum with an intermediate group variably described as a myoclonic variant of LGS or a poor prognostic subgroup of MAE (15). See Table 22.1.

West Syndrome

WS is present in 2 to 5 per 100,000 children (37) and consists of a triad that includes IS, psychomotor developmental arrest, and a unique EEG abnormality referred to as hypsarrhythmia (high-voltage, random, asynchronous background with multifocal spikes and sharp waves) that often precedes or evolves to LGS (see Chapter 17) (Fig. 22.3). A history of IS may occur in up to 20% to 40% of children with LGS though in some patients different EEG patterns may exist (see Chapter 17) (4,10–13,18). Many associations among IS, MISF, and LGS exist. For example patients with Down syndrome may have IS and hypsarrhythmia on the EEG that transitions to EGE and MISF or to LGS with epilepsy that occurs in approximately 5% of patients (38).

In patients with IS, the presence of hypsarrhythmia may be absent as in the case of Aicardi's syndrome. Additionally, hypsarrhythmia may be seen in other types of severe infantile epileptic encephalopathies without IS. The onset of WS is usually between 4 and 7 months of age with 90% that are associated with neurological abnormalities from underlying structural, genetic, or inborn errors of metabolism present (39). Patients with IS reflect an interaction between early brain development, precise timing of a neurological insult, and a

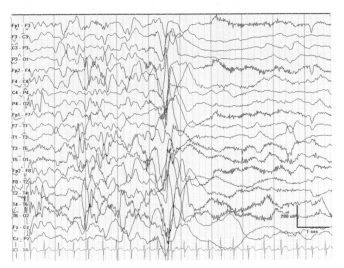

FIGURE 22.3 Infantile spasm depicted on ictal EEG in a 7-month old with cortical dysplasia and left temporal lobe seizures. A 2-week course of ACTH was followed by resolution of hypsarrhythmia and spasms.

pathophysiologic process. WS is often symptomatic; however, an idiopathic form with a multi-factorial genetic predisposition and an X-linked recessive and dominant form have been described (22). The early childhood epileptic encephalopathies do not permit precise classifications of specific groups of patients but rather evoke a spectrum of conditions with significant electroclinical overlap.

Ohtahara syndrome (early infantile epileptic encephalopathy) represents only 0.2% of the early childhood epilepsies with refractory tonic spasms, burst suppression on EEG, and an overall poor prognosis. Seizure onset is within the first 3 months of life and asymmetric tonic seizures and focal seizures occur in approximately one third of patients. Ohtahara syndrome often evolves to WS between 3 and 6 months of age and subsequently into LGS between 1 and 3 years of age (40). The cause is often symptomatic and a high mortality rate is encountered in infancy. Genetic testing may be useful with a high STXBP1 mutation frequency found in this syndrome (22). Another early epileptic encephalopathy is early myoclonic encephalopathy. It presents in the first month with fragmentary myoclonus, massive myoclonia, and multifocal seizures. These patients later develop tonic seizures and their EEG is characterized by a burst suppression pattern. The similarity of the EEG patterns has led authors to question whether Ohtahara syndrome and EME are separate entities (41).

Myoclonic Astatic Epilepsy

Myoclonic astatic epilepsy described by Doose is a childhood EGE syndrome characterized by seizure types that are similar to those seen with LGS including atypical absence, myoclonic, atonic, tonic, and tonic–clonic seizures (5). In contrast to LGS, MAE has more prominent myoclonic seizures and less prominent tonic seizures early in the course of the condition. Partial seizures are rare. MAE usually presents between 7 months and 6 years of age. The characteristic massive myoclonic seizures are brief symmetrical jerks involving the neck, shoulders, and arms followed by an abrupt loss of muscle tone that usually results in a fall (astatic seizure). Patients with MAE may also

TABLE 22.1

SUMMARY OF THE ENCEPHALOPATHIC GENERALIZED EPILEPSY SYNDROMES AND CLINICAL FEATURES

Syndrome vs. Clinical Features	Lennox–Gastaut Syndrome (15,16,19,32)	Myoclonic-Astatic Epilepsy (5,29,44,47)	Severe Myoclonic Epilepsy of Infancy (15,44,45)	Epilepsy with MISF (8,9)	Localization-Related Epilepsy with Secondary Bilateral Synchrony (9,46)	Landau-Kleffner Syndrome and Atypical Benign Partial Epilepsy with CSWS (6,15)
Clinical seizure types	Atypical absence (75%), tonic–atonic seizures (75%), myoclonic (30%), partial (15%) and GTC (7%) seizures	Myoclonic, myoclonic-astatic seizures, partial seizures rare	Febrile seizures followed by afebrile U/L clonic and GTC seizures. Later myoclonic, atypical absence, and complex partial	GTC, tonic, partial, myoclonic, atypical absence, and atonic seizures	Partial, atypical absence, and GTC seizures	Partial seizures, clusters of atonic and myoclonic seizures in ABPE with CSWS. LKS with associated auditory agnosia
MRI	Normal or nonspecific abnormal	Normal	Normal	Normal or abnormal	Normal or abnormal	Usually normal
Interictal EEG pattern	Awake = SSW Asleep = GPFA Background with diffuse slowing often multi-focal spikes	GSW, often mixture of SSW and fast (>3 Hz) GSW	Multi-focal and generalized spikes; PPR in 40%	Multi-focal spikes	Frontal or bifrontal predominant GSW often 3 Hz or <3 Hz	Focal temporal predominant spikes; SSW during sleep
Course	Often severe mental retardation	50% with resolution of seizures in 3 years and 50% with normal IQ	Mental retardation, persistent seizures	Variable	Variable	Possible good outcome if steroid responsive
Prognosis	Progressive deterioration despite broad spectrum AEDs	Often stabilizes with AEDs after the first 3 years	Progressive deterioration initially followed by a static phase	Static	Static; May respond to surgical intervention	Variable; May respond to steroid therapy

Abbreviations: GTC, generalized tonic–clonic; U/L, unilateral; PPR, photoparoxysmal response; GPFA, generalized paroxysmal fast activity; GSW, generalized spike-and-waves; SSW, slow spike-and-waves; AED, antiepileptic drugs.

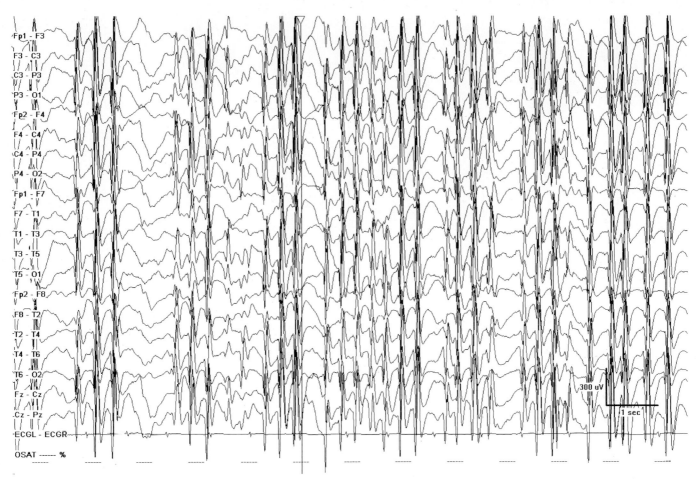

FIGURE 22.4 Generalized spike and wave at varying frequencies in 9-year-old with myoclonic astatic epilepsy.

present with pure atonic seizures, atypical absence, GTC seizures, or with episodes of nonconvulsive status epilepticus. Most patients are neurologically normal at onset and there is a family history of epilepsy in 40% of patients (5). The ictal EEG shows spike or polyspike-and-wave discharges at a frequency of 2 to 4 Hz. The interictal EEG may be normal. When it is abnormal, it may show brief bursts of 3-Hz GSW, 4- to 7-Hz parietal theta, and 4-Hz occipital activity consistently blocked by eye opening (Fig. 22.4) (42). In contrast to the uniformly poor prognosis of LGS, at least half of the patients with MAE will have their seizures cease within 3 years and more than 50% of patients will have a normal IQ in this subgroup (29). Valproic acid (VPA), lamotrigine (LTG), and ethosuximide (ESM) have been generally used for treatment (29) though topiramate (TPM), felbamate (FBM), and rufinamide (RUF) may prove to be useful agents as well since they have demonstrated efficacy in LGS.

A recent cluster analysis of 72 patients with severe cryptogenic childhood generalized epilepsy was conducted (43). The patients clustered into three groups by this analysis. The first group corresponded with MAE and had frequent massive myoclonus, short bursts of 3-Hz GSW, a family history of epilepsy (20%), and a relatively favorable outcome. The second group was similar except for longer bursts of irregular SSW and a lesser amount of 3-Hz GSW, with more frequent myoclonic status epilepticus. This group appeared to correlate with the intermediate group and correspond to an unfavorable variant of MAE or myoclonic variant of LGS. The third group correlated with LGS and had a greater incidence of atypical absence seizures in addition to subtle tonic seizures, less myoclonus, a limited family history of epilepsy, and an abrupt onset of MR with EEG features including long bursts of SSW. The second and third groups had a poor outcome. This study emphasized the presence of distinct groups of childhood epileptic encephalopathies and the difficulty with classification (43).

Dravet Syndrome

Severe myoclonic epilepsy of infancy (Dravet syndrome) is a childhood epileptic encephalopathy that usually presents with prolonged febrile seizures during the first year of life. During the second and third years of life, myoclonic seizures and atypical absences subsequently appear. The myoclonic seizures may be massive and associated with falls. Tonic–clonic and partial seizures are also common. Tonic seizures are rare and when present they are infrequent. The EEG often is normal initially and only shows SSW during atypical absence seizures. Over time, focal abnormalities develop and spike- and polyspike-and-wave discharges are seen associated with the myoclonic seizures. Early photosensitivity may be present in 40% of patients (44). Although the myoclonic seizures may resolve, other seizure types persist and there is a progressive cognitive deterioration accounting for a poor prognosis.

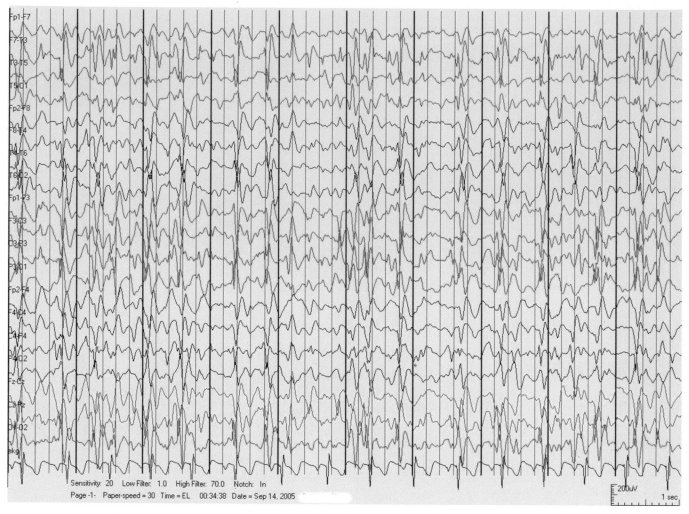

FIGURE 22.5 Electrical status epilepticus of slow sleep in a 9-year old with Landau–Kleffner syndrome. Borrowed from Demos Publishers, In: *Handbook of EEG*, Tatum WO, Husain A, Benbadis SR, Kaplan PW, eds., 2008:104.

Dravet syndrome usually occurs in sporadic patients and heterozygous de novo SCN1A mutations have been found in 33% to 100% of patients (22,45).

Atypical Benign Partial Epilepsy with Continuous Spike and Wave of Sleep

This syndrome appears to be at the malignant end of the spectrum for children who manifest partial epilepsy in childhood. A benign partial epilepsy may exist with a more malignant representation with continuous spike-and-wave of sleep and has been termed "pseudo-LGS" (see Chapter 23) (15). Atypical benign partial epilepsy with continuous spike-and-waves in sleep may present with clusters of myoclonic and atonic seizures lasting 2 to 4 weeks in patients between 2 and 6 years of age. These clusters are separated by seizure-free periods (6), and in contrast to LGS, tonic seizures do not occur. The EEG shows diffuse slow spike and wave discharges during sleep (Fig. 22.5). Central spikes are usually prominent with this syndrome similar to other forms of more benign focal epilepsy. Remission occurs before age 15, but patients may be left cognitively impaired (6).

Localization-Related Epilepsy with Secondary Bilateral Synchrony

Focal epilepsy with secondary bilateral synchrony is best identified when there is a focal EEG spike that leads into a generalized discharge. Because of the limitations of surface-scalp EEG recording, there may be variability in the presence of a preceding focal discharge before the generalized burst in seen. Characterization of the discharges shows that they tend to have a frontal predominance and often discharge irregularly at 2 to 2.5 Hz. The interval between the focal discharge and the onset of the generalized discharge is very brief but is greater than the mean callosal transmission time and may further decrease in duration as the discharge continues (9). Since the primary focus may not be discernable on routine EEG, it may give the false appearance of a generalized discharge. Foci most likely to create this phenomenon are most often seen in the frontal lobes but can be seen elsewhere along the midline of the cerebrum (46). Furthermore, clinical seizures associated with this phenomenon may imitate absence seizures further providing a challenge to differentiate a generalized from focal seizure. There is optimism that the new technique of magnetoencephalography may help in identifying the focal origin of patients with epilepsy and burst of secondary bilateral synchrony on EEG (47).

Angelman and Rett Syndrome

Angelman syndrome (AS) is characterized by severe developmental delay, absent speech, paroxysms of laughter, a puppet-like gait with ataxia, and jerky movements (also known as the happy puppet syndrome), in addition to other distinctive clinical features. Patients with AS also have intractable epilepsy and EEG characteristics that may be confused with LGS (48). Seizure types that may be observed include atypical absence, myoclonic, clonic, and complex partial seizures. Characteristic EEG findings are diffuse, bilateral, frontally predominant, high-amplitude delta waves with a notched or triphasiform slow wave that appears as SSW complexes with a notched appearance of the sharp waves that are superimposed upon the slower delta activity. The frequency may be 2 to 2.5 Hz and resembles the SSW that is seen in LGS (Fig. 22.6). There are not usually clear sharp waves unless the patient is having atypical absence seizures, and the findings have been referred to as "ill-defined slow-spike-and wave" (48). The 10-Hz GPFA seen in LGS is not seen in AS (48). Other EEG features with AS include a generalized or posterior-dominant high amplitude (>200 microvolts) theta rhythm that may be elicited by eye closure and reveal high voltage delta activity intermixed with sharp waves. AS is associated with deletions in chromosome 15q11–q13 in 70% of patients (49). Other genetic causes include UBE3A mutations, uni-parental disomy, or methylation imprint abnormalities (49).

Rett syndrome is encountered between 6 months and 3 years of age and only in females. Rett syndrome is characterized by cognitive regression, autistic features, microcephaly, ataxia, and hand-wringing movements in addition to multiple seizure types that include absence, myotonic, and atonic seizures (49), thus mimicking LGS. The EEG may show progressive slowing of the background activity with needle-like central spikes that are activated by somatosensory stimulation. A unique feature includes

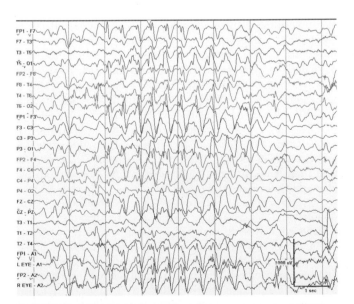

FIGURE 22.6 Ill defined slow spike-and-wave on interictal EEG in a 4-year-old with Angelman syndrome. (EEG courtesy of Maria Gieron-Korthals, MD)

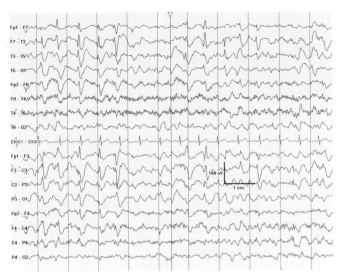

FIGURE 22.7 Slow spike-and-wave in an 8-year-old with Rett syndrome. (EEG courtesy of Selim R. Benbadis, MD)

a 4- to 6-Hz rhythmic theta pattern maximal centrally (50). It may also present with SSW (Fig. 22.7).

Severe Epilepsy With Multiple Independent Spike Foci

EGE with MISF has been proposed as an independent entity (51) that is clinically related to LGS with MR and intractable epilepsy. Three or more epileptic foci are present with at least one in each hemisphere. In patients with this EEG finding, more than 50% of patients had more than one type of seizure and 50% were having daily seizures (8). This is especially true when the spikes occurred at least every 10 seconds (8). When EGE is present, a variety of seizures including GTC, focal, tonic, myoclonic, atypical absence, and atonic seizures may be seen. EGE with MISF has extensive overlap with the other epileptic encephalopathies and may frequently transition in an age-dependent fashion to other epilepsies including LGS, Ohtahara's epileptic encephalopathy, and WS (51). It may also be seen in 10% to 20% of symptomatic LGS patients as they age, but rarely in those with the cryptogenic form (52). Like LGS, EGE with MISF may be seen in patients with extensive bilateral cerebral pathology and manifests severe intractable epilepsy. When the EEG features of MISF are present a more variable prognosis for mental normalcy is present than in patients with LGS, with one third of patients mentally normal (8).

DIAGNOSTIC EVALUATION

Neuroimaging is essential due to the many diverse structural lesions that may cause EGE and LGS and impact diagnosis and treatment. It is helpful to have specific neuroimaging protocols that are designed to detect neuronal migrational disorders that might further implicate a potentially surgically remediable localization remediable epilepsy (53). Even when high-resolution brain MRI is performed, it may be the presence of focal IEDs that lead to the discovery of subtle regions of gray-white junction blurring or abnormal cortical thickening that are the only signs of cortical dysplasia.

PET scans of the brain obtained in patients with LGS (54) have yielded variable findings and may reflect the varying etiologies. However, FDG-PET brain scans have proven useful in resective epilepsy surgery (55) when a localization-related epilepsy with secondary bilateral synchrony is the cause of the epileptic encephalopathy.

The importance of the EEG in the evaluation of patients with EGE and LGS has long proven to be the cornerstone to the diagnosis of patients with epileptic encephalopathies (20) and has been discussed. Hypsarrhythmia, SSW, GPFA, MISF, and interictal disturbances of the waking background are notorious features that may indicate the predisposition for a severe intractable EGE or LGS. Video-EEG monitoring may be helpful to further classify the ictal electroclinical behavior (56) such that additional treatment options become more likely considerations, yet it is the clinical history and associated features that characterize the individual entities within the clinical spectrum of epileptic encephalopathies.

Metabolic and genetic evaluations without a clinical direction suspected from the history, physical, and neuroimaging is presently of low yield. Specific genetic analyses may become more commonplace as the genetic basis for different cortical malformations becomes known. Conditions such as lissencephaly, double-cortex syndrome, and bilateral perisylvian polymicrogyria have been linked to an EGE- or LGS-like picture and genetic testing may prove to be confirmatory (57). Early in the course of the epilepsy when this evaluation is done, mitochondrial disorders and neuronal ceroid lipofuscinosis may present similarly, and appropriate biochemical evaluations should be considered. Additionally, molecular genetic studies have identified causative genes and loci for a number of early malignant epileptic encephalopathies creating the possibility of genetic testing (22) both for diagnosis and differential diagnosis. For example, SCN1A channel defects may present with a clinical scenario suggesting generalized epilepsy with febrile seizures plus or severe myoclonic epilepsy of infancy which may be confused with LGS. However, febrile seizures will often be absent in LGS, and the EEG in Dravet syndrome will not typically demonstrate SSW. Further evaluation for aminoacidopathies, organic acidopathies, urea cycle defects, chromosomal abnormalities should be performed where appropriate. Lumbar puncture should be used in cases of suspected infectious and metabolic etiologies (especially mitochondrial and neurotransmitter deficiencies).

TREATMENT

The treatment of patients with EGE and LGS includes efforts at managing the underlying cause of the associated cognitive or behavioral dysfunction, attempting to control seizures and providing support for the family or caretakers involved with their care.

AEDs are the mainstay of therapy for patients with EGE even though they often demonstrate intractability to medication. The multiple seizure types associated with LGS often require broad spectrum AEDs singly or in combinations. VPA, LTG, and TPM are the most widely used agents and are useful AEDs for EGE and LGS at the present time (15,58). FBM has been shown to have a significant effect on both seizure reduction as well as demonstrating a favorable neurocognitive profile. It is considered a proven AED in the treatments of LGS,

but its use has been limited by the occurrence of hepatic failure and aplastic anemia (59). Recently, randomized controlled clinical drug trials of RUF, a novel AED, have been completed and approved for use as an adjunctive treatment for patients with LGS (60) as it demonstrated efficacy in the treatment of tonic, atonic, and atypical absence seizures associated with LGS but did not have a significant effect on focal seizures in LGS. Many other medications have purported benefit including levetiracetam, clonazepam, and clobazam. Clobazapam may be preferable to clonazepam given a lesser likelihood to cause sedation. It is often tempting to continue adding or increase the dose of AEDs since seizures are rarely adequately controlled. Although AEDs can decrease the number of seizures, oversedation may paradoxically worsen the seizures. Over sedation may be as damaging to development and gaining functional skills as the recurrent seizures. In clinical practice, simplifying AEDs may surprisingly improve seizure control and functionality (4). In particular, benzodiazepines use may evoke sedation and may provoke atypical absence and tonic status epilepticus (30,31).

VPA or valproate is the traditional broad spectrum AED that is often initially employed when treating patients with EGE and particularly patients with cryptogenic LGS. There is evidence that some patients in this group may overlap with MAE and demonstrate a favorable response with seizure reduction (36). Valproate is efficacious for myoclonic, absence, and atonic seizures. It often is used in polypharmaceutical combinations in LGS increasing the risk of serious hepatotoxicity especially in the early childhood years (15). Despite the fact that historically it is considered a drug of choice for LGS (61,62), there are no large-scale double-blinded studies in LGS (23).

LTG is a broad spectrum AED that typically has minimal adverse effects upon cognition and behavior, but requires slow dose titration to avoid a potentially severe drug-induced rash. A double-blind placebo-controlled clinical trial found that 33% of patients with LGS had a 50% decrease in the number of generalized seizures (including atypical absence, tonic, myoclonic, and atonic) (63). The effect was most marked in tonic–clonic and atonic seizures and was less helpful for atypical absence (63). There was no increase in adverse effects as compared to placebo except for an increase in respiratory infections. From a practical standpoint, it is difficult to use it as an initial drug because of the slow titration. The risk of rash is greater in the presence of VPA and a longer titration process is required when using this drug in those currently treated with VPA. In this AED regimen, VPA inhibits the metabolism of LTG and leads to greater serum concentrations at lower doses when compared with those that employ only enzyme-inducing AEDs, though VPA and LTG may reflect a combination that demonstrates synergy beyond the simple additive effects (15).

TPM is a broad spectrum AED with initial randomized, double-blind, placebo-controlled trial demonstrating 33% of patients with a greater than 50% reduction in total number of seizures (64). An open label extension of the same study utilizing an average of close to 10 mg/kg/day showed a greater than 50% decrease in drop attacks in 55% of the patients including 15% with elimination of drop attacks (65). Another RCT also demonstrated the greatest efficacy in reducing drop attacks and major motor seizures (tonic and tonic–clonic) (66). The primary adverse events are somnolence, dizziness, psychomotor slowing, and oligohydrosis seen in children prompting attention to adequate hydration with use.

FBM is now a third line AED that is reserved for situations in which other AEDs have demonstrated inefficacy. Initial studies showed a 44% decrease in atonic seizures and a 26% decrease in total seizures during the maintenance phase of the FBM trials in LGS. Parental reports of increased alertness and improved verbal output were noted very early in its use (67). Now, it has more limited use due to the risk of liver failure in children (approximately 1 in 30,000). There is also a risk of about 127 per million exposures for aplastic anemia but no cases were seen under the age of 13 (59).

Rufinamide has shown efficacy in the tonic, atonic, and atypical absence seizures associated with LGS but not with partial seizures in this syndrome. The initial study of LGS patients over 4 years showed a 33% decrease in total seizure frequency and a 42% decrease in drop attacks. The most serious side effect noted in the trials was mild CNS adverse events and hypersensitivity reactions (60).

Other drugs that have been studied in small studies include levetiracetam, zonisamide, clobazam, nitrazepam, acetazolamide, and amantidine (33). In a study of six patients, levetiracetam showed significant reductions in myoclonic, atonic, and atypical absence, but not tonic seizures (68). Post-marketing experience of zonisamide is suggestive that it is helpful in reduction of seizures in LGS (69). The 1,4-benzodiazepines—clonazepam, nitrazepam, and diazepam—have also been used extensively in LGS. In one study of 14 patients, adjunctive nitrazepam resulted in a 41% reduction in seizures (70). Clobazam, a 1,5-benzodiazepine, may be associated with less sedation. Ethosuximide occasionally demonstrates benefit in patients with atypical absence but also myoclonic and atonic seizures as well (33). Intravenous immunoglobulin has previously been used successfully in patients with LGS (71). Involvement of immunogenetic mechanisms in triggering or maintaining some cases of LGS is hypothesized, and an association between LGS and HLA B7 has been described (72). Corticosteroids and ACTH may be effective early in the treatment of cryptogenic LGS though steroids usually have a limited role due to the high rates of relapse following discontinuation though they may be used in pulse doses for episodes of nonconvulsive status epilepticus (33).

NONMEDICAL THERAPIES

The ketogenic diet (KD) is a specialized high-fat, low-carbohydrate diet that may be useful for EGE and LGS and may be particularly helpful in decreasing the number of atonic seizures and should be considered an option when medical therapy is ineffective (see Chapter 69) (73). The use of the KD and a reduction in the number of AEDs may be useful not only for seizure frequency but also for functionality. In one prospective multicenter observational study of children with intractable EGE, 10% were seizure-free after 1 year on the KD and another 30% had >90% improvement of seizure control (74). There is some evidence that adults with refractory epilepsy may benefit from the diet even when less restrictions are used with the modified Atkins diet (75).

Surgical options are usually palliative with corpus callosotomy and vagus nerve stimulation (VNS) the most frequently utilized (see chapter 91). Corpus callosotomy is a surgical procedure that disconnects the anterior two third to three fourth of the cerebral hemispheres to prevent seizure propagation to eliminate the risk of falls and injury by reducing spread of generalized seizures (see chapter 88). Partial callosotomy is effective in 50% to 75% of cases while complete callosotomy may reach 80% to 90% reduction of drop attacks associated with generalized tonic and atonic seizures that require transcallosal propagation to affect both hemispheres to result in falls. In severely mentally retarded patients, a complete callosotomy may offer improved efficacy when compared with partial corpus callosotomy (76). Disconnection syndrome is the most serious side-effect from callosotomy with an inability to transfer sensory information from one hemisphere to another and motor and coordination difficulties in the non-dominant limbs.

Another surgical procedure used to treat larger focal areas of epileptogenicity residing within "eloquent" areas of cortex is multiple subpial transaction (MST). MST was designed to interrupt horizontal intracortical fibers to contain neocortical synchronously interacting regions of the brain to minimize seizure spread that leads to clinical seizures. Application of MST as a solitary procedure for patients with epileptic encephalopathies is rarely performed though it has been used in patients with Landau–Kleffner syndrome that are capable of manifesting SSW. As discussed above, if a focal lesion can be found then the syndrome of partial seizures with secondary bilateral synchrony should be considered since there have even been reports of successful resolution of LGS following focal resection (77,78).

Some epilepsy centers initially use VNS prior to corpus callosotomy (79). Vagal nerve stimulation can be helpful in LGS although it does not appear to have the same efficacy as it does in partial seizures (80). In a multicenter retrospective study of VNS in LGS patients, an average reduction of 44% was reported after 6 months (81). A recent study demonstrated greater efficacy of callosotomy compared to VNS for GTC seizures though the risk of complications in the callosotomy group were greater and therefore the balance of potential benefits of VNS as opposed to callosotomy must be weighted against the greater risk (82).

Other alternative treatments have also been suggested including herbal remedies and homeopathic treatments that have become available for patients with LGS on the Internet (83). Substantiation of efficacy in randomized controlled clinical trials remains to be elucidated.

PROGNOSIS

The prognosis of the EGEs and of LGS overall is poor. Few patients lead independent lives as an adult as a result of daily seizures, cognitive, or behavioral abnormalities. Refractory seizures are the rule, and the prognosis for normal intellectual function rarely occurs (10). An onset before age 3 is more likely to be associated with MR with the majority of individuals requiring special classes or sheltered workshop environments. Some patients show deterioration of previously established function especially when seizures are frequent (52). Though tonic seizures may persist, the SSW pattern may resolve and rarely newer forms of seizure semiologies will evolve to dominate the clinical profile such as partial seizures. Approximately half of symptomatic LGS and one third of the cryptogenic form lose the electroclinical characteristics of

LGS evolving into another form of EGE, epilepsy with MISF, or LRE (52). Patients with LGS and tonic seizures, GPFA, or non-convulsive status epilepticus usually have the same seizure types persisting in adulthood. In contrast, those with atypical absence or myoclonic seizures carry a more hopeful prognosis and are more likely to evolve to manifest multi-focal or focal seizures (33). Patients with an early age of onset, frequent disabling seizures, repeated episodes of status epilepticus, and a preceding history of IS associated with WS have a relatively worse prognosis for normal cognitive development (84).

CONCLUSION

There are few groups of patients as challenging as those with EGE and LGS. Seizures are usually refractory to treatment, and the overall prognosis for normal cognitive development is poor. It is crucial to distinguish patients with EGE from those with LRE who may possess a surgically remediable condition or those with a more favorable prognosis such as MAE. Similarly, identifying refractory epilepsies with a genetic foundation such as AS, Rett syndrome, or SCN1A mutations with poor prognoses is also important to provide genetic counseling and helpful to prevent unnecessary diagnostic evaluations. In EGE, the benefit of treatment with AEDs with respect to the goal of seizure reduction must be realistically balanced with the risks of overmedication. When AEDs are ineffective and injury is recurrent, alternative therapies such as KD, VNS, and corpus callosotomy should also be considered (79). Last but not least, support for caretakers and families of patients with EGE and LGS is crucial as refractory seizures that cause injury create considerable anguish for caretakers and family alike and protective measures should be considered at home and also at school. While protective helmets may help prevent injury, they stigmatize patients with uncontrolled seizures and an effort should be made to seek the least intrusive methods to balance safety with psychosocial development. Despite our seemingly futile efforts toward seizure control and assistance with growth and development, patients with EGE and LGS represent an important group to understand and serve in that their success as human beings need to be measured using a different scale than those patients with normal cognitive function and absent comorbidity.

References

1. Gibbs FA, Gibbs EL, Lennox WG. Influence of the blood sugar level on the wave and spike formation in Petit Mal epilepsy. *Arch Neurol Psychiatry.* 1939;41:1111–1116.
2. Lennox WG, The petit mal epilepsies. *JAMA* 1945;129:1069–1074.
3. Gastaut H, Roger J, Soulayrol R, et al. Childhood epileptic encephalopathy with diffuse slow spike-waves (otherwise known as "petit Mal Variant") or Lennox Syndrome. *Epilepsia.* 1966;7:139–179.
4. Markand ON. Lennox-Gastaut Syndrome (Childhood epileptic encephalopathy). *J Clin Neurophysiol.* 2003;20:426–441.
5. Doose H, Gerken H, Leonhardt R, et al. Centrencephalic myoclonic-astatic petit mal: clinical and genetic investigations. *Neuropediatrie.* 1970;2:59–78.
6. Aicardi J, Chevrie JJ. Atypical benign partial epilepsy of childhood. *Develop Med Child Neurol.* 1982;24:281–292.
7. Dravet C, Roger J, Bureau M, et al. Myoclonic epilepsies in childhood. In: Akimoto H, Kazamatsur H, Seino M et al., eds. *Advances in Epilepsy,* XIII Epilepsy International Symposium. New York: Raven Press; 135–140.
8. Blume WT. Clinical and electroencephalographic correlates of the multiple independent spike foci pattern in children. *Ann Neurol.* 1978;4:541–547.
9. Beaumanoir A, Mira L. Secondary bilateral synchrony: significant EEG pattern in frontal lobe seizures in Frontal seizures and epilepsies in children. In: Beaumanoir A, Andermann F, Mira L, Zifkin B. eds. John Libbey Eurotext; 2003:195–205.
10. Camfield P, Camfield C. Long term prognosis for symptomatic (secondarily) generalized epilepsies: a population based study. *Epilepsia.* 2007;48: 1128–1132.
11. Trevatham E, Murphy CC, Yeargin-Allsopp M. Prevalence and Descriptive Epidemiology of Lennox-Gastaut Syndrome among Atlanta Children. *Epilepsia.* 1997;38:1283–1288.
12. Rantal H, Putkonen T. Occurrence, outcome, and prognostic factors on infantile spasms and Lennox-Gastaut Syndrome. *Epilepsia.* 1999;40: 286–289.
13. Heiskala H. Community-based study of Lennox-Gastaut Syndrome. *Epilepsia.* 1997;38:526–531.
14. Crumrine PK. Lennox Gastaut Syndrome. *J Child Neurol.* 2002;17(suppl 1): S70–S75.
15. Arzimanoglou A, Guerrini R, Aicardi J. *Lennox-Gastaut Syndrome in Aicardi's Epilepsy in Children.* 3rd ed. Lippincott Williams & Wilkins, 2004:38–50.
16. Chevrie JJ, Aicardi J. Childhood epileptic encephalopathy with slow spike-wave: a statistical study of 80 cases. *Epilepsia.* 1972;13:259–271.
17. Ohtahara S, Ohtsuka Y, Yoshinaga H, et al., Lennox-Gastaut Syndrome:etiological considerations in Lennox-Gastaut Syndrome in The Lennox-Gastaut Syndrome. In: Niedermeyer E, Degen R. eds. New York: Alan R. Liss; 1988:47–63.
18. Lombroso CT. A prospective study of infantile spasms: clinical and therapeutic correlations. *Epilepsia.* 1983;24:135–158.
19. Roger J, Dravet C, Bureau M. The Lennox-Gastaut Syndrome. *Clev Clinic J Med.* 1989;56(supp):S172–S180.
20. Dravet C, Roger J. The Lennox-Gastaut syndrome: historical aspects from 1966 to 1987 in The Lennox-Gastaut Syndrome. In: Niedermeyer E, Degen R. eds. New York: Alan R. Liss; 1988:9–23.
21. Aicardi J, Chevrie JJ. Myoclonic epilepsies of childhood. *Neuropediatrie.* 1971;3:177–190.
22. Deprez L, Jansen A, De Jonghe P. Genetics of epilepsy syndromes starting in the first year of life. *Neurology.* 2009;72:273–281.
23. Arzimanoglou A, French J, Blume WT, et al. Lennox-Gastaut syndrome: a consensus approach on diagnosis, assessment, management, and trial methodology. *Lancet Neurol.* 2009;8:82–93.
24. Egli M, Mothersill I, O'Kane M, et al. The Axial spasm-the predominant type of drop seizure in patients with secondary generalized epilepsy. *Epilepsia.* 1985;26:401–415.
25. Ikeno T, Shigematsu H, Miyakoshi M, et al. An analytic study of epileptic falls. *Epilepsia.* 1985;26:612–621.
26. Markand ON. Slow spike-wave activity in EEG and associated clinical features: often called "Lennox" or Lennox-Gastaut" syndrome. *Neurology.* 1977;27:746–757.
27. Blume WT, David RB, Gomez MR. Generalized sharp and slow wave complexes-associated clinical features and long term follow up. *Brain.* 1973;96:289–306.
28. Bonanni P, Parmeggiani L, Guerrini R. Different neurophysiologic patterns of myoclonus characterize Lennox-Gastaut syndrome and myoclonic astatic epilepsy. *Epilepsia.* 2002;43:609–615.
29. Beaumanoir A, Foletti G, Magistris M, et al. Status epilepticus in Lennox-Gastaut Syndrome in The Lennox-Gastaut Syndrome. In: Niedermeyer E, Degen R. eds. New York: Alan R. Liss; 1988:283–300.
30. Bittencourt PRM, Richens A. Anticonvulsant-induced status epilepticus in Lennox-Gastaut syndrome. *Epilepsia.* 1981;22:129–134.
31. Dimario FJ, Clancy RR. Paradoxical precipitation of tonic seizures by lorazepam in a child with atypical absence seizures. *Pediatr Neurol.* 1988;4:249–251.
32. Trevatham E. Infantile spasms and Lennox-Gastaut Syndrome. *J Child Neurol.* 2002;17:2S9–2S22.
33. Farrell K, Tatum WO. Encephalopathic Generalized Epilepsy and Lennox-Gastaut Syndrome. The Treatment of Epilepsy; Practice and Principals. 4th ed. In: Wyllie E, ed. Baltimore: Lippincott, Williams & Williams; 2006:429–440. Chapter 33.
34. Blume WT. Pathogenesis of Lennox-Gastaut Syndrome: Considerations and hypothesis. *Epileptic disord.* 2001;3:183–196.
35. Brenner RP, Atkinson R. Generalized paroxysmal fast activity: electroencephalographic and clinical features. *Ann Neurol.* 1982;11:386–390.
36. Ohtsuka Y, Yoshinaga H, Kobayashi K, et al. Diagnostic issues and treatment of cryptogenic or symptomatic generalized epilepsies. *Epilepsy Res.* 2006;70(supp):S132–S140.
37. Wong M, Trevathan E. Infantile spasms. *Pediatr Neurol.* 2001;24:89–98.
38. Stafstrom CE, Patxot OF, Gilmore HE, et al Seizures in children with Down syndrome: etiology, characteristics and outcome. *Dev Med Child Neurol.* 1991;33:191–200.
39. Hrachovy RA, Glaze DG, Frost JD Jr. A retrospective study of spontaneous remission and long-term outcome in patients with infantile spasms. *Epilepsia.* 1991;32:212–214.
40. Ohtahara S, Yamotogi Y. Epileptic encephalopathies in early infancy with suppression burst. *J Clin Neurophysiol.* 2003;20:398–407.
41. Djukic A, Lado FA, Shinnar S, et al. Are early myoclonic epilepsy (EME) and the Ohtahara Syndrome (EIEE) truly independent of each other?. *Epilepsy Res.* 2006;70S:S68–S76.

42. Oguni H, Tanaka T, Hayashi K, et al. Treatment and long term prognosis of myoclonic-astatic epilepsy of early childhood. *Neuropediatrics.* 2002;33:122–132.

43. Kaminska A, Ickowicz A, Plouin P, et al. Delineation of cryptogenic Lennox-Gastaut syndrome and myoclonic astatic epilepsy using multiple correspondence analysis. *Epilepsy Res.* 1999;36:15–29.

44. Guerrini R, Bonanni P, Marini C, et al. The myoclonic epilepsies in the treatment of epilepsy: Principles and Practices. In: Wyllie E,Gupta A, Lachhwani DK. eds. Lippincott Williams and Wilkins; 2006:407–428.

45. Wolff M, Casse-Perrot C, Dravet C. Severe myoclonic epilepsy of infants (Dravet Syndrome): Natural history and neuropsychological findings. *Epilepsia.* 2006;47(suppl 2):45–48.

46. Blume WT, Pillay N. Electroencephalographic and clinical correlates of secondary bilateral synchrony. *Epilepsia.* 1985;26:636–641.

47. Tanaka N, Kamada K, Takeuchi F, et al. Magnetoencephalographic analyis of secondary bilateral synchrony. *J Neuroimaging.* 2005;15:89–91.

48. Valente KD, Andrade JQ, Grossman RM, et al. Angelman Syndrome: Difficulties in EEG pattern recognition and possible misinterpretations. *Epilepsia.* 2003;44:1051–1063.

49. Jedele KB. The overlapping spectrum of Rett and Angelman Syndromes: a clinical review. *Semin Pediatr Neurol.* 2007;14:108–117.

50. Glaze DG. Neurophysiology of Rett Syndrome. *Ment Retard Dev Disabil Res Rev.* 2002;8(2):66–71.

51. Yamatogi Y, Ohtahara S. Multiple independent spike foci and epilepsy, with special reference to a new epileptic syndrome of "severe epilepsy with multiple independent spike foci". *Epilepsy research.* 2007;70(supp):S96–S104.

52. Oguni h, Hayashi K, Osawa M. Long term prognosis of Lennox-Gastaut Syndrome. *Epilepsia.* 37(supp 3):44–47.

53. Tatum WO IV, Benbadis SR, Hussain A, et al. Ictal EEG Remains The Prominent Predictor Of Seizure Free Outcome After Temporal Lobectomy In Epileptic Patients With Normal Brain MRI. *Seizure.* 2008;17:631–636.

54. Chugani HT, Mezziotta JC, Engel J, et al. The Lennox-Gastaut syndrome: Metabolic subtypes 2-deoxy-2-floro-d-glucose positron emission tomography. *Ann Neurol.* 1987;21:4–13.

55. Goffin K, Dedeurwaerdere S, Van Laere K, et al. Neuronuclear assessment of patients with epilepsy. *Semin Nucl Med.* 2008;38(4):227–239.

56. Tatum WO 4th. Long-Term EEG Monitoring: A Clinical Approach to Electrophysiology. *J Clin Neurophysiol.* 2001;18(5):442–455.

57. Guerrini R. Genetic malformations of the cerebral cortex and epilepsy. *Epilepsia.* 2005;46(supp1):32–37.

58. French JA, Kanner AM, Bautista J, et al. Efficacy and tolerability of the new antiepileptic drugs II: treatment of refractory epilepsy: report of the of the therapeutics and technology assessment committee of the American Academy of neurology and American epilepsy Society. *Neurology.* 2004;62:1261–1273.

59. Pellock JM, Faught E, Leppik IE, et al. Felbamate: consensus of current clinical experience. *Epilepsy Research.* 2006;71:89–101.

60. Arroyo S. Rufinamide. *Neurotherapeutics.* 2007;4:155–162.

61. Wheless JW, Clarke DF. Treatment of Pediatric epilepsy: expert opinion. *J Child Neurol.* 2005;20:S1–S6.

62. Wheless JW, Clarke DF, Arzimanoglou A, et al. Treatment of Pediatric Epilepsy: European expert opinion. *Epileptic Disord.* 2007;9:353–412.

63. Motte J, Trevathan E, Arvidsson JFV and the Lamictal Study group. Lamotrigine for generalized seizures associated with the Lennox Gastaut Syndrome. *N Engl J Med.* 1997;337:1807–1812.

64. Sachedo RC, Glauser TA, Ritter F et al. A double-blind, randomized trial of topiramate in Lennox-Gastaut syndrome. *Neurology.* 1999;52:1882–1887.

65. Glauser TA, Levisohn PM, Ritter F, et al. Topiramate in Lennox-Gastaut syndrome: open-label treatment of patients completing a randomized controlled trial. Topiramate YL study group. *Epilepsia.* 2000;suppl 1:S86–S90.

66. Coppola G, Caliendo G, Veggiotti P, et al. Topiramate as add-on drug in children, adolescents and young adults with Lennox-Gastaut syndrome: an Italian multicentre study. *Epilepsy Research.* 2002;51:147–153.

67. The felbamate study group in Lennox Gastaut syndrome. Efficacy of Felbamate in Childhood Epileptic Encephalopathy (Lennox-Gastaut Syndrome). *N Engl J Med.* 1993;328:29–33.

68. De los Reyes EC, Sharp GB, Williams JP. Levetiracetam in the treatment of Lennox Gastaut syndrome. *Pediatr Neurol.* 2004;30:254–256.

69. Iinuma K, Haginoya K. Clinical efficacy of zonisamide in childhood epilepsy after long term treatment: a postmarketing, multi-institutional survey. *Seizure.* 2004;13(suppl 1):S34–S39.

70. Hosain SA, Green NS, Solomon GE, et al. Nitrazepam for the treatment of Lennox-Gastaut syndrome. *Pediatr Neurol.* 2003;28:16–19.

71. van Rijckevorsel-Harmant K, Delire M, Rucquoy-Ponsar M. Treatment of idiopathic West and Lennox-Gastaut syndromes by intravenous administration of human polyvalent immunoglobulins. *European Archives of Psychiatry and Neurological Sciences.* 1986;236(2):119–122.

72. Smeraldi A, Scorza Smeraldi R, Cazullo CL, et al. Immunogenitics of the Lennox-Gastaut SYndome: frequency of HLA antigens and haplotypes in patients and first degree relatives. *Epilepsia.* 1975;16:699–703.

73. Freeman JM, Vining EPG, Pillas DJ, et al. The efficacy the ketogenic diet-1998: a prospective evaluation of intervention in 150 children. *Pediatrics.* 1998;102:1358–1363.

74. Vining EPG, Freeman JM, Balaban-Gil K, et al. A multi-center study of the efficacy of the ketogenic diet. *Arch Neurol.* 1998;55:1433–1437.

75. Freeman JM, Kossoff EH, Hartman AL. The ketogenic diet: one decade later. *Pediatrics.* 2007;119(3):535–543.

76. Maehara T, Shimizu H. Surgical outcome of corpus callostomy in patients with drop attacks. *Epilepsia.* 2008;42(1):67–71.

77. Quarato PP, Di Gennaro G, Manfredi M, et al. Atypical Lennox-Gastaut syndrome successfully treated with removal of parietal dysembryionic tumour. *Seizure.* 2002;11:325–329.

78. You SJ, Lee J-K, Ko, T-S. Epilepsy surgery in a patient with Lennox-Gastaut syndrome and cortical dysplasia. *Brain and Dev.* 2007;29:167–170.

79. Benbadis SR, Tatum WO, Vale FL. When drugs don't work: an algorithmic approach to medically intractable epilepsy. *Neurology.* 2000;55(12):1780–1784.

80. Rychlicki F, Zampoli N, Trigani R, et al. Vagus nerve stimulation: clinical experience in drug resistant pediatric epileptic patients. *Seizure.* 2006;15:483–490.

81. Helmers SL, Wheless JW, Frost M, et al. Vagal nerve stimulation in Pediatric patients with refractory epilepsy: retrospective study. *J Child Neurol.* 2001;16:843–848.

82. Nei M, O'Connor M, Liporace J, et al. Refractory generalized seizures: response to corpus callosotomy and vagus nerve stimulation. *Epilepsia.* 2006;47(1):115–122.

83. The Lennox-Gastaut syndrome. http://www.lennoxgastaut-options.com, accessed 2/2/09

84. Dulac O, Engel J. Lennox Gastaut Syndrome. ILAE Update; last updated April 30, 2005 at http://www.ilae-epilepsy.org/Visitors/Centre/ctf/lennox_gastaut.cfm (accessed 1/25/09).

CHAPTER 23 ■ CONTINUOUS SPIKE WAVE OF SLOW SLEEP AND LANDAU–KLEFFNER SYNDROME

MOHAMAD A. MIKATI AND SARA M. WINCHESTER

EPILEPTIC APHASIA: OVERVIEW

There are three types of mechanisms by which epilepsy can cause aphasia: (1) ictal, in which the aphasia is a manifestation of a focal seizure involving the speech areas; (2) interictal, in the which the aphasia is due to the direct effect of interictal spike-wave discharges; and (3) paraictal, in the which the aphasia is secondary to an epileptic encephalopathy. In the latter, the discharges can be present predominantly or exclusively in sleep, but the effect of the encephalopathy extends into wakefulness (1).

Ictal Aphasia

Ictal aphasia often occurs in left frontal or left temporal simple or complex partial seizures. In addition, nonconvulsive status epilepticus has presented as a subacute progressive aphasia in patients with epilepsy with acquired lesions such as cysticercosis or astrocytoma in adults and children (2–4). An example is that of a 6.5-year-old boy with a history of complex partial seizures who, after the addition of lamotrigine, developed severe oromotor apraxia with difficulty in chewing, swallowing, and speech. These symptoms constitute the opercular syndrome. This syndrome resolved over a 1-week time period following the substitution of phenobarbital for lamotrigine (5).

Interictal Aphasia

Patients with benign epilepsy with centrotemporal spikes (BECTS) have been reported to have a number of cognitive and speech abnormalities that correlate with the interictal discharges and then resolve with the disappearance of these discharges. For example, in one study of 20 patients with BECTS, 13 patients had language dysfunction, in particular in reading, spelling, auditory verbal learning, auditory discrimination, and expressive dysfunction. Moreover, language dysfunction was associated with spike frequency greater than 10 spikes/min (6). Croona and colleagues found normalization of cognitive dysfunction after resolution of spikes in patients with BECTS (7); similarly, Lindgren and colleagues identified no major cognitive deficits after the resolution of electroencephalogram (EEG) findings in patients with BECTS (8). BECTS may also cause an opercular syndrome in rare instances. For instance, a 5-year-old girl with BECTS developed fluctuating but persistent oromotor apraxia, drooling, dysarthria, and dysphagia over the course of 1 year. Her EEG demonstrated a marked increase in interictal awake and sleep discharges, which became bilateral. Here fluoro-deoxyglucose-positron emission tomography (FDG-PET) showed a bilateral increase in uptake in the opercular regions. Following the adjustment of her antiepileptic regimen (clonazepam in place of carbamazepine), the patient demonstrated both clinical recovery and normalization of the EEG and PET (9).

Paraictal Aphasia

This phenomenon occurs in Landau–Kleffner syndrome (LKS) and is part of the global impairment in epilepsy with continuous spikes and waves during slow sleep. LKS and continuous spike wave of slow sleep (CSWS) are two rare epileptic encephalopathies which can cause cognitive dysfunction and speech and behavioral disturbances. Previous reviews of these disorders such as the one by Neville and Cross in the previous edition of this book have noted the significant overlap between these two conditions, in that CSWS has various clinical manifestations including LKS. However, LKS is generally considered to have less prominent EEG findings that do not fulfill all criteria for CSWS (10,11). This chapter will explore the similarities and differences between the two syndromes.

DEFINITIONS AND GENERAL OVERVIEW

Landau–Kleffner Syndrome

The ILAE defined this syndrome as "a childhood disorder in which acquired aphasia, multifocal spikes, and spike and wave discharges are associated" (12). LKS was absent in earlier classification schemes from the ILAE in 1969 and 1981 as encephalopathies were not included. The general clinical presentation is that of verbal auditory agnosia, loss of language skills and behavioral problems, usually presenting between 3 and 8 years of age. Various seizure types may be present, and they generally respond well to antiepileptic therapy. EEG demonstrates paroxysmal spikes and spike and slow waves that are often multifocal and most commonly seen in temporal or temporoparietal-occipital regions. Activation of discharges occurs in sleep, and continuous spikes and spike waves during slow sleep are present in as many as 80% of patients.

Landau–Kleffner Variant

These patients do not have all of the classic features of LKS but have prominent behavioral problems with autistic features.

Continuous Spikes and Waves During Slow Sleep (as an EEG Finding)

Spike-wave activity constitutes >85% of slow-wave sleep time (13). It is found in multiple epilepsy syndromes. Synonyms include subclinical status epilepticus of sleep in children as when it was first described in 1971 (14), as well as electrographic status epilepticus during sleep (ESES) (15). However, some investigators have cautioned against using CSWS and ESES as synonyms; rather, ESES is used by some to describe the EEG abnormalities while the phrase "continuous spikes and waves during slow sleep" is used to designate the epilepsy syndrome as detailed below (16). In this chapter, we will use the term CSWS when referring to the EEG findings and CSWSS or "continuous spikes and waves during slow sleep syndrome" to refer to the epilepsy syndrome involving that EEG finding.

Epilepsy with Continuous Spikes and Waves During Slow Sleep. This epilepsy syndrome consists of neuropsychological and behavioral changes secondary to spikes and waves during slow sleep and is associated with both generalized and partial seizures during sleep and primarily atypical absences during wakefulness. Although the seizures tend to improve over time in patients with CSWSS, neuropsychological deficits may persist and affect quality of life.

The spike wave focus in CSWS is usually anterior in contrast to the temporal and posterior focus in LKS. This localization correlates with the clinical presentations of global impairments manifested by patients with CSWSS and the auditory agnosia evident in those with LKS.

General Principles of Therapy For Epileptic Aphasias

Therapy of ictal aphasia is achieved with traditional antiepileptic drugs or epilepsy surgery if appropriate. Therapy of interictal aphasia also includes traditional medications; although only case reports and case series currently support their use, prospective controlled studies are needed. Treatment of paraictal aphasia consists of traditional antiepileptic medications, immunotherapy, and surgical approaches, which will be discussed in this chapter.

CONTINUOUS SPIKE WAVES OF SLOW SLEEP SYNDROME AND LANDAU–KLEFFNER SYNDROME

Epidemiology and Clinical Presentation

Both CSWSS and LKS are rare. CSWSS was first described in 1971. Although the prevalence of CSWSS is unknown, Morikawa and colleagues found an incidence of 0.5% in 12,854 children reviewed at their center over 10 years, which has been corroborated by other researchers (17,18). Similarly in LKS, first described in 1957 (19), the prevalence is also unknown. However, 81 cases were reported between 1957 and 1980 and 117 between 1981 and 1991. Certainly there are many more cases of LKS than have been reported.

Epileptologists have noted that CSWSS and LKS have many clinical similarities. In both instances, children generally demonstrate regression after a period of normal development. In CSWSS, most patients have normal neuropsychological and motor development prior to the onset of CSWS as an EEG finding. When CSWS develops, most patients demonstrate a deterioration of language that can be accompanied by behavioral changes and rarely psychosis, temporospatial disorientation, a marked impairment in IQ, reduced attention span, aggression, and hyperkinesis. The pattern of neuropsychological deficits may vary among patients, possibly related to the location and duration of CSWS. Neuropsychological deterioration is one of the prominent clinical signs of CSWSS, but motor impairment and seizures may also be present (20). The most disabling motor deficits include dystonia, dyspraxia and ataxia, and negative myoclonus. The epileptic manifestations of CSWSS will be described later in this chapter.

Although considered a diagnosis of children, CSWSS has been identified in an adult in a recent case report of a 21-year-old male admitted for video-EEG and seizure exacerbations with outbursts of anger. Focal slow wave activity in the right temporal region and CSWS were observed during 3 days of monitoring; this finding resolved after a change in his antiepileptic regimen (21).

CSWS may occur in children with other pathologies such as hydrocephalus or brain tumor. In a recent case report of nine children with early-onset hydrocephalus and seizures, CSWS was present and associated with neurocognitive and motor deterioration. Hyperkinesia, aggressiveness, and poor socialization were present, and one third of the children also had reduced attention span, deterioration of language, and temporospatial discrimination. Two patients had negative myoclonus. Antiepileptic drug regimens were modified, resulting in improvement in the clinical picture. Thus, this report illustrates the importance of performing periodic EEG recordings during sleep in children with hydrocephalus who exhibit behavioral and language deterioration (22).

Patients with LKS present with loss of expressive speech and verbal agnosia usually between the ages of 3 and 8 years, although patients as young as 2 years and as old as 14 years have been identified. Both CSWSS and LKS demonstrate a preponderance of male patients, specifically with a ratio of 2:1 in LKS. Family and medical history are usually noncontributory in LKS. However, some authors have noted that in as many as 13% of reported cases of LKS, the patient had some prior language abnormality in contrast to the strict definition of the syndrome which requires prior normal development (23,24). Case reports of patients with CSWSS have implicated a possible unknown genetic mechanism in that a pair of affected monozygotic twins has been identified. Familial seizure disorders, including febrile convulsions, have been identified in 15% of patients with CSWS (25,26).

In one review by Rousselle and Revol (27) of 209 cases from the literature, children were classified into four groups depending on prior development and clinical presentation. The first group, consisting of 35 children, initially had a normal neurological exam, except for one child, and all presented with severe epilepsy without any significant neuropsychological deterioration. The second group of 33 children presented with language deterioration and were classified as LKS. The third group of children encompassed 99 children who were initially normal neurologically but then had global or selective neuropsychological deterioration without alteration of language function. These were consistent with the CSWSS. The final group consisting of 42 children had either focal or diffuse brain lesions and unknown clinical manifestations. The authors then correlated the clinical impairment in these four groups with the duration and the location of the electrographic abnormalities, which supported prior hypotheses that the neuropsychological deficits and acquired aphasia were the consequences of the EEG findings during sleep. For instance, children in group one had a mean duration of 6 months of CSWS and a centrotemporal focus of EEG findings, an area, presumably, without cognitive role. Those in group two with LKS exhibited a temporal lobe prominence of abnormalities and ESES for at least 18 months. Those with global deterioration in the third and fourth groups had a frontal prominence of EEG abnormalities and CSWS for at least 2 years (27).

In patients with LKS, anxiety can occur as a reaction to the loss of understanding of spoken language. In some patients, the auditory agnosia is insidious and can present over the course of a year, initially manifesting as word deafness. Children may not respond to parents' commands, even those issued in a loud voice. The agnosia can worsen to the point that children are unable to recognize familiar sounds in their environment, such as a ringing bell or a telephone. Rarely parents may report sudden worsening or loss of language after a clinical seizure. Initially parents suspect that the child has a hearing impairment, but no abnormalities are found in audiograms or brainstem auditory-evoked responses. However, there may be delays in long-latency cortical-evoked responses, implicating the posterior temporal regions of the brain. In addition, permanent extinction of one ear contralateral to the involved temporal cortex is shown with dichotic listening tasks. Word deafness can progress to the point that the child does not respond at all. Problems in expression, including frequent or continuous misarticulations, telegraphic speech, flowing jargon, or even complete mutism, may occur. Written language in older children may be preserved or impaired (28). The type of aphasia may change over time, and no strict correlation has been observed between the EEG abnormalities and the type of aphasia demonstrated (29).

The language problems of LKS may resemble those of the autistic spectrum disorders. However, there are some clear differences that aid in distinguishing these entities. Autistic children have difficulty in the development of spoken language and with starting a conversation. Their language is typically stereotyped, repetitive, and characteristic. Sometimes autistic children will have seizures and frequent EEG discharges, further confusing the distinction between the two syndromes. Moreover, it is also known that at least one third of autistic children will have neurodevelopmental deterioration involving language, sociability, and playing and thinking skills.

However, the differences between LKS and autistic patients lie in the age of presentation and the extent and types of language deficits. For instance, those with autism will typically experience language regression before the age of 3 and will typically lose single words. Those children with LKS present at an older age (typically 5 to 7 years old) and thus have a more dramatic presentation in that they lose phrases or whole sentences and more vocabulary as they have had time to develop more language. In addition, children with LKS do not tend to have the difficulties with reciprocal social interactions nor the limited, stereotyped interests and behaviors manifested by children on the autistic spectrum.

Children who fulfill at least some of the clinical and electrographic criteria of LKS, but who also have behavioral difficulties more typical of the autistic spectrum disorders, are characterized as having the Landau–Kleffner variant. In addition, speech loss with autistic symptoms caused by epilepsy due to a focal lesion has been reported in a few cases. DeLong and Heinz described four infants with bilateral hippocampal sclerosis with episodes of status epilepticus and severe infantile autism (30). Gillberg and colleagues described a patient with tuberous sclerosis, autism, and continuous epileptiform activity emanating from the right parieto-occipital and temporal areas (31). Mikati et al. recently reported a case detailed below with a right temporal ganglioglioma that fulfilled the criteria of LKS and autism (32).

Behavioral difficulties are identified in some series in at least half of the children with classical LKS (33). These difficulties cannot be ascribed simply to the children's frustration at being unable to communicate many of their needs; rather, the severity and type of behavioral disturbance suggests another etiology. Hyperactivity, impulsivity, and aggression may be encountered. Sleep, and in particular settling down at bedtime, is difficult (11). In addition, as many as two thirds of children with LKS may exhibit motor problems that encompass organizational difficulties, ataxia, bulbar symptoms, and dystonia, making activities of daily living more difficult for them (34,35).

Epileptic Manifestations

Seventy percent of patients with LKS have seizures. One third of them have one seizure or a single status epilepticus event, usually at the onset of the syndrome. The other patients usually have occasional seizures between 5 and 10 years. Sporadic seizures persist in one fifth of the patients after the age of 10. However, seizures rarely occur after the age of 15. The predominant seizure type in LKS is a nocturnal simple partial seizure. Complex partial seizures can occur infrequently, but atonic seizures are common. More rare seizure types encountered include generalized tonic–clonic seizures, atypical absence, and myoclonic-astatic seizures. Prognosis is not determined by the type or frequency of seizures.

Similarly, in CSWSS, seizures are not the major clinical feature, and often present months or years prior to the diagnosis. Focal or generalized tonic–clonic seizures, especially common at night, are seen. "Drop attacks" or atonic seizures occur in about half of the patients and may precede the electrographic abnormalities (17). Tassinari and colleagues have observed that the seizure semiology may change after the EEG findings are first discovered (20). They have proposed three classifications of patients with CSWSS based on seizure patterns: one group with rare nocturnal seizures comprising 11% of patients, a second group with unilateral partial motor seizures

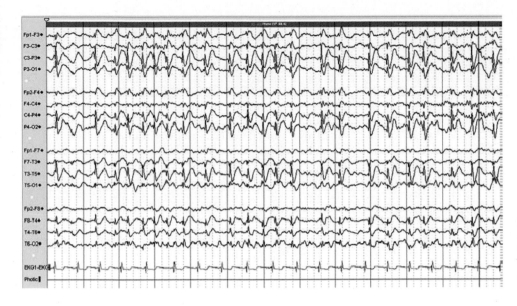

FIGURE 23.1 The EEG of a 6-year-old girl with LKS showing essentially continuous predominantly left-sided spike slow-wave discharges with phase reversals over C3 and T3 in sleep.

or generalized tonic–clonic seizures occurring mainly during sleep without events during wakefulness in 44.5% of patients, and a third group (also 44.5%) with rare nocturnal seizures but with atypical absence seizures that may include atonic or tonic components causing sudden falls (36).

EEG Findings

In LKS, focal or multifocal epileptic discharges commonly occur in the temporal areas (Fig. 23.1), although localization to the frontal lobes has been reported in one third of patients in one series (35). Studies have implicated the temporal lobe as being the site origin of the discharges in LKS, in particular the superior temporal gyrus and into the sylvian fissure. However, EEG foci may also encompass multiple and extrasylvian locations (37). Paroxysmal activity is rarely precipitated by hyperventilation or by photic stimulation but is consistently enhanced during sleep, often leading to continuous spikes and waves during slow sleep. Although common, the presence of CSWS is not essential to diagnose LKS as studies have shown that this EEG pattern occurs in a variable percentage of up to 80%, but not in all, of the patients fulfilling the criteria of LKS. One study noted that presence of epileptiform activity in slow-wave sleep in patients with LKS was variable, occurring in 85% of slow-wave sleep in 20% of patients (which meets definition for CSWS). An additional 26% of patients had epileptiform activity in 50 to 80% of sleep, and discharges were present in less than 50% of sleep for the remaining 54% of the patients (35). It is important to note that the epileptiform abnormalities seen in the EEG during slow-wave sleep in LKS patients may temporarily abate; thus, a single normal tracing during sleep does not exclude this diagnosis (38).

Patients with CSWSS demonstrate spike-and-slow-wave activity that is bilateral and mainly generalized. The continuous spike-wave discharges occur at 1.5 to 2.5 Hz and persist during slow-wave sleep, particularly in the first sleep cycle (39).

A recent review of children with CSWS was undertaken by Van Hirtum-Das and colleagues. They analyzed 1497 EEG

records of children admitted to UCLA for overnight-video-EEG monitoring during a 5-year period. Of the records analyzed, 102 met criteria for CSWS. Clinical information from 90 patients revealed that 18 of them met criteria for LKS. The authors noted that of children who did not fit diagnostic criteria for LKS, a spike-wave index of greater than 50% was more likely to be associated with global developmental problems than a spike wave index of less than 50%. Children with generalized discharges were more likely to have severe or global developmental disturbance than those with focal abnormalities, although this finding did not reach significance (40).

Diagnosis and Differential Diagnosis

Essentials for the diagnosis of LKS include (1) auditory agnosia with language regression and (2) epileptiform abnormalities that worsen during sleep. Ancillary testing is not required to diagnose the syndrome, although brain magnetic resonance imaging (MRI) is performed to rule out focal lesions. Twenty to thirty percent of children will not have clinical seizures at the time of their diagnosis of LKS. Some authors have suggested two variant forms of LKS: one with mild primary language delay and typical regression after the age of 2 and a second form seen in those with a lesion, usually temporal. Children younger than 2 years with regression of speech are typically excluded from the diagnosis of LKS even if they demonstrate the typical epileptiform abnormalities (11).

The diagnosis of CSWSS as an epilepsy syndrome is also based upon the clinical presentation and the EEG findings. Tassinari proposed the following criteria for the syndrome of CSWS: (1) neuropsychological impairment seen as global or selective regression of cognitive or expressive functions such as acquired aphasia, (2) motor impairment in the form of ataxia, dyspraxia, dystonia, or a unilateral deficit, (3) epilepsy with focal (partial motor seizures) or generalized seizures (tonic–clonic or absence), complex partial seizures or epileptic falls, and (4) electrographic status epilepticus occurring during at least 85% of slow sleep (20). In addition, there was a previous criterion proposed in earlier reports that the EEG abnormality should persist on three or more records for at least 1 month (14). Whether all these criteria must be present to make the diagnosis is debatable: Some patients may not have the clinical seizures or some of the motor manifestations but may have the other findings as well as a clinical course and response to therapy that are fully consistent with this syndrome.

It is crucial to distinguish LKS, Landau–Kleffner variant, and CSWSS from each other and from autism and benign rolandic epilepsy with centrotemporal spikes (BECTS) that exacerbates during sleep. As discussed above, CSWSS resembles LKS clinically, but the difference between them arises from the EEG (which might not show continuous spikes and waves during slow sleep in LKS) and from the general mental deficiency and neuropsychological deficits in CSWSS in contrast to the, relatively isolated, serious comprehension problems (auditory agnosia) in LKS. Moreover, the spike focus in LKS is usually temporal in contrast to the frontal focus in CSWSS. The course of the two syndromes differs in that patients with CSWSS tend to suffer from global cognitive abnormalities whereas those with LKS have deficits primarily in the spheres of behavior and speech.

Care must also be taken to differentiate these disorders from BECTS with exacerbation during sleep. In rare cases of BECTS, the strong activation during sleep of the centrotemporal EEG spike-and-wave activity results in cognitive decline, speech difficulty, and attention disorders. EEG in the typical patient with BECTS displays normal background rhythms with spike foci that may be unilateral or bilateral. The EEG record as a rule shows typical morphology of high-amplitude and diphasic waveforms. Usually, however, the deficits are not severe enough and demonstrate differences from those seen in LKS and CSWSS as described below.

The seizure types found in patients with BECTS are typically simple partial seizures that include speech arrest, excessive drooling, twitching of the face, stiffening of the tongue, or other sensorimotor phenomena of the orofacial region. Less frequently, complex partial seizures, generalized seizures, or complex partial seizures with secondary generalization may be observed. When regression is present, it typically does not consist of verbal or auditory agnosia. Most patients have normal cognition and have a good long-term outcome. However, some patients may develop oromotor dysfunction, neuropsychological deficits, or attention deficits with learning disorders. These outcomes may be more common in patients with BECTS who already had atypical features. Atypical features include leg jerking, unilateral body sensations, ictal blindness, epigastric pain, lateral body torsion, diurnal seizures only, status epilepticus, developmental delay, and attention deficit disorder. Neuropsychological deficits may consist of cognitive dysfunction, auditory-verbal and visuospatial memory problems, and behavioral problems. BECTS may be exacerbated by some antiepileptic drugs, leading to continuous spikes and waves during slow sleep as an EEG finding. Patients may develop the atypical features over time. Finally, a small number of patients with BECTS develop LKS years later.

Laboratory and Radiologic Studies

Imaging, including computed tomography (CT) brain and or MRI brain, is usually performed. Cerebrospinal fluid analysis may be performed as well. In one series of 67 patients with CSWS, structural abnormalities on brain MRI were present in half of the patients (33/67). The most common radiographic abnormalities seen were cortical dysplasia, congenital stroke, diffuse atrophy, white matter changes, and abnormal or delayed myelination. Those children with radiographic abnormalities were more likely to have developmental delay (40). In some patients, multilobar polymicrogyria has been associated with CSWS, and these patients were more likely to have atonic seizures but not to have apparent cognitive deficits at the time of diagnosis (41).

In contrast, children with LKS usually have normal imaging and CSF studies. Rarely there may be elevations in CSF protein or IgG, white matter changes on brain MRI, or structural abnormalities. Occasionally, some enlargement or asymmetry of the temporal horns can be present, and this finding

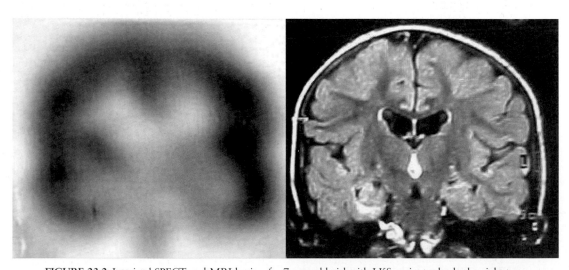

FIGURE 23.2 Interictal SPECT and MRI brain of a 7-year-old girl with LKS variant who had a right temporal lobe ganglioglioma. Despite a distinctly localized lesion in the right medial temporal lobe, the perfusion abnormality involves hypoperfusion of the whole of the right temporal and parietal lobes as compared to the left. The asymmetric temporoparietal perfusion demonstrated in this interictal SPECT has been described in other patients with LKS.

has been attributed to long-term epileptic activity. Various studies using single-photon emission computed tomography (SPECT) and PET in patients with LKS have demonstrated abnormalities in perfusion and glucose metabolism in the temporal lobe. These findings have included hyper- or hypometabolism in the middle temporal gyri on FDG-PET. SPECT scans have also shown abnormalities in the temporal lobe consisting of hypo- or hyperperfusion. Hyperperfusion has been identified during times of active seizure discharges or during clinical epileptic seizures. Hypoperfusion and asymmetry in perfusion of the temporoparietal regions between the two sides (Fig. 23.2) have also been reported at other times (42,43). The exact relationship between the aphasia seen in LKS and changes in glucose metabolism in the temporal lobe is not known as these features are also present in patients with epilepsy who do not manifest aphasia. Bilateral volume reduction of the superior temporal areas in LKS has also been reported (Fig. 23.3) (44).

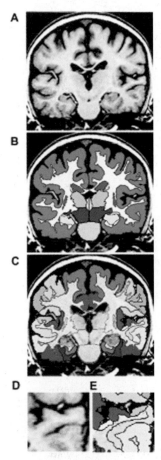

FIGURE 23.3 Demonstration of bilateral volume reduction of the superior temporal areas in Landau–Kleffner syndrome. Slices of T1-weighted fast-spoiled gradient-recalled (FSPGR) images, segmented structures, and parcellation units are shown at the level of Heschl gyrus, basal ganglia, amygdala, hippocampus, and thalamus. (**A**) T1-weighted FSPGR images; (**B**) segmented structures; (**C**) parcellation units; (**D**) enlarged T1-weighted FSPGR images of Heschl gyrus and surroundings; and (**E**) enlarged parcellation units of Heschl gyrus and surroundings. Heschl gyrus, dark blue; planum polare, light yellow; planum temporale, dark green; superior temporal gyrus posterior, light green; middle temporal gyrus, light blue; insula, brown; parieto-operculum cortex, light brown. (From Takeoka M, Riviello JJ Jr., Duffy FH, et al. Bilateral volume reduction of the superior temporal areas in Landau-Kleffner syndrome. *Neurology.* 2004;63(7):1152–1153.)

Etiology and Pathogenesis

It appears that LKS is a syndrome of multiple etiologies that are yet to be elucidated fully. This syndrome first was attributed to encephalitis because initial reports indicated the presence of encephalitic changes in a biopsy taken from the cortex of a patient with LKS. However, subsequent investigations could not confirm the presence of encephalitic changes in pathologic specimens from other patients. Autoimmune mechanisms have been proposed as well. Autoantibodies against brain-derived neurotrophic factor, neuronal antigens, myelin, and brain endothelial cells were found in the sera of some patients with LKS. In addition, IgM antiendothelial cell autoantibodies were found by Connolly and colleagues in the sera of children with LKS compared with healthy children (45). In support of an immunologic mechanism, in at least some of the LKS patients, is our experience in 11 patients with this syndrome who were given intravenous immunoglobulin (IVIG); the two patients who did respond were found to have a high IgG index in their cerebrospinal fluid in contrast to the patients who did not respond to the therapy (46). Various case reports have implicated genetic predisposition, cerebral arteritis, toxoplasmosis, neurocysticercosis, temporal astrocytoma, temporal ganglioglioma, *Haemophilus influenzae* meningitis, subacute sclerosing panencephalitis, inflammatory demyelinating disease, and abnormal zinc metabolism. A recent case report identified a patient with LKS who had a right temporal ganglioglioma causing secondary falsely localizing left temporal lobe CSWS with a clinical picture of Landau–Kleffner variant; the patient responded to resection (32). Mitochondrial respiratory chain defects have been identified in two patients with LKS in one group of children with epilepsy syndromes (47).

Over the past 5 years, recent data have provided substantial insights into the pathophysiology of LKS and CSWSS. Shouse and colleagues developed an amygdala kindling model of kittens that resembles continuous spikes and waves during slow sleep in its electrical activity (48). The mechanisms leading to persistent spike-wave activity in this model and in patients with CSWSS and LKS appear to involve cortical rather than subcortical synchronization. In both LKS and CSWSS, there is a bilateral or unilateral increase in metabolism in the temporal cortex in sleep that often persists into wakefulness and becomes normal or decreased after recovery. The thalamus does not show such abnormalities. This finding suggests that the mechanisms of neuronal synchronization occurring in CSWSS and LKS are different from those of primary generalized epilepsy and involve cortical rather than thalamocortical-mediated synchronization. Furthermore, functional maturation and pruning of synapses occur in a sequential fashion in different areas of the developing brain: first in the occipital areas, then in the temporal areas, and finally in the frontal areas (49). Maximal synaptic density in the visual cortex occurs at about 1 year of age and in the auditory cortex at approximately 4 years of age. The timing of occurrence of LKS with the abnormal discharges that are maximal over the temporal area coincides with the time of occurrence of functional maturation of temporal speech areas in childhood. Thus, it has been hypothesized that the continuous discharges and abnormally increased neuronal activity impair pruning and consequently result in long-term speech deficits (28).

Treatment and Overall Course

General Principles of Therapy

Patients with CSWSS and LKS require the support of a multidisciplinary team including a speech therapist, neuropsychologist, and a pediatric neurologist. Issues addressed by this team include seizures, speech and neuropsychological dysfunction, and behavioral problems. Families and patients require integration of medical and neuropsychological services as well as support services including speech therapy and social work. Family and parent support groups may be helpful.

Therapy of LKS and CSWSS is controversial given the lack of controlled clinical trials. Figure 23.4 shows the approach we have been using in the management of these two disorders. The therapeutic approaches used are based on open-label data, usually collected from case reports with small numbers of patients. Therapy consists of pharmacologic treatment and surgical treatment. Pharmacologic intervention includes anticonvulsants, corticosteroids, adrenocorticotrophic hormone (ACTH), and IVIG. Steroid therapy and high-dose benzodiazepines are most commonly used now. It is important to address all of the symptoms of the disorder, in particular seizures, speech problems, and behavior. Management of seizures is more straight forward in most cases. It is important to note that due to the unpredictable remissions and fluctuating course of LKS, it is difficult to assess the effectiveness of any treatment.

Antiepileptic Drugs

Conventional antiepileptic drugs are effective in controlling the seizures of patients with LKS; however, their effect on aphasia is not consistent. Recently some studies have noted that the use of repeated high doses of diazepam resolved the electrical abnormality and improved cognitive and speech functions but that tolerance to the drug is an issue. DeNegri et al. reported that a regimen of a high dosage of oral diazepam (0.75 mg/kg/day with a blood level of 100 to 400 ng/mL) given for six short cycles (3 to 4 weeks) was successful in treating ESES in patients, including one with LKS (50). In a subsequent study published in abstract form, Riviello and his group reported the administration of rectal or oral diazepam 1 mg/kg/dose (up to a maximum of 40 mg) for patients with LKS or CSWS on two consecutive nights with continuous video-EEG monitoring for 2 days and pulse oximetry for 4 h following the diazepam dose. The patients were then administered diazepam 0.5 mg/kg/day (up to a maximum of 20 mg) for 3 to 4 weeks, followed by a slow taper (2.5 mg/month). Eleven of the 13 patients responded to treatment in that their language and EEG improved within a month. We believe that this treatment should be used very early in the management, or possibly as the initial management, of children with LKS.

Valproate (10 to 50 mg/kg/day) (51–53), clobazam (1 to 1.6 mg/kg/day) (51), and ethosuximide (20 mg/kg/day) were reported to be effective in stopping seizures and in reducing language problems in about half of the patients who received them (51). Valproate at a dose of 20 mg/kg/day was reported to be effective in improving the speech problems, especially in those patients whose aphasia started earlier (53). The use of ethosuximide (20 mg/kg/day) combined with either valproic acid, phenobarbital, carbamazepine, or a benzodiazepine, and that of vigabatrin combined with ethosuximide, carbamazepine, or clonazepam were also reported to be effective in

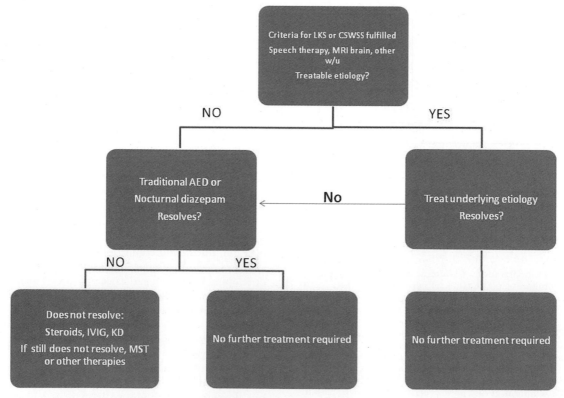

FIGURE 23.4 Proposed algorithm for treatment of LKS and CSWSS based on a protocol at the authors' institution. Other centers may have different protocols.

some patients with LKS (54). However, it is not recommended to use carbamazepine in patients with LKS because it was often found to worsen their condition, even if these patients have focal motor seizures. Lamotrigine monotherapy improved cognitive functions and language in some patients (54). Nicardipine (0.5 to 2 mg/kg/day) combined with conventional antiepileptic drugs was reported to be effective in some patients with LKS (55). Felbamate given as polytherapy or as monotherapy (60 mg/kg/day) was able to dramatically improve language skills and EEG abnormalities in some patients (56). Sulthiame and levetiracetam (35 to 60 mg/kg/day) in some patients as well as levetiracetam in one patient have been reported to be effective in the treatment of LKS (57). Vigabatrin was reported to produce dramatic improvement in speech and seizures in a case of LKS (58). The 4:1 ketogenic diet (four parts saturated fats and one part proteins and carbohydrates) was reported to be an effective treatment of patients with acquired epileptic aphasia. Valproate and ethosuximide have also been found to be helpful in patients with CSWSS (25).

In a recent study by Kramer and colleagues of 34 patients with CSWSS (the study did not include LKS), levetiracetam and clobazam were found to be the most efficacious antiepileptic drugs. Forty one percent responded to levetiracetam, 31% responded to clobazam, and 17% responded to sulthiame. Valproate, lamotrigine, topiramate, and ethosuximide showed no efficacy. High-dose diazepam was efficacious in 37%, but all the children had a temporary response (59).

Corticosteroids and ACTH

Corticosteroids and ACTH (50 to 80 units/day given for 4 weeks to 3 months) have been reported to be useful in improving language, cognitive, and behavioral problems. For example, ACTH given at 20 units/day for 1 to 2 weeks improved EEG abnormalities, clinical seizures, and behavior and speech problems in a recent case report of five children (60). Although it is not known which regimen is most effective (51,61–70), the therapy was found to be more effective when used earlier in the course, and long-term low-dose therapy was continued in the patients as relapses were common after the initial treatment.

Prednisone is given orally (2 to 3 mg/kg for 1 to 2 months and then tapered according to response) or given at a dose that ranges from 30 to 60 mg/day (51,61–65). Dexamethasone has been given to patients with LKS in a dose of 4 mg/day for 2 weeks and then tapered after that. Steroids have been helpful in children with CSWS, in that 65% responded (59).

Intravenous methylprednisolone given as 20 mg/kg daily for 3 days and then every 4 days then repeated three times, followed by oral prednisolone 2 mg/kg daily for 1 month or given as 500 mg over 3 h daily for 5 days followed by 250 mg infusion over 2 h once a month was reported to be effective in a few patients resistant to other therapies (66,67). An additional study by You demonstrated that treatment with prednisolone 2 mg/kg/day for 6 weeks followed by a 2-week weaning period did improve seizure frequency in children with refractory epilepsy, including LKS (71). Treatment with steroids usually needs to be prolonged for several months or for more than a year to avoid relapses. This prolonged steroid therapy can cause several side effects, including avascular necrosis of the hip, hypertension, behavioral abnormalities, gastric ulcers, hyperglycemia, and immunosuppression. Side effects can be lessened with every-other-day dosing or weekend pulse dosing.

Intravenous Immunoglobulin

IVIG is a useful option in the therapy of LKS and CSWSS because occasional cases respond to this treatment. Historically, IVIG has been used in West syndrome, Lennox–Gastaut syndrome, and more recently in LKS and CSWS (72). The usual protocol for intractable seizures is 2 g/kg of IVIG in divided doses over 4 days followed by 1 g/kg/day every 4 weeks for 6 months. However, in LKS the patients who respond tend to do so within days of initiation of the IVIG and need IVIG at the time of the exacerbations of their aphasia. Whether long-term therapy with IVIG is needed and how long is not clear. A high cerebrospinal fluid IgG index may be a prognostic indicator as stated above. In our experience although only a minority of children show a definite remarkable and long-term response to this therapy (about 20% of patients), the children who do so initially have a quick and dramatic change starting around day 3 of the infusion. This eventually results in the remission of speech difficulties within a few days to a few weeks. After such an initial and remarkable improvement, these patients can have relapses a few months apart but can still respond to additional courses of IVIG in the same quick and remarkable manner (73–75).

Surgery

Multiple subpial transection (MST) is a procedure that has been reported to improve the profile of patients with LKS who have failed multiple medical therapies (76). This procedure involves sectioning the horizontal interneurons, thereby hopefully decreasing the epileptic discharges from the speech cortex while simultaneously preserving the area's physiologic functions. Multiple subpial transection in some reports has eradicated continuous spike waves during sleep and ameliorated language function of those children as well. In a position paper by Cross et al., MST was considered the surgical procedure of choice in LKS as recommended by the ILAE Subcommission for Pediatric Epilepsy Surgery (77). However, this procedure should only be performed at specialized centers thoroughly familiar with this problem. Many experts still view it as a mostly experimental procedure. Patients in general must fulfill several restrictive criteria prior to undergoing the surgery, including a normal developmental history of language and cognition prior to onset of language dysfunction, normal nonverbal cognitive function, unilateral intra- and perisylvian epileptogenic zone, and duration continuous spikes and waves during slow sleep of lesser than 3 years. Vagal nerve stimulation is another type of surgery that may help patients with LKS with refractory seizures. It was reported to decrease seizure frequency by half in three of six children in one study. One study found benefit in the procedure in patients with seizures, CSWS, and pure language regression but who did not have autistic features or global cognitive impairment. Significant benefit has not been established in other studies in patients with CSWS and autistic features (76). Effects on aphasia still need to be determined. It also remains to be proven whether the extent of improvement in patients who have undergone multiple subpial transection affects the quality of life or long-term outcome. In children who have CSWS in conjunction with other pathologies, epilepsy surgery may be beneficial. For instance, one case report detailed the story of a 5-year-old child with right congenital hemiparesis due to prenatal left MCA infarction. He had focal epilepsy since the age of 3 months, but then had rapid cognitive and behavioral regression with a frontal syndrome between the age of 4 and 5 years. EEG recordings during sleep revealed CSWS. Hemispherectomy resulted in remission of the clinical seizures and resolution of the CSWS on EEG, with subsequent partial remission of the neurocognitive issues (78). In other cases focal resection of localized lesions has resulted in similar improvements (32).

Speech Therapy

Interventions to improve speech dysfunction have included sign language, a daily diary of consecutive pictures of the classroom routine, auditory training starting with environmental sounds, and a "graphic conversation" technique. Despite appropriate treatment, some patients with LKS may still have problems related to processing of oral language. Case reports exist of children with LKS who have learned sign language; using sign language does not appear to impair ability to regain oral language. Interestingly, ability of children with LKS to learn a new linguistic code such as sign language may indicate that higher order language areas are preserved in this syndrome (79).

Behavioral modification techniques and medications may also be required. Features of attention deficit hyperactivity disorder may respond to methylphenidate, amphetamine, or atomoxetine. Impulsivity and aggressive behavior may require clonidine, behavioral modification techniques, or consultation with a child psychiatrist. Anxiety may be alleviated with selective serotonin reuptake inhibitors. Sleep difficulties have been treated with melatonin or short-acting benzodiazepines. It should be noted that side effects secondary to antiepileptic medications may exacerbate features of LKS, such as valproate worsening irritability, particularly in combination with corticosteroids. Parents and other caregivers as well as school personnel will require education regarding the management decisions. Some authors have noted behavioral improvements after appropriate medical treatment of the seizures or after MST (80). One recent case–control study found high rates of psychiatric diagnoses in cases of children with BECTS and CSWSS using the Schedule for Affective Disorders and Schizophrenia in School-Age Children (K-SADS) and advocated consultation of a psychiatrist when treating these children (81).

General Course and Prognosis

CSWSS is usually seen in younger children, and potential for resolution of the EEG findings and clinical seizures is good. Most children do not have further seizures as they reach adolescence; this improvement may precede the resolution of EEG abnormalities in 30% of patients or coincide with the resolution in another 40% of patients. Finally, 40% of children stop having seizures after the EEG improves. However, this guideline is not absolute as case reports exist of adults with nearly CSWS that were present for at least 4 years (82). Experts have cautioned that prognosis "at best remains guarded" due to potential for neuropsychological deficits. Some studies have noted partial but significant epint improvement after resolution of the EEG findings with at least half of patients with CSWS

having nearly average neuropsychological outcome with ability to live independently (83,84). Duration of the abnormal EEG findings in children with CSWSS has been correlated with residual intellectual deficit at follow-up (59). In fact, longer duration of the CSWS in children with LKS and CSWSS may be the major predictor of poor outcome. Some experts have postulated that abnormal neuronal activity during a critical period for synaptogenesis may result in abnormal proliferation and neuronal connections, potentially explaining the neuropsychological deficits that develop (85).

Children with LKS can recover completely from aphasia months or years after the onset of the syndrome. Others, who constitute approximately one half of patients, recover partially or suffer from permanent aphasia. Some cases are characterized by periods of fluctuating relapses and remissions. Prognosis is affected by many factors, such as age at onset, type of language deficit, frequency and topography of EEG abnormalities, epilepsy duration, and effectiveness and side effects of antiepileptic drugs. Outcomes range from permanent aphasia to complete recovery. Moreover, the prognosis is better when the onset of language deficits occurs after the age of 6 and when speech therapy is started at an early stage of the illness. Verbal agnosia has been shown recently to significantly affect quality of life (86).

The relationship between age at onset of language deficits and end result is contrary to the situation of childhood aphasia after structural injury. The older the patient with LKS, the greater the chance of language improvement. In aphasia associated with a lesion, the older the age at which the lesion appears, the lower the probability of language improvement. Improvement in EEG often precedes improvement in LKS-associated language disorders but does not guarantee the most favorable outcome. In fact some have found a strong relationship between the manifestation of language problems and EEG changes where speech and EEG improved simultaneously, whereas others did not find such a relationship.

CONCLUSIONS

There is increasing recognition of the clinical spectrum of epilepsies associated with aphasia and of the underlying pathophysiologic mechanisms. There have also been recent advances in identifying more effective therapeutic strategies for these disorders. However, a significant group of patients are left with permanent deficits in critical spheres of cognition and communication which can impact their quality of life. The discovery of more effective therapies depends on further understanding of the underlying pathophysiology as well as further trials, including hopefully controlled and multicenter clinical therapeutic investigations.

References

1. Hirsch E, Valenti MP, Rudolf G, et al. Landau Kleffner syndrome is not an eponymic badge of ignorance. *Epilepsy Res.* 2006;70(Suppl 1):S239–S247.
2. Otero E, Cordova S, Diaz F, et al. Acquired epileptic aphasia (the Landau-Kleffner syndrome) due to neurocysticercosis. *Epilepsia.* 1989;30: 569–572.
3. Solomon G, Carson D, Pavlakis S, et al. Intracranial EEG monitoring in Landau-Kleffner syndrome associated with left temporal lobe astrocytoma. *Epilepsia.* 1993;34:557–560.
4. Chung PW, Seo DW, Kwon JC, et al. Nonconvulsive status epilepticus presenting as a subacute progressive aphasia. *Seizure.* 2002;11:449–454.

5. Shuper A, Stahl B, Mimouni M. Transient opercular syndrome: a manifestation of uncontrolled epileptic activity. *Acta Neurol Scand.* 2000;101:335–338.
6. Staden U, Isaacs E, Boyd SG, et al. Language dysfunction in children with rolandic epilepsy. *Neuropediatrics.* 1998;29:242–248.
7. Croona C, Kihlgren M, Lundberg S, et al. Neuropyschological findings in children with benign childhood epilepsy with centrotemporal spikes. *Dev Med Child Neurol.* 1999;41:813–818.
8. Lindgren S, Kilhlgren M, Melin L, et al. Development of cognitive functions in children with rolandic epilepsy. *Epilepsy Behav.* 2004;5:903–910.
9. Tachikawa E, Oguni H, Shirakawa S, et al. Acquired epileptiform opercular syndrome: a case report and results of single photon emission computed tomography and computer-assisted electroencephalographic analysis. *Brain Dev.* 2001;23:246–250.
10. Cross JH, Jackson GP, Neville BCR, et al. Fortnightly review: epilepsy in childhood. *BMJ.* 1997;315:924–930.
11. Neville BCR, Cross JH. Continuous spike wave of slow sleep and Landau-Kleffner syndrome. In: Wyllie E, et al. eds. *Epilepsy Syndromes: Diagnosis and Treatment. The Treatment of Epilepsy: Principles and Practice.* Philadelphia: Lippincott, Williams, and Wilkins; 2005:455–462.
12. Commission on Classification and Terminology of the International League against Epilepsy. Proposal for revised classification of epilepsies and epileptic syndromes. *Epilepsia.* 1989;30:389–399.
13. Tassinari CA. The Lennox Gastaut syndrome—nosology and differential diagnosis. *Folia Psychiatr Neurol Jpn.* 1985;39:237–239.
14. Patry G, Lyagoubi S, Tassinari CA. Subclinical "electrical status epilepticus" induced by sleep in children. A clinical and electroencephalographic study of six cases. *Arch Neurol.* 1971;24:242–252.
15. Tassinari CA, Daniele O, Gambarelli F, et al. [Excessive 7–14-sec positive spikes during REM sleep in monozygotic non-epileptic twins with speech retardation.] *Rev Electroencephalogr Neurophysiol Clin.* 1977;7:192–193.
16. Galanopoulou AS, Bojko A, Lado F, et al. The spectrum of neuropsychiatric abnormalities associated with electrical status epilepticus in sleep. *Brain Dev.* 2000;22:279–295.
17. Morikawa T, Seino M, Watanabe Y, et al. Clinical relevance of continuous spike waves during slow wave sleep. In: Manelis S, Bental E, Loeber JN, et al. eds. *Advances in Epileptology.* New York: Raven Press; 1989:359–363.
18. Kramer U, Nevo M, Neufeld Y, et al. Epidemiology of epilepsy in childhood; a cohort of 440 consecutive patients. *Pediatr Neurol.* 1998;18:46–50.
19. Landau WM, Klettner RF. Syndrome of acquired aphasia with convulsive disorder in children. *Neurology.* 1957;7:523–530.
20. Tassinari CA, Rubboli G, Volpi L, et al. Encephalopathy with electrical status epilepticus during slow sleep or ESES syndrome including the acquired aphasia. *Clin Neurophysiol.* 2000;111:S94–S102.
21. Bensalem-Owen MK, Fakhoury TA. Continuous spikes and waves during slow sleep in an adult. *Epilepsy Behav.* 2008;12(3):489–491.
22. Caraballo RH, Bongiorni L, Cersosimo R, et al. Epileptic encephalopathy with continuous spikes and waves during sleep in children with shunted hydrocephalus: a study of nine cases. *Epilepsia.* 2008;49(9):1520–1527.
23. Bureau M. Outstanding cases of CSWS and LKS: analysis of the data sheets provided by the participants. In: Beaumanoir A, Bureau M, Deonna T, et al., eds. *Continuous Spikes and Waves During Slow Sleep. Electrical Status Epilepticus During Slow Sleep: Acquired Epileptic Aphasia and Related Xonditions.* London: John Libbey; 1995:213–216.
24. Beaumanoir A. The Landau Kleffner syndrome. In: Beaumanoir A, Bureau M, Deonna T, et al., eds. *Epileptic Syndromes in Infancy, Childhood and Adolescence.* London: John Libbey; 1992:231–244.
25. Case reports. In: Beaumanoir A, Bureau M, Deonna T, et al., eds. *Continuous Spike Waves During Slow Sleep. Electrical Status Epilepticus During Slow Sleep: Acquired Epileptic Apharsia and Related Conditions.* London: John Libbey; 1995:169–210.
26. Tassinari CA, Rubboli G, Volpi L, et al. Electrical status epilepticus during slow sleep (ESES or CSWS) including aquired epileptic aphasia (Landau-Kleffner syndrome). In: Roger J, Bureau M, Dravet C, et al., eds. *Epileptic Syndromes in Infancy, Childhood, and Adolescence.* London: John Libbey; 265–283.
27. Rouselle C, Revol M. Relations between cognitive functions and CSWS. In: Beaumanoir A, Bureau M, Deonna T, et al., eds. *Continuous Spikes and Waves During Slow Sleep. Electrical Status Epilepticus During Slow Sleep: Acquired Epileptic Aphasia and Related Conditions.* London: John Libbey; 1995:123–133.
28. Maquet P, Hirsch E, Metz-Lutz MN, et al. Regional cerebral glucose metabolism in children with deterioration of one or more cognitive functions and continuous spike and wave discharges in sleep. *Brain.* 1995;118:1497–1520.
29. Rapin I, Mattis S, Rowan AJ, et al. Verbal auditory agnosia and seizures in children. *Dev Med Child Neurol.* 1977;19:192–207.
30. DeLong GR, Heinz FR. The clinical syndrome of early-life hippocampal sclerosis. *Ann Neurol.* 1997;42:11–17.
31. Gillberg C, Uvebrant P, Carlsson G, et al. Autism and epilepsy (and tuberous sclerosis?) in two pre-adolescent boys: neuropsychiatric aspects before and after surgery. *J Intellect Disabil Res.* 1996;40:75–81.
32. Mikati MA, El-Bitar MK, Najjar MW, et al. A child with refractory complex partial seizures, right temporal ganglioglioma, contralateral continuous electrical status epilepticus, and a secondary Landau-Kleffner autistic syndrome. *Epilepsy Behav.* December 12, 2008 [Epub ahead of print].
33. Neville BG, Burch VM, Cass H, et al. Behavioural aspects of Landau-Kleffner syndrome. In: Gillberg C, O'Brien G, eds. *Developmental Disability and Behaviour.* London: Cambridge University Press; 2000:56–63.
34. Neville BG, Burch VM, Cass H, et al. Motor disorders in Landau Kleffner syndrome. *Epilepsia.* 1998;(Suppl 6):123.
35. Hirsch E, Maquet P, Metz-Lutz MN, et al. The eponym "Landau Kleffner syndrome" should not be restricted to childhood acquired aphasia with epilepsy. In: Beaumanoir A, Bureau M, Deonna T, et al., eds. *Continuous Spike and Wave During Slow Sleep. Electrical Status Epilepticus During Slow Sleep. Acquired Epileptic Aphasia and Related Conditions.* London: John Libbey; 1995:57–62.
36. Dalla Bernardina B, Fontana E, Michelizza B, et al. Partial epilepsies of childhood, bilateral synchronization, continuous spike waves during slow sleep. In: Manelis S, Bental E, Loeber JN, eds. *Advances in Epileptology.* New York: Raven Press; 1989:295–302.
37. Paetau R, Grandstrom ML, Blomstedt G, et al. Magnetoencephalography in presurgical evaluation of children with Landau Kleffner syndrome. *Epilepsia.* 1999;40:326–335.
38. Deonna T, Roulet E. Acquired epileptic aphasia (AEA): definition of the syndrome and current problems. In: Beaumanoir A, Bureau M, Deonna T, et al., eds. *Continuous Spikes and Waves During Slow Sleep. Electrical Status Epilepticus During Slow Sleep; Acquired Epileptic Aphasia and Related Conditions.* London: John Libbey; 1995:37–45.
39. Genton P, Guerrini R, Bureau M, et al. Continuous focal discharges during REM sleep in a case of Landau Kleffner syndrome: a three year follow up. In: Beaumanoir A, Bureau M, Deonna T, et al., eds. *Continuous Spikes and Waves During Slow Sleep. Electrical Status Epilepticus During Slow Sleep; Acquired Epileptic Aphasia and Related Conditions.* London: John Libbey; 1995:155–159.
40. Van Hirtum-Das M, Licht EA, Koh S, et al. Children with ESES: variability in the syndrome. *Epilepsy Res.* 2006;70(Suppl 1):S248–S258.
41. Guerrini R, Genton P, Bureau M, et al. Multilobar polymicrogyria, intractable drop attac seizures and sleep-related electrical status epilepticus. *Neurology.* 1998;51:504–512.
42. O'Tuama LA, Urion DK, Janicek MJ, et al. Regional cerebral perfusion in Landau-Kleffner syndrome and related childhood aphasias. *J Nucl Med.* 1992;33:1758–1765.
43. Harbord MG, Singh R, Morony S. SPECT abnormalities in Landau-Kleffner syndrome. *J Clin Neurosci.* 1999;6:9–16.
44. Takeoka M, Riviello JJ Jr., Duffy FH, et al. Bilateral volume reduction of the superior temporal areas in Landau-Kleffner syndrome. *Neurology.* 2004;63(7):1152–1153.
45. Connolly AM, Chez M, Streif EM, et al. Brain-derived neurotrophic factor and autoantibodies to neural antigens in sera of children with autistic spectrum disorders, Landau-Kleffner syndrome, and epilepsy. *Biol Psychiatry.* 2006;59(4):354–363.
46. Mikati MA, Shamseddine AN. Management of Landau-Kleffner syndrome. *Paediatr Drugs.* 2005;7:377–389.
47. Lee YM, Kang HC, Lee JS, et al. Mitochondrial respiratory chain defects: underlying etiology in various epileptic conditions. *Epilepsia.* 2008;49(4):685–690.
48. Shouse MN, Scordato JC, Farber PR. Ontogeny of feline temporal lobe epilepsy in amygdala-kindled kittens: an update. *Brain Res.* 2004;1027:126–143.
49. Huttenlocher PR, Dabholkar AS. Regional differences in synaptogenesis in human cerebral cortex. *J Comp Neurol.* 1997;387:167–178.
50. De Negri M, Baglietto MG, Battaglia FM, et al. Treatment of electrical status epilepticus by short diazepam (DZP) cycles after DZP rectal bolus test. *Brain Dev.* 1995;17:330–333.
51. Marescaux C, Hirsch E, Finck S, et al. Landau-Kleffner syndrome: a pharmacologic study of five cases. *Epilepsia.* 1990;31:768–777.
52. Bharani S, Trivedi C, Shendurnikar N, et al. Landau-Kleffner syndrome. *Indian J Pediatr.* 2001;68:567–569.
53. Holmes GL, Riviello JJ Jr. Treatment of childhood idiopathic language deterioration with valproate. *Epilepsy Behav.* 2001;2:272–276.
54. Rossi PG, Parmeggiani A, Posar A, et al. Landau-Kleffner syndrome (Landau-Kleffner syndrome): long-term follow-up and links with electrical status epilepticus during sleep (electrographic status epilepticus during sleep). *Brain Dev.* 1999;21:90–98.
55. Pascual-Castroviejo I. Nicardipine in the treatment of acquired epilepsy and aphasia. *Dev Med Child Neurol.* 1990;32:930.
56. Glauser TA, Olberding LS, Titanic MK, et al. Felbamate in the treatment of acquired epileptic aphasia. *Epilepsy Res.* 1995;20:85–89.
57. Kossoff EH, Boatman D, Freeman JM. Landau-Kleffner syndrome responsive to levetiracetam. *Epilepsy Behav.* 2003;4:471–475.
58. Appleton R, Hughes A, Beirne M, et al. Vigabatrin in the Landau-Kleffner syndrome. *Dev Med Child Neurol.* 1993;35:457–459.
59. Kramer U, Sagi L, Goldberg-Stern H, et al. Clinical spectrum and medical treatment of children with electrical status epilepticus in sleep (ESES). *Epilepsia.* November 2008 [Epub ahead of print].
60. Lena S, Judit N, Rozalia K. Adrenocorticotropic hormone therapy in acquired childhood epileptic aphasia. *Ideggyogy Sz.* 2008;61(11–12):409–416 [article in Hungarian, abstract in English].

61. Lerman P, Lerman-Sagie T, Kivity S. Effects of early corticosteroid therapy for Landau-Kleffner syndrome. *Dev Med Child Neurol*. 1991;33:257–260.

62. Guerreiro MM, Camargo EE, Kato M, et al. Brain single photon emission computed tomography imaging in Landau-Kleffner syndrome. *Epilepsia*. 1996;37:60–67.

63. Coutinho do Santos LH, Antoniuk SA, Rodrigues M, et al. Landau-Kleffner syndrome. Study of four cases. *Arq Neuro-Psiquiatr*. 2002;60:239–241.

64. Uldall P, Sahlholdt L, Alving J. Landau-Kleffner syndrome with onset at 18 months old and an initial diagnosis of pervasive developmental disorder. *Eur J Pediatr Neurol*. 2000;4:81–86.

65. Sinclair DB, Snyder TJ. Corticosteroids for the treatment of Landau-Kleffner syndrome and continuous spike-wave discharge during sleep. *Pedatri Neurol*. 2005;32:300–306.

66. Aykut-Bingol C, Arman A, Tokol O, et al. Pulse methylprednisolone therapy in Landau-Kleffner syndrome. *J Epilepsy*. 1996;9:189–191.

67. Tsuru T, Mori M, Mizuguchi M, et al. Effects of high-dose intravenous corticosteroid therapy in Landau-Kleffner syndrome. *Pediatr Neurol*. 2000;22:145–147.

68. Perniola T, Margari L, Buttiglione M, et al. A case of Landau-Kleffner syndrome secondary to inflammatory demyelinating disease. *Epilepsia*. 1993;34:551–556.

69. Tutuncuoglu S, Serdaroglu G, Kadioglu B. Landau-Kleffner syndrome beginning with stuttering: case report. *J Child Neurol*. 2002;17:785–788.

70. Raybarman C. Landau-Kleffner syndrome: a case report. *Neurol India*. 2002;50:212–213.

71. You SJ, Jung DE, Kim HD, et al. Efficacy and prognosis of a short course of prednisolone therapy for pediatric epilepsy. *Eur J Paediatr Neurol*. 2008;12(4):314–320.

72. Mikati MA, Kurdi R. Immunotherapy in Epilepsy. In: Wheless J, Willmore LJ, Brumback R. *Advanced Therapy in Epilepsy*. 2009; BC Decker. In publication.

73. Fayad, MN, Choueiri R, Mikati M. Landau-Kleffner syndrome: consistent response to repeated intravenous gammaglobulin doses: a case report. *Epilepsia*. 1997;38:489–494.

74. Lagae LG, Silberstein J, Gillis PL, et al. Successful use of intravenous immunoglobulins in Landau-Kleffner syndrome. *Pediatr Neurol*. 1998;18:165–168.

75. Mikati MA, Saab R. Successful use of intravenous immunoglobulin as initial monotherapy in Landau-Kleffner syndrome. *Epilepsia*. 2000;41:880–886.

76. Neville BG, Harkness W, Cross JH, et al. Surgical treatment of severe autistic regression in childhood epilepsy. *Pediatr Neurol*. 1997;16:137–140.

77. Cross H, Jayakar P, Nordli D, et al. Proposed criteria for referral and evaluation of children for epilepsy surgery: recommendations of the Subcommission for Pediatric Epilepsy Surgery. *Epilepsia*. 2006;47:952–959.

78. Kallay C, Mayor-Dubois C, Maeder-Ingvar M, et al. Reversible acquired epileptic frontal syndrome and CSWS suppression in a child with congenital hemiparesis treated by hemispherotomy. *Eur J Paediatr Neurol*. October 20, 2008 [Epub ahead of print].

79. Perez ER, Davidoff V. Sign language in childhood epileptic aphasia (Landau-Kleffner syndrome). *Dev Med Child Neurol*. 2001;43(11):739–744.

80. Besag FM. Behavioral aspects of pediatric epilepsy syndromes. *Epilepsy Behav*. 2004;(Suppl 1):S3–S13.

81. Taner Y, Erdogan-Bakar E, Turanli G, et al. Psychiatric evaluation of children with CWSW (continuous spikes and waves during slow sleep) and BRE (benign childhood epilepsy with centrotemporal spikes/rolandic epilepsy) compared to children with absence epilepsy and healthy controls. *Turk J Pediatr*. 2007;49(4):397–403.

82. Mariotti P, Della Marca G, Iuvone L, et al. Is ESES/CSWS a strictly age-related disorder? *Clin Neurophysiol*. 2000;111:452–456.

83. Tassinari CA, Bureau M, Dravet C, et al. Epilepsy with continuous spikes and waves during slow sleep—otherwise described as ESES (electrical status epilepticus during slow sleep). In: Roger J, Bureau M, Dravet C, et al., eds. *Epileptic Syndromes in Infancy, Childhood, and Adolescence*. London: John Libbey; 1992:245–256.

84. Mira L, Oxilia B, Van Lierde A. Cognitive assessment of children with CSWS syndrome: a critical review of data from 155 cases submitted to the Venice colloquium. In: Beaumanoir A, Bureau M, Deonna T, et al., eds. *Continuous Spike Waves During Slow Sleep. Electrical Status Epilepticus During Slow Sleep: Acquired Epileptic Aphasia and Related Conditions*. London: John Libbey; 1995:229–242.

85. Nickels K, Wirrell E. Electrical status epilepticus in sleep. *Semin Pediatr Neurol*. 2008;15(2):50–60.

86. Duran MH, Gumaraes CA, Medeiros LL, et al. Landau-Kleffner syndrome: long-term follow-up. *Brain Dev*. 2009;31(1):58–63.

CHAPTER 24 ■ EPILEPSY WITH REFLEX SEIZURES

BENJAMIN ZIFKIN AND FREDERICK ANDERMANN

DEFINITION AND CLASSIFICATION

The seizures of reflex epilepsy are reliably precipitated by some identifiable factor (1). The International League Against Epilepsy (2) describes reflex epilepsies as "epilepsies characterized by specific modes of seizure precipitation." The recent classification proposal (3) redefines reflex epilepsy syndromes as "syndromes in which all epileptic seizures are precipitated by sensory stimuli." Reflex seizures that occur in focal and generalized epilepsy syndromes that are also associated with spontaneous seizures are generally listed as seizure types, for example, photosensitive seizures in patients with juvenile myoclonic epilepsy (JME). Reflex seizures may be classified as occurring in generalized or in focal epilepsy syndromes (4). Reflex seizures can also be classified according to the seizure trigger. Reflex seizures may not differ in semiology from those encountered in other forms of epilepsy but understanding of the seizure trigger is important in the management of the patient and study of the mechanisms of epileptogenicity. Seizures triggered by factors such as alcohol withdrawal are not included among reflex seizures.

The use of the term reflex has been controversial. Hall (5) first applied it to epilepsy in 1850. Arguing that no reflex arc is involved in reflex epilepsy, others proposed terms such as sensory precipitation (6,7) or stimulus sensitive epilepsies (8). Wieser (9) noted that sensory precipitation epilepsy is a misnomer because some reflex seizures are not precipitated by sensory stimuli. Most authorities retain reflex epilepsy to mean that a certain stimulus regularly elicits an observable response in the form of abnormal, paroxysmal, electroencephalographic (EEG) activity associated with or without a clinical seizure. Although some investigators restrict the term reflex epilepsy to cases in which a certain stimulus always induces seizures (10), it may include cases in which spontaneous seizures also occur or instances in which the epileptogenic stimulus does not invariably induce an attack (11), which often occurs in patients taking antiepileptic drugs. The term "epilepsy with reflex seizures," although more cumbersome, perhaps better reflects clinical reality and more accurately describes cases with reflex and spontaneous attacks.

Reflex seizures have long fascinated epileptologists. Apart from epileptic photosensitivity to flickering light, cases of reflex epilepsy are relatively rare and permit glimpses into the mechanisms of epileptogenesis and the organization of cognitive function. The identification of a patient with reflex epilepsy depends on the physician's awareness and on the observations of the patient and witnesses. The epileptogenic trigger must occur often enough in everyday life so that the patient suspects its relation to the resulting seizures. If the trigger is ubiquitous, however, the seizures appear to occur by chance or with no obvious antecedent. Many triggers have been recognized and studied. This chapter reviews the neurophysiology of reflex epilepsy from the available human and animal studies. We also discuss clinical features of reflex seizures classified by the triggering stimulus.

BASIC MECHANISMS OF REFLEX EPILEPSY

There are two types of animal model of reflex epilepsy. In the first, irritative cortical lesions are created and their activation by specific stimuli is studied. The second model involves naturally occurring reflex epilepsies or seizures induced by specific sensory stimulation in genetically predisposed animals.

The first approach has been used since 1929, when Clementi (12) induced convulsions with intermittent photic stimulation (IPS) after applying strychnine to the visual cortex. This technique also demonstrated that strychninization of auditory (13), gustatory (14), and olfactory cortex (15) produced focal irritative lesions that may produce seizures with the appropriate afferent stimulus. EEG studies showed that the clinical seizures (chewing movements), which were induced by photic stimulation in rabbits with strychnine lesions of the visual cortex, resulted from rapid transmission of the epileptic discharge from the visual cortex to masticatory areas (16). The EEG spread of paroxysmal discharge from visual cortex may also occur in the fronto-rolandic areas during seizures (17). The ictal EEG spread was thought to represent cortico-cortical conduction (12,17), although later work with pentylenetetrazol also implicated thalamic relays (18) and demonstrated spread of the visual-evoked potential to the brainstem reticular formation (19). Hunter and Ingvar (20) identified a subcortical pathway involving the thalamus and reticular system and an independent cortico-cortical system for radiation of visual-evoked responses to the frontal lobe. In cats and monkeys, the fronto-rolandic region was also shown to receive spreading-evoked paroxysmal activity from auditory and other stimuli (21,22).

The second approach, the study of naturally occurring or induced reflex seizures in genetically susceptible animals, has been pursued in domestic fowls and chickens with photosensitivity (23,24), rodents susceptible to sound-induced convulsions (25), the E1 mouse sensitive to vestibular stimulation (26), and the Mongolian gerbil sensitive to a variety of stimuli (27,28).

The only species in which the reflex seizures and EEG findings are similar to those in humans is the baboon Papio papio (29), except that the light-induced epileptic discharges in baboons occur in the fronto-rolandic area rather than in the occipital lobe (30). EEG, visual-evoked potentials, intracerebral recording, and lesion and pharmacologic studies show that visual afferents are necessary to trigger fronto-rolandic light-induced epileptic discharges. The occipital lobe does not generate this abnormal activity but sends cortico-cortical visual afferents to hyperexcitable frontal cortex, which is responsible for the epileptiform activity (31). The interhemispheric synchronization of the light-induced paroxysmal EEG activity and seizures depends mainly on the corpus callosum and not on the brain stem. Brain stem reticular activation depends initially on frontal cortical mechanisms until a seizure is about to begin, at which point the cortex can no longer control reticular activation. The genetically determined hyperexcitability may be related to cortical biochemical abnormalities, involving regulation of extracellular calcium concentration (32,33) or an imbalance between excitatory and inhibitory neurotransmitter amino acids (34) similar to those described in feline generalized penicillin epilepsy and in human epilepsy (35).

In human epileptic photosensitivity, generalized epileptiform activity and clinical seizures can be activated by the localized occipital trigger. Studies in photosensitive patients who are also pattern-sensitive suggest that generalized seizures and EEG paroxysmal activity can occur in these subjects if normal excitation of visual cortex involves a certain "critical mass" of cortical area with synchronization and subsequent spreading of excitation (36–39). We (40) suggested that a similar mechanism involving recruitment of a critical mass of parietal rather than visual cortex is responsible for generalized seizures induced by thinking or by spatial tasks. Studies of reading epilepsy also suggest that increased task difficulty, complexity, or duration increases the chance of EEG or clinical activation (41,42).

Wieser proposed a neurophysiologic model for critical mass (9), referring to the group 1 and group 2 epileptic neurons of the chronic experimental epileptic focus described by Wyler and Ward (43). Group 1 neurons produce abundant, spontaneous, high-frequency bursts of action potentials. Group 2 neurons have a variable interspike interval, and their spontaneous epileptic activity is less marked. Moreover, these properties are influenced by external stimuli that can promote or inhibit the incorporation of group 2 neurons into the effective quantity of epileptic tissue and thus trigger or inhibit a seizure. The stimuli effective in eliciting reflex seizures would act on this population of neurons, recruiting them into the highly epileptic group 1 neuron pool to form the critical mass needed to produce epileptogenic EEG activity or clinical seizures. This mechanism also can explain conditioning (44) and deconditioning (45) of reflex epileptic responses. A further generalizing system also must be postulated to account for the seizures observed with photic or cognitive stimulation, analogous to the cortico-cortical pathways linking occipital cortex with fronto-rolandic cortex in *Papio papio*. A role for reticulothalamic structures has been suggested but seems unnecessary, at least in certain animal models in which cortico-cortical spread of evoked epileptic activity persists after mesencephalic and diencephalic ablation (20).

Patients with reflex seizures may report that emotion plays a role in seizure induction and, sometimes, in seizure inhibition. Gras et al. (46) emphasized the influence of emotional content in activating EEG spikes in a patient with reading epilepsy. An emotional component was also obvious in several cases of musicogenic and eating epilepsy. Fenwick (47)

described psychogenic seizures as epileptic seizures generated by an action of mind, self-induced attacks (e.g., by thinking sad thoughts), and those unintentionally triggered by specific mental activity such as thinking. This use of the term psychogenic seizures, common in European epileptology, does not refer to nonepileptic events. Fenwick related seizure induction and inhibition in some individuals with or without typical reflex seizures to the neuronal excitation and inhibition accompanying mental activity. He also referred to the alumina cream model, with recruitment of group 2 neurons and evoked change in neuronal activity surrounding the seizure focus as factors in seizure occurrence, spread, and inhibition.

Wolf (48) believed that two pathophysiologic theories have arisen in the discussion of reflex epilepsies. For primary reading epilepsy he observed that seizure evocation would depend on involvement of the multiple processes used for reading, an activity involving both hemispheres, with a functional rather than a topographic anatomy. "Maximal interactive neuronal performance is at least a facilitating factor," (48) he wrote and suggested that the functional complexity of the epileptogenic tasks leads to seizure precipitation. He contrasted this with the suggestion described previously that the latency, dependence on task duration and complexity, and influence of nonspecific factors such as attention and arousal often observed in these seizures depend on the ad hoc recruitment of a critical mass of epileptogenic tissue to produce a clinical seizure or paroxysmal EEG activity in response to the different characteristics of an effective triggering stimulus. In seizures induced by reading, thinking, photic response, and pattern-sensitivity, the relatively localized trigger induces generalized or bilateral EEG abnormalities and seizures. The recruitment that produces these seizures, however, need not be confined to physically contiguous brain tissue or fixed neuronal links. Instead, it may depend on activity of a function-related network of both established and plastic links between brain regions, modified by the effects of factors such as arousal. These two approaches share much common ground.

Disorders of cortical development may be present in some patients with reflex seizures. Reportedly normal imaging may be misleading; subtle changes or dysplastic lesions may be missed without special magnetic resonance imaging (MRI) techniques or may only be found in a surgical pathology specimen (49–52).

REFLEX EPILEPSY WITH VISUAL TRIGGERS

Epilepsy with reflex seizures evoked by visual stimuli is the most common reflex epilepsy. Of the several abnormal EEG responses to laboratory IPS described, only generalized paroxysmal epileptiform discharges (e.g., spikes, polyspikes, spike and wave complexes) are clearly linked to epilepsy in humans. About 5% of patients with epilepsy show this response to IPS (53,54). Photosensitivity is genetically determined (55) but studies of the epileptic response to IPS are complicated by the age and sex dependence of the phenomenon, which occurs most frequently in adolescents and women, and by differences in how IPS is performed. An expert panel has recommended a protocol for performing IPS and guidelines for interpreting the EEG responses. This is shown in a review with video (56).

Recent detailed studies on subjects known to have visually induced seizures examined whether color modulation could be an independent factor in human epileptic photosensitivity. Among photosensitive epilepsy patients sensitive to flash and pattern stimulation, 25/43 were sensitive to color stimulation, particularly at frequencies below 30 per sec. Red was the most effective color and red-blue was the most provocative alternating stimulus. They concluded that "color sensitivity follows two different mechanisms: one, dependent on color modulation, plays a role at lower frequencies (5 to 30 Hz). Another, dependent on single-color light intensity modulation correlates to white light sensitivity and is activated at higher frequencies." This also suggests a mechanism to explain observations that colored spectacles adapted to the patient's color sensitivity may be useful for treatment (57).

Sensitivity to IPS is customarily divided into three groups: patients with light-induced seizures only, patients with photosensitivity and other seizure types, and asymptomatic individuals with isolated photosensitivity. Kasteleijn-Nolst Trenité (58) has shown that more than half of known photosensitive patients questioned immediately after stimulation denied having had brief but clear-cut seizures induced by IPS and documented by video-EEG monitoring. Photosensitive epilepsy may be classified into two major groups, depending on whether the seizures are induced by flickering light. Further classification of photosensitive epilepsy into sub-groups is as follows:

Seizures induced by flicker
    Pure photosensitive epilepsy including idiopathic photosensitive occipital epilepsy
    Photosensitive epilepsy with spontaneous seizures
    Self-induced seizures
Visually evoked seizures not induced by flicker
    Pattern-sensitive seizures
    Seizures induced by eye closure
    Self-induced seizures

Pure Photosensitive Epilepsy

Pure photosensitive epilepsy is characterized by generalized seizures provoked exclusively by a flickering light source. According to Jeavons (59), 40% of photosensitive patients have this variety of epilepsy, and television is the most common precipitating factor. Video games may trigger these seizures, although not all such events represent pure photosensitive epilepsy (60,61). Other typical environmental stimuli include discothèque lights and sunlight reflected from snow or the sea or interrupted by roadside structures or trees. Rotating helicopter rotors and tower-mounted wind turbines, which can reflect or break up light into flicker, also present risk (62,63).

Pure photosensitive epilepsy is typically a disorder of adolescence, with a female predominance. Reviews of the topic have been provided by several authors (53,54,56,58,64). The seizures are generalized tonic–clonic in 84% patients (65), absences in 6%, partial motor seizures (possibly asymmetric myoclonus in some cases) in 2.5%, and myoclonic seizures in 1.5% of patients. Subtle myoclonic seizures may go unnoticed until an obvious seizure occurs. The developmental and neurologic examinations are normal. The resting EEG may be normal in about one half of patients, but spike-and-wave complexes may be seen with eye closure. IPS evokes a photoconvulsive response in virtually all patients. Depending on the photic stimulus and on the patient's degree of photosensitivity, the clinical response ranges from subtle eyelid myoclonus to a generalized tonic–clonic convulsion.

Pure photosensitive epilepsy is typically conceptualized as a variety of idiopathic generalized epilepsy, but cases occur in which EEG and clinical evidence favors the occipital lobe origin, as predicted by theoretical and animal models (66,67). IPS can also induce clear-cut partial seizures originating in the occipital lobe (68,69). As in more typical photosensitive subjects, environmental triggers include television and video games. Many of these patients have idiopathic photosensitive occipital lobe epilepsy, a relatively benign, age-related syndrome without spontaneous seizures, although cases with occipital lesions have been reported, including patients with celiac disease. The clinical seizure pattern depends on the pattern of spread. The visual stimulus triggers initial visual symptoms that may be followed by versive movements and motor seizures; however, migraine-like symptoms of throbbing headache, nausea, and sometimes vomiting are common and can lead to delayed or incorrect diagnosis.

Photosensitivity with Spontaneous Seizures

Jeavons and Harding (65) found that about one third of their photosensitive patients with environmentally precipitated attacks also had spontaneous seizures similar to those of pure photosensitive epilepsy. Spike-and-wave activity was common in the resting EEG patterns of patients with spontaneous seizures, and only 39% of patients had normal resting EEGs. Photosensitivity may accompany idiopathic generalized epilepsies, especially JME, and is associated with onset in childhood and adolescence, normal intellectual development and neurologic examination, normal EEG background rhythm, and generally good response to treatment with valproate. Photosensitive benign myoclonic epilepsy may also begin in infants, with a generally good prognosis though the events may be overlooked by the parents for some time before diagnosis (70). Photosensitivity also may occur with severe myoclonic epilepsy of infancy (Dravet syndrome) or with disesases associated with progressive myoclonic epilepsy like Lafora disease, Unverricht–Lundborg disease, and the neuronal ceroid lipofuscinoses (71). Photosensitivity is usual in eyelid myoclonia with absences (EMA) but not in benign occipital epilepsies of childhood of the Gastaut or Panayiotopoulos types despite the florid EEG abnormalities (71).

Pure photosensitive epilepsy may be treated by avoiding or modifying environmental light stimuli, increasing the distance from the television set, watching a small screen in a well-lighted room, using a remote control so that the set need not be approached, and monocular viewing or the use of polarized spectacles to block one eye should provide protection (59,72). Colored spectacles may be useful in selected cases (73,74). Drug treatment is needed if these measures are impractical or unsuccessful, if photosensitivity is severe, or if spontaneous attacks occur. The drug of choice is valproate, which in one study (75) abolished photosensitivity in 54% of patients and markedly reduced it in a further 24%. Lamotrigine, topiramate, ethosuximide, benzodiazepines such as clobazam (76), and levetiracetam (58) also may be useful. Quesney et al. (77) proposed a dopaminergic mechanism in human epileptic photosensitivity based on the transient abolition of photosensitivity with apomorphine, and bromocriptine and parenteral L-dopa have been reported to alleviate photosensitivity (78,79). About one fourth of patients with pure photosensitive epilepsy lose their photosensitivity by 25 years (80). Because this resolution usually occurs only in the third decade, withdrawal of treatment too early may lead to seizure recurrence; serial EEG recording to determine the photosensitivity range may be helpful in assessing and during follow-up (58).

Seizures with Self-Induced Flicker

Reports of self-induced epileptic attacks using visual sensitivity antedated the discovery of the photoconvulsive EEG response (81). Regarded as rare, self-induction was reported particularly in mentally retarded children and adolescents, with a female preponderance (53,54,82,83). More recent information, however, shows that although some affected patients are retarded, most are not (84–86). When carefully sought, the syndrome is not rare; it was found in about 40% of photosensitive patients studied by Kasteleijn-Nolst Trenité et al. (84). The EEG usually shows spontaneous generalized spikes or spike and wave complexes, and about 75% of patients are sensitive to IPS. The self-induced seizures are usually myoclonic, especially with palpebral myoclonus, or absences, and some patients have EMA. Patients induce seizures with maneuvers that cause flicker, such as waving a hand with fingers spread apart in front of their eyes or gazing at a vertically rolling television image. Monitoring (86,87) shows that these behaviors, once thought to be part of the seizure, precede the attacks and are responsible for inducing them. The compulsive nature of this behavior has been observed often and has been likened to self-stimulation (88) in experimental animals. Patients have reported intensely pleasant sensations and relief of stress with self-induced photosensitive absence seizures (85,86). Frank sexual arousal has been described (89,90). Patients are often unwilling to give up their seizures, and noncompliance with standard, well-tolerated antiepileptic drugs is common (84,85). Treatment is difficult, however, even in compliant patients (83). Drugs that suppress self-stimulation in animals, such as chlorpromazine and pimozide, may block the pleasurable response without affecting the response to IPS and have partially reduced or completely terminated self-induction (83,91). The effectiveness of valproate in reducing or abolishing photosensitivity has resulted in virtual disappearance of this form of self-induction, which is now encountered in patients for whom the drug has not been prescribed and in those with inadequate drug levels for any reason. Many patients appear not to want treatment for their self-induced attacks.

VISUALLY EVOKED SEIZURES NOT INDUCED BY FLICKER

Pattern-Sensitive Seizures

Absences, myoclonus, or more rarely, tonic–clonic seizures may occur in response to epileptogenic patterns. These are striped and include common objects such as the television screen at short distances, curtains or wallpaper, escalator steps, and striped clothing. Pattern sensitivity is seen in about 70% of photosensitive patients tested with patterned IPS in the EEG laboratory, but sensitivity to stationary striped patterns affects only about 30% (38). However, clinical pattern sensitivity is rare, and patients often may not make the association, the family may be unaware of it, and physicians may not enquire about it.

Wilkins et al. (37,39,92–94) studied the properties of epileptogenic patterns, isolating visual arc size, brightness, contrast, orientation, duty cycle, and sensitivity to movement and binocularity. They concluded that the seizures involve excitation and synchronization of a sufficiently large number of cells in the primary visual cortex with subsequent generalization. We can compare this with the previously described animal experiments and Wieser's theory. Pattern sensitivity optimally requires binocular viewing, and treatment may be aided by avoidance of environmental stimuli (admittedly often impractical) as well as by alternating occlusion of one eye with polarizing spectacles, and increased distance from the television set. Spontaneous attacks or a high degree of pattern sensitivity requires antiepileptic drug treatment, as described earlier.

Seizures Induced by Eye Closure

Although eye closure may evoke paroxysmal activity in photosensitive patients, especially those with EMA, seizures induced by eye closure are unusual. They are rare in patients not sensitive to simple flash IPS. Seizures with eye closure are typically absences or myoclonic attacks and are not specific for any one cause. They must be distinguished from rare seizures occurring with eyes closed or with loss of central fixation. Panayiotopoulos et al. (95,96) studied these extensively and described the syndromes in which they occur.

Self-Induced Seizures

Photosensitive patients may induce seizures with maneuvers that do not produce flicker. These attacks are similar to flicker-induced seizures, but the inducing behaviors are not. Pattern-sensitive patients may be irresistibly drawn to television screens, which they must approach closely to resolve the epileptogenic pattern of vibrating lines, or they may spend hours gazing through venetian blinds or at other sources of pattern stimulation. Those sensitive to eye closure have been observed to use forceful slow upward gaze with eyelid flutter (97,98) to induce paroxysmal EEG discharge and, at times, frank seizures. These patients are often children, who describe the responses as pleasant: "as nice as being hugged, but not as nice as eating pudding" (C. D. Binnie, personal communication). We have observed that these tonic eyeball movements are always associated with spike-and-wave activity in young individuals. As they mature, their movements may persist but no longer elicit epileptiform activity and can be likened to a tic learned in response to positive reinforcement. These observations and the compulsive seizure-inducing behavior of many such patients suggest that, as in flicker-induced seizures, the self-induced attacks give pleasure or relieve stress. Experience suggests that treatment is similarly difficult (83).

SEIZURES INDUCED BY TELEVISION AND OTHER ELECTRONIC SCREENS

Television is probably the most common environmental trigger of photosensitive seizures. A television screen produces flicker at the mains frequency, generating IPS at 60 Hz in North America and 50 Hz in Europe. Jeavons and Harding (65) found that photosensitivity was more common at the lower frequency, which partly explained the higher incidence of television-induced seizures in Europe than in North America. Television-induced seizures, however, are not related to alternating current (AC) frequency flicker alone. Wilkins et al. (93,94) described two types of television-sensitive patients: those sensitive to IPS at 50 Hz, who apparently were sensitive to whole-screen flicker even at distances greater than 1 m from the screen, and patients not sensitive to the mains frequency flicker but who responded to the vibrating pattern of interleaved lines at half the AC frequency, which can be discerned only near the screen. They emphasized that increased distance from the screen decreased the ability to resolve the line pattern and that a small screen evoked less epileptiform activity than a large one. Binocular viewing was also needed to trigger attacks.

Not suprisingly, domestic video games using the home television screen viewed at close distances for long periods and sometimes under conditions of sleep deprivation and possible alcohol or nonmedical drug use can trigger seizures in predisposed individuals, some of whom were not known to be photosensitive. Some individuals are not photosensitive and may have seizures by chance or induced by thinking or other factors. These events, however, have caused many patients with epilepsy to believe erroneously that they are at risk from video games and they need accurate information about their personal risk (99).

Not all seizures triggered by television and similar screens fit this pattern. Seizures can be triggered even at greater distances and by noninterlaced screens without flicker, and flashing or patterned screen content is implicated in such episodes including that from video games. Nevertheless, the 50/25 Hz frequency appears to be a powerful determinant of screen sensitivity, and in countries with 50 Hz AC, special 100-Hz television sets have been shown to reduce the risk of attacks (100). Other preventive measures include watching a small screen from afar in a well-lighted room, using a remote control to avoid approaching the set, and covering one eye and looking away if the picture flickers or if myoclonia occurs (101).

Broadcasting of certain forms of flashing or patterned screen content has been responsible for outbreaks of photosensitive seizures, most notably in Japan where 685 people, mostly children and young adults with no history of epilepsy, were hospitalized after viewing a cartoon (102). The details of triggering factors in screen images have been summarized (103) and were used to develop broadcast standards in the United Kingdom and Japan, which now reduce this risk. Electronic filters have also been proposed (104). Further outbreaks are to be expected if viewers, especially mass audiences of adolescents, are exposed to such screen content when guidelines do not exist or are violated (105).

SEIZURES INDUCED BY COMPLEX NONVISUAL ACTIVITY

Reflex epilepsy with nonvisual stimuli is rare though reflex seizures with JME are more common than was previously thought. Seizures may be classified as those with relatively simple somatosensory triggers and those triggered by complex activity, such as thinking, eating, or listening to music.

Seizures Induced by Thinking

Wilkins et al. (40) introduced the term seizures induced by thinking to describe a patient who reported seizures induced by mental arithmetic but who proved also to be sensitive to tasks involving manipulation of spatial information with or without any motor activity. Other complex mental activities have been reported to trigger seizures, such as card games and board games, such as checkers (British, draughts), or making complex decisions. A rather consistent electroclinical syndrome emerges, most succinctly called seizures induced by thinking, reviewed in Andermann et al. (106).

About 80% of patients have more than one trigger, but because EEG monitoring of detailed neuropsychological testing was not always performed, this may be an underestimate. Reading is not usually an effective trigger, and unlike reading epilepsy, most patients also have apparently spontaneous attacks. The seizures are typically generalized myoclonus, absences, or tonic–clonic attacks, and the induced EEG abnormalities are almost always generalized spike-and-wave or polyspike-and-wave activity. Focal spiking is found only in about 10% of patients, and photosensitivity is seen in about 25%. Although numbers are small, most subjects are men. The mean age of onset is 15 years. Family histories of epilepsy are neither typical nor helpful in the diagnosis. Avoidance of triggering stimuli is practical only when activation is related to cards or other games, but drugs effective in idiopathic generalized epilepsies have been most useful. Epileptogenic tasks in these patients involve the processing of spatial information and possibly sequential decisions. The generalized seizures and EEG discharges may depend on initial involvement of parietal or, possibly, frontal cortex and subsequent generalization, much as pattern-sensitive seizures depend on initial activation of primary visual cortex. Recent studies provide more detail on the cerebral representation of calculation and spatial thought and document a bilateral functional network activated by such tasks (107).

Praxis-Induced Seizures

Japanese investigators (108) have described praxis-induced seizures as myoclonic seizures, absences, or generalized convulsions triggered by activities as in seizures induced by thinking but with the difference that precipitation depends on using a part of the body to perform the task (e.g., typing). Hand or finger movements without "action-programming activity" (defined as "higher mental activity requiring hand movement" and apparently synonymous with praxis) are not effective triggers (109). EEG responses consist of bisynchronous spike or polyspike-and-wave bursts at times predominant over centroparietal regions. Most subjects have JME; some had another idiopathic-generalized epilepsy syndrome. None had clear-cut localization-related epilepsy. In its milder forms, such as the morning myoclonic jerk of the arm manipulating a utensil (M. Seino, personal communication, 1999), this phenomenon resembles cortical reflex myoclonus as part of a "continuum of epileptic activity centered on the sensorimotor cortex" (110). It also appears to be another manifestation of triggering of a generalized or bilateral epileptiform response by a local or functional trigger (111), in this case requiring participation of the rolandic region of one or both hemispheres which may be regionally hyperexcitable in JME (112). The seizures of idiopathic generalized epilepsy may involve only selected thalamocortical networks (113) and this seems especially so in JME (114).

Reading Epilepsy

Bickford et al. (115) first identified primary and secondary forms of reading epilepsy. The primary form consists of attacks triggered exclusively by reading, without spontaneous seizures. Age at onset is typically between 12 and 25 years. Patients report characteristic jaw jerks or clicks. If reading continues, a generalized convulsion may occur. Prolonged reading-induced partial seizures with ictal dyslexia, bilateral myoclonic seizures, and absences have been reported. The resting EEG pattern is normal, but during reading, abnormal paroxysmal activity is recorded, often consisting of sharp theta activity that may be generalized (97,115–118) or localized to either temporoparietal region, especially on the dominant side (119–121). These abnormalities frequently are correlated with the jaw jerks and monitoring also shows perioral reflex myoclonus similar to that seen in JME. Bilateral or asymmetric myoclonic attacks or jerks of the arms and head also similar to those of JME may also occur with bilaterally synchronous spike-and-wave activity.

Patients with primary reading epilepsy are typically developmentally normal, with normal neurologic examinations. No structural lesions have been demonstrated. A family history of epilepsy is common, and familial reading epilepsy has been reported (120–122). Patients with secondary reading epilepsy also have spontaneous seizures without jaw jerking and often have an abnormal baseline EEG. Primary reading epilepsy was classified as an idiopathic, age-related, localization-related epilepsy but recent opinion is less certain as to its focal nature (3). Attacks are induced by reading and may be produced easily for study in sensitive subjects. Functional magnetic resonance imaging has shown (123) activations in most subjects in areas overlapping or adjacent to those physiologically activated during language and facial motor tasks, including subcortical structures as also noted by Archer et al. (124). Reading epilepsy seems to be an example of activation of a hyperexcitable network, which can produce seizures when sufficient critical mass is incorporated by adequate stimuli to produce a seizure, at times a seizure of apparently generalized epilepsy. We have noted that it may rely on both existing and reorganized functional links between brain regions and need not be confined to physically contiguous brain sites or established neuronal links.

The triggering stimulus in reading epilepsy is unknown. Bickford et al. (115) proposed that normal sensory stimuli influenced some hyperexcitable cortical focus. Critchley et al. (119) emphasized several factors: the visual pattern of printed words, attention, proprioceptive input from jaw and extraocular muscles, and conditioning. Forster (45) theorized that the seizures were evoked by higher cognitive functions; however, patients with primary reading epilepsy are not photosensitive, deny other precipitating cognitive stimuli, and do not appear to have thinking-induced seizures. Patients with the latter almost always deny activation by reading. A single patient with otherwise clear-cut primary reading epilepsy reported induction by card playing while drinking beer (125). Comprehension of the material being read is essential in some cases and irrelevant in others, suggesting that attention is not sufficient to precipitate seizures. Studies suggest that increased difficulty, complexity, or duration of a task increases the chance of EEG or clinical activation (41,42). Functional imaging has shown that these seizures result from activation of parts of a speech and language network in both hemispheres (126), confirming that the hyperexcitable neuronal tissue forming the critical mass is not necessarily contiguous but is functionally linked, as discussed by Salek-Haddadi et al. (123) and by Rémillard et al. (127). A mechanism similar to that in pattern-sensitive epilepsy, in which generalized activity is activated by the occipital cortical stimuli, may operate in some cases of primary reading epilepsy in which bilateral myoclonic attacks or bilaterally synchronous epileptiform activity is triggered. Primary reading epilepsy generally responds well to valproate, and benzodiazepines or lamotrigine are expected to be useful as well, but patients often decline treatment especially if they have only jaw jerks.

Language-Induced Epilepsy

Geschwind and Sherwin (128) described a patient whose seizures were induced by three components of language: speaking, reading, and writing. Some other cases have been reported since. Similar to those in primary reading epilepsy, the seizures consist of jaw jerks, with focal (116,129–131) or generalized (128) abnormal paroxysmal EEG activity during language tasks. In some patients, isolated components of language were the only effective seizure triggers. Writing (132,133), typing (134), listening to spoken language (135), and singing or recitation (136) have been reported as isolated triggers. Writing or speaking may activate patients with reading epilepsy (131,137), and exceptionally, reading epilepsy occurred in a patient who was also activated by card games (125). We consider activation by drawing (138) to be part of seizures induced by thinking, and other patients believed to have language-induced epilepsy may have thinking-induced seizures. This heterogeneity suggests that the definition of a language-induced epilepsy is not clear-cut. Cases may form part of relatively more stereotyped syndromes of reading epilepsy, whose definition should be broadened. Alternatively, Koutroumanidis et al. (126) suggested that primary reading epilepsy might be classified as a variant of a more broadly defined language-induced epilepsy. The association of reflex language-induced epilepsy and idiopathic generalized epilepsy was explored by Valenti et al. (139) and is of interest since some patients with reading epilepsy also seem to have an underlying generalized epilepsy.

Musicogenic Epilepsy

The rare musicogenic epilepsy consists of seizures provoked by hearing music. The music that triggers seizures is often remarkably specific in any one patient and no consistent epileptogenic features of musical sound can be identified. A startle effect is not required. Many patients have spontaneous attacks as well. Some attacks can be provoked by music and by nonmusical sounds such as ringing or whirring noises. In some patients, an effective musical stimulus often induces emotional and autonomic manifestations before the clinical seizure begins. Patients may report triggers with personal emotional significance. However, in some patients, the triggers have no particular connotations (140), while in others they may (141). Triggers without particular emotional significance can induce the typical autonomic features before the clinical attack (142,143). Establishment of the seizure as a conditioned response has also been suggested (97,140,142,144), but this view is not generally accepted (145). A case with self-induction possibly motivated by emotional factors has been described (146). Musicogenic attacks may appear only in adulthood, often in the context of a preexisting symptomatic localization-related epilepsy. Many case reports antedate intensive monitoring and modern imaging, but the seizures appear to be simple or complex partial, and epileptiform EEG abnormalities are recorded focally from either temporal lobe but more frequently over the right side. Mesial temporal and lateral temporal seizure onsets have been documented (147).

The pathophysiology of musicogenic epilepsy is obscure. Studies in epileptic subjects not sensitive to music show that musical stimuli may have widespread effects on neuronal activity in human temporal lobes, extending well beyond the rather restricted primary auditory area (148); that different components of music have different effects, possibly with specialized lateralization and localization; and that the effects of music differ from those of speech (149,150). Components of musical stimuli such as melodic contour and perception of unfamiliar pitch patterns are processed by cortical subsystems rather than by a nonspecific music area of the brain (151–153). Functional imaging of musical perception has been reviewed (154). Wieser et al. (155) suggested a right temporal predominance for musicogenic seizures. Right anterior and mesial hyperperfusion during ictal single-photon emission computed tomography has been documented (154,156) and later detailed coregistration functional imaging supported a privileged role for right temporolimbic activation (157). Zifkin and Zatorre (158) note that more complex musical processing tasks activate more cortical and subcortical territory bilaterally, although with right hemisphere predominance. Hyperexcitable cortical areas could be stimulated to different degrees and extents by different musical stimuli in patients sensitive to these triggers. Gloor (159) suggested that responses to limbic stimulation in epileptic subjects depend on widespread neuronal matrices linked through connections which have become strengthened through repeated use of interest in considering the delay from seizure onset to the development of sensitivity to music and the extent of the networks involved in musical perception.

The extreme specificity of the stimulus in some patients and the delay from stimulus to seizure onset can be useful in preventing attacks but these seizures usually occur in patients with partial seizures, and appropriate antiepileptic drugs are generally required. Intractable seizures should prompt evaluation for surgical treatment.

Seizures Induced By Eating (Eating Epilepsy)

Boudouresques and Gastaut (160) first described eating epilepsy in four patients who experienced seizures after a heavy meal. Gastric distention may have been at least partly responsible for the attacks (161), but many such seizures occurred early in the meal and were unrelated to gastric distention (162,163). The clinical characteristics are usually stereotyped in individual patients but there are few common features among patients. Some patients have seizures at the very sight or smell of food, whereas others have them only in the middle of a meal or shortly afterward. In some patients, the seizures may be associated with the emotional or autonomic components of eating; in others, they are associated with sensory afferents from tongue or pharynx. These seizures have also been documented in young children, in whom they can be mistaken for gastroesophageal reflux (164).

Seizures with eating are almost always related to a symptomatic partial epilepsy. Cases in which the seizures were generalized from onset are exceptional (165). Rémillard et al. (127) suggested that seizures in patients with temporolimbic epilepsy are activated by eating from the beginning of their seizure disorder and continue to have most seizures with meals. In contrast, patients with localized extralimbic, usually postcentral, seizure onset develop reflex activation of seizures later in their course, with less constant triggering by eating and more prominent spontaneous seizures. These patients typically have more obvious lesions and findings on neurologic examination.

The mechanism of eating epilepsy is unclear. Several investigators suggest that interaction of limbic and extralimbic cortices (166) and contributions from subcortical structures, such as hypothalamus (160,167,168), are particularly important. Other proposed triggering mechanisms include a conditioned response, mastication (167), stimulation of the esophagus (169), and satisfaction of a basic drive (164). Rémillard et al. (127) suggested that seizures with extralimbic, suprasylvian onset, often involving obvious structural lesions, may be activated by specific thalamocortical afferents. That obvious combinations of several stimuli are required in some cases (170,171) added to the circumstantial evidence favoring an interaction among cortical areas and diencephalic structures, which in other cases could involve less obvious combinations of stimuli. When the abnormal cortex is located in regions responding to proprioceptive and other sensory afferents (especially lingual, buccal, or pharyngeal) activated by the extensive sensory input generated by a complex behavior such as eating, patients may be more sensitive to the physical manipulation of food, texture, temperature, and chewing. They may also have seizures induced by activities such as brushing teeth. These patients have extralimbic seizure onset. This mechanism may be similar to that described for other proprioceptive or somatosensory-induced seizures (110). A similar mechanism, but with afferents recruiting hyperexcitable temporolimbic structures, may also operate in subjects with temporolimbic seizure onset, who may be more sensitive to gustatory, olfactory, affective, or emotional stimuli or to stimuli arising from more distal parts of the gut. Alerting stimuli have been reported to abolish attacks (172), providing further circumstantial evidence for the participation of an increasing cortical mass and of subcortical influences in some cases of reflex epilepsy.

The extraordinarily high frequency of seizures associated with meals in Sri Lanka (173) may be ascribed to the inclusion of all attacks occurring from 0.5 h before to 0.5 h after eating. This does not correspond to eating epilepsy as defined here.

Proprioceptive-Induced Seizures and Startle Epilepsy

Proprioceptive-induced seizures include those that appear to be evoked by active or passive movements. Gowers (174) first described seizures induced by movement in humans, and they have been characterized as movement-induced seizures. Studies in the monkey by Chauvel and Lamarche (175) suggest that proprioception is the most important trigger and that the term movement-induced seizures is incorrect. Spontaneous and reflex seizures were observed with a chronic alumina focus in the cortical foot area. Reflex motor attacks were triggered by active or passive movement of the contralateral limb and by tapping the hindlimb tendons. The stimuli activating proprioceptive afferents to a hyperexcitable cortical area triggered seizures. Seizures could not be elicited in the curarized animal. In humans, focal reflex or posture-induced seizures can be transiently observed in patients with nonketotic hyperglycemia, resolving only with metabolic correction. Interictal focal neurologic deficits are seen as evidence of underlying cortical dysfunction (171,176). Proprioceptive afferents, rather than the observed movements, are implicated in seizure precipitation in animal studies and probably in humans (177), although the case reported by Gabor (178) is a possible exception. Arseni et al. (179) and Oller-Daurella and Dini (180) have confirmed the epileptic nature of these attacks.

Startle epilepsy involves seizures induced by sudden and unexpected stimuli (181,182). Typically lateralized and tonic, the seizures are often associated with developmental delay, gross neurologic signs, such as hemiplegia, and cerebral lesions (183–185). Computed tomography scans often show unilateral or bilateral mesial frontal lesions (180); patients with normal scans have had dysplastic lesions identified on magnetic resonance imaging (186). Electroencephalograms with depth electrodes have shown initial ictal discharge in the supplementary motor area (187) and mesial frontal cortex (188). These represent a symptomatic localization-related epilepsy and are often medically intractable. Most patients have other spontaneous seizures.

Proprioceptive-induced seizures can be confused with nonepileptic conditions. Clinical and EEG findings should permit differentiation of startle epilepsy from startle disease or hyperekplexia and from other excessive startle disorders (189–191) and should exclude cataplexy and myoclonic epilepsy syndromes. Apparent movement-induced seizures without startle must be distinguished from paroxysmal kinesi-

genic choreoathetosis, in which movements are clearly tonic and choreoathetoid, consciousness is preserved, and the EEG pattern remains normal during attacks (192).

Seizures Triggered by Somatosensory Stimulation

Seizures may be induced by tapping or rubbing individual regions of the body (110). These are partial seizures, often with initial localized sensory symptoms and tonic features, and typically occur in patients with lesions involving postrolandic cortex. A well-defined trigger zone may be found as in patients whose seizures are triggered by brushing the teeth (193). Drugs for partial seizures are needed, but the seizures may be intractable and require evaluation for surgery.

Reflex drop attacks elicited by walking (194) are seen rarely in patients with reflex interictal spikes evoked by percussion of the foot (195). We consider these to be a variety of seizures induced by proprioceptive stimulation. They are interesting because, unexpectedly, individuals with the interictal-evoked spikes do not usually have such attacks. This disorder probably represents a form of idiopathic localization-related epilepsy of childhood, distinct because of the parietal lobe involvement, though underlying dysplastic lesions cannot be excluded. Participation of a more elaborate network for motor programming cannot be excluded in some cases especially if the effective stimulus seems restricted to activities such as walking (196).

Touch-Evoked Seizures

Seizures can be evoked by simple touch (i.e., "tap" seizures), apparently unrelated to proprioceptive afferents (197,198), although startle may be important. These reflex-generalized myoclonic attacks and associated bilateral spike-and-wave EEG discharges occur without evidence of lateralized lesions; the family history may be positive (199). These typically occur in normal infants and toddlers and can represent an idiopathic and relatively benign generalized myoclonic epilepsy syndrome rather than a progressive myoclonic encephalopathy (200,201). They usually respond to valproate, but prolonged treatment may not be needed.

Hot Water Epilepsy

Seizures triggered by immersion in hot water were first described in 1945 (202). The condition is rare in Japan, the Americas, and Europe but seems more common in India (203,204). Little EEG documentation is available, but the epileptic nature of these attacks has been confirmed in some patients (205,206). Indian patients are typically boys, with a mean age at onset of 13.4 years and who are reported to have complex partial or generalized tonic–clonic seizures during ritual bathing when jugs of hot water are poured over the head. Startle and vasovagal events cannot be excluded in many cases nor can they be discounted in some North American, European, and Japanese reports. These cases typically involve younger children than in India, with complex partial seizures occurring as soon as the child is immersed in hot water;

sensitivity often diminishes with time (207). A mechanism involving defective thermoregulation has been proposed, and some of the attacks may be a form of situation-related seizure with age-dependent occurrence similar to febrile convulsions (202). However, many Turkish subjects have interictal temporal EEG abnormalities and complex partial seizures (208); spontaneous seizures have been reported in most Turkish subjects if the reflex attacks begin after early childhood (209).

Miscellaneous Reflex Seizures

Other unusual reflex stimuli have been described, usually as occasional case reports but more recently with improved EEG and radiologic documentation. Vestibular stimuli have been reported to induce seizures. It is important to exclude startle effects with caloric stimulation, for example, and to take into account the time required for caloric stimulation to be effective (210).

Klass and Daly reported the extraordinary case of a child with generalized seizures self-induced by looking at his own hand. By 4 years of age, medications were withdrawn, and no further seizures, reflex or otherwise, occurred in 26 years of follow-up (211). The EEG was said to be normal. A similar case has been reported (45).

CONCLUSIONS

Reflex seizures and reflex epilepsy continue to challenge and puzzle neurologists and neurophysiologists. Intensive monitoring and advances in imaging have helped to clarify some of the mechanisms involved in these cases, which must represent some of nature's more complex experiments. Continued progress depends on the skill and imagination of neurologists and at least as much on their patients, to whom these studies are really dedicated.

References

1. Wilkins AJ. http://privatewww.essex.ac.uk/~arnold/epilepsy.html
2. Commission on Classification and Terminology of the International League Against Epilepsy. Proposal for revised classification of epilepsies and epileptic syndromes. *Epilepsia.* 1989;30:389–399.
3. Engel J Jr. A proposed diagnostic scheme for people with epileptic seizures and with epilepsy: report of the ILAE Task Force on Classification and Terminology. *Epilepsia.* 2001;42:796–803.
4. Engel J Jr. Report of the ILAE Classification Core Group. *Epilepsia.* 2006;47:1558–1568.
5. Hall M. *Synopsis of the Diastaltic Nervous System.* London: Joseph Mallet; 1850:112.
6. Gastaut H. Reflex mechanisms in the genesis of epilepsy. *Epilepsia.* 1962;3:457–460.
7. Penfield W, Erickson T. *Epilepsy and Cerebral Localization.* Springfield, IL: Charles C Thomas; 1941:28.
8. Commission on Classification and Terminology of the International League Against Epilepsy. Proposal for classification of epilepsies and epileptic syndromes. *Epilepsia.* 1985;26:268–278.
9. Wieser HG. Seizure-inducing and preventing mechanisms. In: Beaumanoir A, Gastaut H, Naquet R, eds. *Reflex Seizures and Reflex Epilepsies.* Geneva: Editions Médecine et Hygiène; 1989:49–60.
10. Henner K. Reflex epileptic mechanisms: conceptions and experiences of a clinical neurologist. *Epilepsia.* 1962;3:236–250.
11. Beaumanoir A, Gastaut H, Naquet R, eds. *Reflex Seizures and Reflex Epilepsies.* Geneva: Editions Médecine et Hygiène; 1989:554.
12. Clementi A. Stricninizzazione della sfera corticale visiva ed epilessia sperimentale da stimoli luminosi. *Arch Fisiol.* 1929;27:356–387.
13. Clementi A. Stricninizzazione della sfera corticale visiva ed epilessia sperimentale da stimoli acustici. *Arch Fisiol.* 1929;27:388–414.
14. Clementi A. Sfera gustativa della corteccia cerebrale del cane ed epilessia sperimentale riflessa a tipo sensoriale gustativo. *Boll Soc Ital Biol.* 1935;10:902–904.
15. Moruzzi G. *L'Epilessia sperimentale.* Bologna, Italy: Nicolo Zanichelli; 1946:128.
16. Terzian H, Terzuolo C. Richerche electrofisiologiche sull'epilessia fotica di Clementi. *Arch Fisiol.* 1951;5:301–320.
17. Fulchignoni S. Contributo alla conoscenza dell'epilessia sperimentale riflessa per stimoli luminosi. *Riv Pat Nerv Ment.* 1938;51:154.
18. Gastaut H, Hunter J. An experimental study of the mechanism of photic activation in idiopathic epilepsy. *Electroencephalogr Clin Neurophysiol.* 1950;2:263–287.
19. Gastaut H. L'épilepsie photogénique. *Rev Prat.* 1951;1:105–109.
20. Hunter J, Ingvar D. Pathways mediating metrazol-induced irradiation of visual impulses. *Electroencephalogr Clin Neurophysiol.* 1955;7:39–60.
21. Bignall KE, Imbert M. Polysensory and corticocortical projections to the frontal lobe of squirrel and rhesus monkey. *Electroencephalogr Clin Neurophysiol.* 1969;26:206–215.
22. Buser P, Ascher P, Bruner J, et al. Aspects of sensory motor reverberations to acoustic and visual stimuli: the role of primary specific cortical areas. In: Moruzzi G, Fessard A, Jasper HH, eds. *Brain Mechanisms. Progress in Brain Research.* Amsterdam: Elsevier; 1963;1:294–322.
23. Crichlow EC, Crawford RD. Epileptiform seizures in domestic fowl, II: intermittent light stimulation and the electroencephalogram. *Can J Physiol Pharmacol.* 1974;52:424–429.
24. Johnson DD, Davis HL. Drug responses and brain biochemistry of the Epi mutant chicken. In: Ookawa T, ed. *The Brain and Behavior of the Fowl.* Tokyo: Japan Scientific Society Press; 1983:281–296.
25. Chapman AG, Meldrum BS. Epilepsy-prone mice: genetically determined sound-induced seizures. In: Jobe PC, Laird HE II, eds. *Neurotransmitters and Epilepsy.* Clifton, NJ: Humana Press; 1987.
26. Seyfried TN, Glaser GH. A review of mouse mutants as genetic models of epilepsy. *Epilepsia.* 1985;26:143–150.
27. Löscher W, Schmidt D. Which animal models should be used in the search for new antiepileptic drugs: a proposal based on experimental and clinical considerations. *Epilepsy Res.* 1988;2:145–181.
28. Loskota WJ, Lomax P, Rich ST. The gerbil as a model for the study of the epilepsies: seizure patterns and ontogenesis. *Epilepsia.* 1974;15:109–119.
29. Killam KF, Killam EK, Naquet R. An animal model of light sensitive epilepsy. *Electroencephalogr Clin Neurophysiol.* 1967;22(suppl):497–513.
30. Killam KF, Killam EK, Naquet R. Mise en évidence chez certains singes d'un syndrome myoclonique. *C R Acad Sci (Paris).* 1966;262:1010–1012.
31. Menini C, Silva-Barrat C. The photosensitive epilepsy of the baboon. A model of generalized reflex epilepsy. In: Zifkin BG, Andermann F, Beaumanoir A, et al., eds. *Reflex Epilepsies and Reflex Seizures: Advances in Neurology,* vol 75. Philadelphia: Lippincott–Raven Press; 1998:29–47.
32. DeSarro GB, Nistico G, Meldrum BS. Anticonvulsant properties of flunarizine on reflex and generalized models of epilepsy. *Neuropharmacology.* 1986;25:695–701.
33. Pumain R, Menini C, Heinemann U, et al. Chemical synaptic transmission is not necessary for epileptic seizures to persist in the baboon Papio papio. *Exp Neurol.* 1985;89:250–258.
34. Lloyd KG, Scatton B, Voltz C, et al. Cerebrospinal fluid amino acid and monoamine metabolite levels of Papio papio: correlation with photosensitivity. *Brain Res.* 1986;363:390–394.
35. Gloor P, Metrakos J, Metrakos K, et al. Neurophysiological, genetic and biochemical nature of the epileptic diathesis. In: Broughton RJ, ed. *Henri Gastaut and the Marseilles School's Contribution to the Neurosciences.* Amsterdam: Elsevier; 1982:45–56.
36. Binnie CD, Findlay J, Wilkins AJ. Mechanisms of epileptogenesis in photosensitive epilepsy implied by the effects of moving patterns. *Electroencephalogr Clin Neurophysiol.* 1985;61:1–6.
37. Wilkins AJ, Andermann F, Ives J. Stripes, complex cells and seizures: an attempt to determine the locus and nature of the trigger mechanism in pattern-sensitive epilepsy. *Brain.* 1975;98:365–380.
38. Wilkins AJ, Binnie CD, Darby CE. Visually induced seizures. *Prog Neurobiol.* 1980;15:85–117.
39. Wilkins AJ, Binnie CD, Darby CE. Interhemispheric differences in photosensitive epilepsy, I: pattern sensitivity threshold. *Electroencephalogr Clin Neurophysiol.* 1981;52:461–468.
40. Wilkins AJ, Zifkin B, Andermann F, et al. Seizures induced by thinking. *Ann Neurol.* 1982;11:608–612.
41. Christie S, Guberman A, Tansley BW, et al. Primary reading epilepsy: investigation of critical seizure-provoking stimuli. *Epilepsia.* 1988; 29:288–293.
42. Wolf P, Mayer T, Reker M. Reading epilepsy: report of five new cases and further considerations on the pathophysiology. *Seizure.* 1998;7:271–279.
43. Wyler AR, Ward AA Jr. Epileptic neurons. In: Lockard JS, Ward AA Jr, eds. *Epilepsy: A Window to Brain Mechanisms.* New York: Raven Press; 1980:51–68.
44. Gastaut H, Régis H, Dongier S, et al. Conditionnement électroencéphalographique des décharges épileptiques et notion d'épilepsie réflexo-conditionnée. *Rev Neurol.* 1956;94:829–835.
45. Forster FM. *Reflex Epilepsy, Behavioral Therapy and Conditional Reflexes.* Springfield, IL: Charles C Thomas; 1977:318.

46. Gras P, Grosmaire N, Giroud M, et al. Exploration d'un cas d'épilepsie à la lecture par EEG avec électrodes sphénoïdales: rôle des régions temporales dans le déclenchement émotionnel des crises. *Neurophysiol Clin.* 1992;22:313–320.

47. Fenwick P. Self-generation of seizures by an action of mind. In: Zifkin BG, Andermann F, Beaumanoir A, et al., eds. *Reflex Epilepsies and Reflex Seizures: Advances in Neurology*, vol 75. Philadelphia: Lippincott–Raven Press; 1998:87–92.

48. Wolf P. From seizures to syndromes. In: Wolf P, ed. *Epileptic Seizures and Syndromes*. London: John Libbey; 1994:39–40.

49. Woermann FG, Free SL, Koepp MJ, et al. Abnormal cerebral structure in juvenile myoclonic epilepsy demonstrated with voxel-based analysis of MRI. *Brain.* 1999;122:2111–2118.

50. Martinez O, Reisin R, Zifkin BG, et al. Evidence for reflex activation of experiential complex partial seizures. *Neurology.* 2000;56:121–123.

51. Palmini A, Halasz P, Scheffer IE, et al. Reflex seizures in patients with malformations of cortical development and refractory epilepsy. *Epilepsia.* 2005;46:1224–1234.

52. Malone S, Miller I, Jakayar P, et al. MRI-negative frontal lobe epilepsy with ipsilateral akinesia and reflex activation. *Epileptic Disord.* 2008;10:349–355.

53. Kasteleijn-Nolst Trenité DG. Photosensitivity in epilepsy: electrophysiological and clinical correlates. *Acta Neurol Scand.* 1989;125(suppl):31–49.

54. Newmark ME, Penry JK. *Photosensitivity and Epilepsy: A Review*. New York: Raven Press; 1979:220.

55. Waltz S, Christen HJ, Doose H. The different patterns of the photoparoxysmal response–a genetic study. *Electroencephalogr Clin Neurophysiol.* 1992;83:138–145.

56. Zifkin BG, Kasteleijn-Nolst Trenité D. Reflex epilepsy and reflex seizures of the visual system: a clinical review. *Epileptic Disord.* 2000;2:129–136.

57. Parra J, Lopes da Silva FH, Stroink H, et al. Is colour modulation an independent factor in human visual photosensitivity? *Brain.* 2007;130:1679–1689.

58. Kasteleijn-Nolst Trenité DGA. Reflex seizures induced by intermittent light stimulation. In: Zifkin BG, Andermann F, Beaumanoir A, et al., eds. *Reflex Epilepsies and Reflex Seizures. Advances in Neurology*, vol 75. Philadelphia: Lippincott–Raven Press; 1998:99–121.

59. Jeavons PM. Photosensitive epilepsy. In: Laidlaw J, Richens A, eds. *A Textbook of Epilepsy.* 2nd ed. Edinburgh: Churchill Livingstone; 1982:195–210.

60. DeMarco P, Ghersini L. Videogames and epilepsy. *Dev Med Child Neurol.* 1985;27:519–521.

61. Kasteleijn-Nolst Trenité DGA, Dekker E, Spekreijse S, et al. Role of television, video games and computers in epileptic photosensitive patients: preliminary results. *Epilepsia.* 1994;35(suppl 7):37.

62. Cushman JT, Floccare DJ. Flicker illness: An underrecognized but preventable complication of helicopter transport. *Prehosp Emerg Care.* 2007;11(1):85–88.

63. Harding G, Harding P, Wilkins A. Wind turbines, flicker, and photosensitive epilepsy: Characterizing the flashing that may precipitate seizures and optimizing guidelines to prevent them. *Epilepsia.* 2008;49:1095–1098.

64. Harding GFA, Jeavons PM. *Photosensitive Epilepsy*. London: Mac Keith Press; 1994.

65. Jeavons PM, Harding GFA. Photosensitive epilepsy. In: *Clinics in Developmental Medicine.* London: Heinemann Medical; 1975:56–121.

66. Aso K, Watanabe K, Negoro T, et al. Photosensitive partial seizure: the origin of abnormal discharges. *J Epilepsy.* 1988;1:87–93.

67. Rubboli G, Michelucci R, Ambrosetto G, et al. Le crisi indotte dalla televisione: epilessia generalizzata od occipitale? *Boll Lega Ital Epil.* 1988;6263:207–208.

68. Guerrini R, Bonanni P, Parmeggiani L, et al. Induction of partial seizures by visual stimulation. In: Zifkin BG, Andermann F, Beaumanoir A, et al., eds. *Reflex Epilepsies and Reflex Seizures: Advances in Neurology.* vol 75. Philadelphia: Lippincott–Raven Press; 1998:159–178.

69. Hennessy M, Binnie CD. Photogenic partial seizures. *Epilepsia.* 2000;41:59–64.

70. Capovilla G, Beccaria F, Gambardella A, et al. Photosensitive benign myoclonic epilepsy in infancy. *Epilepsia.* 2007;48:96–100.

71. Berkovic SF, Andermann F, Carpenter S, et al. Progressive myoclonus epilepsies: specific causes and diagnosis. *N Engl J Med.* 1986;315:296–305.

72. Wilkins AJ, Darby CE, Binnie CD. Optical treatment of photosensitive epilepsy. *Electroencephalogr Clin Neurophysiol.* 1977;43:577.

73. Wilkins AJ, Baker A, Amin D, et al. Treatment of photosensitive epilepsy using coloured glasses. *Seizure.* 1999;8:444–449.

74. Capovilla G, Gambardella A, Rubboli G, et al. Suppressive efficacy by a commercially available blue lens on PPR in 610 photosensitive epilepsy patients. *Epilepsia.* 2006;47:529–533.

75. Harding GFA, Herrick CE, Jeavons PM. A controlled study of the effect of sodium valproate on photosensitive epilepsy and its prognosis. *Epilepsia.* 1979;19:555–565.

76. Chapman AG, Horton RW, Meldrum BS. Anticonvulsant action of a 1,5 benzodiazepine, clobazam, in reflex epilepsy. *Epilepsia.* 1978;19:293–299.

77. Quesney LF, Andermann F, Gloor P. Dopaminergic mechanism in generalized photosensitive epilepsy. *Neurology.* 1981;31:1542–1544.

78. Clemens B. Dopamine agonist treatment of self-induced pattern-sensitive epilepsy: a case report. *Epilepsy Res.* 1988;2:340–343.

79. Morimoto T, Hayakawa T, Sugie H, et al. Epileptic seizures precipitated by constant light, movement in daily life, and hot water immersion. *Epilepsia.* 1985;26:237–242.

80. Harding GF, Edson A, Jeavons PM. Persistence of photosensitivity. *Epilepsia.* 1997;38:663–669.

81. Radovici A, Misirliou V, Gluckman M. Épilepsie réflexe provoquée par éxcitations optiques des rayons solaires. *Rev Neurol.* 1932;1:1305–1308.

82. Andermann K, Berman S, Cooke PM, et al. Self-induced epilepsy. A collection of self-induced epilepsy cases compared with some other photoconvulsive cases. *Arch Neurol.* 1962;6:49–65.

83. Binnie CD. Self-induction of seizures: the ultimate noncompliance. *Epilepsy Res.* 1988;1(suppl):153–158.

84. Kasteleijn-Nolst Trenité DG, Binnie CD, Overweg J, et al. Treatment of self-induction in epileptic patients: who wants it? In: Beaumanoir A, Gastaut H, Naquet R, eds. *Reflex Seizures and Reflex Epilepsies.* Geneva: Editions Médecine et Hygiène; 1989:439–446.

85. Lerman P, Kivity S. Self-induced photogenic epilepsy: a report of 14 cases. In: Beaumanoir A, Gastaut H, Naquet R, eds. *Reflex Seizures and Reflex Epilepsies.* Geneva: Editions Médecine et Hygiène; 1989:379–384.

86. Tassinari CA, Rubboli G, Rizzi R, et al. Self-induction of visually induced seizures. In: Zifkin BG, Andermann F, Beaumanoir A, et al., eds. *Reflex Epilepsies and Reflex Seizures: Advances in Neurology.* vol 75. Philadelphia: Lippincott–Raven Press; 1998:179–192.

87. Watanabe K, Negoro T, Matsumoto A, et al. Self-induced photogenic epilepsy in infants. *Arch Neurol.* 1985;42:406–407.

88. Olds J, Milner P. Positive reinforcement produced by electrical stimulation of septal area and other areas of rat brain. *J Comp Physiol Psychol.* 1954;47:419–427.

89. Ehret R, Schneider E. Photogene Epilepsie mit suchtartiger Selbstauslosung kleiner Anfälle und wiederholten Sexualdelikten. *Arch Psychiatr Nervenkr.* 1961;202:75–94.

90. Faught E, Falgout J, Nidiffer FD. Self-induced photosensitive absence seizures with ictal pleasure. *Arch Neurol.* 1986;43:408–410.

91. Overweg J, Binnie CD. Pharmacotherapy of self-induced seizures. In: *The 12th Epilepsy International Symposium.* Copenhagen, Denmark, 1980 (abstract).

92. Wilkins AJ, Binnie CD, Darby CE, et al. Epileptic and nonepileptic sensitivity to light. In: Beaumanoir A, Gastaut H, Naquet R, eds. *Reflex Seizures and Reflex Epilepsies.* Geneva: Editions Médecine et Hygiène; 1989:153–162.

93. Wilkins AJ, Darby CE, Binnie CD. Neurophysiological aspects of pattern-sensitive epilepsy. *Brain.* 1979;102:125.

94. Wilkins AJ, Darby CE, Binnie CD, et al. Television epilepsy: the role of pattern. *Electroencephalogr Clin Neurophysiol.* 1979;47:163–171.

95. Panayiotopoulos CP. Fixation-off, scotosensitive, and other visual-related epilepsies. In: Zifkin BG, Andermann F, Beaumanoir A, et al., eds. *Reflex Epilepsies and Reflex Seizures: Advances in Neurology.* vol 75. Philadelphia: Lippincott–Raven Press; 1998:139–157.

96. Giannakodimos S, Panayiotopoulos CP. Eyelid myoclonia with absences in adults: a clinical and video-EEG study. *Epilepsia.* 1996;37:36–44.

97. Gastaut H, Tassinari CA. Triggering mechanisms in epilepsy: the electroclinical point of view. *Epilepsia.* 1966;7:85–138.

98. Green JB. Self-induced seizures: clinical and electroencephalographic studies. *Arch Neurol.* 1966;15:579–586.

99. Millett CJ, Fish DR, Thompson PJ. A survey of epilepsy-patient perceptions of video-game material/electronic screens and other factors as seizure precipitants. *Seizure.* 1997;6:457–459.

100. Ricci S, Vigevano F, Manfredi M, et al. Epilepsy provoked by television and video games: safety of 100 Hz screens. *Neurology.* 1998;50:790–793.

101. Binnie CD, Wilkins AJ. Visually induced seizures not caused by flicker (intermittent light stimulation). In: Zifkin BG, Andermann F, Beaumanoir A, et al., eds. *Reflex Epilepsies and Reflex Seizures: Advances in Neurology.* vol 75. Philadelphia: Lippincott–Raven Press; 1998:123–138.

102. Ishida S, Yamashita Y, Matsuishi T, et al. Photosensitive seizures provoked while viewing "Pocket Monsters," a made-for-television animation program in Japan. *Epilepsia.* 1998;39:1340–1344.

103. Wilkins AJ, Emmett J, Harding GFA. Characterizing the patterned images that precipitate seizures and optimizing guidelines to prevent them. *Epilepsia.* 2005;46:1212–1218.

104. Takahashi T, Kamijo K, Takaki Y, et al. Suppressive efficacies by adaptive temporal filtering system on photoparoxysmal response elicited by flickering pattern stimulation. *Epilepsia.* 2002;43:530–534.

105. Harding GFA. TV can be bad for your health. *Nat Med.* 1998;4:265–267.

106. Andermann F, Zifkin BG, Andermann E. Epilepsy induced by thinking and spatial tasks. In: Zifkin BG, et al., eds. *Reflex Epilepsies and Reflex Seizures: Advances in Neurology.* vol 75. Philadelphia: Lippincott-Raven Press; 1998:263–272.

107. Stanescu-Cosson R, Pinel P, van De Moortele PF, et al. Understanding dissociations in dyscalculia: a brain imaging study of the impact of number size on the cerebral networks for exact and approximate calculation. *Brain.* 2000;123:2240–1218.

108. Inoue Y, Seino M, Tanaka M, et al. Praxis-induced epilepsy. In: Wolf P, ed. *Epileptic Seizures and Syndromes.* London: John Libbey; 1994:81–91.

109. Matsuoka H, Takahashi T, Sasaki M, et al. Neuropsychological EEG activation in patients with epilepsy. *Brain.* 2000;123:318–330.
110. Vignal J-P, Biraben A, Chauvel PY, et al. Reflex partial seizures of sensorimotor cortex (including cortical reflex myoclonus and startle epilepsy). In: Zifkin BG, Andermann F, Beaumanoir A, et al., eds. *Reflex Epilepsies and Reflex Seizures: Advances in Neurology.* vol 75. Philadelphia: Lippincott–Raven Press; 1998:207–226.
111. Ferlazzo E, Zifkin BG, Andermann E, et al. Cortical triggers in generalized reflex seizures and epilepsies. *Brain.* 2005;128:700–710.
112. Wolf P. Regional manifestation of idiopathic epilepsy. Introduction. In: Wolf P, ed. *Epileptic Seizures and Syndromes.* London: John Libbey; 1994:265–267.
113. Blumenfeld H. From molecules to networks: cortical/subcortical interactions in the pathophysiology of idiopathic generalized epilepsy. *Epilepsia.* 2003;44(suppl 2):7–15.
114. Lin K, Carrete H Jr, Lin J, et al. Magnetic resonance spectroscopy reveals an epileptic network in juvenile myoclonic epilepsy. *Epilepsia* Published Online: February 12, 2009 4:07PM DOI: 10.1111/j.1528-1167.2008.01948.x
115. Bickford RG, Whelan JL, Klass DW, et al. Reading epilepsy: clinical and electroencephalographic studies of a new syndrome. *Trans Am Neurol Assoc.* 1956;81:100–102.
116. Stoupel N. On the reflex epilepsies: epilepsy caused by reading. *Electroencephalogr Clin Neurophysiol.* 1968;25:416–417.
117. Kartsounis LD. Comprehension as the effective trigger in a case of primary reading epilepsy. *J Neurol Neurosurg Psychiatry.* 1988;51:128–130.
118. Newman PK, Longley BP. Reading epilepsy. *Arch Neurol.* 1984;41:13–14.
119. Critchley M, Cobb W, Sears TA. On reading epilepsy. *Epilepsia.* 1959;1:403–417.
120. Daly RF, Forster FM. Inheritance of reading epilepsy. *Neurology.* 1975;25:1051–1054.
121. Ramani V. Reading epilepsy. In: Zifkin BG, Andermann F, Beaumanoir A, et al., eds. *Reflex Epilepsies and Reflex Seizures: Advances in Neurology.* vol 75. Philadelphia: Lippincott–Raven Press; 1998:241–262.
122. Matthews WB, Wright FK. Hereditary primary reading epilepsy. *Neurology.* 1967;17:919–921.
123. Salek-Haddadi A, Mayer T, Hamandi K, et al. Imaging seizure activity: a combined EEG/EMG-fMRI study in reading epilepsy. *Epilepsia.* 2009;50:256–264.
124. Archer JS, Briellmann RS, Syngeniotis A, et al. Spike-triggered fMRI in reading epilepsy: involvement of left frontal cortex working memory area. *Neurology.* 2003;60:415–421.
125. Bingel A. Reading epilepsy. *Neurology.* 1957;7:752–756.
126. Koutroumanidis M, Koepp MJ, Richardson MP, et al. The variants of reading epilepsy. A clinical and video-EEG study of 17 patients with reading-induced seizures. *Brain.* 1998;121:1409–1427.
127. Rémillard GM, Zifkin BG, Andermann F. Seizures induced by eating. In: Zifkin BG, Andermann F, Beaumanoir A, et al., eds. *Reflex Epilepsies and Reflex Seizures: Advances in Neurology.* vol 75. Philadelphia: Lippincott–Raven Press; 1998:227–240.
128. Geschwind N, Sherwin I. Language-induced epilepsy. *Arch Neurol.* 1967;16:25–31.
129. Bennett DR, Mavor H, Jarcho LW. Language-induced epilepsy: report of a case. *Electroencephalogr Clin Neurophysiol.* 1971;30:159.
130. Brooks JE, Jirauch PM. Primary reading epilepsy: a misnomer. *Arch Neurol.* 1971;25:97–104.
131. Lee SI, Sutherling WW, Persing JA, et al. Language-induced seizures: a case of cortical origin. *Arch Neurol.* 1980;37:433–436.
132. Asbury AK, Prensky AL. Graphogenic epilepsy. *Trans Am Neurol Assoc.* 1963;88:193–194.
133. Sharbrough FW, Westmoreland B. Writing epilepsy. *Electroencephalogr Clin Neurophysiol.* 1977;43:506.
134. Cirignotta F, Zucconi M, Mondini S, et al. Writing epilepsy. *Clin Electroencephalogr.* 1986;17:21–23.
135. Tsuzuki H, Kasuga I. Paroxysmal discharges triggered by hearing spoken language. *Epilepsia.* 1978;19:147–154.
136. Herskowitz J, Rosman NP, Geschwind N. Seizures induced by singing and recitation: a unique form of reflex epilepsy in childhood. *Arch Neurol.* 1984;41:1102–1103.
137. Saenz Lope E, Herranz-Tanarro FJ, Masdeu JC. Primary reading epilepsy. *Epilepsia.* 1985;26:649–656.
138. Brenner RP, Seelinger DF. Drawing-induced seizures. *Arch Neurol.* 1979;36:515–516.
139. Valenti MP, Rudolf G, Carré S, et al. Language-induced epilepsy, acquired stuttering, and idiopathic generalized epilepsy: phenotypic study of one family. *Epilepsia.* 2006;47:766–772.
140. Brien SE, Murray TJ. Musicogenic epilepsy. *Can Med Assoc J.* 1984;131:1255–1258.
141. Jallon P, Heraut LA, Vanelle JM. Musicogenic epilepsy. In: Beaumanoir A, Gastaut H, Naquet R, eds. *Reflex Seizures and Reflex Epilepsies.* Geneva: Editions Médecine et Hygiène; 1989:269–274.
142. Critchley M. Musicogenic epilepsy. *Brain.* 1937;60:13–27.
143. Scott D. Musicogenic epilepsy. In: Critchley M, Henson RA, eds. *Music and the Brain.* London: Heinemann Medical; 1977:354–364.
144. Forster FM, Booker HE, Gascon G. Conditioning in musicogenic epilepsy. *Trans Am Neurol Assoc.* 1967;92:236–237.
145. Forster FM. The classification and conditioning treatment of the reflex epilepsies. *Int J Neurol.* 1972;9:73–86.
146. Daly DD, Barry MJ Jr. Musicogenic epilepsy: report of three cases. *Psychosom Med.* 1957;19:399–408.
147. Tayah TF, Abou-Khalil B, Gilliam FG, et al. Musicogenic seizures can arise from multiple temporal lobe foci: intracranial EEG analyses of three patients. *Epilepsia.* 2006;47:1402–1406.
148. Liegeois-Chauvel C, Musolino A, Chauvel P. Localization of the primary auditory area in man. *Brain.* 1991;114:139–151.
149. Creutzfeldt O, Ojemann G. Neuronal activity in the human lateral temporal lobe, III: activity changes during music. *Exp Brain Res.* 1989;77:490–498.
150. Wieser HG, Mazzola G. Musical consonances and dissonances: are they distinguished independently by the right and left hippocampi? *Neuropsychologia.* 1986;24:805–812.
151. Peretz I, Kolinsky R, Tramo M, et al. Functional dissociations following bilateral lesions of auditory cortex. *Brain.* 1994;117:1283–1301.
152. Zatorre RJ. Discrimination and recognition of tonal melodies after unilateral cerebral excisions. *Neuropsychologia.* 1985;23:31–41.
153. Zatorre RJ, Evans AC, Meyer E. Neural mechanisms underlying melodic perception and memory for pitch. *J Neurosci.* 1994;14:1908–1919.
154. Johnsrude IS, Giraud AL, Frackowiak RSJ. Functional imaging of the auditory system: the use of positron emission tomography. *Audiol Neurootol.* 2002;7:251–276.
155. Wieser HG, Hungerbühler H, Siegel AM, et al. Musicogenic epilepsy: review of the literature and case report with ictal single photon emission computed tomography. *Epilepsia.* 1997;38:200–207.
156. Genc BO, Genc E, Tastekin G, et al. Musicogenic epilepsy with ictal single photon emission computed tomography (SPECT): could these cases contribute to our knowledge of music processing? *Eur J Neurol.* 2001;8:191–194.
157. Cho JW, Seo DW, Joo EY, et al. Neural correlates of musicogenic epilepsy:SISCOM and FDG-PET. *Epilepsy Research.* 2007;77:169–173.
158. Zifkin BG, Zatorre R. Musicogenic epilepsy. In: Zifkin BG, Andermann F, Beaumanoir A, et al., eds. *Reflex Epilepsies and Reflex Seizures: Advances in Neurology.* vol 75. Philadelphia: Lippincott–Raven Press; 1998:273–281.
159. Gloor P. Experiential phenomena of temporal lobe epilepsy. Facts and hypotheses. *Brain.* 1990;113:1673–1694.
160. Boudouresques J, Gastaut H. Le mécanisme réflexe de certaines épilepsies temporales. *Rev Neurol.* 1954;90:157–158.
161. Gastaut H, Poirier F. Experimental, or "reflex," induction of seizures: report of a case of abdominal (enteric) epilepsy. *Epilepsia.* 1964;5:256–270.
162. Hernandez-Cossio O, Diaz G, Hernandez-Fustes O. A case of eating epilepsy. In: Beaumanoir A, Gastaut H, Naquet R, eds. *Reflex Seizures and Reflex Epilepsies.* Geneva: Editions Médecine et Hygiène; 1989:301–304.
163. Loiseau P, Guyot M, Loiseau H, et al. Eating seizures. *Epilepsia.* 1986;27:161–163.
164. Plouin P, Ponsot C, Jalin C. Eating seizures in a three year old child. In: Beaumanoir A, Gastaut H, Naquet R, eds. *Reflex Seizures and Reflex Epilepsies.* Geneva: Editions Médecine et Hygiène; 1989:309–313.
165. Cirignotta F, Marcacci G, Lugaresi E. Epileptic seizures precipitated by eating. *Epilepsia.* 1977;18:445–449.
166. Fiol ME, Leppik IE, Pretzel K. Eating epilepsy: EEG and clinical study. *Epilepsia.* 1986;27:441–445.
167. Robertson WC, Fariello RG. Eating epilepsy with a deep forebrain glioma. *Ann Neurol.* 1979;6:271–273.
168. Scollo-Lavizzari G, Hess R. Sensory precipitation of epileptic seizures: report on two unusual cases. *Epilepsia.* 1967;8:157–161.
169. Forster FM. Epilepsy associated with eating. *Trans Am Neurol Assoc.* 1971;96:106–107.
170. Aguglia U, Tinuper P. Eating seizures. *Eur Neurol.* 1983;22:227–231.
171. Reder AT, Wright FS. Epilepsy evoked by eating: the role of peripheral input. *Neurology.* 1982;32:1065–1069.
172. Ganga A, Sechi GP, Porcella V, et al. Eating seizures and distraction-arousal functions. *Eur Neurol.* 1988;28:167–170.
173. Senanayake N. Eating epilepsy—a reappraisal. *Epilepsy Res.* 1990;5:74–79.
174. Gowers WR. *Epilepsy and Other Chronic Convulsive Diseases: Their Causes, Symptoms and Treatment.* London: JA Churchill; 1901:320.
175. Chauvel P, Lamarche M. Analyse d'une 'épilepsie du mouvement' chez un singe porteur d'un foyer rolandique. *Neurochirurgie.* 1975;21:121–137.
176. Singh BM, Gupta DR, Strobos RJ. Nonketotic hyperglycemia and epilepsia partialis continua. *Arch Neurol.* 1973;29:187–190.
177. Rosen I, Fehling C, Sedgwick M, et al. Focal reflex epilepsy with myoclonus: electrophysiological investigation and therapeutic implications. *Electroencephalogr Clin Neurophysiol.* 1977;42:95–106.
178. Gabor AJ. Focal seizures induced by movement without sensory feedback mechanisms. *Electroencephalogr Clin Neurophysiol.* 1974;36:403–408.
179. Arseni C, Stoica I, Serbanescu T. Electroclinical investigations on the role of proprioceptive stimuli in the onset and arrest of convulsive epileptic paroxysms. *Epilepsia.* 1967;8:162–170.
180. Oller-FV L, Dini J. Las crisis epilepticas desencadenadas por movimientos voluntarios. *Med Clin.* 1970;54:189–196.
181. Aguglia U, Tinuper P, Gastaut H. Startle-induced epileptic seizures. *Epilepsia.* 1984;25:712–720.

182. Alajouanine T, Gastaut H. La syncinésie-sursaut et l'épilepsie-sursaut à déclenchement sensoriel ou sensitif inopiné. *Rev Neurol.* 1955;93:29–41.

183. Falconer MA, Driver MV, Serafetinides EA. Seizures induced by movement: report of a case relieved by operation. *J Neurol Neurosurg Psychiatry.* 1963;26:300–307.

184. Lishman WA, Symonds CP, Whitty CWM, et al. Seizures induced by movement. *Brain.* 1962;85:93–108.

185. Whitty CWM, Lishman WA, Fitzgibbon JP. Seizures induced by movement: a form of reflex epilepsy. *Lancet.* 1964;1:1403–1405.

186. Manford MR, Fish DR, Shorvon SD. Startle provoked epileptic seizures: features in 19 patients. *J Neurol Neurosurg Psychiatry.* 1996;61:151–156.

187. Bancaud J, Talairach J, Lamarche M, et al. Hypothèses neuro-physiopathologiques sur l'épilepsie-sursaut chez l'homme. *Rev Neurol.* 1975;131:559–571.

188. Bancaud J, Talairach J, Bonis A. Physiopathogénie des épilepsies-sursaut (à propos d'une épilepsie de l'aire motrice supplémentaire). *Rev Neurol.* 1967;117:441–453.

189. Andermann F, Andermann E. Excessive startle syndromes: startle disease, jumping, and startle epilepsy. *Adv Neurol.* 1986;43:321–338.

190. Gastaut H, Villeneuve A. The startle disease or hyperekplexia: pathological surprise reaction. *J Neurol Sci.* 1967;5:523–542.

191. Saenz-Lope E, Herranz-Tanarro FJ, Masdeu JC, et al. Hyperekplexia: a syndrome of pathological startle responses. *Ann Neurol.* 1984;15:36–41.

192. Bhatia KP. The paroxysmal dyskinesias. *J Neurol.* 1999;246:149–155.

193. D'Souza WJ, O'Brien TJ, Murphy M, et al. Toothbrushing-induced epilepsy with structural lesions in the primary somatosensory area. *Neurology.* 2007;68:769–771.

194. Di Capua M, Vigevano F, Tassinari CA. Drop seizures reflex to walking. In: Beaumanoir A, Gastaut H, Naquet R, eds. *Reflex Seizures and Reflex Epilepsies.* Geneva: Editions Médecine et Hygiène; 1989:83–88.

195. DeMarco P, Tassinari CA. Extreme somatosensory evoked potential (ESEP): an EEG sign forecasting a possible occurrence of seizures in children. *Epilepsia.* 1981;22:569–575.

196. Iriarte J, Sanchez-Carpintero R, Schlumberger E, et al. Gait epilepsy: a case report of gait-induced seizures. *Epilepsia.* 2001;42:1087–1090.

197. Ravindran M. Single case study: contact epilepsy: a rare form of reflex epilepsy. *J Nerv Ment Dis.* 1978;166:219–221.

198. Schmidt G, Todt H. Durch taktile und viscerale Reize ausgeloste Reflexepilepsie beim Kind. *Kinderartzl Praxis.* 1979;47:482–487.

199. Ricci S, Cusmai R, Fusco L, et al. Reflex myoclonic epilepsy of the first year of life. *Epilepsia.* 1993;34(suppl 6):47 (abstr).

200. Deonna T. Reflex seizures with somatosensory precipitation: clinical and electroencephalographic patterns and differential diagnosis, with emphasis on reflex myoclonic epilepsy of infancy. In: Zifkin BG, Andermann F, Beaumanoir A, et al., eds. *Reflex Epilepsies and Reflex Seizures: Advances in Neurology.* vol 75. Philadelphia: Lippincott–Raven Press; 1998:193–206.

201. Revol M, Isnard H, Beaumanoir A, et al. Touch evoked myoclonic seizures in infancy. In: Beaumanoir A, Gastaut H, Naquet R, eds. *Reflex Seizures and Reflex Epilepsies.* Geneva: Editions Médecine et Hygiène; 1989:103–108.

202. Allen IM. Observations on cases of reflex epilepsy. *N Z Med J.* 1945;44:135–142.

203. Satishchandra P, Ullal GR, Shankar SK. Hot water epilepsy. In: Zifkin BG, Andermann F, Beaumanoir A, et al., eds. *Reflex Epilepsies and Reflex Seizures: Advances in Neurology.* vol 75. Philadelphia: Lippincott–Raven Press; 1998:283–293.

204. Szymonowicz W, Meloff KL. Hot water epilepsy. *Can J Neurol Sci.* 1978;5:247–251.

205. Roos RAC, van Dijk JG. Reflex epilepsy induced by immersion in hot water. *Eur Neurol.* 1988;28:6–10.

206. Shaw NJ, Livingston JH, Minus RA, et al. Epilepsy precipitated by bathing. *Dev Med Child Neurol.* 1988;30:108–114.

207. Ioos C, Fohlen M, Villeneuve N, et al. Hot water epilepsy: a benign and unrecognized form. *J Child Neurol.* 2000;15:125–128.

208. Yalçin AD, Toydemir HE, Forta H. Hot water epilepsy: clinical and electroencephalographic features of 25 cases. *Epilepsy Behav.* 2006;9:89–94.

209. Bebek N, Gurses C, Gokyigit A, et al. Hot water epilepsy: clinical and electrophysiologic findings based on 21 cases. *Epilepsia.* 2001;42:1180–1184.

210. Karbowski K. Epileptic seizures induced by vestibular and auditory stimuli. In: Beaumanoir A, Gastaut H, Naquet R, eds. *Reflex Seizures and Reflex Epilepsies.* Geneva: Editions Médecine et Hygiène; 1989:255–260.

211. Klass DW. Self-induced seizures: long-term follow-up of two unusual cases. In: Beaumanoir A, Gastaut H, Naquet R, eds. *Reflex Seizures and Reflex Epilepsies.* Geneva: Editions Médecine et Hygiène; 1989:369–378.

CHAPTER 25 ■ RASMUSSEN ENCEPHALITIS (CHRONIC FOCAL ENCEPHALITIS)

FRANÇOIS DUBEAU

Rasmussen encephalitis (RE) is a progressive disorder of child-hood, associated with hemispheric atrophy, severe focal epilepsy, intellectual decline, and hemiparesis. Neuropathologic features described in the surgical specimens show characteristics of chronic inflammation such as perivascular and leptomeningeal lymphocytic infiltration, microglial nodules, astrocytosis, and neuronal degeneration. There are variants of this syndrome with regard to age at onset, staging, localization, progression, and outcome. Treatment options are limited. Antiepileptic drugs (AEDs) usually show no significant benefit. Immunotherapy trials (undertaken mostly during the 1990s) showed modest transient improvement in symptoms and disease progression in some patients. Only hemispherectomy seems to produce persistent relief of seizures and functional improvement.

The disorder was first described by Dr. Theodore Rasmussen in 1958, who, together with Jerzy Olszewski and Donald Lloyd-Smith, published the clinical and histopathologic features of three patients with focal seizures caused by chronic focal encephalitis (1). The original proband, FS, a 10-year-old boy, was referred in 1945 to Dr. Wilder Penfield by Dr. Edgar Fincher, chief of neurosurgery at Emory University in Atlanta, Georgia, because of intractable right-sided focal motor seizures starting at 6 years of age (2). FS developed a right hemiparesis and underwent, between 1941 and 1956, three surgical interventions (two at the Montreal Neurological Hospital and Institute [MNHI]) at 7, 10, and 21 years of age in an attempt to control the evolution of the disease. In the first chapter of the monograph on chronic encephalitis published by Dr. Frederick Andermann in 1991, Dr. Rasmussen reported a letter by Dr. Fincher to Dr. Penfield (dated 1956) urging him to consider a more extensive cortical excision and concluded, "I note in your discussion that you list the cause as unknown, but if this young-ster doesn't have a chronic low-grade encephalitic process which has likely, by now, burned itself out, I will buy you a new hat." The last intervention was a left hemispherectomy performed by Dr. Rasmussen, and histology showed sparse perivascular inflammation and glial nodules. FS remained seizure-free until his last follow-up at 51 years of age. He was mildly retarded and had a fixed right hemiplegia. He developed hydrocephalus as a late complication of the surgical procedure and required a shunt. Dr. Penfield, who was consulted in this case, remained skeptical of the postulate that the syndrome was a primary inflammatory disorder, and he raised most of the issues that continue to be debated: if it is an encephalitic process, would it not involve both hemispheres? Is the encephalitic process the result of recurrent seizures caused by a small focal lesion in one hemisphere? Why it is that epileptic seizures are destructive in one case and not in another? Dr. Rasmussen himself recognized that Fincher's 1941 diagnosis of chronic encephalitis in FS's case was made 14 years

before case 2 of the original 1958 report (1). The story does not say, however, if Dr. Penfield had to provide his colleague and friend Dr. Fincher with a new hat (3).

This diagnosis, later recognized as "Rasmussen encephali-tis (RE) or syndrome," became the subject of extensive discus-sion in the literature, initially debating the best timing for surgery and best surgical approaches, and, more recently, the etiology and pathogenesis of this unusual and enigmatic dis-ease. A large number of publications can now be found in the literature, and two international symposia were held in Montreal, first in 1988 and again in 2002. In 2004, a European Consensus Group proposed formal diagnostic crite-ria and therapeutic avenues for the management of RE patients (4). The obvious interest for this disease, which is usually described in children, was initially driven by the sever-ity and inescapability of its course, which rapidly led to its description as a prototype of "catastrophic epilepsy." Physicians and scientists became interested due to the unusual pathogenesis and evolution of the syndrome and are now try-ing to reconcile the apparent focal nature of the disease with the postulated viral and autoimmune etiologies that may or may not be mutually exclusive. This chapter reviews and updates a number of issues regarding RE, particularly the putative humoral and cellular immune mechanisms of the dis-ease, the variability of the clinical presentations, and the indi-cations and rationale of new medical therapies, such as immunomodulation and receptor-directed pharmacotherapy.

CLINICAL PRESENTATIONS

Typical Course

In the early stages of the disease, the major issue is diagnosis. A combination of characteristic clinical, electrophysiologic, and imaging findings aids in the diagnosis. The 48 patients studied at the MNHI were collected over a period of 30 years and consisted mostly of referrals from outside Canada. Although now easier to recognize, this disease remains rare. During the last decade, an additional 10 patients at the MNHI were studied; a small number compared to the 100 to 150 inpatients with intractable focal epilepsy due to other causes studied each year at the center. Typically, the disease starts in healthy children between 1 and 13 years (mean age, 6.8 years) with 80% developing seizures before the age of 10 years (5). There is no difference in incidence between the sexes. In approximately half the patients, a history of infectious or inflammatory episode was described 6 months prior to the onset of seizures.

The first sign of the disease is the development of seizures. They are usually partial or secondarily generalized tonic–clonic seizures; 20% of patients in the MNHI series presented with status epilepticus as the first manifestation. Early seizures could be polymorphic with variable semiology, but motor manifestations are almost always reported. Other variable semiology of seizures with somatosensory, autonomic, visual, and psychic features has been described (5,6). The seizures rapidly become refractory, with little response to AEDs. Epilepsia partialis continua (EPC) and other forms of focal seizures are particularly unresponsive to AEDs (7–11). A review of the AED therapy in 25 patients of the MNHI series revealed that no specific agent or combination therapy appeared to be more effective or less toxic than other regimens (9). Our experience with newer AEDs in seven other patients with RE did not support improved effectiveness or tolerability for the new agents. The new AEDs—levetiracetam, topiramate, and even felbamate—may theoretically have a role in the treatment of RE, because levetiracetam has efficacy in treating cortical myoclonus (12,13) and topiramate and felbamate have a direct effect on glutamate receptors and release of N-methyl-D-glutamine (NMDA) (14).

A variety of seizure types develop over time. The most common are focal motor and EPC (in 56% of the patients), with scalp electroencephalogram (EEG) patterns suggesting perirolandic onset. Secondarily generalized motor seizures are also common in many patients, but these appear to be easier to control with AEDs. Other, less frequent types of motor seizures include jacksonian march (12%), posturing (25%), or versive movements of the head and eyes (13%), suggesting involvement of the primary motor, premotor, and supplementary motor areas. Drop attacks, however, are rare. Focal seizures with somatosensory (22% of the patients), visual (16%), or auditory (2%) manifestations are less frequent and appear later in the course of the disease, suggesting that the epileptogenic process has migrated from frontocentral regions to more posterior cortical areas.

Oguni and colleagues (5) divided the progression of the disease into three stages: *stage 1*, from the onset of the seizures and before the development of a fixed hemiparesis (3 months to 10 years; mean duration 2.8 years); *stage 2*, from the development of a fixed hemiparesis (occurring in all 48 patients) to the completion of neurologic deterioration, including intellectual decline (85%), visual (49%) and sensory (29%) cortical deficits, and speech problems (dysarthria 23%, dysphasia 19%) dependent or independent of the burden of seizure activity (2 months to 10 years; mean duration 3.7 years); and *stage 3*, stabilization of the condition in which further progression no longer occurs, and even the seizures tend to decrease in severity and frequency.

Bien and colleagues (15) presented the clinical natural history of RE in parallel with the time course of brain destruction as measured by serial magnetic resonance imaging (MRI), in a series of 13 patients studied histologically. They separated the progression of the disease into *prodromal* (during this stage patients had rare seizures and minimal neurological deterioration), *acute* (a period of intense seizure occurrence, neurological deterioration and atrophy of the brain), and *residual* (with a marked reduction in seizure frequency) stages comparable to the three stages of Oguni and colleagues. However, Bien and coworkers distinguished two patterns of disease depending on the age at onset of the disorder: one with an earlier and more severe disorder starting during childhood (mean age at first seizure, 4.4 years; range, 1.6 to 6.4 years) and a second with a more protracted and milder course starting during adolescence or adult life (mean age at first seizure, 21.9 years; range, 6.4 to 40.9 years), the second pattern representing a now well-described variant of RE (16–20).

Clinical Variants of Rasmussen Encephalitis

RE has been known for more than 50 years. After the initial description, it became clear that the disease is clinically heterogeneous despite the pathologic hallmark of nonspecific chronic inflammation in the affected hemisphere. This heterogeneity may be explained by different etiologies (viral, viral- and nonviral-mediated autoimmune disease), by different reactions of the host's immune system to exogenous or endogenous insults (age, genetic background, presence of another lesion, or "double pathology"), and by the modulating effect of a variety of antiviral, immunosuppressant, and immunomodulatory agents, or receptor-directed pharmacotherapy used in variable combinations and durations to treat these patients. Atypical or unusual clinical features include early onset (usually younger than 2 years of age) with rapid progression of the disease; bilateral cerebral involvement; relatively late onset during adolescence or adult life with slow progression; atypical anatomic location of the initial brain MRI findings; focal and chronic protracted, subcortical, or even multifocal variants of RE; and double pathology.

Bilateral Hemispheric Involvement

Usually the disease affects only one hemisphere, and most autopsy studies available confirmed unilateral cerebral involvement (21). Over time, however, there may be some contralateral ventricular enlargement and cortical atrophy attributed either to the effect of recurrent seizures and secondary epileptogenesis or to Wallerian changes (22). Patients with definite bilateral inflammatory involvement are exceptional and such involvement has been described in no more than 18 patients (17,23–30) including 6 with atypical or doubtful bilateral RE. Bilateral disease tends to occur in children with early onset (before age 2 years), but is also described in the late-onset adolescent or adult forms. A small number had received high-dose steroids or an intrathecal antiviral agent, which suggested that early aggressive immunologic therapy may have predisposed them to contralateral spread of the disease. Thus, there seems to be an early onset variant of RE in which there is an increased risk of bilateral disease, a more malignant course, and a high mortality. Bilateral RE may be related to immaturity of the immune system or, in rare instances, to a possible adverse effect of immunotherapy.

Late-Onset Adolescent and Adult Variants

In the previous edition of this book, we evaluated the proportion of late-onset RE to be approximately 10% of the total number of patients. A thorough review of the literature seems to confirm that the adolescent or adult variant is more common than initially thought. From 1960 to 2008, we identified at least 29 papers in which over 60 cases of late-onset RE were reported (15–20,30–49,59). In the MNHI series, 9 (16%) of 55 patients collected between 1945 and 2000 started to have seizures after the age of 12 years. The largest series, described by Hart and colleagues (20), included 13 adults and adolescents collected from five centers. In comparison with the childhood form, late-onset RE has a more variable evolution (5,13,18,45), a generally more insidious onset of focal neurologic defects and cognitive impairment, and an increased incidence of occipital involvement (23% in the series described by Hart and coworkers vs. 7% in children younger than 12 years in the MNHI series). Hemiparesis and hemispheric atrophy are often late and may not be as severe when compared with the more typical childhood form (13). Occasionally, the outcome in late-onset RE is similar to or worse than in children (17,31,32), but because of the generally more benign and protracted course, early hemispherectomy seems less appropriate in this group of patients in whom neurologic deficits are usually less pronounced. Moreover, because of a lack of plasticity in adults, the decision for hemispherectomy is complicated because of potential risk of new irreversible postoperative deficits in the form of severe motor, visual, and speech and language (dominant hemisphere) impairments.

Focal and Chronic Protracted Variants

There are rare reports of patients with RE whose seizures were relatively well controlled with AEDs or focal resections, and in whom the neurologic status stabilized spontaneously (20,35,38,48,50,51). Rasmussen had already suggested the existence of a "nonprogressive focal form of encephalitis." With Aguilar, he reviewed 512 surgical specimens from 449 patients and found 32 cases with histologic evidence suggesting the presence of active encephalitis (16). Twelve demonstrated progressive neurologic deterioration compatible with RE, and 20 (4.4%) showed no or mild neurologic deterioration. In his review of patients who underwent temporal resections for intractable focal seizures, Laxer (50) found five patients (3.8% of a series of 160 patients) with what he thought was a benign, focal, nonprogressive form of RE. These patients (children or adults) with no evidence of progression are indistinguishable clinically from those with refractory seizures due to other causes, including mesial temporal sclerosis (38,50).

Delayed Seizures Onset Variant

In two recent papers, Korn-Lubetzki and colleagues (52) and Bien and colleagues (53) described five children with RE and delayed seizure onset. They all had slowly progressive hemiparesis, contralateral brain atrophy, and four had pathological features characteristic of RE. Mean age at disease onset was 6.1 (4.8 to 7) years. Two children had seizures 0.5 and 0.6 years after disease onset and the other three were still seizure-free at the time of the report (1.3 to 1.9 years after disease onset). Interestingly, the authors could demonstrate that the progression of the hematrophy in these five patients was similar to the one observed in RE cases with seizures. These two studies re-emphasized the fact that patients with RE may present a more insidious course and the disease should be suspected in cases with new onset progressive unilateral neurological deficits.

Basal Ganglia Involvement

EPC and other types of focal motor seizures are a common finding in patients with RE. Chorea, athetosis, or dystonia were infrequently described and may have been overlooked because of the preponderance of the epileptic manifestations and of the hemiparesis. In 27 of the 48 patients of the MNHI series who had EPC, 9 additionally had writhing or choreiform movements, and a diagnosis of Sydenham chorea was made in 3 of the patients early in the disease course (5). Matthews and colleagues (54) described a 10-year-old girl with a 1-year history of progressive right-sided hemiparesis, EPC, and secondary generalized seizures. MRI showed diffuse cortical and subcortical changes maximum in the perisylvian frontotemporoparietal area. At examination, she had choreic movements of the right arm and hand in addition to EPC. Tien and colleagues (55) were the first to describe atrophy of the caudate and putamen with abnormal high signals and severe left hemispheric atrophy in an 8.5-year-old girl with intractable focal motor seizures. They interpreted these findings as the result of gliosis and chronic brain damage. Topçu and colleagues (10) described a patient who developed hemidystonia as a result of involvement of the contralateral basal ganglia. The movement disorder appeared 3 years after the onset of seizures. A rather typical subsequent evolution suggested RE. The movement disorder started during intravenous immunoglobulin (IVIg) and interferon therapy, and did not respond to anticholinergic drugs or to a frontal resection. Ben-Zeev and colleagues (56), Koehn and Zupanc (57), Frucht (39), Lascelles and colleagues (58), and, finally, Kinay and colleagues (49) each reported a case of RE whose clinical presentation was dominated by a hemidyskinesia, with EPC in three of those patients, and progressive hemiparesis. Two cases showed selective frontal cortical and caudate atrophy on MRI; one developed progressive left basal ganglia atrophy and later focal frontotemporoparietal atrophy; one had only pronounced right caudate, globus pallidus, and putamen atrophy; and one showed progressive right frontoinsular and later diffuse hemispheric atrophy with also progressive atrophy of the right caudate head and putamen. In the case of Frucht, IVIg dramatically improved both the hyperkinetic movements and the EPC, but the effect was transient, suggesting a common neuroanatomic mechanism or humoral autoimmune process. In a series of 21 patients with RE, Bhatjiwale and colleagues (59) looked specifically at the involvement of the basal ganglia. Fifteen (71%) patients showed mild to severe basal ganglia involvement on imaging in three different patterns: predominantly cortical in six cases, predominantly basal ganglia in six cases, and both cortical and basal ganglia involvement in three cases. In five cases, the changes found in the basal ganglia were static, whereas in the others there was steady progression. The caudate nucleus was generally more prominently involved, usually in association with frontal atrophy. Five cases also showed putaminal involvement, always with temporoinsular atrophy. Interestingly, two of the six patients with prominent basal ganglia involvement had dystonia as a presenting feature. The authors postulated that the disease may proceed from different foci, including cases where RE seems to start in deep gray matter. Similar findings were recently described by the Italian Study Group on RE (60), which found basal ganglia atrophy in 9 of 13 patients studied. They suggested that atrophy of the basal ganglia represents only secondary change because of disconnection from the affected overlying frontal and insular cortex.

Brainstem Variant

McDonald and colleagues (61) recently reported a 3-year-old boy with RE manifested by chronic brainstem encephalitis. After a prolonged febrile seizure associated with an acute varicella infection, he developed recurrent partial motor seizures, EPC, and left hemiparesis within a few weeks. After a few more weeks, signs of brainstem involvement appeared; repeated MRI showed increased signal in the pons, but a complete infectious and inflammatory evaluation, including brain biopsy, was negative. He died 14 months after the onset of his illness. Neuropathologic findings in the brainstem were typical of those found in RE. Bilateral mesial temporal sclerosis was also present. The authors proposed that this case represents a rare focal form of RE with primarily involvement of the brainstem, and hemiparesis and mesial temporal sclerosis resulting from seizure activity. This was an isolated case report in a complicated patient, and existence of this variant was then questionable. However, recently, a case of adult-onset RE was described with a relatively typical evolution with EPC, focal motor seizures, progressive impaired motor function of the right hemibody and progressive atrophy of the left hemisphere maximal in the perisylvian regions (47). The diagnosis of RE was confirmed 2.5 years after onset by a brain biopsy and the disease progressed in spite of IVIg. The patient rapidly became hemiplegic but also seizure-free at about the same time. One year later, the patient was admitted because of swallowing problems, palatal paresis, and a dysarthria. MRI showed a progression of the left hemispheric atrophy and an increase in signal extending in the left mesencephalon and pons but sparing the medulla, without contrast enhancement. Authors suggested that the brainstem involvement represented a late relapse of disease activity involving the brainstem.

Multifocal Variant

Maeda and colleagues (62) described a 6-year-old girl with typical RE. One year following the onset of seizures, MRI-FLAIR (fluid attenuated inversion recovery) sequences showed multiple high-signal-intensity areas in the right hemisphere, and a methionine-PET (positron emission tomography) performed at the same time exhibited multifocal methionine uptake areas concordant with the MRI lesions, suggesting multiple independent sites of chronic inflammation. The authors proposed that the inflammatory process in RE may spread from multifocal lesions and not necessarily originate from localized temporal, insular, or frontocentral lesions, as usually described, before spreading across adjacent regions to the entire hemisphere.

Double Pathology

A small number of reports have documented coexisting brain pathologies with RE: a tumor (anaplastic astrocytoma, ganglioglioma, anaplastic ependymoma) in three patients (63–65), dysgenetic tissue in four patients (21,63,66,67), multifocal perivasculitis in seven patients (21), and cavernous angiomas with signs of vasculitis in two patients (21,63). Double pathology in RE supports the theory of focal disruption (trauma, infection, or other pathology) of the blood–brain barrier (BBB), allowing access of antibodies produced by the host to neurons expressing the target receptor and production of focal inflammation (3,68). So far, however, only one case of double pathology provided reasonable support for this hypothesis (67). Strongly positive anti-GluR3 (glutamate receptor 3 subunit) antibodies were measured in one case of RE with concomitant cortical dysplasia in a 2.5-year-old girl with catastrophic epilepsy starting at age 2 years. She underwent a right, partial frontal lobectomy, plasmapheresis, and therapy with IVIg with a transient response, and, finally, a right functional hemispherectomy with good seizure control. GluR3 antibodies were measured serially throughout the course of her treatment and correlated with her clinical status. They were undetectable 1 year after her last surgery.

There are also reports of coexisting autoimmune diseases such as Parry–Romberg syndrome (69–72) or linear scleroderma (72–74), and systemic lupus erythematosus (40) with changes mimicking RE. A case of adult-onset RE associated with a typical narcolepsy syndrome in a previously healthy 40-year-old man was recently reported (41). The patient over the course of a few months developed narcolepsy with confirmatory polysomnography, an histocompatibility leukocyte antigen (HLA) type DQB1*0602, and no detectable cerebrospinal fluid (CSF) hypocretin. Within 2 years, he also developed refractory temporal lobe seizures, and brain MRI initially normal, showed progressive T2 signal changes in the left temporal, insular, and inferior frontal regions sparing the hypothalamus and brainstem. Pathology from a first partial temporal lobe resection was consistent with RE. Over the next 5 years, the patient remained refractory to antiepileptic medication but showed no progressive neurologic deficits or further MRI anomalies and still normal hypothalamus and brainstem. The authors suggested that these two co-occurring rare conditions could be explained by a common autoimmune process affecting the cortex and the hypothalamic hypocretin neurons. In another case, the coexistence of a postviral acute disseminated encephalomyelitis progressing 6 months later to EPC with clinical and imaging features of a RE was described in a 15-year-old boy (75). As both disorders have an immunologic basis, the authors again proposed that they represented manifestations of a common autoimmune disorder of the central nervous system (CNS). Recently, the association of RE and CNS granulomatous disease with mutations NOD2/CARD15 was described in a 12-year-old girl (76). After a severe course with typical features of RE and two sequential biopsies that supported the two diagnosis, the child was found to have three mutations in the NOD2/CARD15 gene. The family history was positive for a paternal uncle with Crohn disease and a paternal grandfather with inflammatory arthritis. Moreover, her clinical manifestations, the seizures, the hemiparesis, and the MRI lesions improved dramatically after she received infliximab, a TNFα inhibitor. Finally, the association of RE and Behcet disease have been described in the same family (a son and his father, respectively) suggesting a common genetic susceptibility to develop autoimmune conditions (49). Inflammatory changes suggestive of RE have also been observed in disorders with impaired immunity such as agammaglobulinemia (77) and multiple endocrinopathies, chronic mucocutaneous candidiasis, and impaired cellular immunity (78). The occurrence of two conditions presumably caused by impaired immunity in the same individual may strengthen the view that immune-mediated mechanisms are responsible for the development of RE.

Finally, the rare association of uveitis (three cases) or choroiditis (one case) with typical features of RE has led to the speculation that a viral infection may have been responsible for both (31,79,80). In all cases, the ocular pathology was ipsilateral to the involved hemisphere that showed chronic encephalitis. In three cases (31,79), the uveitis or choroiditis was detected 2 to 4 months after epilepsy onset. In one case (80), ocular diagnosis preceded the onset of chronic encephalitis. In light of these cases, it was hypothesized that a primary ocular infection, in particular a viral infection with herpes simplex virus (HSV), varicella-zoster virus (VZV), Epstein–Barr virus (EBV), cytomegalovirus (CMV), measles, or rubella, followed by vascular or neurotropic spread to the brain, was a possible mechanism for development of RE.

ELECTROENCEPHALOGRAPHY

Few studies specifically reported the EEG changes associated with RE (6,81–85), and even fewer tried to correlate the clinical and EEG features of the disease over time (6,86–88). So and Gloor (85) reported the scalp and perioperative (ECoG, electrocorticogram) EEG findings in the MNHI series of patients with RE. They summarized the EEG features as (i) disturbance of background activity in all except one patient with more severe slowing and relative depression of background rhythms in the diseased hemisphere; polymorphic or rhythmic delta activity was found in all (more commonly bilateral with lateralized preponderance); (ii) interictal epileptiform activity in 94% of patients, rarely focal (more commonly multifocal and lateralized to one hemisphere or bilateral independent, but strongly lateralized discharges with or without bilateral synchrony); (iii) clinical or subclinical seizure onsets were variable and occasionally focal, but more often poorly localized, lateralized, bilateral, or even generalized; and (iv) no clear electroclinical correlation apparent in many of the recorded clinical seizures, in particular in EPC. The electrographic lateralization of these abnormalities (focal slowing, progressive unilateral deterioration of background activity, ictal, and multifocal interictal hemispheric epileptiform activity) was sufficiently concordant with the clinical lateralization to provide essential information about the abnormal hemisphere in 90% of the cases. These EEG features, indicative of a widespread destructive and epileptogenic process, in the specific clinical context of catastrophic epilepsy and worsening neurologic deficits involving one hemisphere, suggest the diagnosis of chronic encephalitis.

The evolution of the EEG was studied longitudinally in a small number of patients (6,85–88). The studies showed progression of the EEG abnormalities. At the onset of the disease, EEG abnormalities tended to be lateralized and nonspecific, with unilateral slowing of background activity. As the disease progressed, it tended to become bilateral and widespread, multifocal or synchronous, suggesting a more diffuse hemispheric process, but not always confined to one hemisphere. It is not clear if this late bilateralization of the EEG abnormalities represented functional interference, secondary epileptogenesis, or, much less likely, inflammatory process directly involving the contralateral hemisphere.

Finally, a case report of persistant ictal EEG discharges after a functional hemispherectomy suggests that the inflammatory process may continue even in a disconnected hemisphere (89).

IMAGING

Anatomic Imaging

Imaging studies, although not specific, are extremely important for the diagnosis of RE. Typically, they show progressive, lateralized atrophy coupled with localized or lateralized functional abnormalities (6,8,15,55,59,60,66,90–94). Brain MR studies early in the course of the illness may be normal, rapidly followed by a combination of characteristic features that parallel the clinical and electrophysiological deteriorations, reflecting the nature of the pathologic process. Recent studies using serial MRIs in a relatively large number of patients with RE provided better insight into the early, progressive, and late gray and white matter changes expected in this disease: cortical swelling, atrophy of cortical gray matter and deep gray matter nuclei, particularly the caudate, a hyperintense signal in gray and white matter, and secondary changes (6,15,59,60,94,95). In the early phase of the disease, when the MRI still appears normal, a few studies demonstrated abnormalities of perfusion or metabolism by single-photon-emission computed tomography (SPECT) or PET, suggesting that these imaging procedures may aid in early identification of the disease and of the abnormal hemisphere (55,93,96–100). In some studies, PET was found to detect lesions sooner and depict their extent better than concomitant MRI (99,100). However, even on MR scans obtained early in the course, the cortex can show focal hyperintense signals on T2 or FLAIR sequences (60) and may appear swollen. This can be explained by brain edema at the onset of inflammation (94) or, alternatively, by recurrent focal seizures (101). Bien and colleagues (94) compared MR images with surgical specimens obtained from 10 RE patients. In those areas with increased signal, the number of T cells, microglial nodules, and glial fibrillary acidic antigen (GFAP) positive astrocytes was increased compared to areas showing more atrophy and no increased signal. They demonstrated that the densities of T cells, microglial nodules, and astrocytes were inversely correlated to disease duration. Very early signal change in the white matter (within 4 months) is also frequent, usually focal, with or without swelling (60). Later, progressive atrophy of the affected hemisphere occurs, reflecting the manner in which the disease spreads, and with most of the hemispheric volume loss occurring during the first 2 years

(15,60,94). The cortical atrophy is initially either temporal, frontoinsular, or frontocentral, and, more rarely, parietooccipital, later spreading across the hemisphere. Basal ganglia involvement, mostly of the putamen and caudate, is also characteristic and may be a result of direct damage by the pathologic process or secondary to changes caused by disconnection of the basal ganglia from the affected overlying frontocentral and insular cortices (59,60). MRI brain volumetry studies performed in a large series of patients with RE confirmed that the unaffected contralateral hemisphere also undergoes progressive tissue loss although at a lower rate and with a much lesser magnitude compare to the affected hemisphere (22). Other secondary changes usually associated with severe hemispheric tissue loss are atrophy of the brainstem, particularly of the cerebral peduncle and pons, thinning of the corpus callosum, and atrophy of the contralateral cerebellar hemisphere (60). Surprisingly, gadolinium enhancement on MRI is rarely observed (36,60,66,93,94,102,103). Finally, the finding of calcifications is atypical and should raise doubts on the diagnosis of RE (59,104). The European consensus group suggested cranial computed tomography (CT) to document or exclude calcifications (4).

Functional Imaging

Several studies, often case reports, have emphasized the utility of functional imaging such as PET, SPECT, and proton magnetic resonance spectroscopy (MRS) in the diagnosis and follow-up. Functional abnormalities may be useful in cases in which MRI is normal, usually at the onset of the disease or when structural imaging fails to provide satisfactory localizing information. Combined anatomic and functional neuroimaging may serve to focus the diagnostic work-up, hasten brain biopsy for definitive diagnosis, or define the appropriate surgical approach. It may be useful to follow the evolution of the disease or the result of treatment. Finally, functional studies may provide insight into the cortical reorganization of speech areas and of motor and somatosensory cortices.

Fiorella and colleagues (93) reviewed 2-deoxy-2-[^{18}F]-fluoro-D-glucose PET (FDG-PET) and MRI studies of 11 patients with surgically proven RE. All had diffuse, unilateral cerebral hypometabolism on PET images, closely correlated with the distribution of cerebral atrophy on MRI. Even subtle diffuse atrophic changes were accompanied by marked decreases in cerebral glucose use that, according to the authors, increased diagnostic confidence and aided in the identification of the abnormal hemisphere. During ictal studies, patients had multiple foci of hypermetabolism, indicative of multifocal seizure activity within the affected hemisphere, and never showed such changes in the contralateral one. Similar findings had been reported in smaller series (55,60,97,102,105–108). Although MRI alone is generally sufficient to identify the affected hemisphere, FDG-PET confirms the findings in each case. Blood flow or perfusion studies using Oxygen-15 PET showed a similar correlation, with regions of perfusion change corresponding with structural MRI changes (97). Using a specific radioligand ([^{11}C]*(R)*-PK11195) for peripheral benzodiazepine-binding sites on cells of mononuclear phagocyte lineage, Banati and colleagues (109) demonstrated in vivo the widespread activation of microglia in three patients, which is usually found by neuropathologic study. Also, a [^{11}C]methionine PET demonstrated in a 6-year-old girl with RE multifocal uptake regions, which corresponded to high signal intensity areas described on FLAIR MRI and suggesting sites of underlying inflammation (62).

SPECT was used to study regional blood flow in a number of patients (8,10,60,89,90,96,98,105,107,110–116). The findings may be of some help and more sensitive than anatomic neuroimaging early in the disease, but are nonspecific. As with FDG-PET, the regions of functional change usually correlate with anatomic abnormalities. Interictal SPECT scans reveal diminished perfusion in a large zone surrounding the epileptic area shown on electroencephalography. This hypoperfusion may show some variability depending on fluctuation of the epileptic activity. Ictal studies often show zones of hyperperfusion representing likely areas of more intense seizure activity. Sequential scans may be helpful to follow the progression of the disease (90) or the effect of a treatment (113).

MRS has been used in a number of patients with RE (54,60,113,117–124). Localized proton MRS was described for the first time in two patients by Matthews and colleagues (54). They showed reduced *N*-acetylaspartate (NAA) concentrations—a compound exclusively found in neurons and their processes—in diseased areas in both patients, suggesting neuronal loss. In addition, MRS showed increased lactate in a patient with EPC, probably the result of excessive and repetitive seizure activity. These findings were confirmed by Peeling and Sutherland (117) and by Cendes and colleagues (118). Peeling and Sutherland also showed that the concentration of NAA in vitro (MRS on tissue obtained from surgical patients) was reduced in proportion to the severity and extent of the encephalitis. Cendes and colleagues did sequential studies at 1 year in three patients and demonstrated progression of the MRS changes. They noted that those changes were more widespread than the structural changes seen on anatomic MRI. Tekgul and colleagues (124) also did sequential NAA/Cr ratios in three patients with RE and demonstrated progressive reduction of the ratios related to the duration and progressive course of the disease. They measured interleukin-6 (a proinflammatory cytokine produced by astrocytes and microglial cells) response in the CSF and serum and found that the magnitude of the responses in the CSF was correlated with the severity of neuronal damage as measured by MRS. Overall, the studies using NAA indicate that MRS can identify and quantify neuronal damage and loss throughout the affected hemisphere, including areas that appear anatomically normal. In addition to NAA and lactate, other compounds measured included choline, creatine, *myo*-inositol, glutamine, and glutamate. Choline is usually elevated, which probably indicates demyelination and increased membrane turnover (98,118,119,122). *Myo*-inositol, a glial cell marker, was found to be elevated in a small number of patients (98,120,122,123), indicating glial proliferation or prominent gliotic activity. Hypothetically, *myo*-inositol signal should increase with the progression of the disease. Lactate was almost always elevated, and this increase probably results from ongoing or repetitive focal epileptic activity rather than being a marker of the inflammatory process itself (117–119,121). The largest peaks in lactate were usually detected in patients with EPC. Glutamine and glutamate levels were also elevated in two patients so far, a finding of interest considering the potential role of excitatory neurotransmitters in the disease (98).

ETIOLOGY AND PATHOGENESIS

The etiology and pathogenesis of RE remain unknown. Typical histologic findings reported in surgical or autopsy specimens are perivascular lymphocytic cuffing, proliferation of microglial nodules, neuronal loss, and gliosis in the affected hemisphere. The microglial nodules are associated with frequent nonspecific neuronophagia and occur particularly near perivascular cuffs of lymphocytes and monocytes. There is some evidence of spongiosis, but this is not as widespread as in the true spongiform encephalopathies. Lesions tend to extend in a confluent rather than a multifocal manner. Finally, the main inflammatory changes are found in the cortex and their intensity is inversely correlated with disease duration, with slow progress toward a "burnt-out" stage (15,21,125). A recent neuropathology study of 45 hemispherectomies in RE patients (125) showed the multifocality (contradicting the previous impression of a centrifugal pattern of the cortical pathology) and heterogeneity of the pathological changes in each patient, findings consistent with a progressive process of neuronal damage (at multiple times and in various sites). Pathological changes were from early inflammation to extensive neuronal cell death and cavitation, and the presence of T lymphocytes and neuroglial reactions suggested an immune-mediated process involving the cerebral cortex and white matter. Three mechanisms or processes, not mutually exclusive, have been proposed to explain the initiation and unusual evolution of this rare clinical syndrome: first, *viral infections directly inducing CNS injury*; second, *a viral-triggered autoimmune CNS process*; and third, *a primary autoimmune CNS process*. It is also possible that RE has a noninflammatory origin, and that the observed inflammation merely represents a response to injury.

The observation of the type of inflammatory process found within the lesions has led over the last few years to multifaceted approaches to uncover a possible infectious or immune-mediated (humoral or cellular) etiology. Epidemiologic studies have not identified a genetic, environmental (geographical or seasonal), or clustering effect, and failed to demonstrate any association between exposure to various factors, including viruses, and the subsequent development of RE. In many cases, there is no apparent increase in pre-existent febrile convulsions, or immediately preceding or associated infectious illness. Serologic studies to detect antecedent viral infection have been contradictory or inconclusive (17,126–135); the search for a pathogenic virus has so far mostly focused on the herpes virus family; and direct brain tissue analysis has also yielded inconsistent results (17,130,131,134–137). Expression of the interferon-induced MxA protein was tested negative in several cases of RE also arguing against a viral etiology (138). The role of an infectious agent, and the *viral hypothesis*, in the causation of RE, remains, at best, uncertain. It should be noted, however, that a few patients were reported to improve with antiviral therapy (25,139–141).

Systemic (50–55,58) and CSF compartment immune responses still fail to indicate clear evidence of either ongoing or deficient immune reactivity (142). A primary role for pathogenic antibodies in the etiology of RE was proposed after Rogers and colleagues (143) described rabbits immunized with fusion proteins containing a portion of the GluR3. Those animals developed intractable seizures, and, on histopathologic examination, their brains showed changes characteristic of RE with perivascular lymphocytic infiltrate and microglial nodules. The subsequent finding of autoantibodies to GluR3 in the sera of some affected patients with RE led to the definition of a *GluR3 autoantibody hypothesis* and allowed new speculation into its pathogenesis. GluR3 autoantibodies may cause damage to the brain, and eventually epilepsy, by excitotoxic mechanisms. In the animal model, GluR3 autoantibodies appear to activate the excitatory receptor that leads to massive influx of ions, neuronal cell death, local inflammation, and further disruption of the BBB, allowing entrance of more autoantibodies (68,144,145). Another proposed mechanism suggests that GluR3 autoantibodies can cause damage by activating complement cascades that lead to neuronal cell death and inflammation (146,147). These hypotheses prompted a number of open-labeled therapeutic attempts to modulate the immune system of patients, especially by removing or annihilating the circulating pathogenic factors presumably responsible for the disease (68,143,146–150). Among cases with no detectable anti-GluR3 antibodies, several were also described to respond well to immunosuppressive treatments (3,19). Other reports in several patients showed no response to plasma exchange (19,148). Finally, more recent work shows that anti-GluR3 antibodies are not specific for RE but can be detected in other neurological disorders, particularly in non-RE patients with catastrophic epilepsy. Since the sensitivity of detection is low for the RE population and the presence of GluR3 antibodies does not distinguish RE from other forms of epilepsy, the anti-GluR3 antibody test is not useful for a diagnosis of RE (151–159).

In one study, GluR3 antibodies were found in serum of 5/6 and CSF of 4/4 patients with RE and serum of 12/71 patients with other epilepsies (160). Some patients also harbored additional autoimmune antibodies (in serum of 5/6 patients with RE, e.g., anti-GAD [glutamic acid decarboxylase], anti-cardiolipin, anti-dsDNA, anti-RNP [anti-ribonucleoprotein], anti-SS-A [antinucluear antibody; anti-RO]). In another study, the same group (161) found elevated levels of GluR3B in the serum of two monozygotic twins, one with presumed RE and the other healthy. More interestingly, they also found in both twins elevated titers of anti-dsDNA, anti-GAD, anti-cardiolipin, anti-RNP, anti-SS-A, and anti-beta2GPI, and elevated levels of different cytokines; the antibodies tended to be more elevated in RE twin and the cytokines more elevated in the healthy one. The reasons for such findings are unknown but the authors speculated that they represented immune responses to a common injury leading one twin to an immune or autoimmune epilepsy disorder. Whether GluR3 autoantibodies in severe forms of epilepsy are responsible for the seizures or whether they result from an underlying degenerative or inflammatory process is still unclear. Passive transfer of the disease into naïve animals remains unsuccessful so far, and additional animal models of this illness are lacking. In a recent review paper, Levite and Ganor (162) summarized the up-to-date evidence concerning GluR autoantibodies in human diseases including epilepsy.

Various other autoantibodies against neural molecules were described in RE: autoantibodies against munc-18 (163,164), neuronal acetylcholine receptor α_7 subunit (159, 165,166), anti-GAD (160,167), and NMDA receptor NR2 subunit isoforms

NR2A through NR2D, specifically GluR epsilon$_2$ (43,168,169), have been reported in some patients. Again, however, these autoantibodies could be detected in neurological diseases other than RE, confirming that none of the described autoantibodies is specifically associated with this disease, and that a variety of autoantibodies to neuronal and synaptic structures can be found that may contribute to the inflammatory process, or represent an epiphenomenon of an activated immune system. Takahashi and colleagues (168) showed that GluR epsilon$_2$ were present only in patients with EPC (15 patients, including 10 with histologically proven or clinical RE, 3 with acute encephalitis/encephalopathy, and 2 with nonprogressive EPC), and antibodies were directed primarily against cytoplasmic epitopes, suggesting the involvement of T-cell–mediated autoimmunity. To summarize, it may very well be that the antibodies are related to epilepsy rather than specific for RE and are markers for neuronal damage rather than causative (170,171).

Recent reports indeed suggested that a T-cell–mediated inflammatory response may be another initiating or perpetuating mechanism in RE. Active inflammatory brain lesions contain large numbers of T lymphocytes (172). These are recruited early within the lesions, suggesting that a T-cell–dependent immune response contributes to the onset and evolution of the disease. Li and colleagues (173) analyzed T-cell receptor expression in the lesions of patients with RE and found that the local immune response includes restricted T-cell populations that are likely to have expanded from a small number of precursor T cells, responding themselves to discrete antigenic epitopes. However, the nature of the antigen that triggers such a response is unknown. Nevertheless, recent work provides further credence to the hypothesis that a T-cell–mediated cytotoxic reaction (CD8$^+$ T-cell cytotoxicity) induces damage, correlating with activation of the granzyme B pathway, and apoptotic death of cortical neurons in RE (157,174,175). In an attempt to combine existing knowledge, these investigators (175) proposed a new scheme of pathogenesis: an initial unihemispheric focal event leading to BBB opening, the onset of a cytotoxic T-cell response, and then spreading of the immune attack across the affected hemisphere. First, a focal event initiates the process (e.g., infection, trauma, immune-mediated brain damage, even focal seizure activity) and an immune reaction with antigen presentation in the CNS and entry of cytotoxic T lymphocytes into the CNS across the disrupted BBB. Second, activated cytotoxic T lymphocytes attack CNS neurons while the inflammatory process, together with the release of cytokines, causes a spread of the inflammatory reaction and recruitment of more activated cytotoxic T lymphocytes. Third, the generation of potentially antigenic fragments, including GluR3 and others to be identified, gives rise to autoantibodies (176), and may lead to an antibody-mediated "second wave of attack." More recently, the same investigators added to this scheme of pathogenesis that astrocytic apoptosis and loss are also features of RE (177). They suggested a specific attack by cytotoxic T lymphocytes responsible for astrocytic degeneration, which in turn would contribute to more neuronal dysfunction and death.

CRITERIA FOR (EARLY) DIAGNOSIS

The clinical changes of RE are nonspecific, particularly at the beginning of the disease, and clearly at this stage the major issue is diagnosis. We now have better diagnostic criteria that

can lead to early diagnosis (Table 25.1) (4,6,15,23,60,94, 178,179). The onset in a previously healthy child is of a rapidly increasing frequency and severity of simple focal,

TABLE 25.1

CRITERIA FOR (EARLY) DIAGNOSIS OF RASMUSSEN ENCEPHALITIS

Clinical	• Refractory focal motor seizures rapidly increasing in frequency and severity, and often polymorphic • EPC • Motor, progressive hemiparesis, and cognitive deterioration
Electroencephalography	• Focal or regional slow wave activity contralateral to motor manifestations • Multifocal, usually lateralized, interictal, and ictal epileptiform discharges • Progressive, lateralized impoverishment of background activity
Imaging	• *MRI*: focal cortical swelling with hyperintensity and white matter signal hyperintensity, insular cortical atrophy, atrophy of the head of caudate nucleus, and progressive gray and white matter atrophy, unilateral. No gadolinium enhancement and no calcifications on head CT. • *PET*: unilateral, hemispheric, but during early stage may be restricted to frontal and temporal regions, glucose hypometabolism • *SPECT*: unilateral interictal hemispheric hypoperfusion and ictal multifocal hyperperfusion • *MRS*: unilateral reduced NAA, and increased lactate, choline, myoinositol and glutamine/glutamate
Blood	• None, except inconsistent finding of anti-GluR3 antibodies
CSF	• None, except sometimes presence of oligoclonal bands and inconsistent elevated levels of anti-GluR3 antibodies
Histopathology	• Microglial nodules, perivascular lymphocytic infiltration, neuron degeneration, and spongy degeneration • Combination of active and remote, multifocal, intracortical, and white matter lesions

Abbreviations: CT, computed tomography; GluR3, glutamate receptor 3 subunit; MRI, magnetic resonance imaging; MRS, magnetic resonance spectroscopy; NAA, *N*-acetylaspartate; PET, positron emission tomography; SPECT, single-photon-emission computed tomography; CSF, cerebrospinal fluid.

usually motor, seizures often followed by a postictal deficit. This, and a lack of evidence of anatomic abnormalities on early brain MRI, should raise suspicion regarding the diagnosis of RE. Further course and evaluation with scalp EEG showing unilateral findings with focal or regional slowing, deterioration of background activity, multifocal interictal epileptiform discharges, and seizure onset or EPC, particularly corresponding to the cortical motor area, are major neurophysiologic features in favor of RE. Early MRI characteristics include the association of focal white matter hyperintensity and cortical swelling with hyperintense signal, particularly in the insular and peri-insular regions. This is followed by hemispheric atrophy that is usually predominant in the peri-insular and frontal regions, and the head of the caudate nucleus contralateral to the clinical manifestations. Gadolinium enhancement is unusual in RE and calcifications are not present. Functional imaging studies may reveal abnormalities before any visible structural changes. Typically, FDG-PET shows diffuse hemispheric glucose hypometabolism. SPECT shows unilateral interictal hypoperfusion and ictal multifocal areas of hyperperfusion confirming the lateralized hemispheric nature of the lesion and its extent. MRS may also help in the early detection of brain damage and shows a lateralized decrease in NAA intensity relative to creatine, suggesting neuronal loss or damage in one hemisphere. No laboratory test can support the diagnosis of RE. There is no consistent systemic and CSF response that may contribute to the diagnosis, and, in fact, the most common feature is the lack of cellular or protein response including oligoclonal bands in the CSF of patients with RE. Brain biopsy is often used as a diagnostic tool in many centers for confirming the diagnosis. However, histologic findings in RE are nonspecific chronic inflammatory changes that may be subtle enough to be missed by an inexperienced pathologist. Furthermore, the brain involvement may be patchy, and a normal biopsy, particularly when obtained from stereotactic small needles, does not rule out the diagnosis of RE. In some experienced centers, brain biopsy is not routinely done, and clinical evolution in association with scalp electroencephalography and brain MRI are considered diagnostic of RE. Granata and colleagues (6) suggested that the association of refractory focal seizures with predominantly motor component and with contralateral focal EEG and neuroimaging changes could allow a diagnosis of RE 4 to 6 months after the appearance of the first symptoms.

The differential diagnosis is large encompassing progressive, unilateral, neurological disorders due to inflammatory or infectious processes; developmental, metabolic, or degenerative diseases; and neoplastic, paraneoplastic, vascular, or even toxic neuropathogeneses (4). It includes focal cortical dysplasia and tuberous sclerosis; mitochondrial encephalopathy, such as mitochondrial encephalopathy with lactic acidosis and stroke-like episodes (MELAS); brain tumors; focal unihemispheric cerebral vasculitis; degenerative cortical gray matter diseases; and some forms of meningoencephalitis or disseminated encephalomyelitis. Although several diagnostic criteria have been proposed, especially for an early diagnosis of RE, the correct identification of patients with this disease remains a matter of experience, particularly if specific investigative or therapeutic interventions are considered. When a constellation of clinical and laboratory findings highlights the possibility of RE, close follow-up is necessary to assess progression of the disease and eventually confirm its diagnosis.

MEDICAL AND SURGICAL TREATMENTS

The typical evolution of RE is characterized by the development of intractable seizures, progressive neurologic deficits, and intellectual impairment. AEDs quite consistently fail to provide any significant improvement in seizures. This has led clinicians to try a variety of empiric treatments, including antiviral agents and immunomodulatory or immunosuppressive therapies. Surgery, and specifically hemispherectomy, appears to be successful in arresting the disease process. However, the ensuing neurologic deficits due to surgery usually lead to reluctance to carry out this procedure until significant hemiparesis or other functional deficits have already occurred. Apart from the surgical treatment, there is however no established treatment for RE. With the increasing experience and knowledge of the pathogenesis of RE, immunomodulatory treatment now have a more rationale basis and clearer indications for their use. These therapies should probably be considered at the early stages of the disease to halt its progression; in cases where surgery is not possible, for instance when important functional brain areas are involved; or in severe bilateral or other unusual variants of RE.

Repetitive transcranial magnetic stimulation by reducing cortical excitability can suppress, at least momentarily, seizure activity and hence may be a useful noninvasive palliative tool in some cases; only one case has been reported (180) and clearly further explorations are needed. Botulinum toxin was marginally used in attempts to control focal seizures or hyperkinetic movements in RE. To date, only two patients were reported with such treatment (181,182). Finally, to our knowledge, no patient with RE showed significant benefit from either vagal nerve or deep brain stimulation.

Antiepileptic Drug Therapy

Guidelines for AED treatment in RE are difficult to define and have always been empirical. No AED, or any polytherapy regimen, has been proven to be superior (9), and the choice of the ideal AED rests on its clinical efficacy and side-effect profile. Because of the nature of this disease, the danger of overtreatment is high. AED pharmacokinetics, toxicity, and interactions may be better determinants of AED selection and combination therapy. EPC is particularly difficult to treat, but AEDs can reduce the frequency and severity of other focal and secondarily generalized seizures. Since the author's original report on AED efficacy in RE (9), several new agents have been introduced. Drugs such as topiramate and felbamate that act on excitatory neurotransmitters or those that may affect cortically generated myoclonus, like levetiracetam in EPC, may have a more specific role in the treatment.

Antiviral Therapy

Most treatments directed at aborting the progression of the disease were based on the assumption that RE is either an infectious, a viral, or an autoimmune disorder. Examples of antiviral treatments are scarce, and only two reports (25,140) are published: one on the treatment of four patients with ganciclovir, a potent anticytomegalovirus drug, and another on the treatment of a single patient with zidovudine. Although definite improvement was documented in four of the five patients, no further reports using antiviral agents in RE have been published.

Immune Therapy

Evidence implicating humoral and cellular immune responses in the pathophysiology of RE has led to various therapeutic initiatives. A number of case reports and small series suggesting potential therapeutic roles of immune-directed interventions have now been published. These include interferon, steroids, IVIg, plasmapheresis, selective immunoglobulin G immunoadsorption by protein A, and immunosuppression or immunomodulation with drugs such as cyclophosphamide, azathioprine, tacrolimus, rituximab, and even thalidomide. Rarely, such approaches have been associated with sustained cessation of seizure activity and arrest in the progression of the inflammatory process. In the majority of the cases, only transient or partial improvements because of immunomodulator or immunosuppressor use have been noted. Of potential importance is the observation that, to date, the more aggressive immune therapies have been deferred to later stages of the disease, where the burden of the disease is considered to outweigh the toxicity of these interventions. The challenge is to develop safe therapeutic protocols that can be tested in patients soon after the diagnosis, and at a time when less damage has occurred and the process may have a better chance to respond to therapy. Eventually, regimens that strike the proper balance between safety and efficacy in typical RE could be applied to the more unusual variants.

Interferon-α

Intraventricular interferon-α has been tried in only two children (139,141) with the rationale that interferons have both immunomodulating (enhancement of phagocytic activity of macrophages and augmentation of the cytotoxicity of target-specific lymphocytes) and antiviral activity (inhibition of viral replication in virus-infected cells). In both cases, improvement of the epileptic and neurologic syndromes was observed.

Steroids

Relatively low- and high-dose steroid regimens were used either alone or in association with other agents such as IVIg. Initial reports were somewhat discouraging (8,77), but eventually the use of high-dose intravenous (IV) boluses led to encouraging results. When applied during the first year of the disease, pulse IV steroids were effective in suppressing, at least temporarily, the inflammatory process (19,23,24,113). The proposed modes of action of steroids include an antiepileptic effect, an improvement of BBB function—and hence reduction of entry into the brain of potentially deleterious toxic or immune mediators—and a direct anti-inflammatory effect. Because of a less favorable response and of the adverse effects of prolonged high-dose steroids, Hart and colleagues (23) suggested the use of IVIg as initial treatment followed by high-dose steroids, or both, to control seizures and improve the end point of the disease. More recently, Granata and colleagues have proposed a protocol for administration of immunomodulatory treatments in children sand adults with RE (40). Corticosteroids were given alone or in combination with

plasmapharesis, IVIg, protein A Ig immnunoadsorption, or cyclophosphamide with positive but time-limited clinical responses in 11 of 15 patients. The long-term efficacy of steroids in RE remains unknown, but they may be effective when used in pulses to stop status epilepticus (23,40). Also, one has to weight the risks of long-term steroid therapy and maybe more importantly of delaying unduly the most appropriate treatment for this severe condition, which, in the majority of the patients, remains in the long run, surgery of the affected hemisphere (183).

Immunoglobulin

The use of IVIg in RE was first described by Walsh (184) in a 9-year-old child who received repeated infusions of IVIg over a period of several months with initial improvement, but later followed by protracted deterioration and cessation of the treatment. Eight subsequent studies reported the effect of IVIg, alone or in combination, with other treatment modalities (19,23,34,37,40,113,185,186). These reports show similar results with initial benefit, but with a much less clear-cut, long-term effect. They indicate variable results, ranging from no benefit to significant improvement, maintained in a single case for a period of close to 4 years (185). IVIg is usually much better tolerated than steroids. The basis for a potential therapeutic effect of immunoglobulin in RE is not known, but may reflect the functions of natural antibodies in maintaining immune homeostasis in healthy people (187). Leach and colleagues (34) showed a delayed but more persistent response in two adults and suggested that IVIg is more effective in adults than in children. They also proposed that IVIg may have a disease-modifying effect. This phenomenon is probably real, but, to date, no one has shown that the early use of immune therapy can modify the long-term course of RE. In a recent report (188), guidelines on the use of IVIg for neurologic conditions were presented by a Canadian expert panel. The expert panel stated that in view of the seriousness of potential adverse events and current lack of data surrounding their frequency, IVIg should be prescribed only for appropriate clinical indications for which there is a known benefit. They identified five reports of IVIg use for RE and recommended that IVIg may be an option as a short-term measure for patients with RE.

Plasmapheresis and Selective IgG Immunoadsorption

Plasma exchange is used with the assumption that circulating factors, likely autoantibodies, are pathogenic in at least some patients (19,40,143,148–150). The majority of patients treated with apheresis showed repeated, and at times dramatic, but transient responses. Because of the lack of long-term efficacy and the complications, plasma exchange should probably be used as adjunctive therapy and may be especially useful in patients with acute deterioration, such as status epilepticus.

Immunosuppressive and Immunomodulation Therapy

Immunosuppressants are used in other autoimmune disorders and also in the prevention and treatment of transplant rejection. They act against the activation of T cells, which, in view of the recent findings of cytotoxic T-lymphocyte–mediated damage in RE (157,173,175), may lead to their acquiring a more prominent role in medical treatment.

Few studies reported on the use of cyclophosphamide in no more than half-a-dozen patients (19,40,148). It was proposed that intermittent cyclophosphamide may well replace steroid therapy because it is associated with less risk of systemic complications. The experience in this small number of patients suggests that neither acute nor chronic use of cyclophosphamide produces significant change on seizure frequency or disease progression.

Seven patients with RE were treated with oral tacrolimus (median follow-up, 25.4 mo) with superior outcome regarding neurologic function and progression rate of atrophy but no better seizure outcome compared to 12 untreated RE patients (189). There were no major side effects.

Following demonstration of antibodies directed against brain tissue in RE and the real but modest effects on disease with immunomodulation (steroids, IVIg, plasmapharesis and immunosuppressants), a pilot study is now on going with rituximab to directly attack the B cells thought to be involved in the process (190).

Thalidomide was used for the first time by Ravencroft and colleagues (191) in a 7-year-old male with RE and high level of CSF tumor TNFα, and a dramatic and sustained clinical response. This prompted a second case report of a 13-year-old girl with a refractory RE since age 5 in whom thalidomide was administered because of a life-threatening condition (192). Prior to thalidomide administration, she received sequentially acyclovir, IVIg, IV and oral steroids, a partial left parasagittal frontoparietal resection, plasma exchanges, and cyclophosphamide. After thalidomide was started, she rapidly improved and during the following 3 years received oral thalidomide 300 mg/day (in addition to valproic acid, clonazepam, piracetam) with a significant and sustained reduction in the frequency and intensity of her seizures. She only developed a moderate neutropenia attributed to the drug.

Surgery

The only effective surgical procedure seems to be the resection or disconnection of the affected hemisphere (92,193–195). Alternative procedures such as partial corticectomies, subpial transection, and callosal section have limited results and do not render patients seizure-free (8,196–200). The recent publication by Kossoff and colleagues (195) clearly demonstrated the benefits of hemispherectomy in children with RE. They showed that 91% of 46 children (mean age at surgery, 9.2 years) with severe RE who underwent hemispherectomy (in the majority hemidecortication) between 1975 and 2002 became seizure-free (65%) or had nondisabling seizures (26%) that often did not require medications. Patients were walking independently, and all were talking at the time of their most recent follow-up, with relatively minor or moderate residual speech problems. Twenty-one had left-sided pathology (presumably involving the dominant hemisphere) with a mean age at surgery of 8.8 years.

Hemispherectomy, hemidecortication, functional hemispherectomy, or hemispherotomy have proven efficacy for control of seizures in patients with RE (40,92,193–195,199, 201–208). The decision on how early in the course of the disease surgery should be undertaken depends on the certainty of the diagnosis, the severity and frequency of the seizures, and the impact on the psychosocial development of the patient. The natural evolution of the disease and the severity of the epilepsy often justify early intervention, even prior to maximal neurologic deficit. Finally, involvement of the dominant hemisphere by the disease process provides important observations on brain plasticity, especially on the shift of language (4,202,203,209–219). Recent reports looking at language outcomes after long-term RE, serial Amytal tests, functional MRI studies, and hemispherectomy illustrate the great plasticity of the child's brain and the ability of the nondominant hemisphere to take over some language function even at a relatively late age. The decision about such a radical procedure requires considerable time and thought, and the psychological preparation of the patients and their families is essential (92,209,220,221).

CONCLUSION AND FUTURE PERSPECTIVES

Rasmussen encephalitis, although a rare disorder, is now much better delineated and understood by the wider clinical and scientific community. However, the early recognition of the disease in a naïve patient continues to be a challenge. Although confirmation of the clinical diagnosis of RE rests on pathologic findings, in vivo combinations of diagnostic approaches such as clinical course, scalp EEG findings, and high-resolution MRI suggest the diagnosis with a high degree of accuracy. The syndrome, however, appears more clinically heterogeneous than initially thought; localized, protracted, or slowly progressive forms of the disease have now been described, suggesting that distinct pathophysiologic mechanisms may be at play. Evidence implicating immune responses in the pathophysiology of RE has accumulated involving both B- and T-cell–mediated processes, but the mechanisms by which the immune system is activated remain to be elucidated. The identification of autoantigens provides evidence that RE can be associated with an immune attack on synaptic antigens and impaired synaptic function leading to seizures and cell death. In addition, T-cell–mediated cytotoxicity may lead to neuronal damage and apoptotic death. Identification of the initiating event (possibly the antigen that triggered the autoimmune response) and of the sequence of immune reactivities occurring in the course of the disease will hopefully allow timely and specific short- or long-term immunotherapy. Patients with RE, however, usually present with rapid progression, and questions on the type and timing of surgical intervention are still being raised. It seems clear that most will fare better with earlier surgery, and only hemispherectomy techniques can provide definitive and satisfactory results with good seizure, cognitive, and psychosocial outcome.

ACKNOWLEDGMENT

I thank Dr. Frederick Andermann and Dr. Amit Bar-Or for thoughtful comments.

References

1. Rasmussen T, Olszewski J, Lloyd-Smith D. Focal seizures due to chronic localized encephalitis. *Neurology.* 1958;8:435–445.
2. Rasmussen T. Chronic encephalitis and seizures: historical introduction. In: Andermann F, ed. *Encephalitis and Epilepsy: Rasmussen's Syndrome.* London: Butterworth-Heinemann; 1991:1–4.

3. Antel JP, Rasmussen T. Rasmussen's encephalitis and the new hat. *Neurology.* 1996;46:9–11.

4. Bien CG, Granata T, Antozzi C, et al. Pathogenesis, diagnosis and treatment of Rasmussen encephalitis: A European consensus statement. *Brain.* 2005;128:454–471.

5. Oguni H, Andermann F, Rasmussen T. The natural history of the syndrome of chronic encephalitis and epilepsy: A study of the MNHI series of forty-eight cases. In: Andermann F, ed. *Encephalitis and Epilepsy: Rasmussen's Syndrome.* London: Butterworth-Heinemann; 1991:7–35.

6. Granata T, Gobbi G, Spreafico R, et al. Rasmussen's encephalitis. Early characteristics allow diagnosis. *Neurology.* 2003;60:422–425.

7. Gupta PC, Roy S, Tandon PN. Progressive epilepsy due to chronic persistent encephalitis. Report of 4 cases. *J Neurol Sci.* 1974;22:105–120.

8. Piatt JH Jr, Hwang PA, Armstrong DC, et al. Chronic focal encephalitis (Rasmussen syndrome): six cases. *Epilepsia.* 1988;29:268–279.

9. Dubeau F, Sherwin A. Pharmacologic principles in the management of chronic focal encephalitis. In: Andermann F, ed. *Encephalitis and Epilepsy: Rasmussen's Syndrome.* London: Butterworth- Heinemann; 1991:179–192.

10. Topçu M, Turanli G, Aynaci FM, et al. Rasmussen's encephalitis in childhood. *Child Nerv Syst.* 1999;15:395–402.

11. Sinha S, Satishchandra P. Epilepsia partialis continua over last 14 years: experience from a tertiary care center from south India. *Epilepsy Res.* 2007;74:55–59.

12. Genton P, Gelisse P. Antimyoclonic effect of levetiracetam. *Epileptic Disord.* 2000;2:209–212.

13. Frucht SJ, Louis ED, Chuang C, et al. A pilot tolerability and efficacy study of levetiracetam in patients with chronic myoclonus. *Neurology.* 2001;57:1112–1114.

14. Moshé SL. Mechanisms of action of anticonvulsant agents. *Neurology.* 2000;55(Suppl 1):S32–S40.

15. Bien CG, Widman G, Urbach H, et al. The natural history of Rasmussen's encephalitis. *Brain.* 2002;125:1751–1759.

16. Aguilar MJ, Rasmussen T. Role of encephalitis in pathogenesis of epilepsy. *Arch Neurol.* 1960;2:663–676.

17. McLachlan RS, Girvin JP, Blume WT, et al. Rasmussen's chronic encephalitis in adults. *Arch Neurol.* 1993;50:269–274.

18. Larner AJ, Smith SJ, Duncan JS, et al. Late-onset Rasmussen's syndrome with first seizure during pregnancy. *Eur Neurol.* 1995;35:172.

19. Krauss GL, Campbell ML, Roche KW, et al. Chronic steroid-responsive encephalitis without autoantibodies to glutamate receptor GluR3. *Neurology.* 1996;46:247–249.

20. Hart YM, Andermann F, Fish DR, et al. Chronic encephalitis and epilepsy in adults and adolescents: a variant of Rasmussen's syndrome? *Neurology.* 1997;48:418–424.

21. Robitaille Y. Neuropathological aspects of chronic encephalitis. In: Andermann F, ed. *Encephalitis and Epilepsy: Rasmussen's Syndrome.* London: Butterworth-Heinemann; 1991:79–110.

22. Larionov S, König R, Urbach H, et al. MRI brain volumetry in rasmussen encephalitis: The fate of affected and "unaffected" hemispheres. *Neurology.* 2005;64:885–887.

23. Hart YM, Cortez M, Andermann F, et al. Medical treatment of Rasmussen's syndrome (chronic encephalitis and epilepsy): effect of high-dose steroids or immunoglobulins in 19 patients. *Neurology.* 1994;44:1030–1036.

24. Chinchilla D, Dulac O, Robain O, et al. Reappraisal of Rasmussen's syndrome with special emphasis on treatment with high dose of steroids. *J Neurol Neurosurg Psychiatry.* 1994;57:1325–1333.

25. De Toledo JC, Smith DB. Partially successful treatment of Rasmussen's encephalitis with zidovudine: symptomatic improvement followed by involvement of the contralateral hemisphere. *Epilepsia.* 1994;35:352–355.

26. Takahashi Y, Kubota H, Fujiwara T, et al. Epilepsia partialis continua of childhood involving bilateral brain hemispheres. *Acta Neurol Scand.* 1997;96:345–352.

27. Silver K, Andermann F, Meagher-Villemure K. Familial alternating epilepsia partialis continua with chronic encephalitis: another variant of Rasmussen syndrome? *Arch Neurol.* 1998;55:733–736.

28. Tobias SM, Robitaille Y, Hickey WF, et al. Bilateral Rasmussen encephalitis: postmortem documentation in a five-year-old. *Epilepsia.* 2003;44:127–130.

29. Andermann F, Farrell K. Early onset Rasmussen syndrome: a malignant, often bilateral form of the disorder. *Epilepsy Res.* 2006;70:S259–S262.

30. deLeva MF, Varrone A, Filla A, et al. Neuroimaging follow up in a case of Rasmussen encephalitis with dyskinesias. *Mov Disord.* 2007;22:2117–2121.

31. Gray F, Serdaru M, Baron H, et al. Chronic localised encephalitis (Rasmussen's) in an adult with epilepsia partialis continua. *J Neurol Neurosurg Psychiatry.* 1987;50:747–751.

32. Stephen LJ, Brodie MJ. An islander with seizures. *Scott Med J.* 1998;43:183–184.

33. Coral LC, Haas LJ. Probable Rasmussen's syndrome: case report [Portuguese]. *Arq Neuropsiquiatr.* 1999;57:1032–1035.

34. Leach JP, Chadwick DW, Miles JB, et al. Improvement in adult onset Rasmussen's encephalitis with long-term immunomodulatory therapy. *Neurology.* 1999;52:738–742.

35. Yeh PS, Lin CN, Lin HJ, et al. Chronic focal encephalitis (Rasmussen's syndrome) in an adult. *J Formos Med Assoc.* 2000;99:568–571.

36. Vadlamudi L, Galton CJ, Jeavons SJ, et al. Rasmussen's syndrome in a 54-year-old female: more support for an adult variant. *J Clin Neurosci.* 2000;7:154–156.

37. Villani F, Spreafico R, Farina L, et al. Immunomodulatory therapy in an adult patient with Rasmussen's encephalitis. *Neurology.* 2001;56:248–250.

38. Hennessy MJ, Koutroumanidis M, Dean AF, et al. Chronic encephalitis and temporal lobe epilepsy: a variant of Rasmussen's syndrome? *Neurology.* 2001;56:678–681.

39. Frucht S. Dystonia, athetosis, and epilepsia partialis continua in a patient with late-onset Rasmussen's encephalitis. *Mov Disord.* 2002;17:609–612.

40. Granata T, Fusco L, Gobbi G, et al. Experience with immunomodulatory treatments in Rasmussen's encephalitis. *Neurology.* 2003;61:1807–1810.

41. Lagrange AH, Blaivas M, Gomez-Hassan D, et al. Rasmussen's syndrome and new-onset narcolepsy, cataplexy, and epilepsy in an adult. *Epilepsy Behav.* 2003;4:788–792.

42. Wennberg R, Nag S, McAndrews MP, et al. Chronic (Rasmussen's) encephalitis in an adult. *Can J Neurol Sci.* 2003;30:263–265.

43. Takahashi Y, Mori H, Mishina M, et al. Autoantibodies and cell-mediated autoimmunity to NMDA-type GluRε2 patients with Rasmussen's encephalitis and chronic progressive epilepsia partialis continua. *Epilepsia.* 2005;46:S152–S158.

44. Hunter GRW, Donat J, Pryse-Phillips W, et al. Rasmussen's encephalitis in a 58-year-old female: still a variant? *Can J Neurol Sci.* 2006;33:302–305.

45. Villani F, Pincherle A, Antozzi C, et al. Adult-onset Rasmussen's encephalitis: anatomical-electrographic-clinical features of 7 italian cases. *Epilepsia.* 2006;47:S41–S46.

46. Jallon-Rivière V, Dupont S, Bertran F, et al. le syndrome de Rasmussen à début tardif: caractéristiques cliniques et thérapeutiques [Paris]. *Rev Neurol.* 2007;163:573–580.

47. Queseda CM, Urbach H, Elger CE, et al. Rasmussen encephalitis with ipsilateral brain stem involvement in an adult patient. *J Neurol Neurosurg Psychiatry.* 2007;78:200–201.

48. Gambardella A, Andermann F, Shorvon, et al. Limited chronic focal encephalitis. *Neurology.* 2008;70:374–377.

49. Kinay D, Bebek N, Vanli E, et al. Rasmussen's encephalitis and Behcet's disease: autoimmune disorders in first degree relatives. *Epileptic Disord.* 2008;10:319–324.

50. Laxer KD. Temporal lobe epilepsy with inflammatory changes. In: Andermann F, ed. *Encephalitis and Epilepsy: Rasmussen's Syndrome.* London: Butterworth-Heinemann; 1991:135–140.

51. Nayak D, Abraham M, Chandrasekharan K, et al. Lingual epilepsia partialis continua in Rasmussen's encephalitis. *Epileptic Disord.* 2006;8:114–117.

52. Korn-Lubetzki I, Bien CG, Bauer J, et al. Rasmussen encephalitis with active inflammation and delayed seizures onset. *Neurology.* 2004;62:984–986.

53. Bien CG, Elger CE, Leitner Y, et al. Slowly progressive hemiparesis in childhood as a consequence of Rasmussen encephalitis without or with delayed-onset seizures. *Europ J Neurol.* 2007;14:387–390.

54. Matthews PM, Andermann F, Arnold DL. A proton magnetic resonance spectroscopy study of focal epilepsy in humans. *Neurology.* 1990;40:985–989.

55. Tien RD, Ashdown BC, Lewis DV Jr, et al. Rasmussen's encephalitis: neuroimaging findings in four patients. *Am J Roentgenol.* 1992;158:1329–1332.

56. Ben-Zeev B, Nass D, Polack S, et al. Progressive unilateral basal ganglia atrophy and hemidystonia: a new form of chronic focal encephalitis. *Neurology.* 1999;S2:A42.

57. Koehn MA, Zupanc ML. Unusual presentation and MRI findings in Rasmussen's syndrome. *Pediatr Neurol.* 1999;21:839–842.

58. Lascelles K, Dean AF, Robinson RO. Rasmussen's encephalitis followed by lupus erythematosus. *Dev Med Child Neurol.* 2002;44:572–574.

59. Bhatjiwale MG, Polkey C, Cox TC, et al. Rasmussen's encephalitis: neuroimaging findings in 21 patients with a closer look at the basal ganglia. *Pediatr Neurosurg.* 1998;29:142–148.

60. Chiapparini L, Granata T, Farina L, et al. Diagnostic imaging in 13 cases of Rasmussen's encephalitis: can early MRI suggest the diagnosis? *Neuroradiology.* 2003;45:171–183.

61. McDonald D, Farrell MA, McMenamin J. Rasmussen's syndrome associated with chronic brain stem encephalitis. *Eur J Paediatr Neurol.* 2001;5:203–206.

62. Maeda Y, Oguni H, Saitou Y, et al. Rasmussen syndrome: multifocal spread of inflammation suggested from MRI and PET findings. *Epilepsia.* 2003;44:1118–1121.

63. Hart Y, Andermann F, Robitaille Y, et al. Double pathology in Rasmussen's syndrome: a window on the etiology? *Neurology.* 1998;50:731–735.

64. Firlik KS, Adelson PD, Hamilton RL. Coexistence of a ganglioglioma and Rasmussen's encephalitis. *Pediatr Neurosurg.* 1999;30:278–282.

65. Kumar R, Wani AA, Reddy J, et al. Development of anaplastic ependymoma in Rasmussen's encephalitis: review of the literature and case report. *Childs Nerv Syst.* 2006;22:416–419.

66. Yacubian EM, Rosemberg S, Marie SK, et al. Double pathology in Rasmussen's encephalitis: etiological considerations. *Epilepsia.* 1996;37: 495–500.

67. Palmer CA, Geyer JD, Keating JM, et al. Rasmussen's encephalitis with concomitant cortical dysplasia: the role of GluR3. *Epilepsia.* 1999;40:242–247.

68. Twyman RE, Gahring LC, Spiess J, et al. Glutamate receptor antibodies activate a subset of receptors and reveal an agonist binding site. *Neuron.* 1995;14:755–762.

69. Straube A, Padovan CS, Seelos K. Parry-Romberg syndrome and Rasmussen syndrome: only an incidental similarity? *Nervenarzt.* 2001;72:641–646.

70. Shah JR, Juhasz C, Kupsky WJ, et al. Rasmussen encephalitis associated with Parry-Romberg syndrome. *Neurology.* 2003;61:395–397.

71. Paprocka J, Jamroz E, Adamek D, et al. Difficulties in differentiation of Parry-Romberg syndrome, unilateral facial sclerodermia and Rasmussen syndrome. *Childs Ner Syst.* 2006;22:409–415.

72. Carreño M, Donaire A, Barceló MI, et al. Parry Romberg síndrome and linear scleroderma in coup de sabre mimicking Rasmussen encephalitis. *Neurology.* 2007;68:1308–1310.

73. Pupillo G, Andermann F, Dubeau F. Linear scleroderma and intractable epilepsy: neuropathologic evidence for a chronic inflammatory process. *Ann Neurol.* 1996;39:277–278.

74. Stone J, Franks AJ, Guthrie JA, et al. Scleroderma 'en coup de sabre': pathological evidence of intracerebral inflammation. *J Neurol Neurosurg Psychiatry.* 2001;70:382–385.

75. Ramaswamy V, Sinclair DB, Wheatley BM, et al. Epilepsia partialis continua: acute disseminated encephalomyelitis or Rasmussen's encephalitis? *Pediatr Neurol.* 2005;32:341–345.

76. Goyal M, Cohen ML, Bangert BA, et al. Rasmussen syndrome and CNS granulomatous disease with NOD2/CARD15 mutations. *Neurology.* 2007;69:640–643.

77. Lyon G, Griscelli C, Fernandez-Alvarez E, et al. Chronic progressive encephalitis in children with X-linked hypogammaglobulinemia. *Neuropaediatrie.* 1980;11:57–71.

78. Gupta PC, Rapin I, Houroupian DS, et al. Smoldering encephalitis in children. *Neuropediatrics.* 1984;15:191–197.

79. Harvey AS, Andermann F, Hopkins IJ, et al. Chronic encephalitis (Rasmussen's syndrome) and ipsilateral uveitis. *Ann Neurol.* 1992;32:826–829.

80. Fukuda T, Oguni H, Yanagaki S, et al. Chronic localized encephalitis (Rasmussen's syndrome) preceded by ipsilateral uveitis: a case report. *Epilepsia.* 1994;35:1328 1331.

81. Bancaud J, Bonis A, Trottier S, et al. Continuous partial epilepsy: syndrome and disease [French]. *Rev Neurol.* 1982;138:803–814.

82. Bancaud J. Kojewnikow's syndrome (epilepsia partialis continua) in children. In: Roger J, Dravet C, Bureau M, et al., eds. *Epileptic Syndromes in Infancy, Childhood and Adolescence.* 2nd ed. London: John Libbey; 1992:363–379.

83. Dulac O, Dravet C, Plouin P, et al. Nosological aspects of epilepsia partialis continua in children [French]. *Arch Fr Pediatr.* 1983;40:689–695.

84. Hwang PA, Piatt J, Cyr L, et al. The EEG of Rasmussen's encephalitis. *Electromyogr Clin Neurophysiol.* 1988;69:51P–52P.

85. So NK, Gloor P. Electroencephalographic and electrocorticographic findings in chronic encephalitis of the Rasmussen type. In: Andermann F, ed. *Encephalitis and Epilepsy: Rasmussen's Syndrome.* London: Butterworth-Heinemann; 1991:37–45.

86. Campovilla G, Paladin F, Dalla Bernardina B. Rasmussen's syndrome: longitudinal EEG study from the first seizure to epilepsia partialis continua. *Epilepsia.* 1997;38:483–488.

87. Andrews PI, McNamara JO, Lewis DV. Clinical and electroencephalographic correlates in Rasmussen's encephalitis. *Epilepsia.* 1997;38: 189–194.

88. Beaumanoir A, Grioni D, Kullman G, et al. EEG anomalies in the prodromic phase of Rasmussen's syndrome. Report of two cases [French]. *Neurophysiol Clin.* 1997;27:25–32.

89. Thomas P, Zifkin B, Ghetau G, et al. Persistence of ictal activity after functional hemispherectomy in Rasmussen syndrome. *Neurology.* 2003;60: 140–142.

90. English R, Soper N, Shepstone BJ, et al. Five patients with Rasmussen's syndrome investigated by single-photon-emission computed tomography. *Nucl Med Commun.* 1989;10:5–14.

91. Tampieri D, Melanson D, Ethier R. Imaging of chronic encephalitis. In: Andermann F, ed. *Encephalitis and Epilepsy: Rasmussen's Syndrome.* London: Butterworth-Heinemann; 1991:47–69.

92. Vining EP, Freeman JM, Brandt J, et al. Progressive unilateral encephalopathy of childhood (Rasmussen's syndrome): a reappraisal. *Epilepsia.* 1993;34:639–650.

93. Fiorella DJ, Provenzale JM, Coleman RE, et al. 18F-fluorodeoxyglucose positron emission tomography and MR imaging findings in Rasmussen encephalitis. *Am J Neuroradiol.* 2001;22:1291–1299.

94. Bien CG, Urbach H, Deckert M, et al. Diagnosis and staging of Rasmussen's encephalitis by serial MRI and histopathology. *Neurology.* 2002;58:250–257.

95. Takeoka M, Kim F, Caviness VS, et al. MRI volumetric analysis in Rasmussen encephalitis: A longitudinal study. *Epilepsia.* 2003;44:247–251.

96. Burke GJ, Fifer SA, Yoder J. Early detection of Rasmussen's syndrome by brain SPECT imaging. *Clin Nucl Med.* 1992;17:730–731.

97. Kaiboriboon K, Cortese C, Hogan RE. Magnetic resonance and positron emission tomography changes during the clinical progression of Rasmussen encephalitis. *J Neuroimaging.* 2000;10:122–125.

98. Geller E, Faerber EN, Legido A, et al. Rasmussen encephalitis: complementary role of multitechnique neuroimaging. *Am J Neuroradiol.* 1998;19:445–449.

99. Lee J, Juhasz C, Kaddurah AK, et al. Patterns of cerebral glucose metabolism in early and late stages of Rasmussen's syndrome. *J Child Neurol.* 2001;16:798–805.

100. Fogarasi A, Hegyi M, Neuwirth M, et al. Comparative evaluation of concomitant structural changes and functional neuroimages in Rasmussen's encephalitis. *J Neuroimaging.* 2003;13:339–345.

101. Sammaritano M, Andermann F, Melanson D, et al. Prolonged focal cerebral edema associated with partial status epilepticus. *Epilepsia.* 1985;26:334–339.

102. Zupanc ML, Handler EG, Levine RL, et al. Rasmussen encephalitis: epilepsia partialis continua secondary to chronic encephalitis. *Pediatr Neurol.* 1990;6:397–401.

103. Nakasu S, Isozumi T, Yamamoto A, et al. Serial magnetic resonance imaging findings of Rasmussen's encephalitis. *Neurol Med Chir.* 1997;37:924–928.

104. Derry C, Dale RC, Thom M, et al. Unihemispheric cerebral vasculitis mimicking Rasmussen's encephalitis. *Neurology.* 2002;58:327–328.

105. Hwang PA, Gilday DL, Spire JP, et al. Chronic focal encephalitis of Rasmussen: functional neuroimaging studies with positron emission tomography and single-photon emission computed tomography scanning. In: Andermann F, ed. *Encephalitis and Epilepsy: Rasmussen's Syndrome.* London: Butterworth-Heinemann; 1991:61–72.

106. Hajek M, Antonini A, Leenders KL, et al. Epilepsia partialis continua studied by PET. *Epilepsy Res.* 1991;9:44–48.

107. Duprez TPJ, Grandin C, Gadisseux JF, et al. MR-monitored remitting-relapsing pattern of cortical involvement in Rasmussen syndrome: comparative evaluation of serial MR and PET/SPECT features. *J Comput Assist Tomogr.* 1997;21:900–904.

108. Shetty-Alva N, Novotny EJ, Shetty T, et al. Positron emission tomography in Rasmussen's encephalitis. *Pediatr Neurol.* 2007;36:112–114.

109. Banati RB, Guerra GW, Myers R, et al. [^{11}C](*R*)-PK11195 positron emission tomography imaging of activated microglia in vivo in Rasmussen's encephalitis. *Neurology.* 1999;53:2199–2203.

110. Aguilar Rebolledo F, Rojas Bautista J, Villanueva Perez R, et al. SPECT-99mTc-HMPAO in a case of epilepsia partialis continua and focal encephalitis [Spanish]. *Rev Invest Clin.* 1996;48:199–205.

111. Yacubian EMT, Sueli KNM, Valério RMF, et al. Neuroimaging findings in Rasmussen's syndrome. *J Neuroimaging.* 1997;7:16–22.

112. Paladin F, Capovilla G, Bonazza A, et al. Utility of Tc 99m HMPAO SPECT in the early diagnosis of Rasmussen's syndrome. *Ital J Neurol Sci.* 1998;19:217–220.

113. Vinjamuri S, Leach JP, Hart IK. Serial perfusion brain tomographic scans detect reversible focal ischemia in Rasmussen's encephalitis. *Postgrad Med J.* 2000;76:33–40.

114. Ishibashi H, Simos PG, Wheless JW, et al. Multimodality functional imaging evaluation in a patient with Rasmussen's encephalitis. *Brain Dev.* 2002;24:239–244.

115. Hartley LM, Harkness W, Harding B, et al. Correlation of SPECT with pathology and seizure outcome in children undergoing epilepsy surgery. *Dev Med Child Neurol.* 2002;44:676–680.

116. Borneo JG, Hamilton M, Vezina W, et al. Utility of ictal SPECT in the presurgical evaluation of Rasmussen's encephalitis. *Can J Neurol Sci.* 2006;33:107–110.

117. Peeling J, Sutherland G. 1H magnetic resonance spectroscopy of extracts of human epileptic neocortex and hippocampus. *Neurology.* 1993;43:589–594.

118. Cendes F, Andermann F, Silver K, et al. Imaging of axonal damage in vivo in Rasmussen's syndrome. *Brain.* 1995;118:753–758.

119. Sundgren PC, Burtsher IM, Lundgren J, et al. MRI and proton spectroscopy in a child with Rasmussen's encephalitis. Case report. *Neuroradiology.* 1999;41:935–940.

120. Tükdogan-Sözüer D, Özek MM, Sav A, et al. Serial MRI and MRS studies with unusual findings in Rasmussen's encephalitis. *Eur Radiol.* 2000;10:962–966.

121. Park YD, Allison JD, Weiss KL, et al. Proton magnetic resonance spectroscopic observations of epilepsia partialis continua in children. *J Child Neurol.* 2000;15:729–733.

122. Sener RN. Rasmussen's encephalitis: proton MR spectroscopy and diffusion MR findings. *J Neuroradiol.* 2000;27:179–184.

123. Sener RN. Diffusion MRI and spectroscopy in Rasmussen's encephalitis. *Eur Radiol.* 2003;13:2186–2191.

124. Tekgul H, Polat M, Kitis O, et al. T-Cell subsets and interleukin-6 response in Rasmussen's encephalitis. *Pediatr Neurol.* 2005;33:39–45.

125. Pardo CA, Vining EPG, Guo L, et al. The pathology of Rasmussen syndrome: stages of cortical involvement and neuropathological studies in 45 hemispherectomies. *Epilepsia.* 2004;45:516–526.

126. Friedman H, Ch'ien L, Parham D. Virus in brain of child with hemiplegia, hemiconvulsions, and epilepsy. *Lancet.* 1977;2:666.

127. Riikonen R. Cytomegalovirus infection and infantile spasms. *Dev Med Child Neurol.* 1978;20:570–579.

128. Mizuno Y, Chou SM, Estes ML, et al. Chronic localized encephalitis (Rasmussen's) with focal cerebral seizures revisited. *J Neuropathol Exp Neurol.* 1985;44:351.

129. Asher DM, Gadjusek DC. Virologic studies in chronic encephalitis. In: Andermann F, ed. *Encephalitis and Epilepsy: Rasmussen's Syndrome.* London: Butterworth-Heinemann; 1991:147–158.

130. Walter GF, Renella RR. Epstein-Barr virus in brain and Rasmussen's encephalitis. *Lancet.* 1989;1:279–280.

131. Power C, Poland SD, Blume WT, et al. Cytomegalovirus and Rasmussen's encephalitis. *Lancet.* 1990;336:1282–1284.

132. Farrell MA, Cheng L, Cornford ME, et al. Cytomegalovirus and Rasmussen's encephalitis. *Lancet.* 1991;337:1551–1552.

133. Vinters HV, Wang R, Wiley CA. Herpesviruses in chronic encephalitis associated with intractable childhood epilepsy. *Hum Pathol.* 1993;24: 871–879.

134. Atkins MR, Terrell W, Hulette CM. Rasmussen's syndrome: a study of potential viral etiology. *Clin Neuropathol.* 1995;14:7–12.

135. Jay V, Becker LE, Otsubo H, et al. Chronic encephalitis and epilepsy (Rasmussen's encephalitis): detection of cytomegalovirus and herpes simplex virus 1 by the polymerase chain reaction and *in situ* hybridization. *Neurology.* 1995;45:108–117.

136. Prayson RA, Frater JL. Rasmussen encephalitis. A clinicopathologic and immunohistochemical study of seven patients. *Am J Clin Pathol.* 2002; 117:776–782.

137. Eeg-Olofsson O, Bergström T, Andermann F, et al. Herpesviral DNA in brain tissue from patients with temporal lobe epilepsy. *Acta Neurol Scand.* 2004;109:169–174.

138. Lampe JB, Schneider-Schaulies S, Aguzzi A. Expression of the interferon-induced MxA protein in vrial encephalitis. *Neuropathol Appl Neubiol.* 2003;29:273–279.

139. Maria BL, Ringdahl DM, Mickle JP, et al. Intraventricular alpha interferon therapy for Rasmussen's syndrome. *Can J Neurol Sci.* 1993; 20:333–336.

140. McLachlan RS, Levin S, Blume WT. Treatment of Rasmussen's syndrome with ganciclovir. *Neurology.* 1996;47:925–928.

141. Dabbagh O, Gascon G, Crowell J, et al. Intraventricular interferon-α stops seizures in Rasmussen's encephalitis: a case report. *Epilepsia.* 1997;38:1045–1049.

142. Grenier Y, Antel JP, Osterland CK. Immunologic studies in chronic encephalitis of Rasmussen. In: Andermann F, ed. *Encephalitis and Epilepsy: Rasmussen's Syndrome.* London: Butterworth-Heinemann; 1991:125–134.

143. Rogers SW, Andrews PI, Garhing LC, et al. Autoantibodies to glutamate receptor GluR3 in Rasmussen's encephalitis. *Science.* 1994;265:648–651.

144. Levite M, Fleidervish IA, Schwarz A, et al. Autoantibodies to the glutamate receptor kill neurons via activation of the receptor ion channel. *J Autoimmun.* 1999;13:61–72.

145. Levite M, Hermelin A. Autoimmunity to the glutamate receptor in mice-a model for Rasmussen's encephalitis? *J Autoimmun.* 1999;13:73–82.

146. He XP, Patel M, Whitney KD, et al. Glutamate receptor GluR3 antibodies and death of cortical cells. *Neuron.* 1998;20:153–163.

147. Whitney KD, Andrews JM, McNamara JO. Immunoglobulin G and complement immunoreactivity in the cerebral cortex of patients with Rasmussen's encephalitis. *Neurology.* 1999;53:699–708.

148. Andrews PI, Ditcher MA, Berkovic SF, et al. Plasmapheresis in Rasmussen's encephalitis. *Neurology.* 1996;46:242–246.

149. Palcoux JB, Carla H, Tardieu M, et al. Plasma exchange in Rasmussen's encephalitis. *Ther Apher.* 1997;1:79–82.

150. Antozzi C, Granata T, Aurisano N, et al. Long-term selective IgG immunoadsorption improves Rasmussen's encephalitis. *Neurology.* 1998;51:302–305.

151. Paas J. The pathophysiological mechanism underlying Rasmussen's encephalitis. *Trends Neurosci.* 1998;21:468–469.

152. Palace J, Lang B. Epilepsy: an autoimmune disease? *J Neurol Neurosurg Psychiatry.* 2000;69:711–714.

153. Aarli JA. Rasmussen's encephalitis: a challenge to neuroimmunology [editorial]. *Curr Opin Neurol.* 2000;13:297–299.

154. Wiendl H, Bien CG, Bernasconi P, et al. GluR3 antibodies: prevalence in focal epilepsy but no specificity for Rasmussen's encephalitis. *Neurology.* 2001;57:1511–1514.

155. Baranzini SE, Laxer K, Saketkhoo R, et al. Analysis of antibody gene rearrangement, usage, and specificity in chronic focal encephalitis. *Neurology.* 2002;58:709–716.

156. Mantegazza R, Bernasconi P, Baggi F, et al. Antibodies against GluR3 peptides are not specific for Rasmussen's encephalitis but are also present in epilepsy patients with severe, early onset disease and intractable seizures. *J Neuroimmunol.* 2002;131:179–185.

157. Bien CG, Bauer J, Deckwerth TL, et al. Destruction of neurons by cytotoxic T cells: a new pathogenic mechanism in rasmussen's encephalitis. *Ann Neurol.* 2002;51:311–318.

158. Bernasconi P, Cipelletti B, Passerini L, et al. Similar binding to glutamate receptors by Rasmussen and partial epilepsy patients' sera. *Neurology.* 2002;59:1998–2001.

159. Watson R, Jiang Y, Bermudez I, et al. Absence of antibodies to glutamate receptor type 3 (GluR3) in Rasmussen encephalitis. *Neurology.* 2004;63:43–50.

160. Ganor Y, Goldberg-Stern H, Amron D, et al. Autoimmune epilepsy: some epilepsy patients harbor autoantibodies to glutamate receptors and dsDNA on both sides of the Bloo-brain Barriers, which may kill neurons and decrease in brain fluids after hemispherotomy. *Clinl Dev Immunol.* 2004;11:241–252.

161. Ganor Y, Freilinger M, Dulac O, et al. Monozygotic twins discordant for epilepsy differ in the levels of potentially pathogenic autoantibodies and cytokines. *Autoimmunity.* 2005;38:139–150.

162. Levite M, Ganor Y. Autoantibodies to glutamate receptors can damage the brain in epilepsy, systemic lupus erythematous and encephalitis. *Expert Rev Neurother.* 2008;8:1141–1160.

163. Yang R, Puranam RS, Butler LS, et al. Autoimmunity to munc-18 in Rasmussen's encephalitis. *Neuron.* 2000;28:375–383.

164. Alvarez-Barón E, Bien CG, Schramm J, et al. Autoantibodies to munc18, cerebral plasma cells and B-lymphocytes in Rasmussen encephalitis. *Epilepsy Res.* 2008;80:93–97.

165. Watson R, Lang B, Bermudez I, et al. Autoantibodies in Rasmussen's encephalitis. *J Neuroimmunol.* 2001;118:148.

166. Watson R, Jepson JEC, Bermudez I, et al. α7-Acetylcholine receptor antibodies in two patients with Rasmussen encephalitis. *Neurology.* 2005; 65:1802–1804.

167. Herranz AC, Sánchez Pérez I, Aparicio Meix JM, et al. Sindrome de Rasmussen: una enfermedad autoimmune [Barc]. *An Pediatr.* 2003;59: 187–189.

168. Takahashi Y, Mori H, Mishina M, et al. Autoantibodies to NMDA receptor in patients with chronic forms of epilepsia partialis continua. *Neurology.* 2003;61:891–896.

169. Kumakura A, Miyajima T, Fujii T, et al. A patient with epilepsia partialis continua with anti-glutamate receptor ε2 antibodies. *Pediatr Neurol.* 2003;29:160–163.

170. Levite M. Autoimmune epilepsy. *Nat Immunol.* 2002;3:500.

171. Lang B, Dale RC, Vincent A. New autoantibody mediated disorders of the central nervous system. *Curr Opin Neurol.* 2003;16:351–357.

172. Farrell MA, Droogan O, Secor DL, et al. Chronic encephalitis associated with epilepsy: immunohistochemical and ultrastructural studies. *Acta Neuropathol.* 1995;89:313–321.

173. Li Y, Uccelli A, Laxer KD, et al. Local-clonal expansion of infiltrating T lymphocytes in chronic encephalitis of Rasmussen. *J Immunol.* 1997;158: 1428–1437.

174. Gahring LC, Carlson NG, Meyer EL, et al. Cutting edge: granzyme B proteolysis of a neuronal glutamate receptor generates an autoantigen and is modulated by glycosylation. *J Immunol.* 2001;166:1433–1438.

175. Bauer J, Bien CG, Lassmann H. Rasmussen's encephalitis: a role for autoimmune cytotoxic T lymphocytes. *Curr Opin Neurol.* 2002;15: 197–200.

176. Bien CG, Elger CE, Wiendl H. Advances in pathogenic concepts and therapeutic agents in Rasmussen's encephalitis. *Expert Opin Investig Drugs.* 2002;11:981–989.

177. Bauer J, Elger CE, Hans VH, et al. Astrocytes are a specific immunological target in Rasmussen's encephalitis. *Ann Neurol.* 2007;62:67–80.

178. Bahi-Buisson N, Nabbout R, Plouin P, et al. Avancées actuelles sur le concept pathogéniques et thérapeutiques de l'encéphalite de Rasmussen [Paris]. *Rev Neurol.* 2005;161:395–405.

179. Hart Y. Rasmussen's encephalitis. *Epiletic Disord.* 2004;6:133–144.

180. Rotenberg A, Cabacar D, Bae EH, et al. Transient supression of seizures by repetitive transcranial magnetic stimulation in a case of Rasmussen's encephalitis. *Epilepsy Behav.* 2008;13:260–262.

181. Lozsadi DA, Hart IK, Moore AP. Botulinum toxin A improves involuntary limb movements in Rasmussen syndrome. *Neurology.* 2004;62: 1233–1234.

182. Browner N, Azher SN, Jankovic J. Botulinum toxin treatment of facial myoclonus in suspected Rasmussen encephalitis. *Movt Disord.* 2006;21: 1500–1502.

183. Daniel RT, Villemure JG. Experience with immunomodulatory treatments in Rasmussen's encephalitis. *Neurology.* 2004;63:1761–1762.

184. Walsh PJ. Treatment of Rasmussen's syndrome with intravenous gamma-globulin. In: Andermann F, ed. *Encephalitis and Epilepsy: Rasmussen's Syndrome.* London: Butterworth-Heinemann; 1991:201–204.

185. Wise MS, Rutledge SL, Kuzniecky RI. Rasmussen syndrome and long-term response to gamma globulin. *Pediatr Neurol.* 1996;14:149–152.

186. Caraballo R, Tenembaum S, Cersosimo R, et al. Rasmussen syndrome [Spanish]. *Rev Neurol.* 1998;26:978–983.

187. Gold R, Stangel M, Dalakas MC. Drug insight: the use of intravenous immunoglobulin in neurology: therapeutic considerations and practical issues [review]. *Nat Clin Pract Neurol.* 2007;3:36–44.

188. Feasby T, Benstead T, Brouwers M, et al. Guidelines on the use of intravenous globulin for neurological conditions. *Transfus Med Rev* 2007;21:S57–S107.

189. Bien CG, Gleissner U, Sassen R, et al. An open study of tacrolimus therapy in Rasmussen encephalitis. *Neurology.* 2004;62:2106–2109.

190. Laxer KD. A pilot study of the use of Rituximab in the treatment of chronic focal encephalitis. *Clinical Trials.* 2008;192.

191. Ravenscroft A, Schoemen JF, Pretorious ML, et al. Rasmussen's encephalitis: case presentation and discussion on the role of specific immune modulation [abstract]. *Brain Dev.* 1998;20:398.
192. Marjanovic BD, Stojanov LM, Zdravkovic DS, et al. Rasmussen syndrome and long-term response to thalidomide. *Pediatr Neurol.* 2003;29:151–156.
193. Villemure JG, Andermann F, Rasmussen TB. Hemispherectomy for the treatment of epilepsy due to chronic encephalitis. In: Andermann F, ed. *Encephalitis and Epilepsy: Rasmussen's Syndrome.* London: Butterworth-Heinemann; 1991:235–244.
194. DeLalande O, Pinard JM, Jalin O, et al. Surgical results of hemispherotomy. *Epilepsia.* 1995;36(Suppl 3):241.
195. Kossoff EH, Vining EPG, Pillas DJ, et al. Hemispherectomy for intractable unihemispheric epilepsy. Etiology and outcome. *Neurology.* 2003;61:887–890.
196. Olivier A. Corticectomy for the treatment of seizures due to chronic encephalitis. In: Andermann F, ed. *Encephalitis and Epilepsy: Rasmussen's Syndrome.* London: Butterworth-Heinemann; 1991:205–212.
197. Spencer SS, Spencer DD. Corpus callosotomy in chronic encephalitis. In: Andermann F, ed. *Encephalitis and Epilepsy: Rasmussen's Syndrome.* London: Butterworth-Heinemann; 1991:213–218.
198. Morrell F, Whisler WW, Cremin Smith M. Multiple subpial transection in Rasmussen's encephalitis. In: Andermann F, ed. *Encephalitis and Epilepsy: Rasmussen's Syndrome.* London: Butterworth-Heinemann; 1991:219–234.
199. Honavar M, Janota I, Polkey CE. Rasmussen's encephalitis in surgery for epilepsy. *Dev Med Child Neurol.* 1992;34:3–14.
200. Sawhney IMS, Robertson IJA, Polkey CE, et al. Multiple subpial transaction: a review of 21 cases. *J Neurol Neurosurg Psychiatry.* 1995;58:344–349.
201. Devlin AM, Cross JH, Harkness W, et al. Clinical outcomes of hemispherectomy for epilepsy in childhood and adolescence. *Brain.* 2003;126:556–566.
202. Jonas R, Nguyen S, Hu B, et al. Cerebral hemispherectomy: hospital course, seizure, developmental, language, and motor outcomes. *Neurology.* 2004;62:1712–1721.
203. Pulsifer MB, Brandt J, Salorio CF, et al. The cognitive outcome of hemispherectomy in 71 children. *Epilepsia.* 2004;45:243–254.
204. Cook SW, Nguyen ST, Hu BS, et al. Cerebral hemispherectomy in pediatric patients with epilepsy: comparison of three techniques by pathological substrates in 115 patients. *J Neurosurg Pediatr.* 2004;100:125–141.
205. Koh S, Mathern GW, Glasser G, et al. Status epilepticus and frequent seizures: incidence and clinical characteristics in pediatric surgery patients. *Epilepsia.* 2005;46:1950–1954.
206. Tubbs RS, Nimjee SM, Oakes WJ. Long-term follow-up in children with functional hemispherectomy for Rasmussen's encephalitis. *Childs Nerv Syst.* 2005;21:461–465.
207. Basheer SN, Connolly MB, Lautzenhiser A, et al. Hemispheric surgery in children with refractory epilepsy: Seizure outcome, complications, and adaptative function. *Epilepsia.* 2007;48:133–140.
208. Delalande O, Bulteau C, Dellatolas G, et al. Vertical parasagittal hemispherotomy: Surgical procedures and clinical long-term outcomes in a population of 83 children. *Neurosurgery.* 2007;60:S19–S32.
209. Guimarães CA, Souza EAP, Montenegro MA, et al. Rasmussen's encephalitis. The relevance of neuropsychological assessment in patient's treatment and follow up. *Arq Neuropsiquiatr.* 2002;60:378–381.
210. Taylor LB. Neuropsychological assessment of patients with chronic encephalitis. In: Andermann F, ed. *Encephalitis and Epilepsy: Rasmussen's Syndrome.* London: Butterworth-Heinemann; 1991:111–124.
211. Boatman D, Freeman J, Vining E, et al. Language recovery after left hemispherectomy in children with late-onset seizures. *Ann Neurol.* 1999;46:579–586.
212. Curtiss S, de Bode S. Age and etiology as predictors of language outcome following hemispherectomy. *Dev Neurosci.* 1999;21:174–181.
213. Curtiss S, de Bode S, Mathern GW. Spoken language outcomes after hemispherectomy: factoring in etiology. *Brain Lang.* 2001;79:379–396.
214. Telfeian AE, Berqvist C, Danielak C, et al. Recovery of language after left hemispherectomy in a sixteen-year-old girl with late-onset seizures. *Pediatr Neurosurg.* 2002;37:19–21.
215. Hertz-Pannier L, Chiron C, Jambaqué I, et al. Late plasticity for language in a child's non-dominant hemisphere. A pre- and post-surgery fMRI study. *Brain.* 2002;125:361–372.
216. Boatman D, Vining EP, Freeman J, et al. Auditory processing studied prospectively in two hemidecorticectomy patients. *J Child Neurol.* 2003;18:228–232.
217. Rosa C, Lassonde M. Spécialisation hémisphérique. Développement et plasticité. In: Hommet C, Jambaqué I, Billard C, et al., eds. *Neuropsychologie de l'enfant et troubles du développement.* Marseille: Solal editeurs; 2005:11–35.
218. Voets NL, Adcock JE, Flitney DE, et al. Distinct right frontal lobe activation in language processing following left hemisphere injury. *Brain.* 2006;129:754–766.
219. Bulteau C, Dorfmuller G, Fohlen M, et al. Évaluation à long terme des déconnexions hémisphériques. *Neurochirurgie.* 2008;54:358–361.
220. Freeman JM. Rasmussen's syndrome: progressive autoimmune multi-focal encephalopathy. *Pediatr Neurol.* 2005;32:295–299.
221. Vining EPG. Struggling with Rasmussen's syndrome. *Epilepsy Curr.* 2006;6:20–21.

CHAPTER 26 ■ HIPPOCAMPAL SCLEROSIS AND DUAL PATHOLOGY

LUIGI D'ARGENZIO AND J. HELEN CROSS

HISTORICAL BACKGROUND

Hippocampal sclerosis (HS) was first described by Bouchet and Cazauvielh in 1825. They described hippocampal atrophy on a pathological examination of a patient who had died of seizures (1). In 1880, Sommer made the first microscopical description of HS, describing the finding of pyramidal neurons unhomogeneously destroyed, lacking mainly in the CA1 and prosubiculum areas, with the CA2 to CA4 subfields left relatively spared (2). In the mid-1900s a rational surgical therapy was proposed for HS, after ictal discharges had been demonstrated arising from the affected area in individuals with presumed temporal lobe epilepsy (3). Later, the term mesial temporal sclerosis (MTS) was used to define the histopathological complex of alterations in the amygdala, uncus, and temporal lobe, often associated with HS (4).

HIPPOCAMPAL SCLEROSIS

The hippocampus is part of the limbic lobe and it is situated in the mesial part of the temporal lobe, arched around the mesencephalon. It is divided in three parts (i.e., head, body, and tail) and is formed by a bilaminar archicortical structure divided in six layers. The inner structure is called Cornu Ammonis (CA; Ammon's horn) and contains four subfields, CA1 to CA4 (Fig. 26.1).

The classical histological description of HS includes a distinctive pattern of neuronal loss, gliosis, and reorganization not found in other neurological diseases (5,6). The neuronal loss and gliosis primarily involve the hippocampal sectors CA1, CA3, and CA4, with relative sparing of CA2 (Fig. 26.2). The hilar region and dentate granule cells containing somatostatin and neuropeptide Y are particularly vulnerable, whereas GABA neurons are rather preserved. Axons of dentate granule cells (mossy fibers) form aberrant excitatory feedback synapses on the dendritic spines of the same cells (7). Cell loss can extend into adjacent entorinal cortex and amygdala.

HS can be reliably detected in vivo using magnetic resonance imaging (MRI). Features include hippocampal atrophy with increased signal on T_2-weighted images or fluid attenuated inversion recovery (FLAIR) and decreased signal on T_1-weighted images, particularly using coronal sections perpendicular to the long axis of the hippocampus (Fig. 26.3). MRI sensitivity in the detection of HS is about 80% to 90% increasing as the neuronal cells decrease. A correct identification of HS by MRI is achievable in 90% of cases with a neuronal decrease of about 50%. However, MRI specificity is not as high as its sensitivity. Absence of unilateral atrophy is not sufficient to exclude HS (8,9).

Controversies in Etiology

The prevalence and incidence of HS in the general population is not known (10). As the prevalence of epilepsy ranges from 2.7 to 6.8 per 1000 (11), and HS is believed to cause about 20% of all epilepsies in adults (12), an overall prevalence of 0.5 to 1.3 per 1000 in adult population might be assumed.

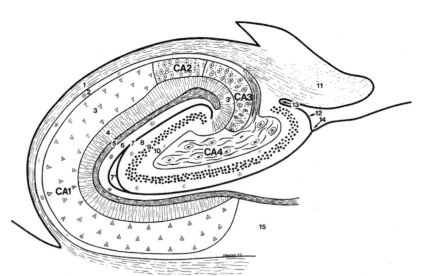

FIGURE 26.1 Structure of the hippocampus, coronal section. CA1 to CA4, fields of cornu ammonis. Cornu ammonis: 1, alveus; 2, stratum oriens; 3, stratum pyramidale; 3′, stratum lucindum; 4, stratum radiatum; 5, stratum lacunosum; 6, stratum moleculare; 7, vestigial hippocampal sulcus (note a residual cavity); 7′, gyrus dentatus; 8, stratum molecular; 9, stratum granulosum; 10, polymorphic layer; 11, fimbria; 12, margo denticulatus; 13, fimbriodentate sulcus; 14, superficial hippocampal sulcus; 15, subiculum.

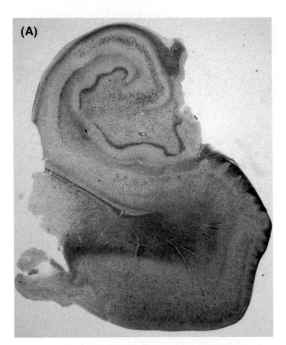
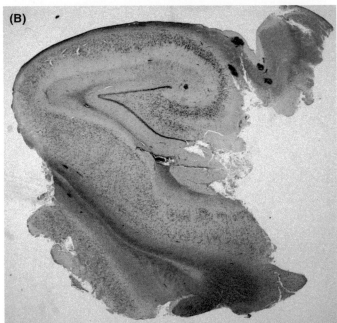

FIGURE 26.2 Appearance of the hippocampus in hippocampal sclerosis at the interface between CA2 and CA1 regions. There is a marked loss of neurons in the CA1 region with gliosis (**A**) compared to a normal hippocampus (**B**).

However, in a general nonepileptic population, unilateral HS has been found incidentally in about 14% of MRI scans (13). Thus, unilateral volumetric reduction of hippocampus is, to some extent, independent from the presentation of epilepsy. Most of the epidemiological data on HS, however, comes from surgical series in both adults and children. In adult epilepsy neurosurgical series, HS is responsible for about 86% of surgical procedures (14). In pediatric neurosurgical series, HS represents a less frequent etiology (about 6%) with pathologies such as low-grade tumors and cortical malformation being relatively more common as a cause of temporal lobe epilepsy (15,16). However, in a series of newly diagnosed children with temporal lobe epilepsy, HS has a much higher representation, suggesting that not all go on to drug resistance or that intractability manifests in later life (17,18). Many adults coming to surgery, however, have had a history of epilepsy for many years, often originating in childhood, suggesting that earlier referral would have been beneficial.

The etiology and pathogenesis of HS remains unclear. Initial reports identified mechanical insults or cerebral infections as having a possible pathogenic role (19–21). Even in the presence of some evidence that vascular insults or viral infections could damage hippocampal areas in animal models, no consistent clinical data exist to support that these antecedents may be relevant in humans (22–24). Several authors have identified in adult surgical series a previous history of febrile seizures (FS) and status epilepticus (SE) during the first years of life as the most common antecedent and possible cause for HS. This gains further support from the early animal studies in baboons where HS was induced by SE even when systemic parameters such as temperature and blood pressure were controlled (25). However, in pediatric series these associations are not so consistent, recognizing that both may be a presenting feature of underlying idiopathic epilepsy (26–28). FS are a common type of seizure among children before the age of

5 years with an incidence of about 7% and a prevalence of 2% to 5% (29,30). The incidence of subsequent mesial temporal lobe epilepsy (MTLE) in adolescent with previous FS is low. Further, it is recognized that there appears to be a "latent" period to the presentation of temporal lobe epilepsy following the antecedent (31,32). It is not surprising, therefore, that population-based studies and prospective studies on FS have failed to demonstrate an association with HS, if indeed it is relevant (33–35). Although, about 10% to 40% of surgical adult patients with HS have had a previous history of FS, epidemiological study has revealed a prevalence of epilepsy after simple FS (1%) to be comparable to that of the general population (0.4%), whereas this rises to 22% following "complex" FS where seizures are unilateral or prolonged (4,31,33,36).

SE is a rare life-threatening epileptic condition that affects about 10 to 20 per 100,000 children per year, with an overall mortality rate of 11% (37,38). Even if different definitions of SE have been used, and heterogeneous disorders could be classified as nonconvulsive SE, a previous history of SE is found in about 40% of patients with HS. The clinical presentation of MTLE is usually later in patients with previous SE than in those with a history of FS (31).

The presumption has been that HS is the consequence of earlier damage from prolonged FS or SE. This may produce hippocampal alterations as a consequence of their ongoing epileptic activity, as the time frame of their clinical presentation is usually during the first years of life, when the cortex, and hippocampal areas in particular, might be more susceptible to such damage. Alternatively, there may need to be an underlying predisposition for such to occur. Several issues about etiology, therefore, remain. The incidence of HS and MTLE is low in children who suffered from FS and/or SE. It is still debated which are, if any, the characteristics to distinguish those with a later onset of HS from those who appear to present with no antecedent. Prospective imaging studies performing sequential

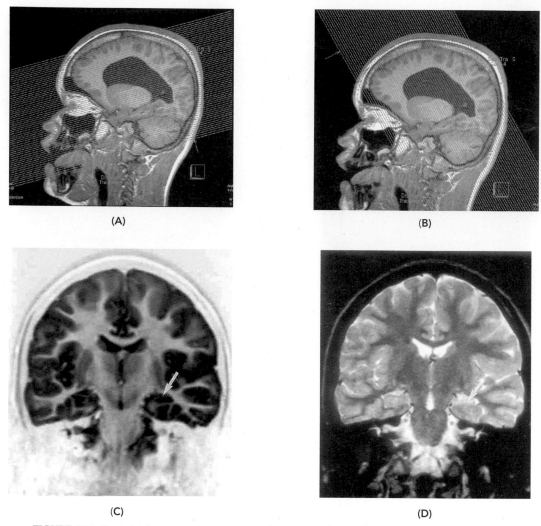

FIGURE 26.3 Optimized magnetic resonance imaging to view abnormalities of the hippocampus. Slices taken orientated at an angle parallel (see **A**) and perpendicular (see **B**) to the axis of the hippocampus. T_1 sequence (**C**) demonstrating small left hippocampus with low signal form within *(arrow)*, with high signal seen on T_2 sequence (**D**) *(arrow)*.

images in a population of children experiencing their first episode of SE have demonstrated changes in the hippocampus in a proportion (39,40). An ongoing multicenter study is currently prospectively following a subgroup of patients with febrile SE. Even if there are not conclusive results on the onset of MTLE in this cohort, short-term outcome has been shown to be different compared with those with shorter FS, suggesting that there could be a particular subgroup of children experiencing FS in whom this is either a marker of a pre-existing damage and/or a cause of additional damage to an already vulnerable brain (41,42). Indeed, previous data suggest hippocampi in these children could be acutely sensitive to prolonged insults, and a unilateral loss of volume could be evidenced a few months after the event. Furthermore, differences in clinical presentation, shorter latency period, and slight different postsurgical outcome in a pediatric population, compared with adult series, has raised the question whether there might be different subpopulation of patients with heterogeneous etiologies that end in a common pathway leading to hippocampal neural loss and subsequent intractable epilepsy (43,44).

Although, some authors have suggested that there could not be a specific cause for HS detected by neuroimaging or at surgery, some propose that a causal relation between early insults and the later development of MTLE might be artificial in retrospective studies, whereas others speculate HS could be a consequence instead of the cause of intractable seizures (45–47). Pre-existing subtle brain lesions, in fact, might predispose both to complex febrile convulsions and to later epilepsy. There may also be a developmental contribution to the likelihood of HS being present. Extrahippocampal seizures have been associated with neural loss and mossy fiber sprouting, and subtle abnormalities on MRI have been identified in the hippocampus consistent with seizure-induced injury (48–50). However, recent findings in an experimental animal model found the immature brain to be more protected than the adult one to seizure-induced damage. Further, in children with extratemporal seizures with onset before 6 months of age, hippocampi do not tend to have any sign of neural loss, suggesting a possible protective effect in the very young (26,51).

Diagnosis

The habitual clinical seizures that occur in about 90% of patients with MTLE consist of focal seizures, usually with an aura, mainly abdominal (nausea, pressure, butterflies, rising epigastric sensation). Less common reports include fear, dreamy states, olfactory and gustatory hallucinations, as well as ictal language impairment (52). Focal seizures involve impairment of consciousness (staring, motor arrest, or restlessness) with usually oroalimentary (chewing, swallowing, lip smacking, licking) and ipsilateral appendicular automatisms (fiddling, fumbling, picking, tapping, patting, scratching the face). Autonomic phenomena (pupillary dilatation, cardiovascular symptoms, pallor) are also frequent. Such features may be less distinct in the small child. Seizure duration is usually of 2 to 3 min with possible secondary generalization. Although seizure semiology may change over time, about 10% of patients may never present with secondary generalization, in particular those who receive an appropriate antiepileptic drugs (AEDs) treatment (53,54). Postictal symptoms include aphasia, mainly with dominant-hemisphere lesions, drowsiness, confusion, and rarely contralateral Todd's hemiparesis. It must be emphasized however that, even if these symptoms and signs are suggestive of MTLE, they do not exclude seizures arising from other cortical areas.

Interictal scalp EEG in patients with histologically proven HS show anterior temporal spikes and sharp waves, while posterior and extratemporal discharges are likely to be caused by other pathologies (55,56). Distinctive anterior temporal rhythmic theta or alpha activity within 30 sec prior to the first subjective or objective indication of a seizure is strongly associated with HS. Correct lateralization of the seizure onset is achieved in about 80% of the cases (57,58). The remaining 20% of patients could have bilateral or independent onset. Full neuropsychological evaluation, with functional imaging if required, is part of any presurgical evaluation in order to determine any cognitive, predominately memory/language deficit and predict any possible consequence of surgery. Wada testing or language mapping in selected patients may be required but is largely precluded now by functional language MRI (see Chapter 79).

A subset of patients could present contradictory electroencephalogram (EEG)–MRI localization of the epileptic focus. If this is the case, invasive monitoring or functional imaging could be indicated to localize the epileptogenic area. 2-deoxy-2-[18F]-fluoro-D-glucose positron emission tomography (FDG-PET) usually demonstrates up to 100% sensitivity for HS, showing a unilateral interictal hypo- or ictal hypermetabolism. However, specificity of PET for HS is limited, as the presence of hypometabolism does not correlate necessarily with HS (59). Ictal SPECT may also contribute to seizure lateralization (60,61). Invasive recording can be avoided in most patients and it is usually performed when scalp EEG and other investigation (e.g., lack of atrophy on MRI) fail or are not sufficient to lateralize seizure onset.

The rate of psychiatric disorder amongst adults and children coming to surgery for HS remains high. Adult patients with MTLE evaluated for surgical treatment demonstrate a psychiatric comorbidity in about 50% of cases, these being commonly of a nonpsychotic nature (62–64). About 80% of children, however, with temporal lobe epilepsy who undergo surgical resection have been shown to have a psychiatric diagnosis (67). Autistic spectrum disorders are seen in about 40% of the cases, as well as other behavioral problems, such as attention deficit/hyperactivity disorder or oppositional defiant disorder, are less frequent but still more prevalent in these children than in general population. After surgery, resolution of psychiatric disorders is not guaranteed, and indeed such may still evolve over time in adults and children. It is, therefore, important for individuals to be counselled with regard to this preoperatively (65).

Management

Medical treatment is still the first therapeutic approach at the onset of the epilepsy but often fails to achieve seizure freedom or reduction in seizure frequency. About 10% to 42% of patients on a medical treatment have been reported to become seizure-free for at least 1 year, but significant periods of seizure control and even remission can be possible before intractability is evident (66,67). Some authors have reported that about 25% of adult patients could become seizure-free and 38% have a significant reduction in seizure frequency if treated with appropriate AEDs (68).

Although drug-resistant epilepsy lacks a standard definition, there is some evidence that seizure freedom is highly unlikely after failure of two AEDs. Patients with HS are likely to be intractable in about 90% of the cases (69). Surgical resection represents the treatment of choice for individuals experiencing ongoing seizures with HS. This approach is highly effective for medically intractable patients, and should be proposed as early as possible, since ongoing seizures can greatly impact on patient's quality of life (see Chapter 82) (70).

The most commonly performed surgical procedure is the anterior temporal lobectomy (ATL) in which the anterior part of middle and inferior temporal gyri is resected. If HS is on the dominant hemisphere, usually a modified resection is performed in order to spare the language function. The affected hippocampus has to be completely removed to gain a good surgical outcome (although this is not usually possible), and this does not further impair the neuropsychological functions (71). An alternative procedure is the selective amygdalohippocampectomy (SAH) in which the amygdala, the parahippocampal gyrus, and the hippocampus are resected, while the lateral ventricle is spared. The two procedures seem to be equally effective for adults in seizure control with an overall postsurgical Engel class I outcome at 1-year follow-up of 68% versus 76% for ATL and SAH, respectively (72).

Although surgery for HS is amenable also during early childhood, these cases are rare, and this approach has traditionally been delayed until late childhood or adolescent. This could account for the relatively lower proportion of cases in surgical series (16), but also relatively higher proportions of other pathologies. Therefore, few data are available for surgical outcome after ATL or SAH in the pediatric population, and where evident seizure-free rates are similar to those of the adult series (15). Those available have also, however, determined candidates on the basis of adult criteria, for example, cognitively normal individuals (86). The true spectrum of children who may benefit from surgery is, therefore, relatively under-reported (65). Dual pathology may also be relatively over-represented in the pediatric age group (see Dual Pathology) (15,73).

Predictors of Postsurgical Outcome in HS

Several factors have been investigated to predict the surgical outcome. In adult surgical series, an earlier age at onset of epilepsy has been related to a most severe histological grade of HS and to a poorer postsurgical outcome (74). This evidence might have at least two different possible explanations: on the one hand, an earlier seizures presentation could reflect a more catastrophic epilepsy type, or, on the contrary, it could be the result of more prolonged epilepsy duration, as most of patients in adult series undergo surgical procedures decades after epilepsy onset (75). Duration of epilepsy is not correlated either to the severity of neuronal loss or with the volumetric reduction of hippocampal structures, once the age at seizure onset is taken into account (74,76). Furthermore, early onset MTLE might be akin to a peculiar subgroup of patients. Previous exposure to different initial precipitating injuries, when present, could also modify surgical outcome. Presence of FS, though a negative prognostic factor for drug control of seizures, is likely to predict a more favorable outcome after surgery (68,75,77–79). Idiopathic HS, however, has worse postsurgical prognosis.

Data from the presurgical evaluation may indicate the likelihood of seizure freedom following surgery. Ictal localization or even lateralization of seizures on scalp EEG, consistent with positive MRI for hippocampal atrophy, predicts seizure control following temporal lobectomy in more than 90% of patients, while in HS MRI-negative patients the outcome is worse (80,81). Furthermore, bilateral FDG-PET abnormalities in unilateral MRI affected patients are related to bilaterally independent epileptic foci and to worse surgical outcome (82). On the contrary, discordance between functional and anatomical data, absence of a clear lesion at MRI, and the subsequent use of intracranial monitoring predict poor seizure outcome (77).

DUAL PATHOLOGY

Dual pathology defines the finding of coexistent HS and other histological alteration such as neoplasms, porencephalic cysts, periventricular heterotopias, and other pathologies (e.g., vascular/ischemic insults, Sturge–Weber syndrome, Rasmussen encephalitis) (Fig. 26.4). The most frequently associated lesions are cortical dysgenesis, in particular type II focal cortical dysplasia (FCD) (83,84). This case definition usually excludes the presence of HS and lesions in temporal lobe in the same patients, as it is difficult to distinguish between pathologies that could directly or indirectly affect the hippocampal neurons.

The prevalence of dual pathology is difficult to assess. Currently, this diagnosis is confirmed in about 5% to 20% of adult surgical candidates, and this rate is likely to increase with decreasing age at presentation (85,86). However, these rates refer to presurgical identification of coexistent lesions using MRI: the low predictive positive value of this technique in determining the presence of either HS in diagnosed extratemporal lesions or subtle FCD in diagnosed HS might underestimate the real prevalence of dual pathology, in particular in pediatric series (26,87). The use of postacquisition analysis may help in identifying subtle alterations of cortical architecture and has been related to poor surgical outcome, but this approach still lacks a clinical framework (27).

The possible etiology of HS in dual pathology is still debated. In contrast to those coming to surgery for primary HS, FS, and SE do not seem to be relevant (26,73). The pattern and severity of hippocampal atrophy seem to be related to associated extratemporal lesions, with less severe neuronal loss associated with acquired lesions (i.e., gliomas, hamartomas) than with developmental lesions (i.e., FCD, cortical heterotopia) (84,88). Thus, it is still unclear if patients with

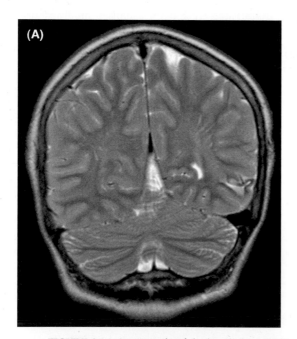 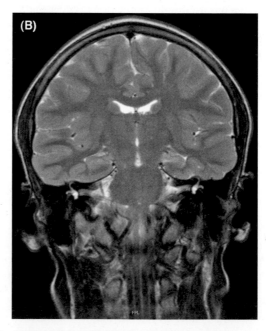

FIGURE 26.4 An example of dual pathology. MRI of a 14-year-old boy who had experienced a small intracerebral bleed in the course of chemotherapy treatment for leukemia at age 8 years; he had developed seizures with temporal lobe semiology. MRI at 14 years revealed a small cavity with low signal on T_2 in the posterior left temporal lobe (**A**) *(arrow)* with also additional evidence of left hippocampal sclerosis (**B**) *(arrow)*.

dual pathology represent a distinctive group of subjects with dissimilar causal and prognostic factors, or if in this group the extratemporal pathology is more detectable than in those patients in which the HS is the only visible lesion.

Virtually all patients reported as having dual pathology present with intractable epilepsy, for which surgery represents elective treatment (69). Individuals with extratemporal cortical subtle abnormalities are about 13 times more likely to have seizures after surgery compared with those who do not have such evidence (27). Therefore, the surgical approach for dual pathology is slightly different from classic HS, as the resection of both lesions is a prerequisite for a good seizure outcome (86).

CONCLUSION

HS remains an important cause of drug-resistant epilepsy in adults; its contribution to pediatric epilepsy is probably greater than appreciated. Debate continues as to the etiology of this pathology, although genetic predisposition and injury appear contributory. Moreover, it may be that multiple etiologies are responsible, resulting in HS as a final common pathway. Where seizures continue, and appear to come from one side, surgery is the optimal treatment of choice.

References

1. Bouchet C, Cazauvielh Y. De l'èpilepsie considèrèe dan ses rapports avec l'aliènation mentale. *Arch Gen Med Par.* 1825;9:510–542.
2. Sommer W. Erkrankung des Ammonshorns als atiologisches Moment der Epilepsie. *Arch f Psychiat Berl.* 1880;10:631–675.
3. Bailey P, Gibbs FA. The surgical treatment of psychomotor epilepsy. *J Am Med Assoc.* 1951;145:365–370.
4. Falconer MA, Taylor DC. Surgical treatment of drug-resistant epilepsy due to mesial temporal sclerosis. Etiology and significance. *Arch Neurol.* 1968;19:353–361.
5. Babb TL. Synaptic reorganizations in human and rat hippocampal epilepsy. *Adv Neurol.* 1999;79:763–779.
6. Lüders H. *Textbook of Epilepsy Surgery.* London: Informa Healthcare; 2008.
7. Proper EA, Oestreicher AB, Jansen GH, et al. Immunohistochemical characterization of mossy fibre sprouting in the hippocampus of patients with pharmaco-resistant temporal lobe epilepsy. *Brain.* 2000;123(Pt 1):19–30.
8. Jackson GD, Berkovic SF, Duncan JS, et al. Optimizing the diagnosis of hippocampal sclerosis using MR imaging. *Am J Neuroradiol.* 1993;14:753–762.
9. Kuzniecky RI, Knowlton RC. Neuroimaging of epilepsy. *Semin Neurol.* 2002;22:279–288.
10. Panayiotopoulos CP, International League against Epilepsy. *The Epilepsies: Seizures, Syndromes and Management : Based on the ILAE Classifications and Practice Parameter Guidelines.* Oxfordshire, UK: Bladon Medical Publishing; 2005.
11. Hauser WA, Annegers JF, Kurland LT. Prevalence of epilepsy in Rochester, Minnesota: 1940–1980. *Epilepsia.* 1991;32:429–445.
12. Wiebe S. Epidemiology of temporal lobe epilepsy. *Can J Neurol Sci.* 2000;27(suppl 1):S6–S10.
13. Benbadis SR, Wallace J, Reed Murtagh F. MRI evidence of mesial temporal sclerosis in subjects without seizures. *Seizure.* 2002;11:340–343.
14. Vickrey BG, Hays RD, Rausch R, et al. Outcomes in 248 patients who had diagnostic evaluations for epilepsy surgery. *Lancet.* 1995;346:1445–1449.
15. Wyllie E, Comair YG, Kotagal P, et al. Seizure outcome after epilepsy surgery in children and adolescents. *Ann Neurol.* 1998;44:740–748.
16. Harvey AS, Cross JH, Shinnar S, et al. Defining the spectrum of international practice in pediatric epilepsy surgery patients. *Epilepsia.* 2008; 49:146–155.
17. Davidson S, Falconer MA. Outcome of surgery in 40 children with temporal-lobe epilepsy. *Lancet.* 1975;1:1260–1263.
18. Grattan-Smith JD, Harvey AS, Desmond PM, et al. Hippocampal sclerosis in children with intractable temporal lobe epilepsy: detection with MR imaging. *Am J Roentgenol.* 1993;161:1045–1048.
19. Cavanagh JB, Meyer A. Aetiological aspects of Ammon's horn sclerosis associated with temporal lobe epilepsy. *Br Med J.* 1956;2:1403–1407.
20. Earle KM, Baldwin M, Penfield W. Incisural sclerosis and temporal lobe seizures produced by hippocampal herniation at birth. *AMA Arch Neurol Psychiatry.* 1953;69:27–42.
21. Armstrong DD. The neuropathology of temporal lobe epilepsy. *J Neuropathol Exp Neurol.* 1993;52:433–443.
22. Squier W, Salisbury H, Sisodiya S. Stroke in the developing brain and intractable epilepsy: effect of timing on hippocampal sclerosis. *Dev Med Child Neurol.* 2003;45:580–585.
23. Theodore WH, Epstein L, Gaillard WD, et al. Human herpes virus 6B: a possible role in epilepsy? *Epilepsia.* 2008;49:1828–1837.
24. Wu HM, Huang CC, Chen SH, et al. Herpes simplex virus type 1 inoculation enhances hippocampal excitability and seizure susceptibility in mice. *Eur J Neurosci.* 2003;18:3294–3304.
25. Meldrum BS, Vigouroux RA, Rage P, et al. Hippocampal lesions produced by prolonged seizures in paralyzed artificially ventilated baboons. *Experientia.* 1973;29:561–563.
26. Riney CJ, Harding B, Harkness WJ, et al. Hippocampal sclerosis in children with lesional epilepsy is influenced by age at seizure onset. *Epilepsia.* 2006;47:159–166.
27. Sisodiya SM, Moran N, Free SL, et al. Correlation of widespread preoperative magnetic resonance imaging changes with unsuccessful surgery for hippocampal sclerosis. *Ann Neurol.* 1997;41:490–496.
28. Scheffer IE, Berkovic SF. Generalized epilepsy with febrile seizures plus. A genetic disorder with heterogeneous clinical phenotypes. *Brain.* 1997; 120(Pt 3):479–490.
29. Vestergaard M, Pedersen CB, Sidenius P, et al. The long-term risk of epilepsy after febrile seizures in susceptible subgroups. *Am J Epidemiol.* 2007;165:911–918.
30. Sillanpaa M, Camfield P, Camfield C, et al. Incidence of febrile seizures in Finland: prospective population-based study. *Pediatr Neurol.* 2008;38:391–394.
31. Mathern GW, Babb TL, Vickrey BG, et al. The clinical-pathogenic mechanisms of hippocampal neuron loss and surgical outcomes in temporal lobe epilepsy. *Brain.* 1995;118(Pt 1):105–118.
32. Offringa M, Bossuyt PM, Lubsen J, et al. Risk factors for seizure recurrence in children with febrile seizures: a pooled analysis of individual patient data from five studies. *J Pediatr.* 1994;124:574–584.
33. Berg AT, Shinnar S, Levy SR, et al. Childhood-onset epilepsy with and without preceding febrile seizures. *Neurology.* 1999;53:1742–1748.
34. Camfield P, Camfield C, Gordon K, et al. What types of epilepsy are preceded by febrile seizures? A population-based study of children. *Dev Med Child Neurol.* 1994;36:887–892.
35. Verity CM, Golding J. Risk of epilepsy after febrile convulsions: a national cohort study. *Br Med J.* 1991;303:1373–1376.
36. Verity CM. Do seizures damage the brain? The epidemiological evidence. *Arch Dis Child.* 1998;78:78–84.
37. Arzimanoglou A. Outcome of status epilepticus in children. *Epilepsia.* 2007;48(suppl 8):91–93.
38. Rosenow F, Hamer HM, Knake S. The epidemiology of convulsive and nonconvulsive status epilepticus. *Epilepsia.* 2007;48(suppl 8):82–84.
39. Scott RC, King MD, Gadian DG, et al. Hippocampal abnormalities after prolonged febrile convulsion: a longitudinal MRI study. *Brain.* 2003;126:2551–2557.
40. Scott RC, King MD, Gadian DG, et al. Prolonged febrile seizures are associated with hippocampal vasogenic edema and developmental changes. *Epilepsia.* 2006;47:1493–1498.
41. Shinnar S, Pellock JM, Berg AT, et al. Short-term outcomes of children with febrile status epilepticus. *Epilepsia.* 2001;42:47–53.
42. Shinnar S, Hesdorffer DC, Nordli DR Jr., et al. Phenomenology of prolonged febrile seizures: results of the FEBSTAT study. *Neurology.* 2008;71:170–176.
43. Scott RC, Gadian DG, Cross JH, et al. Quantitative magnetic resonance characterization of mesial temporal sclerosis in childhood. *Neurology.* 2001;56:1659–1665.
44. Fung CW, Scott RC, Harding B, et al. Clinical spectrum of paediatric patients with mesial temporal lobe epilepsy: hippocampal sclerosis and post-surgical outcome. *Epilepsia.* 2005;46:54–55.
45. Cavazos JE, Das I, Sutula TP. Neuronal loss induced in limbic pathways by kindling: evidence for induction of hippocampal sclerosis by repeated brief seizures. *J Neurosci.* 1994;14:3106–3121.
46. Robinson RJ. Febrile convulsions. *Br Med J.* 1991;303:1345–1346.
47. Mathern GW, Adelson PD, Cahan LD, et al. Hippocampal neuron damage in human epilepsy: Meyer's hypothesis revisited. *Prog Brain Res.* 2002;135:237–251.
48. Mathern GW, Babb TL, Mischel PS, et al. Childhood generalized and mesial temporal epilepsies demonstrate different amounts and patterns of hippocampal neuron loss and mossy fibre synaptic reorganization. *Brain.* 1996;119(Pt 3):965–987.
49. Scott RC, Cross JH, Gadian DG, et al. Abnormalities in hippocampi remote from the seizure focus: a T2 relaxometry study. *Brain.* 2003;126:1968–1974.
50. Lindsay J, Ounsted C, Richards P. Long-term outcome in children with temporal lobe seizures. I: Social outcome and childhood factors. *Dev Med Child Neurol.* 1979;21:285–298.
51. Sperber EF, Haas KZ, Stanton PK, et al. Resistance of the immature hippocampus to seizure-induced synaptic reorganization. *Brain Res Dev Brain Res.* 1991;60:88–93.
52. French JA, Williamson PD, Thadani VM, et al. Characteristics of medial temporal lobe epilepsy: I. Results of history and physical examination. *Ann Neurol.* 1993;34:774–780.

53. Wieser HG. ILAE Commission Report. Mesial temporal lobe epilepsy with hippocampal sclerosis. *Epilepsia.* 2004;45:695–714.

54. Fogarasi A, Tuxhorn I, Janszky J, et al. Age-dependent seizure semiology in temporal lobe epilepsy. *Epilepsia.* 2007;48:1697–1702.

55. Williamson PD, French JA, Thadani VM, et al. Characteristics of medial temporal lobe epilepsy: II. Interictal and ictal scalp electroencephalography, neuropsychological testing, neuroimaging, surgical results, and pathology. *Ann Neurol.* 1993;34:781–787.

56. Hamer HM, Najm I, Mohamed A, et al. Interictal epileptiform discharges in temporal lobe epilepsy due to hippocampal sclerosis versus medial temporal lobe tumors. *Epilepsia.* 1999;40:1261–1268.

57. Dericioglu N, Saygi S. Ictal scalp EEG findings in patients with mesial temporal lobe epilepsy. *Clin EEG Neurosci.* 2008;39:20–27.

58. Foldvary N, Klem G, Hammel J, et al. The localizing value of ictal EEG in focal epilepsy. *Neurology.* 2001;57:2022–2028.

59. Willmann O, Wennberg R, May T, et al. The contribution of 18F-FDG PET in preoperative epilepsy surgery evaluation for patients with temporal lobe epilepsy: a meta-analysis. *Seizure.* 2007;16:509–520.

60. Spanaki MV, Spencer SS, Corsi M, et al. Sensitivity and specificity of quantitative difference SPECT analysis in seizure localization. *J Nucl Med.* 1999;40:730–736.

61. Van Paesschen W. Ictal SPECT. *Epilepsia.* 2004;45(suppl 4):35–40.

62. Foong J, Flugel D. Psychiatric outcome of surgery for temporal lobe epilepsy and presurgical considerations. *Epilepsy Res.* 2007;75:84–96.

63. Manchanda R, Schaefer B, McLachlan RS, et al. Psychiatric disorders in candidates for surgery for epilepsy. *J Neurol Neurosurg Psychiatry.* 1996;61:82–89.

64. Matsuura M, Oana Y, Kato M, et al. A multicenter study on the prevalence of psychiatric disorders among new referrals for epilepsy in Japan. *Epilepsia.* 2003;44:107–114.

65. McLellan A, Davies S, Heyman I, et al. Psychopathology in children with epilepsy before and after temporal lobe resection. *Dev Med Child Neurol.* 2005;47:666–672.

66. Berg AT, Langfitt J, Shinnar S, et al. How long does it take for partial epilepsy to become intractable? *Neurology.* 2003;60:186–190.

67. Stephen LJ, Kwan P, Brodie MJ. Does the cause of localisation-related epilepsy influence the response to antiepileptic drug treatment? *Epilepsia.* 2001;42:357–362.

68. Kim WJ, Park SC, Lee SJ, et al. The prognosis for control of seizures with medications in patients with MRI evidence for mesial temporal sclerosis. *Epilepsia.* 1999;40:290–293.

69. Semah F, Lamy C, Demeret S. Hippocampal sclerosis and other hippocampal abnormalities in the early identification of candidates for epilepsy surgery. *Arch Neurol.* 2002;59:1042–1043.

70. Duchowny M, Levin B, Jayakar P, et al. Temporal lobectomy in early childhood. *Epilepsia.* 1992;33:298–303.

71. Hermann B, Davies K, Foley K, et al. Visual confrontation naming outcome after standard left anterior temporal lobectomy with sparing versus resection of the superior temporal gyrus: a randomized prospective clinical trial. *Epilepsia.* 1999;40:1070–1076.

72. Arruda F, Cendes F, Andermann F, et al. Mesial atrophy and outcome after amygdalohippocampectomy or temporal lobe removal. *Ann Neurol.* 1996;40:446–450.

73. Maton B, Jayakar P, Resnick T, et al. Surgery for medically intractable temporal lobe epilepsy during early life. *Epilepsia.* 2008;49:80–87.

74. Davies KG, Hermann BP, Dohan FC Jr., et al. Relationship of hippocampal sclerosis to duration and age of onset of epilepsy, and childhood febrile seizures in temporal lobectomy patients. *Epilepsy Res.* 1996;24:119–126.

75. Elsharkawy AE, Alabbasi AH, Pannek H, et al. Long-term outcome after temporal lobe epilepsy surgery in 434 consecutive adult patients. *J Neurosurg.* 2009;110:1135–1146.

76. Cendes F, Andermann F, Gloor P, et al. Atrophy of mesial structures in patients with temporal lobe epilepsy: cause or consequence of repeated seizures? *Ann Neurol.* 1993;34:795–801.

77. Tonini C, Beghi E, Berg AT, et al. Predictors of epilepsy surgery outcome: a meta-analysis. *Epilepsy Res.* 2004;62:75–87.

78. Pittau F, Bisulli F, Mai R, et al. Prognostic factors in patients with mesial temporal lobe epilepsy. *Epilepsia.* 2009;50(suppl 1):41–44.

79. Janszky J, Schulz R, Ebner A. Clinical features and surgical outcome of medial temporal lobe epilepsy with a history of complex febrile convulsions. *Epilepsy Res.* 2003;55:1–8.

80. Spencer SS. When should temporal-lobe epilepsy be treated surgically? *Lancet Neurol.* 2002;1:375–382.

81. Jack CR Jr., Sharbrough FW, Cascino GD, et al. Magnetic resonance image-based hippocampal volumetry: correlation with outcome after temporal lobectomy. *Ann Neurol.* 1992;31:138–146.

82. Koutroumanidis M, Hennessy MJ, Seed PT, et al. Significance of interictal bilateral temporal hypometabolism in temporal lobe epilepsy. *Neurology.* 2000;54:1811–1821.

83. Fauser S, Schulze-Bonhage A, Honegger J, et al. Focal cortical dysplasias: surgical outcome in 67 patients in relation to histological subtypes and dual pathology. *Brain.* 2004;127:2406–2418.

84. Levesque MF, Nakasato N, Vinters HV, et al. Surgical treatment of limbic epilepsy associated with extrahippocampal lesions: the problem of dual pathology. *J Neurosurg.* 1991;75:364–370.

85. Kutsy RL. Focal extratemporal epilepsy: clinical features, EEG patterns, and surgical approach. *J Neurol Sci.* 1999;166:1–15.

86. Li LM, Cendes F, Andermann F, et al. Surgical outcome in patients with epilepsy and dual pathology. *Brain.* 1999;122(Pt 5):799–805.

87. Mohamed A, Wyllie E, Ruggieri P, et al. Temporal lobe epilepsy due to hippocampal sclerosis in pediatric candidates for epilepsy surgery. *Neurology.* 2001;56:1643–1649.

88. de Lanerolle NC, Kim JH, Williamson A, et al. A retrospective analysis of hippocampal pathology in human temporal lobe epilepsy: evidence for distinctive patient subcategories. *Epilepsia.* 2003;44:677–687.

CHAPTER 27 ■ MALFORMATIONS OF CORTICAL DEVELOPMENT AND EPILEPSY

GHAYDA MIRZAA, RUBEN KUZNIECKY, AND RENZO GUERRINI

The formation and development of the human cerebral cortex is a complex dynamic process that can be broken down into partially overlapping stages that occur over the span of several gestational weeks (1). During the first stage, stem cells proliferate and differentiate into young neurons or glial cells deep in the forebrain, with the ventricular and subventricular zones lining the cerebral cavity. During the second stage, neurons migrate away from their place of origin toward the pial surface and settle within the cortical plate. When neurons reach their destination, they order themselves into specific "architectonic" patterns and this third phase involves final organization within the typical six layers of cortex, associated with synaptogenesis and apoptosis.

Any disruption of this process, whether by genetic or environmental factors, may result in malformations of cortical development (MCD). Until the advent of high-resolution neuroimaging and the recent increase in the treatment of neocortical epilepsy by surgery, these disorders were much less commonly known. Magnetic resonance imaging (MRI) has allowed MCD to be identified earlier in life, leading to improved diagnosis, knowledge of the clinical consequences, and rapid progress in understanding their pathogenesis. This chapter reviews common cortical malformations associated with epilepsy.

CLASSIFICATION

The first classification scheme for MCD, proposed in 1996, was based on the first developmental step (cell proliferation, neuronal migration, cortical organization) at which the developmental process was disturbed (2). Since then, increasing recognition of MCD and ongoing improvement in imaging techniques, molecular biology techniques, and knowledge of mechanisms of brain development have resulted in continual and rapid improvement of the understanding of these disorders. The most recent update to the classification scheme was proposed in 2005 (3). This genotype-based scheme allows for a better conceptual understanding of these disorders (Table 27.1). Table 27.2 presents the most updated list of genes/loci identified in relation to MCD (40). The nomenclature and classification will undoubtedly continue to evolve during the upcoming years.

MALFORMATIONS OF CORTICAL DEVELOPMENT

Accurate diagnosis relies on recognition of the malformation on brain imaging studies; assessment of the prognosis and genetic counseling depend on the specific diagnosis. In the following sections, the genetic, imaging, and functional aspects of some of the most common MCD will be discussed with special emphasis on epilepsy associated with these disorders.

MCD DUE TO ABNORMAL PROLIFERATION/APOPTOSIS (ABNORMALITIES OF BRAIN SIZE)

Malformations in this group are characterized by an increase or decrease in the number of neurons and glia with corresponding changes in brain size, designated as either microcephaly or megalencephaly (MEG). No abnormal cell types are seen. The most common types of microcephaly and MEG are not typically included under brain malformations because brain structure appears grossly normal; however, detailed studies of neuronal cell types have not been described.

Microcephaly Syndromes

Microcephaly, as a primary abnormality, is best defined as a head circumference of three standard deviations or more below the mean. When congenital microcephaly is the only abnormality on evaluation, the disorder is called primary microcephaly, or microcephaly vera (41,42) though these terms are often little understood.

Most of these patients fall into two groups (43). The first group comprises children with extreme microcephaly but only moderate neurologic problems, usually only moderate mental retardation without spasticity or epilepsy. Several genes associated with this phenotype have been identified (see Table 27.2).

The second and more important group from an epilepsy standpoint consists of primary microcephaly with severe spasticity and epilepsy (43–46). Abnormal reflexes and generalized spasticity are evident antenatally. Subsequent poor feeding and recurrent vomiting lead to poor weight gain, severe developmental delay, with consequent profound mental retardation and spastic quadriparesis. Early onset intractable epilepsy is common. In addition to a simplified gyral pattern, MRI of the brain may show enlarged extra-axial spaces, delayed myelination, agenesis of the corpus callosum, or severe hypoplasia of the brainstem and cerebellum. This clinical spectrum suggests pathogenetically heterogenous conditions, and several genes have been identified (see Table 27.2).

Children with severe congenital microcephaly are often incorrectly diagnosed as having lissencephaly (LIS) because of a reduced number of broad gyri; however the cortex is not

TABLE 27.1

CLASSIFICATION SCHEME FOR MALFORMATIONS OF CORTICAL DEVELOPMENT[a]

I. Malformations due to abnormal neuronal and glial proliferation or apoptosis
   A. Decreased proliferation/increased apoptosis or increased proliferation/decreased apoptosis—abnormalities of brain size
     1. Microcephaly with normal to thin cortex
     2. Microlisssencephaly (extreme microcephaly with thick cortex)
     3. Microcephaly with extensive polymicrogyria
     4. Macrocephalies
   B. Abnormal proliferation (abnormal cell types)
     1. Non-neoplastic
       a. Cortical hamartomas of tuberous sclerosis
       b. Cortical dysplasia with balloon cells
       c. Hemimegalencephaly
     2. Neoplastic (associated with disordered cortex)
       a. Dysembryoplastic neuroepithelial tumor
       b. Ganglioglioma
       c. Gangliocytoma
II. Malformations due to abnormal neuronal migration
   A. Lissencephaly/subcortical band heterotopia spectrum
   B. Cobblesone complex/congenital muscular dystrophy syndromes
   C. Heterotopias
     1. Subependymal (periventricular)
     2. Subcortical (other than band heterotopias)
     3. Marginal glioneuronal
III. Malformations due to abnormal cortical organization (including late neuronal migration)
   A. Polymicrogyria and schizencephaly
     1. Bilateral polymicrogyria syndromes
     2. Schizencephaly (polymicrogyria with clefts)
     3. Polymicrogyria or schizencephaly as part of multiple congenital anomaly/mental retardation syndromes
   B. Cortical dysplasia with balloon cells
   C. Microdysgenesis
IV. Malformations of cortical development, not otherwise classified
   A. Malformations secondary to inborn errors of metabolism
     1. Mitochondrial and pyruvate metabolic disorders
     2. Peroxisomal disorders
   B. Other unclassified malformations
     1. Sublobar dysplasia
     2. Others

[a]Each main category is expanded in additional tables in Ref. 3.

thick as in true LIS (Fig. 27.1), and genetic tests for LIS are always normal. A few patients with severe congenital microcephaly and a thick cortex are designated to have microlissencephaly (47); these children also have intractable epilepsy. Most syndromes with severe congenital microcephaly have autosomal recessive inheritance.

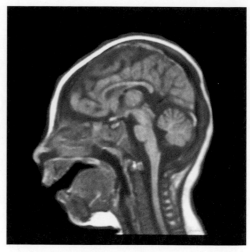

FIGURE 27.1 Microcephaly. Sagittal MRI demonstrates microcephaly (<3SD) with relative preservation of normal sulcal cerebral anatomy.

Megalencephaly Syndromes

MEG occurs as a mild familial variant with normal brain structure, but is otherwise an uncommon brain malformation that may be associated with developmental and neurological problems (48). The clinical findings have been variable but are usually mild to moderate, particularly with the familial form. A subset of patients has severe mental retardation, intractable epilepsy, and other neurologic abnormalities (48); however, the basis for this difference is not clear and a few distinct subtypes have been described. Several MEG syndromes with cortical malformations and severe epilepsy are likely underrecognized (see Table 27.2).

MCD DUE TO ABNORMAL PROLIFERATION (ABNORMAL CELL TYPES)

Malformations in this group are characterized by abnormal neurons and, often, glia. All of these are localized malformations. In some, abnormal cell types have been classified neoplastic, although the malignant potential is low. The most common of these is tuberous sclerosis complex reviewed in (Chapter 31).

Hemimegalencephaly

Hemimegalencephaly (HMEG) is a brain malformation characterized by the presence of an enlarged and dysplastic cerebral hemisphere (Fig. 27.2). The overgrowth may occasionally involve part of the hemisphere or the entire hemisphere in addition to a part of the contralateral one as well. Macroscopically, the involved hemisphere is enlarged with cortical dysgenesis, white matter hypertrophy, and a dilated and dysmorphic lateral ventricle. There is no clear predilection for right or left sides (49). The microscopic features of HMEG vary significantly and may include polymicrogyria (PMG), heterotopic gray matter, cortical dysplasia (cortical dyslamination,

TABLE 27.2

GENETIC MALFORMATIONS OF CORTICAL DEVELOPMENT

Malformations and syndromes	Gene	Locus	Refs
Malformations due to abnormal neuronal and glial proliferation or apoptosis			
Decreased proliferation/increased apoptosis or increased proliferation/decreased apoptosis—abnormalities of brain size			
Microcephaly (MIC)			
Moderate phenotype: MIC group 1	ASPM, MCPH1	9q34, 15q, 19q13	
MIC, severe phenotype			
Amish, lethal MIC	SLC25A19	17q25.3	
MIC with heterotopias	ARFGEF2	20q13.13	
MIC group 2, other types	—	—	
Seckel syndrome	ATR	3q22-q24	
Microlissencephaly (MLIS)			
MLIS group a, *a = p*	—	—	
Barth MLIS syndrome (group b), *a = p*	—	—	
Megalencephaly (MEG)			
MEG, isolated	—	—	
Macrocephaly-capillary malformation (M-CM) syndrome	—	—	
MEG with megacorpus callosum	—	—	
MEG polymicrogyria (PMG) polydactyly–hydrocephalus	—	—	
Abnormal proliferation (abnormal cell types)			
Focal cortical dysplasia			
Tuberous sclerosis	TSC1	9q34.13	(4)
Tuberous sclerosis	TSC2	16p13.3	(5)
Hemimegalencephaly (HMEG)			
HMEG, isolated	—	—	
Epidermal nevus syndrome	—	—	
Hypomelanosis of Ito	—	—	
Klippel–Trenaunay syndrome	—	—	
Neuromelanosis	—	—	
Proteus syndrome	—	—	
Malformations due to abnormal neuronal migration			
Lissencephaly (LIS)			
Classic LIS			
Baraitser–Winter Syndrome, *a > p*	—	—	
Miller–Dieker Syndrome (MDS), *a = p*	LIS1 + YWHAE	17P13.3	(6)
Isolated LIS sequence, *a = p, a > p*	DCX	Xq22.3-q23	(7)
Isolated LIS sequence, *a = p, p > a*	LIS1	17p13.3	(8)
Subcortical band heterotopias, *a = p, a > p*	DCX	Xq22.3-q23	(7)
LIS with cerebellar hypoplasia (LCH)			
LCH group a, *a = p, a > p, p > a*	LIS1, DCX	17p13.3, Xq22.3-q23	
LCH group b, *a > p*	RELN	7q22.1	(9)
	VLDLR	9p24.2	(10)
LCH group d, *a = p*	—	—	
LIS with ACC			
XLAG, *p > a*	ARX	Xp22.1	(11)
LIS with agenesis of the corpus callosum (ACC), other types	—	—	
Cobblestone cortical malformations (AR)			
Fukuyama congenital muscular dystrophy or Walker–Warburg syndrome (WWS)	FCMD	9q31.2	(12)
Muscle–eye–brain (MEB) disease or WWS	FKRP	19q13.32	(13)

(Continued)

TABLE 27.2 (Continued)

Malformations and syndromes	Gene	Locus	Refs
MEB	*LARGE*	22q12.3	(14)
MEB	*POMGnT1*	1p34.1	(15)
MEB or WWS	*POMT1*	9q34.13	(16)
MEB or WWS	*POMT2*	14q24.3	(17)
Bilateral frontoparietal cobblestone malformation (previously polymicrogyria)	*GPR56*	16q13	(18)
Heterotopia (XL, AD)			
Classical bilateral periventricular nodular heterotopia (PNH)	*FLNA*	Xq28	(19)
Ehlers–Danlos syndrome and PNH	*FLNA*	Xq28	(19)
Facial dysmorphisms, severe constipation, and PNH	*FLNA*	Xq28	(20)
Fragile-X syndrome and PNH	*FMR1*	Xq27.3	(21)
Williams syndrome and PNH	—	7q11.23	(22)
PNH with limb abnormalities (limb reduction abnormality or syndactyly)	—	Xq28	(23)
Agenesis of the corpus callosum and PNH	—	1p36.22-pter	(24)
Agenesis of the corpus callosum, polymicrogyria, and PNH	—	6q26-qter	(25)
PNH	—	5p15.1	(26)
PNH	—	5p15.33	(26)
PNH	—	4p15	(27)
Heterotopia (AR)			
Microcephaly and PNH	*ARFGEF2*	20p13	(28)
Donnai–Barrow syndrome and PNH	*LRP2*		(27)
CEDNIK syndrome	*SNAP29*	22q11.2	(29)
Malformations due to abnormal cortical organization			
Polymicrogyria (XL, AD)			
Rolandic seizures, oromotor dyspraxia	*SRPX2*	Xq22	(30)
Agenesis of the corpus callosum (ACC), microcephaly, and polymicrogyria (PMG)	*TBR2*	3p21	(31)
Aniridia plus	*PAX6*	11p13	(32)
PMG	—	1p36.3-pter	(33)
Microcephaly, PMG	—	1q44-qter	(34)
Facial dysmorphism and PMG	—	2p16.1-p23	(35)
Microcephaly, hydrocephalus, and PMG	—	4q21-q22	(36)
PMG	—	21q2	(37)
DiGeorge syndrome	—	22q11.2	(4)
Polymicrogyria (AR)			
Goldberg–Shprintzen syndrome	*KIAA1279*	10q21.3	(38)
Microsyndrome	*RAB3GAP1*	2q21.3	(39)

bizarre enlarged neurons, balloon cells), blurring of the gray–white junction, and an increase in the number of neurons and astrocytes (50–52).

HMEG is most often an isolated congenital abnormality, but is sporadically associated with neurocutaneous and overgrowth syndromes. Neurocutaneous associations include the linear nevus sebaceous syndrome (53) (where 50% have associated HMEG), hypomelanosis of Ito (54), tuberous sclerosis (55), and neurofibromatosis (56).

The etiology of HMEG remains unknown with no clear environmental associations or chromosomal abnormalities. It is generally assumed that HMEG results from a defect leading to excessive proliferation of both neurons and astrocytes, and the known associations of HMEG with other disorders of cellular proliferation (such as [tuberous sclerosis (TSC) and neurofibromatosis (NF)]) support this hypothesis.

The clinical triad of HMEG is typically (i) intractable partial seizures starting from the neonatal period or early infancy, (ii) unilateral neurologic signs (hemiparesis, hemianopia), and (iii) developmental delay (57). Seizures are typically partial and are almost always intractable to medical therapy. Infantile spasms, tonic seizures, or electroclinical features of Ohtahara syndrome (58) or West syndrome may occur.

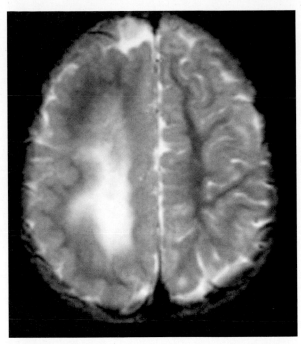

FIGURE 27.2 Hemimegalencephaly. Axial MRI shows large hemisphere with white matter changes. Note the smooth cortex in the posterior region.

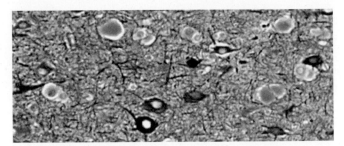

FIGURE 27.3 Focal cortical dysplasia. Silver staining showing irregular arrangement of big neurons and pale brown balloon cells.

The MRI appearance is characteristic. The enlargement of at least one lobe that may range from mild to severe is present in all patients. In some, enlargement may be localized to the frontal or temporoparietal regions. The gray matter is almost uniformly abnormal showing areas of thickening and simplification or overfolding, resembling pachygyria or PMG, respectively. The underlying hemispheric white matter is usually abnormal with abnormal signal characteristics and/or alteration in volume (increased or decreased) in some individuals. Heterotopia is commonly seen, and the ventricular system is enlarged in most patients. Electroencephalographic abnormalities are often extensive throughout the abnormal hemisphere and a suppression burst pattern can be observed early on in the most severe cases.

Predictors of poor outcome are severity of hemiparesis, smoothness of the cortical surface on MRI, and abnormal activity on electroencephalography (EEG). Both the epilepsy and the developmental delay may be improved in selected patients by anatomical or functional hemispherectomy (59,60).

Focal Cortical Dysplasia

The term focal cortical dysplasia (FCD) (59,60) designates a spectrum of abnormalities of the laminar structure of the cortex, variably associated with cytopathological features including giant (or cytomegalic) neurons, dysmorphic neurons, and balloon cells (61,62) (Fig. 27.3). Despite attempts to classify FCD based on subtle histological characteristics (61,62), no consistent nomenclature has been reached. One existing system is based on the presence or absence of abnormal cells, primarily balloon cells or large dysmorphic neurons (with FCD without balloon cells called type 1 and with balloon cells type 2). FCD shows a spectrum of severity in terms of its gross morphology, topography, and microscopic

features. At the mildest end of the spectrum is "microdysgenesis," which is poorly defined and refers to subtle developmental cortical abnormalities including neuronal heterotopias, undulations of cortical layering, or neuronal clusters amongst cell sparse areas (63). Microdysgenesis has been found at autopsy more commonly in those with epilepsy compared to controls without epilepsy or other neurological disorders (64) as well as in surgical specimens from patients with medically intractable epilepsy (63,65). Despite this, it remains unclear what degree of microdysgenesis may fall within the normal spectrum (66).

According to the prevailing hypothesis, FCD originates from abnormal migration, maturation, and cell death during ontogenesis (67,68). The close cytoarchitectural similarities between FCD and the cortical tubers of tuberous sclerosis (TS) prompted the hypothesis of a common pathogenetic basis (69), and a study has supported the role of TSC1 gene in the pathogenesis of FCD (69), although this remains yet to be confirmed. Moreover, histopathologic similarities between FCD, HMEG, and the dysembryoplastic neuroepithelial tumors (70), two highly epileptogenic developmental lesions, further support the hypothesis of a developmental origin. A link has been postulated between FCD and perinatal or early postnatal brain injury, with subsequent cell differentiation in the scarred area (70,71).

The most common clinical sequelae of FCD are seizures, developmental delay or intellectual disability, and focal neurologic deficits (72–74). Related epilepsy is usually focal, intractable, and often complicated by focal status epilepticus. FCD has been shown to be intrinsically epileptogenic both in vivo using corticography during epilepsy surgery (75) and in vitro using cortex resected from patients with intractable epilepsy (76,77).

FCD is rarely visible by computerized tomography (CT) and the mildest malformations can be cryptic to MRI. Other lesions can be detected by blurring of the cortex–white matter junction on T1-weighted images as well as cortical thickening or abnormal T2 or fluid attenuated inversion recovery (FLAIR) hyperintensity in the white matter of a gyrus or in the depth of a sulcus (78). When a band of abnormal signal intensity is seen extending from the cortex to the superolateral margin of the lateral ventricle (Fig. 27.4), the lesion is called transmantle dysplasia.

Cortical Dysplasia with Neoplastic Changes

Several low-grade, primarily neuronal, neoplasms are associated with cortical dysplasia, including dysembryoplastic neuroepithelial tumors, ganglioglioma, and gangliocytoma.

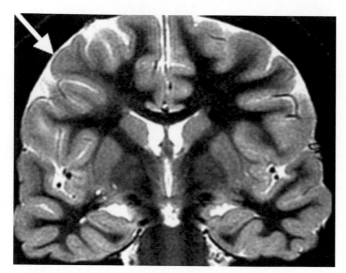

FIGURE 27.4 Coronal T2W MRI showing an area of irregular corti-cal folding *(arrow)* with blurring of the gray–white matter junction and underlying increased signal intensità in the white matter, extend-ing from the subcortex to the ventricular wall. This combination of findings is consistent with focal cortical displasia.

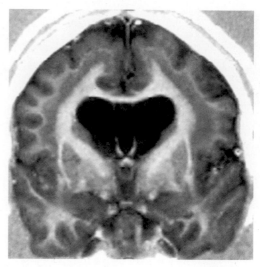

FIGURE 27.5 DCX mutation in a female. Coronal T1W image shows typical subcortical band heterotopia with relative preservation of cortical anatomy.

Controversy continues over their proper classification. These neoplasms occur most often in children and young adults, and the frequency of these neoplasms in epilepsy surgical series is approximately 5% to 8%. The tumors are most often located in the temporal lobes, where residual heterotopic neurons in the white matter are also common (79,80), but can be seen elsewhere. Patients usually present with partial seizures that are difficult to control with anticonvulsant drugs. Surgical treatment is highly effective in most cases if the lesion is com-pletely resected.

MALFORMATIONS DUE TO ABNORMAL NEURONAL MIGRATION (NEURONAL MIGRATION DISORDERS)

Lissencephaly and Subcortical Band Heterotopia

LIS is characterized by absent (agyria) or decreased (pachy-gyria) convolutions, producing cortical thickness and a smooth cerebral surface (81). Several types of LIS have been recog-nized. The most common, classical (or type 1) LIS, features a very thick cortex (10 to 20 mm vs. the normal 4 mm) and no other brain malformations. The cytoarchitecture consists of four primitive layers, rather than the normal six (82–84). From the cortical surface inwards, these consist of (i) a poorly defined marginal zone with increased cellularity, (ii) a superfi-cial cortical gray zone with diffusely scattered neurons, (iii) a relatively neuron-sparse zone, and (iv) a deep cortical gray zone with neurons often oriented in columns (85).

Subcortical band heterotopia (SBH) consists of bands of gray matter interposed in the white matter between the cortex and the lateral ventricles (Fig. 27.5) (86). LIS and SBH com-prise a single malformation. This conclusion is based on observations of rare patients with areas of LIS that merge into

SBH and of multiple families with X-linked LIS in males and SBH in females (87–90).

Two major genes have been associated with classical LIS and SBH. The *LIS1* gene is responsible for the autosomal form of *LIS1* (91), while the doublecortin gene *(DCX or XLIS)* is X-linked (92,93). Although either gene can result in either LIS or SBH, most cases of classical LIS are due to deletions or mutations of *LIS1* (94), whereas most cases of SBH are due to mutations of *DCX* (7). *LIS1*-related LIS is more severe in the posterior brain regions ($p > a$ gradient) (Fig. 27.6), whereas *DCX*-related LIS is more severe in the anterior brain ($a > p$ gradient).

Children with classical LIS often appear normal as new-borns but sometimes have apnea, poor feeding, or hypotonia. Seizures are uncommon during the first few days of life, but typically begin before 6 months of age. The epileptic spectrum

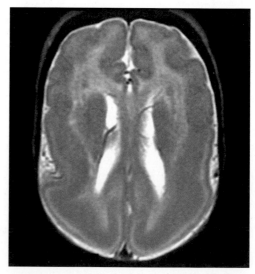

FIGURE 27.6 Lissencephaly. *LIS1* mutation. MRI shows the typical smooth cortex with predominant changes in the posterior regions with the sparse layer seen in the cortex.

is homogenous. In the first year of life, approximately 80% of children present with infantile spasms, often appearing initially as hypsarrhythmia on EEG. The infantile spasms respond at first to corticotrophin or other anticonvulsants in majority of children, but in the long-term, almost all of these children will have frequent seizures and many meet criteria for Lennox–Gastaut syndrome (Chapter 22). Profound mental retardation, early hypotonia, mild spastic quadriplegia, and opisthotonus also are seen. Many patients require a gastrostomy because of poor nutrition and repeated episodes of aspiration and pneumonia (95).

In contrast, patients with SBH and the rare patients with partial LIS have mild to moderate mental retardation (although normal intelligence and severe mental retardation occur), minimal pyramidal signs, and dysarthria (96–98). Seizures usually begin during childhood but may appear much later, and multiple types occur that may be difficult to control; however frequency and severity vary. Epilepsy may be an independent factor to cognitive delay. EEG usually shows generalized spike–wave discharges or multifocal abnormalities (96,99,100). The neurologic outcome depends on the thickness of the heterotopic band on MRI.

Lissencephaly Syndromes and Genes

The most common LIS syndromes include isolated LIS sequence (DCX in males, LIS1 and rarely TUBA1A), SBHs (DCX in females and rarely in males, and LIS1), Miller–Dieker syndrome (MDS) (codeletion of LIS1 and YWHAE), several types of LIS with cerebellar hypoplasia (including mild LIS with cerebellar hypoplasia "group b" [RELN and VLDLR]), and X-linked LIS with abnormal genitalia (ARX). Table 27.3 lists the frequency of the identified mutations in these syndromes. Careful review of brain imaging and clinical features can distinguish these syndromes and usually the causative gene (see Table 27.2).

Isolated lissencephaly sequence (ILIS) consists of classic LIS with a mild facial dysmorphism including mild bitemporal hallowing and small jaw (95,101). ILIS associated with mutations of the X-linked DCX gene is characterized by either severe LIS with no apparent gradient or an $a > p$ gradient and a normal facial appearance (102,103), whereas mutations or deletions of the LIS1 gene produce LIS with $p > a$ gradient (see Fig. 27.6). Facial appearance may be normal or have subtle dysmorphism similar to MDS but much milder (6,95).

MDS consists of classic LIS, facial dysmorphism, and variable other birth defects such as heart malformations and omphalocele. Characteristic dysmorphic facial features include prominent forehead, bitemporal hollowing, short nose with upturned nares, protuberant upper lip with then vermilion border, and small jaw. The brain malformation characteristic of MDS is severe LIS with no apparent gradient, or rarely a $p > a$ gradient similar to ILIS with LIS mutations (6,104). All patients have large deletions of chromosome 17p13 that include LIS1 and YWHAE. About 60% to 70% of deletions are detected by karyotype; the remainder are detectable by fluorescence in situ hybridization (FISH) (6,104).

LIS with cerebellar hypoplasia (LCH) affects a small percentage of patients with LIS syndromes. Group a, the most common type, resembles isolated LIS syndrome but with the addition of mild cerebellar vermis hypoplasia. Some patients have mutations of DCX or LIS1 but much less frequently than patients with typical ILIS. Group b consists of moderate LIS with an $a > p$ gradient, moderate 8 to 10 mm cortical thickness, a globular hippocampus, and a small afoliar cerebellum. Some patients with these imaging findings have mutations of RELN (105–107).

X-linked LIS with abnormal genitalia (XLAG) is a variant LIS in genotypic males with a $p > a$ gradient and intermediate 8 to 10 mm cortical thickness, usually complete agenesis of the corpus callosum, often cavitated or indistinct basal ganglia, severe postnatal microcephaly, and ambiguous or severely hypoplastic genitalia. Affected children have profound mental retardation, hypothalamic dysfunction with poor temperature regulation, intractable epilepsy typically beginning on the first day of life, infancy-onset dyskinesia that may be difficult to distinguish from seizures, and chronic diarrhea (11,108). Female relatives, including some mothers, have isolated agenesis of the corpus callosum. Mutations of the ARX gene have been found in almost all patients (11,109).

TABLE 27.3

FREQUENCY OF MUTATIONS IN LISSENCEPHALY AND SUBCORTICAL BAND HETEROTOPIA SYNDROMES

Syndrome	Gene or locus				
	ARX	DCX	LIS1	Del 17p	RELN
ILS	0	~12	~24	~40	0
LCH	Rare	~25	~15	0[a]	Rare
MDS	0	0	0	All[b]	0
SBH	0	~80	Rare	Rare	0
XLAG	95	0	0	0	0

LIS, lissencephaly; SBH, subcortical band heterotopias; ILS, isolated lissencephaly sequence; LCH, lissencephaly with cerebellar hypoplasia; MDS, Miller–Dieker syndrome; XLAG, X-linked lissencephaly with abnormal genitalia.
[a]Deletion of 17 p 13.3 could be seen in lissencephaly group a (mild vermis hypoplasia).
[b]Miller–Dieker syndrome is partly defined by the deletion.

Cobblestone Brain Malformations (Cobblestone Complex)

Cobblestone complex (previously type 2 or cobblestone LIS) is a severe brain malformation consisting of cobblestone cortex, abnormal white matter (Fig. 27.7), enlarged ventricles often with hydrocephalus, small brainstem, and small dysplastic cerebellum (110–115). In the most severely affected patients, the brain surface is smooth, which led to the designation as LIS, although less severe cobblestone malformations have an irregular, pebbled surface rather than a smooth surface. Severe expression may include progressive hydrocephalus, large posterior fossa cysts (atypical for Dandy–Walker malformation), and occipital cephaloceles. Eye malformations are frequent, and congenital muscular dystrophy is probably always present.

The cobblestone malformation has been observed in three genetic syndromes, although they may clearly overlap: Fukuyama congenital muscular dystrophy, muscle–eye–brain (MEB) disease, and Walker–Warburg syndrome (WWS). All share a clinical course of severe to profound mental retardation, severe hypotonia, mild distal spasticity, and often poor vision.

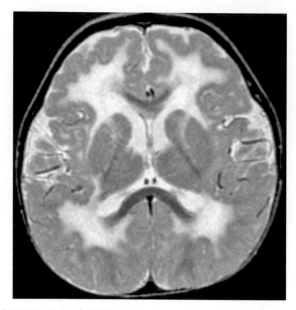

FIGURE 27.7 Axial T2W MRI shows extensive white matter changes and polymicrogyria typical of cobblestone lissencephaly due to a Fukutin mutation.

Fukuyama congenital muscular dystrophy consists of relatively mild cobblestone complex, moderate to severe mental retardation and epilepsy, and severe congenital muscular dystrophy with progressive weakness, joint contractures, and elevated serum levels of creatine kinase (116,117). The causative FCMD gene was identified, as also a common founder mutation of this gene in the Japanese population (12,118).

MEB disease consists of moderate cobblestone dysplasia with moderate to severe mental retardation, epilepsy, complex eye abnormalities (including retinal and choroidal hypoplasia, optic nerve pallor, high-grade myopia, anterior chamber-angle abnormalities, glaucoma, iris hypoplasia, cataracts and rare colobomas (119)), and congenital muscular dystrophy or myopathy with weakness, contractures, and elevated serum levels of creatine kinase. Mutations of three genes, FKRP, LARGE, and POMGnT1, have been found.

WWS includes LIS and the most severe brainstem and cerebellar malformations of any of the cobblestone group. Most patients have hydrocephalus, and approximately 25% have occipital cephaloceles (110,111). All patients have profound mental retardation, epilepsy, and eye abnormalities similar to those of MEB disease and the same congenital muscular dystrophy or myopathy with elevated serum levels of creatine kinase and contractures. Mutations of POMGnT1 do not appear to cause WWS (110,111). However, mutations of POMT1 and FCMD have been found in a few patients (15,120,121).

Heterotopia

Heterotopia is defined as groups of cells found in inappropriate location in the correct tissue of origin. There are three main groups of heterotopias: periventricular (usually nodular), subcortical (either nodular or laminar), and leptomeningeal, of which only the first two can be detected by imaging. Periventricular nodular heterotopia (PNH) is by far the most frequent. Subcortical nodular heterotopia (SNH) is relatively frequent and is often accompanied by irregular folding of the overlying cortex. This malformation is usually detected when performing a brain MRI scan after seizure onset, since it produces no neurological signs or cognitive impairment. Its etiology and genetic bases, if any, remain unknown. SBH is a mild form of LIS and is classified in that group. We will consider here periventricular heterotopia, which is by far the most frequent and best known form of nodular heterotopia.

Periventricular Nodular Heterotopia

PNH consists of nodules of gray matter located along the lateral ventricles with a total failure of migration of some neurons (3); it ranges from isolated, single to confluent bilateral nodules. The overlying cortex may show an abnormal organization (122), and the heterotopias may show some rudimentary lamination and a variety of neuronal types (123).

The most frequent manifestation of PNH is epilepsy, occurring in 80% to 90% of patients, with most having various types of partial seizures, which are usually intractable (124). Studies using depth electrodes in patients with PNH and epilepsy have shown the nodules to be intrinsically epileptogenic (125), and temporal lobe surgery for patients with PNH and associated hippocampal sclerosis has generally been unsuccessful (126).

In typical PNH, the MRI will show nodular masses of gray matter that lie adjacent to the lateral ventricles and often protrude into the lumen (Fig. 27.8). The signal intensity is identical to that of cortical gray matter. Functional studies using FDG-PET and HMPAO-SPECT have shown changes in metabolic activity and perfusion to be almost identical in the heterotopic nodules and normal overlying cortex (127). Most are located along the lateral ventricular walls, although they may occasionally be seen posteriorly or medially. The nodules may be single or multiple, unilateral or bilateral, large or small, and symmetric or asymmetric. They may be contiguous or separated to resemble "pearls on a string." PNH differ from the subependymal nodules of TSC, which are usually smaller, fewer, inhomogeneous, calcified, and have signal intensity resembling white matter. PNH may be associated with additional brain anomalies such as cerebellar vermis hypoplasia, and is the most common MCD found in association with hippocampal sclerosis (65). Unilateral or focal PNH may occur in combination with SNH

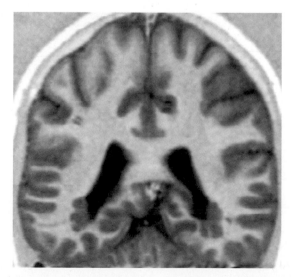

FIGURE 27.8 Coronal T1W MRI shows gray matter heterotopia lining the posterior ventricular system.

or in association with other MCDs such as PMG (122,128,129). Typical bilateral PNH may be associated with mild to moderate hypoplasia of the corpus callosum or cerebellum, the latter primarily involving the vermis. Usually, PNH is limited to the periventricular region but may occasionally form a larger mass that may deform or displace the lateral ventricle.

Mutations in the FLNA gene were identified in families having multiple affected members with bilateral PNH (130). FLNA is located on the long arm of the X-chromosome, and (131,133) mutations in males are thought to be lethal, thus explaining the female predominance of PNH. Although approximately 80% of familial cases of PNH have FLNA mutations, mutations have been detected in only approximately 20% of sporadic PNH patients (131). Those with mutations usually have a typical bilateral PNH pattern (132), with most patients with atypical PNH not having FLNA mutation (131,133). An autosomal recessive form of PNH with microcephaly has been found to be due to mutations in the ARFGEF2 gene in a small number of children from consanguineous parents (19). It is likely that PNH is a genetically heterogeneous disorder secondary to abnormalities of genes involved in neuroblast proliferation or initiation of neuroblast migration.

MALFORMATIONS DUE TO ABNORMAL CORTICAL ORGANIZATION

Polymicrogyria

Polymicrogryria (PMG) refers to a cerebral cortex with excessive microscopic gyration, and is probably one of the most common of the MCD. The imaging appearance of PMG varies with the patient's age (28). In newborns and young infants, the malformed cortex is very thin with multiple, very small undulations. After myelination, PMG appears as thickened cortex with irregular cortex–white matter junction (134).

PMG is a common cortical malformation and is associated with a wide number of patterns and syndromes and with mutations in several genes. Its pathogenesis is not understood. Brain pathology demonstrates abnormal development or loss of neurons in middle and deep cortical layers (135), variably associated with an unlayered cortical structure (136).

The clinical sequelae of PMG are highly variable depending on the extent and location of the PMG, the presence of other brain malformations, and the influence of complications such as epilepsy. In addition, PMG is reported as an occasional component in multiple different syndromes or disorders including metabolic disorders, chromosome deletion syndromes, and multiple congenital anomaly syndromes. These patients may have a wide spectrum of clinical problems other than those attributable to the PMG. Some patients with PMG have fewer clinical problems than would be expected for the location and extent of cortex involved. The most common form of PMG involves the perisylvian regions in a bilateral and rather symmetric pattern (Fig. 27.9). The combination of bilateral perisylvian PMG (BPP) associated with oromotor dysfunction and a seizure disorder has been called the "congenital bilateral perisylvian syndrome," and is the best described syndrome with PMG. Patients with BPP typically have oromotor dysfunction including difficulties with tongue (tongue protrusion and side to side movement), facial and pharyngeal motor function resulting in problems with speech production, sucking and swallowing, excessive drooling, and facial diplegia. They may also have an expressive dysphasia in addition to dysarthria. More severely affected patients have minimal or no expressive speech necessitating the use of alternate methods of communication such as signing. On examination, there is facial diplegia, limited tongue movements, a brisk jaw jerk, and frequent absence of the gag reflex (137). In patients presenting in childhood there may be other abnormalities including arthrogryposis, hemiplegia, and hearing loss, although there is limited pediatric data available (138). There may be mild to moderate intellectual disability in up to 75% of the cases (137). Motor dysfunction may include limb spasticity, although this is rarely severe if present. Other patterns of PMG have been described including unilateral perisylvian PMG (139), bilateral frontal PMG (140), bilateral frontoparietal PMG (141), bilateral parasagittal parieto-occipital PMG (142), bilateral parieto-occipital PMG (143), multilobar PMG

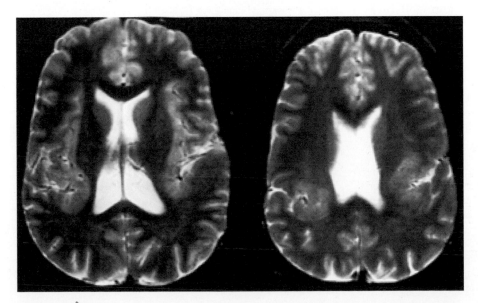

FIGURE 27.9 Congenital Bilateral Perisylvian Syndrome (CBPS). The axial T2W MRI shows perisylvian polymicrogyria. The lesions are often asymmetric.

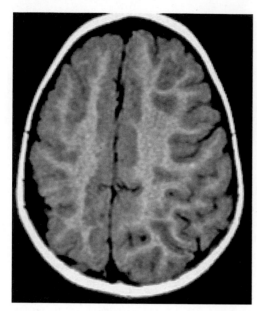

FIGURE 27.10 Unilateral polymicrogyria. Axial T1W image shows evidence of hemispheric atropy and underlying PMG. Note the changes are centered on the central region.

(Fig. 27.10) (144), and bilateral generalized PMG (145). The clinical features of these rarer forms of PMG vary from those seen in BPP, although epilepsy and some degree of developmental delay are common accompaniments.

The frequency of epilepsy in PMG is 60% to 85% (137,146,147), although seizure onset may not occur until the second decade, however, usually between the ages of 4 and 12 (148). Seizure types include atypical absence (62%), atonic and tonic drop attacks (73%), generalized tonic–clonic seizures (35%), and partial seizures (26%) (148). Occasionally, patients develop bilateral facial motor seizures with retained awareness. A small number of patients may present with infantile spasms (146,148,149) in contrast to patients with LIS, TSC, or FCD in which the frequency of spasms is higher. EEG typically shows generalized spike-wave or multifocal discharges with a centroparietal emphasis (148). Seizures may be daily and intractable in at least 50% of patients (148).

Using CT and low field strength MRI, PMG is difficult to discern and may only appear as thickened cortex (150–153). The only role for CT in the evaluation of PMG is to assess for evidence of calcification which is seen in PMG resulting from congenital cytomegalovirus (CMV) infection. Using high-quality 1.5T MRI with appropriate age-specific protocols, it is now possible to reliably differentiate PMG from other MCD (154). Polymicrogyric cortex often appears mildly thickened (6 to 10 mm) on imaging due to cortical overfolding rather than true cortical thickening. With better imaging (such as inversion recovery) using thin contiguous slices, microgyri and microsulci may be appreciated. Diffusely abnormal white matter signal should raise the question of an in utero infection (such as CMV) or a peroxisomal disorder (155–157). Other developmental anomalies may also be seen including ventricular enlargement or dysmorphism and abnormalities of the corpus callosum and cerebellum, although the patterns and prevalence of these associated brain malformations are poorly documented.

Few topics in the field of MCD have generated as much discussion as the etiology and pathogenesis of PMG. Initial

theories of PMG suggested that it was the result of a vascular defect such as arterial ischemia. Numerous etiologies, both genetic and nongenetic, have since been reported in association with PMG. Nongenetic causes other than hypoxia or hypoperfusion mainly relate to congenital infections including cytomegalovirus (155,158–160). There are a multitude of reports of PMG in association with genetic factors, either as part of a known genetic disease or a multiple congenital anomaly syndrome, in association with a structural chromosomal abnormality, or in families with multiple affected members and/or consanguinity. There is an association of PMG with some metabolic diseases including Zellweger syndrome, although the pathological changes differ from typical PMG (157,161,162). Zellweger syndrome has been found to be due to mutations in the PEX family of genes (163,164). Despite the long-held assumption that most forms of PMG are the result of a nongenetic insult, familial cases and examples of PMG occurring in other genetic syndromes and structural chromosomal abnormalities are now abundant in the literature, as reviewed in Jansen and Andermann (165). All modes of inheritance have been suggested although an X-linked inheritance pattern appears most frequent (166). The gene for bilateral frontoparietal PMG has been identified as GPR56, yet the function of this gene in cortical development is unclear (167). Mutations in the gene SRPX2 have been found in one family with BPP (168), but thus far mutations in this gene have not been identified in other patients with BPP. PMG is also reported as a component of several chromosomal deletion syndromes, particularly the 22q11.2 deletion syndromes such as the DiGeorge and velocardiofacial syndromes (30).

References

1. Gleeson JG, Walsh CA. Neuronal migration disorders: from genetic diseases to developmental mechanisms. *Trends Neurosci.* 2000;23(8):352–359.
2. Barkovich AJ, Kuzniecky R, Dobyns WB, et al. A classification scheme for malformations of cortical development. *Neuropediatrics.* 1996;27:59–63.
3. Barkovich AJ, Kuzniecky R, Jackson GD, et al. A developmental and genetic classification for malformations of cortical development. *Neurology.* 2005;65:1873–1887.
4. Van Slegtenhort M, de Hoogt R, Hermans C, et al. Identification of the tuberous sclerosis gene TSC1 on chromosome 9q34. *Science.* 1997;227 (5327):805–808.
5. European Chromosome 16 Tuberous Sclerosis Consortium. Identification and characterization of the tuberous sclerosis gene on chromosome 16. *Cell.* 1993;75(7):1305–1315.
6. Cardoso C, Leventer RJ, Ward HL, et al. Refinement of a 400-kb critical region allows genotypic differentiation between isolated lissencephaly, Miller-Dieker syndrome, and other phenotypes secondary to deletions of 17p13.3. *Am J Hum Genet.* 2003;72:918–930.
7. Matsumoto N, Leventer RJ, Kuc JA, et al. Mutation analysis of the DCX gene and genotype/phenotype correlation in subcortical band heterotopia. *Eur J Hum Genet.* 2001;9:5–12.
8. Cardoso C, Leventer RJ, Dowling JJ, et al. Clinical and molecular basis of classical lissencephaly: mutations in the LIS1 gene (PAFAH1B1). *Hum Mutat.* 2002;19(1):4–15.
9. Zaki M, Shehab M, El-Aleem AA, et al. Identification of a novel recessive RELN mutation using a homozygous balanced reciprocal translocation. *Am J Med Genet A.* 2007;143A(9):939–944.
10. Boycott KM, Flavelle S, Bureau A, et al. Homozygous deletion of the very low density lipoprotein receptor gene causes autosomal recessive cerebellar hypoplasia with cerebral gyral simplification. *Am J Hum Genet.* 2005;77(3):477–483.
11. Kato M, Das S, Petras K, et al. Mutations of ARX are associated with striking pleiotropy and consistent genotype-phenotype correlation. *Hum Mutat.* 2004;23:147–159.
12. Kondo-Iida E, Kobayashi K, Watanabe M, et al. Novel mutations and genotype-phenotype relationships in 107 families with Fukuyama-type congenital muscular dystrophy (FCMD). *Hum Mol Genet.* 1999;8:2303–2309.
13. Beltran-Valero de Bernabé D, Voit T, Longman C, et al. Mutations in the FKRP gene can cause muscle-eye-brain disease and Walker-Warburg syndrome. *J Med Genet.* 2004;41(5):e61.

14. Longman C, Brockington M, Torelli S, et al. Mutations in the human LARGE gene cause MDC1D, a novel form of congenital muscular dystrophy with severe mental retardation and abnormal glycosylation of alpha-dystroglycan. *Hum Mol Genet.* 2003;12(21):2853–2861.

15. Beltran-Valero De Bernabe D, Currier S, Steinbrecher A, et al. Mutations in the O-mannosyltransferase gene POMT1 give rise to the severe neuronal migration disorder Walker-Warburg syndrome. *Am J Hum Genet.* 2002;71:1033–1043.

16. van Reeuwijk J, Maugenre S, van den Elzen C, et al. The expanding phenotype of POMT1 mutations: from Walker-Warburg syndrome to congenital muscular dystrophy, microcephaly, and mental retardation. *Hum Mutat.* 2006;27(5):453–459.

17. van Reeuwijk J, Janssen M, van den Elzen C, et al. POMT2 mutations cause alpha-dystroglycan hypoglycosylation and Walker-Warburg syndrome. *Med Genet.* 2005;42(12):907–912.

18. Piao X, Chang BS, Bodell A, et al. Genotype-phenotype analysis of human frontoparietal polymicrogyria syndromes. *Ann Neurol.* 2005;58(5):680–687.

19. Sheen VL, Ganesh VS, Topcu M, et al. Mutations in ARFGEF2 implicate vesicle trafficking in neural progenitor proliferation and migration in the human cerebral cortex. *Nat Genet.* 2004;36:69–76.

20. Hehr U, Hehr A, Uyanik G, et al. A filamin A splice mutation resulting in a syndrome of facial dysmorphism, periventricular nodular heterotopia, and severe constipation reminiscent of cerebro-fronto-facial syndrome. *J Med Genet.* 2006;43(6):541–544.

21. Moro F, Pisano T, Bernardina BD, et al. Periventricular heterotopia in fragile X syndrome. *Neurology.* 2006;67(4):713–715.

22. Ferland RJ, Gaitanis JN, Apse K, et al. Periventricular nodular heterotopia and Williams syndrome. *Am J Med Genet A.* 2006;140(12):1305–1311.

23. Fink JM, Dobyns WB, Guerrini R, et al. Identification of a duplication of Xq28 associated with bilateral periventricular nodular heterotopia. *Am J Hum Genet.* 1997;61(2):379–387.

24. Neal J, Apse K, Sahin M, et al. Deletion of chromosome 1p36 is associated with periventricular nodular heterotopia. *Am J Med Genet A.* 2006;140(15):1692–1695.

25. Eash D, Waggoner D, Chung J, et al. Calibration of 6q subtelomere deletions to define genotype/phenotype correlations. *Clin Genet.* 2005;67(5):396–403.

26. Sheen VL, Wheless JW, Bodell A, et al. Periventricular heterotopia associated with chromosome 5p anomalies. *Neurology.* 2003;60(6):1033–1036.

27. Gawlik-Kuklinska K, Wierzba J, Wozniak A, et al. Periventricular heterotopia in a boy with interstitial deletion of chromosome 4p. *Eur J Med Genet.* 2008;51(2):165–171.

28. Takanashi J, Barkovich AJ. The changing MR imaging appearance of polymicrogyria; a consequence of myelination. *Am J Neuroradiol.* 2003;24:788–793.

29. Sprecher E, Ishida-Yamamoto A, Mizrahi-Koren M, et al. A mutation in SNAP29, coding for a SNARE protein involved in intracellular trafficking, causes a novel neurocutaneous syndrome characterized by cerebral dysgenesis, neuropathy, ichthyosis, and palmoplantar keratoderma. *Am J Hum Genet.* 2005;77(2):242–251.

30. Robin NH, Taylor CJ, Donald-McGinn DM, et al. Polymicrogyria and deletion 22q11.2 syndrome: window to the etiology of a common cortical malformation. *Am J Med Genet A.* 2006;140:2416–2425.

31. Baala L, Briault S, Etchevers HC, et al. Homozygous silencing of T-box transcription factor EOMES leads to microcephaly with polymicrogyria and corpus callosum agenesis. *Nat Genet.* 2007;39(4):454–456.

32. Glaser T, Jepeal L, Edwards JG, et al. PAX6 gene dosage effect in a family with congenital cataracts, aniridia, anophthalmia and central nervous system defects. *Nat Genet.* 1994;7(4):463–471. Erratum in: *Nat Genet.* 1994;8(2):203.

33. Ribeiro Mdo C, Gama de Sousa S, Freitas MM, et al. Bilateral perisylvian polymicrogyria and chromosome 1 anomaly. *Pediatr Neurol.* 2007;36(6):418–420.

34. Zollino M, Colosimo C, Zuffardi O, et al. Cryptic t(1;12)(q44;p13.3) translocation in a previously described syndrome with polymicrogyria, segregating as an apparently X-linked trait. *Am J Med Genet A.* 2003;117A(1):65–71.

35. Dobyns WB, Mirzaa G, Christian SL, et al. Consistent chromosome abnormalities identify novel polymicrogyria loci in 1p36.3, 2p16.1-p23.1, 4q21.21-q22.1, 6q26-q27, and 21q2. *Am J Med Genet A.* 2008;146A(13):1637–1654.

36. Nowaczyk MJ, Teshima IE, Siegel-Bartelt J, et al. Deletion 4q21/4q22 syndrome: two patients with de novo 4q21.3q23 and 4q13.2q23 deletions. *Am J Med Genet.* 1997;69(4):400–405.

37. Yao G, Chen XN, Flores-Sarnat L, et al. Deletion of chromosome 21 disturbs human brain morphogenesis. *Genet Med.* 2006;8(1):1–7.

38. Brooks AS, Bertoli-Avella AM, Burzynski GM, et al. Homozygous nonsense mutations in KIAA1279 are associated with malformations of the central and enteric nervous systems. *Am J Hum Genet.* 2005;77(1):120–126.

39. Aligianis IA, Johnson CA, Gissen P, et al. Mutations of the catalytic subunit of RAB3GAP cause Warburg Micro syndrome. *Nat Genet.* 2005;37(3):221–223.

40. Guerrini R, Dobyns WB, Barkovich J. Abnormal development of the human cerebral cortex: genetics, functional consequences and treatment options. *Trends Neurosci.* 2008;31(3):154–162.

41. Opitz JM, Holt MC. Microcephaly: general considerations and aids to nosology. *J Craniofac Genet Dev Biol.* 1990;10:175–204.

42. Tolmie JL, McNay M, Stephenson JBP, et al. Microcephaly: genetic counseling and antenatal diagnosis after birth of an affected child. *Am J Med Genet.* 1987;27:583–594.

43. Dobyns WB. Primary microcephaly: new approaches for an old disorder. *Am J Med Genet.* 2002;112:315–317.

44. Barkovich AJ, Ferriero DM, Barr RM, et al. Microlissencephaly: a heterogenous malformation of cortical development. *Neuropediatrics.* 1998;29:113–119.

45. Sztriha L, Al-Ghazali LI, Varady E, et al. Autosomal recessive micrencephaly with simplified gyral pattern, abnormal myelination and arthrogryposis. *Neuropediatrics.* 1999;30:141–145.

46. Ten Donkelaar HJ, Wesseling P, Semmekrot BA, et al. Severe, non X-linked congenital microcephaly with absence of the pyramidal tracts in two siblings. *Acta Neuropathol (Berl).* 1999;98:203–211.

47. Dobyns WB, Barkovich AJ. Microcephaly with simplified gyral pattern (oligogyric microcephaly) and microlissencephaly: reply. *Neuropediatrics.* 1999;30:104–106.

48. DeMeyer W. Megalencephaly in children: clinical syndromes, genetic patterns, and differential diagnosis from other causes of megalocephaly. *Neurology.* 1972;22:634–643.

49. Barkovich AJ, Chuang SH. Unilateral megalencephaly: correlation of MR imaging and pathologic characteristics. *Am J Neuroradiol.* 1990;11:523–531.

50. Robain O, Floquet C, Heldt N, et al. Hemimegalencephaly: a clinicopathological study of four cases. *Neuropathol Appl Neurobiol.* 1988;14:125–135.

51. De Rosa MJ, Secor DL, Barsom M, et al. Neuropathologic findings in surgically treated hemimegalencephaly: immunohistochemical, morphometric, and ultrastructural study. *Acta Neuropathol (Berl).* 1992;84:250–260.

52. Bosman C, Boldrini R, Dimitri L, et al. Hemimegalencephaly: histological, immunohistochemical, ultrastructural and cytofluorimetric study of six patients. *Childs Nerv Syst.* 1996;12:765–775.

53. Dobyns WB, Garg BP. Vascular abnormalities in epidermal nevus syndrome. *Neurology.* 1991;41:276–278.

54. Peserico A, Battistella PA, Bertoli P, et al. Unilateral hypomelanosis of Ito with hemimegalencephaly. *Acta Paediatr Scand.* 1988;77:446–447.

55. Maloof J, Sledz K, Hogg JP, et al. Unilateral megalencephaly and tuberous sclerosis: related disorders? *J Child Neurol.* 1994;9:443–446.

56. Ross GW, Miller JQ, Persing JA, et al. Hemimegalencephaly, hemifacial hypertrophy and intracranial lipoma: a variant of neurofibromatosis. *Neurofibromatosis.* 1989;2:69–77.

57. Trounce JQ, Rutter N, Mellor DH. Hemimegalencephaly: diagnosis and treatment. *Dev Med Child Neurol.* 1991;33:261–266.

58. Ohtsuka Y, Ohno S, Oka E. Electroclinical characteristics of hemimegalencephaly. *Pediatr Neurol.* 1999;20:390–393.

59. Devlin AM, Cross JH, Harkness W, et al. Clinical outcomes of hemispherectomy for epilepsy in childhood and adolescence. *Brain.* 2003;126(Pt 3):556–566.

60. Maher CO, Cohen-Gadol AA, Raffel C. Cortical resection for epilepsy in children with linear sebaceous nevus syndrome. *Pediatr Neurosurg.* 2003;39:129–135.

61. Palmini A, Najm I, Avanzini G, et al. Terminology and classification of the cortical dysplasias. *Neurology.* 2004;62:S2–S8.

62. Tassi L, et al. Focal cortical dysplasia: neuropathological subtypes, EEG, neuroimaging and surgical outcome. *Brain.* 2002;125:1719–1732.

63. Hardiman O, Burke T, Phillips J, et al. Microdysgenesis in resected temporal neocortex: incidence and clinical significance in focal epilepsy. *Neurology.* 1988;38:1041–1047.

64. Meencke HJ, Veith G. Migration disturbances in epilepsy. *Epilepsy Res Suppl.* 1992;9:31–39; discussion 39–40.

65. Raymond AA, Fish DR, Sisodiya SM, et al. Abnormalities of gyration, heterotopias, tuberous sclerosis, focal cortical dysplasia, microdysgenesis, dysembryoplastic neuroepithelial tumour and dysgenesis of the archicortex in epilepsy. Clinical, EEG and neuroimaging features in 100 adult patients. *Brain.* 1995;118(Pt 3):629–660.

66. Meencke HJ, Veith G. The relevance of slight migrational disturbances (microdysgenesis) to the etiology of the epilepsies. *Adv Neurol.* 1999;79:123–131.

67. Ying Z, Gonzalez-Martinez J, Tilelli C, et al. Expression of neural stem cell surface marker CD133 in balloon cells of human focal cortical dysplasia. *Epilepsia.* 2005;46:1716–1723.

68. Najm IM, Tilelli CQ, Oghlakian R, et al. Pathophysiological mechanisms of focal cortical dysplasia: a critical review of human tissue studies and animal models. *Epilepsia.* 2007;48(suppl 2):21–32.

69. Becker AJ, Urbach H, Scheffler B, et al. Focal cortical dysplasia of Taylor's balloon cell type: mutational analysis of the TSC1 gene indicates a pathogenic relationship to tuberous sclerosis. *Ann Neurol.* 2002;52:29–37.

70. Golden JA, Harding BN. *Pathology and Genetics: Developmental Neuropathology.* Basel, Switzerland: ISN Neuropath Press; 2004.

71. Marin-Padilla M, Parisi JE, Armstrong DL, et al. Shaken infant syndrome: developmental neuropathology, progressive cortical dysplasia, and epilepsy. *Acta Neuropathol.* 2002;103:321–332.

72. Wyllie E, Baumgartner C, Prayson R, et al. The clinical spectrum of focal cortical dysplasia and epilepsy. *J Epilepsy.* 1994;7:303–312.

73. Mackay MT, Becker LE, Chuang SH, et al. Malformations of cortical development with balloon cells: Clinical and radiologic correlates. *Neurology.* 2003;60:580–587.

74. Barkovich AJ, Kjos BO. Nonlissencephalic cortical dysplasias: correlation of imaging findings with clinical deficits. *Am J Neuroradiol.* 1992;13:95–103.

75. Palmini A, Gambardella A, Andermann F, et al. Instrinsic epileptogenicity of human dysplastic cortex as suggested by corticography and surgical results. *Ann Neurol.* 1995;37:476–487.

76. Mattia D, Olivier A, Avoli M. Seizure-like discharges recorded in human dysplastic neocortex maintained in vitro. *Neurology.* 1995;45:1391–1395.

77. Avoli M, Louvel J, Mattia D, et al. Epileptiform synchronization in the human dysplastic cortex. *Epileptic Disord.* 2003;5(suppl 2):S45–S50.

78. Colombo N, Tassi L, Galli C, et al. Focal cortical dysplasias: MR imaging, histopathologic and clinical correlations in surgically treated patients with epilepsy. *Am J Neuroradiol.* 2003;24:724–733.

79. Emery JA, Roper SN, Rojianni AM. White matter neuronal heterotopias in temporal lobe epilepsy: a morphometric and immunohistochemical study. *J. Neuropathol Exp Neurol.* 1997;56:1276–1282

80. Rojiani AM, Emery JA, Anderson KJ, et al. Distribution of heterotopic neurons in normal hemispheric white matter: a morphometric analysis. *J Neuropathol Exp Neurol.* 1996;55:178–183.

81. Friede, RL. *Developmental Neuropathology.* New York: Springer-Verlag; 1989:577.

82. Harding B, Copp AJ. Malformations. In: Greenfield JD, Lantos PL, Graham DI, eds. *Greenfield's Neuropathology.* 7th ed. Vol 1. London: Arnold; 2002.

83. Crome L. Pachygyria. *J Pathol Bacteriol.* 1956;71:335–352.

84. Norman MG, McGillivray BC, Kalousek DK, et al. *Congenital Malformations of the Brain: Pathological, Embryological, Clinical, Radiologic and Genetic Aspects.* New York: Oxford University Press; 1995.

85. Forman MS, Squier W, Dobyns WB, et al. Genotypically defined lissencephalies show distinct pathologies. *J Neuropathol Exp Neurol.* 2005;64:847–857.

86. Barkovich AJ. Congenital malformations of the brain and skull. In: Barkovich A, ed. *Pediatric Neuroimaging.* 3rd ed. Philadelphia: Lippincott William & Wilkins; 2000:251–381.

87. Pilz DT, Kuc J, Matsumoto N, et al. Subcortical band heterotopia in rare affected males can be caused by missense mutations in DCX (XLIS) or LIS1. *Hum Mol Genet.* 1999;8:1757–1760.

88. des Portes V, Pinard JM, Smadja D, et al. Dominant X linked subcortical laminar heterotopia and lissencephaly syndrome (XSCLH/LIS): evidence for the occurrence of mutation in males and mapping of a potential locus in XQ22. *J Med Genet.* 1997;34:177–183.

89. Matell M. Ein Fall von Heterotopie der frauen Substanz in de beiden Hemispheren des Grosshirns. *Arch Psychiatr Nerven.* 1893;25:124–136.

90. Ross ME, Allen KM, Srivastava AK, et al. Linkage and physical mapping of x-linked lissencephaly/sbh (XLIS): a gene causing neuronal migration defects in human brain. *Hum Mol Genet.* 1997;6:555–562.

91. Reiner O, Carrozzo R, Shen Y, et al. Isolation of a Miller-Dieker lissencephaly gene containing G-protein beta-subunit-like repeats. *Nature.* 1993;364:717–721.

92. des Portes V, Francis F, Pinard JM, et al. Doublecortin is the major gene causing X-linked subcortical laminar heterotopia (SCLH). *Hum Mol Genet.* 1998;7:1063–1070.

93. Gleeson JG, Allen KM, Fox JW, et al. Doublecortin, a brain-specific gene mutated in human X-linked lissencephaly and double cortex syndrome, encodes a putative signaling protein. *Cell.* 1998;92:63–72.

94. Mei D, Lewis R, Parrini E, et al. High frequency of genomic deletions and a duplication in the LIS1 gene in lissencephaly: implications for molecular diagnosis. *J Med Genet.* 2008;45:355–361.

95. Dobyns WB, Elias ER, Newlin AC, et al. Causal heterogeneity in isolated lissencephaly. *Neurology.* 1992;42:1375–1388.

96. D'Agostino MD, Bernasconi A, Das S, et al. Subcortical band heterotopia (SBH) in males: clinical, imaging and genetic findings in comparison with females. *Brain.* 2002;125(Pt 11):2507–2522.

97. Dobyns WB, Andermann E, Andermann F, et al. X-linked malformations of neuronal migration. *Neurology.* 1996;47:331–339.

98. Barkovich AJ, Guerrini R, Battaglia G, et al. Band heterotopia: correlation of outcome with magnetic resonance imaging parameters. *Ann Neurol.* 1994;36:609–617.

99. Battaglia A. Seizures and dysplasias of cerebral cortex in dysmorphic syndromes. In: Guerrini R, Andermann F, Canapicchi R, et al., eds. *Dysplasias of Cerebral Cortex and Epilepsy.* Philadelphia: Lippincott-Raven; 1996:199–209.

100. Palmini A, Andermann F, Aicardi J, et al. Diffuse cortical dysplasia, or the 'double cortex' syndrome: the clinical and epileptic spectrum in 10 patients. *Neurology.* 1991;41:1656–1662.

101. Dobyns WB, Stratton RF, Greenberg F. Syndromes with lissencephaly. I: Miller-Dieker and Norman-Roberts syndromes and isolated lissencephaly. *Am J Med Genet.* 1984;18:509–526.

102. Dobyns WB, Truwit CL, Ross ME, et al. Differences in the gyral pattern distinguish chromosome 17-linked and X-linked lissencephaly. *Neurology.* 1999;22;53:270–277.

103. Pilz DT, Matsumoto N, Minerath S, et al. LIS1 and XLIS (DCX) mutations cause most classical lissencephaly, but different patterns of malformation. *Hum Mol Genet.* 1998;7:2029–2037.

104. Dobyns WB, Curry CJR, Hoyme HE, et al. Clinical and molecular diagnosis of Miller-Dieker syndrome. *Am J Hum Genet.* 1991;48:584–594.

105. Hong SE, Shugart YY, Huang DT, et al. Autosomal recessive lissencephaly with cerebellar hypoplasia is associated human RELN mutations. *Nat Genet.* 2000;26:93–96.

106. Kato M, Takizawa N, Yamada S, et al. Diffuse pachygyria with cerebellar hypoplasia: a milder form of microlissencephaly or a new genetic syndrome? *Ann Neurol.* 1999;46:660–663.

107. Hourihane JO, Bennett CP, Chaudhuri R, et al. A sibship with a neuronal migration defect, cerebellar hypoplasia and congenital lymphedema. *Neuropediatrics.* 1993;24:43–46.

108. Dobyns WB, Berry-Kravis E, Havernick NJ, et al. X-linked lissencephaly with absent corpus callosum and ambiguous genitalia. *Am J Med Genet.* 1999;86(4):331–337.

109. Kitamura K, Yanazawa M, Sugiyama N, et al. Mutation of ARX causes abnormal development of forebrain and testes in mice and X-linked lissencephaly with abnormal genitalia in humans. *Nat Genet.* 2002;32:359–369.

110. Dobyns WB, Kirkpatrick JB, Hittner HM, et al. Syndromes with lissencephaly. II: Walker-Warburg and cerebro-oculo-muscular syndromes and a new syndrome with type II lissencephaly. *Am J Med Genet.* 1985;22:157–195.

111. Dobyns WB, Pagon RA, Armstrong D, et al. Diagnostic criteria for Walker-Warburg syndrome. *Am J Med Genet.* 1989;32:195–210.

112. Dubowitz V. 22nd ENMC sponsored workshop on congenital muscular dystrophy held in Baarn, The Netherlands, 14–16 May 1993. *Neuromuscul Disord.* 1994;4:75–81.

113. Haltia M, Leivo I, Somer H, et al. Muscle-eye-brain disease: a neuropathological study. *Ann Neurol.* 1997;41:173–180.

114. Takada K, Nakamura H, Takashima S. Cortical dysplasia in Fukuyama congenital muscular dystrophy (FCMD): a Golgi and angioarchitectonic analysis. *Acta Neuropathol.* 1988;76:170–178.

115. Walker AE. Lissencephaly. *Arch Neurol Psychiatry.* 1942;48:13–29.

116. Osawa M, Arai Y, Ikenaka H, et al. Fukuyama congenital progressive muscular dystrophy. *Acta Pediatr Jpn.* 1991;33:261–269.

117. Fukuyama Y, Osawa M. A genetic study of the Fukuyama type congenital muscular dystrophy. *Brain Dev.* 1984;6:373–390.

118. Kobayashi K, Nakahori Y, Miyake M, et al. An ancient retrotransposal insertion causes Fukuyama type congenital muscular dystrophy. *Nature.* 1998;394:388–392.

119. Santavuori P, Somer H, Sainio K, et al. Muscle-eye-brain disease (MEB). *Brain Dev.* 1989;11:147–153.

120. Beltran-Valero De Bernabe D, van Bokhoven H, van Beusekom E, et al. A homozygous nonsense mutation in the Fukutin gene causes a Walker-Warburg syndrome phenotype. *J Med Genet.* 2003;40:845–848.

121. Silan F, Yoshioka M, Kobayashi K, et al. A new mutation of the Fukutin gene in a non-Japanese patient. *Ann Neurol.* 2003;53:392–396.

122. Hannan AJ, Servotte S, Katsnelson A, et al. Characterization of nodular neuronal heterotopia in children. *Brain.* 1999;122(Pt 2):219–238.

123. Kakita A, Hayahi S, Moro F, et al. Bilateral periventricular nodular heterotopia due to filamin 1 gene mutation: widespread glomeruloid microvascular anomaly and dysplastic cytoarchitecture in the cerebral cortex. *Acta Neuropathol.* 2002;104:649–657.

124. Dubeau F, Tampieri D, Lee N, et al. Periventricular and subcortical nodular heterotopia. A study of 33 patients. *Brain.* 1995;118(Pt 5):1273–1287.

125. Kothare SV, VanLandingham K, Armon C, et al. Seizure onset from periventricular nodular heterotopias: depth- electrode study. *Neurology.* 1998;51:1723–1727.

126. Li LM, Dubeau F, Andermann F, et al. Periventricular nodular heterotopia and intractable temporal lobe epilepsy: poor outcome after temporal lobe resection. *Ann Neurol.* 1997;41:662–668.

127. Morioka T, Nishio S, Sasaki M, et al. Functional imaging in periventricular nodular heterotopia with the use of FDG-PET and HMPAO-SPECT. *Neurosurg Rev.* 1999;22:41–44.

128. Leventer RJ, Phelan EM, Coleman LT, et al. Clinical and imaging features of cortical malformations in childhood. *Neurology.* 1999;53:715–722.

129. Soto Ares G, Hamon-Kerautret M, Houlette C, et al. Unusual MRI findings in grey matter heterotopia. *Neuroradiology.* 1998;40:81–87.

130. Fox JW, Lamperti ED, Eksioglu YZ, et al. Mutations in filamin 1 prevent migration of cerebral cortical neurons in human periventricular heterotopia. *Neuron.* 1998;21:1315–1325.

131. Sheen VL, Dixon PH, Fox JW, et al. Mutations in the X-linked filamin 1 gene cause periventricular nodular heterotopia in males as well as in females. *Hum Mol Genet.* 2001;10:1775–1783.

132. Poussaint TY, Fox JW, Dobyns WB, et al. Periventricular nodular heterotopia in patients with filamin-1 gene mutations: neuroimaging findings. *Pediatr Radiol.* 2000;30:748–755.

133. Parrini E, Ramazzotti A, Dobyns WB, et al. Periventricular heterotopia: phenotypic heterogeneity and correlation with Filamin A mutations. *Brain.* 2006;129(Pt 7):1892–1906.
134. Guerrini R, Dobyns WB, Barkovich AJ. Abnormal development of the human cerebral cortex: genetics, functional consequences and treatment options. *Trends Neurosci.* 2008;31:154–162.
135. Englund C, Fink A, Lau C, et al. Pax6, Tbr2, and Tbr1 are expressed sequentially by radial glia, intermediate progenitor cells, and postmitotic neurons in developing neocortex. *J Neurosci.* 2005;25:247–251.
136. Harding B, Copp A. Malformations of the nervous system. In: Graham J, Lantons PL, eds. *Greenfields Neuropathlogy.* London-Melbourne-Auckland: Edward Arnold; 1997:521–538.
137. Kuzniecky RI, Andermann F, Guerrini R. Congenital bilateral perisylvian syndrome: study of 31 patients. *Lancet.* 1993;341:608–612.
138. Miller SP, Shevell M, Rosenblatt B, et al. Congenital bilateral perisylvian polymicrogyria presenting as congenital hemiplegia. *Neurology.* 1998;50:1866–1869.
139. Sebire G, Husson B, Dusser A, et al. Congenital unilateral perisylvian syndrome: radiological basis and clinical correlations. *J Neurol Neurosurg Psychiatry.* 1996;61:52–56.
140. Guerrini R, Barkovich AJ, Sztriha L, et al. Bilateral frontal polymicrogyria: a newly recognized brain malformation syndrome. *Neurology.* 2000;54:909–913.
141. Chang BS, Piao X, Bodell A, et al. Bilateral frontoparietal polymicrogyria: clinical and radiological features in 10 families with linkage to chromosome 16. *Ann Neurol.* 2003;53:596–606.
142. Guerrini R, Dubeau F, Dulac O, et al. Bilateral parasagittal parietooccipital polymicrogyria and epilepsy. *Ann Neurol.* 1997;41:65–73.
143. Ferrie CD, Jackson GD, Giannakodimos S, et al. Posterior agyria-pachygyria with polymicrogyria: evidence for an inherited neuronal migration disorder. *Neurology.* 1995;45:150–153.
144. Guerrini R, Genton P, Bureau M, et al. Multilobar polymicrogyria, intractable drop attack seizures, and sleep- related electrical status epilepticus. *Neurology.* 1998;51:504–512.
145. Chang BS, Piao X, Giannini C, et al. Bilateral generalized polymicrogyria (BGP): a distinct syndrome of cortical malformation. *Neurology.* 2004;62:1722–1728.
146. Gropman AL, Barkovich AJ, Vezina LG, et al. Pediatric congenital bilateral perisylvian syndrome: clinical and MRI features in 12 patients. *Neuropediatrics.* 1997;28:198–203.
147. Barkovich AJ, Hevner R, Guerrini R. Syndromes of bilateral symmetrical polymicrogyria. *Am J Neuroradiol.* 1999;20:1814–1821.
148. Kuzniecky RI, Andermann F, Guerrini R, et al. The epileptic spectrum in the congenital bilateral perisylvian syndrome. *Neurology.* 1994;44: 379–385.
149. Kuzniecky R, Andermann F, Guerrini R. Infantile spasms: an early epileptic manifestation in some patients with the congenital bilateral perisylvian syndrome. *J Child Neurol.* 1994;9:420–423.
150. Byrd SE, Osborn RE, Bohan TP, et al. The CT and MR evaluation of migrational disorders of the brain. Part II. Schizencephaly, heterotopia and polymicrogyria. *Pediatr Radiol.* 1989;19:219–222.
151. Barkovich AJ, Chuang SH, Norman D. MR of neuronal migration anomalies. *Am J Neuroradiol.* 1987;8:1009–1017.
152. Kuzniecky RI, Andermann F, CBPS Study Group. The congenital bilateral perisylvian syndrome: imaging findings in a multicenter study. *Am J Neuroradiol.* 1994;15:139–144.
153. Barkovich AJ, Kuzniecky RI. Neuroimaging of focal malformations of cortical development. *J Clin Neurophysiol.* 1996;13:481–494.
154. Raybaud C, Gerard N, Canto-Moreira N, et al. High-definition magnetic resonance imaging identification of cortical dysplasias: micropolygyria versus lissencphaly. In: Guerrini R, Andermann F, Canapicchi R, et al., eds. *Dysplasias of Cerebral Cortex and Epilepsy.* 1st ed. Philadelphia, PA: Lipincott-Raven; 1996:131–143.
155. Barkovich AJ, Lindan CE. Congenital cytomegalovirus infection of the brain: imaging analysis and embryologic considerations. *Am J Neuroradiol.* 1994;15:703–715.
156. van der Knaap MS, Valk J. The MR spectrum of peroxisomal disorders. *Neuroradiology.* 1991;33:30–37.
157. Barkovich AJ, Peck WW. MR of Zellweger syndrome. *Am J Neuroradiol.* 1997;18:1163–1170.
158. Iannetti P, Nigro G, Spalice A, et al. Cytomegalovirus infection and schizencephaly: case reports. *Ann Neurol.* 1998;43:123–127.
159. Hayward JC, Titelbaum DS, Clancy RR, et al. Lissencephaly-pachygyria associated with congenital cytomegalovirus infection. *J Child Neurol.* 1991;6:109–114.
160. Crome L, France NE. Microgyria and cytomegalic inclusion disease in infancy. *J Clin Pathol.* 1959;12:427.
161. Zellweger H. The cerebro-hepato-renal (Zellweger) syndrome and other peroxisomal disorders. *Dev Med Child Neurol.* 1987;29:821–829.
162. Kaufmann WE, Theda C, Naidu S, et al. Neuronal migration abnormality in peroxisomal bifunctional enzyme defect. *Ann Neurol.* 1996; 39:268–271.
163. Shimozawa N, Suzuki Y, Zhang Z, et al. Identification of PEX3 as the gene mutated in a zellweger syndrome patient lacking peroxisomal remnant structures. *Hum Mol Genet.* 2000;9:1995–1999.
164. Raymond GV. Peroxisomal disorders. *Curr Opin Neurol.* 2001;14: 783–787.
165. Jansen A, Andermann E. Genetics of the polymicrogyria syndromes. *J Med Genet.* 2005;42:369–378.
166. Guerreiro MM, Andermann E, Guerrini R, et al. Familial perisylvian polymicrogyria: a new familial syndrome of cortical maldevelopment. *Ann Neurol.* 2000;48:39–48.
167. Piao X, Hill RS, Bodell A, et al. G protein-coupled receptor-dependent development of human frontal cortex. *Science.* 2004;303:2033–2036.
168. Roll P, Rudolf G, Pereira S, et al. SRPX2 mutations in disorders of language cortex and cognition. *Hum Mol Genet.* 2006;15:1195–1207.

CHAPTER 28 ■ BRAIN TUMORS AND EPILEPSY

LARA JEHI

Multiple epidemiological studies established the frequent coexistence of brain tumors and epilepsy. Recently, significant insights into the mechanisms of epileptogenesis were derived from studying the intricate relationship between the two conditions. This chapter will discuss the following:

1. Current data on the prevalence and incidence of epilepsy in brain tumor patients, and vice-versa
2. Clinical characteristics of patients with brain tumor and epilepsy
3. Various proposed mechanisms of epileptogenesis in brain tumor patients
4. Medical as well as surgical treatment of brain tumor patients with epilepsy

EPIDEMIOLOGY

Up to 38% of patients with a primary and 20% of those with a secondary brain tumor initially seek medical attention following a seizure (1). On the other hand, brain tumors cause about 10% to 15% of all adult-onset and 0.2% to 6% of all childhood-onset epilepsies (2–4).

Major tumor characteristics that determine the likelihood of developing epilepsy include tumor type, grade, and location. As a general rule, the lower the grade of the tumor, the closer it is to the cortex, and the more connected it is to potentially epileptogenic structures (e.g., hippocampus, primary motor cortex, etc.), the higher are the chances of it producing seizures. The following statistics illustrate these concepts: first, while only 30% to 60% of high-grade gliomas (5,6) and 20% of primary central nervous system (CNS) lymphoma (7) lead to epilepsy, seizures occur in up to 40% of patients with meningiomas (8) and in more than 80% of those with low-grade gliomas (9,10). Second, among patients with a low-grade glioma, cortical location and oligodendroglioma and oligoastrocytoma subtypes are significantly more associated with epilepsy when compared to deeper midline locations and astrocytoma, respectively (10). Third, while tumors represent up to 56.3% of epilepsy etiologies in the temporal lobe epilepsy literature (11), they proportionally only account for half as many (27%) extratemporal lobe epilepsies (12). In one series of 147 patients with newly diagnosed brain tumors, primary location of the tumor also correlated with seizure risk: parietal (80%), temporal (74%), frontal (62%), and occipital (0%) (1). Infratentorial and sellar tumors rarely cause seizures unless they extend into the cerebral hemispheres (3). Careful consideration of these epidemiological observations, as well as detailed analyses of clinical variables and basic science investigations, improved our understanding of various mechanisms of epileptogenicity and facilitated the development of targeted treatments.

Table 28.1 summarizes the prevalence of various tumor types encountered in series of medically intractable, chronic epilepsy. Table 28.2 summarizes the prevalence of seizures in various types of brain tumors.

CLINICAL CHARACTERISTICS

Most tumor-related seizures first appear early in the course of the disease, usually as a presenting manifestation (9). In 10% to 30% of brain tumor patients, epilepsy develops later in the disease course (4,9). In brain tumor patients presenting with seizures, age and presence of associated neurological deficits may correlate with tumor grade: children and adolescents usually have no associated neurological deficits and generally have a low-grade tumor, whereas middle-aged or elderly people often have other associated neurological deficits on presentation and end up with the diagnosis of a high-grade brain neoplasm (3,17,18).

Both focal and generalized seizures occur in the setting of brain tumors (9,10,15,19,20). Even isolated auras have been reported as the only epileptic manifestation of temporal lobe tumors (21). Therefore, in any given patient, seizure semiology is mainly determined by the location of the tumor and its connectivity. However, certain general remarks may be noted. First, seizures that start earlier in the course of a brain tumor are more likely to be generalized: Hildebrand et al. (9) found that while 50% of "early seizures" occurring at or soon after brain tumor diagnosis were generalized and 40% were focal, the converse was true when seizures occurred during the later follow-up phases, with about 75% being focal and only 20% being generalized. Second, in certain special situations, seizure semiology carries a specific tumor-related diagnostic correlation such as with gelastic seizures and hypothalamic hamartomas.

The observations made above are likely due to distinctly different mechanisms of epileptogenicity that will be detailed later. In brief though, younger patients are statistically more likely to have small, slow-growing tumors (developmental tumors, low-grade gliomas, etc.) that take their time to develop focal and remote cellular and pathway changes sufficient to develop epileptogenicity without causing major local tissue damage. As such, patients with low-grade temporal lobe tumors, for example, might not have palpable deficits on a traditional neurological examination, would develop seizures later in the course of the tumor progression, and would have more complex partial seizures related to dysfunction of the limbic network. On the other hand, an older patient with a glioblastoma multiforme would have a larger rapidly growing tumor, causing significant local tissue damage with associated neurological deficits and seizures starting earlier in the tumor disease course as a result of abrupt tissue necrosis.

TABLE 28.1

TUMOR TYPES ENCOUNTERED IN MEDICALLY INTRACTABLE EPILEPSY

All intractable tumoral epilepsies

				Tumor types				
Study	Ganglioglioma	DNET[a] (%)	Pilocytic astrocytoma (%)	Oligodendroglioma (%)	Oligoastrocytoma (%)	Fibrillary astrocytoma (%)	PXA[a] (%)	Other (%)
Zentner et al. (13) (N = 146)	45	13	14	10	7	10	0.5	0.5
Morris et al. (14) (N = 124)	40	12	2	8	5	23	1	10
Bourgeois et al. (15) (N = 98)	11	23	N/A	24	15	21	0	4
Tumoral temporal lobe epilepsy								
Plate et al. (11) (N = 126)	13	N/A	10	12	10	18	9	26
Zaatreh et al. (23) (N = 68)	21	6	N/A	18	N/A	46[b]	N/A	9
Tumoral extratemporal lobe epilepsy								
Frater et al. (12) (N = 37)	19	16	N/A	11	3	35[b]	N/A	16

[a]DNET, dysembryoplastic neuroepithelial tumor; PXA, pleomorphic xanthoastrocytoma.
[b]Nonspecifically referred to as low-grade astrocytoma.

TABLE 28.2

SEIZURE FREQUENCY IN VARIOUS BRAIN TUMOR
TYPES

Tumor	Seizure frequency (%)
Dysembryoplastic neuroepithelial tumor (4,16)	100
Ganglioglioma (3)	80–90
Low-grade astrocytoma (3)	75
Meningioma (8)	27–60
Glioblastoma multiforme (3)	29–50
Primary CNS lymphoma (3,7)	10–20

Regardless of the tumor type, patients who present with
seizures as the initial symptom of a brain tumor are at higher
risk of later developing epilepsy (recurrent seizures), even with
prophylactic trials of antiepileptic drug (AED) treatment
(22,23). Furthermore, up to 50% of those tumor-related epilepsies may become medically intractable, a risk which is significantly higher than that seen with other epilepsies (9,20,24).

PROPOSED MECHANISMS OF EPILEPTOGENESIS

The development of epilepsy in a brain tumor patient is probably a multifactorial phenomenon. So, even though we will discuss multiple proposed mechanisms of epileptogenicity in
brain tumors, it is important to remember that those mechanisms are not mutually exclusive, and that in any given patient,
epilepsy is likely due to an interplay of all of those variables.

Role of Tumor Type

High-grade tumors may lead to epilepsy by abruptly damaging local tissue, causing tissue necrosis and hemosiderin deposition, and increasing excitability of local and immediately
surrounding cortex (4,18,25). Chronic intractable epilepsy is,
however, most often caused by lower grade tumors, specifically low-grade gliomas and developmental tumors—mainly
gangliogliomas and dysembryoplastic neuroepithelial tumors
(DNET) (11,12,13–15,26,27). These developmental tumors
are surrounded by dysplastic cortex in 25% to 70% of cases
(12,14,28,29), or may be associated with coexistent hippocampal sclerosis (6,30). In such a setting of "dual pathology," seizures may be mainly or independently arising from
the dysplasia or hippocampal sclerosis, and not necessarily the
tumor. A practical and important implication of that is the
inability to control seizures surgically in patients with chronic
intractable epilepsy due to such dual pathology unless both
"lesions" are resected.

Role of Peritumoral Morphological Changes

A brain tumor disrupts the tissue around it and causes a variety of morphological changes that facilitate excitability and

thus increase epileptogenicity. Those changes include aberrant
neuronal migration, enhanced intercellular communication
through increased expression of gap junctions, changes in
synaptic vesicles, and increased local concentrations of glutamate and lactate (3,4,25,31). Synaptic transmission, including
GABA receptor signaling, may be underexpressed in brain
tumor tissues compared with control tissue, further increasing
excitability (32).

In addition to the above microscopic and molecular
changes, gross tumor-related effects include mass effect, local
edema, and increased pressure. Also, local infiltrative tumor
growth may cause local irritation and epileptogenicity, presumably through inducing tissue hypoxia (33).

Role of Changes to the Microenvironment

Tumors have increased metabolic requirements, and even with
increased angiogenesis, eventually lead to intra- and peritu-
moral hypoxia. This alkalinizes the interstitial pH and causes
glial cell swelling and damage, increasing neuronal excitability
and facilitating epileptogenic activity (4,34). The risk of
epilepsy further increases because of increased inward-sodium
currents at the level of the astrocytic cell membrane. This
results from defective intracellular mechanisms for deoxyribonucleic acid (DNA) repair and genetic instability also occurring due to tumor-related hypoxia (3).

Role of Genetic Factors

Some studies have suggested a role for *LGI-1* in tumor-related
epilepsy (3,4). This is a tumor-suppressor gene absent in
glioblastoma multiforme and other high-grade invasive
tumors. It also happens to be responsible for the rare autosomal dominant lateral temporal lobe epilepsy. Some have,
therefore, suggested that it may then be implicated in both
tumor progression and epileptogenesis (3,4).

In addition, LIM-domain-binding 2 (LDB2) transcript,
critical for brain development during embryogenesis, was one
of the strongest reduced mRNAs in gangliogliomas in recent
array analyses. Silencing of LDB2 resulted in substantially
aberrant dendritic arborization in cultured developing primary hippocampal neurons. This characterizes yet another
molecular mechanism operating in gangliogliomas, contributing to the development of dysplastic neurons and an aberrant
neuronal network (35).

Role of Disruption of Functional Network Topology and Secondary Epileptogenesis

Rather than traditional views conceptualizing the brain as a
conglomerate of segregated functional areas, each specifically
dedicated to one function, the modern theory of brain
networks proposes the presence of cortical networks composed
of multiple cortical regions connected via white matter pathways controlling various mainly higher cortical functions, and
requiring a delicate balance between excitability and inhibition
of those multiple pathways to operate correctly (3). A disruption of those "normal networks"—as occurs anatomically with

a tumor—will disturb this balance, leading to multiple consequences, including deafferentation and release of regulatory inhibition on potentially epileptogenic structures (such as the hippocampus), and the appearance of pathological, less stable compensatory networks that may themselves be more excitable and thus potentially epileptogenic. This hypothesis is still being investigated, and further research is needed to clarify the full extent of its impact. It might, however, partly explain, among other things, how an epileptogenic focus arises distant from a tumor (30), and why a procedure that would not basically affect this desynchronization and deafferentation, such as with a simple removal of the tumor via a lesionectomy, may not achieve optimal seizure freedom (36).

It has been suggested that in almost one third of patients with brain tumors and epilepsy, the epileptogenic focus does not correspond to tumor location. This phenomenon is called secondary epileptogenesis, implying that an actively discharging epileptogenic region induces similar paroxysmal activity in regions distant from the original site. This process is mostly seen with low-grade brain tumors located in the temporal lobe, which may have associated hippocampal sclerosis (21). In those cases, the "secondary focus" becomes a completely independent epileptic generator that needs to be also removed to achieve seizure freedom in intractable patients. Since young age and long disease duration have been proposed as being the main risk factors for this secondary epileptogenesis (37), early resection of the primary focus—the tumor—has been promoted to avoid the development of an irreversible secondary focus and was actually shown to correlate with better rates of seizure freedom following resective epilepsy surgery (10,15,37).

TREATMENT OF SEIZURES IN THE SETTING OF BRAIN TUMORS

With seizures occurring so frequently in patients with brain tumors, it is important to be aware of the various treatment options available. Very often, adequate treatment of seizures in such a setting requires a multidisciplinary approach, including the patient's neuro-oncologist, neurosurgeon, and epileptologist. Goals of treatment need to be clarified early on in the treatment course, as well as a clear determination of the risk–benefit ratio of various medical and surgical therapeutic options. For example, aiming at complete seizure freedom in a patient with an inoperable, rapidly growing, glioblastoma multiforme while concomitantly using five different AEDs with their associated side effects, may actually end up being counterproductive, worsening the patient's quality of life. On the other hand, a simple reduction in seizure frequency would likely be an unacceptable treatment goal in a patient with a developmental tumor where resective epilepsy surgery has a high chance of achieving complete seizure freedom with relatively low associated comorbidity.

The following section will review current information available on medical and surgical aspects of the treatment of seizures in the setting of brain tumors.

Medical Treatment

Anticonvulsant medications are the mainstay of epilepsy treatment in any patient with seizures, including one with a brain tumor. However, little is known about the specific efficacy of different AEDs in the setting of a brain neoplasm. As can be concluded from Table 28.3, summarizing most recent major studies addressing this issue, many patients have recurrent seizures (60% to 70%) despite the use of AEDs. First-line AEDs fail in about 60% of patients and, of the remainder, a similar proportion of second-line treatments with monotherapy or polytherapy fails (9). A few retrospective studies have favored the use of valproic acid when compared to phenytoin or carbamazepine in view of the promptness of it achieving a therapeutic level, its enzyme-inhibiting properties that may increase the effectiveness of concomitant chemotherapy, and some potential inherent antitumor effects (3,33). However, it may cause significant bone marrow suppression, especially given its combination with chemotherapy. On the other hand, several prospective studies have recently suggested that either gabapentin (38), levetiracetam (39,40), or topiramate (41) may be effective options for add-on therapy. In one prospective series of 26 patients with primary brain tumors who received add-on levetiracetam, usually in combination with valproic acid, a seizure reduction of more than 50% was observed in 65% of patients (40). In a small prospective series of 14 patients with intractable seizures and brain neoplasms, gabapentin was added to phenytoin, carbamazepine, or clobazam. Reduction in seizure frequency was seen in all patients, and more than 50% became seizure-free (38). In another prospective observational study of 47 glioma patients, initial or add-on therapy with topiramate achieved complete seizure freedom in 56% of patients with a seizure reduction in an additional 20% after a mean follow-up of 16.5 months (41). All three prospective studies report a low incidence of side effects, although those were slightly higher with topiramate when compared to levetiracetam or gabapentin. No head-to-head trials comparing those various AEDs are available.

Table 28.3 summarizes data from some major studies evaluating medical treatment of seizures in brain tumors.

Special Issues Pertaining to Medical Treatment of Epilepsy in Brain Tumors

Medical Intractability of Epilepsy in Brain Tumors

While 20% to 25% of epilepsy patients in general continue to have frequent seizures despite the use of AEDs at adequate serum concentrations, this medical intractability occurs in up to 50% to 60% of patients with seizures and brain tumors (3,9,10,17,20,25,34). This has been attributed to a variety of possible mechanisms. Overexpression of proteins belonging to the multidrug resistance pathway is a frequently discussed mechanism of refractoriness. These proteins are members of the adenosine triphosphate (ATP)-binding cassette transporter family, normally present in the apical membranes of endothelial cells. The multidrug-resistance gene MDR-1 (ABCB1, P-glycoprotein) and multidrug-resistance–related protein (MRP, ABCC1) contribute to the blood–brain and blood–cerebrospinal fluid barriers by controlling the transport of various lipophilic substances in and out of the brain. Many AEDs, including phenytoin, carbamazepine, lamotrigine, felbamate, and phenobarbital, are substrates for MDR-1 products, and are therefore actively eliminated from the intracellular milieu and brain parenchyma when the MDR proteins are overexpressed. Such overexpression has been

TABLE 28.3

SUMMARY OF STUDIES EVALUATING EFFECTIVENESS OF VARIOUS AEDS IN THE SETTING OF SEIZURES IN BRAIN TUMORS

	Study characteristics			Tumor characteristics		AED characteristics		Outcome	
Study	N	Type[a]	Follow-up	Grade	Treatment	Primary drug	Add-on drug	% Seizure-free (%)	% Seizure reduction (%)
Hildebrand et al. (9)	234	R	3–276	High, grade II glioma	Surgery Radiation Chemotherapy	VPA CBZ GBP LTG Others		13	NA
Wick et al. (33)	107	R		High, Low	Surgery Chemotherapy Radiotherapy	PHT VPA CBZ		30[b]	
Wagner et al. (40)	26	P	9.3	High	Radiotherapy Chemotherapy Steroids Surgery	VPA	LEV	20	65
Maschio et al. (39)	19	P	7–50	High	Radiotherapy Chemotherapy Steroids Surgery	LTG VPA TOP OXC	LEV	47	72
Newton et al. (3)	41	R	1–2	High	Radiotherapy Chemotherapy Steroids	PHT CBZ	LEV	59	90
Maschio et al. (41)	47	P	3–48 (16.5)	High, Metastatic, Low	Surgery Steroids Radiotherapy	PHT CBZ PB	TOP	56	76
Perry et al. (38)	14	P	1–6	High	Radiotherapy Steroids	PHT CBZ Clobazam	GBP	57	100

[a]P, prospective; R, retrospective.
[b]70% of patients on CBZ had recurrent seizures, as opposed to 51% of those on PHT and 44% of those on VPA.
CBZ, carbamazepine; PHT, phenytoin; PB, phenobarbital; VPA, valproic acid; TOP, topiramate; LTG, lamotrigine.

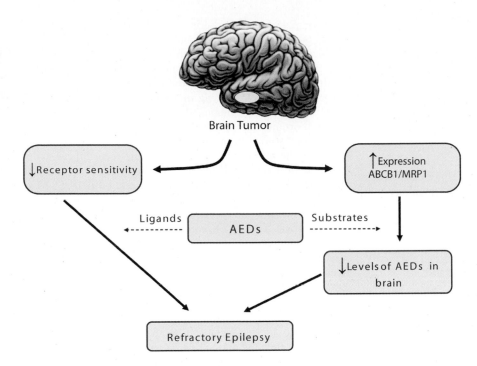

FIGURE 28.1 Decreased receptor sensitivity and increased expression of multidrug resistance proteins play the most important roles in medical refractoriness seen with brain tumors and epilepsy.

found for MDR-1 in cells of patients with gliomas and gangliogliomas (20,25,42), and for another MDR protein, the breast-cancer-resistance protein (BCRP), in endothelial cells of brain tumor specimens from astrocytomas, anaplastic astrocytomas, and glioblastoma multiforme (34). Gabapentin may be transported via a nonspecific transporter out of the brain. However, levetiracetam does not seem to be a substrate for either MDR-1 or other MDR proteins, while the histone deacetylase–inhibiting effects of valproic acid might reduce the expression of P-glycoprotein and MRP-1 raising interest in the potential usefulness of those AEDs in intractable patients (34). This needs to be confirmed by further studies.

Other proposed mechanisms of AED resistance in brain tumors are reduced drug receptor sensitivity, including ion channels, neurotransmitter receptors, and metabolic enzymes involved in the activity of neurotransmitters, as well as reduction in the concentration of several enzyme-inducing AEDs caused by concomitant use of chemotherapeutic agents. Figure 28.1 illustrates the interaction among various proposed mechanisms of resistance to medical therapy.

Issues Related to Interactions between AEDs and Antineoplastic Agents

There is a significant risk for drug–drug interactions during concomitant use of AEDs and chemotherapeutic agents, as both are substrates for the same hepatic metabolic pathways, mainly the cytochrome P450 system. Carbamazepine, phenytoin, phenobarbital, and primidone, and to a lesser extent lamotrigine and topiramate, have prominent cytochrome P450 enzyme-inducing effects, while valproic acid has an inhibitory effect. Induction or inhibition of these enzymes by AEDs can cause a decrease or increase in anticancer drug concentrations, and thus possibly their effectiveness. Similarly, enzyme inhibition or induction by anticancer drugs can lead to toxicity or loss of seizure control (34,43). Newer AEDs such as gabapentin, levetiracetam, and pregabalin do not influence the cytochrome P450 or other metabolic pathways, and theoretically would have a minimal risk for drug–drug interactions with chemotherapeutic agents (4,25).

Dexamethasone is frequently used in the treatment of tumor-associated edema, and also interacts significantly with certain AEDs. It competes with phenytoin for protein binding, raising its blood concentration. Conversely, it may cause the opposite effect of lowering phenytoin's serum concentration by affecting its hepatic metabolism (25).

In summary, significant risks for reduced effectiveness and toxicity exist for both chemotherapeutic agents and enzyme-inducing and -inhibiting AEDs when used concomitantly. The patient should be cautiously observed for side effects, and serum AED blood levels need to be monitored closely.

AED Prophylaxis in Brain Tumors

The American Academy of Neurology published a consensus statement in 2000 recommending that AED prophylaxis should not be used, and current AEDs discontinued, in brain tumor patients who do not have a history of seizures (22). A more recent meta-analysis of controlled clinical trials evaluating the effectiveness of seizure prophylaxis in people with brain tumors, performed between 1966 and 2007, found no difference between the treatment interventions and the control groups in preventing a first seizure in participants with brain tumors concluding that the evidence is neutral, neither for nor against seizure prophylaxis, in people with brain tumors (23). The authors recognized that these conclusions apply only for the older AEDs: phenytoin, phenobarbital, and divalproex sodium (23). Therefore, based on current evidence, the decision to start prophylactic AED use in brain tumor patients should ultimately be guided by assessment of individual risk factors and careful discussion with patients, keeping in mind that there is no strong evidence that any of the currently available AEDs reliably prevent a first seizure in a brain tumor patient.

Surgical Treatment

In general, the following questions are considered when evaluating the surgical management of a patient with tumor-associated epilepsy: does this patient really need surgery now to treat his/her seizures or is medical therapy sufficient? Should any kind of neurophysiological testing be performed prior to surgery? What type of surgery should be offered? Will a lesionectomy be appropriate, or is a more aggressive resection required? How can this patient be counseled about his/her seizure outcome following surgery? Despite extensive literature available on these topics, such decisions remain very much patient-dependent, and a careful consideration of all treatment options, as well as a clear and educated patient informed consent process represent the cornerstones of a successful "outcome." The following segments will briefly address some of the questions raised above.

Timing of Surgery: Now or Later?

A critical piece of information that determines the answer to this question is the type and grade of the tumor in question. Alternatively asked, this question is equivalent to deciding whether the patient needs "tumor surgery" or "epilepsy surgery." In patients with a high-grade brain tumor, or one with a high risk of malignant transformation such as gangliogliomas, surgical removal is an essential part of the tumor treatment, and should be performed regardless of whether it is believed to help with seizures or not in order to improve the patient's quality of life and chances of survival (13,15,18,21,25,44). On the other hand, most developmental tumors and many low-grade tumors may be observed for years from a tumor treatment perspective, or be treated with chemotherapy or radiotherapy. "Tumor surgery" is therefore not required immediately, and the decision to operate would mainly depend on whether a patient's seizures are controlled with AEDs or not. Many epileptologists usually wait until seizures are medically intractable before pursuing surgical tumor removal. However, many studies suggest that a shorter epilepsy duration at the time of tumor resection is an important predictor of postoperative seizure freedom. In a retrospective review of 332 patients following resection of low-grade gliomas, postoperative seizure control was significantly poorer in patients with longer seizure history ($P < 0.001$) (10). In another study evaluating the seizure outcome of 26 children following resection of their DNETs, all patients with epilepsy duration of less than 2 years were seizure-free at 12 months after surgery as opposed to 7/11 of those with longer seizure history (24). Such observations, together with the high risk of intractability in low-grade tumors (1,3,4), support early removal of low-grade brain tumors associated with epilepsy, especially when the tumor is easily surgically accessible (3). At any rate, a careful preoperative attempt at determining the nature of the tumor should be one of the initial steps in evaluating whether a patient needs immediate surgery or not.

Presurgical Neurophysiological Evaluation

In most tumor-related epilepsy surgery patients, preoperative video-EEG evaluations confirm that seizures arise from the lobe involved with the tumor. In one study of children with dysmebryoplastic neuroepithelial tumors, all but one case had ictal onset discharges unilaterally concordant with the tumor location (24). In another series of adult tumor-related epilepsy patients, the epileptogenic focus as determined by interictal and ictal recordings agreed with the involved lobe in 72% of the cases (14). So, why do we need to perform video-EEG evaluations prior to treating the epilepsy of a brain tumor patient by simply removing the tumor? Several hypothetical and evidence-based outcome data support this practice. First, it is important to acknowledge that even though the above-mentioned studies showed seizures arising from the "same lobe" as the tumor, electrocorticographic recordings usually show that the tumors themselves are electrically inert and that epilepsy often arises from the tissue surrounding the tumor (31). Some have even suggested that seizures arise distant from the tumor in up to a third of patients with brain tumors and epilepsy (3,9,30). So, a preoperative video-EEG evaluation may provide evidence for the extent of epileptogenicity in the surrounding brain tissues. Figure 28.2 illustrates a case where a subdural EEG evaluation confirmed ictal onset distal from the tumor and where seizure-freedom was achieved by resecting both the lesion and surrounding cortex. Second, not all brain tumors are epileptogenic and not all "spells" are epileptic, so a video-EEG evaluation may be helpful in confirming the epileptic nature of a patient's spells and characterizing the relationship of the epileptogenic focus to the tumor itself (29). Third, some studies have reported better seizure outcomes with the use of intraoperative electrocorticography in tumor surgery and the resection of intraoperatively identified zones of interictal spiking and ictal onsets (3,13,45). In a study of 35 patients with intractable temporal lobe epilepsy (TLE) related to benign mass lesions, the number of 3-year postoperative seizure-free incidences for the group that underwent lesionectomy plus additional spike-positive site resection equated to 90.9%. In contrast, in the group that underwent a lesionectomy only, 76.9% were seizure-free for 3 years postoperatively (45). However, such results need to be reproduced in larger scale randomized studies. Lastly, when tumors occur in proximity to eloquent cortex, intra- or extraoperative functional mapping is often essential in determining the extent of the surgical resection (46). For all the above reasons, it is recommended to perform a neurophysiological evaluation, preferably at least a video-EEG evaluation with ictal recordings, prior to proceeding to surgery in a brain tumor patient with seizures.

Type of Surgery: Lesionectomy Alone or More Aggressive Resection?

Multiple studies have reported favorable seizure outcomes with complete lesionectomies alone, with seizure-freedom rates ranging from 65% to 80% (21,26,27,47). There is evidence, however, to support more aggressive resections in certain situations. This issue has been investigated most extensively in relation to temporal lobe tumors and epilepsy. In one study of 18 patients who underwent surgical removal of a dysembryoplastic neuroepithelial tumor—12 via temporal lobectomy and six via lesionectomy—temporal lobectomy led to a better seizure outcome (Engel Class I, 83.3%; Engel Class IA, 66.7%) than lesionectomy (Engel Classes I and IA, 33.3%) after a mean follow-up of 10.8 years (16). In another study reporting 41 surgical interventions in 38 adults with dual pathology, including 10 with tumors, lesionectomy plus mesial temporal resection resulted in complete freedom from seizures in 11/15 (73%) patients,

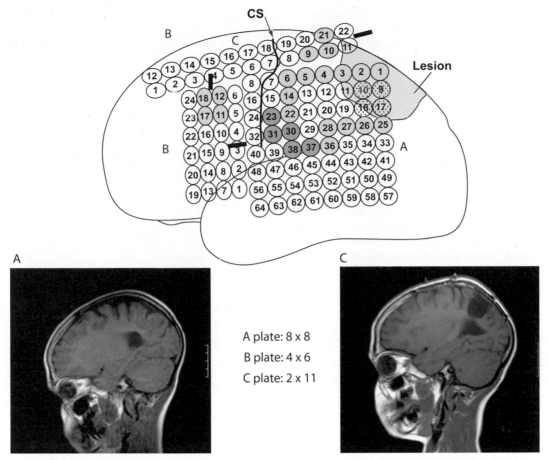

FIGURE 28.2 This figure illustrates the case of a 10-year-old boy with a left parietal low-grade glioma where subdural EEG recordings showed interictal activity diffusely, both proximal and distal to the lesion (light gray), and two different seizure patterns: one arising from the lesion itself (speckled gray) and one arising somewhat distally from the lesion (dark gray). Central sulcus (CS) location is also illustrated. An "extensive lesionectomy" was performed to include areas of identified epileptogenicity rendering the patient seizure-free (follow-up of 2 years). **A** and **C** show the preoperative and postoperative MRI, respectively.

while only 2/10 (20%) patients who had mesial temporal resection alone and 2/16 (12.5%) who had a lesionectomy alone were seizure-free ($P < 0.001$) (48). Such findings have been attributed to the high prevalence of dual pathology in temporal lobe tumors (28,29,49), and to the risk of associated secondary epileptogenesis. This is supported by the persistence of interictal spiking recorded with intraoperative electrocorticography in the hippocampus of 86% of cases and in the amygdala in 64% of the cases after resection of temporal lobe tumors (3). The practice of resecting the mesial temporal structures while resecting the tumor is easy to accept and understand when there is preoperative evidence of dual pathology preoperatively, that is when the hippocampus looks dysmorphic or sclerosed on baseline magnetic resonance imaging (MRI). In such cases, the above-mentioned outcome data prompt most surgical centers to resect the hippocampus, especially if neuropsychologial testing suggests a low risk for postoperative functional decline. The decision becomes more problematic when the hippocampus looks normal on imaging, especially if baseline neuropsychological testing is normal. Currently, it is difficult to justify resecting a dominant normally appearing hippocampus unless there is compelling evidence, such as

with extraoperative depths recordings for example, documenting seizures arising from the mesial structures.

Seizure Outcome

In both temporal and extratemporal epilepsy surgery, a tumoral etiology carries usually a favorable prognosis and is associated with a favorable seizure outcome in as many as 65% to 87% of the cases (10,15,21,26,27,47,50).

Consistently identified favorable prognostic indicators are complete tumor resection and short epilepsy duration at the time of surgery.

In one study evaluating outcomes of 44 patients with ganglioglioma following surgery, 23/23 patients with a gross total tumor removal were seizure-free at last follow-up compared to 1/3 of those with subtotal resections (51). In another review of 332 adults with low-grade glioma, patients with a gross-total resection were 16 times more likely to achieve seizure freedom than after subtotal resection/biopsy alone (10). Residual tumor on postoperative MRI in a cohort of 26 children with DNETs predicted long-term seizure recurrence (24). There is little doubt currently then that a complete resection is the crucial determinant of seizure freedom. Seizure recurrence should prompt an evaluation for tumor recurrence (24,29).

Similarly, a shorter duration of epilepsy at the time of surgery seems to predict more favorable seizure outcomes (10,24,51). This finding may support early tumor removal in the setting of seizures, as discussed previously.

CONCLUSIONS

Tumors constitute a very important cause of chronic intractable epilepsy, and seizures represent a very frequent presenting symptom of brain tumors. Our knowledge of the mechanisms defining the relationship between the two conditions has grown exponentially over the past few years, but a lot remains to be learned. Several medical and surgical treatment options are available, and multiple potential mechanisms of epileptogenicity in brain tumors have been proposed. So, a diagnostic or a treatment approach focused solely on one mechanistic premise will provide an incomplete view of the true disease pathophysiology and likely be unsuccessful.

References

1. Lynam LM, Lyons MK, Drazkowski JF, et al. Frequency of seizures in patients with newly diagnosed brain tumors: a retrospective review. *Clin Neurol Neurosurg.* 2007;109(7):634–638.
2. Ibrahim K, Appleton R. Seizures as the presenting symptom of brain tumours in children. *Seizure.* 2004;13(2):108–112.
3. Brogna C, Gil Robles S, Duffau H. Brain tumors and epilepsy. *Expert Rev Neurother.* 2008;8(6):941–955.
4. van Breemen MS, Wilms EB, Vecht CJ. Epilepsy in patients with brain tumours: epidemiology, mechanisms, and management. *Lancet Neurol.* 2007;6(5):421–430.
5. Scott GM, Gibberd FB. Epilepsy and other factors in the prognosis of gliomas. *Acta Neurol Scand.* 1980;61(4):227–239.
6. Prayson RA. Pathology of epileptogenic neoplasms. In: Lüders HO, ed. *Textbook of Epilepsy Surgery.* 1st ed. United Kingdom: Informa; 2008:1373–1383.
7. Hochberg FH, Miller DC. Primary central nervous system lymphoma. *J Neurosurg.* 1988;68(6):835–853.
8. Lieu AS, Howng SL. Intracranial meningiomas and epilepsy: incidence, prognosis and influencing factors. *Epilepsy Res.* 2000;38(1):45–52.
9. Hildebrand J, Lecaille C, Perennes J, et al. Epileptic seizures during follow-up of patients treated for primary brain tumors. *Neurology.* 2005; 65(2):212–215.
10. Chang EF, Potts MB, Keles GE, et al. Seizure characteristics and control following resection in 332 patients with low-grade gliomas. *J Neurosurg.* 2008;108(2):227–235.
11. Plate KH, Wieser HG, Yasargil MG, et al. Neuropathological findings in 224 patients with temporal lobe epilepsy. *Acta Neuropathol.* 1993; 86(5):433–438.
12. Frater JL, Prayson RA, Morris HH III, et al. Surgical pathologic findings of extratemporal-based intractable epilepsy: a study of 133 consecutive resections. *Arch Pathol Lab Med.* 2000;124(4):545–549.
13. Zentner J, Hufnagel A, Wolf HK, et al. Surgical treatment of neoplasms associated with medically intractable epilepsy. *Neurosurgery.* 1997; 41(2):378–386; discussion 386–387.
14. Morris HH III, Estes ML, Prayson RA, et al. Frequency of different tumor types encountered in the Cleveland Clinic epilepsy surgery program. *Epilepsia.* 1996;37(suppl 5):S96.
15. Bourgeois M, Sainte-Rose C, Lellouch-Tubiana A, et al. Surgery of epilepsy associated with focal lesions in childhood. *J Neurosurg.* 1999;90(5): 833–842.
16. Chan CH, Bittar RG, Davis GA, et al. Long-term seizure outcome following surgery for dysembryoplastic neuroepithelial tumor. *J Neurosurg.* 2006;104(1):62–69.
17. Bromfield EB. Epilepsy in patients with brain tumors and other cancers. *Rev Neurol Dis.* 2004;1(suppl 1):S27–S33.
18. Salmaggi A, Silvani A, Merli R, et al. Multicentre prospective collection of newly diagnosed glioblastoma patients: update on the Lombardia experience. *Neurol Sci.* 2008;29(2):77–83.
19. Hamilton W, Kernick D. Clinical features of primary brain tumours: a case-control study using electronic primary care records. *Br J Gen Pract.* 2007;57(542):695–699.
20. Dupont S. Epilepsy and brain tumors. *Rev Neurol (Paris).* 2008; 164(6–7):517–522.
21. Bauer R, Dobesberger J, Unterhofer C, et al. Outcome of adult patients with temporal lobe tumours and medically refractory focal epilepsy. *Acta Neurochir (Wien).* 2007;149(12):1211–1216; discussion 1216–1217.
22. Glantz MJ, Cole BF, Forsyth PA, et al. Practice parameter: anticonvulsant prophylaxis in patients with newly diagnosed brain tumors. Report of the Quality Standards Subcommittee of the American Academy of Neurology. *Neurology.* 2000;54(10):1886–1893.
23. Tremont-Lukats IW, Ratilal BO, Armstrong T, et al. Antiepileptic drugs for preventing seizures in people with brain tumors. *Cochrane Database Syst Rev.* 2008;2:CD004424.
24. Nolan MA, Sakuta R, Chuang N, et al. Dysembryoplastic neuroepithelial tumors in childhood: long-term outcome and prognostic features. *Neurology.* 2004;62(12):2270–2276.
25. van Breemen MS, Vecht CJ. Optimal seizure management in brain tumor patients. *Curr Neurol Neurosci Rep.* 2005;5(3):207–213.
26. Zaatreh MM, Firlik KS, Spencer DD, et al. Temporal lobe tumoral epilepsy: characteristics and predictors of surgical outcome. *Neurology.* 2003;61(5):636–641.
27. Zaatreh MM, Spencer DD, Thompson JL, et al. Frontal lobe tumoral epilepsy: clinical, neurophysiologic features and predictors of surgical outcome. *Epilepsia.* 2002;43(7):727–733.
28. Prayson RA, Estes ML, Morris HH. Coexistence of neoplasia and cortical dysplasia in patients presenting with seizures. *Epilepsia.* 1993;34(4): 609–615.
29. Jehi LE, Luders HO, Naugle R, et al. Temporal lobe neoplasm and seizures: how deep does the story go? *Epileptic Disord.* 2008;10(1):56–67.
30. Adachi Y, Yagishita A. Gangliogliomas: characteristic imaging findings and role in the temporal lobe epilepsy. *Neuroradiology.* 2008;50(10):829–834.
31. Wolf HK, Roos D, Blumcke I, et al. Perilesional neurochemical changes in focal epilepsies. *Acta Neuropathol.* 1996;91(4):376–384.
32. Aronica E, Boer K, Becker A, et al. Gene expression profile analysis of epilepsy-associated gangliogliomas. *Neuroscience.* 2008;151(1):272–292.
33. Wick W, Menn O, Meisner C, et al. Pharmacotherapy of epileptic seizures in glioma patients: who, when, why and how long? *Onkologie.* 2005;28(8–9):391–396.
34. Vecht CJ, van Breemen M. Optimizing therapy of seizures in patients with brain tumors. *Neurology.* 2006;67(12 suppl 4):S10–S13.
35. Fassunke J, Majores M, Tresch A, et al. Array analysis of epilepsy-associated gangliogliomas reveals expression patterns related to aberrant development of neuronal precursors. *Brain.* 2008;131(Pt 11):3034–3050.
36. Morioka T, Hashiguchi K, Nagata S, et al. Additional hippocampectomy in the surgical management of intractable temporal lobe epilepsy associated with glioneuronal tumor. *Neurol Res.* 2007;29(8):807–815.
37. Morrell F, deToledo-Morrell L. From mirror focus to secondary epileptogenesis in man: an historical review. *Adv Neurol.* 1999;81:11–23.
38. Perry JR, Sawka C. Add-on gabapentin for refractory seizures in patients with brain tumours. *Can J Neurol Sci.* 1996;23(2):128–131.
39. Maschio M, Albani F, Baruzzi A, et al. Levetiracetam therapy in patients with brain tumour and epilepsy. *J Neurooncol.* 2006;80(1):97–100.
40. Wagner GL, Wilms EB, Van Donselaar CA, et al. Levetiracetam: preliminary experience in patients with primary brain tumours. *Seizure.* 2003;12(8):585–586.
41. Maschio M, Dinapoli L, Zarabla A, et al. Outcome and tolerability of topiramate in brain tumor associated epilepsy. *J Neurooncol.* 2008;86(1):61–70.
42. Lazarowski A, Czornyj L, Lubienieki F, et al. ABC transporters during epilepsy and mechanisms underlying multidrug resistance in refractory epilepsy. *Epilepsia.* 2007;48(suppl 5):140–149.
43. Yap KY, Chui WK, Chan A. Drug interactions between chemotherapeutic regimens and antiepileptics. *Clin Ther.* 2008;30(8):1385–1407.
44. Moots PL, Maciunas RJ, Eisert DR, et al. The course of seizure disorders in patients with malignant glioma. *Arch Neurol.* 1995;52(7):717–724.
45. Sugano H, Shimizu H, Sunaga S. Efficacy of intraoperative electrocorticography for assessing seizure outcomes in intractable epilepsy patients with temporal-lobe-mass lesions. *Seizure.* 2007;16(2):120–127.
46. Serletis D, Bernstein M. Prospective study of awake craniotomy used routinely and nonselectively for supratentorial tumors. *J Neurosurg.* 2007;107(1):1–6.
47. Jehi LE, O'Dwyer R, Najm I et al. A longitudinal study of surgical outcome and its determinants following posterior cortex epilepsy surgery. *Epilepsia.* 2009;50(9):2040–2052.
48. Li LM, Cendes F, Andermann F, et al. Surgical outcome in patients with epilepsy and dual pathology. *Brain.* 1999;122(Pt 5):799–805.
49. Takahashi A, Hong SC, Seo DW, et al. Frequent association of cortical dysplasia in dysembryoplastic neuroepithelial tumor treated by epilepsy surgery. *Surg Neurol.* 2005;64(5):419–427.
50. Boesebeck F, Janszky J, Kellinghaus C, et al. Presurgical seizure frequency and tumoral etiology predict the outcome after extratemporal epilepsy surgery. *J Neurol.* 2007;254(8):996–999.
51. Park YS, Kim DS, Shim KW, et al. Factors contributing to resectability and seizure outcomes in 44 patients with ganglioglioma. *Clin Neurol Neurosurg.* 2008;110(7):667–673.

CHAPTER 29 ■ POST-TRAUMATIC EPILEPSY

STEPHAN SCHUELE

EPIDEMIOLOGY

Post-traumatic epilepsy (PTE) accounts for around 200 new cases of epilepsy per 100,000 persons per year (1,2). PTE is the leading cause of epilepsy with onset in young adulthood and the most common cause of acquired epilepsy (3,4). Head trauma underlies 6% of all epilepsies in the general population and accounts for 5% of patients seen at specialized epilepsy centers (5,6).

The cumulative risk of late unprovoked post-traumatic seizures consistent with a diagnosis of PTE varies between 2% and 20% in civilian populations suffering from closed head injuries, and can be as high as 50% in military series after penetrating head injuries (5). Nearly 40% of these late seizures appear within the first 6 months after injury; more than 50% appear by 1 year and 70% to 80% appear by 2 years after the injury (7,8). Although the risk of PTE continues to decline as the postinjury seizure-free interval lengthens, late seizures may begin over 15 years after the initial insult (9–11). The probability of PTE 5 years after traumatic brain injury (TBI) is estimated as 0.7% after mild, 1.2% after moderate, and 10.0% after severe TBI (10). After follow-up for more than 30 years, the probability increases to 2.1% for mild, 4.2% for moderate, and 16.7% for severe TBI. The relative risk (RR) of developing PTE after mild TBI is increased by twofold, moderate TBI by fourfold, and severe TBI by sevenfold or more (Table 29.1) (12,13).

Although the annual incidence of head injury in the general population has not changed in the past 30 years, the number of survivors of severe head injuries has risen, leading to a higher prevalence of patients with PTE (14). In addition, given the high percentage of head injuries of soldiers from the Iraq and Afghanistan wars a markedly increased number of veterans with post-traumatic seizures are anticipated.

PATHOPHYSIOLOGY OF POST-TRAUMATIC SEIZURES

Early Seizures

Early post-traumatic seizures are triggered by the acute trauma or subsequent complications and have to be differentiated from late, unprovoked post-traumatic seizures defining a diagnosis of epilepsy (10). A variety of mechanisms directly related to the initial trauma can trigger symptomatic seizures: The immediate insult after a head injury leads to diffuse axonal injury due to shearing forces and focal brain damage caused by the direct impact to the skull, movement of the brain within the skull (coup and contre coup), or penetrating wounds (15–18). Secondary axonal injury ensues caused by retraction and swelling of the injured axons with distal wallerian degeneration (19). Subsequent brain necrosis may result from cytotoxic processes such as the release of free oxygen radicals and cytokines and the influx of calcium into open ion channels (16,20). Most of these early post-traumatic seizures occur within the first week after injury (10). Complications

---

TABLE 29.1

RISK OF POST-TRAUMATIC EPILEPSY

Risk factors		Cumulative incidence (10)		Relative risk/standardized incidence ratio
		5 yrs	30 yrs	
Closed head injury	Mild	0.7%	2.1%	2.22 [95% CI 2.07–2.38] (13)
				1.5 [95% CI 1.0–2.2] (10)
Multivariate analysis (10)	Moderate	1.2%	4.2%	2.9 [95% CI 1.9–4.1] (10)
• Contusion	Severe	10.0%	16.7%	7.40 [95% CI 6.16–8.89] (13)
• Subdural				
• Skull fracture				17.0 [95% CI 12.3–23.6] (10)
• LOC > 1 d				
• Early seizure				
• Age ≥ 65 yrs				
Penetrating head injury (89)		22–43%	50%	

TABLE 29.2

DEFINITIONS

Seizures	Timing postinjury	Increased risk of epilepsy	Prophylaxis
Impact convulsion	At impact. Nonepileptic	–	For 7 days in patients with *severe* TBI
Early seizure	< 1 week[a]	+	
Immediate seizure	< 24 hrs		
Late seizure	> 1 week[a]	+++	After first late seizure
Post-traumatic seizures	Single or recurrent seizures after TBI, separated by early or late occurrence, not attributable to another obvious cause.		
Post-traumatic epilepsy	Late-onset, recurrent, unprovoked seizures after TBI, not attributable to another obvious cause.		

Degree of TBI	LOC	Skull fracture	Structural brain damage
Mild	< 30 min	–	–
Moderate	> 30 min and < 24 hrs	+/–	–
Severe	> 24 hrs	+	+

[a]4 weeks in patients with additional complications which may cause acute symptomatic seizures.

during the acute recovery phase, for example, hypoxia, increased intracranial pressure, hypotension, ischemia, cerebral edema, intracranial bleeding, electrolyte imbalances, or infections can cause symptomatic seizures several weeks after the injury (Table 29.2) (7,10,21,22). Overall, 90% of seizures within the first 4 weeks after head injury will happen during the first week and more than half of them within the first 24 hours (23,24).

The incidence of early post-traumatic seizures depends on the severity of the injury and is seen in approximately 2.5% of head injury patients in population-based studies and in up to 16% of patients admitted after severe head trauma (7,10,25–31). Moderate to severe head injury, in particular the presence of a subdural or intracerebral hematoma, a depressed skull fracture, a penetrating brain injury, or a cortical contusion, increases the incidence of early seizures up to 30% (10,32,33). With mild head injuries, early seizure often indicates other neurologic or systemic abnormalities and should warrant further evaluation and observation (21,34–36). A structural lesion from the acute injury—for example, an epidural or subdural hematoma—has to be excluded with imaging. On rare occasions, seizures after mild trauma are seen in the context of a pre-existing brain pathology (37,38), a constellation called pseudotraumatic epilepsy (39).

Approximately 10% of patients with early symptomatic seizures develop PTE. Early seizures are associated with an increased risk for late seizures (7,10,25–31). In most cases, the increased risk for PTE is not a direct consequence of the early seizures. Multivariate analysis in a large population-based study demonstrated that the increased risk of late epilepsy can be explained by other factors, for example, the presence of a cerebral contusion or hematoma, skull fracture, or age (10).

The presentation of early post-traumatic seizures is variable. Nonconvulsive, purely electrographic seizures only detectable by continuous electroencephalogram (EEG) monitoring appear to occur frequently. Based on a study with continuous intensive care unit (ICU) EEG monitoring, which included mostly patients with severe head injury, 21 out of 94 patients (22%) had post-traumatic seizures within the first week of injury (40). Only six patients had clinically witnessed generalized tonic–clonic seizures, another four patients showed subtle myoclonic movements with an epileptiform EEG correlate, and more than half of the patients had electrographic seizure without associated clinical signs. Frequent post-traumatic electrographic seizures are associated with episodic increases in intracranial pressure and lactate/pyruvate ratio, and may be a target for aggressive antiepileptic management (41).

Approximately 10% to 20% of early seizures evolve into status epilepticus, more often seen in children (23,42). Generalized convulsive status epilepticus often accompanies underlying secondary complications, such as ischemia or metabolic imbalance. Focal motor status is most common with subdural hematomas or depressed skull fractures and can be refractory to treatment. Patients with early status epilepticus may have a higher risk for late seizures than patients with self-limited early seizures according to one study (43). Patients with early status epilepticus had a 41% 10-year cumulative risk to develop late seizures compared to a 13% risk after brief symptomatic seizures. It remains unclear if this is related to the underlying lesion, the effect of the status itself, or a shared susceptibility for prolonged early seizures and epilepsy in some patients.

Late Seizures and Epileptogenesis

"Through trauma, the brain may be injured by contusion, laceration, compression, and it is well known that these insults may result in epilepsy after a 'silent period of strange ripening.' That period lasts for months or years, but these insults produce epilepsy in the case of one individual and not in the case of another . . . . Our attention should therefore be directed toward the discovery of this mysterious difference" (44,45).

The development of PTE after a latent period has been an intriguing observation and challenge for more than half a century. The "strange ripening" in PTE is a rare example of human epileptogenesis, the process whereby a nonepileptic brain is transformed into a brain able to generate recurrent, unprovoked seizures (46). The window between insult and occurrence of these unprovoked seizures offers a unique opportunity to investigate the potential mechanisms leading to epileptogenesis, to identify biomarkers, and to implement therapeutic interventions that are truly antiepileptic in the sense that they are able to prevent the development of the disease rather than merely suppress the seizures. Most of our understanding of the cellular and molecular mechanisms of epileptogenesis derives from experimental animal models which are not specifically related to traumatic injury: for example, disinhibition and selective loss of inhibitory γ-aminobutyric acid (GABA)ergic neurons and increased glutamatergic excitation have been described in post-traumatic as well as other experimental models of epileptogenesis (47,48).

One can argue that a better understanding and targeting of universal mechanisms of epileptogenicity may preferentially benefit patients with PTE given the prolonged latent period between injury and onset of epilepsy. On the other hand, prevention of PTE may require a more specific target unique to the epileptogenic process following head trauma. One example of a more specific epileptogenic process is early symptomatic seizure or status after head trauma that could cause progressive changes in neural networks and lead the way to spontaneous and recurrent late seizures (49), which may explain at least a portion of the PTEs. Another example is the hemosiderin deposition and formation of free iron radicals typical for head trauma and their high epileptogenic potential, which has been investigated over several decades (50,51).

Two animal models of PTE—the fluid percussion model leading to mesial temporal and the "cortical undercut" model for neocortical epilepsy—have been widely used to investigate epileptogenicity after traumatic brain injury (31,52–54). Based on the fluid percussion model, either a selective loss of hilar interneurons in the dentate gyrus or a relative survival of irritable mossy fibers, may lead to persistent granule cell hyperexcitability (55–57). A more recent study demonstrated that focal brain injury after a single episode of fluid percussion injury is able to trigger spontaneous seizures (58), which originate from the site of injury and become clinically and electrographically more severe over time (59,60).

Isolation of a small cortical region by transecting the white matter with a needle leads to epileptiform activity of the pyramidal cell layer in slice recordings in the "cortical undercut" model. Axonal sprouting of the isolated pyramidal cells is associated with an increased number of excitatory connections (61). Early application of tetrodotoxin after the injury blocks action potentials and prevents the development of evoked and spontaneous epileptiform activity in the neocortical slices (62), suggesting that post-traumatic epileptogenesis may be an activity-dependent process.

Tetrodotoxin given within 3 days of injury was able to prevent the occurrence of late seizures in an animal model of PTE (63). Some seizure medications have also shown antiepileptic properties in a kindling but not a post-traumatic animal model of epilepsy (64).

The process of epileptogenesis and postinjury recovery overlap in time and seem to share some basic mechanisms, including neurogenesis, axonal sprouting, and activity dependence (47). Disease-modifying agents and antiepileptic drugs may, therefore, have a positive (or negative) effect on recovery or epileptogenicity. TBI drug trials aimed to improve injury recovery have not looked at late seizures as an outcome measure or as an adverse effect. There are at least data that seizure medications—including remacemide, topiramate, talampanel, lacosamide, and carisbamate—seem to cause no major benefit nor harm on post-traumatic recovery in animal models (47). The process of epileptogenicity after trauma might be very specific. Effective prevention might need a clear target, appropriate timing, and should not interfere with adaptive processes necessary for functional recovery (48).

TREATMENT OF EARLY AND LATE SEIZURES

A meta-analysis (64) demonstrates the role for phenytoin (RR 0.33; confidence interval [CI], 0.19 to 0.59) and carbamazepine (RR 0.39; CI 0.17 to 0.92) in the prevention of early seizures after head trauma. A Cochrane Database Review of six trials concluded a beneficial effect of antiepileptic drugs (RR 0.34; 95% CI 0.21 to 0.54) for prevention of early seizures; based on the Cochrane estimate, for every 100 patients treated, 10 would be kept seizure-free in the first week (65,66). However, seizure control was not associated with a reduction in mortality or neurological disability or a diminished occurrence of late seizures (pooled RR 1.28; 95% CI 0.90 to 1.81).

On the basis of an analysis of prospective studies (67), the American Academy of Neurology has published recommendations on the use of antiepileptic drug prophylaxis in adults with traumatic brain injury. Their current recommendation is to use short-term phenytoin prophylaxis in adults only with severe brain injury with the goal to prevent early post-traumatic seizures. Phenytoin may be initiated as an intravenous loading dose as soon as possible after the injury. Data on newer antiepileptic medications for the prophylaxis of early seizures after severe head trauma are limited. Levetiracetam has been used in this indication and one observational study suggests that it may be similarly effective as phenytoin with easier use and less side effects (66,68). There are insufficient data to make recommendations on the use of antiepileptic drugs to prevent seizures in children (69–72). Current evidence does not support the routine use of antiepileptic drugs beyond the first 7 days after the injury. Administration of glucocorticoids after brain injury does not prevent late post-traumatic seizures, and early treatment with steroids has been shown to increase seizure activity (73).

Medical prophylaxis of late post-traumatic seizures is currently not recommended. For a long time, phenytoin and phenobarbital were thought to be useful in the prevention of late seizures based on observational studies (74,75), and they were routinely prescribed as a prophylactic medication for the most severely injured patients or those experiencing early post-traumatic seizures for 6 months or more (76). However, more recent randomized, double-blind, prospective evaluations of antiseizure prophylaxis with phenytoin, phenobarbital, carbamazepine, and valproic acid consistently found no benefit (69,77–79), irrespective of the choice of antiepileptic drug (79,80). On the contrary, phenytoin can impair cognition in post-traumatic patients (81) and benzodiazepines and barbiturates may interfere with injury recovery (82).

Late post-traumatic seizures beyond the period of the acute insult reflect permanent changes in the brain and signal the onset of PTE (25,83–85). After a first late unprovoked post-traumatic seizure, the vast majority of patients (86%) experience a second seizure within the following 2 years with the highest risk after a focal injury or coma for over 7 days (85). Treatment initiation in patients after a first late post-traumatic seizure seems appropriate even if the formal diagnosis of epilepsy requiring at least two unprovoked epileptic seizures cannot be made.

POST-TRAUMATIC EPILEPSY RISK FACTORS

Severity of Head Trauma

The risk of developing PTE depends on the severity of the head trauma and the presence of a penetrating injury. The most commonly used criterion for the severity of closed head trauma employed by epidemiologic studies examining civilian populations is based on the duration of loss of consciousness or amnesia and the presence of structural brain damage—the latter based on a focal neurological examination, x-rays showing a depressed skull fracture, or findings on computed tomography (CT) scan (10,12). Correlating with the severity of the TBI and an increased risk of PTE are prolonged coma or amnesia (longer than 24 hours), brain contusion, intracranial hematoma, depressed skull fracture, dural penetration, and, to a lesser extent, linear skull fractures (83,86,87).

The incidence of late post-traumatic seizures after closed head injury depends on the study population and varies between 1.9% and 25.3% (7,10,25,26,28–30). In the series reported by Annegers and Coan (see Table 29.1) (10,88), the RR of seizures was 1.5 (95% CI 1.0 to 2.2) after mild injuries with no increase after 5 years; 2.9 (95% CI 1.9 to 4.1) after moderate injuries; and 17.2 (95% CI 12.3 to 23.6) after severe injuries. In this study, mild trauma was defined by the presence of coma or amnesia for less than 30 minutes and the absence of a skull fracture; moderate head trauma was classified as coma or amnesia lasting between 30 minutes and 24 hours and the presence of a skull fracture in patients without contusion or intracranial hemorrhage; and severe trauma was classified as coma or amnesia for more than 24 hours and/or brain contusion or intracranial hemorrhage (see Table 29.2). According to a recent multicenter study, the highest cumulative probability for PTE after a two-year follow-up is seen with biparietal contusions (66%), dural penetration with bone and metal fragments (63%), multiple intracranial operations (37%), multiple subcortical contusions (33%), subdural hematoma (28%), midline shift >5 mm (26%), and multiple or bilateral contusions (25%) (30).

In military personnel who survive high-velocity penetrating head injuries during warfare, the long-term risk of PTE is consistently estimated at 50% in series examining the major wars of the 20th century (89,90). The ongoing war in Iraq has a lower percentage of penetrating head injuries. On the other hand, head injury caused by explosive devices is one of the signature injuries of the Iraq war, leading in about one third of

injured soldiers to various degrees of closed head injury. In combination with the better injury survival to death ratio (7.0 compared to 1.6 for World War II and 2.8 for the Vietnam War), the high percentage of patients with head injury will likely amount to a significant incidence of post-traumatic seizures.

Early Seizures

An early seizure increases the risk to develop late epilepsy by more than 25% after moderate and severe head injury according to most series (28,33,83,84,87). Mild TBI with early seizures may not carry an increased risk for late epilepsy (88). Late seizures are more likely to begin early (within the first year) if there has been an early seizure.

Age

The influence of age on the development of early seizures is well documented (2,29,83,84). Children younger than age 5 years are more likely than adults to have seizures within the first hour after mild head injury (26,27,42,91). However, early seizures are less predictive of late seizures in children than in adults (7,84).

Patients older than age 65 years are highly vulnerable to more severe brain damage and late PTE from any type of head injury (10,92). Earlier reports suggested an increased vulnerability for the development of late seizures associated with post-traumatic hippocampal sclerosis in children younger than 5 years of age (93,94). These findings have not been confirmed in more recent case series (95–97).

Genetic Factors

The evidence for genetic influences on post-traumatic seizures is conflicting. Some studies (98) reported a higher incidence of seizures in family members of patients with post-traumatic seizures; other research has failed to demonstrate a similar relationship (11,99). According to a recent report, a family history of epilepsy and mild brain injury independently contributed to the risk of epilepsy (13), which supports the concept that genetic factors play a role even in symptomatic focal epilepsies (100,101).

DIAGNOSIS

Clinical Seizures

The full spectrum of seizure semiology can be seen after head trauma. The site of injury and the underlying structural damage determine the type of focal manifestations (9,11,102,103). Early post-traumatic seizures are likely to present as generalized tonic–clonic convulsions even in the presence of focal brain damage (26,34,104). Late seizures mostly have a focal onset (9,102,103) and may develop subsequent to early generalized seizures (11). An interaction between the site of injury and the time when seizures are first noticed has been described. Seizures appear earliest after lesions of the motor area, followed by temporal lobe and those in the frontal or occipital areas (105).

Diagnostic Pitfalls

Nonepileptic Post-Traumatic Seizures

Head trauma is a risk factor for epilepsy but is also strongly associated with nonepileptic seizure disorders—presenting in the setting of a somatoform disorder, factitious disorder, or malingering (106,107). The diagnosis can be challenging, particularly in patients with mild head injury and normal routine EEG and magnetic resonance imaging (MRI).

A recent article published a series of 127 patients diagnosed with intractable post-traumatic seizures who underwent video-EEG (VEEG) monitoring (96,97). VEEG was able to capture typical events in 104 patients (82%) during an average length of stay of 4.6 days (standard deviation [SD] 2.4, median 4). Thirty-six out of the 104 patients (35%) were found to have nonepileptic seizures. There was no difference in the mean duration (19.2 years; SD 11.06, median 18) between onset of seizure-like events and diagnostic referral in patients with epileptic and nonepileptic events. Trauma is a shared risk factor for epileptic and nonepileptic events, but only two patients (1.9%) had both epileptic and nonepileptic seizures.

The majority of patients had focal onset epilepsy: 54% presenting with temporal, 33% frontal, 5% parietal, and 3% with occipital lobe epilepsy. Secondary generalized convulsions were more common for extratemporal compared to temporal lobe onset epilepsy (19% vs. 33%, RR 1.25, $P = 0.01$). Half of the patients with temporal lobe epilepsy had mesial temporal lobe sclerosis, most of them with a head injury after the age of 5 years. Interestingly, six patients thought to have symptomatic focal epilepsy for many years were diagnosed as generalized epilepsy; four of them had features of idiopathic generalized epilepsy. This illustrates that the onset of idiopathic generalized epilepsy during teenage years and the high frequency of minor head injuries during the same age can easily delay the diagnosis of the underlying epilepsy syndrome with significant impact on the medical management and outcome (Fig. 29.1).

Nonepileptic seizures after head trauma pose a particular challenge to the medical community. The risk for developing epilepsy after a mild head injury is low, but may occur even in the presence of a normal interictal EEG and MRI (Fig. 29.2A). On the other hand, nonepileptic seizures are not uncommon after minor head injuries, and a delay in diagnosis and antiepileptic therapy interfers not only with rational treatment, but also negatively affects long-term prognosis (108).

There is no clear relationship between the presence of preinjury mental disorders and post-traumatic nonepileptic seizures. However, a high incidence of new psychiatric conditions including post-traumatic stress disorder, depression, and anxiety in up to 75% of patients can be noted, often associated with dissociative symptoms and complaints.

Up to one third of patients with nonepileptic seizures have a history of head injury, in 78% to 91% mild injuries (106,107). Secondary gain from disability or workman's compensation has a tendency to perpetuate nonepileptic seizure disorders. In regards to disability estimation, nonepileptic seizures can be as disabling as epileptic events. However, the disability claim is based on a completely different diagnostic entity, which may influence the chance of approval. In the setting of workman's compensation, a diagnostic distinction between epileptic and nonepileptic events is paramount to establish a likely causal relationship of the seizures to the injury.

Differentiating epileptic and nonepileptic seizures will pose a diagnostic challenge in Iraq veterans. The high number of mild head injuries is associated with a small but definitive risk for PTE and also bears a high risk of post-traumatic stress disorder (PTSD), which is often combined with somatic complaints including seizure-like episodes (109,110).

Nonconvulsive Seizures and Status Epilepticus

There is limited literature regarding the incidence of late post-traumatic nonconvulsive seizures and status (Fig. 29.2B). Particularly, patients with persistent cognitive impairment after head injuries are at risk of subclinical seizures for a variety of reasons. They have a 20% risk to develop epilepsy and they may not be able to communicate seizure symptoms. The caregivers may confound seizure activity with other causes of impaired or fluctuating cognition and consciousness (21). Patients who are not cognitively impaired do not recognize more than half of their seizures. The accuracy is even lower in complex partial seizures and during nighttime, which raises further concerns of the accuracy of seizure reporting in high-risk population with cognitive impairment (111).

Testing

Imaging

Imaging of the brain has been extremely helpful to predict the risk of seizures after head injury. CT and MRI of the brain aid to determine the underlying etiology, support the diagnosis in patients presenting with seizure-like events and may delineate a focal lesion amenable to surgery.

The presence of a focal brain lesion is a risk factor for the development of early seizures as well as late seizures (84,112). The odds ratio of PTE with a focal lesion on CT or MRI scan lies between 2 and 6 (28,29). However, the severity and localization of traumatic brain lesions on MRI do not appear to correlate with the risk for late seizures (113). The presence of cortical or subcortical hemosiderin alone was also not associated with an increased risk of late seizures (28). Only more detailed characteristics of the lesion itself, for example, the relation of hemosiderin deposition to surrounding gliosis or a history of a surgical intervention, may provide additional information in respect to epileptogenesis and risk of PTE (114). Functional studies, either with diffusion weighted MRI or tomography using radioactive tracers may be more specific in predicting the epileptogenic potential of a structural abnormality (115,116). On the other hand, high field MRI and diffusion tensor imaging may offer a higher sensitivity to detect diffuse axonal injury in patients with mild head trauma (117,118).

Not infrequently and despite a diffuse injury to the closed skull, the epileptogenic process manifests itself in a vulnerable brain region such as the hippocampus (119). Surgical series of anterior temporal resections report that 10% of their patients presented with trauma as the major risk factor for epilepsy (93–95,120). Around half of the patients with PTE undergoing epilepsy surgery have hippocampal sclerosis that can be

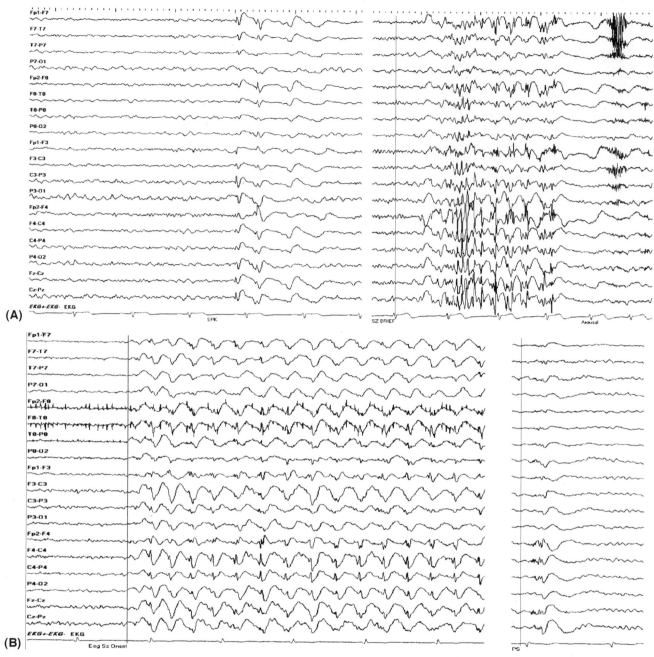

FIGURE 29.1 A and B: Idiopathic generalized epilepsy versus secondary bilateral hypersynchrony. **A** (upper panels): 39-year-old male diagnosed with post-traumatic epilepsy after he was hit with baseball bat at age of 13 years and started to have seizures 1 year later. Diagnosed with post-traumatic epilepsy. Sporadic generalized convulsions throughout his life. Treated with phenobarbital and phenytoin and later switched to carbamazepine. After starting pregabalin, he developed concentration difficulties, stuttering speech, poor concentration. Referred for presurgical workup. VEEG showed interictal generalized spike and waves and polyspikes (*left* and *right* upper panels). Myoclonic jerks associated with generalized EEG pattern were recorded. Seizure-free on valproic acid. Impression: juvenile myoclonic epilepsy. **B** (lower panels): 29-year-old female with minor head trauma at age 13 years when she fell on ice and briefly lost consciousness. Onset of epilepsy age 14. Outside EEG reported as generalized spike-and-wave discharges consistent with idiopathic generalized epilepsy. Seizure-free on carbamazepine for many years. Subacute onset of frequent staring and confusion after carbamazepine was switched to levetiracetam since she wanted to become pregnant. EEG showed a generalized spike-and-wave pattern more prominent over the right hemisphere (lower left panel) consistent nonconvulsive epileptic stupor. Nonconvulsive status persistent despite loading her with valproic acid and levetiracetam, only transient improvement with ativan. EEG status eventually resolved after carbamazepine was resumed. Interictal EEG showed generalized and right frontal spikes and polyspikes (see Fig. 29.2A, lower right panel). Impression: post-traumatic focal epilepsy with secondary bilateral hypersynchrony on EEG.

associated with an additional focal neocortical abnormality in around one third of patients (96,97).

On the other hand, diffuse abnormalities, often global cerebral atrophy, are common in the cases with hippocampal sclerosis. And in surgical patients with PTE, there is always the concern that the obvious MRI lesion only represents the "tip of the iceberg," and that neighboring or remote sites, not visible on MRI, are the actual or future culprit for focal epileptogenicity

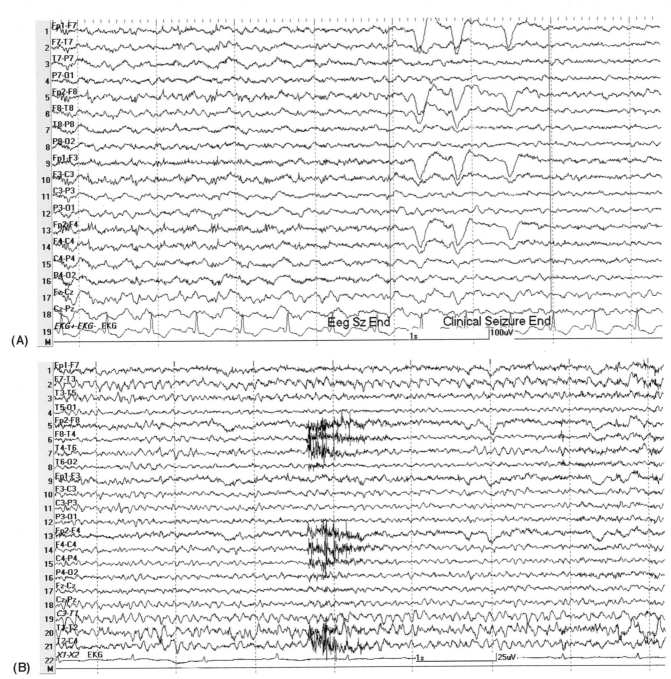

FIGURE 29.2 A and B: Epilepsy after minor head trauma. **A** (upper panel): 50-year-old right-handed male with a mild head injury in 2002 when he hit his head on an iron beam at work. No loss of consciousness. First seizure 6 days later, second event 10 months later, both described as generalized convulsion without warning. Three MRI studies including gradient echo sequence for trauma were normal. Several routine EEGs and prior VEEG monitoring (on medication, no events recorded) were normal, and the concern of nonepileptic seizures was raised. Patient was admitted for second VEEG monitoring. Within 1 day of discontinuing his medications, carbamazepine and phenobarbital, he developed non-convulsive status epilepticus. The EEG shows prolonged episodes of generalized slowing with superimposed paroxysmal fast activity in the bifrontal region, clinically associated with staring, occasional lip smacking, and diffuse myoclonic jerks. EEG and clinical seizure activity resolved after administration of ativan. Impression: post-traumatic epilepsy after concussion without loss of consciousness. **B** (lower panel): 50-year-old male with a first seizure 25 years after a mild head trauma. Subsequent CT scan of the brain showed remote left inferior frontal and bilateral temporal contusions. He was treated with antiepileptic medications for 3 years without recurrence. Two years after stopping the medication, the patient presents with difficulty speaking, brief episodes of unresponsiveness, and ongoing headaches for several days. Routine EEG showed left temporal electrographic seizures lasting around 30 seconds, seen twice during a 30-minute recording, without noticeable clinical changes. Subsequent VEEG showed 6 to 12 seizures per hour which subsided after temporary burst suppression with midazolam. Impression: late post-traumatic epilepsy after minor head trauma presenting with nonconvulsive status epilepticus.

(121). Patients with a neocortical temporal and extratemporal post-traumatic encephalomalacia who are thought to have surgically amenable focal epilepsy based on surface VEEG recording usually require an invasive evaluation to define the precise focus and extent of the epileptogenic lesion. Orbital frontal and anterior temporal–polar cortices are predisposed to injury after closed head injuries and seem to represent areas particularly susceptible for epileptogenic brain injury.

Diagnostic EEG and Video-EEG Monitoring

EEG patterns during the acute phase of head injury are usually nonspecific and reflect systemic factors in addition to the effects of the acute brain damage (122). In that stage, routine EEG might be helpful to predict recovery from coma (123). Interictal epileptiform abnormalities may appear as early as a week after injury (124). Focal EEG activity seen 1 month after head trauma may predict an increased risk of seizures at 1 year after head injury (28). However, in most studies, the EEG during the early phase after injury proved not helpful to predict the development of PTE and seems not an adequate tool to select patients for prophylactic treatment to prevent epileptogenesis and late seizures (104,125,126). The available evidence does not support the use of early EEG changes to predict long-term seizure risk (67). On the other hand, the high risk of subclinical seizures acutely after traumatic brain injury may warrant continuous VEEG monitoring to detect early electrographic seizure activity and provide treatment (40,127).

After the acute recovery phase, routine EEG can be useful to support the diagnosis of epilepsy in patients with late post-traumatic seizures and to distinguish between focal and generalized epilepsy syndromes (104,128). However, overinterpretation of EEG findings can lead to an erroneous diagnosis of epilepsy in patients with nonepileptic seizures and delay the diagnosis and adequate treatment.

Diagnostic VEEG is the gold standard to arrive to a definitive diagnosis in patients with pharmacoresistant seizures for more than a year. Monitoring should be done in a setting where antiepileptic medications can safely be withheld. A recent study in patients with intractable seizures and a history of moderate to severe traumatic brain injury was able to deliver a definitive diagnosis in 82% of patients during an average length of stay of 4.6 days (SD 2.4, median 4) while off antiepileptic medications (96,97). Unfortunately, referral for monitoring was delayed by an average of 19 years after onset of seizures, irrespective if the seizures proved to be epileptic or nonepileptic. Diagnostic VEEG evaluations are not only helpful to differentiate between epileptic and nonepileptic events, but can also influence the choice of medication. Over 5% of patients diagnosed with focal epilepsy may turn out to have an unrecognized generalized epilepsy syndrome (96,97).

TREATMENT

Medical

Seizure remission with medical treatment in patients with post-traumatic seizures ranges from 25% to 40% but with a high risk for seizure recurrence when medications are discontinued. One study described that seizures which develop within the first year after injury are more likely to remit with medication than those that appear later (86). However, the prevailing evidence suggests no significant relation between the occurrence of the first seizure and responsiveness to medication (11,129). Similar to symptomatic epilepsies, a high seizure frequency in the first year of onset predicts future seizure severity and medical intractability (11,130). Seizures that occur after severe head injury or that resist early control tend to persist (85). The chance for spontaneous remission is low, but a medication taper can be justified in selected patients with normal EEG and imaging findings and good response to

initial treatment, who have been seizure-free for at least two years.

Surgical

The selective vulnerability of the hippocampus after blunt head trauma has been well demonstrated in animal models and described in patients with PTE (55). Histopathological examination in a series of temporal lobectomies and trauma as the major risk factor for epilepsy showed neocortical gliosis in all specimens and hippocampal neuronal loss in 94% of the cases. These findings confirm that a blunt head trauma is able to induce hippocampal epilepsy in the absence of other known risk factors (120). The length of the latent period until the onset of recurrent seizures was inversely related to the age at the time of trauma, which is consistent with prior reports suggesting a particular predilection for post-traumatic hippocampal sclerosis below the age of 5 years (93). However, other studies well demonstrated that trauma may lead to hippocampal sclerosis even at a later age (94,96).

Patients with a history of head trauma who undergo temporal resection are less likely to become seizure-free than patients without a history of trauma (55% vs. 40% Engel class Ia) (95). However, these patients may still achieve significant seizure reduction beyond what they can expect from medical management. In a series of 102 patients, 59% of patients with PTE reported a class I outcome with resective surgery after a mean follow-up close to 4 years compared to a 70% class I outcome in all patients undergoing resection. The presence of an isolated focal MRI abnormality—mesial temporal or neocortical—seems critical for a chance of a successful surgical intervention in patients with PTE (94).

FUTURE DIRECTIONS

The study of PTE yields valuable insights into the complex process of epileptogenesis. The role of neuroprotective agents in traumatic brain injury and prospective trials with some new antiepilepsy medications may eventually lead to a reduction in the incidence of PTE. The delayed onset of PTE months or years after the injury offers a unique window for antiepileptic prophylaxis. However, a better understanding of the mechanisms specific to the epileptogenic process after head injuries is required.

The diagnosis of PTE remains a challenge and contributes significantly to treatment failure. More than one third of patients diagnosed with post-traumatic seizures may have nonepileptic events. Early and late post-traumatic epileptic seizures may go unrecognized, particularly in patients with cognitive impairment and altered level of consciousness. Correct determination of the epilepsy syndrome and appropriate choice of medical and surgical management is crucial to improve treatment outcome.

References

1. Annegers JF, Grabow JD, Kurland LT, et al. The incidence, causes, and secular trends of head trauma in olmsted county, minnesota, 1935–1974. *Neurology.* 1980;30(9):912–919.
2. Bruns J Jr, Hauser WA. The epidemiology of traumatic brain injury: a review. *Epilepsia.* 2003;44(suppl 10):2–10.
3. Annegers JF, Rocca WA, Hauser WA. Causes of epilepsy: contributions of the rochester epidemiology project. *Mayo Clin Proc.* 1996;71(6):570–575.

4. Hauser WA, Annegers JF, Rocca WA. Descriptive epidemiology of epilepsy: contributions of population-based studies from rochester, minnesota. *Mayo Clin Proc.* 1996;71(6):576–586.

5. Agrawal A, Timothy J, Pandit L, et al. Post-traumatic epilepsy: an overview. *Clin Neurol Neurosurg.* 2006;108(5):433–439.

6. Hauser WA, Annegers JF, Kurland LT. Incidence of epilepsy and unprovoked seizures in rochester, minnesota: 1935–1984. *Epilepsia.* 1993;34(3):453–468.

7. Annegers JF, Grabow JD, Groover RV, et al. Seizures after head trauma: a population study. *Neurology.* 1980;30(7 Pt 1):683–689.

8. Hughes JR. Post-traumatic epilepsy in the military. *Mil Med.* 1986;151(8):416–419.

9. Walker AE, Erculei F. Post-traumatic epilepsy 15 years later. *Epilepsia.* 1970;11(1):17–26.

10. Annegers JF, Hauser WA, Coan SP, et al. A population-based study of seizures after traumatic brain injuries. *N Engl J Med.* 1998;338(1):20–24.

11. Salazar AM, Jabbari B, Vance SC, et al. Epilepsy after penetrating head injury. I. clinical correlates: a report of the vietnam head injury study. *Neurology.* 1985;35(10):1406–1414.

12. Herman ST. Epilepsy after brain insult: targeting epileptogenesis. *Neurology.* 2002;59(9 suppl 5):S21–S26.

13. Christensen J, Pedersen MG, Pedersen CB, et al. Long-term risk of epilepsy after traumatic brain injury in children and young adults: a population-based cohort study. *Lancet.* 2009;373(9669):1105–1110.

14. Thurman D, Guerrero J. Trends in hospitalization associated with traumatic brain injury. *J Am Med Assoc.* 1999;282(10):954–957.

15. Adams H, Mitchell DE, Graham DI, et al. Diffuse brain damage of immediate impact type. its relationship to 'primary brain-stem damage' in head injury. *Brain.* 1977;100(3):489–502.

16. Miller JD. Head injury. *J Neurol Neurosurg Psychiatry.* 1993;56(5):440–447.

17. Payan H, Toga M, Berard-Badier M. The pathology of post-traumatic epilepsies. *Epilepsia.* 1970;11(1):81–94.

18. Gennarelli TA, Graham DI. Neuropathology. In: Siler JM, McAllister TW, Yudofsky SC, eds. *Textbook of Traumatic Brain Injury.* Washington, DC: American Psychiatric Publishing Inc.; 2005:27–50.

19. Povlishock JT. Traumatically induced axonal injury: pathogenesis and pathobiological implications. *Brain Pathol.* 1992;2(1):1–12.

20. Ikeda Y, Long DM. The molecular basis of brain injury and brain edema: the role of oxygen free radicals. *Neurosurgery.* 1990;27(1):1–11.

21. Yablon SA. Posttraumatic seizures. *Arch Phys Med Rehabil.* 1993;74(9):983–1001.

22. Miller JD, Becker DP. Secondary insults to the injured brain. *J R Coll Surg Edinb.* 1982;27(5):292–298.

23. Pagni CA. Posttraumatic epilepsy. incidence and prophylaxis. *Acta Neurochir Suppl (Wien).* 1990;50:38–47.

24. Jennett B. *Epilepsy After Non-Missile Head Injuries.* Chicago, IL: Year Book Medical Publishers Inc.; 1975.

25. Jennett WB, Lewin W. Traumatic epilepsy after closed head injuries. *J Neurol Neurosurg Psychiatry.* 1960;23:295–301.

26. Desai BT, Whitman S, Coonley-Hoganson R, et al. Seizures and civilian head injuries. *Epilepsia.* 1983;24(3):289–296.

27. Hahn YS, Fuchs S, Flannery AM, et al. Factors influencing posttraumatic seizures in children. *Neurosurgery.* 1988;22(5):864–867.

28. Angeleri F, Majkowski J, Cacchio G, et al. Posttraumatic epilepsy risk factors: one-year prospective study after head injury. *Epilepsia.* 1999;40(9):1222–1230.

29. Asikainen I, Kaste M, Sarna S. Early and late posttraumatic seizures in traumatic brain injury rehabilitation patients: brain injury factors causing late seizures and influence of seizures on long-term outcome. *Epilepsia.* 1999;40(5):584–589.

30. Englander J, Bushnik T, Duong TT, et al. Analyzing risk factors for late posttraumatic seizures: a prospective, multicenter investigation. *Arch Phys Med Rehabil.* 2003;84(3):365–373.

31. Garga N, Lowenstein DH. Posttraumatic epilepsy: a major problem in desperate need of major advances. *Epilepsy Curr.* 2006;6(1):1–5.

32. Lee ST, Lui TN, Wong CW, et al. Early seizures after moderate closed head injury. *Acta Neurochir (Wien).* 1995;137(3–4):151–154.

33. Temkin NR. Risk factors for posttraumatic seizures in adults. *Epilepsia.* 2003;44(suppl 10):18–20.

34. Lee ST, Lui TN. Early seizures after mild closed head injury. *J Neurosurg.* 1992;76(3):435–439.

35. Haydel MJ, Preston CA, Mills TJ, et al. Indications for computed tomography in patients with minor head injury. *N Engl J Med.* 2000;343(2):100–105.

36. Ropper AH, Gorson KC. Clinical practice. concussion. *N Engl J Med.* 2007;356(2):166–172.

37. Clear D, Chadwick DW. Seizures provoked by blows to the head. *Epilepsia.* 2000;41(2):243–244.

38. Wolf P. Minor head trauma unmasking asymptomatic lesions. *Epilepsia.* 2001;42(4):573.

39. Krayenbuhl H, Hess R, Weber G, et al. Pseudo-traumatic epilepsy. *Epilepsia.* 1970;11(1):59–71.

40. Vespa PM, Nuwer MR, Nenov V, et al. Increased incidence and impact of nonconvulsive and convulsive seizures after traumatic brain injury as detected by continuous electroencephalographic monitoring. *J Neurosurg.* 1999;91(5):750–760.

41. Vespa PM, Miller C, McArthur D, et al. Nonconvulsive electrographic seizures after traumatic brain injury result in a delayed, prolonged increase in intracranial pressure and metabolic crisis. *Crit Care Med.* 2007;35(12):2830–2836.

42. Jennett B. Early traumatic epilepsy. incidence and significance after nonmissile injuries. *Arch Neurol.* 1974;30(5):394–398.

43. Hesdorffer DC, Logroscino G, Cascino G, et al. Risk of unprovoked seizure after acute symptomatic seizure: effect of status epilepticus. *Ann Neurol.* 1998;44(6):908–912.

44. Penfield W. Symposium on post-traumatic epilepsy. *Epilepsia.* 1961;2:109–110.

45. Frey LC. Epidemiology of posttraumatic epilepsy: a critical review. *Epilepsia.* 2003;44(suppl 10):11–17.

46. Jensen FE. Posttraumatic epilepsy: treatable epileptogenesis. introduction. *Epilepsia.* 2009;50(suppl 2):1–3.

47. Pitkaenen A, Immonen RJ, Groehn OHK, et al. From traumatic brain injury to posttraumatic epilepsy: what animal models tell us about the process and treatment options. *Epilepsia.* 2009;50(suppl 2):21–29.

48. Prince DA. Epilepsy following cortical injury: cellular and molecular mechanisms as targets for potential prophylaxis. *Epilepsia.* 2009;50(suppl 2):30–40.

49. Lowenstein DH. Recent advances related to basic mechanisms of epileptogenesis. *Epilepsy Res Suppl.* 1996;11:45–60.

50. Willmore LJ, Sypert GW, Munson JB. Recurrent seizures induced by cortical iron injection: A model of posttraumatic epilepsy. *Ann Neurol.* 1978;4(4):329–336.

51. Willmore LJ, Ueda Y. Posttraumatic epilepsy: hemorrhage, free radicals and the molecular regulation of glutamate. *Neurochem Res.* 2009;34(4):688–697.

52. McIntosh TK, Vink R, Noble L, et al. Traumatic brain injury in the rat: characterization of a lateral fluid-percussion model. *Neuroscience.* 1989;28(1):233–244.

53. Laurer HL, McIntosh TK. Experimental models of brain trauma. *Curr Opin Neurol.* 1999;12(6):715–721.

54. Prince DA, Tseng GF. Epileptogenesis in chronically injured cortex: in vitro studies. *J Neurophysiol.* 1993;69(4):1276–1291.

55. Lowenstein DH, Thomas MJ, Smith DH, et al. Selective vulnerability of dentate hilar neurons following traumatic brain injury: a potential mechanistic link between head trauma and disorders of the hippocampus. *J Neurosci.* 1992;12(12):4846–4853.

56. Santhakumar V, Bender R, Frotscher M, et al. Granule cell hyperexcitability in the early post-traumatic dentate gyrus: the 'irritable mossy cell' hypothesis. *J Physiol.* 2000;524(Pt 1):117–134.

57. Sloviter RS. Permanently altered hippocampal structure, excitability, and inhibition after experimental status epilepticus in the rat: the "dormant basket cell" hypothesis and its possible relevance to temporal lobe epilepsy. *Hippocampus.* 1991;1(1):41–66.

58. D'Ambrosio R, Fairbanks JP, Fender JS, et al. Post-traumatic epilepsy following fluid percussion injury in the rat. *Brain.* 2004;127 (Pt 2):304–314.

59. D'Ambrosio R, Fender JS, Fairbanks JP, et al. Progression from frontal-parietal to mesial-temporal epilepsy after fluid percussion injury in the rat. *Brain.* 2005;128(Pt 1):174–188.

60. Kharatishvili I, Nissinen JP, McIntosh TK, et al. A model of posttraumatic epilepsy induced by lateral fluid-percussion brain injury in rats. *Neuroscience.* 2006;140(2):685–697.

61. Salin P, Tseng GF, Hoffman S, et al. Axonal sprouting in layer V pyramidal neurons of chronically injured cerebral cortex. *J Neurosci.* 1995;15(12):8234–8245.

62. Graber KD, Prince DA. Tetrodotoxin prevents posttraumatic epileptogenesis in rats. *Ann Neurol.* 1999;46(2):234–242.

63. Graber KD, Prince DA. A critical period for prevention of posttraumatic neocortical hyperexcitability in rats. *Ann Neurol.* 2004;55(6):860–870.

64. Temkin NR. Antiepileptogenesis and seizure prevention trials with antiepileptic drugs: meta-analysis of controlled trials. *Epilepsia.* 2001;42(4):515–524.

65. Schierhout G, Roberts I. Anti-epileptic drugs for preventing seizures following acute traumatic brain injury. *Cochrane Database Syst Rev.* 2001;(4):CD000173.

66. Haltiner AM, Newell DW, Temkin NR, et al. Side effects and mortality associated with use of phenytoin for early posttraumatic seizure prophylaxis. *J Neurosurg.* 1999;91(4):588–592.

67. Chang BS, Lowenstein DH, Quality Standards Subcommittee of the American Academy of Neurology. Practice parameter: antiepileptic drug prophylaxis in severe traumatic brain injury: report of the quality standards subcommittee of the American Academy of Neurology. *Neurology.* 2003;60(1):10–16.

68. Jones KE, Puccio AM, Harshman KJ, et al. Levetiracetam versus phenytoin for seizure prophylaxis in severe traumatic brain injury. *Neurosurg Focus.* 2008;25(4):E3.

69. Young B, Rapp RP, Norton JA, et al. Failure of prophylactically administered phenytoin to prevent early posttraumatic seizures. *J Neurosurg.* 1983;58(2):231–235.

70. Lewis RJ, Yee L, Inkelis SH, et al. Clinical predictors of post-traumatic seizures in children with head trauma. *Ann Emerg Med.* 1993;22(7):1114–1118.

71. Tilford JM, Simpson PM, Yeh TS, et al. Variation in therapy and outcome for pediatric head trauma patients. *Crit Care Med.* 2001;29(5):1056–1061.

72. Adelson PD, Bratton SL, Carney NA, et al. Guidelines for the acute medical management of severe traumatic brain injury in infants, children, and adolescents. Chapter 19. The role of anti-seizure prophylaxis following severe pediatric traumatic brain injury. *Pediatr Crit Care Med.* 2003;4(3 suppl):S72–S75.

73. Watson NF, Barber JK, Doherty MJ, et al. Does glucocorticoid administration prevent late seizures after head injury? *Epilepsia.* 2004;45(6):690–694.

74. Rish BL, Caveness WF. Relation of prophylactic medication to the occurrence of early seizures following craniocerebral trauma. *J Neurosurg.* 1973;38(2):155–158.

75. Servit Z, Musil F. Prophylactic treatment of posttraumatic epilepsy: results of a long-term follow-up in Czechoslovakia. *Epilepsia.* 1981;22(3):315–320.

76. Rapport RL II, Penry JK. A survey of attitudes toward the pharmacological prophylaxis of posttraumatic epilepsy. *J Neurosurg.* 1973; 38(2):159–166.

77. McQueen JK, Blackwood DH, Harris P, et al. Low risk of late post-traumatic seizures following severe head injury: implications for clinical trials of prophylaxis. *J Neurol Neurosurg Psychiatry.* 1983;46(10):899–904.

78. Glotzner FL, Haubitz I, Miltner F, et al. Seizure prevention using carbamazepine following severe brain injuries. *Neurochirurgia (Stuttg).* 1983;26(3):66–79.

79. Temkin NR, Dikmen SS, Anderson GD, et al. Valproate therapy for prevention of posttraumatic seizures: a randomized trial. *J Neurosurg.* 1999;91(4):593–600.

80. Temkin NR, Dikmen SS, Wilensky AJ, et al. A randomized, double-blind study of phenytoin for the prevention of post-traumatic seizures. *N Engl J Med.* 1990;323(8):497–502.

81. Dikmen SS, Temkin NR, Miller B, et al. Neurobehavioral effects of phenytoin prophylaxis of posttraumatic seizures. *J Am Med Assoc.* 1991; 265(10):1271–1277.

82. Perna R. Brain injury: benzodiazepines, antipsychotics, and functional recovery. *J Head Trauma Rehabil.* 2006;21(1):82–84.

83. Jennett WB. Late epilepsy after blunt head injuries: a clinical study based on 282 cases of traumatic epilepsy. *Ann R Coll Surg Engl.* 1961;29:370–384.

84. De Santis A, Sganzerla E, Spagnoli D, et al. Risk factors for late posttraumatic epilepsy. *Acta Neurochir Suppl (Wien).* 1992;55:64–67.

85. Haltiner AM, Temkin NR, Dikmen SS. Risk of seizure recurrence after the first late posttraumatic seizure. *Arch Phys Med Rehabil.* 1997;78(8):835–840.

86. Jennett B. Epilepsy and acute traumatic intracranial haematoma. *J Neurol Neurosurg Psychiatry.* 1975;38(4):378–381.

87. Weiss GH, Feeney DM, Caveness WF, et al. Prognostic factors for the occurrence of posttraumatic epilepsy. *Arch Neurol.* 1983;40(1):7–10.

88. Annegers JF, Coan SP. The risks of epilepsy after traumatic brain injury. *Seizure.* 2000;9(7):453–457.

89. Salazar A, Aarabi B, Levi L, et al. Posttraumatic epilepsy following craniocerebral missile wounds in recent armed conflicts. In: Aarabi B, Kaufman HH, Dagi TF, et al., eds. *Missile Wounds of the Head and Neck.* Vol 2. Park Ridge, IL: Thieme; 1999:281–292.

90. Lowenstein DH. Epilepsy after head injury: an overview. *Epilepsia.* 2009;50(suppl 2):14–20.

91. Hendrick EB, Harris L. Post-traumatic epilepsy in children. *J Trauma.* 1968;8(4):547–556.

92. Hernesniemi J. Outcome following head injuries in the aged. *Acta Neurochir (Wien).* 1979;49(1–2):67–79.

93. Mathern GW, Babb TL, Vickrey BG, et al. Traumatic compared to nontraumatic clinical-pathologic associations in temporal lobe epilepsy. *Epilepsy Res.* 1994;19(2):129–139.

94. Marks DA, Kim J, Spencer DD, et al. Seizure localization and pathology following head injury in patients with uncontrolled epilepsy. *Neurology.* 1995;45(11):2051–2057.

95. Schuh LA, Henry TR, Fromes G, et al. Influence of head trauma on outcome following anterior temporal lobectomy. *Arch Neurol.* 1998; 55(10):1325–1328.

96. Diaz-Arrastia R, Agostini MA, Frol AB, et al. Neurophysiologic and neuroradiologic features of intractable epilepsy after traumatic brain injury in adults. *Arch Neurol.* 2000;57(11):1611–1616.

97. Hudak AM, Trivedi K, Harper CR, et al. Evaluation of seizure-like episodes in survivors of moderate and severe traumatic brain injury. *J Head Trauma Rehabil.* 2004;19(4):290–295.

98. Evans JH. Post-traumatic epilepsy. *Neurology.* 1962;12:665–674.

99. Schaumann BA, Annegers JF, Johnson SB, et al. Family history of seizures in posttraumatic and alcohol-associated seizure disorders. *Epilepsia.* 1994;35(1):48–52.

100. Kjeldsen MJ, Corey LA, Christensen K, et al. Epileptic seizures and syndromes in twins: the importance of genetic factors. *Epilepsy Res.* 2003;55(1–2):137–146.

101. Luders HO, Turnbull J, Kaffashi F. Are the dichotomies generalized versus focal epilepsies and idiopathic versus symptomatic epilepsies still valid in modern epileptology? *Epilepsia.* 2009;50(6):1336–1343.

102. Russell WR, Whitty CW. Studies in traumatic epilepsy. II. Focal motor and somatic sensory fits: a study of 85 cases. *J Neurol Neurosurg Psychiatry.* 1953;16(2):73–97.

103. Russell WR, Whitty CW. Studies in traumatic epilepsy. 3. Visual fits. *J Neurol Neurosurg Psychiatry.* 1955;18(2):79–96.

104. da Silva AM, Nunes B, Vaz AR, et al. Posttraumatic epilepsy in civilians: clinical and electroencephalographic studies. *Acta Neurochir Suppl (Wien).* 1992;55:56–63.

105. Paillas JE, Paillas N, Bureau M. Post-traumatic epilepsy. Introduction and clinical observations. *Epilepsia.* 1970;11(1):5–15.

106. Barry E, Krumholz A, Bergey GK, et al. Nonepileptic posttraumatic seizures. *Epilepsia.* 1998;39(4):427–431.

107. Westbrook LE, Devinsky O, Geocadin R. Nonepileptic seizures after head injury. *Epilepsia.* 1998;39(9):978–982.

108. Mooney G, Speed J. The association between mild traumatic brain injury and psychiatric conditions. *Brain Inj.* 2001;15(10):865–877.

109. Xydakis MS, Robbins AS, Grant GA. Mild traumatic brain injury in U.S. soldiers returning from iraq. *N Engl J Med.* 2008;358(20):2177.

110. Hoge CW, McGurk D, Thomas JL, et al. Mild traumatic brain injury in U.S. soldiers returning from Iraq. *N Engl J Med.* 2008;358(5): 453–463.

111. Hoppe C, Poepel A, Elger CE. Epilepsy: accuracy of patient seizure counts. *Arch Neurol.* 2007;64(11):1595–1599.

112. D'Alessandro R, Tinuper P, Ferrara R, et al. CT scan prediction of late post-traumatic epilepsy. *J Neurol Neurosurg Psychiatry.* 1982;45(12): 1153–1155.

113. Levin HS, Williams DH, Eisenberg HM, et al. Serial MRI and neurobehavioural findings after mild to moderate closed head injury. *J Neurol Neurosurg Psychiatry.* 1992;55(4):255–262.

114. Messori A, Polonara G, Carle F, et al. Predicting posttraumatic epilepsy with MRI: prospective longitudinal morphologic study in adults. *Epilepsia.* 2005;46(9):1472–1481.

115. Kumar R, Gupta RK, Rao SB, et al. Magnetization transfer and T2 quantitation in normal appearing cortical gray matter and white matter adjacent to focal abnormality in patients with traumatic brain injury. *Magn Reson Imaging.* 2003;21(8):893–899.

116. Mazzini L, Cossa FM, Angelino E, et al. Posttraumatic epilepsy: neuroradiologic and neuropsychological assessment of long-term outcome. *Epilepsia.* 2003;44(4):569–574.

117. Topal NB, Hakyemez B, Erdogan C, et al. MR imaging in the detection of diffuse axonal injury with mild traumatic brain injury. *Neurol Res.* 2008;30(9):974–978.

118. Wang JY, Bakhadirov K, Devous MDS, et al. Diffusion tensor tractography of traumatic diffuse axonal injury. *Arch Neurol.* 2008; 65(5):619–626.

119. Coulter DA, Rafiq A, Shumate M, et al. Brain injury-induced enhanced limbic epileptogenesis: anatomical and physiological parallels to an animal model of temporal lobe epilepsy. *Epilepsy Res.* 1996;26(1): 81–91.

120. Swartz BE, Houser CR, Tomiyasu U, et al. Hippocampal cell loss in posttraumatic human epilepsy. *Epilepsia.* 2006;47(8):1373–1382.

121. Rosenow F, Luders H. Presurgical evaluation of epilepsy. *Brain.* 2001;124(Pt 9):1683–1700.

122. Gutling E, Gonser A, Imhof HG, et al. EEG reactivity in the prognosis of severe head injury. *Neurology.* 1995;45(5):915–918.

123. Facco E. Current topics. The role of EEG in brain injury. *Intensive Care Med.* 1999;25(8):872–877.

124. Courjon JA. Posttraumatic epilepsy in electroclinical practice. In: Walker AE, Caveness WF, Critchley M, eds. *The Late Effects of Head Injury.* Springfield, IL: Charles C Thomas; 1969:215–227.

125. Jennett B, Van De Sande J. EEG prediction of post-traumatic epilepsy. *Epilepsia.* 1975;16(2):251–256.

126. Reisner T, Zeiler K, Wessely P. The value of CT and EEG in cases of posttraumatic epilepsy. *J Neurol.* 1979;221(2):93–100.

127. Scheuer ML. Continuous EEG monitoring in the intensive care unit. *Epilepsia.* 2002;43(suppl 3):114–127.

128. Salinsky M, Kanter R, Dasheiff RM. Effectiveness of multiple EEGs in supporting the diagnosis of epilepsy: an operational curve. *Epilepsia.* 1987;28(4):331–334.

129. Caveness WF, Meirowsky AM, Rish BL, et al. The nature of posttraumatic epilepsy. *J Neurosurg.* 1979;50(5):545–553.

130. MacDonald BK, Johnson AL, Goodridge DM, et al. Factors predicting prognosis of epilepsy after presentation with seizures. *Ann Neurol.* 2000;48(6):833–841.

CHAPTER 30 ■ EPILEPSY IN THE SETTING OF CEREBROVASCULAR DISEASE

STEPHEN HANTUS, NEIL FRIEDMAN, AND BERND POHLMANN-EDEN

Cerebrovascular disease is a significant cause of seizures and a risk factor for the development of epilepsy in all age groups. Stroke is a common cause of morbidity and mortality in the elderly population and is the leading cause of epilepsy in patients older than 60. Seizures occur in 7% to 11% of adult patients who survive strokes, while poststroke epilepsy develops in 2% to 4% (1,2). Cerebrovascular disease is less common in the pediatric population, but early vascular insults are associated with an increased incidence of epilepsy as compared to adult patients. Understanding the prevalence, etiology, and risk factors associated with poststroke seizures and epilepsy is of vital clinical importance, and multiple studies have attempted to address these issues (2–5). The management, prognosis, and treatment of seizures and epilepsy associated with cerebrovascular disease are less well known and will remain an important area for investigation (6).

EPILEPSY IN PEDIATRIC CEREBROVASCULAR DISEASE

The past decade has seen a renewed interest and focus in pediatric stroke. Although relatively uncommon, the reported incidence has increased with better data collection, improved imaging modalities, and better recognition and awareness amongst physicians. An incidence rate of 2.52/100,000 children per year (0.63/100,000 children per year for ischemic stroke) was found in the first North American population–based study of pediatric stroke from 1965 to 1974 (7). Since then, data from the largest cohort of pediatric stroke patients from the prospective Canadian Ischemic Stroke Registry have shown an incidence of 6/100,000 children per year (3.3/100,000 for arterial ischemic stroke [AIS]) (8). The highest incidence occurs in the neonatal period with estimates as high as 20 to 30/100,000 newborns per year, although a recent population-based epidemiologic study from Switzerland using magnetic resonance imaging (MRI) confirmation of neonatal AIS showed a higher incidence of just over 40/100,000 per year or 1 in 2300 live births per year (9).

Perinatal arterial ischemic stroke occurs primarily in term infants and comprises approximately 25% to 30% of all AISs in children (10,11). Two thirds have large vessel infarcts (12) compared with childhood stroke in which more than 50% of strokes involve small vessel territory. The anterior circulation is five times more commonly involved than the posterior circulation and 60% to 65% involve the left middle cerebral artery territory (12–15). Multiple infarcts are seen in 15% to 20% of cases.

Childhood AIS is more common in males (11) and blacks (16), with the mean age of presentation being 4 to 6 years

(10,17–19). Ischemic stroke is more common than hemorrhagic stroke. Stroke remains one of the top 10 causes of death in children (20) with a mortality rate of approximately 10% (21). Outcome, in general, is better than that seen in adults, mostly due to brain plasticity and the absence of ubiquitous underlying degenerative vascular disease such as atherosclerosis. Morbidity, however, remains a serious complication of pediatric stroke, and a majority of survivors will have residual and persistent neurological and/or cognitive impairment. Neurological impairment includes residual hemiparesis in about two thirds of children, visual field deficits, cognitive and behavioral difficulties, and/or epilepsy (22). The recurrence risk for stroke is variable and depends on the underlying etiology, and has been estimated to be 15% to 20% (22). The etiologies of stroke in childhood are multitude, and vary considerably from those seen in adults, with approximately 20% to 30% of cases remaining unresolved.

Seizures are more commonly seen as a heralding symptom in childhood stroke than they are in adult stroke. However, even in childhood stroke, as compared to neonatal stroke, motor deficits are more commonly the presenting neurological symptom than seizures. The reported incidence of stroke-associated seizures and subsequent epilepsy in children with stroke has been highly variable, partly based on few prospective studies, selection bias, small sample size, lack of long-term follow-up, and differing definitions and terminology in the classification of epilepsy. Acute symptomatic seizures at stroke onset occur in ~30% of childhood AISs (reported incidence of 19% to 54%) with epilepsy as a sequelae in ~28% (reported incidence of 7% to 58%) (19,23–30). Data regarding seizure presentation and subsequent epilepsy risk for hemorrhagic stroke in childhood is much less clear, with only few descriptive series. Seizure at onset would appear to be slightly more common than with childhood AIS occurring in ~40% (25,26) with the subsequent risk of epilepsy varying between 10% and 39% (25,26,28).

The situation is different in *perinatal* stroke where seizures are the most frequent presenting neurological symptom, occurring in over 80%. Focal neurological deficits, such as hemiplegia, or generalized symptoms, such as hypotonia or encephalopathy, are uncommon. In a large prospective series (31), 62 of 90 (69%) term infants who presented only with seizures (and without evidence of a more diffuse neonatal encephalopathy) showed MRI evidence of acute focal ischemia (35/62) or hemorrhagic brain injury (27/62). Similarly, in an autopsy series of 592 infants (32), 5.4% were found to have AISs and none showed focal neurological features during the newborn period; however, 17% had neonatal seizures. Twelve to 18% of all neonatal seizures are associated with perinatal infarcts (33–36), tend to be focal (75%), and typically present

371

within the first 72 hours of stroke onset. Generalized and subtle seizures, including apnea, and electrographic seizures (37,38) in the absence of clinical findings may occur. The seizures usually last 3 to 5 days (39,40) in duration and tend to be easy to control medically (39,41,42). Neonatal seizures have been reported in over 70% of the cases of sinovenous thrombosis (43). In the Canadian pediatric ischemic stroke registry, the risk of epilepsy was 20% following an infarct due to sinovenous thrombosis versus 15% when the stroke was due to an AIS. The data, however, of subsequent epilepsy risk following perinatal AIS has been very inconsistent and has varied considerably from 0% to 50% depending on the nature of the study. The overall "mean" from these studies would suggest a risk of about 22% for the subsequent development of epilepsy (22). Fetal stroke appears to predict the earlier onset of epilepsy in one recent large cohort (44).

The electroencephalogram (EEG) in neonatal stroke is highly variable and frequently normal. Abnormalities include focal or generalized slowing; focal, multifocal or bilateral spike or spike-and-wave discharges; low voltage rhythms; and burst suppression. Periodic lateralized epileptiform discharges (PLEDs) have also been reported in neonatal stroke in the term infant (45). The presence of an abnormal background on EEG (22) independent of EEG seizures or epileptiform discharges has been associated with hemiplegia at outcome (12).

For *childhood* AIS, cortical involvement has, not surprisingly, been associated with a subsequent risk for epilepsy (25). Subcortical infarcts (basal ganglia, thalamus) have also been associated with seizures either as an isolated presenting feature or in combination with a hemiplegia (46). The semiology of the seizures is variable and often patients have more than one seizure type including focal motor, complex partial seizures, with or without secondary generalization, and occasionally, primary generalized seizures. Status epilepticus has rarely been reported (47). The occurrence of seizures and/or altered level of consciousness at the initial presentation of childhood AIS has been associated with increased mortality at 6 months or unfavorable neurological outcome (29).

> Infantile hemiplegia offers some of the most typical instances of cortical epilepsy, and it may be well to consider how far it is likely that surgical interference can here be successful—Sir William Osler (48).

Surgical intervention for intractable epilepsy as a consequence of perinatal stroke dates back to the latter part of the 19th century (48,49). The first detailed series of hemispherectomy in children as a treatment option for intractable epilepsy, however, can be traced back to Krynauw in 1950. Histopathology of the resected specimens documented infarcts due to vascular ischemia/stroke as the etiology in a number of his cases (50).

EPILEPSY IN ADULT CEREBROVASCULAR DISEASE

Epidemiology

The reported incidence of poststroke seizure and epilepsy has varied in the literature from 3.3% to 13%, although heterogeneous study designs, inconsistent use of terminology, and variable follow-up periods have made them difficult to interpret (51). The Oxfordshire community stroke project prospectively followed 675 patients with a first stroke for a minimum of 2 years, and found a 7.7% prevalence of poststroke seizures (1). The Seizures After Stroke Study (SASS) prospectively followed 1897 patients for a mean follow-up time of 9 months and found 168 patients with poststroke seizures (8.9%) (2). Multiple studies have also differentiated early, late and recurrent seizures as having different clinical characteristics and prognoses (52–54). A study by Berges et al. retrospectively evaluated 3205 patients and identified 57 patients with early onset seizures (within 2 weeks of the stroke in the study) and 102 patients with late onset seizures (greater than 2 week from the stroke). They found that the later onset seizures were significantly more likely to recur (develop poststroke epilepsy) than the early seizures (53). In a retrospective study of Rochester Minnesota residents, 192 patients were identified with poststroke seizures with 91 patients having acute symptomatic seizures and 101 patients having unprovoked seizures (3). Two key points were made by this study: the acute symptomatic seizures had a much higher 30-day mortality (41.9%) versus the unprovoked seizures (5%), and the recurrence rate was 33% for the acute symptomatic seizure group and 71.5% for the unprovoked seizure group.

The international league against epilepsy (IILAE) has developed definitions for early and late poststroke seizures that have been variably defined in the past:

Acute symptomatic seizure: Epileptic seizure within the first 24 hours after onset of stroke.
Early poststroke seizure: One or more seizures within the first week after the stroke.
Late poststroke seizure: One unprovoked epileptic seizure at least 1 week after the stroke.
Poststroke epilepsy: Two or more unprovoked epileptic seizures at least 1 week after the stroke.

The prevalence of poststroke epilepsy has been reported variably from 2% to 4.1% with follow-up periods ranging from 9 months to 7 years (1,2,52–57). A large prospective study followed 1195 patients for 7 years and found 38 patients (3.2%) with poststroke epilepsy (57).

Status epilepticus also occurs in poststroke patients with an overall prevalence reported at 1.5% of all new onset strokes, which represents 10% of the patients presenting with poststroke seizures (58–60). The number of the patients is small, but these patients tend to have early onset status, nonconvulsive seizures with no apparent clinical signs, and increased mortality.

In conclusion, poststroke seizures occur in 7% to 11% of new onset strokes. Approximately one third of these occur as acute symptomatic or early onset seizures and are predicted to have a higher 30-day mortality and decreased incidence of seizure recurrence. While the unprovoked or late seizures are predicted to have 50% to 70% recurrence rates, and thus frequently develop into poststroke epilepsy. The prevalence of poststroke epilepsy is 2% to 4% in patients with new onset strokes. Status epilepticus occurs after stroke in a smaller portion of patients (1.5%), but is associated with an early onset and high mortality.

Pathophysiology

Much of the pathophysiology of poststroke seizures requires further investigation. Based on animal models, acute symptomatic seizures are thought to arise from the penumbra surrounding the infarction (61). Occlusion of middle cerebral artery blood flow in rats is associated with epileptic spiking over the region of proposed penumbra. The ischemia is hypothesized to release glutamate-causing excitotoxicity and early seizures. Other factors proposed to effect early seizures are deposits of hemosiderin-causing focal cerebral irritability, fluctuations in cerebral ions concentrations, and loss of inhibitory GABAergic circuits (62). The pathogenesis of late seizures and poststroke epilepsy is even less clear. Etiological factors include the formation of a gliotic scar with reorganization of axonal connections, loss of GABAergic pathways, the presence of hemosiderin in cortical neurons, and free radical formation and membrane peroxidation. Another possible trigger of late seizures is recurrent ischemia at the site of the previous stroke. This mechanism was proposed after a series of positron emission tomography (PET) studies demonstrated decreased oxygen metabolism and cerebral blood flow in the area of the old stroke in patients with late seizures. In patients with old strokes and no seizures, the metabolism and cerebral blood flow was not decreased. The authors argue that this effect, seen in late onset seizures, is more likely related to additional ischemia based on Cobalt PET that selectively shows acute ischemic changes. The same changes were not seen in patients who developed recurrent seizures (poststroke epilepsy) suggesting that the effect was not due to seizure alone (60,63).

Predictors of Poststroke Epilepsy

A number of clinical factors have been proposed to predict which patients would develop poststroke seizures and epilepsy. Cortical location, stroke severity, and hemorrhagic stroke all were shown to be independent risk factors on multivariate analysis (1,2,52,56,57). In additional to localization to the cortex, an island of spared cortex, infarct with irregular borders, temporal-parietal location, and posterior cerebral artery infarcts have all been hypothesized to increase the risk of poststroke epilepsy (64).

Diagnostic Studies in Poststroke Epilepsy

The value of EEG in predicting poststroke seizures and epilepsy has been controversial (65). In a retrospective study of 110 patients who developed poststroke seizures (12 early seizures, 98 late seizures), EEGs were compared after stroke, after the first seizure to a control group of stroke patients without seizures. PLEDs have been associated with increased risk of seizures in prior studies and were also predictive in this study. However, PLEDs were only recorded in 5.8% of patients who would later develop seizures, and none in the control group without seizures. Thus, PLEDs were predictive (more often with early seizures), but were rarely observed. Frontal Intermittent Rhythmic Delta (FIRDA) was observed in 24.6% of the seizure group, compared to 1.1% of the control group. Diffuse slowing also occurred more frequently in the seizure group (21.7%) than in the control group (5.1%). Focal slowing was equally represented in both groups. Normal EEGs were seen in only 8.5% of the seizure group, while 53.8% of the control group was normal. The authors concluded that PLEDs, FIRDA, and diffuse slowing are the typical EEG findings of early seizures, while FIRDA and diffuse slowing may

suggest an increased risk to develop late onset seizures. The findings of a normal EEG poststroke would suggest decreased risk of developing late onset seizures (65). In a prospective study of 100 patients who received continuous EEG after acute stroke, 17% were found to have epileptiform discharges or seizures (66). Stroke severity (measured by National Institute of Health Stroke Scale [NIHSS]) was the only independent predictor of epileptiform discharges and/or seizures on continuous EEG (CEEG). In a study of 102 patients with nontraumatic intra-cerebral hemorrhage (ICH) who underwent continuous EEG monitoring, 32% were found to be having seizures (67). In addition, patients who expanded their hemorrhage by 30% or more were twice as likely to have electrographic seizures. Many of the seizures recorded were without clinical signs. Cortical location and severity of the ICH were related to increased seizure risk. PLEDs were associated with increased mortality. Twenty-eight percent of the seizures were recorded after 24 hours, but only 5% were recorded after 48 hours. In conclusion, poststroke EEG may be useful in prediction of future seizures if PLEDs, FIRDA, or diffuse slowing are noted, and CEEG may be of value in high-risk patients with severe ischemic stroke and ICHs.

Treatment

The treatment of poststroke seizures and epilepsy has been controversial.[6] In animal models of ischemia, antiepileptic medications have been shown to have a neuroprotective effect; however, the same has not been demonstrated in humans (68). First generation antiepileptics (phenytoin, phenobarbital, and benzodiazepines) were shown to worsen functional recovery in animal models of stroke (69). Unfortunately, there are no randomized controlled trials of treatment for patients with poststroke seizures or epilepsy. The risk of seizure recurrence after an early seizure has been reported from 13% to 43%. This is similar to the recurrence risk of 24% that is quoted to patients with a single seizure and normal imaging and EEG studies. However, the risk of recurrent seizures after a single late onset seizure is in the range of 54% to 66%, thus some have advocated treatment with antiepileptic drugs (AEDs) after even a single late onset seizure, while others prefer to treat after a second unprovoked seizure (51,60,70). When medications are used, these seizures tend to respond to monotherapy with relatively rare recurrence (most notably due to noncompliance). Though no studies have been conducted in poststroke epilepsy patients per se, a study compared lamotrogine, gabapentin, and carbamazepine in the elderly (with stroke the most likely etiology of the majority of seizures) (71). Seizure control was similar among all three drugs, but tolerability favored lamotrigine and gabapentin. Decreased interactions with other medications are an added advantage of the newer AEDs when considering medications for poststroke epilepsy.

References

1. Burn J, Dennis M, Bamford J, et al. Epileptic seizures after a first stroke: The oxfordshire community stroke project. *Br Med J.* 1997;315(7122): 1582–1587.
2. Bladin CF, Alexandrov AV, Bellavance A, et al., for the Seizures After Stroke Study Group. Seizures after stroke: A prospective multicenter study. *Arch Neurol.* 2000;57(11):1617–1622.

3. Hesdorffer DC, Benn EK, Cascino GD, et al. Is a first acute symptomatic seizure epilepsy? mortality and risk for recurrent seizure. *Epilepsia.* 2009;50(5):1102–1108.

4. Ferro JM, Pinto F. Poststroke epilepsy: Epidemiology, pathophysiology and management. *Drugs Aging.* 2004;21(10):639–653.

5. Burneo JG, Fang J, Saposnik G, for the Investigators of the Registry of the Canadian Stroke Network. Impact of seizures on morbidity and mortality after stroke: a Canadian multi-centre cohort study. *Eur J Neurol.* 2009.(E-pub ahead of print); PMID: 19686350; ISSN: 1471-0552.

6. Labovitz DL, Hauser WA. Preventing stroke-related seizures: When should anticonvulsant drugs be started? *Neurology.* 2003;60(3):365–366.

7. Schoenberg BS, Mellinger JF, Schoenberg DG. Cerebrovascular disease in infants and children: A study of incidence, clinical features, and survival. *Neurology.* 1978;28:763–768.

8. de Veber G, Roach ES, Riela AR, et al. Stroke in children: recognition, treatment, and future directions. *Semin Pediatr Neurol.* 2000;7:309–317.

9. Schulzke S, Weber P, Luetschg J, et al. Incidence and diagnosis of unilateral arterial cerebral infarction in newborn infants. *J Perinat Med.* 2005; 33:170–175.

10. de Veber GA, MacGregor D, Curtis R, et al. Neurologic outcome in survivors of childhood arterial ischemic stroke and sinovenous thrombosis. *J Child Neurol.* 2000;15:316–324.

11. Golomb MR, Fullerton HJ, Nowak-Gottl U, et al., for the International Pediatric Stroke Study Group. Male predominance in childhood ischemic stroke. Findings from the international pediatric stroke study. *Stroke.* 2008;40(1):52–57.

12. Mercuri E, Rutherford M, Cowan F, et al. Early prognostic indicators of outcome in infants with neonatal cerebral infarction: a clinical, electroencephalogram, and magnetic resonance imaging study. *Pediatrics.* 1999; 103:39–46.

13. Perlman JM, Rollins NK, Evans D. Neonatal stroke: clinical characteristics and cerebral blood flow velocity measurements. *Pediatr Neurol.* 1994; 11:281–284.

14. Filipek PA, Krishnamoorthy KS, Davis KR, et al. Focal cerebral infarction in the newborn: a distinct entity. *Pediatr Neurol.* 1987;3:141–147.

15. Gunther G, Junker R, Strater R, et al. Symptomatic ischemic stroke in full-term neonates: role of acquired and genetic prothrombotic risk factors. *Stroke.* 2000;31:2437–2441.

16. Fullerton HJ, Wu YW, Zhao S, et al. Risk of stroke in children: ethnic and gender disparities. *Neurology.* 2003;61:189–194.

17. Ganesan V, Prengler M, McShane MA, et al. Investigation of risk factors in children with arterial ischemic stroke. *Ann Neurol.* 2003;53:167–173.

18. Steinlin M, Pfister I, Pavlovic J, et al. The first three years of the swiss neuropaediatric stroke registry (SNPSR): a population-based study of incidence, symptoms and risk factors. *Neuropediatrics.* 2005;36:90–97.

19. De Schryver EL, Kappelle LJ, Jennekens-Schinkel A, et al. Prognosis of ischemic stroke in childhood: a long-term follow-up study. *Dev Med Child Neurol.* 2000;42:313–318.

20. Arias E, Anderson RN, Kung HC, et al. Deaths: final data for 2001. *Natl Vital Stat Rep.* 2003;52:1–115.

21. Lynch JK, Han CJ. Pediatric stroke: what do we know and what do we need to know? *Semin Neurol.* 2005;25:410–423.

22. Friedman NR. Pediatric stroke: past, present and future. *Adv Pediatr.* 2009;56:271–299.

23. Isler W. Stroke in childhood and adolescence. *Eur Neurol.* 1984;23: 421–424.

24. Lanska MJ, Lanska DJ, Horwitz SJ, et al. Presentation, clinical course, and outcome of childhood stroke. *Pediatr Neurol.* 1991;7:333–341.

25. Yang JS, Park YD, Hartlage PL. Seizures associated with stroke in childhood. *Pediatr Neurol.* 1995;12:136–138.

26. Giroud M, Lemesle M, Madinier G, et al. Stroke in children under 16 years of age. Clinical and etiological difference with adults. *Acta Neurol Scand.* 1997;96:401–406.

27. Ganesan V, Hogan A, Shack N, et al. Outcome after ischaemic stroke in childhood. *Dev Med Child Neurol.* 2000;42:455–461.

28. Lanthier S, Carmant L, David M, et al. Stroke in children: the coexistence of multiple risk factors predicts poor outcome. *Neurology.* 2000;54: 371–378.

29. Delsing BJ, Catsman-Berrevoets CE, Appel IM. Early prognostic indicators of outcome in ischemic childhood stroke. *Pediatr Neurol.* 2001;24:283–289.

30. Barnes C, Newall F, Furmedge J, et al. Arterial ischaemic stroke in children. *J Paediatr Child Health.* 2004;40:384–387.

31. Cowan F, Rutherford M, Groenendaal F, et al. Origin and timing of brain lesions in term infants with neonatal encephalopathy. *Lancet.* 2003;361: 736–742.

32. Barmada MA, Moossy J, Shuman RM. Cerebral infarcts with arterial occlusion in neonates. *Ann Neurol.* 1979;6:495–502.

33. Estan J, Hope P. Unilateral neonatal cerebral infarction in full term infants. *Arch Dis Child Fetal Neonatal Ed.* 1997;76:F88–F93.

34. Levy SR, Abroms IF, Marshall PC, et al. Seizures and cerebral infarction in the full-term newborn. *Ann Neurol.* 1985;17:366–370.

35. Aso K, Scher MS, Barmada MA. Cerebral infarcts and seizures in the neonate. *J Child Neurol.* 1990;5:224–228.

36. Tekgul H, Gauvreau K, Soul J, et al. The current etiologic profile and neurodevelopmental outcome of seizures in term newborn infants. *Pediatrics.* 2006;117:1270–1280.

37. Clancy R, Malin S, Laraque D, et al. Focal motor seizures heralding stroke in full-term neonates. *Am J Dis Child.* 1985;139:601–606.

38. Scher MS, Wiznitzer M, Bangert BA. Cerebral infarctions in the fetus and neonate: maternal-placental-fetal considerations. *Clin Perinatol.* 2002;29: 693–724, vi–vii.

39. Fujimoto S, Yokochi K, Togari H, et al. Neonatal cerebral infarction: symptoms, CT findings and prognosis. *Brain Dev.* 1992;14:48–52.

40. Jan MM, Camfield PR. Outcome of neonatal stroke in full-term infants without significant birth asphyxia. *Eur J Pediatr.* 1998;157:846–848.

41. Trauner DA, Chase C, Walker P, et al. Neurologic profiles of infants and children after perinatal stroke. *Pediatr Neurol.* 1993;9:383–386.

42. Sran SK, Baumann RJ. Outcome of neonatal strokes. *Am J Dis Child.* 1988;142:1086–1088.

43. de Veber G, Andrew M, Adams C, et al. Cerebral sinovenous thrombosis in children. *N Engl J Med.* 2001;345:417–423.

44. Golomb MR, Garg BP, Carvalho KS, et al. Perinatal stroke and the risk of developing childhood epilepsy. *J Pediatr.* 2007;151:409–413, 413.e1–413.e2.

45. Rando T, Ricci D, Mercuri E, et al. Periodic lateralized epileptiform discharges (PLEDs) as early indicator of stroke in full-term newborns. *Neuropediatrics.* 2000;31:202–205.

46. Brower MC, Rollins N, Roach ES. Basal ganglia and thalamic infarction in children, cause and clinical features. *Arch Neurol.* 1996;53:1252–1256.

47. Mancini J, Girard N, Chabrol B, et al. Ischemic cerebrovascular disease in children: retrospective study of 35 patients. *J Child Neurol.* 1997;12: 193–199.

48. Osler W. *The Cerebral Palsies of Children.* London: MacKeith; 1987.

49. Sachs B, Peterson F. A study of cerebral palsies of early life, based upon an analysis of one hundred and forty cases. *J Nerv Ment Dis.* 1890;17: 295–332.

50. Krynauw RA. Infantile hemiplegia treated by removing one cerebral hemisphere. *J Neurol Neurosurg Psychiatry.* 1950;13:243–267.

51. Slapø GD, Lossius MI, Gjerstad L. Poststroke epilepsy: occurrence, predictors and treatment. *Exp Rev Neurother.* 2006;6(12):1801–1809.

52. Lamy C, Domigo V, Semah F, et al. Early and late seizures after cryptogenic ischemic stroke in young adults. *Neurology.* 2003;60(3):400–404.

53. Berges S, Moulin T, Berger E, et al. Seizures and epilepsy following strokes: recurrence factors. *Eur Neurol.* 2000;43(1):3–8.

54. Giroud M, Gras P, Fayolle H, et al. Early seizures after acute stroke: a study of 1,640 cases. *Epilepsia.* 1994;35(5):959–964.

55. So EL, Annegers JF, Hauser WA, et al. Population-based study of seizure disorders after cerebral infarction. *Neurology.* 1996;46(2):350–355.

56. Lossius MI, Ronning OM, Mowinckel P, et al. Incidence and predictors for post-stroke epilepsy. A prospective controlled trial. The Akershus stroke study. *Eur J Neurol.* 2002;9(4):365–368.

57. Kammersgaard LP, Olsen TS. Poststroke epilepsy in the copenhagen stroke study: incidence and predictors. *J Stroke Cerebrovasc Dis.* 2005;14(5): 210–214.

58. Velioglu SK, Ozmenoglu M, Boz C, et al. Status epilepticus after stroke. *Stroke.* 2001;32(5):1169–1172.

59. Afsar N, Kaya D, Aktan S, et al. Stroke and status epilepticus: stroke type, type of status epilepticus, and prognosis. *Seizure.* 2003;12(1):23–27.

60. De Reuck J, Van Maele G. Status epilepticus in stroke patients. *Eur Neurol.* 2009;62(3):171–175.

61. Hartings JA, Williams AJ, Tortella FC. Occurrence of nonconvulsive seizures, periodic epileptiform discharges, and intermittent rhythmic delta activity in rat focal ischemia. *Exp Neurol.* 2003;179(2):139–149.

62. Ferro JM, Canhao P, Bousser M, et al, for the ISCVT Investigators. Early seizures in cerebral vein and dural sinus thrombosis: risk factors and role of antiepileptics. *Stroke.* 2008;39(4):1152–1158.

63. De Reuck J, Vonck K, Santens P, et al. Cobalt-55 positron emission tomography in late-onset epileptic seizures after thrombo-embolic middle cerebral artery infarction. *J Neurol Sci.* 2000;181(1–2):13–18.

64. De Reuck J, Claeys I, Martens S, et al. Computed tomographic changes of the brain and clinical outcome of patients with seizures and epilepsy after an ischaemic hemispheric stroke. *Eur J Neurol.* 2006;13(4): 402–407.

65. De Reuck J, Goethals M, Claeys I, et al. EEG findings after a cerebral territorial infarct in patients who develop early- and late-onset seizures. *Eur Neurol.* 2006;55(4):209–213.

66. Carrera E, Michel P, Despland P, et al. Continuous assessment of electrical epileptic activity in acute stroke. *Neurology.* 2006;67(1):99–104.

67. Claassen J, Jette N, Chum F, et al. Electrographic seizures and periodic discharges after intracerebral hemorrhage. *Neurology.* 2007;69(13): 1356–1365.

68. Crumrine RC, Bergstrand K, Cooper AT, et al. Lamotrigine protects hippocampal CA1 neurons from ischemic damage after cardiac arrest. *Stroke.* 1997;28(11):2230–2237.

69. Brailowsky S, Knight RT, Efron R. Phenytoin increases the severity of cortical hemiplegia in rats. *Brain Res.* 1986;376(1):71–77.

70. Ryvlin P, Montavont A, Nighoghossian N. Optimizing therapy of seizures in stroke patients. *Neurology.* 2006;67(12 Suppl 4):S3–S9.

71. Rowan AJ, Ramsay RE, Collins JF, et al. the VA Cooperative Study 428 Group. New onset geriatric epilepsy: a randomized study of gabapentin, lamotrigine, and carbamazepine. *Neurology.* 2005;64(11):1868–1873.

CHAPTER 31 ■ EPILEPSY IN THE SETTING OF NEUROCUTANEOUS SYNDROMES

AJAY GUPTA

Neurocutaneous syndromes are genetically and clinically heterogeneous congenital diseases with common characteristics of distinct cutaneous stigmata in association with neurologic disease and involvement of various organs and systems. Cutaneous findings, noted by the patient, family, or a family physician, are usually the tip-off for suspecting a neurocutaneous disease. In a few of the neurocutaneous syndromes, epilepsy is the most common presenting symptom. Identification and chronic management of these patients with complex epilepsy issues often fall into the hands of neurologists and epileptologists, who sometimes, lead a team of various specialists in a multidisciplinary clinic model to provide disease-based clinical care. Recognition of neurocutaneous syndromes associated with epilepsy is therefore of critical importance for neurologists and epileptologists. Accurate early diagnosis is vital to counsel the patient and the family regarding chronicity of the condition, choose appropriate antiepileptic drugs for epilepsy, ensure timely selection of candidates for epilepsy surgery, guide testing and consulting for coexisting morbidities, and, when appropriate, refer for genetic testing and counseling. In this chapter, we will discuss diagnosis and treatment of such conditions. While our focus will be on the diagnosis and treatment of epilepsy in these conditions, we will touch upon important aspects of comorbid neuropsychiatric conditions, and other organ system involvement that impact decision making for medical and surgical treatment of epilepsy. Clinical, radiographic, and pathologic findings are presented in the pictorial atlas (Chapter 5).

TUBEROUS SCLEROSIS COMPLEX

Tuberous sclerosis complex (TSC) is a multisystem genetic disease with an autosomal dominant pattern of inheritance. The prevalence of this disease is reported to be 1 in 6000 to 10,000 (1). Seizures are one of the most common presenting symptoms in TSC, and most patients with TSC develop life-long refractory epilepsy. The classic Vogt triad of mental retardation, seizures, and adenoma sebaceum that was used to diagnose TSC in the pre-MRI and gene testing era is found in only 29% of TSC patients (2). Diagnostic criteria for clinical diagnosis of TSC have been developed and are clinically useful (3). However, TSC remains a disease with extremely variable expression, and approximately 7% of the patients with TSC1 or TSC2 mutation may not meet diagnostic criteria for TSC, and 15% of patients who meet the criteria for TSC may not have detectable mutation in TSC1 or TSC2 (4). Approximately 60% of the patients are the only family members affected, suggesting a new spontaneous mutation (5). Mutations in two genes have been identified in patients with TSC. TSC1 is located at chromosome 9q34 and encodes a protein called hamartin. TSC2 is located at chromosome 16p13.3 and encodes a protein called tuberin. Although located on different chromosomes, the two genes code two proteins that work in the same biochemical pathway, the mTOR (mammalian target of rapamycin) pathway that is critical to cell cycle regulation. Pathogenic mutations in the TSC1 or TSC2 genes activate the mTOR cascade, resulting in abnormal growth and proliferation in various organs and systems. An understanding of this mechanism provided a unique opportunity to test rapamycin as a potential therapeutic agent targeting TSC-related diseases in various organs and systems (6–8). Although most patients have mutations localizable to either TSC1 or TSC2 by currently available testing, 15% of patients may not have a detectable known mutation (9). Such patients should be screened for TSC2 deletions. Sporadic mutations are more common in the TSC2 gene. Mutations of TSC1 seem to result in less severe phenotypic expression. Specifically, TSC1 patients appear to have fewer seizures, fewer intracranial lesions, and less severe mental retardation (9). Both parents of a child who has TSC should be examined for evidence of the disease. When the index case has an identified pathogenic mutation, family members at risk could be screened by looking for that specific mutation. In a case with no identifiable mutations, the family screening could begin by testing of the biologic parents by means of a complete physical including a Wood's lamp examination, dilated eye examination, magnetic resonance imaging (MRI) of the head, and renal ultrasonography. If the biological parents have no evidence of TSC, the recurrence risk for their next child is low due to a remote possibility of gonadal mosaicism; if either parent has the disease, the risk for another affected child is 50%.

Epilepsy and Neurologic Manifestations in TSC

Seizures are one of the most common presentations in TSC and occur in up to 80% patients with TSC. Most patients of TSC with seizures tend to present early in life, and 70% TSC patients develop epilepsy by the age of 1 year (2,10). A typical patient is an infant who presents with infantile spasms with no prenatal and perinatal adverse events (11,12). Life-long neurologic morbidity of TSC is usually defined early in life by intractable epilepsy and global cognitive delay that typically go hand in hand. Early onset of epilepsy is one of the important risk factors for continuing seizures and cognitive disability later in life (2,13). Most infants with epileptic spasms, despite going into remission with antiepileptic treatment (vigabatrin, ACTH, or other medications), develop complex partial, focal motor, tonic or generalized tonic–clonic seizures later in life. It is generally accepted that most seizures in TSC are partial onset seizures from one or more cortical tubers. Infrequently, a TSC patient may present with seizures later in teenage years or adulthood with exclusively partial seizures (2,13,14).

EEG has no specificity to the diagnosis of TSC. A variety of abnormal findings could be seen during the interictal period including a picture of hypsarrhythmia during infancy and Lennox–Gastaut syndrome in older children and adults. Westmoreland found that 88% of TSC patients had abnormal recordings; 75% had epileptiform discharges, and focal slowing occurred in 13%. The epileptiform discharges were multifocal in 25% and focal in 23%; hypsarrhythmia occurred in 19% and generalized spike–wave discharges in 8% (14). Approximately 70% of focal spikes were in the temporal lobe. A variety of seizure onset (ictal EEG) could be observed ranging from exclusively well-localized focal seizures with partial semiology to generalized or nonlocalized ictal EEG onset with generalized motor or bland seizures. It remains unclear if the threshold of epileptogenicity from the tuber(s) changes over a life time. It is also not known if and how multiple epileptogenic tubers interact with each other leading to an unpredictable course of epilepsy. Cusmai and coworkers reported that during follow-up EEG, although some epileptic foci disappeared (usually occipital foci), others became evident, especially in the frontal regions (consistent with posterior–anterior migration of epileptic foci in childhood) (15). The study also found that, although there was no correlation between the number of EEG foci and the number of cortical tubers, in 25 of 26 patients in their series, there was an EEG and MRI topographic correlation between at least one large tuber (larger than 10 mm in the axial plane and 30 mm in the coronal plane) and an EEG focus. Secondary bilateral synchrony appeared in 35% of children with tuberous sclerosis after the age of 2 years, especially during drowsiness and sleep (15,16).

Fifty percent to 65% of TSC patients have mild to moderate mental retardation. Intelligence quotient (IQ) appears to be bimodally distributed in patients with tuberous sclerosis. On the good side of the spectrum are the few patients who have no or infrequent seizures beginning after early childhood with no or mild learning disabilities and an IQ that is lower than siblings without TSC. On the guarded side of the spectrum are TSC patients who present with infantile spasms or catastrophic epilepsy with onset before 12 months of age who end up with moderate to severe mental retardation, limited or no speech, and inability to ambulate (17). Autism is commonly described in TSC patients and is reported in 25% to 50% of patients. Between 26% and 58% of children with tuberous sclerosis and infantile spasms have autism, compared with 13% of patients with infantile spasms who do not have tuberous sclerosis (17–19). The association between autism and tuberous sclerosis therefore appears to be more than coincidental. Both the number of tubers and their topography seem to play an important role in the cognitive outcome. The persistence of epileptic foci in anterior and posterior areas is thought to be important in the development of autistic traits, such as severe disability in verbal and nonverbal communication, stereotypies, and complete indifference to social interaction. Patients with multiple cortical lesions

are likely to have developmental delay and intractable seizures. However, it is not possible to predict neurocognitive function or burden of epilepsy in an individual TSC patient by brain MRI alone. Patients with TSC also have other neuropsychiatric morbidity in the form of high frequency of hyperactive and aggressive behavior, and rarely self-mutilation (18). Subependymal giant cell astrocytomas (SEGAs) may grow and obstruct the cerebrospinal fluid (CSF) flow presenting with symptoms and signs of hydrocephalus requiring tumor excision with or without placement of ventriculo–peritoneal shunt.

Nonneurologic Lesions in TSC

TSC patients have a multitude of cutaneous lesions such as hypomelanic macules (ash leaf spots), adenoma sebaceum (facial angiofibromas), forehead plaques, shagreen patches, and ungual or subungual fibromas. In Gomez's series of 300 patients with TSC, skin lesions were seen in 96%, followed by seizures in 84%, retinal hamartomas in 47%, and mental impairment in 45% (2). Patients with TSC may have many visceral lesions including: cardiac rhabdomyomas, phakomas in the eyes (retinal hamartoma), renal cysts and angiomyolipomas, hepatic cysts, and pulmonary lymphangiomyomatosis.

Brain Involvement and Neuroimaging in TSC

TSC is associated with a variety of brain lesions, and these are: cortical tubers, white matter lesions, subependymal nodules (SENs), and SEGAs (20,21). Histologically, each of the four types of intracranial lesions are composed of clusters of giant cells with varying degrees of neuronal and astrocytic differentiation, and the presence of cells that are transitional forms between these two types. On unenhanced brain computed tomography (CT), cortical and subcortical white matter lesions in TSC appear hypodense and may be mistaken for a remote insult; however, the presence of multiple lesions and associated calcified SEN usually clarify the diagnosis. Many unsuspecting patients are identified to have TSC for the first time by a brain CT done as a part of the evaluation for an unrelated question (e.g., in the emergency room after a head trauma).

While brain CT is helpful in noticing calcified lesions in TSC, brain MRI is the neuroimaging procedure of choice to elicit the extent of all lesions. Age is an important factor in interpretation of brain MRI in TSC. Cortical tubers are hyperintense on T2 and flair sequences, and hypointense on T1 sequences in patients with mature myelination. In newborn and infants with immature myelination, the tubers are hyperintense to unmyelinated white matter on T1 sequences and appear hypointense on T2-weighted images. This effect of immature myelination on the brain MRI findings in infants with TSC is felt to be secondary to the increased water content in unmyelinated regions of the brain. There is evidence to suggest that cortical tuber count and location is associated with increased risk of infantile spasms (22). There also appears to be a correlation between increased number of tubers, development of early seizures and developmental delay.

There are three types of white matter lesions in TSC (20,21). These are, in the order of common occurrence; thin linear bands extending radially from the ventricular surface to cortical tubers, wedge-shaped bands with apices near ventricles, and amorphous lesions in the deep white matter. The white matter lesions tend to be predominant in frontal lobes.

SENs are often near the caudate head or caudothalamic groove. They are variable in appearance and signal intensity. SENs do not usually obstruct CSF flow, but may uncommonly do so by mechanical pressure against the foramen of Monro. SENs may rarely enhance on gadolinium administration in a nodular or ring-like fashion, and enhancement is better appreciated at higher signal strengths. When small, SENs are better seen on CT than MRI because of the presence of calcification.

SEGAs are slow-growing tumors. They are typically located near the foramen of Monro and are believed to originate from SEN. However, rarely SEGAs may also appear in other locations in the brain. Typically, there is no edema in brain parenchyma adjacent to the SEGA. Most SEGAs are benign, although there are rare cases of malignant degeneration. The symptoms of SEGAs are mainly due to their location (22). TSC patients with a SEGA often present with acute or chronic increased intracranial pressure, suggesting chronic or intermittent obstruction at the level of the foramen of Monro. The incidence of SEGAs in various studies on TSC is reported to be 1.7% to 26%. A recent series in a moderate sized group of patients reported 8.2% (23). SEGAs are generally iso- to hypointense to brain parenchyma on T1-weighted images and hyperintense on T2-weighted images. SEGAs are heterogeneous in appearance. Flow voids may be identified within these lesions. They often have internal susceptibility artifact reflecting hemorrhage or calcification. SEGAs usually show contrast enhancement. A SEGA should be suspected, and periodic screening scans are indicated if SENs show increased size and contrast enhancement.

Medical Treatment of Epilepsy in TSC

The first-line treatment for seizures is antiepileptic medications. Many case series and randomized clinical trials show that vigabatrin is particularly effective in the treatment for infantile spasms and partial seizures during infancy in TSC (24–26). Vigabatrin may cause irreversible peripheral field visual defects after long-term use, and most experts agree not to use vigabatrin beyond 6 to 12 months of treatment. Adrenocorticotropin (ACTH) provides an alternative treatment; the response of children with tuberous sclerosis and infantile spasms to corticotropin is similar to the response of children with cryptogenic infantile spasms; however, those with tuberous sclerosis have a higher relapse rate. Vigabatrin may be superior compared to ACTH considering the similar or marginally better rate and rapidity of seizure remission, ease of oral administration, lack of serious side effects in the short term, and significantly low cost of treatment (24–26). Many experts use vigabatrin as the first-line drug in infantile seizures in the setting of TSC. Other antiepileptic treatments could be used in TSC following the general guidelines of partial versus generalized seizures. However, one should keep in mind that most seizures in patients with TSC are partial in origin despite an overwhelming electroclinical picture of generalized epileptic encephalopathy, therefore, not contraindicating antiepileptic drugs that are effective only for partial epilepsy are not

contraindicated. Coexisting renal morbidity in TSC warrants cautious use of topiramate and zonisamide, and ketogenic diet. Extra caution is required for monitoring preexisting neuropsychiatric and behavior issues that may paradoxically show worsening with antiepileptic drug(s). Vagal nerve stimulation has also been used in few refractory patients that were not candidates for surgery (27).

Surgical Treatment and Outcome of Epilepsy in TSC

Like any other refractory partial epilepsy, when medical treatment fails, evaluation for the possibility of epilepsy surgery should be considered early in every patient with TSC (28). Frequency of medical intractability of seizures is higher in TSC and reported to be approximately 50% in patients with tuberous sclerosis and partial epilepsy (13). Seizure freedom or effective control of debilitating seizures after epilepsy surgery would likely improve quality of life in patients and families with TSC. However, two key rules for planning surgical strategy, localization of the epileptogenic zone (EZ) and minimizing risk of a permanent new postoperative deficit(s), pose additional challenges unique to TSC. These challenges emanate from multiple factors, often age related, and are in complex interaction with each other. First, the presence of multiple bilateral tubers, sometimes partially or nearly confluent, on the brain MRI portrays a possibility of multiple epileptogenic lesions. The tubers often intermingle with white matter abnormalities and defy accurate identification of margins even on a high-resolution brain MRI making anatomical delineation for surgery inaccurate. Second, the patient is frequently a child or a cognitively disabled young adult with stereotypic nonfocal seizure semiology (epileptic spasms, bland seizures with behavior arrest, tonic or atonic seizures with falls) and a scalp video EEG that often shows overwhelming generalized or multiregional interictal abnormalities and nonlocalizable ictal onset. Considering recent reports of a single epileptogenic lesion on the brain MRI leading to generalized and multiregional interictal and ictal abnormalities on scalp EEG, a scenario of multiple epileptogenic lesions with such an EEG appears to be an insurmountable condition for epilepsy surgery (Chapter 90). Third, young age along with cognitive delay and behavior issues render cooperation for noninvasive mapping of eloquent functions, whenever necessary, challenging or even impractical. And lastly, lack of long-term longitudinal postoperative outcome studies make family counseling before surgery imprecise as there is always a potential concern for emergence of epileptogenicity from the nonresected tubers. No wonder, in the quest for a successful surgical strategy in TSC, multiple presurgical investigative tools in various combinations and recipes have been reported in the published case series from various centers (28).

Use of multimodal presurgical tools such as 18F-flurodeoxyglucose (FDG) positron emission tomography (PET), alpha-[(11)C] methyl-L-tryptophan (AMT) PET, ictal single photon emission computed tomography (SPECT), and magnetoencephalogram (MEG) coregistered to the brain MRI have been used in varying combinations with claims of success; however, there is no perfect formula in identification of the epileptogenic tuber, and neither has any tool(s), alone or in combination, been shown to improve the rate of seizure freedom after surgery (28–34). A logical step-by-step investigation tailored to each patient remains the cornerstone of presurgical evaluation in TSC. Recently, in patients with an unidentifiable EZ (epileptogenic tuber[s]) on multimodal, noninvasive investigations, bilateral subdural and depth electrode implantation encompassing wide regions of brain bilaterally followed by a focused search for the epileptogenic tuber(s) with staged resection(s) has been reported from one center (35). Palliative procedures, such as corpus callosotomy or partial or complete resection of the "most" epileptogenic tuber (cause of most frequent or most severe seizures), could also help in some patients with TSC where surgery is done to minimize injuries, abolish the most disabling seizures with falls and loss of consciousness, and prevent episodes of life-threatening status epilepticus.

Published series on epilepsy surgery in TSC have reported high rates of success in alleviating or significantly improving seizures in most patients who undergo surgery. In a systematic review of literature published between 1960 and 2006, Jansen et al. (2007) reviewed a sample of 177 TSC patients who underwent epilepsy surgery and were subjects in 25 published articles in peer-reviewed journals. Not surprisingly, authors found these observational case series incomparable due to extreme variability in the collection and reporting of data (36). However, in a composite analysis, 75% TSC patients were either seizure free (57%; 0.1 to 47 [mean 3.7] years follow-up) or >90% improved in seizure frequency (18%; 0.5 to 20 [mean 4.2] years follow-up). Such high success rates after surgery in TSC parallel seizure outcome after a single lesion extratemporal lobe epilepsy surgery. Also of interest was the finding that a large number of TSC patients who underwent surgery had generalized and multiregional interictal scalp EEG abnormalities (48%) and nonlocalizable ictal onset (46%) findings; however, the presence of focal versus nonfocal scalp EEG abnormalities had no statistically significant relationship to seizure remission after surgery (36). Obviously, these patients were selected for epilepsy surgery based on other (not studied in the paper) criteria(s), such as semiology, functional deficits, dominant tuber(s) on the brain MRI, nuclear imaging studies, or MEG, again highlighting the point that generalized and multiregional EEG abnormalities on the scalp video EEG does not preclude surgical candidacy in a child with a solitary or multiple lesions (such as in TSC).

The investigation to find the culprit tuber (and define the EZ) is therefore, best individualized to each patient considering all aspects of their clinical condition and goals of epilepsy surgery. No formula fits all TSC patients. Every TSC patient with refractory epilepsy should undergo presurgical evaluation using a customized approach.

STURGE–WEBER SYNDROME

Sturge–Weber syndrome (SWS) or Sturge–Weber–Dimitri syndrome is also known as encephalotrigeminal angiomatosis or encephalofacial angiomatosis. SWS was first described in 1879 by Sturge, who thought that the neurologic features of the syndrome resulted from a nevoid condition of the brain similar to that affecting the face. Volland in 1912 and Weber in 1922 described the intracranial calcifications, and Dimitri was the first to report a case with calcifications seen on skull roentgenogram. SWS is a sporadic disease presumed to be caused by somatic mutation. Prevalence of SWS is estimated

in one study to be 1 in 50,000. Characteristic clinical features of SWS are unilateral facial portwine stain (PWS), ipsilateral pial angiomatosis, epilepsy, stroke-like episodes, and glaucoma. Neurologic manifestations include seizures, varying degrees of mental retardation, migraine-like headaches, intermittent or progressive stroke-like episodes with focal deficits such as hemiparesis, hemiatrophy, aphasia, and hemianopsia (21,37).

Chronic cortical ischemia from angiomatous malformation leading to calcification and laminar cortical necrosis have been proposed as likely mechanisms of brain injury. During the sixth week of intrauterine life, the primitive embryonal vascular plexus develops around the cephalic portion of the neural tube and under the ectoderm in the region destined to be the facial skin. In SWS, it is hypothesized that the vascular plexus fails to regress, as it should in the embryo in the ninth week, resulting in angiomatosis of related tissues (38). The intracranial lesion is thought to be due to proliferation of leptomeningeal vessels in the subarachnoid space that causes shunting of blood away from the brain tissue resulting in decreased blood flow, decreased venous return (venous stasis), and consequent focal hypoxia leading to cellular death. This is seen radiographically as gliosis, volume loss, and calcification.

Epilepsy and Neurologic Manifestations in SWS

Seizures are the most common neurologic presentation and occur in 75% to 80% of children with SWS. Only 10% to 20% of children with unilateral portwine nevus of the forehead have a leptomeningeal angioma. Typically, SWS involve occipital and posterior parietal lobes ipsilateral to the portwine nevus, but it can affect other cranial regions and both cerebral hemispheres. Bilateral brain lesions occur in 15% of children. Bilateral hemispheric involvement increases the risk of seizure. The age range of onset of seizure varies between birth and 23 years with median age of 6 months (39). The risk of developing seizures is highest in the first 2 years of life and occurs earlier in patients with bilateral disease. The most common type of seizure is a partial seizure, usually a focal motor with hemitonic, hemiclonic semiology. Secondarily generalized seizures are also uncommonly seen, usually later in childhood and adolescence. There is also an increased incidence of prolonged seizures or status epilepticus in SWS patients. In many SWS patients, seizures tend to cycle with relapsing clusters over few days, and then remitting for many days to weeks. Fever and infection may trigger the onset of seizure clusters in many children. Seizures frequently accompany stroke-like episodes. Onset of a motor deficit may precede a cluster or prolonged seizures rather than seizures followed by Todd paralysis; however, this distinction could be difficult in children. Hemiparesis is often discovered for the first time around the seizure clusters before it becomes an obvious permanent deficit. It remains unclear if fixed hemiparesis is a stuttering progressive hemiparesis that occurs due to acute (seizures, stroke-like episodes) over chronic (hypoxia from leptomeningeal angiomatosis) injury, raising the question of SWS being a progressive disease. Fixed hemiparesis contralateral to the facial angioma eventually occurs in 50% children. Transient episodes of hemiplegia, not related to clinical or EEG evidence of seizure activity, may also occur. As a general rule, children with SWS do not exhibit significant mental retardation in the absence of seizures. Hemiparesis and hemisensory loss increase in frequency with age. Hemianopsia is often present by the time hemiparesis is manifested. SWS patients may also have associated migraine-like headache, attention deficit disorder, and mild to severe cognitive impairment (39,40). Sixty percent to 80% of SWS patients have some degree of mental retardation, and 47% to 60% are reported to have moderate to severe mental retardation in two studies. Bilateral hemispheric involvement usually shows increased severity of mental retardation (41). Intensity of seizures rather than age of onset or hemiparesis were correlated with the presence and severity of mental retardation (42).

EEG could serve as a noninvasive tool for diagnosis of brain involvement in newborns and young infants who have not yet developed neurologic symptoms and signs. Commonly seen EEG abnormalities are slowing and attenuation of background activity on one (ipsilateral to the disease) or both (likely bilateral disease) sides, epileptiform spikes coexisting with background abnormalities, and only epileptiform spikes without background abnormalities. Few patients may have bilateral independent or generalized spike discharges. Quantitative EEG (qEEG) has been claimed to provide an objective measure of EEG asymmetry that correlates with clinical status and brain asymmetry seen on MRI (43).

Nonneurologic Lesion in SWS

The hallmark cutaneous lesion of SWS is the unilateral facial capillary angioma (i.e., PWS or nevus flammeus) in the distribution of cranial nerve V. The dermatologic lesion of a facial PWS is usually present during birth. It is a flat lesion of variable size, involving the upper eyelid and forehead. The size of cutaneous angioma does not predict the size of intracranial angioma. It is unilateral in 70% cases, almost always ipsilateral to the brain involvement. Usually it is in the V1 distribution with variable V2 and V3 involvement. Patients with V1 involvement are at risk for neuro-ocular lesions. Some experts feel that facial angioma is not a sine qua non, and up to 5% of patients with SWS do not have facial angiomas. Nevi may be found on the nape of neck above or below the hairline, upper trunk, or even the extremities, and hence may escape recognition on a cursory examination. Even when facial angiomas are bilateral, intracranial involvement tends to be unilateral or dominant (asymmetric) on one side (21,41).

Glaucoma is diagnosed in 15% of SWS patients at birth, 61% in the first year of life, and 72% by the age of 5 years (39). Presence of vascular malformation in the distribution of V1 segment increases the probability of glaucoma. The presence of buphthalmos and amblyopia in newborns with SWS may suggest glaucoma. There may be associated vascular abnormality in the conjuctiva, sclera, retina, and choroid. In SWS, glaucoma is usually found with ipsilateral choroidal angiomas. This elevated intraocular pressure may be due to elevated episcleral venous pressure (44). Dilated episcleral and retinal vessels are present with V1 involvement. There is increased incidence of retinal detachment secondary to hemorrhages from the choroidal hemangiomas. Eye involvement may result in acute or chronic or acute on chronic visual loss that may not be readily apparent in a young infant without an opthalmologic examination by an expert.

Brain Involvement and Neuroimaging in SWS

Characteristics brain MRI findings in SWS are enhancement of the leptomeningeal angioma, enlarged transmedullary veins, choroid plexus hypertrophy, white matter abnormalities, calcification, and patchy parenchymal gliosis (neuronal loss) (Chapter 5). However, the brain MRI may only show subtle or no abnormalities in young infants who are, at a later date, shown to have SWS. Unenhanced CT scan of the brain, although routinely not done, may show cortical calcification typically described as "tram track or gyriform" appearance. Calcification may be absent or minimal in neonates and infants. On brain MRI, calcified lesions are best visualized on gradient or susceptibility sequences where they exhibit gyriform susceptibility artifact (low signal areas). Contrary to what might be anticipated intuitively, neither MR venography nor MR angiography are generally helpful in assessing SWS (21).

Medical Treatment of Epilepsy in SWS

Broad spectrum antiepileptic medications that are effective in partial seizures may control seizures. Onset of epilepsy before 2 years of age increases the risk of mental retardation and refractory epilepsy. Clinical progression may have a stuttering course with unpredictable periods of rapid worsening, episodes of intense seizure clusters and status epilepticus, and stroke-like episodes as discussed in the previous section (39,43). There is a higher risk for neurologic complications in widespread or bihemispheric disease. Aspirin 3 to 5 mg/kg/day is often recommended for patients with SWS as primary prevention or secondary prevention (after first stroke-like episode), but its efficacy is controversial, and there have been no controlled trials. In one case series, patients who received prophylactic aspirin were found to have 65% fewer strokes than those who did not (45). Due to low risk, it may be prudent to use aspirin under close monitoring. Regular evaluation by an ophthalmologist is recommended, particularly in those patients with choroidal lesions. Medical and surgical treatment of glaucoma includes beta-blockers, carbonic anhydrase ophthalmic drops, and surgery. Salvaging (or preventing) visual loss by aggressive glaucoma management has important implications for future epilepsy surgery that likely involves ipsilateral posterior quadrant resection with permanent postoperative contralateral hemianopsia (37).

Surgical Treatment and Outcome of Epilepsy in SWS

About 50% patients of SWS may have medically refractory epilepsy. Epilepsy in SWS is amenable to surgical treatment in most refractory patients with SWS (37). Peterman and associates followed 25 patients with SWS for more than 5 years and reported spontaneous remission or controlled epilepsy in nearly half (40). In medically refractory patients, presurgical evaluation should be promptly considered. General principles of pediatric epilepsy surgery apply to SWS children (Chapter 90). The timing of surgery is important. Considering that in some SWS patients, the disease may be progressive; some experts argue that early resective surgery may be useful in halting the progressive brain involvement, neurologic deficits, and cognitive impairment. Visually guided complete excision of the angiomatous cortex with or without the guidance of intraoperative electrocorticography is generally considered the primary surgical strategy. Extensive hemispheric resection and hemispherectomy could be considered in children with extensive unilateral brain involvement and a fixed hemiparesis. The completeness of resection or disconnection of diseased tissue is an important factor in achieving epilepsy control. Seventy percent to 80% patients may be seizure free or significantly improved (>75% to 90% seizure reduction) after surgery, and early surgery may improve developmental outcome in refractory patients. The prognosis for intellectual outcome is better in patients who underwent surgery earlier (preferably before the age of 3 years) compared with those who were operated on later (37,46–50). In patients with bihemispheric disease and intractable generalized seizures, corpus callosotomy could be considered. However, very few patients with SWS have undergone this procedure (51).

LESS COMMON NEUROCUTANEOUS SYNDROMES

Epidermal Nevus Syndrome

Epidermal nevus syndrome (ENS) is a sporadic neurocutaneous disorder without any known familial cases. Somatic mutation is postulated as the underlying genetic mechanism. The defining cutaneous feature of ENS are congenital epidermal nevi that are usually raised (palpable), and may be band-like, round, oval, or linear in configuration. Cutaneous lesions may be subtle to detect due to their skin-like color and velvety appearance in infancy; however, they may become verrucous orange or brown later in life. A wide variety of epidermal congenital lesions have been linked to ENS, such as linear sebaceous nevus (of Jadassohn), nevus verrucosus, ichthyosis hystrix, nevus unius lateris, and inflammatory linear verrucous epidermal nevus. The cutaneous lesions may differ somewhat in histology. Characteristically, the dermis is not involved, and there is thickening and hyperkeratosis of the epidermis with hyperplasia of the sebaceous glands. Some investigators prefer to group the cutaneous lesions together, whereas others maintain that these are separate entities on the basis of histologic differences (52). The potential for malignant transformation exists after puberty. Heterogeneity of cutaneous findings in ENS is not just limited to skin, brain involvement also tend to be variable ranging from focal cortical dysplasia to hemispheric dysplasia and hemimegalencephaly (53). In this chapter, we use the term *epidermal nevus syndrome* to encompass all these entities. Besides cutaneous manifestations, there is a wide spectrum of clinical presentation involving multiple organs and systems. Ocular, dental, and skeletal abnormalities, as well as malignancies, have been reported. Ocular involvement reported in approximately 25% of cases include microphthalmia, proptosis, choristomas (including dermoids and epidermoids), cataracts, and colobomas (54).

Brain Involvement, Epilepsy, and Its Treatment in ENS

Pathogenesis of brain involvement is postulated to be vascular dysplasia and migrational anomalies. Brain involvement is usually ipsilateral or asymmetric bilateral (worse ipsilateral) to the cutaneous findings. However, there is no consistent relationship between side of nevus and CNS abnormality. Various types of brain malformations and migration abnormalities are reported; however, classical involvement of the brain is in the form of hemimegalencephaly (17 out of 60 patients in Pavone study) (53,55–57). In a series of 60 patients, Solomon and Esterly reported moderate to severe CNS involvement in 30 patients (50%) (52). Reported clinical, EEG, and imaging findings include mental retardation, seizures, hyperkinesis, hydrocephalus, porencephaly, cortical atrophy, nonfunctioning cerebral venous sinuses, hemimacrocephaly or macrocephaly, hemimegalencephaly, infantile spasms with hypsarrhythmia or hemihypsarrhythmia, and other seizure types such as myoclonic, complex partial, partial motor, and generalized seizures (53,55–58). In other words, ENS has a wide spectrum of findings; however, in general, the neurologic involvement is severe. Seizure onset is usually within the first year of life. Seizures are usually daily, catastrophic and fail to respond to medical treatment. Pediatric epilepsy surgery (Chapter 90) principles should again guide the testing, timing, and surgical strategy. Anatomic or functional hemispherectomy is the treatment of choice in patients with hemimegalencephaly (59). Important considerations before epilepsy surgery in ENS patients include careful examination and investigations to elicit the clinical severity of other organ/system involvement in the patient. Counseling of parents is critical as the long-term outlook for neurocognitive development is guarded in ENS. Histopathologic examination of the brain resected in epilepsy surgery cases has shown a spectrum of dysplastic abnormalities, including diffuse cortical dysplasia, gyral fusion, pial glioneuronal hamartomas, cortical astrocytosis, and foci of microcalcification.

Neurofibromatosis 1

In neurofibromatosis type 1 (NF1), seizures occur in 3% to 5% of individuals, a rate that is slightly higher than in the general population. Korf and associates found that 21 (5.4%) of 359 children with neurofibromatosis had seizures (60). A variety of seizure types, including infantile spasms, absence, generalized convulsions, and complex partial seizures, have been reported (60–63). Seizures were due to tumors (hamartomas), cortical malformations, and mesial temporal sclerosis. Complex partial seizures appear to be the most common type, and have been reported in the absence of obvious structural lesions. Cognitive impairment is often present in those NF1 patients who have seizures. Age of presentation varied from 4 days to over 20 years.

RARE NEUROCUTANEOUS CONDITIONS WITH EPILEPSY

Incontinentia Pigmenti

Incontinentia pigmenti, which occurs almost exclusively in females (X-linked dominant condition), presents in the neonatal period with erythematous bullous lesions that become crusted and pigmented. Children with this disorder may develop seizures (13.3%), mental retardation (12.3%), or spasticity (11.4%). A variety of dysplastic brain MRI findings may be seen (64).

Hypomelanosis of Ito

Seizures and mental retardation are also seen in approximately two thirds of children with hypomelanosis of Ito, in which irregular, hypopigmented skin lesions along the embryonal lines of dermatologic fusion are seen. Seizures are more severe in early onset cases and consist of infantile spasms or myoclonic seizures. Choroidal atrophy, corneal opacities, deafness, dental anomalies, hemihypertrophy, hypotonia, and macrocephaly may also be seen (65,66). Reported CT and brain MRI findings include cerebral atrophy, porencephaly, and low-density areas in the white matter. Autopsy showed gray matter heterotopias and abnormal cortical lamination in a patient in one series indicative of abnormalities in neuronal migration (66).

Neurocutaneous Melanosis

Neurocutaneous melanosis (NM) is a rare disorder in which patients have congenital cutaneous nevi and leptomeningeal melanosis leading to CNS manifestations (67–70). Patients have multiple congenital cutaneous nevi, the largest of which typically measures greater than 5 cm. A 2.5% risk of developing NM with CNS involvement is quoted in patients with large congenital melanocytic nevi (67). NM may be lethal early in life, but some patients survive into their 20s. NM patients usually present with seizures or increased intracranial pressure. Cranial nerve palsy, hemiparesis, myelopathy, or psychiatric disorders may coexist. NM is believed to be a sporadic neurocutaneous disorder and is not transmitted as a single gene disorder. Most common brain MRI findings in NM patients are T1 shortening (increased signal) in temporal lobe and infratentorial brain on noncontrast exams. There is variable ventriculomegaly. There may be thickening of leptomeninges of brain and spine as demonstrated on contrast enhancement. Leptomeninges may appear to be normal on T1- and T2-weighted sequences. Usually there is leptomeningeal enhancement; however, cases have been described without the leptomeningeal involvement. There may also be pachymeningeal (dural) involvement (68–70).

References

1. Wiederholt WC, Gomez MR, Kurland LT. Incidence and prevalence of tuberous sclerosis in Rochester, Minnesota, 1950 through 1982. *Neurology.* 1985;35(4):600–603.
2. Gomez MR. Neurologic and psychiatric features. In: Gomez MR, ed. *Tuberous Sclerosis.* New York, NY: Ravon Press; 1988:21–36.
3. Roach ES, Gomez MR, Northrup H. Tuberous sclerosis complex consensus conference: Revised clinical diagnostic criteria. *J Child Neurol.* 1998;13(12):624–628.
4. Jozwiak S, Schwartz RA, Janniger CK, et al. Usefulness of diagnostic criteria of tuberous sclerosis complex in pediatric patients. *J Child Neurol.* 2000;15(10):652–659.
5. Fleury P, de Groot WP, Delleman JW, et al. Tuberous sclerosis: The incidence of sporadic cases versus familial cases. *Brain Dev.* 1980;2(2):107–117.
6. Franz DN, Leonard J, Tudor C, et al. Rapamycin causes regression of astrocytomas in tuberous sclerosis complex. *Ann Neurol.* 2006;59(3):490–498.
7. Bissler JJ, McCormack FX, Young LR, et al. Sirolimus for angiomyolipoma in tuberous sclerosis complex or lymphangioleiomyomatosis. *N Engl J Med.* 2008;358(2):140–151.
8. Paul E, Thiele E. Efficacy of sirolimus in treating tuberous sclerosis and lymphangioleiomyomatosis. *N Engl J Med.* 2008;358(2):190–192.
9. Dabora SL, Jozwiak S, Franz DN, et al. Mutational analysis in a cohort of 224 tuberous sclerosis patients indicates increased severity of TSC2, compared with TSC1, disease in multiple organs. *Am J Hum Genet.* 2001;68(1):64–80.
10. Webb DW, Fryer AE, Osborne JP. Morbidity associated with tuberous sclerosis: A population study. *Dev Med Child Neurol.* 1996;38(2):146–155.
11. Hunt A. Tuberous sclerosis: A survey of 97 cases. I: Seizures, pertussis immunisation and handicap. *Dev Med Child Neurol.* 1983;25(3):346–349.
12. Pampiglione G, Moynahan EJ. The tuberous sclerosis syndrome: Clinical and EEG studies in 100 children. *J Neurol Neurosurg Psychiatry.* 1976;39(7):666–673.
13. Yamamoto N, Watanabe K, Negoro T, et al. Long-term prognosis of tuberous sclerosis with epilepsy in children. *Brain Dev.* 1987;9(3):292–295.
14. Westmoreland BF. Electroencephalographic experience at the mayo clinic. In: Gomez MR, ed. *Tuberous Sclerosis.* New York, NY: Ravon Press; 1988:37–50.
15. Cusmai R, Chiron C, Curatolo P, et al. Topographic comparative study of magnetic resonance imaging and electroencephalography in 34 children with tuberous sclerosis. *Epilepsia.* 1990;31(6):747–755.
16. Ganji S, Hellman CD. Tuberous sclerosis: Long-term follow-up and longitudinal electroencephalographic study. *Clin Electroencephalogr.* 1985;16(4):219–224.
17. Joinson C, O'Callaghan FJ, Osborne JP, et al. Learning disability and epilepsy in an epidemiological sample of individuals with tuberous sclerosis complex. *Psychol Med.* 2003;33(2):335–344.
18. Hunt A, Dennis J. Psychiatric disorder among children with tuberous sclerosis. *Dev Med Child Neurol.* 1987;29(2):190–198.
19. Jambaque I, Cusmai R, Curatolo P, et al. Neuropsychological aspects of tuberous sclerosis in relation to epilepsy and MRI findings. *Dev Med Child Neurol.* 1991;33(8):698–705.
20. Roach ES, Williams DP, Laster DW. Magnetic resonance imaging in tuberous sclerosis. *Arch Neurol.* 1987;44(3):301–303.
21. Moon D, Gupta A. Magnetic resonance imaging in neurocutaneous syndromes. In: Luders HO, ed. *Textbook of Epilepsy Surgery.* 3rd ed. London, UK: Informa Healthcare; 2008:721–730.
22. Doherty C, Goh S, Young Poussaint T, et al. Prognostic significance of tuber count and location in tuberous sclerosis complex. *J Child Neurol.* 2005;20(10):837–841.
23. Goh S, Butler W, Thiele EA. Subependymal giant cell tumors in tuberous sclerosis complex. *Neurology.* 2004;63(8):1457–1461.
24. Lux AL, Edwards SW, Osborne JP, et al. Randomized trial of vigabatrin in patients with infantile spasms. *Neurology.* 2002;59(4):648.
25. Elterman RD, Shields WD, Mansfield KA, et al. US Infantile Spasms Vigabatrin Study Group. Randomized trial of vigabatrin in patients with infantile spasms. *Neurology.* 2001;57(8):1416–1421.
26. Hancock E, Osborne JP, Milner P. The treatment of west syndrome: A cochrane review of the literature to December 2000. *Brain Dev.* 2001;23(7):624–634.
27. Parain D, Penniello MJ, Berquen P, et al. Vagal nerve stimulation in tuberous sclerosis complex patients. *Pediatr Neurol.* 2001;25(3):213–216.
28. Gupta A. "Epilepsy surgery recipes galore": In quest for the epileptogenic tuber in tuberous sclerosis complex. *Epileptic Disord.* 2009;11(1):80–81.
29. Kamimura T, Tohyama J, Oishi M, et al. Magnetoencephalography in patients with tuberous sclerosis and localization-related epilepsy. *Epilepsia.* 2006;47(6):991–997.
30. Koh S, Jayakar P, Resnick T, et al. The localizing value of ictal SPECT in children with tuberous sclerosis complex and refractory partial epilepsy. *Epileptic Disord.* 1999;1(1):41–46.
31. Chandra PS, Salamon N, Huang J, et al. FDG-PET/MRI coregistration and diffusion-tensor imaging distinguish epileptogenic tubers and cortex in patients with tuberous sclerosis complex: A preliminary report. *Epilepsia.* 2006;47(9):1543–1549.
32. Kagawa K, Chugani DC, Asano E, et al. Epilepsy surgery outcome in children with tuberous sclerosis complex evaluated with alpha-[11C]methyl-L-tryptophan positron emission tomography (PET). *J Child Neurol.* 2005;20(5):429–438.
33. Fedi M, Reutens DC, Andermann F, et al. Alpha-[11C]-methyl-L-tryptophan PET identifies the epileptogenic tuber and correlates with interictal spike frequency. *Epilepsy Res.* 2003;52(3):203–213.
34. Asano E, Chugani DC, Muzik O, et al. Multimodality imaging for improved detection of epileptogenic foci in tuberous sclerosis complex. *Neurology.* 2000;54(10):1976–1984.
35. Weiner HL, Carlson C, Ridgway EB, et al. Epilepsy surgery in young children with tuberous sclerosis: Results of a novel approach. *Pediatrics.* 2006;117(5):1494–1502.
36. Jansen FE, van Huffelen AC, Algra A, et al. Epilepsy surgery in tuberous sclerosis: A systematic review. *Epilepsia.* 2007;48(8):1477–1484.
37. Tripathi AK, Gupta A. Sturge–Weber syndrome. In: Chapman K, Rho JM, eds. *Pediatric Epilepsy Case Studies.* 1st ed. Boca Raton, FL: CRC Press; 2008:153–160.

38. Di Rocco C, Tamburrini G. Sturge–Weber syndrome. *Childs Nerv Syst.* 2006;22(8):909–921.

39. Sujansky E, Conradi S. Sturge–Weber syndrome: Age of onset of seizures and glaucoma and the prognosis for affected children. *J Child Neurol.* 1995;10(1):49–58.

40. Peterman AF, Hayles AB, Dockerty MB, et al. Encephalotrigeminal angiomatosis (Sturge–Weber disease); clinical study of thirty-five cases. *J Am Med Assoc.* 1958;167(18):2169–2176.

41. Bebin EM, Gomez MR. Prognosis in Sturge–Weber disease: Comparison of unihemispheric and bihemispheric involvement. *J Child Neurol.* 1988;3(3): 181–184.

42. Kramer U, Kahana E, Shorer Z, et al. Outcome of infants with unilateral Sturge–Weber syndrome and early onset seizures. *Dev Med Child Neurol.* 2000;42(11):756–759.

43. Hatfield LA, Crone NE, Kossoff EH, et al. Quantitative EEG asymmetry correlates with clinical severity in unilateral Sturge–Weber syndrome. *Epilepsia.* 2007;48(1):191–195.

44. Phelps CD. The pathogenesis of glaucoma in Sturge–Weber syndrome. *Ophthalmology.* 1978;85(3):276–286.

45. Maria BL, Neufeld JA, Rosainz LC, et al. Central nervous system structure and function in Sturge–Weber syndrome: Evidence of neurologic and radiologic progression. *J Child Neurol.* 1998;13(12):606–618.

46. Ito M, Sato K, Ohnuki A, et al. Sturge–Weber disease: Operative indications and surgical results. *Brain Dev.* 1990;12(5):473–477.

47. Hoffman HJ, Hendrick EB, Dennis M, et al. Hemispherectomy for Sturge–Weber syndrome. *Childs Brain.* 1979;5(3):233–248.

48. Falconer MA, Rushworth RG. Treatment of encephalotrigeminal angiomatosis (Sturge–Weber disease) by hemispherectomy. *Arch Dis Child.* 1960;35:433–447.

49. Bourgeois M, Crimmins DW, de Oliveira RS, et al. Surgical treatment of epilepsy in Sturge–Weber syndrome in children. *J Neurosurg.* 2007;106(1 suppl):20–28.

50. Kossoff EH, Buck C, Freeman JM. Outcomes of 32 hemispherectomies for Sturge–Weber syndrome worldwide. *Neurology.* 2002;59(11):1735–1738.

51. Nordgren RE, Reeves AG, Viguera AC, et al. Corpus callosotomy for intractable seizures in the pediatric age group. *Arch Neurol.* 1991;48(4): 364–372.

52. Solomon LM, Esterly NB. Epidermal and other congenital organoid nevi. *Curr Probl Pediatr.* 1975;6(1):1–56.

53. Gurecki PJ, Holden KR, Sahn EE, et al. Developmental neural abnormalities and seizures in epidermal nevus syndrome. *Dev Med Child Neurol.* 1996;38(8):716–723.

54. Traboulsi EI, Zin A, Massicotte SJ, et al. Posterior scleral choristoma in the organoid nevus syndrome (linear nevus sebaceus of jadassohn). *Ophthalmology.* 1999;106(11):2126–2130.

55. Pavone L, Curatolo P, Rizzo R, et al. Epidermal nevus syndrome: A neurologic variant with hemimegalencephaly, gyral malformation, mental retardation, seizures, and facial hemihypertrophy. *Neurology.* 1991;41 (2 Pt 1):266–271.

56. Baker RS, Ross PA, Baumann RJ. Neurologic complications of the epidermal nevus syndrome. *Arch Neurol.* 1987;44(2):227–232.

57. Herbst BA, Cohen ME. Linea nevus sebaceus. A neurocutaneous syndrome associated with infantile spasms. *Arch Neurol.* 1971;24(4):317–322.

58. Chalhub EG, Volpe JJ, Gado MH. Linear nevus sebaceous syndrome associated with porencephaly and nonfunctioning major cerebral venous sinuses. *Neurology.* 1975;25(9):857–860.

59. Loddenkemper T, Alexopoulos AV, Kotagal P, et al. Epilepsy surgery in epidermal nevus syndrome variant with hemimegalencephaly and intractable seizures. *J Neurol.* 2008;255(11):1829–1831.

60. Korf BR, Carrazana E, Holmes GL. Patterns of seizures observed in association with neurofibromatosis 1. *Epilepsia.* 1993;34(4):616–620.

61. Balestri P, Vivarelli R, Grosso S, et al. Malformations of cortical development in neurofibromatosis type 1. *Neurology.* 2003;61(12): 1799–1801.

62. Vivarelli R, Grosso S, Calabrese F, et al. Epilepsy in neurofibromatosis 1. *J Child Neurol.* 2003;18(5):338–342.

63. Korf BR. Neuroimaging in children with neurofibromatosis type 1. *J Pediatr.* 1993;122(5 pt 1):834–835.

64. Cohen BA. Incontinentia pigmenti. *Neurol Clin.* 1987;5(3):361–377.

65. Gordon N. Hypomelanosis of ito (incontinentia pigmenti achromians). *Dev Med Child Neurol.* 1994;36(3):271–274.

66. Glover MT, Brett EM, Atherton DJ. Hypomelanosis of ito: Spectrum of the disease. *J Pediatr.* 1989;115(1):75–80.

67. Bittencourt FV, Marghoob AA, Kopf AW, et al. Large congenital melanocytic nevi and the risk for development of malignant melanoma and neurocutaneous melanocytosis. *Pediatrics.* 2000;106(4):736–741.

68. Kadonaga JN, Frieden IJ. Neurocutaneous melanosis: Definition and review of the literature. *J Am Acad Dermatol.* 1991;24(5 pt 1):747–755.

69. Chu WC, Lee V, Chan YL, et al. Neurocutaneous melanomatosis with a rapidly deteriorating course. *AJNR Am J Neuroradiol.* 2003;24(2): 287–290.

70. Byrd SE, Darling CF, Tomita T, et al. MR imaging of symptomatic neurocutaneous melanosis in children. *Pediatr Radiol.* 1997;27(1):39–44.

CHAPTER 32 ■ EPILEPSY IN THE SETTING OF INHERITED METABOLIC AND MITOCHONDRIAL DISORDERS

SUMIT PARIKH, DOUGLAS R. NORDLI JR., AND DARRYL C. DE VIVO

There are more than 11,000 well-recognized and well-characterized inherited disorders in humans, with many of them associated with seizures and epilepsy. The daunting task for the clinician is to recognize these important diagnoses in the patient with epilepsy so that optimal medical treatment, family counseling, and prognosis can be provided. Often, the presentation is not distinct enough to allow precise identification of the disorder on the basis of clinical criteria alone. Instead, the physician must observe a patient over a period of time and begin screening tests to detect abnormalities suggestive of the underlying disorder. These abnormalities point the way toward further diagnostic evaluations, which may culminate in the definitive diagnosis of the inherited disorder and actual detection of the defective gene. In other circumstances, important clues are present when a child is first seen, but these features can be easily overlooked if the clinical data are not synthesized and analyzed in an orderly way.

In general, the scalp electroencephalogram (EEG) has low specificity but high sensitivity for diagnosing, determining severity, and monitoring brain dysfunction over a period of time in children of all ages. Although various electroencephalographic patterns are reported in the literature as being typical of an inborn error of metabolism, rarity of metabolic disorders, ascertainment bias, and limited repertoire of possible EEG findings in the face of enormous variability in spectrum and severity of metabolic disorders reduce the usefulness of EEG in suggesting a specific diagnosis. EEG may, however, supplement clinical assessment and other test results in shortening the list of possible diagnoses.

How can clinicians mentally organize this wealth of material? One method is to group diseases according to categories on the basis of the subcellular organelle involved: mitochondrial, lysosomal, peroxisomal, and so on. Another method is to group diseases according to metabolic or catabolic pathways, such as organic aciduria, aminoaciduria, and fatty acid oxidation. However, the clinical presentation within these groups may be diverse and dissimilar. Another method of grouping is to organize diseases according to their clinical presentation. This can be performed by age, but many different disorders are responsible for seizures and epilepsy within any defined age group. Diseases may also be organized on the basis of specific characteristics of the seizures and the epilepsy syndromes. As each metabolic and mitochondrial disorder may present along a biologic spectrum, with more severe involvement presenting earlier and in a more devastating fashion, various epilepsy syndrome presentations can occur due to the same disorder. Early myoclonic epilepsy, West syndrome, and progressive myoclonus epilepsy are three well-recognized epilepsy syndromes in which there is a high likelihood of an inborn error of metabolism. In other instances, metabolic and mitochondrial diseases can masquerade as forms of cryptogenic epilepsy. Once the etiology is established, the epilepsy classification will change to symptomatic, generalized epilepsy caused by a specific disorder (e.g., secondary to phenylketonuria [PKU]).

In the organization of this chapter, we group the various disorders first by their age at onset (early infancy or later infancy and childhood onset) followed by the metabolic process or organelle affected. We also list, in tabular form (Table 32.1), the various cryptogenic or symptomatic epilepsy syndromes that might be mistaken for these disorders. In addition, we discuss clinical and EEG features of certain disorders that may provide clues to the underlying etiology. We also review the appropriate screening tests that may be performed, where applicable, followed by more definitive diagnostic procedures. Genetic information is listed for each condition when known.

For an up-to-date review of an individual metabolic disease, its genetics or to find a lab where an analyte or gene test can be sent, we recommend visiting the NIH GeneReviews site at http://www.genetests.org.

METABOLIC DISORDERS IN THE NEWBORN AND YOUNG INFANT

Disorders of Neurotransmitter Synthesis and Removal

Tetrahydrobiopterin and Guanine Triphosphate Cyclohydrolase Deficiency

Tetrahydrobiopterin (BH4) is a cofactor for the enzymes involved in converting tyrosine and tryptophan to levodopa and serotonin. Deficiencies in BH4 lead to disruptions in the neurotransmitter amines, levodopa, and serotonin. It is one of several disorders of neurotransmitter production. Defects most commonly occur due to abnormalities of guanine triphosphate cyclohydrolase (GTPCH), the first enzyme involved in the multistep process of converting GTP to BH4. However, defects in other enzymes in the pathway have also been identified.

GCH1 is the gene involved in GTPCH enzyme formation. Autosomal dominant mutations lead to early onset

TABLE 32.1

METABOLIC DISEASES MASQUERADING AS EPILEPSY SYNDROMES

Neonatal seizures
- Organic acidurias
- Urea cycle defects
- Peroxisomal disorders: Zellweger syndrome
- Molybdenum cofactor deficiency/sulfite oxidase deficiency
- Pyridoxine, pyridoxal phosphate, or folinic acid responsive epilepsy
- Mitochondrial disorders
- Disorders of biotin metabolism
- Glucose transporter defect (Glut-1 deficiency)
- Disorders of fructose metabolism

Early myoclonic encephalopathy/early infantile epileptic encephalopathy
- Glycine encephalopathy (nonketotic hyperglycinemia)
- Serine deficiency (3-phosphoglycerate dehydrogenase deficiency)
- Creatine synthesis or transport disorders
- Organic acidurias, especially propionic academia
- Mitochondrial disorders, especially those leading to Leigh syndrome
- D-glycine acidemia

Cryptogenic epilepsies with progressive neurologic decline
- GM1 and GM2 gangliosidoses
- Neuronal ceroid lipofuscinosis
- Infantile neuroaxonal dystrophy
- Glut-1 deficiency
- Late-onset multiple carboxylase deficiency
- Disorders of cerebral and peripheral folate metabolism
- Disorders of neurotransmitter synthesis
- Arginase deficiency (urea cycle defect)
- Amino and organic acidurias (variant phenotypes)
- Sialidoses

West syndrome, generalized
- Pyruvate dehydrogenase deficiency
- Pyruvate carboxylase deficiency
- Congenital disorder of glycosylation type III
- Organic and amino acidurias

Progressive myoclonus epilepsies
- Lafora disease (EPM2A/B gene mutations)
- Unverricht–Lundborg disease (EPM1 gene mutations)
- Mitochondrial diseases including MERRF/MELAS, and POLG1 gene mutations
- Dentatorubral–pallidoluysian atrophy
- Neuronal ceroid lipofuscinosis
- GM1 and GM2 gangliosidoses
- Sialidoses

MERRF, myoclonic epilepsy with ragged-red fibers; MELAS, mitochondrial encephalomyopathy with lactic acidosis and stroke-like episodes.

dopa-responsive dystonia (Segawa disease), and autosomal recessive mutations lead to a neonatal onset encephalopathy. Genetic testing for *GCH1* mutations and several other enzyme deficiencies in the BH4 synthesis pathway is now available (1).

Symptoms typically involve variable and fluctuating levels of psychomotor retardation, convulsions, microcephaly, swallowing difficulties, truncal hypotonia, limb hypertonia, involuntary movements, and oculogyric crises. Some of these symptoms begin shortly after infancy. A diurnal pattern of worsening of symptoms may be described. Of clinical note, other enzyme abnormalities both before and after BH4 production (including α-amino decarboxylase deficiency [AADC] involved in converting levodopa to active dopamine) can lead to identical symptoms (2).

Diagnosis of all of the neurotransmitter disorders is typically made by measuring levels of spinal fluid neurotransmitter metabolites (5-hydroxyindoleacetic acid [HIAA] and homovanillic acid [HVA]) and precursors (biopterin, neopterin, and 3-methyl-dopa). Elevations in plasma and cerebrospinal fluid (CSF) phenylalanine may be seen in the amino acid profile of some patients but this finding is frequently not present (2).

Treatment includes tetrahydrobiopterin supplementation, and pharmacotherapy with levodopa–carbidopa, or 5-hydroxytryptophan. In AADC deficiency a dopamine agonist and monoamine oxidase-inhibitor are used. Treatment is beneficial to varying degrees (3).

Glycine Encephalopathy (formerly Nonketotic Hyperglycinemia)

In this autosomal recessive inborn error of amino acid metabolism, large amounts of glycine accumulate in the body, especially the brain, because of a defect in the multienzyme complex for glycine cleavage. The enzyme system is confined to the mitochondria and is composed of four protein components (designated P, H, T, and L), three of which have a gene identified. GLDC, localized to 9p22, is the most common gene affected, with mutations leading to abnormal functioning of the P protein (4).

The pathophysiology of nonketotic hyperglycinemia (NKH) has not been fully elucidated, but the elevated glycine is believed to impact the central nervous system (CNS) via its role as an inhibitory transmitter in the brainstem and spinal cord, and an excitatory transmitter in the cortex. The majority of cases present within the first 48 hours of life with lethargy, respiratory difficulties, apnea, and seizures that are often myoclonic or characterized as infantile spasms. Cortical malformations or corpus callosum defects may be present. A burst-suppression EEG pattern with variable intervals between the bursts alternating with epochs of greater continuity is characteristic. The combination of early-onset seizures with prominent myoclonias and variable burst-suppression EEG is also called early myoclonic epilepsy (EME), as described by Aicardi. Glycine encephalopathy is an important cause of EME evolving to hypsarrhythmia, although this is more commonly observed in Ohtahara syndrome. Ohtahara syndrome is thought by some authorities to be more commonly associated with structural abnormalities and not as highly associated with errors of metabolism (2).

Later onset forms of this disease have also been described, with patients having varying degrees of epilepsy, retardation, and movement abnormalities. An adolescent/adult onset form presents with associated spastic paraparesis and optic atrophy (5).

Laboratory testing reveals elevations of glycine in the plasma, urine, and CSF amino acid profile. The absence of excess ketones in the blood and urine, and of abnormal organic acids in the urine, helps to differentiate NKH from other conditions associated with hyperglycinemia, such as propionic and methylmalonic acidemia. The ratio of CSF to serum glycine is also helpful, as it is significantly elevated in patients with NKH. Genetic sequencing for the three known loci is clinically available (6).

There is no effective long-term treatment for this disorder. High doses of benzoate may reduce CSF glycine and improve seizure control, but it does not appear to stop the development of mental retardation (7,8). Because benzoate treatment may deplete carnitine levels, carnitine supplementation is recommended when benzoate is used (9). Dextromethorphan, an N-methyl-D-aspartic acid (NMDA) antagonist has been tried for this condition as well. Valproic acid should be avoided because it induces hyperglycinemia. Strychnine, a glycine antagonist, and diazepam have been reported to blunt seizures, but have not influenced the long-term outcome (10). Prognosis is poor, with progressive microcephaly and intractable epilepsy. Even when treated, death often occurs within the first few months to years of life (11).

A transient form of NKH exists with similar early clinical and biochemical findings. In this condition, glycine concentrations normalize between 2 and 8 weeks of life, and prognosis is favorable (12).

Serine and 3-Phosphoglycerate Dehydrogenase Deficiency

3-Phosphoglycerate dehydrogenase (PHGDH) deficiency is an autosomal recessive condition that results in impaired L-serine biosynthesis due to a mutation in the *PHGDH* gene (1p12). Serine is the precursor of D-serine and glycine, both potent neurotransmitters. Serine also has a role in myelin production (13).

Typically there is a pre- or perinatal onset of symptoms including congenital microcephaly, intractable seizures, spastic quadraparesis, and profound cognitive delays. The magnetic resonance imaging (MRI) may show white matter lesions. The condition is often misdiagnosed as cerebral palsy. Reduced serine levels are found in CSF amino acid specimens though glycine levels are not always low. Plasma serine and glycine levels may only be low in fasting specimens but are not reliable indicators as they may also be normal (14).

Enzyme activity can be measured in skin fibroblasts. Genetic testing is clinically available. Treatment involves supportive care and L-serine supplementation (15).

Succinic Semialdehyde Dehydrogenase Deficiency

Succinic semialdehyde dehydrogenase (SSADH) deficiency is an autosomal recessive disorder impairing γ-aminobutyric acid (GABA) catabolism. The enzyme is involved in the second and final step of GABA degradation. GABA, an inhibitory neurotransmitter, accumulates (16). The *ALDH5A1* (6p22) gene encodes this enzyme and mutations here account for over 97% of cases (17).

The disorder is slowly progressive with an infancy to childhood onset. Seizures occur in more than 50% of patients.

Other symptoms include varying degrees of ataxia, hypotonia, speech delay, and mental retardation. A movement disorder with hyperkinetic movements, choreoathetosis, dystonia, and myoclonus can be seen with earlier onset, more severe disease. Aggressive behaviors and self-injury may also occur (18).

Diagnosis is initially made by finding elevations of 4-hydroxybutyric (4HB) acid in urine organic acids, plasma, or CSF. Of clinical note, the 4HB peak can be easily missed on routine organic acid analysis due to its coeluting with a large urea peak. Thus, one must ensure that the lab processing the specimen is monitoring for this ion. Variable elevations of glycine can be seen in the amino acid profile. Confirmatory gene sequencing is clinically available. The EEG may show generalized background slowing and spike discharges (19).

Treatment of this disorder is symptom based. Vigabatrin, an irreversible inhibitor of GABA transaminase, has been used in some individuals with positive responses (including increased socialization, behavioral improvement, increased alertness, and reduced ataxia), treatment with this agent has worsened symptoms in others. Valproate use is contraindicated as it may inhibit residual SSADH enzyme activity (20–22).

Vitamin and Mineral Metabolism-Related Diseases

Pyridoxine (and Folinic Acid) Responsive Epilepsy

In pyridoxine responsive epilepsy, refractory seizures typically develop within the first several days of life. These may be characterized by infantile spasms or have a variety of partial, myoclonic, and atonic features. Atypical presentations include a later onset of seizures, seizures that initially respond to treatment and then become intractable, and seizures with only a partial initial response to pyridoxine.

The disorder occurs due to a mutation in the *ALDH7A1* gene (5q31). The *ALDH7A1* gene encodes for a protein antiquitin, which is involved in pyridoxine metabolism. When antiquitin is not functional, pyridoxine metabolism is impaired (23). Pyridoxine plays several critical roles, including the conversion of levodopa to dopamine and glutamate inactivation via glutamic acid decarboxylase.

Diagnosis has typically been made clinically, with seizures abating after a high dose of IV pyridoxine (100 to 500 mg). The initial EEG is characterized by generalized bursts of high-voltage delta activity interspersed with spike and sharp waves and periods of asynchronous attenuation. After treatment there is conversion of the EEG to a burst-suppression pattern, and later normalization with subsequent doses. This change occurs within minutes and may persist for hours, or even a day (24). Confirmatory testing is via spinal fluid analysis, as described below. Testing for *ALDH7A1* mutations is clinically available.

A recent clinical and genetic link has been made between folinic acid responsive epilepsy, pyridoxine responsive epilepsy, and *ALDH7A1* mutations, thus leading one to conclude that folinic acid and pyridoxine responsive seizures are one and the same. Previously it was believed that folinic acid responsive epilepsy was a rare yet separate metabolic epileptic encephalopathy with a diagnosis made by identifying a characteristic peak of a yet unknown compound in spinal fluid neurotransmitter analysis (25).

More recently a patient with folinic acid responsive epilepsy was found to respond to pyridoxine supplementation (26). Eventually, individuals with folinic acid responsive epilepsy were identified as having *ALDH7A1* mutations and patients identified as having pyridoxine-dependent epilepsy (mutation confirmed cases) were found to have the characteristic folinic acid responsive peak identified in their CSF (27).

In evaluating these patients, plasma, urine, and spinal fluid levels of pipecolic acid may also be elevated though this chemical is not a reliable biomarker (28). A link also exists to elevated urinary concentration of α-aminoadipic semialdehyde (α-AASA), though this compound is not routinely measured (23). The characteristic peak of this yet unidentified compound is found when spinal fluid neurotransmitter testing is run. Spinal fluid folate levels are normal in this condition. As the link between folinic acid and pyridoxine responsive epilepsy is secure, routine CSF analysis for diagnosis is crucial. Early treatment is also critical, as it improves developmental outcome. Maintenance therapy with pyridoxine and folinic acid is necessary. Onset of disease may extend beyond the newborn period, making this disorder a consideration in older infants with refractory seizures as well (29,30). Due to pyridoxine and folic acid's relatively decreased ability to cross the blood–brain barrier, treatment with pyridoxal 5-phosphate and folinic acid is recommended.

Pyridoxal-L-Phosphate Responsive Epilepsy

Some neonates and children with an epileptic encephalopathy seemed to respond to pyridoxal-L-phosphate (PLP) supplementation as opposed to pyridoxine. Further research showed that some of these individuals have defect in an enzyme pyridoxal/PLP—pyridox(am)ine 5′-phosphate oxidase (PNPO) required for the synthesis of intracellular PLP from dietary pyridoxine. Eventually, the *PNPO* gene (17q21.2) was identified and these mutations were confirmed as the cause of this relatively rare condition. The clinical presentation in these children is similar to those with pyridoxine-dependent epilepsy and disorders of neurotransmitter metabolism as described above. Treatment, however, requires PLP as opposed to pyridoxine (31).

Molybdenum Cofactor Deficiency and Sulfite Oxidase Deficiency

The rare conditions of molybdenum cofactor deficiency (MOCOD) and sulfite oxidase deficiency present shortly after birth, also with a progressive encephalopathy, feeding difficulties, hypotonia, and refractory partial, myoclonic, or apparently generalized seizures. Dysmorphic features, lens dislocation, and hepatomegaly are all characteristic findings (32). The two conditions have an essentially identical clinical phenotype, likely due to both conditions leading to the loss of sulfite oxidase function. As typical of all of these diseases, later onset and relatively milder and varying phenotypes have been described in the literature.

Molybdenum cofactor is critically needed for the proper function of three enzymes: sulfite oxidase, xanthine dehydrogenase, and aldehyde oxidase. Sulfite oxidase converts sulfite to sulfate. Xanthine dehydrogenase converts xanthine to hypoxanthine to eventually form uric acid. Aldehyde dehydrogenase is involved in the reverse reaction of hypoxanthine to xanthine (33).

MOCOD is due to mutations in one of two genes, *MOCS1*, at 6p21.3 or *MOCS2*, at 5q11 (34). Sulfite oxidase deficiency is typically due to mutations in the *SUOX* gene on chromosome 12 (35).

The EEG in these patients may show multifocal paroxysms and a burst-suppression pattern. Neuroimaging may show poor differentiation between the gray and white matter, severe cerebral and cerebellar atrophy, and multiple cystic cavities in the white matter. Diagnosis is made by a variety of methods. Since MOCOD and isolated sulfite oxidase deficiency both result in high levels of urinary sulfites, a sulfite dipstick on a fresh urine sample may detect abnormalities, though this test has a high false-negative rate (36,37). Plasma uric acid levels may be low in MOCOD, but not sulfite oxidase deficiency. Both disorders will lead to an accumulation of urine *S*-sulfocysteine. The two disorders can be distinguished on laboratory testing as elevations of urine purines and pyrimidines (xanthine and hypoxanthine) occur in MOCOD but not in sulfite oxidase deficiency. The enzyme deficiencies can be demonstrated in cultured fibroblasts and liver tissue. Genetic testing is clinically available. No effective treatment has been identified and prognosis is poor, with death occurring within the first days to weeks of life (38).

Cerebral Folate Deficiency

Folate is concentrated in the nervous system, and the CSF concentrations of folate are higher than the serum concentrations. Deficiencies in cerebral folate lead to a slowly progressive encephalopathy, with intractable seizures. If it occurs in conjunction with systemic folate deficiency, megaloblastic anemia, mouth ulceration, diarrhea, and failure to thrive may also be seen. Neuroimaging may reveal calcifications in the occipital lobes and basal ganglia (39).

Reductions in cerebral folate can occur due to systemic disease, gut malabsorption syndromes such as colitis, primary mitochondrial disorders (40), other metabolic diseases (see Section "Methylenetetrahydrofolate Reductase Deficiency"), and certain genetic syndromes (Rett syndrome) (41).

A primary disorder of cerebral folate has also been identified that occurs due to lactose-mediated autoantibodies forming to the cerebral folate receptor (42). This condition is different from folinic acid responsive epilepsy described above.

The disorder is typically diagnosed by finding low levels of methyltetrahydrofolate (MTHF) in CSF. Normal amino and organic acids analysis and normal plasma folate levels help exclude other potentially treatable causes. If another syndromic, metabolic, or systemic cause of low cerebral folate is not identified, specialized testing for folate autoantibodies is clinically available (42).

Treatment involves supplementation with IV and oral folate. Folinic acid may be used since it has better blood–brain barrier penetration than folic acid. If lactose-mediated autoantibodies are identified, a lactose-free diet is also recommended (43). Outcome is still poor.

Methylenetetrahydrofolate Reductase Deficiency

Methylenetetrahydrofolate reductase deficiency (1p36.3) is the most common inborn error of folate metabolism (44). The metabolic defect results from insufficient production of 5-MTHF, which is needed for the remethylation of homocysteine to methionine, because of a deficiency in methylenetetrahydrofolate reductase. In affected individuals, a progressive neurologic syndrome develops in infancy. Children with this disorder have acquired microcephaly and seizures characterized by intractable infantile spasms, generalized atonic and myoclonic seizures, and focal motor seizures. EEG findings vary from diffuse slowing of background activity to continuous spike–wave complexes or multifocal spikes. The early-onset form differs from the late-onset form. The latter presents with progressive motor deterioration, schizophrenia-like psychiatric symptoms, and recurrent strokes; seizures are uncommon. Homocystinuria and elevated serum concentrations of homocysteine with reduced or normal serum methionine are the main biochemical features. Homocystinuria can be caused by several other amino acid disorders as well. Dietary supplementation with folic acid, betaine, and methionine has proven beneficial. In the acute setting, high-dose methionine has been effective in stopping seizures (45).

Defects in methionine biosynthesis are also associated with seizures. Convulsions are frequent and are predominantly generalized, although myoclonic seizures with hypsarrhythmia have been reported. Diagnostic laboratory findings are megaloblastic anemia, homocystinuria, decreased methionine, and normal folate and cobalamin concentrations in the absence of methylmalonic aciduria (45).

Inborn Errors of Creatine Metabolism

Creatine represents a storage depot of adenosine triphosphate (ATP) for various tissues including the brain. Depletion of cerebral creatine due to inborn errors in synthesis or transport leads to a progressive encephalopathy and epilepsy. Creatine forms via a two-step enzymatic path, with arginine converted to guanidinoacetate via arginine:glycine amidinotransferase (AGAT) and then to creatine via guanidinoacetate N-methyltransferase (GAMT). Deficiencies in both enzymes have been identified and the genetic loci for AGAT and GAMT are known. Creatine, once formed, is transported into the cell via a specific transporter and abnormalities in creatine transport can also occur due to defects in the SLC6A8 gene at Xq28 (46).

Development can be delayed from the beginning or after a regression beginning between 3 months and 2 years of age. Seizures may present in the first months of life with generalized tonic–clonic, astatic, absence, myoclonic, or partial events. Multifocal epileptiform discharges have been reported on the EEGs of affected individuals (47). Other clinical features may include dystonia, dyskinesias, microcephaly, and autistic behaviors (48).

A mild form presenting with severe speech delay, mild autism, and infrequent seizures has also been identified (49).

Diagnosis is typically via quantifying urine, plasma, and/or spinal fluid guanidinoacetate and creatine. Low creatinine is not a reliable marker of the condition. Brain magnetic resonance spectroscopy (MRS) shows a reduced creatine peak (50).

Supplementation with creatine monohydrate (350 mg/kg per day to 2 g/kg per day) has led to improvement in affected individuals though not in patients with creatine transporter disorders (46).

Early-Onset Multiple Carboxylase Deficiency (Holocarboxylase Synthetase Deficiency)

Early-onset multiple carboxylase deficiency presents in the first week of life with lethargy, respiratory abnormalities, irritability, poor feeding, and emesis. A skin rash is present in more than 50% of patients. Generalized tonic convulsions, partial motor seizures, and multifocal myoclonic jerks develop

in 25% to 50% of cases. This disease is tested for in the neonate in certain states via expanded newborn screening and can often be treated prior to symptom onset. A deficiency in the enzyme holocarboxylase synthetase (HLCS) leads to a decrease in holocarboxylase. As this enzyme links biotin to four carboxylases in the mitochondria and one in the cytosol, an inactivity of all carboxylases results. The HLCS gene locus is 21q22.1. Although rare, this condition is very important to recognize because prompt treatment with biotin may result in dramatic improvement. Laboratory findings demonstrate ketoacidosis and a characteristic pattern on organic acid analysis. Hyperammonemia may be seen with acute episodes. Electrographically, a burst-suppression pattern or multifocal spikes are observed. Definitive diagnosis can be made by enzyme assays, and gene sequencing. Treatment with biotin (10 mg/day) produces clinical improvement (51).

Late-Onset Multiple Carboxylase Deficiency (Biotinidase Deficiency)

This disease is also screened for in certain states via expanded newborn screening. The disorder involves the body's ability to recycle biotin via biotinidase. The BTD gene has been identified at the 3p25 locus (52).

When not diagnosed early, seizures are a prominent feature occurring in 50% to 75% of affected children. In fact, seizures are the presenting feature in 38% of patients and may be generalized tonic–clonic, partial, myoclonic, or infantile spasms. Symptoms often begin at 3 to 6 months of age, with hypotonia and developmental delay. Seborrheic or atopic dermatitis and alopecia are common. As the disease progresses, ataxia, optic atrophy, and sensorineural hearing loss develop. Later onset and/or milder phenotypes exist due to partial enzyme deficiency. EEG findings may include a suppression-burst pattern, absence of physiologic sleep patterns, poorly organized and slow waking background activity, and frequent spike and spike-slow-wave discharges (53).

Diagnosis is typically made via abnormalities in urine organic acid and plasma acylcarnitine analysis. Biotinidase enzyme activity can be measured in leukocytes and cultured fibroblasts. Genetic sequencing is clinically available. As this is a treatable condition, screening followed by a therapeutic trial with high-dose oral biotin should be considered in infants with developmental delay and persistent seizures of unknown etiology (2).

Menkes Disease (Kinky Hair Disease)

An X-linked disorder of copper absorption, Menkes disease was first described by Menkes and colleagues in 1962. Defects in the copper transporting ATPase gene (ATP7A, Xq12–q13) impairs intestinal copper absorption, reduces copper export from tissues, and decreases the activity of copper-dependent enzymes, including dopamine β-hydroxylase (54).

A characteristic twisting of the hair shaft, resulting in "kinky hair" of the head and eyebrows, is noted on microscopic examination of the poorly pigmented hairs. Affected boys may be premature and may have neonatal hyperbilirubinemia or hypothermia. Progressive neurologic deterioration with spasticity is present by 3 months of age, and children may have associated bone and urinary tract abnormalities as well. The disease has a rapidly fatal course.

Seizures are a prominent feature in Menkes disease, with intractable generalized or focal convulsions. Infantile spasms have also been reported (55). Stimulation-induced myoclonic jerks may be present. Multifocal spike and slow-wave activity can be seen on the EEG, sometimes resembling hypsarrhythmia (56).

Laboratory testing reveals extremely low serum copper and ceruloplasmin levels. Elevations in CSF lactate may be seen, and there is low total copper content in the brain. Neuroimaging may show brain atrophy, focal areas of necrosis, and subdural collections. Brain magnetic resonance angiography (MRA) shows dilated and tortuous intracranial blood vessels. Genetic testing of the *ATP7A* gene via sequencing and deletion analysis identifies almost all patients with Menkes (54).

There is no fully effective treatment. Daily copper injections may be beneficial if administered early in the course of the disease.

Phenotypic overlap exists between Menkes disease and occipital horn syndrome (57). It is now known that both Menkes and occipital horn syndrome conditions are allelic due to mutations in the same gene (57).

Disorders of Carbohydrate Metabolism

Glut-1 Transporter Deficiency Syndrome

The Glut-1 transporter deficiency syndrome was first described in 1991 (58). The autosomal dominant condition results from a loss of functional glucose transporters, encoded by the SLC2A gene, that mediate glucose transport across the blood–brain barrier (59). Clinical features include developmental delay, ataxia, hypotonia, infantile seizures, and acquired microcephaly. There is a reduction in the CSF-to-blood glucose ratio to half of normal (typically, CSF glucose is less than 40 mg/dL). In addition, a low lactate concentration might be seen. Additional confirmation of impaired glucose transport can be performed through assays in erythrocytes (60) and clinical genetic testing is available.

Seizures, specifically neonatal ones, are often the first identified feature of this syndrome though patients with later onset and mild epilepsy have been described. Typical seizure types include absence, myoclonic, astatic, generalized tonic–clonic, and partial–complex. About 10% of patients have no clinical seizures. A normal EEG is commonly seen between seizures, although generalized 2.5- to 4-Hz spike–wave discharges are observed in more than one third of children older than 2 years of age (61).

Affected individuals without the classic clinical features have been identified and a screening for lumbar puncture should be considered in those with refractory epilepsy (62). Seizures tend to be refractory to anti-epilepsy drugs (AEDs). Early initiation of the ketogenic diet is effective in the treatment of seizures as well as overall disease progression, as it provides an alternative cerebral energy source (63).

Recently, paroxysmal exertional dyskinesia (PED) has been recognized as an allelic variant of Glut-1 deficiency (64,65). Some patients with PED also have epilepsy. The condition appears to be phenotypically milder clinically with less striking hypoglycorrhachia (66).

Other Disorders

Fructose 1,6-bisphosphatase deficiency, a rare, potentially life-threatening disorder of gluconeogenesis, presents within the first few days of life with respiratory abnormalities, hypotonia, lethargy, hepatomegaly, irritability, and convulsions. Laboratory findings reveal lactic acidosis, ketosis, hypoglycemia, elevated plasma concentrations of alanine, and the presence of abnormal urinary organic acids with glycerol and glycerol-3-phosphate (67). The *FBP1* gene is located at 9q22.2–q22.3 (68). Neurologic sequelae can be prevented by avoidance of hypoglycemia.

Hereditary fructose intolerance (fructose 1,6-biphosphate aldolase deficiency) may be seen in the neonatal period in infants who are formula fed and given fructose or sucrose early in life. Symptoms include profound hypoglycemia, emesis, and convulsions. If the disease is readily diagnosed, fructose and sucrose can be eliminated from the diet before significant cerebral injury occurs (67).

Mitochondrial Disorders

Disorders of energy metabolism typically present with later onset epilepsy outside of the immediate newborn period. However there are exceptions to the rule, especially when discussing the dizzying and ever-growing array of mitochondrial phenotypes.

Mitochondria are the cell's energy factories, though they also have a key role in initiating apoptosis, and reactive oxygen species formation and removal. When not functioning properly, organs most dependent on cellular energy show symptoms—especially the brain. While multiorgan involvement and lactic acidosis were initially described as sine qua nons of the disease, these findings are not reliably present and the vast majority of patients do not present with the classically described syndromes. These phenotypes, such as MELAS, MERRF and at least 10 others, created order to a set of novel and often unrelated symptoms prior to our current knowledge of the disease. We now know that almost any unexplained neurologic symptom can be due to mitochondrial dysfunction, especially refractory epilepsy. The epilepsy may occur in isolation, or with other neurologic problems including optic nerve disease, retinal pigmentary changes, hearing loss, developmental delays, neuropathy, and myopathy. Myoclonic epilepsy has been associated with mitochondrial disease, but patients with almost any seizure type, including generalized epilepsy are seen (69).

These conditions typically occur due to genetic abnormalities leading to aberrant mitochondrial function. Over 2000 nuclear DNA (nDNA) genes are involved in mitochondrial formation and function, along with maternally inherited mitochondrial DNA (mtDNA) providing an additional 37 genes. Thus, most cases of mitochondrial disease are autosomal recessive in inheritance and less than 20% have a maternal mtDNA-based inheritance pattern. However, less than 5% of nDNA genes leading to mitochondrial disease have been identified. Diagnostic testing initially involves looking for a combination of biochemical abnormalities in plasma amino acids, acylcarnitines, lactate, pyruvate, and urine organic acids. Additional layers of diagnostic evidence are added by functional analysis of mitochondrial enzyme activity and other ultrastructural and proteomic studies in tissue (most reliably muscle, though skin fibroblasts, liver or heart tissue can be studied). These studies allow for focused genetic testing in select cases (70).

Treatment varies and includes preventing worsening during metabolic or physiologic stresses, avoiding mitochondrial toxins and poisons, use of select cofactors and supplements, and providing symptomatic care.

Pyruvate Dehydrogenase Deficiency

The mitochondrial pyruvate dehydrogenase (PHD) complex is composed of three enzymes: pyruvate decarboxylase (E1), dihydrolipoyl transacetylase (E2), and dihydrolipoyl dehydrogenase (E3). The E1 enzyme is itself a complex structure, a heterotetramer of two α and two β-subunits. The E1 α-subunit is particularly important, as it contains the E1 active site. Mutations in the *PDHA1* gene (Xp22.2–p22.1) encoding for this region are the most common cause of PDH deficiency (71).

Pyruvate dehydrogenase deficiency has a wide variety of clinical presentations, ranging from acute lactic acidosis in infancy with severe neurologic impairment in affected males, to a slowly progressive neurodegenerative disorder in some males and more commonly females. Structural abnormalities, such as agenesis of the corpus callosum, are often present on neuroimaging (72). Epilepsy frequently occurs and includes infantile spasms and myoclonic seizures. EEG findings include multifocal slow spike-wave discharges (73).

Pyruvate Carboxylase Deficiency

Pyruvate carboxylase is a biotin-responsive enzyme that converts pyruvate to oxaloacetate in the citric acid cycle. Two predominant clinical presentations occur with pyruvate carboxylase deficiency. The neonatal type (type B) manifests with severe lactic acidemia and death in the first few months of life. The infantile and juvenile type (type A) begins in the first 6 months of life with episodes of lactic acidemia precipitated by an infection. Developmental delay, failure to thrive, hypotonia, and seizures, including infantile spasms with hypsarrhythmia, may be seen (74). A benign form (type C) also has been described with recurrent metabolic acidosis and normal neurologic development (75). Mosaicism of the phenotypes mitigates a prolonged survival (76).

Seizures are related to the energy dysfunction that occurs secondary to Krebs cycle dysfunction. Treatment with the ketogenic diet or corticotropins may markedly exacerbate the disorder and should be avoided (77,78).

Leigh Syndrome

Leigh syndrome (subacute necrotizing encephalomyelopathy) is both a clinical and radiologic phenotype and may be related to various metabolic defects, including syndromic and nonsyndromic mitochondrial disease, and pyruvate dehydrogenase deficiency. Biochemical defects in nuclear and mitochondrially encoded complexes 1 to 5 have been identified with this condition. It is genetically heterogeneous, and depending on the etiology, may be autosomal recessive or dominant, X-linked or maternally inherited (79).

The clinical presentation is often acute to subacute, involving regression, progressive hypotonia, lactic acidosis, and failure to thrive. The disease progresses with spasticity, abnormal eye movements, and central respiratory failure. The neuroimaging shows bilateral, fairly symmetric, basal ganglia, thalamic, midbrain lesions that can fluctuate in severity. Varying degrees of white matter lesions may also be present along with cortical and cerebellar atrophy (80).

A variety of different seizures, including focal and generalized seizures, have been described (81). Infantile spasms and hypsarrhythmia may occur (82,83). In addition, there have been cases of epilepsia partialis continua (84). EEG features do not appear to be distinctive enough to contribute to the clinical diagnosis of Leigh syndrome (85).

Disorders of Amino and Organic Acids Metabolism

Amino and organic acids predominantly form from the catabolism of proteins and carbohydrates. Any enzymatic defect in these metabolic pathways leads to an accumulation of potentially acidic compounds, and partial inhibition of the citric acid and urea cycles. Acidosis and hyperammonemia ensues leading to encephalopathy and at times, seizures. These disorders, when most severe (a severe enzyme deficiency), typically present in the newborn period, especially after an infant is exposed to a protein or carbohydrate challenge in the diet. For some, this means after feeding in the 1st day, while for others it is after the introduction of solid foods. Regardless of the type of amino or organic acid disorder, the acute presentation is often the same. Milder enzyme deficiencies may present with a later sudden-onset epileptic encephalopathy (later infancy, childhood, or in the adult years) in the midst of a physiologic stressor (illness, surgery, fasting) that leads to accelerated catabolism. Thus, many of these metabolic disorders should be considered in a patient with an acute to subacute epileptic encephalopathy of later onset as well when an etiology for the problem remains unknown. With the advent and increased utilization of expanded newborn screening (NBS) in states across this country, and internationally, many "classic" inborn errors of metabolism are now diagnosed and treated before they lead to neurologic symptoms. Conditions such as PKU, propionic, or methylmalonic acidemia, and other relatively well-known amino or organic acid and fat metabolism disorders have become chronic conditions with improved neurologic outcomes due to early diagnosis and preventative care. However, there is no "standardized" national NBS protocol and the diseases screened for still vary from state to state and country to country. Thus, while many inborn errors of metabolism may now be excluded by the extended newborn screen, familiarity with the diseases screened for in one's area is useful. As genetic knowledge of these conditions has evolved, we have moved from making an analyte-based diagnosis from blood and urine testing to confirmatory molecular genetic diagnostic studies. The treatment for all of these diseases is often very similar in the acute encephalopathy period—correct any metabolic derangements (acidosis/hyperammonemia), stop the introduction of the toxic substance by making the patient NPO, stop catabolism with dextrose-containing fluids, and prescribe any metabolic scavengers if available.

Below we discuss a few of the disorders where seizures are a prominent feature.

Phenylketonuria

One of the most frequent autosomal inborn errors of metabolism, occurring in 1 in 10,000 to 15,000 live births, PKU is caused by a deficiency in hepatic phenylalanine hydroxylase (86). As a consequence of the metabolic defect, toxic levels of the essential amino acid phenylalanine accumulate.

Currently, diagnosis is typically made with NBS, and in fact, this was the condition that led to the advent of NBS by Dr. Robert Guthrie in the 1960s. NBS is able to diagnose a 100% of these patients. If the patient has not received NBS, routine amino acid analysis in plasma will identify elevated phenylalanine (87).

PKU occurs due to mutations in the *PAH* gene (12q23.2). Mutations in this gene account for more than 99% of the cases (88).

If untreated, severe mental retardation, behavioral disturbances, psychosis, and acquired microcephaly can result. Seizures are present in 25% of affected children. The majority of children with PKU (80% to 95%) are also found to have abnormalities on the EEG. An age-related distribution of EEG findings and seizure types has been observed since a 1957 report by Low and associates (89). Infantile spasms and hypsarrhythmia predominate in the young infant. As the children mature, tonic–clonic and myoclonic seizures become more frequent, and the EEG evolves to mild diffuse background slowing, focal sharp waves, and irregular generalized spike and slow waves (90,91). Donker and colleagues showed proportionate increases in delta activity as levels rose during phenylalanine loading (92).

Primary treatment is a phenylalanine-free diet. With early detection and institution of this diet, the neurologic sequelae of hyperphenylalaninemia can be prevented or significantly minimized (93).

Maple Syrup Urine Disease

Maple syrup urine disease (MSUD) is an autosomal recessive condition due to a defect in the branched-chain α-keto acid dehydrogenase complex (BCKAD), and was first reported by Menkes and colleagues in 1954 (94).

The enzyme defect leads to accumulation of the branched-chain amino acids—valine, leucine, isoleucine—and their keto acids in body tissues and fluids. This disease is now tested for in most extended NBS panels and diagnosed prior to the onset of symptoms.

The BCKAD enzyme complex has four components, and three genes (*BCKDHA*/19q13.1–q13.2, *BCKDHB*/6p22–p21, and *DBT*/1p31) have been identified with mutations in them leading to over 95% of cases (95).

Feeding difficulties, irritability, and lethargy are observed during the first few weeks of life. If left untreated, these signs may progress to stupor, apnea, opisthotonos, myoclonic jerks, and partial and generalized seizures. A characteristic odor can be detected in the urine and cerumen, but this may not be detectable until several weeks after birth. Milder variants of MSUD present with poor growth, irritability, or developmental delays later in infancy or childhood (2).

Laboratory testing reveals a metabolic acidosis and elevated blood and urine ketones. Hypoglycemia and hyperammonemia are rarely present in this disease. Ferric chloride testing of the urine causes a gray–green reaction, and the 2,4-dinitrophenylhydrazine test is positive. A marked elevation in branched-chain amino acids/branched-chain keto acids in the plasma, urine, and CSF amino acid profile is observed, and the presence of L-alloisoleucine is pathognomonic for this condition. Definitive testing can be performed by enzyme assay and molecular genetic studies (96).

The EEG shows diffuse slowing and a loss of reactivity to auditory stimuli. The "comblike rhythm" characteristic of maple syrup urine disease was initially reported by Trottier and associates in 1975, when bursts of a central mu-like rhythm were observed in four affected patients (97). Tharp described resolution of this pattern in an affected infant when dietary therapy was initiated (98). Korein and coworkers observed a paroxysmal spike and spike–wave response to photic stimulation in 7 of 15 affected patients (97).

Pathologic studies reveal diffuse myelin loss and increased total brain lipid content. Cystic degeneration of the white matter associated with gliosis is observed. Disordered neuronal migration may occur with heterotopias and disrupted cortical lamination.

Acute treatment is aimed at counteracting the effects of hypoglycemia, acidosis, and ending catabolism. Dialysis or exchange transfusion rarely is necessary. Dietary therapy with protein restriction, thiamine supplementation, and elimination of branched-chain amino acids from the diet is the mainstay of treatment (96).

Histidinemia

Histidinemia or histidase deficiency is also associated with infantile spasms and myoclonic seizures. Other features include developmental delay and an exaggerated startle response. A diet low in histidine may be partially beneficial.

Isovaleric Acidemia

This condition is screened for by extended NBS. Symptoms develop during the neonatal period in half of the children with isovaleric aciduria (gene locus 15q14–q15). The presentation typically involves poor feeding, vomiting, dehydration, and a progressive encephalopathy manifested by lethargy, tremors, seizures, and coma. Depressed platelets and leukocytes may be seen, and the urine odor has been described as similar to that of "sweaty feet." Cerebral edema is present, and seizures are most often partial motor or generalized tonic. The EEG shows dysmature features during sleep. Distinctive biochemical findings include metabolic acidosis, ketosis, lactic acidosis, and hyperammonemia. High urine concentrations of isovaleryl-glycine in urine organic acids and isovalerylcarnitine in acylcarnitine analysis is diagnostic. Genetic testing is clinically available (99).

Propionic Acidemia

This condition is screened for by extended NBS. The symptoms of propionic acidemia also appear during the neonatal period, with 20% of affected newborns having seizures as the first symptom. Characteristic features include vomiting, lethargy, ketosis, neutropenia, periodic thrombocytopenia, hypogammaglobulinemia, developmental retardation, and intolerance to protein. Patients may have very puffy cheeks and an exaggerated cupid bow upper lip. Mutations have been identified in both the α-subunit (13q32) and β-subunit (3q21–q22) of propionyl coenzyme A (CoA) carboxylase (100). Generalized seizures are typical, although partial seizures have also been reported. The EEG shows background disorganization, with marked frontotemporal and occipital slow-wave activity. In 40% of children, myoclonic seizures develop in later infancy, and older children may have atypical absence seizures. Biochemical findings include metabolic acidosis, ketosis, and elevation of branched-chain amino acids and propionic acid (101).

Methylmalonic Acidemia

This condition is screened for by extended NBS. Methylmalonic acidemia may be caused by deficiencies of the enzyme methylmalonyl-CoA mutase or adenosylcobalamin synthetic enzymes. Methylmalonic acidemia occurs in association with homocystinuria in the combined deficiency of methylmalonic-CoA mutase and methyltetrahydrofolate: homocysteine methyltransferase (102,103). Forms responsive to vitamin B$_{12}$ have been reported (104). Stomatitis, glossitis, developmental delay, failure to thrive, and seizures are the major features. Lesions of the globus pallidus on computed tomography or MRI are characteristic.

Diffuse tonic seizures and partial seizures with secondary generalization are the most frequent seizure types. Seizures may be characterized by eyelid clonus with simultaneous upward deviation of the eyes. In a review of 22 patients, Stigsby and collaborators described abnormalities on the EEG in seven patients, consisting of multifocal spike discharges and depressed background activity in two, excessive generalized slowing in two, and mild background slowing with lack of sleep spindles in three (101). Two children were reported to have myoclonus and a hypsarrhythmic EEG pattern (105).

3-Methylglutaconic Aciduria

This condition is screened for by extended NBS. Severe developmental delay, progressive encephalopathy, and seizures are features of 3-methylglutaconic aciduria with normal 3-methylglutaconyl-CoA hydratase. This disorder results from a mutation on chromosome 9 in the gene encoding the enzyme 3-methylglutaconyl-CoA hydratase. Seizures occur in one third of cases, and infantile spasms have been reported early in the course of the disorder. The typical organic acid abnormality includes marked elevations in 3-methylglutaconic acid and 3-methylglutaric acid in the urine (106).

3-Hydroxy-3-Methylglutaric Aciduria

This condition is screened for by extended NBS. Seizures are the presenting symptom in 10% of patients with 3-hydroxy-3-methylglutaric aciduria, a disorder caused by a deficiency in the enzyme that mediates the final step of leucine degradation and plays a pivotal role in hepatic ketone body production. The odor of the urine may resemble that of a cat. The chromosome location for this disorder is 1pter-p33 (107).

Glutaric Acidemia Type I

This condition is screened for by extended NBS. Glutaric acidemia type I is a more common autosomal recessive disorder of lysine metabolism that is caused by a deficiency in glutaryl-CoA dehydrogenase (19p13.2). Seizures are often the first clinical sign of metabolic decompensation after a febrile illness. Vigabatrin, L-carnitine, baclofen, and riboflavin supplementation have been suggested (108).

Urea Cycle Disorders

Urea cycle disorders (UCDs) occur due to partial or complete deficiencies of enzymes involved in the body's attempt to remove waste nitrogen that forms from protein and carbohydrate catabolism. The incidence of these disorders is as high as 1:25,000, though later onset diseases from partial defects are often underdiagnosed. All of these disorders are autosomal recessive except for ornithine transcarbamylase (OTC) deficiency which is X-linked dominant, but can present in both males and females. OTC is the most common of these disorders, accounting for over 50% of patients with UCDs (109).

The clinical manifestations of most of these disorders are similar and result, at least in part, from ammonia elevations. Typically, affected newborns present with poor feeding, emesis, hyperventilation, lethargy, or convulsions 1 to 5 days after birth. These signs lead to deepening coma, with decorticate and decerebrate posturing and progressive loss of brainstem function. Brain imaging and pathology reveal cerebral edema with pronounced astrocytic swelling (110).

Later onset disease due to partial enzyme deficiencies can present with progressive spasticity of the lower extremity, episodic vomiting, or episodic fluctuating encephalopathy with or without seizures. Some individuals may be symptom free until in the midst of a physiologic stressor that leads to an acute metabolic decompensation (111).

The clinical diagnosis is confirmed by elevations in serum ammonia, absence of urine ketones, and respiratory alkalosis. In contrast, metabolic acidosis and ketosis frequently occur with disorders of organic acid or pyruvate metabolism. Characteristic findings in plasma amino and urine organic acids, along with measurements of urine orotic acid can help differentiate among the various enzymatic defects. Measurements of plasma citrulline and argininosuccinic acid, may also be helpful. Definitive diagnosis is established via gene sequencing if the enzymatic defect is identified by screening biochemical tests in blood and urine. If the enzyme defect needs further defining or confirmation, biochemical analysis in skin fibroblasts or liver can be performed (112).

The EEG shows a low-voltage pattern, with diffuse slowing and multifocal epileptiform discharges (113). Two patients studied by Verma and coworkers in 1984 demonstrated episodes of sustained monorhythmic theta activity (114). In patients with acute neonatal citrullinemia, a burst-suppression pattern has been described (115).

In the acute setting, hemodialysis has been used to reduce serum ammonia and can be lifesaving. Protein restriction and medical therapy aimed at lowering serum ammonia are recommended in the long-term management of these children. Liver transplantation has been successful in reducing ammonia levels in patients and in reversing neurologic deficits in adults with milder disease (116,117).

Fatty Acid Oxidation Defects

The multienzyme, multistep process of fatty acid oxidation, also occurs inside the mitochondria. Deficiencies of any of the enzymes involved, including carnitine palmitoyltransferase types I and II, may present in the newborn period (118). The infantile type of carnitine palmitoyltransferase II deficiency presents as severe attacks of hypoketotic hypoglycemia, sometimes associated with cardiac damage, culminating in sudden death. A deficiency in carnitine acylcarnitine translocase also may produce seizures, apnea, and bradycardia in the neonatal period. Seizures may occur in other defects of fatty acid oxidation, most notably in short-chain acyl-CoA dehydrogenase deficiency (119).

Peroxisomal Disorders

Peroxisomes play an important role in the body's ability to break down very-long-chain-fatty acids (VLCFA) via omega-oxidation and phytanic and pristanic acid production. Phytanic and pristanic acid are involved in the synthesis of bile acids, plasmalogens, and pipecolic acid (120).

Disorders of the peroxisome have been divided into three categories: (i) disorders of peroxisomal biogenesis (Zellweger syndrome spectrum [ZSS]), (ii) disorders of a single peroxisomal enzyme (X-linked adrenoleukodystrophy [XALD], acyl-coenzyme A [acyl-CoA] oxidase deficiency); and (iii) disorders with deficiencies of multiple peroxisomal enzymes (rhizomelic chondrodysplasia punctata). The discussion that follows is limited to ZSS and acyl-CoA oxidase deficiency. XALD is discussed with the later-onset conditions.

Zellweger Syndrome Spectrum

The Zellweger syndrome spectrum (ZSS) is the most common peroxisomal disorder in early infancy, with an estimated incidence of 1:50,000. This disorder was previously categorized as three distinct diseases (ZS, neonatal adrenoleukodystrophy, and infantile Refsum disease), but is now known to be a single condition with a varying spectrum of phenotypic severity. The ZSS phenotype is caused by mutations in any of several different genes involved in peroxisome biogenesis, of which at least 12 have been identified, named *PEX* 1–12. *PEX1* mutations are the most common cause of ZSS (121).

Diagnosis is made via sending a peroxisomal panel which measures plasma levels of VLCFA, phytanic and pristanic acid, and plasmalogens. VLCFA can be the initial screening test, though one must keep in mind that the degree of elevation may vary and that false-negatives can occur (122). Confirmatory molecular genetic testing is available as well.

Dysmorphic features may be noted shortly after birth. Within the first week to several months of life, the affected child develops encephalopathy, hypotonia, and hyporeflexia. Seizures occur in 80% of patients, including partial, generalized tonic–clonic (rare), and myoclonic seizures, and atypical flexor spasms. Multisystem abnormalities of the brain, kidneys, liver, skeletal system, and eyes may occur. Eye abnormalities include cataracts, glaucoma, corneal clouding, optic nerve hypoplasia, pigmentary retinal degeneration, and Brushfield spots. The presence of the latter, along with hypotonia and a dysmorphic appearance, may cause confusion in the diagnosis of Down syndrome versus ZSS. Findings on neuroimaging can include pachygyria or polymicrogyria localized to the opercular region and cerebellar heterotopias (123).

Patients with ZSS have partial motor seizures originating in the arms, legs, or face. The seizures do not culminate in generalized seizures and are easily controlled with medication. The interictal EEG of patients with ZS shows infrequent bilateral independent multifocal spikes, predominantly in the frontal motor cortex and surrounding regions. Less frequently, hypsarrhythmia is observed (124).

Presently, only symptomatic treatment is available for this condition.

Acyl-Coenzyme A Oxidase Deficiency

Acyl-CoA oxidase deficiency was initially described in two siblings by Poll-The and colleagues (125). Clinical features included hypotonia, pigmentary retinopathy, hearing loss, developmental delay, adrenocortical insufficiency, absence of dysmorphic features, and onset of seizures shortly after birth. A deficiency in acyl-CoA oxidase was identified, resulting from a deletion in its coding gene (17q25). In children with acyl-CoA oxidase deficiency, serum VLCFA levels are elevated, whereas pipecolic acid levels are normal. Cortical malformations are generally absent, and the interictal EEG may show continuous diffuse high-voltage theta activity (126).

Storage Disease

Tay–Sachs Disease and Sandhoff Disease

GM2 gangliosidosis is an autosomal recessive lysosomal disorder that invariably includes seizures as a prominent feature. The infantile forms of GM2 gangliosidosis include Tay–Sachs disease, caused by a deficiency in hexosaminidase A (Hex A), and Sandhoff disease, caused by a deficiency in Hex A and B. The enzymatic defect leads to intraneuronal accumulation of GM2 ganglioside. Tay–Sachs disease does not have any extraneural involvement and the clinical presentation is that of a progressive encephalopathy (2).

The *HEXA* gene is localized to chromosome 15 (15q23–q24), and mutations are found more commonly in the Ashkenazi Jewish population of Eastern or Central European descent. The overall incidence in the general population (1 in 112,000 live births) increases to 1 in 3900 in this defined group (127).

Development appears to be normal until 4 to 6 months of age, when hypotonia and loss of motor skills are evident. Within the next several months to years, spasticity, blindness, and macrocephaly develop. The classic cherry-red spot is present in the ocular fundi of more than 90% of patients. Seizures become prominent, with frequent partial motor, complex partial, and atypical absence seizures that respond poorly to medication. Myoclonic jerks are frequent and are often triggered by an exaggerated startle response to noise (2).

The EEG is normal early in the course of disease. Gradually, background activity slows, with bursts of high-voltage delta activity and very fast central spikes. Diffuse spike and sharp-wave activity may be noted with acoustically induced myoclonic seizures. As the disease progresses, EEG amplitude declines (128).

Enzymatic studies in leukocytes and skin fibroblasts reveal an isolated absence or deficiency in hexosaminidase A activity. Clinical genetic testing is available. Prenatal diagnosis and carrier detection for high-risk populations are also available (2).

Sandhoff disease is associated with a mutation of the β-subunit of hexosaminidase, (*HEXB*) located on chromosome 5 (5q13) (129). Unlike Tay–Sachs disease, there is no association with a particular ethnic group. Clinical presentation is similar to that of Tay–Sachs; however, distinguishing features in some patients include hepatosplenomegaly and skeletal involvement. Enzymatic testing demonstrates the diminished activity of hexosaminidase A and B. Detection of N-acetylglucosamine-containing oligosaccharides in the urine and foam cells in the bone marrow is also diagnostic. As with Tay–Sachs disease, no treatment is immediately available (2).

Krabbe Disease (Globoid Cell Leukodystrophy)

Another lysosomal disorder occurring in this age group is globoid cell leukodystrophy (Krabbe disease) due to a deficiency of galactocerebrosidase enzyme activity (GALC). The *GALC* gene is located at chromosome 14q31 (130).

Depending on the severity of the enzyme deficiency, there are four phenotypic presentations of the disorder: (i) with an infantile onset, before the age of 6 months; (ii) a late infantile onset, between ages 6 months and 3 years; (iii) a juvenile onset, between ages 3 and 7 years; and (iv) adult onset beginning after 7 years of age. The majority of cases begin within the first 3 to 6 months of life with irritability, poor feeding, emesis, and rigidity. Muscular spasms induced by stimulation are prominent. Blindness and optic atrophy ensue. Initially, increased tendon reflexes are present and then gradually diminish as breakdown of peripheral myelin occurs (131).

Partial or generalized clonic or tonic seizures, as well as infantile spasms, are seen, which may be difficult to distinguish from muscular spasms (132). In contrast to what is observed in many classic white matter diseases, seizures occur early in the course of Krabbe disease in 50% to 75% of infants with the disorder. EEG characteristics include a hypsarrhythmia-like pattern with irregular slow activity and multifocal discharges of lower amplitude than that typically seen with West syndrome. In a 1969 study of seven infants by Kliemann and coworkers, six children had prominent β activity occurring independently in the posterior temporal regions and vertex that was superimposed over slower, high-amplitude waves. This activity was observed to be state-dependent and to occur in long runs without any apparent clinical manifestations. In the terminal stages of the disease, little electrical activity is detected (133).

Diagnosis is made by measuring GALC enzyme activity in leukocytes or skin fibroblasts, followed by confirmatory gene sequencing. The disease is relentlessly progressive, with death by 1 to 2 years of age (131).

GM1 Gangliosidosis Types I and II

GM1 gangliosidosis occurs due to lysosomal β-galactosidase (GLB) deficiency, and mutations in the *GLB1* gene localized to chromosome 3 (3p21.33). GLB deficiency leads to the accumulation of GM1 ganglioside and degradation products in nerve cells and other tissues. In the infantile onset form of the condition, the affected child is initially normal and then has regression of development at 3 to 6 months of age, with rapid neurologic deterioration. Seizures develop by 2 years of age. Clinical features may include coarse facial features, hepatomegaly, bone deformities (dysostosis multiplex), visual abnormalities, hypotonia, progressive microcephaly, and hematologic abnormalities. A macular cherry-red spot can be seen. Diagnosis is determined by findings of reduced GLB enzyme activity in leukocytes or skin fibroblasts, urine galactose-containing oligosaccharides in association with elevated keratan sulfate, vacuolization in blood lymphocytes or bone marrow, and by distinctive findings on long bone and spine radiographs. Definitive testing by molecular genetics is also available (134).

Neurologic deterioration in the juvenile form of GM1 gangliosidosis type II is generally slower than in type I. Cerebral manifestations with regression of developmental milestones and visual symptoms are typically present by 2 to 4 years of age (134).

EEG features of both forms include background slowing, with increasing, irregular slow activity as the disease progresses.

In type II, a fluctuating 4- to 5-cycle temporal rhythmic discharge has been observed (135).

Progressive Encephalopathy with Edema, Hypsarrhythmia, and Optic Atrophy

Progressive encephalopathy with edema, hypsarrhythmia, and optic atrophy (PEHO) syndrome, described by Salonen and associates in 1991, is characterized by infantile spasms, arrest of psychomotor development, hypotonia, hypsarrhythmia, edema, and optic atrophy (136). Characteristic features include epicanthal folds, midfacial hypoplasia, protruding ears, gingival hypertrophy, micrognathia, and tapering fingers. Edema develops over the limbs and face. The progressive decline seen with this disease suggests a metabolic defect, although no biochemical marker has been identified. Based on the pattern of inheritance associated with the disease, it is presumed to be an autosomal recessive disorder. Neuroimaging shows progressive brain atrophy and abnormal myelination. Hypoplasia of the corpus callosum has been reported. Seizures generally begin as infantile spasms with associated hypsarrhythmia on the EEG. Later, other seizure types may be seen, including tonic, tonic–clonic, and absence seizures. The EEG may evolve to a slow spike-wave pattern. Prognosis is poor in children with this disorder, with survival only into adolescence (137).

METABOLIC DISORDERS OF LATE INFANCY, CHILDHOOD, AND ADOLESCENCE

While many of the previously discussed disorders can have a later onset of symptoms, there are several disorders that classically begin outside of the newborn and early infancy period. A few of these disorders are discussed below.

Storage Disorders

Neuronal Ceroid Lipofuscinoses

The neuronal ceroid lipofuscinoses (NCL) are a group of diseases that result in storage of lipopigments in the brain and other tissues. At least five clinical subtypes have been reported, as well as rare, atypical forms, and most are transmitted as autosomal recessive traits. The disorder can present at any age, from infancy through adulthood.

The condition occurs due to a genetic defect leading to impaired lysosomal function and intra- and extra-lysosomal storage. Thus far seven genes (*CLN* 1, 2, 3, 4, 5, 6, and 8) have been identified, leading to the various phenotypes though depending on the type of mutation, there is significant overlap between age of onset and symptoms (138).

Evaluation for this condition typically begins with quantification of palmitoyl-protein thioesterase (PPT1) and tripeptidyl-peptidase (TPP1) enzyme levels in leukocytes. Based on the enzyme deficieny found and age of onset, targeted gene sequencing is performed. If enzyme levels are normal or the patient has an adult onset of symptoms, electron microscopy of skin for characteristic abnormalities and/or lymphocytes for vacuoles is recommended. This approach has evolved from the previous one of obtaining a skin biopsy as the diagnostic test in all patients. In rare instances, storage product identification in cells from a rectal suction or conjunctival biopsy is necessary. With advances in genetic knowledge this type of testing is now infrequent (139).

Visual loss is a feature of almost all except the adult form of NCL either as the presenting symptom or occurring months to years after disease onset. The infantile form typically presents between 6 and 24 months of age with developmental regression, myoclonus, ataxia, and visual failure. Other features include incoordination of limb movements, acquired microcephaly, and optic atrophy. Seizures are prominent, including myoclonic jerks and astatic, atonic, or generalized seizures. EEG features aid in the diagnosis, with an early attenuation and progressive loss of the background. Neuroimaging may show progressive cerebral and cerebellar atrophy (140).

The late infantile form has epilepsy beginning between the ages of 2 and 4 years, followed by cognitive decline, ataxia, and eventually visual failure with optic atrophy. Early development is normal or may be mildly delayed. Multiple seizure types develop as well, with staring spells and generalized tonic–clonic, myoclonic, and atonic components. As the disease progresses, irregular myoclonic jerks evoked by proprioceptive stimuli, voluntary movement, or emotional fluctuations become prominent. A characteristic EEG pattern of occipital spikes on low-frequency photic stimulation is observed. Giant visual evoked responses and somatosensory evoked potentials are seen as well. Juvenile-onset disease presents with visual loss between the ages of 4 and 10 years. Epilepsy begins a year to several years later, with multiple seizure types. The treatment of these conditions is symptomatic. Life span varies from several years to adulthood depending on the severity of the enzyme defect (140).

Metachromatic Leukodystrophy

Metachromatic leukodystrophy is the result of a deficiency of arylsulfatase A (ASA), leading to an accumulation of lipid sulfatide. A late infantile, juvenile, and adult onset subtypes occur with about half of patients presenting between the ages of 1 and 2 years. Hypotonia, weakness, and unsteady gait suggestive of a neuropathy or myopathy are the most common presenting symptoms with the late-infantile form. These symptoms are followed by a progressive decline in mental and motor skills (141).

Partial seizures develop late in the clinical course in 25% of patients with the late-infantile form of metachromatic leukodystrophy and in 50% to 60% of patients with the juvenile-onset form (142,143). A progression from normal EEG features to diffuse slowing with epileptiform discharges correlates well with clinical decline (144). Bone marrow transplantation, especially if prior to the onset of neurologic symptoms, may be beneficial in some patients and may be accompanied by improvements in clinical neurophysiologic studies (145).

Diagnosis is made by quantifying ASA enzyme activity in leukocytes or cultured skin fibroblasts. Urine sulfatide activity can be measured. Molecular genetic testing of the *ARSA* gene (22q13.3–qter) is clinically available. Treatment is symptomatic (146).

Mucopolysaccharidoses

The mucopolysaccharidoses are a family of lysosomal storage disorders caused by a deficiency in several enzymes involved in the degradation of glycosaminoglycans. The various mucopolysaccharidoses share many clinical features, including a progressive course, multisystem involvement, organ enlargement, dysostosis multiplex, and abnormal facial features (147).

A subtype with a primarily neurologic phenotype is Sanfilippo syndrome (mucopolysaccharidosis type III), in which only heparan sulfate is excreted in the urine; four different subtypes have been described, each associated with a different enzymatic defect. The gene locus is 17q25.3 (148).

Generalized seizures develop in about 40% of patients with Sanfilippo syndrome, but these are often easily controlled with AEDs. Progressive dementia and severe behavioral disorders are other features. In a careful study of one patient, the EEG showed lack of normal sleep staging, absence of vertex waves and sleep spindles, and an unusual alteration of low-amplitude fast activity (12 to 15 Hz) with generalized slowing (149). Bone marrow transplantation was successful in several cases but not useful in others. Enzyme replacement therapy is available for some of these conditions (150).

Sialidosis Type I

Sialidosis type I, an autosomal recessive disorder of late childhood to adolescence, is characterized by progressive visual loss, polymyoclonus, and seizures. The myoclonus can be debilitating and is stimulated by voluntary movement, sensory stimulation, or excitement. Increased myoclonus with cigarette smoking and menstruation has been reported. As the disease progresses, cognitive decline, cerebellar ataxia, and blindness with optic atrophy occur. Dysmorphic features, bony abnormalities, and hepatosplenomegaly are absent. The EEG contains rhythmic spiking over the vertex, with a positive polarity overlying a low-voltage background (151). Neuroimaging shows diffuse cerebral and cerebellar atrophy. Diagnosis can be made by detection of an increase in sialic acid—containing oligosaccharides in the urine, vacuolated lymphocytes in the peripheral blood, and foamy histiocytes in bone marrow smears. Enzyme assays for deficiency of α-neuraminidase, the structural components of which are encoded on chromosome 10, offer definitive diagnosis. The gene defect has been localized to 6p21.3 (152).

Sialidosis Type II (Galactosialidosis)

Sialidosis type II, the juvenile form of this group of disorders, has features similar to those of sialidosis type I. Distinguishing characteristics are the less prominent myoclonic activity and the additional clinical features of coarse facies, corneal clouding, dysostosis multiplex, and hearing loss. Inheritance is autosomal recessive, and a higher incidence of this form of the disease is found in Japan. In the majority of cases, a partial deficiency of β-galactosidase can be seen in addition to neuraminidase deficiency (galactosialidosis), which may be the result of a defect in protective protein; the gene locus coding for this protein is 20q13.1. The electroencephalogram contains moderate-voltage generalized 4 to 6 per second paroxysms (153).

Gaucher Disease Type III

Three types of Gaucher diseases are known: type I, a chronic form with adult onset; type II, a rare form associated with infantile demise; and type III, a chronic form with neurologic involvement. These disorders result from a mutation in the gene encoding acid β-glucosidase (1q21), which leads to accumulation of glucosylceramide in the lysosomes of cells in the reticuloendothelial system (154). In the rare type III form, hepatosplenomegaly may be present from birth or early infancy, which may cause type III to be confused with the more common type I form of Gaucher disease. When neurologic symptoms develop in childhood to early adulthood, type III can be clearly distinguished from type I, in which cerebral features are absent. Frequent myoclonic jerks and tonic–clonic seizures ultimately develop. A supranuclear palsy of horizontal gaze is present in the majority of cases and is an important diagnostic sign. Generalized rigidity, progressive cognitive decline, and facial grimacing may be present. Paroxysmal EEG abnormalities may be seen prior to the onset of convulsions, with worsening as the disease progresses; diffuse polyspikes and spike–wave discharges are also seen. The most characteristic EEG findings are rhythmic trains of spike or sharp waves at 6 to 10 per second (155). The diagnosis can be made by the clinical findings in combination with Gaucher cells detected in the bone marrow. Another laboratory abnormality is an elevated serum acid phosphatase. Unlike type I disease, which is prevalent in the Ashkenazi Jewish population, type III is reported predominantly in Sweden. A multimodal approach is suggested with enzyme replacement therapy and deoxynojirimycin analogs aimed at blocking the synthesis of glucocerebroside to lessen the systemic manifestations. Therapeutic trials with bone marrow transplantation have shown some success in improving CNS manifestations of Gaucher disease type III (156).

Neuroaxonal Dystrophies

Axonal dystrophies include infantile neuroaxonal dystrophy, pantothenate kinase-associated neurodegeneration (formerly Hallervorden–Spatz disease), and Schindler disease. Pantothenate kinase-associated neurodegeneration is not discussed here, as seizures are not a prominent feature.

Infantile neuroaxonal dystrophy (Seitelberger disease) is an autosomal recessive disorder affecting both the central and the peripheral nervous systems. Characteristic pathologic features of axonal spheroids within the peripheral and central nervous systems are seen. Clinical features begin between 1 and 2 years of age with psychomotor regression, hypotonia, and development of a progressive motor sensory neuropathy. Seizures occur in one third of patients, with onset of convulsions after 3 years of age. The EEG finding of high-amplitude fast activity (16 to 24 Hz), unaltered by eye opening or closure, is characteristic of all children with this disorder, regardless of the occurrence of seizures. During sleep, the fast activity may persist, and K complexes are typically absent (157). Seizure types described with infantile neuroaxonal dystrophy include myoclonic and tonic (158,159). A video-EEG case report by Wakai and associates described tonic spasms and an electrographic correlate of a diffuse, 1-second, high-voltage slow complex, followed by desynchronization suggestive of infantile spasms (160).

Schindler disease results from a deficiency in α-N-acetylgalactosaminidase (22q11). Affected patients appear normal at birth, but progressive neurologic decline becomes evident in the second year. Manifestations include spasticity, cerebellar signs, and extrapyramidal dysfunction. Generalized tonic–clonic seizures and myoclonic jerks are common. EEG abnormalities include diffuse and multifocal spikes and spike–wave complexes (161).

Mitochondrial Diseases

An overview of mitochondrial disease has been outlined in the earlier portion of this chapter.

POLG1 Disease, Including Childhood-Onset Epilepsia Partialis Continua, and Alpers Disease

The mitochondrial DNA polymerase gamma (*POLG1*) is a nuclear DNA gene required for mtDNA replication. Over the past several years mutations of this gene have been linked to a wide-array of growing phenotypes. While many of these phenotypes do not have seizures as their primary or only feature, a phenotype with epilepsia partialis continua as the initial and often only manifestation is known as is a form with progressive myoclonic epilepsy (162).

POLG1 mutations have also been identified as the principal cause of Alpers disease (163). Alpers and Alpers–Huttenlocher diseases are characterized by a rapidly progressive encephalopathy with intractable seizures and diffuse neuronal degeneration. Seizures are often partial complex or myoclonic though they can evolve to include multiple types. The EEG may show rhythmic slowing, predominating either in the posterior or anterior derivations, sometimes admixed with periodic brush-like patterns (164). Varying amounts of liver disease is also present. Symptoms may begin at any age and liver disease may not be present for years. Encephalopathy and liver disease can stabilize with partial resolution of symptoms. Disease onset after exposure to valproate and valproate-related worsening of existing symptoms is characteristic of this condition (165,166).

MERRF and MELAS

While we now understand that most patients with mitochondrial disease do not present syndromically or with maternally inherited disease, the initially described conditions designated by acronyms remain an important cause of mitochondrial disease and epilepsy. Two of these syndromic presentations of mitochondrial disease are described below.

Onset of myoclonic epilepsy with ragged-red fibers (MERRF) occurs before 20 years of age, with ataxia and seizures that are predominantly myoclonic. Affected individuals may have short stature, neurosensory hearing loss, optic atrophy, myopathy, or encephalopathy. EEG findings may include background slowing, focal epileptiform discharges, and atypical spike or sharp and slow-wave discharges that have a variable association with the myoclonic jerks. Suppression of these discharges during sleep is characteristic. As with many of the progressive myoclonus epilepsies, giant somatosensory evoked potentials are observed. Lactic acidosis and the presence of ragged-red fibers on muscle biopsy are common features of the diagnosis. The inheritance pattern is compatible with maternal transmission. In the majority of cases, a point mutation at position 8344 of the mitochondrial gene for transfer ribonucleic acid (tRNA)-lysine has been identified (167).

Classically, mitochondrial encephalopathy with lactic acidosis and stroke-like episodes (MELAS) presents in childhood with the sudden onset of stroke-like episodes. Migraine-like headaches, progressive deafness, seizures, cognitive decline, and myopathic features may accompany these symptoms.

Epilepsia partialis continua can be seen, and seizures often evolve into partial or generalized status epilepticus. Myoclonic seizures are prominent in individuals with MELAS. In the acute stage following a stroke-like episode, 10 of 11 EEG showed focal high-voltage delta waves with polyspikes. These discharges were interpreted as ictal phenomena. Later, focal spikes or sharp waves and 14- and 6-Hz positive bursts were frequently recorded. The observed seizures were characterized by focal clonic and myoclonic movements with migrainous headache. Lactic acid is elevated in the blood, and ragged-red fibers are present on muscle biopsy. Four-point mutations are predominantly seen with MELAS. Three of these (3243, 3250, and 3271) affect the mitochondrial DNA gene of tRNA-leucine. The other mutation involves a coding region of complex I of the respiratory chain (168).

Dentatorubral–Pallidoluysian Atrophy

Dentatorubral–pallidoluysian atrophy (DRPLA) is a rare autosomal dominant disease due to a trinucleotide (CAG) expansion of the *ATN1* gene on chromosome 12p (12p13.31). Clinical manifestations are dependent on the length of the unstable trinucleotide repeats and vary from a juvenile-onset progressive myoclonic epilepsy to an adult-onset syndrome with ataxia, dementia, and choreoathetosis. The juvenile form can also be variable in its presentation. In general, symptoms begin in infancy to early childhood with myoclonus, ataxia, dementia, opsoclonus, or seizures that can be generalized tonic–clonic, atypical absence, or atonic. Pathologic features are striking, with neuronal loss and gliosis in the dentatorubral and pallidoluysian structures (169).

The EEG characteristically shows bursts of slowing, irregular spike-wave discharges, and multifocal paroxysmal discharges. A photoparoxysmal response is seen, and myoclonic seizures can often be triggered by photic stimulation (170).

Congenital Disorders of Glycosylation

Congenital disorders of glycosylation (CDG) are multisystemic diseases characterized by a defect in the synthesis of *N*-linked glycoproteins and glycolipids. CDGs are divided into types, depending on whether the defects impair lipid-linked oligosaccharide assembly and transfer (CDG-I) or alter trimming of the protein-bound oligosaccharide or the addition of sugars to it (CDG-II) (171).

CDG type Ia, phosphomannomutase-2 deficiency, is the best characterized and most common of these syndromes (gene *PMM2*, 16p13.3–p13.2). The most common symptoms include infant-onset failure to thrive and hepatopathy. Developmental delays, cerebellar hypoplasia, ataxia, progressive neuropathy involving the legs, retinal degeneration, and skeletal deformities are also common. Subcutaneous tissue changes with an odd distribution of fat, retracted nipples, and odd facies, including almond-shaped eyes, have been described. Imaging studies reveal cerebellar hypoplasia. A unique pattern of coagulation changes is associated with the syndrome, including depression of factor XI, antithrombin III, protein C, and, to a lesser extent, protein S and heparin cofactor II. These changes may account for stroke-like

episodes observed in affected children. Clinical neurophysiologic studies demonstrate interictal epileptiform discharges and giant somatosensory evoked potentials. Screening for this condition includes assessing glycosylation status via mass spectroscopy (and previously via isoelectric focusing of transferrin isoforms) (172).

Many other CDG subtypes have now also been described (173).

Disorders of Peroxisome Metabolism

X-linked Adrenoleukodystrophy

XALD is an X-linked genetic defect in one of the peroxisomal membrane transport proteins. The condition occurs due to mutations in the *ABCD* gene (Xq28) and leads to three varied phenotypes. The childhood onset form begins in early school age with attention deficit and cognitive regression.

Partial motor seizures, often with secondary generalization, and generalized tonic–clonic seizures can occur. Status epilepticus has been the initial presenting symptom, and epilepsia partialis continua has also been reported. Diagnosis is made by quantifying VLCFA in plasma, followed by gene sequencing and confirmation (174).

The EEG is characteristic, with high-voltage polymorphic delta activity and loss of faster frequencies over the posterior regions (175).

Adrenomyeloneuropathy and isolated Addison disease presentations account for the other phenotypes and are typically not associated with epilepsy.

Progressive Myoclonic Epilepsies

The progressive myoclonic epilepsies are a collection of disorders presenting with the triad of myoclonic seizures, tonic–clonic seizures, and neurologic dysfunction that often manifests as dementia and ataxia. Onset generally begins in childhood through adolescence, though they may begin later in life. If myoclonic features are not prominent, children with this syndrome may be erroneously diagnosed with Lennox–Gastaut syndrome. For this reason, a careful history to detect myoclonic features is important in children with intellectual deterioration and frequent seizures (176).

Previously discussed disorders that can lead to this phenotype include mitochondrial cytopathies (especially *POLG1* mutations, MERRF, and MELAS), sialidoses, some of the other lysosomal diseases, DRPLA, and NCL. The two disorders below are listed separately since they are atypical storage diseases and are routinely tested for via direct molecular genetic testing nowadays.

Lafora Body Disease

Although the biochemical error in Lafora body disease remains unknown, this autosomal recessively inherited disease occurs due to mutations in either the *EPM2A* (6q24) or *EPM2B* (6p22.3) genes (177).

Symptoms typically begin in the teen years, with focal, multiregional, or generalized myoclonus. The myoclonus is brought out by action, touch, light, and stress. Generalized tonic–clonic seizures may also occur. A prior childhood history of an isolated febrile or afebrile seizure may exist. Cognitive symptoms may lag by months or years and initially include visual hallucinations, personality changes, confusion, and ataxia. The visual hallucinations frequently represent occipital seizures (178).

Generalized bursts of spikes and polyspikes superimposed on a normal background may be seen initially on the EEG. The presence of spikes in the posterior quadrant is a distinguishing feature that suggests the diagnosis with the appropriate clinical scenario (179). As the disease progresses, the EEG becomes increasingly disorganized. A photoconvulsive response can be seen with photic stimulation.

On neuroimaging, cerebellar atrophy is occasionally observed. Intracytoplasmic inclusion bodies (Lafora bodies) are seen on electron microscopy of a skin, liver, or muscle biopsy. A negative biopsy does not exclude the diagnosis. Molecular genetic testing is the preferred route of diagnosis. There is no effective treatment for this disorder, and the average life span after onset is 2 to 10 years (178).

Unverricht–Lundborg Disease (Baltic Myoclonus)

This autosomal recessive progressive encephalopathy is characterized by relentless myoclonus and generalized seizures due to defective function of the cystatin B protein due to mutations in the *CSTB* gene (21q22.3). Testing for a common dodecamer repeat (that leads to over 90% of cases) and several point mutations is clinically available (180).

Onset is in childhood or adolescence with seizures that are predominantly myoclonic and frequently occur after awakening. Absence and atonic seizures are also observed. Myoclonus can become quite disabling, interfering with speech and swallowing, and is often provoked by voluntary movement and excitement. Cognition is generally retained, although a mild decline may be observed later in the disease course. A labile affect and depression are commonly seen. Cerebellar ataxia, tremors, hyporeflexia, wasting of the distal musculature, and signs of chronic denervation on electromyography may be seen as the disease progresses (181).

The EEG reveals progressive slowing, with generalized 3- to-5-per-second spike–wave-like bursts that are frontally predominant. Paroxysmal flicker responses and generalized spikes and polyspikes are seen with photic stimulation (182,183). Although this disorder occurs worldwide, it has an especially high incidence in Finland, Estonia, and areas of the Mediterranean.

Phenytoin and AEDs predominantly affecting sodium channels will worsen symptoms (184). Death occurs in the third to fourth decade of life.

Disorders of Amino Acid Metabolism

Homocystinuria

Disorders of transsulfuration include cystathionine β-synthase deficiency, the most frequent cause of homocystinuria; the gene locus is 21q22.3 (185). The condition is screened for in extended newborn testing in many states. Mental retardation, behavioral disturbances, and seizures are manifestations of CNS involvement; ectopia lentis, osteoporosis, Marfanoid habitus, and scoliosis are other common clinical findings (186). Some patients respond to pyridoxine therapy. Generalized seizures occur in about 20% of patients with pyridoxine-nonresponsive homocystinuria and in 16% of patients with the pyridoxine-responsive form. EEG features are relatively nonspecific, with slowing and focal interictal epileptiform discharges that may ameliorate with treatment (187). Thromboembolism, malar flush, and livedo reticularis reflect vascular system involvement. Biochemical abnormalities include homocystinemia, methioninemia, decreased cystine concentration, and homocystinuria.

DIAGNOSTIC INVESTIGATION IN METABOLIC AND MITOCHONDRIAL DISORDERS

The diagnosis of genetically determined metabolic diseases can be complicated for many reasons. We suggest that a genetic metabolic basis be considered for all unexplained epileptic conditions of infancy or childhood until proven otherwise. Routine interrogation of blood, urine, and CSF samples as discussed in this chapter will be informative in a significant subset of patients and alternative treatment options may emerge.

The classic aminoacidopathies and organic acidurias, once suspected, can easily be diagnosed via appropriate blood or urine measurements. However, the diagnosis of a rare condition such as CDG may require specific glycosylation testing in a specialized research laboratory. Before obtaining appropriate metabolic, biochemical, or tissue specimens, the physician should try to formulate a differential diagnosis. Age at onset, type of epilepsy, associated clinical findings, family history, ethnicity, and neurologic examination continue to be the most important considerations in initial diagnostic possibilities. Neurologists experienced in metabolic disorders can often narrow the list of possible disorders at the first clinical encounter. Therefore, a consultation with a metabolic specialist is useful before or after initial screening tests are performed in such patients.

The presence of macular cherry-red spots, abnormal appearance of the hair, or a peculiar distribution of fat over the posterior flanks or thighs immediately suggests a diagnosis of Tay–Sachs disease, Menkes disease, or CDG, respectively. Deceleration of head growth during infancy, with consequent acquired microcephaly, may imply Glut-1 transporter deficiency, another defect of energy metabolism, the infantile form of neuronal ceroid lipofuscinosis, or Rett syndrome, among other possibilities. Dislocated lenses and a seizure followed by a stroke are characteristic of homocystinuria. Seizures with stroke-like episodes also suggest CDG, mitochondrial disorders, OTC deficiency, and glycolytic disorders. Genetically determined metabolic diseases often have a saltatory historical pattern in contrast to neurodegenerative diseases, which are inexorably progressive.

Evaluation in the Absence of Overt Clinical Clues

In certain circumstances, the underlying problem will not be intuitively obvious and the patient's disorder may masquerade as a form of cryptogenic epilepsy.

Certain screening tests can be used to help narrow the differential diagnosis. A complete blood cell count with differential and platelet count should be obtained in every case. Bone marrow depression occurs in the organic acidemias, and the peripheral smear may reveal important clues such as a macrocytic anemia or vacuolated lymphocytes. A complete serum chemistry profile will uncover acidosis, and electrolyte disturbances or specific organ dysfunction. A low blood urea nitrogen may suggest a defect involving the urea cycle. Calcium and magnesium concentrations should be determined in every case. A low uric acid concentration raises the possibility of molybdenum cofactor deficiency. Ammonia elevations, when mild, point toward amino and organic acidopathies, and urea cycle defects when marked. Quantitative measurement of plasma amino acids and urine organic acids provide diagnostic clues about disorders of amino and organic metabolism, mitochondrial disease, urea cycle disorders and disorders of vitamin metabolism.

When faced with refractory epilepsy without an etiology at any age, spinal fluid analysis is mandatory to exclude certain treatable causes of the epilepsy. An elevated CSF protein concentration is characteristic of demyelinating and inflammatory conditions, including certain mitochondrial disorders, metachromatic leukodystrophy and globoid cell leukodystrophy. A low CSF glucose concentration is consistent with hypoglycemia caused by a defect of gluconeogenesis or Glut-1 transporter defects. Lactate and pyruvate values are elevated in CSF disorders of cerebral energy metabolism, including pyruvate dehydrogenase deficiency, pyruvate carboxylase deficiency, numerous disturbances of the respiratory chain, certain defects of neurotransmitter synthesis and Menkes disease. A low CSF lactate value may be seen in Glut-1 transporter defects. CSF amino acids can provide additional information in disorders of ammonia, amino acid, organic acid, and mitochondrial metabolism. Elevations in threonine can be seen in pyridoxal 5-phosphate-dependent seizures. Elevations in glycine may point toward glycine encephalopathy (NKHG). Abnormally low serine concentrations point to PHGD deficiency.

Spinal fluid neurotransmitter analysis should also be routine in these circumstances. This testing includes measuring the neurotransmitter amines, biopterin, neopterin, and 5-MTHF levels. A low CSF 5-MTHF concentration suggests a defect involving folate metabolism, whether due to systemic disease, another inborn error of metabolism or primary cerebral folate deficiency. Abnormal CSF dopamine, and serotonin metabolites, along with biopterin and neopterin help diagnose disorders of neurotransmitter synthesis. In addition, if an unknown diagnostic marker compound appears on high-performance liquid chromatograms (routinely performed as part of spinal fluid neurotransmitter testing), the finding is diagnostic of pyridoxine and folinic acid responsive epilepsy due to *ALDH7A1* mutations.

More focused testing for specific disorders may also be needed. These include transferrin isoform analysis via mass spectroscopy (previously isoelectric focusing) for disorders of *N*-glycosylation, urine *S*-sulfocysteine for sulfite oxidase or molybdenum cofactor deficiency, lysosomal enzyme analysis in leukocytes for various storage disorders or palmitoyl-protein thioesterase 1 (PPT1), and tripeptidyl peptidase 1 (TPP1) levels in leukocytes for the neuronal ceroid lipofuscinoses. A peroxisomal panel in blood or at least VLCFA levels will help diagnose ZSS and XALD. In addition, urine oligosaccharides, sialic acid levels, and glycosaminoglycans help better elucidate the cause of certain storage disorders. Urine guanidinoacetate and creatine levels are sent for diagnosing disorders of creatine synthesis. Urine and spinal fluid pipecolic acid levels are elevated at times in pyridoxine-dependent epilepsy and peroxisomal disease.

Tissue biopsy specimens also provide important information in establishing a diagnosis. Specimens of skin, peripheral nerve, and skeletal muscle may provide useful clues as well. These tissues can be sent for electron microscopy, histopathologic staining, and selective biochemical analysis. Only rarely are a liver or brain biopsy necessary. Rectal and conjunctival biopsies are infrequently performed.

At times, but less frequently, the EEG features may be sufficiently distinctive to suggest the diagnosis of a limited number of conditions (Table 32.2). In other disorders, the EEG features can help narrow the differential diagnosis. For example, a burst-suppression pattern is seen in patients with NKH,

---

TABLE 32.2

ELECTROENCEPHALOGRAPHIC PATTERNS AND THEIR ASSOCIATED DISORDERS

Electroencephalogram pattern	Disorder
Comblike rhythm	Maple syrup urine disease, propionic acidemia
Fast central spikes	Tay–Sachs disease
Rhythmic vertex-positive spikes	Sialidosis type I
Vanishing electroencephalogram	Infantile neuronal ceroid lipofuscinosis type I
High-amplitude 16- to 24-Hz activity	Infantile neuroaxonal dystrophy
Diminished spikes during sleep	Progressive myoclonus epilepsy
Giant somatosensory evoked potentials	Progressive myoclonus epilepsy
Marked photosensitivity	Progressive myoclonus epilepsy and neuronal ceroid lipofuscinosis, particularly type II
Burst-suppression pattern	Neonatal citrullinemia, nonketotic hyperglycinemia, propionic acidemia, Leigh syndrome, D-glycine acidemia, molybdenum cofactor deficiency, Menkes disease, holocarboxylase synthetase deficiency, neonatal adrenoleukodystrophy
Hypsarrhythmia	Zellweger syndrome, neonatal adrenoleukodystrophy, neuroaxonal dystrophy, nonketotic hyperglycinemia, phenylketonuria, congenital defect of glycosylation type III

PKU, maple syrup urine disease, and molybdenum cofactor/sulfite oxidase deficiency, in addition to other disorders. Some distinctive EEG features include a comblike rhythm with 7- to 9-Hz central activity, which is seen in patients with maple syrup urine disease and propionic acidemia; vertex-positive polyspikes, seen in sialidosis type I; bioccipital polymorphic delta activity, seen in X-linked adrenoleukodystrophy; and 16- to 24-Hz invariant activity, seen in those with infantile neuroaxonal dystrophy.

Brain imaging provides important information, although findings are rarely specific. Progressive atrophy is associated with neuronal ceroid lipofuscinosis, mitochondrial diseases, and certain storage disorders. White matter signal abnormalities are characteristic of peroxisomal disease (especially XALD), storage disorders, some mitochondrial diseases, disorders of neurotransmitter synthesis, MOCOD, disorders of creatine transport and synthesis, and some organic acidurias. Calcification of the cerebral cortex and basal ganglia is seen with many inherited metabolic diseases. Brain MRA may show abnormal dilatation and tortuosity of intracranial blood vessels in patients with Menkes disease. Brain MRS may demonstrate elevated lactate levels in those with various mitochondrial diseases, elevated N-acetylaspartic acid in patients with Canavan disease, or depressed creatine levels in those with inborn errors of creatine metabolism.

When the clinician is asked to evaluate a child with a progressive encephalopathy manifesting with seizures and no overt clinical clues, a screening paradigm must be used. There is seemingly no limit to the number of tests that can be performed, and the financial burden of these investigations can quickly become considerable. Accordingly, we propose the following screening tests, which should be tailored to the age and symptoms at presentation.

To some extent, the differential diagnosis can be pared down by calling to mind a discrete list of diseases for each of the different epilepsy syndromes (see Table 32.1). Nevertheless, it is likely that screening evaluations will need to be performed. Table 32.3 presents metabolic diseases associated with seizures and common biochemical abnormalities. Table 32.4 presents treatable or modifiable metabolic disorders that should not be overlooked.

General Studies

- Complete blood cell count with differential
- Electrolytes, CO_2, BUN/creatinine, and liver enzymes (Chem-20)
- Uric acid levels in blood and urine
- Blood ammonia
- Blood lactate/pyruvate
- Plasma amino acids
- Plasma acylcarnitines
- Urine organic acids
- Electroencephalography
- MRI and MRS

Additional Tests to Consider

- VLCFA and/or peroxisomal panel (which also checks phytanic and pristanic acid levels)

TABLE 32.3

METABOLIC DISEASES AND BIOCHEMICAL ABNORMALITIES

Seizures and metabolic acidosis
- Pyruvate dehydrogenase complex deficiency
- Pyruvate carboxylase deficiency
- Mitochondrial encephalomyopathies
- Amino and organic acidurias
- Multiple carboxylase deficiency disorders

Seizures and hypoglycemia
- Glycogen storage diseases
- Fructose 1,6-bisphosphatase deficiency
- Hereditary fructose intolerance
- Galactosemia
- Organic acidemias
- Disorders of N-glycosylation

Seizures and hyperammonemia
- Urea cycle defects, including hyperammonemia–hyperornithinemia–homocitrullinuria disorder
- Biotinidase deficiency
- Organic acidurias
- Fatty acid oxidation disorders
  - Carnitine palmitoyltransferase type I deficiency
- Mitochondrial cytopathies

- Lysosomal enzyme analysis in leukocytes
- Biotinidase level, followed by biotin administration
- CSF for:
  - Routine studies, especially glucose, lactate, and pyruvate; a concomitant pre-LP plasma glucose sample is needed for comparison to accurately evaluate for GLUT1 disease, CSF and plasma glucose should be obtained on fasting specimens with the patient not receiving dextrose-containing IV fluids.
  - Amino acids; a concomitant pre-LP plasma amino acid sample is needed for comparison
  - Neurotransmitter levels including biogenic amines (dopamine and serotonin metabolites), neopterin, and biopterin. This testing automatically screens for the unknown peak seen in cases of pyridoxine-dependent/folinic acid-responsive epilepsy (this testing can even be obtained after performing a therapeutic trial of pyridoxine, folinic acid, or pyridoxal 5-phosphate)
  - 5-MTHF for cerebral folate deficiency
  - Pyridoxal 5-phosphate for PNPO deficiency
  - Succinyladenosine for adenylosuccinase deficiency (a disorder of purine/pyrimidine metabolism)
- PPT1/TPP1 levels for neuronal ceroid lipofuscinosis (recommended prior to obtaining skin biopsies)
- Transferrin glycosylation studies via mass spectroscopy (previously transferrin isoelectric focusing)
- Serum copper/ceruloplasmin
- Urine guanidinoacetate and creatine for disorders of creatine synthesis or transport
- Urine S-sulfocysteine for sulfite oxidase and/or molybdenum cofactor deficiency
- Urine oligosaccharides and/or mucopolysaccharides
- Urine purine/pyrimidine analysis

TABLE 32.4

TREATABLE OR MODIFIABLE METABOLIC DISORDERS

Category	Disorder	Screening Test(s)	Notes
Common disorders	Amino and organic acidopathies Mitochondrial cytopathies Fatty acid oxidation disorders Urea cycle disorder Biotinidase deficiency	Amino acids, plasma Organic acids, urine Lactate/pyruvate Acylcarnitines, plasma Ammonia Biotinidase activity	Fasting or preprandial specimens preferred; urine amino acids and urine acylcarnitines should be obtained selectively
Require spinal fluid for diagnosis	Glut-1 transporter Defects	CSF glucose	Obtain pre-LP plasma glucose for comparison
	Glycine encephalopathy (NKHG)	CSF amino acids	Obtain pre-LP plasma amino acids for comparison
	Serine deficiency (PHGDH deficiency)	CSF amino acids	Obtain pre-LP plasma amino acids for comparison
	Pyridoxine and folinic acid responsive epilepsy	Identification of an unknown compound peak when CSF neurotransmitter amines are tested	Plasma, urine, and CSF pipecolic acid and CSF threonine may also be elevated
	Defects of neurotransmitter synthesis	CSF neurotransmitter amines, biopterin, and neopterin	
	Cerebral folate deficiency	CSF methyltetrahydrofolate	Need plasma folate for comparison
	Pyridoxal phosphate responsive epilepsy	CSF pyridoxal phosphate level	CSF threonine may also be elevated
Less common disorders	Disorders of creatine synthesis	Urine guanidinoacetate Brain MRS	Plasma levels may also be obtained
	Sulfite oxidase/molybdenum cofactor deficiency	Uric acid, plasma Urine S-sulfocysteine	Uric acid is normal in sulfite oxidase deficiency
	Disorders of copper metabolism	Plasma copper and ceruloplasmin	24-hour urine collections may be needed
	Thyroid transporter defects	T3, free T4 and TSH	TSH alone is not an accurate screening tool

Selective

- Skin biopsy for
  - Electron microscopy
  - Fibroblast culture with fibroblasts sent for enzymatic assays (mitochondrial disorders, neuronal ceroid lipofuscinoses, Lafora body disease, PDH and PC deficiencies, lysosomal storage disease)
- Muscle biopsy (mitochondrial disorders)
- Nerve biopsy (neuroaxonal dystrophy)
- MRS (mitochondrial disorders and disorders of creatine synthesis and transport)
- Bone marrow for Gaucher cells

Focused Genetic Testing

- Chromosome micro- or oligo-array analysis (comparative genomic hybridization)
- Methylation studies of chromosome 15q12 for Prader–Willi/Angelman syndrome followed by *UBE3A* gene sequencing if Angelman syndrome is suspected
- Rett/*MECP2* and *CDKL5* gene sequencing and deletion analysis

- *EPM1* (Unverricht–Lundborg/Baltic myoclonus) and *EPM2A/B* (Lafora body) testing for PME
- Select nDNA and mtDNA gene analysis for mitochondrial disease
- *POLG1* gene sequencing for brain–liver disease (Alpers phenotype) or epilepsia partialis continua

TREATMENT OF METABOLIC AND MITOCHONDRIAL DISORDERS

The treatment of seizures associated with inherited metabolic and mitochondrial diseases should focus on the metabolic disturbance. Seizures associated with hypoglycemia, hyponatremia, hypocalcemia, and hypomagnesemia respond best to correction of these disturbances and should be treated with appropriate replacement therapy. Dietary treatment is beneficial for many inherited metabolic diseases, including defects of the urea cycle, defects of fatty acid oxidation, gluconeogenic defects, aminoacidopathies, organic acidurias, and the Glut-1 deficiency syndrome and can lead to a better neurologic outcome if started early.

In particular, the ketogenic diet is effective in controlling seizures in patients with the Glut-1 deficiency syndrome, and it improves cognitive outcome in patients with pyruvate dehydrogenase deficiency (E1). Blood ketones should be monitored directly and every effort should be made to maintain a significant ketonemia with blood B-hydroxybutyrate values around 5 mM. Urine ketone measures can be misleading and falsely reassuring.

PKU can be well treated with a diet low in phenylalanine. Protein restriction is recommended for defects of the urea cycle, and fat restriction is advised for defects involving fatty acid oxidation. Pyridoxine-dependent epilepsy and other vitamin-responsive syndromes respond to prompt administration of the specific vitamin or cofactor. A lactose-free diet aids those with primary cerebral folate deficiency. Enzyme protein replacement has proved effective in patients with Gaucher disease. Bone marrow transplantation has been used to treat patients with mucopolysaccharidoses and adrenoleukodystrophy. Some patients with urea cycle defects, gangliosidoses, or leukodystrophies have improved with liver transplantation.

A general rule of thumb in regards to acute treatment when any metabolic disorder leading to epilepsy is suspected as follows:

- Make the patient NPO; this prevents the intake of any potentially harmful compound in the diet
- Begin dextrose-containing IV fluids; dextrose is used here as a dietary substrate and not just to prevent hypoglycemia. It is also a metabolic signal to the body to end catabolism. A high glucose delivery (D10 or D20) can also be used with insulin if needed. Insulin also serves as a metabolic signal to the body to end catabolism and helps maintain normoglycemia
- Correct any electrolyte disturbances
- Prevent fasting and dehydration by administering IV fluids
- Avoid medications that may worsen acidosis including lactated ringers, and valproic acid (when possible)
- Begin empiric trials of pyridoxine, pyridoxal phosphate, biotinidase, and folinic acid while awaiting test results
- Consider beginning IV levocarnitine while awaiting test results

Conventional AEDs may be useful adjuncts to the specific treatment of a metabolic disorder but are often ineffective when used alone. In some circumstances, patients with metabolic derangements or neurodegenerative disorders may worsen with AED treatment that may be contraindicated—for example, phenytoin in patients with Unverricht–Lundborg disease; corticotropin and ketogenic diet in those with pyruvate carboxylase deficiency; ketogenic diet in patients with organic acidurias; and valproate in individuals with urea cycle, fatty acid oxidation, and mitochondrial defects. Metabolites of valproate interfere with β-oxidation, and valproate use depletes carnitine stores. Valproate is also an inhibitor of mitochondrial complex 1 and 4 and can lead to a fatal hepatopathy in patients with mitochondrial *POLG1* gene mutations. Valproate, topiramate, zonisamide, and acetazolamide are relatively contraindicated with the ketogenic diet. Kidney stones are a complication associated with the ketogenic diet, as well as with acetazolamide, zonisamide, and topiramate use. Carnitine should be considered as a supplement in patients with any metabolic disorder that presents with seizures, particularly when valproate is used. An experimental report of inhibited glucose transport with phenobarbital raises concern for its use in patients with Glut-1 deficiency syndrome.

CONCLUSIONS

Seizures are often part of the clinical picture of inherited metabolic disorders, particularly when these conditions first appear during the neonatal period or infancy. Unfortunately, the clinical presentation of seizures is seldom distinctive enough to allow immediate diagnosis. Nevertheless, the timing of onset, certain characteristic clinical features, family history, and EEG findings may facilitate recognition of the more common diagnoses (see Table 32.1). Why seizures commonly accompany some metabolic diseases and infrequently occur in others is only partially understood, but certain correlations are intuitively obvious. Defects in energy metabolism are commonly associated with seizures—for example, the Glut-1 deficiency syndrome, other hypoglycemic syndromes, and defects of pyruvate metabolism; the Krebs cycle; and the respiratory chain. Also, seizures frequently accompany inherited metabolic disorders that affect neurotransmission, such as glycine encephalopathy, pyridoxine-dependent epilepsy, and GABA transaminase deficiency. A more fundamental common mechanism may be operative in many of these conditions. For example, an alteration in the ratio of glutamic acid to GABA may exist in disorders associated with cerebral energy failure and in conditions affecting the GABA shunt. Any inherited metabolic condition in which the extracellular glutamate concentration is elevated and the extracellular GABA concentration is lowered would lower the seizure threshold. Recent studies have confirmed this speculation in patients with symptomatic hypoglycemia, NKH, and pyridoxine-dependent epilepsy.

In contrast, defects of fatty acid oxidation are less likely to be associated with epilepsy. Fatty acids do not serve as oxidizable fuels for brain metabolism. Brain function is compromised mainly when the patient is subjected to fasting and hypoketotic hypoglycemia develops. Under these conditions, the brain is deprived of its two primary fuels, glucose and ketone bodies, and disturbed consciousness and seizures may occur. An exception is short-chain acyl-CoA dehydrogenase deficiency, which is frequently associated with seizures in the absence of hypoglycemia.

Metabolic diseases provide some important insights into the neurochemical determinants of the epileptic state. Alterations of neurotransmission and ion channels are common themes in the pathophysiology of these diverse metabolic conditions. All infants and young children seen with unexplained seizure disorders (cryptogenic epilepsy), and adolescents and adults with unexplained epilepsy that began in childhood should be evaluated for an inherited metabolic disorder. Careful study of patients will continue to identify novel inherited metabolic disorders and lead to more direct and effective treatments of these conditions.

References

1. Horvath GA, Stockler-Ipsiroglu SG, Salvarinova-Zivkovic R, et al. Autosomal recessive GTP cyclohydrolase I deficiency without hyperphenylalaninemia: Evidence of a phenotypic continuum between dominant and recessive forms. *Mol Genet Metab.* 2008;94:127–131.
2. Valle D, Scriver CR, Beaudet A, et al. *Metabolic and Molecular Bases of Inherited Disease.* 8th ed. New York: McGraw-Hill; 2004.
3. Jaggi L, Zurfluh MR, Schuler A, et al. Outcome and long-term follow-up of 36 patients with tetrahydrobiopterin deficiency. *Mol Genet Metab.* 2008;93:295–305.

4. Toone JR, Applegarth DA, Coulter-Mackie MB, et al. Biochemical and molecular investigations of patients with nonketotic hyperglycinemia. *Mol Genet Metab.* 2000;70:116–121.

5. Dinopoulos A, Matsubara Y, Kure S. Atypical variants of nonketotic hyperglycinemia. *Mol Genet Metab.* 2005;86:61–69.

6. Applegarth DA, Toone JR. Nonketotic hyperglycinemia (glycine encephalopathy): Laboratory diagnosis. *Mol Genet Metab.* 2001;74: 139–146.

7. Hamosh A, Maher JF, Bellus GA, et al. Long-term use of high-dose benzoate and dextromethorphan for the treatment of nonketotic hyperglycinemia. *J Pediatr.* 1998;132:709–713.

8. Zammarchi E, Donati MA, Ciani F, et al. Failure of early dextromethorphan and sodium benzoate therapy in an infant with nonketotic hyperglycinemia. *Neuropediatrics.* 1994;25:274–276.

9. Van Hove JL, Kishnani P, Muenzer J, et al. Benzoate therapy and carnitine deficiency in non-ketotic hyperglycinemia. *Am J Med Genet.* 1995;59: 444–453.

10. Matalon R, Naidu S, Hughes JR, et al. Nonketotic hyperglycinemia: Treatment with diazepam—a competitor for glycine receptors. *Pediatrics.* 1983;71:581–584.

11. Boneh A, Degani Y, Harari M. Prognostic clues and outcome of early treatment of nonketotic hyperglycinemia. *Pediatr Neurol.* 1996;15: 137–141.

12. Schiffmann R, Kaye EM, Willis JK, III, et al. Transient neonatal hyperglycinemia. *Ann Neurol.* 1989;25:201–203.

13. Pind S, Slominski E, Mauthe J, et al. V490M, a common mutation in 3-phosphoglycerate dehydrogenase deficiency, causes enzyme deficiency by decreasing the yield of mature enzyme. *J Biol Chem.* 2002;277:7136–7143.

14. de Koning TJ, Klomp LW. Serine-deficiency syndromes. *Curr Opin Neurol.* 2004;17:197–204.

15. Jaeken J. Genetic disorders of gamma-aminobutyric acid, glycine, and serine as causes of epilepsy. *J Child Neurol.* 2002;17(suppl 3):3S84–S87; discussion 3S88.

16. Jakobs C, Bojasch M, Monch E, et al. Urinary excretion of gamma-hydroxybutyric acid in a patient with neurological abnormalities. The probability of a new inborn error of metabolism. *Clin Chim Acta.* 1981;111:169–178.

17. Trettel F, Malaspina P, Jodice C, et al. Human succinic semialdehyde dehydrogenase: Molecular cloning and chromosomal localization. *Adv Exp Med Biol.* 1997;414:253–260.

18. Pearl PL, Gibson KM, Acosta MT, et al. Clinical spectrum of succinic semialdehyde dehydrogenase deficiency. *Neurology.* 2003;60:1413–1417.

19. Pearl PL, Capp PK, Novotny EJ, et al. Inherited disorders of neurotransmitters in children and adults. *Clin Biochem.* 2005;38:1051–1058.

20. Gibson KM, Doskey AE, Rabier D, et al. Differing clinical presentation of succinic semialdehyde dehydrogenase deficiency in adolescent siblings from Lifu Island, New Caledonia. *J Inherit Metab Dis.* 1997;20:370–374.

21. Gropman A. Vigabatrin and newer interventions in succinic semialdehyde dehydrogenase deficiency. *Ann Neurol.* 2003;54(suppl 6):S66–S72.

22. Pearl PL, Gibson KM, Cortez MA, et al. Succinic semialdehyde dehydrogenase deficiency: Lessons from mice and men. *J Inherit Metab Dis.* 2009;32:343–352.

23. Mills PB, Struys E, Jakobs C, et al. Mutations in antiquitin in individuals with pyridoxine-dependent seizures. *Nat Med.* 2006;12:307–309.

24. Wang PJ, Lee WT, Hwu WL, et al. The controversy regarding diagnostic criteria for early myoclonic encephalopathy. *Brain Dev.* 1998;20:530–535.

25. Torres OA, Miller VS, Buist NM, et al. Folinic acid-responsive neonatal seizures. *J Child Neurol.* 1999;14:529–532.

26. Nicolai J, van Kranen-Mastenbroek VH, Wevers RA, et al. Folinic acid-responsive seizures initially responsive to pyridoxine. *Pediatr Neurol.* 2006;34:164–167.

27. Gallagher RC, Van Hove JL, Scharer G, et al. Folinic acid-responsive seizures are identical to pyridoxine-dependent epilepsy. *Ann Neurol.* 2009;65:550–556.

28. Plecko B, Hikel C, Korenke GC, et al. Pipecolic acid as a diagnostic marker of pyridoxine-dependent epilepsy. *Neuropediatrics.* 2005;36:200–205.

29. Chou ML, Wang HS, Hung PC, et al. Late-onset pyridoxine-dependent seizures: Report of two cases. *Zhonghua Min Guo Xiao Er Ke Yi Xue Hui Za Zhi.* 1995;36:434–437.

30. Goutieres F, Aicardi J. Atypical presentations of pyridoxine-dependent seizures: A treatable cause of intractable epilepsy in infants. *Ann Neurol.* 1985;17:117–120.

31. Mills PB, Surtees RA, Champion MP, et al. Neonatal epileptic encephalopathy caused by mutations in the PNPO gene encoding pyridox(am)ine 5'-phosphate oxidase. *Hum Mol Genet.* 2005;14:1077–1086.

32. Johnson JL, Waud WR, Rajagopalan KV, et al. Inborn errors of molybdenum metabolism: Combined deficiencies of sulfite oxidase and xanthine dehydrogenase in a patient lacking the molybdenum cofactor. *Proc Natl Acad Sci USA.* 1980;77:3715–3719.

33. Shalata A, Mandel H, Reiss J, et al. Localization of a gene for molybdenum cofactor deficiency, on the short arm of chromosome 6, by homozygosity mapping. *Am J Hum Genet.* 1998;63:148–154.

34. Reiss J, Dorche C, Stallmeyer B, et al. Human molybdopterin synthase gene: Genomic structure and mutations in molybdenum cofactor deficiency type B. *Am J Hum Genet.* 1999;64:706–711.

35. Johnson JL, Coyne KE, Garrett RM, et al. Isolated sulfite oxidase deficiency: Identification of 12 novel SUOX mutations in 10 patients. *Hum Mutat.* 2002;20:74.

36. Slot HM, Overweg-Plandsoen WC, Bakker HD, et al. Molybdenum-cofactor deficiency: An easily missed cause of neonatal convulsions. *Neuropediatrics.* 1993;24:139–142.

37. Shih VE, Carney MM, Mandell R. A simple screening test for sulfite oxidase deficiency: Detection of urinary thiosulfate by a modification of sorbo's method. *Clin Chim Acta.* 1979;95:143–145.

38. Rupar CA, Gillett J, Gordon BA, et al. Isolated sulfite oxidase deficiency. *Neuropediatrics.* 1996;27:299–304.

39. Lanzkowsky P. Congenital malabsorption of folate. *Am J Med.* 1970;48:580–583.

40. Garcia-Cazorla A, Quadros EV, Nascimento A, et al. Mitochondrial diseases associated with cerebral folate deficiency. *Neurology.* 2008;70: 1360–1362.

41. Ramaekers VT, Sequeira JM, Artuch R, et al. Folate receptor autoantibodies and spinal fluid 5-methyltetrahydrofolate deficiency in rett syndrome. *Neuropediatrics.* 2007;38:179–183.

42. Ramaekers VT, Rothenberg SP, Sequeira JM, et al. Autoantibodies to folate receptors in the cerebral folate deficiency syndrome. *N Engl J Med.* 2005;352:1985–1991.

43. Ramaekers VT, Sequeira JM, Blau N, et al. A milk-free diet downregulates folate receptor autoimmunity in cerebral folate deficiency syndrome. *Dev Med Child Neurol.* 2008;50:346–352.

44. Goyette P, Pai A, Milos R, et al. Gene structure of human and mouse methylenetetrahydrofolate reductase (MTHFR). *Mamm Genome.* 1998;9:652–656.

45. Abeling NG, van Gennip AH, Blom H, et al. Rapid diagnosis and methionine administration: Basis for a favourable outcome in a patient with methylene tetrahydrofolate reductase deficiency. *J Inherit Metab Dis.* 1999;22:240–242.

46. Stockler S, Schutz PW, Salomons GS. Cerebral creatine deficiency syndromes: Clinical aspects, treatment and pathophysiology. *Subcell Biochem.* 2007;46:149–166.

47. Leuzzi V. Inborn errors of creatine metabolism and epilepsy: Clinical features, diagnosis, and treatment. *J Child Neurol.* 2002;17(suppl 3): 3S89–S97; discussion 3S97.

48. Sykut-Cegielska J, Gradowska W, Mercimek-Mahmutoglu S, et al. Biochemical and clinical characteristics of creatine deficiency syndromes. *Acta Biochim Pol.* 2004;51:875–882.

49. Vodopiutz J, Item CB, Hausler M, et al. Severe speech delay as the presenting symptom of guanidinoacetate methyltransferase deficiency. *J Child Neurol.* 2007;22:773–774.

50. Carducci C, Birarelli M, Leuzzi V, et al. Guanidinoacetate and creatine plus creatinine assessment in physiologic fluids: An effective diagnostic tool for the biochemical diagnosis of arginine: Glycine amidinotransferase and guanidinoacetate methyltransferase deficiencies. *Clin Chem.* 2002;48:1772–1778.

51. Aoki Y, Li X, Sakamoto O, et al. Identification and characterization of mutations in patients with holocarboxylase synthetase deficiency. *Hum Genet.* 1999;104:143–148.

52. Hymes J, Stanley CM, Wolf B. Mutations in BTD causing biotinidase deficiency. *Hum Mutat.* 2001;18:375–381.

53. Salbert BA, Pellock JM, Wolf B. Characterization of seizures associated with biotinidase deficiency. *Neurology.* 1993;43:1351–1355.

54. Cecchi C, Biasotto M, Tosi M, et al. The mottled mouse as a model for human menkes disease: Identification of mutations in the Atp7a gene. *Hum Mol Genet.* 1997;6:425–433.

55. Sfaello I, Castelnau P, Blanc N, et al. Infantile spasms and menkes disease. *Epileptic Disord.* 2000;2:227–230.

56. Sztriha L, Janaky M, Kiss J, et al. Electrophysiological and 99mTc-HMPAO-SPECT studies in menkes disease. *Brain Dev.* 1994;16:224–228.

57. Tumer Z, Horn N. Menkes disease: Underlying genetic defect and new diagnostic possibilities. *J Inherit Metab Dis.* 1998;21:604–612.

58. De Vivo DC, Trifiletti RR, Jacobson RI, et al. Defective glucose transport across the blood–brain barrier as a cause of persistent hypoglycorrhachia, seizures, and developmental delay. *N Engl J Med.* 1991;325:703–709.

59. Wang D, Kranz-Eble P, De Vivo DC. Mutational analysis of GLUT1 (SLC2A1) in glut-1 deficiency syndrome. *Hum Mutat.* 2000;16:224–231.

60. Klepper J, Garcia-Alvarez M, O'Driscoll KR, et al. Erythrocyte 3-O-methyl-D-glucose uptake assay for diagnosis of glucose-transporter-protein syndrome. *J Clin Lab Anal.* 1999;13:116–121.

61. Leary LD, Wang D, Nordli DR Jr, et al. Seizure characterization and electroencephalographic features in glut-1 deficiency syndrome. *Epilepsia.* 2003;44:701–707.

62. Brockmann K, Wang D, Korenke CG, et al. Autosomal dominant glut-1 deficiency syndrome and familial epilepsy. *Ann Neurol.* 2001;50:476–485.

63. Klepper J, Scheffer H, Leiendecker B, et al. Seizure control and acceptance of the ketogenic diet in GLUT1 deficiency syndrome: A 2- to 5-year follow-up of 15 children enrolled prospectively. *Neuropediatrics.* 2005;36:302–308.

64. Suls A, Dedeken P, Goffin K, et al. Paroxysmal exercise-induced dyskinesia and epilepsy is due to mutations in SLC2A1, encoding the glucose transporter GLUT1. *Brain.* 2008;131:1831–1844.

65. Weber YG, Storch A, Wuttke TV, et al. GLUT1 mutations are a cause of paroxysmal exertion-induced dyskinesias and induce hemolytic anemia by a cation leak. *J Clin Invest.* 2008;118:2157–2168.

66. De Vivo DC, Wang D. Glut1 deficiency: CSF glucose. How low is too low? *Rev Neurol (Paris).* 2008;164:877–880.

67. van den Berghe G. Disorders of gluconeogenesis. *J Inherit Metab Dis.* 1996;19:470–477.

68. el-Maghrabi MR, Lange AJ, Jiang W, et al. Human fructose-1,6-bisphosphatase gene (FBP1): Exon–intron organization, localization to chromosome bands 9q22.2–q22.3, and mutation screening in subjects with fructose-1,6-bisphosphatase deficiency. *Genomics.* 1995;27:520–525.

69. DiMauro S, Schon EA. Mitochondrial disorders in the nervous system. *Annu Rev Neurosci.* 2008;31:91–123.

70. Haas RH, Parikh S, Falk MJ, et al. The in-depth evaluation of suspected mitochondrial disease. *Mol Genet Metab.* 2008;94:16–37.

71. Chun K, MacKay N, Petrova-Benedict R, et al. Mutations in the X-linked E1 alpha subunit of pyruvate dehydrogenase: Exon skipping, insertion of duplicate sequence, and missense mutations leading to the deficiency of the pyruvate dehydrogenase complex. *Am J Hum Genet.* 1995;56: 558–569.

72. Brown GK, Otero LJ, LeGris M, et al. Pyruvate dehydrogenase deficiency. *J Med Genet.* 1994;31:875–879.

73. Otero LJ, Brown GK, Silver K, et al. Association of cerebral dysgenesis and lactic acidemia with X-linked PDH E1 alpha subunit mutations in females. *Pediatr Neurol.* 1995;13:327–332.

74. Robinson BH, Oei J, Saudubray JM, et al. The French and North American phenotypes of pyruvate carboxylase deficiency, correlation with biotin containing protein by 3H-biotin incorporation, 35S-streptavidin labeling, and northern blotting with a cloned cDNA probe. *Am J Hum Genet.* 1987;40:50–59.

75. Van Coster RN, Fernhoff PM, De Vivo DC. Pyruvate carboxylase deficiency: A benign variant with normal development. *Pediatr Res.* 1991;30:1–4.

76. Wang D, Yang H, De Braganca KC, et al. The molecular basis of pyruvate carboxylase deficiency: Mosaicism correlates with prolonged survival. *Mol Genet Metab.* 2008;95:31–38.

77. DeVivo DC, Haymond MW, Leckie MP, et al. The clinical and biochemical implications of pyruvate carboxylase deficiency. *J Clin Endocrinol Metab.* 1977;45:1281–1296.

78. Rutledge SL, Snead OC III, Kelly DR, et al. Pyruvate carboxylase deficiency: Acute exacerbation after ACTH treatment of infantile spasms. *Pediatr Neurol.* 1989;5:249–252.

79. DiMauro S, De Vivo DC. Genetic heterogeneity in Leigh syndrome. *Ann Neurol.* 1996;40:5–7.

80. Leigh D. Subacute necrotizing encephalomyelopathy in an infant. *J Neurol Neurosurg Psychiatry.* 1951;14:216–221.

81. DiMauro S, Ricci E, Hirano M, et al. Epilepsy in mitochondrial encephalomyopathies. *Epilepsy Res Suppl.* 1991;4:173–180.

82. Kamoshita S, Mizutani I, Fukuyama Y. Leigh's subacute necrotizing encephalomyelopathy in a child with infantile spasms and hypsarrhythmia. *Dev Med Child Neurol.* 1970;12:430–435.

83. Tsao CY, Luquette M, Rusin JA, et al. Leigh syndrome, cytochrome C oxidase deficiency and hypsarrhythmia with infantile spasms. *Clin Electroencephalogr.* 1997;28:214–217.

84. Elia M, Musumeci SA, Ferri R, et al. Leigh syndrome and partial deficit of cytochrome c oxidase associated with epilepsia partialis continua. *Brain Dev.* 1996;18:207–211.

85. Van Erven PM, Colon EJ, Gabreels FJ, et al. Neurophysiological studies in the Leigh syndrome. *Brain Dev.* 1986;8:590–595.

86. O'Connell P, Lathrop GM, Law M, et al. A primary genetic linkage map for human chromosome 12. *Genomics.* 1987;1:93–102.

87. Scriver CR. The PAH gene, phenylketonuria, and a paradigm shift. *Hum Mutat.* 2007;28:831–845.

88. DiLella AG, Kwok SC, Ledley FD, et al. Molecular structure and polymorphic map of the human phenylalanine hydroxylase gene. *Biochemistry.* 1986;25:743–749.

89. Low NL, Bosma JF, Armstrong MD. Studies on phenylketonuria. VI. EEG studies in phenylketonuria. *AMA Arch Neurol Psychiatry.* 1957;77: 359–365.

90. Pietz J, Schmidt E, Matthis P, et al. EEGs in phenylketonuria. I: Follow-up to adulthood; II: Short-term diet-related changes in EEGs and cognitive function. *Dev Med Child Neurol.* 1993;35:54–64.

91. Swaiman K. F. Aminoacidopathies and organic acidemias resulting from deficiency of enzyme activity and transport abnormalities. In: Swaiman KF, Ashwal S, Ferriero DF, eds. *Pediatric Neurology.* 4th ed. St. Louis: Mosby; 2006.

92. Donker DN, Reits D, Van Sprang FJ, et al. Computer analysis of the EEG as an aid in the evaluation of dietetic treatment in phenylketonuria. *Electroencephalogr Clin Neurophysiol.* 1979;46:205–213.

93. Medical Research Council. Recommendations on the dietary management of phenylketonuria. report of medical research council working party on phenylketonuria. *Arch Dis Child.* 1993;68:426–427.

94. Menkes JH, Hurst PL, Craig JM. A new syndrome: Progressive familial infantile cerebral dysfunction associated with an unusual urinary substance. *Pediatrics.* 1954;14:462–467.

95. Nellis MM, Kasinski A, Carlson M, et al. Relationship of causative genetic mutations in maple syrup urine disease with their clinical expression. *Mol Genet Metab.* 2003;80:189–195.

96. Morton DH, Strauss KA, Robinson DL, et al. Diagnosis and treatment of maple syrup disease: A study of 36 patients. *Pediatrics.* 2002;109: 999–1008.

97. Korein J, Sansaricq C, Kalmijn M, et al. Maple syrup urine disease: Clinical, EEG, and plasma amino acid correlations with a theoretical mechanism of acute neurotoxicity. *Int J Neurosci.* 1994;79:21–45.

98. Tharp BR. Unique EEG pattern (comb-like rhythm) in neonatal maple syrup urine disease. *Pediatr Neurol.* 1992;8:65–68.

99. Sidbury JB, Jr, Smith EK, Harlan W. An inborn error of short-chain fatty acid metabolism: The odor-of-sweaty-feet syndrome. *J Pediatr.* 1967;70: 8–15.

100. Kennerknecht I, Klett C, Hameister H. Assignment of the human gene propionyl coenzyme A carboxylase, alpha-chain (PCCA) to chromosome 13q32 by in situ hybridization. *Genomics.* 1992;14:550–551.

101. Stigsby B, Yarworth SM, Rahbeeni Z, et al. Neurophysiologic correlates of organic acidemias: A survey of 107 patients. *Brain Dev.* 1994; 16(suppl):125–144.

102. Bartholomew DW, Batshaw ML, Allen RH, et al. Therapeutic approaches to cobalamin-C methylmalonic acidemia and homocystinuria. *J Pediatr.* 1988;112:32–39.

103. Enns GM, Barkovich AJ, Rosenblatt DS, et al. Progressive neurological deterioration and MRI changes in cblC methylmalonic acidaemia treated with hydroxocobalamin. *J Inherit Metab Dis.* 1999;22:599–607.

104. Mahoney MJ, Bick D. Recent advances in the inherited methylmalonic acidemias. *Acta Paediatr Scand.* 1987;76:689–696.

105. Guevara-Campos J, Gonzalez-de-Guevara L, Medina-Atopo M. Methylmalonic aciduria associated with myoclonic convulsions, psychomotor retardation and hypsarrhythmia. *Rev Neurol.* 2003;36:735–737.

106. Gibson KM, Wappner RS, Jooste S, et al. Variable clinical presentation in three patients with 3-methylglutaconyl-coenzyme A hydratase deficiency. *J Inherit Metab Dis.* 1998;21:631–638.

107. Wang S, Nadeau JH, Duncan A, et al. 3-Hydroxy-3-methylglutaryl coenzyme A lyase (HL): Cloning and characterization of a mouse liver HL cDNA and subchromosomal mapping of the human and mouse HL genes. *Mamm Genome.* 1993;4:382–387.

108. Hoffmann GF, Zschocke J. Glutaric aciduria type I: From clinical, biochemical and molecular diversity to successful therapy. *J Inherit Metab Dis.* 1999;22:381–391.

109. Tuchman M, Lee B, Lichter-Konecki U, et al. Cross-sectional multicenter study of patients with urea cycle disorders in the United States. *Mol Genet Metab.* 2008;94:397–402.

110. Bachmann C. Inherited hyperammonemias. In: Blau N, Duran M, Blaskovics ME, et al., eds. *Physician's Guide to the Laboratory Diagnosis of Metabolic Diseases.* 2nd ed. Berlin: Springer; 2003.

111. Lien J, Nyhan WL, Barshop BA. Fatal initial adult-onset presentation of urea cycle defect. *Arch Neurol.* 2007;64:1777–1779.

112. Summar M. Current strategies for the management of neonatal urea cycle disorders. *J Pediatr.* 2001;138:S30–S39.

113. Garcia-Alvarez M, Nordli DR, DeVivo DC, eds. Inherited metabolic disorders. In: Engel J Jr, Pedley TA, Aicardi J, et al., eds. *Epilepsy: A Comprehensive Textbook.* 2nd ed. Philadelphia: Lippincott Williams & Wilkins; 2007.

114. Verma NP, Hart ZH, Kooi KA. Electroencephalographic findings in urea-cycle disorders. *Electroencephalogr Clin Neurophysiol.* 1984;57: 105–112.

115. Naidu S, Niedermeyer E, Aalto A. Degenerative disorders of the central nervous system. In: Niedermeyer E, LopesDaSilva F, eds. *Electroencephalography: Basic Principles, Clinical Applications, and Related Fields.* 5th ed. Baltimore: Lippincott Williams & Wilkins; 2004.

116. Todo S, Starzl TE, Tzakis A, et al. Orthotopic liver transplantation for urea cycle enzyme deficiency. *Hepatology.* 1992;15:419–422.

117. Yazaki M, Ikeda S, Takei Y, et al. Complete neurological recovery of an adult patient with type II citrullinemia after living related partial liver transplantation. *Transplantation.* 1996;62:1679–1684.

118. Bonnefont JP, Djouadi F, Prip-Buus C, et al. Carnitine palmitoyltransferases 1 and 2: Biochemical, molecular and medical aspects. *Mol Aspects Med.* 2004;25:495–520.

119. Tein I. Role of carnitine and fatty acid oxidation and its defects in infantile epilepsy. *J Child Neurol.* 2002;17(suppl 3):3S57–3S82; discussion 3S82–3S83.

120. Depreter M, Espeel M, Roels F. Human peroxisomal disorders. *Microsc Res Tech.* 2003;61:203–223.

121. Moser AB, Rasmussen M, Naidu S, et al. Phenotype of patients with peroxisomal disorders subdivided into sixteen complementation groups. *J Pediatr.* 1995;127:13–22.

122. Soorani-Lunsing RJ, van Spronsen FJ, Stolte-Dijkstra I, et al. Normal very-long-chain fatty acids in peroxisomal D-bifunctional protein deficiency: A diagnostic pitfall. *J Inherit Metab Dis.* 2005;28:1172–1174.

123. Steinberg SJ, Elcioglu N, Slade CM, et al. Peroxisomal disorders: Clinical and biochemical studies in 15 children and prenatal diagnosis in 7 families. *Am J Med Genet.* 1999;85:502–510.

124. Takahashi Y, Suzuki Y, Kumazaki K, et al. Epilepsy in peroxisomal diseases. *Epilepsia.* 1997;38:182–188.

125. Poll-The BT, Roels F, Ogier H, et al. A new peroxisomal disorder with enlarged peroxisomes and a specific deficiency of acyl-CoA oxidase (pseudo-neonatal adrenoleukodystrophy). *Am J Hum Genet.* 1988;42:422–434.

126. Ferdinandusse S, Denis S, Hogenhout EM, et al. Clinical, biochemical, and mutational spectrum of peroxisomal acyl-coenzyme A oxidase deficiency. *Hum Mutat.* 2007;28:904–912.

127. Nakai H, Byers MG, Nowak NJ, et al. Assignment of beta-hexosaminidase A alpha-subunit to human chromosomal region 15q23–q24. *Cytogenet Cell Genet.* 1991;56:164.

128. Cobb W, Martin F, Pampiglione G. Cerebral lipidosis: An electroencephalographic study. *Brain.* 1952;75:343–357.

129. Yamanaka S, Johnson ON, Norflus F, et al. Structure and expression of the mouse beta-hexosaminidase genes, hexa and hexb. *Genomics.* 1994;21:588–596.

130. Zakharova E, Boukina TM. Gene symbol: GALC disease: Krabbe disease. *Hum Genet.* 2008;124:299.

131. Suzuki K. Globoid cell leukodystrophy (Krabbe's disease): Update. *J Child Neurol.* 2003;18:595–603.

132. Blom S, Hagberg B. EEG findings in late infantile metachromatic and globoid cell leucodystrophy. *Electroencephalogr Clin Neurophysiol.* 1967;22:253–259.

133. Kliemann FA, Harden A, Pampiglione G. Some E.E.G. observations in patients with Krabbe's disease. *Dev Med Child Neurol.* 1969;11:475–484.

134. Brunetti-Pierri N, Scaglia F. GM1 gangliosidosis: Review of clinical, molecular, and therapeutic aspects. *Mol Genet Metab.* 2008;94:391–396.

135. Harden A, Martinovic Z, Pampiglione G. Neurophysiological studies in GM1, gangliosidosis. *Ital J Neurol Sci.* 1982;3:201–206.

136. Salonen R, Somer M, Haltia M, et al. Progressive encephalopathy with edema, hypsarrhythmia, and optic atrophy (PEHO syndrome). *Clin Genet.* 1991;39:287–293.

137. Somer M, Sainio K. Epilepsy and the electroencephalogram in progressive encephalopathy with edema, hypsarrhythmia, and optic atrophy (the PEHO syndrome). *Epilepsia.* 1993;34:727–731.

138. Wisniewski KE, Zhong N, Philippart M. Pheno/genotypic correlations of neuronal ceroid lipofuscinoses. *Neurology.* 2001;57:576–581.

139. Beaudoin D, Hagenzieker J, Jack R. Neuronal ceroid lipofuscinosis: What are the roles of electron microscopy, DNA and enzyme analysis in diagnosis? *J Histotechnol.* 2004;27:237–243.

140. Jalanko A, Braulke T. Neuronal ceroid lipofuscinoses. *Biochim Biophys Acta.* 2009;1793:697–709.

141. Gieselmann V. Metachromatic leukodystrophy: Recent research developments. *J Child Neurol.* 2003;18:591–594.

142. Balslev T, Cortez MA, Blaser SI, Haslam RH. Recurrent seizures in metachromatic leukodystrophy. *Pediatr Neurol.* 1997;17:150–154.

143. Fukumizu M, Matsui K, Hanaoka S, et al. Partial seizures in two cases of metachromatic leukodystrophy: Electrophysiologic and neuroradiologic findings. *J Child Neurol.* 1992;7:381–386.

144. Wang PJ, Hwu WL, Shen YZ. Epileptic seizures and electroencephalographic evolution in genetic leukodystrophies. *J Clin Neurophysiol.* 2001;18:25–32.

145. Solders G, Celsing G, Hagenfeldt L, et al. Improved peripheral nerve conduction, EEG and verbal IQ after bone marrow transplantation for adult metachromatic leukodystrophy. *Bone Marrow Transplant.* 1998;22:1119–1122.

146. Lugowska A, Wlodarski P, Ploski R, et al. Molecular and clinical consequences of novel mutations in the arylsulfatase A gene. *Clin Genet.* 2009;75:57–64.

147. Muenzer J. The mucopolysaccharidoses: A heterogeneous group of disorders with variable pediatric presentations. *J Pediatr.* 2004;144:S27–S34.

148. Zhang W, Huiping S. Gene symbol: SGSH disease: Sanfilippo syndrome type A. *Hum Genet.* 2008;124:323.

149. Kriel RL, Hauser WA, Sung JH, et al. Neuroanatomical and electroencephalographic correlations in sanfilippo syndrome, type A. *Arch Neurol.* 1978;35:838–843.

150. Pastores GM. Laronidase (aldurazyme): Enzyme replacement therapy for mucopolysaccharidosis type I. *Expert Opin Biol Ther.* 2008;8:1003–1009.

151. Engel J, Jr, Rapin I, Giblin DR. Electrophysiological studies in two patients with cherry red spot—myoclonus syndrome. *Epilepsia.* 1977;18:73–87.

152. Pshezhetsky AV, Richard C, Michaud L, et al. Cloning, expression and chromosomal mapping of human lysosomal sialidase and characterization of mutations in sialidosis. *Nat Genet.* 1997;15:316–320.

153. Okamura-Oho Y, Zhang S, Callahan JW. The biochemistry and clinical features of galactosialidosis. *Biochim Biophys Acta.* 1994;1225:244–254.

154. Ginns EI, Choudary PV, Tsuji S, et al. Gene mapping and leader polypeptide sequence of human glucocerebrosidase: Implications for Gaucher disease. *Proc Natl Acad Sci USA.* 1985;82:7101–7105.

155. Nishimura R, Omos-Lau N, Ajmone-Marsan C, et al. Electroencephalographic findings in Gaucher disease. *Neurology.* 1980;30:152–159.

156. Krivit W, Peters C, Shapiro EG. Bone marrow transplantation as effective treatment of central nervous system disease in globoid cell leukodystrophy, metachromatic leukodystrophy, adrenoleukodystrophy, mannosidosis, fucosidosis, aspartylglucosaminuria, hurler, maroteaux-lamy, and sly syndromes, and Gaucher disease type III. *Curr Opin Neurol.* 1999;12:167–176.

157. Ferriss GS, Happel LT, Duncan MC. Cerebral cortical isolation in infantile neuroaxonal dystrophy. *Electroencephalogr Clin Neurophysiol.* 1977;43:168–182.

158. Butzer JF, Schochet SS, Jr, Bell WE. Infantile neuroaxonal dystrophy: An electron microscopic study of a case clinically resembling neuronal ceroid-lipofuscinosis. *Acta Neuropathol.* 1975;31:35–43.

159. Wakai S, Asanuma H, Tachi N, et al. Infantile neuroaxonal dystrophy: Axonal changes in biopsied muscle tissue. *Pediatr Neurol.* 1993;9:309–311.

160. Wakai S, Asanuma H, Hayasaka H, et al. Ictal video-EEG analysis of infantile neuroaxonal dystrophy. *Epilepsia.* 1994;35:823–826.

161. Desnick RJ, Wang AM. Schindler disease: An inherited neuroaxonal dystrophy due to alpha-N-acetylgalactosaminidase deficiency. *J Inherit Metab Dis.* 1990;13:549–559.

162. Engelsen BA, Tzoulis C, Karlsen B, et al. POLG1 mutations cause a syndromic epilepsy with occipital lobe predilection. *Brain.* 2008;131:818–828.

163. Chan SS, Copeland WC. DNA polymerase gamma and mitochondrial disease: Understanding the consequence of POLG mutations. *Biochim Biophys Acta.* 2009;1787:312–319.

164. Boyd SG, Harden A, Egger J, et al. Progressive neuronal degeneration of childhood with liver disease ("alpers' disease"): Characteristic neurophysiological features. *Neuropediatrics.* 1986;17:75–80.

165. Wolf NI, Rahman S, Schmitt B, et al. Status epilepticus in children with alpers' disease caused by POLG1 mutations: EEG and MRI features. *Epilepsia.* 2008;50:1596–1607.

166. McFarland R, Hudson G, Taylor RW, et al. Reversible valproate hepatotoxicity due to mutations in mitochondrial DNA polymerase gamma (POLG1). *Arch Dis Child.* 2008;93:151–153.

167. Finsterer J. Genetic, pathogenetic, and phenotypic implications of the mitochondrial A3243G tRNALeu(UUR) mutation. *Acta Neurol Scand.* 2007;116:1–14.

168. Berkovic SF, Shoubridge EA, Andermann F, et al. Clinical spectrum of mitochondrial DNA mutation at base pair 8344. *Lancet.* 1991;338:457.

169. Ikeuchi T, Koide R, Onodera O, et al. Dentatorubral-pallidoluysian atrophy (DRPLA): Molecular basis for wide clinical features of DRPLA. *Clin Neurosci.* 1995;3:23–27.

170. Saitoh S, Momoi MY, Yamagata T, et al. Clinical and electroencephalographic findings in juvenile type DRPLA. *Pediatr Neurol.* 1998;18:265–268.

171. Freeze HH. Update and perspectives on congenital disorders of glycosylation. *Glycobiology.* 2001;11:129R–143R.

172. Petersen MB, Brostrom K, Stibler H, et al. Early manifestations of the carbohydrate-deficient glycoprotein syndrome. *J Pediatr.* 1993;122:66–70.

173. Freeze HH. Genetic defects in the human glycome. *Nat Rev Genet.* 2006;7:537–551.

174. Bezman L, Moser AB, Raymond GV, et al. Adrenoleukodystrophy: Incidence, new mutation rate, and results of extended family screening. *Ann Neurol.* 2001;49:512–517.

175. Mamoli B, Graf M, Toifl K. EEG, pattern-evoked potentials and nerve conduction velocity in a family with adrenoleucodystrophy. *Electroencephalogr Clin Neurophysiol.* 1979;47:411–419.

176. Berkovic SF, Cochius J, Andermann E, et al. Progressive myoclonus epilepsies: Clinical and genetic aspects. *Epilepsia.* 1993;34(suppl 3):S19–S30.

177. Ganesh S, Puri R, Singh S, et al. Recent advances in the molecular basis of Lafora's progressive myoclonus epilepsy. *J Hum Genet.* 2006;51:1–8.

178. Minassian BA. Progressive myoclonus epilepsy with polyglucosan bodies: Lafora disease. *Adv Neurol.* 2002;89:199–210.

179. Ponsford S, Pye IF, Elliot EJ. Posterior paroxysmal discharge: An aid to early diagnosis in Lafora disease. *J R Soc Med.* 1993;86:597–599.

180. Joensuu T, Kuronen M, Alakurtti K, et al. Cystatin B: Mutation detection, alternative splicing and expression in progressive myoclonus epilepsy of Unverricht–Lundborg type (EPM1) patients. *Eur J Hum Genet.* 2007;15:185–193.

181. Magaudda A, Ferlazzo E, Nguyen VH, et al. Unverricht–Lundborg disease, a condition with self-limited progression: Long-term follow-up of 20 patients. *Epilepsia.* 2006;47:860–866.

182. Berkovic SF, So NK, Andermann F. Progressive myoclonus epilepsies: Clinical and neurophysiological diagnosis. *J Clin Neurophysiol.* 1991;8:261–274.

183. Koskiniemi M, Toivakka E, Donner M. Progressive myoclonus epilepsy. electroencephalographical findings. *Acta Neurol Scand.* 1974;50:333–359.

184. Medina MT, Martinez-Juarez IE, Duron RM, et al. Treatment of myoclonic epilepsies of childhood, adolescence, and adulthood. *Adv Neurol.* 2005;95:307–323.

185. Munke M, Kraus JP, Ohura T, et al. The gene for cystathionine beta-synthase (CBS) maps to the subtelomeric region on human chromosome 21q and to proximal mouse chromosome 17. *Am J Hum Genet.* 1988;42:550–559.

186. Mudd SH, Skovby F, Levy HL, et al. The natural history of homocystinuria due to cystathionine beta-synthase deficiency. *Am J Hum Genet.* 1985;37:1–31.

187. Del Giudice E, Striano S, Andria G. Electroencephalographic abnormalities in homocystinuria due to cystathionine synthase deficiency. *Clin Neurol Neurosurg.* 1983;85:165–168.

CHAPTER 33 ■ NEONATAL SEIZURES

KEVIN E. CHAPMAN, ELI M. MIZRAHI, AND ROBERT R. CLANCY

Neonatal seizures are a classic and ominous neurologic sign that can arise in any newborn infant. Their significance lies in their high incidence, association with acute neonatal encephalopathies, substantial mortality, neurologic morbidity, and the concern that seizures per se could extend the acute brain injury. Seizures in the neonate differ clinically and electrographically from those in mature infants and children. Diagnostic and treatment decisions remain limited by a paucity of rigorous scientific data for this population. This chapter reviews the significance of neonatal seizures, the pathophysiologic basis of clinical, electroclinical, and electrographic seizures, prognostic expectations, and etiologies, and surveys current treatment options that might themselves pose a risk to the developing brain.

HISTORICAL BACKGROUND

The appearance of "seizures," "fits," or "convulsions" in newborn infants has been known since antiquity. *Seizure* is derived from a Greek word implying a sudden "attack of disease." The invention of the electroencephalograph (EEG) by Hans Berger allowed investigators to discover the epileptic mechanisms that underlie seizure expression in mature individuals. It was naturally assumed that clinical seizures in neonates were always associated with abnormal, excessive, paroxysmal electrical discharges arising from repetitive neuronal firing in the cerebral cortex. Despite the identification of electroclinical correlations of seizures in mature individuals, progress in understanding the nosology of neonatal seizures was only recently notable. Although some neonatal seizures

are accompanied by simultaneous epileptic discharges seen on EEG, not every clinical event in a neonate presenting as an abrupt "attack" is truly epileptic, and the relationship between neonatal seizures and the conventional connotations of the term *epilepsy* demands careful scrutiny. Thus, seizures in the neonate are now distributed into three classes (Fig. 33.1). "Electroclinical" seizures are abnormal, clinically observable events that are consistently founded on a specific epileptic mechanism and coincide with an obvious electrographic seizure during simultaneous EEG monitoring. "Clinical-only" seizures refer to other abnormal-appearing abrupt clinical events that are not associated with simultaneous electrographic seizure activity during EEG monitoring; they may be considered a type of *nonepileptic* seizure; "EEG-only" seizures lack definite clinical seizure activity; they are also called "subclinical" or "occult."

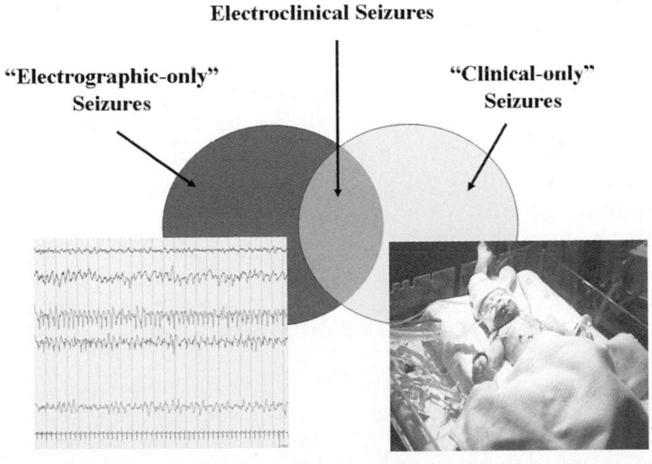

SIGNIFICANCE OF NEONATAL SEIZURES

Incidence

The incidence of seizures in the first 28 days of life, one of the highest risk periods for seizures in humans, ranges between 1% and 5%. Depending on the methodology used, seizures occur at a rate of 1.5 to 5.5 per 1000 neonates (1–7), most within the first week of life (4). Incidence varies with specific risk factors. Lanska and colleagues (4) reported the incidence of seizures in all neonates to be 3.5 per 1000, but 57.5 per 1000 in very-low-birth-weight (<1500 g) infants, 4.4 per 1000 in low-birth-weight (1500 to 2499 g) infants, and 2.8 per 1000 in normal-birth-weight (2500 to 3999 g) infants. Scher and colleagues (8,9) described seizures in 3.9% of neonates younger than 30 weeks conceptional age and in 1.5% of those older than 30 conceptional weeks.

The human newborn is especially vulnerable to a wide range of toxic or metabolic conditions. Sepsis, meningitis, hypoxic–ischemic encephalopathy (HIE), hypoglycemia, and hyperbilirubinemia are capable of eliciting seizures. This may explain, in part, the frequent occurrence of brain-damaging events in the first 30 days of life. While most neonatal seizures commonly result from an underlying acute illness, some are reversible, indicating a potentially *treatable* condition. For example, the presence of hypocalcemia, hypomagnesemia, hypoglycemia, pyridoxine deficiency, or sepsis-meningitis may be heralded by neonatal seizures.

It is now well established that the neonatal brain itself may be especially prone to seizures when injured. One suspected mechanism of enhanced seizure susceptibility in the newborn

FIGURE 33.1. Three types of "seizures" in the newborn: "electrographic only," "electroclinical," and "clinical only."

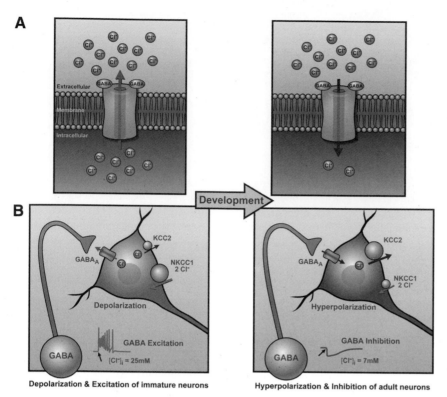

FIGURE 33.2. Developmental changes in chloride homeostasis during development. **A:** During development, the intracellular chloride concentration decreases. In the immature neurons, efflux of the negatively charged chloride ions produces inward electric current and depolarization. In the mature neurons, chloride enters the cell and produces outward electric current and hyperpolarization. **B:** Developmental change in the intracellular chloride is due to the changes in the expression of the two major chloride cotransporters, KCC2 and NKCC1. Chloride extruder KCC2 is expressed late in development, whereas NKCC1, which accumulates chloride in the cell, is more expressed in the immature neurons. (Adapted from Ben-ari Y, Gaiarsa J, Tyzio R, et al. GABA: a pioneer transmitter that excites immature neurons and generates primitive oscillations. *Physiol Rev.* 2007;87:1215–1284, with permission.)

is the relative imbalance between inhibition and excitation. Compared with more mature brains, the neonatal brain exhibits delayed maturation of inhibitory circuits and precocious maturation of excitatory circuits (10). This "imbalance" reflects a desirable and natural aspect of early central nervous system (CNS) development characterized by exuberant growth of excitatory synapses (10) coupled with activity-dependent pruning that is necessary for the prodigious rate of novel learning that faces all neonates. Moreover, according to studies in the neonatal rat, γ-aminobutyric acid (GABA)—the major inhibitory neurotransmitter in the mature brain—may exert paradoxically *excitatory* effects in early CNS development (11,12).

A developmentally dependent cation chloride cotransporter channel (KCC2)—which extrudes chloride into the extracellular space—does not reach mature levels in the rat hippocampus until after the third postnatal week (Fig. 33.2). Instead, early in development, the NKCC1 transporter predominates and actively transports chloride into the neuron. Thus, when the ligand-dependent $GABA_A$ receptor is activated in the immature rat, extracellular chloride follows its electrochemical gradient out of the neuron and paradoxically depolarizes it. After the appearance of KCC2, the intracellular concentration of chloride is kept low, and activation of the $GABA_A$ receptor allows chloride to run along its electrochemical gradient into the neuron. This leads to hyperpolarization and allows for the inhibitory action of the receptor (13,14). Current electrophysiological evidence suggests that this excitatory-to-inhibitory switch in the rat hippocampus is complete by postnatal day 14 (15,16), an age that may reflect the developmental state of a human toddler. Interestingly, oxytocin has been suggested to induce the switch in GABA from excitatory to inhibitory through downregulation of NKCC1. An oxytocin receptor antagonist administered prior

to delivery prevented the expected switch to GABA hyperpolarization and exacerbated anoxic injury in perinatal rat pups (17).

The paradoxically excitatory effect of GABA during the neonatal period potentially contributes to the refractoriness of neonatal seizures to phenobarbital and benzodiazepines. In some experimental models of induced neonatal seizures, inhibition of the NKCC1 transporter with bumetanide alters chloride transport and significantly enhances the anticonvulsant effects of phenobarbital in neonatal rat hippocampi (18). Clinical studies using bumetanide have been proposed and are in the planning stages.

Glutamatergic receptors also regulate excitability in the immature neuron and undergo developmental changes that contribute to the propensity of the neonate to seizures. Glutamate receptors are classified according to their sensitivity to various ligands: N-methyl-D-aspartate (NMDA), α-amino-3-hydroxy-5-methyl-4-isoxazolepropionic acid (AMPA), and kainate. These receptors can have various functional properties based on their subunit composition that changes during development. NMDA receptors in immature neurons express primarily the NR2B subunit that prolongs the duration of the excitatory postsynaptic potential. Increased expression of the NR2C, NR2D, and NR3A subunits confer a reduced sensitivity to blockade by magnesium, resulting in increased excitability (19).

Prognostic Significance

Neonatal seizures are a powerful prognostic indicator of mortality and neurologic morbidity. The summary report from Bergman and associates (2) of 1667 patients noted an overall mortality of 24.7% before 1969 and 18% after 1970. Volpe (20) cited a mortality rate of 40% before 1969 and 15% after

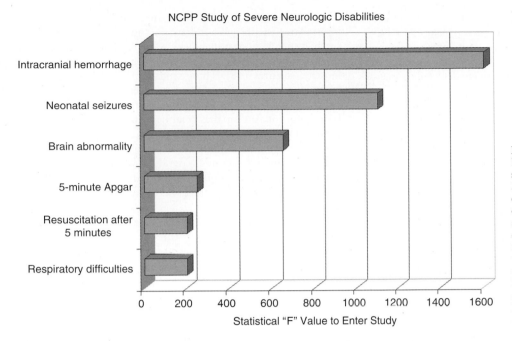

NCPP Study of Severe Neurologic Disabilities

FIGURE 33.3. The National Collaborative Perinatal Population (NCPP) study prospectively followed more than 34,000 mothers to identify perinatal events associated with adverse outcomes. Fifty neonates were found with subsequent severe neurologic handicaps. Six independent variables, including neonatal seizures, were associated with such neurologically devastating outcomes. (Adapted from Nelson KB, Broman SH. Perinatal risk factors in children with serious motor and mental handicaps. *Ann Neurol.* 1977;2: 371–377, with permission.)

1969. According to Lombroso (21), mortality decreased modestly from about 20% previously to 16% in the early 1980s. These improvements probably reflect better obstetrical management and modern neonatal intensive care. All of these studies relied on seizure diagnosis by clinical criteria and did not require EEG confirmation.

Survivors of neonatal seizures face an exceptionally high risk for cerebral palsy, often with mental retardation and chronic postnatal epilepsy. The National Collaborative Perinatal Population (NCPP) study (22,23) examined numerous clinical perinatal factors for their association with severe mental retardation, cerebral palsy, and microcephaly (Fig. 33.3). The clinical diagnosis of "neonatal seizures" was independently and significantly associated with these adverse outcomes and eclipsed only by "intracranial hemorrhage" in forecasting them. Neurologic functioning may even be impaired in those who appear "normal" after neonatal seizures (24).

Contemporary studies of the prognosis after neonatal seizures have emphasized the inclusion of infants whose seizure type was confirmed by EEG monitoring. Outcome has been assessed in terms of survival, neurologic disability, developmental delay, and postnatal epilepsy. Ortibus and colleagues (25) reported that 28% died; 22% of survivors were neurologically normal at an average of 17 months of age; 14% had mild abnormalities; and 36% were severely abnormal. In 2007, Pisani and colleagues (26) identified 106 consecutively admitted neonates with video-EEG confirmed seizures over a 5-year period. The mortality rate was 19% with a favorable outcome found in only 34% of patients. Cerebral palsy was identified in 37%, developmental delay in 34%, and 21% had postnatal epilepsy at 24 months of follow-up.

Preliminary results of the Neonatal Seizures Clinical Research Centers from 1992 to 1997 have been reported (27). Of the 207 full-term infants with video-EEG-confirmed seizures who were prospectively enrolled, 28% died. Two-year follow-up data were available for 122 patients, or 86% of the survivors. Abnormal neurologic findings were noted in

42%. A Mental Developmental Index (MDI) score below 80 was present in 55%, a Psychomotor Developmental Index (PDI) score less than 80 in 50%, and chronic postnatal epilepsy in 26%.

Whether seizures themselves adversely affect the developing brain is difficult to determine from clinical studies. Seizure *burden* may appear to influence outcome because some infants who experience brief, infrequent seizures may have relatively good long-term outcomes, whereas those with prolonged seizures often do not fare as well. However, easily controlled or self-limited seizures may be the result of transient, successfully treated, or benign CNS disorders of neonates, while medically refractory neonatal seizures may stem from more sustained, less treatable, or more severe brain disorders. Legido and associates (28) studied 40 neonates with electrographic seizures detected on randomly timed routine EEG examinations and monitored them for cerebral palsy, mental retardation, and epilepsy. Overall neurologic outcome was more favorable in those with two or fewer seizures per hour than in those with more than that number. In the subgroup with seizures caused by asphyxia, cerebral palsy was more frequent when more than five seizures occurred per hour. However, these results might equally reflect more severe underlying injuries that triggered both the additional short-term seizures and greater morbidity on long-term follow-up.

Attempting a balanced approach, McBride and coworkers (29) followed up 68 high-risk neonates with birth asphyxia, meningitis, and other stressors linked to neonatal seizures. All infants underwent long-term EEG monitoring. Forty developed electrographic seizures, while 28 did not. Based on logistic regression analysis, electrographic neonatal seizures were significantly correlated with death and cerebral palsy. One study found that patients with neonatal status epilepticus were at a higher risk for severe neurologic disability and postnatal epilepsy than those with fewer seizures (22). Other investigators (30), using proton magnetic resonance spectroscopy

(^{1}H-MRS), found an association of measures of seizure severity with impaired cerebral metabolism measured by lactate/choline and compromised neuronal integrity measured by N-acetylaspartate/choline, and suggested this as evidence of brain injury not limited to structural damage detected by magnetic resonance imaging (MRI).

Neonatal Seizures May Be Inherently Harmful

Neonatal seizures may be intrinsically harmful to the brain (31). Most seizures were long assumed to be the innocuous, albeit conspicuous, result of an acute injury, and the subsequent long-term neurodevelopmental abnormalities the result of their underlying causes, not the seizures themselves. Basic laboratory studies focused on the effects of seizures on the developing brain have not resolved the controversy (32–36). Immature animals are more resistant than older animals to some seizure-induced injury (37). The immature brain may be resistant to acute seizure-induced cell loss (34); however, functional abnormalities such as impairment of visual–spatial memory and reduced seizure threshold (38) occur after seizures, and seizures have been noted to induce changes in brain development, including altered neurogenesis (39), synaptogenesis, synaptic pruning, neuronal migration, and the sequential expression of genes including neurotransmitter receptors and transporters (40,41).

While neonatal seizures seem to induce little histologic damage to the brain (37), studies have revealed that recurrent seizures can produce long-lasting changes in the developing brain, making them more prone to epilepsy and impairing future learning and behavior. Holmes and colleagues (42) documented impaired spatial learning and memory, decreased activity levels, significantly lower threshold to pentylenetetrazol-induced seizures, and sprouting of CA3 mossy fibers in adult rats that had recurrent neonatal seizures compared to those without neonatal seizures.

Alterations in receptor subunit expression have been implicated as a cause for some of the changes following neonatal seizures. Status epilepticus induced in neonatal rats produced decreased expression of the AMPA receptor GluR2 subunit and increased susceptibility to kainate-induced seizures later in life (43). A recent study demonstrated that a single episode of seizures in neonatal rat pups (at P7) produced long-lasting alterations in excitatory glutametergic synapses that impaired working memory in adulthood (44). The single episode of recurrent seizures over a 3-hour period reduced NMDA receptor NR2A subunit expression and shifted GluR1 subunits to intracellular pools, making them unavailable for incorporation into postsynaptic membranes (44). Recurrent neonatal seizures likewise produced decreased NR2A expression (45).

The most frequent clinical setting for the occurrence of neonatal seizures in both term and preterm neonates is following hypoxic–ischemic injury (20). A rodent study of hypoxia-induced seizures demonstrated a decrease in GluR2 receptor expression allowing an increase in calcium influx that may contribute to the chronic epileptogenic effects of hypoxia-induced neonatal seizures (46). Treatment with AMPA receptor antagonists, but not NMDA receptor or GABA$_A$ receptor antagonists, after hypoxia-induced seizures in neonatal rats reduced the susceptibility to seizures and seizure-induced injury later in life (47). Likewise, topiramate—which acts mechanistically in part by blocking AMPA/kainate receptors—exerts anticonvulsant activity against perinatal hypoxia-induced seizures (48). These studies highlight the potential utility of topiramate in neonates with seizures associated with hypoxic–ischemic encephalopathy, but the lack of an intravenous formulation makes treatment in critically ill children challenging (49). A concern with recurrent neonatal seizures is the concept that "seizures beget seizures"—with recurrent seizures inducing secondary ictal onset zones. An elegant study by Khalilov and colleagues (50) attempted to determine if GABA or NMDA signaling was required for creation of a secondary epileptogenic focus. They dissected two intact neonatal hippocampi with their connecting commissural fibers and placed them in three contiguous chambers. Recurrent seizures were induced in one hippocampus with repeated doses of kainate that eventually propagated to the other hippocampus and established a secondary epileptogenic focus. Addition of an NMDA receptor antagonist to the seizure naïve hippocampus (not stimulated with kainate) inhibited the creation of a "mirror-focus." Interestingly, GABAergic synapses in this system became excitatory in the secondary focus, which is known to be an important contributor to epileptogenesis in the neonatal hippocampus. This study again supports the possible role of NMDA receptor antagonists in the clinical treatment of neonatal seizures.

Finally, neonatal seizures in rats alter the subsequent composition of the GABA$_A$ receptor. Each GABA$_A$ receptor is a pentamer in which five subunits assemble into a functional ligand-gated receptor (Fig. 33.4). Six subunit classes may comprise the pentamer: six variants of alpha, three of beta, three of gamma, one of delta, one of epsilon, and three of rho. The specific composition of an individual GABA$_A$ receptor depends on developmental age. In the studies of Zhang and associates (12), rats with neonatal seizures had a substantially higher proportion of the α_1 GABA$_A$ subunit than did control animals (Fig. 33.5) (51). Higher levels of the α_1 GABA$_A$ subunit may provide a protective role in decreasing the severity or frequency of seizures later in life following earlier neonatal seizures (52).

CLASSIFICATION AND CLINICAL FEATURES OF NEONATAL SEIZURES

Application of a syndromic classification to neonatal seizures is limited when considered in light of the classification of the International League Against Epilepsy (ILAE) (53,54). Almost all neonatal seizures are thought to be symptomatic, an acute reaction, or consequence of a specific etiology. The ILAE addresses only five neonatal syndromes: benign neonatal convulsions, benign familial neonatal convulsions (BFNC), early myoclonic encephalopathy (EME), early infantile epileptic encephalopathy (EIEE), and migrating partial seizures of infancy. These are discussed later.

Seizures in the neonate are uniquely different from those in older infants and children. These differences are based on mechanisms of epileptogenesis, the developmental state of the immature brain, and the relatively greater importance of nonepileptic mechanisms of seizure generation in this age

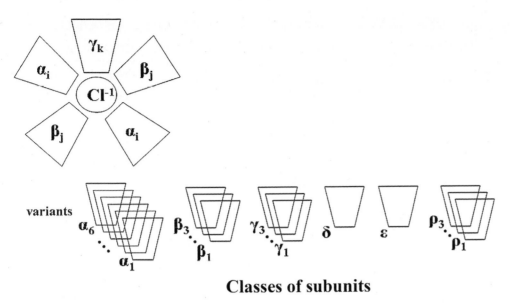

Classes of subunits

FIGURE 33.4. γ-Aminobutyric acid is a pentamer structure composed of six possible classes of subunits. The subunits themselves may have multiple variants that are expressed at different developmental ages.

group. Neonatal seizures may be classified by (i) clinical manifestations, (ii) the relationship between clinical seizures and electrical activity on the electroencephalogram, and (iii) seizure pathophysiology.

Clinical Classifications

A number of clinical classifications of neonatal seizures have been published (55–62). Early classifications focused on the *clinical* differences between seizures in neonates and those in older children: neonatal seizures were reported to be clonic or tonic, not tonic–clonic; when focal, they were either unifocal or multifocal. Later classifications included the term *myoclonus*. Another distinguishing feature of neonatal seizures is the occurrence of events described initially as "anarchic" (55) and thereafter "minimal" (57) or "subtle" (58). These events included oral–buccal–lingual movements such as sucking and chewing; movements of progression,

such as bicycling of the legs and swimming movements of the arms; and random eye movements. First considered epileptic in origin, they were later deemed to be exaggerated reflex behaviors and thus were called "brainstem release phenomena" or "motor automatisms" (60). Table 33.1 lists the clinical characteristics of neonatal seizures according to a current classification scheme (63) that can be applied through observation.

Electroclinical Associations

Neonatal seizures may also be classified by the temporal relationship of clinical events to electrical seizures recorded on scalp electroencephalograms. In an electroclinical seizure, the clinical event overlaps with electrographic seizure activity. Some clinical-only events characterized as neonatal seizures may occur without any EEG seizure activity. Electrical-only seizures (also called subclinical or occult) occur in the absence of any clinical events.

Seizure Pathophysiology

Seizures may be classified as epileptic or nonepileptic (Table 33.2). Some clinical neonatal seizures are clearly epileptic, occurring in close association with EEG seizure activity, involving clinical events that can be neither provoked by stimulation nor suppressed by restraint, and directly triggered by hypersynchronous cortical neuronal discharges. The following properties of the developing brain intensify seizure initiation, maintenance, and propagation: increases in cellular and synaptic excitation and a tendency to enhance propagation of an epileptic discharge (35,64–66). The clinical events that are most clearly epileptic in origin are focal clonic, focal tonic, some types of myoclonic, and rarely spasms (see Tables 33.1 and 33.2). Electrical-only seizures are, by definition, epileptic.

Best considered nonepileptic in origin (60,67) are events that occur in the absence of electrical seizure activity but that have clinical characteristics resembling reflex behaviors.

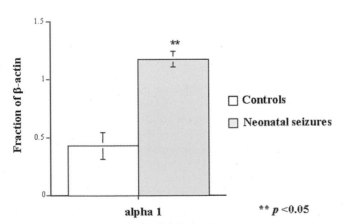

FIGURE 33.5. Rat pups subjected to seizures had significant differences in α-aminobutyric acid subunit composition in later life compared with control animals. (Adapted from Brooks-Kayal AR, Shumate MD, Jim H, et al. Gamma-aminobutyric acid(A) receptor subunit expression predicts functional changes in hippocampal dentate granule cells during postnatal development. *J Neurochem.* 2001;77:1266–1278, with permission.)

TABLE 33.1

CLINICAL CHARACTERISTICS, CLASSIFICATION, AND PRESUMED PATHOPHYSIOLOGY OF NEONATAL SEIZURES

Classification	Characteristics	Pathophysiologic basis
Focal clonic	Repetitive, rhythmic contraction of muscle groups of the limbs, face, or trunk	Epileptic
	May be unifocal or multifocal	
	May occur synchronously or asynchronously in muscle groups on one side of the body	
	May occur simultaneously but asynchronously on both sides	
	Cannot be suppressed by restraint	
Focal tonic	Sustained posturing of single limbs	Epileptic
	Sustained asymmetric posturing of the trunk	
	Sustained eye deviation	
	Cannot be provoked by stimulation or suppressed by restraint	
Generalized tonic	Sustained symmetric posturing of limbs, trunk, and neck	Presumed nonepileptic
	May be flexor, extensor, or mixed extensor/flexor	
	May be provoked or intensified by stimulation	
	May be suppressed by restraint or repositioning	
Myoclonic	Random, single, rapid contractions of muscle groups of the limbs, face, or trunk	Epileptic or nonepileptic
	Typically not repetitive or may recur at a slow rate	
	May be generalized, focal, or fragmentary	
	May be provoked by stimulation	
Spasms	May be flexor, extensor, or mixed extensor/flexor	Epileptic
	May occur in clusters	
	Cannot be provoked by stimulation or suppressed by restraint	
Motor automatisms ocular signs	Random, roving eye movements or nystagmus (distinct from tonic eye deviation)	Nonepileptic
	May be provoked or intensified by tactile stimulation	
Oral–buccal–lingual movements	Sucking, chewing, tongue protrusions	Nonepileptic
	May be provoked or intensified by stimulation	
Progression movements	Rowing or swimming movements	Nonepileptic
	Pedaling or bicycling movements of the legs	
	May be provoked or intensified by stimulation	
	May be suppressed by restraint or repositioning	
Complex purposeless movements	Sudden arousal with transient increased random activity of limbs	Nonepileptic
	May be provoked or intensified by stimulation	

Such clinical events, whether provoked by stimulation or arising spontaneously, can be suppressed or altered by restraining or repositioning the infant. The clinical events may grow in intensity with increases in the repetition rate of stimulation (temporal summation) or the sites of simultaneous stimulation (spatial summation). Some types of myoclonic events, generalized tonic posturing, and motor automatisms can be classified as "nonepileptic" (see Tables 33.1 and 33.2).

Paroxysmal clinical changes related to the autonomic nervous system have been proposed as manifestations of seizures. These include stereotyped, episodic alterations in heart rate, respiration, and blood pressure (59,68,69). Skin flushing, salivation, apnea (70,71), and pupillary dilation may also be autonomic signs of seizures, but they are usually associated with other clinical manifestations, except in the therapeutically paralyzed infant (60).

Electrographic Seizures

Although visual observation is critical to the detection of clinical neonatal seizures, the electroencephalogram offers the most important means of confirmation and characterization. Infants with normal background activity are much less likely to develop seizures than are those with significant background abnormalities (72).

Interictal Background and Prediction Value

The ongoing cerebral electrical activity is the stage on which the drama of the episodic electrographic seizure unfolds. In many ways, the integrity of the EEG background is more

TABLE 33.2

CLASSIFICATION OF NEONATAL SEIZURES BY
ELECTROCLINICAL FINDINGS

Clinical seizures with a consistent electrocortical signature
(epileptic)
Focal clonic
   Unifocal
   Multifocal
   Hemiconvulsive
   Axial
Focal tonic
   Asymmetric truncal posturing
   Limb posturing
   Sustained eye deviation
Myoclonic
   Generalized
   Focal
Spasms
   Flexor
   Extensor
   Mixed extensor/flexor
Clinical seizures without a consistent electrocortical signature
(presumed nonepileptic)
Myoclonic
   Generalized
   Focal
   Fragmentary
Generalized tonic
   Flexor
   Extensor
   Mixed extensor/flexor
Motor automatisms
   Oral–buccal–lingual movements
   Ocular signs
   Progression movements
   Complex purposeless movements
Electrical seizures without clinical seizure activity

critical than the mere presence or absence of the seizures themselves. For example, with or without electrographic seizures, an extremely abnormal EEG background (burst suppression (73) or isoelectric recording) inherently conveys a sense of profound electrophysiologic disruption and forecasts an exceedingly high risk for death or adverse neurologic outcome. Conversely, a nearly normal interictal EEG background suggests relatively preserved neurologic health despite the intrusion of the seizures.

The interictal background also occasionally can offer clues to seizure etiology. Persistently focal sharp waves may suggest a restricted injury such as localized subarachnoid hemorrhage, contusion, or stroke, whereas multifocal sharp waves suggest diffuse dysfunction. Hypocalcemia is a consideration if a well-maintained background features excessive bilateral central spikes. Inborn errors of metabolism, such as maple-syrup urine disease, are sometimes associated with distinctive vertex wicket spikes. Pseudoperiodic discharges raise the suspicion of herpes simplex virus encephalitis or a localized acute destructive lesion such as stroke or hemorrhage. A grossly abnormal electroencephalogram in the absence of any obviously acquired disease suggests cerebral dysgenesis.

Interictal EEG spikes per se have uncertain diagnostic significance (74). Interictal focal sharp waves and spikes are not typically considered indicators of epileptogenesis in the same way as they are in older children and adults. Compared with those of age-matched neonates without seizures (75,76), the interictal records of infants with electroencephalogram-confirmed seizures have background abnormalities, excessive numbers of "spikes" (lasting <200 msec) compared with sharp waves (lasting >200 msec), excessive occurrence of spikes or sharp waves per minute, and a tendency for "runs," "bursts," or "trains" of repetitive sharp waves. However, only a few infants with confirmed seizures exhibit all of these interictal characteristics, and many show no excessive spikes or sharp waves.

Characteristics

At the heart of the epileptic process is the abnormal, excessive, repetitive electrical firing of neurons. Affected neurons lose their autonomy and are engulfed by the synchronized bursts of repeated electrical discharges. Sustained trains of action potentials arise in the affected neurons, which repeatedly fire and eventually propagate beyond their site of origin. At the conclusion of the ictus, inhibitory influences terminate the electrophysiologic cascade and end the seizure. Electrographic seizures in the neonate have varied appearances and are relatively rare before 34 to 35 weeks conceptional age. The morphology, spatial distribution, and temporal behavior of the seizure discharges may differ within and between individuals. Despite the differences between the term and preterm neonatal brain, the variety of types of electrographic seizures does not differ between them (77).

Morphology. An electrographic seizure is a discrete abnormal event lasting at least 10 seconds, with a definite beginning, middle, and end (78). No single morphologic pattern characterizes a seizure (Fig. 33.6). Even in the same patient, the ictal EEG activity may appear pleomorphic. The "typical" neonatal seizure begins as low-amplitude, rhythmic, or sinusoidal waveforms or spike or sharp waves. As the seizure evolves, the amplitude of the ictal activity increases, while its frequency slows (79). Spikes or sharp waves are not necessarily present. Instead, rhythmic activity of any frequency (delta, theta, alpha, or beta) can make up the ictal patterns at the scalp surface.

Spatial Distribution. In older children generalized seizures may appear simultaneously, synchronously, and symmetrically in both hemispheres. In the neonatal brain, which lacks the physiologic organization necessary for such exquisite orchestration, individual seizures always arise focally, for example, first appearing in the left temporal region (T_3), migrating to adjacent electrode sites FP_3, C_3, or O_1, and finally engaging the entire hemisphere (so-called hemiconvulsive seizure); seizures may also migrate from one hemisphere to another (63). Occasionally, simultaneous focal seizures may appear to behave independently, spreading to all brain regions, and superficially masquerading as a "generalized seizure." However, the ictal patterns are not those of the truly generalized seizures, which usually are composed of spike or polyspike slow-wave discharges.

Although diffuse causes of encephalopathy such as meningitis, hypoglycemia, or hypoxia–ischemia may be expected to produce generalized seizures, each seizure instead arises from a restricted area of cortex. Multiple seizures that each originate from different scalp regions are called "multifocal-onset seizures"; those that arise from the same scalp location are unifocal onset and raise the possibility of a localized structural abnormality such as a stroke (78), reflecting the restricted functional disturbance.

Temporal Profile. The typical duration of an electrographic neonatal seizure is about 1 to 2 minutes and is followed by an interictal period of variable length (Fig. 33.7). These temporal characteristics were obtained from relatively brief tracings randomly selected during a variety of acute encephalopathies (9). Few studies comprehensively describe the natural history of electrographic seizures during continuous monitoring from the onset of acute neurologic illness. Solitary, prolonged electrographic seizures are rare in newborn infants; more than 90% of those seizures recorded in one study lasted less than 30 minutes (77). Repetitive brief serial seizures are much more characteristic than prolonged seizures lasting many hours.

Special Ictal Electroencephalographic Morphologies. Some ictal patterns unique to the neonatal period are associated with severe encephalopathies. Electrical seizures of the depressed brain are long, low in voltage, and highly localized. They may be unifocal or multifocal and show little tendency to spread or modulate. Not associated with clinical seizures, they occur when the EEG background is depressed and undifferentiated, and suggest a poor prognosis. Alpha (α) seizure activity (80–82) is characterized by sudden, transient, rhythmic activity in the α frequency range (8 to 12 Hz) in the temporal or central region, unaccompanied by clinical events. An α discharge usually indicates a severe encephalopathy and poor prognosis.

Video-EEG monitoring has been the basis of clinical investigations into the classification, therapy, and prognosis of neonatal seizures (83–86), but is not widely available for routine use. Attended EEG with simultaneous observation by trained electroneurodiagnostic technologists remains the conventional method of monitoring newborns with seizures.

Amplitude-integrated EEG. Amplitude-integrated EEG (aEEG) is becoming increasingly used in the neonatal intensive care unit setting for bedside evaluation of cerebral activity. While various

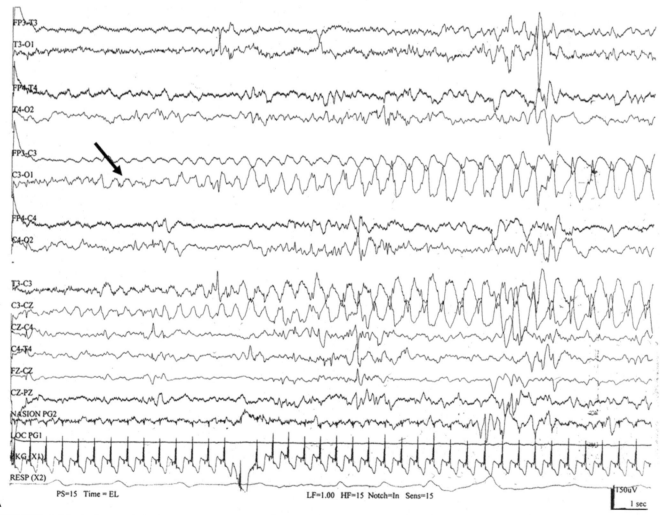

FIGURE 33.6. No single morphologic pattern characterizes electrographic neonatal seizures; rather, their distinctive behavior as a discrete, evolving electrographic event identifies them as ictal. **A:** A focal seizure arises from C_3 (*arrow*) as low-amplitude, rhythmic theta activity that gradually changes to higher-amplitude delta activity. (*continued on next page*)

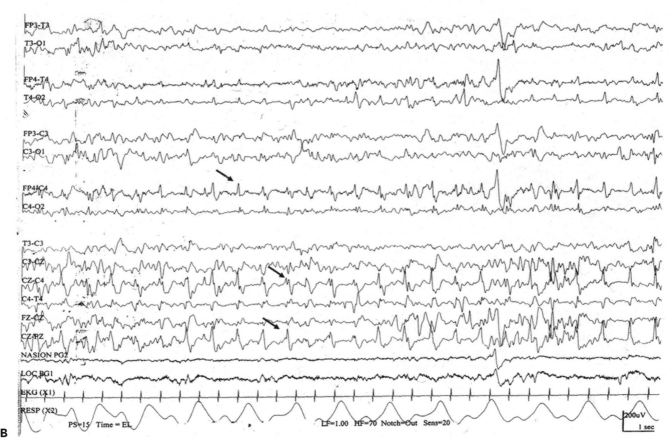

B

FIGURE 33.6. (*continued*) **B:** An electrographic seizure is in progress as repetitive spikes in the right frontopolar, central, and midline vertex regions (*arrows*).

techniques are available, two electrodes are commonly used to acquire data that are then processed and compressed to provide a simple trend of the background EEG activity in those regions (Fig. 33.8). Advantages over conventional EEG include widespread availability, ease of application, and the lack of dependence on specially trained neurophysiologists.

The compressed data provides information about the background of the EEG that can be used for prognostic purposes, including inclusion in therapeutic neuroprotection (e.g., cerebral head cooling) (87). Neonatal seizures can be detected with aEEG as sudden elevations of the margins of the background tracing (Fig. 33.9). Studies comparing neonatal seizure detection between aEEG and conventional EEG demonstrate that only 22% to 57% of *infants* with seizures are accurately identified by neonatologist readers. These readers correctly detected 12% to 38% of the seizures confirmed by conventional EEG (Table 33.3) (88,89). Certain seizure characteristics influence their identification: amplitude, duration, number of seizures

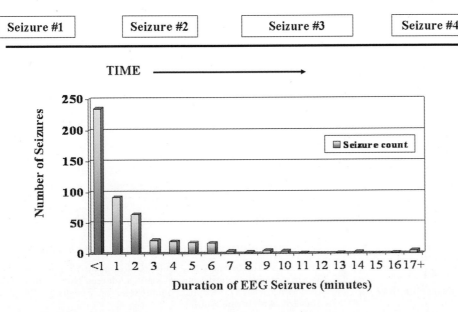

FIGURE 33.7. In most neonates with electrographic seizures, the electroencephalogram shows a series of brief ictal events, typically lasting less than 2 minutes, followed by varying-length interictal periods. The histogram shows the distribution of durations (minutes) of 487 electroencephalographic seizures recorded from 42 neonates. (Adapted from Clancy RR, Legido A. The exact ictal and interictal duration of electroencephalographic neonatal seizures. *Epilepsia.* 1978;28:537–541, with permission.)

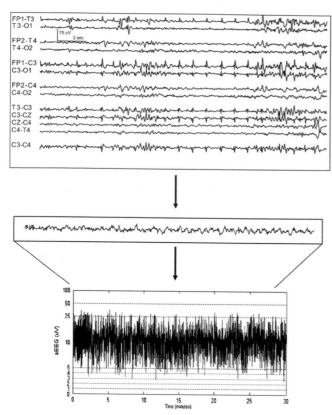

FIGURE 33.8. The routine neonatal EEG examination typically displays 12 or more channels from the full array of the 10–20 system. Cerebral function monitors, such as aEEG, use a single channel from a pair of scalp electrodes (commonly the left and right parietal regions) and then processes the raw EEG to a compressed display, which is very useful for reviewing long-term trends.

TABLE 33.3

COMPARISONS OF CONVENTIONAL AND AMPLITUDE-INTEGRATED EEG FOR SEIZURE DETECTION

Diagnostic tool	Neonates with seizures (%)	EEG seizures per neonate (%)
Conventional EEG ("gold standard")	100	100
Single channel of "raw" EEG (C3 → C4)	94	78
aEEG of single-channel EEG (C3 → C4)	22–57	12–38
Single channel of "raw" EEG at the forehead (Fp3 → Fp4)	66	46

by vecuronium or pancuronium, clinical recognition is useless. It would be useful to develop measures of the "burden" of electrographic seizures in individual infants.

There is an obvious hierarchy to measures of seizure burden. The simplest measure is to simply consider them "present" or "absent." However, the number of recorded electrographic seizures varies widely, even in a similar context. For example, during 48 hours of video-EEG monitoring after newborn heart surgery, 11.5% of 183 newborns were "seizure positive" with one or more electrographic seizures detected; but total seizure *counts* varied from 1 to 217 (Fig. 33.11) (85). Because individual electrographic seizures also vary in length, another measure of EEG seizure burden is to describe the *percentage* of time in which seizure activity is present in any brain region. This can range from a 0% if no seizures are captured to 100% if the entire record demonstrates seizure activity anywhere in the brain. Unfortunately, there is only a modest (albeit statistically significant) correlation between seizure counts and the percentages of the recordings showing seizure activity (89). The most detailed measure of seizure burden incorporates knowledge of their spatial distribution. Individual electrographic seizures may remain confined to their area of origin or may spread substantially to other regions (91). This varies considerably among individual neonates (Fig. 33.12) (85). Simple seizure counts or measuring

per hour, and the spatial restrictions imparted by sampling just 1 or 2 electrode pairs (89). Clearly, aEEG cannot supplant conventional EEG but can provide very useful complementary information that may guide decision making at the bedside in real time.

Measures of Electrographic Seizure "Burden". Most electrographic neonatal seizures do not provoke distinctive clinical signs (90) (Fig. 33.10), and, in infants iatrogenically paralyzed

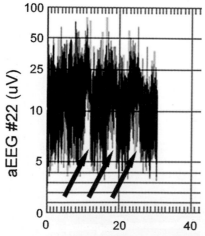

FIGURE 33.9. Thirty-minute aEEG in a term infant with three captured seizures (*arrows*).

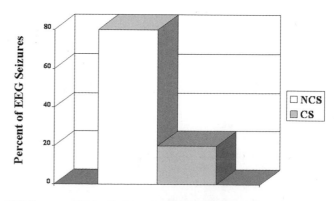

NCS = no clinical signs; CS = definite clinical signs.

FIGURE 33.10. In one study, only 20% of electrographic neonatal seizures produce definite clinical signs. (Adapted from Clancy RR, Legido A, Lewis D. Occult neonatal seizures. *Epilepsia.* 1988;29: 256–261, with permission.)

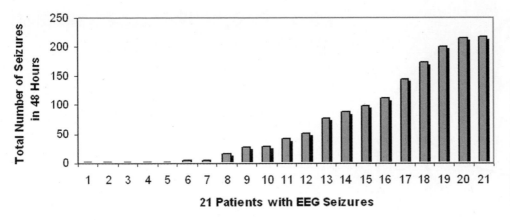

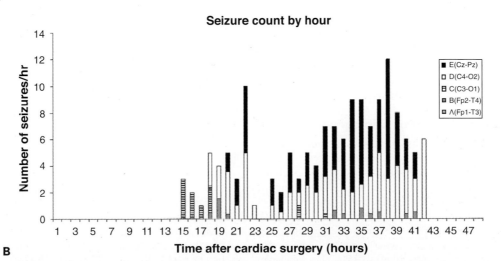

FIGURE 33.11. Distribution of the total number of electrographic neonatal seizures during 48 hours of electroencephalograph monitoring after newborn heart surgery. From 1 to 217 seizures occurred during the study period. (Adapted from Sharif U, Ichord R, Saymor JW, et al. Electrographic neonatal seizures after newborn heart surgery. *Epilepsia.* 2003;44: 164.)

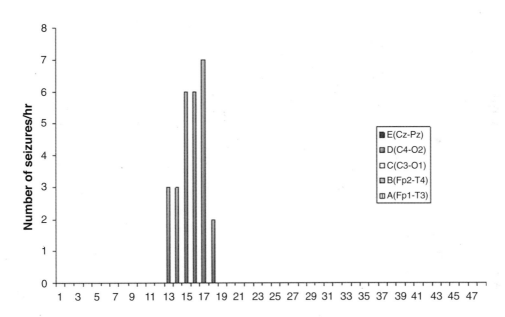

FIGURE 33.12. The spatial distribution of electroencephalographic (EEG) seizures varies among neonates. **A:** All EEG seizures begin in a single brain region (C_4–O_2). **B:** EEG seizures begin in four locations (C_z–P_z, C_4–O_2, C_3–O_1, and Fp_2–T_4). (Adapted from Sharif U, Ichord R, Saymor JW, et al. Electrographic neonatal seizures after newborn heart surgery. *Epilepsia.* 2003;44:164.)

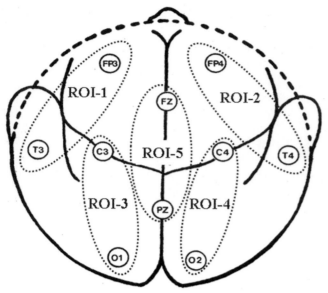

FIGURE 33.13. The entire array of the standard neonatal electroencephalogram can be reduced to five nonoverlapping regions of interest that identify the spatial characteristics of electroencephalographic seizures.

the percentage of time with seizures does not provide information about their *spatial* distribution. One approach to measure EEG seizure burden, temporal–spatial analysis, reduces the entire neonatal electroencephalogram into five nonoverlapping areas of interest (92): the left and right frontotemporal areas; the left and right centro-occipital areas; and one midline region (Fig. 33.13). The percentage of ictal time at each of these five regions gives the most comprehensive picture of the geographic distribution of seizure burden. Future investigations may determine whether a "dose–response" curve exists between this fuller, temporal–spatial measure of seizure burden and eventual long-term neurodevelopmental follow-up.

Etiologic Factors

Acute or chronic conditions can give rise to seizures. In most cases, specific causes can be determined after analysis of clinical and laboratory information (Table 33.4). Table 33.5 lists potential causes of neonatal seizures, but only a few are discussed in detail.

Acute Causes

Hypoxic–Ischemic Etiologies

Probably the most common cause of neonatal seizures, "acute neonatal encephalopathy" (93) is characterized by depressed mental status (lethargy or coma); seizures; axial and appendicular hypotonia with an overall reduction in spontaneous motor activity; and clear evidence of bulbar dysfunction with poor sucking, and swallowing, and an inexpressive face (94). Care should be taken to separate this generic designation from neonatal HIE. Not every infant who is acutely encephalopathic has suffered hypoxia–ischemia (95). The American College of Obstetricians and Gynecologists Task Force on Neonatal Encephalopathy and Cerebral Palsy suggests four

TABLE 33.4

DATA TO DETERMINE THE ETIOLOGY OF NEONATAL SEIZURES

Clinical	Complete history, general physical and neurologic examinations, eye examination
Neuroimaging	Computerized tomographic or magnetic resonance imaging
Blood tests	Arterial blood gases and pH
	Sodium, glucose, calcium, magnesium, ammonia, lactate and pyruvate, serum amino acids
	Comprehensive "neogen" panel[a]
	TORCH (toxoplasmosis, other infections, rubella, cytomegalovirus, and herpes simplex) titers
	Biotin
Urine tests	Reducing substances, sulfites, organic acids
	Toxicologic screen
Cerebrospinal fluid tests	Red and white blood cell counts
	Glucose and protein
	Culture
	Neurotransmitter profile[b]

[a]Varies by US states.
[b]In the proper clinical context.

diagnostic criteria for HIE: (i) evidence of metabolic acidosis in fetal umbilical cord arterial blood obtained at delivery (pH value less than 7 and base deficit greater than 12 mmol/L); (ii) early onset of severe or moderate neonatal encephalopathy in infants born at 34 or more weeks of gestation; (iii) subsequent cerebral palsy of the spastic quadriplegic or dyskinetic type; and (iv) exclusion of other identifiable etiologies such as trauma, coagulation disorders, infectious conditions, or genetic disorders (96). These four conditions should occur in the context of a "sentinel" hypoxic event immediately before or during labor, such as uterine rupture, abruption of the placenta, or prolapse of the umbilical cord. There should also be a sudden and sustained fetal bradycardia or the absence of fetal heart rate variability; persistent, late, or variable decelerations; Apgar scores of 0 to 3 after 5 minutes; and, in most, multisystem involvement within 72 hours of birth. Examples of multisystem malfunction (97) include acute renal tubular necrosis, elevated values of liver function tests, necrotizing enterocolitis from bowel ischemia, and depressed blood-cell lines (e.g., thrombocytopenia) because of ischemic injury of the bone marrow (98). Early imaging studies should show acute diffuse cerebral abnormalities consistent with hypoxia–ischemia.

Other conditions that can clinically mimic acute neonatal HIE are some inborn errors of metabolism, pyridoxine dependency, stroke, coagulopathies, sinovenous thrombosis, and "fetal sepsis syndrome" (99–102), which can occur with sepsis or chorioamnionitis (103,104). The latter is suspected in a mother with abdominal pain and tenderness, fever, leukocytosis, and foul-smelling amniotic fluid, and can be confirmed by

TABLE 33.5

ETIOLOGIES OF NEONATAL SEIZURES

Acute	Chronic
Acute neonatal encephalopathy (includes classic hypoxic–ischemic encephalopathy, both ante- and intrapartum)	Isolated cerebral dysgenesis, e.g., lissencephaly, hemimegalencephaly
Arterial ischemic stroke	Cerebral dysgenesis associated with inborn errors of metabolism
Sinovenous thrombosis	Chronic infection (TORCH [toxoplasmosis, other infections, rubella, cytomegalovirus, and herpes simplex] syndromes)
Extracorporeal membrane oxygenation	Neurocutaneous syndromes
Congenital heart disease	• Incontinentia pigmenti (Bloch–Sulzberger syndrome)
Vein of Galen malformation	• Hypomelanosis of Ito
Giant arteriovenous malformation	• Sturge–Weber syndrome
Hypertensive encephalopathy	• Tuberous sclerosis
Intracranial hemorrhage (subdural subarachnoid, intraventricular, intraparenchymal)	• Linear sebaceous nevus (epidermal nevus syndrome)
Trauma (intrapartum and nonaccidental)	Genetic conditions
Infections (sepsis, meningitis, encephalitis)	• 22Q11 microdeletion
Transient, simple metabolic disorders	• ARX (aristaless-related homeobox) mutations
Inborn errors of metabolism (including pyridoxine-dependent seizures)	Specific very early onset epilepsy syndromes
Intoxication	• Fifth-day fits (benign neonatal convulsions)
	• Benign familial neonatal seizures
	• Early myoclonic encephalopathy
	• Early infantile epileptic encephalopathy
	• Migrating partial seizures of infancy

pathologic examination of the placenta and umbilical cord (105).

Perinatal stroke is defined as a cerebrovascular event occurring between 28 weeks of gestation and 7 days of age. The incidence is 1 in 4000 live births (106). There are two main clinical presentations: (i) acute appearance of neonatal seizures, hypotonia, feeding difficulties, and, rarely, hemiparesis (78,105,107,108) (Fig. 33.14) and (ii) later discovery of stroke through the gradual appreciation of a congenital hemiparesis or the onset of a partial seizure disorder in an infant apparently healthy at birth. Risk factors include congenital heart defects (CHDs), blood and lipid disorders, infection, placental disorders, vasculopathy, trauma, dehydration, and extracorporeal membrane oxygenation (ECMO).

Cerebral sinovenous thrombosis is estimated to occur at a rate of 0.67 cases per 100,000 children per year (108–111) in neonates and older children. The neonatal presentation most frequently includes seizures (57% to 71%) and other nonspecific CNS signs such as lethargy (35% to 58%), but only infrequently frank hemiparesis (109,112) (Fig. 33.15). Maternal risk factors associated with thrombosis included preeclampsia/hypertension, gestational diabetes, and meconium aspiration or meconium stained placenta (112). The sagittal and transverse sinuses are most commonly involved, but multiple sinus thromboses also occur. The reported outcomes include a variable mortality rates from 2% to 13%; 21% developed normally while 60% had cognitive impairment, 64% had motor impairment, and 40% had epilepsy (112,113).

Extracorporeal membrane oxygenation (ECMO) is an effective therapy for newborn infants with life-threatening respiratory failure unresponsive to maximum conventional medical support. However, the procedure requires ligations of the right common carotid artery and right jugular vein at a time when the infants' underlying lung disease may render them particularly vulnerable to the effects of diffuse CNS hypoxia–ischemia. The high rate of subsequent neurologic morbidity among survivors raises the possibility that ECMO itself may contribute to ischemic-reperfusion brain injuries (114). A high proportion of survivors have MRI-identified focal parenchymal brain lesions, often announced by seizures during ECMO. Cerebral hemorrhage and infarction have been reported in 28% to 52% of ECMO-treated infants (115). CHDs enhance the risk for neonatal seizures (116), which can arise preoperatively or postoperatively. Some of these infants find it difficult to make the transition from intrauterine to extrauterine life, exhibiting depressed Apgar scores and persistent hypoxia leading to hypotension, acidosis, and multisystem failure including encephalopathy with seizures. CHDs also may be associated with the presence of other midline somatic defects including CNS anomalies. Seizures can arise from concurrent cerebral dysgenesis as well (117). Strokes may occur from multiple mechanisms including right to left intracardiac shunting or embolization during cardiac catheterization. Hypocalcemia may trigger seizures in the setting of DiGeorge syndrome. However, seizures usually arise *after* newborn heart surgery; they do not occur at random, but, rather, are influenced by suspected or confirmed genetic disorders, aortic arch obstruction, or the need for prolonged deep hypothermic circulatory arrest (118). This population is especially valuable for neuroprotection trials, because the child's

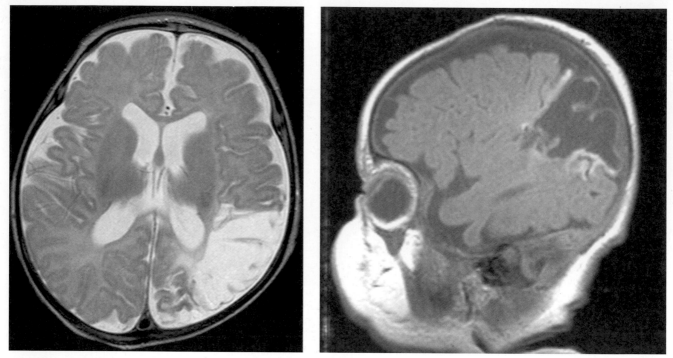

FIGURE 33.14. Arterial ischemic stroke in the distribution of the left middle cerebral artery in a 41-week estimated-gestational-age infant with a prothrombotic disorder.

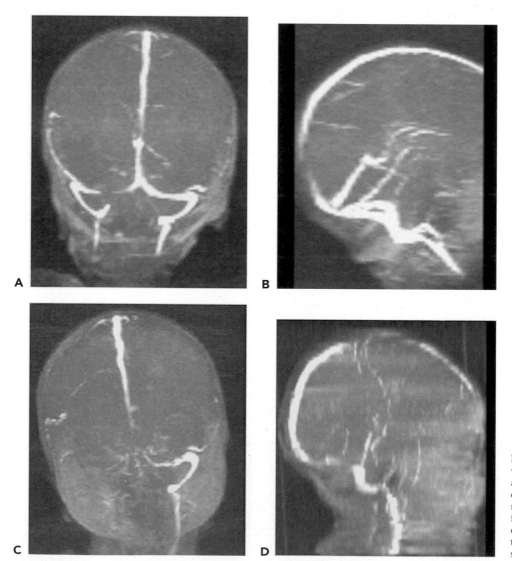

FIGURE 33.15. Magnetic resonance venogram of a 2-week-old term infant admitted for seizures, lethargy, and dehydration. **A,B:** Thrombosis of the right transverse sinus was noted on the first day of hospitalization. **C,D:** By day 10, the thromboses had extended to the sigmoid, jugular, and straight sinuses.

status can be determined before surgery (119). The hypothesis is that if a neuroprotective agent administered preoperatively prevents seizures, the child has benefited from the neuroprotection afforded by the intervention.

Metabolic Etiologies

Hypoglycemia, hyponatremia, hypernatremia, hypocalcemia, hypomagnesemia, and acute hyperbilirubinemia (acute kernicterus) can be associated with neonatal seizures. These conditions are detectable by simple screening tests (see Table 33.4).

Hypoglycemia may itself cause brain damage independent of the seizures. Causes of hypoglycemia that should be evaluated in children include simple prematurity, maternal diabetes, nesidioblastosis, galactosemia, defects of gluconeogenesis, glycogen storage diseases, and respiratory chain defects. Glucose transporter type I syndrome (GLUT I deficiency) is characterized by infantile seizures that usually begin between 6 and 12 weeks of life, developmental delay, ataxia, and progressive microcephaly (120–122). Affected newborns appear normal at birth. Neonatal seizures, initially rare, increase in frequency as the developmental delay becomes evident. The resultant diminution in transported glucose at the blood–brain barrier markedly reduces brain and cerebrospinal fluid values. Genetic studies implicate numerous mutations. The ketogenic diet is one treatment modality since it provides an alternate form of fuel for the CNS.

Inborn Errors of Metabolism

For a detailed discussion, see Chapter 32. The discussion below is limited to the diagnosis of common neonatal conditions amenable to treatment with a specific intervention.

Maple-syrup urine disease, ketotic and nonketotic hyperglycinemia, and urea cycle disorders may all induce a severe acute encephalopathy with seizures. Maple syrup urine disease produces an inability to decarboxylate branched-chain amino acids such as leucine, isoleucine, and valine. After receiving a protein load from a milk feeding, the neonate develops a shrill cry, progressive obtundation, hypotonia punctuated with episodic posturing, and seizures. Urine testing for 2,4-dinitrophenylhydrazine (DNPH) shows positive results, and hypoglycemia may appear from the elevated leucine.

Nonketotic hyperglycinemia has a catastrophic clinical presentation (aptly named glycine encephalopathy) with intractable seizures, coma, hiccups, apnea, pupil-sparing ophthalmoparesis, spontaneous and stimulus-provoked myoclonus, and a burst-suppression pattern on electroencephalography. Glycine levels are elevated in the blood and cerebrospinal fluid. The disorder represents an inability to cleave glycine, which is both an excitatory and inhibitory neurotransmitter. Treatment involves an N-methyl-D-aspartate antagonist, as well as magnesium, sodium benzoate, and dextromethorphan.

The ketotic hyperglycinemias, propionic and methylmalonic acidemias, present with overwhelming multisystem failure and dehydration, ketoacidosis, and fulminant CNS signs such as seizures, vomiting, and coma. Diagnosis is made by serum amino acid surveys and measurement of specific enzyme activity.

Carbamoylphosphate synthetase deficiency, ornithine carbamyl transferase deficiency, citrullinemia, and arginosuccinic acidemia are among the large number of urea-cycle abnormalities, and each cause neonatal seizures in the first days or weeks of life. Coma and prominent bulbar dysfunction are

noted with ophthalmoparesis, fixed pupils, absent gag reflex, poor sucking, and apnea. The degree of serum ammonia elevation may correlate with the discontinuity in the abnormal EEG backgrounds (123).

Biotinidase deficiency may produce alopecia, seborrheic dermatitis, developmental delay, hypotonia, and ataxia. Seizures may begin as early as the first week of life. The diagnosis is made by measurement of blood levels of biotinidase activity. Oral administration of free biotin daily is the treatment.

Pyridoxine-dependent seizures (124,125) usually arise between birth and 3 months of age, although atypical cases have been reported up to 3 years. Some seizures can be appreciated in utero (126), especially if a previous pregnancy had been similarly affected with this autosomal recessive disorder. Parental consanguinity is not uncommon. The neonate presents with agitation, irritability, jitteriness, diminished sleep, and intractable clonic seizures. The EEG patterns are entirely nonspecific and include abnormal backgrounds, excessive multifocal sharp waves, and focal electrographic seizures evolving to hypsarrhythmia later in the first year. The diagnosis is made when seizures immediately cease and epileptiform EEG activity disappears within a few hours of the intravenous administration of 50 to 100 mg of pyridoxine. Lifelong therapy with pyridoxine 50 to 100 mg/day is necessary. Despite early treatment, some neonates are eventually retarded and show MRI evidence of a leukodystrophy. Mutations in α-aminoadipic semialdehyde (α-AASA) dehydrogenase (antiquitin) leading to inactivation of pyridoxal phosphate (PLP) have been found in multiple individuals with pyridoxine-dependent seizures (127). PLP is an essential cofactor in multiple enzymatic reactions, including the formation of GABA. Elevations of urinary α-AASA can be used as a screening tool for identifying individuals with antiquitin mutations. However, this should not substitute for a pyridoxine trial, especially in the acute setting.

Folinic acid–responsive neonatal seizures were first described by Hyland as the unexpected appearance of seizures in term infants during the first few hours or days of life (128). Subsequently intractable, the seizures were associated with severe developmental delay, progressive atrophy on MRI examination, and frequent bouts of status epilepticus. The patients did not respond to intravenous pyridoxine. Analysis of cerebrospinal fluid by means of high-performance liquid chromatography with electrochemical detection consistently revealed an as yet unidentified compound, now used as the marker for this condition. Seizures ceased and the EEG pattern improved after the administration of 2.5 mg of folinic acid twice daily. Some cases of folinic acid–responsive seizures were initially responsive to pyridoxine (129). Gallagher and colleagues (130) identified the biochemical marker for folinic acid–responsive seizures in two individuals who were controlled with pyridoxine. They identified gene mutations in antiquitin in those two individuals along with seven other individuals with folinic acid–responsive seizures. The authors suggest that the two conditions are allelic and recommend considering treating patients with α-AASA dehydrogenase deficiency with both pyridoxine and folinic acid.

The molybdenum cofactor is essential for the proper functioning of the enzymes sulfite oxidase and xanthine dehydrogenase. Deficiency of the cofactor and isolated sulfite oxidase deficiency are autosomal recessive errors that produce severe neurologic symptoms resulting from a lack of sulfite oxidase activity (129–133). The presentation includes poor feeding, an abnormally pitched cry, jitteriness, and intractable seizures. A fresh urine sample shows positive results of a sulfite test and elevated levels of xanthine and hypoxanthine, coupled with depressed concentrations of uric acid. This array of chemical malfunction can arise from mutations in three molybdenum cofactors or in gephyrin. Synthesis of molybdenum cofactor requires the activities of at least six gene products including gephyrin (134), a polypeptide responsible for the clustering of inhibitory glycine receptors and postsynaptic membranes in the rat CNS. Mutations in sulfite oxidase are found in patients with isolated sulfite oxidase deficiency. There is no effective treatment, and prognosis for neurologic recovery and survival is poor.

Neonatal Intoxications

Lidocaine or mepivacaine inadvertently injected into the fetal scalp during local pudendal analgesia for the mother, cocaine, heroin (135), amphetamines, propoxyphene, and theophylline also may cause seizures.

Chronic Causes

Cerebral Dysgenesis

Some neonatal seizures result from long-standing disorders, such as cerebral dysgenesis, neurocutaneous syndromes, genetic disorders, or very early onset epilepsy. An MRI scan should be performed early to uncover cerebral dysgenesis (136). In lissencephaly or hemimegalencephaly (Fig. 33.16), no acute cause for seizures such as neonatal depression or birth trauma is present, and the infant appears outwardly well yet experiences seizures. The identification of cerebral

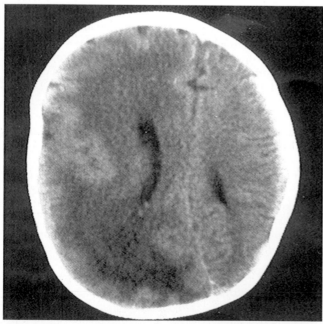

FIGURE 33.16. Computed tomography scan of the head showing right hemimegalencephaly with dysplastic and enlarged right cerebral hemisphere. Brain magnetic resonance imaging provides better resolution and definition of the abnormality and reveals subtle involvement of the contralateral hemisphere.

dysgenesis on neuroimaging should not dissuade the clinician from seeking evidence of inborn errors of metabolism, as both may coexist (e.g., cytochrome oxidase deficiency; glutaric aciduria types I and II; 3-hydroxyisobutaric aciduria; 3-methylglutaconic aciduria; 3-ketothiolase deficiency; sulfite oxidase deficiency; pyruvate dehydrogenase deficiency; neonatal adrenoleukodystrophy; fumaric aciduria; long ketotic hyperglycinemia; and Zellweger syndrome) (137).

TORCH Infections

Chronic TORCH (toxoplasmosis, other infections, rubella, cytomegalovirus, and herpes virus) infections can be identified by ophthalmologic changes, microcephaly, periventricular calcifications on neuroimaging, and appropriate serological blood tests. Congenital infections acquired before the fourth month of gestation may cause an acquired form of migration defect and give rise to "dysgenetic" patterns on computed tomography (CT) or MRI scanning (138).

Neurocutaneous Syndromes

Among the neurocutaneous syndromes that may give rise to neonatal seizures is familial incontinentia pigmenti, a mixed syndrome of different mosaicisms (139). This X-linked dominant state is presumably lethal in males. Perinatal inflammatory vesicles are followed by verrucous patches that produce a distinctive pattern of hyperpigmentation and finally dermal scarring. The cause is a mutation in the *NEMO* (NFκB essential modulator) gene located on Xq28 that renders cells susceptible to apoptosis when exposed to tumor necrosis factor alpha (TNFα) (140). Bloch–Sulzberger syndrome is an earlier described synonym. In contrast to the familial form, sporadic incontinentia pigmenti maps to Xp11 and is considered its "negative" pattern. Better known as hypomelanosis of Ito, its cutaneous lesions appear as areas of hypopigmentation.

Tuberous sclerosis may create neonatal seizures in two basic ways (141): first, through cortical tubers, which in the neonate may be easier to appreciate on CT scan than on MRI, and second, embolic stroke from intracardiac tumors. In the neonate, the classic neurocutaneous signs are often not apparent, except for hypomelanotic macules noted at or soon after birth; however, these may be evident only on skin examination under a Wood's lamp.

Linear sebaceous nevi are a family of disorders with distinctive raised, waxy, sometimes verrucous nevi on the scalp or face, associated with hemihypertrophy, hemimegalencephaly, and neonatal seizures (142).

Sturge–Weber syndrome is a sporadic syndrome featuring the distinctive port wine stain and associated vascular anomaly over the cortical surface. It may manifest with neonatal seizures.

Epilepsy Syndromes of Early Infantile Onset

In the 1970s, French neurologists coined the "fifth-day fits" (benign neonatal convulsions) to describe an electroclinical syndrome in which seizures unexpectedly arose between the fourth and sixth days of life (143). The seizures were usually partial clonic, often with apnea and status epilepticus. More than half had a distinctive "theta pointu alternant" pattern in which the bursts of cerebral electrical activity in the discontinuous parts of the record showed sharply contoured theta waves, especially in the central regions. This EEG pattern has also been recognized in patients with unmistakable HIE.

Benign *familial* neonatal convulsions (BFNC) were the first idiopathic epilepsy syndrome discovered to be caused by a single gene mutation (144,145). Partial seizures unexpectedly begin by the third day of life in neurologically normal-appearing patients, 10% to 15% of whom progress to epilepsy. Three known genetic defects are responsible for this disorder (144). BFNC type I has a defective gene *KCNQ2* at chromosomal locus 20q13.3 with an aberrant α subunit of the voltage-gated potassium channel. Type II has an abnormal *KCNQ3* gene, located on 8q24, and also codes for an aberrant α subunit of the voltage-gated potassium channel. BFNC with myokymia (146) has been reported as a separate mutation of *KCNQ2*, also on 20q13.3. Some so-called benign familial neonatal–infantile seizures (147,148), which typically appear in the first year of life, present with neonatal seizures. These are associated with the aberrant gene *SCN2A*, located on 2q24, that represents a defective α subunit of the voltage-gated sodium channel (144).

Migrating partial seizures in infancy constitute a constellation of unprovoked, alternating electroclinical seizures and subsequent neurodevelopmental devastation that was described in 1995 by Coppola and associates (149). Although multifocal neonatal seizures are not uncommon after infections, metabolic disorders, and hypoxia–ischemia, they can also accompany cerebral dysgenesis and some other neonatal seizure syndromes. In migrating partial seizures in infancy, healthy infants without cerebral dysplasia display multifocal partial seizures that arise independently and sequentially from both hemispheres (Fig. 33.17) within the first 6 months of life and progress through a period of intractability, ultimately

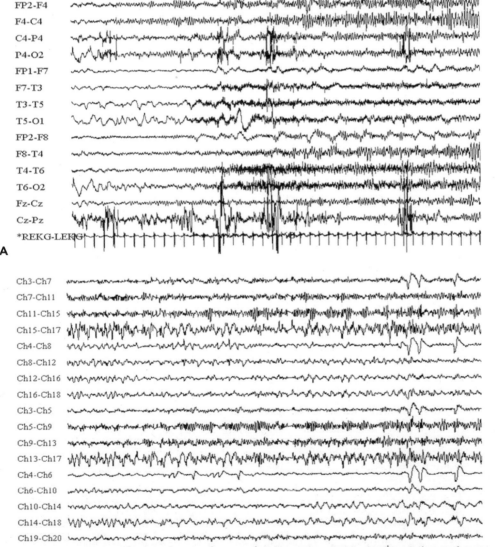

FIGURE 33.17. Migrating partial seizures in infancy. Seizure originating from the right hemisphere (**A**), followed by one arising from the left hemisphere (**B**) (odd channel numbers represent the left hemisphere and even channel numbers represent the right hemisphere). Note that the time axis of the electroencephalogram rhythm strip is slightly compressed. The time and amplitude calibration bar appears at the top of the figure: 1 second and 50 μV. (Adapted from Marsh E, Melamed S, Clancy R. Migrating partial seizures in early infancy: expanding the phenotype of a rare neonatal seizure type. *Epilepsia.* 2003;44:305, with permission.)

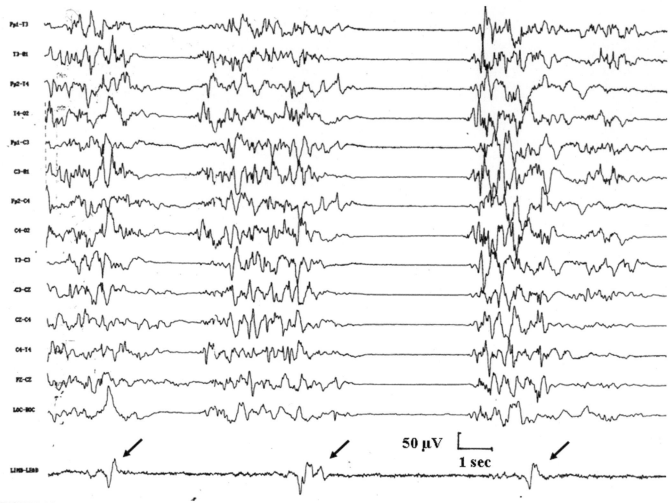

FIGURE 33.18. Burst-suppression electroencephalographic pattern of early myoclonic epilepsy. The abnormal myoclonic movements, detected by the bottom electromyographic channel (*arrows*), occur during the "burst" periods of the tracing.

leading to severe psychomotor retardation. As described in the original paper and later case reports, prognosis was very poor, with 28% mortality and the majority of survivors profoundly retarded and nonambulatory; however, later patients have fared somewhat better (150).

First described by Aicardi and Goutieres (151), EME is characterized by maternal reports of sustained, rhythmic fetal kicking, oligohydramnios or polyhydramnios, normal Apgar scores, and seizure onset from the first day of life to several months (typical age, 16 days). Clinical seizures include erratic fragments of *myoclonic* activity, massive myoclonia, stimulus-sensitive myoclonia, and partial seizures. Electroencephalograms are eventually markedly abnormal, frequently with a burst-suppression background. The myoclonic limb movements tend to occur during the burst periods of the burst suppression activity (Fig. 33.18). All patients are completely resistant to antiepileptic drugs (AEDs). Other clinical features are progressive decline in head circumference percentiles, bulbar signs (especially apnea), feeding difficulties, cleft or high-arched palate, and severe psychomotor delay. Progressive cerebral atrophy is evident on neuroimaging scans (152). A recent case report identified a disruption of the tyrosine protein kinase receptor ErbB4 in a patient with EME (153).

Early infantile epileptic encephalopathy (EIEE), also known as Ohtahara syndrome, is characterized by intractable *tonic* seizures in the setting of a severe encephalopathy and a burst-suppression background pattern (154). In fact, the EEG findings alone appear similar to those of EME, and there is discussion that they may represent a spectrum of disease (155). Many infants with EIEE harbor overt cerebral dysgenesis or cortical dysplasias. Survivors often develop typical infantile spasms with hypsarrhythmia and Lennox–Gastaut syndrome accompanied by multifocal spikes on the electroencephalogram. Cases of EIEE have been found in patients with ARX mutations (156). Recently 5 of 13 patients with EIEE were found to have mutations in the gene encoding syntaxin binding protein 1 (*STXBP1*) (157). The *STXBP1* gene plays an important role in synaptic vesicle release.

TREATMENT

Despite the decades-long recognition of neonatal seizures, treatment recommendations rest almost entirely on conventional wisdom and traditional practices. Because AEDs are used to treat neonatal seizures of *epileptic* origin, initial consideration is given to the clinical and EEG features of the events. Discussion has also centered on the advisability of treating all epileptic neonatal seizures, as some are brief, infrequent, and self-limited. On the one hand, if the burden of seizures will be minimal, the infant need not be exposed to acute and long-term drug therapy. On the other hand, epileptic neonatal seizures that are long, frequent, and not self-limited are treated acutely and vigorously with AEDs.

No studies unequivocally demonstrate the efficacy of barbiturates in the treatment of neonatal seizures. In a randomized, controlled study (158), thiopental was administered soon after perinatal asphyxia. Seizures were diagnosed by clinical signs and occurred in 76% of treated infants and in 73% of a control (placebo) group. High doses of phenobarbital given after perinatal asphyxia resulted in a lower rate of recurrent seizures compared to placebo, although the difference was not statistically significant (159). Another randomized study using phenobarbital prophylactically in neonates with perinatal asphyxia found a statistically significant decrease in the incidence of neonatal seizures compared with placebo control (160). This study has some limitations, including a small number of patients with seizures and lack of EEG data for clinical confirmation or identification of electrographic seizures. In another study of 31 acutely ill neonates with electrographic seizures detected during continuous electroencephalograph monitoring, only 2 had a complete cessation of both clinical and EEG seizures with AEDs (161). Six had an equivocal electroclinical response. Clinical seizures stopped in 13, although the electrographic seizures persisted. The remaining 10 had persistent electroclinical seizures. Two studies (84,91) reported a mixed response of electroclinical seizures to phenobarbital. In a comparison study (162), electrographic seizures ceased in 43% of the group treated with phenobarbital and in 45% of the group given phenytoin; however, the lack of a placebo control precluded determination of absolute efficacy. Video-EEG monitoring demonstrated cessation of seizures in 11 of 22 infants after administration of 40 mg/kg phenobarbital (84). The choice of a second-line drug for nonresponders was limited to lignocaine or benzodiazepines. According to a recent Cochrane review (163), ". . . at the present time, anticonvulsant therapy determined in the immediate period following perinatal asphyxia cannot be recommended for routine clinical practice, other than in the treatment of prolonged or frequent clinical seizures." In addition, another Cochrane review noted (164), ". . . there is little evidence from randomised controlled trials to support the use of any of the anticonvulsants currently used in the neonatal period."

In summary, despite the frequent empiric selection of phenobarbital in clinical practice for the treatment of neonatal seizures, evidence of its efficacy is limited, and animal studies raise concern that phenobarbital itself may have deleterious effects on the young nervous system (see Potential Deleterious Effects of Antiepileptic Drug Administration on the Immature CNS). A joint venture by the National Institutes of Health and the Food and Drug Administration, the "newborn drug development initiative," fosters the performance of ethical, well-controlled trials of pharmaceutical agents used in neonatal neurology, cardiology, anesthesia, pain management, and related disorders. Few drugs for use in the newborn have been subjected to adequately powered, randomized, placebo-controlled investigations to demonstrate real safety and efficacy. Drugs with potential for the treatment of neonatal seizures are no exception.

Nevertheless, in ordinary clinical practice, it is common to administer AEDs in an effort to reduce or eliminate seizures in the newborn. Early studies of neonatal seizures recommended loading doses of phenobarbital 15 to 20 mg/kg, with the intention of generating serum levels between 15 and 20 μg/mL, and followed by maintenance doses of 3 to 4 mg/kg/day. In the comparative study with phenytoin (162,165), phenobarbital doses were chosen to achieve *free* (unbound) concentrations of 25 μg/mL. This was accomplished by incubating the infant's blood with phenobarbital to determine drug binding. Plasma binding of phenobarbital in neonates varies from 0% to 45%. The "mg/kg" dose needed to provide a free plasma-bound level of 25 μg/mL is calculated by the formula: plasma-bound dose = (25 mg/kg) × Vd (L/kg)/(% free binding). For phenobarbital, the volume of distribution is assumed to be 1 L/kg.

The "mg/kg" dose of phenytoin should be calculated to achieve, but not exceed, free concentrations of 3 μg/mL (162,165). The dosing formula: (3 μg/kg) × Vd (L/kg)/(% free binding) assumes a volume of distribution of 1 L/kg. Phenytoin has nonlinear pharmacokinetics: steady-state plasma concentrations at one dosing schedule do not predict those at another schedule (166,167). There are also variable rates of hepatic metabolism, decreases in elimination rates during the first weeks of life, and variable bioavailability with different generic preparations. A redistribution of the AED after the initial dose decreases brain concentrations thereafter; thus, dosage must be tailored to the individual patient after therapy begins.

Phenytoin should be given by direct intravenous infusion at a rate no faster than 1 mg/kg/min. Serum binding of the drug is unpredictable in critically ill neonates, and excessively rapid administration or high concentrations can result in serious or lethal cardiac arrhythmias. Furthermore, phenytoin is strongly alkalotic and may lead to local venous thrombosis or tissue irritation. The use of fosphenytoin may reduce these risks.

While phenobarbital remains first-line therapy for neonatal seizures, there is some debate about second-line therapy. In two surveys of pediatric epileptologists in the United States and Europe, phenobarbital was identified as the treatment of choice, while intravenous benzodiazepines and fosphenytoin or phenytoin were also considered first-line therapy (168,169). In a treatment review of five neonatal intensive care units in the United States (170), phenobarbital was the most common first-line AED (82%) followed by lorazepam (9%) and phenytoin (2%). Second-line therapy after treatment failure to the first was most frequently lorazepam (50%), phenytoin (39%), and phenobarbital (20%).

Benzodiazepines, typically lorazepam (0.15 mg/kg) and diazepam (0.3 mg/kg), can be effective therapies for refractory patients. Side effects of acute administration include hypotension and respiratory depression. Alternative or adjuvant AEDs have also been empirically prescribed for refractory neonatal seizures. Clonazepam, lidocaine (171–173), and midazolam (174,175) are administered intravenously; carbamazepine (176), primidone (177), valproate (178), vigabatrin (179), and lamotrigine (180) are given orally.

The administration of antiepileptic medications may terminate the clinical manifestation of the seizure while the electrographic discharge continues (161,162). This disconnect is often termed uncoupling and poses serious concerns for the clinician and researchers in determining response rates to AEDs. Scher and colleagues found 58% of patients continued

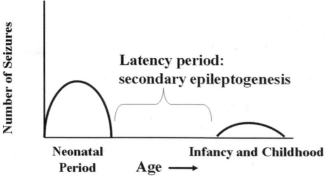

FIGURE 33.19. Acute neonatal seizures are often followed by chronic postnatal epilepsy. A latent period, during which secondary epileptogenesis develops, gives rise to spontaneous, unprovoked seizures.

experiencing electrographic seizures after an administered AED had stopped their clinical seizures (181). This phenomenon may be explained by the caudal–rostral maturational switch from NKCC1 to KCC2, allowing medications to be more effective against brainstem and spinal cord neurons before more rostral structures (14). The relatively high rates of uncoupling stresses the importance of EEG documentation of resolution of neonatal seizures.

Chronic Postnatal Epilepsy and the Need for Long-Term Treatment

Chronic postnatal epilepsy is relatively common in the wake of neonatal seizures (Fig. 33.19). For many patients, permanent, fixed brain injuries, such as resolving stroke, ischemia, or traumatic lesions, serve as the nidus for future epilepsy. As mentioned, repeated neonatal seizures may have "instructed" the brain how to have future seizures, resulting in a persistent lowering of the seizure threshold (38) and the development of chronic epilepsy. In infants with EME or EIEE, neonatal seizures represent the beginning of very early onset epilepsy, which persists by its nature. The most common occurrence, however, is epilepsy after neonatal seizures triggered by acute neonatal conditions.

Ellenberg and colleagues (182) found that approximately 20% of survivors of neonatal seizures experienced one or more seizures up to 7 years of age; nearly two thirds of the seizures occur within the first 6 months of life. Other researchers (8,25–27,91) reported rates ranging from 17% to 30%. The 56% noted by Clancy and colleagues (28,183) may be explained by the population's relatively serious risk factors for CNS dysfunction. Partial and generalized seizures characterize postneonatal epilepsy and do not seem to be preventable by the long-term administration of AEDs after neonatal seizures.

Not all neonates require extended therapy after acute seizures have been controlled, although no criteria for long-term maintenance AED use have been sufficiently studied. For chronic therapy, either phenobarbital or phenytoin 3 to 4 mg/kg/day is given and serum levels are monitored. Reported schedules for discontinuation of maintenance therapy range from 1 week to 12 months after the last seizure (184); one currently used schedule withdraws AEDs 2 weeks after the last seizure (185).

Potential Deleterious Effects of Antiepileptic Drug Administration on the Immature CNS

AEDs prevent or interrupt electrographic seizures by the blockade of voltage-dependent sodium channels and glutamatergic excitatory neurotransmission and enhancing of GABA-mediated inhibition. However, in this critical time of early brain development, suppression of synaptic transmission may have incidental undesirable consequences, because neuronal and synaptic pruning are activity dependent. Since the 1970s, it has been known that rat pups fed phenobarbital have later reductions in brain weight and in total brain cell count (186). How AEDs may harm the developing rat brain remains under investigation, but evidence suggests that these drugs may trigger apoptotic neurodegeneration in the rodent forebrain and suppress an endogenous neuroprotective system already in place (187). The clinical impact of these findings is less certain. Most neonates are given phenobarbital because of seizures, and it is difficult to determine how much of any long-term aftermath is the result of the seizures' underlying etiology, the attacks themselves, or the medications administered to suppress them. Some neonates receive phenobarbital for other reasons, such as to provide sedation or to accelerate hepatic maturity in neonatal hyperbilirubinemia and appear to experience no ill effects. Likewise, benzodiazepines are commonly administered for sedation or to reduce agitation, and no obvious adverse effects are associated with their use, although careful studies are lacking.

References

1. Eriksson M, Zetterstrom R. Neonatal convulsions: incidence and causes in the Stockholm area. *Acta Paediatr Scand.* 1979;68:807–811.
2. Bergman I, Painter MJ, Hirsch RP. Outcomes in neonates with convulsions treated in an intensive care unit. *Ann Neurol.* 1983;14:642.
3. Spellacy W, Peterson P, Winegar A. Neonatal seizures after cesarean section: higher risk with labor. *Am J Obstet Gynecol.* 1987;157:377–379.
4. Lanska MJ, Lanska DJ, Baumann RJ, et al. A population-based study of neonatal seizures in Fayette County, Kentucky. *Neurology.* 1995;45:724–732.
5. Ronen G, Penney S. The epidemiology of clinical neonatal seizures in Newfoundland, Canada. *Ann Neurol.* 1995;38:518–519.
6. Ronen GM, Penney S, Andrews W. The epidemiology of clinical neonatal seizures in Newfoundland: a population-based study. *J Pediatr.* 1999;134:71–75.
7. Saliba RM, Annegers JF, Waller DK, et al. Incidence of neonatal seizures in Harris County, Texas, 1992–1994. *Am J Epidemiol.* 1996;150:763–769.
8. Scher M, Aso K, Beggarly M, et al. Electrographic seizures in preterm and full-term neonates: clinical correlates, associated brain lesions and risk for neurologic sequelae. *Pediatrics.* 1993;91:128–134.
9. Scher M, Hamid M, Steppe D, et al. Ictal and interictal electrographic seizure durations in preterm and term neonates. *Epilepsia.* 1993;34:284–288.
10. Johnston MV. Selective vulnerability in the neonatal brain. *Ann Neurol.* 1998;44:155–156.
11. Zhang G, Hsu FC, Raol YH, et al. Selective alterations of GABA A receptor subunit expression and function in hippocampal dentate granule cells after seizures in the developing brain. *Epilepsia.* 2001;42:224.
12. Zhang G, Raol YH, Hsu FC, et al. Effects of status epilepticus on hippocampal GABA$_A$ receptors are age-dependent. *Neuroscience.* 2004;125:299–303.
13. Staley K. Enhancement of the excitatory actions of GABA by barbiturates and benzodiazepines. *Neurosci Lett.* 1992;146:105–107.
14. Dzhala VI, Talos DM, Sdrulla DA, et al. NKCC1 transporter facilitates seizures in the developing brain. *Nat Med.* 2005;11:1205–1213.
15. Khazipov R, Khalilov I, Tyzio R, et al. Developmental changes in GABAergic actions and seizure susceptibility in the rat hippocampus. *Eur J Neurosci.* 2004;19:590–600.

16. Tyzio R, Holmes GL, Ben-Ari Y, et al. Timing of the developmental switch in GABA$_A$ mediated signaling from excitation to inhibition in CA3 rat hippocampus using gramicidin perforated patch and extracellular recordings. *Epilepsia.* 2007;48(suppl 5):96–105.

17. Tyzio R, Cossart R, Khalilov I, et al. Maternal oxytocin triggers a transient inhibitory switch in GABA in the fetal brain during delivery. *Science.* 2006;314:1788–1792.

18. Dzhala VI, Brumback AC, Staley KJ. Bumetanide enhances Phenobarbital efficacy in a neonatal seizure model. *Ann Neurol.* 2008;63:222–235.

19. Silverstein FS, Jensen FE. Neonatal seizures. *Ann Neurol.* 2007;62: 112–120.

20. Volpe J. Neonatal seizures. In: *Neurology of the Newborn.* 5th ed. Philadelphia: Saunders; 2008:203–244.

21. Lombroso CT. Prognosis in neonatal seizures. *Adv Neurol.* 1983;34:101.

22. Ellenberg JH, Nelson KB. Cluster of perinatal events identifying infants at high risk for death or disability. *J Pediatr.* 1988;113:546–552.

23. Nelson KB, Broman SH. Perinatal risk factors in children with serious motor and mental handicaps. *Ann Neurol.* 1977;2:371–377.

24. Temple CM, Dennis J, Carney R, et al. Neonatal seizures: long-term outcome and cognitive development among "normal" survivors. *Dev Med Child Neurol.* 1995;37:109–118.

25. Ortibus EL, Sum JM, Hahn JS. Predictive value of EEG for outcome and epilepsy following neonatal seizures. *Electroencephalogr Clin Neurophysiol.* 1996;98:175–185.

26. Pisani F, Cerminara C, Fusco C, et al. Neonatal status epilepticus vs recurrent neonatal seizures: clinical findings and outcome. *Neurology.* 2007; 69:2177–2185.

27. Mizrahi EM, Clancy R, Dunn JK, et al. Neurologic impairment, developmental delay and post-natal seizures two years after video-EEG documented seizures in near-term and full-term neonates: report of the Clinical Research Centers for Neonatal Seizures. *Epilepsia.* 2001;102:47.

28. Legido A, Clancy RR, Berman PH. Neurologic outcome after electroencephalographically proven neonatal seizures. *Pediatrics.* 1991;88: 583–596.

29. McBride MC, Laroia N, Guillet R. Electrographic seizures in neonates correlate with poor neurodevelopmental outcome. *Neurology.* 2000;55: 506–513.

30. Miller SP, Weiss J, Barnwell A, et al. Seizure-associated brain injury in term newborns with perinatal asphyxia. *Neurology.* 2002;58:542–548.

31. Schmid R, Tandon P, Stafstrom CE, et al. Effects of neonatal seizures on subsequent seizure-induced brain injury. *Neurology.* 1999;53:1754–1761.

32. Wasterlain CG, Plum F. Retardation of behavioral landmarks after neonatal seizures in rats. *Trans Am Neurol Assoc.* 1973;98:320–321.

33. Wasterlain CG. Neonatal seizures and brain growth. *Neuropadiatrie.* 1978;9:213–228.

34. Wasterlain C, Niquet J, Thompson K, et al. Seizure-induced neuronal death in the immature brain. *Prog Brain Res.* 2002;135:335–353.

35. Holmes G. Epilepsy in the developing brain. *Epilepsia.* 1997;38:12–30.

36. Yager JY, Armstrong EA, Miyashita H, et al. Prolonged neonatal seizures exacerbate hypoxic-ischemic brain damage: correlation with cerebral energy metabolism and excitatory amino acid release. *Dev Neurosci.* 2002;24:367–381.

37. Haas KZ, Sperber EF, Opanashuk LA, et al. Resistance of immature hippocampus to morphologic and physiologic alterations following status epilepticus or kindling. *Hippocampus.* 2001;11:615–625.

38. Mazarati A, Bragin A, Baldwin R, et al. Epileptogenesis after self-sustaining status epilepticus. *Epilepsia.* 2002;43:74–80.

39. Sankar R, Shin D, Liu H, et al. Granule cell neurogenesis after status epilepticus in the immature rat brain. *Epilepsia.* 2000;41:S53–S56.

40. McCabe BK, Silveira DC, Cilio MR, et al. Reduced neurogenesis after neonatal seizures. *J Neurosci.* 2001;21:2094–2103.

41. Fando JL, Conn M, Wasterlain CG. Brain protein synthesis during neonatal seizures: an experimental study. *Exp Neurol.* 1979;63:220–228.

42. Holmes GL, Gairsa JL, Chevassus-Au-Louis N, et al. Consequences of neonatal seizures in the rat: morphological and behavioral effects. *Ann Neurol.* 1998;44:845–857.

43. Zhang G, Raol YH, Hsu FC, et al. Long-term alterations in glutamate receptor and transporter expression following early-life seizures are associated with increased seizure susceptibility. *J Neurochem.* 2004;88: 91–101.

44. Cornejo BJ, Mesches MH, Coultrap S, et al. A single episode of neonatal seizures permanently alters glutamatergic synapses. *Ann Neurol.* 2007;61: 411–426.

45. Swann JW, Le JT, Lam TT, et al. The impact of chronic network hyperexcitability on developing glutamatergic synapses. *Eur J Neurosci.* 2007;26: 975–991.

46. Sanchez RM, Koh S, Rio C, et al. Decreased glutamate receptor 2 expression and enhanced epileptogenesis in immature rat hippocampus after perinatal hypoxia-induced seizures. *J Neurosci.* 2001;21: 8154–8163.

47. Koh S, Tibayan FD, Simpson JN, et al. NBQX or topiramate treatment after perinatal hypoxia-induced seizures prevents later increases in seizure-induced neuronal injury. *Epilepsia.* 2004;45:569–575.

48. Koh S, Jensen FE. Topiramate blocks perinatal hypoxia-induced seizures in rat pups. *Ann Neurol.* 2001;50:366–372.

49. Sankar R, Painter MJ. Neonatal seizures: after all of these years we still love what doesn't work. *Neurology.* 2005;64:776–777.

50. Khalilov I, Holmes GL, Benari Y. In vitro formation of a secondary epileptogenic mirror focus by interhippocampal propogation of seizures. *Nat Neurosc.* 2003;6:1079–1085.

51. Brooks-Kayal AR, Shumate MD, Jin H, et al. Gamma-aminobutyric acid(A) receptor subunit expression predicts functional changes in hippocampal dentate granule cells during postnatal development. *J Neurochem.* 2001;77:1266–1278.

52. Raol YH, Lund IV, Bandyopadhyay S, et al. Enhancing GABA$_A$ receptor α1 subunit levels in hippocampal dentate gyrus inhibits epilepsy development in an animal model of temporal lobe epilepsy. *J Neurosc.* 2006;26: 11342–11346.

53. Commission on Classification and Terminology of the International League Against Epilepsy. Proposal for revised classification of epilepsies and epileptic syndromes. *Epilepsia.* 1989;30:389–399.

54. ILAE Regional Commission. A proposed diagnostic scheme for people with epileptic seizures and with epilepsy: report of the ILAE Task Force on Classification and Terminology. *Epilepsia.* 2001;42:796–803.

55. Dreyfus-Brisac C, Monod N. Electroclinical studies of status epilepticus and convulsions in the newborn. In: Kellaway P, Petersen I, eds. *Neurological and Electroencephalographic Correlative Studies in Infancy.* New York: Grune and Stratton; 1964:250–272.

56. Rose A, Lombroso C. A study of clinical, pathological and electroencephalographic features in 137 full-term babies with a long-term follow up. *Pediatrics.* 1970;45:404–425.

57. Lombroso C. Seizures in the newborn. In: Vinken P, Bruyn G, eds. *The Epilepsies. Handbook of Clinical Neurophysiology.* Vol 15. Amsterdam: North Holland; 1974:189–218.

58. Volpe J. Neonatal seizures. *N Engl J Med.* 1973;289:413–416.

59. Watanabe K, Hara K, Miyazaki S. Electroclinical studies of seizures in the newborn. *Folia Psychiatr Neurol Jpn.* 1977;31:383–392.

60. Mizrahi EM, Kellaway P. Characterization and classification of neonatal seizures. *Neurology.* 1987;37:1837–1844.

61. Volpe J. Neonatal seizures: current concepts and revised classification. *Pediatrics.* 1989;84:422–428.

62. Scher MS. Neonatal seizure classification: a fetal perspective concerning childhood epilepsy. *Epilepsy Res.* 2006;70:41–57.

63. Mizrahi EM, Kellaway P. *Diagnosis and Management of Neonatal Seizures.* Philadelphia: Lippincott-Raven; 1998.

64. Hablitz J, Lee W, Prince D. NMDA receptor involvement in epileptogenesis in the immature neocortex. *Epilepsy Res Suppl.* 1992;8:139–145.

65. Prince D. Basic mechanisms of focal epileptogenesis. In: Avanzini G, Fariello R, Heinemann U, et al., eds. *Epileptogenic and Excitotoxic Mechanisms.* London: John Libbey; 1993:17–27.

66. Schwartzkroin P. Plasticity and repair in the immature central nervous system. In: Schwartzkroin P, Moshe SL, Nobels JL, eds. *Brain Development and Epilepsy.* New York: Oxford University Press; 1995:234–267.

67. Kellaway P, Hrachovy R. Status epilepticus in newborns: a perspective on neonatal seizures. In: Delgado-Escueta A, Wasterlain C, Treiman D, et al., eds. *Advances in Neurology.* New York: Raven Press; 1983:93–99.

68. Lou H, Friss-Hansen B. Arterial blood pressure elevations during motor activity and epileptic seizures in the newborn. *Acta Paediatr Scand.* 1979;68:803–806.

69. Goldberg R, Goldman S, Ramsay R. Detection of seizure activity in the paralyzed neonate using continuous monitoring. *Pediatrics.* 1982;69: 583–586.

70. Donati F, Schaffler L, Vassella F. Prolonged epileptic apneas in a newborn: a case report with ictal EEG recording. *Neuropediatrics.* 1995;26: 223–225.

71. Watanabe K, Hara K, Miyazaki S, et al. Apneic seizures in the newborn. *Am J Dis Child.* 1982;136:980–984.

72. Laroia N, Guillet R, Burchfiel J, et al. EEG background as predictor of electrographic seizures in high-risk neonates. *Epilepsia.* 1998;39:545–551.

73. Menache C, Bourgeois B, Volpe J. Prognostic value of neonatal discontinuous EEG. *Pediatr Neurol.* 2002;27:93–101.

74. Hrachovy R, Mizrahi EM, Kellaway P. Electroencephalography of the newborn. In: Daly D, Pedley T, eds. *Current Practice of Clinical Electroencephalography.* 2nd ed. New York: Raven Press; 1990:201–242.

75. Clancy R. Interictal sharp EEG transients in neonatal seizures. *J Child Neurol.* 1989;4:30–38.

76. Clancy R, Bergqvist AC, Dlugos D. Neonatal electroencephalography. In: Ebersole JS, Pedley T, eds. *Current Practice of Clinical Electroencephalography.* 3rd ed. Philadelphia: Lippincott-Raven; 2003: 160–234.

77. Patrizi S, Holmes GL, Orzalesi M, et al. Neonatal seizure: characteristics of EEG ictal activity in preterm and fullterm infants. *Brain Dev.* 2003;25: 427–437.

78. Clancy R, Malin S, Laraque D, et al. Focal motor seizures heralding stroke in full-term neonates. *Am J Dis Child.* 1985;139:601–606.

79. Clancy RR, Legido A. The exact ictal and interictal duration of electroencephalographic neonatal seizures. *Epilepsia.* 1987;28:537–541.

80. Knauss T, Carlson C. Neonatal paroxysmal monorhythmic alpha activity. *Arch Neurol.* 1978;35:104–107.

81. Willis J, Gould JB. Periodic alpha seizures with apnea in a newborn. *Dev Med Child Neurol.* 1980;22:214–222.

82. Watanabe K, Kuroyanagi M, Hara K, et al. Neonatal seizures and subsequent epilepsy. *Brain Dev.* 1982;4:341–346.

83. Mizrahi EM. Neonatal seizures: problems in diagnosis and classification. *Epilepsia.* 1987;28:S46–S55.

84. Boylan GB, Rennie JM, Pressler RM, et al. Phenobarbitone, neonatal seizures, and video-EEG. *Arch Dis Child Fetal Neonat Ed.* 2002;86:F165–F170.

85. Sharif U, Ichord R, Gaynor JW, et al. Electrographic neonatal seizures after newborn heart surgery. *Epilepsia.* 2003;44:164.

86. Bye AM, Cunningham CA, Chee KY, et al. Outcome of neonates with electrographically identified seizures, or at risk of seizures. *Pediatr Neurol.* 1997;16:225–231.

87. Gluckman PD, Wyatt JS, Azzopardi D, et al. Selective head cooling with mild systemic hypothermia after neonatal encephalopathy: multicentre ransomised trial. *Lancet.* 2005;365:663–670.

88. Rennie JM, Chorley G, Boylan GB, et al. Non-expert use of the cerebral function monitor for neonatal seizure detection. *Arch Dis Child Fetal Neonatal Ed.* 2004;89:37–40.

89. Shellhaas RA, Soaita AI, Clancy RR. Sensitivity of amplitude-integrated electroencephalography for neonatal seizure detection. *Pediatrics.* 2007;120:770–777.

90. Clancy R, Legido A, Lewis D. Occult neonatal seizures. *Epilepsia.* 1988;29:256–261.

91. Bye AM, Flanagan D. Spatial and temporal characteristics of neonatal seizures. *Epilepsia.* 1995;36:1009–1016.

92. Clancy RR. The contribution of EEG to the understanding of neonatal seizures. *Epilepsia.* 1996;37:S52–S59.

93. Leviton A, Nelson KB. Problems with definitions and classifications of newborn encephalopathy. *Pediatr Neurol.* 1992;8:85–90.

94. Durham SR, Clancy R, Leuthardt E, et al. CHOP Infant Coma Scale ("infant face scale"): a novel coma scale for children less than two years of age. *J Neurotrauma.* 2000;17:729–737.

95. Graham EM, Holcroft CJ, Blakemore KJ. Evidence of intrapartum hypoxia-ischemia is not present in the majority of cases of neonatal seizures. *J Matern Fetal Neonat Med.* 2002;12:123–126.

96. ACOG Task Force on Neonatal Encephalopathy and Cerebral Palsy. *Neonatal Encephalopathy and Cerebral Palsy: Defining the Pathogenesis and Pathophysiology.* Washington, DC: American College of Obstetricians and Gynecologists; 2002:73–80.

97. Martin-Ancel A, Garcia-Alix A, Gaya F, et al. Multiple organ involvement in perinatal asphyxia. *J Pediatr.* 1995;127:786–793.

98. Phelan JP, Korst LM, Ahn MO, et al. Neonatal nucleated red blood cell and lymphocyte counts in fetal brain injury. *Obstet Gynecol.* 1998;91:485–489.

99. Dammann O, Leviton A. Maternal intrauterine infection, cytokines, and brain damage in the preterm newborn. *Pediatr Res.* 1997;42:1–8.

100. Grether J, Nelson KB. Maternal infection and cerebral palsy in infants of normal birth weight. *JAMA.* 1997;278:207–211.

101. Kadhim H, Tabarki B, Verellen G, et al. Inflammatory cytokines in the pathogenesis of periventricular leukomalacia. *Neurology.* 2001;56:1278–1284.

102. Svigos JM. The fetal inflammatory response syndrome and cerebral palsy: yet another challenge and dilemma for the obstetrician. *Aust NZ Obstet Gynaecol.* 2001;41:170–176.

103. Baud O, Emilie D, Pelletier E, et al. Amniotic fluid concentrations of interleukin-1beta, interleukin-6 and TNF-alpha in chorioamnionitis before 32 weeks of gestation: histological associations and neonatal outcome. *Br J Obstet Gynaecol.* 1999;106:72–77.

104. Wu YW, Colford JM, Jr. Chorioamnionitis as a risk factor for cerebral palsy: a meta-analysis. *JAMA.* 2000;284:1417–1424.

105. Ment LR, Duncan CC, Ehrenkranz RA. Perinatal cerebral infarction. *Ann Neurol.* 1984;16:559–568.

106. deVeber G, Monagle P, Chan A, et al. Prothrombotic disorders in infants and children with cerebral thromboembolism. *Arch Neurol.* 1998;55:1539–1543.

107. Perlman JM, Rollins NK, Evans D. Neonatal stroke: clinical characteristics and cerebral blood flow velocity measurements. *Pediatr Neurol.* 1994;11:281–284.

108. Sreenan C, Bhargava R, Robertson CM. Cerebral infarction in the term newborn: clinical presentation and long-term outcome. *J Pediatr.* 2000;137:351–355.

109. deVeber G, Andrew M, Canadian Pediatric Ischemic Stroke Study Group. Cerebral sinovenous thrombosis in children. *N Engl J Med.* 2001;345:417–423.

110. Barron TF, Gusnard DA, Zimmerman R, et al. Cerebral venous thrombosis in neonates and children. *Pediatr Neurol.* 1992;8:112–116.

111. Rivkin MJ, Anderson ML, Kaye EM. Neonatal idiopathic cerebral venous thrombosis: an unrecognized cause of transient seizures or lethargy. *Ann Neurol.* 1992;32:51–56.

112. Fitzgerald KC, Williams LS, Garg BP, et al. Cerebral sinovenous thrombosis in the neonate. *Arch Neurol.* 2006;63:405–409.

113. Wasay M, Dai AI, Ansari M, et al. Cerebral venous sinus thrombosis in children: a multicenter cohort from the United States. *J Child Neurol.* 2008;23:23–31.

114. Korinthenberg R, Kachel W, Koelfen W, et al. Neurological findings in newborn infants after extracorporeal membrane oxygenation, with special reference to the EEG. *Dev Med Child Neurol.* 1993;35:249–257.

115. Lago P, Rebsamen S, Clancy R, et al. MRI, MRA and neurodevelopmental outcome following neonatal ECMO. *Pediatr Neurol.* 1995;12:294–304.

116. Clancy R. The neurology of hypoplastic left heart syndrome. In: Rychik J, Wenovsky G, eds. *The Hypoplastic Left Heart Syndrome.* Boston: Kluwer Academic; 2003:251–273.

117. Natowicz M, Chatten J, Clancy R. Genetic disorders and major extracardiac anomalies associated with the hypoplastic left heart syndrome. *Pediatrics.* 1988;82:698–706.

118. Clancy RR, McGaurn S, Wernovsky G, et al. Risk of seizures in survivors of newborn heart surgery using deep hypothermic circulatory arrest. *Pediatrics.* 2001;111:592–601.

119. Clancy RR, McGaurn SA, Goin JE, et al. Allopurinol neuro-cardiac protection trial in infants undergoing heart surgery utilizing deep hypothermic circulatory arrest. *Pediatrics.* 2001;107:61–70.

120. De Vivo DC, Trifiletti RR, Jacobson RI, et al. Defective glucose transport across the blood–brain barrier as a cause of persistent hypoglycorrhachia, seizures and developmental delay. *N Engl J Med.* 1991;325:703–709.

121. Fishman RA. The glucose-transporter protein and glucopenic brain injury. *N Engl J Med.* 1991;325:731–732.

122. Maher F, Vannucci S, Simpson I. Glucose transporter proteins in the brain. *FASEB J.* 1994;8:1003–1011.

123. Clancy R, Chung HJ. EEG changes during recovery from acute severe neonatal citrullinemia. *Electroencephalogr Clin Neurophysiol.* 1991;78:222–227.

124. Pettit RE. Pyridoxine dependency seizures: report of a case with unusual features. *J Child Neurol.* 1987;2:38–41.

125. Coker SB. Post-neonatal vitamin B6–dependent epilepsy. *Pediatrics.* 1992;90:221–223.

126. Osiovich H, Barrington K. Prenatal ultrasound diagnosis of seizures. *Am J Perinatol.* 1996;13:499–501.

127. Mills PB, Struys E, Jakobs C, et al. Mutation in antiquin in individuals with pyridoxine-dependent seizures. *Nat Med.* 2006;12:307–309.

128. Torres OA, Miller VS, Buist NM, et al. Folinic acid-responsive neonatal seizures. *J Child Neurol.* 1999;14:529–532.

129. Nicolai J, van Kranen-Mastenbroek VH, Wevers RA, et al. Folinic acid-responsive seizures initially responsive to pyridoxine. *Pediatr Neurol.* 2006;34:164–167.

130. Gallagher RC, Van Hove JL, Scharer G, et al. Folinic-acid responsive seizures are identical to pyridoxine-dependent epilepsy. *Ann Neurol.* 2009;65:550–556.

131. Slot HMJ, Overweg-Plandsoen WCG, Bakker HD, et al. Molybdenum-cofactor deficiency: an easily missed cause of neonatal convulsions. *Neuropediatrics.* 1993;24:139–142.

132. Arnold GL, Greene CL, Stout JP, et al. Molybdenum cofactor deficiency. *J Pediatr.* 1993;123:595–598.

133. Johnson JL. Prenatal diagnosis of molybdenum cofactor deficiency and isolated sulfite oxidase deficiency. *Proc Natl Acad Sci U S A.* 2002;23:6–8.

134. Stallmeyer B, Schwartz G, Sculze J, et al. The neurotransmitter receptor-anchoring protein gephyrin reconstitutes molybdenum cofactor biosynthesis in bacteria, plants and mammalian cells. *Proc Natl Acad Sci U S A.* 1998;96:1333–1338.

135. Herzlinger RA, Kandall SR, Vaughan HG, Jr. Neonatal seizures associated with narcotic withdrawal. *J Pediatr.* 1977;91:638–641.

136. Porter BE, Brooks-Kayal AR, Golden JA. Disorders of cortical development and epilepsy. *Arch Neurol.* 2002;59:361–365.

137. Tharp BR. Neonatal seizures and syndromes. *Epilepsia.* 2002;43:2–10.

138. Hayward JC, Titelbaum D, Clancy R, et al. Lissencephaly-pachygyria associated with congenital cytomegalovirus infection. *J Child Neurol.* 1991;6:109.

139. Bachevalier F, Marchal C, Di Cesare MP, et al. Lethal neurological involvement during incontinentia pigmenti. *Ann Dermatol Venereol.* 2003;130:1139–1142.

140. Nelson DL. NEMO, NFκB signalling and incontinentia pigmenti. *Curr Opin Genet Dev.* 2006;16:282–288.

141. Miller SP, Tasch T, Sylvain M, et al. Tuberous sclerosis complex and neonatal seizures. *J Child Neurol.* 1998;13:619–623.

142. Clancy R, Kurtz M, Baker D. Neurological manifestations of the organoid nevus syndrome. *Arch Neurol.* 1985;42:236–240.

143. Dehan M, Navelet Y, d'Allest AM, et al. Quelques precisions sur le syndrome des convulsions du cinquième jour de vie. *Arch Fr Pediatr.* 1982;39:405–407.

144. George AJ. Molecular basis of inherited epilepsy. *Arch Neurol.* 2004;61:473–478.

145. Cooper EC, Jan LY. Ion channel genes and human neurological disease: recent progress, prospects and challenges. *Proc Natl Acad Sci U S A.* 1998;96:4759–4766.

146. Dedek K, Kunath B, Kananura C, et al. Myokymia and neonatal epilepsy caused by a mutation in the voltage sensor of the KCNQ2 K+ channel. *Proc Natl Acad Sci U S A.* 2001;98:12272–12277.

147. Watanabe K, Yamoto N, Negoro T. Benign complex partial epilepsies in infancy. *Pediatr Neurol.* 1987;3:208–211.

148. Herlenius E, Heron SE, Grinton BE, et al. SCN2A mutations and benign familial neonatal-infantile seizures: the phenotypic spectrum. *Epilepsia.* 2007;48:1138–1142.

149. Coppola G, Plouin P, Chiron C, et al. Migrating partial seizures in infancy: a malignant disorder with developmental arrest. *Epilepsia.* 1995;36: 1017–1024.

150. Marsh E, Melamed S, Clancy R. Migrating partial seizures in early infancy: expanding the phenotype of a rare neonatal seizure type. *Epilepsia.* 2005;46:568–572.

151. Aicardi J, Goutieres F. Encephalopathie myoclonique neonatale. *Rev Electroencephalogr Neurophysiol Clin.* 1978;8:99–101.

152. Clancy R, Chung HJ, Hayward JC, et al. Early myoclonic epileptic encephalopathy. *Ann Neurol.* 1990;28:472–473.

153. Backx L, Ceulemans B, Vermeesch JR, et al. Early myoclonic encephalopathy caused by a disruption of the neuregulin-1 receptor ErbB4. *Eur J Hum Genet.* 2009;17:378–382.

154. Ohtahara S, Ishida T, Oka E, et al. On the specific age-dependent epileptic syndrome. The early-infantile epileptic encephalopathy with suppression-burst. *No To Hattatsu.* 1976;8:270–280.

155. Djukic A, Lado FA, Shinnar S, et al. Are early myoclonic encephalopathy (EME) and the Ohtahara syndrome (EIEE) independent of each other? *Epilepsy Res.* 2006;70:68–76.

156. Kato M, Saitoh S, Kamei A, et al. A longer polyalanine expansion mutation in the ARX gene causes early infantile epileptic encephalopathy with suppression-burst pattern (Ohtahara syndrome). *Am J Hum Genet.* 2007;81:361–366.

157. Saitsu H, Kato M, Mizuguchi T, et al. *De novo* mutations in the gene encoding STXBP1 (MUNC18-1) cause early infantile epileptic encephalopathy. *Nat Genet.* 2008;40:782–788.

158. Goldberg RN, Moscoso P, Bauer CR, et al. Use of barbiturate therapy in severe perinatal asphyxia: a randomized controlled trial. *J Pediatr.* 1986; 109:851–856.

159. Hall RT, Hall FK, Daily DK. High-dose phenobarbital therapy in term newborn infants with severe perinatal asphyxia: a randomized, prospective study with three-year follow-up. *J Pediatr.* 1998;132:345–348.

160. Singh D, Kumar P, Narang A. A randomized controlled trial of phenobarbital in neonates with hypoxic ischemic encephalopathy. *J Matern Fetal Neonatal Med.* 2005;18:391–395.

161. Connell J, Oozeer R, de Vries L, et al. Clinical and EEG response to anticonvulsants in neonatal seizures. *Arch Dis Child.* 1989;64:459–464.

162. Painter MJ, Scher MS, Stein AD, et al. Phenobarbital compared with phenytoin for the treatment of neonatal seizures. *N Engl J Med.* 1999;341:485–489.

163. Evans DJ, Levene MI, Tsakmakis M. Anticonvulsants for preventing mortality and morbidity in full term newborns with perinatal asphyxia. *Cochrane Database Syst Rev.* 2007;(3):CD001240.

164. Booth D, Evans DJ. Anticonvulsants for neonates with seizures. *Cochrane Database Syst Rev.* 2004;(3):CD004218.

165. Painter MJ, Alvin J. Neonatal seizures. *Curr Treat Options Neurol.* 2001; 3:237–248.

166. Bourgeois B, Dodson W. Phenytoin elimination in newborns. *Neurology.* 1983;33:173–178.

167. Dodson W. Antiepileptic drug utilization in pediatric patients. *Epilepsia.* 1984;25:S132–S139.

168. Wheless JW, Clarke DF, Carpenter D. Treatment of pediatric epilepsy: expert opinion. *J Child Neurol.* 2005;20:S1–S56.

169. Wheless JW, Clarke DF, Arzimanoglou A, et al. Treatment of pediatric epilepsy: European expert opinion. *Epileptic Disord.* 2007;9:353–412.

170. Bartha AI, Shen J, Katz KH, et al. Neonatal seizures: multicenter variability in current treatment practices. *Pediatr Neurol.* 2007;37:85–90.

171. Hellstrom-Westas L, Westgren U, Rosen I, et al. Lidocaine for treatment of severe seizures in newborn infants, I: clinical effects and cerebral electrical activity monitoring. *Acta Paediatr Scand.* 1988;77:79–84.

172. Norell E, Gamstorp I. Neonatal seizures: effect of lidocaine. *Acta Paediatr Scand Suppl.* 1970;206(suppl):97–98.

173. Malingré MM, Van Rooij LG, Rademaker CM, et al. Development of an optimal lidocaine infusion strategy for neonatal seizures. *Eur J Pediatr.* 2006;165:598–604.

174. Sheth RD, Buckley DJ, Gutierrez AR, et al. Midazolam in the treatment of refractory neonatal seizures. *Clin Neuropharmacol.* 1996;19:165–170.

175. Castro Conde JR, Hernández Borges AA, Doménech Martínez E, et al. Midazolam in neonatal seizures with no response to Phenobarbital. *Neurology.* 2005;64:876–879.

176. Macintosh D, Baird-Lampert J. Is carbamazepine an alternative maintenance therapy for neonatal seizures? *Dev Pharmacol Ther.* 1987;10: 100–106.

177. Sapin J, Riviello JJ, Grover W. Efficacy of primidone for seizure control in neonates and young infants. *Pediatr Neurol.* 1988;4:292–295.

178. Gal P, Otis K, Gilman J, et al. Valproic acid efficacy, toxicity and pharmacokinetics in neonates with intractable seizures. *Neurology.* 1988;38: 467–471.

179. Aicardi J, Mumford J, Dumas C. Vigabatrin as initial therapy for infantile spasms: a European retrospective survey. *Epilepsia.* 1996;37:638–642.

180. Barr P, Buettiker V, Anthony J. Efficacy of lamotrigine in refractory neonatal seizures. *Pediatr Neurol.* 1999;20:161–163.

181. Scher MS, Alvin J, Gaus L, et al. Uncoupling of EEG-clinical neonatal seizures after antiepileptic drug use. *Pediatr Neurol.* 2003;28:277–280.

182. Ellenberg JH, Hirtz D, Nelson KB. Age at onset of seizures in young children. *Ann Neurol.* 1984;15:127–134.

183. Clancy RR, Legido A. Postnatal epilepsy after EEG-confirmed neonatal seizures. *Epilepsia.* 1991;32:69–76.

184. Boer H, Gal P. Neonatal seizures: a survey of current practice. *Clin Pediatr.* 1982;21:453–457.

185. Fenichel G. Paroxysmal disorders. In: *Clinical Pediatric Neurology.* 3rd ed. Philadelphia: WB Saunders; 2001:1–45.

186. Daval J-L, Pereira de Vasconcelos A, Lartaud I. Development of mammalian cultured neurons following exposure to anticonvulsant drugs. In: Wasterlain CG, Vert P, eds. *Neonatal Seizures.* New York: Raven Press; 1990:295–301.

187. Bittigau P, Sifringer M, Genz K. Antiepileptic drugs and apoptotic neurodegeneration in the developing brain. *Proc Natl Acad Sci U S A.* 2002; 99:15089–15094.

CHAPTER 34 ■ FEBRILE SEIZURES

MICHAEL DUCHOWNY

Almost three decades ago, Livingston (1) observed that children with febrile seizures fared considerably better than those with epileptic convulsions not activated by fever; their prognosis with respect to epilepsy was uniformly more favorable, and they were more likely to be neurologically normal. Febrile seizures are now recognized as a relatively benign, age-dependent epilepsy syndrome and the most prevalent form of seizure in early life.

The National Institutes of Health (NIH) Consensus Development Conference on the Management of Febrile Seizures defined a febrile seizure as "an event in infancy or childhood, usually occurring between 3 months and 5 years of age, associated with fever but without evidence of intracranial infection or defined cause" (2). This definition is useful because it emphasizes age specificity and the absence of underlying brain abnormalities. It also implies that febrile seizures are not true epilepsy, because affected individuals are not predisposed to recurrent afebrile episodes.

In clinical practice, however, the NIH definition must be interpreted with caution. Intracranial infection may not be readily apparent, especially in very young infants. Although few medical practitioners advocate extensive testing in a healthy child with a brief nonfocal febrile seizure, an infant or child in febrile status epilepticus requires immediate medical attention.

Familiarity with the clinical manifestations and long-term prognosis of febrile seizures is essential in caring for affected individuals. Epidemiologic studies have been especially useful in identifying features of the seizure or the patient that involve adverse consequences. Understanding these factors forms the basis of proper seizure management and family counseling.

PREDISPOSING FACTORS

Genetics

There is no consensus regarding the mode of inheritance of febrile seizures or their clinical expression. Autosomal dominant (3), autosomal recessive (4), and polygenic theories (5,6) have all been formulated.

Febrile seizures are approximately two to three times more common among family members of affected children than in the general population (3,7). Affected parents increase the risk for the occurrence of febrile seizures in siblings. The risk increases when both parents are affected and is increased further in proportion to the number of febrile seizures experienced by the proband (8). A higher incidence of afebrile epilepsy has been found in first-degree relatives of patients with febrile seizures (8,9). Conversely, the occurrence of febrile seizures in first-degree relatives is itself a risk factor for febrile seizure recurrence (10). Siblings have the greatest

risk, followed by offspring, nieces, and nephews (8). Coexistence of febrile seizures and epilepsy increases the risk for both disorders in siblings (8). Temporal lobe seizures are more likely to begin early but remit permanently if a first-degree relative has experienced a febrile seizure (11). A single gene is held responsible, because the siblings of patients with temporal lobe and febrile seizures have a similar incidence of febrile seizures alone.

The incidence of febrile seizures also varies according to geographic region and race. Parents and siblings of Asian children are at considerably higher risk for febrile seizures than are Western families. Sibling risk approaches 30% if one parent has had a febrile seizure. The difference in frequency of febrile seizures in Asian compared with European or North American families suggests a strong, genetically determined population effect (12).

Linkage studies in a number of large pedigrees have identified several mutations in sodium channel subunit genes (13). Putative febrile seizure loci include FEB 1 (chromosome 8q13–21), FEB 2 (chromosome 19p), FEB 3 (chromosome 2q23–24), and FEB 4 (chromosome 5q14–15 and 5q14–23) (14–16). All affected individuals present with recurrent febrile seizures by 3 years of age, with no evidence of structural brain pathology or intracranial infection. Although most individuals are predisposed to later afebrile seizures, families mapping to the FEB 3 locus have significantly higher rates of later epilepsy compared with that reported in general population studies or in families with febrile seizures (17). Linkage studies in large kindreds have recently identified two novel loci on chromosomes 21q22 (18) and chromosome 3q26.2-26.33 (19). The human *SEZ-6* gene is related to the occurrence and development of FS and may be a good candidate gene for epilepsy (20). Although a recent report suggests that a splice variant in the A allele of the *SCNA1* gene is common and a relevant risk factor for FS (21), a subsequent study failed to replicate the original observation (21a).

Genetic linkage between febrile seizures and absence epilepsy has also been described (22). A new locus for febrile seizures was identified on chromosome 3P in a four-generational study of 51 French family members. The association of benign familial infantile seizures and febrile seizures with linkage on chromosome 16 has also reported (23).

Despite the identification of multiple febrile seizure loci and mutated genes, little evidence points to their direct contribution toward the majority of febrile seizures reported in the most affected individuals. This probably reflects the marked heterogeneous clinical manifestations of febrile seizures and their lack of association with known genetic loci (24). Furthermore, family pedigrees of most known febrile seizure phenotypes are atypical of "common" febrile seizures, in that mutation-specific febrile seizures often have an extended age of onset and offset, and predispose individuals to later afebrile seizures. Pal and associates (25) used a case-control study design to identify specific phenotypic subgroups of febrile seizures and reduce clinical heterogeneity. In a comparison of 83 patients with febrile seizures who had a first-degree family history and 101 control patients with febrile seizures who lacked affected family members, the investigators found that a first-degree family history of febrile seizures and the later occurrence of afebrile seizures were specifically and independently associated with an increased risk for febrile seizure recurrence.

Age

The onset of febrile seizures generally follows a bell-shaped pattern. Ninety percent of these seizures occur within the first 3 years of life (26), 4% before 6 months, and 6% after 3 years of age. Approximately 50% appear during the second year of life, with a peak incidence between 18 and 24 months (26).

Febrile seizures occurring before 6 months of age should always raise the level of suspicion of infectious causes; bacterial meningitis must be excluded by examination of the cerebrospinal fluid (CSF) in patients of this age group. Febrile seizures after 5 years of age also should be managed cautiously, because benign causes are less common in older children.

The limited age range in febrile seizures has never been satisfactorily explained. Immaturity of central neurotransmission may play a role but should affect other childhood seizure types equally. Prostaglandin E_2, but not homovanillic or 5-hydroxyindoleacetic acid, is increased in lumbar CSF following febrile seizures in humans (27,28). Hyperthermia-induced convulsions in the developing rat can alter nicotinic and muscarinic cholinergic function (29). The maximum changes occur 55 days after the last convulsion, suggesting the importance of secondary factors.

Fever

Febrile seizures typically occur relatively early in an infectious illness, usually during the rising phase of the temperature curve. Rectal temperatures at this time may exceed 39.2°C (102.6°F), and approximately one fourth of seizures occur at temperatures above 40.2°C (104.4°F). The contribution of the rate of rise versus the final temperature reached in inducing the seizure has been debated (30). However, despite the implicit relationship between fever and seizure activation, temperature itself probably does not lower the seizure threshold. The incidence of febrile seizures does not increase in proportion to temperature elevation, and febrile seizures are generally uncommon in the later stages of a persistent illness. Moreover, children between the ages of 6 and 18 months who experience a fever higher than 40°C (104°F) have a sevenfold reduction in seizure recurrence compared with children with a fever below 40°C (104°F) (31). A brief duration of fever before the initial febrile seizure has been linked to an increased risk for seizure recurrence (32).

Febrile seizures typically are associated with common childhood illnesses, most frequently viral upper respiratory tract, middle ear, and gastrointestinal infections. Bacterial infections, including bacteremia, pneumonia, sepsis, and meningitis, are rare concomitants of febrile seizures. None of the common viral or bacterial childhood infectious illnesses appears to be uniquely capable of activating febrile seizures.

Febrile seizures in conjunction with shigellosis constitute the most frequent extraintestinal manifestation of this infection (33). A direct neurotoxic effect of the *Shigella* bacterium on seizure threshold has been proposed.

Immunization-related seizures also manifest with fever, usually within 24 hours of DTP vaccination and 8 to 14 days after MMR inoculation (34,35). Approximately one fourth of immunization-related seizures are related to administration of diphtheria–pertussis–tetanus (DPT) vaccine, and one fourth follow measles immunization. Data from the National Collaborative Perinatal Project indicate that age of onset, personal and family history, and clinical presentation of postimmunization seizures resemble those of febrile seizures from infectious causes (36). The risk of DPT-induced febrile seizures increases if a family member has had an afebrile seizure (37,38). These shared features suggest that infectious and immunization-related febrile seizures are expressions of a unitary condition.

Associated Factors

Ancillary factors related to underlying illness or fever may be implicated in the pathogenesis of febrile convulsions, usually with little supportive evidence. Direct viral invasion of brain tissue has been proposed (39), but children with proven viral infections appear no more likely to experience seizure recurrence than do uninfected children (40). Electrolyte disturbances are said to lower seizure threshold, but this mechanism remains relatively unsupported (41). Transient pyridoxine deficiency seems unlikely, and the association of *Shigella* infection and febrile seizures has prompted a search for an epileptogenic neurotoxin.

Proinflammatory cytokines have recently been implicated in the pathogenesis of febrile seizures. Interleukin (IL)-1β, tumor necrosis factor-α, and nitrite levels are all increased in the CSF of children with a febrile seizure (42). Increased secretion of IL-6 and IL-10 by liposaccharide-stimulated mononuclear cells is higher in patients with a history of previous febrile seizures (43).

Girls younger than 18 months of age have a slightly higher risk than boys of experiencing more frequent and severe febrile seizures (44,45). Ounsted (46) proposed that an excess of boys from one-sex sibships may explain the male predominance that has been observed in some studies (46,47) but not in others (26).

TYPES OF FEBRILE SEIZURES

Simple Febrile Convulsions

Simple febrile convulsions are solitary events, lasting less than 15 minutes and lacking focality. They occur in neurologically normal children and are not associated with persistent deficits. The source of the fever is always outside the central nervous system (CNS).

Between 80% and 90% of all febrile seizures are simple episodes (26,48,49). This figure is probably an underestimate, because most published series are hospital based and thus weighted toward children with complex risk factors (50).

Despite their common occurrence, the sporadic nature and brief duration of febrile seizures make analysis difficult. Descriptions provided by parents and emergency department personnel are retrospective and probably not entirely accurate. Video-electroencephalographic studies of afebrile generalized seizures, for example, often reveal subtle atonic or myoclonic components that were omitted in the witnessed accounts. Lack of objectivity notwithstanding, febrile seizures are described as tonic, clonic, or tonic–clonic events that usually begin without warning and display upward eye deviation as consciousness is lost. Atonic forms are rare, and postictal depression is generally brief.

Electroencephalography has not been particularly useful in the evaluation of simple febrile seizures. Although paroxysmal and nonspecific electroencephalographic (EEG) abnormalities are often evident within 24 hours of seizure onset, they have little prognostic significance. Slow-wave activity occurs in up to one third of patients (51), and is often bilateral and prominent in the posterior regions (47). Twenty percent of patients, usually older than 2.5 years of age, have generalized spike-and-wave discharges on the electroencephalogram.

In a longitudinal study of 89 patients with febrile seizures followed until puberty, Doose and associates (52) identified three patterns of EEG abnormality: rhythms of 4 to 7 Hz, generalized spike-and-wave discharges, and photosensitivity. None were specific for febrile seizures because all had been described in generalized epilepsies as well. Genetic factors probably account for the age-related expression of these EEG patterns in benign, simple febrile seizures.

Because seizures in the setting of a febrile illness may result from CNS infection, trauma, or electrolyte disturbance, laboratory investigation is usually warranted even when findings on the physical examination are normal. The diagnostic yield of such studies is usually well below 2%, however, and difficult to justify (53). The skull roentgenogram and lumbar puncture are even less likely to contribute useful information in healthy children (54), and the rare seizure caused by electrolyte disturbance usually can be diagnosed from the patient's history. The confirmation of viral meningitis by lumbar puncture does not alter long-term management.

The evaluation of simple febrile seizures should therefore rely primarily on careful history taking, and judicious laboratory and radiologic testing. This approach, which is particularly important in children who are normal, has been underscored in an editorial (55) stating that "children who have their first febrile convulsion need no more tests than the clinical findings dictate." An exception is the requirement for CSF examination in all patients younger than 6 months of age who lack any of the classic signs of bacterial meningitis. The rule that all children younger than 18 months of age with a first febrile seizure should always undergo CSF examination is probably excessive, and each child should be evaluated individually. When meningitis is suspected clinically, lumbar puncture should be performed promptly in the physician's office or emergency department.

Hospitalization is rarely necessary following a simple febrile seizure. Testing can usually be performed in an outpatient setting because risk of seizure recurrence is low. Even so, pediatricians may hospitalize patients who can be sent home safely. In 1975, 24% of practicing pediatricians routinely admitted children after a first febrile seizure; a decade later, 20% still followed this practice (56). However, a more recent evaluation (57) found a decline in the rate of admission with the decision to admit most frequently occurring in those with prolonged seizures.

Complex Febrile Seizures

The concept of a "complex" febrile seizure originated with epidemiologic studies indicating that several patient- and seizure-related variables predicted higher rates of subsequent epilepsy: seizure duration longer than 15 minutes, focal seizure manifestations, seizure recurrence within 24 hours, abnormal neurologic status, and afebrile seizures in a parent or sibling (58). Six percent of patients with two or more risk factors developed afebrile epilepsy by the age of 7 years, compared with only 0.9% if risk factors were absent (58).

Studies conducted at the Mayo Clinic also reveal a less favorable prognosis for patients with complex febrile seizures (49). Seventeen percent of neurologically impaired children with complex febrile seizure manifestations developed epilepsy by the third decade, compared with 2.5% of children who lacked risk factors. The occurrence of focal, recurrent, and prolonged seizures raised the risk for afebrile episodes to nearly 50%.

Children with complex febrile convulsions may subsequently exhibit a variety of afebrile seizure patterns. The National Collaborative Perinatal Project (48) found generalized tonic–clonic seizures to be the most frequent and absence or myoclonic seizures less common. In the Mayo Clinic experience (59), 29 cases of afebrile epilepsy developed in a cohort of 666 patients with febrile seizures. Seizures were classified as focal in 16 patients and of temporal origin in 10 patients. Generalized tonic–clonic seizures were reported in 12 patients, 3 of whom also had absence seizures. One patient had unclassifiable seizures. In a retrospective analysis of 504 children with epilepsy, Camfield and colleagues (60) found a 14.9% incidence of prior febrile seizures. Febrile seizures most often preceded generalized tonic–clonic afebrile seizures and were regarded as fundamentally indicative of reduced seizure threshold.

Complex febrile seizures must be managed more aggressively than simple episodes. Meningitis must be excluded by timely performance of CSF examination, and neuroimaging studies are indicated to detect structural lesions. However, the risk of a lesion requiring neurosurgical intervention is extremely low (61). In acute bacterial meningitis, focal febrile seizures may accompany cortical vein or sagittal sinus thrombosis. In North America, parasitic disease and brain abscess are uncommon causes of complex febrile seizures.

Although children with complex febrile seizures may be expected to show a higher rate of abnormal EEG recordings than normal, confirmatory data are sparse. Studies of febrile seizures rarely include EEG findings, although this type of information would enhance the value of electroencephalography in the management of patients with febrile seizures.

Febrile Status Epilepticus

Although most febrile seizures are self-limited, prolonged episodes and febrile status epilepticus are not rare. The reported occurrence of epilepsy, brain damage, or death following febrile status epilepticus further underscores its serious nature. Of 1706 children with febrile seizures followed in the National Collaborative Perinatal Project, 8% experienced seizures for longer than 15 minutes, and 4% had seizures for longer than 30 minutes (48). Febrile status epilepticus accounted for approximately 25% of all cases of status epilepticus in children (37,62), and is often the initial presentation of chronic epilepsy (48).

The phenomenology of prolonged febrile seizures has been investigated in a prospective multi-center study examining the consequences of febrile status epilepticus in children aged 1 month through 5 years (63). Most episodes were focal, occurred in very young children and usually were the first febrile seizure. Seizure duration in this group was typically very prolonged suggesting that the longer the seizure continued, the less likely it was to spontaneously cease.

Children with febrile status epilepticus are typically mentally and physically normal but compared to children with simple febrile seizures, are more likely to demonstrate abnormalities on MRI including cortical dysplasia and subcortical focal hyperintensities (64). As with simple febrile seizures, common childhood infectious diseases and immunizations are the primary cause of the fever. An association between female sex and febrile status epilepticus has been observed in some studies (65), whereas others (26,32,63) have found a slight male predominance. Younger age strongly predisposes patients toward prolonged unilateral febrile seizures (66).

Postmortem studies of patients dying of febrile status epilepticus reveal widespread neuronal necrosis of the cortex, basal ganglia, thalamus, cerebellum, and temporolimbic structures (67). Rare inflammatory changes suggest that seizures and anoxia, rather than infection, are the primary causes of mortality (47,67,68).

Prospective studies reveal that the risk for death or permanent neurologic impairment following febrile status epilepticus is negligible (48,69). The tendency for febrile status epilepticus to recur is especially low in neurologically normal children (70), and mortality in this group has markedly declined. None of the 1706 patients followed in the National Collaborative Perinatal Project died as a consequence of febrile seizures, a finding confirmed by others (70).

A few infants present with severe febrile hemiconvulsive status that is followed by permanent hemiplegia. After a variable seizure-free interval, they develop chronic focal epilepsy that can persist for many years. This presentation, called the hemiconvulsion–hemiplegia–epilepsy (HHE) syndrome, was described by Gastaut and associates (71), who regarded it as distinct from other prenatal or perinatal causes of infantile hemiplegia and epilepsy.

The HHE syndrome usually manifests before the age of 2 years as status epilepticus lasting from hours to days. Seizures may be triggered by any of the benign childhood infections or they may be idiopathic in nature. Hemiconvulsions are typical at onset, but generalized patterns usually predominate as the seizure progresses. Postictal unresponsiveness may be prolonged.

After the ictus, the child has a variable degree of residual spastic hemiparesis. Recovery of motor function depends on the severity and topography of the damage and the age at which it is acquired. The later emergence of afebrile seizures changes the designation of the hemiconvulsion–hemiplegia syndrome into the HHE syndrome. Recurrent and often medically resistant seizures may persist for years thereafter. Complex partial seizures are the most prevalent form of later epilepsy. Some patients with the HHE syndrome and intractable disabling partial seizures may achieve freedom from seizures after cortical resection or hemispherectomy. Histopathologic analysis reveals atrophy and gliosis throughout the involved hemisphere, with prominent sclerosis of mesial temporal structures. Improvements in the acute treatment of patients with status epilepticus have made the HHE syndrome rare.

RISK ASSESSMENT IN FEBRILE SEIZURES

Febrile Seizure Recurrence

Approximately one third of patients with febrile seizures experience additional attacks; of this group, one-half will have a third seizure (72,73) and 9% experience more than three attacks (58).

Age of onset is the most important predictor of febrile seizure recurrence. One-half of all infants younger than 1 year of age at the time of their first febrile seizure will have a recurrence, compared with 20% of children older than 3 years of age. Young age at onset, a history of febrile seizures in first-degree relatives, low-grade fever in the emergency department, and brief interval between fever onset and seizure presentation are strong independent predictors of febrile seizure recurrence (74). Recurrences generally occur within 1 year but are no more likely in children who had a complex febrile seizure than in those who experienced a simple febrile seizure.

In those with a subsequent febrile episode (75), approximately one-half of all recurrent febrile seizures occur within the 2 hours following onset of fever. Young age at onset and high temperature favor recurrence.

Children with multiple risk factors experience the highest rates of febrile seizure recurrence. The presence of two or more risk factors is associated with a 30% or greater recurrence risk, whereas three risk factors are associated with a 60% or greater recurrence risk (74). Subsequent febrile seizures are more likely to be prolonged when the initial febrile seizure is prolonged (76). Febrile seizure recurrence is not more likely in children with abnormal neurodevelopmental status (76).

Epilepsy and Association with Hippocampal Sclerosis

Between 1.5% and 4.6% of children with febrile seizures go on to develop afebrile seizures (77–80). Although this rate is significantly higher than in the general population, it reflects primarily infants and children with one or more complex febrile seizures (58,81). The presence of a neurodevelopmental abnormality, a family history of epilepsy, and prolonged duration of fever are also definite risk factors (82). The forms of later epilepsy are varied and similar to the seizure pattern encountered in children without a history of febrile seizures.

The mechanism by which individuals with febrile seizures are predisposed to later epilepsy is much less clear. Prolonged febrile convulsions in early infancy may precede a variety of seizures but are particularly common in children who develop intractable seizures of temporal lobe origin (83). Histopathologic studies of temporal lobectomy specimens demonstrate hippocampal sclerosis (HS) in approximately half of all surgical cases. HS is hypothesized to result from asphyxia during prolonged febrile seizures, especially febrile status epilepticus (84,85). Prolonged childhood febrile seizures are known to increase cerebral metabolic demand and to induce systemic changes, including hypoxia, hypoglycemia, and arterial hypotension (86). Hyperpyrexia may increase cerebral metabolic rate by as much as 25% (87). Neuronal changes are observed in the neocortex, thalamus, and hippocampus in paralyzed and ventilated seizing animals with controlled systemic factors (86). For reasons that are unclear, there is a significant predominance of right-sided HS in patients with a history of febrile seizures (88).

The association between prolonged febrile seizures and later HS continues to be controversial. Provenzale et al. (89) found that markedly intense hippocampal signal in children with febrile status epilepticus was highly associated with subsequent HS. Theodore et al. (90) noted reduced cerebral volumes after complex febrile seizures suggesting that damage is even more widespread than the hippocampus alone. However, in a long-term follow-up study of 24 patients with a prolonged first febrile seizure, Tarkka and colleagues (91) found no reduction in mean hippocampal volumes compared with a control group with a simple febrile seizure and no later epilepsy. Bower and coworkers (92) investigated patients with proven HS and febrile seizures, and did not find a relationship between hippocampal volume reduction and history of febrile seizures. These larger series contrast with well-documented, individual prospective case studies linking prolonged febrile seizures to subsequent hippocampal swelling, atrophy, and sclerosis (93,94). Prolonged febrile seizures that predispose individuals to HS occur in clusters of unilateral or generalized febrile status, with unilateral ictal EEG discharges and prolonged postictal unresponsiveness.

It is also possible that prolonged febrile seizures act in combination with later afebrile seizures to influence the development of HS. Theodore and associates (90) investigated hippocampal volumes in patients with medically uncontrolled temporal lobe epilepsy and found that individuals with a history of complex or prolonged febrile seizures had smaller ipsilateral hippocampal volumes than did those without a history of febrile seizures. Epilepsy duration had a significant effect on ipsilateral hippocampal volume, suggesting that damage to the hippocampus after a first prolonged febrile seizure may be progressive. Experimental studies of febrile seizures suggest that progressive hippocampal changes could be modulated through alteration of activity-dependent regulation of cyclic nucleotide-gated channels (95).

The clinical and experimental sequelae of prolonged febrile seizures are difficult to reconcile with epidemiologic data indicating that most severe attacks do not produce long-lasting consequences. Febrile seizures should therefore be considered to represent a continuum of brain dysfunction ranging from very mild local cellular changes to severe generalized damage or hemiatrophy.

Neuroimaging studies further support the concept of selective hippocampal vulnerability to prolonged or recurrent febrile seizures in susceptible individuals (96). Confirmed MRI evidence of hippocampal damage was identified in 6 of 15 infants with focal or lateralized complex febrile seizures and in none of 12 infants with generalized febrile seizures (97). Signs of preexisting hippocampal abnormalities and electrographic seizure discharges in the temporal lobe in several infants suggest primary febrile seizure onset in the temporal lobe. Hippocampal volumetry reveals smaller total volumes and a larger right-to-left ratio in children with complex febrile seizures than in controls (98). Increasing duration of the seizure is inversely associated with ipsilateral, but not contralateral, hippocampal volume, suggesting that the deleterious effects of persistent seizures remain localized to the epileptogenic zone (90).

A complex relationship exists among age, sex, and hemispheric vulnerability in children who develop temporal lobe seizures after prolonged febrile convulsions. Left-sided HS is more common following prolonged febrile seizures in the first year of life but is rare after 2 years of age, whereas right-sided HS is equally prevalent throughout the first 4 years of life (99,100). The risk for HS in both sexes is highest in the first year of life, but declines gradually in boys and precipitously in girls. These observations suggest differential rates of vulnerability for each cerebral hemisphere in both sexes.

Genetic Predisposition

Genetic factors may contribute to the development of epilepsy in some individuals with febrile seizures. Temporal lobe seizures are more likely to begin early but remit permanently if a first-degree relative has experienced a febrile seizure (11). A single gene is held responsible, because the siblings of patients with temporal lobe and febrile seizures have a similar incidence of febrile seizures alone.

The autosomal dominantly inherited syndrome of generalized epilepsy with febrile seizures plus (GEFS+) was first described in a large kindred from rural Victoria, Australia (101). The clinical phenotype includes those with febrile seizures in early childhood who develop persistent febrile seizures beyond age 6 years and individuals with a variety of heterogeneous afebrile generalized seizure phenotypes. Seizures typically cease by midadolescence.

GEFS+ demonstrates an autosomal-dominant mode of inheritance. In GEFS+ families, a mutation in the voltage-gated sodium channel β_1 subunit (SCN1B) gene at chromosome 19q13.1 and two mutations of the same α_1 subunit (SCN1A) gene at chromosome 2q24 have been identified (102–106). Rather than being a rare disorder, the GEFS+ phenotype has now been identified in multiple families with generalized epilepsy and febrile seizures (107). To date, six loci for GEFS+ have been defined including a recently reported linkage to a 13-Mb interval on chromosome 8p23–21 in five French families (108). The phenotypically heterogeneous nature of the later epilepsy is attested to by the recently recognized association of the SCN1A mutation to partial as well as generalized seizures (109). Several large kindreds with autosomal-dominant temporal lobe epilepsy and febrile seizures that do not show linkage to candidate regions for familial partial epilepsy and febrile seizures have also been described (110,111).

Mutations in the gene encoding the gamma-2 subunit of the $GABA_A$ receptor (GABRG2) have now been described in

GEFS+ (112). Additional *GABRG2* alleles that alter current desensitization and reduce benzodiazepine enhancement have also been characterized (113).

The spectrum of genetic epilepsies associated with febrile seizures is expanding. Severe myoclonic epilepsy of infancy, also known as Dravet syndrome, is a malignant epileptic encephalopathy that typically presents in the first year of life with prolonged febrile seizures (114). Febrile seizures may be generalized or focal and typically first occur between 5 and 7 months. Initial development and EEG studies are normal, making early diagnosis extremely challenging. Other seizure types and developmental regression subsequently intervene between the ages of 1 and 4 years. Myoclonic seizures are often mild or absent, or disappear after a relatively brief period. Ataxia and pyramidal signs evolve later in some patients and can progressively restrict ambulation. Intellectual functioning is almost always severely impaired. The adult presentation of Dravet syndrome without early onset febrile seizures has recently been described (115).

A high proportion of family members of individuals with Dravet syndrome exhibit various seizure types. It has been suggested that Dravet syndrome should be included within the phenotypic continuum of GEFS+, but at the severe end of the spectrum (116). Missense mutations in the gene that encodes the neuronal voltage-gated *SCN1A* in families of GEFS+ patients has been identified in approximately one third of patients with Dravet syndrome (117,118). A greater frequency of unilateral motor seizures occurs in patients carrying this mutation (118).

Treatment of Dravet syndrome patients is often challenging. Multiple antiepileptic drugs including stiripentol have been advocated (119). Levetiracetam has been advocated as add-on therapy (120).

Human Herpes Virus 6B

Human herpes virus 6 (HHV6) is a common childhood infectious agent responsible for roseola infantum and several severe infectious syndromes. In immunocompromised patients, reactivation of viral activity may lead to severe limbic encephalitis. Examination of temporal lobectomy specimens reveals a high incidence of active HHV6B replication in hippocampal astrocytes (121). This association points to a possible link between early viral infection, complex or prolonged febrile seizures and later HS.

FEBRILE SEIZURES AND LATER NEUROPSYCHOLOGICAL STATUS

The consequences of febrile seizures on later intellectual functioning and behavior have been extensively studied. Although some children with febrile seizures can manifest cognitive sequelae, virtually all had neurologic deficits that predated their convulsions (122). A cohort of 381 children with simple and complex febrile seizures was compared with a control group with respect to academic progress, intelligence, and behavior; no differences were observed between the groups in any of the measures (123).

Two large, longitudinal, population-based studies provide strong evidence that febrile seizures do not adversely affect neuropsychological status. Ellenberg and Nelson (69) studied intellectual and academic function following febrile seizures in 431 sibling pairs 7 years of age who were part of the National Collaborative Perinatal Project. Children with febrile seizures and normal intelligence achieved reading and spelling milestones at rates similar to those of their seizure-free siblings. Poor academic performance on the Wide Range Achievement Test was equally common in patients with febrile seizures and sibling controls. The National Child Development Study, completed in the United Kingdom, also found that children with febrile seizures did not differ from controls in behavior, height, head circumference, or academic achievement (78,124).

THERAPY

The American Academy of Pediatrics, through its Committee on Quality Improvement, published two practice parameters dealing with the evaluation of the child with a first febrile seizure and the long-term treatment of the child with simple febrile seizures in 1996 and 1999, respectively (125,126). These publications provided an analytic framework for the evaluation and treatment of patients with febrile seizures. Pertinent evidence on individual therapeutic agents, including study results and dosing guidelines was supplied. These practice parameters were further reviewed and expanded in 2000 and 2008 (127,128). Recommendation for the management of febrile seizures has also been issued by Italian League Against Epilepsy (129). The guidelines are similar to the American Academy of Pediatrics and stress the benign prognosis and need for conservative management. Implementation of febrile seizure guidelines in pediatric emergency departments positively modifies clinical management and patient welfare (130).

The role of lumbar puncture in very young patients with febrile seizures has recently been evaluated. In a retrospective cohort review of 706 pediatric patients aged 6 to 18 months being evaluated for a first febrile seizure in an emergency department, lumbar puncture was performed in 271 (38%) children (131). CSF white blood cell count was elevated in only 10 cases (3.8%) and no patient was diagnosed with bacterial meningitis. These findings suggest that the American Academy of Pediatrics recommendations to strongly consider lumbar puncture in this age group may need to be reconsidered.

Although current evidence demonstrates that antipyretic agents do not reduce the risk of febrile seizure recurrence (126,127), parents should be taught the importance of prompt use of antipyretics and tepid sponge bathing to control fever and make the child more comfortable. Unfortunately, fever may be recognized only after the onset of convulsion; therefore, attention must be directed to other signs of infection, such as anorexia, diarrhea, or rash (26). Bacterial infections should be treated with the appropriate antibiotic agents.

Prophylactic antiepileptic drug (AED) therapy should be withheld, as the benefits of treatment do not outweigh the risks. Recurrent febrile seizures and later afebrile epilepsy, the major sequelae of a febrile seizure, are both rare. Despite their anxiety, family members should be counseled about the merits of withholding prophylactic treatment. Parents must come to regard simple febrile seizures as a benign disorder that remits with time.

The use of AEDs can sometimes be considered following the occurrence of complex febrile seizures that carry an increased risk for later epilepsy. However, even seemingly life-threatening seizures must be evaluated cautiously. As neurologic impairment and death are extremely unlikely, even after febrile status epilepticus, most children do not require the use of long-term medication. The NIH consensus panel found that high-risk patients with two risk factors (e.g., abnormalities on neurologic examination, prolonged focal seizure, family history of epilepsy) still had only a 13% chance of developing epilepsy. Moreover, even though phenobarbital reduced febrile seizure recurrence, there is no firm evidence that the prevention of recurrent febrile seizures diminishes the risk for later epilepsy.

Febrile seizures often cease by the time a child is examined; prolonged episodes can be terminated with the use of parenteral diazepam, lorazepam, or phenobarbital. Phenobarbital, valproic acid, and diazepam all prevent febrile seizure recurrence (132–137), but slow oral absorption necessitates long-term administration and renders these agents ineffective in short attacks. Therapeutic levels of phenytoin and carbamazepine do not prevent recurrent febrile seizures, although phenytoin may decrease seizure severity (138).

Phenobarbital administration has been associated with rash, sedation, and dysarthria. Hyperactivity, behavioral disorders, irritability, and sleep abnormalities occur in up to 40% of patients, and may provoke parental resistance to medication and noncompliance. Most behavior problems appear shortly after therapy is initiated, are idiosyncratic, and resolve with discontinuation of barbiturates (139).

The long-term effects on cognitive functioning of prolonged barbiturate therapy remain controversial. Prolonged administration was reported not to impair cognitive function (140–142), but serum levels were rarely recorded in these studies, and the populations were highly variable with respect to seizure type, degree of control, and administration of other AEDs. In one study (143), children with febrile seizures receiving daily doses of phenobarbital were compared with carefully matched controls. No differences in performance were apparent on the Wechsler Preschool and Primary Scales of Intelligence, Matching Familiar Figures Test, or Children's Embedded Figures Test (143).

Farwell and colleagues (144) performed the most comprehensive evaluation of phenobarbital administration on intelligence and found an 8-point discrepancy between patients and controls on the Stanford-Binet Scales of Intelligence administered up to 2.5 years after treatment. Barbiturate levels were unrelated to intelligence quotient (IQ) scores, and no difference was detected in the incidence of behavioral problems. Phenobarbital also had no effect on febrile seizure recurrence. Only 25% of the eligible study children completed IQ testing, however, and long-term compliance with medication could not be enforced.

Rectally administered diazepam gel is currently the agent of choice for short-term prophylaxis of febrile seizures (145). Parents are easily instructed on its safe administration. Used intermittently, rectal diazepam gel is equally effective as continuous phenobarbital and terminates most febrile seizures immediately (53,143,146–148). Respiratory depression is a potential concern but is rarely encountered in clinical practice, and tolerance is not associated with infrequent use. Buccal midazolam is as effective as rectal diazepam (149) and intravenous midazolam is as effective as diazepam for controlling seizures in a prehospital setting (150). Nasal midazolam offers rapid seizure termination and can be administered

by parents or caretakers of children with recurrent febrile seizures (151).

Intermittent diazepam has rekindled interest in simple febrile seizure prevention. In one study (152), the number of recurrent seizures was reduced in nearly 50% of all children receiving diazepam at fever onset, compared with those receiving placebo. Intermittent therapy for acute seizures is particularly well received by family members because of the considerable anxiety that is provoked. Preventive agents are thus chosen by most parents (153). Rectal diazepam affords primary control over a stressful emergency, thereby improving the quality of life in more than half of affected families (148).

CONCLUSIONS

The syndrome of febrile seizures is the most common seizure presentation in infancy and early childhood. Most events are self-limited and carry only a modest risk for febrile seizure recurrence. Febrile seizures are thus a genetically predetermined, age-dependent response to fever and not an epilepsy. Treatment with prophylactic AEDs is not indicated.

Fewer than 10% of patients with febrile seizures experience severe or recurrent attacks. Risk factors for complex episodes are known, and the likelihood of developing epilepsy remains at less than 5%. Diagnostic procedures or treatment should be considered only on an individual basis; febrile status epilepticus must be treated as a medical emergency. Underlying neurologic disorders require investigation, and "epileptic seizures exacerbated by fever" should be distinguished from febrile seizures per se. Rectal diazepam gel is now considered the agent of choice for acute febrile seizure termination. It is important to counsel families about the benign and genetic nature of febrile seizures and to provide reassurance about the excellent long-term prognosis. There is no evidence that prophylactic administration of AEDs prevents the occurrence of later epilepsy.

References

1. Livingston S. *Comprehensive Management of Epilepsy in Infancy, Childhood and Adolescence.* Springfield, IL: Charles C Thomas; 1972.
2. National Institutes of Health. Consensus Development Conference on Febrile Seizures. Proceedings. *Epilepsia.* 1981;22:377–381.
3. Frantzen E, Lennox-Buchthal M, Nygaard A, et al. A genetic study of febrile convulsions. *Neurology.* 1970;20:909–917.
4. Gastaut H. On genetic transmission of epilepsies. *Epilepsia.* 1969;10:3–6.
5. Tsuboi T. Polygenic inheritance of epilepsy and febrile convulsions: analysis based on a computational model. *Br J Psychiatry.* 1976;129:239–242.
6. Tsuboi T, Endo S. Febrile convulsions followed by nonfebrile convulsions: a clinical, electroencephalographic and follow-up study. *Neuropadiatrie.* 1977;8:209–223.
7. Nelson KB, Ellenberg JH. Prenatal and perinatal antecedents of febrile seizures. *Ann Neurol.* 1990;27:127–131.
8. Hauser WA, Annegers JF, Anderson VE, et al. The risk of seizure disorders among relatives of children with febrile convulsions. *Neurology.* 1985;35:1268–1273.
9. Metrakos JD, Metrakos K. Genetic factors in epilepsy. *Mod Probl Pharmacopsychiatry.* 1970;44:77–86.
10. Rantala H, Uhari M. Risk factors for recurrences of febrile convulsions. *Acta Neurol Scand.* 1994;90:207–210.
11. Lindsay J, Ounsted C, Richards P. Long-term outcome in children with temporal lobe seizures. IV. Genetic factors, febrile convulsions and the remission of seizures. *Dev Med Child Neurol.* 1980;22:429–439.
12. Fukuyama YK, Kagawa K, Tanaka KA. A genetic study of febrile convulsions. *Eur Neurol.* 1979;18:166–182.
13. Iwasaki N, Nakayama J, Hamano K, et al. Molecular genetics of febrile seizures. *Epilepsia.* 2002;43(suppl 9):32–35.

14. Nakayama J, Hamano K, Iwasaki N, et al. Significant evidence for linkage of febrile seizures to chromosome 5q14-q15. *Hum Mol Genet.* 2000;9:87–91.

15. Lopes-Cendes I, Scheffer IE, Berkovic SF, et al. A new locus for generalized epilepsy with febrile seizures plus maps to chromosome 2. *Am J Hum Genet.* 2000;66:698–701.

16. Deprez L, Claes LR, Claeys KG, et al. Genome-wide linkage of febrile seizures and epilepsy to the FEB4 locus at 5q14.3-q23.1 and no MASS1 mutation. *Hum Genet.* 2006;118:618–625.

17. Peiffer A, Thompson J, Charlier C, et al. A locus for febrile seizures (FEB3) maps to chromosome 2q23–24. *Ann Neurol.* 1999;46:671–678.

18. Hedera P, Ma S, Blair MA, et al. Identification of a novel locus for febrile seizures and epilepsy on chromosome 21q22. *Epilepsia.* 2006;47: 1622–1628.

19. Dai XH, Chen WW, Wang X, et al. A novel genetic locus for familial febrile seizures and epilepsy on chromosome 3q26.2-q26.33. *Hum Genet.* 2008;124:423–429.

20. Yu Z-L, Jiang J-M, Wu, D-H, et al. Febrile seizures are associated with mutation of seizure-related (SEZ)6, a brain-specific gene. *J Neurosci Res.* 2007;85:166–172.

21. Schlachter K, Gruber-Sedlmayr U, Stogmann E, et al. A splice site variant in the SCN1A gene confers risk of febrile seizures. *Neurology.* 2009;72: 974–978.

21a. Petrovski S, Scheffer IE, Sisodiya SM, et al. Lack of replication of association between *SCN1A* SNP and febrile seizures. *Neurology.* 2009;73: 1928–1930.

22. Nabbout R, Baulac S, Desguerre I, et al. New locus for febrile seizures with absence epilepsy on 3p and a possible modifier gene on 18p. *Neurology.* 2007;68:1374–1381.

23. Weber YG, Jacob M, Lerche H. A BFIS like syndrome with later onset and febrile seizures: suggestive linkage to chromosome 16p11.2–16q12.1 *Epilepsia.* 2008;49:1959–1964.

24. Racacho LJ, McLachlan RS, Ebers GC, et al. Evidence favoring genetic heterogeneity for febrile convulsions. *Epilepsia.* 2000;41:132–139.

25. Pal DK, Kugler SL, Mandelbaum DE, et al. Phenotypic features of familial febrile seizures: case-control study. *Neurology.* 2003;60:410–414.

26. Verity CM, Butler NR, Golding J. Febrile convulsions in a national cohort followed up from birth. I. Prevalence and recurrence in the first five years of life. *Br Med J.* 1985;290:1307–1310.

27. Habel A, Yates CM, McQueen JK, et al. Homovanillic acid and 5-hydroxyindoleacetic acid in lumbar cerebrospinal fluid in children with afebrile and febrile convulsions. *Neurology.* 1981;31:488–491.

28. Loscher W, Siemes H. Increased concentration of prostaglandin E-2 in cerebrospinal fluid of children with febrile convulsions. *Epilepsia.* 1988;29:307–310.

29. McCaughran JA Jr, Edwards E, Schechter N. Experimental febrile convulsions in the developing rat: effects on the cholinergic system. *Epilepsia.* 1984;25:250–258.

30. Berg AT. Are febrile seizures provoked by a rapid rise in temperature? *Am J Dis Child.* 1993;147:1101–1103.

31. El-Radhi AS, Withana K, Banajeh S. Recurrence rate of febrile convulsion related to the degree of pyrexia during the first attack. *Clin Pediatr (Phila).* 1986;25:311–313.

32. Berg AT, Shinnar S, Hauser WA, et al. A prospective study of recurrent febrile seizures. *N Engl J Med.* 1992;327:1122–1127.

33. Lahat E, Katz Y, Bistritzer T, et al. Recurrent seizures in children with *Shigella*-associated convulsions. *Ann Neurol.* 1990;28:393–395.

34. Cody CL, Baraff LJ, Cherry JD, et al. Nature and rates of adverse reactions associated with DTP and DT immunizations in infants and children. *Pediatrics.* 1981;68:650–660.

35. Barlow WE, Davis RL, Glasser JW, et al. The risk of seizures after receipt of whole-cell pertussis or measles, mumps, and rubella vaccine. *N Engl J Med.* 2001;345:656–661.

36. Hirtz DG, Nelson KB, Ellenberg JH. Seizures following childhood immunizations. *J Pediatr.* 1983;102:14–18.

37. Maytal J, Shinnar S, Moshe SL, et al. Low morbidity and mortality of status epilepticus in children. *Pediatrics.* 1989;83:323–331.

38. Livengood JR, Mullen JR, White JW, et al. Family history of convulsions and use of pertussis vaccine. *J Pediatr.* 1989;115:527–531.

39. Lewis HM, Parry JV, Parry RP, et al. Role of viruses in febrile convulsions. *Arch Dis Child.* 1979;54:869–876.

40. Rantala H, Uhari M, Tuokko H. Viral infections and recurrences of febrile convulsions. *J Pediatr.* 1990;116:195–199.

41. Wallace SJ. Factors predisposing to a complicated initial febrile convulsion. *Arch Dis Child.* 1975;50:943–947.

42. Haspolat S, Mihci E, Coskun M, et al. Interleukin-1beta, tumor necrosis factor-alpha, and nitrite levels in febrile seizures. *J Child Neurol.* 2002;17:749–751.

43. Straussberg R, Amir J, Harel L, et al. Pro- and anti-inflammatory cytokines in children with febrile convulsions. *Pediatr Neurol.* 2001; 24:49–53.

44. Millichap JG. *Febrile Convulsions.* New York: Macmillan; 1968.

45. Taylor DC, Ounsted C. Age, sex, and hemispheric vulnerability in the outcome of seizures in response to fever. In: Brierley JB, Meldrum BS, eds. *Brain Hypoxia. Clinics in Developmental Medicine.* Vol. 39/40. London: Heinemann; 1971:266–273.

46. Ounsted C. The sex ratio in convulsive disorders with a note on single-sex sib-ships. *J Neurol Neurosurg Psychiatry.* 1953;16:267–274.

47. Lennox-Buchthal MA. Febrile convulsions. A reappraisal. *Electro-Encephalogr Clin Neurophysiol.* 1973;32(suppl):1–138.

48. Nelson KB, Ellenberg JH. Prognosis in children with febrile seizures. *Pediatrics.* 1978;61:720–727.

49. Annegers JF, Hauser WA, Shirts SB, et al. Factors prognostic of unprovoked seizures after febrile convulsions. *N Engl J Med.* 1987;316: 493–498.

50. Ellenberg JH, Nelson KB. Sample selection and the natural history of disease. Studies of febrile seizures. *JAMA.* 1980;243:1337–1340.

51. Frantzen E, Lennox-Buchthal M, Nygaard A. Longitudinal EEG and clinical study of children with febrile convulsions. *Electroencephalogr Clin Neurophysiol.* 1968;24:197–212.

52. Doose H, Ritter K, Volzke E. EEG longitudinal studies in febrile convulsions. Genetic aspects. *Neuropediatrics.* 1983;14:81–87.

53. Jaffe M, Bar-Joseph G, Tirosh E. Fever and convulsions—indications for laboratory investigations. *Pediatrics.* 1981;67:729–731.

54. Kudrajavcev T. Skull x-rays and lumbar puncture in a young child presenting with a seizure and fever. In: Nelson KB, Ellenberg JH, eds. *Febrile Seizures.* New York: Raven Press; 1981:221–229.

55. Febrile convulsions: a suitable case for treatment [editorial]? *Lancet.* 1980;2:680–681.

56. Hirtz DG, Lee YJ, Ellenberg JH, et al. Survey on the management of febrile seizures. *Am J Dis Child.* 1986;140:909–914.

57. Hampers LC, Thompson DA, Bajaj L, et al. Febrile seizures: measuring adherence to AAP guidelines among community ED physicians. *Pediatr Emerg Care.* 2006;22:465–469.

58. Nelson KB, Ellenberg JH. Predictors of epilepsy in children who have experienced febrile seizures. *N Engl J Med.* 1976;295:1029–1033.

59. Annegers JF, Hauser WA, Elveback LR, et al. The risk of epilepsy following febrile convulsions. *Neurology.* 1979;29:297–303.

60. Camfield P, Camfield C, Gordon K, et al. What types of epilepsy are preceded by febrile seizures? A population-based study of children. *Dev Med Child Neurol.* 1994;36:887–892.

61. Teng D, Dayan P, Tyler S, et al. Risk of intracranial pathologic conditions requiring emergency intervention after a first complex febrile seizure among children. *Pediatrics.* 2006;117:528–530.

62. Aicardi J, Chevrie JJ. Convulsive status epilepticus in infants and children. A study of 239 cases. *Epilepsia.* 1970;11:187–197.

63. Shinnar S, Hesdorffer DC, Nordli DC, et al. Phenomenology of prolonged febrile seizures: results of the FEBSTAT study. *Neurology.* 2008;71: 170–176.

64. Hesdorffer DC, Chan S, Tian H, et al. Are MRI-detected brain abnormalities associated with febrile seizure type? *Epilepsia.* 2008;49:765–771.

65. Chevrie JJ, Aicardi J. Duration and lateralization of febrile convulsions. Etiological factors. *Epilepsia.* 1975;16:781–789.

66. Herlitz GP. Studien über die Sogenannten initalen Fieber-krampfe bei Kindern. *Acta Paediatr Scand.* 1941;29(suppl 1):1–142.

67. Fowler M. Brain damage after febrile convulsions. *Arch Dis Child.* 1957;32:67–76.

68. Zimmerman HM. The histopathology of convulsive disorders in children. *J Pediatr.* 1938;13:859–890.

69. Ellenberg JH, Nelson KB. Febrile seizures and later intellectual performance. *Arch Neurol.* 1978;35:17–21.

70. Maytal J, Shinnar S. Febrile status epilepticus. *Pediatrics.* 1990;86: 611–616.

71. Gastaut H, Poirier F, Payan H, et al. HHE syndrome, hemiconvulsions, hemiplegia, epilepsy. *Epilepsia.* 1959;1:418–447.

72. Berg AT, Shinnar S, Hauser WA, et al. Predictors of recurrent febrile seizures: a meta-analytic review. *J Pediatr.* 1990;116:329–337.

73. Van den Berg BJ. Studies on convulsive disorders in young children. 3. Recurrence of febrile convulsions. *Epilepsia.* 1974;15:177–190.

74. Berg AT, Shinnar S, Darefsky AS, et al. Predictors of recurrent febrile seizures. A prospective cohort study. *Arch Pediatr Adolesc Med.* 1997; 151:371–378.

75. Van Stuijvenberg M, Steyerberg EW, Derksen-Lubsen G, et al. Temperature, age, and recurrence of febrile seizures. *Arch Pediatr Adolesc Med.* 1998;152:1170–1175.

76. Berg AT, Shinnar S. Complex febrile seizures. *Epilepsia.* 1996;37: 126–133.

77. Hauser WA, Kurland LT. The epidemiology of epilepsy in Rochester, Minnesota, 1935 through 1967. *Epilepsia.* 1975;16:1–66.

78. Ross EM, Peckham CS, West PB, et al. Epilepsy in childhood: findings from the National Child Development Study. *Br Med J.* 1980;280:207–210.

79. Ueoka K, Nagano H, Kumanomidou U, et al. Clinical and electroencephalographic study in febrile convulsions with special reference to follow-up study. *Brain Dev.* 1979;1:196.

80. Van der Berg BJ, Yerushalmy J. Studies on convulsive disorders in young children. I. Incidence of febrile and nonfebrile convulsions by age and other factors. *Pediatr Res.* 1969;3:298–304.

81. Wallace SJ. Recurrence of febrile convulsions. *Arch Dis Child.* 1974;49:763–765.

82. Shinnar S, Glauser TA. Febrile seizures. *J Child Neurol.* 2002;17(suppl 1): S44–S52.

83. Wallace SJ. Spontaneous fits after convulsions with fever. *Arch Dis Child.* 1977;52:192–196.

84. Falconer MA. Genetic and related aetological factors in temporal lobe epilepsy. *Epilepsia.* 1971;12:13–31.

85. Rasmussen T. Relative significance of isolated infantile convulsions as a primary cause of focal epilepsy. *Epilepsia.* 1979;20:395–401.

86. Meldrum BS. Secondary pathology of febrile and experimental convulsions. In: Brazier MAB, Coceani F, eds. *Brain Dysfunction in Infantile Febrile Convulsions.* New York: Raven Press; 1976.

87. Nemoto EM, Frankel HM. Cerebral oxygenation and metabolism during progressive hyperthermia. *Am J Physiol.* 1970;219:1784–1788.

88. Janszky J, Woermann FG, Barsi P, et al. Right hippocampal sclerosis is more common than left after febrile seizures. *Neurology.* 2003;60:1209–1210.

89. Provenzale JM, Barboriak DP, VanKandingham K, et al. Hippocampal MRI signal intensity after febrile status epilepticus is predictive of subsequent mesial temporal sclerosis. *Am J Roentgenol.* 2008;190:976–983.

90. Theodore WH, Bhatia S, Hatta J, et al. Hippocampal atrophy, epilepsy duration, and febrile seizures in patients with partial seizures. *Neurology.* 1999;52:132–136.

91. Tarkka R. Paakko E, Pyhtinen J, et al. Febrile seizures and mesial temporal sclerosis: No association in a long-term follow-up study. *Neurology.* 2003;60:215–218.

92. Bower SP, Kilpatrick CJ, Vogrin SJ. Degree of hippocampal atrophy is not related to a history of febrile seizures in patients with proved hippocampal sclerosis. *J Neurol Neurosurg Psychiatry.* 2000;69:733–738.

93. Schulz R, Ebner A. Prolonged febrile convulsions and mesial temporal lobe epilepsy in an identical twin. *Neurology.* 2001;57:318–320.

94. Sokol DK, Demyer WE, Edwards-Brown M, et al. From swelling to sclerosis: acute change in mesial hippocampus after prolonged febrile seizure. *Seizure.* 2003;12:237–240.

95. Brewster A, Bender RA, Chen Y, et al. Developmental febrile seizures modulate hippocampal gene expression of hyperpolarization-activated channels in an isoform- and cell-specific manner. *J Neurosci.* 2002;22:4591–4599.

96. Salanova V, Markand O, Worth R, et al. FDG-PET and MRI in temporal lobe epilepsy: relationship to febrile seizures, hippocampal sclerosis and outcome. *Acta Neurol Scand.* 1998;97:146–153.

97. VanLandingham KE, Heinz ER, Cavazos JE, et al. Magnetic resonance imaging evidence of hippocampal injury after prolonged focal febrile convulsions. *Ann Neurol.* 1998;43:413–426.

98. Szabó CA, Wyllie E, Siavalas EL, et al. Hippocampal volumetry in children 6 years or younger: assessment of children with and without complex febrile seizures. *Epilepsy Res.* 1999;33:1–9.

99. Taylor DC. Differential rates of cerebral maturation between sexes and between hemispheres. Evidence from epilepsy. *Lancet.* 1969;2:140–142.

100. Taylor DC, Ounsted C. Biological mechanisms influencing the outcome of seizures in response to fever. *Epilepsia.* 1971;12:33–45.

101. Scheffer IE, Berkovic SF. Generalized epilepsy with febrile seizures plus. A genetic disorder with heterogeneous clinical phenotypes. *Brain.* 1997;120:479–490.

102. Wallace RH, Wang DW, Singh R, et al. Febrile seizures and generalized epilepsy associated with a mutation in the Na+-channel beta 1 subunit gene SCN1B. *Nat Genet.* 1998;19:366–370.

103. Wallace RH, Scheffer JE, Parasivam G. Generalized epilepsy with febrile seizures plus: mutation of the sodium channel subunit SCN1B. *Neurology.* 2002;58:1426–1429.

104. Sugawara T, Mazaki-Miyazaki E, Ito M, et al. Nav1.1 mutations cause febrile seizures associated with afebrile partial seizures. *Neurology.* 2001;57:703–705.

105. Lerche H, Jurkat-Rott K, Lehmann-Horn F. Ion channels and epilepsy. *Am J Med Genet.* 2001;106:146–159.

106. Ito M, Nagafuji H, Okazawa H, et al. Autosomal dominant epilepsy with febrile seizures plus with missense mutations of the (Na+)-channel alpha 1 subunit gene, SCN1A. *Epilepsy Res.* 2002;48:15–23.

107. Singh R, Scheffer IE, Crossland K, et al. Generalized epilepsy with febrile seizures plus: a common childhood-onset genetic epilepsy syndrome. *Ann Neurol.* 1999;45:75–81.

108. Baulac S, Gourfinkel-An I, Couarch P, et al. A novel locus for generalized epilepsy with febrile seizures plus in French families. *Arch Neurol.* 2008;65:943–951.

109. Abou-Khalil B, Ge O, Desai R, et al. Partial and generalized epilepsy with febrile seizures plus and a novel SCN1A mutation. *Neurology.* 2001;57:2265–2272.

110. Ward N, Evanson J, Cockerell OC. Idiopathic familial temporal lobe epilepsy with febrile convulsions. *Seizure.* 2002;11:16–19.

111. Depondt C, Van Paesschen W, Matthijs G, et al. Familial temporal lobe epilepsy with febrile seizures. *Neurology.* 2002;58:1429–1433.

112. Baulac S, Huberfeld G, Gourfinkel-An I, et al. First genetic evidence of GABA(A) receptor dysfunction in epilepsy: a mutation in the gamma2-subunit gene. *Nat Genet.* 2001;28(1):46–48.

113. Audenaert D, Schwartz E, Claeys KG, et al. A novel GABRG2 mutation associated with febrile seizures. *Neurology.* 2006;67:687–690.

114. Dravet C, Bureau M, Oguni H, et al. Severe myoclonic epilepsy in infancy: Dravet syndrome. *Adv Neurol.* 2005;95:71–102.

115. Jansen FE, Sadleir LG, Harkin LA, et al. Severe myoclonic epilepsy of infancy (Dravet syndrome): recognition and diagnosis in adults. *Neurology.* 2006;2224–2226.

116. Singh R, Andermann E, Whitehouse WP, et al. Severe myoclonic epilepsy of infancy: extended spectrum of GEFS+? *Epilepsia.* 2001;42:837–844.

117. Claes L, Del Favero J, Ceulemans B, et al. De novo mutations in the sodium-channel gene SCN1A cause severe myoclonic epilepsy of infancy. *Am J Hum Genet.* 2001;68:1327–1332.

118. Nabbout R, Kozlovski A, Gennaro E, et al. Absence of mutations in major GEFS+ genes in myoclonic astatic epilepsy. *Epilepsy Res.* 2003;56:127–133.

119. Ceulemans B, Boel M, Claes L, et al. Severe myoclonic epilepsy in infancy: toward an optimal treatment. *J Child Neurol.* 2004;19:516–521.

120. Striano P, Coppola A, Pezzala M, et al. An open-label trial of levetiracetam in severe myoclonic epilepsy of infancy. *Neurology.* 2007;69:250–254.

121. Theodore W, Epstein L, Gaillard WD, et al. Human herpes virus 6B: a possible role in epilepsy? *Epilepsia.* 2008;45:149–158.

122. Wallace SJ. Neurological and intellectual deficits: convulsions with fever viewed as acute indications of life-long developmental defects. In: Brazier MAB, Coceani F, eds. *Brain Dysfunction in Infantile Febrile Convulsions.* New York: Raven Press; 1976:259–277.

123. Verity CM, Greenwood R, Golding J. Long-term intellectual and behavioral outcomes of children with febrile convulsions. *N Engl J Med.* 1998;338:1723–1728.

124. Wolf SM. Controversies in the treatment of febrile convulsions. *Neurology.* 1979;29:287–290.

125. American Academy of Pediatrics. Practice parameter: the neurodiagnostic evaluation of the child with a first simple febrile seizure. Provisional Committee on Quality Improvement, Subcommittee on Febrile Seizures. *Pediatrics.* 1996;97:769–772.

126. American Academy of Pediatrics. Practice parameter: long-term treatment of the child with simple febrile seizures. Committee on Quality Improvement, Subcommittee on Febrile Seizures. *Pediatrics.* 1999;103:1307–1309.

127. Baumann RJ, Duffner PK. Treatment of children with simple febrile seizures: the AAP practice parameter. American Academy of Pediatrics. *Pediatr Neurol.* 2000;23:11–17.

128. American Academy of Pediatrics. Febrile seizures: clinical practice guideline for the long-term management of the child with simple febrile seizures. Steering committee on quality improvement and management, subcommittee on febrile seizures. *Pediatrics.* 2008;121:1281–1286.

129. Capovilla G, Mastangelo M, Romeo A, et al. Recommendations for the management of "febrile seizures". Steering committee on quality improvement and management, subcommittee on febrile seizures. Ad hoc task force of LICE guidelines commission. *Epilepsia.* 2009;50(suppl 1):2–6.

130. Callegaro S, Titomanlio T, Donega S, et al. Implementation of a febrile seizure guideline in two pediatric emergency departments. *Pediatr Neurol.* 2009;40:78–83.

131. Kimia AA, Campraro AJ, Hummel D, et al. Utility of lumbar puncture for first simple febrile seizure among children 6 tp 18 months of age. *Pediatrics.* 2009;123:6–12.

132. Faero O, Kastrup KW, Lykkegaard Nielsen E, et al. Successful prophylaxis of febrile convulsions with phenobarbital. *Epilepsia.* 1972;13:279–285.

133. Lee K, Taudorf K, Hvorslev V. Prophylactic treatment with valproic acid or diazepam in children with febrile convulsions. *Acta Paediatr Scand.* 1986;75:593–597.

134. Mamelle N, Mamelle JC, Plasse JC, et al. Prevention of recurrent febrile convulsions—a randomized therapeutic assay: sodium valproate, phenobarbital and placebo. *Neuropediatrics.* 1984;15:37–42.

135. Ngwane E, Bower B. Continuous sodium valproate or phenobarbitone in the prevention of "simple" febrile convulsions. Comparison by a double-blind trial. *Arch Dis Child.* 1980;55:171–174.

136. Wallace SJ, Smith JA. Successful prophylaxis against febrile convulsions with valproic acid or phenobarbitone. *Br Med J.* 1980;280:353–354.

137. Wallace SJ, Smith JA. Prophylaxis against febrile convulsions. *Br Med J.* 1980;280:863–864.

138. Melchior JC, Buchthal F, Lennox-Buchthal M. The ineffectiveness of diphenylhydantoin in preventing febrile convulsions in the age of greatest risk, under three years. *Epilepsia.* 1971;12:55–62.

139. Wolf SM, Forsythe A. Behavior disturbance, phenobarbital, and febrile seizures. *Pediatrics.* 1978;61:728–731.

140. Chaudhry M, Pond DA. Mental deterioration in epileptic children. *J Neurol Neurosurg Psychiatry.* 1961;24:213–219.

141. Holdsworth L, Whitmore K. A study of children with epilepsy attending ordinary schools. I. Their seizure patterns, progress and behaviour in school. *Dev Med Child Neurol.* 1974;16:746–758.

142. Wapner I, Thurston DL, Holowach J. Phenobarbital. Its effect on learning in epileptic children. *JAMA.* 1962;182:937.

143. Wolf SM, Forsythe A, Stunden AA, et al. Long-term effect of phenobarbital on cognitive function in children with febrile convulsions. *Pediatrics.* 1981;68:820–823.

144. Farwell JR, Lee YJ, Hirtz DG, et al. Phenobarbital for febrile seizures—effects on intelligence and on seizure recurrence. *N Engl J Med.* 1990;322:364–369.
145. Dreifuss FE, Rosman NP, Cloyd JC, et al. A comparison of rectal diazepam gel and placebo for acute repetitive seizures. *N Engl J Med.* 1998;338:1869–1875.
146. Knudsen FU. Effective short-term diazepam prophylaxis in febrile convulsions. *J Pediatr.* 1985;106:487–490.
147. Knudsen FU, Vestermark S. Prophylactic diazepam or phenobarbitone in febrile convulsions: a prospective, controlled study. *Arch Dis Child.* 1978;53:660–663.
148. Kriel RL, Cloyd JC, Hadsall RS, et al. Home use of rectal diazepam for cluster and prolonged seizures: efficacy, adverse reactions, quality of life, and cost analysis. *Pediatr Neurol.* 1991;7:13–17.
149. Scott RC, Besag FM, Neville BG. Buccal midazolam and rectal diazepam for treatment of prolonged seizures in childhood and adolescence: a randomised trial. *Lancet.* 1999;353:623–626.
150. Rainbow J, Browne GJ, Lam LT. Controlling seizures in the prehospital setting: diazepam or midazolam? *J Paediatr Child Health.* 2002;38:582–586.
151. Lehat E, Goldman M, Barr J, et al. Comparison of intranasal midazolam with intravenous diazepam for treating febrile seizures in children: prospective randomised study. *Br Med J.* 2000;321:83–86.
152. Rosman NP, Colton T, Labazzo J, et al. A controlled trial of diazepam administered during febrile illnesses to prevent recurrence of febrile seizures. *N Engl J Med.* 1993;329:79–84.
153. Millichap JG, Colliver JA. Management of febrile seizures: survey of current practice and phenobarbital usage. *Pediatr Neurol.* 1991;7:243–248.

CHAPTER 35 ■ SEIZURES ASSOCIATED WITH NONNEUROLOGIC MEDICAL CONDITIONS

STEPHAN EISENSCHENK, JEAN CIBULA, AND ROBIN L. GILMORE

Seizures frequently arise during the course of medical illnesses that do not primarily affect the central nervous system (CNS). The truism that appropriate treatment depends on correct diagnosis emphasizes the importance of the differential diagnosis. A patient's history, including a review of medications and physical examination, should be informed by a consideration of the seizures as a symptom of CNS dysfunction. The urgency to pursue a diagnosis is related to the time of presentation following the seizure. The evaluation of a patient presenting 24 hours after a single seizure is paced by other manifestations of CNS dysfunction. In a neurologically intact patient without progressive symptoms, quick (within days), but not emergent (within hours), evaluation may be appropriate. Within the first 24 hours, vital signs, level of consciousness, and focality on examination determine urgency. The need for emergent neuroimaging studies and lumbar puncture depends on the likelihood of intracranial lesion, CNS or systemic infection, a patient's metabolic state, and the possibility of intoxication. In a patient who presents more than 1 week after an initial seizure, recurrent attacks establish the diagnosis of epilepsy.

Several factors predispose a patient to seizures, including (i) changes in blood–brain barrier permeability as a result of infection, hypoxia, dysautoregulation of cerebral blood flow, or microdeposition of hemorrhage or edema secondary to vascular endothelial damage; (ii) alteration of neuronal excitability by exogenous or endogenous substances, such as excitatory and inhibitory neurotransmitters; (iii) inability of glial cells to regulate the neuronal extracellular environment; (iv) electrolyte imbalances; (v) hypoxia-ischemia; and (vi) direct and remote effects of neoplasm (1). Some patients without epilepsy may be genetically prone to seizures secondary to systemic factors.

Understanding the interaction of other organ systems is necessary for the appropriate management of seizures. In patients with hepatic or renal dysfunction, changes in pharmacokinetics induced by metabolic dysfunction alter treatment with antiepileptic drugs (AEDs). In cases of hepatic dysfunction, plasma concentrations must be correlated with serum albumin and protein levels and, if possible, free (unbound) levels. Patients with hepatic and renal failure may have normal serum and albumin levels, but altered protein binding, resulting in elevated concentrations of free drug (2).

METABOLIC DISORDERS

Metabolic disorders, although often suspected during outpatient evaluation of new-onset seizures, are found in <10% of patients and usually involve glucose metabolism (3). In the hospital setting, disorders of electrolytes and fluid balance predominate. Encephalopathies may be associated with electrolyte disturbances, hypocalcemia, hypercalcemia, hypoglycemia, hypothyroidism, thyrotoxic storm, adverse effects of drugs, organ failure, and many other conditions.

Hyponatremia

Because electrolyte disturbances are usually secondary processes, effective management of associated seizures begins with identification and treatment of the primary disorder in conjunction with cautious correction of the electrolyte disturbance. Hyponatremia, defined as a serum sodium level lower than 115 mEq/L, is one of the most frequently reported metabolic abnormalities, affecting 2.5% of hospitalized patients (4). Neurologic symptoms occur often in patients with acute hyponatremia (5,6), and convulsions in this setting have a mortality rate estimated to exceed 50% (7). Correction to levels higher than 120 mEq/L is essential; however, the rate of correction is controversial. Rapid correction of hyponatremia is associated with central pontine myelinolysis, manifested as pseudobulbar palsy and spastic quadriparesis (8). Originally described in patients with alcoholism and malnutrition, the condition was later observed in dehydrated patients undergoing rehydration (9), and in one small study (10) was accompanied in each patient by a recent rapid increase in serum sodium levels. Pathologic features include symmetrical, noninflammatory demyelination in the basis pontis, with relative neuronal and axonal sparing. In animal models of central pontine myelinolysis, rapid correction of sustained vasopressin-induced hyponatremia with hypertonic saline was followed by demyelination (11). Some authorities consider a correction of more than 12 mEq/L per day to be unnecessarily aggressive (10).

Levels of serum sodium are most commonly reduced as a result of either sodium depletion or water "intoxication," or both (7); these are examples of hypo-osmolar hyponatremia. Hyponatremia with normal osmolality is rare, but may accompany hyperlipidemia or hyperproteinemia. Hyperosmolar hyponatremia occurs in such hyperosmolar states as hyperglycemia and is discussed later in this chapter. Hypo-osmolar hyponatremia may occur with normal extracellular fluid volume, hypovolemia, or hypervolemia (12). Hypo-osmolar hyponatremia with hypovolemia may follow renal (diuretic use, Addison disease) or extrarenal (vomiting, diarrhea, or "third spacing") loss. The syndrome of inappropriate antidiuretic hormone secretion, hypothyroidism, and some psychotropic agents may lead to hypo-osmolar hyponatremia with normal volume. Hypo-osmolar hyponatremia with hypervolemia, frequently seen with clinical edema, occurs in patients with cardiac failure, nephrotic syndrome, and acute or chronic renal failure. The therapeutic implications of these conditions are significant, because appropriate treatment for normovolemic or hypervolemic hyperosmolar hyponatremia is water restriction. Hypovolemic hyponatremia is managed by replacement of water and sodium (12).

Finally, hyponatremia is sometimes considered to be an iatrogenic effect of prescribed medications, including diuretics, carbamazepine, oxcarbazepine, and serotonin reuptake inhibitors (13). Hyponatremia can also be a complication of abuse of illicit substances, such as 3,4-methylenedioxymethamphetamine (MDMA, or "ecstasy") (14,15).

Hypocalcemia

Although seizures resulting from severe hypocalcemia (<6 mg/dL) are relatively uncommon, they occur in approximately 25% of patients who present as medical emergencies (16). Severe, acute hypocalcemia most often follows thyroid or parathyroid surgery. Late-onset hypocalcemia with seizures may appear years after extensive thyroid surgery (17); the condition is believed to be rare and is not well understood. Hypocalcemia frequently complicates renal failure and acute pancreatitis (7), and may also occur along with vitamin D deficiency and renal tubular acidosis. Nutritional rickets is still reported, although rarely in the United States, occasionally with hypocalcemic seizures (18). Tetany is the most common neuromuscular accompaniment of hypocalcemia (19). Manifesting as spontaneous, irregular, repetitive action potentials that originate in peripheral nerves, tetany is sometimes confused with seizure activity. Latent tetany may be unmasked by hyperventilation or regional ischemia (Trousseau test). In the average adult, an intravenous (IV) bolus of 15 mL of 10% calcium gluconate solution (a calcium concentration of 9 mg/mL) administered slowly, along with cardiac monitoring, followed by infusion of the equivalent of 10 mL/hour of the same solution, should relieve seizures (20).

Hypomagnesemia

Hypomagnesemia is associated with seizures, but usually only at levels lower than 0.8 mEq/L (21). Because a related hypocalcemia may be produced by a decrease in, or end-organ resistance to, circulating levels of parathyroid hormone, magnesium levels should be measured in the patient with hypocalcemia who does not respond to calcium supplementation. Convulsions are treated with intramuscular injections of 50% magnesium sulfate every 6 hours. Because transient hypermagnesemia may induce respiratory muscle paralysis (21), IV injections of calcium gluconate should be administered concurrently.

Hypophosphatemia

Profound hypophosphatemia may accompany alcohol withdrawal, diabetic ketoacidosis, long-term intake of phosphate-binding antacids, recovery from extensive burns, hyperalimentation, and severe respiratory alkalosis. A sequence of symptoms consistent with metabolic encephalopathy involves irritability, apprehension, muscle weakness, numbness, paresthesias, dysarthria, confusion, obtundation, convulsive seizures, and coma (22). Generalized tonic–clonic seizures have been noted at phosphate levels lower than 1 mg/dL, and affected patients may not respond to AED therapy (23).

Disturbances of Glucose Metabolism

Hypoglycemia and nonketotic hyperglycemia may be associated with focal seizures; such seizures do not occur with ketotic hyperglycemia, however, probably because of the anticonvulsant action of the ketosis (24). Ketosis also involves intracellular acidosis with enhanced activity of glutamic acid decarboxylase, which leads to an increase in γ-aminobutyric acid and a corresponding increase in seizure threshold.

Nonketotic hyperglycemia, with or without hyperosmolarity, may produce seizures and in animal models increases seizure frequency through brain dehydration, provided a cortical lesion is present (25). Focal motor seizures and epilepsia partialis continua, well-known complications of nonketotic hyperglycemia, occur in approximately 20% of patients (26).

Rarely, patients with focal seizures associated with nonketotic hyperglycemia may have reflex- or posture-induced epilepsy provoked by active or passive movement of an extremity (27,28), and usually have nonreflex seizures as well, related perhaps to an underlying focal cerebral ischemia. Such seizures are refractory to conventional anticonvulsant treatment. In fact, phenytoin may further increase the serum glucose level by inhibiting insulin release (29). Thus, correction of the underlying metabolic disturbance is of utmost importance.

Hypoglycemia is particularly seizure provoking and is most frequently related to insulin or oral hypoglycemic agents, although occasionally the etiology may not be obvious. Another common cause is the use of drugs that interact with oral hypoglycemic agents (30). Islet cell dysmaturation syndrome, characterized by islet cell hyperplasia, pancreatic adenomatosis, and nesidioblastosis, is associated with infantile hyperinsulinemic hypoglycemia. Bjerke and coworkers (31) reported on 11 infants with this condition, eight of whom presented with hypoglycemic seizures. Five infants had preoperative neurologic impairment. All showed improvement postoperatively, but only one infant had normal findings on neurologic examination. Early diagnosis is a decisive factor in averting long-term complications; treatment entails resection of the pancreas.

Hypoparathyroidism

Seizures occur in 30% to 70% of patients with hypoparathyroidism, usually along with tetany and hypocalcemia. They may be generalized tonic–clonic, focal motor, or, less frequently, atypical absence and akinetic seizures. Restoration of normal calcium levels is necessary. Because AEDs may partially suppress seizures, as well as tetany and the Trousseau sign, hypocalcemia must be considered.

Thyroid Disorders

Hyperthyroidism is associated only rarely with seizures, although generalized and focal seizures have occurred in 10% of patients with thyrotoxicosis (32). Typically, thyrotoxicosis may be associated with nervousness, diaphoresis, heat intolerance, palpitations, tremor, and fatigue. Hashimoto thyroiditis often coexists with other autoimmune disorders (33), such as Hashimoto encephalopathy, a steroid-responsive relapsing condition (34) that produces seizures even in euthyroid patients (35).

Seizures have been reported in patients with myxedema. As many as 20% to 25% of patients with myxedemic coma have generalized convulsions. Patients with hypothyroidism may have obstructive sleep apnea (36) with hypoxic seizures (37).

Adrenal Disorders

Seizures are uncommon with adrenal insufficiency but may occur in patients with pheochromocytoma (38). More commonly, a pheochromocytoma-induced hypertensive crisis may trigger a hypertensive encephalopathy, characterized by altered mental status, focal neurologic signs and symptoms, and/or seizures. Other neurologic complications include stroke caused by cerebral infarction or an embolic event secondary to a mural thrombus from a dilated cardiomyopathy. Intracerebral hemorrhage may also occur because of uncontrolled hypertension. Additional symptoms are tremor, nausea, anxiety, sense of impending doom, epigastric pain, flank pain, constipation or diarrhea, and weight loss. These spells may last minutes to an hour. Blood pressure is almost always markedly elevated during the episode.

Uremia

A change in mental status is the hallmark of uremic encephalopathy, which also involves simultaneous neural depression (obtundation) and neural excitation (twitching, myoclonus, generalized seizures). Epileptic seizures occur in up to one fourth of patients with uremia, and the reasons are quite varied.

Phenytoin is the AED usually administered to nontransplanted patients with uremia (see "Transplantation and Seizures"). Critical changes in the pharmacokinetics of AEDs include (i) increased volume of distribution, producing lowered plasma drug levels; (ii) decreased protein binding, creating higher free-drug levels; and (iii) increased hepatic enzyme oxygenation, yielding increased plasma elimination (2). Because patients with uremia have plasma-protein–binding abnormalities and because phenytoin is highly plasma bound, drug administration is different from that in nonuremic patients. In one study, a 2 mg/kg IV dose produced a level of 1.4 μg/mL in patients with uremia, compared with 2.9 μg/mL in control patients (39). In nonuremic patients, up to 10% of phenytoin is not protein bound, whereas in uremic patients, as much as 75% may not be protein bound. Thus, free phenytoin levels (between 1 and 2 μg/mL) should be used instead of total phenytoin levels to assess therapeutic efficacy (40). With gabapentin, pregabalin, and levetiracetam, which is eliminated solely via renal excretion, the usual total dose should be reduced equivalently to the reduction in creatinine clearance (41–43).

The treatment of renal failure may also lead to dialysis dysequilibrium, characterized by headache, nausea, and irritability, which may progress to seizures, coma, and death attributable to the entry of free water into the brain, with resultant edema. Dialysis dementia, caused by the toxic effects of aluminum, is now rare. Renal transplant recipients may experience cerebrovascular disease, opportunistic infections, or malignant neoplasms, particularly primary lymphoma of the brain.

In uremic patients with renal insufficiency, adverse reactions to antibiotics are a common cause of seizures (44). Patients may have focal motor or generalized seizures, or myoclonus. In uremia, reduced protein binding increases the free fraction of highly protein-bound drugs in serum (and therefore in the CNS). Raised concentrations of neurotoxic agents, such as cephalosporins, may increase seizure susceptibility, which may be enhanced further by the altered blood–brain barrier.

The hemodialysis patient represents a special challenge because of decreased concentrations of dialyzable AEDs. Plasma protein binding determines how effectively a drug can be dialyzed. The more protein bound a drug, the less dialyzable it is (45). Hence, levels of a drug such as phenobarbital (40% to 60% protein bound) will decrease during dialysis more than will levels of valproic acid (80% to 95% bound). One way, albeit cumbersome, to avoid "losing" an agent is to dialyze against a dialysate containing the drug. Another option, if seizures occur near the time of dialysis, is to use a highly protein-bound drug, such as valproic acid. For special considerations in the kidney transplant patient, see "Transplantation and Seizures."

Inborn Errors of Metabolism

Metabolic errors, either inborn or acquired, occur most often in early childhood. Phenylketonuria is the most common of several aminoacidopathies that may be associated with infantile spasms, and myoclonic or tonic–clonic seizures occur in one fourth of these patients (46). Evidence of hypsarrhythmia may be seen on the electroencephalogram (EEG), but a high proportion of patients have abnormal EEGs without seizures.

Although hereditary fructose intolerance does not usually involve neurologic impairment, as does untreated phenylketonuria, a small number of children experience seizures that are sometimes related to prolonged hypoglycemia (47).

Because excess ammonia is excreted as urea, disorders of the urea cycle, such as hyperammonemia, may be associated with symptoms ranging from coma and seizures to mild, nonspecific aberrations in neurologic function (46).

Various storage diseases result from abnormal accumulation of normal substrates and their catabolic products within lysosomes. The absence or inefficiency of lysosomal enzymes in such conditions as sphingolipidoses, mucopolysaccharidoses, mucolipidoses, glycogen storage diseases, and glycoproteinoses may give rise to seizures (46).

Purine syndromes and hyperuricemia are not usually associated with seizure disorders unless mental retardation or dementia coexists. Allopurinol is an important adjunctive treatment in some patients.

TABLE 35.1

SAFE AND UNSAFE AGENTS IN PATIENTS WITH PORPHYRIA

Safe agents	Unsafe agents
Acetaminophen	Barbiturates
Acetazolamide	Carbamazepine
Allopurinol	Chloramphenicol
Aminoglycosides	Chlordiazepoxide
Amitriptyline	Diphenhydramine
Aspirin	Enalapril
Atropine	Ergot compounds
Bromides	Erythromycin
Bupivacaine	Ethanol
Chloral hydrate	Flucloxacillin
Chlorpromazine	Flufenamic acid
Codeine	Griseofulvin
Corticosteroids	Hydrochlorothiazide
Diazepam	Imipramine
Gabapentin	Lisinopril
Heparin	Methyldopa
Insulin	Metoclopramide
Levetiracetam	Nifedipine
Meclizine	Oral contraceptives
Meperidine	Pentazocine
Morphine	Phenytoin
Penicillins (see unsafe agents	Piroxicam
for exceptions)	Pivampicillin
Procaine	Progesterone
Prochlorperazine	Pyrazinamide
Promethazine	Rifampin
Propoxyphene	Sulfonamides
Propranolol	Theophylline
Propylthiouracil	Valproic acid
Quinidine	Verapamil
Streptomycin	Oral contraceptives
Temazepam	
Tetracycline	
Thyroxine	
Trifluoperazine	
Warfarin	

Adapted from Gorchein A. Drug treatment in acute porphyria. *Br J Clin Pharmacol.* 1997;44:427–434, with permission.

Porphyria

The disorders of heme biosynthesis are classified into two groups: erythropoietic and hepatic. Seizures and other neurologic manifestations occur only in the hepatic group, which comprises acute intermittent porphyria, hereditary coproporphyria, and variegate porphyria (48). Seizures affect approximately 15% of patients, usually during an acute attack (49) often precipitated by an iatrogenically introduced offending agent. The generalized (occasionally focal) seizures may begin up to 28 days after exposure to the agent. The epileptogenic mechanism is not well understood. Some authors have suggested that δ-aminolevulinic acid and porphobilinogen, both structurally similar to the neurotransmitters glutamate and α-aminobutyric acid (GABA), are toxic to the nervous system, although clinical evidence refutes this contention (48).

A cornerstone of the treatment is the provision of a major portion of daily caloric requirements by carbohydrates to lower porphyrin excretion. Glucose prevents induction of hepatic δ-aminolevulinic acid synthetase in symptomatic patients, as does IV hematin. Porphyrogenic drugs, such as phenytoin, barbiturates, carbamazepine, succinimides, and oxazolidinediones, should be avoided. Drugs are considered unsafe if they induce experimental porphyria in animals. Using chick-embryo hepatocyte culture, Reynolds and Miska (49) found that carbamazepine, clonazepam, and valproate increased porphyrin to levels comparable with those achieved with phenobarbital and phenytoin. Bromides are recommended for the long-term management (50), and diazepam, paraldehyde, and IV magnesium sulfate therapy for the acute treatment of seizures (51). Serum bromide levels should be maintained between 60 and 90 μg/dL. Many side effects and a long half-life make bromides difficult to use. Bromides are excreted by the kidney, and paraldehyde is excreted unchanged by the lungs (the remainder by the liver). Larson and colleagues (52) reported on one patient with intractable epilepsy who was safely managed with low-dose clonazepam and a high-carbohydrate diet after phenytoin and carbamazepine use had independently precipitated attacks. In two separate studies, gabapentin controlled complex partial and secondarily generalized seizures in patients with porphyria (53,54). Because gabapentin is excreted unmetabolized by the kidneys, it does not induce hepatic microsomal enzymes (55) and should not worsen hepatic cellular dysfunction. Vigabatrin, which also does not induce hepatic metabolism, may be a useful antiseizure medication in patients with porphyria. Table 35.1 lists agents that are safe and unsafe to use in patients with porphyria (56).

OXYGEN DEPRIVATION

Perinatal Anoxia and Hypoxia

Whether it occurs in utero, during delivery, or in the neonatal period, significant anoxia can extensively damage the CNS, leading to chronic, usually secondarily generalized, epilepsy most commonly associated with mental retardation or other neurologic impairment. Neonatal seizures carry a risk for increased mortality, probably from the underlying brain disease rather than from the seizures themselves (57).

In the neonatal period, subtle, frequently refractory seizures may occur, as well as tonic, focal clonic, myoclonic seizures and multifocal clonic jerks. Not all paroxysmal events are seizures; however, some are brainstem release phenomena. Continuous video–electroencephalographic monitoring has made the diagnosis of these disorders more accurate and has led to improved treatment, including the avoidance of inappropriate AED use.

Because the initial insult usually occurs in utero, ventilation, cerebral perfusion, and adequate glucose levels must be maintained as preventive measures. Vigorous AED treatment is recommended because of the potential for additional brain injury, but opinions vary as to the degree of vigor to be applied. Arguments for aggressive therapy have been based on the realization that seizures may compromise ventilation and increase systemic blood pressure and cerebral perfusion, leading to hemorrhagic infarction, intraventricular hemorrhage, or both (58,59). Seizures may also result in cellular starvation through exhaustion of cerebral glucose and high-energy phosphate compounds. Experimental studies demonstrate that seizures decrease brain protein levels, deoxyribonucleic acid (DNA), ribonucleic acid (RNA), and cell content. Treatment of anoxic seizures in the newborn is reviewed in Chapter 33.

As the infant matures, the seizure type changes. Infantile spasms and hypsarrhythmia may occur in patients 2 to 12 months of age.

Adult Anoxia and Hypoxia

In adults, anoxic or posthypoxic seizures are residuals of cardiac arrest, respiratory failure, anesthetic misadventure, carbon monoxide poisoning, or near-drowning. Precipitating cardiac sources typically are related to embolic stroke, 13% of which involve seizures (60) or hypoperfusion or hyperperfusion of the cerebral cortex (2). Approximately 0.5% of patients who have undergone coronary bypass surgery experience seizures without evidence of focal CNS injury (61). In patients with respiratory disorder, acute hypercapnia may lower seizure threshold, whereas chronic stable hypoxia and hypercapnia rarely cause seizures. Subacute bacterial endocarditis can lead to septic emboli and intracranial mycotic aneurysms, which can produce seizures either from focal ischemia or from rupture and subarachnoid hemorrhage. Syncopal myoclonus and convulsive syncope may result from transient hypoxia.

Seizures may involve only minimal facial or axial movement (62), although nonconvulsive status epilepticus typically signifies a poor prognosis (63,64). Myoclonic status epilepticus or generalized myoclonic seizures that occur repetitively for 30 minutes are usually refractory to medical treatment (65). Concern has been raised that myoclonic status epilepticus may produce progressive neurologic injury in comatose patients resuscitated from cardiac arrest (65). When postanoxic myoclonic status epilepticus is associated with cranial areflexia, eye opening at the onset of myoclonic jerks, and EEG patterns indicating poor prognosis, the outlook for neurologic recovery is grim (66).

Treatment is directed mainly toward preventing a critical degree of hypoxic injury. Barbiturate medication and reduction of cerebral metabolic requirements by continuous hypothermia may prevent the delayed worsening (67). Frequently, the seizures cease after 3 to 5 days. Postanoxic seizures are frequently myoclonic. Phenobarbital 300 mg/day, clonazepam 8 to 12 mg/day in three divided doses, and 4-hydroxytryptophan 100 to 400 mg/day have been recommended (68), as has valproic acid (69).

ALCOHOL

Generalized tonic–clonic seizures occur during the first 48 hours of withdrawal from alcohol in intoxicated patients and are most common 12 to 24 hours after binge drinking (70). Seizures that occur more than 6 days following abstinence should not be ascribed to withdrawal. Interictal EEG findings are usually normal. Partial seizures often result from CNS infection or cerebral cicatrix caused by remote head trauma. (Recent occult head trauma, including subdural hematoma, should be considered in any alcoholic patient.) Although the incidence of alcoholism in patients with seizures is not higher than in the general population, alcoholic individuals do have a higher incidence of seizures (71).

The treatment depends on associated conditions, but replacement of alcohol is generally not recommended. To prevent the development of Wernicke–Korsakoff syndrome, thiamine should be administered prior to IV glucose. Magnesium deficiency should be corrected, as reduced levels may interfere with the action of thiamine. Preferred treatment is with benzodiazepines or paraldehyde. Paraldehyde may be administered in doses of 0.1 to 0.2 mL/kg orally or rectally every 2 to 4 hours. Diazepam, lorazepam, clorazepate, and chlordiazepoxide in conventional dosages are equally useful (72).

INFECTIONS

Infection is associated with seizures, both directly via parenchymal invasion by the pathogen and indirectly via neurotoxins. Direct parenchymal infections may be bacterial, fungal, mycobacterial, viral, spirochetal, or parasitic. Neurodegenerative disorders, such as Creutzfeldt–Jakob disease and subacute sclerosing panencephalitis, can also result from CNS infection.

Meningitis

Patients with seizures, headache, or fever (even low grade) should undergo lumbar puncture once a mass lesion has been excluded. In the infant with diffuse, very high intracranial pressure, lumbar puncture should be delayed until antibiotics and pressure-reducing measures are initiated. The pathogenic cause of bacterial meningitis varies with age: In newborns, *Escherichia coli* and group B streptococcus are most common; in children 2 months to 12 years of age, *Haemophilus influenzae*, *Streptococcus pneumoniae*, and *Neisseria meningitidis* are usual; in children older than 12 years of age and in adults, *S. pneumoniae* and *N. meningitidis* are found most often; in adults older than 50 years of age, *H. influenzae* is increasingly being reported. In infants, geriatric patients, and the immunocompromised, *Listeria monocytogenes* must also be considered.

Encephalitis

The herpes simplex variety is the most common form of encephalitis associated with seizures (73). Fever, headache, and confusion are punctuated by both complex partial and generalized seizures. The propensity of the virus for the temporal lobe is well known. Equine encephalitides, St. Louis encephalitis, and rabies also produce seizures. Rabies is distinguished from other viruses by dysphagia, dysarthria, facial numbness, and facial muscle spasm.

Diazepam or lorazepam may be used for the acute control of seizures caused by meningitis or encephalitis. Seizures persisting for more than 1 day or the development of status epilepticus indicates the need for maintenance AED therapy—phenytoin in adults, in children, and phenobarbital in infants.

Nonbacterial Chronic Meningitis

Lyme disease, a tick-borne spirochetosis, is associated with meningitis, encephalitis, and cranial or radicular neuropathies in up to 20% of patients. Seizures are not a prominent feature. Treatment consists of high-dose IV penicillin G in addition to AEDs (74).

Neurosyphilis is another spirochetal cause of seizures, which occasionally are the initial manifestation of syphilitic meningitis. In the early 20th century, 15% of patients with adult-onset seizures had underlying neurosyphilis. The incidence decreased dramatically over the years; however, the recent upsurge in primary syphilis among younger individuals is reflected in the report that seizures occur in approximately 25% of patients with symptomatic neurosyphilis. The diagnosis rests on the demonstration of positive serologic findings and clinical symptoms, but the signs are not pathognomonic and often overlap with those of other diseases. IV penicillin remains the treatment of choice. Sarcoidosis should also be considered in patients with nonbacterial meningitis and seizures.

Opportunistic CNS Infections

Acquired immunodeficiency syndrome (AIDS) is associated with several unique neurologic disorders, and seizures may play a major role when opportunistic infections or metabolic abnormalities, especially cerebral toxoplasmosis or cryptococcal meningitis, occur. *L. monocytogenes* should also be considered in immunocompromised patients. Metabolic abnormalities, particularly uremia and hypomagnesemia, predispose patients infected with the human immunodeficiency virus (HIV) to seizures. New-onset epilepsy partialis continua as an early manifestation of progressive multifocal leukoencephalopathy in patients with HIV-1 infection has been reported (75). CNS lymphoma in HIV-infected patients may also give rise to seizures.

Parasitic CNS Infections

In some areas, neurocysticercosis is the most commonly diagnosed cause of partial seizures. The adult pork tapeworm resides in the human small bowel after ingestion of infected meat. The oncospheres (hatched ova) penetrate the gut wall and develop into encysted larval forms, usually in brain or skeletal muscle. Computed tomography (CT) scans reveal calcified lesions, cysts with little or no enhancement, and usually no sign of increased intracranial pressure. In the past, treatment involved the use of only praziquantel 50 mg/kg/day for 15 days or albendazole 15 mg/kg/day. However, while undergoing therapy, most patients had clinical exacerbations, including worsening seizures, attributed to inflammation with cyst expansion caused by the death of cysticerci. For this reason, treatment with the antihelminthic drug and steroids has been advocated.

Antihelminthic agents by themselves do not change the course of neurocysticercosis or its associated epilepsy. A trial of antihelminthic agents combined with steroids or steroids alone showed comparable efficacy in terms of patients who were cyst-free at 1 year or seizure-free during follow-up (76).

Hydatid disease of the CNS (echinococcal infection) may result from exposure to dogs and sheep. Echinococcal cysts destroy bone, and a large proportion of such cysts are found in vertebrae. On CT scans, echinococcal brain cysts are fewer and larger than the cysts associated with cysticercosis. Treatment is usually surgical, largely because mebendazole and flubendazole have been associated with disease progression in up to 25% of patients. Nonetheless, adjuvant chemotherapy may be warranted in some cases (77).

Trichinosis may be encountered wherever undercooked trichina-infected pork is consumed. Complications of CNS migration include seizures, meningoencephalitis, and focal neurologic signs; eosinophilia is common during acute infection. Muscle biopsy may be necessary for diagnosis (73).

Cerebral malaria is similar to neurosyphilis, in that almost every neurologic sign and symptom has been attributed to the disorder. Diagnosis requires characteristic forms in the peripheral blood smear. Treatment depends on whether chloroquine resistance is present in the geographic region of infection.

Toxoplasmosis is a parasitic infection that affects adults, children, and infants. Use of immunosuppressive agents in patients with malignancies or transplants (see related sections later in this chapter), as well as recognition of AIDS, has emphasized the need to reconsider the neurologic sequelae of toxoplasmosis. Diagnosis may be elusive. Cerebrospinal fluid may reveal normal findings or mild pleocytosis (78). Serologic data may be difficult to interpret because encephalitis caused by *Toxoplasma gondii* may occur in patients who reactivate latent organisms and do not develop the serologic response of acute infection. CT scanning may reveal typical lesions. Therapy includes pyrimethamine and sulfadiazine or trisulfapyrimidines.

Cytomegalovirus retinitis, the most common ocular opportunistic infection in patients with AIDS (79), is increasingly being treated with a combination of foscarnet and ganciclovir. Foscarnet is also used to treat cytomegalovirus esophagitis associated with AIDS, but seizures have occurred with this agent, possibly as a result of changes in ionized calcium concentrations (80).

Systemic Infections

Systemic infection involving hypoxia (e.g., pneumonia) or metabolic changes may give rise to seizures. Through an indirect, poorly understood mechanism, seizures are prominent in two serious gastrointestinal (GI) infections: shigellosis and cholera. Ashkenazi and associates (80) demonstrated that the Shiga toxin is not essential for the development of the neurologic manifestations of shigellosis and that other toxic products may play a role.

Zvulunov and colleagues (82) examined 111 children who had convulsions with shigellosis and were followed for 3 to 18 years. No deaths or persistent motor deficits occurred. Only one child developed epilepsy by the age of 8 years; 15.7% of the children had recurrent febrile seizures. Poor co-ordination of fine hand movements was noted in 3.3% of the 92 children who had no preexisting neurologic abnormality. The convulsions associated with shigellosis have a favorable prognosis and do not necessitate long-term follow-up or treatment.

Most clinical manifestations of cholera are caused by fluid loss. Seizures, which are the most common CNS complication, occasionally occur both before and after treatment, and may result from hypoglycemia or overcorrection of electrolyte abnormalities. The cornerstone of treatment, however, is fluid replacement. Up to 3% of body weight, or 30 mL/kg, should be administered during the first hour, followed by 7% for the next 5 to 6 hours. Lactated Ringer solution given intravenously with potassium chloride or isotonic saline and sodium lactate (in a 2:1 ratio) is used. Adjunctive treatment with a broad-spectrum antibiotic shortens the duration of diarrhea and hastens the excretion of *Vibrio cholerae*.

The seizures associated with shigellosis and cholera infection may share a common pathogenesis. Depletion of hepatic glycogen and resultant hypoglycemia are typically reported in children with these illnesses (83).

GASTROINTESTINAL DISEASE AND SEIZURES

In nontropical sprue, or celiac disease, damage to the small bowel by gluten-containing foods leads to chronic malabsorption. Approximately 10% of patients have significant neurologic manifestations, with the most frequent neurologic complication being seizures (reported in 1% to 10% of patients), which are often associated with bilateral occipital calcifications (84,85). Possible mechanisms include deficiencies of calcium, magnesium, and vitamins; genetic factors (86); and isolated CNS vasculitis (87). Malabsorption may be occult, and seizures may be the dominant feature. Strict gluten exclusion usually produces a rapid response.

Inflammatory bowel disease (ulcerative colitis and Crohn disease) is associated with a low incidence of focal or generalized seizures. Unsurprisingly, generalized seizures frequently accompany infection or dehydration. In approximately 50% of all patients with focal seizures, a vascular basis is suspected (88).

Whipple disease is a multisystem granulomatous disorder caused by *Tropheryma whippelii* (89). Approximately 10% of patients have dementia, ataxia, or oculomotor abnormalities; as many as 25% have seizures (90). Early treatment is important, as untreated patients with CNS involvement usually die within 12 months (91). Some patients develop cerebral manifestations after successful antibiotic treatment of GI symptoms (92). Although several agents that cross the blood–brain barrier, such as chloramphenicol and penicillin, have been suggested for treatment (93), a high incidence of CNS relapse led Keinath and coworkers (94) to recommend penicillin 1.2 million units and streptomycin 1.0 g/day for 10 to 14 days, followed by trimethoprim–sulfamethoxazole 1 double-strength tablet twice a day for 1 year. Treatment of the underlying disease may not prevent seizures, however, in which case AEDs in a suspension or elixir are usually required because malabsorption is a significant problem (95).

Hepatic Encephalopathy

Wilson disease, acquired hepatocerebral degeneration, Reye syndrome, and fulminant hepatic failure, among other disorders, may lead to hepatic encephalopathy. Manifestations progress through four stages. Stage 1 is incipient encephalopathy. In stage 2, mental status deteriorates and asterixis develops. In stage 3, focal or generalized seizures may occur. Stage 4 is marked by coma and decerebrate posturing.

The incidence of seizures varies from 2% to 33% (96). Hypoglycemia complicating liver failure may be responsible for some seizures. Hyperammonemia is associated with seizures and may contribute to the encephalopathy of primary hyperammonemic disorders; treatments that reduce ammonia levels also ameliorate the encephalopathy (96). Therapy should be directed toward the etiology of the hepatic failure; levels of GI protein and lactulose must be reduced. Long-term use of AEDs is not usually required unless there is a known predisposition to seizures (e.g., previous cerebral injury). Little experience with the use of AEDs has actually been reported. Those AEDs with sedative effects may precipitate coma and are generally contraindicated. Phenytoin and gabapentin are reasonable choices, but valproic acid and its salt should be avoided.

INTOXICATION AND DRUG-RELATED SEIZURES

This section is *not* to be used as a guide to the management of drug intoxication. Rather, it reviews specific instances of intoxication during which intractable seizures sometimes develop.

Prescription Medication-Induced Seizures

Many medications provoke seizures in both epileptic and nonepileptic patients (Table 35.2). Predisposing factors include family history of seizures, concurrent illness, and high-dose intrathecal and IV administration. The convulsions are usually generalized with or without focal features; status epilepticus may occur in up to 15% of patients (97). Because many medical conditions result from polypharmacy, drug-induced seizures may be more common in geriatric patients.

Intoxication from treatment with tricyclic antidepressants (TCAs) has led to generalized tonic–clonic seizures; in fact, seizures may occur at therapeutic levels in approximately 1% of patients (98). Because desipramine is believed to have a lower risk for precipitating seizures than other drugs in this class, the agent is preferred in patients with known seizure disorders (99). Barbiturates are relatively contraindicated, and amitriptyline and imipramine depress the level of consciousness. Diazepam or paraldehyde is preferred. Physostigmine may reverse the neurologic manifestations of TCA reactions; however, because it may also cause asystole, hypotension, hypersalivation, and convulsions, this agent should not be used to treat tricyclic-induced seizures. The combination of chlomipramine with valproic acid may result in elevation of chlomipramine levels with associated seizures (100).

TABLE 35.2

AGENTS REPORTED TO INDUCE SEIZURES

Analgesics	Alfentanil, fentanyl, mefenamic acid, meperidine, pentazocine, propoxyphene, tramadol
Antibiotics	Ampicillin, carbenicillin, cephalosporins, imipenem, isoniazid, lindane, metronidazole, nalidixic acid, oxacillin, penicillin, pyrimethamine, ticarcillin
Antidepressants	Amitriptyline, bupropion, doxepin, fluoxetine, imipramine, maprotiline, mianserin, nomifensine, nortriptyline, paroxetine, sertraline, trazadone, venlafaxine
Antineoplastic agents	Busulfan, carmustine (BCNU), chlorambucil, cytosine arabinoside, methotrexate, vincristine
Antipsychotics	Clozapine, clomipramine, chlorpromazine, fluphenazine, haloperidol, olanzapine, perphenazine, pimozide, prochlorperazine, quetiapine, respiridone, thioridazine, trifluoperazine
Bronchial agents	Aminophylline, theophylline
General anesthetics	Enflurane, ketamine, methohexital
Local anesthetics	Bupivacaine, lidocaine, procaine
Sympathomimetics	Ephedrine, phenylpropanolamine, terbutaline
Others	Alcohol, amphetamines, anticholinergics, antihistamines, aqueous iodinated contrast agents, atenolol, baclofen, chloroquine, copper toxicity, cyclosporine, domperidone, ergonovine, flumazenil, folic acid, foscarnet, gangcyclovir, hyperbaric oxygen, insulin, lithium, mefloquine, methylphenidate, methylxanthines, oxytocin, phencyclidine, ritonavir, tacrolimus (FK506)

Fluoxetine, sertraline, and other selective serotonin reuptake inhibitors (SSRIs) have an associated seizure risk of approximately 0.2%. The SSRIs may have an antiepileptic effect at therapeutic doses (101). Fluvoxamine overdose has also been reported to provoke status epilepticus (102). When combined with other serotonergic agents or monoamine oxidase inhibitors, however, they may induce the "serotonin syndrome" of delirium, tremors, and, occasionally, seizures (103). Other symptoms include agitation, myoclonus, hyperreflexia, diaphoresis, shivering, tremor, diarrhea, incoordination, and fever. Venlafaxine, a serotonin and norepinephrine reuptake inhibitor, has emerged as a common cause of drug-induced seizures (104). Linezolid, a new synthetic antimicrobial agent, is an important weapon against methicillin-resistant *Staphylococcus aureus* (MRSA). There are reports of serotonin syndrome developing after concomitant use of linezolid and the SSRI paroxetine, as well as citalopram (105) and mirtazapine (106). Other substances used in combination with SSRIs that have precipitated the serotonin syndrome include St. John's wort (107).

Antipsychotic agents have long been known to precipitate seizures (97). Both the phenothiazines and haloperidol have been implicated, but the potential is greater with phenothiazines, and seizures occur more frequently with increasing dosage (108). Clozapine, an atypical antipsychotic agent (dibenzodiazepine class) used for the treatment of intractable schizophrenia, may also be useful for tremor and psychosis in patients with Parkinson disease (109,110). As with other antipsychotic agents, the incidence of seizures increases with increasing dosage (111). If reduction of dosage is not practical, phenytoin or valproate may be added; however, carbamazepine should be avoided because antipsychotic agents may induce agranulocytosis. Lithium may also precipitate seizures (112).

The use of theophylline and other methylxanthines may lead to generalized tonic–clonic seizures; rarely, patients may experience seizures with nontoxic levels of theophylline. Seizures resulting from overdosage are best treated with IV diazepam. Massive overdosage may induce hypocalcemia and other electrolyte abnormalities (113).

Lidocaine precipitates seizures, usually in the setting of congestive heart failure, shock, or hepatic insufficiency. General anesthetics, such as ketamine and enflurane, are also implicated (see "Central Anticholinergic Syndrome"). Alfentanil is a potent short-acting opioid agent that may induce clinical and electroencephalographic seizures (114).

Verapamil intoxication may be associated with seizures through the mechanism of hypocalcemia, although hypoxia also may play a role (115). Other calcium-channel blockers have not been reported to produce this adverse effect. Meperidine, pentazocine, and propoxyphene, among other analgesic drugs, infrequently cause seizures (116).

Many antiparasitic agents and antimicrobials, particularly penicillins and cephalosporins in high concentrations, are known seizure precipitants. It should be noted that some antibiotics, such as the fluoroquinolones, may lower the seizure threshold. Carbapenem antimicrobials also have significant neurotoxic potential, with meropenem perhaps having the lowest incidence (117,118). Lindane, an antiparasitic shampoo active against head lice (*Pediculosis capitis*), has a rare association with generalized, self-limited seizures; it is best to use another agent should reinfestation occur. Seizures have not been reported with permethrin, another antipediculosis agent.

Severe isoniazid intoxication involves coma, severe, intractable seizures, and metabolic acidosis. Ingestion of >80 mg/kg of body weight produces severe CNS symptoms that are rapidly reversed with IV administration of pyridoxine at 1 mg per every 1 mg of isoniazid (119). Conventional doses of short-acting barbiturates, phenytoin, or diazepam are also recommended to potentiate the effect of pyridoxine (120).

Recreational Drug-Induced Seizures

Alldredge and associates (121) retrospectively identified 49 cases of recreational drug-induced seizures in 47 patients seen between 1975 and 1987. Most patients experienced a single generalized tonic–clonic attack associated with acute drug intoxication, but seven patients had multiple seizures and two had status epilepticus. The recreational drugs implicated were cocaine (32 cases), amphetamines, heroin, and phencyclidine; a combination of drugs was responsible for 11 cases. Seizures occurred independently of the route of administration and were reported in both first-time and chronic abusers. A total of 10 patients (21%) reported prior seizures, all temporally associated with drug abuse. Except for one patient who experienced prolonged status epilepticus causing a fixed neurologic deficit, most patients had no obvious short-term neurologic sequelae (121). Marijuana is unlikely to alter the seizure threshold (122). Patients with seizures who test positive for marijuana on toxicologic screening should be investigated for other illicit drug and alcohol use.

Cocaine, a biologic compound that is one of the most abused recreational drugs in the United States, commonly gives rise to tremors and generalized seizures. Seizures can develop immediately following drug administration, without other toxic signs. Convulsions and death can occur within minutes of overdose. Pascual-Leone and coworkers (123) retrospectively studied 474 patients with medical complications related to acute cocaine intoxication. Of 403 patients who had no seizure history, approximately 10% had seizures within 90 minutes of cocaine use. The majority of seizures were single and generalized, induced by IV or "crack" cocaine, and were not associated with any lasting neurologic deficits. Most of the focal or repetitive attacks involved an acute intracerebral complication or concurrent use of other drugs. Of 71 patients with previous noncocaine-related seizures, 17% presented with cocaine-induced seizures, most of which were multiple and of the same type as they had regularly experienced (123).

The treatment of choice for recreational drug-induced seizures is diazepam or lorazepam. Bicarbonate for acidosis, artificial ventilation, and cardiac monitoring are also useful, depending on the duration of the seizures. Urinary acidification accelerates excretion of the drug. Chlorpromazine has also been recommended because it raised, rather than lowered, the seizure threshold in cocaine-intoxicated primates (124). The use of TCAs decreases vasoconstrictor and cardiac action (125).

Acute overdose of amphetamine causes excitement, chest pain, hypertension, tachycardia, and sweating, followed by delirium, hallucinations, hyperpnea, cardiac arrhythmias, hyperpyrexia, seizures, coma, and death. Because chlorpromazine prolongs the half-life of amphetamine, phenothiazines and haloperidol have been recommended; if signs of atropinization are present, neither should be used. Barbiturates can aggravate delirium. Seizures are treated with diazepam or, if long-term antiepileptic therapy is indicated, with phenytoin. Acidification of urine may enhance drug excretion.

Methamphetamine is a synthetic agent with toxic effects, including seizures, that are similar to those with amphetamine and cocaine (126). The amphetamine derivative (MDMA) stimulates the release and inhibits the reuptake of serotonin (5-HT) and other neurotransmitters, such as dopamine, to a lesser extent. Mild versions of the serotonin syndrome often develop, when hyperthermia, mental confusion, and hyperkinesia predominate (126). MDMA may also cause seizures in conjunction with rhabdomyolysis and hepatic dysfunction (127).

γ-Hydroxybutyric acid (GHB), or sodium oxybate, is an agent that is approved for use in patients with narcolepsy who experience episodes of cataplexy, a condition characterized by the acute onset of weakness or paralyzed muscles triggered by an intense emotion. It is now also a popular agent among recreational drug users. GHB is a naturally occurring substance in the human brain. Its abuse potential is secondary to its ability to induce a euphoric state without a hangover effect. Additional effects of increased sensuality and disinhibition further explain the popularity of the agent. Abusers will often ingest sufficient quantities to lead to a severely depressed level of consciousness. It is not uncommon to observe seizures in these cases. With acute overdose, patients have experienced delirium and transient respiratory depression, which can be fatal (129).

GHB is believed to bind to $GABA_B$ and GHB-specific receptors. It blocks dopamine release at the synapse and produces an increase in intracellular dopamine. This is followed by a time-dependent leakage of dopamine from the neuron. GHB reportedly lengthens slow-wave sleep. The toxicity of GHB is dose-dependent and can result in nausea, vomiting, hypotonia, bradycardia, hypothermia, random clonic movements, coma, respiratory depression, and apnea. Combining GHB with other depressants or psychoactive compounds may exacerbate its effects. Other subjective effects reportedly include euphoria, hallucinations, relaxation, and disinhibition. Deaths involving solely the use of GHB appear to be rare and have involved the "recreational abuse" of the drug for its "euphoric" effects. GHB abuse frequently involves the use of other substances, such as alcohol or MDMA (130).

CENTRAL ANTICHOLINERGIC SYNDROME

Many drugs used as anesthetic agents and in the intensive care unit may cause seizures. Although a discussion of each agent is beyond the scope of this chapter, we review the central anticholinergic syndrome (131), a common disorder associated with blockade of central cholinergic neurotransmission, whose symptoms are identical to those of atropine intoxication: seizures, agitation, hallucinations, disorientation, stupor, coma, and respiratory depression. Such disturbances may be induced by opiates, ketamine, etomidate, propofol, nitrous oxide, and halogenated inhalation anesthetics, as well as by such H_2-blocking agents as cimetidine. An individual predisposition exists for central anticholinergic syndrome that is unpredictable from laboratory findings or other signs. The postanesthetic syndrome can be prevented by administration of physostigmine during anesthesia.

OTHER SEIZURE PRECIPITANTS

Heavy metal intoxication, especially with lead and mercury, is a well-known seizure precipitant. Ingestion of lead from paint and inhalation of lead oxide are specific hazards among young children. Hyperbaric oxygenation provokes seizures, possibly as a toxic effect of oxygen itself. Some antineoplastic agents, such as chlorambucil and methotrexate, precipitate seizures. Table 35.2 lists other agents reported to induce seizures (132).

Increasingly utilized prophylactically and as alternative medicine, many herbs and other alternative treatments may increase the risk for seizures (133). This may be through intrinsic proconvulsive effects of contamination by heavy metals. These include cyanobacteria (aka spirulina, blue–green algae), ephedra (ma huang), ginkobiloba, pennyroyal, primrose oil, sage, star anise, star fruit, and wormwood. In addition, many herbs may have an effect on AED concentrations via the cytochrome P450 and P-glycoprotein systems.

More recently, there has also been concern that seizures may also be induced following consumption of energy drinks and supplements. It has been proposed that large consumption of compounds rich in caffeine, taurine, and guarana seed extract may provoke seizures (134).

ECLAMPSIA

A condition unique to pregnancy and puerperium, eclampsia is characterized by convulsions following a preeclamptic state involving hypertension, proteinuria, edema, and coagulopathy, as well as headache, drowsiness, and hyper-reflexia. Eclampsia is associated with a maternal mortality of 1% to 2% and a rate of complications of 35% (135). In the United States, magnesium sulfate is the chosen therapy, whereas in the United Kingdom, such conventional AEDs as phenytoin and diazepam are used (136,137). The antiepileptic action of magnesium sulfate is accompanied by hypotension, weakness, ataxia, respiratory depression, and coma. The recommended "therapeutic level" is 3.29 μmol/L; however, weakness and ataxia appear at 3.5 to 5.0 μmol/L, and respiratory depression at 5.0 μmol/L (138). Kaplan and associates (139) argue that magnesium sulfate is not a proven AED; even at therapeutic levels, 12% of patients continued to have seizures in one study (140). The use of magnesium sulfate or conventional AEDs for preeclamptic or eclamptic seizures remains controversial. Because eclamptic seizures are clinically and electrographically indistinguishable from other generalized tonic–clonic attacks, the use of established AEDs, such as diazepam, lorazepam, and phenytoin, is recommended (139). In a recent randomized study of 2138 women with hypertension during labor (141), no eclamptic convulsions occurred in women receiving magnesium sulfate, whereas seizures were frequent with phenytoin use. Methodological problems, however, involved the route of administration of the second phenytoin dose after loading and the low therapeutic phenytoin level at the time of the seizure.

Magnesium sulfate has a beneficial effect on factors leading to eclampsia and can reverse cerebral arterial vasoconstriction (142). By the time a neurologist is consulted, however, the patient will have received magnesium sulfate and will require additional treatment to control seizures.

MALIGNANCY

Mechanisms for induction of seizures in patients with cancer include direct invasion of cortex or leptomeninges, metabolic derangements, opportunistic infection, and chemotherapeutic agents (143). Limbic encephalitis is a paraneoplastic syndrome seen in patients with small-cell carcinoma or, less commonly, Hodgkin disease. Patients usually present with amnestic dementia, affective disturbance, and sometimes a personality change. During the illness, both complex partial and generalized seizures may occur. Paraneoplastic limbic encephalitis associated with anti-Hu (antineuronal nuclear antibody type 1) antibodies may present with seizures and precede the diagnosis of cancer (144). If the etiology of new-onset seizures is not defined in a patient with known cancer, frequent neuroimaging studies should assess the individual for metastatic disease.

Opsoclonus–myoclonus syndrome (myoclonic infantile encephalopathy) occurs most frequently in young children (mean age, 18 months). Approximately half of the cases have been reported in patients with neuroblastoma, but only approximately 3% of all neuroblastoma cases are complicated by the syndrome. Opsoclonus–myoclonus syndrome has been reported with carcinoma but occurs idiopathically as well. Because the idiopathic and paraneoplastic syndromes are indistinguishable clinically, opsoclonus–myoclonus syndrome should always prompt a search for neuroblastoma. Symptoms respond to steroid or corticotropin therapy. In the majority of cases, successful treatment of the neuroblastoma leads to remission; however, the syndrome may reappear with or without tumor recurrence (145).

VASCULITIS

Seizures as a manifestation of vasculitis may occur as a feature of encephalopathy, as a focal neurologic deficit, or in association with renal failure (146). The incidence of seizures increases with the duration and severity of the underlying vasculitis (147), and ranges from 24% to 45% (148). The relationship of the seizure disorder to the underlying disease may not always be clear, however. A confounding feature of AED therapy is the occurrence of drug-induced systemic lupus erythematosus (149). Although this association has been challenged—the seizures were believed to be an initial manifestation of lupus—phenytoin-associated lupus and spontaneous lupus do have different loci of immunoregulation (150). Systemic necrotizing vasculitis and granulomatous vasculitis rarely present with seizures. Among patients with giant-cell arteritis with nonocular signs, seizures occur in 1.5% (150). Behçet disease is associated with neurologic involvement in 10% to 25% of patients. Onset is usually acute, and seizures occasionally occur.

TRANSPLANTATION AND SEIZURES

Organ transplantation has led to newly recognized CNS disorders and new manifestations of old disorders. Seizures in patients anticipating or having undergone transplantation may be difficult to manage for several reasons: (i) these individuals are frequently metabolically stressed; (ii) preexisting diseases and preceding therapies may have affected the CNS (e.g., candidates for bone marrow transplantation may have received L-asparaginase, which is associated with acute intracerebral hemorrhage and infarction, and ischemic seizures); and (iii) immunosuppressive agents, particularly cyclosporine and tacrolimus (FK506), may themselves provoke seizures.

Some transplant patients appear to have an increased risk for seizures. Wijdicks and colleagues (151) concluded that most new-onset seizures in 630 patients undergoing orthotopic liver transplantation resulted from immunosuppressant neurotoxicity (cyclosporine and FK506) and did not indicate a poor outcome. Vaughn and coworkers (152) reported that of 85 patients who had received a lung transplant, 22 had seizures (including 15 of 18 patients with cystic fibrosis); in patients younger than age 25 years, particularly those given IV methylprednisolone to prevent rejection, the seizure risk was increased. Bone marrow transplant recipients with human leukocyte antigen mismatch and unrelated donor material have an enhanced risk for seizures from cyclosporine neurotoxicity (153). Foscarnet, used to treat cytomegalovirus hepatitis following bone marrow transplantation (154), may also precipitate seizures (80). For the acute management of prolonged seizures, benzodiazepines are least likely to induce the enzyme system responsible for metabolizing immunosuppressant drugs (155).

Long-term management of transplant recipients with seizures is determined after the etiology has been ascertained. Because allograft survival is decreased with phenytoin or phenobarbital and steroids (156), the use of AEDs has been discouraged (157). The half-lives of prednisolone and, probably, cyclosporine (155) are decreased when phenobarbital, phenytoin, or carbamazepine are administered. Valproic acid is a reasonable choice, except in hepatic transplantation patients and in bone marrow transplantation patients during engraftment.

Gabapentin may be useful in patients undergoing hepatic or bone marrow transplantation. The agent eliminated renally as unchanged drug from the systemic circulation, with very little gabapentin protein bound, and probably has fewer drug interactions than other AEDs. Gabapentin use in patients with renal failure must be modified, however.

Phenytoin should be considered for patients with partial seizures, except during bone marrow engraftment, when carbamazepine is also relatively contraindicated because of toxic hematologic side effects. During the 2- to 6-week period of engraftment, phenobarbital is acceptable. When AEDs other than valproic acid or gabapentin are used, the doses of immunosuppressive agents should be increased to ensure therapeutic immunosuppression. Cyclosporine levels should be determined. Experience with other AEDs, such as lamotrigine and topiramate, in these settings is limited.

POSTERIOR REVERSIBLE ENCEPHALOPATHY SYNDROME

The clinical syndrome of posterior reversible encephalopathy syndrome (PRES) involves headache, encephalopathy, visual symptoms, and seizures. Conditions that may predispose to develop PRES include pre-eclampsia/eclampsia, post-transplantation, immune suppression, infection, autoimmune disease, chemotherapy, dialysis, and multiple metabolic disorders. Seizures have been noted relatively frequently in PRES. Clinical seizures occurred in more than 85% of cases of which there were multiple seizures in more than one third of patients. Although infrequent, patients may also present with status epilepticus. Of those patients that recover, it is rare that they will have recurrent seizures (158,159).

References

1. Delanty N, Vaughan CJ, French JA. Medical causes of seizures. *Lancet.* 1998;352:383–390.
2. Boggs JG. Seizures in medically complex patients. *Epilepsia.* 1997; 38(suppl 4):S55–S59.
3. Turnbull TL, Vanden Hoek TL, Howes DS, et al. Utility of laboratory studies in the emergency department patient with a new-onset seizure. *Ann Emerg Med.* 1990;19:373–377.
4. Anderson RJ, Chung HM, Kluge R, et al. Hyponatremia: a prospective analysis of its epidemiology and the pathogenetic role of vasopressin. *Ann Intern Med.* 1985;102:164–168.
5. Arieff AI, Guisardo R. Effects on the central nervous system of hypernatremic and hyponatremic states. *Kidney Int.* 1976;10:104–116.
6. Daggett P, Deanfield J, Moss F. Neurological aspects of hyponatremia. *Postgrad Med J.* 1982;58:737–740.
7. Riggs JE. Neurologic manifestations of fluid and electrolyte disturbances. *Neurol Clin.* 1989;7:509–523.
8. Adams RD, Victor M, Mancall EL. Central pontine myelinolysis: a hitherto undescribed disease occurring in alcoholic and malnourished patients. *AMA Arch Neurol Psychiatry.* 1959;81:154–172.
9. Paguirigan A, Lefken EB. Central pontine myelinolysis. *Neurology.* 1969;19:1007–1011.
10. Norenberg MD, Leslie KO, Robertson AS. Association between rise in serum sodium and central pontine myelinolysis. *Ann Neurol.* 1982;11: 128–135.
11. Kleinschmidt-DeMasters BK, Norenberg MD. Neuropathologic observations in electrolyte-induced myelinolysis in the rat. *J Neuropathol Exp Neurol.* 1962;41:67–80.
12. Rossi NF, Schrier RW. Hyponatremic states. In: Maxwell MH, Cleeman CR, Narins RG, eds. *Clinical Disorders of Fluid and Electrolyte Metabolism.* 5th ed. New York: McGraw-Hill; 1987:461–470.
13. Schmidt D, Sachdeo R. Oxcarbazepine for treatment of partial epilepsy: a review and recommendations for clinical use. *Epilepsy Behav.* 2000;1: 396–405.
14. Sue YM, Lee YL, Huang JJ. Acute hyponatremia, seizure, and rhabdomyolysis after ecstasy use. *J Toxicol Clin Toxicol.* 2002;40:931–932.
15. Hartung TK, Schofield E, Short AI, et al. Hyponatraemic states following 3,4-methylenedioxymethamphetamine (MDMA, "ecstasy") ingestion. *Quart J Med.* 2002;95:431–437.
16. Gupta MM. Medical emergencies associated with disorders of calcium homeostasis. *J Assoc Physicians India.* 1989;37:629–631.
17. Halperin I, Nubiola A, Vendrell J, et al. Late-onset hypocalcemia appearing years after thyroid surgery. *J Endocrinol Invest.* 1989;12:419–422.
18. Pugliese MT, Blumberg DL, Hludzinski J, et al. Nutritional rickets in suburbia. *J Am Coll Nutr.* 1998;17:637–641.
19. Layzer RB. *Neuromuscular Manifestations of Systemic Disease.* Philadelphia: FA Davis; 1985:58–62.
20. Riggs JE. Electrolyte disturbances. In: Johnson RT, ed. *Current Therapy in Neurologic Disease.* Philadelphia: BC Decker; 1985:325–328.
21. Whang R. Clinical disorders of magnesium metabolism. *Compr Ther.* 1997;23:168–173.
22. Silvis SE, Paragas PD. Paresthesias, weakness, seizures, and hypophosphatemia in patients receiving hyperalimentation. *Gastroenterology.* 1972;62:513–520.
23. Knochel JP. The pathophysiology and clinical characteristics of severe hypophosphatemia. *Arch Intern Med.* 1977;137:203–220.
24. Singh BM, Strobos RJ. Epilepsia partialis continua associated with nonketotic hyperglycemia: clinical and biochemical profile of 21 patients. *Ann Neurol.* 1980;8:155–160.
25. Vastola EF, Maccario M, Homan RO. Activation of epileptogenic foci by hyperosmolality. *Neurology.* 1967;17:520–526.
26. Singh BM, Gupta DR, Strobos RJ. Nonketotic hyperglycemia and epilepsia partialis continua. *Arch Neurol.* 1973;29:189–190.
27. Brick J, Gutrecht J, Ringel R. Reflex epilepsy and nonketotic hyperglycemia in the elderly: a specific neuroendocrine syndrome. *Neurology.* 1989;39:394–399.
28. Venna N, Sabin T. Tonic focal seizures in nonketotic hyperglycemia of diabetes mellitus. *Arch Neurol.* 1981;38:512–514.
29. Guisado R, Arieff AI. Neurologic manifestations of diabetic comas: correlation with biochemical alterations of the brain. *Metabolism.* 1975;24: 665–679.
30. Juurlink DN, Mamdani M, Kopp A, et al. Drug–drug interactions among elderly patients hospitalized for drug toxicity. *J Am Med Assoc.* 2003;289:1652–1658.
31. Bjerke HS, Kelly RE Jr, Geffner ME, et al. Surgical management of islet cell dysmaturation syndrome in young children. *Surg Gynecol Obstet.* 1990;171:321–325.
32. Jabbari B, Huott AD. Seizures in thyrotoxicosis. *Epilepsia.* 1980;21: 91–96.
33. Henderson LM, Behan PO, Aarli J, et al. Hashimoto's encephalopathy: a new neuroimmunological syndrome. *Ann Neurol.* 1987;22:140–141.
34. Shaw PJ, Walls TJ, Newman PK, et al. Hashimoto's encephalopathy: a steroid-responsive disorder associated with high anti-thyroid antibody titers—report of 5 cases. *Neurology.* 1991;41:228–233.
35. Henchey R, Cibula J, Helveston W, et al. Electroencephalographic findings in Hashimoto's encephalopathy. *Neurology.* 1995;45:977–981.
36. Rajagopal KR, Abbrecht PH, Derderian SS, et al. Obstructive sleep apnea in hypothyroidism. *Ann Intern Med.* 1984;101:491–494.
37. Gilmore RL, Falace P, Kanga J, et al. Sleep-disordered breathing in Mobius syndrome. *J Child Neurol.* 1991;6:73–77.
38. Kaplan PW. Metabolic and endocrine disorders resembling seizures. In: Engel J Jr, Pedley T, eds. *Epilepsy: A Comprehensive Textbook.* Philadelphia: Lippincott-Raven; 1997:2661–2770.
39. Odar-Cederlof I, Borga O. Kinetics of diphenylhydantoin in uraemic patients: consequence of decreased plasma protein binding. *Eur J Clin Pharmacol.* 1974;7:31–37.

40. Lockwood AH. Neurologic complications of renal disease. *Neurol Clin.* 1989;7:617–627.
41. Beydoun VA, Uthman BM, Sackellares JC. Gabapentin: pharmacokinetics, efficacy, and safety. *Clin Neuropharmacol.* 1995;18:469–481.
42. Ben-Menachem E. Pregabalin pharmacology and its relevance to clinical practice. *Epilepsia.* 2004;45(suppl 6):13–18.
43. Radtke RA. Pharmacokinetics of levetiracetam. *Epilepsia.* 2001; 42(suppl 4):24 27.
44. Manian FA, Stone WJ, Alford RH. Adverse antibiotic effects associated with renal insufficiency. *Rev Infect Dis.* 1990;12:236–249.
45. Knoben JE, Anderson PO. *Handbook of Clinical Drug Data.* 6th ed. Hamilton, IL: Drug Intelligence; 1989:36–54.
46. Cassidy G, Corbett J. Learning disorders. In: Engel J Jr, Pedley T, eds. *Epilepsy: A Comprehensive Textbook.* Philadelphia: Lippincott-Raven; 1997:2053–2063.
47. Labrune P, Chatelon S, Huguet P, et al. Unusual cerebral manifestations in hereditary fructose intolerance. *Arch Neurol.* 1990;47:1243–1244.
48. Sergay SM. Management of neurologic exacerbations of hepatic porphyria. *Med Clin North Am.* 1979;63:453–463.
49. Reynolds NC Jr, Miska RM. Safety of anticonvulsants in hepatic porphyrias. *Neurology.* 1981;31:480–484.
50. Bonkowsky HL, Sinclair PR, Emery S, et al. Seizure management in acute hepatic porphyria: risks of valproate and clonazepam. *Neurology.* 1980;30:588–592.
51. Shedlofsky SI, Bonkowshy HL. Seizure management in the hepatic porphyrias: results from a cell-culture model of porphyria [letter]. *Neurology.* 1984;34:399.
52. Larson AW, Wasserstrom WR, Felsher BF, et al. Posttraumatic epilepsy and acute intermittent porphyria: effects of phenytoin, carbamazepine, and clonazepam. *Neurology.* 1978;28:824–828.
53. Krauss GL, Simmons-O'Brien E, Campbell M. Successful treatment of seizures and porphyria with gabapentin. *Neurology.* 1995;45:594–595.
54. Zadra M, Grandi R, Erli LC, et al. Treatment of seizures in acute intermittent porphyria: safety and efficacy of gabapentin. *Seizure.* 1998;7:415–416.
55. Richens A. Clinical pharmacokinetics of gabapentin. In: Chadwick D, ed. *New Trends in Epilepsy Management: The Role of Gabapentin.* London: Royal Society of Medical Services; 1993:41–46.
56. Gorchein A. Drug treatment in acute porphyria. *Br J Clin Pharmacol.* 1997;44:427–434.
57. Mir NA, Faquih AM, Legnain M. Perinatal risk factors in birth asphyxia: relationship of obstetric and neonatal complications to neonatal mortality in 16,365 consecutive live births. *Asia Oceania J Obstet Gynaecol.* 1989;15:351–357.
58. Kreisman NR, Sick TJ, Rosenthal M. Importance of vascular responses in determining cortical oxygenation during recurrent paroxysmal events of varying duration and frequency of repetition. *J Cereb Blood Flow Metab.* 1983;3:330–338.
59. Perlman JM, Herscovitch P, Kreusser KL, et al. Positron emission tomography in the newborn: effect of seizure on regional blood flow in an asphyxiated infant. *Neurology.* 1985;35:244–247.
60. Easton JD, Sherman DG. Management of cerebral embolism of cardiac origin. *Stroke.* 1980;11:433–442.
61. Roach GW, Kanchuger CM, Mangano CM, et al. Adverse cerebral outcomes after coronary bypass surgery. Multicenter Study of Perioperative Ischemia Research Group and the Ischemia Research and Education Foundation Investigators. *N Engl J Med.* 1996;335:1857–1863.
62. Simon RP, Aminoff MJ. Electrographic status epilepticus in fatal anoxic coma. *Ann Neurol.* 1986;20:351–355.
63. Boggs JG, Towne A, Smith J, et al. Frequency of potentially ictal patterns in comatose ICU patients. *Epilepsia.* 1994;35(suppl 8):135.
64. Towne AR, Pellock JM, Ko D, et al. Determinants of mortality in status epilepticus. *Epilepsia.* 1994;35:27–34.
65. Krumholz A, Stern BJ, Weiss HD. Outcome from coma after cardiopulmonary resuscitation: relation to seizures and myoclonus. *Neurology.* 1988;38:401–405.
66. Young GB, Gilbert JJ, Zochodne DW. The significance of myoclonic status epilepticus in postanoxic coma. *Neurology.* 1990;40:1843–1848.
67. Richter JA, Holtman JR, Jr. Barbiturates: their in vivo effects and potential biochemical mechanisms. *Prog Neurobiol.* 1982;18:275–319.
68. Lamsback WJ, Navrozov M. The acquired metabolic disorders of the nervous system. In: Adams RD, Victor M, eds. *Principles of Neurology.* 5th ed. New York: McGraw-Hill; 1993:877–902.
69. Bruni J, Willmore LJ, Wilder BJ. Treatment of post-anoxic intention myoclonus with valproic acid. *Can J Neurol Sci.* 1979;6:39–42.
70. Mattson RH. Seizures associated with alcohol use and alcohol withdrawal. In: Browne TR, Feldman RG, eds. *Epilepsy: Diagnosis and Management.* Boston: Little, Brown; 1983:325–332.
71. Forster FM, Booker H. The epilepsies and convulsive disorders. In: Joynt R, ed. *Clinical Neurology, III.* Philadelphia: JB Lippincott; 1984:1–68.
72. Engel J. *Seizures and Epilepsy.* Philadelphia: FA Davis; 1989:402.
73. Labar DR, Harden C. Infection and inflammatory diseases. In: Engel J, Jr, Pedley T, eds. *Epilepsy: A Comprehensive Textbook.* Philadelphia: Lippincott-Raven; 1997:2587–2596.
74. Garcia-Monaco JC, Benach JL. Lyme neuroborreliosis. *Ann Neurol.* 1995;37:691–702.
75. Ferrari S, Monaco S, Morbin M, et al. HIV-associated PML presenting as epilepsia partialis continua. *J Neurol Sci.* 1998;161:180–184.
76. Carpio A, Santillan F, Leon P, et al. Is the course of neurocysticercosis modified by treatment with antihelminthic agents? *Arch Intern Med.* 1995;155:1982–1988.
77. Kammerer WS, Schantz PM. Echinococcal disease. *Infect Dis Clin North Am.* 1993;7:605–618.
78. Horowitz S, Bentson JR, Benson F, et al. CNS toxoplasmosis in acquired immunodeficiency syndrome. *Arch Neurol.* 1983;40:649–652.
79. Das BN, Weinberg DV, Jampol LM. Cytomegalovirus retinitis. *Br J Hosp Med.* 1994;52:163–166.
80. Lor E, Liu YQ. Neurologic sequelae associated with foscarnet therapy. *Ann Pharmacother.* 1994;28:1035–1037.
81. Ashkenazi S, Cleary KR, Pickering LK, et al. The association of Shiga toxin and other cytotoxins with the neurologic manifestations of shigellosis. *J Infect Dis.* 1990;161:961–965.
82. Zvulunov A, Lerman M, Ashkenazi S, et al. The prognosis of convulsions during childhood shigellosis. *Eur J Pediatr.* 1990;149:293–294.
83. Butler T, Arnold M, Islam M. Depletion of hepatic glycogen in the hypoglycaemia of fatal childhood diarrhoeal illnesses. *Trans R Soc Trop Med Hyg.* 1989;83:839–843.
84. Kieslich M, Errazuriz G, Posselt HG, et al. Brain white-matter lesions in celiac disease: a prospective study of 75 diet-treated patients. *Pediatrics.* 2001;108:E21.
85. Finelli PF, McEntee WJ, Ambler M, et al. Adult celiac disease presenting as cerebellar syndrome. *Neurology.* 1980;30:245–249.
86. Albers JW, Nostrant TT, Riggs JE. Neurologic manifestations of gastrointestinal disease. *Neurol Clin.* 1989;7:525–548.
87. Rush PJ, Inman R, Berstein M, et al. Isolated vasculitis of the central nervous system in a patient with celiac disease. *Am J Med.* 1986;81:1092–1094.
88. Gendelman S, Present D, Janowitz HD. Neurological complications of inflammatory bowel disease (IBD) [abstract]. *Gastroenterology.* 1982;82:1065.
89. Relman DA, Schmidt TM, MacDermott RP, et al. Identification of the uncultured bacillus of Whipple's disease. *N Engl J Med.* 1992;327:293–301.
90. Louis ED, Lynch T, Kaufmann P, et al. Diagnostic guidelines in central nervous system Whipple's disease. *Ann Neurol.* 1996;40:561–568.
91. Johnson L, Diamond I. Cerebral Whipple's disease. Diagnosis by brain biopsy. *Am J Clin Pathol.* 1980;74:486–490.
92. Feurle GE, Volk B, Waldherr R. Cerebral Whipple's disease with negative jejunal histology. *N Engl J Med.* 1979;300:907–908.
93. Ryser RJ, Locksley RM, Eng SC, et al. Reversal of dementia associated with Whipple's disease by trimethoprim-sulfamethoxazole, drugs that penetrate the blood-brain barrier. *Gastroenterology.* 1984;86:745–752.
94. Keinath RD, Merrell DE, Vlietstra R, et al. Antibiotic treatment and relapse in Whipple's disease. Long-term follow-up of 88 patients. *Gastroenterology.* 1985;88:1867–1873.
95. Gerard A, Sarrot-Reynauld F, Liozon E, et al. Neurologic presentation of Whipple disease: report of 12 cases and review of the literature. *Medicine (Baltimore).* 2002;81:443–457.
96. Herlong HF. Hepatic encephalopathy. In: Johnson RT, ed. *Current Therapy in Neurologic Disease, II.* Toronto: BC Decker; 1987:303–306.
97. Messing RO, Closson RG, Simon RP. Drug-induced seizures: a 10-year experience. *Neurology.* 1984;34:1582–1586.
98. Lowry MR, Dunner FJ. Seizures during tricyclic therapy. *Am J Psychiatry.* 1980;137:1461–1462.
99. Richardson JW, III, Richelson R. Antidepressants: clinical update for medical practitioners. *Mayo Clin Proc.* 1984;59:330–337.
100. De Toledo JC, Haddad H, Ramsey RE. Status epilepticus associated with the combination of valproic acid and clomipramine. *Ther Drug Monit.* 1997;19(1):71–73.
101. Favale E, Rubino V, Mainardi P, et al. Anticonvulsant effect of fluoxetine in humans. *Neurology.* 1995;45:1926–1927.
102. Loo H, Plau A, Galinowski A, et al. Epileptogenic action of fluvoxamine. Apropos of a case. *Encephale.* 1987;13(4):231–232.
103. Bodner RA, Lynch T, Lewis L, et al. Serotonin syndrome. *Neurology.* 1995;45:219–223.
104. Mago R, Mahajan R, Thase ME. Medically serious adverse effects of newer antidepressants. *Curr Psychiatry Rep.* 2008;10(3):249–257.
105. Bernard L, Stern R, Lew D, et al. Serotonin syndrome after concomitant treatment with linezolid and citalopram. *Clin Infect Dis.* 2003;36:1197.
106. Ubogu EE, Katirji B. Mirtazapine-induced serotonin syndrome. *Clin Neuropharmacol.* 2003;26:54–57.
107. Dannawi M. Possible serotonin syndrome after combination of buspirone and St. John's wort. *J Psychopharmacol.* 2002;16:401.
108. Logothetis J. Spontaneous epileptic seizures and electroencephalographic changes in the course of phenothiazine therapy. *Neurology.* 1967;17:869–877.
109. Pfeiffer RF, Kang J, Graber B, et al. Clozapine for psychosis in Parkinson's disease. *Mov Disord.* 1990;5:239–242.

110. Friedman JH, Lannun MC. Clozapine-responsive tremor in Parkinson's disease. *Mov Disord.* 1990;5:225–229.

111. Devinsky O, Honigfeld G, Patin J. Clozapine-related seizures. *Neurology.* 1991;41:369–371.

112. Julius SC, Brenner RP. Myoclonic seizures with lithium. *Biol Psychiatry.* 1987;22:1184–1190.

113. Eshleman SH, Shaw LM. Massive theophylline overdose with atypical metabolic abnormalities. *Clin Chem.* 1990;36:398–399.

114. Keene DL, Roberts D, Splinter WM, et al. Alfentanil mediated activation of epileptiform activity in the electrocorticogram during resection of epileptogenic foci. *Can J Neurol Sci.* 1997;24(1):37–39.

115. Hendren WG, Schieber RS, Garrettson LK. Extracorporeal bypass for the treatment of verapamil poisoning. *Ann Emerg Med.* 1989;18:984–987.

116. Blain PG, Lane RJM. Neurologic disorders. In: Davies DM, ed. *Textbook of Adverse Drug Reactions.* 4th ed. New York: Oxford University Press; 1991:535–566.

117. Melhorn AJ, Brown DA. Safety concerns with fluoroqinolones. *Ann Pharmacother.* 1007;41:1859–1866.

118. Norrby SR. Neurotoxicity of carabapenem antibacterials. *Drug Safety.* 1996;15:87–90.

119. Watkins RC, Hambrick EL, Benjamin G, et al. Isoniazid toxicity presenting as seizures and metabolic acidosis. *J Natl Med Assoc.* 1990;2:57–64.

120. Chin L, Sievers ML, Herrier RN, et al. Potentiation of pyridoxine by depressants and anticonvulsants in the treatment of acute isoniazid intoxication in dogs. *Toxicol Appl Pharmacol.* 1981;58:504–509.

121. Alldredge BK, Lowenstein DH, Simon RP. Seizures associated with recreational drug abuse. *Neurology.* 1989;39:1037–1039.

122. Brust JCM, Ng SKC, Hauser AW, et al. Marijuana use and the risk of new onset seizures. *Trans Am Clin Climatol Assoc.* 1992;103:176–181.

123. Pascual-Leone A, Dhuna A, Altafullah I, et al. Cocaine-induced seizures. *Neurology.* 1990;40:404–407.

124. Johnson S, O'Meara M, Young JB. Acute cocaine poisoning. Importance of treating seizures and acidosis. *Am J Med.* 1983;75:1061–1064.

125. Antelman SM, Kocan D, Rowland N, et al. Amitriptyline provides long-lasting immunization against sudden cardiac death from cocaine. *Eur J Pharmacol.* 1981;69:119–120.

126. Jaffe JH. Drug addiction and drug abuse. In: Gilman AG, Goodman LS, Rall TW, et al., eds. *Goodman and Gilman's the Pharmacologic Basis of Therapeutics.* 7th ed. New York: Macmillan; 1985:550–554.

127. Parrott AC. Recreational ecstasy/MDMA, the serotonin syndrome, and serotonergic neurotoxicity. *Pharmacol Biochem Behav.* 2002;71:837–844.

128. Henry JA, Jeffreys KJ, Dawling S. Toxicity and death from 3,4-methylenedioxymethamphetamine ("ecstasy"). *Lancet.* 1992;340:384–387.

129. Li J, Stokes SA, Wockener A. A tale of novel intoxication: seven cases of gamma hydroxybutyric acid overdose. *Ann Emerg Med.* 1998;31:723–728.

130. European Monitoring Centre for Drugs and Drug Addiction Scientific Committee. Report on the Risk Assessment of GHB in the Framework of the Joint Action on New Synthetic Drugs. Lisbon, Portugal: European Center for Drugs and Drug Addiction; 2000.

131. Schneck HJ, Ruprecht J. Central anticholinergic syndrome (CAS) in anesthesia and intensive care. *Acta Anaesthesiol Belg.* 1989;40:219–228.

132. Alper K, Schwartz KA, Kolts RL, et al. Seizure incidence in psychopharmacological clinical trials: an analysis of Food and Drug Administration (FDA) summary basis of approval reports. *Biol Psychiatry.* 2007;62(4):325–354.

133. Samuels N, Finkelstein Y, Singer SR, et al. Herbal medicine and epilepsy: proconvulsive effects and interactions with antiepileptic drugs. *Epilepsia.* 2008;49(3):373–380.

134. Iyadurai SJP, Chung SS. New-onset seizures in adults: possible association with consumption of popular anergy drinks. *Epilepsy Behav.* 2007;10:504–508.

135. Douglas KA, Redman CWG. Eclampsia in the United Kingdom. *Br Med J.* 1994;309:1395–1400.

136. Duley L, Johansen R. Magnesium sulfate for preeclampsia and eclampsia: the evidence so far. *Br J Obstet Gynaecol.* 1994;101:565–567.

137. Hutton JD, James DK, Stirrat GM, et al. Management of severe preeclampsia and eclampsia by UK consultants. *Br J Obstet Gynaecol.* 1992;99:554–556.

138. Dinsdale HB. Does magnesium sulfate treat eclamptic seizures? *Arch Neurol.* 1988;45:1360–1361.

139. Kaplan PW, Lesser RP, Fisher RS, et al. No, magnesium sulfate should not be used in treating eclamptic seizures. *Arch Neurol.* 1988;45:1361–1364.

140. Pritchard JA, Cunningham FG, Pritchard SA. The Parkland Memorial Hospital protocol for treatment of eclampsia. Evaluation of 245 cases. *Am J Obstet Gynecol.* 1984;148:951–963.

141. Lucas MJ, Leveno KJ, Cunningham FG. A comparison of magnesium sulfate with phenytoin for the prevention of eclampsia. *N Engl J Med.* 1995;333:201–205.

142. Belfort MA, Mose KJ, Jr. Effect of magnesium sulfate on maternal brain blood flow in preeclampsia: a randomized, placebo-controlled study. *Am J Obstet Gynecol.* 1992;167:661–666.

143. Stein DA, Chamberlain MC. Evaluation and management of seizures in the patient with cancer. *Oncology.* 1991;5:33–39.

144. Dalmau J, Graus F, Rosenblum MK, et al. Anti-Hu–associated paraneoplastic encephalitis/sensory neuropathy: a clinical study of 71 patients. *Medicine (Baltimore).* 1992;71:59–72.

145. Dropcho E. The remote effects of cancer on the nervous system. *Neurol Clin.* 1989;7:579–603.

146. Bennahum DA, Messner RP. Recent observations on central nervous system lupus erythematosus. *Semin Arthritis Rheum.* 1975;4:253–266.

147. Adelman DC, Saltiel E, Klinenberg JR. The neuropsychiatric manifestations of systemic lupus erythematosus: an overview. *Semin Arthritis Rheum.* 1986;15:185–199.

148. Ellis SG, Verity MA. Central nervous system involvement in systemic lupus erythematosus. A review of neuropathologic findings in 57 cases, 1955–1977. *Semin Arthritis Rheum.* 1979;8:212–221.

149. Alarcon-Segovia D, Palacios R. Differences in immunoregulatory T cell circuits between diphenylhydantoin-related and spontaneously occurring systemic lupus erythematosus. *Arthritis Rheum.* 1981;24:1086–1092.

150. Nadeau S, Watson RT. Neurologic manifestations of vasculitis and collagen vascular syndromes. In: Joynt R, ed. *Clinical Neurology.* Vol 4. Philadelphia: Lippincott-Raven; 1997:1–166.

151. Wijdicks EMF, Plevak DJ, Wiesner RH, et al. Causes and outcome of seizures in liver transplant recipients. *Neurology.* 1996;47:1523–1525.

152. Vaughn BV, Ali II, Olivier KN, et al. Seizures in lung transplant recipients. *Epilepsia.* 1996;37:1175–1179.

153. Zimmer WE, Hourihane JM, Wang HZ, et al. The effect of human leukocyte antigen disparity on cyclosporine neurotoxicity after allogeneic bone marrow transplantation. *Am J Neuroradiol.* 1998;19:601–608.

154. Zomas A, Mehta J, Powles R, et al. Unusual infections following allogeneic bone marrow transplantation for chronic lymphocytic leukemia. *Bone Marrow Transplant.* 1994;14:799–803.

155. Gilmore R. Seizures and antiepileptic drug use in transplant patients. *Neurol Clin.* 1988;6:279–296.

156. McEnery PT, Stempel DA. Commentary: anticonvulsant therapy and renal allograft survival. *J Pediatr.* 1976;88:138–139.

157. Wassner SJ, Malekzadeh MH, Pennisi AJ, et al. Allograft survival in patients receiving anticonvulsant medications. *Clin Nephrol.* 1977;8:293–297.

158. Lee VH, Wijdicks EFM, Manno EM, et al. Clinical spectrum of reversible posterior leukoencephalopathy syndrome. *Arch Neurol.* 2008;65(2):205–221.

159. Bartynski WS. Posterior reversible encephalopathy syndrome, Part 1: fundamental imaging and clinical features. *Am J Neuroradiol.* 2008;29:1036–1042.

CHAPTER 36 ■ EPILEPSY IN PATIENTS WITH MULTIPLE HANDICAPS

JOHN M. PELLOCK

Disabilities associated with the varying etiologies of epilepsy or with the disease itself often lead to multiple handicaps that complicate the diagnosis of epilepsy, render it refractory to treatment, and increase its morbid consequences. Some disabilities are developmental and frequently noted in children. Others are acquired disorders with accompanying behavioral, intellectual, communication, motor, and psychosocial deficits. Mental retardation and cerebral palsy are the most commonly discussed, but autism, attention deficit hyperactivity disorder, learning disabilities, depression, and psychoses all complicate epilepsy as well.

MENTAL RETARDATION

Just as epilepsy is not a solitary disease, mental retardation is not a disease, a syndrome, or a specific medical disorder. In 2002, the American Association on Mental Retardation (1) described a disability originating before age 18 years characterized by significant limitations both in intellectual functioning and adaptive behavior as expressed in conceptual, social, and practical adaptive skills. Five criteria were believed to be essential: (i) the limitation in present functioning must be considered within the context of community environments typical to the individual's age, peers, and culture; (ii) to be valid, an assessment must consider cultural and linguistic diversity, as well as differences in communication, sensory, motor, and behavioral factors; (iii) within an individual, limitations often coexist with strengths; (iv) an important purpose of describing limitations is to develop a profile of needed supports; and (v) with appropriate personalized supports over a sustained period, the life functioning of the person with mental retardation generally will improve. These criteria do not state an intelligence quotient (IQ) measurement as a determining factor, but the 1994 (2) and 2000 (3) editions of the *Diagnostic and Statistical Manual of Mental Disorders* recognized an IQ of approximately 70 or below and further described mild (IQ 50/55 to 70), moderate (IQ 35/40 to 50/55), severe (IQ 20/25 to 35/40), and profound (IQ less than 20/25) categories. An early classification employed IQ levels for educable (50 to 75), trainable (30 to 50), and severely or profoundly retarded (less than 30). A recent trend simplifies the categories to mild (IQs from 50 to 70) and severe (IQs less than 50) (1,4,5). The abilities of a person with mental retardation depend both on intelligence, as measured by formal testing, and social adaptability, which includes interpersonal and group behaviors (4).

The comorbidities of mental retardation include cerebral palsy, autism, epilepsy, and numerous behavioral diagnoses such as attention deficit hyperactivity disorder and oppositional defiant disorder. These comorbid conditions are determined by specific etiologic diagnoses such as chromosomal disorders, neurocutaneous syndromes, central nervous system (CNS) injury, and inherited metabolic disorders (Table 36.1). The overlay of diagnostic categories and etiologies demonstrate that both epilepsy and mental retardation are symptoms of numerous conditions responsible for CNS dysfunction. Not infrequently, the specific cause remains unknown, although advances in neuroimaging, molecular genetics, and metabolic testing may remedy this lack. The relative risk of mental retardation appears to increase with decreasing socioeconomic status (1,4–6).

Severe mental retardation is found in approximately 0.3% to 0.4% of the general population, or in 10% of the mentally retarded. The mild form has an estimated incidence of 20 to 30 cases per 1000 livebirths, or 2% to 3% of the population, and is more frequent in males. Approximately 50% of all persons with cerebral palsy have mental retardation (7). Compared with the general population, children with developmental delay and those with a diagnosis of mental retardation are at an increased risk for epilepsy. The incidence of childhood-onset epilepsy associated with mental retardation and cerebral palsy ranges from 15% to 38% (8). The highest rates of epilepsy are found in children with severe developmental disability and multiple handicaps; coexisting cerebral palsy and mental retardation increase the likelihood of epilepsy twofold, compared with either condition alone (8). In these children, intellectual disability results primarily from the underlying brain disease, not from epilepsy (9); however, continued frequent, repetitive, and uncontrolled seizures may produce additional neuropsychological deficits.

The management of epilepsy in the multihandicapped patient begins with careful evaluation and classification. Treatment, though usually pharmacologic, may be etiologically specific in the presence of metabolic disease, involve surgery when malformations or brain foci can be localized, or use diet or vagus nerve stimulation. Practice guidelines from the American Academy of Neurology have addressed the initial evaluation of the patient with mental retardation or global developmental delay (10). Differential diagnoses to be considered will depend on clinical findings and history (see Table 36.1). Some refractory epilepsy syndromes—especially encephalopathic epilepsies such as Lennox–Gastaut syndrome, infantile spasms (West syndrome), and malignant partial epilepsy—are more common in the multihandicapped patient than in the general population. Comorbid epilepsy and mental retardation is characterized by multiple, yet poorly described, seizure types, long-standing epilepsy, frequent polytherapy, increased use of sedating antiepileptic drugs (AEDs),

`TABLE 36.1`

MENTAL RETARDATION: CATEGORIES OF CAUSES

Sociocultural or environmental
- Nutritional deprivation

Developmental or cerebral dysgenesis
- Anencephaly
- Neural tube defects
- Encephalocele
- Holoprosencephaly
- Lissencephaly
- Micrencephaly
- Megalencephaly
- Hydranencephaly
- Porencephaly
- Schizencephaly

Chromosomal or genetic
- X-linked syndromes
- Multiple minor congenital anomaly syndromes
- Contiguous gene syndromes
- Single-gene disorders

Metabolic
- Perinatal and postnatal hypoxic-ischemic encephalopathy
- Hypoglycemia
- Severe hypernatremia
- Enzyme defects

Prematurity
- Intracranial hemorrhage
- Hydrocephalus
- Periventricular leukomalacia
- Periventricular hemorrhagic infarction

Traumatic brain injury
- Physical abuse, maternal trauma, birth trauma

Endocrine
- Hypothyroidism

- Hyperthyroidism
- Hypoparathyroidism

Nutritional
- Severe prenatal and postnatal protein malnutrition
- Periconceptual folate deficiency
- Vitamin and essential element deficiency

Infection
- Toxoplasmosis
- Syphilis
- Rubella
- Cytomegalovirus
- Herpes simplex virus
- Streptococcus
- Human immunodeficiency virus

Neuromuscular disorder
- Myotonic dystrophy
- Dystrophinopathy
- Cerebro-ocular muscular dystrophy

Toxic exposures
- Heavy-metal poisoning
- Alcohol-related birth defects
- Ionizing radiation
- Drug embryopathies
- Teratogens

Cerebrovascular
- Hemorrhage
- Multiple infarctions
- Venous sinus thrombosis

Neurocutaneous syndromes
- Neurofibromatoses
- Tuberous sclerosis

From Roeleveld N, Zielhuis GA, Gabreels F. The prevalence of mental retardation: a critical review of recent literature. *Dev Med Child Neurol.* 1997;39:125–132, with permission.

and sometimes frequent changes in therapy. In other patients, therapy has remained unchanged for years, despite uncontrolled seizures and new drugs and modalities, increasing the risk of status epilepticus and seizure clusters. Although many etiologies of epilepsy and mental retardation are long-standing, the new onset of seizures in a person with mental retardation or other neurologic handicap requires a complete reevaluation, including brain imaging studies, because of the equivalent or heightened risk of stroke, neoplasm, and head trauma compared with the general population. Treatment of these individuals is discussed in the following sections.

CEREBRAL PALSY

Cerebral palsy frequently shares an etiology with epilepsy, and the disorders often coexist. The term *cerebral palsy* is applied to a heterogenous group of nonprogressive or static motor disorders of CNS origin that occur early in life (11). Incidence is

about 2.5 cases per 1000 livebirths, higher in twins and triplets (12). Early studies suggested an approximately 28% incidence of epilepsy in persons with cerebral palsy, but more recent epidemiologic studies place the combined incidence at 0.8 cases per 1000 livebirths. Individuals with severe cerebral palsy and those with both mental retardation and cerebral palsy run a high risk of epilepsy (8).

Cerebral palsy can be classified into four clinical types: hemiplegic, diplegic, tetraplegic, and dystonic or athetoid. The hemiplegic form manifests as a motor deficit in the second to third month of life and is usually linked to porencephaly or loss of brain volume in a territory of major cerebral vessels (12). Partial epilepsy is thus frequent in these patients. Spastic diplegia is associated with prematurity; newborns or neonates weighing less than 1500 g are at greatest risk. Underlying periventricular leukomalacia is often seen. The less common tetraplegic cerebral palsy results from global ischemia or widespread brain malformation, and usually involves secondarily generalized epilepsy with multiple seizure types. Dystonic cerebral palsy is often secondary to brain injury of the basal ganglia in the last trimester of gestation; kernicterus or hypoxic ischemic damage is a frequent accompaniment (12).

The diagnostic evaluation of children with cerebral palsy parallels that for mental retardation. Perhaps the most important determination is that the motor deficit is static, nonprogressive, and long-standing. The American Academy of Neurology recommends neuroimaging studies; other testing should depend on findings from history, physical examination, and imaging (13). Worsening cerebral palsy should prompt a complete diagnostic reevaluation. Cerebral palsy and epilepsy associated with hydrocephalus managed with ventricular shunting, worsening epilepsy, motor signs, or deterioration in intellectual ability or behavior mandate reevaluation for shunt malfunction and other complications. Initiation or discontinuation of medications for spasticity, movement disorders, or maladaptive behaviors may significantly affect the frequency of seizures.

The appearance of epilepsy in the population with cerebral palsy can vary significantly. Seizures usually have an earlier onset in individuals with severe cerebral palsy than in those with milder forms. The ability to control seizures is frequently related to the severity of the motor deficit. Fewer children with symptomatic or cryptogenic epilepsy associated with cerebral palsy can eventually discontinue AEDs. In one study

(12,14), 30 (54%) of 56 children with a significant neurologic handicap had recurrent seizures on withdrawal of AEDs, compared with an overall recurrence rate of 31%.

AUTISM

Autism is a heterogeneous, pervasive developmental disorder that portends lifelong disability (Table 36.2) (2,15,16). Markedly abnormal or impaired development in social interaction and communication skills, evident in the first 3 years of life, affect language and behavior (15,16). Affected children typically do not demonstrate the normal attachment to and interest in parents, caregivers, and peers and also may show little separation anxiety. Children with autistic spectrum disorders may exhibit echolalia and verbal repetition, along with abnormalities in pitch, intonation, rate, and rhythm, as well as frequent stereotypic self-stimulating movements and a fascination for toys or objects with repetitive motion (17). The more recent identification and inclusion of autism in Rett, Fragile X, and Angelman syndromes suggest a higher incidence than previously reported (18,19). Epidemiologic studies indicate rates as high as six cases per 1000 children (18), with a 3:1 higher incidence in boys. When cases of Asperger syndrome are included, a ratio as high as 15:1 can be seen (20).

TABLE 36.2

DIAGNOSTIC CRITERIA FOR AUTISTIC DISORDER (299.00)

A. A total of six (or more) items from (1), (2), and (3), with two from (1), and at least one each from (2) and (3).

1. Qualitative impairment in social interaction, manifest by at least two of the following:
   - Marked impairment in the use of multiple nonverbal behaviors, such as eye-to-eye gaze, facial expression, body postures, and gestures, to regulate social interaction
   - Failure to develop peer relationships appropriate to developmental level
   - Lack of spontaneous seeking to share enjoyment, interests, or achievements with other people (e.g., by lack of showing, bringing, or pointing out objects of interest)
   - Lack of social or emotional reciprocity

2. Qualitative impairment in communication, as manifest by at least one of the following:
   - Delay in, or total lack of, the development of spoken language (not accompanied by an attempt to compensate through alternative modes of communication such as gesture or mime)
   - In individuals with adequate speech, marked impairment in the ability to initiate or sustain a conversation with others
   - Stereotyped and repetitive use of language, or idiosyncratic language
   - Lack of varied, spontaneous make-believe, or social imitative play appropriate to developmental level

3. Restrictive repetitive and stereotypic patterns of behavior, interests, and activities, as manifested by at least one of the following:
   - Encompassing preoccupation with one or more stereotyped and restricted patterns of interest that is abnormal either in intensity or focus
   - Apparently inflexible adherence to specific nonfunctional routines or rituals
   - Stereotyped and repetitive motor mannerisms (e.g., hand or finger flapping or twisting, or complex whole-body movements)
   - Persistent preoccupation with parts of objects

B. Delays or abnormal functioning in at least one of the following areas, with onset prior to age 3 years:
   1. Social interaction
   2. Language as used in social communication
   3. Symbolic or imaginative play

C. The disturbance is not better accounted for by Rett disorder or childhood disintegrative disorder.

   The other pervasive developmental disorders include Asperger disorder, Rett syndrome, childhood disintegrative disorder, pervasive developmental disorder-not otherwise specified (PDD NOS), or atypical autism.

Reprinted from the *Diagnostic and Statistical Manual of Mental Disorders.* 4th ed. Washington, DC: American Psychiatric Association, 1994:70–71, with permission.

Despite multiple etiologies of autistic spectrum disorder, a specific cause is not identified in up to 90% of patients (17). Underlying diagnoses include phenylketonuria, congenital infections (rubella, cytomegalovirus), tuberous sclerosis, and Fragile X and Rett syndromes. Early onset of epilepsy, particularly infantile spasms, predicts a high risk for autistic spectrum disorder (21). Functional abnormalities in cerebellar, cortical, and basal ganglia have been suggested. Electroencephalographic (EEG) abnormalities are present in 27% to 65% of individuals; prolonged recordings commonly demonstrate paroxysmal epileptiform activity (22,23). Correlation of EEG abnormalities and clinical seizures is not absolute, even in patients with apparent language arrest, verbal auditory agnosia, and autistic regression associated with Landau–Kleffner syndrome (24–26). Whether ongoing seizures contribute to autistic regression remains controversial (27). Approximately 70% to 75% of persons with autism have IQ scores below 70 and thus are classified as mentally retarded; 25% to 35% develop some form of epilepsy, with seizures more likely in individuals with low IQs. Hyperactivity, impulsivity, short attention span, oversensitivity to sound and touch, various preoccupations, and self-stimulatory behaviors are common. Difficulties with transition, along with obsessions and compulsions, frequently need specific treatments. The diagnostic evaluation of the patient with suspected autism requires detailed history taking and developmental screening, along with observation. The American Academy of Neurology evidence-based guidelines suggest extensive use of checklists for autism in toddlers, screening questionnaires, audiologic testing, and screening for lead exposure. Specific genetic and metabolic tests, and screening for other toxins or infections may be indicated. Electroencephalography may be performed if epilepsy is suspected. Brain imaging studies, although rarely helpful, may be ordered in specific cases. Psychological, developmental, and speech and language assessments, along with educational testing, are critical (16).

Treatment of the autistic individual comprises behavioral approaches, education, and cognitive and language training. Early interventions may be critical. Medications that affect serotonergic and dopaminergic systems have been used, along with specific agents for abnormal behaviors or seizures. Classic and atypical neuroleptic drugs, together with selective serotonin uptake inhibitors (SSRIs), are advantageous in individual patients (18). Newer members of these classes appear not to reduce seizure threshold with fewer deleterious effects. Medications for hyperactivity and inattention may also ameliorate stereotypic behaviors. Stimulants and atomoxetine rarely exacerbate seizures; however, high doses of bupropion may aggravate epilepsy or induce new-onset seizures. The use of anticonvulsants to control behavioral outbursts and affective dysregulation has gained in popularity. The clinician who treats autistic individuals with epilepsy must be aware of the medications that can afford symptomatic relief of maladaptive behavior and consider drug interactions and toxic reactions, as well as possible decreases or exacerbations of seizures either directly or indirectly through altered sleep–wake patterns.

LANDAU–KLEFFNER SYNDROME

Landau and Kleffner first described the syndrome of acquired aphasia in childhood associated with a convulsive disorder (28), in which a previously normal child, usually male, between the ages of 3 and 7 years, deteriorates and almost seems unable to hear because of verbal auditory agnosia that may progress to mutism. Except for the language impairment, these children are intellectually normal but exhibit behavioral disturbances such as hyperactivity, attention deficit, and, rarely, psychosis. Many clinical variants have been noted, but Landau–Kleffner syndrome should be distinguished from autistic regression and disintegrative epileptiform disorder (Table 36.3) (29). Seizures occur in approximately 75% of patients before or after onset of aphasia. The EEG recording consists of a variety of nonspecific generalized and focal abnormalities that increase during sleep, progressing to continuous spike-and-wave rhythms during slow-wave sleep. Treatment includes traditional AEDs, steroids or corticotropin, immunoglobulins, and calcium-channel blockers; multiple subpial transactions may be performed. The outcome is generally poor for language recovery and normalization of behavior but seizures generally are controlled. Continuous spike-and-wave rhythms in slow-wave sleep portend a less favorable outcome (30,31).

TABLE 36.3

COMPARISON OF LANDAU–KLEFFNER SYNDROME, AUTISTIC EPILEPTIFORM REGRESSION, AND DISINTEGRATIVE EPILEPTIFORM DISORDER

	Aphasia	Social	Cognitive	Abnormal electroencephalogram	Prior normal development
Acquired epileptiform aphasia (Landau–Kleffner syndrome)	Yes	No	No	Yes	Yes
Autistic regression	Yes	Yes	No	No	Yes or no
Autistic epileptiform regression	Yes	Yes	No	Yes	Yes or no
Disintegrative disorder	Yes	Yes	Yes	No	Yes until age 2 years
Disintegrative epileptiform disorder	Yes	Yes	Yes	Yes	Yes until age 2 years

Adapted from Nass R, Gross A. Landau–Kleffner syndrome and its variants. In: Devinsky E, Westbrook LE, eds. *Epilepsy and Developmental Disabilities.* Boston: Butterworth-Heinemann; 2002:79–92, with permission.

DIAGNOSTIC EVALUATION

If the patient with multiple handicaps is not young and the epilepsy is not of recent onset, the diagnostic evaluation is challenging. These patients present with numerous disabilities, multiple but poorly described, refractory seizures, and frequent bouts of status epilepticus. Lifelong AED use, including polytherapy, may produce a tolerance to side effects. Documentation to help identify the interactions of all factors often is inadequate, and the ictal events are rarely witnessed. Stereotypic behaviors are frequently misinterpreted as seizures, and periods of inattention or short-lived motor activity are not recognized as ictal events or are not even noted. Reevaluation requires a chronologic approach to determine etiology, accurate diagnosis of the epilepsy syndrome, and insight into therapeutic success and failure. Observational records noting not only total number of seizures but their characteristics, length, and time of appearance, during both wakefulness and sleep, can be useful.

If diagnostic studies are not available for review, the EEG and magnetic resonance imaging (MRI) should be repeated. When indicated, expanded "newborn metabolic screens" and genetic testing for specific syndromes of epilepsy and developmental abnormalities should be considered, particularly in those with early onset seizures (32). The need for sedation in many of these individuals who cannot fully cooperate entails an additional risk, and the process of obtaining informed consent should include a frank explanation of risks and benefits given to the patient and legal guardian. Aberrant behavior and heavy sedation may limit the full diagnostic scope of prolonged EEG monitoring, including assessment of waking background activity; however, the actual recording of events may be impossible without the patient's cooperation or this type of record. A meticulous medical history and collaboration with caregivers may yield the most useful information about the patient during and after the ictal event. Interictal electroencephalographs and those performed as soon as possible after the presumptive seizure also may be helpful. Video recordings of events that occur at home, school, or elsewhere are extremely valuable, even without simultaneous electroencephalography.

THERAPY

The treatment of seizures in children and adults with developmental disability and multiple handicaps follows the same principles that govern therapy for other patients with epilepsy; however, frequent comorbidity, including both motor and intellectual deficits, is a complicating factor. Epilepsy in this population is most likely cryptogenic or symptomatic, rarely idiopathic. Refractory disease is common, and only a small percentage of these patients become seizure-free with or without AEDs (12,14,33–37). In addition to both partial and generalized seizures, status epilepticus and seizure clusters occur frequently. Along with long-term administration of AEDs for seizure control, plans for intermittent or acute emergent therapy for prolonged or clustered seizures, perhaps using rectally administered diazepam or other benzodiazepines (37,38), should be in place (38–40). Medical personnel and caregivers must devise guidelines for *intermittent* use of benzodiazepines to avoid inadvertent long-term administration and consequent decreased efficacy as rescue therapy.

The AED of choice depends on its efficacy against a specific seizure type balanced by tolerability and lack of adverse effects, including not exacerbating other seizure types (38). Figure 36.1 lists suggested medications for specific seizure types. Vagus nerve stimulation, ketogenic diet, and surgery should be considered when appropriate. Although most patients benefit from a reduction in drug dosage during treatment with the ketogenic diet, the interactions with drugs and metabolic effects of this nonpharmacologic method must be carefully monitored.

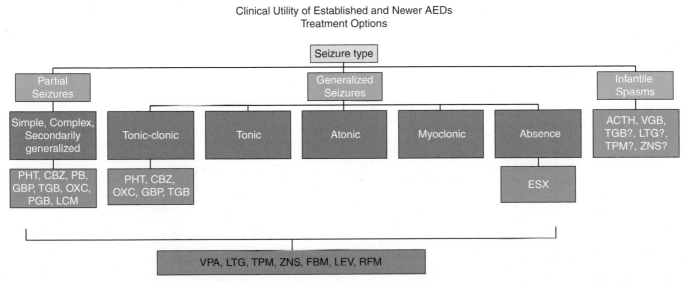

FIGURE 36.1 Treatment options for specific seizure types. ACTH, adrenocorticotrophic hormone; CBZ, carbamazepine; ESX, ethosuximide; FBM, felbamate; GBP, gabapentin; LCM, lacosemide; LTG, lamotrigine; LEV, levetiracetam; OXC, oxcarbazepine; PB, phenobarbital; PHT, phenytoin; PGB, pregabalin; RFM, rufinamide; TGB, tiagabine; TPM, topiramate; VGB, vigabatrin; VPA, valproic acid; ZNS, zonisamide.

Behavioral disturbances are particularly difficult to manage (41). In children and adults with autistic spectrum disorder, some medications that ameliorate behavior affect serotonin and dopamine, including atypical neuroleptics, stimulants, and related compounds that targeted hyperactive behavior, antidepressants, and antianxiety agents (18). Significant differences in their mechanisms of action make it difficult to explain why AEDs are efficacious in autistic spectrum disorders and other behavioral states (18). Mentally retarded individuals appear more likely than other patients to demonstrate aberrant behaviors, including significant aggressiveness, in response to a number of AEDs and psychotropic agents. Two trials in children with partial seizures demonstrate the interaction between previous behavioral states and side-effect profiles. One study of gabapentin as monotherapy for children with benign epilepsy with centrotemporal spikes reported a low incidence of behavioral side effects (38), whereas gabapentin as adjunctive therapy produced a much higher rate of negative behavior, especially in patients with mental retardation (42). Among AEDs introduced since 1990, felbamate, gabapentin, lamotrigine, topiramate, levetiracetam, oxcarbazepine, zonisamide, and vigabatrin have produced, at least in case reports, aberrant behavior in persons with behavioral comorbidity, including those with mental retardation (38). Even if comorbid conditions are not present, most AEDs can affect cognitive function and behavior, particularly with rapid titration or use of high doses (43). Careful titration and monotherapy are recommended whenever possible. Barbiturates and benzodiazepines classically have been associated with mental obtundation, depressive symptoms, and behavioral problems, but their discontinuation will sometimes aggravate negative behaviors (44,45). Increased acting out and belligerence may appear as part of the "brightening" process that can occur with conversion to newer, less sedative AEDs. Thus, changes in therapy should be made slowly with careful clinical monitoring (38).

Polytherapy should be avoided, or, if unavoidable, reduced (36,46–48), as an excessive drug burden complicates the assessment of efficacy and tolerability. In addition to behavioral and cognitive adverse effects, drug interactions can result in cumulative toxic reactions. Complicating the reduction in polypharmacy is the belief that any change in medication will exacerbate seizure frequency. Although this occasionally may occur in an individual patient, long-term studies suggest that polypharmacy can be reduced successfully, especially when a newer AED is substituted for a traditional medication (36,38,46–48). In one study of 244 mentally retarded patients with epilepsy who were followed up for 10 years, monotherapy could be increased in 36.5% to 58.1% with no evident loss of seizure control (36). Total discontinuation of AED therapy may be more difficult (14,34,36,37), however, involving a risk of seizure recurrence that ranges from 40% to 50% (14,36). Length of seizure freedom during AED therapy and degree of mental handicap are reasonable indicators of success (14). Identification of the epilepsy syndrome may also aid in predicting successful AED withdrawal.

Therapy for the multihandicapped individual comprises several components: physical, occupational, speech, language, educational, vocational, and psychological (49–51). Unwanted effects of therapy must also be considered. In addition to specific AEDs (46), other medications may exert a negative effect on seizures. Barbiturates and benzodiazepines have a long association with rebound or withdrawal seizures; stability may return when these drugs are replaced (37). High doses of antidepressants have been linked to increased incidences of seizures in clinical trials (52): bupropion 2.2%, clomipramine 1.66%, and maprotiline 15.6% (41). The seizure risk with SSRIs is lower, ranging from 0.04% to 0.3%. For patients with epilepsy, recommended antidepressants are SSRIs, antidepressants with multiple sites of action (e.g., nefazodone and venlafaxine), monoamine oxidase inhibitors, and tricyclic antidepressants (41,52). Psychostimulants and the new agent, atomoxetine, appear unlikely to exacerbate seizures, but the subject is controversial (53); use of these agents in the management of attentional disorders and hyperactivity is not contraindicated (41,53). Sometimes, reduction in dosage of an AED prescribed primarily for a behavior disorder, such as valproate or lamotrigine used to treat bipolar symptoms, will exacerbate seizures. The physician treating a patient with multiple handicaps must appreciate this potential unwanted effect.

Adverse effects extend beyond behavioral abnormalities and neurotoxic reactions. Bone health, contracture formation, weight regulation, gastrointestinal disturbances, gynecologic concerns, and drug interactions affect not only the treatment of epilepsy but also medications prescribed for other comorbidities (44,46). Many of these patients cannot properly express or describe their complaints. Increased irritability or changes in behavior may often be the only sign of significant abnormality in this group.

CONCLUSIONS

The treatment of the multihandicapped child or adult with epilepsy must be tailored to the individual patient. A careful assessment of all comorbid conditions must be part of the intake evaluation, which should include the natural history of the epilepsy and previous treatment. New-onset seizures or seizures that have changed in type or intensity warrant a complete evaluation. Frequently, the best indicator of a good response to an AED will be the past success. A medication may have been changed because of the hope for improved control of epilepsy or behavior with a newer AED. A return to tried-and-true therapy may be the best approach. The comorbid treatment and the epilepsy treatment will each affect the other. Similarly, management of comorbidities besides epilepsy will greatly improve the total outcome and quality of life. Understanding the difficulties in diagnosis and treatment of individuals with multiple handicaps and the inter-relationship between epilepsy and comorbidities and their treatments is essential.

References

1. American Association on Mental Retardation. *Mental Retardation: Definition, Classification and Systems of Support.* 10th ed. Annapolis Junction, MD: AAMR Publications; 2002.
2. American Psychiatric Association. *Diagnostic and Statistical Manual of Mental Disorders.* 4th ed. Washington, DC: American Psychiatric Association; 1994:70–71.
3. American Psychiatric Association. *Diagnostic and Statistical Manual of Mental Disorders.* 4th ed. text revision. Washington, DC: American Psychiatric Association; 2000.
4. Roeleveld N, Zielhuis GA, Gabreels F. The prevalence of mental retardation: a critical review of recent literature. *Dev Med Child Neurol.* 1997;39:125–132.

5. Weinstein B, Steedman JG, Miller G, et al. *Mental Retardation*. San Diego, CA: Medlink Neurology; 2004.

6. Kiely M. The prevalence of mental retardation. *Epidemiol Rev*. 1987;9: 194–228.

7. Miller G. Cerebral palsies. In: Miller G, Ramer JC, eds. *Static Encephalopathies of Infancy and Childhood*. New York: Raven Press; 1992:11–26.

8. Shinnar S, Pellock JM. Update on the epidemiology and prognosis of pediatric epilepsy. *J Child Neurol*. 2002;17(suppl 1):S4–S17.

9. Dodson WE. Epilepsy, cerebral palsy and IQ. In: Pellock JM, Dodson WE, Bourgeois BFD, eds. *Pediatric Epilepsy. Diagnosis and Therapy*. New York: Demos; 2002:613–627.

10. Shevell M, Aswal S, Donley D, et al. Practice parameter: evaluation of the child with global developmental delay. *Neurology*. 2003;60:367–380.

11. Badawi N, Watson L, Petterson B, et al. What constitutes cerebral palsy? *Dev Med Child Neurol*. 1998;40:847–851.

12. Camfield C, Camfield P, Watson L. Cerebral palsy in children with epilepsy. In: Devinsky O, Westbrooke LE, eds. *Epilepsy and Developmental Disabilities*. Boston: Butterworth-Heinemann; 2002:33–40.

13. Ashwal S, Russman BS, Blaseo PA, et al. Practice parameter: diagnostic assessment of the child with cerebral palsy. *Neurology*. 2004;62:851–863.

14. Camfield P, Camfield C. Initiating and discontinuing antiepileptic drugs in children with neurologic handicaps and epilepsy. In: Devinsky O, Westbrook LE, eds. *Epilepsy and Developmental Disabilities*. Boston: Butterworth-Heinemann; 2002:281–286.

15. Filipek PA, Accardo PJ, Baranek GT, et al. The screening and diagnosis of autistic spectrum disorders. *J Autism Dev Disord*. 1999;29:437–482.

16. Filipek PA, Accardo PJ, Ashwal S, et al. Practice parameter: screening and diagnosis of autism: report for the Quality Standards Subcommittee of the American Academy of Neurology and the Child Neurology Society. *Neurology*. 2000;55:468–479.

17. Spratt EG, Macias MM, Lee DO. *Autistic Spectrum Disorders*. San Diego, CA: Medlink Neurology; 2004.

18. Parlermo MT, Curatolo P. Pharmacologic treatment of autism. *J Child Neurol*. 2004;19:155–164.

19. Ehlers S, Gillberg C. The epidemiology of Asperger's syndrome: a total population study. *J Child Psychol Psychiatry*. 1993;34:1327–1350.

20. Baird G, Charman T, Baron-Cohen S, et al. A screening instrument for autism at 18 months of age: a 6-year follow-up study. *J Child Psychol Psychiatry*. 2000;39:694–702.

21. Saemundsen E. Ludviqsson P, Rafnsson V. Risk of autistic spectrum disorders after infantile spasms: a population based study nested in a cohort with seizures in the first year of life. *Epilepsia*. 2008;49:1865–1870.

22. Minshew N. Indices of neural function in autism: clinical and biologic implications. *Pediatrics*. 1991;87:774–780.

23. Yaylali I, Tuchman R, Jayakar P. Comparison of the utility of routine versus prolonged EEG recordings in children with language regression [abstract]. Presented at the American Clinical Neurophysiology Society Annual Meeting, Boston, MA, September, 1996.

24. Tuchman RF. Acquired epileptiform aphasia. *Semin Pediatr Neurol*. 1997;4:93–101.

25. Shinnar S, Rapin I, Arnold S, et al. Language regression in childhood. *Pediatr Neurol*. 2001;24:183–189.

26. Nass R, Devinsky O. Autistic regression with rolandic spikes. *Neuropsychiatry Neuropsychol Behav Neurol*. 1999;12:193–197.

27. Rapin I. Autism in search of a home in the brain. *Neurology*. 1999;52: 902–904.

28. Landau W. Landau–Kleffner syndrome. An eponymic badge of ignorance. *Arch Neurol*. 1992;49:353.

29. Nass R, Gross A. Landau–Kleffner syndrome and its variants. In: Devinsky E, Westbrook LE, eds. *Epilepsy and Developmental Disabilities*. Boston: Butterworth-Heinemann; 2002:79–92.

30. Nass R, Gross A, Wisoff J, et al. Outcome of multiple subpial transections for autistic epileptiform regression. *Pediatr Neurol*. 1999;21: 464–470.

31. Rossi PG, Parmeggiani A, Posar A, et al. Landau–Kleffner syndrome (LKS): long-term follow-up and links with electrical status epilepticus during sleep (ESES). *Brain Dev*. 1999;21:90–98.

32. Deprez L, Jansen A, DeJonghe P. Genetics of epilepsy syndromes starting in the first year of life. *Neurology*. 2009;72:273–281.

33. Bourgeois BFD. Controlling seizures in children with developmental disabilities: an overview. In: Devinsky E, Westbrook LE, eds. *Epilepsy and Developmental Disabilities*. Boston: Butterworth-Heinemann; 2002: 273–280.

34. Steffenburg U, Hedstrom A, Lindroth A, et al. Intractable epilepsy in a population-based series of mentally retarded children. *Epilepsia*. 1998;39: 767–775.

35. Aicardi J, Shorvon SD. Intractable epilepsy. In: Engel JJ, Pedley TA, eds. *Epilepsy: A Comprehensive Textbook*. Philadelphia: Lippincott-Raven; 1997:1325–1331.

36. Pellock JM, Hunt PA. A decade of modern epilepsy therapy in institutionalized mentally retarded patients. *Epilepsy Res*. 1996;25:263–268.

37. Mirza EU, Credeur LH, Penry JK. Results of antiepileptic drug reduction in patients with multiple handicaps and epilepsy. *Drug Invest*. 1993;5: 320–326.

38. Pellock JM, Morton LD. Treatment of epilepsy in the multiply handicapped. *Ment Retard Dev Disabil Res Rev*. 2000;6:309–323.

39. Dreifuss F, Rosman N, Cloyd J, et al. A comparison of rectal diazepam gel and placebo for acute repetitive seizures. *N Engl J Med* 1998;338: 1869–1875.

40. Pellock JM, Leszczyszyn DJ. Status epilepticus. In: Devinsky E, Westbrook LE, eds. *Epilepsy and Developmental Disabilities*. Boston: Butterworth-Heinemann; 2002:93–110.

41. Pellock JM. Understanding co-morbidities affecting children with epilepsy. *Neurology*. 2004;62(suppl 2):S17–S23.

42. Khurana DS, Riviello J, Helmers S, et al. Efficacy of gabapentin therapy in children with refractory seizures. *J Pediatr*. 1996;128:829–833.

43. Meador KJ. Cognitive outcomes and predictive factors in epilepsy. *Neurology*. 2002;58(suppl 5):S21–S26.

44. Brent DA, Crumrine PK, Varma RR, et al. Phenobarbital treatment and major depressive disorder in children with epilepsy. *Pediatrics*. 1987;80: 909–917.

45. Theodore WH, Porter RJ. Removal of sedative-hypnotic antiepileptic drugs from the regimen of patients with intractable epilepsy. *Ann Neurol*. 1983;13:320–324.

46. Perucca E, Beghi E, Dulac O, et al. Assessing risk to benefit ratio in antiepileptic drug therapy. *Epilepsy Res*. 2000;41:107–139.

47. Schmidt D. Reduction of two-drug therapy in intractable epilepsy. *Epilepsia*. 1983;24:368–376.

48. Albright P, Bruni J. Reduction of polytherapy in epileptic patients. *Arch Neurol*. 1985;42:797–799.

49. Michaud LJ, American Academy of Pediatrics Committee on Children With Disabilities. Prescribing therapy services for children with motor disabilities. *Pediatrics*. 2004;113:1836–1838.

50. Tara HL, American Academy of Pediatrics Committee on School Health. School-based mental health services. *Pediatrics*. 2004;113: 1839–1845.

51. Devinsky O, Westbrook LE, eds. *Epilepsy and Developmental Disabilities*. Boston: Butterworth-Heinemann; 2002.

52. Harden CL, Goldstein MA. Mood disorders in patients with epilepsy: epidemiology and management. *CNS Drugs*. 2002;16:291–302.

53. Feldman H, Crumrine P, Handen BL, et al. Methylphenidate in children with seizures and attention-deficit disorder. *Am J Dis Child*. 1989;143: 1081–1086.

CHAPTER 37 ■ EPILEPSY IN THE ELDERLY

ILO E. LEPPIK AND ANGELA K. BIRNBAUM

The elderly, often defined as those 65 years or older, are the most rapidly growing segment of the US population; and demographic trends project that their numbers will increase from an estimated 40 million in 2010 to 71.5 million in 2030 (1). Notably, the incidence (new cases) of epilepsy is significantly higher in this population than in any other (2,3). In 1995 alone, approximately 181,000 US persons developed epilepsy, 68,000 of whom were over age 65 (4). High rates of epilepsy in the elderly have also been reported from the Netherlands and Finland (5,6). Thus, due to the projected increase in the number of elderly persons, as well as their propensity to develop epilepsy, these individuals will represent an increasingly large group of patients needing expert care pertaining to this disorder.

DEFINITION OF EPILEPSY AND SEIZURES

Currently, there is a debate within the medical community regarding the precise definition of epilepsy (7). Until recently, it has been accepted that persons should not be diagnosed with epilepsy until an individual experienced two or more seizures. However, in light of current diagnostic tools, brain pathologies can be more readily identified. Epidemiologic studies have shown that persons with certain conditions, such as stroke or brain tumor, have a high probability of experiencing additional seizures after an initial ictal event. Therefore, it has been proposed that epilepsy be defined as a condition of the central nervous system (CNS) predisposed to recurrent seizures (8). Thus, the occurrence of a single seizure associated with a specific pathology may be considered sufficient to initiate treatment to prevent future seizures. This is of particular importance to the geriatrician due to the fact that many persons within this age group suffering from seizures possess an identifiable brain pathology that corresponds with a known risk for future seizures.

CAUSES

Within the elderly population, the most common identifiable cause of epileptic seizures is a previous stroke, which accounts for 30% to 40% of all epileptic seizure cases (2). In a prospective study of 1897 patients suffering from stroke, seizures occurred in 168 (8.9%) persons during a 9-month follow-up period (9). Of the 265 persons within the study who suffered a hemorrhagic stroke, 28 (10.6%) suffered a seizure. Of the 1632 persons within the study who suffered an ischemic stoke, 140 (8.6%) suffered a seizure (9). Thus, those who suffered a hemorrhagic stroke had an increased risk for a seizure

as compared to those who suffered an ischemic stroke. During the 9 months of follow-up in this study, epilepsy, as defined by the onset of a second seizure, occurred in 47 out of 1897 (2.5%) persons. A longer observation period might have detected a higher rate. Some retrospective studies have indicated that the eventual risk of experiencing seizures after suffering a stroke may be as high as 20% (10). It has been estimated that each year more than 730,000 US persons suffer from stroke. Accordingly, the incidence of seizures after stroke may exceed 36,000 cases per year (10).

Of particular note is the fact that a transient ischemic attack (TIA) will sometimes lead to simple partial seizures whose pattern is similar to the deficit of the TIA. This may create confusion and concern that another TIA is occurring. The key differential feature, however, is that simple partial seizures rarely last more than a few minutes, whereas TIAs last much longer.

Brain tumor, head injury, and Alzheimer's disease are other major causes of epilepsy in the elderly. It is suspected that those persons with Alzheimer's disease who experience brief periods of increased confusion may be having unrecognized partial complex seizures. Most problematic, though, is that in a large number of cases the precise cause cannot be determined and the etiology is termed cryptogenic (crypt = hidden; genic = cause).

DIAGNOSIS

The diagnosis of epilepsy is difficult in the elderly. In the Veteran's Affairs (VA) Cooperative Study #428, a large portion of subjects with epilepsy had been initially misdiagnosed (11). Because most seizures in the elderly are caused by a focal area of damage to the brain, the most common seizure types are localization related. Complex partial seizures are the most common seizure type, accounting for nearly 40% of all seizures in the elderly population (12). Both simple and complex may spread and develop into generalized tonic–clonic seizures.

When diagnosing epilepsy, a clear distinction must be made between epileptic seizures—those arising from brain pathology—and nonepileptic seizures—those arising within a normal brain due to an alteration in physiology, such as hypoxia. Therefore, it is necessary that other causes of seizure activity, such as cardiac insufficiency, metabolic conditions, convulsive syncope (micturation syncope, cough syncope), be eliminated as possible effectors before it can be concluded that the ictal event was an epileptic seizure.

Evaluation after a single seizure must therefore be comprehensive. A thorough history must be obtained, focusing on events of the previous day or days, in order to identify any precipitating or predisposing factors that may have led to the onset. Because epileptic seizures are usually unprovoked, an electrocardiogram (EKG) should be utilized in order to rule out possible cardiac conditions. Also, laboratory tests for metabolic disorders should be done, as well as a review of prescription drugs, over-the-counter agents, and natural products being used by the patient. Specifically, it should be noted that many natural products designed to simulate weight loss or improve memory may have proconvulsant properties. Further, withdrawal from CNS depressants such as benzodiazepines or alcohol provoke seizures and stimulants such as methamphetamine and cocaine may cause convulsions. Unfortunately, abuse of drugs is not absent in the elderly, and a drug screen should be considered.

CT and MRI

The use of cortical imaging studies is highly predictive of seizures (13). Thus, structural studies, such as computed tomography (CT) that screen for intracerebral hemorrhage, brain tumor, and encephalomalacia, should be performed.

CT scans serve as an appropriate imaging tool for the initial emergency study. Because of its X-ray modality, it is capable of detecting tissue contrasts; therefore, it is effective in locating blood, areas of encephalomalacia, and calcified lesions. CT, however, is often unable to appropriately visualize glial tumors or any small changes that may be occurring within the hippocampus. Detection of these lesions require magnetic resonance imaging (MRI), which is more appropriate for noticing subtle changes in brain tissue and should be requested if an obvious pathology is not detected by the initial CT scan.

Electroencephalogram

Electroencephalograms (EEGs) serve many useful roles in the diagnosis of epilepsy. Detection of interictal patterns can confirm the presence of physiologically abnormal brain, solidifying the diagnosis of an epileptic as opposed to a nonepileptic seizure; additionally, these patterns can also provide information on the severity of the epilepsy. Further, EEGs are also able to identify the epileptogenic region, providing additional clues to the etiology of the patient's disorder. Persons who experience periodic lateralized epileptiform discharges (PLEDs) after a stroke are also prone to develop seizures; and, those with focal spikes have a 78% risk (14). It is recommended that an EKG rhythm strip be obtained during an EEG in order to help identify artifacts and to provide additional evidence to exclude a cardiac cause for the seizure.

COMPLEX ISSUES

Problems faced by the elderly suffering from epilepsy are different and more complex than those faced by younger adults also suffering from the same disorder. These problems involve medical complexities—for example, correct diagnoses, selection of the most appropriate medication(s), and presence of comorbid illnesses—as well as other societal factors such as emotional stability and economic responsibilities.

FALLS, FRACTURES, AND BONE HEALTH

The presence of epilepsy increases the risk for falls and fractures by two- to sixfold. Osteoporosis and bone fractures are commonly seen in the elderly population and thus an elderly person with epilepsy is at increased risk. Lack of exercise, inadequate nutrition, impairment of mobility, and neurological conditions leading to poor balance and protective reflexes may all play a role. Large prospective studies in women and men have associated use of both phenytoin and gabapentin with decreased bone mineral density (15,16). The fact that nonenzyme-inducing antiepileptic drugs (AEDs) such as gabapentin and valproate both affect bone mineral density while carbamazepine, a strong inducer, does not, brings into question the commonly held belief that the influence of AEDs on bone health is only through vitamin D metabolism. However, vitamin D supplementation is recommended for all elderly, with or without epilepsy. Not well studied is the possible influence of AED toxicity (ataxia, neuropathy, nystagmus, sedation) on falls. Because the elderly are more sensitive to AED side effects, care should be taken to avoid AED concentrations in the higher range effective for younger adults, and levels below the usually effective range may be appropriate.

THE ELDERLY ARE NOT A HOMOGENEOUS POPULATION

Like the pediatric population, the elderly does not represent a single cohort. Thus, broad statements about these persons may not be relevant to each individual patient. Just as medical issues involving persons up to 18 years of age cannot be properly interpreted without using *newborn*, *infant*, *child*, and *adolescent* subcategories, elderly persons should also be subdivided into appropriate cohorts. A widely used system divides this group into the *young-old* (65 to 74 years of age), the *middle-old* or *old* (75 to 84 years of age), and the *old-old* (≥85 years of age). However, because these persons develop health issues at different times, further subdivisions, such as the elderly healthy who have epilepsy (EH), the elderly with multiple medical problems (EMMP), and the frail elderly (FE), those usually found residing in nursing homes (NHs), have also been proposed (Table 37.1) (17).

Adding to the complexity are the major differences between the community-dwelling elderly, those living independently, and the elderly residing within NHs. Drug side effects,

TABLE 37.1

CATEGORIZATION OF ELDERLY WITH EPILEPSY

Young-old healthy EH	Middle-old healthy EH	Old-old healthy EH
Young-old multiple medical problems EMMP	Middle-old multiple medical problems EMMP	Old-old multiple medical problems EMMP
Young-old frail FE	Middle-old frail FE	Old-old frail FE

Modified from Leppik IE. Introduction to the International Geriatric Epilepsy Symposium (IGES). *Epilepsy Res.* 2006;68(suppl 1):S1–S4.

efficacy, absorption, and other factors may be markedly different between a 93-year-old healthy person living independently and a 68-year-old frail person residing in an NH. Also, issues regarding health care delivery will likely differ between the community-dwelling elderly and those residing within an NH. Thus, studies should be designed to address specific populations, and reports should specify the populations studied (18).

Also seen as significantly problematic is the selection of an appropriate AED, which requires the consideration of many factors. Such factors include: changes in organ function, increased susceptibility to adverse effects, use of other medications known to interact with AEDs, and economic limitations associated with the respective patient. Further, pharmaceutical treatment within the elderly carries greater risks than in younger persons. In addition to their use in epilepsy, AEDs are prescribed for a variety of other disorders affecting the elderly, including pain and psychiatric disorders. AEDs rank fifth among all drug categories in their capacity to illicit adverse reactions (19). Yet, very little research has been done within this vulnerable population and only general recommendations can be made at this time.

AED Use in Community-Dwelling Elderly

The largest study of AED use in US community-dwelling elderly was coordinated by Berlowitz (20,21). This study's cohort identified 1,130,155 veterans ≥65 years of age from the VA national database between 1997 and 1999. Of these persons, 20,558 (1.8%) were identified as having epilepsy by exhibiting an ICD-9-CM representative of this condition. Approximately 80% of the studied persons were receiving one AED, whereas 20% were being treated with two or more. Phenytoin was used as monotherapy by almost 70% of the cohort, whereas phenobarbital was used as monotherapy by approximately 10%. Another 5% were using phenobarbital in combination with phenytoin, though not exclusively. Carbamazepine was used by just more than 10% and newer AEDs (gabapentin and lamotrigine) were used by less than 10% (21). Levetiracetam was not available at the time of the survey. Smaller studies of AED use in community-dwelling non-VA elderly patients have shown similar distributions of AED use, with phenytoin as, by far, the most widely used AED in the United States by this population. These studies done almost a decade ago from this writing may not reflect current practice.

Pharmacoepidemiology of AED Use in Nursing Homes

As people age, their need for NH care increases due to greater frailty and the likely onset of age-related diseases. For patients ≥65 years of age, there is a lifetime risk of 43% to 46% of becoming an NH resident (22). Accordingly, at any one time 4.5% of the US elderly population resides within an NH (23).

In any research concerning NHs, it is necessary to make distinctions between *residents* and *admissions*. A *resident* cohort includes all residents in the facility at a specified time, and usually represents a cross-sectional sample that consists of a mixture of newly admitted residents and those who have

been in the NH for different periods of time. In contrast, an *admission* cohort includes all people admitted to a facility during a specified time period (24).

In a study of US NH *residents* residing within various facilities during the spring of 1995 (24), the mean age of the 21,551 studied persons was 83.78 years of age (SD = 8.13 years). The sample had the following age group distribution: *young-old* 15%, *middle-old* or *old* 36%, and *old-old* 49%. This distribution is similar to the data provided by the U.S. Census Bureau which, in 2000, noted the admittance of 1,555,800 persons to NH facilities (23). Of the residents in the Garrard et al. NH sample, 10.5% had one or more AED orders on the day of study and 9.2% had a seizure indication (epilepsy or seizure disorder) documented in their chart. Phenytoin was used by 6.2% of the residents, followed by carbamazepine (1.8%), phenobarbital (1.7%), clonazepam (1.2%), valproic acid (VPA; 0.9%), and all other AEDs combined (1.2%). These percentages exceed 10.5% due to AED polytherapy. If these results are extrapolated to all 1,557,800 US elderly NH residents in 2000 (23), then as many as 163,569 people were likely to have been receiving at least one AED. In the Garrard et al. study, age was inversely related to AED use. Of the *young-old* cohort, 23.7% were prescribed an AED—16.4% for seizure indication and 7.3% for other. Of the *middle-old* or *old*, 12.2% were prescribed an AED—8.3% for seizure indication and 3.9% for other. However, of the *old-old* cohort only, 5.8% were prescribed an AED—3.7% for seizure indication and 2.1% for other. Notably, this finding was unexpected due to the upward curve in the incidence of epilepsy/seizure disorder as it relates to advancing age in the community-dwelling elderly. Thus, one of the major findings concerning AED use in US NHs is that the *young-old* are three to four times more likely to be prescribed an AED than the *old-old*, either prior to or after admission. A similar pattern was reported from a study in Italy (25).

In a study of NH *admissions* using a longitudinal design to explore AED use at the time of admission, two study groups were used: the first representing all persons aged ≥65 years admitted between January 1 and March 31, 1999 to one of the 510 Beverly Enterprises NH facilities in 31 US states (N = 10,318); while the second represented a follow-up cohort (n = 9516) of those in the admissions group who were not using an AED at the time of NH admission (24). The cohort not receiving AEDs at the time of admission was followed for 3 months or until NH discharge—whichever occurred first—after their initial admission date. Approximately 8% (n = 802) of the admissions group used one or more AEDs at entry, and among these, greater than half (58%) had an epilepsy/seizure disorder indication. The AEDs used by newly admitted individuals with an epilepsy/seizure disorder (n = 585) included phenytoin (n = 315; 54%), VPA (n = 57; 10%), carbamazepine (n = 52; 9%), and gabapentin (n = 27; 5%).

Among the 9516 residents within the follow-up cohort of the Garrard et al. study who were not using an AED at admission, 260 (3%) were started on an AED within 3 months of admission. Factors associated with the initiation of AEDs during this period included epilepsy/seizure, manic depression (bipolar disease), age group, cognitive performance (minimum data set cognition scale [MDS-COGS]), and peripheral vascular disease (PVD). Thus, many persons admitted without a diagnosis of epilepsy were diagnosed as such after entry, and the incidence of newly diagnosed epilepsy after admission to

TABLE 37.2

FREQUENCY OF USE OF COMEDICATIONS WITH
POTENTIAL PHARMACOKINETIC OR PHARMACODY-
NAMIC INTERACTIONS WITH ANTIEPILEPTIC
DRUGS IN 4,291 NURSING HOME RESIDENTS

Drug category	% use with AEDs
Antidepressants	18.9
Antipsychotics	12.7
Benzodiazepams	22.4
Thyroid supplements	14.0
Antacids	8.0
Calcium Channel Blockers	6.9
Warfarin	5.9
Cimetidine	2.5

From Lackner TE, Cloyd JC, Thomas LW, et al. Antiepileptic drug use
in nursing home residents: effect of age, gender, and comedication on
patterns of use. *Epilepsia.* 1998;39(10):1083–1087.

the NH far exceeds numbers relevant to other age group populations. A crude estimate would be 600/100,000 per 3 months,
or four to six times that reported for community-dwelling
elderly. AEDs used by those in the cohort that had AEDs
started after admission and who had an epilepsy/seizure indication were: phenytoin 48%, gabapentin 13%, carbamazepine
12%, VPA 8%, phenobarbital 7%, and other 12%. There was
also an inverse relationship between age group and initiation
of an AED. Compared to the *young-old*, those in the *middle-
old* or *old* age group were 33% less likely to have been prescribed an AED, whereas the *old-old* were 50% less likely to
have been prescribed an AED (24).

Another issue is that many elderly persons are taking other
potentially interfering drugs (Table 37.2). In addition to
AEDs, the average elderly NH patient takes six medications
concomitantly, greatly increasing the risk for side effects and
drug–drug interactions (26).

CLINICAL PHARMACOLOGY OF AEDs IN THE ELDERLY

The theoretical basis for expecting age-related changes in drug
pharmacokinetics were described many years ago but have not
been widely applied to AEDs. Drug concentration at the site
of action determines the magnitude of both desired and toxic
responses. The unbound drug concentration in serum is in
direct equilibrium with the concentration at the site of action
and provides the best correlation to drug response (27). Total
serum drug concentration is useful for monitoring therapy
when the drug is not highly protein-bound (less than 75%), or
when the ratio of unbound to total drug concentration
remains relatively stable. Three of the major AEDs (VPA,
phenytoin, and carbamazepine, respectively) are highly protein-bound, and protein binding is frequently altered.

Age-related physiologic changes that appear to have the
greatest effect on AED pharmacokinetics involve protein binding and a reduction in liver volume and blood flow (28–30).
Reduced serum albumin and increased AAG (1-acid glycoprotein) concentrations in the elderly may alter protein binding

of some drugs (27–29). By age 65, many individuals have low
normal albumin concentrations or are considered hypoalbu-
minemic. Albumin concentration may be further reduced by
conditions such as malnutrition, renal insufficiency, and
rheumatoid arthritis. The concentration of AAG, a reactant
serum protein, increases with age, and further elevations occur
during pathophysiologic stress, such as stroke, heart failure,
trauma, infection, myocardial infarction, surgery, and chronic
obstructive pulmonary disease (29).

Administration of enzyme-inducing AEDs also increases
AAG (31). When the concentration of AAG rises, the binding
of weakly alkaline and neutral drugs such as carbamazepine
to AAG can increase, causing higher total serum drug concentrations and decreased unbound drug concentrations. Because
of the complexity of confounding variables and the lack of
correlation between simple measures of liver function and
drug metabolism, the effect of age on hepatic drug metabolism
remains largely unknown (32,33). Interestingly, genetic determinants of hepatic isoenzymes may be more important than
age in determining a person's clearance (34).

Renal clearance is the major route of elimination for a
number of newer AEDs. It is well known that an elderly person's renal capacity decreases by approximately 10% per
decade (35). However, there exists a substantial amount of
individual variability because clearance is also highly dependent upon the patient's general state of health (36).

Despite the theoretical effects of age-related physiologic
changes on drug disposition and the widespread use of AEDs
in the elderly, few studies on AED pharmacokinetics in the
elderly have been published. The available reports generally
involve single-dose evaluations in small samples of the *young-
old*. Also, there is a lack of data regarding AED pharmacokinetics in the *oldest-old*, those individuals who may be at greatest risk for therapeutic failure and adverse reactions.

VARIABILITY OF AED LEVELS IN NURSING HOMES

Studies have shown that in compliant young patients, the variability of AED concentrations over time is relatively small.
One study showed that in institutionalized younger adults, the
variability between serial phenytoin measurements over time
was on the order of 10%. Within the same study, compliant clinic
patients experienced variability of approximately 20% (37).
Approximately 5% to 10% of this variability may be due to
interlaboratory variability in measurement of drug concentrations, although laboratories not following rigid quality control
standards may experience even larger amounts of variability.
The remainder of noted variability could arise from day-to-day
alterations in absorption, metabolism, or differences in AED
dose content. The variability for carbamazepine is on the
order of 25%, possibly due to its shorter half-life, which may
increase sample time variability (38).

A small study found that phenytoin levels may fluctuate in
the NH elderly (39). This was confirmed in an analysis of serial phenytoin levels from NH patients across the United States
who had experienced no change in dose, formulation, or medication (40). Some patients experienced a difference in concentration of two- to threefold from the lowest to the highest
level. Interestingly, some had very little fluctuation and were
similar to that of the younger adults previously mentioned.

Similar but less severe fluctuations were also observed for carbamazepine and VPA (41a, 41). These findings suggest that *elderly frail* NH residents may experience a greater variability in absorption of drugs. Factors that contribute to this variability in concentration must be identified and strategies should be developed in order to minimize this phenomenon.

CLINICAL TRIALS OF AEDs IN THE ELDERLY

All major AEDs have an FDA indication for use for the seizure types most likely to be encountered in the elderly. However, there is little data relating specifically to these drugs in the elderly, and those that are available have been limited to the community-dwelling elderly. An analysis from the VA cooperative study of carbamazepine and valproate found that elderly patients often had seizure control associated with lower AED levels than those seen in younger subjects. Notably, these elderly patients also experienced side effects at lower levels compared with the levels in younger subjects (42).

A multicenter, double-blind, randomized comparison between lamotrigine and carbamazepine in newly diagnosed epileptic elderly patients (mean = 77 years of age) in the United Kingdom showed that the main difference between the two groups was the rate of dropout due to adverse events, with lamotrigine incurring an 18% dropout rate compared to that of carbamazepine which incurred a 42% dropout rate (43). The VA Cooperative Study #428, an 18-center, parallel, double-blind trial on the use of gabapentin, lamotrigine, and carbamazepine, in patients ≥60 years of age found that drug efficacy did not differ, but the main finding favoring the two newer AEDs was better tolerability than carbamazepine (11).

CHOOSING AEDs FOR THE ELDERLY

At the present time, there is little data regarding the clinical use of AEDs in the elderly. The paucity of information makes it very difficult to recommend specific AEDs with any confidence that outcomes will be optimal. A drug that is optimal for the EH group may not be appropriate for the EMMP or FE groups due to the differences in pharmacokinetic or pharmacodynamic properties in these populations.

To date, phenytoin is still the most commonly used AED in both the community-dwelling and NH elderly within the United States, although expert opinion may disagree with this practice (21). In the following sections, discussion is based first on the most commonly used AEDs for which there is more data, and is then followed by an alphabetical review of newer AEDs. Table 37.3 provides a summary of the properties of most AEDs.

Phenytoin

Phenytoin is effective for localization-related epilepsies, and thus has an efficacy profile appropriate for the elderly. Evidence for this can be gathered from a VA cooperative study, which included elderly patients, that found phenytoin to be as effective as carbamazepine, phenobarbital, and primidone and that phenytoin and carbamazepine were better tolerated (44). Phenytoin has a narrow therapeutic range, is approximately 90% bound to serum albumin, and undergoes saturable metabolism, which has the effect of producing nonlinear changes in serum concentrations when the dose is changed or absorption is altered. Clinical studies in elderly patients have shown decreases in phenytoin binding to albumin and increases in free fraction. The binding of phenytoin to serum proteins correlates with the albumin concentration, which is typically low normal to subnormal in the elderly. One study compared the pharmacokinetics of phenytoin at steady state after oral administration in 34 elderly (60 to 79 years of age) persons, 32 middle-aged (40 to 59 years of age) persons, and 26 younger adult (20 to 39 years of age) persons with epilepsy (45). All subjects had normal albumin concentrations and liver function, and received no other medications, including other AEDs known to alter hepatic metabolism. The maximum rate of metabolism (V_{max}) declined with age, and significantly lower values of V_{max} were seen in the elderly group compared to the younger adults (45). Other earlier and smaller studies have also shown that phenytoin metabolism is reduced in the elderly. Therefore, lower maintenance doses of phenytoin may be needed to attain desired unbound serum concentrations. Relatively small changes in dose (<10%) are recommended when making dosing adjustments. Thus, in the elderly a starting daily dose of 3 mg/kg appears to be appropriate, rather than the 5 mg/kg/day used in younger adults (46). A study using stable labeled (nonradioactive) phenytoin to precisely measure half-life showed that the half-life in healthy elderly was similar to that of younger adults (34). NH studies revealed that residents were taking daily phenytoin doses lower than younger adults when measured by mg/day, but the doses expressed as mg/kg/day were similar to those used in younger adults (41). These data suggest that metabolism may not decrease greatly with age and that use of lower doses in the NH elderly may reflect age-related changes to the therapeutic or toxic effects with advancing age. A 3 mg/kg dose is only 160 mg/day for a 52-kg woman or 200 mg/day for a 66-kg man. A gender effect was found in the NH population as women required higher doses of PHT than men to achieve similar serum concentrations (41).

Due to the high protein binding of phenytoin, unbound phenytoin concentrations may be a better indicator of efficacy and toxicity than total concentrations. Measurement of unbound phenytoin concentrations is essential for elderly patients who have: (i) decreased serum albumin concentration; (ii) total phenytoin concentrations that are near the upper boundary of the therapeutic range; (iii) total concentrations that decline over time; (iv) a low total concentration relative to the daily dose; or (v) total concentrations that do not correlate with clinical response. A range of 5 mg/L to 15 mg/L total may be more appropriate as a therapeutic range for the elderly (46).

Phenytoin has many drug–drug interactions and should be used cautiously in EMMP patients receiving other medications. VPA, which is also highly protein bound, competes with phenytoin for albumin-binding sites and inhibits phenytoin's metabolism. Carbamazepine induces phenytoin metabolism and necessitates higher phenytoin doses. There is also some indication that serotonin selective reuptake inhibitor (SSRI) antidepressants may inhibit the cytochrome 2C family of

TABLE 37.3

AED PHARMACOKINETICS IN THE ELDERLY

Drug	Protein binding	Elimination	Comments
Carbamazepine	75–85%	Hepatic CYP 3A4/5	Causes hyponatremia
			Levels increased by erythromycin, propoxyphene and grapefruit juice
			Decreases levels of calcium channel blockers (dilitiazem, verapamil)
			Decreases effect of warfarin
			Decreases tricyclic antidepressant levels
Felbamate	<10%	Hepatic	
Gabapentin	<10%	Renal	Elimination correlates with creatinine clearance
			No drug interactions
Lamotrigine	55%	hepatic-glucuronide conjugation	Levels decreased by inducing agents—carbamazepine, phenytoin, some hormones, and others yet to be determined
			Levels increased by valproate
Levetiracetam	<10%	Renal	Very water soluble, IV formulation available
			No drug interactions
Oxcarbazepine	40%	Hepatic	Causes hyponatremia
Phenobarbital	50%	Hepatic renal	Induces metabolism of many drugs
Phenytoin	80–93%	Hepatic CYP 2C9 CYP 2C19	Protein binding decreased with reduced serum albumin and renal failure
			Decreases levels of calcium-channel blockers (dilitiazem, verapamil)
			Complicated interaction with warfarin
			Decreases tricyclic antidepressant levels
			Interacts with diabetes and arthritis medications
			Decreases effectiveness of cancer chemotherapy
Topiramate	9–17%	Hepatic and renal	Inhibits CYP 2C19 and increase serum
			Phenytoin and other drug levels
			Induces CYP-3A4 isoenzymes
Valproic acid	87–95%	Hepatic multiple pathways	Protein binding decreased in elderly
			Inhibits glucuronidation and may increase levels of lamotrigine and other drugs
			Decreases platelet function
Zonisamide	40%	Hepatic CYP 3A4	Weight loss and nephrolithiasis are issues

P450 enzymes responsible for metabolizing phenytoin (47). Fluoxetine and norfluoxetine are more potent inhibitors of this enzyme, followed by sertraline and paroxetine. The latter two serotonin selective reuptake inhibitor (SSRI) antidepressants may prove to be a safer choice in the elderly. Coumadin also has a very complicated interaction with phenytoin and often doses of both need to be manipulated (46).

Phenytoin has some effects on cognitive functioning, especially at higher phenytoin serum concentrations (48). However, it is not known if the elderly will be more sensitive to this problem. In addition, phenytoin may cause imbalance and ataxia. It is likely that EMMP patients, especially those with CNS disorders, may be more sensitive to this medication (49). In a study involving elderly persons, among the various lifestyle, demographic, and health factors which contributed to an increased risk, phenytoin was the only drug which was associated with a significant increase in fractures (50). However, this study could not determine if this was due to falls from ataxia or seizures, or was an effect due to bone changes.

Phenytoin is also known to be a mild blocker of cardiac conduction and should be used cautiously in persons with conduction defects, especially heart blocks. In spite of its limitations, phenytoin is the least expensive major AED. This, as well as its long record of use, may account for it presently being the most widely used AED.

Carbamazepine

Carbamazepine is effective for localization-related epilepsies, and thus has an efficacy profile appropriate for the elderly. Evidence from two large VA studies showed it to be as effective as phenytoin, phenobarbital, primidone, and valproate, but better tolerated than the latter three (44,51). Two studies of new-onset epilepsy in the community-dwelling elderly found carbamazepine to be as effective as lamotrigine, but noted that it had a higher incidence of side effects (11,43).

The apparent clearance of carbamazepine has been reported to be 20% to 40% lower in the elderly as compared to adults (52,53). A population analysis of patients from ambulatory neurology clinics at three medical centers also showed that the apparent oral clearance of carbamazepine was 25% lower in those patients who were greater than

70 years old (38). Decreases in clearance result in prolonged half-life elimination. These changes in carbamazepine pharmacokinetics indicate that lower and less frequent dosing in elderly patients may be appropriate. Lower doses of carbamazepine have been observed in older (>85 years) elderly NH residents as compared to elderly in the younger age group (65 to 74 years); however, doses were similar after adjusting for a patients' weight (40a). Observed carbamazepine concentrations in the Birnbaum study were lower or below the suggested therapeutic range used in treating younger adults.

Carbamazepine has some significant drug–drug interactions with medications that inhibit the cytochrome P450 enzyme, CYP3A4, responsible for carbamazepine metabolism. Among the inhibitors are erythromycin, fluoxetine, ketoconazole, propoxyphene, and cimetidine. At least one food (grapefruit juice) has been identified to interact with carbamazepine causing increases in its serum concentrations. Elderly healthy patients will need to be cautioned about these interactions, and should be instructed to inform the physician whenever they are beginning a new medication, including any over-the-counter medications. Many other drug interactions do occur, so carbamazepine is one AED that will need to be used cautiously in EMMP patients receiving other medications.

Carbamazepine also induces the CYP3A4 system, reducing the effectiveness of other drugs. St. John's Wort, an herbal remedy used for depression, is a powerful inducer of CYP3A4 and may significantly lower the concentration of carbamazepine.

Carbamazepine has some effects on cognitive functioning, especially at higher levels. However, it is not known if the elderly will be more sensitive to this problem. In addition, carbamazepine may cause imbalance and ataxia. It is possible that EMMP patients, especially those with CNS disorders, may be more sensitive to these effects. One of the major concerns with carbamazepine is its effect on sodium levels (54). Hyponatremia is a well-known phenomenon seen with carbamazepine use, and may cause significant problems in younger adults, especially if there is polydypsia. The hyponatremia associated with carbamazepine is more pronounced as a person becomes older (55). This may become more problematic if a person is on a salt restriction diet or a diuretic. Because of the mild neutropenia associated with carbamazepine use in younger adults, the effects of this AED on hematopoietic parameters in the elderly will need to be studied. Carbamazepine is also known to affect cardiac rhythms, and should be used cautiously, if at all, in persons with rhythm disturbances.

One of the pharmacokinetic problems of carbamazepine is its short half-life. This requires it to be taken multiple times in a day. In the elderly, however, the half-life may be longer, and slow-release formulations may overcome the need to dose multiple times each day and may overcome some of the side-effect problems associated with a rapid time to a high peak (short T_{max} and high C_{max}).

Phenobarbital

Phenobarbital is effective for localization-related epilepsies, and has an efficacy profile appropriate for the elderly. However, a VA cooperative study demonstrated that phenobarbital and primidone are not as well tolerated when compared to carbamazepine or phenytoin (44). Thus, although phenobarbital is the least expensive of all AEDs, its side-effects profile, which may worsen cognition and depression, make it an undesirable drug for the elderly, especially in the NH setting where declines in cognition are already present.

Valproic Acid

Only a few studies have compared the pharmacokinetics of VPA in young and old patients (56,57). Total VPA clearance is similar in young and elderly individuals; however, unbound clearance is higher in the elderly. In a study of steady-state VPA pharmacokinetics in six young adult and six elderly volunteers (68 to 89 years), the average unbound fraction of VPA was 9.5% in the elderly compared with 6.6% in younger subjects (57).

Much like phenytoin, VPA is associated with reduced protein binding and unbound clearance in the elderly. As a result, the desired clinical response may be achieved with a lower dose. A nationwide elderly NH study showed that valproic acid (VPA) dose and total VPA concentrations decrease within elderly age groups (58). The apparent clearance of VPA in elderly NH residents has also been shown to be 27% lower in women, 41% greater with the coadministration of an inducer such as carbamazepine or phenytoin, and to be 25% greater when the syrup formulation was used (41b). Because the serum elimination half-life may be prolonged, the dosing interval can be extended. If the albumin concentration has fallen or the patient's clinical response does not correlate with total drug concentration, measurement of the unbound drug should be considered. Because of its effects on mood stabilization, it may be especially appropriate for elderly patients with a dual diagnosis.

Felbamate

Felbamate is effective for localization-related epilepsies and appears to have a broader spectrum of effectiveness than some of the other AEDs. Elderly subjects had a lower mean clearance (31.2 vs. 25.1 mL/min; 90% CI: 11.4 to –0.9; $P = 0.02$) than adults in a study involving 24 elderly healthy volunteers (59). Felbamate is primarily metabolized by the liver and is known to have a number of drug–drug interactions, both inhibitory and inductive, and therefore may not be a good choice for EMMP patients.

Gabapentin

Gabapentin is effective for localization-related epilepsies, and has an efficacy profile appropriate for the elderly. Gabapentin is not metabolized by the liver, but rather renally excreted; therefore, there are no drug–drug interactions (60). Thus it may be especially useful in EMMP patients. There is, however, a reduction of renal function that correlates with advancing age, so doses may need to be adjusted in both EH and EMMP patients. Levels must be monitored after initiation and doses adjusted accordingly. However, gabapentin does appear to have some sedative side effects, especially at higher levels, and the elderly may be more sensitive to this problem.

Gabapentin has a short half-life that requires it to be given multiple times a day. In the elderly, however, the half-life may be longer due to a reduction in renal elimination. Because gabapentin is effective in treating neuralgic pain, it may be additionally beneficial for someone suffering from both epilepsy and pain.

The VA Cooperative Study #428 compared carbamazepine with gabapentin and lamotrigine. Efficacies were similar but withdrawal related to side effects was highest for carbamazepine (11), suggesting that the newer AEDs may be better tolerated.

Lamotrigine

Lamotrigine is effective for localization-related epilepsies, and has an efficacy profile appropriate for the elderly. However, very few studies regarding lamotrigine and its effects on the elderly have been published. Lamotrigine is primarily metabolized by the liver using the glucuronidation pathway, which unlike the P450 system, is thought to be less affected by age (61). Data from a population pharmacokinetic study of 163 epilepsy patients, which only included 30 subjects greater than 65 years of age, 10 subjects between 70 and 76 years of age and no subjects from the old-old age group showed that age did not affect lamotrigine apparent clearance (62). Based on a study of 150 elderly subjects, the drop out rate due to adverse events was lower with lamotrigine (18%) than with carbamazepine (42%). The difference was attributable to the finding that lamotrigine subjects had fewer rashes (lamotrigine 3%, carbamazepine 19%) and fewer complaints of somnolence (lamotrigine 12%, carbamazepine 29%) (43). Clinicians may want to consider other factors when dosing elderly lamotrigine patients. Elderly community-dwelling epilepsy patients aged 59 to 92 years from the VA Cooperative Study #428 showed that lamotrigine apparent clearance can be affected by blood urea nitrogen and serum creatinine ratio, weight, and phenytoin use (63).

Lamotrigine clearance is increased by approximately two to three times with coadministration of phenytoin and carbamazepine, whereas lamotrigine clearance decreases twofold with coadministration of VPA (64). However, these drug interaction studies included very few elderly subjects. Therefore, the extent of the changes in clearance with administration of comedications in the elderly is not known, and caution may need to be observed in EMMP patients who are on other drugs.

Levetiracetam

Levetiracetam has been approved as adjunctive therapy for partial-onset seizures in adults. Levetiracetam is extremely water soluble, which allows for rapid and complete absorption after oral administration. Levetiracetam is not metabolized by the liver, and thus is free of auto-induction kinetics and drug–drug interactions. Lack of protein binding (<10%) also avoids the problems of displacing highly protein-bound drugs and the monitoring of unbound concentrations. The lack of drug interactions makes levetiracetam useful for treating elderly epilepsy patients, particularly those patients who have other illnesses and are taking other medications (65). Notably, the manufacturer reports a decrease of 38% in total body clearance and an increased half-life up to 2.5 hours longer in elderly subjects (age 61 to 88 years) who exhibited creatinine clearances ranging from 30 to 74 mL/min. However, doses do need to be adjusted depending on the renal function of the patient as measured by serum creatinine and levetiracetam concentrations (66).

One prospective phase 4 study indicates a favorable efficacy profile in the elderly (67). Levetiracetam also appears to have a favorable safety profile. It was initially studied as a potential agent for treating cognitive disorders in the elderly, and thus a considerable amount of data regarding its tolerability in this age group is available. Analysis of 3252 elderly persons involved in studies of levetiracetam for epilepsy and other conditions demonstrated that levetiracetam was well tolerated by the elderly (68).

Oxcarbazepine

Oxcarbazepine is rapidly metabolized by first-pass metabolism to 10-hydroxcarbazepine (10-OH-carbazepine or MHD); MHD is considered the active compound. MHD is further metabolized by glucuronidation and excreted by the kidneys (69). The most extensive elderly oxcarbazepine study involved low doses of oxcarbazepine given to 12 young and 12 elderly healthy male volunteers and 12 young and 12 elderly female volunteers. At low doses of oxcarbazepine (300 to 600 mg/day), a significantly higher maximum concentration, higher area under the curve parameters, and a lower elimination rate constant were observed in the elderly volunteers (70).

Oxcarbazepine can affect the cytochrome P450 system by inducing the metabolism of the CYP3A4 enzyme that is responsible for the metabolism of dihydropyridine calcium antagonists and many other substances using this pathway (71,72). However, oxcarbazepine appears to have a more powerful effect on sodium balance than carbamazepine and this effect has been shown to increase with age resulting in more pronounced hyponatremia in this age group (55).

Pregabalin

Pregabalin is related to gabapentin but is more potent, with doses of only one-fifth those of gabapentin needed for therapeutic effect. Its absorption also appears to be more predictable because of the lower amounts transported across the intestinal system. Although it may prove to be a favorable AED for the elderly, its cost and lack of experimental and clinical data may limit its use.

Tiagabine

Tiagabine is effective for localization-related epilepsies, has an efficacy profile appropriate for the elderly, and is primarily metabolized by the liver (CYP3A4). Comedications that affect CYP3A4 substrates will also affect the metabolism of tiagabine, giving it a drug interaction profile similar to carbamazepine. A major feature of tiagabine is its potency; usually, effective doses are 20 to 60 mg/day, and effective concentrations are 100 to 300 ng/mL, or as much as100-fold lower than other AEDs.

Topiramate

Topiramate is effective for localization-related epilepsies, and thus has an efficacy profile appropriate for the elderly. Topiramate is approximately 20% bound to serum proteins and is both metabolized by the liver and excreted unchanged in the urine. The enzymes involved in topiramate's metabolism have not been identified; however, the cytochrome P450 system may be involved. Topiramate clearance may decrease with age, causing higher than expected serum concentrations with doses that are used in younger adults. In addition, topiramate metabolism can be induced in the presence of inducing comedications such as carbamazepine and phenytoin (73). There is also some indication that topiramate can inhibit CYP2C19 activity (74); thus, levels will need to be monitored in order to ensure that the topiramate dose given does not result in higher than expected serum concentrations. Topiramate does have effects on cognitive functioning, especially at higher levels. However, it is not known if the elderly will be more sensitive to this problem.

Zonisamide

Zonisamide is effective for localization-related epilepsies (75). Protein binding is approximately 40% and its major elimination pathway is hepatic as a substrate of CYP 3A4. It may thus have interactions with other drugs using this pathway. In addition to the usual side effects of AEDs of somnolence and dizziness, zonisamide may be associated with weight loss. It has an association with the development of renal calculi in approximately 1% to 2% of persons during chronic use (76).

DRUG INTERACTIONS WITH NON-AEDs

Comedications are frequently used by patients in NHs receiving AEDs (see Table 37.2). Thus, it is imperative to note that concomitant medications taken by elderly patients can alter the absorption, distribution, and metabolism of AEDs, thereby increasing the risk of toxicity or therapeutic failure.

Calcium-containing antacids and sucralfate reduce the absorption of phenytoin (77,78). The absorption of phenytoin, carbamazepine, and valproate may be reduced significantly by oral antineoplastic drugs that damage gastrointestinal cells (48,80). In addition, phenytoin concentrations may be lowered by intravenously administered antineoplastic agents (80). The use of folic acid for treatment of megaloblastic anemia may decrease serum concentrations of phenytoin and enteral feedings can also lower serum concentrations in patients receiving orally administered phenytoin (81).

Many drugs displace AEDs from plasma proteins, an effect that is especially serious when the interacting drug also inhibits the metabolism of the displaced drug; this occurs when valproate interacts with phenytoin. Several drugs used on a short-term basis (including propoxyphene and erythromycin) or as a maintenance therapy (such as cimetidine, diltiazem, fluoxetine, and verapamil) significantly inhibit the metabolism of one or more AEDs that are metabolized by the P450 system. Certain agents can induce the P450 system or other enzymes, causing an increase in drug metabolism.

The most commonly prescribed inducers of drug metabolism are phenytoin, phenobarbital, carbamazepine, and primidone. Ethanol, when used chronically, also induces drug metabolism (82).

The interaction between antipsychotic drugs and AEDs is complex. Hepatic metabolism of certain antipsychotics such as haloperidol can be increased by carbamazepine, resulting in diminished psychotropic response. Antipsychotic medications, especially chlorpromazine, promazine, trifluoperazine, and perphenazine can reduce the threshold for seizures; and, the risk of seizure is directly proportional to the total number of psychotropic medications being taken, their doses, any abrupt increases in doses, and the presence of organized brain pathology (83). The epileptic patient taking antipsychotic drugs may need a higher dose of antiepileptic medication to control seizures. In contrast, CNS depressants are likely to lower the maximum dose of AEDs that can be administered before toxic symptoms occur.

DOSING

Compliance is a potential challenge in the elderly due to multiple medications, memory problems, and visual issues. In general, twice daily dosing is preferable. In long-term care facilities, drug adherence may be less of an issue than with community-dwelling elderly patients; however, reductions in staff time spent on the multiple administrations of medicines may help to reduce errors and cost.

CONCLUSIONS

Elderly epileptic patients face issues that may alter the approach of AED treatments. Information obtained from studies of younger adults may at times be applicable to the elderly, but not in all instances. Thus, two major conclusions which deserve special consideration can be reached at this time. First, AED levels may fluctuate significantly in the elderly NH population and dose changes based on a single level may exacerbate these already unstable levels. This is particularly true for the older AEDs, but whether the newer or water soluble AEDs are better still needs to be demonstrated. Second, although age may influence hepatic clearance, earlier studies may have overestimated the degree of this effect; accordingly, the genetic makeup of a patient's isoenzymes may play a much greater role than previously suspected. Of the newer AEDs, gabapentin, lamotrigine, and levetiracetam are the most widely researched and utilized. As drug patents expire, costs may lessen and lead to increasing use. However, much more research is needed in order to determine the best treatments for EH, EMMP, and FE cohorts.

References

1. Administration on Aging. *A Profile of Older Americans*. Washington, DC: U.S. Department of Health and Human Services; 2005.
2. Hauser W, Hesdorffer D. *Epilepsy, Frequency, Causes and Consequences*. New York, NY: Demos Publications; 1990:51.
3. Hauser WA, Annegers JF, Rocca WA. Descriptive epidemiology of epilepsy: contributions of population-based studies from Rochester, Minnesota. *Mayo Clin Proc.* 1996;71(6):576–586.
4. Epilepsy Foundation of America. *Epilepsy, a Report to the Nation*. Landover MD: Epilepsy Foundation of America; 1999.

5. de la Court A, Breteler MM, Meinardi H, et al. Prevalence of epilepsy in the elderly: the Rotterdam Study. *Epilepsia.* 1996;37(2):141–147.

6. Sillanpaa M, Kalviainen R, Klaukka T, et al. Temporal changes in the incidence of epilepsy in Finland: nationwide study. *Epilepsy Res.* 2006; 71(2–3):206–215.

7. Fisher RS, Leppik I. Debate: When does a seizure imply epilepsy? *Epilepsia.* 2008;49(suppl 9):7–12.

8. Fisher RS, van Emde Boas W, Blume W, et al. Epileptic seizures and epilepsy: definitions proposed by the International League Against Epilepsy (ILAE) and the International Bureau for Epilepsy (IBE). *Epilepsia.* 2005;46(4):470–472.

9. Bladin CF, Alexandrov AV, Bellavance A, et al. Seizures after stroke: a prospective multicenter study. *Arch Neurol.* 2000;57(11):1617–1622.

10. Silverman IE, Restrepo L, Mathews GC. Poststroke seizures. *Arch Neurol.* 2002;59(2):195–201.

11. Rowan AJ, Ramsay RE, Collins JF, et al. New onset geriatric epilepsy: a randomized study of gabapentin, lamotrigine, and carbamazepine. *Neurology.* 2005;64(11):1868–1873.

12. Hauser WA. Seizure disorders: the changes with age. *Epilepsia.* 1992; 33(suppl 4):S6–S14.

13. Gupta SR, Naheedy MH, Elias D, et al. Postinfarction seizures. A clinical study. *Stroke.* 1988;19(12):1477–1481.

14. Holmes GL. The electroencephalogram as a predictor of seizures following cerebral infarction. *Clin Electroencephalogr.* 1980;11(2):83–86.

15. Ensrud KE, Walczak TS, Blackwell T, et al. Antiepileptic drug use increases rates of bone loss in older women: a prospective study. *Neurology.* 2004;62:2051–2057.

16. Ensrud KE, Walczak TS, Blackwell TL, et al. Antiepileptic drug use and rates of hip bone loss in older men: a prospective study. *Neurology.* 2008;71:723–730.

17. Leppik IE. Introduction to the International Geriatric Epilepsy Symposium (IGES). *Epilepsy Res.* 2006;68(suppl 1):S1–S4.

18. Leppik IE, Brodie MJ, Saetre ER, et al. Outcomes research: clinical trials in the elderly. *Epilepsy Res.* 2006;68(suppl 1):S71–S76.

19. Moore SA, Teal TW. Adverse drug reaction surveillance in the geriatric population: a preliminary review. *Proceedings of the Drug Information Association Workshop Geriatric Drug Use: Clinical and Social Perspectives.* Washington, DC: Pergamon Press; 1985.

20. Perucca E, Berlowitz D, Birnbaum A, et al. Pharmacological and clinical aspects of antiepileptic drug use in the elderly. *Epilepsy Res.* 2006; 68(suppl 1):S49–S63.

21. Pugh M, Cramer J, Knoefel J, et al. Potentially inappropriate antiepileptic drugs for elderly patients with epilepsy. *J Am. Geriatr Soc.* 2003;52: 417–422.

22. Kemper P, Murtaugh CM. Lifetime use of nursing home care. *N Engl J Med.* 1991;324(9):595–600.

23. Hetzel L, Smith A. *The 65 Years and Over Population: 2000. Census 2000 Brief.* Washington, DC: Census Bureau; 2001:C2KBR/01-10.

24. Garrard J, Harms S, Hardie N, et al. Antiepileptic drug use in nursing home admissions. *Ann Neurol.* 2003;54(1):75–85.

25. Galimberti CA, Magri F, Magnani B, et al. Antiepileptic drug use and epileptic seizures in elderly nursing home residents: a survey in the province of Pavia, Northern Italy. *Epilepsy Res.* 2006;68(1):1–8.

26. Lackner TE, Cloyd JC, Thomas LW, et al. Antiepileptic drug use in nursing home residents: effect of age, gender, and comedication on patterns of use. *Epilepsia.* 1998;39(10):1083–1087.

27. Wallace S, Verbeeck R. Effect of age and sex on the plasma binding of acidic and basic drugs. *Clin Pharmacokinet.* 1987;12:91–97.

28. Greenblatt DJ. Reduced serum albumin concentration in the elderly: a report from the Boston Collaborative Drug Surveillance Program. *J Am Geriatr Soc.* 1979;27(1):20–22.

29. Verbeeck RK, Cardinal JA, Wallace SM. Effect of age and sex on the plasma binding of acidic and basic drugs. *Eur J Clin Pharmacol.* 1984;27(1):91–97.

30. Wynne HA, Cope LH, Mutch E, et al. The effect of age upon liver volume and apparent liver blood flow in healthy man. *Hepatology.* 1989;9(2):297–301.

31. Tiula E, Neuvonen PJ. Antiepileptic drugs and alpha 1-acid glycoprotein. *N Engl J Med.* 1982;307(18):1148.

32. Cusack BJ. Drug metabolism in the elderly. *J Clin Pharmacol.* 1988;28 (6):571–576.

33. Dawling S, Crome P. Clinical pharmacokinetic considerations in the elderly. An update. *Clin Pharmacokinet.* 1989;17(4):236–263.

34. Ahn JE, Cloyd JC, Brundage RC, et al. Phenytoin half-life and clearance during maintenance therapy in adults and elderly patients with epilepsy. *Neurology.* 2008;71(1):38–43.

35. Rowe JW, Andres R, Tobin JD, et al. The effect of age on creatinine clearance in men: a cross-sectional and longitudinal study. *J Gerontol.* 1976;31(2):155–163.

36. Fehrman-Ekholm I, Skeppholm L. Renal function in the elderly (>70 years old) measured by means of iohexol clearance, serum creatinine, serum urea and estimated clearance. *Scand J Urol Nephrol.* 2004;38(1):73–77.

37. Leppik IE, Cloyd JD, Sawchuk RJ, et al. Compliance and variability of plasma phenytoin levels in epileptic patients. *Ther Drug Mon.* 1979;1: 475–483.

38. Graves NM, Brundage RC, Wen Y, et al. Population pharmacokinetics of carbamazepine in adults with epilepsy. *Pharmacotherapy.* 1998;18(2):273–281.

39. Mooradian AD, Hernandez L, Tamai IC, et al. Variability of serum phenytoin concentrations in nursing home patients. *Arch Intern Med.* 1989; 149(4):890–892.

40. Birnbaum A, Hardie NA, Leppik IE, et al. Variability of total phenytoin serum concentrations within elderly nursing home residents. *Neurology.* 2003;60(4):555–559.

40a. Birnbaum AK, Conway JM, Hardie NA, et al. Carbamazepine dose-concentration relationship in elderly home residents. *Epilepsy Res.* 2007; 77:31–35.

41. Birnbaum AK, Hardie NA, Conway JM, et al. Phenytoin use in elderly nursing home residents. *Am J Geriatr Pharmacother.* 2003;1(2):90–95.

41a. Leppik IE, Conway JC, Strege MA, et al. Intra-individual variability of carbamazepine and valproic acid serum concentrations in elderly nursing home residents. Presented in American Academy of Neurology annual meeting, April 13, 2010.

41b. Birnbaum AK, Ahn JE, Brundage RC, et al. Population pharmacokinetics of valproic acid concentrations in elderly nursing home residents. *Ther Drug Monit.* 2007;29(5):571–575.

42. Ramsay R, Rowan A, Slater J, et al. Effect of age on epilepsy and its treatment results from the VA Cooperative Study. *Epilepsia.* 1994;35(suppl 8):91.

43. Brodie MJ, Overstall PW, Giorgi L. Multicentre, double-blind, randomised comparison between lamotrigine and carbamazepine in elderly patients with newly diagnosed epilepsy. The UK Lamotrigine Elderly Study Group. *Epilepsy Res.* 1999;37(1):81–87.

44. Mattson RH, Cramer JA, Collins JF, et al. Comparison of carbamazepine, phenobarbital, phenytoin, and primidone in partial and secondarily generalized tonic-clonic seizures. *N Engl J Med.* 1985;313(3):145–151.

45. Bauer LA, Blouin RA. Age and phenytoin kinetics in adult epileptics. *Clin Pharmacol Ther.* 1982;31(3):301–304.

46. Leppik IE. *Contemporary Diagnosis and Management of the Patient with Epilepsy.* 6th ed. Newton, PA: Handbooks in Healthcare; 2006.

47. Nelson MH, Birnbaum AK, Remmel RP. Inhibition of phenytoin hydroxylation in human liver microsomes by several selective serotonin re-uptake inhibitors. *Epilepsy Res.* 2001;44(1):71–82.

48. Thompson P, Huppert FA, Trimble M. Phenytoin and cognitive function: effects on normal volunteers and implications for epilepsy. *Br J Clin Psychol.* 1981;20(Pt 3):155–162.

49. Bourdet SV, Gidal BE, Alldredge BK. Pharmacologic management of epilepsy in the elderly. *J Am Pharm Assoc (Wash).* 2001;41(3):421–436.

50. Bohannon AD, Hanlon JT, Landerman R, et al. Association of race and other potential risk factors with nonvertebral fractures in community-dwelling elderly women. *Am J Epidemiol.* 1999;149(11):1002–1009.

51. Mattson RH, Cramer JA, Collins JF. A comparison of valproate with carbamazepine for the treatment of complex partial seizures and secondarily generalized tonic-clonic seizures in adults. The Department of Veterans Affairs Epilepsy Cooperative Study No. 264 Group. *N Engl J Med.* 1992;327(11):765–771.

52. Cloyd JC, Lackner TE, Leppik IE. Antiepileptics in the elderly. Pharmacoepidemiology and pharmacokinetics. *Arch Fam Med.* 1994; 3(7):589–598.

53. Graves NM, Holmes GB, Leppik IE. Compliant populations: variability in serum concentrations. *Epilepsy Res Suppl.* 1988;1:91–99.

54. Henry DA, Lawson DH, Reavey P, et al. Hyponatraemia during carbamazepine treatment. *Br Med J.* 1977;1(6053):83–84.

55. Dong X, Leppik IE, White J, et al. Hyponatremia from oxcarbazepine and carbamazepine. *Neurology.* 2005;65(12):1976–1978.

56. Bryson SM, Verma N, Scott PJ, et al. Pharmacokinetics of valproic acid in young and elderly subjects. *Br J Clin Pharmacol.* 1983;16(1):104–105.

57. Perucca E, Grimaldi R, Gatti G, et al. Pharmacokinetics of valproic acid in the elderly. *Br J Clin Pharmacol.* 1984;17(6):665–669.

58. Birnbaum AK, Hardie NA, Conway JM, et al. Valproic acid doses, concentrations, and clearances in elderly nursing home residents. *Epilepsy Res.* 2004;62(2–3):157–162.

59. Richens A, Banfield CR, Salfi M, et al. Single and multiple dose pharmacokinetics of felbamate in the elderly. *Br J Clin Pharmacol.* 1997;44(2):129–134.

60. Richens A. Clinical pharmacokinetics of gabapentin. In: Chadwick D, ed. *New Trends in Epilepsy Management: The Role of Gabapentin.* London, England: Royal Society of Medicine Services; 1993:41–46.

61. Peck AW. Clinical pharmacology of lamotrigine. *Epilepsia.* 1991;32 (suppl 2):S9–S12.

62. Hussein Z, Posner J. Population pharmacokinetics of lamotrigine monotherapy in patients with epilepsy: retrospective analysis of routine monitoring data. *Br J Clin Pharmacol.* 1997;43(5):457–465.

63. Punyawudho B, Ramsay RE, Macias FM, et al. Population pharmacokinetics of lamotrigine in elderly patients. *J Clin Pharmacol.* 2008;48:455–463.

64. Yuen AW, Land G, Weatherley BC, et al. Sodium valproate acutely inhibits lamotrigine metabolism. *Br J Clin Pharmacol.* 1992;33(5):511–513.

65. Patsalos PN, Sander JW. Newer antiepileptic drugs. Towards an improved risk-benefit ratio. *Drug Saf.* 1994;11(1):37–67.

66. French J. Use of levetiracetam in special populations. *Epilepsia.* 2001;42(suppl 4):40–43.

67. Morrell MJ, Leppik I, French J, et al. The KEEPER trial: levetiracetam adjunctive treatment of partial-onset seizures in an open-label community-based study. *Epilepsy Res.* 2003;54(2–3):153–161.

68. Cramer JA, Leppik IE, Rue KD, et al. Tolerability of levetiracetam in elderly patients with CNS disorders. *Epilepsy Res.* 2003;56(2–3):135–145.

69. Faigle JW, Menge GP. Metabolic characteristics of oxcarbazepine (Trileptal) and their beneficial implications for enzyme induction and drug interactions. *Behav Neurol.* 1990;3:21–30.

70. van Heiningen PN, Eve MD, Oosterhuis B, et al. The influence of age on the pharmacokinetics of the antiepileptic agent oxcarbazepine. *Clin Pharmacol Ther.* 1991;50 (4):410–419.

71. Klosterskov Jensen P, Saano V, Haring P, et al. Possible interaction between oxcarbazepine and an oral contraceptive. *Epilepsia.* 1992;33(6):1149–1152.

72. Zaccara G, Gangemi PF, Bendoni L, et al. Influence of single and repeated doses of oxcarbazepine on the pharmacokinetic profile of felodipine. *Ther Drug Monit.* 1993;15(1):39–42.

73. Sachdeo RC, Sachdeo SK, Walker SA, et al. Steady-state pharmacokinetics of topiramate and carbamazepine in patients with epilepsy during monotherapy and concomitant therapy. *Epilepsia.* 1996;37(8):774–780.

74. Levy R, Bishop F, Streeter A, et al. Explanation and prediction of drug interactions with topiramate using a CYP450 inhibition spectrum. *Epilepsia.* 1995;36(suppl 4):47.

75. Leppik IE, Willmore LJ, Homan RW, et al. Efficacy and safety of zonisamide: results of a multicenter study. *Epilepsy Res.* 1993;14: 165–173.

76. Wroe O. Zonisamide and renal calculi in patients with epilepsy: how big an issue? *Curr Med Res Opin.* 2007;23(8):1765–1773.

77. Nation RL, Evans AM, Milne RW. Pharmacokinetic drug interactions with phenytoin (Part I). *Clin Pharmacokinet.* 1990;18(1):37–60.

78. Nation RL, Evans AM, Milne RW. Pharmacokinetic drug interactions with phenytoin (Part II). *Clin Pharmacokinet.* 1990;18(2):131–50.

79. Bollini P, Riva R, Albani F, et al. Decreased phenytoin level during antineoplastic therapy: a case report. *Epilepsia.* 1983;24(1):75–78.

80. Neef C, de Voogd-van der Straaten I. An interaction between cytostatic and anticonvulsant drugs. *Clin Pharmacol Ther.* 1988;43(4):372–375.

81. Haley CJ, Nelson J. Phenytoin-enteral feeding interaction. *Dicp Ann Pharmacother.* 1989;23(10):796–798.

82. Sandor P, Sellers EM, Dumbrell M, et al. Effect of short- and long-term alcohol use on phenytoin kinetics in chronic alcoholics. *Clin Pharmacol Ther.* 1981;30(3):390–397.

83. Cold JA, Wells BG, Froemming JH. Seizure activity associated with antipsychotic therapy. *Dicp - Ann Pharmacother.* 1990;24(6): 601–606.

CHAPTER 38 ■ STATUS EPILEPTICUS

HOWARD P. GOODKIN AND JAMES J. RIVIELLO JR.

Status epilepticus (SE) is a life-threatening medical emergency that requires prompt recognition and immediate treatment. SE is not a disease in itself but rather a manifestation of either a primary central nervous system (CNS) insult or a systemic disorder with secondary CNS effects. It is important to identify and specifically treat the precipitating cause, thus preventing ongoing neurologic injury and seizure recurrence. A team approach, with an organized and systematic treatment regimen, planned in advance, is needed, including one for patients with refractory status epilepticus (RSE). It is imperative that treatment of SE rigorously adheres to basic neuroresuscitation principles—the ABCs (airway, breathing, circulation). Although the initial approach is standard, once a patient is stabilized, management must be individualized with the goal of terminating the seizure and treating the underlying condition.

DEFINITION

SE can present in many different forms that range from the easily recognized, prolonged, overt, generalized convulsive SE to the more difficult to recognize nonconvulsive SE (NCSE) that is characterized by a prolonged continuous ictal electrographic discharge pattern, with or without obvious clinical signs. Given the broad range of clinical presentations and that the underlying mechanism that causes these prolonged seizures is not completely known, it has been difficult to develop definition and classification systems that are well-accepted, comprehensive, mechanistic, and clinically useful.

At first, Gastaut's classic operational definition of SE as "an epileptic seizure that is sufficiently prolonged or repeated at sufficiently brief intervals so as to produce an unvarying and enduring epilepticus condition" (1) may seem vague, cumbersome, and insufficient as it fails to provide adequate guidance to the clinician. However, it has the advantage of allowing for a dynamic interpretation.

Other proposed recent operational definitions have attempted to be more precise by including a time duration (2,3). However, the basis for the time chosen has varied. As experimental studies demonstrated that homeostatic mechanisms fail after 30 minutes of continuous seizure activity, resulting in an increase in the risk of neuronal injury, the Working Group on Status Epilepticus of the Epilepsy Foundation of America (EFA) defined SE as >30 minutes of either continuous seizure activity or two or more sequential seizures without full recovery of consciousness (4). In defining SE, others have chosen to emphasize the need for the prompt care of the patient and to define the seizure duration required to fulfill the definition of SE in the 5- to 10-minute range (5). It is expected that future definitions of SE will continue to better define the mechanisms that underlie the self-sustained nature of these prolonged seizures.

CLASSIFICATION

Multiple schemas for the classification of SE have been proposed. Traditionally, the International Classification of Epileptic Seizures separates the prolonged, continuous, or repetitive seizures of SE from the self-limited seizure and classifies SE into two broad categories—either generalized or focal (partial)—based on a combination of the electrographic pattern and seizure semiology (6–11).

In contrast, other proposed classification schemas have placed an emphasis on seizure semiology. One recent proposal divided SE into the categories of aura status, autonomic status, dyscognitive status, motor status (simple motor and complex motor), and special status (e.g., hypomotor status) (12). A more familiar predominantly semiologically based SE classification system divides SE into the two broad categories of convulsive, and nonconvulsive (13). However, the division between convulsive SE and NCSE may not be so obvious as subtle convulsive SE or NCSE—characterized by no obvious clinical signs despite marked impairment of consciousness and bilateral EEG discharges—may evolve from convulsive SE or follow its unsuccessful treatment.

In a study of 458 patients from the Netherlands (1980 to 1987) (14–16), generalized convulsive SE occurred in 346 (77%); NCSE in 65 (13%); and simple partial SE in 47 (10%). Of patients with NCSE, 40 had complex partial SE and 25 had absence SE. In this study, within the NCSE group of patients, focal signs occurred more often with complex partial SE, a fluctuating consciousness was more common with absence SE, and the majority of patients in both groups had prior epilepsy (14). With simple partial SE, 46 patients had somatomotor features and one had aphasia with hallucinations (15).

As future classification systems are developed, psychogenic nonepileptic SE which occurs in adults (17) and children (18,19) should likely be included as a special category to assure clinical recognition of these events. Pseudo-SE may occur as an expression of Munchausen's syndrome (factitious disorder by proxy) (20).

THE CLINICAL AND ELECTROGRAPHIC STAGES OF STATUS EPILEPTICUS

The clinical stages of SE include the premonitory (prodromal) stage; the incipient stage (0 to 5 minutes); the early stage (5 to 30 minutes); the "transition stage" to the late or established stage (30 to 60 minutes); the refractory stage (longer than 60 to 90 minutes) (21); and the postictal stage (Table 38.1).

TABLE 38.1

STAGES OF STATUS EPILEPTICUS

Premonitory	
Incipient[a]	0 to 5 minutes
Early[a]	5 to 30 minutes
Transition	from early to established
Established (late)	30 to 60 minutes
Refractory	after 60 minutes
Postictal	

[a]Special circumstances of the early and incipient stages for which early anesthetic therapy should be considered are listed in Table 38.2.

TABLE 38.2

SPECIAL CIRCUMSTANCES OF THE EARLY STAGE

Postoperative patients, especially cardiac surgery and neurosurgery
Head trauma, brain tumor, increased intracranial pressure
CNS infections (meningitis, encephalitis, brain abscess)
Organ failure, especially hepatic or multisystem failure
Hyperthermia, malignant hyperthermia, hyperthyroidism
Metabolic disorders prone to increased intracranial pressure, diabetic ketoacidosis, or organic acid disorders

The premonitory stage consists of confusion, myoclonus, or increasing seizure frequency; the early stage consists of continuous seizure activity; and the refractory stage may consist of subtle generalized convulsive SE or NCSE. It has now become clear that the "transition" stage from the early to late stages of SE is not fixed in time and may vary depending on the underlying etiology. SE should not be considered refractory if therapy has been inadequate.

A predictable sequence of EEG progression occurs during the clinical stages in experimental models and humans: (i) discrete seizures with interictal slowing; (ii) waxing and waning of ictal discharges; (iii) continuous ictal discharges; (iv) continuous ictal discharges punctuated by flat periods; and (v) periodic epileptiform discharges (PEDs) on a flat background (Fig. 38.1) (22). However, every episode of SE does not pass through every one of these defined stages (23) (Fig. 38.2). The PED stage may also consist of either lateralized (PLED) or bilateral (BPED) patterns (22). The response to treatment appears to depend on electrographic stage (see "Trends in Patients with Status Epilepticus"). In one study (22), discrete seizures were all controlled with diazepam (six of six patients), whereas in the PED stage, the seizure stopped in only one of six patients and overt clinical seizures were converted to either subtle or electrographic seizures in five of the six patients.

TRENDS IN PATIENTS WITH STATUS EPILEPTICUS

As prolonged seizures are unlikely to spontaneously cease, the overall trend in SE has been to decrease the time duration required for diagnosis and to treat as soon as possible. Although the EFA Working Group defined SE as a seizure duration >30 minutes, the Working Group recommended treatment as soon as 10 minutes after seizure onset (4). Lowenstein and colleagues (5) proposed an operational definition for generalized convulsive SE in adults and older children (>5 years of age) of ≥5 minutes of either a continuous seizure or two or more discrete seizures between which there is incomplete recovery of consciousness. In treatment studies, the Veterans Affairs (VA) Cooperative Study (24), which compared various first-line antiepileptic drugs (AEDs), treatment for SE was initiated at 10 minutes, and the San Francisco Prehospital Treatment study used 5 minutes (25). Beran has questioned waiting even as long as 5 minutes to treat an ongoing seizure as these time windows are based on the inherent

risk of ongoing seizure activity (26). Similarly, Lowenstein and Alldredge had recommended immediately proceeding to anesthesia in the special case of SE developing while in the intensive care unit (ICU) (2). Table 38.2 lists other special circumstances for which immediate seizure control during the early stage or even the incipient stage of SE (see Table 38.1) is recommended (27).

Clinical data characterizing the duration of a typical seizure support this trend. A typical clinical seizure rarely lasts as long as 5 minutes. A typical generalized tonic–clonic seizure lasts 31 to 51 seconds, with a postictal phase of a few seconds to 4 minutes (28). In an inpatient study, mean seizure duration was 62 seconds, with a range of 16 to 108 seconds (29). In partial seizures in children, the typical duration was 97 seconds (30). In a prospective study of new onset seizures in children, the frequency distribution of seizure duration was best described as the sum of two groups: one with a mean of 3.6 minutes (76% of cases) and the other with a mean of 31 minutes (24% of cases); if the seizure duration was 5 to 10 minutes, it was unlikely to cease spontaneously within the next few minutes (31).

The trend for prompt treatment during the early stage is also supported by clinical and experimental studies characterizing the treatment of SE. In the prospective VA Cooperative Study, the first-line treatment of the shorter duration, overt, generalized SE was more successful than the first-line treatment of the more prolonged subtle SE, independent of treatment arm. In addition, in post hoc analysis, it was demonstrated that when the first-line AEDs failed, there was only a 5.3% response to a third AED (21). Although the response rate to treatment with a third AED was higher (58%) in a retrospective study of 83 episodes of SE in 74 patients treated at Columbia University (32), it has been posited that this difference reflected earlier treatment.

A time-dependent efficacy of treatment has also been observed in experimental models of SE. Following induction of SE with the combination of lithium and the cholinergic agonist pilocarpine, diazepam was effective in controlling SE shortly after onset but was effective in only 17% of rats in the late stages of SE (33). This finding was later confirmed in a second model of SE for both diazepam and phenytoin (34). This decrease in the benzodiazepine response occurs rapidly after the onset of SE and in young animals with ages corresponding to a human toddler (35–37). Diazepam and the other benzodiazepines enhance the function of a subset of benzodiazepine-sensitive $GABA_A$ receptors. Recent studies (38–41) have demonstrated that the surface expression of these receptors declines during SE and have proffered that

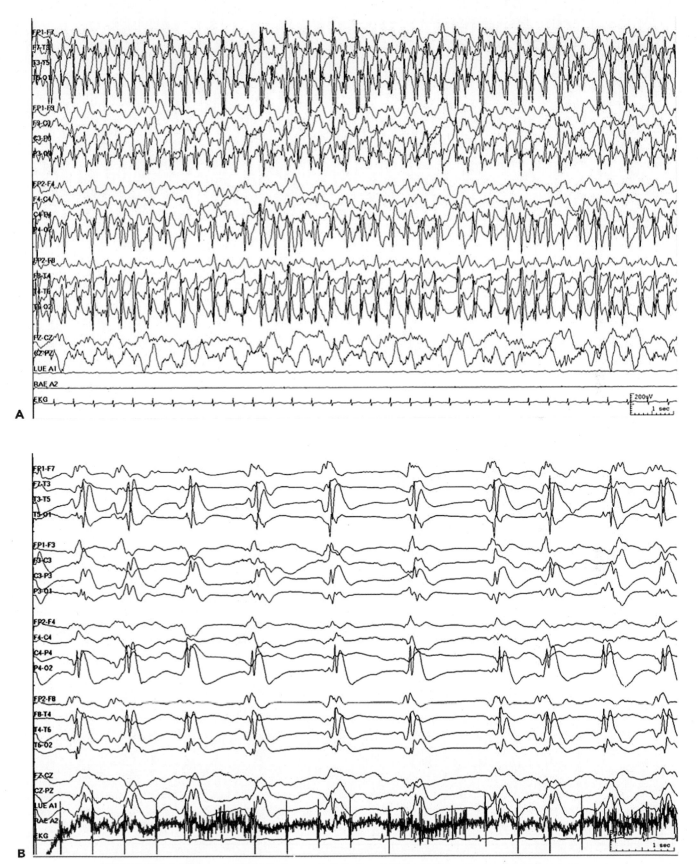

FIGURE 38.1 A: Continuous ictal discharges. **B:** Periodic epileptiform discharges on a flat background.

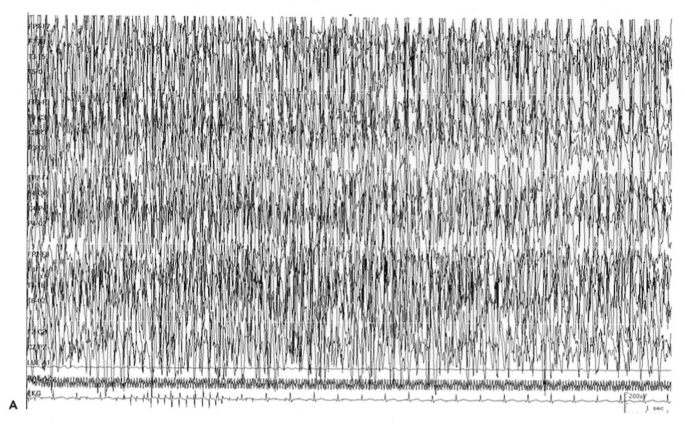

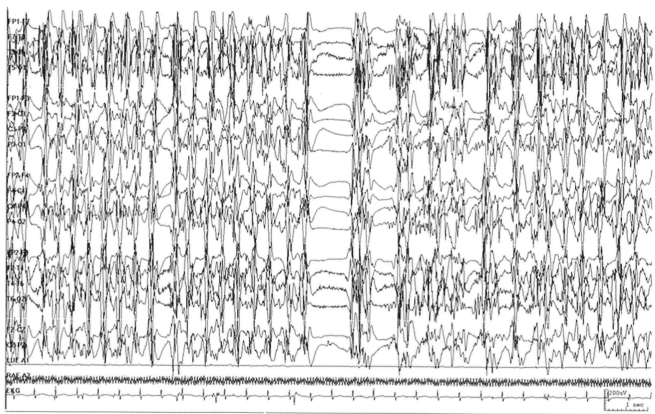

FIGURE 38.2 Same patient, different seizure. **A:** Continuous ictal discharge. **B:** Continuous ictal discharges punctuated by flat periods.

this reduction in surface expression, which is the result of activity-dependent, subunit-specific trafficking of $GABA_A$ receptors, partially accounts for the time-dependent efficacy of the first-line agents.

PATHOPHYSIOLOGY

Mechanistically, SE occurs when there is a failure of factors that "normally" terminate seizures (5,42). What are these pathophysiologic mechanisms? SE results from decreased cerebral inhibition, excessive cerebral excitation, or a combination of both. A rapid modification in the properties of $GABA_A$ receptors (35,43) through mechanisms such as altered receptor trafficking (see Section "Trends in Patients with Status Epilepticus") likely contributes to the reduction in inhibition.

Excessive excitation itself may cause neuronal injury and cell death, referred to as excitotoxic injury. This has been demonstrated in experimental models, such as in kainic acid–induced limbic seizures (44), but its occurrence in humans has been questioned. An outbreak of domoic acid poisoning, an excitotoxic agent, with acute symptoms, including SE, was associated with neuronal loss and astrocytosis that was greatest in the hippocampus and amygdala; this is similar to the seizures induced by kainic acid (45,46). A survivor developed epilepsy and, after death, autopsy revealed hippocampal sclerosis (47).

Prolonged seizures in anesthetized baboons cause irreversible neuronal injury (48,49). Lothman outlined the alterations in systemic and brain metabolism occurring with prolonged SE (50): decreased brain oxygen tension, mismatch between the sustained increase in oxygen and glucose utilization and a fall in cerebral blood flow, and depletion of brain glucose and oxygen. In the incipient or early stages of SE, brain compensatory mechanisms may protect against neuronal injury. However, at some point the ability to compensate for neuronal injury is exhausted, and the risk of neuronal injury increases. This point defines the transition stage from early to late (established) SE. During all stages, the ability to compensate requires adequate airway and good breathing, circulation, and cerebral blood flow.

EPIDEMIOLOGY OF STATUS EPILEPTICUS

There have been two large, population-based studies in the United States—one performed in Richmond, Virginia (51), and the other in Rochester, Minnesota (52). These two studies estimate that 60,000 to 150,000 episodes of SE occur per year in the United States resulting in approximately 55,000 deaths per year. Overall, SE accounts for 1% to 8% of hospital admissions for epilepsy. Between 4% and 16% of patients with epilepsy will have at least one episode of SE, with one third of the cases occurring as the presenting symptom in patients with a first unprovoked seizure, one third in patients with established epilepsy, and one third in those with no history of epilepsy (53).

The incidence has varied by location: the rate in the study performed in Richmond was 41/100,000 (51) and the rate in Rochester study was 18/100,000 (52); but in the study performed in California (54), the overall rate of generalized

convulsive SE was lower (6.2/100,000). However, across these studies, the higher incidence rates have occurred at the extremes of life. In the California study, the incidence rate for children <5 years of age was 7.5/100,000 and the incidence rate for the elderly was 22.3/100,000. Overall, a lower incidence has been reported from Europe; the incidence rate was 9.9/100,000 in Switzerland (55), 15.8/100,000 in Germany (56), and 13.1/100,000 in Bologna (57).

In children, SE is most common in the very young, especially those <2 years of age (58). In the community-based prospective North London Status Epilepticus in Childhood Surveillance Study (NLSTEPSS), the incidence of SE during childhood was from 17 to 23/100,000 per year (59). For children with epilepsy, SE typically occurs within 2 years of the onset of epilepsy (60), and recurrent SE is more likely with an underlying neurologic disorder (61).

ETIOLOGY OF STATUS EPILEPTICUS

Seizures are also classified according to etiology, and SE classification has been expanded to include symptomatic, remote symptomatic, remote symptomatic with acute precipitant, progressive encephalopathy, cryptogenic, idiopathic, and febrile SE (62).

In several studies of adult SE, trauma, tumor, and vascular disease were the most frequently identified causes, although idiopathic and unknown causes were also common (63–66). Etiology also differs among centers and by ages. In San Francisco, noncompliance with AEDs and alcohol withdrawal were the two most common etiologies (Table 38.3) (63,66), whereas cerebrovascular damage was the most common etiology in Richmond (67).

For children in North London, the age-adjusted incidence for acute symptomatic SE was 16.9% in those less than one year of age, 2.5% in those 1 to 4 years of age, and 0.1% in those 5 to 15 years of age. The incidence of an acute on

TABLE 38.3

ETIOLOGY IN THE SAN FRANCISCO STUDIES: CHANGES OVER TIME

Etiology	1980 (number of cases)	1993 (number of cases)
Anticonvulsant withdrawal	27	48
Alcohol-related	15	43
Drug intoxication	10	14
CNS infection	4	12
Refractory epilepsy	—	10
Trauma	3	8
Tumor	4	7
Metabolic disorders	8	7
Stroke	15	6
Cardiac arrest	4	6
Unknown	15	8

CNS, central nervous system.
From Refs. 63 and 66.

TABLE 38.4

COMPARISON OF ETIOLOGY IN CHILDREN AND
ADULTS IN THE RICHMOND STUDY

Etiology	% of children (<16 years)	% of adults (>16 years)
Cerebrovascular	3.3	25.2
Medication change	19.8	18.9
Anoxia	5.3	10.7
EtOH/drug-related	2.4	12.2
Metabolic	8.2	8.8
Unknown	9.3	8.1
Fever/infection	35.7	4.6
Trauma	3.5	4.6
Tumor	0.7	4.3
CNS infection	4.8	1.8
Congenital	7.0	0.8

CNS, central nervous system.
From DeLorenzo RJ, Towne AR, Pellock JM, et al. Status epilepticus in
children, adults, and the elderly. *Epilepsia*. 1992;33(suppl 4):S15–S25,
with permission.

remote (remote symptomatic with an acute precipitant) was
6%, 5.3%, and 0.7%, respectively. A prolonged febrile seizure
occurred in 4.1/100,000; acute symptomatic causes in
2.2/100,000; remote symptomatic in 2.3/100,000; acute on
remote in 2.1/100,000; idiopathic in 1.4/100,000; cryptogenic
in 0.2/100,000; and unclassified in 1/100,000 (59).

As the Richmond study included adults and children, the
etiologies in these two groups at one center can be directly
compared (Table 38.4). In adults, cerebrovascular disease
was the most common etiology, occurring in 25.2% versus
only 3.3% in children, whereas in children, fever or infection
was the most common cause, occurring in 35.7% versus only
4.6% in adults. Medication change was a major cause in
both adults and children—20% in children versus 19% in
adults (67). The incidence of tumors was higher in older
studies (64,65).

PROGNOSIS OF PATIENT WITH STATUS EPILEPTICUS

Although many people survive an episode of SE with no or
limited untoward effects, SE is life-threatening and is associated with long-term neurologic sequelae. The prognosis of SE
depends on etiology, duration (2), and age (58).

The mortality rate in modern, general SE series ranges
from 4% (68) to 37% (69) and is higher with an acute precipitant (69). An acute precipitant is more likely when there
is no prior history of epilepsy (69,70), but may also be
responsible for death in persons with known epilepsy with
SE. In one series, 63% of patients survived, 28.6% died
from the underlying cause, 6.6% died from other causes,
and 1.8% died from the SE itself (69). For the 74 patients
retrospectively studied at Columbia (71), the mortality rate
was 21% (14/85) and was higher with acute symptomatic
seizures and older ages. Interestingly, in a study limited only
to patients with *de novo* SE (72), SE occurring in patients

already hospitalized, the mortality was very high—61%
(25/41).

Short-term and long-term mortalities were compared using
data from the Rochester study (73–75): mortality was 19%
(38/201) within the first 30 days, but cumulative mortality
was 43% over 10 years (73). The long-term mortality risk
increased with an SE duration >24 hours, acute symptomatic
etiology, and myoclonic SE (73).

In the Richmond study, the mortality rate was 32% when
the duration was >60 minutes versus only 2.7% when the
duration was 30 to 59 minutes (76). Other factors associated
with a high mortality rate in the Richmond study included
anoxia and older age, whereas a low mortality rate was associated with alcohol and AED withdrawal (76).

In the Netherlands study (16), prognosis of patients with
generalized convulsive SE was related to treatment adequacy.
A favorable outcome occurred in 263 of 346 patients (76%),
with outcome related to cause, duration >4 hours, more
than one medical complication, and quality of care. In order
to analyze the treatment effects, therapy was classified as
insufficient if the wrong AED dose or route was used, if an
unnecessary delay occurred, if mechanical ventilation was
not used despite respiratory insufficiency or medical complications, or if neuromuscular paralysis was used without electroencephalogram (EEG) monitoring (in order to detect
seizure activity). The most common reason for classifying
therapy as insufficient was an inadequate AED dose. In the
patients with a favorable outcome (n = 263), therapy was
classified as good or sufficient in 85.6%, and considered
insufficient in only 10.3%; in those with sequelae (n = 45),
therapy was inadequate in 22.2%. When the morbidity was
from SE itself, insufficient therapy occurred in 50% of
patients. With the occurrence of death (n = 38), therapy was
sufficient in 44.7% of patients, and in cases of death due to
SE itself, therapy was considered insufficient in 62% of
patients (16).

The mortality rate in pediatric SE ranges from 3% to 11%,
and is also related to etiology and age (68,77–82). In one
study, the mortality was 4%, occurring only with acute symptomatic or progressive symptomatic etiologies (77). In
NLSTEPSS, the overall mortality was 3%. In the Richmond
study, for children ranging in age from 0 months to 16 years
(n = 598), the overall mortality rate was 6.2% (37 of 598).
The highest rates occurred during the first 6 months of life
(24%; 18 of 75) and between 6 and 12 months of age (9%; 5
of 54) with a lower rate (1%; 4 of 469) in children older than
1 year (83). The difference likely reflects a higher incidence of
symptomatic SE in the youngest children. With respect to
morbidity following SE in children, a Canadian study of SE
reported 34% of 40 children with an SE duration of 30 to 720
minutes had subsequent neurodevelopmental deterioration
(84). Even in children with febrile SE, speech deficits have
been reported (85).

An increase in morbidity and mortality has also been
reported with NCSE, which is related to SE duration (36
hours to >72 hours) (86). However, this increased morbidity
with NCSE is controversial (87–89). Following cardiopulmonary resuscitation, SE, status myoclonus, and myoclonic
SE are predictive of a poor outcome (90). On EEG, burst-
suppression (91) and PEDs are predictive of a poor outcome
(92), whereas a normal EEG is associated with a good prognosis (93).

MANAGEMENT OF STATUS EPILEPTICUS

The initial management of patients with SE begins with the ABCs—airway, breathing, and circulation (Table 38.5). Diagnostic studies are then selected, depending on a patient's history and physical examination (not all studies need to be obtained for every patient). Serum glucose should be checked immediately with Dextrostix (Bayer Corporation, West Haven, Connecticut) to rapidly diagnose hypoglycemia. A complete blood count may be helpful for diagnosing infection, although leukocytosis may occur with SE. Electrolytes, calcium, phosphorous, and magnesium values may also be helpful. Lumbar puncture (LP) should be considered in the febrile patient, although cerebrospinal fluid (CSF) pleocytosis may occur without infection, presumably due to a breakdown in the blood-brain barrier (94). In one study, the highest CSF white blood cell count from SE alone (no acute insult) was 28×10^6/L (95). If there is concern about increased intracranial pressure or a structural lesion, LP can be deferred until neuroimaging is performed. If there is evidence of infection, antibiotics can be administered prior to LP. In those taking an

TABLE 38.5

IMMEDIATE MANAGEMENT OF STATUS EPILEPTICUS

The ABCs

Stabilize and maintain the Airway; position head to avoid airway obstruction

Establish Breathing (i.e., ventilation): administer oxygen by nasal cannula or mask

Maintain the Circulation: start intravenous (IV) line

Monitor the Vital Signs: pulse (ECG monitoring), respiratory rate, blood pressure, temperature, pulse oximetry, check Dexstrostix

Start intravenous (IV) line

Use normal saline

Consider thiamine 100 mg; followed by 50 mL of D50%

Determine what studies are needed

Consider CBC, electrolytes, calcium, phosphorus, magnesium; AED levels, toxicology

Lumbar puncture (especially if febrile)

Neuroimaging, cranial CAT scan or MRI

EEG, if diagnosis initially in doubt

Points from history:

Has an AED been given (prehospital treatment or inpatient), is patient on any AEDs (especially phenobarbital or phenytoin), or are there any allergies, or has the patient ever had Stevens–Johnson syndrome?

Characteristics of past seizures: is there a history of status epilepticus?

Are treatable causes present (any acute precipitants)?

Fever or illness, head trauma, possible electrolyte imbalance, intoxications, toxin exposure?

Are chronic medical conditions present or is patient on steroid therapy? (If so, needs stress coverage)

ECG, electrocardiogram; CBC, complete blood count; AED, antiepileptic drug; CAT, computerized axial tomography; MRI, magnetic resonance imaging; EEG, electroencephalography.

AED, levels should be obtained as low AED levels may contribute to the development of SE in both adults and children (96,97). A practice parameter on the diagnostic assessment of the child with SE has been produced (98). When done, electrolytes or glucose were abnormal in 6%; blood cultures were abnormal in 2.5%; a CNS infection was found in 12.5%; an ingestion was found in 3.6%; an inborn error of metabolism was found in 4.2%; and AED levels were low in 32%.

Neuroimaging options include cranial computed axial tomography (CAT) scan and magnetic resonance imaging (MRI). CAT scans are readily available on an emergency basis and should identify all disorders demanding immediate intervention, such as tumor or hydrocephalus, but may not show the early phases of infarction. CAT scan and MRI may detect focal changes, which may be transient (99) and secondary to a focal seizure (suggesting the origin of focus). Of the two, MRI is the more sensitive technique. Although these lesions may mimic those of ischemic stroke, they are reported to cross vascular territories (100). Changes in diffusion-weighted images and the apparent diffusion coefficient (ADC) may occur suggesting both cytotoxic and vasogenic edema (101). Progressive changes also occur, such as hippocampal atrophy and sclerosis, or global atrophy (102,103). In a fatal case of unexplained SE, high signal lesions in the mesial temporal lobes and hippocampal neuronal loss were reported (104). In general, neuroimaging should be performed in all patients with new-onset SE, especially if there is no prior history of epilepsy.

Intoxication with certain agents, particularly theophylline (70,72,105) and isoniazid (INH) (106), which may involve acidosis (107) and is treated with pyridoxine (vitamin B_6) (108), may predispose individuals to generalized convulsive SE or NCSE. Immunosuppressants such as cyclosporine (109) or tacrolimus, and ifosfamide (110) may predispose individuals to NCSE, which may also occur when phenytoin or carbamazepine is used in patients with idiopathic generalized epilepsy (111); lithium (112), tiagabine (113), and amoxapine (114) may also be implicated. Fatal SE has occurred with flumazenil, therefore caution should be exercised in patients with a history of seizures, chronic benzodiazepine use, or when a mixed overdose is suspected (115).

An EEG is not initially needed for treatment. Indications for emergency EEG include unexplained altered awareness (to exclude NCSE) (Fig. 38.3); the use of neuromuscular paralysis in a patient with SE; high-dose suppressive therapy for refractory SE; and no return to baseline or improvement in mental status following control of overt convulsive movements (to exclude ongoing subtle SE) (116). NCSE occurs in 14% of adults (117) and 26% of children (118) in whom generalized convulsive SE has been controlled after treatment. NCSE was detected in 8% of all comatose patients (91). Therefore, the EEG should be used when the diagnosis is in doubt, especially in patients with pseudoseizures.

ANTIEPILEPTIC DRUG THERAPY FOR STATUS EPILEPTICUS

Treatment should be aimed at controlling SE as soon as possible, particularly before brain compensatory mechanisms fail. Despite adequate oxygenation and ventilation, such failure has been reported within 30 to 60 minutes in experimental SE (50) and within 30 to 45 minutes in humans (2). Systemic and

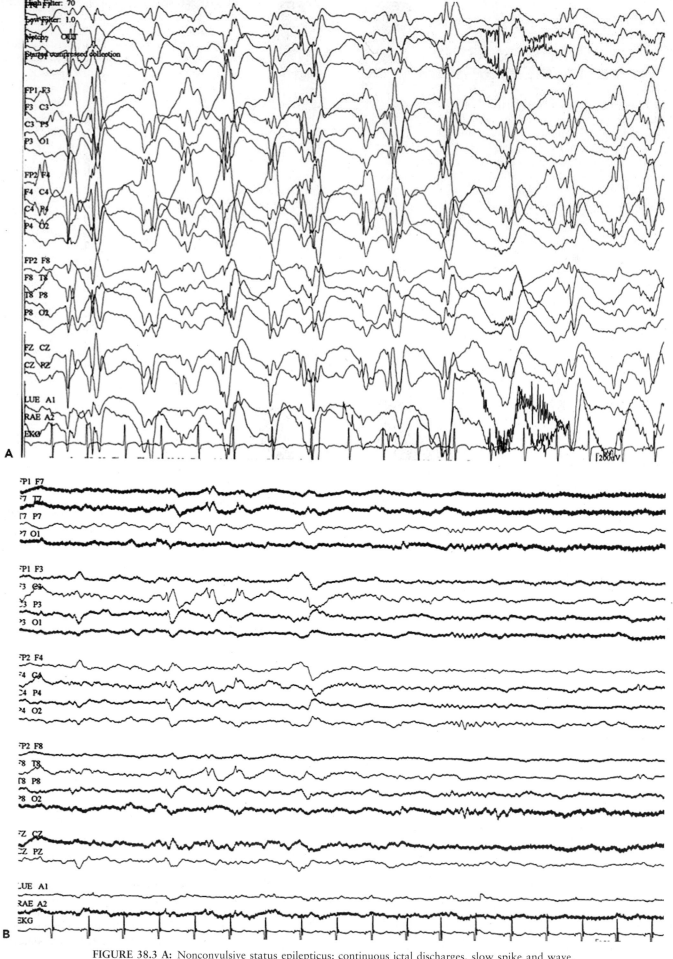

FIGURE 38.3 A: Nonconvulsive status epilepticus: continuous ictal discharges, slow spike and wave, with altered awareness. **B:** Nonconvulsive status epilepticus: electroencephalogram after lorazepam, now with improved awareness.

metabolic changes occur early, with increases in blood pressure, lactate and glucose levels. Both respiratory and metabolic acidosis may develop, although the former is more common (119). Initially, brain parenchymal oxygenation, lactate, glucose, and oxygen utilization remain stable, cerebral blood flow increases, but cerebral glucose slightly decreases. In later stages, blood pressure may be normal or decrease slightly, glucose may decrease, and hyperthermia and respiratory compromise may occur, leading to hypoxia and hypercarbia. Brain parenchymal oxygenation, cerebral blood flow, and brain glucose decrease all contribute to an energy mismatch (50). Neuron-specific enolase, a marker of brain injury, is elevated in the serum following both convulsive and NCSE (120,121).

Neuronal injury may occur in the absence of metabolic derangement. In paralyzed and ventilated baboons given bicuculline, a $GABA_A$ receptor competitive antagonist, to induce electrographic SE (48,49), neuronal loss was observed in the neocortex and hippocampus. Brain lesions following flurothyl-induced SE in the paralyzed and well-oxygenated rat include hypermetabolic infarction of the substantia nigra (122). In humans, neuronal loss was seen following SE in three patients without hypotension, hypoxemia, hypoglycemia, or hyperthermia (123).

Most of the AEDs used to treat SE have the potential for respiratory and cardiac depression, especially when administered by a loading dose (124). Therefore, protecting the airway, controlling ventilation, and monitoring cardiac and hemodynamic function are mandatory. Intravenous (IV) administration is the preferred route for the treatment of SE, especially in the inpatient setting, but if IV access is difficult, intramuscular (IM), rectal, or intranasal routes have been used. The rectal route may be useful if IV access is difficult or if concern exists regarding side effects, particularly respiratory depression. Diazepam is the most widely used rectal AED.

Primary Antiepileptic Drugs for Status Epilepticus

The benzodiazepines (e.g., lorazepam and diazepam), phenytoin or its prodrug form fosphenytoin, and phenobarbital are the current drugs of first choice for the initial therapy in patients with SE (Table 38.6). However, some advocate the early use of the secondary agents (e.g., valproic acid, levetiracetam, anesthetics).

Treatment of SE is typically initiated with a benzodiazepine. Of diazepam and lorazepam, diazepam has a more rapid onset of action because of greater lipid solubility (124), but it may need to be followed by another AED because seizure recurrence is common. This is especially true with acute symptomatic SE. In one study, only nine of 20 patients maintained seizure control for >2 hours (125), and in another study, only five of 15 patients maintained good seizure control for 24 hours (126). Because of a smaller volume of distribution, lorazepam has longer anticonvulsant activity than diazepam (127), with less respiratory depression and sedation. In addition, the rate of seizure recurrence with lorazepam is less than that with diazepam (128). Lorazepam has been used in both adults and children (129,130). In a double-blind study of lorazepam 4 mg versus diazepam 10 mg, seizures were controlled in 89% of episodes with lorazepam versus 76% with diazepam, with similar times of onset and adverse events (131). Midazolam may be administered IM if there is no IV access, and has been associated with less sedation and respiratory depression (132).

Phenytoin may be administered by an IV loading dose in normal saline (it precipitates with dextrose), at 20 mg/kg (15 mg/kg in the elderly), which rapidly achieves a therapeutic level without respiratory depression or sedation and can also provide maintenance therapy (133–135). This lack of sedation is important for monitoring mental status, such as in patients with head trauma. The infusion rate should be no faster than 1 mg/kg/min in a child (not to exceed 25 mg/min), 50 mg/min in an adult, and 20 mg/min in the elderly. Pulse and blood pressure should be monitored. If hypotension develops, the infusion rate should be decreased. In adults, a therapeutic level should be maintained for up to 24 hours after a loading dose has been administered (133), but may not last as long in children (136). A level obtained 2 hours after loading may help guide the timing of maintenance therapy with phenytoin (136).

IV phenytoin has an alkaline pH and contains solvents that can cause vascular irritation, cardiac depression, and hypotension. The purple glove syndrome, consisting of distal limb edema, discoloration, and pain, may occur following IV phenytoin infiltration; treatment may require fasciotomies and amputation. In one series, purple glove syndrome occurred in nine of 152 patients (137); in a prospective series, it occurred in only three of 179 patients (138). The syndrome has also been reported following oral dosing in a child (139).

The phosphate ester prodrug of phenytoin, fosphenytoin, is dosed as phenytoin equivalent (PE) at 20 mg PE/kg. It can be administered in a dextrose solution. Fosphenytoin is water soluble and may be given by the IM route, with paresthesias

TABLE 38.6

FIRST-LINE INTRAVENOUS ANTIEPILEPTIC DRUGS

AED	Dose	Rate	Max
Lorazepam	0.1 mg/kg	2 mg/min (2–5)	8 mg
Diazepam	0.2 mg/kg	5 mg/min	16–20 mg
Fosphenytoin	20 mg PE/kg	up to 3 mg PE/kg/min	150 mg/min (adult)
Phenytoin	20 mg/kg	up to 1 mg/kg/min	50 mg/min (adult)
			25 mg/min (child)
			20 mg/min (elderly)
Phenobarbital	20 mg/kg	1 mg/kg/min	100 mg/min (adult)
			30 mg/min (child)

and injection-site pruritus as possible adverse effects. Bioavailability is 100% compared to phenytoin, and the conversion half-life is 7 to 15 minutes (140). Fosphenytoin is rapidly converted to phenytoin by serum and tissue alkaline phosphatases (141). It may be difficult to maintain therapeutic levels in infants, and additional doses may be required (142); subtherapeutic free phenytoin levels also occur in older children (143). A 2-hour phenytoin level is suggested to ensure conversion (143). Side effects are more likely in patients with hypoalbuminemia, renal failure, or hepatic failure, and in the elderly, because of the presence of higher free phenytoin levels. In these patients; the infusion rate should be decreased by 25% to 50% (140). The only advantage of IV phenytoin over IV fosphenytoin is significantly lower cost.

Phenobarbital has been used to treat SE in all age groups. Although still considered the agent of choice for neonatal seizures, its efficacy is equivalent to that of phenytoin (144). Respiratory depression and sedation occur, and caution is advised, especially when phenobarbital is administered in combination with other sedative AEDs (such as benzodiazepines). In a randomized trial of diazepam and phenytoin versus phenobarbital (10 mg/kg IV), phenobarbital had a shorter median seizure time (5 minutes vs. 9 minutes) and response latency (5.5 minutes vs. 15 minutes), with a similar incidence of intubation, hypotension, and arrhythmia (145). The loading dose for phenobarbital is 15 to 20 mg/kg, administered at a rate no higher than 100 mg/min in older children and adults and 20 mg/kg in neonates and infants (143).

The landmark VA Cooperative Study (24) compared the efficacy of various first-line agents—lorazepam (0.1 mg/kg), phenobarbital (15 mg/kg), diazepam (0.15 mg/kg) plus phenytoin (18 mg/kg), and phenytoin alone (18 mg/kg)—in the treatment of SE with successful treatment defined as control of seizure activity within 20 minutes (25). Treatment efficacy of overt generalized convulsive SE was similar with lorazepam (65%), phenobarbital (58%), and diazepam plus phenytoin (56%), whereas phenytoin alone was associated with lower efficacy (44%). This may be related to a 4.7-minute infusion time with lorazepam versus 33 minutes with phenytoin alone.

Second-Line Agents for Status Epilepticus

Sodium valproate (VPA) has been available in IV form since 1995 (Depacon, Abbott Laboratories, North Chicago, Ill) (146). Although it is not yet approved by the U.S. Food and Drug Administration (FDA) for the treatment of SE, doses of 15 to 33 mg/kg have been administered safely in adults (147–156) at a rate of 20 to 50 mg/min (148). In a review of 13 elderly patients with SE and hypotension, a mean loading dose of 25 mg/kg at 35 mg/min was associated with no change in blood pressure (149). In one study, an infusion rate of 3 mg/kg/min was associated with hypotension in two of 72 patients (152).

Two studies have evaluated IV phenytoin versus IV VPA as first-line therapy for SE. They first used IV VPA, 30 mg/kg over 15 minutes, or IV PHT, 18 mg/kg at a rate of 50 mg/minute; if SE continued, the other AED was used (157). Used as initial therapy, SE was controlled in 66% with VPA versus 42% with PHT; in the refractory patients, VPA was effective in 79% versus 25% with PHT. The side effects were similar. In the second study (158), there was equal efficacy

(88% for both) with side effects of 12% with PHT versus none with VPA. In diazepam-resistant SE, 31/41 (76%) episodes of SE were controlled with a 25 mg/kg loading dose over 30 minutes. The probability of successful treatment with VPA was time-dependent: if the VPA was given early (within 3 hours), next-line therapy with anesthesia was required in only 5%, but when VPA was given later, anesthesia was needed in 60% (159).

In children, loading doses of 10 to 30 mg/kg have been used, with most using the higher-dose ranges; an infusion rate of 1 mg/kg/hour was not associated with serious side effects (153). A 20-mg/kg loading dose should produce a serum level of 75 mg/L (154). Valproate is safe in adults and children (147,152,156). One study reported on 48 IV VPA doses, mean 22 mg/kg (range 7.5 to 41.5 mg/kg), with a mean infusion rate of 5 mg/minute, with only one adverse event—burning at the infusion site (160). Hypotension occurred in one child at an infusion rate of 30 mg/kg/hour (0.5 mg/kg/min) (155). A loading dose of 10 to 25 mg/kg over 30 minutes has been used in neonates (161).

Levetiracetam is now available in an IV preparation and has been used to control SE, typically as second-line therapy. The pharmacokinetic profile is similar for IV and oral levetiracetam with no difference following an oral or IV dose of 500 to 1500 mg in adults (162). Levetiracetam levels peak within 2 hours, a steady state is achieved within 2 days, and there are no significant drug interactions (163). IV levetiracetam with a mean loading dose of 944 mg (range 250 to 1500 mg) controlled 16/18 episodes of SE following benzodiazepine failure (164). A 20 mg/kg loading dose followed by 15 mg/kg b.i.d, after 6 hours, controlled SE in 82% overall and in 11/12 (92%) as first-line therapy (165). A total of 2/50 (4%) developed thrombocytopenia. In nine children with acute seizure exacerbations or refractory SE, a loading dose of 10 to 30 mg/kg was given over 30 minutes, with a mean dose of 228 mg/kg/day. One child had an increase of seizures, and no agitation or behavioral problems occurred (166).

Treatment Guidelines for Status Epilepticus

Standard treatment guidelines are needed in advance for all medical emergencies in order to improve the quality of emergency care (167,168). The treatment guideline can then be analyzed, and modified, if needed. To this end, there are a few randomized clinical trials, the EFA Working Group timetable (4), treatment surveys, and various societies' treatment guidelines that can assist in this process. A survey of the United Kingdom (UK) Intensive Care Society revealed that only 12% of the respondents used a specific protocol (169), and that first-line therapy was frequently with a benzodiazepine plus phenytoin. In a United States survey of neurologists and intensivists ($N = 106$), 76% used lorazepam first, with 95% using phenobarbital or phenytoin if lorazepam failed (170). A survey of epileptologists was conducted to establish consensus guidelines for first-line, second-line, and third-line treatment options for epilepsy syndromes (171). A treatment of choice was determined if selected by >50% of respondents. Lorazepam was considered the treatment of choice for generalized convulsive, focal, and absence SE, with diazepam or phenytoin considered first-line treatment for generalized convulsive SE and focal SE;

diazepam and sodium valproate were considered first-line treatment for absence epilepsy (171).

Prior to the VA Cooperative Study, the EFA Working Group suggested either lorazepam or diazepam as first-line therapy, but now lorazepam is initially used by many (2,170,171). European guidelines have used either lorazepam or diazepam for first-line therapy. Most guidelines still use either phenytoin or phenobarbital if a benzodiazepine fails, but there is increasing use of either VPA or levetiracetam. We use 0.1 mg /kg lorazepam initially for children, at a maximum dose of 4 mg when IV access is available; if IV access is not available, diazepam or lorazepam can be administered rectally, or fosphenytoin or midazolam via the IM route. However, although there are theoretical reasons to support the use of lorazepam over diazepam (as discussed in "Primary Antiepileptic Drugs for Status Epilepticus"), a review of randomized clinical trials in children found no evidence that treatment with IV lorazepam was better than treatment with diazepam (172).

Treatment of Refractory Status Epilepticus

Refractory SE occurs when seizures persist despite adequate treatment. By this time, the airway should be protected, ventilation should be controlled with intubation, and transfer to the critical care unit should already be in progress. Such care requires a team approach among providers. The mortality in adults with refractory SE varies from 39% to 48% (173) and in children, from 16% to 43.5% (62,174,175). Etiology is a very important determinant, with a higher mortality among symptomatic patients (16,32,62,69,71). In children, our data demonstrate that etiology is related to prognosis (62).

If convulsive activity has stopped but mental status does not improve, NCSE must be excluded, which occurs in 14% of adults (117), 25% of children (118), and 8% of those with unexplained coma (91). An immediate EEG is performed, if available; if not available, additional empiric AED therapy must be considered. If SE persists for >1 hour despite adequate doses of conventional AEDs, then high-dose suppressive therapy with IV anesthetic agents should be used (Table 38.7). The treatment goal is to stop SE immediately and to prevent seizure recurrence. Pentobarbital has been the most widely used agent under these circumstances (176–182), administered at 2 to 10 mg/kg followed by a continuous infusion. Midazolam has a shorter half-life and is associated with less sedation (132,183–188). High-dose phenobarbital is also used; it is associated with less cardiovascular depression than pentobarbital (189,190) but has a longer half-life.

Other agents used include benzodiazepines (191,192), thiopental (193), lidocaine (194–196), inhalational anesthetics such as isoflurane (Forane, Baxter Pharmaceuticals, Deerfield, Ill) (197,198), and propofol (199). Propofol has two main advantages: a rapid onset and a short duration of action. One study with pentobarbital and propofol in adults showed equal efficacy, but propofol controlled SE in 2.6 minutes versus 123 minutes with pentobarbital (199). Another study in children with RSE reported an efficacy of 64% with propofol versus 55% with thiopental, and no side effects with propofol, with infusion rates less than 5 mg/kg/hour (200,201). Propofol may cause metabolic acidosis with prolonged use in children (202,203). In adults, deaths have

TABLE 38.7

AGENTS USED IN REFRACTORY STATUS EPILEPTICUS

Intravenous
  Pentobarbital
  Midazolam
  Thiopental
  Propofol
  Phenobarbital
  Diazepam
  Lorazepam
  Ketamine
  Lidocaine
  Chlormethizaole
  Etomidate
  Magnesium (especially for eclampsia)
Rectal
  Paraldehyde
  Chloral hydrate
Other
  Hypothermia, with pentobarbital
  Inhalational agents, especially isoflurane
  Vagus Nerve Stimulation (VNS)

occurred with high propofol infusion rates (204); this is known as propofol infusion syndrome (205). Even in an adult study that showed equal efficacy for seizure control, a 57% mortality rate was reported with propofol, versus only 17% with midazolam (183). Therefore, propofol should be used with caution, especially in children and ideally for a short time only, and the infusion rate should not exceed 67 μg/kg/min (206). Immediate control can be achieved and then another agent used if long-term suppression is needed. Ketamine may be of value, since it is potentially a neuroprotective agent (207–209). Chlormethiazole (210), etomidate (211), and clonazepam (212) are used in Europe; paraldehyde (213) and chloral hydrate (214) may be administered rectally, although paraldehyde is no longer available in the United States. Hypothermia (215) and vagus nerve stimulation (216) have also been used.

To date, no prospective study has been conducted in patients with refractory SE. In a systematic review of refractory SE treatment with pentobarbital, propofol, or midazolam (217), pentobarbital was associated with better seizure control than the other two agents. In the UK survey (N = 408), if first-line treatment failed, 142 (35%) of the respondents used a benzodiazepine infusion and 130 (32%) used a general anesthetic. If seizures continued, 333 (82%) used thiopentone and 56 (14%) used propofol (169). Based on the consensus guidelines, the drug of choice for "therapeutic coma" in patients with generalized convulsive SE and focal SE was pentobarbital, and first-line agents were midazolam and propofol; for absence seizures, pentobarbital was the drug of choice, with no other first-line options, and midazolam was considered second-line therapy (171). In the US survey, when generalized convulsive SE was refractory to two AEDs, 43% of respondents used phenobarbital, 16% used valproate, and 19% gave one of three agents (pentobarbital, midazolam, or propofol) by continuous infusion (170).

The goal is to control refractory SE and prevent seizure recurrence. Typically, seizures are controlled within 1 hour of beginning a continuous infusion (217). A systematic review (217) defined the following responses to treatment when seizures were not controlled: immediate (acute) treatment failure (clinical or electrographic seizures from 60 minutes to 6 hours after the initial loading dose), breakthrough seizures (any clinical or EEG seizure after the first 6 hours), withdrawal seizures (seizures occurring within 48 hours of discontinuing or tapering treatment), or changed therapy (switched AED because of poor seizure control).

Whether clinical seizures alone or both clinical and electrographic seizures need complete control is controversial (218,219). In this situation, many clinicians use high-dose suppressive therapy with a burst-suppression pattern on EEG, aiming for complete control of both the clinical and electrographic seizures. Some aim only for control of clinical seizures (without EEG monitoring). In the US survey, the titration goal with a continuous infusion was burst suppression in 56% of respondents versus elimination of seizures in 41% (170), whereas in a European survey, up to 70% titrated the EEG to a burst-suppression pattern (220). However, the outcome is not related to the extent of EEG burst suppression and is more dependent on etiology (221).

Even if a burst-suppression pattern is the goal, the degree of suppression needed is unclear. We have used a burst-suppression pattern as the clinical end point, aiming for an interburst interval of at least 5 seconds in duration (62,222). In an analysis of the depth of EEG suppression with barbiturate anesthetics (pentobarbital or thiopental) in adults, persistent seizure control was better with electrocerebral inactivity on EEG (17 of 20) versus a burst-suppression pattern (six of 12 patients) (223,224). Using a midazolam infusion to eliminate all clinical and electrographic seizures and reaching burst suppression only if needed, acute treatment failure occurred in 18% of episodes, breakthrough seizures in 56%, and post treatment seizures in 68% (187). In the systematic review, breakthrough seizures occurred less frequently with titration to EEG background suppression (53%) versus titration to seizure suppression only (4%). However, hypotension occurred more often with titration to background suppression (217).

Prolonged high-dose suppressive therapy can be used (62,225), usually with various AED combinations. High-dose suppressive therapy is used initially for a short time (12 to 24 hours); the infusion is then tapered, and if SE recurs, the sequence restarts (51,62,222). Mirski and colleagues recommended prolonged therapy with a potentially good prognosis: a healthy patient (no premorbid illness), a self-limited disease, and with neuroimaging not indicating a poor prognosis (226). Bramstedt and colleagues (227) recommended ethically with-holding suppressive therapy if only expected to sustain organic life. We have treated children for prolonged periods of up to 146 days (62,225) and a 26-year-old with encephalitis was treated for 11 months (228). In our experience with children, no survivor of acute symptomatic refractory SE (*n* = 7) returned to baseline, and all subsequently developed refractory epilepsy; seizure recurrence was reported upon drug tapering in two children, and within 1 to 16 months in the other five (225). In our entire group with refractory SE, 32% returned to baseline (62), and in the adult systematic review, only 29% (48 of 164 patients) returned to baseline (217).

Infectious or inflammatory disorders appear to predispose to refractory SE. In our series, 7/22 had "presumed encephalitis" (62,225). Kramer also reported severe RSE from "presumed encephalitis" (229). Holtkamp reported encephalitis as a predictor for RSE (230) and referred to this as a "malignant variant" (231), and Wilder–Smith defined the syndrome of New Onset Refractory Status Epilepticus (232). Characteristic features include female gender, young age, previous good health, CSF pleocytosis, antecedent febrile illness, and prolonged treatment (32 day average). We reported complete seizure control during suppression in 5/7 in this group, with then a seizure recurrence and the development of refractory epilepsy ranging from 1 to 16 months later (225). The occurrence of this latent period raises the question if either neuroprotective, anti-epileptic, or even immunomodulatory agents might be helpful in this situation.

Several specific repetitive disorders have been reported in SE: stimulus-induced rhythmic, periodic, or ictal discharges (SIRPIDS) (233) and cycling seizures (234). Acute encephalitis with refractory, repetitive partial seizures has been described in children with encephalitis (235,236). These have an abrupt onset in the setting of a fever following an antecedent infection, are brief, focal seizures, occur with an escalating frequency, and are resistant to standard anticonvulsants and require high-dose suppressive therapy for control.

Prehospital Treatment

Since the advent of intrarectally administered AEDs, the premonitory or early stage can now be treated (237–239), although other routes of administration are also used. The prospective San Francisco Prehospital Treatment study (*N* = 205) showed lorazepam was more effective than diazepam in terminating SE (59% response with lorazepam vs. 43% response with diazepam, and 21% response with placebo; *P* = 0.001) (25). In a retrospective study of 38 children with generalized convulsive SE, use of prehospital diazepam (0.6 mg rectally) was associated with a shorter seizure duration (32 minutes vs. 60 minutes) and a reduced likelihood of seizure recurrence in the emergency department (58% vs. 85%), with no difference with respect to intubation (240). Rectal diazepam can be administered at home for the treatment of SE or serial seizures; the maximum dose is 20 mg. A rectal gel preparation, Diastat (Valeant Pharmaceuticals, Also Viejo, CA), is available, which is easier to administer (241–243). Although only approved by the FDA for the treatment of selected, refractory, patients on stable regimens of AEDs for the treatment of seizure exacerbation, Diastat is used as a therapeutic remedy for SE at home. IV benzodiazepines are still preferable for the treatment of inpatients. Lorazepam can be administered sublingually (244) and midazolam can be given by intranasal or buccal mucosa routes (245), with rapid buccal absorption documented by serum levels and EEG beta activity (246). The efficacy of intranasal midazolam (0.2 mg/kg) is equivalent to that of IV diazepam (0.3 mg/kg) for the treatment of prolonged febrile seizures (247), and buccal midazolam (10 mg) and rectal diazepam (10 mg) have shown equal efficacy for seizures >5 minutes (245). Paraldehyde is included in a UK pediatric treatment protocol (168), but as previously noted, it is no longer available in the United States.

TABLE 38.8

A SUGGESTED TIMETABLE FOR THE TREATMENT OF STATUS EPILEPTICUS

Time (min)	Action
0–5	Diagnose status epilepticus by observing continuing seizure activity
	Give oxygen by nasal cannula or mask; position head for optimal airway patency
	Obtain vital signs and pulse oximetry
	Establish IV line; draw venous blood samples for glucose level, serum chemistries, hematology studies, toxicology screens, and AED levels (if applicable).
	If hypoglycemia is established, or blood glucose measurement not available, administer glucose; in adults, give thiamine first (100 mg), followed by 50 mL of 50% glucose by direct push into IV line; in children, give 2 mL/kg of 25% glucose
5	If seizure continues, give lorazepam 0.1 mg/kg, at 2 mg/min
10–20	If seizure continues, give fosphenytoin 20 mg PE/kg, or if not available, phenytoin 20 mg/kg (in children, give a second dose of lorazepam 0.1 mg/kg, before giving fosphenytoin or phenytoin)
20	Give phenobarbital 20 mg/kg
30	Give additional fosphenytoin 10 mg PE/kg
40	IV valproate 40 mg/kg
40–60	Intravenous anesthesia: pentobarbital 5 to 15 mg/kg loading dose midazolam 0.2 mg/kg loading dose propofol 1–2 mg/kg loading dose thiopental 5 mg/kg all followed by intravenous infusions

AED, antiepileptic drug.
Modified from Refs. 2, 3, and 250.

Emergency Department or Inpatient Treatment

Lorazepam 0.1 mg/kg should be administered initially. A suggested treatment sequence follows, as outlined in Table 38.8 (248–250).

References

1. Gastaut H. Classification of status epilepticus. *Adv Neurol.* 1983;34:15–35.
2. Lowenstein DH, Alldredge BK. Status epilepticus. *N Engl J Med.* 1998;338:970–976.
3. Delgado-Escueta AV, Wasterlain C, Treiman DM, et al. Current concepts in neurology: management of status epilepticus. *N Engl J Med.* 1982;306:1337–1340.
4. Treatment of Convulsive Status Epilepticus. Recommendations of the Epilepsy Foundation of America's Working Group on Status Epilepticus. *J Am Med Assoc.* 1993;270:854–859.
5. Lowenstein DH, Bleck T, Macdonald RL. It's time to revise the definition of status epilepticus. *Epilepsia.* 1999;40:120–122.
6. Arnautova EN, Nesmeianova TN. A Proposed international classification of epileptic seizures. *Epilepsia.* 1964;5:297–306.
7. Gastaut H. Clinical and electroencephalographical classification of epileptic seizures. *Epilepsia.* 1970;11:102–113.
8. Proposal for Revised Clinical and Electroencephalographic Classification of Epileptic Seizures. From the commission on classification and terminology of the international league against epilepsy. *Epilepsia.* 1981;22:489–501.
9. Proposal for Classification of Epilepsies and Epileptic Syndromes. Commission on classification and terminology of the international league against epilepsy. *Epilepsia.* 1985;26:268–278.
10. Proposal for Revised Classification of Epilepsies and Epileptic Syndromes. Commission on classification and terminology of the international league against epilepsy. *Epilepsia.* 1989;30:389–399.
11. Engel J Jr. A proposed diagnostic scheme for people with epileptic seizures and with epilepsy: report of the ILAE Task Force on Classification and Terminology. *Epilepsia.* 2001;42:796–803.
12. Rona S, Rosenow F, Arnold S, et al. A semiological classification of status epilepticus. *Epileptic Disord.* 2005;7:5–12.
13. Treiman DM, Delgado-Escueta AV. Status epilepticus. In: Thompson RA, Green RA, Green JR, eds. *Critical Care of Neurological and Neurosurgical Emergencies.* New York: Raven Press; 1980:53–99.
14. Scholtes FB, Renier WO, Meinardi H. Non-convulsive status epilepticus: causes, treatment, and outcome in 65 patients. *J Neurol Neurosurg Psychiatry.* 1996;61:93–95.
15. Scholtes FB, Renier WO, Meinardi H. Simple partial status epilepticus: causes, treatment, and outcome in 47 patients. *J Neurol Neurosurg Psychiatry.* 1996;61:90–92.
16. Scholtes FB, Renier WO, Meinardi H. Generalized convulsive status epilepticus: causes, therapy, and outcome in 346 patients. *Epilepsia.* 1994;35:1104–1112.
17. Pakalnis A, Drake ME Jr, Phillips B. Neuropsychiatric aspects of psychogenic status epilepticus. *Neurology.* 1991;41:1104–1106.
18. Tuxhorn IE, Fischbach HS. Pseudostatus epilepticus in childhood. *Pediatr Neurol.* 2002;27:407–409.
19. Pakalnis A, Paolicchi J, Gilles E. Psychogenic status epilepticus in children: psychiatric and other risk factors. *Neurology.* 2000;54:969–970.
20. Savard G, Andermann F, Teitelbaum J, et al. Epileptic Munchausen's syndrome: a form of pseudoseizures distinct from hysteria and malingering. *Neurology.* 1988;38:1628–1629.
21. Shorvon S. *Status Epilepticus: Its Clinical Features and Treatment in Children and Adults.* New York: Cambridge University Press; 1994.
22. Treiman DM, Walton NY, Kendrick C. A progressive sequence of electroencephalographic changes during generalized convulsive status epilepticus. *Epilepsy Res.* 1990;5:49–60.
23. Lowenstein DH, Aminoff MJ. Clinical and EEG features of status epilepticus in comatose patients. *Neurology.* 1992;42:100–104.
24. Treiman DM, Meyers PD, Walton NY, et al. A comparison of four treatments for generalized convulsive status epilepticus. Veterans Affairs Status Epilepticus Cooperative Study Group. *N Engl J Med.* 1998;339:792–798.
25. Alldredge BK, Gelb AM, Isaacs SM, et al. A comparison of lorazepam, diazepam, and placebo for the treatment of out-of-hospital status epilepticus. *N Engl J Med.* 2001;345:631–637.
26. Beran RG. An alternative perspective on the management of status epilepticus. *Epilepsy Behav.* 2008;12:349–353.
27. Riviello JJ Jr, Holmes GL. The treatment of status epilepticus. *Semin Pediatr Neurol.* 2004;11:129–138.
28. Gastaut H, Broughton R. *Epileptic Seizures: Clinical and Electrographic Features, Diagnosis, and Treatment.* Springfield, IL: Charles C. Thomas; 1972.
29. Theodore WH, Porter RJ, Albert P, et al. The secondarily generalized tonic-clonic seizure: a videotape analysis. *Neurology.* 1994;44:1403–1407.
30. Holmes GL. Partial complex seizures in children: an analysis of 69 seizures in 24 patients using EEG FM radiotelemetry and videotape recording. *Electroencephalogr Clin Neurophysiol.* 1984;57:13–20.
31. Shinnar S, Berg AT, Moshe SL, et al. How long do new-onset seizures in children last? *Ann Neurol.* 2001;49:659–664.
32. Mayer SA, Claassen J, Lokin J, et al. Refractory status epilepticus: frequency, risk factors, and impact on outcome. *Arch Neurol.* 2002;59:205–210.

33. Walton NY, Treiman DM. Response of status epilepticus induced by lithium and pilocarpine to treatment with diazepam. *Exp Neurol.* 1988; 101:267–275.

34. Mazarati AM, Baldwin RA, Sankar R, et al. Time-dependent decrease in the effectiveness of antiepileptic drugs during the course of self-sustaining status epilepticus. *Brain Res.* 1998;814:179–185.

35. Kapur J, Macdonald RL. Rapid seizure-induced reduction of benzodiazepine and Zn²⁺ sensitivity of hippocampal dentate granule cell GABAA receptors. *J Neurosci.* 1997;17:7532–7540.

36. Jones DM, Esmaeil N, Maren S, et al. Characterization of pharmacoresistance to benzodiazepines in the rat Li-pilocarpine model of status epilepticus. *Epilepsy Res.* 2002;50:301–312.

37. Goodkin HP, Liu X, Holmes GL. Diazepam terminates brief but not prolonged seizures in young, naive rats. *Epilepsia.* 2003;44:1109–1112.

38. Goodkin HP, Joshi S, Mtchedlishvili Z, et al. Subunit-specific trafficking of GABA(A) receptors during status epilepticus. *J Neurosci.* 2008;28: 2527–2538.

39. Goodkin HP, Yeh JL, Kapur J. Status epilepticus increases the intracellular accumulation of GABAA receptors. *J Neurosci.* 2005;25:5511–5520.

40. Naylor DE, Liu H, Wasterlain CG. Trafficking of GABA(A) receptors, loss of inhibition, and a mechanism for pharmacoresistance in status epilepticus. *J Neurosci.* 2005;25:7724–7733.

41. Terunuma M, Xu J, Vithlani M, et al. Deficits in phosphorylation of GABA(A) receptors by intimately associated protein kinase C activity underlie compromised synaptic inhibition during status epilepticus. *J Neurosci.* 2008;28:376–384.

42. Meldrum BS. The revised operational definition of generalised tonic-clonic (TC) status epilepticus in adults. *Epilepsia.* 1999;40:123–124.

43. Kapur J, Coulter DA. Experimental status epilepticus alters gamma-aminobutyric acid type A receptor function in CA1 pyramidal neurons. *Ann Neurol.* 1995;38:893–900.

44. Lothman EW, Collins RC, Ferrendelli JA. Kainic acid-induced limbic seizures: electrophysiologic studies. *Neurology.* 1981;31:806–812.

45. Perl TM, Bedard L, Kosatsky T, et al. An outbreak of toxic encephalopathy caused by eating mussels contaminated with domoic acid. *N Engl J Med.* 1990;322:1775–1780.

46. Teitelbaum JS, Zatorre RJ, Carpenter S, et al. Neurologic sequelae of domoic acid intoxication due to the ingestion of contaminated mussels. *N Engl J Med.* 1990;322:1781–1787.

47. Cendes F, Andermann F, Carpenter S, et al. Temporal lobe epilepsy caused by domoic acid intoxication: evidence for glutamate receptor-mediated excitotoxicity in humans. *Ann Neurol.* 1995;37:123–126.

48. Meldrum BS. Metabolic factors during prolonged seizures and their relation to nerve cell death. *Adv Neurol.* 1983;34:261–275.

49. Meldrum BS, Brierley JB. Prolonged epileptic seizures in primates. Ischemic cell change and its relation to ictal physiological events. *Arch Neurol.* 1973;28:10–17.

50. Lothman E. The biochemical basis and pathophysiology of status epilepticus. *Neurology.* 1990;40:13–23.

51. DeLorenzo RJ, Hauser WA, Towne AR, et al. A prospective, population-based epidemiologic study of status epilepticus in Richmond, Virginia. *Neurology.* 1996;46:1029–1035.

52. Hesdorffer DC, Logroscino G, Cascino G, et al. Incidence of status epilepticus in Rochester, Minnesota, 1965–1984. *Neurology.* 1998;50:735–741.

53. Hauser WA. Status epilepticus: epidemiologic considerations. *Neurology.* 1990;40:9–13.

54. Wu YW, Shek DW, Garcia PA, et al. Incidence and mortality of generalized convulsive status epilepticus in California. *Neurology.* 2002;58: 1070–1076.

55. Coeytaux A, Jallon P, Galobardes B, et al. Incidence of status epilepticus in French-speaking Switzerland (EPISTAR). *Neurology.* 2000;55: 693–697.

56. Knake S, Rosenow F, Vescovi M, et al. Incidence of status epilepticus in adults in Germany: a prospective, population-based study. *Epilepsia.* 2001;42:714–718.

57. Vignatelli L, Tonon C, D'Alessandro R. Incidence and short-term prognosis of status epilepticus in adults in Bologna, Italy. *Epilepsia.* 2003;44: 964–968.

58. Shinnar S, Pellock JM, Moshe SL, et al. In whom does status epilepticus occur: age-related differences in children. *Epilepsia.* 1997;38:907–914.

59. Chin RF, Neville BG, Peckham C, et al. Incidence, cause, and short-term outcome of convulsive status epilepticus in childhood: prospective population-based study. *Lancet.* 2006;368:222–229.

60. Sillanpaa M, Shinnar S. Status epilepticus in a population-based cohort with childhood-onset epilepsy in Finland. *Ann Neurol.* 2002;52:303–310.

61. Shinnar S, Maytal J, Krasnoff L, et al. Recurrent status epilepticus in children. *Ann Neurol.* 1992;31:598–604.

62. Sahin M, Menache CC, Holmes GL, et al. Outcome of severe refractory status epilepticus in children. *Epilepsia.* 2001;42:1461–1467.

63. Lowenstein DH, Alldredge BK. Status epilepticus at an urban public hospital in the 1980s. *Neurology.* 1993;43:483–488.

64. Rowan AJ, Scott DF. Major status epilepticus. A series of 42 patients. *Acta Neurol Scand.* 1970;46:573–584.

65. Oxbury JM, Whitty CW. Causes and consequences of status epilepticus in adults. A study of 86 cases. *Brain.* 1971;94:733–744.

66. Aminoff MJ, Simon RP. Status epilepticus. Causes, clinical features and consequences in 98 patients. *Am J Med.* 1980;69:657–666.

67. DeLorenzo RJ, Towne AR, Pellock JM, et al. Status epilepticus in children, adults, and the elderly. *Epilepsia.* 1992;33(suppl 4):S15–S25.

68. Aicardi J, Chevrie JJ. Convulsive status epilepticus in infants and children. A study of 239 cases. *Epilepsia.* 1970;11:187–197.

69. Barry E, Hauser WA. Status epilepticus: the interaction of epilepsy and acute brain disease. *Neurology.* 1993;43:1473–1478.

70. Dunn DW. Status epilepticus in children: etiology, clinical features, and outcome. *J Child Neurol.* 1988;3:167–173.

71. Claassen J, Lokin JK, Fitzsimmons BF, et al. Predictors of functional disability and mortality after status epilepticus. *Neurology.* 2002;58:139–142.

72. Delanty N, French JA, Labar DR, et al. Status epilepticus arising de novo in hospitalized patients: an analysis of 41 patients. *Seizure.* 2001;10: 116–119.

73. Logroscino G, Hesdorffer DC, Cascino GD, et al. Long-term mortality after a first episode of status epilepticus. *Neurology.* 2002;58:537–541.

74. Logroscino G, Hesdorffer DC, Cascino G, et al. Time trends in incidence, mortality, and case-fatality after first episode of status epilepticus. *Epilepsia.* 2001;42:1031–1035.

75. Logroscino G, Hesdorffer DC, Cascino G, et al. Short-term mortality after a first episode of status epilepticus. *Epilepsia.* 1997;38:1344–1349.

76. Towne AR, Pellock JM, Ko D, et al. Determinants of mortality in status epilepticus. *Epilepsia.* 1994;35:27–34.

77. Maytal J, Shinnar S, Moshe SL, et al. Low morbidity and mortality of status epilepticus in children. *Pediatrics.* 1989;83:323–331.

78. Yager JY, Cheang M, Seshia SS. Status epilepticus in children. *Can J Neurol Sci.* 1988;15:402–405.

79. Eriksson KJ, Koivikko MJ. Status epilepticus in children: aetiology, treatment, and outcome. *Dev Med Child Neurol.*, 1997;39:652–658.

80. Phillips SA, Shanahan RJ. Etiology and mortality of status epilepticus in children. A recent update. *Arch Neurol.* 1989;46:74–76.

81. Fujiwara T, Ishida S, Miyakoshi M, et al. Status epilepticus in childhood: a retrospective study of initial convulsive status and subsequent epilepsies. *Folia Psychiatr Neurol Jpn.* 1979;33:337–344.

82. Vigevano F, DiPauua M, Fusco C, et al. Status epilepticus in infancy and childhood. *Pediatr Neurosci.* 1985;1:101–112.

83. Morton LD, Garnett LK, Towne AR, et al. Mortality of status epilepticus in the first year of life. *Epilepsia.* 2001;42:165.

84. Barnard C, Wirrell E. Does status epilepticus in children cause developmental deterioration and exacerbation of epilepsy? *J Child Neurol.* 1999; 14:787–794.

85. van Esch A, Ramlal IR, van Steensel-Moll HA, et al. Outcome after febrile status epilepticus. *Dev Med Child Neurol.* 1996;38:19–24.

86. Krumholz A, Sung GY, Fisher RS, et al. Complex partial status epilepticus accompanied by serious morbidity and mortality. *Neurology.* 1995;45: 1499–1504.

87. Krumholz A. Epidemiology and evidence for morbidity of nonconvulsive status epilepticus. *J Clin Neurophysiol.* 1999;16:314–322.

88. Jordan KG. Nonconvulsive status epilepticus in acute brain injury. *J Clin Neurophysiol.* 1999;16:332–340.

89. Drislane FW. Evidence against permanent neurologic damage from nonconvulsive status epilepticus. *J Clin Neurophysiol.* 1999;16:323–331.

90. Krumholz A, Stern BJ, Weiss HD. Outcome from coma after cardiopulmonary resuscitation: relation to seizures and myoclonus. *Neurology.* 1988;38:401–405.

91. Towne AR, Waterhouse EJ, Boggs JG, et al. Prevalence of nonconvulsive status epilepticus in comatose patients. *Neurology.* 2000;54:340–345.

92. Nei M, Lee JM, Shanker VL, et al. The EEG and prognosis in status epilepticus. *Epilepsia.* 1999;40:157–163.

93. Jaitly R, Sgro JA, Towne AR, et al. Prognostic value of EEG monitoring after status epilepticus: a prospective adult study. *J Clin Neurophysiol.* 1997;14:326–334.

94. Schmidley JW, Simon RP. Postictal pleocytosis. *Ann Neurol.* 1981;9: 81–84.

95. Barry E, Hauser WA. Pleocytosis after status epilepticus. *Arch Neurol.* 1994;51:190–193.

96. Maytal J, Novak G, Ascher C, et al. Status epilepticus in children with epilepsy: the role of antiepileptic drug levels in prevention. *Pediatrics.* 1996;98:1119–1121.

97. Barry E, Hauser WA. Status epilepticus and antiepileptic medication levels. *Neurology.* 1994;44:47–50.

98. Riviello JJ Jr, Ashwal S, Hirtz D, et al. Practice parameter: diagnostic assessment of the child with status epilepticus (an evidence-based review): report of the Quality Standards Subcommittee of the American Academy of Neurology and the Practice Committee of the Child Neurology Society. *Neurology.* 2006;67:1542–1550.

99. Kramer RE, Luders H, Lesser RP, et al. Transient focal abnormalities of neuroimaging studies during focal status epilepticus. *Epilepsia.* 1987;28: 528–532.

100. Lansberg MG, O'Brien MW, Norbash AM, et al. MRI abnormalities associated with partial status epilepticus. *Neurology.* 1999;52:1021–1027.

101. Senn P, Lovblad KO, Zutter D, et al. Changes on diffusion-weighted MRI with focal motor status epilepticus: case report. *Neuroradiology.* 2003; 45:246–249.

102. Perez ER, Maeder P, Villemure KM, et al. Acquired hippocampal damage after temporal lobe seizures in 2 infants. *Ann Neurol.* 2000;48:384–387.

103. Scott RC, Gadian DG, King MD, et al. Magnetic resonance imaging findings within 5 days of status epilepticus in childhood. *Brain.* 2002;125:1951–1959.

104. Nixon J, Bateman D, Moss T. An MRI and neuropathological study of a case of fatal status epilepticus. *Seizure.* 2001;10:588–591.

105. Itoh Y, Nagaki S, Kuyama N, et al. A case of acute theophylline intoxication with repeated status convulsivus. *Brain Dev.* 1999;31:559–564.

106. Caksen H, Odabas D, Erol M, et al. Do not overlook acute isoniazid poisoning in children with status epilepticus. *J Child Neurol.* 2003;18:142–143.

107. Hankins DG, Saxena K, Faville RJ Jr, et al. Profound acidosis caused by isoniazid ingestion. *Am J Emerg Med.* 1987;5:165–166.

108. Wason S, Lacouture PG, Lovejoy FH Jr. Single high-dose pyridoxine treatment for isoniazid overdose. *J Am Med Assoc.* 1981;246:1102–1104.

109. Gleeson JG, duPlessis AJ, Barnes PD, et al. Cyclosporin A acute encephalopathy and seizure syndrome in childhood: clinical features and risk of seizure recurrence. *J Child Neurol.* 1998;13:336–344.

110. Primavera A, Audenino D, Cocito L. Ifosfamide encephalopathy and nonconvulsive status epilepticus. *Can J Neurol Sci.* 2002;29:180–183.

111. Osorio I, Reed RC, Peltzer JN. Refractory idiopathic absence status epilepticus: A probable paradoxical effect of phenytoin and carbamazepine. *Epilepsia.* 2000;41:887–894.

112. Gansaeuer M, Alsaadi TM. Lithium intoxication mimicking clinical and electrographic features of status epilepticus: a case report and review of the literature. *Clin Electroencephalogr.* 2003;34:28–31.

113. Ostrovskiy D, Spanaki MV, Morris GL, III. Tiagabine overdose can induce convulsive status epilepticus. *Epilepsia.* 2002;43:773–774.

114. Litovitz TL, Troutman WG. Amoxapine overdose. Seizures and fatalities. *J Am Med Assoc.* 1983;250:1069–1071.

115. Haverkos GP, DiSalvo RP, Imhoff TE. Fatal seizures after flumazenil administration in a patient with mixed overdose. *Ann Pharmacother.* 1994;28:1347–1349.

116. Privitera MD, Strawsburg RH. Electroencephalographic monitoring in the emergency department. *Emerg Med Clin North Am.* 1994;12:1089–1100.

117. DeLorenzo RJ, Waterhouse EJ, Towne AR, et al. Persistent nonconvulsive status epilepticus after the control of convulsive status epilepticus. *Epilepsia.* 1998;39:833–840.

118. Tay SK, Hirsch LJ, Leary L, et al. Nonconvulsive status epilepticus in children: clinical and EEG characteristics. *Epilepsia.* 2006;47:1504–1509.

119. Wijdicks EF, Hubmayr RD. Acute acid-base disorders associated with status epilepticus. *Mayo Clin Proc.* 1994;69:1044–1046.

120. DeGiorgio CM, Correale JD, Gott PS, et al. Serum neuron-specific enolase in human status epilepticus. *Neurology.* 1995;45:1134–1137.

121. Rabinowicz AL, Correale JD, Bracht KA, et al. Neuron-specific enolase is increased after nonconvulsive status epilepticus. *Epilepsia.* 1995;36:475–479.

122. Nevander G, Ingvar M, Auer R, et al. Status epilepticus in well-oxygenated rats causes neuronal necrosis. *Ann Neurol.* 1985;18:281–290.

123. Fujikawa DG, Itabashi HH, Wu A, et al. Status epilepticus-induced neuronal loss in humans without systemic complications or epilepsy. *Epilepsia.* 2000;41:981–991.

124. Browne TR. The pharmacokinetics of agents used to treat status epilepticus. *Neurology.* 1990;40:28–32.

125. Prensky AL, Raff MC, Moore MJ, et al. Intravenous diazepam in the treatment of prolonged seizure activity. *N Engl J Med.* 1967;276:779–784.

126. Sawyer GT, Webster DD, Schut LJ. Treatment of uncontrolled seizure activity with diazepam. *J Am Med Assoc.* 1968;203:913–918.

127. Treiman DM. The role of benzodiazepines in the management of status epilepticus. *Neurology.* 1990;40:32–42.

128. Cock HR, Schapira AH. A comparison of lorazepam and diazepam as initial therapy in convulsive status epilepticus. *Quart J Med.* 2002;95:225–231.

129. Walker JE, Homan RW, Vasko MR, et al. Lorazepam in status epilepticus. *Ann Neurol.* 1979;6:207–213.

130. Lacey DJ, Singer WD, Horwitz SJ, et al. Lorazepam therapy of status epilepticus in children and adolescents. *J Pediatr.* 1986;108:771–774.

131. Leppik IE, Derivan AT, Homan RW, et al. Double-blind study of lorazepam and diazepam in status epilepticus. *J Am Med Assoc.* 1983;249:1452–1454.

132. Kumar A, Bleck TP. Intravenous midazolam for the treatment of refractory status epilepticus. *Crit Care Med.* 1992;20:483–488.

133. Cranford RE, Leppik IE, Patrick B, et al. Intravenous phenytoin: clinical and pharmacokinetic aspects. *Neurology.* 1978;28:874–880.

134. Cloyd JC, Gumnit RJ, McLain LW Jr. Status epilepticus. The role of intravenous phenytoin. *J Am Med Assoc.* 1980;244:1479–1481.

135. Salem RB, Wilder BJ, Yost RL, et al. Rapid infusion of phenytoin sodium loading doses. *Am J Hosp Pharm.* 1981;38:354–357.

136. Riviello JJ, Jr, Roe EJ, Jr, Sapin JI, et al. Timing of maintenance phenytoin therapy after intravenous loading dose. *Pediatr Neurol.* 1991;7:262–265.

137. O'Brien TJ, Cascino GD, So EL, et al. Incidence and clinical consequence of the purple glove syndrome in patients receiving intravenous phenytoin. *Neurology.* 1998;51:1034–1039.

138. Burneo JG, Anandan JV, Barkley GL. A prospective study of the incidence of the purple glove syndrome. *Epilepsia.* 2001;42:1156–1159.

139. Yoshikawa H, Abe T, Oda Y. Purple glove syndrome caused by oral administration of phenytoin. *J Child Neurol.* 2000;15:762.

140. Fischer JH, Patel TV, Fischer PA. Fosphenytoin: clinical pharmacokinetics and comparative advantages in the acute treatment of seizures. *Clin Pharmacokinet.* 2003;42:33–58.

141. Browne TR. Fosphenytoin (Cerebyx). *Clin Neuropharmacol.* 1997;20:1–12.

142. Takeoka M, Krishnamoorthy KS, Soman TB, et al. Fosphenytoin in infants. *J Child Neurol.* 1998;13:537–540.

143. Koul R, Deleu D. Subtherapeutic free phenytoin levels following fosphenytoin therapy in status epilepticus. *Neurology.* 2002;58:147–148.

144. Painter MJ, Scher MS, Stein AD, et al. Phenobarbital compared with phenytoin for the treatment of neonatal seizures. *N Engl J Med.* 1999;341:485–489.

145. Shaner DM, McCurdy SA, Herring MO, et al. Treatment of status epilepticus: a prospective comparison of diazepam and phenytoin versus phenobarbital and optional phenytoin. *Neurology.* 1988;38:202–207.

146. Devinsky O, Leppik I, Willmore LJ, et al. Safety of intravenous valproate. *Ann Neurol.* 1995;38:670–674.

147. Venkataraman V, Wheless JW. Safety of rapid intravenous infusion of valproate loading doses in epilepsy patients. *Epilepsy Res.* 1999;35:147–153.

148. Naritoku DK, Mueed S. Intravenous loading of valproate for epilepsy. *Clin Neuropharmacol.* 1999;22:102–106.

149. Sinha S, Naritoku DK. Intravenous valproate is well tolerated in unstable patients with status epilepticus. *Neurology.* 2000;55:722–724.

150. Chez MG, Hammer MS, Loeffel M, et al. Clinical experience of three pediatric and one adult case of spike-and-wave status epilepticus treated with injectable valproic acid. *J Child Neurol.* 1999;14:239–242.

151. Kaplan PW. Intravenous valproate treatment of generalized nonconvulsive status epilepticus. *Clin Electroencephalogr.* 1999;30:1–4.

152. Ramsay RE, Cantrell D, Collins SD, et al. Safety and tolerance of rapidly infused Depacon. A randomized trial in subjects with epilepsy. *Epilepsy Res.* 2003;52:189–201.

153. Campistol J, Fernandez A, Ortega J. Status epilepticus in children. Experience with intravenous valproate. Update of treatment guidelines. *Rev Neurol.* 1999;29:359–365.

154. Hovinga CA, Chicella MF, Rose DF, et al. Use of intravenous valproate in three pediatric patients with nonconvulsive or convulsive status epilepticus. *Ann Pharmacother.* 1999;33:579–584.

155. White JR, Santos CS. Intravenous valproate associated with significant hypotension in the treatment of status epilepticus. *J Child Neurol.* 1999;14:822–823.

156. Yu KT, Mills S, Thompson N, et al. Safety and efficacy of intravenous valproate in pediatric status epilepticus and acute repetitive seizures. *Epilepsia.* 2003;44:724–726.

157. Misra UK, Kalita J, Patel R. Sodium valproate vs phenytoin in status epilepticus: a pilot study. *Neurology.* 2006;67:340–342.

158. Gilad R, Izkovitz N, Dabby R, et al. Treatment of status epilepticus and acute repetitive seizures with i.v. valproic acid vs phenytoin. *Acta Neurol Scand.* 2008;118:296–300.

159. Olsen KB, Tauboll E, Gjerstad L. Valproate is an effective, well-tolerated drug for treatment of status epilepticus/serial attacks in adults. *Acta Neurologica Scandinavica. Supplementum.* 2007;187:51–54.

160. Morton LD, O'Hara KA, Coots BP, et al. Safety of rapid intravenous valproate infusion in pediatric patients. *Pediatr Neurol.* 2007;36:81–83.

161. Alfonso I, Alvarez LA, Gilman J, et al. Intravenous valproate dosing in neonates. *J Child Neurol.* 2000;15:827–829.

162. Ramael S, De Smedt F, Toublanc N, et al. Single-dose bioavailability of levetiracetam intravenous infusion relative to oral tablets and multiple-dose pharmacokinetics and tolerability of levetiracetam intravenous infusion compared with placebo in healthy subjects. *Clin Ther.* 2006;28:734–744.

163. Patsalos PN, Ghattaura S, Ratnaraj N, et al. In situ metabolism of levetiracetam in blood of patients with epilepsy. *Epilepsia.* 2006;47:1818–1821.

164. Knake S, Gruener J, Hattemer K, et al. Intravenous levetiracetam in the treatment of benzodiazepine refractory status epilepticus. *J Neurol Neurosurg Psychiatry.* 2008;79:588–589.

165. Ruegg S, Naegelin Y, Hardmeier M, et al. Intravenous levetiracetam: treatment experience with the first 50 critically ill patients. *Epilepsy Behav.* 2008;12:477–480.

166. Deposiario-Cabacar DT, Peters J, Pong AW, et al. High-dose intravenous levetiracetam for acute seizure exacerbation in children with intractable epilepsy. *Epilepsia.* [Epub February 12, 2010].

167. Appleton R, Choonara I, Martland T, et al. The treatment of convulsive status epilepticus in children. The Status Epilepticus Working Party, Members of the Status Epilepticus Working Party. *Arch Dis Child.* 2000;83:415–419.

168. Shephard SM. Management of status epilepticus. *Emerg Med Clin North Am.* 1994;12:941–961.

169. Walker MC, Smith SJ, Shorvon SD. The intensive care treatment of convulsive status epilepticus in the UK. Results of a national survey and recommendations. *Anaesthesia.* 1995;50:130–135.

170. Claassen J, Hirsch LJ, Mayer SA. Treatment of status epilepticus: a survey of neurologists. *J Neurol Sci.* 2003;211:37–41.

171. Karceski S, Morrell MJ, Carpenter D. Treatment of epilepsy in adults: expert opinion, 2005. *Epilepsy Behav.* 2005;7(suppl 1):S1–S64.

172. Appleton R, Martland T, Phillips B. Drug management for acute tonic-clonic convulsions including convulsive status epilepticus in children. *Cochrane Database Syst Rev.* 2002:CD001905.

173. Bleck TP. Advances in the management of refractory status epilepticus. *Crit Care Med.* 1993;21:955–957.

174. Gilbert DL, Gartside PS, Glauser TA. Efficacy and mortality in treatment of refractory generalized convulsive status epilepticus in children: a meta-analysis. *J Child Neurol.* 1999;14:602–609.

175. Kim SJ, Lee DY, Kim JS. Neurologic outcomes of pediatric epileptic patients with pentobarbital coma. *Pediatr Neurol.* 2001;25:217–220.

176. Lowenstein DH, Aminoff MJ, Simon RP. Barbiturate anesthesia in the treatment of status epilepticus: clinical experience with 14 patients. *Neurology.* 1988;38:395–400.

177. Yaffe K, Lowenstein DH. Prognostic factors of pentobarbital therapy for refractory generalized status epilepticus. *Neurology.* 1993;43:895–900.

178. Young GB, Blume WT, Bolton CF, et al. Anesthetic barbiturates in refractory status epilepticus. *Can J Neurol Sci.* 1980;7:291–292.

179. Van Ness PC. Pentobarbital and EEG burst suppression in treatment of status epilepticus refractory to benzodiazepines and phenytoin. *Epilepsia.* 1990;31:61–67.

180. Young RS, Ropper AH, Hawkes D, et al. Pentobarbital in refractory status epilepticus. *Pediatr Pharmacol.* 1983;3:63–67.

181. Rashkin MC, Youngs C, Penovich P. Pentobarbital treatment of refractory status epilepticus. *Neurology.* 1987;37:500–503.

182. Osorio I, Reed RC. Treatment of refractory generalized tonic-clonic status epilepticus with pentobarbital anesthesia after high-dose phenytoin. *Epilepsia.* 1989;30:464–471.

183. Prasad A, Worrall BB, Bertram EH, et al. Propofol and midazolam in the treatment of refractory status epilepticus. *Epilepsia.* 2001;42:380–386.

184. Parent JM, Lowenstein DH. Treatment of refractory generalized status epilepticus with continuous infusion of midazolam. *Neurology.* 1994;44:1837–1840.

185. Rivera R, Segnini M, Baltodano A, et al. Midazolam in the treatment of status epilepticus in children. *Crit Care Med.* 1993;21:991–994.

186. Holmes GL, Riviello JJ Jr. Midazolam and pentobarbital for refractory status epilepticus. *Pediatr Neurol.* 1999;20:259–264.

187. Claassen J, Hirsch LJ, Emerson RG, et al. Continuous EEG monitoring and midazolam infusion for refractory nonconvulsive status epilepticus. *Neurology.* 2001;57:1036–1042.

188. Ulvi H, Yoldas T, Mungen B, et al. Continuous infusion of midazolam in the treatment of refractory generalized convulsive status epilepticus. *Neurol Sci.* 2002;23:177–182.

189. Crawford TO, Mitchell WG, Fishman LS, et al. Very-high-dose phenobarbital for refractory status epilepticus in children. *Neurology.* 1988;38:1035–1040.

190. Sudoh A, Sugai K, Miyamoto T, et al. Non-intravenous high-dose phenobarbital therapy for status epilepticus refractory to continuous infusion of midazolam or pentobarbital: report of three cases. *Brain Dev.* 2002;34:23–29.

191. Singhi S, Banerjee S, Singhi P. Refractory status epilepticus in children: role of continuous diazepam infusion. *J Child Neurol.* 1998;13:23–26.

192. Singhi S, Murthy A, Singhi P, et al. Continuous midazolam versus diazepam infusion for refractory convulsive status epilepticus. *J Child Neurol.* 2002;17:106–110.

193. Parviainen I, Uusaro A, Kalviainen R, et al. High-dose thiopental in the treatment of refractory status epilepticus in intensive care unit. *Neurology.* 2002;59:1249–1251.

194. De Giorgio CM, Altman K, Hamilton-Byrd E, et al. Lidocaine in refractory status epilepticus: confirmation of efficacy with continuous EEG monitoring. *Epilepsia.* 1992;33:913–916.

195. Pascual J, Ciudad J, Berciano J. Role of lidocaine (lignocaine) in managing status epilepticus. *J Neurol Neurosurg Psychiatry.* 1992;55:49–51.

196. Sata Y, Aihara M, Hatakeyama K, et al. Efficacy and side effects of lidocaine by intravenous drip infusion in children with intractable seizures. *Brain Dev.* 1997;29:39–44.

197. Kofke WA, Snider MT, Young RS, et al. Prolonged low flow isoflurane anesthesia for status epilepticus. *Anesthesiology.* 1985;62:653–656.

198. Ropper AH, Kofke WA, Bromfield EB, et al. Comparison of isoflurane, halothane, and nitrous oxide in status epilepticus. *Ann Neurol.* 1986;19:98–99.

199. Stecker MM, Kramer TH, Raps EC, et al. Treatment of refractory status epilepticus with propofol: clinical and pharmacokinetic findings. *Epilepsia.* 1998;39:18–26.

200. Schor NF, Riviello JJ Jr. Treatment with propofol: the new status quo for status epilepticus? *Neurology.* 2005;65:506–507.

201. van Gestel JP, Blusse van Oud-Alblas HJ, Malingre M, et al. Propofol and thiopental for refractory status epilepticus in children. *Neurology.* 2005;65:591–592.

202. Parke TJ, Stevens JE, Rice AS, et al. Metabolic acidosis and fatal myocardial failure after propofol infusion in children: five case reports. *Br Med J.* 1992;305:613–616.

203. Hanna JP, Ramundo ML. Rhabdomyolysis and hypoxia associated with prolonged propofol infusion in children. *Neurology.* 1998;50: 301–303.

204. Stelow EB, Johari VP, Smith SA, et al. Propofol-associated rhabdomyolysis with cardiac involvement in adults: chemical and anatomic findings. *Clin Chem.* 2000;46:577–581.

205. Vasile B, Rasulo F, Candiani A, et al. The pathophysiology of propofol infusion syndrome: a simple name for a complex syndrome. *Intensive Care Med.* 2003;29:1417–1425.

206. Cornfield DN, Tegtmeyer K, Nelson MD, et al. Continuous propofol infusion in 142 critically ill children. *Pediatrics.* 2002;110:1177–1181.

207. Borris DJ, Bertram EH, Kapur J. Ketamine controls prolonged status epilepticus. *Epilepsy Res.* 2000;42:117–122.

208. Fujikawa DG. Neuroprotective effect of ketamine administered after status epilepticus onset. *Epilepsia.* 1995;36:186–195.

209. Sheth RD, Gidal BE. Refractory status epilepticus: response to ketamine. *Neurology.* 1998;51:1765–1766.

210. Browne TR. Paraldehyde, chlormethiazole, and lidocaine for treatment of status epilepticus. *Adv Neurol.* 1983;34:509–517.

211. Yeoman P, Hutchinson A, Byrne A, et al. Etomidate infusions for the control of refractory status epilepticus. *Intensive Care Med.* 1989;15:255–259.

212. Congdon PJ, Forsythe WI. Intravenous clonazepam in the treatment of status epilepticus in children. *Epilepsia.* 1980;21:97–102.

213. Curless RG, Holzman BH, Ramsay RE. Paraldehyde therapy in childhood status epilepticus. *Arch Neurol.* 1983;40:477–480.

214. Lampl Y, Eshel Y, Gilad R, et al. Chloral hydrate in intractable status epilepticus. *Ann Emerg Med.* 1990;19:674–676.

215. Orlowski JP, Erenberg G, Lueders H, et al. Hypothermia and barbiturate coma for refractory status epilepticus. *Crit Care Med.* 1984;12:367–372.

216. Winston KR, Levisohn P, Miller BR, et al. Vagal nerve stimulation for status epilepticus. *Pediatr Neurosurg.* 2001;34:190–192.

217. Claassen J, Hirsch LJ, Emerson RG, et al. Treatment of refractory status epilepticus with pentobarbital, propofol, or midazolam: a systematic review. *Epilepsia.* 2002;43:146–153.

218. Bleck TP. Management approaches to prolonged seizures and status epilepticus. *Epilepsia.* 1999;40(suppl 1):S59–S63.

219. Bleck TP. Refractory status epilepticus in 2001. *Arch Neurol.* 2002;59:188–189.

220. Holtkamp M, Masuhr F, Harms L, et al. The management of refractory generalised convulsive and complex partial status epilepticus in three European countries: a survey among epileptologists and critical care neurologists. *J Neurol Neurosurg Psychiatry.* 2003;74:1095–1099.

221. Rossetti AO, Logroscino G, Bromfield EB. Refractory status epilepticus: effect of treatment aggressiveness on prognosis. *Arch Neurol.* 2005;62:1698–1702.

222. Sahin M, Riviello JJ Jr. Prolonged treatment of refractory status epilepticus in a child. *J Child Neurol.* 2001;16:147–150.

223. Krishnamurthy KB, Drislane FW. Relapse and survival after barbiturate anesthetic treatment of refractory status epilepticus. *Epilepsia.* 1996;37:863–867.

224. Krishnamurthy KB, Drislane FW. Depth of EEG suppression and outcome in barbiturate anesthetic treatment for refractory status epilepticus. *Epilepsia.* 1999;40:759–762.

225. Sahin M, Menache CC, Holmes GL, et al. Prolonged treatment for acute symptomatic refractory status epilepticus: outcome in children. *Neurology.* 2003;61:398–401.

226. Mirski MA, Williams MA, Hanley DF. Prolonged pentobarbital and phenobarbital coma for refractory generalized status epilepticus. *Crit Care Med.* 1995;23:400–404.

227. Bramstedt KA, Morris HH, Tanner A. Now we lay them down to sleep: ethical issues with the use of pharmacologic coma for adult status epilepticus. *Epilepsy Behav.* 2004;5:752–755.

228. Ohori N, Fujioka Y, Ohta M. Experience in managing refractory status epilepticus caused by viral encephalitis under long-term anesthesia with barbiturate: a case report. *Rinsho Shinkeigaku.* 1998;38:474–477.

229. Kramer U, Shorer Z, Ben-Zeev B, et al. Severe refractory status epilepticus owing to presumed encephalitis. *J Child Neurol.* 2005;20:184–187.

230. Holtkamp M, Othman J, Buchheim K, et al. Predictors and prognosis of refractory status epilepticus treated in a neurological intensive care unit. *J Neurol Neurosurg Psychiatry.* 2005;76:534–539.

231. Holtkamp M, Othman J, Buchheim K, et al. A "malignant" variant of status epilepticus. *Arch Neurol.* 2005;62:1428–1431.

232. Wilder-Smith EP, Lim EC, Teoh HL, et al. The NORSE (new-onset refractory status epilepticus) syndrome: defining a disease entity. *Ann Acad Med Singapore.* 2005;34:417–420.

233. Hirsch LJ, Claassen J, Mayer SA, et al. Stimulus-induced rhythmic, periodic, or ictal discharges (SIRPIDs): a common EEG phenomenon in the critically ill. *Epilepsia.* 2004;45:109–123.

234. Friedman DE, Schevon C, Emerson RG, et al. Cyclic electrographic seizures in critically ill patients. *Epilepsia.* 2008;49:281–287.

235. Sakuma H. Acute encephalitis with refractory, repetitive partial seizures. *Brain Dev.* 2009;31:510–514.

236. Shyu CS, Lee HF, Chi CS, et al. Acute encephalitis with refractory, repetitive partial seizures. *Brain Dev.* 2008;30:356–361.

237. Kriel RL, Cloyd JC, Hadsall RS, et al. Home use of rectal diazepam for cluster and prolonged seizures: efficacy, adverse reactions, quality of life, and cost analysis. *Pediatr Neurol.* 1991;7:13–17.

238. Graves NM, Kriel RL. Rectal administration of antiepileptic drugs in children. *Pediatr Neurol.* 1987;3:321–326.
239. Woody RC, Laney SM. Rectal anticonvulsants in pediatric practice. *Pediatr Emerg Care.* 1988;4:112–116.
240. Alldredge BK, Wall DB, Ferriero DM. Effect of prehospital treatment on the outcome of status epilepticus in children. *Pediatr Neurol.* 1995;12:213–216.
241. Dreifuss FE, Rosman NP, Cloyd JC, et al. A comparison of rectal diazepam gel and placebo for acute repetitive seizures. *N Engl J Med.* 1998;338:1869–1875.
242. Cloyd JC, Lalonde RL, Beniak TE, et al. A single-blind, crossover comparison of the pharmacokinetics and cognitive effects of a new diazepam rectal gel with intravenous diazepam. *Epilepsia.* 1998;39:520–526.
243. Cereghino JJ, Mitchell WG, Murphy J, et al. Treating repetitive seizures with a rectal diazepam formulation: a randomized study. The North American Diastat Study Group. *Neurology.* 1998;51:1274–1282.
244. Yager JY, Seshia SS. Sublingual lorazepam in childhood serial seizures. *Am J Dis Child.* 1988;142:931–932.
245. Holmes GL. Buccal route for benzodiazepines in treatment of seizures? *Lancet.* 1999;353:608–609.
246. Scott RC, Besag FM, Neville BG. Buccal midazolam and rectal diazepam for treatment of prolonged seizures in childhood and adolescence: a randomised trial. *Lancet.* 1999;353:623–626.
247. Lahat E, Goldman M, Barr J, et al. Comparison of intranasal midazolam with intravenous diazepam for treating febrile seizures in children: prospective randomised study. *BMJ.* 2000;321:83–86.
248. Kalviainen R. Status epilepticus treatment guidelines. *Epilepsia.* 2007;48(suppl 8):99–102.
249. Meierkord H, Boon P, Engelsen B, et al. EFNS guideline on the management of status epilepticus. *Eur J Neurol.* 2006;13:445–450.
250. Hirsch LJ, Claassen J. The current state of treatment of status epilepticus. *Curr Neurol Neurosci Rep.* 2002;2:345–356.

CHAPTER 39 ■ PSYCHOGENIC NONEPILEPTIC ATTACKS

SELIM R. BENBADIS

Psychogenic nonepileptic seizures are commonly seen at epilepsy centers, where they represent 15% to 30% of patients referred for refractory seizures (1,2). They are probably common in the general population, with an estimated prevalence of 2 to 33 per 100,000, making this problem nearly as common as multiple sclerosis or trigeminal neuralgia. Thus, however uncomfortable they may be, neurologists and epileptologists will have to deal with this issue. In addition to being common, psychogenic nonepileptic attacks (PNEA) may represent a challenge, both in diagnosis and in management.

TERMINOLOGY

The terminology on the topic has been variable and confusing. Strictly speaking, terms like pseudoseizures, nonepileptic seizures, and nonepileptic events include both psychogenic and *nonpsychogenic* (i.e., organic) episodes that mimic epileptic seizures. Examples of nonpsychogenic episodes include syncope (the most common), paroxysmal movement disorders (e.g., dystonia), cataplexy, complicated migraines, and (in children) breath-holding spells and shuddering attacks. On the other hand, terms like psychogenic or hysterical seizures refer to a subset of nonepileptic seizures that adds the very important connotation of a psychological origin. In other words, *nonepileptic* is not synonymous with *psychogenic*. Because the term psychogenic seizures could possibly be interpreted as epileptic seizures triggered by psychological factor, *psychogenic nonepileptic seizures* (PNES) has become the preferred term (3). However, the word "seizure" here creates much confusion among patients and families, and we advocate the phrase psychogenic nonepileptic attacks (PNEA), which will be used throughout this chapter (for discussion, please see references 3a and 3b).

THE MISDIAGNOSIS OF EPILEPSY

The erroneous diagnosis of epilepsy is relatively common. A very consistent finding is that about a quarter of patients previously diagnosed with epilepsy and who are not responding to drugs are found to be misdiagnosed. This is true in both in referral epilepsy clinics and in epilepsy monitoring units (2,4,5). Most patients misdiagnosed as epilepsy are eventually shown to have PNEA or (more rarely) syncope (2–7). Occasionally, other paroxysmal conditions can be misdiagnosed as epilepsy (8), but PNEA are by far the most common condition. Unfortunately, once the diagnosis of "seizures" is made, it is easily perpetuated without being questioned and is difficult to undo, which explains the usual diagnostic delay (9,10) and its cost (11–14). It is a disconcerting fact that despite the ability to make a diagnosis of PNEA with near-certainty, the delay in diagnosis remains long at about 7 to 10 years (9,10), indicating that neurologists may not have a high enough index of suspicion when drugs fail. This chapter will first review the steps involved in making the diagnosis, and will then turn to management considerations.

SUSPECTING THE DIAGNOSIS

PNEA are initially suspected in the clinic, on the basis of the history and examination. A number of "red flags" are useful in clinical practice, and should raise the suspicion that "seizures" may be psychogenic rather than epileptic. Of course, resistance to antiepileptic drugs (AEDs) can be the first clue, and is usually the reason for referral to the epilepsy center. Most (about 80%) patients with PNEA have been treated with AEDs for some time before the correct diagnosis is made (15). This is because the diagnosis of epilepsy is usually based solely on the history and may be difficult. A very high frequency of "seizures" that is completely unaffected by AEDs (i.e., no difference whether on or off AEDs) should suggest the possibility of a psychogenic etiology. The presence of specific triggers that are unusual for epilepsy can be very suggestive of PNEA, and this should be specifically asked about during history taking (Table 39.1). For example emotional triggers ("stress" or "getting upset") are commonly reported in PNEA. Other triggers that suggest PNEA can include pain, certain movements, sounds, lights, etc., especially if they are alleged to *consistently* trigger a "seizure." The circumstances in which attacks occur can be very helpful. PNEA (like other psychogenic symptoms) tend to occur in the presence of an "audience," and occurrence in the physician's office or the waiting room or during the exam is suggestive of PNEA (16). Similarly, PNEA tend to not occur in sleep, although they may seem to be reported as doing so (17,18). If the historian and witnesses are astute enough, the detailed description of the spells often includes characteristics that are inconsistent with epileptic seizures. In particular, some characteristics of the motor ("convulsive") phenomena are associated with PNEA (see "EEG–video monitoring"). However, witnesses' accounts are rarely detailed enough to describe these accurately, and in fact even seizures witnessed by physicians and thought to be epileptic often turn out to be PNEA. The past medical history can be useful. Coexisting poorly defined (probably psychogenic) conditions such as "fibromyalgia" and unexplained "chronic pain" are associated with psychogenic

TABLE 39.1

CLUES THAT SUPPORT A DIAGNOSIS OF PNEA

History
  Events that are resistant to AED therapy
  Events that occur at a high frequency
  Unusual triggers
  Events occur in the presence of an "audience"
  Events occur in the physician's waiting room
  Past medical history includes
    Chronic pain or "fibromyalgia"
    Other poorly documented clinical syndromes (chronic
      fatigue syndrome, Lyme disease)
  Floridly positive review of systems
Physical examination
  Over-dramatization or hysterical features
  Give-way weakness
  Tight-roping
  Event occurs during the examination
Video–EEG
  Event semiology
    Gradual onset and gradual termination
    Side-to-side head movements and other asynchronous
      movements (e.g., bicycling)
    Pelvic thrusting
    Opisthotonic posturing
    Stuttering
    Eye closure
    Whispering during the postictal period
  Pseudosleep
  Toy stuffed animal brought with the patient to the
    monitoring unit

symptoms, with a high predictive value of 70% to 80% (16,19,20). Most likely other "fashionable" unsubstantiated diagnoses such as "chronic fatigue" or Lyme disease have the same value. Similarly, a florid review of systems suggests somatization (21). The psychosocial history, with evidence for maladaptive behaviors or associated psychiatric diagnoses, should raise the suspicion of PNEA. The examination, paying particular attention to mental status evaluation including the general demeanor and appropriate level of concern, overdramatization or hysterical features, can be very telling. Lastly, the examination often uncovers histrionic behaviors such as give-way weakness or tight-roping. Performing the examination can in itself act as an "activation" in suggestible patients, making a spell more likely to occur during the history taking or examination (16). Occasionally, patients with PNEA present with pseudostatus. Compared to status epilepticus, patients with pseudostatus are younger, have port systems implanted more frequently, receive higher doses of benzodiazepines, and have lower serum creatine kinase (CK) levels (22).

By contrast to the above, certain symptoms, when present, argue in favor of epileptic seizures and should warrant caution. These include significant postictal confusion, incontinence, and (most important) significant injury (23–27). Although some injuries have been reported in PNEA, data

that describe injuries in patients with PNEA are largely based on patients' self-reports (28). In particular, tongue biting is highly specific to generalized tonic–clonic seizures (24), and thus is a very helpful sign when present. Postictal stertorous breathing is quite specific for convulsive epileptic seizures (29,30), as is postictal nose rubbing (31). Some of the signs associated with seizures, such as tongue biting, falling, or incontinence, can be *reported* by patients with PNEA (32). Obviously symptoms like incontinence, tongue biting, and injuries are much more specific if they are *documented* rather than *reported*. Similarly, the prevalence of a history of sleep events is similar in PNEA and epilepsy, and is of no value in discriminating between the two, although a history of events occurring exclusively during sleep does suggest epileptic seizures (33). Again, *documented* occurrence out of sleep is not the same as *reported* occurrence out of sleep.

CONFIRMING THE DIAGNOSIS

EEG and Ambulatory EEG

Because of its low sensitivity, routine EEG of course is not very helpful in making a diagnosis of PNEA. However, the presence of repeated normal EEGs, especially in light of frequent attacks and resistance to medications, certainly can be viewed as a "red flag" (34). Ambulatory EEG is increasingly used, is cost-effective, and can contribute to the diagnosis by recording the habitual episode and documenting the absence of EEG changes. However, because ictal EEG can only be interpreted in the context of the video, and because of the difficulties in conveying this diagnosis (see the section "Management"), it should always be confirmed by EEG–video monitoring.

EEG–Video Monitoring

This is the gold standard for diagnosis (2,8,12,14,17,23, 27,32,35,36), and is in fact indicated in all patients who continue to have frequent seizures despite medications (37). In the hands of experienced epileptologists, the combined electroclinical analysis of both the clinical semiology of the "ictus" and the ictal EEG findings allow a definitive diagnosis in nearly all cases. If an attack is recorded, the diagnosis is usually easy, and it is exceptional that this question (PNEA vs. epilepsy) cannot be answered. Further, most patients have their first event in the first 2 days (2,35,36).

The principle of EEG–video monitoring is to record an episode and demonstrate that (i) there is no change in the EEG during the clinical event and (ii) the clinical spell is not consistent with seizure types that can be unaccompanied by EEG changes. Ictal EEG has limitations because it may be negative in "simple partial" seizures (38,39) and in some "complex partial" ones, especially frontal (27,35,40). Ictal EEG may also be uninterpretable or difficult if movements generate excessive artifact (see "Pitfalls of EEG–Video").

Analysis of the ictal semiology (i.e., video) is at least as important as the ictal EEG, as it often shows behaviors that are obviously nonorganic and incompatible with epileptic seizures. Certain characteristics of the motor phenomena are strongly associated with PNEA. These include a very gradual onset or termination, pseudosleep, discontinuous (stop-and-go), irregular or asynchronous (out-of-phase) activity including side-to-side head movement, pelvic thrusting, opisthotonic posturing, stuttering, and weeping (17,18,23,25,27,41–44). A particularly useful sign is preserved awareness during bilateral motor activity, since unresponsiveness is almost always present during bilateral motor activity, with the notable exception of supplementary motor area seizures (40,45). Other useful symptoms have been described more recently and have a helpful association with (reasonable specificity for) PNEA. Although this has been questioned (46), ictal eye closure is relatively specific PNEA (47), especially when *prolonged and with complete unresponsiveness*. Postictal behaviors that are "overdramatic" such as whispering voice or partial motor responses have a strong association with PNEA (48). Lastly, bringing a toy stuffed animal into the epilepsy monitoring unit (EMU) may have some diagnostic value, as it is more common in patients with PNEA than in those with epilepsy (49).

Inductions

Provocative techniques, activation procedures, or "inductions" can be extremely useful for the diagnosis of PNEA, particularly when the diagnosis remains uncertain and no spontaneous attacks occur during monitoring. Many epilepsy centers use some sort of provocative technique to aid in the diagnosis of PNEA (50,51). Intravenous (IV) saline injection has traditionally been the most commonly used (52–55), but various other techniques have been described (56–60), which may be preferable (see below).

The principle behind provocative techniques is suggestibility, which is a feature of somatoform disorders in general. For example, in psychogenic movement disorders, where the diagnosis rests solely on phenomenology (i.e., there is no equivalent of the EEG), response to placebo or suggestion is considered a strong diagnostic criterion for psychogenic mechanism (61,62).

There are many advantages to the use of provocative techniques. First, when carefully studied and using simultaneous EEG, their specificity approaches 100% (63). Second, there are difficult situations in which the combination of semiology (video) and EEG does not allow one to conclude that an episode is psychogenic in origin. As mentioned above, two relatively common scenarios are (i) the ictal EEG is uninterpretable due to movement-related artifacts and (ii) the ictal EEG is normal but the symptoms are consistent with a "simple partial" seizure. In these situations, the very presence of suggestibility (i.e., suggestion triggers the episode in question) is the strongest argument to support a psychogenic etiology. Third, at least theoretically, nonepileptic is not quite synonymous with psychogenic. The combination of a recorded attack with normal ictal EEG makes the diagnosis of a nonepileptic spell, but does not in itself categorize it as psychogenic. On the other hand, a positive induction does stamp the episode as psychogenic, and even difficult-to-convince lay people and attorneys understand this concept. Fourth, there is a strong economic argument for the use of these techniques, especially with the constraints imposed by third-party payers. When spontaneous attacks do not occur in the allotted time for monitoring, the evaluation may be inconclusive. In this situation, provocative techniques often turn an inconclusive evaluation into a diagnostic one.

The main limitation of provocative techniques is that they raise ethical concerns. Several valid ethical arguments against placebo induction have been raised and acknowledged, mak-

ing these techniques a little controversial (50,51,64–67). Of main concern is the fact that physicians cannot honestly disclose the content of the syringe (for IV saline) or cannot say that the maneuver (e.g., tuning fork or patch) induces seizures. Even if the term "seizures" is then used in a broader sense, encompassing PNEA, a degree of disingenuousness persists. The problem is particularly acute when a placebo is used, which results in deceptive "beating around the bush." Thus, techniques that do not use placebo may be preferable, which circumvents these ethical problems while retaining similar diagnostic value (56,59,67,68). The best documented technique uses a combination of hyperventilation, photic stimulation, and strong verbal suggestion (56,59,68). If hyperventilation is contraindicated or ill-advised, counting aloud with arms raised will work equally well. The sensitivity is comparable to other methods, ranging from 60% to 90%. One major advantage of this technique is that hyperventilation and photic stimulation truly induce seizures, so that deception is not inherent to the procedure. Indeed these maneuvers are performed during most EEGs, so that most patients will have undergone them previously. For this reason, patients or their families are not intrigued by the induction technique and do not ask about it (59,67). In fact a comparable provocative technique using "psychiatric interview" was found not harmful and even useful by patients (56). Provocative techniques should only be performed with EEG–video monitoring. Without the use of a placebo, provocative techniques are similar to other clinical maneuvers performed during the neurologic examination when nonorganic symptoms are suspected. Much of the objections against inductions are theoretical and are far outweighed by the practical consequences of perpetuating a wrong diagnosis of epilepsy (67).

Pitfalls of EEG–Video

As already mentioned, the most obvious limitation of ictal EEG is that it may be negative in some partial seizures (38,39,40,45). Knowing what type of clinical seizures may be unaccompanied by ictal EEG changes, therefore, is critical in avoiding errors. The most common type of seizures that are unaccompanied by ictal EEG changes are those without impairment of awareness, that is, "simple partial" seizures. This includes all simple partial seizures with *subjective* phenomena, that is, auras, which can involve the five senses as well as psychic or experiential sensations. Motor "simple partial" seizures include focal clonic seizures and brief tonic seizures such as those typical of frontal lobe seizures. These are typically brief (5 to 30 seconds) and tonic and may be "hypermotor," but not usually as dramatically flailing or thrashing as PNEA. Ictal EEG may also be uninterpretable or difficult to read if movements generate excessive artifact. In such situations, it can be impossible to "prove" that such episodes are psychogenic. For example, brief episodes of deja-vu or fear or tonic stiffening with no EEG changes can never be *proven* to be psychogenic. Arguments in favor of PNEA include the fact that the events never progress to clear seizures and suggestibility (triggering them with placebo maneuvers). Lastly, a very solid rule is that psychogenic events do not occur out of sleep, so that attacks that arise out of EEG-verified sleep are always organic (epileptic seizures or parasomnias). Epileptic seizures with altered awareness and no EEG changes are very rare but exist, and if the clinical events are strongly suggestive of seizures, it is best to err on the side of treating them as epileptic.

Of course, lack of ictal EEG changes only indicates that the episodes are nonepileptic, and nonepileptic does not always mean psychogenic. Other diagnoses organic symptoms must be considered before making a diagnosis of PNEA. The most common ones to consider are syncope for episodes that occur when awake and parasomnias for episodes that occur in sleep.

A common misconception is that a recorded episode with a negative EEG is all it takes to make a diagnosis of PNEA. This is grossly inaccurate. A "negative" EEG can only be interpreted *in the context* of the semiology of the attack in question. Thus, both the video and EEG must be available. (In fact the diagnosis would probably be more accurate with video alone than with EEG alone.)

When used properly, EEG–video allows the diagnosis of paroxysmal seizure-like events, and in particular the diagnosis of PNEA, with a high degree of confidence. However, in a study of interrater reliability for the diagnosis of PNEA by EEG-video monitoring (69), agreement was only moderate. Although this may be related to limitations of the study (diagnosis based on EEG-video alone, artificial nature of the forced choice paradigm, single episode), it highlights the difficulties and subjective components inherent to this diagnosis. Further, a closer look at their data reveals that in 12 of 22 patients, there was agreement in ≥19 reviewers, and in 17 of 22 patients, there was agreement in ≥17 reviewers. These data suggest that the diagnosis is not difficult in most patients, but that there are a few difficult ones that account for an only moderate overall agreement.

Short-Term Outpatient EEG–Video With Activation

An extension of the use of inductions is that, when patients are strongly suspected to have PNEA on clinical grounds, they can undergo outpatient "EEG–video with activation." This can be very cost-effective while retaining the same specificity and reasonably high sensitivity, as demonstrated in several studies (68,70,71), including a study in the Veterans Administration (VA) population (72).

Postictal laboratory tests can be useful in clinical settings where EEG–video is not readily available, but their sensitivity and specificity are not high enough compared to EEG–video to be of great value (73). These include prolactin (PRL), creatine kinase (CK), and serum-specific enolase. Surprisingly, PRL was the subject of a recent AAN practice parameter (74). As mentioned above, CK levels can be useful in pseudostatus (22).

DIFFICULT AND SPECIAL ISSUES IN DIAGNOSIS

Previous Abnormal EEG

This is a very common problem. Many patients with PNEA seen at epilepsy centers have had previous EEGs interpreted as epileptiform. In this situation, it is essential to obtain and review the actual tracing previously read as epileptiform, since no amount of normal subsequent EEGs will "cancel" the previous abnormal one. When reviewed, the vast majority will turn out to show overinterpreted normal variants (35,75–77). By far the most common errors in EEG interpretation, and the main source of over-reading, are benign temporal sharp tran-

sients or "wicket spikes" (75,76). Unfortunately, obtaining prior EEGs can be difficult. First, records are not always available or accessible, and second, digital EEG systems are not compatible among each other. In this regard, software that allows one to read any digital EEG format is very valuable, although most digital EEG now can be provided with stand-alone software on the same CD or DVD. The same errors in diagnosis occur for benign nonspecific episodic symptoms not even suggestive of seizures (e.g., light-headedness, dizziness, weakness, and numbness), resulting in the (mis)diagnosis of seizures being *entirely* based on the (over-read) EEG.

In children, coexisting benign focal epileptiform discharges (BFEDC) on EEG are a common "red herring." Such discharges are frequently seen in asymptomatic children, and do not necessarily confirm that the reported episodes are epileptic. When the symptoms are mismatched with the expected manifestations of BFEDC, for example in children with medically refractory "convulsions" or staring spells, video–EEG is indicated.

Coexisting Epilepsy

There is a widely held belief that many or most patients with PNEA also have epilepsy. A careful review of the literature shows that this belief is inaccurate. Reports that have found high percentages of patients with PNEA to also have epilepsy are based on loose criteria (such as "abnormal EEG"), whereas those that required definite evidence for coexisting epilepsy found percentages between 9% and 15% (78,79). Patients with coexisting PNEA and epilepsy are generally of younger age, have a higher percentage of spontaneous events during monitoring, a shorter disease duration, a longer time to PNEA diagnosis, and a lower percentage lost at follow-up (80). They also present obvious management difficulties.

Older Patients

PNEA, like other psychogenic symptoms, tend to begin in younger patients, but they do occur in older patients and even begin in older patients commonly (81,82).

Coexisting Organic Disease

A related phenomenon is that seizures are especially likely to be overdiagnosed as epileptic in patients with other organic neurologic diseases, for example, multiple sclerosis, stroke, or antecedent brain surgery (83). For example, in patients with moderate-to-severe traumatic brain injury diagnosed with post-traumatic epilepsy, 30% are found to have PNEA instead (84). Thus, as is the general rule, if seizures do not respond to medications, a diagnosis of PNEA should be considered despite the coexistence of organic disease. PNEA after some kind of head injury are particularly thorny because they often involve litigation.

PNEA after Epilepsy Surgery

PNEA may occur after epilepsy surgery (85–87), and should always be considered if seizures recur and are somewhat different than preoperatively. PNEA tend to occur within a month after surgery (86). Risk factors include neurologic dysfunction in the right hemisphere, seizure onset after adolescence, low intelligence quotient (IQ), serious preoperative psychopathologic conditions, and major surgical complications (86,87).

Epilepsy Surgery in Patients with PNEA

Occasionally, patients evaluated for resective epilepsy surgery also have PNEA, especially triggered by activation procedures. In the right circumstances, this is not a contraindication to surgery (88). If the epilepsy is refractory and severe, then it may be appropriate to perform surgery to improve the patient's medical condition and provide relief from the burden of seizures and high-dose antiepileptic medication, while approaching the PNEA with psychiatric intervention.

Pseudosyncope

Seizure-like episodes that are characterized by limp loss of consciousness mimic syncope rather than seizures, and are better described as pseudosyncope. The clinical red flags that lead to suspecting them are similar to PNEA. Most likely, a high proportion of "syncope of unknown origin" are psychogenic, but are never diagnosed because such patients see cardiologists rather than neurologists and are rarely sent for EEG–video monitoring. When recorded in the EMU, the diagnosis of psychogenic syncope is not difficult since these episodes can be induced by suggestion, and "true" syncope shows a reliable series of ictal EEG changes (89).

Other "Unexpected PNEA"

As outlined above, PNEA can be found when relatively unexpected in patients who are *assumed* to have epilepsy—such as after head injury (84)—elderly (81,82), patients awarded seizure dogs (90), and patients referred specifically for vagus nerve stimulation (VNS) (91). Therefore, it is always best to verify the diagnosis when episodes are frequent and red flags exist.

PSYCHOPATHOLOGY

PNEA are by definition a psychiatric disorder. According to the Diagnostic and Statistical Manual of Mental Disorders (DSM) classification (92), physical symptoms caused by psychological causes can fall under three categories: somatoform disorders, factitious disorders, and malingering. Somatoform disorders are by definition the unconscious production of physical symptoms due to psychological factors, which means that symptoms are not under voluntary control, that is, the patient is not faking and not intentionally trying to deceive. Somatoform disorders are subdivided into several disorders depending on the characteristics of the physical symptoms and their time course. The two somatoform disorders relevant to PNEA are conversion disorder and somatization disorder. In fact, the DSM IV has a subcategory of conversion disorder specifically termed *conversion disorder with seizures*. By contrast to the unconscious (unintentional) production of symptoms of the somatoform disorders (including conversion), factitious disorder and malingering imply that the patient is purposely deceiving the physician, that is, faking the symptoms. The difference between the two (factitious disorder and

malingering) is that in malingering the reason for doing so is tangible and rationally understandable (albeit possibly reprehensible), while in factitious disorder the motivation is a pathologic need for the sick role. An important corollary, therefore, is that malingering is not considered a mental illness whereas factitious disorder is (92).

It is generally accepted that most patients with PNEA fall under the somatoform category (unconscious production of symptoms), rather than the intentional faking type (malingering and factitious). However, while the DSM classification is simple in theory, it is nearly impossible to know if a given patient is faking. Intentional faking can only be diagnosed in some circumstances by catching a person in the act of faking (e.g., self-inflicting injuries, ingesting medications or eye drops to cause signs, putting blood in the urine to simulate hematuria). Malingering may be underdiagnosed, partly because the "diagnosis" of malingering is essentially an accusation.

From a practical point of view, the role of the neurologists and other medical specialists is to determine whether there is an organic disease. Once the symptoms are shown to be psychogenic, the exact psychiatric diagnosis and its treatment should be best handled by mental health professionals.

The role of antecedent sexual trauma or abuse is thought to be important in the psychopathology of psychogenic seizures and psychogenic symptoms in general. A history of abuse may be more frequent in convulsive rather than limp type of PNEA (93). Overall about three quarters of patients report antecedent traumatic factors, in order of frequency: sexual abuse (33%), physical abuse (26%), bereavement (19%), health-related trauma (8%), and accident or assault (8%).

Antecedent trauma is associated with a later age at onset and with the presence of other medically unexplained symptoms. Sexual abuse, in particular, is associated with physical abuse, self-harm, and medically unexplained symptoms (94). Patients who report a history of sexual abuse may have earlier onset PNEA and more features suggestive of epilepsy (convulsive and more severe attacks, nocturnal attacks, injuries, incontinence), more emotional triggers, prodromes, and flashbacks. They also had more severe psychiatric diagnoses, more social security benefits, and were less often in cohabiting relationships (95).

Patients with PNEA perform similarly on measures of effort compared to intractable epilepsy patients (96,97), supporting the notion that the vast majority are not in the consciously faking category. In addition, Minnesota Multiphasic Personality Inventory (MMPI) findings are also poor in discriminating between patients with PNEA and those with intractable seizures (98). Thus, while psychological profiles may be useful for treatment strategies, they are not particularly helpful for diagnosis.

PROGNOSIS

Overall, outcome in adults is tenuous (99–101). After 10 years of symptoms, over half of patients continue to have "seizures" and remain dependent on social security. Outcome is better in patients with greater educational attainments, younger onset and diagnosis, attacks with less dramatic features, fewer additional somatoform complaints, lower dissociation scores, lower scores of the higher order personality dimensions "inhibitedness," "emotional dysregulation," and "compulsivity" (100,101). The limp or catatonic type may have a better prognosis than the convulsive or thrashing type (102). Quality of life is severely affected in patients with PNEA (103). It should be noted that PNEA patients tend to have more side effects from AED (104), and in addition to oral AED, they can suffer from intensive care unit (ICU) complications (105). In addition, improvement in the seizure-like attacks does not necessarily translate in to overall improvement or productivity, as the underlying psychopathology may not be improved (106). Duration of the illness is probably the single most important prognostic factor in PNEA, that is, the longer patients have been treated for epilepsy, the worse the prognosis (10,102,107). Thus, obtaining a definite diagnosis of PNEA early in the course is critical.

Outcome of PNEA is overall better in children and adolescents (108), probably because the duration of illness is short, and the psychopathology or stressors are different from those in adults (107,109). School refusal and family discord may be significant factors. Serious mood disorders and ongoing sexual or physical abuse are common in children with PNEA and should be sought in every case.

MANAGEMENT

Role of the Neurologist or Epileptologist

The role of the neurologist or epileptologist does not end when the diagnosis of PNEA is made. In fact, arguably the most important step in initiating treatment is in the delivery of the diagnosis to patients and families (10,110–112). Unless patients and families understand and accept the diagnosis, they will not comply with the recommendations. Therefore, communicating the diagnosis is critical. In fact, patients' understanding and reactions to the diagnosis have an impact on outcome (10). Most patients have carried a diagnosis of epilepsy, so the reactions typically include disbelief and denial as well as anger and hostility ("Are you accusing me of faking?" "Are you saying that I am crazy?"). Written information can be useful in supplementing verbal explanations, but unfortunately patient information material for psychogenic symptoms is rather scarce. Amazingly, the American Psychiatric Association (APA) (http://www.psych.org/) and its patient/community information site (http://www.healthyminds.org/links.cfm) have abundant and professional patient education materials on a broad spectrum of topics, but none on conversion disorder and somatoform disorders (113,114) (Table 39.2). Some written patient education is available (115).

As already mentioned, PNEA, like conversion disorder and somatoform disorders in general, should be handled by mental health professionals. In reality, however, these disorders are largely neglected by the mental health community (114). Although individual efforts exist and slow progress is being made (116–119), leading institutions like the APA appear to be "hiding" from these disorders or be "in denial" (114). Articles on somatoform disorders are also rare in the psychiatric literature.

Delivery of the diagnosis is where the failure and breakdown occur, and this is the main obstacle to effective treatment. Typically, physicians are uncomfortable with this diagnosis, and tend to be uneasy formulating a conclusion. Reports frequently remain vague and fail to give clear conclusions, leaving the clinician hanging (e.g., "there was no EEG change during the episode" or "there is no evidence for epilepsy" or "seizures

TABLE 39.2

FACT SHEETS AND PAMPHLETS AVAILABLE AT THE APA WEB SITES[a]

Addiction
Anxiety disorders
Bipolar disorder
Choosing a psychiatrist
College students and alcohol abuse
Common childhood disorders
Confidentiality
Depression
Disasters: mental health, students, and colleges
Domestic violence
Eating disorders
Funerals and memorials
Gay, lesbian, and bisexual issues
Insanity defense FAQ
Managed care
Media violence
Obsessive–compulsive disorder
Panic disorder
Patients bill of rights
Phobias
Postpartum depression
Posttraumatic stress disorder
Psychiatric dimensions of HIV and AIDS
Psychiatric hospitalization
Seasonal affective disorder
Schizophrenia
Storm disaster
Teen suicide
What is mental illness?

Note the remarkable absence of any information related to somatoform disorders, somatization disorder, conversion, factitious disorder, etc.
HIV, human immunodeficiency virus; AIDS, acquired immune deficiency syndrome.
[a]http://www.psych.org and http://www.healthyminds.org (APA's consumer website).
Adapted from the APA websites (http://www.psych.org and http://www.healthyminds.org), with permission.

were nonepileptic"), and no explanations are given to patients and families. In these situations, patients often continue to be treated for epilepsy, possibly with the understanding that the test was inconclusive. The diagnosis should be explained *clearly*, using unambiguous terms that patients can understand, such as "psychological, stress-induced, and emotional." The physician delivering the diagnosis must be compassionate (remembering that most patients are not faking), but firm and confident (avoiding "wishy-washy" and confusing terms).

The neurologist should also continue to be involved and not "abandon" the patient. The neurologist can assist in weaning AEDs, and may be of assistance in addressing issues like driving and disability. In regards to driving, there are very few data available, and there is no evidence that patients with PNEA have an increased risk of motor vehicle accident (MVA) (120), probably for the same reason that they do not usually sustain serious injuries. Nevertheless, caution is warranted, and each case should be decided individually and jointly by the neurologist and the mental health professional. Another thorny issue is that of disability. PNEA can be truly disabling, and this should be made clear. However, logic dictates that in these cases disability should be filed and justified on the basis of a *psychiatric diagnosis*, not a neurological one. Another reason for the neurologist to continue following these patients is that one should keep an open mind about the possibility of coexisting epilepsy.

Role of the Mental Health Professional

Psychogenic symptoms are by definition a psychiatric disease, and mental health professionals should treat it. Treatment includes psychotherapy and adjunctive medications for coexisting anxiety or depression (116–119,121). Unfortunately, mental health services are not always easily available, especially for the noninsured. Another obstacle is that psychiatrists tend to be skeptical about the diagnosis of psychogenic symptoms, and even for PNEA where EEG–video monitoring allows a near certain diagnosis, they tend to not believe the diagnosis (114,122). A useful approach to combat this skepticism is to provide the treating psychiatrist with the video recordings of the PNEA, as these can be more convincing than written reports.

PNEA IN CHILDREN

Although PNEA are more common in adolescence, they may occur in children as young as 5 or 6 years of age. Most of what has been said here applies to children as well as to adults. However, there are certain features specific to children. First, the differential diagnosis of seizures is broader in children, with many nonepileptic, nonpsychogenic conditions to be considered (8,123). In addition, children also have nonepileptic staring spells, which are behavioral inattention that is misinterpreted by adults (124). The gender difference of female predominance is not seen until adolescence (124,125) and PNEA are as common in preadolescent boys as in girls. As already described, BFEDC of childhood are a common confounding feature on interictal EEG, and outcome of PNEA is overall better in children and adolescents than in adults (108).

A key concern for children with PNEA is that serious underlying psychosocial stressors, such as sexual or physical abuse, may be active at the time of diagnosis and require acute intervention (109). Family discord, school avoidance, and social difficulties may also play a role. As in adults, depression or anxiety may be important features, but their presentation is different in the pediatric population. Video–EEG confirmation provides a powerful tool for the pediatric neurologist who must confidently convey the diagnosis to the child and his parents, teachers, and mental health providers.

CONCLUSION: A MORE GENERAL PERSPECTIVE ON PSYCHOGENIC SYMPTOMS

The literature on PNEA often implies that PNEA represent a unique disorder. In reality, PNEA are but one type of somatoform disorder. How the psychopathology is expressed (PNEA, paralysis, diarrhea, or pain) is only different in the diagnostic aspects. Fundamentally, the underlying psychopathology, its prognosis, and its management, are no different for PNEA than they are for other psychogenic symptoms. Whatever the manifestations, psychogenic symptoms represent a challenge both in diagnosis and in management.

Psychogenic (nonorganic, "functional") symptoms are common in medicine. Conservative estimates consider that at least 10% of all medical services are provided for psychogenic symptoms. They are also common in neurology, representing about 9% of inpatient neurology admissions (126), and probably an even higher percentage of outpatient visits. Common neurologic symptoms that are found to be psychogenic include paralysis, mutism, visual symptoms, sensory symptoms, movement disorders, gait or balance problems, and pain (126–128). Several neurologic symptoms, signs or maneuvers have been described to help differentiate organic from nonorganic symptoms. For example, limb weakness is often evaluated by eliciting the Hoover's test. Other examples include looking for "give-way" weakness and alleged blindness with preserved optokinetic nystagmus. More generally, the neurologic examination often tries to elicit symptoms or signs that do not make neuroanatomical sense, for example, facial numbness affecting the angle of the jaw, gait with astasia-abasia or "tight-roping."

Every medical specialty has its share of symptoms that can be psychogenic. In gastroenterology, these include vomiting, dysphagia, abdominal pain, and diarrhea. In cardiology, chest pain that is noncardiac is traditionally referred to as "musculoskeletal" chest pain but is probably psychogenic. Symptoms that can be psychogenic in other specialties include shortness of breath and cough in pulmonary medicine, psychogenic globus or dysphonia in otolaryngology, excoriations in dermatology, erectile dysfunction in urology, and blindness or convergence spasms in ophthalmology. Pain syndromes for which a psychogenic component is likely include tension headaches, chronic back pain, limb pain, rectal pain, and sexual organs pain. Of course, pain being by definition entirely subjective, so it is extremely difficult, and perhaps impossible, to ever confidently say that pain is "psychogenic." It could even be argued that all pains are psychogenic, and thus psychogenic pain is one of the most "uncomfortable" diagnoses to make. In addition to isolated symptoms, some syndromes are considered to be at least partly psychogenic by some, and possibly entirely psychogenic (i.e., without any organic basis) by others. These controversial but "fashionable" diagnoses include fibromyalgia, fibrositis, myofascial pain, chronic fatigue, irritable bowel syndrome, and multiple chemical sensitivity.

Among psychogenic symptoms, PNEA are unique in one principal characteristic. With video–EEG monitoring, they can be diagnosed with near-certainty. This is in sharp contrast to other psychogenic symptoms, which are almost always a diagnosis of exclusion. This feature allows a clarity and confidence of diagnosis that may assist in the critical step of convincing the patient and family of the nonorganic nature of the PNEA.

References

1. Benbadis SR, Hauser WA. An estimate of the prevalence of psychogenic nonepileptic seizures. *Seizure.* 2000;9:280–281.
2. Benbadis SR, Heriaud L, O'Neill E, et al. Outcome of prolonged EEG-video monitoring at a typical referral epilepsy center. *Epilepsia.* 2004;45:1150–1153.

3. Gates J. Nonepileptic seizures: time for progress. *Epilepsy Behav.* 2000;1:2–6.
3a. Benbadis S. It's not just semantics: "Psychogenic nonepileptic 'seizures' or 'attacks'?" *Neurology.* 2010;75:in press.
3b. LaFrance W Jr. It's not just semantics: "Psychogenic nonepileptic 'seizures' or 'attacks'?" *Neurology.* 2010;75:in press.
4. Smith D, Defalla BA, Chadwick DW. The misdiagnosis of epilepsy and the management of refractory epilepsy in a specialist clinic. *Quart J Med.* 1999;92:15–23.
5. Scheepers B, Clough P, Pickles C. The misdiagnosis of epilepsy: findings of a population study. *Seizure.* 1998;7:403–406.
6. Eiris Punal J, Rodriguez-Nunez A, Fernandez-Martinez N, et al. Usefulness of the head-upright tilt test for distinguishing syncope and epilepsy in children. *Epilepsia.* 2001;42:709–713.
7. Zaidi A, Clough P, Cooper P, et al. Misdiagnosis of epilepsy: many seizure-like attacks have a cardiovascular cause. *J Am Coll Cardiol.* 2000;36:181–184.
8. Benbadis SR. Differential diagnosis of epilepsy. *Continuum Lifelong Learning Neurol.* 2007;13(4):48–70 (published by the American Academy of Neurology).
9. Reuber M, Fernandez G, Bauer J, et al. Diagnostic delay in psychogenic nonepileptic seizures. *Neurology.* 2002;58:493–495.
10. Carton S, Thompson PJ, Duncan JS. Non-epileptic seizures: patients' understanding and reaction to the diagnosis and impact on outcome. *Seizure.* 2003;12:287–294.
11. Nowack WJ. Epilepsy: a costly misdiagnosis. *Clin Electroencephalogr.* 1997;28:225–228.
12. Martin RC, Gilliam FG, Kilgore M, et al. Improved health care resource utilization following video-EEG-confirmed diagnosis of nonepileptic psychogenic seizures. *Seizure.* 1998;7:385–390.
13. Juarez-Garcia A, Stokes T, Shaw B, et al. The costs of epilepsy misdiagnosis in England and Wales. *Seizure.* 2006;15:598–605.
14. Lafrance WC Jr, Benbadis SR. Avoiding the costs of unrecognized psychological nonepileptic seizures. *Neurology.* 2006;66:1620–1621.
15. Benbadis SR. How many patients with pseudoseizures receive antiepileptic drugs prior to diagnosis? *Eur Neurol.* 1999;41:114–115.
16. Benbadis SR. A spell in the epilepsy clinic and a history of "chronic pain" or "fibromyalgia" independently predict a diagnosis of psychogenic seizures. *Epilepsy Behav.* 2005;6:264–265.
17. Benbadis SR, Lancman ME, King LM, et al. Preictal pseudosleep: a new finding in psychogenic seizures. *Neurology.* 1996;47:63–67.
18. Thacker K, Devinsky O, Perrine K, et al. Nonepileptic seizures during apparent sleep. *Ann Neurol.* 1993;33:414–418.
19. Benbadis SR. Association between chronic pain or fibromyalgia and psychogenic seizures. *Am J Prev Med.* 2005;15:117–119.
20. Koganti M, Zvirbulis D, Yonker P, et al. Coexistence of headache and other chronic pain syndromes in patients with psychogenic non epileptic and epileptic seizures. Abstract 1.103, Presented at the annual meeting of the American Epilepsy Society, December 2008; Seattle, WA.
21. Benbadis S. Hypergraphia and the diagnosis of psychogenic attacks. *Neurology.* 2006;67:904.
22. Holtkamp M, Othman J, Buchheim K, et al. Diagnosis of psychogenic nonepileptic status epilepticus in the emergency setting. *Neurology.* 2006;66:1727–1729.
23. Desai BT, Porter RJ, Penry JK. Psychogenic seizures: a study of 42 attacks in six patients, with intensive monitoring. *Arch Neurol.* 1982;39:202–209.
24. Benbadis SR, Wolgamuth BR, Goren H, et al. F Value of tongue biting in the diagnosis of seizures. *Arch Intern Med.* 1995;155:2346–2349.
25. Guberman A. Psychogenic pseudoseizures in non-epileptic patients. *Can J Psychiatry.* 1982;27:401–404.
26. Hoefnagels WAJ, Padberg GW, Overweg J, et al. Transient loss of consciousness: the value of the history for distinguishing seizure from syncope. *J Neurol.* 1991;238:39–43.
27. Meierkord H, Will B, Fish D, et al. The clinical features and prognosis of pseudoseizures diagnosed using video-EEG telemetry. *Neurology.* 1991;41:1643–1646.
28. Peguero E, Abou-Khalil B, Fakhoury T, et al. Self-injury and incontinence in psychogenic seizures. *Epilepsia.* 1995;36:586–591.
29. Sen A, Scott C, Sisodiya SM. Stertorous breathing is a reliably identified sign that helps in the differentiation of epileptic from psychogenic non-epileptic convulsions: an audit. *Epilepsy Res.* 2007;77:62–64.
30. Azar NJ, Tayah TF, Wang L, et al. Postictal breathing pattern distinguishes epileptic from nonepileptic convulsive seizures. *Epilepsia.* 2008;49:132–137.
31. Geyer JD, Payne TA, Faught E, et al. Postictal nose-rubbing in the diagnosis, lateralization, and localization of seizures. *Neurology.* 1999;52:743–745.
32. de Timary P, Fouchet P, Sylin M, et al. Non-epileptic seizures: delayed diagnosis in patients presenting with electroencephalographic (EEG) or clinical signs of epileptic seizures. *Seizure.* 2002;11:193–197.
33. Duncan R, Oto M, Russell AJC, et al. Pseudosleep events in patients with psychogenic non-epileptic seizures: prevalence and associations. *J Neurol Neurosurg Psychiatry.* 2004;75:1009–1012.
34. Davis BJ. Predicting nonepileptic seizures utilizing seizure frequency, EEG, and response to medication. *Eur Neurol.* 2004;51:153–156.
35. Benbadis SR. The EEG in nonepileptic seizures. *J Clin Neurophysiol.* 2006;23:340–352.
36. Lobello K, Morgenlander JC, Radtke RA, et al. Video/EEG monitoring in the evaluation of paroxysmal behavioral events: duration, effectiveness, and limitations. *Epilepsy Behav.* 2006;8:261–266.
37. Benbadis SR, Tatum WO IV, Vale FL. When drugs don't work: an algorithmic approach to medically intractable epilepsy. *Neurology.* 2000;55:1780–1784.
38. Devinski O, Sato S, Kufta CV, et al. Electroencephalographic studies of simple partial seizures with subdural electrode recordings. *Neurology.* 1989;39:527–533.
39. Sperling MR, O'Connor MJ. Auras and subclinical seizures: characteristics and prognostic significance. *Ann Neurol.* 1990;28:320–328.
40. Kanner AM, Morris HH, Lüders H, et al. Supplementary motor seizures mimicking pseudoseizures: some clinical differences. *Neurology.* 1990;40:1404–1407.
41. Gates JR, Ramani V, Whalen S, et al. Ictal characteristics of pseudoseizures. *Arch Neurol.* 1985;42:1183–1187.
42. Gulick TA, Spinks RP, King DW. Pseudoseizures: ictal phenomena. *Neurology.* 1982;32:24–30.
43. Bergen D, Ristanovic R. Weeping as a common element of pseudoseizures. *Arch Neurol.* 1993;50:1059–1060.
44. Vossler DG, Haltiner AM, Schepp SK, et al. Ictal stuttering: a sign suggestive of psychogenic nonepileptic seizures. *Neurology.* 2004;63:516–519.
45. Morris HH, Dinner DS, Lüders H, et al. Supplementary motor seizures: clinical and electroencephalographic findings. *Neurology.* 1988;38:1075–1082.
46. Syed TU, Arozullah AM, Suciu GP, et al. Do observer and self-reports of ictal eye closure predict psychogenic nonepileptic seizures? *Epilepsia.* 2008;49:898–904.
47. Chung SS, Gerber P, Kirlin KA. Ictal eye closure is a reliable indicator for psychogenic nonepileptic seizures. *Neurology.* 2006;66:1730–1731.
48. Chabolla DR, Shih JJ. Postictal behaviors associated with psychogenic nonepileptic seizures. *Epilepsy Behav.* 2006;9:307–311.
49. Burneo JG, Martin R, Powell T, et al. Teddy bears: an observational finding in patients with non-epileptic events. *Neurology.* 2003;61:714–715.
50. Schachter SC, Brown F, Rowan AJ. Provocative testing for nonepileptic seizures: attitudes and practices in the United States among American Epilepsy Society members. *J Epilepsy.* 1996;9:249–252.
51. Stagno SJ, Smith ML. Use of induction procedures in diagnosing psychogenic seizures. *J Epilepsy.* 1996;9:153–158.
52. Walczak TS, Williams DT, Berten W. Utility and reliability of placebo infusion in the evaluation of patients with seizures. *Neurology.* 1994;44:394–399.
53. Cohen RJ, Suter G. Hysterical seizures: suggestion as a provocative EEG test. *Ann Neurol.* 1982;11:391–395.
54. Bazil CW, Kothari M, Luciano D. Provocation of nonepileptic seizures by suggestion in a general seizure population. *Epilepsia.* 1994;35:768–770.
55. Slater JD, Brown MC, Jacobs W, et al. Induction of pseudoseizures with intravenous saline placebo. *Epilepsia.* 1995;36:580–585.
56. Cohen LM, Howard GF III, Bongar B. Provocation of pseudoseizures by psychiatric interview during EEG and video monitoring. *Int J Psychiatry Med.* 1992;22:131–140.
57. Luther JS, McNamara JO, Carwile S, et al. Pseudoepileptic seizures: methods and video analysis to aid diagnosis. *Ann Neurol.* 1982;12:458–462.
58. Riley TL, Berndt T. The role of the EEG technologist in delineating pseudoseizures. *Am J EEG Technol.* 1980;20:89–96.
59. Benbadis SR, Johnson K, Anthony K, et al. Induction of psychogenic nonepileptic seizures without placebo. *Neurology.* 2000;55:1904–1905.
60. Benbadis SR, LaFrance WC Jr. Clinical features and the role of video-EEG monitoring. In: Schachter SC, LaFrance WC Jr, eds. *Gates and Rowan's Nonepileptic Seizures.* 3rd ed. Cambridge, NY: Cambridge University Press; 2010: 38–50.
61. Fahn S, Williams D. Psychogenic dystonia. *Adv Neurol.* 1988;50:431–455.
62. Hinson VK, Haren WB. Psychogenic movement disorders. *Lancet Neurol.* 2006;5:695–700.
63. Lancman ME, Asconape JJ, Craven WJ, et al. Predictive value of induction of psychogenic seizures by suggestion. *Ann Neurol.* 1994;35:359–361.
64. Benbadis SR. Provocative techniques should be used for the diagnosis of psychogenic nonepileptic seizures. *Arch Neurol.* 2001;58:2063–2065.
65. Gates JR. Provocative testing should not be used for nonepileptic seizures. *Arch Neurol.* 2001;58:2065–2066.
66. Leeman B. Provocative techniques should not be used for the diagnosis of psychogenic nonepileptic seizures. *Epilepsy Behav.* 2009;15:110–114; discussion 115–118.
67. Benbadis SR. Provocative techniques should be used for the diagnosis of psychogenic nonepileptic seizures. *Epilepsy Behav.* 2009;15:106–109.
68. McGonigal A, Oto M, Russell AJ, et al. Outpatient video EEG recording in the diagnosis of non-epileptic seizures: a randomized controlled trial of simple suggestion techniques. *J Neurol Neurosurg Psychiatry.* 2002;72:549–551.
69. Benbadis SR, Lafrance WC, Korabathina K, et al. Interrater reliability of EEG-video monitoring. *Neurology.* 2009;73:843–846.
70. Bhatia M, Sinha PK, Jain S, et al. Usefulness of short-term video EEG recording with saline induction in pseudoseizures. *Acta Neurol Scand.* 1997;95:363–366.

71. Benbadis SR, Siegrist K, Tatum WO, et al. Short-term outpatient EEG video with induction in the diagnosis of psychogenic seizures. *Neurology.* 2004;63:1728–1730.

72. Varela HL, Taylor DS, Benbadis SR. Short-term outpatient EEG-video monitoring with induction in a veterans administration population. *J Clin Neurophysiol.* 2007;24:390–391.

73. Willert C, Spitzer C, Kusserow S, et al. Serum neuron-specific enolase, prolactin, and creatine kinase after epileptic and psychogenic non-epileptic seizures. *Acta Neurol Scand.* 2004;109:318–323.

74. Sandstrom SA, Anschel DJ. Use of serum prolactin in diagnosing epileptic seizures: report of the Therapeutics and Technology Assessment Subcommittee of the American Academy of Neurology. *Neurology.* 2006;67:544–545.

75. Benbadis SR, Tatum WO. Over-interpetation of EEGs and misdiagnosis of epilepsy. *J Clin Neurophysiol.* 2003;20:42–44.

76. Benbadis SR, Lin K. Errors in EEG interpretation and misdiagnosis of epilepsy. Which EEG patterns are overread? *Eur Neurol.* 2008;59(5):267–271.

77. Benbadis SR. Errors in EEGs and the misdiagnosis of epilepsy: importance, causes, consequences, and proposed remedies. *Epilepsy Behav.* 2007;11:257–262.

78. Benbadis SR, Agrawal V, Tatum WO IV. How many patients with psychogenic nonepileptic seizures also have epilepsy? *Neurology.* 2001;57:915–917.

79. Lesser RP, Lueders H, Dinner DS. Evidence for epilepsy is rare in patients with psychogenic seizures. *Neurology.* 1983;33:502–504.

80. Mari F, Di Bonaventura C, Vanacore N, et al. Video-EEG study of psychogenic nonepileptic seizures: differential characteristics in patients with and without epilepsy. *Epilepsia.* 2006;47(suppl 5):64–67.

81. Duncan R, Oto M, Martin E, et al. Late onset psychogenic nonepileptic attacks. *Neurology.* 2006;66:1644–1647.

82. Behrouz R, Benbadis SR. Late-onset psychogenic nonepileptic seizures. *Epilepsy Behav.* 2006;8:649–650.

83. Reuber M, Kral T, Kurthen M, et al. New-onset psychogenic seizures after intracranial neurosurgery. *Acta Neurochir.* 2002;144:901–907.

84. Hudak AM, Trivedi K, Harper CR, et al. Evaluation of seizure-like episodes in survivors of moderate and severe traumatic brain injury. *J Head Trauma Rehabil.* 2004;19:290–295.

85. Davies KG, Blumer DP, Lobo S, et al. De Novo nonepileptic seizures after cranial surgery for epilepsy: incidence and risk factors. *Epilepsy Behav.* 2000;1:436–443.

86. Glosser G, Roberts D, Glosser DS. Nonepileptic seizure after resective epilepsy surgery. *Epilepsia.* 1999;40:1750–1754.

87. Ney GC, Barr WB, Napolitano C, et al. New-onset psychogenic seizures after surgery for epilepsy. *Arch Neurol.* 1998;55:726–730.

88. Reuber M, Kurthen M, Fernandez G, et al. Epilepsy surgery in patients with additional psychogenic seizures. *Arch Neurol.* 2002;59:82–86.

89. Benbadis SR, Chichkova R. Psychogenic pseudosyncope: an underestimated and provable diagnosis. *Epilepsy Behav.* 2006;9:106–110.

90. Krauss GL, Choi JS, Lesser RP. Pseudoseizure dogs. *Neurology.* 2007;68:308–309.

91. Attarian H, Dowling J, Carter J, et al. Video EEG monitoring prior to vagal nerve stimulator implantation. *Neurology.* 2003;61:402–403.

92. American Psychiatric Association. *Diagnostic and Statistical Manual of Mental Disorders: DSM-IV.* 4th ed. Washington, DC: American Psychiatric Association; 1994.

93. Abubakr A, Kablinger A, Caldito G. Psychogenic seizures: clinical features and psychological analysis. *Epilepsy Behav.* 2003;4:241–245.

94. Duncan R, Oto M. Predictors of antecedent factors in psychogenic nonepileptic attacks: multivariate analysis. *Neurology.* 2008;71:1000–1005.

95. Selkirk M, Duncan R, Oto M, et al. Clinical differences between patients with nonepileptic seizures who report antecedent sexual abuse and those who do not. *Epilepsia.* 2008;49:1446–1450.

96. Cragar DE, Berry DT, Fakhoury TA, et al. Performance of patients with epilepsy or psychogenic non-epileptic seizures on four measures of effort. *Clin Neuropsychol.* 2006;20:552–566.

97. Dodrill CB. Do patients with psychogenic nonepileptic seizures produce trustworthy findings on neuropsychological tests? *Epilepsia.* 2008;49:691–695.

98. Cragar DE, Schmitt FA, Berry DT, et al. A comparison of MMPI-2 decision rules in the diagnosis of nonepileptic seizures. *J Clin Exp Neuropsychol.* 2003;25:793–804.

99. Lancman ME, Brotherton TA, Asconape JJ, et al. Psychogenic seizures in adults: a longitudinal analysis. *Seizure.* 1993;2:281–286.

100. Reuber M, Pukrop R, Bauer J, et al. Outcome in psychogenic nonepileptic seizures: 1 to 10-year follow-up in 164 patients. *Ann Neurol.* 2003;53:305–311.

101. Arain AM, Hamadani AM, Islam S, et al. Predictors of early seizure remission after diagnosis of psychogenic nonepileptic seizures. *Epilepsy Behav.* 2007;11:409–412.

102. Selwa LM, Geyer J, Nikakhtar N, et al. Nonepileptic seizure outcome varies by type of spell and duration of illness. *Epilepsia.* 2000;41:1330–1334.

103. Szaflarski JP, Hughes C, Szaflarski M, et al. Quality of life in psychogenic nonepileptic seizures. *Epilepsia.* 2003;44:236–242.

104. Reeves AL, McAuley JW, Moore JL, et al. Medication use, self-reported drug allergies, and estimated medication cost in patients with epileptic versus nonepileptic seizures. *J Epilepsy.* 1998;11:191–194.

105. Reuber M, Baker GA, Gill R, et al. Failure to recognize psychogenic nonepileptic seizures may cause death. *Neurology.* 2004;62:834–835.

106. Reuber M, Mitchell AJ, Howlett S, et al. Measuring outcome in psychogenic nonepileptic seizures: how relevant is seizure remission? *Epilepsia.* 2005;46:1788–1795.

107. Gudmundsson O, Prendergast M, Foreman D, et al. Outcome of pseudoseizures in children and adolescents: a 6-year symptom survival analysis. *Dev Med Child Neurol.* 2001;43:547–551.

108. Wyllie E, Friedman D, Lüders H, et al. Outcome of psychogenic seizures in children and adolescents compared with adults. *Neurology.* 1991;41:742–744.

109. Wyllie E, Glazer J, Benbadis S, et al. Psychiatric features of children and adolescents with pseudoseizures. *Arch Pediatr Adolesc Med.* 1999;153:244–248.

110. Benbadis SR, Friedman AL, Kosalko J, et al. Psychogenic seizures: a guide for patients and families. *J Neurosci Nurs.* 1994;26:306–308.

111. McCahill ME. Somatoform and related disorders: delivery of diagnosis as first step. *Am Fam Physician.* 1995;52:193–203.

112. Shen W, Bowman ES, Markand ON. Presenting the diagnosis of pseudoseizure. *Neurology.* 1990;40:756–759.

113. American Psychiatric Association. Available at: http://www.psych.org/ and http://www.healthyminds.org/links.cfm. Accessed December 2008.

114. Benbadis SR. The problem of psychogenic symptoms: is the psychiatric community in denial? *Epilepsy Behav.* 2005;6:9–14.

115. Benbadis SR, Heriaud L. Psychogenic nonepileptic seizures: a guide for patients and families. Available at: http://health.usf.edu/NR/rdonlyres/C4AD7955-E93A-4702-BB3A-C5F5A5381B44/0/PNESbrochure.pdf. Accessed April 28, 2010

116. LaFrance WC Jr, Alper K, Babcock D, et al, for the NES Treatment Workshop participants. Nonepileptic seizures treatment workshop summary. *Epilepsy Behav.* 2006;8:451–461.

117. LaFrance WC Jr, Rusch MD, Machan JT. What is "treatment as usual" for nonepileptic seizures? *Epilepsy Behav.* 2008;12:388–394.

118. LaFrance WC Jr, Blum AS, Miller IW, et al. Methodological issues in conducting treatment trials for psychological nonepileptic seizures. *J Neuropsychiatry Clin Neurosci.* 2007;19:391–398.

119. LaFrance WC Jr. Treating patients with functional symptoms: one size does not fit all. *J Psychosom Res.* 2007;63:633–635.

120. Benbadis SR, Blustein JN, Sunstad L. Should patients with pseudoseizures be allowed to drive? *Epilepsia.* 2000;41:895–897.

121. Kuyk J, Siffels MC, Bakvis P, et al. Psychological treatment of patients with psychogenic non-epileptic seizures: an outcome study. *Seizure.* 2008;17:595–603.

122. Harden CL, Burgut FT, Kanner AM. The diagnostic significance of video-EEG monitoring findings on pseudoseizure patients differs between neurologists and psychiatrists. *Epilepsia.* 2003;44:453–456.

123. Wyllie E, Benbadis S, Kotagal P. Psychogenic seizures and other nonepileptic paroxysmal events in children. *Epilepsy Behav.* 2002;3:46–50.

124. Rosenow F, Wyllie E, Kotagal P, et al. Staring spells in children: descriptive features distinguishing epileptic and nonepileptic events. *J Pediatr.* 1998;133:660–663.

125. Kotagal P, Costa M, Wyllie E, et al. Paroxysmal nonepileptic events in children and adolescents. *Pediatrics.* 2002;110(4):e46.

126. Lempert T, Dietrich M, Huppert D, et al. Psychogenic disorders in neurology: frequency and clinical spectrum. *Acta Neurol Scand.* 1990;82:335–340.

127. Keane JR. Hysterical gait disorder: 60 cases. *Neurology.* 1989;39:586–589.

128. Kapfhammer HP, Dobmeier P, Mayer C, et al. Conversion syndromes in neurology. A psychopathological and psychodynamic differentiation of conversion disorder, somatization disorder and factitious disorder. *Psychother Psychosom Med Psychol.* 1998;48:463–474.

CHAPTER 40 ■ OTHER NONEPILEPTIC PAROXYSMAL DISORDERS

JOHN M. PELLOCK

A number of conditions cause intermittent and recurring symptoms that suggest epilepsy. Although seizures must be considered in the differential diagnosis, the clinical characteristics sometimes clearly differentiate these disorders and true seizures. These so-called nonepileptic paroxysmal disorders tend to recur episodically. They must not be confused with seizures because treatment with antiepileptic drugs is usually unnecessary and unsuccessful, drug use may risk the development of adverse effects, and alternative etiologies may be overlooked (1–6).

For the clinician dealing with a paroxysmal disorder, the patient's age and an accurate description of the event, including the time of occurrence (during wakefulness or sleep), can lead to the correct diagnosis (7,8). Nevertheless, some nonepileptic symptoms can be present in a patient who also has epilepsy, and unusual repetitive movements can be misdiagnosed as seizures when the actual seizures have been controlled by medication. Prensky (7) classified such symptoms as unusual movements, loss of tone or consciousness, respiratory derangements, perceptual disturbances, behavior disorders, and episodic behaviors related to disease states (Table 40.1).

The following overview of nonepileptic paroxysmal disorders is organized by age, type, and time of occurrence. Psychogenic nonepileptic seizures are discussed in Chapter 39.

INFANCY

Sleep

At least two paroxysmal behaviors may be confused with seizures: repetitive episodes of head banging while the infant is falling asleep and benign neonatal myoclonus usually occurring during sleep.

Head Banging (Rhythmic Movement Disorder)

Rhythmic movement disorder, such as repetitive motion of the head, trunk, or extremities, usually occurs as a parasomnia

---

TABLE 40.1

COMMON SYMPTOMS OF NONEPILEPTIFORM PAROXYSMAL DISORDERS

Unusual movement	Respiratory derangements	Behavior disorders
Jitteriness, tremor	Apnea	Night terrors
Masturbation	Breath holding	Sleepwalking
Shuddering	Hyperventilation	Nightmares
Benign sleep myoclonus	Perceptual disturbances	Rage
Startle responses	Dizziness	Confusion
Paroxysmal torticollis	Vertigo	Fear
Self-stimulation	Headache	Acute psychotic symptoms
Head banging (rhythmic movement disorder)	Abdominal pain	Fugue
Tics (Tourette syndrome)	Episodic features of specific disorders	Phobia
Paroxysmal dyskinesias	Ataxia	Panic attacks
Pseudoseizures	Tetralogy spells	Hallucinations
Eye movement	Hydrocephalic spells	Autism
Head nodding	Cardiac arrhythmias	Munchausen by proxy
Loss of tone or consciousness	Hypoglycemia	
Syncope	Hypocalcemia	
Drop attacks	Periodic paralysis	
Narcolepsy/cataplexy	Hyperthyroidism	
Attention deficit	Gastroesophageal reflux	
Acute hemiplegia	Rumination	
	Drug poisoning	
	Cerebrovascular events	

during the transition from wakefulness to sleep or from sustained sleep (9). Head banging can last from 15 to 30 minutes as the infant drifts off to sleep and, unlike similar daytime activity, is usually not related to emotional disturbance, frustration, or anger. No abnormal electroencephalographic (EEG) findings are noted. These benign movements usually disappear within 1 year of onset, typically by the second or third year of life, without treatment (7,9).

Benign Neonatal Myoclonus

Rapid and forceful myoclonic movements may involve one extremity or many parts of the body. Occurring during sleep in early infancy, these bilateral, asynchronous, and asymmetric movements usually migrate from one muscle group to another. Unlike seizures, their rhythmic jerking is not prolonged, although clusters of these movements may occur episodically in all stages of sleep. Attacks are usually only a few minutes long but may last for hours. This myoclonus is not stimulus sensitive, and EEG shows no epileptiform activity. The movements stop as the infant is awakened and should never be seen in a fully awake and alert state. No treatment is required, but clonazepam or other benzodiazepines have been suggested in children who demonstrate a large amount of benign myoclonic activity. The movements typically disappear over several months (10).

Wakefulness

Jitteriness

Neonates and young infants demonstrate this rapid generalized tremulousness, which in neonates may be severe enough to be mistaken for clonic seizures. The infants are alert, and the movements may be decreased by passive flexion or repositioning of the extremities. Although jitteriness may occur spontaneously, it is typically provoked or increased by stimulation. Because neonatal jitteriness may be caused by certain pathologic states, jittery newborns are more likely than normal infants to experience seizures and their EEG tracings may show abnormalities. Central nervous system dysfunction is the suspected etiology, but hypoxic–ischemic insults, metabolic encephalopathies such as hypoglycemia and hypocalcemia, drug intoxication or withdrawal, and intracranial hemorrhage are implicated. The more benign forms of jitteriness usually decrease without specific therapy. Prognosis depends on the etiology, and in neonates with severe, prolonged jitteriness may be guarded. Nevertheless, in 38 full-term infants who were jittery after 6 weeks of age, the movements resolved at a mean age of 7.2 months; 92% had normal findings on neurodevelopmental examinations at age 3 years (11). Sedative agents may be used, but their adverse effects usually increase the irritability (11,12).

Head Banging or Rolling and Body Rocking

Head banging, head rolling, and body rocking often occur in awake infants (7). In older infants, head banging may be part of a temper tantrum. Head rolling and body rocking seemingly are pleasurable forms of self-stimulation and may be related to masturbation. If the infants are touched or their attention is diverted, the repetitive movements cease. They are more common in irritable, excessively active, mentally retarded infants (7). Nevertheless, most of this activity decreases during the second year. Particularly bothersome movements may be diminished by behavior-modification techniques, but drug treatment usually is unnecessary.

Masturbation

Infantile masturbation may mimic abdominal pain or seizures in infant girls, who may sit with their legs held tightly together or straddle the bars of the crib or playpen and rock back and forth. Distracting stimuli usually stop these movements, which disappear in several months. Masturbation in older children is less likely to be confused with seizure activity. In some mentally retarded children, however, self-stimulation can also be associated with a fugue state. Because these children are difficult to arouse during the activity, seizures are commonly suspected (13).

Benign Myoclonus of Early Infancy

Myoclonic movements occur in awake children and may resemble infantile spasms but are not associated with EEG abnormalities. Infants are usually healthy, with no evidence of neurologic deterioration. The myoclonic episodes abate without treatment after a few months (14).

Spasmodic Torticollis

Spasmodic torticollis is a disorder characterized by sudden, repetitive episodes of head tilting or turning to one side with rotation of the face to the opposite side. The episodes may last from minutes to days, during which children are irritable and uncomfortable but alert and responsive. Although behavior may be episodic while the attack continues, EEG findings remain normal. Nystagmus is not associated with this disorder. The etiology is unknown, although dystonia and labyrinthine imbalance have been proposed. A family history of torticollis or migraine may be present. Tonic or rotary movements also may be seen with gastroesophageal reflux (Sandifer syndrome), but they will be longer and less paroxysmal than torticollis without reflux (15–18).

The differential diagnosis includes congenital, inflammatory, and neoplastic conditions of the posterior fossa, cervical cord, spine, and neck in which the episodes of torticollis are sustained, lacking the usual on-and-off variability. An evaluation is necessary, but spasmodic torticollis usually subsides without treatment during the first few years of life.

Spasmus Nutans

Head nodding, head tilt, and nystagmus comprise spasmus nutans. Head nodding or intermittent nystagmus (or both) is usually noted at 4 to 12 months of age; nystagmus may be more prominent in one eye. The symptoms can vary depending on position, direction of gaze, and time of day. The children are clinically alert, and although symptoms may fluctuate throughout the day, episodic alterations in level of consciousness do not occur. Spasmus nutans usually remits spontaneously within 1 or 2 years after onset but may last as long as 8 years. Minor EEG abnormalities may be noted, but classic epileptiform paroxysms are not associated. Because mass lesions of the optic chiasm or third ventricle have been noted in a small number of these infants, computed tomography or magnetic resonance imaging studies generally should be performed (19). It is difficult to distinguish eye movements persisting into later childhood or adulthood from congenital nystagmus (19–21).

Opsoclonus

Opsoclonus is a rare abnormality characterized by rapid, conjugate, multidirectional, oscillating eye movements that are usually continuous but may vary in intensity. Because of this variation and occasionally associated myoclonic movements, generalized or partial seizures may be suspected. The children remain responsive and alert. Opsoclonus usually implies a neurologic disorder such as ataxia myoclonus or myoclonus. Children who develop these signs early in life may have a paraneoplastic syndrome caused by an underlying neuroblastoma (22–24). This triad of opsoclonus, myoclonus, and encephalopathy is termed Kinsbourne encephalopathy (dancing eyes, dancing feet) and responds to removal of the neural crest tumor or treatment with corticosteroids or corticotropin (25). Other forms of episodic ataxia may be seen in later infancy and childhood associated with nystagmus, but rarely true opsoclonus (8).

Rumination

Rumination attacks involve hyperextension of the neck, repetitive swallowing, and protrusion of the tongue and are secondary to an abnormality of esophageal peristalsis. Episodes typically follow or accompany feeding. The child is alert but sometimes seems under stress and uncomfortable. Variable feeding techniques are helpful in this disorder, which resolves as the child matures (26).

Startle Disease or Hyperekplexia

A rare familial disorder with major and minor forms, startle disease (or hyperekplexia) involves a seemingly hyperactive startle reflex, sometimes so exaggerated that it causes falling. In the major form, the infant becomes stiff when handled, and episodes of severe hypertonia cause apnea and bradycardia. Forced flexion of the neck or hips may interrupt these episodes. Also noted, along with transient hypertonia, are falling attacks without loss of consciousness, ataxia, generalized hyperreflexia, episodic shaking of the limbs resembling clonus, and excessive startle. The minor form, in which startle responses are less consistent and not associated with other findings, may represent an augmented normal startle reflex (27). The interictal electroencephalogram shows normal results, but a spike may be associated with a startle attack. Whether this discharge represents an evoked response to the stimulus or an artifact is a subject of debate. The disorder must be distinguished from so-called startle epilepsy, in which a startle is followed by a partial or generalized seizure, which suggests a defect in inhibitory regulation of brainstem centers (28,29). The prognosis in hyperekplexia is variable (27). Seizures do not develop after this benign disorder; however, clonazepam and valproic acid have been used to treat its associated startle, stiffness, jerking, and falling (30,31).

Shuddering Attacks

Shuddering attacks far exceed the normal shivering seen in most older infants and children. A very rapid tremor involves the head, arms, trunk, and even the legs; the upper extremities are adducted and flexed at the elbows or, less often, adducted and extended. The episodes may begin as early as 4 months of age, decreasing gradually in frequency and intensity before age 10 years. Treatment with antiepileptic drugs does not modify the attacks. Except for the artifact, results of electroencephalography are normal. Essential tremor may be more common in the families of children with shuddering spells than in unaffected families (32,33).

Alternating Hemiplegia

Alternating hemiplegia of childhood may be confused with epilepsy because of the paroxysmal episodes of weakness, hypertonicity, or dystonia. Presenting as tonic or dystonic events, these intermittent attacks may alternate from side to side and at times progress to quadriplegia. They usually occur at least monthly and may be part of a larger neurologic syndrome in children with delayed or retarded development who also have seizures, ataxia, and choreoathetosis. Attacks begin before 18 months of age and can be precipitated by emotional factors or fatigue. The hemiplegic episodes may last minutes or hours, and the etiology and mechanism are unknown. Although anticonvulsants and typical migraine treatments are unsuccessful, flunarizine, a calcium-channel blocker (5 mg/kg/day), has been reported to reduce recurrences (34,35).

Respiratory Derangements and Syncope

Primary breathing disorders usually occur without associated epilepsy. At times, however, respiratory symptoms may be confused with epilepsy, or, rarely, tonic stiffening, clonic jerks or seizures may follow primary apnea (36). An electroencephalogram or polysomnogram recorded during the event may easily distinguish a respiratory abnormality associated with true seizures from one completely independent of epilepsy.

Infant Apnea or Apparent Life-Threatening Events

Apnea usually occurs during sleep and may be associated with centrally mediated hypoventilation, airway obstruction, aspiration, or congenital hypoventilation. Formerly called (near) sudden infant death syndrome, these symptoms now are referred to as *apparent life-threatening events*. In central apnea, chest and abdominal movements decrease simultaneously with a drop in air flow. In obstructive apnea, movements of the chest or abdomen (or both) continue, but there is diminished air flow. Central apnea presumably results from a disturbance of the respiratory centers, whereas obstructive apnea is a peripheral event; some infants have a mixed form of the disorder. A few jerks may occur with the apneic episodes but do not represent epileptic myoclonus. The apnea that follows a seizure is a form of central apnea with postictal hypoventilation. Primary apnea, however, is only rarely followed by seizures (37,38).

The etiology and characteristics vary among infants. Apnea of prematurity responds to treatment with xanthine derivatives. In older infants with primary central apnea, elevated cerebrospinal fluid levels of β-endorphin have been reported, and treatment with the opioid antagonist naltrexone has been successful (39). The role of home cardiopulmonary monitors is controversial. Parents should be encouraged to follow the recommendations of the American Academy of Pediatrics that healthy term infants be put to sleep on their back or side to decrease the risk of apnea and possible sudden infant death syndrome (40).

Although apnea occurs less often when the child is fully awake, it may be associated with gastroesophageal reflux (41,42). Aspiration may follow. Reflux is frequently accompanied by staring or flailing or posturing of the trunk or extremities, perhaps in response to the pain of acidic contents washing back into the esophagus. Gastroesophageal reflux is more common when infants are laid supine after feeding. Diagnosis is established by radiologic demonstration of reflux or by abnormal esophageal pH levels. Reflux is treated by upright positioning of the baby during and after feeding (43), thickened feedings, the use of agents to alter sphincter tone, and fundal plication.

Cyanotic Breath-Holding Spells

Although common between the ages of 6 months and 6 years, cyanotic infant syncope (breath-holding spells) is frequently confused with tonic seizures (44). Typically precipitated by fear, frustration, or minor injury, the spells involve vigorous crying, following which the child stops breathing, often in expiration. Cyanosis occurs within several seconds, followed by loss of consciousness, limpness, and falling. Prolonged hypoxia may cause tonic stiffening or brief clonic jerking of the body. After 1 or 2 minutes of unresponsiveness, consciousness returns quickly, although the infant may be briefly tired or irritable. The crucial diagnostic point is the history of an external event, however minor, precipitating the episode. The electroencephalogram does not show interictal epileptiform discharges but may reveal slowing or suppression during the anoxic event. The pathophysiologic mechanism is not well understood, but correction of any underlying anemia may reduce the attacks (45). Children with pallid breath-holding spells have autonomic dysregulation caused by parasympathetic disturbance distinct from that found in cyanotic breath-holding (46). Although the episodes appear unpleasant for the child, they do not result in neurologic damage. Antiepileptic medication may be appropriate for the rare patients with frequent postsyncopal generalized tonic–clonic seizures triggered by the anoxia.

Pallid Syncope

Precipitated by injury or fright, sometimes trivial, pallid infant syncope occurs in response to transient cardiac asystole in infants with a hypersensitive cardioinhibitory reflex. Minimal crying, perhaps only a gasp, and no obvious apnea precede loss of consciousness. The child collapses limply and subsequently may have posturing or clonic movements before regaining consciousness after a few minutes (44,47–49). The asystolic episodes can be produced by ocular compression, but this procedure is risky and of uncertain clinical utility. As with cyanotic breath-holding spells, the key to diagnosis is the association with precipitating events.

The long-term prognosis is benign. Most children require no treatment, although atropine has been recommended for frequent pallid attacks or those followed by generalized tonic–clonic seizures (50). A trial of the anticholinergic drug atropine sulfate 0.01 mg/kg every 24 hours in divided doses (maximum 0.4 mg/day) may increase heart rate by blocking vagal input. Atropine should not be prescribed during very hot weather because hyperpyrexia may occur.

CHILDREN

Sleep

Myoclonus

Nocturnal myoclonic movements, called "sleep starts" or "hypnic jerks" and associated with a sensation of falling, are less common in older children and adolescents than in infants (10). The subtle involuntary jerks of the extremities or the entire body occur while the child is falling asleep or being aroused. Repetitive rhythmic jerking is uncommon, although several series of jerks can occur during the night. The jerks are not associated with epileptiform activity, but a sensory evoked response or evidence of arousal may be present on the electroencephalogram (51–54).

Periodic repetitive movements that resemble myoclonus are seen in deeper stages of sleep and may arouse the patient so that daytime drowsiness is noted. These movements are more common in rapid eye movement (REM) than in nonrapid eye movement (NREM) sleep, and are clearly distinguished from epilepsy on sleep polysomnographic recordings.

Hypnagogic Paroxysmal Dystonia

In hypnagogic paroxysmal dystonia, an extremely rare disorder, sleep may be briefly interrupted by seemingly severe dystonic movements of the limbs lasting a few minutes and accompanied by crying out. No EEG abnormality is noted. Carbamazepine may decrease the attacks. It is not clear whether some or all patients with this clinical syndrome actually have seizures arising from the supplementary motor area (52,55).

Nightmares

Nightmares occur during REM sleep and are rarely confused with seizures. Although children may be restless during the dream, they usually do not scream out, sit up, or have the marked motor symptoms, autonomic activity, and extreme sorrow seen with night terrors. Incontinence may be present, however. Remembrance of the content of nightmares may lead to a fear of sleeping alone. An electroencephalogram recorded during these events shows no abnormalities (7).

Night Terrors (Pavor Nocturnus)

Night terrors, most common in children between the ages of 5 and 12 years, begin from 30 minutes to several hours after sleep onset, usually in stage III or IV of slow-wave sleep. Diaphoretic and with dilated pupils, the children sit up in bed, crying or screaming inconsolably for several minutes before calming down. Sleep resumes after the attack, and the event is not recalled. No treatment is recommended (56,57).

Sleepwalking

Approximately 15% of all children experience at least one episode of sleepwalking or somnambulism, which usually occurs 1 to 3 hours after sleep onset (stages III and IV). The etiology is unknown, but a familial prevalence is noted. Mumbling and sleep-talking, the child walks about in a trance and returns to bed. Semi-purposeful activity such as dressing, opening doors, eating, and touching objects during an episode of somnambulism may be confused with the automatisms of complex partial seizures. The eyes are open, and the child rarely walks into objects. Amnesia follows, and no violence occurs during the event. Treatment usually is not required, except for protecting the wandering child during the night. Benzodiazepine therapy may be helpful in frequent or prolonged attacks (3,58,59).

Wakefulness

Myoclonus

In many normal, awake children, anxiety or exercise may cause an occasional isolated myoclonic jerk. Treatment is rarely necessary.

Multifocal myoclonus may occur in patients with progressive degenerative diseases or during an acute encephalopathy. It may be difficult to distinguish these movements from chorea, and these two disorders may coexist with some encephalopathic illnesses. Myoclonus persists in sleep, whereas chorea usually disappears during sleep (7).

Chorea

Usually seen as rapid jerks of the distal portions of the extremities, choreiform movements may affect muscles of the face, tongue, and proximal portions of the extremities. When associated with athetosis, chorea involves slower, more writhing movements of distal portions of the extremities. The jerks may be so fluid or continuous that they are camouflaged. Acute chorea may accompany metabolic disorders but is more likely in patients recovering from illnesses such as encephalitis. Other causes are Sydenham chorea seen with β-hemolytic streptococcal infection, drug ingestion, and mass lesions or stroke involving the basal ganglia. Treatment depends primarily on the etiology, but movements may respond to haloperidol or a benzodiazepine such as clonazepam (60,61).

Tics

Like chorea, most tics are present during wakefulness and disappear with sleep. They usually involve one or more muscle groups, are stereotypic and repetitive, and appear suddenly and intermittently. Movements may be simple or complex, rhythmic or irregular. Facial twitches, head shaking, eye blinking, sniffling, throat clearing, and shoulder shrugging are typical, although more complex facial distortions, arm swaying, and jumping have been noted. These purposeless movements cannot be completely controlled, but they may be inhibited voluntarily for brief periods and are frequently exacerbated by stress or startle (62–64).

In Tourette syndrome, complex vocal and motor tics are frequently associated with learning disabilities, hyperactivity, attention deficits, and compulsive behaviors. The incidence of simple and complex tics is high in relatives of these patients. The disorder varies in severity but tends to be lifelong, although it may stabilize or improve slightly in adolescence or early adulthood. Combinations of behavior therapy and medical treatment of tics and compulsive behavior are indicated. Haloperidol, pimozide, and clonidine have been used successfully for behavior control. Stimulants such as methylphenidate may initially exacerbate tics (62–64).

Paroxysmal Dyskinesias

Paroxysmal dyskinesias are rare disorders characterized by repetitive episodes of relatively severe dystonia or choreoathetosis (or both). Multiple brief attacks occur daily, precipitated by startle, stress, movement, or arousal from sleep (65). Consciousness is preserved, but discomfort is evident. Both sporadic and familial types have been described. Kinesigenic dyskinesia frequently is associated with the onset of movement as well as with prior hypoxic injury, hypoglycemia, and thyrotoxicosis. Alcohol, caffeine, excitement, stress, and fatigue may exacerbate attacks of paroxysmal dystonic choreoathetosis, a familial form of the disorder. Although the electroencephalogram displays normal findings during the episodes, the paroxysmal dystonic form responds to antiepileptic drugs such as carbamazepine (65–68).

Stereotypic Movements

Other repetitive movements have been mistaken for seizures, especially in neurologically impaired children. Donat and Wright (69) noted head shaking and nodding, lateral and vertical nystagmus, staring, tongue thrusting, chewing movements, periodic hyperventilation, tonic postures, tics, and excessive startle reactions in these patients, many of whom had been treated unnecessarily for epilepsy. Self-stimulatory behaviors such as rhythmic hand shaking, body rocking, and head swaying, performed during apparent unawareness of surroundings, also are common in mentally retarded children without representing or being associated with seizures. Rett syndrome should be suspected when repetitive "hand-washing" movements are noted in retarded girls (70). Deaf or blind children frequently resort to self-stimulation such as hitting their ears or poking at their eyes or ears, which has been misidentified as epilepsy. Behavior training is frequently more successful than medication in controlling these movements (69).

Head Nodding

Head nodding or head drops may be of epileptic or nonepileptic origin. A study by Brunquell and colleagues (71) showed that epileptic head drops were associated with ictal changes in facial expression and subtle myoclonic extremity movements. Rapid drops followed by slow recovery indicated seizures. When the recovery and drop phases were of similar velocity or when repetitive head bobbing occurred, nonepileptic conditions were much more common.

Staring Spells

When ordinary daydreaming or inattentive periods are repetitive and children do not respond to being called, the behaviors may be classified as absence (petit mal) attacks. During innocent daydreaming, posture is maintained and automatisms do not occur. Staring spells are usually nonepileptic in normal children with normal EEG findings, when parents report preserved responsiveness to touch, body rocking, or identification without limb twitches, upward eye movements, interrupted play, or urinary incontinence (72). Children with attention deficit hyperactivity disorder sometimes have staring spells that resemble absence or complex partial seizures. Although unresponsive to verbal stimuli, these children generally become alert immediately on being touched and frequently recall what was said during the staring spell. During these spells, the electroencephalogram pattern is normal. Attention deficit hyperactivity disorder affects 3% to 10% of children and has a male predominance. Stimulants are most widely used, but other medications may be necessary to ameliorate behavior in refractory cases. Antiepileptic drugs usually are ineffective (52,73–76).

Headaches

Recurrent headaches are rarely the sole manifestation of seizures; however, postictal headaches are not uncommon, especially following a generalized convulsion. Headaches also may precede seizures. As an isolated ictal symptom, headache occurs most frequently in children with complex partial seizures (77). Children with ictal headaches experience sudden diffuse pain, often have a history of cerebral injury, derive no relief from sleep, and lack a family history of migraine. Distinguishing headache from paroxysmal recurrent migraine may be difficult in young children when the headache's throbbing unilateral nature is absent or not readily apparent. Migraine, however, is more prevalent than epilepsy. In addition, ictal electroencephalograms during migraine usually show slowing, whereas those during epilepsy demonstrate a clear paroxysmal change. Associated gastrointestinal disturbance and a strong family history of migraine help establish the appropriate diagnosis (77–83).

Epilepsy and migraine can coexist. Children with migraine have a 3% to 7% incidence of epilepsy, and as many as 20% exhibit paroxysmal discharges on interictal electroencephalograms (80). Up to 60% of children with migraine obtain significant relief with antiepileptic medication (82,83). Other variants of migraine that may be confused with seizures include cyclic vomiting (abdominal pain), acute confusional states, and benign paroxysmal vertigo.

Recurrent Abdominal Pain

Recurrent abdominal pain may be associated with vomiting, pallor, or even fever and has been noted in migraine and epilepsy. Usually, these complaints indicate neither diagnosis, although some children with recurrent abdominal pain or vomiting may experience migraine later in life (7,84). About 7% to 76% of children with recurrent abdominal pain exhibit interictal paroxysmal EEG changes. Approximately 15% of these patients have a diagnosis of seizures, and more than 40% have recurrent headaches (7). A family history of migraine is found in approximately 20% (82). Although most of these children do not respond to antiepileptic drugs, approximately 20% obtain relief from antimigraine medications such as β-blockers or tricyclic antidepressants (7,80,84).

Confusional Migraine

Migraine may present in an unusual and sometimes bizarre fashion as confusion, hyperactivity, partial or total amnesia, disorientation, impaired responsiveness, lethargy, and vomiting (85). These episodes must be distinguished from toxic or metabolic encephalopathy, encephalitis, acute psychosis, head trauma, and sepsis as well as from an ictal or postictal confusional state. Confusional migraine usually persists for several hours, less commonly for days, and spontaneously clears following sleep. The diagnosis is usually made following the episode when the patient or family reports severe headache or visual symptoms heralding the onset of the event or a history of similar events. During and soon after the episodes, an electroencephalogram may demonstrate regional slowing, a nondiagnostic finding.

Benign Paroxysmal Vertigo

Benign paroxysmal vertigo consists of brief recurrent episodes of disequilibrium of variable duration that may be misinterpreted as seizures. Lasting from minutes to hours, the attacks of vertigo occur as often as two to three times per week but rarely as infrequently as every 2 to 3 months. Tinnitus, hearing loss, and brainstem signs have been implicated as causes, but the onset is sudden, and the child usually is unable to walk. Extreme distress and nausea are noted, but the child remains alert and responsive during attacks. Nystagmus or torticollis is frequently observed, but between attacks, examination and electroencephalography reveal normal results. A minority of children show dysfunction on vestibular testing, but show no abnormalities on audiograms. A family history of migraine is common, and most of these children experience migraines later in life. No treatment is indicated because the attacks do not respond well to either antiepileptic or antimigraine medications. Benign paroxysmal vertigo usually subsides by ages 6 to 8 years (52,86,87).

Stool-Withholding Activity and Constipation

Children may have sudden interruption of activity and assume a motionless posture with slight truncal flexion when experiencing discomfort from withholding stool (88). The withholding behavior, which may be mistaken for absence or tonic seizures, evolves as a way to prevent the painful passage of stool that is large and hard because of chronic constipation. Small jerks of the limbs may be misperceived as myoclonus, and the child may have fecal incontinence. The behavior resolves with treatment of the chronic constipation.

Rage Attacks

The episodic dyscontrol syndrome, or recurrent attacks of rage following minimal provocation, may be seen in children with or without epilepsy. The behavior often seems completely out of character. Rage may be more common in hyperactive children or those with conduct and personality disorders. Similar dyscontrol and near rage have been seen following head injury with frontal or temporal lobe lesions. Ictal rage is rare, unprovoked, and usually not directed toward an individual. Following attacks of rage and the appearance of near psychosis, the child resumes a normal state and may recall the episode and feel remorseful. Behavior frequently can be modified during the event. Depending on the cause of the associated syndrome, β-blockers (89), stimulant drugs, and carbamazepine along with other antiepileptic drugs have been used to control outbursts (90).

Munchausen Syndrome by Proxy

Munchausen syndrome, or factitious disorder, describes a consistent simulation of illness leading to unnecessary investigations and treatments. When a parent or caregiver pursues such a deception using a child, the situation is called Munchausen syndrome by proxy. Infants may be brought to child neurologists with parental reports suggesting apnea, seizures, or cyanosis; older children may be described to have episodes of loss of consciousness, convulsions, ataxia, headache, hyperactivity, chorea, weakness, gait difficulties, or paralysis. Accompanying symptoms may include gastrointestinal disorders or a history of unusual accidents and

TABLE 40.2

CLINICAL FEATURES OF MUNCHAUSEN SYNDROME BY PROXY

Persistent and recurrent unexplained illness

Clinical signs at variance with the child's health status

Unusual or remarkable signs or symptoms

Signs and symptoms not recurring in parent's absence

Mother or caregiver overattentive or refuses to leave the hospital

Mother or caregiver not appropriately concerned about prognosis

Lack of anticipated response of clinical syndrome

"Rare" clinical syndrome

injuries that are poorly explained and almost never observed by anyone but the parent(s) (Table 40.2). Sometimes the child also becomes persuaded of the reality of the "illness" and develops independent factitious symptoms such as psychogenic seizures.

The perpetrator is often the mother, who appears initially to be a model parent but has a pathologic need for the child to be sick (91–93). Usually young, articulate, and middle class, she has an unnatural attachment to her child, coexisting personality disorder, and somatizing behavior. The mother often has some medical training, for example, as a nurse. Families are usually dysfunctional. The parent's exaggerated and constant need for illness and medical intervention may lead to the child's death.

Treatment is similar to that of child abuse and typically involves a pediatrician, child psychiatrist, nurse, and social workers. The child is separated from the parents, and details of the history are corroborated. Medical and neurologic evaluations rule out specific disease processes. Admission of a child with paroxysmal symptoms to an epilepsy monitoring unit may help to demonstrate this behavior in both mother and child (94).

Future serious psychologic disturbances are a significant possibility. Good relationships with the nonabusive father, successful short-term foster parenting before return to the mother or long-term placement with the same foster parents, long-term treatment or successful remarriage of the mother, and early adoption are associated with more favorable outcome for the child (95).

LATE CHILDHOOD, ADOLESCENCE, AND ADULTHOOD

Wakefulness

Syncope

Syncope is common in adolescents or older children and usually can be distinguished from seizures by description. Warning signs of lightheadedness, dizziness, and visual dimming ("graying out" or "browning out") occur in most patients. Nausea is common before or after the event, and a feeling of heat or cold and profuse sweating are frequent accompaniments. A particular stimulus such as the sight of blood with vasovagal syncope,

TABLE 40.3

CAUSES OF SYNCOPE

Vasovagal	Fear
	Pain
	Unpleasant sights
Reflex	Cough
	Micturition
	Swallowing
	Carotid sinus pressure
Decreased venous return	Orthostatic
	Soldier syncope (standing at attention)
	With Valsalva maneuver
Decreased blood volume	
No clear precipitating event	
Cardiac	Arrhythmia
	Obstructive outflow
Cerebrovascular insufficiency	
Familial	
Undetermined cause	

From Prensky AL. Migraine and migrainous variant in pediatric patients. *Pediatr Clin North Am.* 1976;23:461–471, with permission.

minor trauma, or being in a warm, crowded place often elicits the attack. Orthostatic syncope may follow prolonged standing or sudden change in posture. The family history may disclose similar events (96). Reflex syncope may be seen with coughing, swallowing, or micturition (97). Table 40.3 lists frequent causes of syncope. A few clonic jerks or incontinence occurring late in syncope complicates the picture, but a full history usually elucidates the cause (81).

Physical examination frequently yields normal results, although supine and standing blood pressure measurements may implicate or rule out an orthostatic cause. A reduction in blood pressure of more than 15 points or sinus bradycardia (or both) on rapid standing is highly suggestive of orthostatic hypotension. A search for arrhythmia and murmur is warranted, as cardiac causes of syncope are primarily obstructive lesions or arrhythmias not otherwise clinically evident (97,98). Syncope associated with ophthalmoplegia, retinitis pigmentosa, deafness, ataxia, or seeming myopathy mandates an urgent evaluation for heart block (Kearns–Sayre syndrome) (99).

Electrocardiographic monitoring and echocardiography are frequently more valuable than electroencephalography in establishing the diagnosis. Tilt-table testing may be helpful in this regard (100,101).

Narcolepsy and Cataplexy

Narcolepsy is a state of excessive daytime drowsiness causing rapid brief sleep, sometimes during conversation or play; the patient usually awakens refreshed. Narcolepsy also includes sleep paralysis (transient episodes of inability to move on awakening) and brief hallucinations on arousal along with cataplexy, although not all patients demonstrate the complete syndrome. Measurement of sleep latency through electroencephalogram recordings reveals the appearance of REM sleep within 10 minutes in narcoleptic patients. Narcolepsy may be treated with a stimulant drug (102–104).

Cataplexy produces a sudden loss of tone with a drop to the ground in response to an unexpected touch or emotional stimulus such as laughter. Consciousness is not lost during these brief attacks. Coexistent narcolepsy is common.

Basilar Migraine

Most common in adolescent girls, basilar migraine begins with a sudden loss of consciousness followed by severe occipital or vertex headache. Dizziness, vertigo, bilateral visual loss, and, less often, diplopia, dysarthria, and bilateral paresthesias, may occur. A history of headache or a family history of migraine is helpful in making the diagnosis. Of note, interictal paroxysmal EEG discharges are not uncommon in this population. Children may respond to classic migraine therapy or antiepileptic drugs (105,106). Ergot alkaloids and triptans are generally not recommended (78).

Tremor

An involuntary movement characterized by rhythmic oscillations of a particular part of the body, tremor may appear at rest or with only certain movements. Consequently, it is occasionally mistaken for seizure activity, particularly when the movement is severe and proximal such as in the "wing-beating tremor" of Wilson disease or related basal ganglia disorders. Tremors disappear during sleep. Examination at rest and during activities, possibly by manipulating the affected body part while observing the tremor, usually can define the movement by varying or obliterating the tremor. The electroencephalogram is unchanged as the tremor escalates and diminishes (107).

Panic Disorders

Panic attacks may occur as acute events associated with a chronic anxiety disorder or in patients suffering from depression or schizophrenia. These attacks last for minutes to hours and are accompanied by palpitations, sweating, dizziness or vertigo, and feelings of unreality. The following symptoms also have been noted: dyspnea or smothering sensations, unsteadiness or faintness, palpitations or tachycardia, trembling or shaking, choking, nausea or abdominal distress, depersonalization or derealization, numbness or tingling, flushes or chills, chest pain or discomfort, and fears of dying, aura, going crazy, or losing control. An electroencephalogram recorded at the time of the attacks differentiates ictal fear and nonepileptic panic attacks (108).

Panic disorders involve spontaneous panic attacks and may be associated with agoraphobia. Although they may begin in adolescence, the average age at onset is in the late 1920s. Psychiatric therapy is indicated (109).

Acute fugue, phobias, hallucinations, and autistic behaviors may seem to represent seizures; however, associated features and EEG findings usually distinguish these behavioral disorders from epilepsy.

DISEASE-RELATED BEHAVIORS

Several disease states include recurrent symptoms that are misdiagnosed as epilepsy. Episodes of cyanosis, dyspnea, and unconsciousness followed by a convulsion may occur in as

many as 10% to 20% of children with congenital heart disease, particularly those with significant hypoxemia. In "tet" spells, young children with tetralogy of Fallot squat nearly motionless during exercise as their cardiac reserve recovers (110).

Children and adults with shunted hydrocephalus may have seizures, although these are not usual (111). Obstruction associated with the third ventricle or aqueduct may cause the bobble-head doll syndrome (two to four head oscillations per second) in mentally retarded children (112). In hydrocephalic patients treated by ventricular shunting, acute decompensation may increase seizure frequency or give rise to symptoms misdiagnosed as seizures. So-called hydrocephalic attacks, characterized by tonic, opisthotonic postures frequently associated with a generalized tremor, are caused by increased intracranial pressure and herniation. Head tilt or dystonia also may indicate increased intracranial pressure, a posterior fossa mass, or a Chiari malformation. Urgent evaluation for malfunctioning shunt or increased intracranial pressure is warranted with any of these symptoms.

The episodic nature of periodic paralysis may lead to misidentification of the symptoms as epilepsy. Familial and sporadic cases typically are associated with disorders of sodium and potassium metabolism. Acetazolamide is useful in some forms of the disorder (113).

Cerebrovascular disorders of various types and etiologies may have transient recurrent symptoms and thus are confused with epilepsy. The exact clinical presentation of cerebrovascular disorders in both children and adults depends primarily on the size and location of the brain lesion and on the etiology of the vascular compromise (114,115). Transient ischemic attacks, episodes of ischemic neurologic deficits lasting less than 24 hours, are typically caused by small emboli or local hemodynamic factors that temporarily prevent adequate brain perfusion. Symptoms begin suddenly following an embolus, with the deficit reaching maximum severity almost immediately. Function returns several minutes or hours after the onset of symptoms. Symptomatology is characteristically separated into carotid artery syndromes with symptoms of middle cerebral artery, anterior cerebral, and lacunar deficits. The latter are most common in adults with longstanding hypertension and may be characterized by pure motor hemiparesis or monoparesis and isolated hemianesthesia. Vertebrobasilar syndromes, especially transient ischemic attacks, may be mistaken for epilepsy because of recurrence and duration and may present with ataxia, dysarthria, nausea, vomiting, vertigo, and even coma. Homonymous hemianopsia may result from posterior cerebral artery occlusion. The subclavian steal syndrome is associated with stenosis or occlusion of the subclavian artery proximal to the origin of the vertebral artery. Retrograde flow through the vertebral artery into the poststenotic subclavian artery may occur. Vertigo, ataxia, syncope, and visual disturbance occur intermittently when blood is diverted into the distal subclavian artery. Vigorous exercise of the arms tends to produce symptoms. The brachial and radial pulses in the affected extremity are absent or diminished.

The etiology of cerebral embolism includes cardiopulmonary disorders, traumatic injuries to blood vessels like dissection, and congenital or inflammatory arterial disorders. Besides blood products, air emboli, foreign-body embolism with pellets, needles, or talcum, or fat emboli may be noted. In adults, carotid and vertebrobasilar occlusion with or without embolization is typically associated with systemic cerebrovascular disease. In younger black patients, sickle cell disease always must be considered as an etiology of cerebrovascular symptoms. It is sometimes difficult to distinguish between transient ischemic attacks and brief seizures in these patients who have multiple areas of infarction. Because strokes may occur on the basis of both large- and small-vessel abnormalities associated with sickle cell disease, symptoms may vary.

Transient global amnesia deserves special mention as a symptom that may or may not be related to epilepsy. Multiple authors argue that it is either of vascular origin or related to seizures. Recurrent attacks may occur in up to 25% of cases. Attacks, however, last hours rather than minutes, and the most frequently observed EEG changes are small sharp spikes of questionable significance (116).

CONCLUSIONS

A variety of paroxysmal happenings may be confused with epilepsy. A careful medical history with description of events before, during, and after the spell; age of onset; time of occurrence; and clinical course aided by a through physical examination frequently clarify the nature of these episodes. Home video recordings of the episodes may be extremely helpful. The routine or specialized use of electroencephalography or polysomnography provides further characterization. Dual diagnoses are possible. Abnormal findings on neurologic examination are not uncommon in patients with these nonepileptic events. Previously noted interictal EEG abnormalities should be reviewed to modify the interpretation of false-positive records (117).

References

1. Chutorian AM. Paroxysmal disorders of childhood. In: Rudolph AM, ed. *Rudolph's Pediatrics.* 10th ed. Norwalk, CT: Appleton & Lange; 1991: 1785–1792.
2. Gomez MR, Klass DW. Seizures and other paroxysmal disorders in infants and children. *Curr Probl Pediatr.* 1972;2:2–37.
3. Pedley TA. Differential diagnosis of episodic symptoms. *Epilepsia.* 1983; 24(suppl 1):S31–S44.
4. Rabe EF. Recurrent paroxysmal nonepileptic disorders. *Curr Probl Pediatr.* 1974;4:3–31.
5. Rothner AD. Not everything that shakes is epilepsy. *Cleve Clin J Med.* 1989;56(suppl 2):206–213.
6. So NK, Andermann F. Differential diagnosis. In: Engel J, Pedley TA, eds. *Differential Diagnosis in Epilepsy: A Comprehensive Textbook.* Philadelphia, PA: Lippincott-Raven; 1998:791–797.
7. Prensky AL. An approach to the child with paroxysmal phenomenon with emphasis on nonepileptic disorders. In: Pellock JW, Dodson WE, Bourgeois B, eds. *Pediatric Epilepsy: Diagnosis and Therapy.* 2nd ed. New York: Demos; 2001:97–116.
8. Obeid M, Mikati MA. Expanding spectrum of paroxysmal events in children: potential mimickers of epilepsy. *Pediatr Neurol.* 2007;27:309–316.
9. Hoban TF. Rhythmic movement disorder in children. *CNS Spectr.* 2003;8:135–138.
10. Daoust-Roy J, Seshia SS. Benign neonatal sleep myoclonus. A differential diagnosis of neonatal seizures. *Am J Dis Child.* 1992;146:681.
11. Shuper A, Zalzberg J, Weitz R, et al. Jitteriness beyond the neonatal period: a benign pattern of movement in infancy. *J Child Neurol.* 1991;6: 243–245.
12. Parker S, Zuckerman B, Bauchner H, et al. Jitteriness in full-term neonates: prevalence and correlates. *Pediatrics.* 1990;85:17–23.
13. Fleisher DR, Morrison A. Masturbation mimicking abdominal pain or seizures in young girls. *J Pediatr.* 1990;116:810–814.
14. Lombroso CT, Fejerman N. Benign myoclonus of early infancy. *Ann Neurol.* 1977;1:138–143.
15. Deonna T, Martin D. Benign paroxysmal torticollis in infancy. *Arch Dis Child.* 1981;56:956–959.
16. Gilbert GT. Familial spasmodic torticollis. *Neurology.* 1977;27:11–13.
17. Kinsbourne M. Hiatus hernia with contortions of the neck. *Lancet.* 1964;1:10–58.
18. Ramenofsky ML, Buyse M, Goldberg MJ, et al. Gastroesophageal reflux and torticollis. *J Bone Joint Surg (Am).* 1978;60:1140–1141.
19. King RA, Nelson LB, Wagner RS. Spasmus nutans. *Arch Ophthalmol.* 1986;104:1501–1504.
20. Hoefnagel D, Biery B. Spasmus nutans. *Dev Med Child Neurol.* 1968;10: 32–35.
21. Jayalaksmi P, McNair Scott TF, Tucker SH, et al. Infantile nystagmus: a prospective study of spasmus nutans, congenital nystagmus, and unclassified nystagmus of infancy. *J Pediatr.* 1970;77:177–187.
22. Dyken P, Kolar O. Dancing eyes, dancing feet: infantile polymyoclonia. *Brain.* 1968;91:305–320.
23. Moe PG, Nellhaus G. Infantile polymyoclonia-opsoclonus syndrome and neural crest tumors. *Neurology.* 1970;20:756–764.
24. Soloman GE, Chutorian AM. Opsoclonus and occult neuroblastoma. *N Engl J Med.* 1968;279:475–477.
25. Bienfang DC. Opsoclonus in infancy. *Arch Ophthalmol.* 1974;91: 203–205.
26. Herbst JJ. Gastroesophageal reflux. *J Pediatr.* 1981;98:859–870.
27. Brown P, Rothwell JC, Thompson PD, et al. The hyperexplexias and their relationship to the normal startle reflex. *Brain.* 1991;114:1903–1928.
28. Aguglia U, Tinaper P, Gastaut H. Startle-induced epileptic seizures. *Epilepsia.* 1984;25:720.
29. SaenzLope E, Herranz FJ, Masdue JC. Startle epilepsy: a clinical study. *Ann Neurol.* 1984;16:78–81.
30. Andermann F, Andermann E. Startle disorders of man: hyperexplexia, jumping and startle epilepsy. *Brain Dev.* 1988;10:213–222.
31. Andermann F, Keene DL, Andermann E, et al. Startle disease or hyperexplexia: further delineation of the syndrome. *Brain.* 1980;103:985–997.
32. Holmes GL, Russman BS. Shuddering attacks. *Am J Dis Child.* 1986; 140:72–73.
33. Vanasse M, Bedard P, Anderson F. Shuddering attacks in children: an early clinical manifestation of essential tremor. *Neurology.* 1976;26:1027–1030.
34. Bourgeois M, Aicardi J, Goutieres F. Alternating hemiplegia of childhood. *J Pediatr.* 1993;122:673–679.
35. Silver K, Andermann F. Alternating hemiplegia of childhood: a study of 10 patients and results of flunarizine treatment. *Neurology.* 1993;43:36–41.
36. Watanabe K, Hara K, Hakamada S, et al. Seizures with apnea in children. *Pediatrics.* 1982;79:87–90.
37. Myer EC. Infant apnea, life threatening events and sudden infant death. In: Myer EC, Pellock JM, eds. *Neurologic Emergencies in Infancy and Childhood.* 2nd ed. New York: Demos; 1992:42–55.
38. Thach BT. Sleep apnea in infancy and childhood. *Med Clin North Am.* 1985;69:1289–1315.
39. Myer EC. Naltrexone therapy of apnea in children with elevated CFS β-endorphin. *Ann Neurol.* 1990;27:75–80.
40. Gibson E, Cullen JA, Spinner S, et al. Infant sleep position following new AAP guidelines. *Pediatrics.* 1995;96:69–72.
41. Herbst JJ, Minton SD, Book LS. Gastroesophageal reflux causing respiratory distress and apnea in newborn infants. *J Pediatr.* 1979;95:763–768.
42. Spitzer AR, Boyle JT, Tuchman DN, et al. Awake apnea associated with gastroesophageal reflux: a specific clinical syndrome. *J Pediatr.* 1984;104: 200–205.
43. Meyers WF, Herbst JJ. Effectiveness of positioning therapy for gastroesophageal reflux. *Pediatrics.* 1982;69:768–772.
44. Lombroso CT, Lerman P. Breath-holding spells (cyanotic and pallid infantile syncope). *Pediatrics.* 1967;39:563–581.
45. Colina KF, Abelson HT. Resolution of breath-holding spells with treatment of concomitant anemia. *J Pediatr.* 1995;126:395–397.
46. DiMario FJ, Bauer L, Baxter D. Respiratory sinus arrhythmia in children with severe cyanotic and pallid breath-holding spells. *J Child Neurol.* 1998;13:440–442.
47. Laxdal T, Gomez MR, Reiher J. Cyanotic and pallid syncopal attacks in children (breath-holding spells). *Dev Med Child Neurol.* 1969;11: 755–763.
48. Livingston S. Breath-holding spells in children: differentiation from epileptic attacks. *J Am Med Assoc.* 1970;212:2231–2235.
49. Stephenson J. Reflex anoxic seizures ("white breath-holding"): nonepileptic vagal attacks. *Arch Dis Child.* 1978;53:193–200.
50. McWilliam R, Stephenson J. Atropine treatment of reflex atonic seizures. *Arch Dis Child.* 1984;59:473–485.
51. Coleman RM, Pollak CP, Weitzman ED. Periodic movements in sleep (nocturnal myoclonus): relation to sleep disorders. *Ann Neurol.* 1980;8: 416–421.
52. Holmes GL. *Diagnosis and Management of Seizures in Children.* Philadelphia, PA: WB Saunders; 1987.
53. Mahowald MW, Schenck CH. NREM sleep parasomnias. *Neurol Clin.* 1996;14:675–696.
54. Oswald I. Sudden bodily jerks on falling asleep. *Brain.* 1959;82:92–103.
55. Godbout R, Montplaisir J, Rouleau I. Hypnogenic paroxysmal dystonia: epilepsy or sleep disorder? A case report. *Clin Electroencephalogr.* 1985;16:136–142.
56. DiMario FJ, Emery ES. The natural history of night terrors. *Clin Pediatr.* 1987;26:505–511.
57. Kales A, Kales JD. Sleep disorders: recent findings in the diagnosis and treatment of disturbed sleep. *N Engl J Med.* 1974;290:487–499.

58. Thorpy MJ, Glovinsky PB. Parasomnias. *Psychiatr Clin North Am.* 1987;10:623–639.
59. Vela-Bueno A, Soldatos CR. Episodic sleep disorders (parasomnias). *Semin Neurol.* 1987;7:269–276.
60. Menkes JH. *Textbook of Child Neurology.* Philadelphia, PA: Lea & Febiger; 1990.
61. Nausieda PA, Grossman BJ, Killer WC, et al. Sydenham chorea: an update. *Neurology.* 1980;30:331–334.
62. Erenberg G, Rothner AD. Tourette syndrome: diagnosis and management. *Int Pediatr.* 1987;2:149–153.
63. Golden GS. Tourette syndrome: recent advances. *Neurol Clin.* 1990;8:705–714.
64. Singer HS, Rosenberg LA. Development of behavioral and emotional problems in Tourette syndrome. *Pediatr Neurol.* 1989;5:41–44.
65. Demirkerian M, Jankovic J. Paroxysmal dyskinesias: clinical features and classification. *Ann Neurol.* 1995;38:571–579.
66. Kertesz A. Paroxysmal kinesigenic choreoathetosis. *Neurology.* 1967;17:680–690.
67. Kinast M, Erenberg G, Rothner AD. Paroxysmal choreoathetosis: report of five cases and review of the literature. *Pediatrics.* 1980;65:74–77.
68. Lance JW. Familial paroxysmal dystonic choreoathetosis and its differentiation from related syndromes. *Ann Neurol.* 1977;2:285–293.
69. Donat JF, Wright FS. Episodic symptoms mistaken for seizures in the neurologically impaired child. *Neurology.* 1990;40:156–157.
70. Percy A, Gillberg C, Hayberg B, et al. Rett syndrome and the autistic disorder. *Neurol Clin.* 1990;8:659–676.
71. Brunquell P, McKeever M, Russman BS. Differentiation of epileptic from nonepileptic head drops in children. *Epilepsia.* 1990;31:401–405.
72. Rosemon F, Wyllie E, Kotagal P, et al. Staring spells in children: descriptive features distinguishing epileptic from nonepileptic events. *J Pediatr.* 1998;133:660–663.
73. Barron T. The child with spells. *Pediatr Clin North Am.* 1991;38:711–724.
74. Shaywitz SE, Shaywitz BA. Attention deficit disorder: current perspectives. *Pediatr Neurol.* 1987;3:129–135.
75. Voeller KKS, ed. Attention deficit hyperactivity disorder (ADHD). *J Child Neurol.* 1991;6(suppl):S1–S131.
76. Weinberg WA, Brumback RA. Primary disorder of vigilance: a novel explanation of inattentiveness, daydreaming, boredom, restlessness, and sleepiness. *J Pediatr.* 1990;116:720–725.
77. D'Alessandro R, Sacquengna T, Pazzaglia P, et al. Headache after partial complex seizures. In: Andermann F, Lugaresi E, eds. *Migraine and Epilepsy.* London: Butterworths; 1987:273–328.
78. Annequuin D, Tourmaire B, Massiou H. Migraine and headache in childhood and adolescence. *Pediatr Clin North Am.* 2000;47:617–631.
79. Barlow CF. *Headaches and Migraine in Children.* London: Spastics International Medical; 1984.
80. Blume WT, Young GB. Ictal pain: unilateral, cephalic and abdominal. In: Andermann F, Lugaresi E, eds. *Migraine and Epilepsy.* London: Butterworths; 1987:238–248.
81. Pratt JL, Fleisher GR. Syncope in children and adolescents. *Pediatr Emerg Care.* 1989;5:80–82.
82. Prensky AL. Migraine and migrainous variant in pediatric patients. *Pediatr Clin North Am.* 1976;23:461–471.
83. Prensky AL, Sommer D. Diagnosis and treatment of migraine in children. *Neurology.* 1979;29:506–510.
84. Hammond J. The late sequelae of recurrent vomiting of childhood. *Dev Med Child Neurol.* 1974;16:15–22.
85. Gascon G, Barlow C. Juvenile migraine presenting as an acute confusional state. *J Pediatr.* 1970;45:628–635.
86. Finkelhor BK, Harker LA. Benign paroxysmal vertigo of childhood. *Laryngoscope.* 1987;97:1161–1163.
87. Parker W. Migraine and the vestibular system in childhood and adolescence. *Am J Otolaryngol.* 1989;10:364–371.
88. Rosenberg AH. Constipation and encopresis. In: Wyllie R, Hyams JS, eds. *Pediatric Gastrointestinal Disease.* Philadelphia, PA: WB Saunders; 1993:198–208.
89. Williams DT, Mehl R, Yudofsky S, et al. The effect of propranolol on uncontrolled rage outbursts in children and adolescents with organic brain dysfunction. *J Am Acad Child Psychiatry.* 1982;21:129–135.
90. Elliott FA. The episodic dyscontrol syndrome and aggression. *Neurol Clin.* 1984;2:113–125.
91. Folks DG. Munchausen's syndrome and other factitious disorders. *Neurol Clin.* 1995;13:267–281.
92. Meadow R. Munchausen syndrome by proxy. *Arch Dis Child.* 1982;57:92–98.
93. Meadow R. Neurological and developmental variants of Munchausen syndrome. *Dev Med Child Neurol.* 1991;33:270–272.
94. Wyllie E, Friedman D, Rothner AD, et al. Psychogenic seizures in children and adolescents: outcome after diagnosis by ictal video and electroencephalographic recording. *Pediatrics.* 1990;85:480–484.
95. Bools CN, Neale BA, Meadow SR. Follow-up of victims of fabricated illness (Munchausen syndrome by proxy). *Arch Dis Child.* 1993;69:625–630.
96. Camfield PR, Camfield CS. Syncope in childhood: a case control clinical study of the familial tendency to faint. *Clin J Neurol Sci.* 1990;17:306–308.
97. Katz RM. Cough syncope in children with asthma. *J Pediatr.* 1970;77:48–51.
98. Ruckman RN. Cardiac causes of syncope. *Pediatr Rev.* 1987;9:101–108.
99. Berenberg RA, Pellock JM, DiMauro S, et al. Lumping or splitting? Ophthalmoplegia plus or Kearns-Sayre syndrome. *Ann Neurol.* 1977;1:37–54.
100. Lerman-Sagie T, Rechavia E, Strasberg B, et al. Head-up tilt for the evaluation of syncope of unknown origin in children. *J Pediatr.* 1991;118:676–679.
101. Thilenius OG, Quinones JA, Husayni TS, et al. Tilt test for diagnosis of unexplained syncope in pediatric patients. *Pediatrics.* 1991;87:334–338.
102. Broughton RJ. Polysomnography: principles and applications in sleep and arousal disorders. In: Niedermeyer E, Lopes da Silva F, eds. *Electroencephalography.* 2nd ed. Baltimore, MD: Urban & Schwarzenberg; 1987:687–724.
103. Kotagal S, Hartse KM, Walsh JK. Characteristics of narcolepsy in preteenaged children. *Pediatrics.* 1990;85:205–209.
104. Wittig R, Zorick F, Roehrs T, et al. Narcolepsy in a 7-year-old child. *J Pediatr.* 1983;102:725–727.
105. Camfield PR, Metrakos K, Andermann F. Basilar migraine, seizures, and severe epileptiform EEG abnormalities: a benign syndrome in adolescents. *Neurology.* 1978;28:584.
106. Golden GS, French JH. Basilar artery migraine in young children. *Pediatrics.* 1975;56:722.
107. Hallett M. Classification and treatment of tremor. *J Am Med Assoc.* 1991;266:1115–1117.
108. American Psychiatric Association. *Diagnostic and Statistical Manual of Mental Disorders.* 3rd ed., rev. Washington, DC: American Psychiatric Association; 1987.
109. Kaplan HI, Sadock BJ, eds. *The Comprehensive Textbook of Psychiatry.* 5th ed. Baltimore, MD: Williams & Wilkins; 1989.
110. Paul MH. Tetralogy of Fallot. In: Rudolph AM, ed. *Rudolph's Pediatrics.* 10th ed. Norwalk, CT: Appleton & Lange; 1991:1397–1398.
111. Hack CH, Enril BG, Donat JF, et al. Seizures in relation to shunt displacement in patients with MMC. *J Pediatr.* 1990;116:57–60.
112. Tomasovic JA, Nelhaus G, Moe PG. The bobblehead doll syndrome: an early sign of hydrocephalus. *Dev Med Child Neurol.* 1975;17:177.
113. Meyers KR, Gilden DH, Rinaldi CF, et al. Periodic muscle weakness, normokalemia, and tubular aggregates. *Neurology.* 1972;22:269.
114. Hachinski V, Norris JW. *Stroke.* Philadelphia, PA: FA Davis; 1985.
115. Roach ES, Riela AR. *Pediatric Cerebrovascular Disorders.* New York: Futura; 1988.
116. Miller JW, Petersen RC, Metter EJ, et al. Transient global amnesia. *Neurology.* 1987;37:733–737.
117. Metrick ME, Ritter FJ, Gates JR, et al. Nonepileptic events in children. *Epilepsia.* 1991;32:322–328.

PART IV ■ ANTIEPILEPTIC MEDICATIONS

CHAPTER 41 ■ ANTIEPILEPTIC DRUG DEVELOPMENT AND EXPERIMENTAL MODELS

H. STEVE WHITE

ANIMAL MODELS FOR ANTIEPILEPTIC DRUG DISCOVERY

All of the currently available antiepileptic drugs (AEDs) approved for the treatment of epilepsy have been identified and developed as a result of their ability to block seizures in rodent seizure and epilepsy models. Since 1993, 12 new AEDs have been developed and made available for patients with epilepsy. These new drugs have provided patients with increased seizure control; are proven to be better tolerated; and display fewer drug–drug interactions. Unfortunately, there continues to be a significant unmet need for the adult patient with therapy-resistant epilepsy and the pediatric patient with catastrophic epilepsy. As such, efforts continue in the hope that more efficacious and less toxic AEDs will be identified for this patient population.

A new AED, regardless of the process by which it is designed, must always demonstrate some degree of efficacy in one or more animal seizure or epilepsy models before it is likely to proceed down the drug development pathway and ultimately validated in well-controlled double-blinded randomized clinical trials. Typically, an investigational drug will be evaluated for its ability to block convulsive seizures in models of generalized and partial seizures. This approach provides the necessary proof-of-concept to support the further development of a new chemical entity. Moreover, it provides an indication of the potential therapeutic spectrum of a new drug; that is, broad versus narrow. The remainder of this chapter will briefly review the approach that is employed in the early identification and characterization of a drugs anticonvulsant profile and discuss efforts to develop new models of refractory epilepsy.

In Vivo Testing

It is important to note that no single laboratory test will establish the presence or absence of anticonvulsant activity or fully predict the clinical utility of an investigational AED. Nonetheless, the animal models that have been developed and utilized since phenytoin (PHT) was first identified using the maximal electroshock seizure model (1), do possess varying degrees of face validity. Historically, the successful identification of PHT using the cat maximal electroshock (MES) test by Merritt and Putnam (1) and its subsequent acceptance as an effective drug for the management of human generalized tonic–clonic seizures provided the validation required to consider the MES test as a useful model of human generalized tonic–clonic seizures. In addition to the MES test, the subcutaneous pentylenetetrazol (sc PTZ) test, and the various forms of the kindling model represent two other important in vivo model systems that have played an important role over the last 40 years in the early identification and characterization of AEDs (2,3).

Advances in our understanding at the molecular and genetic level have led to the development of mouse models with known genetic defects that resemble the human condition. Their availability to the general scientific community has provided greater insight into the role of various molecular targets in ictogenesis and epileptogenesis. Furthermore, these mutant mouse models represent important tools for evaluating the therapeutic potential of an investigational drug in a model system that more closely approximates human epilepsy. To this point, they will likely play an important role in efforts to develop personalized medicines for those patients with a known genetic mutation.

CORRELATION OF ANIMAL ANTICONVULSANT PROFILE AND CLINICAL UTILITY

The MES and Kindled Rat Models

The MES test and the kindling model represent two animal models that have proven to be quite predictive of a drug's potential utility against generalized tonic–clonic and partial seizures, respectively (Table 41.1). As mentioned in "In Vivo Testing," the current era of AED discovery was introduced by Merritt and Putnam in 1937 when they identified the anticonvulsant potential of PHT using the MES model. As summarized in Table 41.1, the pharmacological profile of the MES test supports its utility as a predictive model for human generalized tonic–clonic seizures. In contrast, the lack of any demonstrable efficacy by tiagabine, vigabatrin, and levetiracetam in the MES test argues against the utility of this test as a predictive model of partial seizures.

Over the last 20-plus years, the kindling model of partial epilepsy has been used with increasing frequency in the AED discovery process. Kindling refers to the process through which an initially subconvulsive current, when repeatedly delivered to a limbic brain region such as the amygdala or hippocampus, results in a progressive increase in electrographic and behavioral seizure activity (4). In other words, kindling is

TABLE 41.1

CORRELATION BETWEEN ANTICONVULSANT EFFICACY AND CLINICAL UTILITY OF ANTIEPILEPTIC DRUGS IN EXPERIMENTAL ANIMAL MODELS[a]

Experimental model	Clinical seizure type			
	Tonic and/or clonic generalized seizures	Myoclonic/generalized absence seizures	Generalized absence seizures	Partial seizures
MES (tonic extension)[b]	CBZ, PHT, VPA, PB [FBM, GBP, LCM, LTG, PGB, RUF, TPM, ZNS]			
Sc PTZ (clonic seizures)[b]		ESM, VPA, PB[c], BZD [FBM, GBP, PGB, RUF, TGB[c], VGB[c]]		
Spike–wave discharges[d]			ESM, VPA, BZD [LTG, TPM, LVT]	
Electrical kindling (focal seizures)				CBZ, PHT, VPA, PB, BZD [FBM, GBP, LCM, LTG, TPM, TGB, ZNS, LVT, VGB]
PHT-resistant kindled rat[e]				[LVT, GBP, TPM, FBM, LTG]
6 Hz (44 mA)[f]				VPA [LVT]

[a]BZD, benzodiazepines; CBZ, carbamazepine; ESM, ethosuximide; FBM, felbamate; GBP, gabapentin; LTG, lamotrigine; LVT, levetiracetam; PB, phenobarbital; PHT, phenytoin; LCM, lacosamide; PGB, pregabalin; RUF, rufinamide; TGB, tiagabine; TPM, topiramate; VPA, valproic acid; ZNS, zonisamide; VGB, vigabatrin.
[b]Data summarized from Refs. 5 to 7
[c]PB, TGB, and VGB block clonic seizures induced by sc PTZ but are inactive against generalized absence seizures and may exacerbate spike–wave seizures.
[d]Data summarized from GBL, GAERS, and *lh/lh* spike–wave models (8–11).
[e]Data summarized from Ref. 12.
[f]Data summarized from Ref. 13.
[ ] Second-generation AED.
White HS. Epilepsy and disease modification: animal models for novel drug discovery. In: Rho J, Sankar R, Cavazos J, eds. *Epilepsy: Scientific foundations of Clinical Practice*. In Press, 2009, with permission.

associated with a progressive increase in seizure severity and duration, a decrease in focal seizure threshold, and neuronal degeneration in limbic brain regions that resemble human temporal lobe epilepsy. Unlike the MES and PTZ tests, the pharmacological profile of the kindling model supports its utility as a model of focal epilepsy. In support of this conclusion, the kindled rat model is the one animal model that accurately predicted the clinical utility of levetiracetam (LEV) (see Table 41.1) (5–7). This one example demonstrates the importance of employing a battery of models in an initial screening protocol to avoid inadvertently "missing" a potentially important new therapy. In addition to LEV, the kindling rat model accurately predicts the clinical utility of all of the AEDs currently employed in the treatment of partial epilepsy (see Table 41.1).

The Subcutaneous Pentylenetetrazol (sc PTZ) Seizure Test and Other Models of Spike–Wave Seizures

Positive results obtained in the sc PTZ seizure test have historically been considered suggestive of clinical utility against generalized absence seizures. Based on this argument, phenobarbital, gabapentin, pregabalin, and tiagabine, which are all effective in the sc PTZ test, should all be effective against spike–wave seizures, and lamotrigine (LTG), which is inactive in the sc PTZ test, should be inactive against spike–wave seizures. However, clinical experience has shown that this is an invalid prediction; for example, phenobarbital, gabapentin, pregabalin, and tiagabine are not only ineffective, they all aggravate spike–wave seizure discharge. In contrast, LTG has been found to be effective against absence seizures. Given that the overall utility of the sc PTZ test for predicting activity against human spike–wave seizures is limited, any conclusion concerning a drug's potential clinical efficacy against spike–wave seizures is made, positive findings in the sc PTZ test should be corroborated by positive findings in other models of absence, such as the lethargic (*lh/lh*) mouse (8,9,15), the WAG/Rij rat (8), the genetic absence epileptic rat of Strasbourg (10), the γ-butyrolactone (11) seizure test. In addition to being more predictive, all four of these models also accurately predict the potentiation of spike–wave seizures by drugs that elevate GABA concentrations (e.g., vigabatrin and tiagabine), drugs that directly activate the $GABA_B$ receptor, and the barbiturates.

ASSESSING ADVERSE EFFECTS IN ANIMALS

For the patient with refractory epilepsy, the clinical utility of the currently available AEDs is limited in a large part by a lack of efficacy at doses that do not produce limiting side effects. With respect to assessing central nervous system (CNS)–related adverse effects, preclinical testing includes behavioral observations, activity measurements, and models evaluating the potential impact of an AED on motor function in rodents. Among the latter models, the rotarod test is commonly used to quantify a therapeutic index (TI) (16). The extent by which an AED impairs the ability of an animal to remain on a rotating rod is determined at various dose levels. A TI can be established by comparing the median toxic (TD_{50}) dose of an AED that induces impaired performance of the animals in the rotarod against the median effective (ED_{50}) anticonvulsant dose in the same species.

The validity of using normal animals in an attempt to predict adverse effects in epilepsy patients has been brought into question ever since Löscher and Hönack demonstrated that N-methyl-D-aspartate (NMDA) antagonists produced more ataxia, hyperactivity, and stereotypic behaviors in amygdala kindled rats than they did in normal rats (17). This finding was subsequently confirmed in humans when the potential antiepileptic properties of the competitive NMDA antagonist D-CPPene was tested (18). D-CPPene was shown to be well tolerated in healthy volunteers in doses up to 2000 mg/day; whereas, doses of 500 to 1000 mg/day induced severe adverse effects such as confusion, hallucination, ataxia, impaired concentration, and sedation when used as add-on therapy in eight patients with refractory complex partial epilepsy. Interestingly, similar doses of D-CPPene in healthy volunteers and epilepsy patients produced higher exposure levels in the healthy volunteers versus epilepsy patients. These results suggest that pharmacodynamic factors were responsible for the severe adverse effects observed in patients with epilepsy.

The enhanced susceptibility of fully amygdala kindled rats to the behavioral adverse effects of NMDA antagonists has also been observed with several AEDs (19). Thus, this phenomenon appears to represent a permanent reactivity specific for limbic kindling because it has not been observed after chemical kindling (20). Collectively, these findings suggest that the neuronal substrate is altered in the epileptic brain in such a way that leads to a worsened adverse effect profile of AEDs. These findings underlie the importance of using fully limbic kindled animals (or animals with spontaneous seizures) for assessing the adverse effects of an investigational AED. However, a highly promising AED should not necessarily be discarded because of adverse effects observed in an animal model. This information should be used to guide decisions regarding the advancement of one analog over another when testing a series of structurally related molecules.

STRATEGIES FOR ANTIEPILEPTIC DRUG DISCOVERY

Three different approaches are routinely employed in the identification of new AEDs. These include: (i) random screening of new chemical entities for anticonvulsant activity; (ii) structural

modifications of existing AEDs; and (iii) rational, target-based drug discovery. Over the decades, each of these approaches has contributed to the discovery of new AEDs. Regardless of the approach by which a new drug is synthesized, the first proof-of-concept study almost always involves testing it in one or more of the animal models described above; e.g., the MES, sc PTZ and/or kindling model. With the exception of levetiracetam, all of the currently available AEDs (and those currently in development) have been found to possess activity in one or more of these models.

LEV is the (S)-enantiomer of the ethyl analog of the nootropic drug piracetam. LEV was synthesized in 1974 in an attempt to identify a second-generation agent of piracetam. LEV did not show any consistent nootropic activity but revealed potent and general antiseizure activity in sound-susceptible mice (21). Interestingly, LEV was not active in either of the primary seizure screens routinely employed; for example, the MES and sc PTZ tests (15,22).

A further evaluation found levetiracetam to possess anticonvulsant properties in the amygdala kindled rat and to display a marked and persistent ability to inhibit kindling acquisition (15,22,23). Levetiracetam was also found to be active in a variety of genetic animal models of epilepsy, for example, epilepsy-like mice (24), the audiogenic seizure susceptible rat, and the genetic absence epilepsy in rats from Strasbourg (GAERS) rat model of spike–wave seizures (25). Levetiracetam was also shown to be active in the mouse 6 Hz psychomotor seizure model (13).

The ultimate development of LEV illustrates the limitations of relying solely upon the use of acute seizures evoked by MES and sc PTZ in normal animals as a valid screening procedure to identify drugs for a disease that is characterized by a chronic network hypersynchrony and spontaneous seizures. Levetiracetam further exemplifies that it is important to use a battery of models during random screening of new chemical entities that include animal models with (i) an acquired, kindled, alteration in seizure threshold and (ii) induced or natural mutations associated with an altered seizure threshold or spontaneous seizure expression (26). This does not imply that the acute seizure models are of little value. Fortunately for the patient with epilepsy, these models have yielded several new drugs that have proven to be effective for the treatment of their seizures.

MODELS OF PHARMACORESISTANCE

The models summarized in Table 41.1 have been successfully used to identify effective therapies for the treatment of human epilepsy. Clinical experience has demonstrated that they are effective for a large fraction of the patients with partial, generalized, and secondarily generalized seizures. Unfortunately, there still remains a substantial need for the identification of therapies for the patient with refractory seizures. To this point, one might argue that the models summarized in Table 41.1 are not predictive of efficacy in those patients with highly refractory epilepsy. Thus, the identification and characterization of one or more model systems that would predict efficacy in the pharmacoresistant patient population would be a valuable asset to the epilepsy community. Furthermore, the ability to segregate animals on the basis of their responsiveness or lack of sensitivity to a given AED would: (i) provide a greater understanding of the molecular mechanisms underlying pharmacoresistance; (ii) be useful for studies designed to assess whether it is possible to reverse drug resistance; and (iii) provide for the identification and characterization of surrogate markers that might be able to predict which patient will remit and become pharmacoresistant. The experimental epilepsy community will not know which model is the most relevant until the time a drug is found that markedly reduces the incidence of therapy-resistant epilepsy. Only then will we be able to retrospectively determine which model predicts efficacy against refractory seizures.

At the present time, there are a number of potentially interesting model systems of therapy resistance available. From a model perspective, it is first important to provide some operational definition of AED "pharmacoresistance." The participants of two National Institutes of Health/National Institute of Neurological Disorders and Stroke/American Epilepsy Society (NIH/NINDS/AES)-sponsored Workshops on Animal Models held in 2001 and 2002 agreed that any proposed model of "pharmacoresistant" epilepsy should meet certain criteria; that is, "pharmacoresistance" can be defined as persistent seizure activity that does not respond to monotherapy at tolerable doses with at least two currently available AEDs (27,28). Ideally, it can be hoped that any proposed model will lead to the identification of a new therapy that will ultimately be highly effective in humans resistant to existing AEDs.

In recent years, there have been a number of in vivo model systems characterized that display a phenotype consistent with pharmacoresistant epilepsy (see Ref. 29, for review). These include the PHT-resistant kindled rat (30,31), the LTG-resistant kindled rat (32–35), the 6 Hz psychomotor seizure model of partial epilepsy (13), poststatus epileptic models of temporal lobe epilepsy (36–41), and the methylazoxymethanol acetate (MAM) in utero model of nodular heterotopias (42). All of these models have some utility when attempting to differentiate an investigational drug's anticonvulsant profile from existing AEDs. This is not to imply that other approaches using in vitro systems are of any less value and the reader is referred to Refs. 43 and 44 for review and references. At the present time, none of these models are routinely employed in the search for the truly novel AED. To this point, there needs to be a concerted effort to initiate a process whereby investigational AEDs are routinely and systematically evaluated in one or more of these models. Because it is not known whether efficacy in any of these models will yield a drug candidate that proves to be highly effective in the patient with refractory epilepsy, an effort should be made to employ as many novel models as possible in the early evaluation of a new investigational AED.

The Phenytoin-Resistant Kindled Rat Model

Over the years, Löscher and colleagues have conducted extensive pharmacological evaluations in the kindled rat model. They were among the first to demonstrate that AEDs were less effective against the fully expressed kindled seizure than MES-induced generalized tonic extension seizures (45,46). Furthermore, Rundfeldt and colleagues found that the pharmacological response to a challenge dose of PHT

within a population of kindled rats could be differentiated on the basis of whether a particular rat was a responder or a nonresponder (47). This observation became the cornerstone of numerous studies designed to evaluate the effectiveness of "established" and "investigational" AEDs in PHT responders and nonresponders.

One particular advantage of the PHT-resistant kindled rat is that it permits an investigator to conduct comparative studies in two separate populations of rats; that is, sensitive and resistant. Although more labor-intensive than the acute evoked seizure models (MES, sc PTZ, and others), the kindled rat, unlike the spontaneous seizure models (discussed Post Status Epilepticus Models of Temporal Lobe Epilepsy), does not require continuous video–EEG monitoring.

The Lamotrigine-Resistant Kindled Rat Model

The LTG-resistant kindled rat model of partial epilepsy was first described by Postma and colleagues (32). Unlike the PHT-resistant kindled rat, resistance to LTG is induced when a rat is exposed to a low dose of LTG during the kindling acquisition phase. A similar phenomenon has been observed for carbamazepine (CBZ) (48). Perhaps more important is the observation that LTG-resistant rats are also refractory to CBZ, PHT, and topiramate (TPM) but not valproic acid (VPA) or the investigational AED carisbamate (49) and the KCNQ2 ($K_{v7.2}$) activator retigabine (33–35). In this regard, it might serve as an early model of drug-resistant epilepsy to differentiate novel AEDs from PHT, LTG, CBZ, and TPM for further evaluation in more extensive model systems including the PHT-resistant kindled rat.

The Low-Frequency (6 Hz) Electroshock Seizure Model

In many respects, the 6 Hz seizure model offers many of the same advantages of the MES test. Like the MES test, the 6 Hz seizure can be acutely evoked using standard corneal electroshock. Moreover, it is high throughput and requires minimal technical expertise. The main difference between the 6 Hz and MES tests is the frequency (6 Hz vs. 50 Hz) and duration (3 sec vs. 0.2 sec) of the stimulation employed. The low-frequency, long-duration stimulus results in a seizure that is characterized by immobility, forelimb clonus, Straub tail, and facial automatisms and is thought to more closely model human limbic seizures (13,50,51). Interestingly, the pharmacological profile of the 6 Hz model is somewhat dependent on the intensity of the stimulation (Table 41.2). For example, at a convulsive current (CC) sufficient to induce a prototypical seizure in 97% of the population tested (i.e., the CC_{97}), the 6 Hz seizure test is relatively nondiscriminating; that is, the large majority of AEDs evaluated (PHT, LTG, ethosuximide [ESM], LEV, and VPA) are effective in blocking the acute seizure. As the current intensity is increased to a level that is 1.5 times the CC_{97}, several of the AEDs lose their ability to protect against a 6 Hz seizure at doses that do not cause motor impairment. At a current equivalent to two times the CC_{97}, only VPA and LEV retained their ability to block 6 Hz

TABLE 41.2

EFFECT OF STIMULUS INTENSITY ON THE ANTICONVULSANT EFFICACY OF
PHENYTOIN, LAMOTRIGINE, ETHOSUXIMIDE, LEVETIRACETAM, AND
VALPROIC ACID IN THE 6 HZ SEIZURE TEST

	ED50 (mg/kg, i.p.) and 95% CI[a]		
Antiepileptic drug	22 mA	32 mA	44 mA
Phenytoin	9.4 (4.7–14.9)	>60	>60
Lamotrigine	4.4 (2.2–6.6)	>60	>60
Ethosuximide	86.9 (37.8–156)	167 (114–223)	>600
Levetiracetam	4.6 (1.1–8.7)	19.4 (9.9–36.0)	1089 (787–2650)
Valproic acid	41.5 (16.1–68.8)	126 (94.5–152)	310 (258–335)

[a]Confidence interval (CI) shown in ( ).
From Barton ME, Klein BD, Wolf HH, et al. Pharmacological characterization of the 6 Hz psychomotor
seizure model of partial epilepsy. *Epilepsy Res.* 2001;47:217–227, with permission.

seizures; albeit, the potency of both drugs at two times the CC$_{97}$ was markedly reduced (13). The finding that LEV was found to be active at a specific stimulus intensity where other anticonvulsants display little to no efficacy illustrates the use of the 6 Hz model as a screen for novel anticonvulsant compounds; particularly when one considers that LEV was inactive in the acute seizure models such as the MES and PTZ seizure tests (16). Thus, the incorporation of a simple acute screen that would minimize the chances of "missing" a unique drug like LEV should be an important consideration when setting up an anticonvulsant testing protocol to evaluate investigational AEDs.

Poststatus Epilepticus Models of Temporal Lobe Epilepsy

Poststatus epilepticus models of refractory epilepsy are beginning to emerge as important tools in the differentiation of investigational AEDs. These chronic epilepsy models differ significantly from the AED-resistant kindled rat and the 6 Hz seizure model in that seizures are spontaneously evolving and not evoked. This model yields potentially important information about an AED's relative efficacy compared to existing AEDs and thus provides another level of complexity to the pharmacological evaluation of an investigational drug. The development and characterization of this model for AED testing emerged from a focused effort of the epilepsy community to identify clinically relevant models of chronic epilepsy (27,28). The poststatus models described thus far fulfill one important characteristic of the ideal model system; that is, they display spontaneous recurrent seizures (SRS) (27,28). The poststatus epileptic rat provides an investigator with the opportunity to evaluate the efficacy of a given treatment on seizure frequency, seizure type (i.e., focal or generalized), and the liability for tolerance development following chronic treatment. Unfortunately, drug trials in rats with spontaneous seizures take on another level of complexity. They are extremely laborious and time-consuming and require a greater level of technical expertise. As such there have only been a few

pharmacological studies conducted to date (36,38–41). Having said this, the advantages that this model provides for differentiating a given compound from the established AEDs is well worth the investment. All of these models are being used with increasing frequency in the search for novel AEDs. They can play an important role in efforts to differentiate investigational drugs from existing AEDs. Unfortunately, none of these models have been validated clinically and thus, it is too early to say whether any of these models will lead to the identification of the next-generation AED. Importantly, the use of these models has led to the development of novel drug-testing protocols in animals that more closely resemble human clinical protocols.

BIOMARKERS OF THERAPEUTIC RESPONSE

The selection and use of currently available AEDs is based on an accurate diagnosis and assessment of seizure type. Fortunately, this leads to excellent seizure control in the majority of patients with epilepsy. Unfortunately, for those patients whose seizures are not effectively treated with available therapies, there is no method, at least at the present time, for individualizing the choice of AEDs. Ongoing efforts in pharmacogenomics may someday provide a mechanism for avoiding AEDs in patients at high risk of idiosyncratic reactions or in selecting AEDs for certain genetically defined epilepsy syndromes. In addition, the only way to gauge whether an AED will be effective and well tolerated is to monitor the efficacy of a given therapy in a patient over time. As such, there is a need for biomarkers that reliably predict efficacy, safety, and tolerability of an AED early in its course. The availability of predictive biomarkers would be useful for avoiding ineffective treatments and dose-related or idiosyncratic side effects. While emerging proof-of-concept clinical models such as the photosensitivity model may be useful to screen AEDs before launching lengthy and expensive clinical development programs, they do not yet appear able to predict which patients will benefit from specific AEDs.

Lastly, each of the models of pharmacoresistance described so far provide a biological system that will likely lead to a greater understanding of the mechanisms underlying pharmacoresistant epilepsy. As such, they can be used to test novel approaches designed to overcome or reverse therapy resistance, and to perhaps identify appropriate surrogate markers of pharmacoresistance. One can envision the day when we will be able to identify the patient at risk for developing therapy-resistant epilepsy and institute a prophylactic therapy that prevents the emergence of pharmacoresistance.

CONCLUSION

At the current time, there are no known preventive treatments available and the treatment of epilepsy is purely symptomatic. The identification and characterization of an investigational AED relies entirely on the use of a variety of animal seizure and epilepsy models. Those drugs that were discovered with this approach that displayed a favorable therapeutic window and showed no significant preclinical toxicity were advanced into clinical add-on epilepsy trials with patients with refractory partial seizures. Since 1993, 12 new therapies have been brought to the market for the treatment of epilepsy. Despite the success of this approach, as many as one in three patients with partial-onset seizures still remain refractory to available AEDs. It is not clear whether we will be able to identify a therapy that will provide a greater level of efficacy in this patient population using the current approach. As such, there is a clear need to move beyond the conventional animal models and to explore other animal models and molecular targets by which neuronal hyperexcitability may be reduced. Levetiracetam demonstrated that a new therapy does not have to be effective in the traditional seizure models to be effective in the patient with epilepsy. There is no a priori reason to believe that the truly novel AED that will demonstrate a substantial impact in the treatment of the patient with refractory epilepsy will have an anticonvulsant profile that resembles any of the currently available therapies, including levetiracetam. This implies that the community interested in developing a drug for this patient population will need to take a substantial risk when advancing a novel drug into a clinical trial. Only then will we likely find a therapy that provides the level of efficacy for which patients continue to hope.

References

1. Putnam TJ, Merritt HH. Experimental determination of the anticonvulsant properties of some phenyl derivatives. *Science.* 1937;85:525–526.
2. White HS, Johnson M, Wolf HH, et al. The early identification of anticonvulsant activity: role of the maximal electroshock and subcutaneous pentylenetetrazol seizure models. *Ital J Neurol Sci.* 1995;16:73–77.
3. White HS, Wolf HH, Woodhead JH, et al. The National Institutes of Health Anticonvulsant Drug Development Program: Screening for Efficacy. In: French J, Leppik I, Dichter MA, eds. *Antiepileptic Drug Development. Advances in Neurology.* Vol 76. Philadelphia: Lippincott-Raven Publishers; 1998:29–39.
4. Goddard GV, McIntyre DC, Leech CK. A permanent change in brain function resulting from daily electrical stimulation. *Exp Neurol.* 1969;25:295–330.
5. White HS, Woodhead JH, Wilcox KS, et al. Discovery and preclinical development of antiepileptic drugs. In: Levy RH, Mattson RH, Meldrum B, et al., eds. *Antiepileptic Drugs.* 5th ed. Philadelphia: Lippincott; 2002: 36–48.
6. Bialer M, Johannessen SI, Kupferberg HJ, et al. Progress report on new antiepileptic drugs: a summary of the Eigth Eilat Conference (EILAT VIII). *Epilepsy Res.* 2007;73:1–52.
7. Bialer M, Johannessen SI, Levy RH, et al. Progress report on new antiepileptic drugs: a summary of the Ninth Eilat Conference (EILAT IX). *Epilepsy Res.* 2009;83:1–43.
8. Coenen AM, Van Luijtelaar EL. Genetic animal models for absence epilepsy: a review of the WAG/Rij strain of rats. *Behav Genet.* 2003;33: 635–655.
9. Hosford DA, Clark S, Cao Z, et al. The role of GABA$_B$ receptor activation in absence seizures of lethargic (lh/lh) mice. *Science.* 1992;257:398–401.
10. Marescaux C, Vergnes M. Genetic absence epilepsy in rats from Strasbourg (GAERS). *Ital J Neurol Sci.* 1995;16:113–118.
11. Snead OC. Pharmacological modulation of generalized absence seizures in rodents. *J Neural Transm.* 1992;35:7–19.
12. Loscher W. Animal models of epilepsy for the development of antiepileptogenic and disease-modifying drugs. A comparison of the pharmacology of kindling and models with spontaneous recurrent seizures. *Epilepsy Res.* 2002;50:105–123.
13. Barton ME, Klein BD, Wolf HH, et al. Pharmacological characterization of the 6 Hz psychomotor seizure model of partial epilepsy. *Epilepsy Res.* 2001;47:217–227.
14. White HS. Epilepsy and disease modification: animal models for novel drug discovery. In: Rho J, Sankar R, Cavazos J, eds. *Epilepsy: Scientific foundations of Clinical Practice.* New York, NY: Marcel Dekker Inc.; In Press, 2009.
15. Hosford DA, Wang Y. Utility of the lethargic (lh/lh) mouse model of absence seizures in predicting the effects of lamotrigine, vigabatrin, tiagabine, gabapentin, and topiramate against human absence seizures. *Epilepsia.* 1997;38:408–414.
16. Klitgaard H, Matagne A, Gobert J, et al. Evidence for a unique profile of levetiracetam in rodent models of seizures and epilepsy. *Eur J Pharmacol.* 1998;353:191–206.
17. Loscher W, Honack D. Anticonvulsant and behavioral effects of two novel competitive N-methyl-D-aspartic acid receptor antagonists, CGP 37849 and CGP 39551, in the kindling model of epilepsy. Comparison with MK-801 and carbamazepine. *J Pharmacol Exp Ther.* 1991;256: 432–440.
18. Sveinbjornsdottir S, Sander JW, Upton D, et al. The excitatory amino acid antagonist D-CPP-ene (SDZ EAA-494) in patients with epilepsy. *Epilepsy Res.* 1993;16:165–174.
19. Honack D, Loscher W. Kindling increases the sensitivity of rats to adverse effects of certain antiepileptic drugs. *Epilepsia.* 1995;36:763–771.
20. Klitgaard H, Matagne A, Lamberty Y. Use of epileptic animals for adverse effect testing. *Epilepsy Res.* 2002;50:55–65.
21. Gower AJ, Noyer M, Verloes R, et al. ucb LO59, a novel anti-convulsant drug: pharmacological profile in animals. *Eur J Pharmacol.* 1992;222: 193–203.
22. Loscher W, Honack D. Profile of ucb-L059, a novel anticonvulsant drug, in models of partial and generalized epilepsy in mice and rats. *Eur J Pharmacol.* 1993;232:147–158.
23. Loscher W, Honack D, Rundfeldt C. Antiepileptogenic effects of the novel anticonvulsant levetiracetam (ucb L059) in the kindling model of temporal lobe epilepsy. *J Pharmacol Exp Ther.* 1998;284:474–479.
24. De Deyn PP, Kabatu H, D'Hooge R, et al. Protective effect of ucbL059 against postural stimulation-induced seizures in EL Mice. *Neurosciences.* 1992;18:187–192.
25. Gower AJ, Hirsch E, Boehrer A, et al. Effects of levetiracetam, a novel antiepileptic drug, on convulsant activity in two genetic rat models of epilepsy. *Epilepsy Res.* 1995;22:207–213.
26. Klitgaard H. Levetiracetam: the preclinical profile of a new class of antiepileptic drugs? *Epilepsia.* 2001;42(Suppl 4):13–18.
27. Stables JP, Bertram EH, White HS, et al. Models for epilepsy and epileptogenesis: report from the NIH workshop, Bethesda, Maryland. *Epilepsia.* 2002;43:1410–1420.
28. Stables JP, Bertram E, Dudek FE, et al. Therapy discovery for pharmacoresistant epilepsy and for disease-modifying therapeutics: summary of the NIH/NINDS/AES models II workshop. *Epilepsia.* 2003;44:1472–1478.
29. Loscher W, Jackel R, Czuczwar SJ. Is amygdala kindling in rats a model for drug-resistant partial epilepsy? *Exp Neurol.* 1986;93:211–226.
30. Loscher W, Rundfeldt C, Honack D. Pharmacological characterization of phenytoin-resistant amygdala-kindled rats, a new model of drug-resistant partial epilepsy. *Epilepsy Res.* 1993;15:207–219.
31. Rundfeldt C, Loscher W. Anticonvulsant efficacy and adverse effects of phenytoin during chronic treatment in amygdala-kindled rats. *J Pharmacol Exp Ther.* 1993;266:216–223.
32. Postma T, Krupp E, Li XL, et al. Lamotrigine treatment during amygdala-kindled seizure development fails to inhibit seizures and diminishes subsequent anticonvulsant efficacy. *Epilepsia.* 2000;41:1514–1521.
33. Srivastava A, Woodhead JH, White HS. Effect of lamotrigine, carbamazepine and sodium valproate on lamotrigine-resistant kindled rats. *Epilepsia.* 2003;44:42.
34. Srivastava A, Franklin MR, Palmer BS, et al. Carbamazepine, but not valproate, displays pharmaco-resistance in lamotrigine-resistant amygdala kindled rats. *Epilepsia.* 2004;45:12.
35. Srivastava A, White HS. Retigabine decreases behavioral and electrographic seizures in the lamotrigine-resistant amygdala kindled rat model of pharmacoresistant epilepsy. *Epilepsia.* 2005;46:217–218.

36. Brandt C, Volk HA, Loscher W. Striking differences in individual anticonvulsant response to phenobarbital in rats with spontaneous seizures after status epilepticus. *Epilepsia.* 2004;45:1488–1497.
37. Glien M, Brandt C, Potschka H, et al. Effects of the novel antiepileptic drug levetiracetam on spontaneous recurrent seizures in the rat pilocarpine model of temporal lobe epilepsy. *Epilepsia.* 2002;43:350–357.
38. Grabenstatter HL, Ferraro DJ, Williams PA, et al. Use of chronic epilepsy models in antiepileptic drug discovery: the effect of topiramate on spontaneous motor seizures in rats with kainate-induced epilepsy. *Epilepsia.* 2005;46:8–14.
39. Grabenstatter HL, Dudek FE. The effect of carbamazepine on spontaneous seizures in freely-behaving rats with kainate-induced epilepsy. *Epilepsia.* 2005;46:287.
40. Leite JP, Cavalheiro EA. Effects of conventional antiepileptic drugs in a model of spontaneous recurrent seizures in rats. *Epilepsy Res.* 1995;20: 93–104.
41. van Vliet EA, van Schaik R, Edelbroek PM, et al. Inhibition of the multidrug transporter P-glycoprotein improves seizure control in phenytoin-treated chronic epileptic rats. *Epilepsy Res.* 2006;47:672–680.
42. Smyth MD, Barbaro NM, Baraban SC. Effects of antiepileptic drugs on induced epileptiform activity in a rat model of dysplasia. *Epilepsy Res.* 2002;50:251–264.
43. Dichter MA, Pollared J. Cell culture models for studying epilepsy. In: Pitkanen A, Schwartzkroin PA, Moshe SL, eds. *Models of Seizures and Epilepsy.* New York: Elsevier Academic Press; 2006:23–34.
44. Heinemann U, Kann O, Schuchmann S. An overview of *in vitro* seizure models in acute and organotypic slices. In: Pitkanen A, Schwartzkroin PA, Moshe SL, eds. *Models of Seizures and Epilepsy.* New York: Elsevier Academic Press; 2006:35–44.
45. Loscher W. Experimental models for intractable epilepsy in non-primate animal species. In: Schmidt D, Morselli PL, ed. *Intractable Epilepsy: Experimental and Clinical Aspects.* New York: Raven Press; 1986:25–37.
46. Loscher W. Animal models of drug-refractory epilepsy. In: Pitkanen A, Schwartzkroin PA, Moshe SL, eds. *Models of Seizures and Epilepsy.* New York: Elsevier Academic Press; 2006:551–567.
47. Rundfeldt C, Honack D, Loscher W. Phenytoin potently increases the threshold for focal seizures in amygdala-kindled rats. *Neuropharmacology.* 1990;29:845–851.
48. Weiss SR, Post RM. Development and reversal of contingent inefficacy and tolerance to the anticonvulsant effects of carbamazepine. *Epilepsia.* 1991;32:140–145.
49. White HS, Srivastava A, Klein B, et al. The novel investigational neuromodulator RWJ 333369 displays a broad-spectrum anticonvulsant profile in rodent seizure and epilepsy models. *Epilepsia.* 2006;47:200.
50. Barton ME, Peters SC, Shannon HE. Comparison of the effect of glutamate receptor modulators in the 6 Hz and maximal electroshock seizure models. *Epilepsy Res.* 2003;56:17–26.
51. Brown WC, Schiffman DO, Swinyard EA, et al. Comparative assay of antiepileptic drugs by 'psychomotor' seizure test and minimal electroshock threshold test. *J Pharmacol Exp Ther.* 1953;107:273–283.

CHAPTER 42 ■ PHARMACOKINETICS AND DRUG INTERACTIONS

GAIL D. ANDERSON

Pharmacokinetics is the study of the effect of the body on a drug. The pharmacokinetic parameters determine the relationship between an administered dose and the concentration of the drug in the body. The main pharmacokinetic parameters include absorption, distribution, metabolism, and excretion. Table 42.1 summarizes the pharmacokinetic parameters for the most commonly used antiepileptic drugs (AEDs). Pharmacodynamics is the study of the factors that relate to the efficacy and safety of the drug, and determines the relationship between concentration and effect. The relationship between pharmacokinetics and pharmacodynamics is illustrated in Figure 42.1.

PHARMACOKINETICS PARAMETERS

Absorption

Absorption refers to the passage of the drug from its site of administration into the systemic circulation, and is defined by the rate at which the drug leaves the site of administration and the extent at which it occurs.

Bioavailability (F) is the amount of the administered drug that reaches the systemic circulation. F is dependent on the

TABLE 42.1

PHARMACOKINETIC PARAMETERS OF ANTIEPILEPTIC DRUGS

AED	F (%)	V_d (L/kg)	Protein binding (%)	$T_{1/2}$ (hour)	Routes of elimination renal hepatic isozymes involved (%)	Active metabolite
Carbamazepine	70–80	0.8–2	75	12–17	<1 CYP3A4 (major), CYP1A2, 2C8	Yes
Clobazam	87	0.9–1.4	85–93	10–30	Nk CYP2C19, 3A4	Yes
Clonazepam	90	3.2	85	22–40	<1 CYP3A4	Yes
Ethosuximide	>90	0.6–0.7	0	25–60	20 CYP3A4 (major), 2E1	No
Felbamate	>90	0.7–1.0	22–25	20–23	50 UGT, CYP3A4 (20%), 2E1	No
Gabapentin	30–60	0.85	0	5–9	>90 none	No
Lacosamide	100	0.6	<15	13	40 not identified	No
Lamotrigine	98	0.9–1.3	55	12–60	<1 UGT1A4	No
Levetiracetam	100	0.5–0.7	<10	6–8	66 Amidase	No
Oxcarbazepine	>90	Nk	40–60	1–2.5	<1 Cytosolic arylketone reductase	Yes
MHD	–	0.7–0.8	33–40	8–11	20 UGT	No
Phenobarbital	80–90	0.5–1.0	20–60	36–118	20 Glucosides, CYP2C9, 2C19, 2E1	No
Phenytoin	70–100	0.5–1.0	88–93	7–42	2 CYP2C9 (major), CYP2C19	No
Pregablin	>90	0.5	0	5–6.5	>95 none	No
Primidone	>90	0.4–1.0	20–30	3–7	0 CYPs, isozyme not identified	Yes
Rufinamide	85	0.7	34	6–10	<2 non-CYP dependent hydrolysis	No
Stiripental	25	Nk	99	13	<1 UGT and CYPs, isozymes not identified	No
Tiagabine	90	Nk	96	3–8	<2 CYP3A4 (22%),	No
Topiramate	80	0.6–0.8	9–41	21	30 not identified	No
Valproate	90	0.14–0.23	5–15	6–17	<5 β-oxidation, UGT1A6, 1A9, 2B7, CYP2C9, 2C19	Yes
Vigabatrin	50–60	0.8	0	5–8	>90 none	No
Zonisamide	>90	0.8–1.6	40–60	27–70	35 NAT2 (15%), CYP3A4 (major), CYP2C19	No

CYP, cytochrome P450; UGT, UDP glucuronosyltransferase; NAT, N-acetyltransferase; Nk, not known.

Pharmacokinetics   Pharmacodynamics

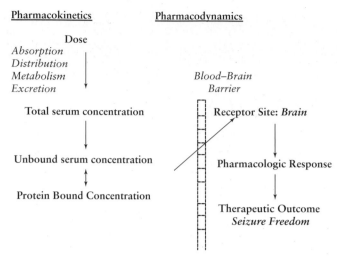

FIGURE 42.1 Relationship between pharmacokinetics and pharmacodynamics.

fraction absorbed through the gastrointestinal (GI) tract plus the fraction lost due to first-pass metabolism (see below). After intravenous (IV) administration, bioavailability is equal to 1.0. Bioavailability for other non-IV formulations is determined by comparing the area of the concentration time curve (AUC) obtained after IV administration of a drug and the AUC obtained after administration by another route (i.e., oral) as shown in Eq. (1), where D is the dose administered:

$$F = \frac{AUC_{oral} \cdot D_{IV}}{AUC_{IV} \cdot D_{oral}} \qquad (1)$$

Most drugs are absorbed by passive diffusion in the GI tract where the rate of absorption is proportional to the drug concentration gradient across the barrier. Other drugs are absorbed by a combination of passive and active transport by proteins that can increase and/or decreased absorption depending on their location and whether they are influx or efflux transporters. For example, the oral absorption of the β-lactam antibiotics is dependent on active transport by the influx transporters for endogenous dipeptides, PEPT1. Conversely, P-glycoprotein (PGP) and other efflux transporters can limit drug absorption by increasing the excretion of drugs into the intestinal lumen from the systemic circulation. The fraction lost in the GI tract can also include metabolism via hydrolysis, glucuronidation, sulfation, and oxidation with CYP3A4 the most dominant cytochrome P450 in the GI tract.

First-pass metabolism of a drug can occur in the GI tract by metabolism as described above and in the liver resulting in a decreased F. Orally administered drugs absorbed from the GI tract reach the liver via the hepatic portal vein prior to entering the systemic circulation. Drugs that are high extraction ratio (ER) drugs (see below) can undergo significant first-pass liver metabolism.

Rate of absorption is generally a first-order process, where the rate of absorption is dependent on the amount of drug; however, some drugs can follow zero-order kinetics with a constant release of drug independent of the amount of drug.

Extended release formulations are used to decrease the frequency of dosing for drugs with rapid elimination to improve convenience and compliance. For extended release drugs, the rate-limiting step in drug elimination is the absorption rate of the drug and not the actual elimination rate. Use of the extended release products can decrease the peak-to-trough fluctuation in serum concentrations and theoretically improve the therapeutic benefit of the drug by decreasing adverse events associated with higher peak concentrations. Other drugs, for example, enteric-coated valproate, are delayed release. The enteric coating improves tolerability by decreasing absorption within the stomach and delaying absorption until the formulation reaches the intestines.

Bioequivalence is defined as chemical, when the drug meets the same chemical and physical standards; biologic, when the administered drug yields similar concentrations in blood; and therapeutic, when the drug provides equal therapeutic benefits in clinical trials. Generic drugs are chemically and biologic equivalent. Manufacturers do not have to prove therapeutic equivalence. There has been a history of problems with generic versions of the older AEDs, specifically carbamazepine and phenytoin, as summarized in several reviews. Nuwer et al. (1) described three pharmacokinetic properties that predisposed the older AEDs to problems with their generic formulations: low water solubility, narrow therapeutic range, and nonlinear pharmacokinetics. Phenytoin is the only older AED that clearly meets all the three criteria. Carbamazepine meets two of three criteria due to its low water solubility and narrow therapeutic range. The nonlinearity due to autoinduction will not influence generic formulation problems. In addition to permeability across the GI, drug absorption from a solid dosage form depends on the release of the drug from the drug product or dissolution. In vitro dissolution can be used to predict in vivo dissolution. The Biopharmaceutics Classification System (BCS) was first developed by Amidon et al. (2) and was designed to correlate a drug's solubility and permeability with the rate and extent of oral drug absorption. A drug is considered to have high solubility when the highest dose strength is soluble in 250 mL or less of aqueous media over a pH range of 1 to 7.5 at 37°C. A drug is considered to be highly permeable when the bioavailability is ≥90%. Drugs are then classified into four BCS classes: high solubility/high permeability (Class I), low solubility/high permeability (Class II), high solubility/low permeability (Class III), and low solubility/low permeability (Class IV). The BCS classification can also provide estimation for the likelihood of problems with generics. Class I drugs are unlikely to demonstrate generic-related problems. For Class I drugs based on BCS classification alone, we can predict that in vitro dissolution testing allows an ability to distinguish between acceptable and unacceptable generic drug products. The BCS classification for the old and newer AEDs is given in Table 42.2. Of the older drugs, carbamazepine, clonazepam, primidone, and phenytoin are not Class I drugs. Of the new AEDs, gabapentin, lamotrigine, levetiracetam, pregabalin, tiagabine, topiramate, and zonisamide are all Class I drugs. Gabapentin is not a Class I drug, due to the transporter-mediated saturable absorption. However, as transport processes occur after dissolution, there is no reason to expect a difference in transporter efficiency with generic products of gabapentin, a highly soluble compound. Felbamate and oxcarbazepine are both Class II drugs. Using the criteria regarding the pharmacokinetic properties that predisposed the older AEDs to bioequivalence problems (low water solubility, narrow therapeutic range, and nonlinear), our current knowledge of the pharmacokinetic properties

TABLE 42.2

BIOPHARMACEUTICAL CLASSIFICATION SYSTEM OF THE AED

AED	Solubility	Permeability	BCS class
Carbamazepine[a]	Low	High	II
Clonazepam[a]	Low	High	II
Ethosuximide	High	High	I
Felbamate	Low	High	II
Gabapentin	High	Low	III
Lamotrigine	High	High	I
Levetiracetam	High	High	I
Oxcarbazepine[a]	Low	High	II
Phenobarbital	High	High	I
Phenytoin[a]	Low	High	II
Pregabalin	High	High	I
Primidone[a]	Low	High	II
Tiagabine	High	High	I
Topiramate	High	High	I
Valproic Acid	High	High	I
Zonisamide	High	High	I

[a]Denotes older AEDs. All other drugs listed are considered to be newer AEDs.
BCS, Biopharmaceutics Classification System.

predicts that the new AEDs should not be predisposed to such problems.

Distribution

Distribution is the process of reversible transfer of drug to and from the site of measurement. Central nervous system distribution is unique due to the blood–brain barrier (BBB). Lipid-soluble and unbound drugs have significantly higher distribution across the BBB then water-soluble and protein-bound drugs. Both influx and efflux transport protein alter brain distribution. PGP is significantly involved in transporting drugs from the brain to the blood and forms an important part of the BBB.

The volume of distribution (V_d) is a measure of the apparent space in the body available to contain the drug. V_d relates the amount of drug in the body to the concentration of drug in the plasma. Therefore, the initial concentration (C_0) attained after administration of a single or bolus dose (D) is dependent on the V_d of the drug. The dose is based on either ideal or total body weight depending on the physiochemical characteristic of the drug. Lipophilic drugs will distribute into adipose tissue and V_d will be dependent on total body weight. In contrast, for water-soluble drugs, V_d is dependent on ideal or lean body weight. V_d can be used to calculate both loading and bolus doses needed to achieve a desired concentration.

$$C_0 = \frac{\text{Dose}}{V_d} \tag{2}$$

The volume of distribution is dependent on plasma volume (V_p), tissue volume (V_t), fraction of drug unbound in plasma

(f_u) and in tissue (f_t) as shown in Eq. (3).

$$V_d = V_p + V_t \frac{f_u}{f_t} \tag{3}$$

Protein Binding

For the AEDs, albumin is the primary binding protein, with the exception of carbamazepine, which is bound to both albumin and alpha$_1$-acid glycoprotein (α_1-AGP). Albumin concentrations are decreased in the neonate, the elderly, in hepatic and renal disease, during pregnancy, and after trauma. α_1-AGP is an acute phase reactive protein and its concentrations are increased in conditions of inflammation and trauma and decreased in neonates. In contrast to albumin, α_1-AGP concentrations are not decreased or increased in the healthy elderly. For the majority of the drugs, protein binding is linear and the percent unbound is a constant within the range of concentrations used clinically. Valproate is the one exception. Valproate is highly protein bound and due to its high molar concentration, valproate saturates albumin-binding sites within the therapeutic range. An increase in the percent unbound as the dose increases results in total valproate concentrations increasing less than proportional with increasing doses. Conversely, unbound valproate concentrations will increase linearly with increasing dose, and total valproate concentrations will no longer reflect unbound or active concentrations.

Elimination Processes

Drugs are eliminated by metabolism and/or excretion of unchanged drug by the kidneys or GI tract. Metabolism occurs predominantly in the liver with the GI, kidneys, lung, and serum as other possible sites of metabolism. For the large majority of drugs, elimination is linear; the elimination rate if proportional to the amount of drug present. For drugs following linear kinetics, clearance is constant and serum concentrations increase proportionally with increasing doses. Unlike other drugs, phenytoin is unique in that its elimination is nonlinear due to saturation of metabolism within the normal dosage range.

This saturation of metabolic processes results in a decreased clearance with increasing doses. For drugs like phenytoin with nonlinear elimination, serum concentrations will increase more than expected with increasing doses.

Clearance is the most useful pharmacokinetic parameter for evaluating an elimination mechanism and in estimation of average steady-state concentrations ($C_{ave,ss}$). Physiologically, clearance is the loss of drug across an organ of elimination and is determined by the blood flow to the organ that metabolizes or eliminates the drug and the efficiency of the organ in extracting the drug. The efficiency is measured by the ER, defined as the ratio of the difference between the concentration into and out of the organ ($C_{in} - C_{out}$) to the concentration entering the organ (C_{in}). Clearance (Cl) is described in terms of the eliminating organ; hepatic clearance (Cl_H) and renal clearance (Cl_R) with total clearance (Cl) determined by the sum of all the partial clearances. After multiple dosing, $C_{ave,ss}$ is dependent on the dose/interval (D/τ), Cl, and F (Eq. 4).

$$C_{ave,ss} = \frac{F \cdot D/\tau}{Cl} \tag{4}$$

The elimination half-life ($T_{1/2}$) is the time required for serum concentrations to decrease by 50% and is independent of dose. As shown in Eq. (5), $T_{1/2}$ is dependent on the clearance and the volume of distribution. It takes four to five $T_{1/2}$'s to eliminate greater than 90% of the drug and to reach steady-state concentrations with multiple dosing irrespective of dose or interval:

$$T_{1/2} = \frac{0.693 \cdot V_d}{Cl} \qquad (5)$$

Excretion

Renal excretion of unchanged drug and metabolites includes the processes of glomerular filtration (GFR), active tubular secretion, and passive reabsorption. For drugs that are predominantly excreted unchanged in the urine, the renal function can be assessed using the serum creatinine to estimate creatinine clearance (CrCl). The clearance of creatinine is dependent on GF rate and tubular secretion. The relationship between the drugs total clearance and CrCl can then be used to estimate doses needed to attain therapeutic concentrations. For most drugs that are significantly excreted unchanged in the urine, the relationship between total clearance and CrCl is linear with the *y*-intercept reflecting the nonrenal portion of the *Cl*. CrCl can be estimated using either the Cockroft–Gault equation or more recently the Modified Diet in Renal Disease Equation (MDRD). The Cockroft–Gault equation estimates CrCl and requires knowledge of the patients' age, sex, and lean body weight (LBW). The MDRD equation was recently developed in a large population of patients with chronic renal failure. The MDRD equation estimates GFR, does not require information on LBW, and also takes into account ethnic differences in renal function. Although either method can be utilized, the relationship between CrCl and dosage for the currently marketed drugs has been developed using an estimation of renal function using Cockroft–Gault equation.

Excretion of drugs into breast milk can occur during lactation. The dose of a drug that the infant receives during breast-feeding is dependent on the amount excreted into the breast milk, the daily volume of milk ingested, and the average plasma concentrations of the mother. The physiochemical properties of a drug will determine how much of the drug will be excreted into the breast milk, including its lipophilicity, protein-binding and ionization properties. The milk to plasma concentration ratio has large inter- and intrasubject variability and is often not known. In contrast, protein binding is usually known and knowledge of the protein-binding properties of a drug can provide a quick and easy tool to estimate exposure of an infant to medication from breast-feeding. Based on an extensive literature review of case reports that included infant concentrations from breast-fed infants exposed to maternal drugs (3), measurable concentrations of drug in the infant did not occur for drugs that were at least 85% protein bound, if there was no placental exposure immediately prior to or during delivery.

Metabolism

Metabolic reactions are primarily catalyzed by the cytochrome P450 (CYP) and UDP glucuronosyltransferase (UGT) enzymes. However, the second- and third-generation AEDs are also metabolized by a variety of other non-CYP/UGT enzymes (see Table 42.1). CYP are a family of multiple enzymes with the individual isozymes being composed of three major families (CYP1, CYP2, and CYP3). Seven primary isozymes are involved in the hepatic metabolism of most drugs: CYP1A2, CYP2A6, CYP2C8/9, CYP2C19, CYP2D6, CYP2E1, and CYP3A4. The most abundant isozyme, CYP3A4, which accounts for approximately 30% of the total hepatic CYP, has the broadest substrate specificity and is involved in the metabolism of more than 50% of all drugs. The UGTs are family of enzymes which catalyze the transfer of a glucuronic acid moiety from a donor cosubstrate UDPGA. The UGT1 family members are capable of glucuronidating a wide range of drugs, xenobiotics, and endobiotics. The UGT2 family of isoforms has long been considered to be more involved in the glucuronidation of endobiotics including steroids and bile acids. UGT2 isozymes seem to favor these types of compound as substrates but can also conjugate drugs. The activity of the metabolic enzymes is dependent on genetic, physiologic, and environmental effects.

Genetic polymorphisms in the expression of CYP1A2, CYP2B6, CYP2C8, CYP2C9, CYP2C19, CYP2D6, CYP3A5, UGT1A1, N-acetyltransferases (NAT2), and thiopurine *S*-methyltransferase (TPMT) have been identified. Poor metabolizers are homozygous for the mutant gene. Extensive metabolizers are either homozygous or heterozygous for the wild-type gene, with heterozygous carriers having intermediate metabolic activity. Ultrametabolizers have multiple copies of the gene; however, this has been described only for the CYP2D6 polymorphism. In addition, the predominant variant of CYP2D6 in Asian and African-American are alleles that have reduced enzyme activity. Overall, there is a large interethnic variability in the proportion of poor metabolizers, intermediate and ultrametabolizers which is beyond the scope of this chapter (4).

The pharmacokinetic hepatic model of elimination is a physiologically based model where hepatic clearance (Cl_H) is dependent on the unbound fraction of the drug in the blood (f_u), activity of the metabolic enzymes (Cl_{int}) and hepatic blood flow (Q_H).

$$Cl_H = \frac{Q_H \cdot (f_u \cdot Cl_{int})}{Q_H + (f_u \cdot Cl_{int})} \qquad (6)$$

For low ER drugs (ER < 0.3), $f_u \cdot Cl_{int} < Q_H$ and clearance is dependent on protein binding and intrinsic clearance. For high ER drugs (ER > 0.7), $f_u \cdot Cl_{int} > Q_H$ and clearance is dependent on Q_H.

Protein Binding and Hepatic Metabolism. Protein-binding effects are only clinically significant for two different types of highly protein-bound drugs that are predominantly eliminated by hepatic elimination. For low ER drugs that undergo dosage adjustment by monitoring total concentrations, total concentrations will underestimate unbound or active concentrations. This has been shown for both phenytoin and valproate in the elderly and in pregnant women with epilepsy. Total concentrations decreased significantly more than unbound concentrations with decreased albumin concentrations. Adjusting doses based on total concentrations would result in higher doses of valproate and phenytoin than needed to maintain therapeutic unbound concentrations. As the teratogenicity of valproate and phenytoin has been found to be dose dependent, minimizing unnecessary dosing increases during pregnancy is desirable. Ideally, unbound concentrations should be measured. Unbound phenytoin concentrations are clinically available and should be utilized whenever possible. Valproate unbound concentrations are not routinely available to the clinician as they may be unreliable due to problems in sample collection. Patients need to be monitored based on clinical measures, that is, change in seizure frequency and/or presence of adverse effects in the case of the AEDs.

For high ER drugs with a narrow therapeutic window and administered by nonoral routes, the AUC of unbound drug can be significantly increased and result in increased pharmacologic effect. The AUC of low ER drugs is independent of protein binding. Of the parenterally available AEDs, only midazolam is a high protein bound, high ER drug.

METHODS TO DETERMINE PHARMACOKINETIC PARAMETERS

Pharmacokinetic parameters are determined using concentration time data by both compartmental and noncompartmental methods of analysis. The majority of drugs are eliminated by a first-order process, that is, elimination rate is dependent on concentration. For the large majority of drugs, serum concentration time data can be modeled using either a one-compartment or a two-compartment model. For one-compartment model, distribution is considered instantaneous, concentrations decline exponentially with time, and a plot of log concentration versus time is linear. For a two-compartment model, the first exponential phase is primarily dependent on distribution into a peripheral compartment and the second exponential phase is dependent on elimination after distribution is complete. The terminal elimination rate constant (β) is determined by linear regression of the log concentration–time data obtained during the terminal exponential phase. The elimination half-life ($T_{1/2}$) is calculated as $0.693/\beta$. Historically, compartmental modeling was performed to determine rate constants of elimination and distribution. The current trend is to utilize noncompartmental analysis. Peak serum concentration (C_{max}) and the time to peak (T_{max}) are obtained by visual inspection of the data. The AUC is calculated by the log-linear trapezoidal method. Clearance is estimated by the ratio of dose to AUC. If the drug is administered orally, an apparent oral clearance (Cl/F) is defined as dose/AUC as bioavailability is unknown or assumed. Renal clearance (Cl_R) is calculated as product of the fraction of the dose excreted unchanged in the urine and Cl.

PHYSIOLOGIC AND PATHOLOGIC EFFECTS ON PHARMACOKINETICS

Age

Gastric pH is increased in neonates, infants, and young children, decreasing to adult values by 2 years of age. The incidence of hypochlorhydria also increases significantly after age 70 years. GI motility is decreased in neonates, reaches adult levels in older infants, and then decreases in the elderly. The bioavailability of drugs given orally that are weak acids, like phenytoin and phenobarbital, may be decreased in infants, young children, and the elderly due to their higher gastric pH. In neonates and infants, the increased total body-water-to-body-fat ratio contributes to an increase in the V_d of hydrophilic drugs, and may require larger mg/kg loading doses of some drugs to achieve therapeutic concentrations. Albumin and α_1-AGP concentrations are decreased in the neonates and young infant. Albumin concentrations alone are decreased in the elderly resulting in decreased protein binding for highly bound drugs. The clinical significance of decreased protein binding is described above for low and high ER drugs. At birth, GFR is approximately 40 mL/min/1.73 m^2 in the full-term neonate and increases steadily to 80% to 90% of adults function by 1 year. From ages 40 to 80 years, kidney function declines at approximately 10% to 20% decrease per decade. Therefore, in general, weight-normalized doses of drugs excreted predominately unchanged by the kidneys need to be reduced in neonates, infants, and elderly. In the past, there was a general assumption that all hepatic drug metabolism was increased in children compared to adults. There is now evidence that the drug metabolism pathways are affected by age separately, depending on the cytochrome P450 isozymes and the conjugation family of enzymes involved in the elimination of the drug (5). Significantly higher weight-corrected doses are needed in children than adults for drugs metabolized by CYP1A2, CYP2C9, and CYP3A4. In contrast, weight-corrected doses for drugs metabolized by CYP2C19, CYP2D6, NAT2, and UGT in children are similar to those in adults. In the elderly, the activity of all of the CYPs are decreased resulting in a need for decreased doses; however, similar to the effects in children, doses of drugs metabolized by the conjugating enzymes, NAT2 and UGT, are not decreased.

Pregnancy

Despite the many physiologic changes that occur during pregnancy that could affect absorption, bioavailability does not appear to be altered. Decreased albumin and α_1-AGP concentrations during pregnancy will result in decreased protein binding for highly bound drugs. The clinical significance of decreased protein binding is described above. Renal clearance and the activity of the CYP3A4, CYP2D6, CYP2C9, and the UGT isozymes are increased during pregnancy, and drugs eliminated by these pathways may need dosage increases during pregnancy. In contrast, CYP1A2 and CYP2C19 activity is decreased, and drugs metabolized by these CYP isozymes may require a decrease in dosage during pregnancy (3).

Renal Disease

The effect of renal disease in addition to declining renal function in the elderly and the immature renal function in neonates and infants all result in decreased clearance for drugs that are predominantly excreted unchanged in the urine. For drugs with both renal and hepatic clearance, the effect of renal dysfunction is proportionate to the fraction of the clearance of the drug dependent on renal clearance. The ability to estimate renal function using serum creatinine provides a method of determining the dose required to maintain a therapeutic effect without toxicity. In addition, to a decreased clearance, renal disease is associated with decreased albumin concentrations which will result in decreased protein binding for highly bound drugs. The clinical significance of decreased protein binding is described above.

Liver Disease

Unlike renal disease, there are no specific markers of liver function that can be used to provide guidance in dosage adjustments. Liver function tests (LFTs) primarily are a measure of the extent of cell death. For example, LFT are significantly increased in acute hepatitis; however, metabolic enzyme function is maintained and doses of drugs eliminated by liver metabolism do not need to be altered. Conversely, acute and chronic cirrhosis results in a decreased ability to metabolize drugs due to effects on the metabolic enzymes and hepatic blood flow. The metabolic enzymes are differentially affected depending on the severity of the cirrhosis with the clearance of drugs metabolized by CYP2C19 affected first during mild liver disease (6). The activity of CYP2C19 is significantly decreased with mild liver disease and remains at a decreased level with increasing severity of disease. The clearance of drugs metabolized by CYP3A4 and CYP2C9 is decreased minimally in mild to moderate liver disease; however, the activity of the enzymes further decreases with increasing severity of the disease. CYP1A2 activity is not altered in mild liver disease; however, activity decreases in moderate liver disease and continues to decrease with the increasing severity of the disease. CYP2D6 activity is not altered in mild or moderate liver disease but does decrease in severe and end-stage liver disease. Clearance of drugs metabolized by CYP2E1 and the conjugating enzymes (UGT, NAT2) are not affected until the patient reaches end-stage liver disease. End-stage liver disease also decreases the renal clearance of drugs. Decreased albumin and α_1-AGP concentrations occur due to decreased synthesis and result in increased free fractions of highly protein-bound drugs.

PHARMACODYNAMIC PARAMETERS

Therapeutic index is the relationship between the dose (or concentration) of the drug required to produce a desired effect versus an undesired effect. The therapeutic or reference range is defined as a range of concentrations within which the probability of the desired clinical response is relatively high and the probability of unacceptable toxicity is relatively low. Table 42.3 summarizes the reference ranges for the AEDs.

Therapeutic drug monitoring (TDM) is widely accepted as a method to improve the effectiveness and safety of the first-generation AEDs, and to identify an individuals' optimum concentration. Like the older AEDs, the new AEDs also have significant pharmacokinetic variability. The use of TDM to individualize drug therapy is based on the general assumptions that (i) there is a relationship between serum concentration and the desired pharmacologic effect and/or toxicity and (ii) the relationship between serum concentration and pharmacologic effect is significantly superior to the relationship between dose and effect. As shown in Figure 42.1, variability in pharmacokinetics of the drug is the primary cause of the lack of

TABLE 42.3

SERUM REFERENCE RANGES FOR AEDS

AED	Reference range	Conversion factor (F) μMol/L = $F \times$ mg/L
Carbamazepine[a]	4–12	4.23
Clobazam[a]	0.03–0.3	3.33
Clonazepam[a]	0.02–0.07	3.17
Ethosuximide	40–100	7.08
Felbamate	30–60	4.20
Gabapentin	2–20	5.84
Lacosamide	Not established	3.96
Lamotrigine	2–20	3.90
Levetiracetam	12–46	5.87
Oxcarbazepine[b]	Not applicable	–
MHD	3–35	3.96
Phenobarbital	10–40	4.31
Phenytoin	10–20	3.96
Pregablin	Not established	4.31
Primidone[a]	5–10	4.58
Rufinamide	10–40	4.20
Stiripental	Not established	4.27
Tiagabine	0.02–0.2	2.66
Topiramate	5–20	2.95
Valproate	50–100	6.93
Vigabatrin	0.8–36	7.74
Zonisamide	10–40	4.71

[a]Active metabolite contributes to activity.
[b]Prodrug: Only concentration of MHD is relevant to reference range.

relationship between dose and concentration at the effect site. Pharmacokinetic variability includes effects on absorption, protein binding, distribution to the receptor site, metabolism, and excretion. Variability can be caused by genetic polymorphisms, age, sex, disease states, and drug interactions. Pharmacodynamic variability can also occur. Unlike the clinical and/or electroencephalographic correlations with serum concentrations of phenytoin, phenobarbital, and ethosuximide, there is only sparse clinical data available for the new AEDs (7). There is experimental evidence of a similar concentration–effect relationship for the new AEDs when compared to the older AEDs. Bialer et al. performed a correlation analysis between effective anticonvulsant dose 50% (ED_{50}) values of a series of old and new AEDs in mice and rats and $C_{ave,ss}$ (8). ED_{50} values were determined in models of maximal electroshock seizure (MES) and in audiogenetic seizure-susceptible mice. A significantly linear relationship was found for $C_{ave,ss}$ and ED_{50} for 11 AEDs. Similar to the therapeutic ranges found clinically, valproate and ethosuximide were the least potent AEDs with the highest therapeutic concentrations. Of the new AEDs evaluated—felbamate, gabapentin, lamotrigine, topiramate, and zonisamide—the ED_{50} serum concentrations were all in the concentration range similar to the old AEDs—carbamazepine, phenobarbital, and phenytoin.

The new AEDs have moderate to high variability in pharmacokinetics as well as intrasubject variability due to comedications (drug interactions), age, pregnancy, and presence of renal or liver disease (7). Similar to the older AEDs, variability in the pharmacokinetics results in a lack of relationship between dose and concentration at the effect site. The experimental data suggest a similar relationship between concentration effect for the new and old AEDs and the substantial interpatient and intrapatient pharmacokinetic variability suggesting that the rational for the widespread use of TDM of the older AEDS is still relevant to the new AEDs (9).

With the addition of generic formulations of the new AEDs, TDM can also play an important role to validate bioequivalence in patients and provide a way to insure patient safety while establishing that generics of AEDs proven to be bioequivalent in population studies are also bioequivalent in individuals.

DRUG INTERACTIONS

AEDs are associated with a wide range of drug interactions. Many of the AEDs are either specific or broad-spectrum inducers and/or inhibitors of metabolic enzymes (Table 42.4).

TABLE 42.4

INDUCTION AND INHIBITION EFFECT OF AEDS ON HEPATIC ENZYMES

AED	Effect	Metabolic enzyme involved[a]
Carbamazepine	Inducer	CYP1A2, CYP2C, CYP3A, UGT
Ethosuximide	No effect	
Felbamate	Inducer	CYP3A4
	Inhibitor	CYP2C19, β-oxidation
Gabapentin	No effect	
Lacosamide	No effect	
Lamotrigine	Inducer	UGT
	Inhibitor	CYP2C19
Levetiracetam	No effect	
Oxcarbazepine	Inducer	CYP3A4
	Inhibitor	CYP2C19
Phenobarbital/ Primidone	Inducer	CYP1A, CYP2A6, CYP2B, CYP2C, CYP3A, UGT
Phenytoin	Inducer	CYP2C, CYP3A, UGT
Pregabalin	No effect	
Stiripental	Inhibitor	CYP1A2, CYP2C9, CYP2C19, CYP2D6, CYP3A4
Tiagabine	No effect	
Topiramate	Inducer	β-oxidation
	Inhibitor	CYP2C19
Valproate	Inhibitor	CYP2C9, UGT, epoxide hydrolase
Vigabatrin	No effect	
Zonisamide	No effect	

[a]The mechanism of the drug interactions reported for clobazam, clonazepam, and rufinamide on serum concentrations of the other AEDs is unknown (see text).

In addition, many of the AEDs are eliminated by pathways that are affected by induction and/or inhibition by other AEDs and non-AEDs (Table 42.5). Drug interactions can occur by pharmacokinetic or pharmacodynamic mechanisms.

Pharmacodynamic interactions occur when the pharmacology of one agent alters the pharmacology or affect of the other drug without altering the serum concentration. Theoretically, the interaction can occur at the receptor or site of action or indirectly by affecting other physiologic mechanisms. However, the most commonly occurring AEDs are pharmacokinetic interactions, where one drug alters the serum concentrations of another. Pharmacokinetic interactions include hepatic enzyme induction and inhibition and protein-binding displacement.

Knowledge of the specific CYP or UGT isozymes involved in the metabolism of the AEDs allows prediction of potential inhibition and induction interactions. Less is known regarding the induction and inhibition potential of the non-CYP and UGT enzymes. The extent of the drug interaction is more difficult to predict than the type of interaction. A large number of patient and drug factors will influence the extent of the induction or inhibition. Intersubject variability in the expression of the CYP and UGT isozymes will influence the fraction of the dose associated with each metabolic pathway that is inhibited. The expression of the isozymes is dependent on both genetic and environmental influences, including concurrent diseases.

Hepatic enzyme induction is generally the result of an increase in the amount of enzyme protein. In most cases, enzyme induction results in an increase in the rate of metabolism of the affected drug, a decrease in the serum concentration of a parent drug, and possibly a loss of clinical efficacy. If the affected drug has an active metabolite, induction can result in increased metabolite concentrations and potentially an increase in the therapeutic effect and toxicity of the drug. Enzyme induction causes major effects on a limited number of extensively metabolized drugs (>75% metabolized) with a low therapeutic index. For the drugs listed in Table 42.6, addition or removal of a broad-spectrum inducer could result in loss of efficacy or toxicity if serum concentrations are not adjusted. Dosage adjustments of approximately 50% to 100%, with careful clinical monitoring, may be required.

The time required for induction depends on both the time to reach steady state of the inducing agent and the rate of synthesis of new enzymes. The amount of enzyme induction is proportional to the dose of the inducing agent. This has been shown for phenytoin, phenobarbital, and carbamazepine. In contrast to the dose relationship, induction is not strictly additive when patients are receiving multiple inducers. Because induction is a gradual process, allowing time for gradual increases in the dose of the affected drug is required. The time course of deinduction is dependent on the rate of degradation of the enzyme and the time required for eliminating the inducing drug. For the AEDs, the rate-limiting step in deinduction is generally dependent on the elimination of the inducing drug. When the inducer is removed, serum concentrations of the affected drug will increase. Serious adverse events can occur if the dose of the affected drug is not reduced. The magnitude and timing of these interactions are critical to allow clinicians to adjust doses in such a way so as to maintain therapeutic effect and avoid toxicity.

Hepatic enzyme inhibition usually occurs because of competition at the enzyme site, and results in a decrease in the rate of metabolism of the affected drug. Clinically, this is associated with an increased serum concentration of the affected drug and

TABLE 42.5

INDUCERS AND INHIBITORS OF CYTOCHROME P450 (CYP) ISOZYMES AND URIDINE DIPHOSPHATE GLUCURONOSYLTRANFERASES (UGT) INVOLVED IN AED METABOLISM

Isozyme	AED substrate	Inducers	Inhibitors[a]
CYP1A2	Carbamazepine	Carbamazepine	Fluvoxamine
		Phenobarbital	
		Phenytoin	
CYP2C8	Carbamazepine	Phenobarbital	
CYP2C9	Carbamazepine	Carbamazepine	Amiodarone, miconazole
	Phenobarbital	Phenobarbital	Cimetidine, propoxyphene
	Phenytoin	Phenytoin	Fluconazole, sulfaphenazole
	Valproate		Gemfibrozil, valproate
CYP2C19	Clobazam	Carbamazepine	Felbamate
	N-desmethylclobazam	Phenobarbital	Fluoxetine
	Diazepam	Phenytoin	Fluvoxamine
	N-desmethyldiazepam		Isoniazid
	Phenobarbital		Ticlopidine
	Phenytoin		
	Valproate		
CYP3A4	Carbamazepine	Carbamazepine	Amprenavir, itraconazole
	Clobazam	Felbamate	Atazanavir, ketoconazole
	Diazepam	Oxcarbazepine	Cimetidine, miconazole
	Ethosuximide	Phenobarbital	Clarithromycin, nelfinavir
	Tiagabine[b]	Phenytoin	Danazol, propoxyphene
		Topiramate	Darunavir, quinupristin
			Diltiazem, ritonavir
			Erythromycin, saquinavir
			Fluconazole, telithromycin
			Grapefruit juice, troleandomycin
			Indinavir, verapamil
			Isoniazid
UGTs	Lamotrigine	Carbamazepine	Valproate
	Lorazepam	Lamotrigine	
	Valproate	Oxcarbazepine	
		Phenobarbital	
		Phenytoin	
		Oral contraceptives	
		Eratopenem, imipenem	
		meropenem, panipenem	

[a]The drugs listed have been shown to be inhibitors of the various CYP and UGT isozymes. Not all interactions have been demonstrated for all drugs. Caution should be exercised with concurrent therapy of known inhibitors and inducers.
[b]The fraction of the clearance associated with the pathway is small; therefore, CYP3A4 inhibitors do not significantly effect tiagabine serum concentrations.

potentially an increased pharmacologic response. The extent of inhibition is dependent on the dose of the inhibitor as the majority of inhibition interactions are competitive. The onset of the interaction is frequently rapid and the extent of the interaction is highly variable. The initial effects of hepatic enzyme inhibition usually occur within 24 hours of addition of the inhibitor, but the time to maximal inhibition will depend on the time needed to achieve steady state of both the affected drug and the inhibiting drug.

Protein-binding displacement interactions result from the displacement of one drug with less affinity for the protein by another drug with greater affinity. Clinically significant interactions occur only with highly protein-bound drugs (>90%). For highly protein-bound drugs that are primarily eliminated by low extraction hepatic metabolism, protein-binding displacement causes a decrease in total serum concentrations of the displaced drug and no change in the unbound drug. Transient increases in unbound drug can be associated with acute toxicity. For most AEDs, total serum concentrations are used for clinical monitoring. Interpretation of total concentrations in the context of protein-binding interactions will result in dosing adjustments that will possibly lead to AED toxicity. In the case of AEDs, phenytoin and valproate are the only drugs involved in clinically important protein-binding interactions.

TABLE 42.6

DRUGS IN WHICH ADDITION OR DISCONTINUATION OF A HEPATIC ENZYME INDUCER COULD CAUSE CLINICALLY SIGNIFICANT EFFECTS

Drug category	Specific drugs
Analgesics	Alfentanyl, methadone
	Fentanyl, morphine
Antidepressant drugs[a]	Amitriptyline, desipramine, nortriptyline
	Amoxapine, doxepine, protriptyline
	Clomipramine, imipramine, trimipramine
Antiepileptic drugs	Carbamazepine, lamotrigine, topiramate
	Clobazam, phenytoin, valproate
	Ethosuximide, tiagabine, zonisamide
	Felbamate
Anti-infectious agents	Itraconazole, mebendazole
	Ketoconazole, voriconazole
Antipsychotic agents	Aripiprazole, risperidone
	Clozapine, quetiapine
	Haloperidol
Antiviral agents	Amprenavir, efavirenz, saquinavir
	Atazanavir, indinavir, tipranavir
	Darunavir, nelfinavir, zidovudine
	Delavirdine, ritonavir
Benzodiazepines	Alprazolam, diazepam, midazolam
	Clonazepam, lorazepam, triazolam
Calcium-channel blockers	Amlodipine, isradipine, nisodipine
	Belpridil, nicardipine, nitrendipine
	Diltiazem, nifedipine, verapamil, felodipine, nimodipine
Cardioactive drugs	Amiodarone, procainamide, quinidine
	Disopyramide, propranolol
Corticosteroids	Cortisone, methylprednisolone
	Betamethasone, prednisolone
	Dexamaethasone, prednisone
	Hydrocortisone, triamcinolone
HMG-CoA reductase inhibitors (statins)	Atorvastatin, lovastatin, simvastatin
Immunosuppressants	Cyclosporine, sirolimus, tacrolimus
Oral anticoagulants	Dicumarol, warfarin
Oral contraceptives	Conjugated estrogens, levonorgestrel
	Ethinyl estradiol, norethindrone
Miscellaneous	Cyclophosphamide,[b] thiotepa[b]
	Theophylline, vincristine

[a]Many antidepressants have active metabolites; therefore the effect of enzyme induction on efficacy is unpredictable.
[b]Increased exposure to active metabolite is associated with increased toxicity.

EFFECT OF AEDS ON OTHER DRUGS

Carbamazepine, phenytoin, phenobarbital, and primidone (via the phenobarbital metabolite) are broad-spectrum inducers of the CYP and UGT isozymes. A list of drugs in which addition or discontinuation of these broad-spectrum hepatic enzyme inducers could cause clinically significant effects is given in Table 42.6. Carbamazepine has been shown to induce the metabolism of drugs that are metabolized by the CYP1A2, CYP2C, CYP3A, and UGTS isozymes (10). Using a gene expression profiling, carbamazepine up-regulated CYP1A, CYP2A, CYP2B, CYP2C, and CYP3A subfamilies; UGT1A; glutathione S-transferase 1A and Z1; sulfotransferase 1A1; and several drug transporters (11). In addition to inducing the metabolism of other drugs, carbamazepine induces its own metabolism. The serum clearance of carbamazepine more than doubles during the initial weeks of therapy. Autoinduction of carbamazepine occurs via induction of CYP3A4 catalyzed metabolism to carbamazepine epoxide (CBZ-epoxide), the active metabolite of carbamazepine. The majority of the induction occurs within 1 week of initiation of carbamazepine and is completed within approximately 3 weeks. The time course of the deinduction is approximately the same. Using midazolam and caffeine as probe substrates for CYP3A4 and CYP1A2, the half-life of induction by carbamazepine were 70 hour and 105 hour, respectively (12).

Phenobarbital increases the metabolism of drugs metabolized by CYP1A, CYP2A6, CYP2B, CYP3A, and UGT isozymes (10,13). The time course of induction and deinduction is primarily dependent on the long elimination half-life of phenobarbital. Induction usually begins in approximately 1 week; with maximal induction occurring 2 to 3 weeks after phenobarbital therapy is initiated. The time course of the deinduction will follow a similar course, as phenobarbital serum concentrations decline over 2 to 3 weeks following removal of drug.

Phenytoin increases the metabolism of drugs that are metabolized by the CYP2C, CYP3A, and UGT isozymes (10,13). Maximal induction occurs approximately 1 to 2 weeks after initiation phenytoin therapy corresponding to the approximate time to steady-state phenytoin concentrations. Theoretically, deinduction requires a similar period of time. Initiation of phenytoin in a patient receiving warfarin requires special consideration. There have been case reports of a hypoprothrombinemic response after phenytoin was given to patients receiving chronic warfarin therapy. Two proposed mechanisms could account for this response. First, when phenytoin therapy is started for a patient stabilized on warfarin therapy, phenytoin may displace warfarin from albumin-binding sites and cause a transient increase in warfarin effect (14). Second, phenytoin initially may competitively inhibit the metabolism of warfarin because both phenytoin and S-warfarin are CYP2C9 substrates. After the initial increased effect of S-warfarin, serum concentrations may decline within 1 to 2 weeks after phenytoin is added because of CYP219 induction. Therefore, an initial decrease and then increase in warfarin dose may be needed in order to maintain the anticoagulation effect desired.

Stiripentol and valproate are both broad-spectrum inhibitors of a variety of metabolic isozymes. Stiripentol is a potent inhibitor of the majority of the CYPs involved in drug metabolism. In vitro studies have demonstrated inhibition of CYP1A2, CYP2C9, CYP2C19, CYP2D6, and CYP3A4. Clinically, stiripentol has been shown to significantly reduce the clearance of many AEDs, including carbamazepine, phenytoin, phenobarbital, and the clearance of the active metabolite of clobazam, N-clobazam z (15). There is a small, but not clinically significant, increase in valproate serum concentrations. As stiripentol inhibits all the major CYPs involved in drug metabolism, caution should be exercised when stiripentol is coadministered with any drug eliminated by predominately CYP catalyzed metabolism.

Valproate is a broad-spectrum inhibitor of hepatic metabolism, including inhibition of CYP2C9, UGT, and epoxide hydrolase, and is a weak inhibitor of CYP1A2 (10). Valproate does not inhibit cyclosporine or oral contraceptives suggesting a lack of inhibition of CYP3A metabolized drugs. Valproate increases the serum concentrations of phenobarbital and phenytoin presumably via inhibition of CYP2C9 (phenytoin, phenobarbital) and N-glucosidation (phenobarbital). Valproate inhibits the glucuronide conjugation of lamotrigine, lorazepam, and zidovudine resulting in significant increases in serum concentrations of the affected drugs (10,13). Valproate is highly protein bound to albumin, and displaces other AEDs (phenytoin, carbamazepine and diazepam) from albumin-binding sites which are only clinical significant for the therapeutic drug monitoring of phenytoin (10).

Lamotrigine is a selective inducer of the UGT isozymes. Lamotrigine autoinduces its own metabolism and decreases valproate serum concentrations by approximately 25% when coadministered with valproate (16). Levonorgestrel concentrations are reduced by approximately 20% and ethinyl estradiol concentrations are unchanged when lamotrigine is coadministered with the combined oral contraceptive (17). There was no change in the serum progesterone concentrations with the combination suggesting that suppression of ovulation was maintained.

Clonazepam, felbamate, oxcarbazepine, rufinamide, and topiramate are inhibitors and inducers of select metabolic enzymes. Clonazepam significantly reduced the clearance of carbamazepine by 22% and increased carbamazepine concentrations suggesting inhibition of CYP3A4 metabolism (18). In contrast, the concentration-to-dose ratio of lamotrigine is significantly lower with coadministration of clonazepam compared to monotherapy (19) suggesting induction of UGT metabolism.

Felbamate is an inhibitor of drugs metabolized by CYP2C19 and β-oxidation and an inducer of drugs metabolized by CYP3A4. An in vitro study in human liver microsomes demonstrated that of the CYPs evaluated, only CYP2C19 metabolized drugs are inhibited (20). This is consistent with clinical experience with felbamate. Felbamate reduces the concentrations of carbamazepine, but increases CBZ-epoxide concentrations, which may require a decrease in carbamazepine dose when felbamate is added. Felbamate also significantly decreases the concentrations of gestodene, the estrogen component in the low dose oral contraceptive. Phenytoin, phenobarbital, and valproate doses may need to be reduced when felbamate therapy is initiated due to inhibition by felbamate of CYP2C19 (phenytoin, phenobarbital) and β-oxidation (valproate) (21).

Oxcarbazepine induces the metabolism of drugs that are catalyzed by CYP3A4 and the UGTs (21). The extent of induction is on the average 46% higher with carbamazepine than with oxcarbazepine (22). Oral contraceptives need to be used cautiously in patients receiving any AED that causes induction of CYP3A4. Two weeks of oxcarbazepine cotherapy with an oral contraceptive resulted in a significant decrease in the serum concentrations of ethinyl estradiol and levonorgestrel (23). Consistent with CYP3A4 induction, a case report found that oxcarbazepine decreased cyclosporine serum concentrations. Felodipine serum concentrations were significantly reduced by coadministration of oxcarbazepine but less than the effect of carbamazepine (21). Inhibition of CYP2C19 results in increases in phenobarbital and phenytoin serum concentrations when oxcarbazepine is added in a dose-dependent manner.

In vitro studies in human liver microsomes have demonstrated that rufinamide does not inhibit model substrates of CYP1A2, CYP2A6, CYP2C9, CYP2C19, CYP2D6, CYP2E1, CYP3A4/5, or CYP4A9/11. In a population pharmacokinetic analysis of safety and efficacy trials (24), rufinamide did not affect the clearance of topiramate or valproate. Rufinamide increased the clearance of carbamazepine and lamotrigine and slightly decreased the clearance of phenobarbital and phenytoin (24). However, all the changes were less than 20% and unlikely to be clinical significant. Rufinamide did not affect the trough serum concentrations of any of the coadministered AEDs including carbamazepine, clobazam, clonazepam, phenobarbital, phenytoin, primidone, oxcarbazepine, or valproate (24).

Topiramate at doses of 50 to 200 mg/day does not interact with oral contraceptives containing ethinyl estradiol and norethindrone (25). Reduced ethinyl estradiol serum concentrations occur with topiramate doses greater than 200 mg/day, suggesting the need for higher doses of oral contraceptives with higher doses of topiramate (23). In some patients, topiramate increases the metabolism of phenytoin by 25%, possibly by inhibiting CYP2C19. The intersubject variability in the phenytoin–topiramate interaction may reflect the intersubject variability in the fraction of phenytoin metabolized by the polymorphically distributed CYP2C9 and CYP2C19. The inhibition spectrum of topiramate was evaluated in human liver microsomes. Topiramate significantly inhibited the model substrate of CYP2C19 with no effect on any of the other CYPs evaluated. The in vitro study was consistent with the inhibitory effect of topiramate on phenytoin and lack of inhibitory effect on the other AEDs (21).

The mechanism of the effects of clobazam on other AEDs is unclear. The concentration-to-dose ratio of lamotrigine is significantly lower with coadministration of clobazam compared to monotherapy (19). In studies of retrospectively collected serum concentrations, clobazam have no significant effect on the concentration-to-dose ratio of carbamazepine, phenobarbital, or phenytoin (26,27). A significant decrease in valproate concentrations was found in one study (26), but not the other (27). In a small group of patients receiving clobazam plus carbamazepine, carbamazepine concentrations did not differ. However, concentrations of CBZ-epoxide and its sequential metabolite, trans-CBZ-diol, were moderately increased compared to concentrations obtained in patients receiving carbamazepine monotherapy. This suggests that clobazam either induces carbamazepine metabolism or inhibits the epoxide hydrolase catalyzed CBZ-epoxide metabolism. Clobazam-induced carbamazepine toxicity associated with significantly increased carbamazepine and CBZ-epoxide concentrations was reported in a patient receiving carbamazepine and topiramate. Similarly, there is a case report of three patients with phenytoin toxicity associated with increased phenytoin concentrations. For both the carbamazepine and phenytoin reports, there was a significant delay in the time course of the interaction implicating the accumulation of the active metabolite of clobazam, N-desmethylclobazam, as the mechanism. Since the interaction does not consistently occur in all patients, the interaction may be dependent on the CYP2C19 genotype. The N-desmethylclobazam/clobazam ratio is sixfold higher in patients homozygous for the CYP2C19 mutant allele (28) which could be responsible for the selective occurrence of the interaction.

Ethosuximide, gabapentin, lacosamide, levetiracetam, pregablin, tiagabine, vigabatrin, and zonisamide are neither inducers nor inhibitors of metabolic enzymes and do not significantly alter the serum concentrations of the other drugs (10,13,21). Neither of the newer agents, eslicarbazepine, which is metabolized via hepatic esterases to the active metabolite S-licarbazepine, nor retigabine, a drug metabolized primarily by acetylation and N-glucuronidation, appear to cause clinically significant pharmacokinetic interactions, although a modest reduction in lamotrigine plasma concentrations when given with retigabine has been suggested.

EFFECT OF OTHER DRUGS ON AEDS

The effect of other drugs on the AEDs can by and large be predicted based on their pharmacokinetic characteristics (see Table 42.1) and knowledge of the specific pathways of elimination (see Table 42.5). Serum concentrations of AEDs that are eliminated predominantly by renal excretion of unchanged drug, gabapentin, pregabalin, and vigabatrin, are not affected by coadministration of other drugs. Serum concentrations of AEDs that are extensively metabolized by CYP and/or UGTs will be decreased in the presence of broad-spectrum and selective enzyme inducers (see Table 42.3). Serum concentrations of AEDs that are eliminated by both renal and hepatic metabolism (felbamate, levetiracetam, and topiramate) will decrease less than those that are predominantly metabolized. The pharmacologic effects of a drug interaction will be more unpredictable for those AEDs with active metabolites, for example, carbamazepine and clobazam, depending on the relative effect of the interaction on parent and/or active metabolite.

Carbamazepine is extensively metabolized to an active metabolite, CBZ-epoxide, which contributes to the therapeutic effects of carbamazepine as well as its neurotoxicity. When considering effects of other drugs on carbamazepine, one must consider the effects on the active metabolite, which is rarely clinically measured. Clinically, the patients may show significant signs of carbamazepine toxicity with what might appear to be small increases in carbamazepine serum concentrations. Valproate inhibits epoxide hydrolase, the enzyme that catalyzes the metabolism of CBZ-epoxide. Increases in serum concentrations of CBZ-epoxide are seen with either an increase or no change in carbamazepine concentrations when valproate is added to carbamazepine therapy. Increased serum concentrations of carbamazepine resulting in carbamazepine toxicity have been reported with several drugs that are potent inhibitors

of CYP3A4 activity. Cases of carbamazepine toxicity with increased carbamazepine serum concentrations have been reported for propoxyphene, danazol, nicotinamide, the macrolide antibiotics (erythromycin, clarithromycin, and troleandomycin), and calcium-channel blockers (verapamil and diltiazem) (10,13). Other known CYP3A4 inhibitors, including several antiviral agents, are given in Table 42.5. Coadministration with carbamazepine often results in reciprocal interactions, that is, carbamazepine decreases the serum concentrations and efficacy of the CYP3A4 inhibitor (see Table 42.2) and the CYP3A4 inhibitor increases the serum concentrations of carbamazepine and results in carbamazepine toxicity (see Table 42.4). St. John's wort, an inducer of CYP3A metabolism, did not significantly affect carbamazepine pharmacokinetics (29). Mechanistically, after the initial autoinduction of CYP3A4 by carbamazepine has occurred in patients, St. John's wort is not able to further increase the CYP3A4 activity.

Clobazam is eliminated predominately by hepatic metabolism to multiple metabolites. The primary metabolite, N-desmethylclobazam (N-clobazam), is active and accumulates to approximately eightfold-higher serum concentrations than clobazam after multiple dosing. Clobazam is metabolized by CYP2C19 and CYP3A4 with CYP2C19, the major enzymes involved in N-clobazam hydroxylation. The ratio of N-clobazam to clobazam was significantly higher in patients receiving phenobarbital, phenytoin, and carbamazepine (27) or concurrent felbamate (30). The concentration-to-dose ratio of N-clobazam and the ratio of N-clobazam to clobazam is significantly higher in patients receiving carbamazepine or phenytoin. Stiripentol inhibits the hydroxylation of N-clobazam, and clobazam doses need to be reduced by half (31).

Clonazepam is extensively metabolized to inactive metabolites by CYP3A4 with less than 1% excreted unchanged in the urine. Carbamazepine increases clonazepam clearance and decreases clonazepam concentrations by 20% to 30% (32). Phenobarbital and phenytoin treatments increased the clearance of a single dose of clonazepam by approximately 20% and 50%, respectively (33).

Ethosuximide is eliminated primarily by hepatic metabolism with major metabolism by CYP3A4 and minor metabolism by CYP2E1 with 20% of the dose excreted unchanged. Valproate and isoniazid have been reported to inhibit the metabolism of ethosuximide and cause small increases in ethosuximide serum concentration; however, a dosage adjustment of ethosuximide usually is not required (10).

Felbamate is eliminated by both renal excretion of unchanged drug (50%), and hepatic metabolism via UGT as a glucuronide conjugate (20%), by CYP3A4 (20%) and CYP2E1. Serum concentrations of felbamate are decreased by carbamazepine, phenytoin, and phenobarbital (21). Erythromycin (a CYP3A4 inhibitor) did not result in a significant increase in felbamate serum concentrations. Due to the small percent of felbamate metabolized by CYP3A4, this is not unexpected. A retrospective evaluation of felbamate serum concentrations found that dose-normalized concentrations of felbamate with concurrent therapy with gabapentin were 37% higher compared to patients receiving monotherapy. A pharmacokinetic study of felbamate and gabapentin has not been done in order to confirm the retrospective observation (21).

Lacosamide is eliminated primarily by renal excretion of unchanged drug and minor metabolism to an O-desmethyl metabolite. In clinical studies, lacosamide concentrations were not altered by coadministered carbamazepine, digoxin, levetiracetam, lamotrigine, metformin, omeprazole, topiramate, valproate, or the combined oral contraceptive containing ethinyl estradiol and levonorgestrel (34). Lamotrigine is extensively metabolized to two N-glucuronide metabolites in a reaction catalyzed by UGT1A4 with only minor renal elimination. Lamotrigine serum concentrations are reduced by carbamazepine, phenytoin, and phenobarbital. In a retrospective analysis, dose-corrected serum concentrations of lamotrigine in patients receiving methsuximide and oxcarbazepine were significantly lower compared to concentration in patients receiving lamotrigine monotherapy (21). The inducing properties of oxcarbazepine were less (29%) compared to carbamazepine (54%). Therefore, replacement of carbamazepine with oxcarbazepine should result in an increase in lamotrigine serum concentrations, and a reduction in lamotrigine dose is necessary. Methsuximide is not a known inducer of UGT; however, a similar decrease in lamotrigine serum concentrations was found in a pharmacokinetic study in 16 patients. Valproate significantly increases lamotrigine serum concentrations presumably by competitively inhibiting lamotrigine glucuronidation. The magnitude of the inhibition is not dependent on the valproate dose or concentration (35). The maximum inhibition of lamotrigine serum clearance at the lowest measured valproate serum concentration is consistent with the approximately 20-fold higher molar concentrations of valproate used as compared to lamotrigine. Lamotrigine concentrations are decreased by ethinyl estradiol containing oral contraceptives. The contraceptive products containing only progestogens do not alter lamotrigine clearance (36). Coadministration of lamotrigine with the combined oral contraceptive results in almost a doubling of lamotrigine concentrations during the first week after the oral contraceptive is stopped (37). Lopinavir/ritonavir decreases lamotrigine concentrations by 50%, presumably due to induction of UGT metabolism (21).

Levetiracetam is eliminated predominantly by renal excretion of unchanged drug (~2/3) and by hydrolysis of the acetamide group, a reaction catalyzed by amidases, an enzyme that is present in a number of tissues. Concentrations of levetiracetam are lower in patients receiving enzyme-inducing drugs and slightly higher in patients also receiving valproate; however, dosage adjustments are not needed (38). The pharmacokinetics of levetiracetam is not altered by coadministration of digoxin, oral contraceptives, or warfarin (21).

Oxcarbazepine is a prodrug which is rapidly converted to an active monohydroxy derivative (MHD) on oral administration, a reaction catalyzed by cytosolic arylketone reductase. MHD is predominately excreted unchanged in the urine or conjugated by UGT and then excreted, with only minor oxidation metabolism to a dihydroxy derivative (DHD). The conversion of oxcarbazepine to MHD appears to be a noninducible pathway. Phenobarbital and phenytoin decrease the serum concentration of MHD presumably due to induction of UGTs. Valproate slightly decreases the elimination of MHD most likely due to inhibition of UGT-catalyzed metabolism (21).

Phenobarbital is eliminated by both renal excretion of unchanged drug and hepatic metabolism. The two primary metabolites of phenobarbital are parahydroxyphenobarbital (PbOH) and phenobarbital N-glucoside. CYP2C9 plays a major role in the formation of PbOH, with minor metabolism

by CYP2C19 and CYP2E1. The diversity of the elimination pathways of phenobarbital and the low protein binding (50%) minimizes the effects of other drugs on phenobarbital. For example, inhibitors of CYP2C9 should alter the formation of PbOH. However, because the fraction of the dose of phenobarbital metabolized by CYP2C9 to PbOH is low (20%), CYP2C9 inhibitors do not cause clinically significant increases in phenobarbital serum concentrations. Valproate causes the only clinically significant increase in phenobarbital serum concentrations because of its broad spectrum of inhibition. Valproate inhibits both major metabolic pathways of phenobarbital, the formation of PbOH and phenobarbital N-glucoside (10).

Phenytoin is eliminated predominately by CYP2C9- and CYP2C19-dependent hepatic metabolism. CYP2C9 and CYP2C19 are polymorphically distributed. Genetic mutations in CYP2C9 result in significantly greater impairment of phenytoin clearance than those of CYP2C19. Clinically significant increases in phenytoin serum concentrations have been demonstrated for inhibitors of CYP2C9 and CYP2C19 enzymes (see Table 42.5). Some commonly used CYP2C9 inhibitors are amiodarone, fluconazole, miconazole, propoxyphene, sulfaphenazole, and valproate. CYP2C19 inhibitors include felbamate, omeprazole, cimetidine, fluoxetine, fluvoxamine, isonizaid, and ticlopidine (10). When carbamazepine and phenytoin are given concurrently, the serum concentrations of both drugs may decrease. Similar to the phenytoin–phenobarbital interactions, phenytoin concentrations may increase in some patients when carbamazepine is added; however, the mechanism is unclear. The effect of valproate on phenytoin is a combination of a protein-binding displacement and enzyme inhibition (39). The interactions result in a disruption of the relationship between unbound and total phenytoin concentrations. Total phenytoin concentrations can increase, decrease, or not change when valproate is added. The unbound phenytoin concentrations, however, will increase. Ideally, unbound phenytoin concentrations should be monitored in a patient receiving both valproate and phenytoin. There is one case report of two patients receiving phenytoin who lost seizure control after Shankhapushpi, an Ayurvedic preparation used for treatment of epilepsy, was added. A follow-up study in rats found that coadministration resulted in a 50% decrease in serum phenytoin concentration (40).

Primidone is metabolized by cytochrome P450 to two active metabolites, phenobarbital and phenylethylmalonamide (PEMA). The CYPs involved have not been identified. A decreased ratio of primidone to phenobarbital occurs with concurrent administration of CYP inducers, phenytoin and carbamazepine (10). Valproate inhibits the formation and elimination of phenobarbital, resulting in variable effects on the primidone–phenobarbital ratio. Isoniazid inhibits the formation of phenobarbital, causing an increased primidone-to-phenobarbital ratio. As both primidone and phenobarbital are active, the clinical significance of the interactions is unclear (10).

Rufinamide is extensively metabolized with less than 2% of the dose excreted in the urine as unchanged drug. The primary metabolic pathway is hydrolysis of the carboxylamide group to an inactive metabolite which is subsequently excreted in the urine (41). In a population pharmacokinetic analysis, concurrent therapy with CYP-enzyme-inducing AEDs increased rufinamide oral clearance by approximately 25%. Valproate reduced the oral clearance of rufinamide by

22% (24). The inhibition effect of valproate on rufinamide in children was significantly greater than in adults (24).

Stiripentol is eliminated extensively by CYP and UGT hepatic metabolism to 13 metabolites and displays Michaelis–Menten nonlinear pharmacokinetics within the range of serum concentrations found clinically. Serum concentrations of stiripentol are significantly decreased in patients receiving concurrent inducing AEDs (15).

Tiagabine is extensively metabolized, with less than 2% excreted unchanged in the urine. CYP3A4 has been identified as the primary isozyme responsible for metabolism of tiagabine to 5-oxo-tigabine (~22% of the dose). In patients treated with CYP-inducing AEDs, tiagabine clearance is significantly increased (21). Inhibitors of CYP3A4 (erythromycin, ketoconazole) significantly decreased the metabolism of tiagabine in vitro. However, in a study in normal subjects, erythromycin did not significantly alter the clearance of tiagabine (21) due to the small fraction of the dose metabolized by CYP3A4. A case report of a 75% increase in tiagabine concentrations with coadministration of gemfibrozil (42), an inhibitor of CYP2C9, suggests a possible role of CYP2C9 in the metabolism of tiagabine.

Topiramate is eliminated by hepatic metabolism and renal excretion of unchanged drug. Concurrent use of enzyme-inducing drugs decreases topiramate serum concentrations by approximately 40% to 50% (43). Valproate does not affect the pharmacokinetics of topiramate (21).

Valproate predominately undergoes hepatic metabolism, with less than 5% of the dose excreted unchanged in the urine. Major metabolism occurs by UGT-catalyzed glucuronide conjugation (UGT1A6, UGT1A9 and UGT2B7) and β-oxidation with minor CYP-dependent metabolism via CYP2C9 and CYP2C19. Valproate concentrations are decreased in the presence of enzyme-inducing AEDs, carbamazepine, phenobarbital, and phenytoin. The carbapenem antibiotics, meropenem, panipenem, eratopenem, and imipenem, significantly decrease valproate concentrations by an average of 34% (44). The effect of meropenem on valproate concentrations in 39 patients led to an electroclinical deterioration in over half of the patients (45). Due to its lack of enzyme-inducing properties, the use of valproate in women taking oral contraceptives has been recommended in the past. However, a recent study has found that total and unbound valproate concentrations are decreased on an average 18% and 30% when women are receiving the combined oral contraceptives (46). Clonazepam and felbamate significantly inhibit valproate metabolism and increase valproate concentrations (10,21). There are case reports of clinically significant decreases in valproate concentrations with coadministration of cisplatin (47) and efavirenz (48).

Vigabatrin cotherapy results in a clinically significant decrease of 25% to 40% in phenytoin serum concentrations in approximately one third of the patients (21). As vigabatrin is not an inducer of CYP metabolism, the mechanism of this interaction is unclear.

Zonisamide is eliminated by a combination of renal excretion of unchanged drug (~35%), metabolism via N-acetylation (~15%), and reduction to 2-sulfamoylacetylphenol (50%). Studies using expressed human CYPs demonstrated that CYP3A4 (major) and CYP3A5 and CYP2C19 are all capable of catalyzing zonisamide reduction. Zonisamide serum clearance is increased in the presence of enzyme-inducing AEDs (carbamazepine, phenytoin, and phenobarbital) (21). Clearance

of retigabine may be modestly increased by phenytoin and carbamazepine.

PHARMACODYNAMIC INTERACTIONS

Classic signs of carbamazepine neurotoxicity (diplopia, dizziness, ataxis) were reported when lamotrigine was added to carbamazepine therapy. In addition, a case report describes four patients who experienced intolerable carbamazepine-related adverse effects when levetiracetam was added to their therapy without an alteration in carbamazepine or carbamazepine epoxide concentrations (49). Similarly, there is an increase in adverse events with cotherapy of lamotrigine and oxcarbazepine without an effect on the pharmacokinetics of either drug (50).

References

1. Nuwer M, Browne T, Dodson W, et al. Generic substitution for antiepileptic drugs. *Neurology.* 1990;40:1647–1651.
2. Amidon GL, Lennernas H, Shah VP, et al. A theoretical basis for a biopharmaceutic drug classification: the correlation of in vitro drug product dissolution and in vivo bioavailability. *Pharm Res.* 1995;12:413–420.
3. Anderson GD. Using pharmacokinetics to predict the effects of pregnancy and maternal-infant transfer of drugs during lactation. *Expert Opin Drug Metabol Toxicol.* 2006;2:947–960.
4. Gardiner SJ, Begg EJ. Pharmacogenetics, drug-metabolizing enzymes, and clinical practice. *Pharmacol Rev.* 2006;58:521–590.
5. Anderson GD, Lynn AM. Optimizing pediatric dosing: a developmental pharmacology approach. *Pharmacotherapy.* 2009;29:680–690.
6. Frye RF, Zgheib NK, Matzke GR, et al. Liver disease selectively modulates cytochrome P450-mediated metabolism. *Clin Pharmacol Ther.* 2006; 80:235–245.
7. Johannessen SI, Tomson T. Pharmacokinetic variability of newer antiepileptic drugs: when is monitoring needed? *Clin Pharmacokinet.* 2006;45:1061–1075.
8. Bialer M, Twyman RE, White HS. Correlation analysis between anticonvulsant ED50 values of antiepileptic drugs in mice and rats and their therapeutic doses and plasma levels. *Epilepsy Behav.* 2004;5:866–872.
9. Anderson GD. Pharmacokinetic, pharmacodynamic, and pharmacogenetic targeted therapy of antiepileptic drugs. *Ther Drug Monit.* 2008;30: 173–180.
10. Anderson G. A mechanistic approach to antiepileptic drug interactions. *Ann Pharmacother.* 1998;32:554–563.
11. Oscarson M, Zanger UM, Rifki OF, et al. Transcriptional profiling of genes induced in the livers of patients treated with carbamazepine. *Clin Pharmacol Ther.* 2006;80:440–456.
12. Magnusson MO, Dahl ML, Cederberg J, et al. Pharmacodynamics of carbamazepine-mediated induction of CYP3A4, CYP1A2, and Pgp as assessed by probe substrates midazolam, caffeine, and digoxin. *Clin Pharmacol Ther.* 2008;84:52–62.
13. Perucca E. Clinically relevant drug interactions with antiepileptic drugs. *Br J Clin Pharmacol.* 2006;61:246–255.
14. Nappi JM. Warfarin and phenytoin interaction. *Ann Intern Med.* 1979; 90:852.
15. Chiron C. Stiripentol. *Neurotherapeutics.* 2007;4:123–125.
16. Anderson GD, Yau MK, Gidal BE, et al. Bidirectional interaction of valproate and lamotrigine in healthy subjects. *Clin Pharmacol Ther.* 1996; 60:145–156.
17. Sidhu J, Job S, Singh S, et al. The pharmacokinetic and pharmacodynamic consequences of the co-administration of lamotrigine and a combined oral contraceptive in healthy female subjects. *Br J Clin Pharmacol.* 2006; 61:191–199.
18. Yukawa E, Nonaka T, Yukawa M, et al. Pharmacoepidemiologic investigation of a clonazepam-carbamazepine interaction by mixed effect modeling using routine clinical pharmacokinetic data in Japanese patients. *J Clin Psychopharmacol.* 2001;21:588–593.
19. Reimers A, Skogvoll E, Sund JK, et al. Lamotrigine in children and adolescents: the impact of age on its serum concentrations and on the extent of drug interactions. *Eur J Clin Pharmacol.* 2007;63:687–692.
20. Glue P, Banfield CR, Perhach JL, et al. Pharmacokinetic interactions with felbamate: in vitro-in vivo correlation. *Clin Pharmacokinet.* 1997; 33:214–224.

21. Hachad H, Ragueneau-Majlessi I, Levy RH. New antiepileptic drugs: review on drug interactions. *Ther Drug Monit.* 2002;24:91–103.

22. Andreasen AH, Brosen K, Damkier P. A comparative pharmacokinetic study in healthy volunteers of the effect of carbamazepine and oxcarbazepine on cyp3a4. *Epilepsia.* 2007;48:490–496.

23. Sabers A. Pharmacokinetic interactions between contraceptives and antiepileptic drugs. *Seizure.* 2008;17:141–144.

24. Perucca E, Cloyd J, Critchley D, et al. Rufinamide: clinical pharmacokinetics and concentration-response relationships in patients with epilepsy. *Epilepsia.* 2008;49:1123–1141.

25. Doose DR, Wang SS, Padmanabhan M, et al. Effect of topiramate or carbamazepine on the pharmacokinetics of an oral contraceptive containing norethindrone and ethinyl estradiol in healthy obese and nonobese female subjects. *Epilepsia.* 2003;44:540–459.

26. Theis JG, Koren G, Daneman R, et al. Interactions of clobazam with conventional antiepileptics in children. *J Child Neurol.* 1997;12:208–213.

27. Sennoune S, Mesdjian E, Bonneton J, et al. Interactions between clobazam and standard antiepileptic drugs in patients with epilepsy. *Ther Drug Monit.* 1992;14:269–274.

28. Kosaki K, Tamura K, Sato R, et al. A major influence of CYP2C19 genotype on the steady-state concentration of N-desmethylclobazam. *Brain Dev.* 2004;26:530–534.

29. Burstein AH, Horton RL, Dunn T, et al. Lack of effect of St John's wort on carbamazepine pharmacokinetics in healthy volunteers. *Clin Pharmacol Ther.* 2000;68:605–612.

30. Contin M, Riva R, Albani F, et al. Effect of felbamate on clobazam and its metabolite kinetics in patients with epilepsy. *Ther Drug Monit.* 1999;21:604–608.

31. Chiron C, Marchand MC, Tran A, et al. Stiripentol in severe myoclonic epilepsy in infancy: a randomised placebo-controlled syndrome-dedicated trial. STICLO study group. *Lancet.* 2000;356:1638–1642.

32. Lai AA, Levy RH, Cutler RE. Time-course of interaction between carbamazepine and clonazepam in normal man. *Clin Pharmacol Ther.* 1978;24:316–323.

33. Khoo KC, Mendels J, Rothbart M, et al. Influence of phenytoin and phenobarbital on the disposition of a single oral dose of clonazepam. *Clin Pharmacol Ther.* 1980;28:368–375.

34. Doty P, Rudd GD, Stoehr T, et al. Lacosamide. *Neurotherapeutics.* 2007;4:145–148.

35. Gidal BE, Anderson GD, Rutecki PR, et al. Lack of an effect of valproate concentration on lamotrigine pharmacokinetics in developmentally disabled patients with epilepsy. *Epilepsy Res.* 2000;42:23–31.

36. Reimers A, Helde G, Brodtkorb E. Ethinyl estradiol, not progestogens, reduces lamotrigine serum concentrations. *Epilepsia.* 2005;46:1414–1417.

37. Christensen J, Petrenaite V, Atterman J, et al. Oral contraceptives induce lamotrigine metabolism: evidence from a double-blind, placebo-controlled trial. *Epilepsia.* 2007;48:484–489.

38. Perucca E, Gidal BE, Baltes E. Effects of antiepileptic comedication on levetiracetam pharmacokinetics: a pooled analysis of data from randomized adjunctive therapy trials. *Epilepsy Res.* 2003;53:47–56.

39. Levy RH, Koch KM. Drug interactions with valproic acid. *Drugs.* 1982;24:543–546.

40. Dandekar UP, Chandra RS, Dalvi SS, et al. Analysis of a clinically important interaction between phenytoin and Shankhapushpi, an Ayurvedic preparation. *J Ethnopharm.* 1992;35:285–288.

41. Bialer M, Johannessen SI, Kupferberg HJ, et al. Progress report on new antiepileptic drugs: a summary of the Fifth Eilat Conference (EILAT V). *Epilepsy Res.* 2001;43:11–58.

42. Burstein AH, Boudreau EA, Theodore WH. Increase in tiagabine serum concentration with coadministration of gemfibrozil. *Ann Pharmacother.* 2009;43:379–382.

43. Britzi M, Perucca E, Soback S, et al. Pharmacokinetic and metabolic investigation of topiramate disposition in healthy subjects in the absence and in the presence of enzyme induction by carbamazepine. *Epilepsia.* 2005;46:378–384.

44. Mori H, Takahashi K, Mizutani T. Interaction between valproic acid and carbapenem antibiotics. *Drug Metab Rev.* 2007;39:647–657.

45. Spriet I, Goyens J, Meersseman W, et al. Interaction between valproate and meropenem: a retrospective study. *Ann Pharmacother.* 2007;41:1130–1136.

46. Galimberti CA, Mazzucchelli I, Arbasino C, et al. Increased apparent oral clearance of valproic acid during intake of combined contraceptive steroids in women with epilepsy. *Epilepsia.* 2006;47:1569–1572.

47. Ikeda H, Murakami T, Takano M, et al. Pharmacokinetic interaction on valproic acid and recurrence of epileptic seizures during chemotherapy in an epileptic patient. *Br J Clin Pharmacol.* 2005;59:593–597.

48. Saraga M, Preisig M, Zullino DF. Reduced valproate plasma levels possible after introduction of efavirenz in a bipolar patient. *Bipolar Disord.* 2006;8:415–417.

49. Besag FM, Berry DJ, Pool F, et al. Carbamazepine toxicity with lamotrigine: pharmacokinetic or pharmacodynamic interaction? *Epilepsia.* 1998;39:183–187.

50. Theis JG, Sidhu J, Palmer J, et al. Lack of pharmacokinetic interaction between oxcarbazepine and lamotrigine. *Neuropsychopharmacology.* 2005;30:2269–2274.

CHAPTER 43 ■ INITIATION AND DISCONTINUATION OF ANTIEPILEPTIC DRUGS

VARDA GROSS TSUR, CHRISTINE O'DELL, AND SHLOMO SHINNAR

Over the past two decades there has been much information about the prognosis of seizure disorders, the effects of antiepileptic drug (AED) therapy on prognosis, and the relative risks of both seizures and AED therapy. This chapter reviews the clinical decision-making in initiating and discontinuing AEDs in children and adults, with particular emphasis on the data regarding the recurrence risk for seizures in different settings and the effect of AEDs on this risk. The risks and benefits of initiating and discontinuing AED therapy are then addressed in the context of an individualized therapeutic approach that emphasizes weighing the risks and benefits of drug therapy versus both the statistical risk of another seizure and the consequences of such an event.

RECURRENCE RISK FOLLOWING A FIRST UNPROVOKED SEIZURE

To develop a rational approach to the management of individuals who present with an initial unprovoked seizure, it is necessary to have some understanding of the natural history and prognosis of the disorder in this setting. Approximately one third to one half of children and adults with seizures will initially present to medical attention following a single seizure (1,2). The remainder will already have a history of prior events at the time of presentation. It is the group who presents with a single seizure that is most relevant to this discussion. In accordance with the International League Against Epilepsy (ILAE) guidelines for epidemiologic research in epilepsy, a first unprovoked seizure is defined as a seizure or flurry of seizures all occurring within 24 hours in a person older than 1 month of age with no prior history of unprovoked seizures (3).

Since 1982, a number of studies have attempted to address the recurrence risk following a first unprovoked seizure using a variety of recruitment and identification techniques (4–23). The reported overall recurrence risk following a first unprovoked seizure in children and adults varies from 27% to 71%. Studies that carefully excluded those with prior seizures report recurrence risks of 27% to 52% (4–18). Higher recurrence risks are, with one exception (19), reported from studies that included subjects who already had recurrent seizures at the time of identification and who were, thus, more properly considered to have newly diagnosed epilepsy.

While there is considerable disparity in the absolute recurrence risk reported in the different studies, the time course of recurrence is remarkably similar among all studies (5). The majority of recurrences occur early, with approximately 50% of recurrences occurring within 6 months of the initial seizure

and over 80% within 2 years of the initial seizure (5,13). Late recurrences are unusual, but they have occurred up to 10 years after the initial seizure (13,14). This time course is true both in studies that report low and high recurrence risks (4,5,7–10, 12–14,19–21).

A relatively small number of factors are associated with a differential recurrence risk. The most important of these are the etiology of the seizure, the electroencephalogram (EEG), and whether the first seizure occurred in wakefulness or sleep. These factors are consistent across most studies regardless of the absolute risk of recurrence reported in the individual study (4,5,7–15,18,20,21). Factors not associated with a significant change in the recurrence risk include the age of onset, the number of seizures in the first 24 hours, and the duration of the initial seizure. The absolute recurrence risks appear similar in children and adults (5), although the consequences of such a recurrence are quite different. Selected risk factors are discussed below.

Etiology

In the ILAE classification, etiology of seizures is classified as remote symptomatic, cryptogenic, or idiopathic (3). Remote symptomatic seizures are those without an immediate cause but with an identifiable prior brain injury or the presence of a static encephalopathy such as mental retardation or cerebral palsy, which are known to be associated with an increased risk of seizures. Cryptogenic seizures are those occurring in otherwise normal individuals with no clear etiology. Until recently, cryptogenic seizures were also called idiopathic. In the new classification, idiopathic is reserved for seizures occurring in the context of the presumed genetic epilepsies such as benign rolandic and childhood absence (24,25). However, much of the literature on the recurrence risk following a first unprovoked seizure lumps idiopathic and cryptogenic together as idiopathic using the original classification developed by Hauser and coworkers (8).

Not surprisingly, both children and adults with a remote symptomatic first seizure have higher risk of recurrence than those with a cryptogenic first seizure. A meta-analysis of the studies published up to 1990 found that the relative risk of recurrence following a remote symptomatic first seizure was 1.8 (95% confidence interval, 1.5, 2.1) compared to those with a cryptogenic first seizure (5). Comparable findings are reported in more recent studies (13,15,21). Idiopathic first unprovoked seizures occur almost exclusively in children. Although the long-term prognosis of these children is quite favorable, the recurrence risk is actually comparable to those with a remote symptomatic first seizure (13). This is because, by definition, to meet the criteria for an idiopathic first seizure, they must have an abnormal EEG (24,25).

Electroencephalogram

The EEG is an important predictor of recurrence, particularly in cases that are not remote symptomatic and in children (5,7,8,10–13,15–18,21,26). Studies of recurrence risk following a first seizure in childhood have uniformly reported that those with an abnormal EEG have a higher recurrence risk than those with a normal EEG (5,7,12,13,15,21,26). For this reason, the American Academy of Neurology's recently published guideline on the evaluation of children with a first unprovoked seizure considers an EEG to be a standard part of the evaluation (21). A recent guideline on the diagnostic evaluation of adults with a first seizure also recommends an EEG, though the level of evidence is not as strong as in children (27). Epileptiform abnormalities are more important than nonepileptiform ones, but any EEG abnormality increases the recurrence risk in cases that are not remote symptomatic (26). In our study, the risk of seizure recurrence within 24 months for children with an idiopathic/cryptogenic first seizure was 25% for those with a normal EEG, 34% for those with non-epileptiform abnormalities, and 54% for those with epileptiform abnormalities (26). Whereas in our data, any clearly abnormal electroencephalographic patterns—including generalized spike and wave, focal spikes, and focal or generalized slowing—increased the risk of recurrence, Camfield and associates (7) reported that only epileptiform abnormalities substantially increase the risk of recurrence in children. Despite minor disagreements as to which electroencephalographic patterns are most significant, the EEG appears to be the most important predictor of recurrence in children with a cryptogenic/idiopathic first seizure. In addition, it is the EEG that primarily distinguishes whether a neurologically normal child with a first seizure is classified as cryptogenic or idiopathic.

In adults, the data are more controversial. The majority of studies do find an increased recurrence risk associated with an abnormal EEG (5,9,10,18), although one study failed to find a significant effect (11). Hauser and colleagues (8) found that generalized spike-and-wave patterns are predictive of recurrence but not focal spikes. A meta-analysis of these studies concluded that the overall data do support an association between an abnormal EEG and an increased recurrence risk in adults as well (5), although which electroencephalographic patterns besides generalized spike and wave are important remains unclear (5,9,10,18). As the recent guideline points out, an EEG is recommended not only to assess recurrence risk but also to help classify the type of epilepsy and potentially identify a specific syndrome (27).

Sleep State at Time of First Seizure

In adults, seizures that occur at night are associated with a higher recurrence risk than those that occur in the daytime (11). In children, whose sleep patterns may include daytime naps, the association is more clearly between sleep state and recurrence risk rather than time of day (13,28). Interestingly, the association is not just because nocturnal seizures tend to occur in certain epilepsy syndromes. Thus, even children whose EEG has centrotemporal spikes and who meet the criteria for benign rolandic seizures (25) have a higher recurrence risk if the first seizure occurs during sleep than if it occurs while awake (28). Furthermore, if the first seizure occurs during sleep, there is a high likelihood that the second one, should it occur, will also occur during sleep (28). In our series, the 2-year recurrence risk was 53% for children whose initial seizure occurred during sleep compared with a 30% risk for those whose initial seizure occurred while awake (13). On multivariable analysis, etiology, the EEG, and sleep state were the major significant predictors of outcome. From a therapeutic point of view, the implication of a seizure during sleep is unclear. While the recurrence risk is higher, recurrences will tend to occur in sleep. As the major risk of a brief seizure in children or adults is that it may happen at a time or place where the impairment of consciousness will have serious consequences, the morbidity of a seizure during sleep is fairly low in both cases.

Seizure Classification

In some studies, the risk of recurrence following a first unprovoked seizure is higher in subjects with a partial seizure than in those with a generalized first seizure (5). This association is mostly found on univariate analysis and disappears once the effect of etiology and the EEG are accounted for (5,8,12,13). Partial seizures are more common in those with a remote symptomatic first seizure and in children with an abnormal EEG (12). Note that some generalized seizure types, such as absence and myoclonic, very rarely present as a first seizure and so would be excluded from studies of first seizure (16,21). Generalized seizures that present to medical attention at the time of the first seizure are usually tonic–clonic (13).

Duration of Initial Seizure

In children, the duration of the first seizure is not associated with a differential recurrence risk. In our study, 48 (12%) of 407 children (38 cryptogenic/idiopathic, 10 remote symptomatic) presented with status epilepticus (duration longer than 30 min) as their first unprovoked seizure (13). The recurrence risk in these children was not different from that in children whose first seizure was briefer. However, if a recurrence did occur, it was likely to be prolonged (13,29). Of the 24 children with an initial episode of status who experienced a seizure recurrence, 5 (21%) recurred with status. Of the 147 children who presented with an initial brief seizure and experienced a seizure recurrence, only 2 (1%) recurred with status epilepticus ($P < 0.001$). In adults, there is a suggestion that a prolonged first seizure, particularly in remote symptomatic cases, is associated with a higher risk of recurrence (10).

Number of Seizures in 24 Hours

The ILAE definition of a first unprovoked seizure includes a seizure flurry occurring within 24 hours (3). Well-designed prospective studies in both children (13) and adults (30) have found no difference in recurrence risks in patients who present with a cluster of seizures in 1 day compared with those who present with a single seizure. This is not an uncommon event and occurs in about 25% of cases. The data support the epidemiological definition of a cluster as being a single event and do not suggest an increased risk of further seizures.

Treatment Following a First Seizure

Five randomized clinical trials in children and adults examined the efficacy of treatment after a first unprovoked seizure (6,20,31–35). Two well-designed prospective studies which randomized subjects to treatment or placebo following a first unprovoked seizure found that treatment reduced the recurrence risk by approximately half (6,20,31). The larger Italian study included both children and adults (20,31). However, while recurrence risk was reduced, there was no difference in long-term outcomes between the two groups. Equal proportions were in 2-year remission after 5 years of follow-up (31). Although the authors of this study initially recommended treatment following a first seizure, once it became apparent that early treatment did not affect long-term prognosis, they changed their recommendation, suggesting that in the majority of cases treatment should not be recommended before a second seizure occurred (31). In the more recent Multicentre Trial for Early Epilepsy and Single Seizures (MESS), immediate treatment after a first unprovoked seizure reduced the risk of recurrence from 50% to 25%, but did not alter long-term outcome (35,36). In general, the accumulating evidence from a large number of studies indicates that AED therapy is effective in reducing the risk of a recurrent seizure but does not alter the underlying disorder and therefore does not change long-term prognosis (37). Based on these data and assessment of risk-to-benefit, the American Academy of Neurology has issued a practice parameter on AED therapy following a first unprovoked seizure in children and adolescents (34). This parameter recommends that (i) treatment with AEDs is not indicated for the prevention of the development of epilepsy and (ii) treatment with an AED may be considered in circumstances where the benefits of reducing the risk of a second seizure outweigh the risks of pharmacologic and psychosocial side effects. The authors rarely prescribe AEDs after a single seizure. A practice parameter addressing this issue in adults is currently under development, but the epidemiologic data and the data from randomized clinical trials are increasingly in favor of not routinely treating after a single seizure even in adults.

What Happens After Two Seizures?

Two studies in adults (9) and children (14) examined what happens after a second seizure. In adults, the recurrence risk after a second seizure is 70%, leading Hauser and coworkers to conclude that, in adults, once a second seizure has occurred, treatment with AEDs is appropriate (9). In children, the recurrence risk following a second seizure is also approximately 70%. Those with a remote symptomatic etiology and those whose second seizure occurs within 6 months of the first have a higher recurrence risk (14). Interestingly, factors such as an abnormal EEG and sleep state at the time of the seizure, which help to differentiate those who only have one seizure from those who experienced a recurrence, are no longer associated with a differential risk of further seizures once a second seizure occurs (14). Despite the similarities in recurrence risk, the issue of treatment following a second seizure in children is less straightforward than in adults. Many of these children have idiopathic self-limited epilepsy syndromes, such as benign rolandic, where the need for treatment has been questioned (38–40). In addition, the frequency of seizures in this group is low, with only 25% of children who had 2 seizures experiencing 10 or more seizures over a 10-year period (14). Thus, the decision regarding treatment in children with cryptogenic/idiopathic seizures who have a second seizure must be individualized and take into account whether the seizures are part of a benign self-limited syndrome, as well as the frequency of the seizures and the relative risks and benefits of treatment.

WITHDRAWAL OF ANTIEPILEPTIC DRUGS IN THOSE WHO HAVE BEEN SEIZURE-FREE ON ANTIEPILEPTIC DRUG THERAPY

AED therapy effectively controls seizures in the majority of patients with epilepsy. The preponderance of evidence indicates that most patients with epilepsy will become seizure-free on AEDs within a few years of diagnosis (41–48). However, the long-term use of AEDs carries with it significant morbidity. Therefore, the issue of whether one can withdraw AEDs in patients with epilepsy after a seizure-free interval becomes important in the treatment of a vast number of patients.

A large number of prospective and retrospective studies in children and adolescents, involving thousands of subjects, have been done over the past 25 years on the question of remission and relapse rates after withdrawal of AEDs. A smaller but still substantial number of studies dealing with adults have also been reported (42,49–81). A meta-analysis of the available literature reported a pooled risk of relapse of 25% at 1 year and 29% at 2 years following AED withdrawal (51).

In childhood-onset epilepsy, the majority of studies report that 60% to 75% of children and adolescents with epilepsy who have been seizure-free for more than 2 to 4 years on medication will remain so after AEDs are withdrawn (49–52,58–60,62–66,68,73–76,79,81). Exceptionally low recurrence rates of 8% to 12% were reported in studies that limited subject entry to neurologically normal children with normal EEGs, many of whom were followed since the onset of their seizures (67,78).

In the past, it was thought that adult-onset epilepsy had a far less favorable prognosis for remission than childhood-onset epilepsy, and that withdrawal of medications was rarely feasible in this population. Although the prognosis in adults does appear to be worse than in children, newer studies suggest that the differences are smaller than thought. Four years after onset, the majority of adults with new-onset seizures will be at least 2 years seizure-free (46,47). Many adults self-discontinue their medications and are still seizure-free years later (41,81). Studies of withdrawing AEDs in adults report recurrence rates of 28% to 66% (52,55,61,65,68,70,80), which is a much larger range than that reported in pediatric studies. However, it should be noted that studies that reported the lowest recurrence risks (55) limited themselves to patients followed since onset of their seizures and who had absence of other presumed risk factors. In pediatric studies, such selected populations have reported recurrence risks of less than 20%.

The preponderance of data at this time indicates that the recurrence risk following withdrawal of AEDs is somewhat higher in adult-onset epilepsy than in childhood-onset epilepsy with a relative risk of approximately 1.3 (51). However, much of the increased risk reported in some studies is a result of the higher risk of recurrence in adolescent-onset seizures (51,73). Selected populations of adults may have low recurrence risks. Two reports showed no differences in recurrence risks between children and adults (55,80). However, these studies have the highest reported recurrence risks for children (31% to 40%) and the lowest reported recurrence risks for adults (35% to 40%). In addition, their definition of children exceeds the usual limits of the term. In one study, 38% of the subjects had childhood onset but this was defined as onset before 15 years of age (55). Several studies in children have reported that an age of onset older than 10 or 12 years was associated with a higher recurrence risk, presumably because this already reflects early adult-onset epilepsy (53,72–74,78).

The data on adolescents indicate that the recurrence rate is more a function of the age at onset than the age at withdrawal of medications (51,73,74). Studies of childhood-onset epilepsy that included adolescents have reported low recurrence risk (50,51,53,59,67,73,74,76,78). Studies of adolescents and adults that have primarily included adolescent-onset cases have reported recurrence rates similar to those seen in adults (51,55,65,80). One retrospective study limited to adolescents with adolescent-onset seizures reported a recurrence rate of 49% (71). A recent meta-analysis found that adolescent-onset epilepsy has a higher recurrence risk following AED withdrawal than either childhood- (relative risk, 1.79) or adult-onset (relative risk, 1.34) epilepsy (51).

When recurrences do occur after discontinuation of AEDs, they tend to occur early (51,73). The timing of recurrence is similar in studies of both children and adults and is independent of the absolute recurrence risk. Many occur as the medications are being tapered. At least half the recurrences occur within 6 months of medication withdrawal, 60% to 90% of recurrences occur within 1 year of withdrawal, and more than 85% of recurrences occur within 5 years (50,5153,55,59,63–65,67,68,70,73,74,76,80). One series in adults reported that 68% of relapses were during drug withdrawal and an additional 24% occurred during the first year after discontinuation of treatment (70). Although late recurrences do occur, they are uncommon (63,73,82). There is no secondary peak in recurrence risk years after discontinuing medications.

In analyzing recurrence risks following withdrawal of AEDs, one must also consider the recurrence risk of patients who are candidates for medication withdrawal but are maintained on AEDs. Annegers and coworkers (41) found a mean relapse risk of 1.6% per year in patients who were in remission for 5 or more years. Similarly, Oller-Daurella and associates (83) reported a 12.6% recurrence rate in a group of patients who were maintained on AEDs after being in remission for 5 or more years. One large-scale, randomized trial of continued AED therapy versus slow withdrawal in 1013

patients who were seizure-free for 2 or more years found a 22% recurrence rate in those maintained on medications compared with a 42% recurrence rate in those whose medications were withdrawn (69). However, after 2 years, the subsequent recurrence risks were identical, suggesting that the increased risk of recurrence attributable to AED withdrawal occurs only in the first 2 years. Late recurrences occur but are not attributable to AED withdrawal. These relapse rates must also be considered when deciding on whether to continue long-term AED therapy. Interestingly, in a 30-year follow-up study of 178 patients with epilepsy, there was a slightly higher recurrence rate in those patients who remained on AEDs, although the two groups were not randomized and were, therefore, not fully comparable (48).

RISK FACTORS FOR RECURRENCE

Clinically, it is important to identify subgroups with better or less favorable prognoses for maintaining seizure remission off medications. It is essential to quantify the significance of risk factors such as etiology, age of onset, type of seizure, and the EEG; however, different studies give very different results. A discussion of potential risk factors and their significance is presented below.

Etiology and Neurologic Status

Patients with remote symptomatic epilepsy associated with a prior neurologic insult, congenital malformation, motor handicap, brain tumor, mental retardation, progressive metabolic disease, trauma, or stroke are less likely to attain complete seizure control than are those with cryptogenic or idiopathic epilepsy (41,44,48).

Even in patients with remote symptomatic epilepsy who do attain seizure remission while on medications, current data indicate that the relapse rate after discontinuation of AEDs is higher than in those with cryptogenic seizures. In one study of 264 children and adolescents, the cumulative recurrence risk 2 years following withdrawal of medications was 26% in the cryptogenic group and 42% in the neurologically abnormal group ($P < 0.005$) (73). Despite the increased risk of recurrence in the neurologically abnormal group, the majority of this population was successfully withdrawn from AEDs. The severity of mental retardation was an additional prognostic factor within this group.

Similar results have been found in other studies (51,59,63–65). A recent study of the prognosis of epilepsy in children with cerebral palsy and epilepsy (56) found that the majority of these children did not achieve remission. However, of the 69 children who achieved a 2-year seizure remission and had their medication withdrawn, 58% remained seizure-free. The type of cerebral palsy was associated with a differential risk of recurrence. With one exception (66), studies that did not find such an association either had very few (74) remote symptomatic cases or were restricted to those with cryptogenic epilepsy (55,67,70,78,80). A meta-analysis estimated the relative risk of recurrence in those with remote symptomatic epilepsy compared with cryptogenic epilepsy to be 1.55 (51). This applies to all remote symptomatic causes including both mental retardation and cerebral palsy. Within the remote symptomatic group, those with severe mental retardation have the highest recurrence risk (73).

Age

As discussed, adolescent- and adult-onset epilepsy are associated with a somewhat poorer prognosis for successful withdrawal of AED therapy (51,61,65,68,70,71,73), although selected populations may do well (55,80). The discussion that follows focuses on differences within the pediatric age group.

Many studies report that an age of onset younger than 12 years is associated with a lower recurrence risk following discontinuation of medication than an older age of onset (50,51,53,59,65,72–74,78). This corresponds to the known higher remission rates in the younger group (41,44,84).

There is some controversy as to whether a very young age of onset of younger than 2 (59,73,84) or 3 years (58,79) may be a poor prognostic factor. Studies that include large numbers of children with remote symptomatic epilepsy have found a worse prognosis in the very young (59), whereas studies of mostly cryptogenic epilepsy have produced conflicting results (58,66,74,79). In one study that examined this question (73), 73% of the children with age of onset older than 12 years and 45% of those with age of onset younger than 2 years experienced seizure recurrence compared with 26% of those with age of onset between 2 and 12 years ($P < 0.0001$). However, the poorer prognosis in those with a very young age of onset was limited to the remote symptomatic group (73). These data are consistent with the findings of Huttenlocher and coworkers (85) that neurologically abnormal children with seizure onset at younger than 2 years of age had a poor prognosis for entering remission.

There are no convincing data that withdrawing AEDs during puberty is associated with a higher risk of recurrence (39,63,64,74,86). In fact, with the exception of one isolated report (82), studies on the remission of seizures and on withdrawing AEDs (41,63,64,73,74,76) do not show a reproducible pattern that correlates with puberty. The probability of attaining remission and of maintaining remission after medication withdrawal is more a function of the age of onset and the duration of the seizure disorder, without a special role for puberty.

Electroencephalogram

An abnormal interictal EEG, particularly one with epileptiform features, is often cited as a predictor of relapse after AED withdrawal (4,51,74,87–89). Results of actual studies in children and adults, however, are conflicting.

In children, a substantial number of studies found that the EEG prior to discontinuation of AEDs was an important predictor of outcome (39,42,51,59,71–74,76). Interestingly, any electroencephalographic abnormality, not just a frankly epileptiform one, was associated with an increased risk of relapse. In a study that examined specific features of the EEG, the presence of either slowing or spikes was associated with an increased risk and the presence of both in the same patient was associated with a very high risk of recurrence (74). Two studies reported that only certain specific epileptiform patterns, such as irregular generalized spike-and-wave pattern, were associated with an increased recurrence risk following medication withdrawal (42,88).

Further evidence for the importance of the EEG as a predictor of outcome can be inferred from three large studies (50,67,78). Because these studies excluded children with abnormal EEGs and report very low recurrence risks of 8% to 12%, they provide indirect evidence for the importance of the EEG as a predictor of recurrence. However, some studies in children did not find the EEG to be predictive (53,64). The studies which did find the EEG to be predictive were mainly of children with cryptogenic seizures. In studies that specifically analyzed the relationship between the EEG and outcome in both cryptogenic and remote symptomatic cases, the EEG was a significant predictor of outcome only in the cryptogenic group (73).

The EEG prior to treatment may also have some predictive value. Certain electroencephalographic patterns are markers for specific epileptic syndromes, such as benign rolandic epilepsy, childhood absence, or juvenile myoclonic epilepsy, which are thought to have a particularly favorable or unfavorable prognosis for remaining in remission following drug withdrawal (25,39,86,90). Changes in the EEG between the onset of seizures and time of medication withdrawal may also have a prognostic value (55,74).

The number of adult studies that have examined this issue is relatively small. Callaghan and coworkers (55) reported that an abnormal EEG was associated with an increased risk of recurrence. However, several other adult studies reported no such association (70,80). At present, the preponderance of evidence indicates that an abnormal EEG is a predictor of recurrence in children with cryptogenic epilepsy, but not in those with remote symptomatic epilepsy. In adults the data are inconclusive, but suggest that an abnormal EEG is associated with a modest increase in recurrence risk (51,52,89). Whether specific electroencephalographic patterns are associated with an increased recurrence risk is a question that requires further study.

Epilepsy Syndrome

Epilepsy syndromes are known to be associated with a differential prognosis for remission (24,25,91). Syndromes such as benign rolandic epilepsy have a particularly favorable prognosis for remission and for successfully discontinuing AEDs, even if the EEG is still abnormal (73), as EEG normalization occurs later than the clinical disappearance of seizures (24). Juvenile myoclonic epilepsy, while having a favorable prognosis for remission on medications, usually requires prolonged treatment and has a high relapse rate when medications are withdrawn (25,90). Syndromes such as Lennox–Gastaut have a poor prognosis for remission even on medications (25,48,91). Overall, patients with both idiopathic and cryptogenic epilepsy syndromes have a similar prognosis (48,73,91). Interestingly, while specific idiopathic syndromes and the various other generalized epilepsy syndromes have different prognoses, the various nonidiopathic partial epilepsies do not appear to have major differences in the relapse rate following medication withdrawal (73). Unfortunately, there is a paucity of such information as few studies of AED withdrawal provide information by epilepsy syndrome. It is clear that future studies will focus on epilepsy syndrome as a major predictor of long-term prognosis and management, both at the time of diagnosis and when in remission on medications (24,43,73,91).

Other Risk Factors

Other risk factors, such as duration of epilepsy, number of seizures, seizure type, and the medication used, have not been consistently associated with a differential risk of relapse following AED withdrawal in either children or adults.

Duration of epilepsy and number of seizures are closely inter-related. A long duration of epilepsy increases the risk of recurrence, although the magnitude of the effect is small (63,64). One study also reported that having more than 30 generalized tonic–clonic seizures was associated with a high risk of recurrence after discontinuation of therapy (59). In a community-based practice, most people are easily controlled within a short time after therapy is initiated so that these factors will rarely be important (43,47,48).

The specific AED used also has not been consistently associated with the risk of recurrence, although one well-designed study reported an increased recurrence risk in adults who were on valproate compared with those on other AEDs (55). Note that all the published studies on AED withdrawal are reporting the results of AED withdrawal from the old AEDs (barbiturates, phenytoin, carbamazepine, valproate, and ethosuximide). The serum drug level does not seem to have a great impact on recurrence risk. Patients who have not had seizures for several years often have "subtherapeutic" levels, and few have high levels. Available studies show little or no correlation between drug level prior to discontinuation and seizure recurrence and outcome (74), or a very modest effect (59).

Seizure type has also not been consistently associated with recurrence risk, except that children with multiple seizure types have a poorer prognosis (63,64). The data regarding partial seizures are conflicting (51,53,55,59,63–65,68,73, 74,76). Note that specific seizure types may be surrogate markers for epilepsy syndromes with a more favorable or less favorable prognosis. At this time, it is not clear that any specific seizure type is associated with an increased risk of recurrence following discontinuation of medication.

HOW LONG TO TREAT AND HOW RAPIDLY TO TAPER?

Duration of Seizure-Free Interval Prior to Attempting Withdrawal of Antiepileptic Drugs

The chances of remaining seizure-free after medication withdrawal is similar whether a 2-year (50,53,55,65,73,74,76) or a 4-year seizure-free interval (59,63,64,68,73,76) is used. One study that evaluated seizure-free intervals of 1 or more years did find that a longer seizure-free period was associated with a slightly lower recurrence risk (76). However, the higher relapse rates were primarily observed in those who were withdrawn after 1 year. In general, the epidemiologic data do not support the need for treatment beyond 2 years in cases where AED withdrawal is being considered.

A few investigators attempted to withdraw AEDs in children with epilepsy after a seizure-free interval of 1 year or less (57,72,88). A meta-analysis found a pooled relative risk of 1.3 for withdrawal prior to 2 years seizure-free versus 2 or more years seizure-free (89). While the recurrence risks in these studies are somewhat higher than in studies that used a longer seizure-free interval, they do suggest that, in selected populations, a shorter seizure-free interval may be sufficient. The higher recurrence risks reflect the fact that when a less stringent criterion for remission is used, fewer patients are actually in long-term remission. Long-term outcomes are not adversely affected by early discontinuation (72).

Duration of Medication Taper

Once the decision to withdraw AEDs has been made, the clinician needs to decide on how quickly the medications can be withdrawn. Many clinicians have used slow tapering schedules lasting many months or even years, thinking that they would reduce the risk of recurrence. Even the randomized study from the Medical Research Council (MRC) AED Drug Withdrawal Group (68) used a relatively slow taper. There is general agreement that abrupt discontinuation of AEDs is inadvisable in an outpatient setting and may increase the risk of seizure recurrence. Beyond that, there is much heated debate primarily based on mythology. A well-designed, prospective, randomized clinical trial has provided solid data on this issue (75). The study compared a rapid 6-week AED taper with a more gradual 9-month taper in children with epilepsy whose AEDs were being discontinued after a 2-year or longer seizure-free interval. There were no differences in recurrence risk at 2 years between the groups with short and long tapering regimens. This well-designed study should finally settle this long-standing controversy, although specific drugs, such as barbiturates and benzodiazepines, might require slightly longer tapering periods. Note that a long tapering period will not alter the recurrence risk at 2 years, but may delay the recurrence and, thus, tends to prolong the period of uncertainty. Thus, a relatively short taper period is particularly important in adolescents and adults if we advise them to stop driving for 6 months to a year following AED withdrawal.

Prognosis Following Relapse

The majority of patients who relapse after medication withdrawal will become seizure-free and in remission after AEDs are restarted, although not necessarily immediately (48,72,83,92,93). The prognosis for long-term remission appears to be primarily a function of the underlying epilepsy syndrome. The MRC randomized study of medication withdrawal in children and adults found that the prognosis for seizure control after recurrence in patients with previously well-controlled seizures was no different in those who were withdrawn from AED therapy and relapsed and those who relapsed while remaining on AED therapy (93).

WITHDRAWAL OF ANTIEPILEPTIC DRUGS AFTER SUCCESSFUL RESECTIVE SURGERY

Epilepsy surgery is the treatment of choice in suitable patients with refractory epilepsy. Patients with intractable epilepsy who undergo resective surgery are considered a class 1 successful outcome if they are seizure-free following surgery, whether they are on AEDs (94,95). In the past, the tendency was to maintain them on at least one AED indefinitely (95). The issue of whether and for how long patients who are seizure-free following surgery need to remain on chronic AED therapy is receiving increased attention. Several retrospective studies in adults report that approximately 60% of patients with medically refractory epilepsy who become seizure-free after resective surgery remain so when AEDs are withdrawn (96–98). Younger age at surgery was a favorable predictor for seizure freedom after AED discontinuation (99,100). Successful withdrawal of AEDs following resective surgery has also been reported in children (101). Generally, the risks of medication withdrawal in this population appear similar to those seen in those with remote symptomatic epilepsy in remission on medications (51,73). It, therefore, appears reasonable to consider medication withdrawal in patients who are seizure-free following resective surgery (95,98,101). The prognostic factors for successful medication withdrawal are not well defined but appear to be different than for those who become seizure-free with medical therapy (98). The optimal timing for medication withdrawal in this population is not clear.

In principle, one can ask, following a potentially curative procedure, why to wait more than a short seizure-free interval, such as 6 months or a year, before attempting withdrawal in this population (98). Berg et al. (102) reported that many of the relapses in patients who attained at least 1-year seizure, remission occurred while reducing or eliminating the AEDs. The risk of recurrence was not higher than in those who continued AEDs (102,103). The physician should remember that while some patients may be eager to try coming off medication in the belief that they are cured (98), many may be unwilling to jeopardize their newly achieved seizure-free state. The decisions need to be individualized, based on the potential risks and benefits in each case and the personal preferences of the patient.

Further, well-controlled prospective studies are needed to provide rational practice guidelines to inform the clinical decision in this setting.

RISKS OF NOT TREATING OR OF DISCONTINUING ANTIEPILEPTIC DRUGS

The major risk associated with not treating after first seizure or of discontinuing AED therapy is having a seizure recurrence. The potential consequences of the seizure recurrence include both direct consequences and psychosocial impact. There is no convincing evidence that a brief seizure causes brain damage (34,40,104,105). Serious injury from a brief seizure is a relatively uncommon event usually related to the impairment of consciousness or loss of consciousness that occurred at an inopportune time or place (e.g., driving, riding a bicycle, swimming, on a stairway, cooking) (26,40,83). These are much less likely to occur in children who are usually in a supervised environment and are not driving, operating heavy machinery, or cooking. In a study of withdrawing AEDs in 264 children with epilepsy who were seizure-free on medication, there were 100 recurrences (83). Of these, two experienced

status epilepticus as their initial recurrence and have done well after reinitiation of AEDs with no long-term consequences. Five sustained an injury as a result of the initial recurrence, including four with lacerations and one with a broken arm. Thus, the rate of serious injury was quite low. Most reports of serious injuries in patients with epilepsy discuss patients with intractable epilepsy who experience injuries such as burns in the context of frequent seizures (106,107).

Status epilepticus is a concern, particularly in adults. It should be noted that the morbidity of status epilepticus in both children and adults is primarily a function of etiology, and in this clinical setting will be low (105,108–110). Furthermore, the risk of status epilepticus in this population is low and essentially limited to those who have had it before (13,29). While status epilepticus is frequently reported in patients with epilepsy who are noncompliant (108,109), the occurrence of status epilepticus in patients who are withdrawn from their AEDs after a seizure-free interval is very low (74,83).

Some authors, most notably Reynolds, have expressed concern that, in addition to the potential for injury, the consequences of a seizure include a worse long-term prognosis, and thus argue that treatment is indicated even after a single seizure (19,111). This view is largely based on Gower's statement that "The tendency of the disease is toward self-perpetuation; each attack facilitates the occurrence of the next by increasing the instability of the nerve elements" (112), which became the basis for the popular notion that "seizures beget seizures." Current epidemiologic data and data from controlled clinical trials indicate that this is not the case (16,17,31,34,38,93,104,113). Studies in developing countries, where treatment delays are a result of the unavailability of AEDs, show no difference in response rate in those with many prior seizures compared with new-onset patients (38,113). Prognosis is primarily a function of the underlying epilepsy syndrome, and although treatment with AEDs does reduce the risk of subsequent seizures, it does not alter the long-term prognosis for seizure control and remission (16,31,34, 38,113). The decision to treat should, therefore, be made on the grounds that the patient has had a sufficient number of events to justify initiating therapy or is at sufficiently high risk for seizure recurrence to justify continued therapy, and not with the hope of somehow preventing the development of "chronic" epilepsy (34).

Although a seizure may be a dramatic and frightening event, the long-term psychosocial impact of an isolated seizure in children is minimal. In adults, the psychosocial impact can be more serious, and includes the loss of driving privileges and possible adverse effects on employment (114,115). Social stigma of seizures is also much more a concern in adolescents and adults.

RISKS OF INITIATING OR CONTINUING TREATMENT WITH ANTIEPILEPTIC DRUGS

Although effective in controlling seizures, AEDs are associated with a variety of significant side effects that must be considered when deciding to initiate or to continue treatment (Table 43.1). Physicians are generally familiar with systemic

TABLE 43.1

RISKS AND ADVERSE EFFECTS OF ANTIEPILEPTIC DRUG THERAPY AND OF SEIZURES[a]

Risks of antiepileptic drug therapy	Risks of seizures
Systemic toxicity	**Physical injury**
Idiosyncratic	Loss of consciousness
Dose related	Falls
Chronic toxicity	Status epilepticus
	Children and adolescents
	Sports injuries
	Bathing/swimming: drowning
	Adolescents and adults
Teratogenicity	Driving accidents
	Bathing/shower: scalding
	Cooking injuries, burns
	Higher cortical functions
Cognitive impairment	Impairment in postictal state
	Children
Adverse effects on behavior	
	Psychosocial
Need for daily medication	Fear of subsequent seizures
Labeling as chronic illness	Loss of privacy
	Stigma of seizures
	Children and adolescents
	Restrictions on school/social activities
	Adolescents and adults
	Restrictions on driving
	Difficulties providing childcare
	Economic/Temporal
Cost of medications	Time lost because of seizure and
Cost/time of laboratory tests	recovery
Cost/time of physician visits	
	Adolescents and adults
	Discrimination in employment

[a]Some adverse effects of seizures may also occur with antiepileptic drug therapy. Adverse effects listed by age group, such as behavioral effects and bathtub drowning, are meant to indicate the predominant age group in which they occur and do not exclude their occurrence in other age groups.

side effects, including idiosyncratic, acute, and chronic. Idiosyncratic and acute adverse events sufficient to require discontinuation of the drug occur in 15% or more of patients newly treated with an AED, and need to be considered when deciding whether to initiate AED therapy. They are not generally a major concern when deciding whether to continue AEDs in patients who are seizure-free as almost all those patients are on stable drug regimens without evidence of acute toxicity. Chronic toxicity is a concern in both settings. There is evidence that children may be more susceptible to chronic toxicity from AEDs (34,116). In the elderly, an additional concern is drug–drug interaction, as many of these patients are on multiple other medications that also are protein bound and metabolized by the cytochrome P450 system. Adverse effects on many AEDs on bone health are also of increasing concern (117).

It is now recognized that AED therapy is associated with a variety of both cognitive and behavioral adverse effects

(116,118). These are more common in children, and sometimes are difficult to recognize. In particular, children on medications since their preschool years may not be identified as having side effects from medications. Only when medications are stopped does it become apparent that the child's performance was impaired by the drug. Adults can also experience cognitive and behavioral adverse events from AED therapy. Increasingly, studies of new AEDs include measures of neuropsychological function to help address this issue. The reason phenobarbital is no longer considered a first-line drug in adults with epilepsy is not because of its efficacy, which is excellent, but because of the impairment of cognition and behavior associated with its use. Although other agents are less of an issue, all AEDs can have adverse effects on cognition and behavior (116,118).

For women of childbearing age, including adolescents, a discussion of the risks of treatment must include consideration of the potential teratogenicity of these compounds (119–121).

As the major teratogenic effects usually occur in the first few weeks of gestation, often before a woman is aware that she is pregnant, the physician must always consider this issue in advance. It impacts both on the decision to initiate or withdraw AED therapy and on the choice of AED. One must also consider that many pregnancies, particularly in adolescents, are unplanned. Furthermore, enzyme-inducing AEDs may reduce the efficacy of oral contraceptives by inducing the hepatic enzyme systems responsible for their metabolism (119–121). For this reason, we are reluctant to initiate AED therapy in adolescent females and are particularly aggressive in trying to withdraw them from medications after a 2-year seizure-free interval, even if their other risk factors are not favorable.

A hidden side effect of continued AED treatment is that of being labeled (see Table 43.1). People with single seizures or epilepsy who have not had a seizure in many years and are off medications are considered to be healthy both by themselves and society. Those individuals can lead normal lives with very few restrictions. Unless they choose to, they rarely need to disclose that they once had seizures. In contrast, even if a patient only had a single seizure or is seizure-free for many years, being on AED therapy implies chronic illness to both the patient and those around the patient (115–122). Continued use of medication requires ongoing medical care to prescribe and monitor the medication, and establishes that the individual is a patient in need of treatment for a chronic condition. It also implies certain restrictions in driving, and may have an adverse impact on obtaining employment and other social issues. Labeling is a problem in both children and adults. The MRC study reported that psychosocial outcomes were improved in adults who were successfully withdrawn from AED therapy (115). In children and adolescents there is the additional problem that the perception of any chronic illness adversely affects the normal psychosocial maturation process, particularly in adolescents (39,122).

COUNSELING FAMILIES

Decisions on initiating or discontinuing AEDs ultimately depend on a relative assessment of risks and benefits. These are assessed differently by physicians and by patients and their families. Therefore, providing appropriate education and counseling to the patients and their families is critical, regardless of the final therapeutic decision. Both seizures and AED therapy are associated with some risks. Even though patients with good prognostic factors have a lower risk of recurrence, this risk is not zero even if they stay on medications. Conversely, those with poor risk factors may nevertheless maintain remission off medications. The risk of adverse events from AED therapy is essentially independent of the recurrence risk and always needs to be considered, as does the psychosocial impact of both seizures and continued AED therapy. Education assists the patient and family in making an informed decision, helps them to fully participate in the plan of care, and prepares them to deal with psychosocial consequences of the diagnosis. Informed decision-making by the physician, in consultation with the family, maximizes the chances of good long-term outcomes.

Patients and families need to be reassured that the risk of a serious injury or death from an isolated seizure is low. They also need to be counseled about appropriate first aid for seizures and safety information. This is a particular problem for adults, as they are more likely to engage in activities that may predispose them to injury should a seizure occur. Places of employment may or may not be accommodating to the person at risk for a seizure.

A discussion of possible restrictions on activities is also important. Parents will need to be told that most of the child's activities can be continued, although some, such as swimming, may need closer supervision. Adolescents and adults will need specific instructions regarding activities such as swimming, cooking, and driving. Counseling often allays fears and educates the patient and family on safety precautions. This reduces the chance for injury from seizures, if the patient is treated. Educational programs are available for school personnel—teachers, nurses, and students—and information for babysitters is also readily available. Note that, in the case of the child or adult with a first seizure, this discussion is equally applicable whether one decides to initiate AED therapy, as therapy reduces, but does not eliminate, the risk of seizure recurrence.

The information provided must be individualized to both the situation and the sophistication level of the patient and the family. The family of a patient with epilepsy who is seizure-free on medications should be familiar with the side effects of AED therapy and with seizures, and be able to discuss recurrence risks from withdrawing AEDs and the potential consequences. In the case of patients with a first seizure, the discussion needs to be more comprehensive, including first-aid measures in case of a recurrence, potential adverse effects of AEDs, risks of recurrence, impact on long-term prognosis of delaying therapy until after a second seizure, and restrictions on activity that will occur with or without therapy. It may be difficult to accomplish this in one session, especially in the emergency department where the circumstances may not be conducive to a calm discussion of the relative risks and benefits, and where key information on recurrence risks, such as the results of the electroencephalograph or an imaging study, may not be available.

Families will usually be interested in information that will help them manage the illness or specific problems. Lengthy explanations on any one issue may be confusing and are usually not helpful. Children and adults may have fear of accidents, fear of the loss of friends, fear of taking "drugs," and other less well-defined concerns. A parent's perception of the child's disorder will be an important factor in later coping and will ultimately impact on the perception of quality of life. Adults may have to make major lifestyle changes. The practitioner's prejudices regarding treatment options will undoubtedly come into play during these discussions, but the different options need to be discussed. Although more time-consuming than issuing a prescription, this counseling is necessary for both informed decision-making and for favorable long-term outcomes.

A THERAPEUTIC APPROACH

Initiating Antiepileptic Drug Therapy

In children with a first seizure, there is an emerging consensus that treatment after a first unprovoked seizure is usually not indicated (6,7,12–14,34,40,51,116), particularly in neurologically normal children with a brief first seizure (34). We will rarely treat a child with a first unprovoked seizure, even in the presence of risk factors such as a remote symptomatic etiology, an abnormal EEG, or a prolonged first seizure (13,14). In children with infrequent brief seizures, particularly in the context of a self-limited benign childhood epilepsy, many clinicians do not initiate AED therapy even after a second or third seizure (14,16,38–40). This is based on an assessment of the relative risks and benefits of AED therapy in children who will most likely enter remission with or without treatment, and who will most likely continue to have only infrequent seizures (14). However, there is no consensus on this issue.

In adults, the decision to treat or not after a first seizure remains more controversial (9,17,31,111). However, prospective studies show lower recurrence risks than previously thought and a well-designed, prospective, randomized study demonstrated no impact on long-term prognosis from delaying therapy (31,34,37). Therefore, a growing number of clinicians are delaying initiating long-term AED therapy after a single seizure (9,17,31). This is particularly true in young adults who would be committing to long-term therapy and in women of childbearing potential. Following two seizures, the risk of further seizures is approximately 70%, and, in general, AED treatment is indicated (9). The major exception may be a woman who wishes to have children in the immediate future and who has had two brief seizures. In this setting there is no definite answer, and the clinician and the patient must again weigh the relative risks and benefits of initiating therapy at that time or waiting (119–121).

In both children and adults, a thorough evaluation of the patient, including a detailed history and neurologic examination, as well as appropriate laboratory studies, such as an electroencephalograph and an imaging study when indicated, are important (21). Of particular importance is a careful history of prior events that may be seizures (21). A substantial proportion of patients who first come to medical attention with a seizure turn out to have had prior episodes that were also seizures (1,2,12,21). This is particularly true for patients who present with a first convulsive episode and, after a careful history is taken, are found to have had prior nonconvulsive episodes of absence or complex partial seizures. These patients fall into the category of newly diagnosed epilepsy, and not first seizure, and usually need treatment.

Withdrawing Antiepileptic Drug Therapy

The question of continuing or withdrawing AED therapy in a given patient must be considered based on an analysis of the relative risks and benefits. The goal is to achieve the best possible outcome for that patient, whether the ultimate decision is to treat or not. In considering the risks of seizure recurrence, the statistical risk of relapse is only one piece of the puzzle. One must consider not only the mathematical probability of seizure recurrence but the consequences of such a recurrence. The risk of seizure recurrence following medication withdrawal in children is somewhat lower than in adults and, in addition, there are identifiable subgroups with a particularly favorable prognosis. Adverse effects of continued AED therapy are also clearly more an issue with children than with adults, particularly adult males. However, it is in the area of potential consequences of a recurrence that the differences are most pronounced.

The adult who is driving and employed can suffer significant adverse social and economic consequences from having a seizure. In addition, an adult is more likely than a child to have the seizure in a setting where a physical injury may occur as a result of impaired consciousness (e.g., driving, operating machinery, cooking). Therefore, a 30% risk of recurrence, which is very acceptable in most children, may be unacceptable to adults because of the more serious consequences of a recurrence. When these are taken into account, patient preferences clearly depend on age and gender, despite similar statistical risks. In the British MRC AED withdrawal study, the psychosocial outcomes of those who successfully came off AEDs were better, and the statistical risk of recurrence was similar to those seen in children (68,69). However, when other adult patients were counseled based on the results of that study, the majority chose to remain on AED therapy (114). Nevertheless, adults who are seizure-free on their AEDs for 2 or more years should have the option of AED withdrawal discussed, even if the recommendation of the clinician is to remain on medications, as some patients will find the risk-to-benefit ratio favorable (114,123). Women of childbearing age are a special category, where a more aggressive approach to AED withdrawal may be indicated for reasons already discussed (119,121,123). Another category where a more aggressive approach should be considered is young adults of either gender with childhood-onset epilepsy who are still on medications. A chance at AED withdrawal, especially if they do not need to drive, should be considered before committing them to life-long therapy (39).

The reverse argument may be made for young children. In this group, the risk of relapse is smaller and, depending on the degree of parental supervision, the consequences relatively minor, whereas the risks of side effects from medications are greater. It is much safer to withdraw AEDs in this environment than when the patient is an adult. The risk-to-benefit analysis favors attempting medication withdrawal even in those with a higher risk of relapse (39,57,88).

Adolescents are a special case with additional issues. Adolescents with any chronic illness tend to become noncompliant as part of adolescence. We would far rather withdraw AEDs in a controlled fashion and make the explicit contract that if a recurrence occurs both the patient and the clinician know that medications are needed, than have the adolescent drive and then become noncompliant. In adolescent women, issues of teratogenicity also need to be considered, especially as most pregnancies in this age group are unplanned. Even if immediate pregnancy is not a major concern, these young women will soon be entering their childbearing years and decision-making needs to take this into account (119,120). On a risk-to-benefit basis, it is rational to attempt medication withdrawal at least once in adolescents, particularly young women, even if they have risk factors for recurrence. A possible exception to this discussion of adolescents is young men with juvenile myoclonic epilepsy, where there is a very high recurrence risk (25,90). This needs to be discussed with the patient. Even then, however, one attempt at withdrawal may be reasonable as the prognosis may be more variable than previously thought (25,91). In the authors' experience, the majority of adolescents who are offered the choice will choose to attempt medication withdrawal, especially if this choice is presented to them before they are driving.

The clinical data do not demonstrate any significant advantages of waiting more than 2 years before attempting AED withdrawal. The exception to this may be the child with an age-dependent epilepsy, where a longer wait may alter the recurrence risk as the underlying syndrome is more likely to be in remission. However, these are precisely the children with a favorable long-term prognosis where AED withdrawal is often successful even after a brief treatment period (38,57,73, 88,89).

Once the decision to withdraw AED therapy is made, the taper should be fairly rapid, as randomized clinical studies show no advantage to a slow taper (75). A slow taper has the additional disadvantage of prolonging the period of uncertainty. In general, we taper a single AED over 4 to 6 weeks. For the patient on two AEDs, we often first taper one AED and see if the patient can be maintained on monotherapy. If the patient remains seizure-free on monotherapy, then a second withdrawal is attempted with the plan of treating with monotherapy only if there is a recurrence.

CONCLUSION

Given the consequences of long-term drug therapy and its lack of effect on long-term prognosis following a first seizure, we generally do not recommend treatment following a first unprovoked seizure in either children or adults. Following a second seizure, treatment is generally indicated in adults and needs to be considered in children. In children and adolescents who are seizure-free on AEDs for at least 2 years, at least one attempt should be made at medication withdrawal, even if risk factors for recurrence are present. In adults, the risk-to-benefit equation in this setting is less clear, and decisions must be individualized after discussion of the risks and benefits with the patient.

The approach presented in this chapter emphasizes that both seizures and the therapies available carry some risk and that optimal patient care requires careful balancing of these risks and benefits. Assessment of risk requires not only ascertaining the statistical risk of a seizure recurrence or of an adverse event, but also the consequences of such an event. This risk-to-benefit approach is useful not only in deciding whether to initiate or discontinue AED therapy, but also in other treatment decisions. This includes deciding whether to add a second drug, to try experimental drugs or therapies such as the ketogenic diet, or to consider epilepsy surgery. In all cases one must balance the risks and benefits of the proposed alternatives, which may change as new information becomes available. Whatever the decision, it should be made jointly by the medical providers and the patient and family after careful discussion, including not only an assessment of the risks and benefits of treatment but also an understanding that individual patients and clinicians place different values on different outcomes and on the acceptability of certain risks.

References

1. Groupe CAROLE (Coordination Active du Reseau Observatoire Longitudinal de l'Epilepsie). Treatment of newly diagnosed epileptic crises. A French experience. *Rev Neurol (Paris)*. 2001;157:1500–1512.
2. Sander JW, Hart YM, Johnson AL, et al. National General Practice Study of Epilepsy: newly diagnosed epileptic seizures in a general population. *Lancet*. 1990;336:1267–1271.
3. Commission on Epidemiology and Prognosis, International League Against Epilepsy. Guidelines for epidemiologic studies on epilepsy. *Epilepsia*. 1993;34:592–596.
4. Annegers JF, Shirts SB, Hauser WA, et al. Risk of recurrence after an initial unprovoked seizure. *Epilepsia*. 1986;27:43–50.
5. Berg A, Shinnar S. The risk of seizure recurrence following a first unprovoked seizure: a quantitative review. *Neurology*. 1991;41:965–972.
6. Camfield P, Camfield C, Dooley J, et al. A randomized study of carbamazepine versus no medication following a first unprovoked seizure in childhood. *Neurology*. 1989;39:851–852.
7. Camfield PR, Camfield CS, Dooley JM, et al. Epilepsy after a first unprovoked seizure in childhood. *Neurology*. 1985;35:1657–1660.
8. Hauser WA, Anderson VE, Loewenson RB, et al. Seizure recurrence after a first unprovoked seizure. *N Engl J Med*. 1982;307:522–528.
9. Hauser WA, Rich SS, Lee JR, et al. Risk of recurrent seizures after two unprovoked seizures. *N Engl J Med*. 1998;338:429–434.
10. Hauser WA, Rich SS, Annegers JF, et al. Seizure recurrence after a 1st unprovoked seizure: an extended follow-up. *Neurology*. 1990;40: 1163–1170.
11. Hopkins A, Garman A, Clarke C. The first seizure in adult life: value of clinical features, electroencephalography and computerized tomographic scanning in prediction of seizure recurrence. *Lancet*. 1988;1: 721–726.
12. Shinnar S, Berg AT, Moshe SL, et al. The risk of recurrence following a first unprovoked seizure in childhood: a prospective study. *Pediatrics*. 1990;85:1076–1085.
13. Shinnar S, Berg AT, Moshe SL, et al. The risk of seizure recurrence following a first unprovoked afebrile seizure in childhood: an extended follow-up. *Pediatrics*. 1996;98:216–225.
14. Shinnar S, Berg AT, O'Dell C, et al. Predictors of multiple seizures in a cohort of children prospectively followed from the time of their first unprovoked seizure. *Ann Neurol*. 2000;48:140–147.
15. Stroink H, Brouwer OF, Arts WF, et al. The first unprovoked seizure in childhood: a hospital based study of the accuracy of the diagnosis, rate of recurrence, and long term outcome after recurrence. Dutch Study of Epilepsy in Childhood. *J Neurol Neurosurg Psychiatry*. 1998;64: 595–600.
16. van Donselaar CA, Brouwer OF, Geerts AT, et al. Clinical course of untreated tonic-clonic seizures in childhood: prospective, hospital based study. *Br Med J*. 1997;314:401–404.
17. van Donselaar CA, Geerts AT, Schimsheimer RJ. Idiopathic first seizure in adult life: who should be treated? *Br Med J*. 1990;302:620–623.
18. van Donselaar CE, Schimsheimer RJ, Geerts AT, et al. Value of the electroencephalogram in adult patients with untreated idiopathic first seizures. *Arch Neurol*. 1992;49:231–237.
19. Elwes RDC, Chesterman P, Reynolds EH. Prognosis after a first untreated tonic-clonic seizure. *Lancet*. 1985;2:752–753.
20. First Seizure Trial Group. Randomized clinical trial on the efficacy of antiepileptic drugs in reducing the risk of relapse after a first unprovoked tonic-clonic seizure. *Neurology*. 1993;43:478–483.
21. Hirtz D, Ashwal S, Berg A, et al. Practice parameter: evaluating a first nonfebrile seizure in children: report of the Quality Standards Subcommittee of the American Academy of Neurology, the Child Neurology Society and the American Epilepsy Society. *Neurology*. 2000;55:616–623.
22. Hirtz DG, Ellenberg JH, Nelson KB. The risk of recurrence of nonfebrile seizures in children. *Neurology*. 1984;34:637–641.
23. Shinnar S, Berg AT, O'Dell C, et al. Predictors of multiple seizures in a cohort of children prospectively followed from the time of their first unprovoked seizure. *Ann Neurol*. 2000;48:140–147.
24. Commission on Classification and Terminology of the International League Against Epilepsy. Proposal for revised classification of epilepsies and epileptic syndromes. *Epilepsia*. 1989;30:389–399.
25. Roger J, Bureau M, Dravet C, et al., eds. *Epileptic Syndromes in Infancy, Childhood and Adolescence*. 3rd ed. London: John Libbey; 2002.
26. Shinnar S, Kang H, Berg AT, et al. EEG abnormalities in children with a first unprovoked seizure. *Epilepsia*. 1994;35:471–476.
27. Krumholz A, Wiebe S, Gronseth G, et al. Quality Standards Subcommittee of the American Academy of Neurology; American Epilepsy Society. Practice Parameter: evaluating an apparent unprovoked first seizure in adults (an evidence-based review): report of the Quality Standards Subcommittee of the American Academy of Neurology and the American Epilepsy Society. *Neurology*. 2007;69:1996–2007.
28. Shinnar S, Berg AT, Ptachewich Y, et al. Sleep state and the risk of seizure recurrence following a first unprovoked seizure in childhood. *Neurology*. 1993;43:701–706.
29. Shinnar S, Berg AT, Moshe SL, et al. How long do new-onset seizures last? *Ann Neurol*. 2001;49:659–664.
30. Kho LK, Lawn ND, Dunn JW, et al. First seizure presentation: do multiple seizures within 24 hours predict recurrence? *Neurology*. 2006;67: 1047–1049.
31. Musicco M, Beghi E, Solari A, et al. Treatment of first tonic-clonic seizure does not improve the prognosis of epilepsy. *Neurology*. 1997;49: 991–998.
32. Chandra B. First seizure in adults: to treat or not to treat. *Clin Neurol Neurosurg*. 1992;94:S61–S63.
33. Das CP, Sawhney IMS, Lal V, et al. Risk of recurrence of seizures following single unprovoked idiopathic seizure. *Neurol India*. 2000;48:357–360.

34. Hirtz D, Berg A, Bettis D, et al. Practice parameter: treatment of the child with a first unprovoked seizure. Report of the Quality Standards Subcommittee of the American Academy of Neurology and the Practice Committee of the Child Neurology Society. *Neurology.* 2003;60: 166–175.

35. Marson A, Jacoby A, Johnson A, et al. Medical Research Council MESS Study Group. Immediate versus deferred antiepileptic drug treatment for early epilepsy and single seizures: a randomized controlled trial. *Lancet.* 2005;365:2007–2013.

36. Kim LG, Johnson TL, Marson AG, et al. Prediction of risk of seizure recurrence after a single seizure and early epilepsy: further results from the MESS trial. *Lancet Neurol.* 2006;5:317–322.

37. Shinnar S, Berg AT. Does antiepileptic drug therapy prevent the development of "chronic" epilepsy? *Epilepsia.* 1996;37:701–708.

38. Ambrosetto G, Tassinari CA. Antiepileptic drug treatment of benign childhood epilepsy with rolandic spikes: is it necessary? *Epilepsia.* 1990;31:802–805.

39. Shinnar S, O'Dell C. Treatment decisions in childhood seizures. In: Pellock JM, Dodson WE, Bourgeois BF, eds. *Pediatric Epilepsy: Diagnosis and Therapy.* 2nd ed. New York: Demos; 2001:291–300.

40. Freeman JM, Tibbles J, Camfield C, et al. Benign epilepsy of childhood: a speculation and its ramifications. *Pediatrics.* 1987;79:864–868.

41. Annegers JF, Hauser WA, Elveback LR. Remission of seizures and relapse in patients with epilepsy. *Epilepsia.* 1979;20:729–737.

42. Andersson T, Braathen G, Persson A, et al. A comparison between one and three years of treatment in uncomplicated childhood epilepsy: a prospective study, II: the EEG as predictor of outcome after withdrawal of treatment. *Epilepsia.* 1997;38:225–232.

43. Berg AT, Shinnar S, Levy SR, et al. Two-year remission and subsequent relapse in children with newly diagnosed epilepsy. *Epilepsia.* 2001;42: 1553–1562.

44. Brorson LO, Wranne L. Long-term prognosis in childhood epilepsy: survival and seizure prognosis. *Epilepsia.* 1987;28:324–330.

45. Callaghan N, Kenny RA, O'Neill B, et al. A prospective study between carbamazepine, phenytoin and sodium valproate as monotherapy in previously untreated and recently diagnosed patients with epilepsy. *J Neurol Neurosurg Psychiatry.* 1985;48:639–644.

46. Elwes RDC, Johnson AL, Shorvon SD, et al. The prognosis for seizure control in newly diagnosed epilepsy. *N Engl J Med.* 1984;311:944–947.

47. Goodridge DMG, Shorvon SD. Epileptic seizures in a population of 6000, II: treatment and prognosis. *Br Med J.* 1983;287:645–647.

48. Sillanpaa M, Jalava M, Kaleva O, et al. Long-term prognosis of seizures with onset in childhood. *N Engl J Med.* 1998;338:1715–1722.

49. Aldenkamp AP, Alpherts WC, Sandstedt P, et al. Antiepileptic drug-related cognitive complaints in seizure-free children with epilepsy before and after drug discontinuation. *Epilepsia.* 1998;39:1070–1074.

50. Arts WFM, Visser LH, Loonen MCB, et al. Follow-up of 146 children with epilepsy after withdrawal of antiepileptic therapy. *Epilepsia.* 1988;29:244–250.

51. Berg AT, Shinnar S. Relapse following discontinuation of antiepileptic drugs: a meta-analysis. *Neurology.* 1994;44:601–608.

52. Berg AT, Shinnar S, Chadwick D. Discontinuing antiepileptic drugs. In: Engel J Jr, Pedley TA, eds. *Epilepsy: A Comprehensive Textbook.* Philadelphia, PA: Lippincott-Raven; 1997:1275–1284.

53. Bouma PAD, Peters ACB, Arts RJHM, et al. Discontinuation of antiepileptic therapy: a prospective trial in children. *J Neurol Neurosurg Psychiatry.* 1987;50:1579–1583.

54. Braathen G, Andersson T, Gylje H, et al. Comparison between one and three years of treatment in uncomplicated childhood epilepsy: a prospective study, I: outcome in different seizure types. *Epilepsia.* 1996;37: 822–832.

55. Callaghan N, Garrett A, Goggin T. Withdrawal of anticonvulsant drugs in patients free of seizures for two years. *N Engl J Med.* 1988;318:942–946.

56. Delgado MR, Riela AR, Mills J, et al. Discontinuation of antiepileptic drug therapy after two seizure-free years in children with cerebral palsy. *Pediatrics.* 1996;97:192–197.

57. Dooley J, Gordon K, Camfield P, et al. Discontinuation of anticonvulsant therapy in children free of seizures for 1 year: a prospective study. *Neurology.* 1996;46:969–974.

58. Ehrhardt F, Forsythe WI. Prognosis after grand mal seizures: a study of 187 children with three year remissions. *Dev Med Child Neurol.* 1989;31: 633–639.

59. Emerson R, D'Souza BJ, Vining EP, et al. Stopping medication in children with epilepsy: predictors of outcome. *N Engl J Med.* 1981;304: 1125–1129.

60. Galimberti CA, Manni R, Parietti L, et al. Drug withdrawal in patients with epilepsy: prognostic value of the EEG. *Seizure.* 1993;2:213–220.

61. Gerstle de Pasquet E, Bonnevaux de Toma S, Bainy JA, et al. Prognosis of epilepsy, remission of seizures and relapse in 808 adult patients. *Acta Neurol Latinoam.* 1981;27:167–176.

62. Gherpelli JLD, Kok F, dal Forno S, et al. Discontinuing medication in epileptic children: a study of risk factors related to recurrence. *Epilepsia.* 1992;33:681–686.

63. Holowach-Thurston JH, Thurston DL, Hixon BB, et al. Prognosis in childhood epilepsy: additional follow up of 148 children 15 to 23 years after withdrawal of anticonvulsant therapy. *N Engl J Med.* 1982;306: 831–836.

64. Holowach J, Thurston DL, O'Leary J. Prognosis in childhood epilepsy: follow up study of 148 cases in which therapy had been suspended after prolonged anticonvulsant control. *N Engl J Med.* 1972;286:169–174.

65. Juul Jensen P. Frequency of recurrence after discontinuance of anticonvulsant therapy in patients with epileptic seizures: a new follow up study after 5 years. *Epilepsia.* 1968;9:11–16.

66. Mastropaolo C, Tondi M, Carboni F, et al. Prognosis after therapy discontinuation in children with epilepsy. *Neurology.* 1992;32:142–145.

67. Matricardi M, Brinciott M, Benedetti P. Outcome after discontinuation of antiepileptic drug therapy in children with epilepsy. *Epilepsia.* 1989;30: 582–589.

68. Medical Research Council Antiepileptic Drug Withdrawal Study Group. Randomised study of antiepileptic drug withdrawal in patients with remission. *Lancet.* 1991;337:1175–1180.

69. Medical Research Council Antiepileptic Drug Withdrawal Study Group. Prognostic index for recurrence of seizures after remission of epilepsy. *Br Med J.* 1993;306:1374–1378.

70. Overweg J, Binnie CD, Oosting J, et al. Clinical and EEG prediction of seizure recurrence following antiepileptic drug withdrawal. *Epilepsy Res.* 1987;1:272–283.

71. Pestre M, Loiseau P, Dartigues JF, et al. Arret du traitement dans les crises épileptiques de l'adolescence. *Rev Neurol (Paris).* 1987;143:40–46.

72. Peters AC, Brouwer OF, Geerts AT, et al. Randomized prospective study of early discontinuation of antiepileptic drugs in children with epilepsy. *Neurology.* 1998;50:724–730.

73. Shinnar S, Berg AT, Moshe SL, et al. Discontinuing antiepileptic drugs in children with epilepsy: a prospective study. *Ann Neurol.* 1994;35: 534–545.

74. Shinnar S, Vining EPG, Mellits ED, et al. Discontinuing antiepileptic medication in children with epilepsy after two years without seizures: a prospective study. *N Engl J Med.* 1985;313:976–980.

75. Tennison M, Greenwood R, Lewis D, et al. Rate of taper of anti-epileptic drugs and the risk of seizure recurrence in children. *N Engl J Med.* 1994;330:1407–1410.

76. Todt H. The late prognosis of epilepsy in childhood: results of a prospective follow up study. *Epilepsia.* 1984;25:137–144.

77. Tonnby B, Nilsson HL, Aldenkamp AP, et al. Withdrawal of antiepileptic medication in children. Correlation of cognitive function and plasma concentration—the Multicentre "Holmfrid" Study. *Epilepsy Res.* 1994;19: 141–152.

78. Tsuchiya S, Maruyama H, Maruyama K, et al. A follow up study of 1007 epileptic children with anticonvulsant therapy for more than 10 years. *No To Hattatsu.* 1985;17:23–28.

79. Visser LH, Arts WFM, Loonen MCB, et al. Follow-up study of 166 children with epilepsy after withdrawal of anticonvulsant therapy. *Adv Epileptol.* 1987;16:401–404.

80. Wallis WE. Withdrawal of anticonvulsant drugs in seizure free epileptic patients. *Clin Neuropharmacol.* 1987;10:423–433.

81. Verotti A, Morresi S, Basciani F, et al. Discontinuation of antiepileptic drugs in children with partial epilepsy. *Neurology.* 2000;55:1393–1395.

82. Shinnar S, O'Dell C, Maw M, et al. Long-term prognosis of children who relapse after withdrawal of antiepileptic drug therapy. *Epilepsia.* 1999;40(suppl 7):85–86.

83. Oller-Daurella L, Pamies R, Oller FVL. Reduction or discontinuance of antiepileptic drugs in patients seizure free for more than 5 years. In: Janz D, ed. *Epileptology.* Stuttgart, Germany: Thieme; 1976:218–227.

84. Shafer SQ, Hauser WA, Annegers JF, et al. EEG and other early predictors of epilepsy remission: a community study. *Epilepsia.* 1988;29:590–600.

85. Huttenlocher PR, Hapke RJ. A follow up study of intractable seizures in childhood. *Ann Neurol.* 1990;28:699–705.

86. Diamantopoulos N, Crumrine PK. The effect of puberty on the course of epilepsy. *Arch Neurol.* 1986;43:873–876.

87. Forster CH, Schmidberger G. Prognostische Wertigkeit von EEG verlautsuntersuchungen bei Kindern mit anfallsrezidiven nach absetzen der antikonvulsiven Therapie. In: Doose H, Gross Selbeck G, eds. *Epilepsie.* Stuttgart, Germany: Thieme; 1978:252–255.

88. Braathen G, Melander H. Early discontinuation of treatment in children with uncomplicated epilepsy: a prospective study with a model for prediction of outcome. *Epilepsia.* 1997;38:561–569.

89. Sirven JI, Sperling M, Wingerchuk DM. Early versus late antiepileptic drug withdrawal for people with epilepsy in remission. *Cochrane Database Syst Rev.* 2001;(3):CD001902.

90. Delgado-Escueta AV, Enrile-Bacsal F. Juvenile myoclonic epilepsy of Janz. *Neurology.* 1984;34:285–294.

91. Sillanpaa M, Jalava M, Shinnar S. Epilepsy syndromes in patients with childhood-onset epilepsy. *Pediatr Neurol.* 1999;21:533–537.

92. Bouma PA, Peters AC, Brouwer OF. Long term course of childhood epilepsy following relapse after antiepileptic drug withdrawal. *J Neurol Neurosurg Psychiatry.* 2002;72:507–510.

93. Chadwick D, Taylor J, Johnson T. Outcomes after seizure recurrence in people with well-controlled epilepsy and the factors that influence it. The MRC Antiepileptic Drug Withdrawal Group. *Epilepsia*. 1996;37:1043–1050.

94. Commission on Neurosurgery of the International League Against Epilepsy (ILAE) 1997–2001. Proposal for a new classification of outcome with respect to epileptic seizures following epilepsy surgery. *Epilepsia*. 2001;42:282–286.

95. Andermann F, Bourgeois BF, Leppik IE, et al. Postoperative pharmacotherapy and discontinuation of antiepileptic drugs. In: Engel J, ed. *Surgical Treatment of the Epilepsies*. 2nd ed. New York: Raven Press; 1993:679–684.

96. Vickrey BG, Hay RD, Rausch R, et al. Outcome in 248 patients who had diagnostic evaluations for epilepsy surgery. *Lancet*. 1995;346:1445–1449.

97. Maher J, McLachlan RS. Antiepileptic drug treatment following temporal lobectomy. *Neurology*. 1997;48:1368–1374.

98. Schiller Y, Cascino GD, So EL, et al. Discontinuation of antiepileptic drugs after successful epilepsy surgery. *Neurology*. 2000;54:346–349.

99. Lee SY, Lee JY, Kim DW, et al. Factors related to successful antiepileptic drug withdrawal after anterior temporal lobectomy for medial temporal lobe epilepsy. *Seizure*. 2008;17:11–18.

100. Al-Kaylani M, Konard P, Lazeby B, et al. Seizure freedom off antiepileptic drugs after temporal lobe epilepsy surgery. *Seizure*. 2007;16:95–98.

101. Gilliam F, Wyllie E, Kashden J, et al. Epilepsy surgery outcome: case assessment in children. *Neurology*. 1997;48:1368–1374.

102. Berg AT, Vickrey BG, Langfitt JT, et al. Reduction of AEDs in post surgical patients who attain remission. *Epilepsia*. 2006;47(1):64–71.

103. Sperling MR, Nei M, Zangaladze A, et al. Prognosis after late relapse following epilepsy surgery. *Epilepsy Res*. 2008;78:77–81.

104. Berg AT, Shinnar S. Do seizures beget seizures? An assessment of the clinical evidence in humans. *J Clin Neurophysiol*. 1997;14:102–110.

105. Shinnar S, Babb TL. Long term sequelae of status epilepticus. In: Engel J Jr, Pedley TA, eds. *Epilepsy: A Comprehensive Text*. Philadelphia, PA: Lippincott-Raven; 1997:755–763.

106. Neufeld MY, Vishne T, Chistik V, et al. Life-long history of injuries related to seizures. *Epilepsy Res*. 1999;34:123–127.

107. Spitz MC. Injuries and death as a consequence of seizures in people with epilepsy. *Epilepsia*. 1998;39:904–907.

108. DeLorenzo RJ, Hauser WA, Towne AR, et al. A prospective population-based epidemiological study of status epilepticus in Richmond, Virginia. *Neurology*. 1996;46:1029–1035.

109. Dodson WE, DeLorenzo RJ, Pedley TA, et al. The treatment of convulsive status epilepticus: recommendations of the Epilepsy Foundation of America's Working Group on Status Epilepticus. *J Am Med Assoc*. 1993;270:854–859.

110. Maytal J, Shinnar S, Moshe SL, et al. The low morbidity and mortality of status epilepticus in children. *Pediatrics*. 1989;83:323–331.

111. Reynolds EH. Do anticonvulsants alter the natural course of epilepsy? Treatment should be started as early as possible. *Br Med J*. 1995;310:176–177.

112. Gowers WR. *Epilepsy and Other Chronic Convulsive Disorders*. London: J&A Churchill; 1881.

113. Sander JWAS. Some aspects of prognosis in the epilepsies: a review. *Epilepsia*. 1993;34:1007–1016.

114. Jacoby A, Baker G, Chadwick D, et al. The impact of counseling with a practical statistical model on a patient's decision making about treatment for epilepsy: findings from a pilot study. *Epilepsy Res*. 1993;16:207–214.

115. Jacoby A, Johnson A, Chadwick D. Psychosocial outcomes of antiepileptic drug discontinuation. *Epilepsia*. 1992;33:1123–1131.

116. Committee on Drugs, American Academy of Pediatrics. Behavioral and cognitive effects of anticonvulsant therapy. *Pediatrics*. 1995;96:538–540.

117. Petty SJ, Paton LM, O'Brien TJ, et al. Effect of antiepileptic medication on bone mineral measures. *Neurology*. 2005;65:1358–1365.

118. Vining EPG, Mellits ED, Dorsen MM, et al. Psychologic and behavioral effects of antiepileptic drugs in children: a double-blind comparison between phenobarbital and valproic acid. *Pediatrics*. 1987;80:165–174.

119. American Academy of Neurology, Quality Standards Subcommittee. Practice parameter: management issues for women with epilepsy—summary statement. *Neurology*. 1998;51:944–948.

120. Commission on Genetics, Pregnancy and the Child, International League Against Epilepsy. Guidelines for the care of women of childbearing age with epilepsy. *Epilepsia*. 1993;34:588–589.

121. Yerby MS. Teratogenic effects of antiepileptic drugs: what do we advise patients. *Epilepsia*. 1997;38:957–958.

122. Hoare P. Does illness foster dependency: a study of epileptic and diabetic children. *Dev Med Child Neurol*. 1984;26:20–24.

123. American Academy of Neurology, Quality Standards Subcommittee. Practice parameter: a guideline for discontinuing antiepileptic drugs in seizure-free patients—summary statement. *Neurology*. 1996;47:600–602.

CHAPTER 44 ■ HORMONES, CATAMENIAL EPILEPSY, SEXUAL FUNCTION, AND REPRODUCTIVE HEALTH IN EPILEPSY

CYNTHIA HARDEN AND ROBERT MARTINEZ

Reproductive hormones play an important role in epilepsy. Steroid hormones that alter the seizure threshold by altering the overall excitability of neurons are termed neuroactive steroids or neurosteroids. Further, seizures can alter the levels of brain-produced hormones likely through affecting the hypothalamic–pituitary axis. Also, antiepileptic medication themselves can affect reproductive hormones by changing the body's metabolism and by altering protein binding.

This chapter reviews and discusses the relevance and interaction between reproductive hormones and epilepsy with a focus on the action of neurosteroids, alterations in reproductive hormones due to seizures and to antiseizure medications, and then turns to the relevant clinical entities including catamenial epilepsy, sexual and reproductive health for both genders, and reproductive and hormonal concerns for mature women with epilepsy.

THE HORMONE–SEIZURE RELATIONSHIP

Effects of Neurosteroids on Neuronal Excitability

Neurosteroids influence brain excitability (1) and the primary reproductive hormones for women, estrogen and progesterone, establish this effect most clearly (2,3). Fluctuations in these hormones over a reproductive cycle change seizure susceptibility in experimental models of epilepsy (4). The effects of these hormones, as well as another neuroactive reproductive hormone, testosterone, will be considered in the following sections. Neurophysiologic effects of exogenous and endogenous neurosteroid can influence seizures and epilepsy; therefore, this initial discussion provides a basis for some of the clinical entities that follow.

Estrogen

Early whole animal and even human experiments have shown that estrogen activates seizures in experimental models of epilepsy and in human cerebral cortex. Estrogen lowers the electroshock seizure threshold (5–7), creates new cortical seizure foci when applied topically (8), activates pre-existing cortical epileptogenic foci (9), and increases the severity of chemically induced seizures (10,11). Intravenously administered estrogen activated electroencephalographic (EEG) epileptiform activity in some women with partial epilepsy (12).

Initial molecular experiments with estrogen on neuronal excitability demonstrated complex effects, altering excitability through both actions on neuronal membranes and on second messenger systems, each with a specific time course of activity. For example, estrogen reduces the effectiveness of gamma amino butyric acid (GABA)-mediated neuronal inhibition by decreasing chloride conductance through the gamma amino butyric acid A (GABA$_A$)-receptor complex. Longer-latency effects of estrogen on neuronal excitability are exerted through inhibition of GABA synthesis in the arcuate nucleus, the ventromedial nucleus of the hypothalamus, and the centromedial group of the amygdala (13), probably through regulation of messenger ribonucleic acid (mRNA) encoding for glutamic acid decarboxylase (GAD), the rate-limiting enzyme for GABA synthesis (14,15). Estrogen also affects mRNA encoding for GABA$_A$-receptor subunits (16). Estradiol rapidly increases responses of neurons to the excitatory neurotransmitter glutamate through agonist binding sites on the N-methyl-D-aspartate (NMDA)-receptor complex (17–20) and through a G-protein-dependent mechanism on non-NMDA glutamate receptors that activate protein kinase (21).

It has since been concluded that the effects of estrogen in the brain follow two avenues, either through genomic or through nongenomic pathways (22). Both avenues involve estrogen receptors (ERs) which are widely distributed in the brain and expressed in both neurons and glia. The most potent human estrogen is β-estradiol which binds to the ER with the highest affinity (23). There are two confirmed types of intracellular ER in the CNS: ERα and ERβ. Both ER subtypes have a similar binding affinity for β-estradiol but have differential affinity to other estrogens, such as phytoestrogens. Further, ERα and ERβ generally have specific regional distributions within the brain and have cell-specific expression. However, there is a high degree of homology between these receptor types and they can be present even within the same cell type (24).

The classic genomic pathway has a specific time course, with an onset between minutes to hours and a long duration of action. This pathway leads to regulation of protein synthesis by a direct or an indirect mechanism. The direct pathway involves binding of β-estradiol to the intracellular ERs. The β-estradiol–ER complex is then translocated from the cytoplasm to the nucleus and regulates gene expression by binding to the estrogen responsive element (ERE) or to proteosynthesis-regulating proteins. The indirect pathway involves binding of β-estradiol to the membrane ER, and in this pathway proteosynthesis is regulated by activation of the second messenger system.

The nongenomic effects have an onset within seconds and have a short duration of action. These are mediated by the membrane ER or by direct interactions with the NMDA or α-amino-3-hydroxyl-5-methyl-4-isoazole propionic acid (AMPA)/kainate receptors. Through these actions, β-estradiol is integral to cell maturation and nutrition, modulates neuronal excitability, and is overall neuroprotective, promoting cell viability.

An interesting aspect of estrogen as a neurosteroid has recently been discovered, and tempers the outlook of estrogen as a proconvulsant molecule, which were initially appreciated in the studies described above. This complexity has been outlined by Velísková (22) wherein the factors associated with proconvulsant and anticonvulsant effects of estrogen are clarified. Specifically, estrogen dose, route of administration, acute versus chronic administration, natural hormonal milieu, and estrogenic species can alter whether estrogen is proconvulsant or anticonvulsant. An example of a clear dose effect is the following experimental data: in ovariectomized rats, pretreatment with physiological doses of β-estradiol delayed the occurrence of kainic acid–induced seizures (an anticonvulsant effect), whereas 20 μg of β-estradiol did not alter the seizure threshold (25) and 40 μg of β-estradiol was proconvulsant (26).

The route of administration of even physiologic doses estrogen also influences its modulating effects on neuroexcitability. This differential effect may be due to opposing genomic versus nongenomic neurophysiologic actions related to the time course associated with the route of administration. For example, intermittent estrogen injections have an anticonvulsant effect in a kainic-acid model compared to constant release from an estrogen implant which had no effect on seizure onset, for example (25,27).

A clear example of the differentiation in effects of estrogenic species was demonstrated early in this exploration; focal application of β-estradiol on the cerebral cortex had no epileptogenic effects, in contrast to the application of conjugated equine estrogens, predominantly comprising estrone, which produced an epileptogenic focus, suggesting that the mixture of conjugated equine estrogens and estrone has higher proepileptogenic potency compared to β-estradiol (8).

Therefore these experiments indicate that the proconvulsant and anticonvulsant effects of estrogen on seizures are linked to its complex activity in the brain, and further, the examples cited herein have ready extrapolation to the use of estrogen in humans.

Progesterone

In contrast, progesterone has long been known to have a seizure-protective effect, as demonstrated in early studies. High doses induce sedation and anesthesia in rats and in humans (28), primarily as a result of actions of the metabolite pregnanolone. Progesterone reduces spontaneous interictal spikes produced by cortical application of penicillin (29), and suppresses kindling (30) and focal seizures (31) in animals. It also heightens the seizure threshold to chemical convulsants (32,33), elevates the electroshock seizure threshold (7,34), and attenuates ethanol-withdrawal convulsions (32).

The anticonvulsant properties of progesterone (34–39) have since been discovered to be through its conversion to the neurosteroid allopregnanolone (40). Allopregnanolone is formed from progesterone by two sequential A-ring reductions catalyzed by 5α-reductase and 3α-hydroxysteroid oxidoreductase

isoenzymes. Allopregnanolone is a potent, broad-spectrum anticonvulsant agent which is the active anticonvulsant progestin molecule in the diverse animal seizure models (35,41) as described above.

The anticonvulsant action of allopregnanolone is via positive allosteric modulation of many GABA$_A$-receptor isoforms (42). Allopregnanolone and indeed all neurosteriods are highly lipophilic molecules that easily cross the blood–brain barrier and diffuse into cellular membranes. They act on GABA$_A$ receptors through binding to specific sites on the receptors by lateral diffusion or from the cell interior (43) following diffusion into the plasma membrane. GABA$_A$ receptors, the predominant mediators of central nervous system inhibition, are pentameric protein complexes surrounding a central chloride-selective ion channel (44). The major isoforms consist of two α-subunits, two β-subunits, and one γ2-subunit, and are primarily localized to synapses (45).

Neurosteroids affect neuronal excitability by binding to discrete sites on the GABA$_A$ receptors that are located within the transmembrane domains of the α- and β-subunits that compose the receptor (46). Binding to the neurosteroid GABA$_A$ receptor enhances the open probability of the GABA$_A$-receptor chloride channel, so that the mean open time is increased and the mean closed time is decreased (43). This increases the chloride current through the channel, hyperpolarizing the cell and resulting in reduced cellular excitability. Neurosteroids modulate most GABA$_A$-receptor isoforms, which distinguishes their spectrum of action from benzodiazepines, which produce their anticonvulsant and sedative action via only a subset of GABA$_A$ receptors that must contain γ2-subunits and do not contain α4- or α6-subunits (not discussed herein).

It should be appreciated that the GABA$_A$-receptor subunit expression and the receptors composed of these subunits are not static in the cell. The subunit composition is dynamic and undergoes compensatory alterations in response to changes in the endogenous hormonal neurosteroid milieu and to exogenously administered pharmacological agents that modulate GABA$_A$ receptors, such as benzodiazepines (47). For example, prolonged exposure to allopregnanolone in rats causes increased expression of the α4 GABA$_A$-receptor subunit in hippocampus, resulting in decreased benzodiazepine sensitivity of GABA$_A$-receptor currents (48). This dynamic quality has implications for seizure threshold during menstrual cycling, although the alterations in receptor composition are not completely understood. Complicating progesterone picture, both progesterone and allopregnanolone exacerbate seizures in animal models of absence epilepsy (49,50).

Testosterone

The neurophysiologic activity of testosterone is no less complex than the previously discussed reproductive hormones. Androgens are irreversibly converted in the body to two major classes of biologically active metabolites: estrogens, formed through the action of a cytochrome P450 enzyme, aromatase; and the 5α-reduced androgens, formed via reduction of the steroid "A" ring catalyzed by 5α-reductase. Aromatase and 5α-reductase are expressed in a large number of organ systems, including the brain (51). Estrogen has proconvulsant potential, as outlined above, while the 5α-reduced androgens, by contrast, tend to have anticonvulsant effects, at least in part because of their ability to act as substrates for the biosynthesis of 5α-androstan-3α 17β-diol (3α-DIOL). This molecule, which is a member of a family of neurosteroid metabolites that modulate the activity of the GABA$_A$ receptor as described above for allopregnanolone, is synthesized peripherally in prostate, liver, and skin, as well as de novo by glial cells in the brain (52). Several reports support the conclusion that 3α-DIOL inhibits seizures, raising discharge thresholds in the limbic system (53) and inhibiting NMDA-receptor–mediated neuronal excitation (54). The potential importance of 3α-DIOL for the antiseizure effect of circulating androgens is underscored by the lack of demonstrable antiseizure effect of testosterone in 5α-reductase knockout mice (55). In animal models of epilepsy, 3α-DIOL is protective against seizures induced by the GABA$_A$ antagonists, pentylenetetrazole, picrotoxin, and β-carboline ester (52). More recently, two other endogenous testosterone metabolites present in fairly high concentrations in men, androsterone and etiocholanolone, have also been found to have anticonvulsant neurosteroid properties (56). These metabolites are produced via metabolism of 3α-DIOL and 5β-androstan-3α 17β-diol by 17β-hydroxysteroid dehydrogenase.

Consistent with the concept that the androgenic metabolic pathway toward estrogen is proconvulsant, in one recent report evaluating the effect of testosterone on pentylenetetrazole-induced seizures in rats, pretreatment with high doses of the aromatase inhibitor letrozole (which blocks the conversion of testosterone to estrogen) markedly increased the seizure threshold compared to the effect of testosterone alone (57).

Anatomic specificity and changes with maturation in the cortical distribution of steroid hormone receptors may account for some of the differential effects of each steroid hormone on neuronal excitability, endocrine function, and reproductive behavior. ERs are located primarily in the mesial temporal lobe (limbic cortex) and hypothalamus (3,58,59); progesterone and androgen receptors are also diffusely distributed over the cerebral cortex (59–64). Many of estrogen's effects, including the steroid-dependent suppression of GAD, are confined to the CA1 region of the hippocampus (65). Neocortical receptors for estrogen in the immature brain are largely absent after puberty (3,66). Anatomic specificity and varying distribution might account, in part, for changes in seizure expression with changes in reproductive function.

EFFECTS OF SEIZURES AND EPILEPSY ON REPRODUCTIVE HORMONES

The finding that reproductive alterations in epilepsy occur across both genders and all ages from puberty onward suggests that the etiology lies outside the use of specific antiepileptic drugs (AEDs) and points to the feature shared between these persons as a possible etiology, that of having seizures and epilepsy. Epilepsy is a disease of the brain and can affect an important brain structure critical for regulating reproductive and sexual behavior, the hypothalamus. The following section serves as a foundation for how reproductive dysfunction can occur in epilepsy, including an increased rate of anovulatory cycles, sexual dysfunction, poloycystic ovarian syndrome, possibly higher rates of infertility, and early onset of menopause. Catamenial seizure exacerbation is contributed to both by anovulatory cycles and by the neuroactivity of hormones described in the previous section.

The hypothalamic hormone gonadotropic-releasing hormone (GnRH) is released in a pulsatile manner, approximately hourly, and in turn stimulates the pulsatile release of the pituitary gonadotropins follicle-stimulating hormone (FSH) and luteinizing hormone (LH). FSH promotes development of the primary ovarian follicle and secretion of estradiol in the female and spermatogenesis in the male. In females, a midcycle surge of LH stimulates ovulation and formation of the progesterone-secreting corpus luteum. In males, LH stimulates interstitial cell secretion of testosterone and other androgens.

Pituitary release of prolactin is also determined by inhibitory and stimulating factors from the hypothalamus. Prolactin initiates milk synthesis in the mammary glands and affects growth, osmoregulation, and fat and carbohydrate metabolism. Prolactin also inhibits sexual behavior (67) and promotes parental behavior (68). Elevated levels can cause impotence in human males (69).

It has long been appreciated that seizures themselves can alter the level of some hormones, particularly hypothalamic tropic hormones and pituitary gonadotropins (70), as readily evidenced by the finding that generalized and complex partial seizures are associated with a prolactin level spike. Pituitary prolactin increases more than twofold after generalized convulsive seizures, most complex partial seizures, and simple partial seizures involving limbic structures, but in general not after nonepileptic seizures (71–73), although it can increase after syncope. The increase occurs within 5 minutes, is maximal by 15 minutes, and persists for 1 hour (74). Other changes include elevation in corticotropin and cortisol following both convulsions and stimulation of mesial temporal lobe structures.

The limbic cortex modulates the hypothalamic–pituitary–gonadal axis. Regions of limbic cortex, particularly the amygdala, have extensive reciprocal connections with the hypothalamus (75). In the amygdala, the corticomedial nuclear group stimulates hypothalamic release of GnRH, and the basolateral nuclear group inhibits its release (76), depending on which group is affected by excitation of the amygdala. The inhibitory or stimulatory effect ultimately alters release of the corresponding pituitary hormones (77), as does seizure-precipitated release of excitatory and inhibitory neurochemicals (78), which regulate neuroendocrine function.

GnRH-secreting neurons are located primarily in the preoptic area of the anterior hypothalamus and their nerve terminals are found in the lateral portions of the external layer of the median eminence adjacent to the pituitary stalk. They serve specifically to stimulate the release of LH and FSH, and could be considered to be a vulnerable neuronal population in that there are estimated to be between only 800 and 2000 GnRH-secreting neurons. Two reports have documented a significant and selective reduction in GnRH fibers in following seizures induced by whole-animal pilocarpine injection (79), and unilaterally in the hypothalamus by ipsilateral amygdalar kainic acid injection (80). These important experiments clearly indicate a mechanism by which seizures and epilepsy disrupt this finely tuned hormonal feedback system by affecting central nervous system reproductive regulation, which could then adversely modify gonadal steroidogenesis and morphology.

There is also evidence in both women and men with epilepsy that pituitary hormone release is abnormal both interically and postically (81–84). The pulsatile secretion of LH has been found to be altered in female patients with both idiopathic generalized epilepsy (IGE) and local related epilepsy (LRE) (85). A lateralization to the specific alteration has been found, as well as with type of epilepsy. Women with left-sided temporolimbic focus may show an increase of LH pulse frequency whereas women with right-sided temporolimbic focus may show reduced LH pulse frequency (83); women with IGE have increased pulse frequency of LH (86) which may explain why women with IGE have been shown to have more anovulatory cycles than those with LRE (87). A recent report in men with epilepsy documents that pulsatile secretion of LH in temporal lobe epilepsy (TLE) is abnormal in the circadian domain as well as interictally and postically. Interictal effects consisted mainly of loss of circadian fluctuations in LH burst amplitude, whereas postictal effects consisted of altered burst timing (88).

Further, although separating the potential adverse effects of epilepsy treatment versus epilepsy on human reproductive parameters, there is laboratory evidence that gonadal dysfunction occurs in the setting of epilepsy but in the absence of AEDs. In an amazing experiment in female rats that had pilocarpine-induced seizures, an increased incidence of acyclicity was found after 2 to 3 months of observation. Ovarian cysts and weight gain were significantly greater in epileptic than control rats, whether rats maintained cyclicity or not. Serum testosterone was increased in epileptic rats, whereas estradiol, progesterone, and prolactin were not. The results suggest that an epileptic condition in the rats leads to increased body weight, cystic ovaries, and increased testosterone levels, analogous to human polycystic ovarian syndrome (PCOS) (89).

EFFECTS OF ANTIEPILEPTIC DRUGS ON REPRODUCTIVE HORMONES

In general, AEDs decrease or increase biologically active serum reproductive hormone levels due to their effects on hormone metabolism. A fairly consistent finding is that AED inducers of hepatic cytochrome P450 3A4 isoenzymes such as phenobarbital, phenytoin, and carbamazepine alter reproductive hormone levels because they are also substrates for this isoenzyme system. These AEDs also are thought to induce production of sex hormone binding globulin (SHBG), thereby reducing biologically active (free) reproductive hormone serum levels (90–94).

Significant increases in SHBG have been shown with the use of carbamazepine and phenytoin in men with partial epilepsy compared to controls (95), while another report showed nonsignificant increases compared to controls with carbamazepine, oxcarbazepine, and valproate (96). Decreased free testosterone in men has been reported with carbamazepine (95–99), phenytoin (97), oxcarbazepine (96), valproate (97), and partial epilepsy without treatment (95,97). This directional change has been less consistent with valproate, which has also been associated with normal free testosterone levels (96). Further, valproate has been associated with increased testosterone and androgen levels; this action has been thought to be clinically important and possibly a contributing or causal factor in polycystic ovary disease (PCOS). Valproate may increase testosterone levels by two inhibitory mechanisms: (i) direct inhibition of cytochrome 2C19 and (ii) inhibition of aromatase, which is a cytochrome P450 enzyme that converts testosterone to estradiol. Induction of aromatase by the cytochrome P450 enzyme-inducing AEDs is another postulated mechanism by which SHBG levels could increase: increased estradiol levels due to increased conversion of testosterone to estradiol promotes hepatic SHBG production.

It is, therefore, established that hepatic cytochrome P450 3A4 isoenzyme-inducing AEDs can lower free testosterone levels, and further, this alteration has been shown to be reversible. In a report by Lossius et al. (98), seizure-free epilepsy patients appropriate for AED withdrawal from either carbamazepine or valproate were evaluated for changes in reproductive hormone levels four months after discontinuing the AED, comparing the subjects withdrawn from carbamazepine or valproate with those who continued on each treatment. Their main findings were that total testosterone and free androgen index (FAI) (100 × testosterone/sex hormone binding globulin) significantly increased after withdrawal from carbamazepine for both genders. In contrast, withdrawing valproate resulted in decreases in these parameters but the small number of subjects in this subset (<10 within each gender) limits the conclusiveness of this finding. However, 17β-estradiol and progesterone also increased significantly in men after stopping carbamazepine, while there were no significant changes in 17β estradiol progesterone, LH, or FSH levels in women after discontinuation of either carbamazepine or valproate.

The effects of AEDs on reproductive hormone levels may be produced by even subtle pharmacokinetic effects as demonstrated in a report on alterations in reproductive hormone levels in women with epilepsy (WWE) taking carbamazepine or oxcarbazepine, in which both AEDs were associated with relatively low total testosterone level and FAI (99). However, oxcarbazepine-treated subjects had higher dehydroepiandrosterone (DHEA) and androstendione than controls, which may be related to the mild inhibitory effect of oxcarbazepine on the isoenzyme 2C19 metabolic pathway.

AEDs which do not induce cytochrome P450 enzymes have little effect on androgens. In a recent study of persons with epilepsy aged 13 to 80 years randomized to either valproate or lamotrigine monotherapy, no changes in total testosterone of FAI were found after 6 or 12 months of treatment either within each treatment group or by comparing treatment groups (100).

The pharmacokinetic effects on reproductive hormone levels are likely only part of the picture regarding how AEDs can alter reproductive hormone activity; effects of AEDs on brain reproductive hormone receptor activity is also emerging. For example, exposure of human hippocampal tissue from surgical resections to the enzyme-inducing AEDs, carbamazepine and phenytoin, upregulates ER-α receptors and androgen receptors (101). The clinical importance of these changes is unclear but raises the possibility that the AEDs may affect reproductive hormone activity and possibly seizure activity through central hormone receptor activity.

CATAMENIAL EPILEPSY

Background

The word "catamenial" is derived from the Greek word "katamenios" meaning monthly. A monthly cyclic seizure exacerbation has been known and documented since ancient times. First attributed to the cycle of the moon, Galen and Antyllus wrote about the nature between the sun and the moon, and the theory that the moon increases moisture and in turn increases epileptic attacks (102). In 1857, Sir Charles Locock first described the menstrual cycle and its relationship with epilepsy (103). Epileptic seizures usually occur in an unpredictable pattern; however, menstrual exacerbations have documented up to 70% of women with epilepsy. Despite the clear and documented relationship, many clinicians discount the association when brought up by female patients. This is contributed to by the lack of specific treatment for catamenial epilepsy and an incomplete understanding of the cause.

The Normal Menstrual Cycle

The average menstrual cycle is 28 days; however the normal range is 24 to 35 days. For study and investigations, the menstrual cycle is numbered by days with day 1 being the first day of menses. Ovulation starts on day 14. The menstrual cycle has two phases: the follicular phase (days 1 to 13) and luteal phase (days 15 to 28). The follicular phase consists of the ovarian follicles growing and the dominant follicle with the most follicular receptors becoming the ovulatory follicle. Ovulation on day 14 is the release of the oocyte. The nondominant follicles degenerate. In the luteal phase, the dominant follicle forms the corpus luteum, which produces progesterone.

The neuroactive steroids, estrogen (β-estradiol) and progesterone, cycle in a manner important to understand when monthly seizure exacerbations are correlated with the menstrual cycle. Estrogen and progesterone are relatively low at day 1, and estrogen increases slightly throughout the follicular phase but at the end of the follicular phase increases suddenly to surge at its highest point during the menstrual cycle. This is closely followed by the sudden LH peak at day 14, which triggers ovulation within 36 to 40 hours. Estrogen levels drop transiently immediately after the LH surge and are followed by a steady increase to reach a maximum during the midluteal phase. Progesterone secretion then increases throughout the luteal phase as estrogen levels remain at levels much lower than the peak level. Therefore, although progesterone is the most abundant ovarian steroid during the luteal phase, estradiol is also produced in significant quantities. At day 26, just prior to the onset of menstrual bleeding, estrogen and progesterone levels drop precipitously; progesterone levels remain low throughout the follicular phase.

Inadequate Luteal Phase (ILP) Cycles

Abnormal FSH secretion will lead to poor follicular development and therefore poorly functioning corpus luteum, a condition known as inadequate luteal phase (ILP) (104). This results in an anovulatory cycle. Due to the poor corpus luteum development, progesterone production is decreased during the menstrual cycle without any change in estrogen production. Etiologies for ILP include dysregulation in the hypothalamic pituitary axis as previously described to occur in persons with epilepsy, primary ovarian defects, or defects in luteal cell steroidogenesis. They are, though, an uncommon cause of infertility (105). ILP cycles occur in women with epilepsy

more frequently than in control women; in one report, over the 3-month observation period, anovulatory cycles were documented to occur in 11% of cycles in control women, 14% of cycles in women with localization-related epilepsy (LRE), and 27% of cycles in woman with IGE (87).

Biologic Mechanisms

The sensitivity of neurons to the modulating effects of individual steroid hormones changes after puberty and in response to fluctuations in basal levels of steroid hormones over a reproductive cycle (33,106). The pubertal surge in estrogen appears to have a neuronal priming effect. In contrast to its effects in postpubertal rats, estrogen does not alter the rate of amygdala kindling in prepubertal male and female rats. Rats castrated prepubertally have higher seizure thresholds to minimal and maximal electroshock than do animals castrated after puberty (7,107). Several rodent models of epilepsy suggest that the sensitivity of the $GABA_A$-receptor complex to neurosteroids varies so as to maintain homeostatic regulation of brain excitability (4,108,109). In rodents, the threshold dose for seizure onset induced by chemical convulsants (bicuculline, picrotoxin, pentylenetetrazol, and strychnine) changes over the estrus cycle. Female rats in estrus are more sensitive to chemical convulsants than are females in diestrus and males, whereas infusion of a progesterone metabolite increases the seizure threshold more for females in diestrus (108). The differential effects of estrogens on neuronal excitability also depend on cycling status. Excitability is enhanced when female rats in low-estrogen states are given estrogen (diestrus) but not when estrogen is given during a high-estrogen state (diestrus) (110).

In summary, the biologic underpinnings for the enhanced seizure susceptibility in perimenstrual catamenial epilepsy is multifactorial and likely include: (i) withdrawal of the anticonvulsant effects of neurosteroids mediated through their action on $GABA_A$ receptors, (ii) the sudden estrogen peak on the day prior to ovulation, (iii) increased frequency of anovulatory cycles due to hypothalamic–pituitary–gonadal axis dysregulation and consequent low progesterone luteal phases, (iv) alteration in $GABA_A$-receptor subunits and subsequent changes in neuronal inhibition. All of these factors are related to the high levels of circulating neurosteroids during the luteal phase and the natural reduction or withdrawal of progesterone that occurs around the time of menstruation.

Definition

The term catamenial epilepsy refers to the temporal relationship between seizure frequency and menstrual phases. It does not refer to seizure type, localization, or an epilepsy syndrome. However, catamenial epilepsy has been noted to be more common in focal epilepsy compared to generalized epilepsy (111,112).

The incidence of catamenial epilepsy varies from 10% to 78% in studies due to the different criteria used by investigators to meet the term catamenial epilepsy. For example, Duncan et al. (113) defined catamenial epilepsy as the occurrence of 75% of seizures within the 10-day frame from 4 days prior to and 6 days after the onset of menstruation. Only

12.5% of women with epilepsy met this stringent criterion (78% of whom reported menstruation-related seizure exacerbations). However, in another seminal study by Herzog in which the pattern of seizure exacerbation throughout the menstrual cycle was carefully evaluated, it appears that a doubling of seizure frequency during portions of the menstrual cycle emerges as consistent with catamenial seizure exacerbations, and approximately one third of women with epilepsy had a catamenial relationship (114). The seizure patterns discovered in this study are described in the following section and have served as a frame of reference for all further clinical work in this area.

Seizure Patterns

Herzog et al. (114) identified three prevalent patterns of catamenial epilepsy based on seizure diaries and midluteal progesterone levels in a large group of women with epilepsy. Seizure exacerbations clustered at three particular portions of the menstrual cycle. These clusters are known as perimenstrual, periovulatory, and luteal. They had a seizure frequency approximately double to that of other days in a cycle. This suggests that a reliable criterion for catamenial epilepsy is a twofold increase in seizure frequency during the perimenstrual, periovulatory, and luteal phases as described in detail next.

The *perimenstrual* (C1) pattern, most frequently observed pattern, is defined as maximal seizure frequency during the menstrual phase (days 25 to 3) compared to the midfollicular (days 4 to 9) and midluteal (days 16 to 24) phases.

The *periovulatory* (C2) pattern, second most frequently observed, is characterized as maximal seizure frequency during the ovulatory phase (days 10 to 13) compared to the midfollicular and midluteal phases.

In the *luteal* (C3) pattern, maximal seizure frequency occurred during the ovulatory, midluteal, and menstrual phases than during the midfollicular phase in women with ILP cycles; this is the third most frequently observed pattern.

Using the above criteria, one third of women had catamenial epilepsy. These phases also are important in that they coincide with the known physiology of ovarian hormones as described in above sections.

These seizure patterns have been found in subsequent studies; one recent report documents catamenial seizure patterns that correlate with decreased progesterone levels, associating the clinical observation with the neurosteroid levels (115). When comparing women with epilepsy to controls, in general, progesterone levels were lower and the estrogen-to-progesterone ratio higher in the perimenstrual and midluteal phases in patients group compared to the control group. There was a catamenial seizure pattern in 31% of patients (53.8% C1 and 46.15% inadequate luteal phase C3 pattern). Patients with C3 pattern showed lower progesterone levels in the midluteal phase compared to patients with noncatamenial pattern, to those with C1 pattern, or to controls. Patients with C1 pattern had lower progesterone levels than controls in the perimenstrual phase. This study reports progesterone levels as an important indicator of catamenial seizure exacerbation.

Conversely, another study pointed to significant variations in estrogen as an indicator, with little change in progesterone levels between study groups (116). In this study, a significant rise ($P > 0.0001$) of β-estradiol was obtained for catamenial

patients compared to normal subjects as well as noncatamenial patients ($P > 0.02$). Other emerging information supports the role of hormones as a contributor to seizure occurrence and cyclic seizure patterns. For example, Murialdo et al. found no direct correlation with increased seizure frequency and reproductive hormone levels, but generally found a decrease in estrogen and progesterone levels compared to controls (117). However, supporting a role of hormonal influences on seizure exacerbation, they found that women with more frequent seizures in general showed more relevant changes in their sex hormone profile and lower progesterone levels during the luteal phase. Another recent report supports the differentiation of seizure patterns between ovulatory and anovulatory cycles in a large cohort of women with partial epilepsy (118).

Catamenial Epilepsy and Antiepileptic Drug (AED) Contributions

Besides the direct effect hormones have on the cortex contributing to catamenial epilepsy, the levels of AEDs also fluctuate during a menstrual cycle, which can partly explain the cyclic nature. The decrease in circulating estrogen and progesterone premenstrually may induce hepatic isoenzymes utilized for AED metabolism. Therefore, normal hormonal cycling may lower the levels of circulating AEDs, thus increasing the risk of breakthrough seizures (119). Rosciszewska et al. (120) measured AED levels during different phases of the menstrual cycle in 64 women receiving phenytoin alone or in combination with phenobarbital. They found that phenytoin levels on day 28 of the menstrual cycle in women with catamenial seizures were significantly lower than levels in women without cyclic seizure exacerbations. Phenobarbital concentrations, however, did not change significantly. A previous study of phenytoin, phenobarbital, carbamazepine levels taken every other day throughout the menstrual cycle in a small group of women with epilepsy showed no relationship between the seizure frequency and a change in serum levels of the AEDs (121). In another recent report, the relationship between hormone levels and seizure frequency was disputed altogether and confounded by the effects of AEDs; despite globally decreased estrogen, progesterone, and FAI but increased SHBG in serum, actual hormone titers were not significantly correlated with seizure frequency exacerbations in women with epilepsy (122). Hormonal changes were explained by the effect of enzyme-inducing AED polytherapies.

Clearly, the interaction of AEDs, hormone levels, and seizure frequency alterations as they as are related to catamenial epilepsy remains incompletely explored.

Water Balance in Menstrual Cycles and Its Importance in Catamenial Epilepsy

In 1911, drainage of subarachnoid fluid was noted to have some success in treating epilepsy (123). This finding first led to studying the association with excessive water ingestion, as well as vasopressin and increased seizure frequency (124), while negative water balance by fluid restriction was shown to decrease seizure frequency (125). With the association between menstruation and fluid retention already known, it was theorized that water imbalance played a role in perimenstrual seizures.

However, Ansell and Clarke (126) found no significant differences in body weight, sodium metabolism, or total body water in 14 epileptic patients, including seven women with perimenstrual seizures, and 10 healthy controls, or between epileptic women with and without catamenial tendencies.

Management of Catamenial Epilepsy

Most of the following interventions have been described as treatments aimed at the premenstrual seizure exacerbation pattern or C1 as described above, which is the most frequent type of catamenial exacerbation; therefore, it accounts for the occasional success reported with these treatments. It should be kept in mind that only women with regular menstrual periods are good candidates for these interventions, since they must be taken a proscribed number of days after the onset of menstrual bleeding. Usually this is around day 18 to 21 depending on the individual seizure pattern, since the luteal phase is unvaryingly 14 days long.

Acetazolamide

Acetazolamide (AZ) has been shown to be efficacious in catamenial epilepsy for 50 years, despite the evidence being anecdotal. Poser (127) reported AZ at a dose of 250 to 500 mg daily for 5 to 7 days prior to the onset of menses was efficacious in treating seizures without significant side effects. In a case report, Ansell and Clarke (128) showed improvement in two women with cyclic perimenstrual seizures who were treated with 5 mg/kg/day of AZ for 3 days prior to menses. While they attributed the efficacy to be from the diuretic effect of the medication, the two patients' body weight, sodium metabolism, and total body water were not statistically different from women with or without catamenial epilepsy (126).

The initial recommended dose of AZ is 4 mg/kg, with a range of 8 to 30 mg/kg/day (not to exceed 1 g/day) divided up to four doses daily. Common and usually dose-related adverse effects include paresthesias, drowsiness, nausea, malaise, fatigue, and diuresis. AZ has also been known to cause growth suppression in children and aplastic anemia. Patients on AZ have been shown to develop tolerance and thus intermittent treatment 1 week prior to menses until the second day of menstrual bleeding is a reasonable, albeit unproven, treatment regimen.

Benzodiazepines

Benzodiazepines are allosteric modulators of GABA receptors and hence are broad-spectrum antiseizure agents. Their main use is for abortive therapy due to the development of habituation and tolerance with chronic, long-term use. However, they have long been used as a practical and safe intermittent treatment approach for catamenial seizure exacerbations.

Clobazam is the only benzodiazepine studied for the treatment of catamenial epilepsy, and has been shown to be effective (129). Clobazam, at 20 to 30 mg/day, cyclically taken 2 to 4 days premenstrually has been shown to reduce catamenial seizures as well as decrease the tolerance associated with continual use. Clobazam, however, is not available in the United States, but this data does support the use of intermittent benzodiazepines in the treatment of catamenial epilepsy.

Increasing Usual AEDs

Due to the physiologic evidence of decreased AED levels premenstrually, a rationale for temporarily increasing AEDs at specific times in a menstrual cycle seems reasonable. However, clinicians must take care in understanding the medications pharmacokinetics, as only a medication with a linear dose-level relationship should be tried in this manner.

Medroxyprogesterone Acetate (MPA)

MPA is a synthetic progestin-only contraceptive agent. Its mechanism of action toward reducing seizure frequency is currently unknown. Studies have shown that the use of MPA in catamenial epilepsy can reduce seizure frequency by 39% at a 1 year follow-up (130,131). MPA is given as an intramuscular injection and ceases the regular menstrual cycle. The standard dose is 150 mg intramuscularly every 12 weeks. Some clinicians advocate shortening the dosing frequency to every 10 weeks since some AEDs can shorten effectiveness. It is believed that the effectiveness of this medication for catamenial epilepsy stems from the fact that you are halting normal menstruation.

Natural Progesterone

Natural progesterone has been considered the treatment of choice for ILP; however, its natural metabolism to allopregnanolone, a neurosteroid anticonvulsant, makes it another option for seizure control. In 1986, Herzog (132) was first to describe natural progesterone and its use in seizure treatment. In his study, eight women with a diagnosis of temporal lobe epilepsy, as well as ILP, were treated with natural progesterone (given as a vaginal suppository). They were given doses ranging from 50 to 400 mg, and were dosed every 12 hours during the phase of highest seizure frequency. Doses were adjusted to obtain serum levels ranging from 5 to 25 ng/mL about 2 to 6 hours after dosing. The levels of the AEDs that the patients were already taking were also measured and titrated to maintain approved therapeutic levels. The results showed that compared to each patients' baseline, monthly seizure frequency decreased by 68% during the 3-month treatment. Seventy-five percent of women had fewer seizures. The most common side effects were fatigue and depression that resolved with decreasing dosing levels.

In a follow-up study, Herzog (133) studied the use of progesterone lozenges. The study group was 25 women with temporal lobe epilepsy matching the definition for catamenial epilepsy in the perimenstrual ($n = 11$) or luteal ($n = 14$) phases. The women were all started at 200 mg three times daily during their exacerbation phase. The doses were adjusted to obtain normal midluteal progesterone levels. The results show that over a 3-month period, 72% of women reported a decrease in seizure frequency and that the average daily seizure frequency decreased by 55%. In the study group, five women reported no change in seizure frequency. The women with ILP noted a slightly larger decrease in seizure frequency compared to the women with perimenstrual catamenial epilepsy, 59% to 49% respectively. Throughout the trial, two women stopped the study due to side effects. In a 3-year follow-up of the remaining 23 women, the mean reduction in focal and generalized seizures was 54% and 58%, respectively. Three women were reported to be seizure-free (134).

From these studies, it is clear that natural progesterone could play an important role in catamenial epilepsy, and a randomized clinical trial has been performed and is under analysis. As of this writing, natural progesterone is not approved for use in the treatment of seizures; however, it is used as an off-label medication.

SEXUAL DYSFUNCTION IN EPILEPSY

It is clear through the evidence stated earlier in the chapter that epilepsy and the medications used for treatment have a significant effect on the normal hormone balance in human physiology. It is not a stretch to expect that sexual function of men and women with epilepsy could be affected. While this subject is usually avoided by the clinician and the patient alike, it is an important aspect to consider. Epilepsy appears to produce a higher incidence of sexual dysfunction compared to other neurologic diseases. Symptoms manifested are mainly of decreased sexual desire and potency (135). Studies reviewing this topic have shown sexual dysfunction in 30% to 66% of men with epilepsy (136–139) and 14% to 50% of women with epilepsy (135,136,140).

This section will cover in more detail the prevalence, common manifestations, localization, and etiology of sexual dysfunction. First, sexual dysfunction in the normal population will be reviewed.

Sexual Dysfunction in the General Population

Men and woman have different types of sexual dysfunction, which are likely secondary to adaptive issues determined by evolutionary principles. In general, as in most mammalian species, the female is the more heavily invested in the offspring; thus, they are usually more discriminatory and less promiscuous than males. Accordingly, sexual dysfunction in women most often presents with issues in restraint and disinhibition, while men have more issues with sexual stimulation (141).

Sexual Dysfunction in Females

The International Consensus Development Conference on Female Sexual Dysfunction has divided the disorders of women into four categories: (i) sexual desire disorders, (ii) sexual arousal disorders, (iii) orgasmic disorders, and (iv) sexual pain disorders (142). These categories are further divided into subtypes for different durations and etiologies and may have overlap. For example, a patient can have decreased sexual desire postmenopausally; however, the decrease in desire may be at least partly due to dyspareunia from declining estrogen levels as well as decreased testosterone (143).

Sexual Dysfunction in Males

The most prominent types of dysfunction seen in males are ejaculatory and orgasmic disorders such as premature and retrograde ejaculation and anorgasmia (144). Hyposexuality also occurs in males as related to an endocrinopathy. Hypogonadism, androgen deficiency, decreases sexual interest

and erectile function leading to poor quality of life (145). Total and free testosterone levels are indicated in this situation and usually are low. In these situations, testosterone replacement can improve the patient's symptoms. The effects of testosterone replacement tend to decrease over time with use, and also there is not sufficient evidence for long-term safety of testosterone replacement, particularly in mature men regarding the effects on prostate growth (146).

The Amygdala and Sexual Drive: Insights from Epilepsy Surgery

Amygdalar size has been associated with sexual functioning in persons with epilepsy (147). Contralateral amygdala volumes were compared in patients with and without a reported increase in sexual drive after temporal lobectomy and in neurologically normal controls. Patients who reported improvement in sexual functioning after surgery had significantly larger contralateral amygdala volumes than patients with no change or a decrease in sexual drive after surgery and control subjects. This study suggests that the amygdala is an influencing factor in sexual functioning for persons with temporal lobe epilepsy.

These findings may be related to previously reported improvements in sexual functioning after temporal lobectomy. Baird et al. (148) reported that one third of their 58 patients undergoing temporal lobectomy had an increase in sexual activity after surgery, whereas one quarter had decreased postsurgical sexual activity. Change in sexuality was more likely to occur in women and in patients with right-sided resections. This association between change in sexuality after surgery and lateralization supports the findings of Herzog et al. (149), who reported that women with temporal lobe epilepsy of right-sided origin had lower bioactive testosterone levels and more sexual dysfunction than women with left-sided temporal lobe epilepsy and controls. It is possible, therefore, that the lateralization as well as the presence of epileptic discharges is a factor in the impairment of sexual function and its improvement after temporal lobectomy.

Sexual Dysfunction in Both Men and Women with Epilepsy

Early clinical research supports the existence in both women and men with epilepsy of a physiologic impairment of sexual arousal that could lead to inadequate arousal and orgasm, which, for men, differs from the sexual dysfunction in the general population. Morrell et al. (150) measured genital blood flow in 17 women and men with temporal lobe epilepsy and 19 control subjects as they watched either erotic or sexually neutral videos. The increase in genital blood flow in response to visual erotic stimulation was significantly diminished in persons with epilepsy compared with controls. The authors hypothesized that dysfunction of specific regions in the limbic and frontal cortical areas by epileptic activity could be the cause of sexual dysfunction. The effect of AEDs on these results was not assessed.

Living with the stigma of epilepsy also may be detrimental to adequate sexual behavior. According to a survey regarding the quality of life of persons with epilepsy across Europe, many subjects reported low satisfaction with sexual relationships in the context of feeling stigmatized by having epilepsy (151). Therefore, the cause of dysfunction is probably multifactorial, with a psychological component, in the epileptic population (152). Normal development and social interactions may be adversely affected in people with epilepsy due to poor self-esteem and poor interactions with other people for fear of having a seizure in their presence. This, in turn, could lead to feeling sexually unattractive and resulting in poor relationships. Arousal is also affected when patients begin to associate intercourse with seizures due to prior incidences with seizures and sexual activity. It has been shown that acceptance of the psychomotor aspect of a chronic disease correlates with improved sexual function, while poor acceptance correlates with the opposite effect (153).

In addition to alteration in the hypothalamic–pituitary–gonadal axis (154), sexuality in epilepsy may be adversely affected by alterations in the levels of pituitary gonadotropins, prolactin, and the sex steroid hormones (155–157). Reductions in LH and elevated prolactin levels are associated with sexual dysfunction, and adequate amounts of estrogen and progesterone are required for sexual behavior in females (158).

Sexual Dysfunction in Women with Epilepsy

Bergen et al. (159) documented a high prevalence of severe sexual dysfunction in women with epilepsy compared to controls. These investigators evaluated 50 women with epilepsy in a tertiary epilepsy care center, all of whom were taking AEDs; 32 had partial epilepsy and 28 were taking only one AED and 22 were taking two or more AEDs. This group of women with epilepsy was compared with a control group of women of similar age without epilepsy. All of the women were asked two simple questions: (i) how often they had the desire for sex and (ii) how often they had intercourse. Equal proportions of women in both groups had a frequent desire for sex, but a much greater proportion of women with epilepsy than of the comparison group had very infrequent sexual desire. Approximately 20% of the women with epilepsy reported that they "almost never" had sexual desire. Very few of the women in the control group, around 2%, reported such a low level of sexual desire. This bimodal distribution, with a peak at the normal level of "often" having sexual desire and another peak at "never" having sexual desire, persisted for the actual rate of sexual intercourse and for married women with epilepsy. There were no subjects in the control population reporting "never" having sexual desire. The investigators found no correlation with age, type of AEDs used, duration of epilepsy, or seizure type. This study revealed that many women with epilepsy have normal sexuality, but there is a significant fraction who have decreased sexual desire.

Further evidence points to specific orgasmic dysfunction for women with epilepsy. Jensen et al. (160) studied sexuality in 48 women with epilepsy and compared their findings with their own previously reported data on sexuality in persons with diabetes mellitus and healthy controls. There was no difference in sexual desire among the three groups, but 19% of the women with epilepsy had orgasmic dysfunction compared with 11% of the diabetes mellitus group and 8% of the controls ($P = 0.081$). The authors found no correlation

between sexual dysfunction and type and duration of epilepsy or AED use. None of the women with epilepsy had levels of free or total testosterone or testosterone-binding globulin outside the normal range. In a study by Duncan et al. (161) of 195 women with epilepsy, significantly less orgasmic satisfaction was reported by the 159 women who were taking AEDs compared with the 36 untreated women and 48 control women without epilepsy. Sexual Experience Scale scores indicated that the AED-treated women with epilepsy were more "moral" and less open to sexual experiences, but in general, those with regular partners appeared to desire and enjoy intercourse as much as the controls and the untreated women.

In a study of 57 women of reproductive age with epilepsy, decreased patient-reported sexual functioning was associated with phenytoin use, with mild depression, and with low levels of estradiol and dehydroepiandrosterone sulfate (162). In another study of patient-reported sexual functioning and sexual arousability in 116 women with epilepsy, anorgasmia was reported by one third of 17 women with primary generalized epilepsy and 18 of 99 women with LRE (163). Compared with historical controls, the women in this study did not have reduced sexual experience but reported less sexual arousability and more sexual anxiety. The authors concluded that in addition to what appears to be physiologic impairment of sexual functioning, that is, inadequate orgasms or anorgasmia, psychosocial factors are likely to contribute to self-reported sexual dysfunction in women with epilepsy.

Specific AED use has been associated with sexual dysfunction for women with epilepsy. Severely decreased libido and anorgasmia have been reported in women treated with valproate for bipolar disorder (163). The authors postulate that this dysfunction, which appears to be similar to that frequently associated with the use of selective serotonin reuptake inhibitors, may be related to increased serotoninergic transmission. An enhancing effect on the serotoninergic system has been described as a possible mechanism of action of valproate in animal studies (164). Two cases of gabapentin-associated anorgasmia have been reported in women with epilepsy, as well, with no information regarding a possible mechanism of this effect (165).

Sexual Dysfunction in Men with Epilepsy

Sexual difficulties were first associated with AEDs in men in the first Veterans Administration Cooperative Study. In that investigation, in which 622 epilepsy patients were randomized to treatment with primidone, phenobarbital, carbamazepine, or phenytoin, 22% of subjects taking primidone reported decreased libido or impotence, compared to 16% of subjects taking phenobarbital, 13% taking carbamazepine, and 11% taking phenytoin (166). More recently, decreased levels of free testosterone were found in a large group of men with epilepsy ($n = 200$) compared with healthy controls ($n = 105$) (167). However, the ratio of testosterone to LH was decreased only among the patients with temporal lobe epilepsy and not those with IGE. This ratio is an indicator of testicular function, since levels of LH, which stimulates testicular testosterone production, increase in response to low testosterone levels. Therefore, a decreased ratio of testosterone to LH suggests testicular dysfunction and an inability to respond to LH stimulation. Carbamazepine-treated men in this study had the greatest alterations in free testosterone levels and testosterone-to-LH ratio, a finding consistent with the postulated effect of carbamazepine of increasing the hepatic production of SHBG and inducing aromatase, which catalyzes the conversion of testosterone to estradiol. Valproate, on the other hand, which inhibits the conversion of testosterone to estradiol, was associated with normal total testosterone levels and testosterone-to-LH ratio, although free testosterone levels were still significantly decreased (97).

Reproductive functioning was evaluated in another recent study of 85 men with LRE, of whom 25 each took lamotrigine, carbamazepine, or phenytoin for at least 6 months (96). The study also included 10 men with epilepsy not taking AEDs and 25 controls without epilepsy. Sexual function scores, bioactive testosterone levels, and ratio of bioactive testosterone to LH were significantly greater in the control and lamotrigine-treated groups than in the carbamazepine- and phenytoin-treated groups. Carbamazepine and phenytoin were associated with increased SHBG levels as well. Sexual function scores were below the control range in 20% of the patients with epilepsy overall, including 32% of those taking carbamazepine, 24% of those taking phenytoin, 20% of those not taking an AED, and 4% of those taking lamotrigine. The investigators noted that lack of enzyme induction is a factor distinguishing lamotrigine from the other two AEDs used in the study. Further, the expected decline in bioactive testosterone with age was greater than expected in all epilepsy subjects, treated or untreated, suggesting an effect of epilepsy itself on testosterone production.

Lamotrigine has been also reported to be associated with improved sexual functioning in 141 women and men with epilepsy, including 79 who began treatment with lamotrigine as monotherapy and 62 who were switched to lamotrigine treatment from another AED (167).

In a recent evaluation of the sexual development of a large group of male adolescents with epilepsy (*n* = 130), their values for height, testicular volume, and penile length were significantly lower, and pubarche was significantly delayed, in comparison with controls (168). Polytherapy was associated with greater deviation from expected developmental and hormonal values. These findings corroborate others regarding the effects of AEDs and probably epilepsy on sexuality in males and further indicate a longitudinal adverse effect on sexual development in young males.

A recent questionnaire study of men with epilepsy who were started on oxcarbazepine and had some sexual dysfunction prior to starting the medicine found that 80% reported an improvement in their sexual functioning after 12 weeks of treatment (169). These findings indirectly support another recent report that testosterone levels are perhaps a minor factor for sexual functioning in men with epilepsy, and that psychosocial factors are of greater importance (170). Further, the effects of AEDs on sexuality may not be strictly related to effects on testosterone, but may be related to effects in the brain on neurotransmitters important for sexuality, such as serotonin (171).

Right-Sided Epilepsy Has More Impact on Sexuality than Left-Sided Epilepsy

Reports from different aspects of the epilepsy literature suggest that seizures of right temporal origin are particularly associated with reproductive dysfunction and possibly even sexual ictal phenomenon. From the epilepsy surgery literature, Baird et al. reported that one third of their 58 temporal lobectomy patients had an increase in sexual activity after surgery, compared with one quarter of patients having decreased postsurgical sexual activity (148). Change in sexuality was more likely to occur in women and in patients with right-sided resections. This lateralization of change in sexuality after surgery is consistent with a report by Herzog et al. (155) that right temporal epileptic discharges in WWE were associated with hypogonadotropic hypogonadism that included, for many subjects, decreased sexual interest. These findings would suggest, therefore, that right temporal resection could improve sexual functioning.

In a carefully performed questionnaire study of sexual functioning in men and women with either right or left temporal lobe epilepsy, Daniele et al. (172) found that sexual interest specifically was decreased in patients with right temporal lobe epilepsy compared to left for both genders, although most aspects of sexual performance were not different. Ictal sexual behaviors and ictal orgasm have been specifically associated with right temporal epilepsy as well (173).

There is also lateralization in the central regulation of gonadotropin secretion: experimental evidence indicates that the right hypothalamus is predominant in the control of reproductive functioning (174), although lateralized kindling has not clearly been shown to be associated with seizure differences in animal studies (175). Therefore, a body of evidence from divergent sources, both clinical- and laboratory-based, suggests that right-sided epilepsy and right temporal lobe epilepsy specifically may be associated with a risk of sexual and reproductive dysfunction.

Evaluation and Treatment

The difficult task of interviewing patients regarding their sexual functioning is simplified as follows, and adapted from a suggested interview developed by Bartlik et al. (176):

- On a scale of 1 to 10, how would you rate your sex life (10 is best)?
- How would you describe your level of desire?
- Do you masturbate? How often?
- Women—do you lubricate?
- Men—do you have difficulty getting an erection? Do you have morning/nocturnal erections?
- Is achieving orgasm difficult? When you have sex or masturbate, what proportion of the time do you achieve orgasm?
- How pleasurable are your orgasms?
- Men—is ejaculating too soon a problem for you?
- Approximately how long does it take you to achieve an orgasm?
- Do you have pain or discomfort during intercourse?
- How long have you had this problem?
- Does anything make it better or worse?
- Men—do you have a desire for sex but erections and orgasm are not adequate?

A tool frequently used to quantify sexual functioning for either research or clinical practice is the Arizona Sexual Experiences Scale (ASEX) (177). This is a user-friendly 5-item rating scale that quantifies sex drive, arousal, vaginal lubrication/penile erection, ability to reach orgasm, and satisfaction from orgasm. Possible total scores range from 5 to 30, with the higher scores indicating more sexual dysfunction.

Other medications than AEDs may also be associated with sexual dysfunction. Evaluation of sexual dysfunction should include consideration of the contribution of the following comedications associated with adverse sexual side effects:

- Antidepressants
- Antihypertensives
- Antipsychotics
- Chemotherapeutic agents
- Statins
- Diuretics
- Allergy meds

Although evaluation and treatment of sexual dysfunction may be outside the realm of most neurologists, an initial laboratory evaluation would include the following serum levels:

- Testosterone, free and total
- Sex hormone binding globulin
- FSH
- LH
- Prolactin
- Hemoglobin A1C
- TSH

The mainstays of treatment for sexual dysfunction, when obviously treatable causes and contributors such as thyroid disease or medication side effects have been ruled out, remain the phosphodiesterase inhibitors and testosterone replacement. These have only been proven effective for men, and phosphodiesterase inhibitors are only useful for improving erectile dysfunction but not libido or sexual desire, which is mediated largely by testosterone. While the phosphodiesterase inhibitors have been nearly miraculous for men with erectile dysfunction, they have not been reliably effective for women, but may be worth trying depending on the clinical situation. The use of aromatase inhibitors in men with epilepsy has been shown to increase testosterone levels and possibly improve seizures as well; however, this intervention remains incompletely explored (178).

Testosterone is also important for libido, desire, and sexual functioning for women of both premenopausal and postmenopausal years. Testosterone replacement is often useful in women with low testosterone status and sexual dysfunction, and it is becoming more widely accepted as a treatment approach although long-term studies are lacking; the most frequent side effects for women are hirsutism and acne (179).

PREMATURE OVARIAN FAILURE: EARLY ONSET OF PERIMENOPAUSE AND MENOPAUSE

Women with epilepsy appear to have a risk of experiencing an early onset of perimenopausal symptoms, often in the late fourth decade or early fifth decade of life. The mechanism by which this could occur is likely also related to the hypothalamic–pituitary–gonadal axis dysfunction, producing dysregulation of maturation of ovarian follicles and therefore early loss of follicles available for ovulation. One of the first scientific reports of early perimenopause was put forth by

Klein et al. (180), in which 7 of 50 women with epilepsy had symptoms or hormonal findings of premature ovarian failure before age 42 years, compared to 3 of 82 healthy control women, pointing to a risk of early perimenopause four times greater in women with epilepsy than in controls. Furthermore, seizure frequency is related to a risk for earlier menopause (181). Within a group of women with epilepsy, those with only rare seizures (e.g., fewer than 20 in a lifetime) had less risk for earlier menopause and had a normal age at menopause of 50 to 51 years. However, the women who had frequent seizures, occurring at least monthly, experienced earlier menopause, at age 46 to 47 years on average. In this study, there was no relationship between early menopause and specific AED treatments.

CHANGES IN SEIZURES RELATED TO PERIMENOPAUSE AND MENOPAUSE

Although no prospective information is available on the course of epilepsy as WWE progress through perimenopause, menopause, and postmenopause, a cross-sectional evaluation was performed in order to obtain information about the effect of menopause and perimenopause on the course of epilepsy. Further, the survey assessed whether a history of a catamenial seizure pattern would influence this course (182). These questionnaires were sent to women with epilepsy using a mailing list from the local epilepsy consumer advocacy organizations; responses were used from (i) women currently in menopause or perimenopause and (ii) respondents who did not have AED changes during these life epochs. Information was provided regarding the course of their epilepsy and treatment, seizure type, relationship of seizures to menses during their reproductive years, specifically the occurrence of seizures in the week before menses and at the onset of menses (catamenial seizure pattern type 1), and any use of hormone replacement therapy (HRT).

Thirty-nine perimenopausal women with epilepsy as defined by a recent change in menstrual pattern and the occurrence of "hot flushes" were evaluated (182). Nine subjects reported no change in seizures at perimenopause, five reported a decrease in seizure frequency, and the majority of women, 25, reported an increase. Twenty-eight (72%) reported having a catamenial seizure pattern before menopause, and eight (15%) subjects took synthetic HRT. HRT had no significant effect on seizures; however, a history of catamenial seizure pattern was significantly associated with an increase in seizures at perimenopause ($P = 0.02$). It can be postulated that reproductive hormonal changes in perimenopause could contribute to increased seizures through the following mechanism: during perimenopause, estrogen levels remain unchanged or may rise with age until the onset of menopause, presumably in response to the elevated FSH levels. However, the cyclic progesterone elevation during the luteal phase of the menstrual cycle gradually becomes less frequent throughout perimenopause, resulting in increasing rates of anovulatory cycles (183). Therefore, the elevation of the estrogen-to-progesterone ratio may contribute to the increase in seizure frequency at perimenopause.

Forty-two postmenopausal women with epilepsy as defined as 1 year without menses were evaluated (182). There was no overall directional change in seizure frequency within this group: 12 subjects reported no change in seizures at menopause, 17 reported a decrease in seizure frequency, and 13 reported an increase. Sixteen (38%) took synthetic HRT. Sixteen (38%) additional subjects (having some overlap with the HRT group) reported having a catamenial seizure pattern before menopause. HRT was significantly associated with an increase in seizures during perimenopause ($P = 0.001$). A history of catamenial seizure pattern was significantly associated with a decrease in seizures at menopause ($P = 0.013$).

These cross-sectional data suggest that women with epilepsy may be likely to have an increase in seizures at perimenopause, and therefore may need more careful monitoring for the need for AED adjustment or AED change. Further, these findings indicate that catamenial seizure pattern may be associated with seizure increase during perimenopause but seizure decrease after menopause, indicating that subsets of women with epilepsy are especially sensitive to endogenous hormonal changes.

HORMONE REPLACEMENT THERAPY IN WOMEN WITH EPILEPSY

The previous results prompted an evaluation of HRT in women with epilepsy, designed to determine whether adding HRT to the medication regimen of postmenopausal WWE was associated with an increase in seizure frequency. The study design was a double-blind, randomized, placebo-controlled trial of the effect of HRT on seizure frequency in postmenopausal women with epilepsy (184). Women took stable doses of AEDs, and were within 10 years of their last menses. After a 3-month prospective baseline, subjects were randomized to placebo, Prempro (0.625 mg of conjugated equine estrogens plus 2.5 mg of medroxyprogesterone acetate or conjugated equine estrogens [CEE]/MPA) daily, or double-dose CEE/MPA daily for a 3-month treatment period. The results were analyzed by chi-square for trend, comparing the numbers of subjects whose seizure frequency increased on treatment compared to baseline versus the number of subjects whose seizures did not increase across treatment arms.

On HRT treatment compared to placebo, there was a significant trend toward increased seizures in a dose-related manner using several seizure frequency analyses. Five (71%) of seven subjects taking double-dose CEE/MPA had a worsening seizure frequency of at least one seizure type, compared with four (50%) of eight taking single-dose CEE/MPA and one (17%) of six taking placebo ($P = 0.05$). An increase in seizure frequency of the subject's most severe seizure type was associated with increasing CEE/MPA dose ($P = 0.008$). An increase in complex partial seizure frequency also was associated with increasing CEE/MPA dose ($P = 0.05$). Total seizure number approached significance with increasing CEE/MPA ($P = 0.10$) as well.

Two subjects taking lamotrigine had a decrease in lamotrigine levels of 25% to 30% while taking CEE/MPA. This is likely due to induction of uridine diphosphate–glucuronosyltransferase (UGT) 1A4 by ethinyl estradiol, which is the predominant metabolic enzyme for lamotrigine, as occurs with hormonal contraceptives (185). Therefore, although the small

numbers of subjects in this study may limit its generalizability, the results indicate that CEE/MPA is associated with a dose-related increase in seizure frequency in postmenopausal WWE. Further, the lamotrigine clearance may be increased with HRT as well.

As an analogous state to HRT during menopause, laboratory evidence suggests that hormone replacement protects against seizure activity in a rodent postmenopausal seizure model. In a kainate-induced model, estrogen pretreatment had no effect on seizure severity but significantly decreased "spread," neuronal loss, and mortality in ovariectomized rats compared with ovariectomized rats without pretreatment. Progesterone pretreatment in this model had a slightly different effects; it decreased seizure severity and hippocampal damage (27). In the NMDA-induced model, estrogen pretreatment decreased total seizure number in ovariectomized rats compared with ovariectomized rats without pretreatment; and in fact, estrogen replacement restored seizure number to that of the intact state (186). In the lithium–pilocarpine model of status epilepticus, estrogen pretreatment is neuroprotective in ovariectomized rats compared with sham-treated ovariectomized controls (187).

Several factors may explain why these laboratory results cannot be extrapolated to the effects of HRT on menopausal women with epilepsy. The differences in the outcome between the clinical study and the laboratory experiments are readily explained by the factors described above by Velíšková (22), relating estrogen dose and species with being proconvulsant rather than anticonvulsant. First, the doses of HRT used by menopausal women are actually relatively higher than the doses used in these laboratory experiments. Second, the main estrogenic species in CEE is estrone, long shown to be more proconvulsant in humans than estradiol. Finally, it is possible that the synthetic progestin, MPA, used in human studies could account for the adverse effects on seizures. It is widely accepted that progesterone (through the action of its reduced metabolite, allopregnanolone) has anticonvulsant properties (41). However, MPA clearly has a different profile of activity in the brain, in that it is not metabolized to allopregnanolone and is not neuroprotective in rodents (188). In one study of ovariectomized rats with and without estrogen replacement, the effect of progesterone versus MPA pretreatment on kainate-induced seizures produced quite differing results for the two compounds. Both progesterone and MPA blocked the neuroprotective effects of estrogen in these experiments (a result differing from previous experiments for progesterone as well), and seizure severity was worse but not significantly so in the MPA-treated group (189). Therefore, several factors, including the possibility of an adverse effect of MPA on seizures, may account for the divergence of the laboratory and clinical experiments.

Progesterone is readily available in its natural form in the FDA-approved form of Prometrium, therefore this may be a reasonable option as the progestin component when HRT is needed for women with epilepsy, especially since there is evidence that it has active anticonvulsant properties. For the estrogenic component, a simplified estrogen compound, such as 17-β-estradiol could be considered and conjugated equine estrogens should be avoided. Clinicians must consider these options since HRT will be needed for some WWE; sleep deprivation related to "hot flushes" can have an adverse effect on seizure frequency and in such cases, HRT may be beneficial by permitting adequate sleep (190).

POLYCYSTIC OVARIAN SYNDROME (PCOS) AND FERTILITY IN EPILEPSY

PCOS is a major cause of infertility and appears to occur at a higher rate in women with epilepsy than in the general population. The definition and diagnostic criteria for PCOS is still evolving in the endocrine community. A recent task force report from The Androgen Excess and PCOS Society has defined the criteria for the polycystic ovary syndrome as the presence of hyperandrogenism (clinical and/or biochemical), ovarian dysfunction (oligo-anovulation and/or polycystic ovaries), and the exclusion of related disorders (191). The cause of PCOS is also mysterious; current thinking is that PCOS is multigenic in etiology but subject to environmental triggers which are as yet unclear (192). Hypothalamic and pituitary dysregulation may be present in PCOS, as evidenced by elevated LH secretion and an increased ratio of LH to FSH. LH stimulates ovarian steroidogenesis, and elevated LH/FSH will produce follicles that do not fully mature, but become numerous and cystic. Immature follicules are deficient in aromatase, the enzyme which produces estrogen in the ovary by converting it from its precursor, testosterone. In this manner, the PCOS ovarian follicle produces primarily androgens. This abnormal system is disrupted further by the conversion of androgen to estrogen by aromatase in the periphery, producing elevated circulating estrogens, which feedback to the pituitary and disregulate normal LH secretion (193). Therefore, the hypothalamic dysfunction described in persons with epilepsy could possibly contribute to the increased rate of PCOS in women with epilepsy. This elevated LH/FSH ratio has been described in women with epilepsy; in an evaluation of women with LRE and IGE, the LH/FSH ratio for both LRE and IGE was significantly elevated compared to controls; the IGE group had the highest ratio, and 19 of the 35 women in this group used valproate (87).

The rate of PCOS for women in general is approximately 7% (194). The rate of PCOS for women with epilepsy is generally higher than this and in one report of women with focal epilepsy of long duration, PCOS defined as elevated testosterone levels and oligomenorrhea or amenorrhea occurred in 10.6%. No difference was found between women taking carbamazepine (10%), valproate (11.1%), or no AEDs (10.5%) (195).

Isojarvi et al. reported the first association between valproate and cystic ovaries (196). They reported that nearly half of the 28 women with epilepsy treated with valproate monotherapy had amenorrhea, oligomenorrhea, or prolonged menstrual cycles, compared to 19% of the 120 women taking carbamazepine monotherapy. These reports in women with epilepsy indicate an association between epilepsy and PCOS. However, one specific feature necessary for the diagnosis of PCOS is consistently associated with valproate. Valproate induces androgen synthesis in the ovary through several mechanisms. One study using human ovarian thecal cell cultures showed that valproate induced ovarian androgen synthesis by augmenting transcription of steroidogenic genes (197). Another report of ovarian follicles in culture with ovarian thecal and granulosal cells, so as to replicate an ovary, showed that valproate increased testosterone secretion from follicles, but had differing effects based on LH stimulation in the culture and on maturity of the follicles (198). Further, valproate inhibits aromatase, which is the enzyme mediating the conversion of testosterone to estradiol (198). Valproate may cause or imitate PCOS simply through its powerful inhibitory action. There is evidence that valproate inhibits insulin metabolism and in this manner produces higher circulating insulin levels and subsequent weight gain (199). Therefore, weight gain and insulin resistance may be pharmacokinetically mediated side effects of valproate; these metabolic abnormalities are also frequent features of PCOS.

Reduced birth rates have been frequently reported in large cohorts of persons with epilepsy. A population-based study showed that men with epilepsy had a 40% lower birth rate than men without epilepsy and women with epilepsy had a 10% lower birth rate than women without epilepsy (200). Another recent study from the same population showed that adults with active epilepsy had decreased birth rates compared to those who went into remission prior to adulthood (201).

As described in this chapter, there are several reasons to explain decreased fertility in women with epilepsy, including early perimenopause and menopause, increased rates of anovulatory cycles, and a frequent occurrence of PCOS. For men with epilepsy, abnormal spermatogenesis may be a cause for infertility. In 65 men with epilepsy taking carbamazepine, oxcarbazepine, or valproate, abnormalities of sperm morphology, motility, and concentration were significantly more common than in 41 control men (96). In this report, oxcarbazepine had the least detrimental effect on sperm quality. Decreased sexual desire may be a factor for both men and women with epilepsy and obviously could contribute to lower birth rates. It should be appreciated, however, that lowered birth rates are not the same as infertility, which is defined as a condition in which a couple has problem in conceiving, or getting pregnant, after one year of regular sexual intercourse without using any birth control methods. No population-based assessment of birth rates has controlled for confounders such as frequency of intercourse and personal choice to have children or not, which are important considerations for persons with epilepsy. Therefore, the conclusion that persons with epilepsy have a higher risk of infertility cannot be supported by current evidence.

CONCLUSIONS

Epilepsy affects reproductive functioning in persons with epilepsy likely through central mechanisms; seizures and interictal effects on the hypothalamic–pituitary–gonadal axis cause subtle changes over time which are of varying clinical significance, but nonetheless indicate that epilepsy has down-stream repercussions linking the brain to the gonads. In this chapter, the emphasis on neurosteroids and the ongoing attempt to associate basic science evidence with clinical entities reflects the complexity of neuroendocrinology in epilepsy and the ongoing search for appropriate animal models (202). Although much is known and explained in this realm, treatment approaches for reproductive hormone-related problems in epilepsy are still early in development.

References

1. Morrell MJ. Hormones and epilepsy through the lifetime. *Epilepsia.* 1992;33(suppl 4):S49–S61.
2. Woolley CS, Schwartzkroin PA. Hormonal effects on the brain. *Epilepsia.* 1998;39(suppl 8):S2–S8.
3. Pfaff DW, McEwen BS. Actions of estrogens and progestins on nerve cells. *Science.* 1983;219:808–814.
4. Finn DA, Gee KW. The influence of estrus cycle on neurosteroid potency at the gamma-aminobutyric acid receptor complex. *J Pharmacol Exp Ther.* 1993;265:1374–1379.
5. Stitt SL, Kinnard WJ. The effect of certain progestins and estrogens on the threshold of electrically induced seizure patterns. *Neurology.* 1968;18:213–216.
6. Wooley DE, Timiras PS. Estrous and circadian periodicity and electroshock convulsions in rats. *Am J Physiol.* 1962;202:379–382.
7. Wooley DE, Timiras PS. The gonad-brain relationship: effects of female sex hormones and electroshock convulsions in the rat. *Endocrinology.* 1962;70:196–209.
8. Marcus EM, Watson CW, Goldman PL. Effects of steroids on cerebral electrical activity: epileptogenic effects of conjugated estrogens and related compounds in the cat and rabbit. *Arch Neurol.* 1966;15:521–532.
9. Logothetis J, Harner R. Electrocortical activation by estrogens. *Arch Neurol.* 1960;3:290–297.
10. Hom AC, Buterbaugh GG. Estrogen alters the acquisition of seizures kindled by repeated amygdala stimulation or pentylenetetrazol administration in ovariectomized female rats. *Epilepsia.* 1986;27:103–108.
11. Woolley CS. Estradiol facilitates kainic acid-induced, but not flurothyl-induced behavioral seizure activity in adult female rats. *Epilepsia.* 2000;41:510–515.
12. Logothetis J, Harner R, Morrell F, et al. The role of estrogens in catamenial exacerbation of epilepsy. *Neurology.* 1959;9:352–360.
13. Wallis CJ, Luttge WG. Influence of estrogen and progesterone on glutamic acid decarboxylase activity in discrete regions of rat brain. *J Neurochem.* 1980;34:609–613.
14. McCarthy MM, Kaufman LC, Brooks PJ, et al. Estrogen modulation of mRNA for two forms of glutamic acid decarboxylase (GAD) in rat brain. *Neuroscience.* 1993;19:1191.
15. Weiland NG. Glutamic acid decarboxylase messenger ribonucleic acid is regulated by estradiol and progesterone in the hippocampus. *Endocrinology.* 1992;131:2697–2702.
16. Peterson SL, Reeves A, Keller M, et al. Effects of estradiol (E2) and progesterone (P4) on expression of mRNA encoding GABAA receptor subunits. *Neuroscience.* 1993;19:1191.
17. Weiland NG. Estradiol selectively regulates agonist binding sites on the N-methyl-D-aspartate receptor complex in the CA-1 region of the hippocampus. *Endocrinology.* 1992;131:662–668.
18. Smith SS, Waterhouse BD, Chapin JK, et al. Progesterone alters GABA and glutamate responsiveness: a possible mechanism for its anxiolytic action. *Brain Res.* 1987;400:353–359.
19. Smith SS, Waterhouse BD, Woodward DJ. Locally applied progesterone metabolites alter neuronal responsiveness in the cerebellum. *Brain Res Bull.* 1987;18:739–747.
20. Wong M, Moss RL. Patch-clamp analysis of direct steroidal modulation of glutamate receptor-channels. *J Neuroendocrinol.* 1994;6:347–355.
21. Gu Q, Moss RL. 17 Beta-estradiol potentiates kainate-induced currents via activation of the cAMP cascade. *J Neurosci.* 1996;16:3620–3629.
22. Velísková J. Estrogens and epilepsy: why are we so excited. *Neuroscientist.* 2007;13:77–88.
23. Mhyre AJ, Dorsa DM. Estrogen activates rapid signaling in the brain: role of estrogen receptor alpha and estrogen receptor beta in neurons and glia. *Neuroscience.* 2006;138:851–858.
24. Matthews J, Gustafsson JA. Estrogen signaling: a subtle balance between ER alpha and ER beta. *Mol Interv.* 2003;3:281–292.
25. Velísková J, Velísek L, Galanopoulou AS, et al. Neuroprotective effects of estrogens on hippocampal cells in adult female rats after status epilepticus. *Epilepsia.* 2000;41:S30–S35.
26. Reibel S, Andre V, Chassagnon S, et al. Neuroprotective effects of chronic estradiol benzoate treatment on hippocampal cell loss induced by status epilepticus in the female rat. *Neurosci Lett.* 2000;281:79–82.
27. Hoffman GE, Moore N, Fiskum G, et al. Ovarian steroid modulation of seizure severity and hippocampal cell death after kainic acid treatment. *Exp Neurol.* 2003;182:124–134.
28. Harrison NL, Simmonds MA. Modulation of the GABA receptor complex by a steroid anaesthetic. *Brain Res.* 1984;323:287–292.
29. Landgren S, Backstrom T, Kalistratov G. The effect of progesterone on the spontaneous interictal spike evoked by the application of penicillin to the cat's cerebral cortex. *J Neurol Sci.* 1976;36:119–133.
30. Holmes GL, Kloczko N, Weber DA, et al. Anticonvulsant effect of hormones on seizures in animals. In: Porter RJ, Mattson RH, Ward AAM Jr, et al., eds. *Advances in Epileptology. XVth Epilepsy International Symposium.* New York: Raven Press; 1984:265–268.
31. Tauboll E, Lindstrom S. The effect of progesterone and its metabolite 5-alpha-pregnan-3-alpha-ol-20-one on focal epileptic seizures in the cat's visual cortex in vivo. *Epilepsy Res.* 1993;14:17–30.
32. Finn DA, Roberts AJ, Crabbe JC. Neuroactive steroid sensitivity in withdrawal seizure-prone and -resistant mice. *Alcohol Clin Exp Res.* 1995;19:410–415.
33. Wilson MA. Influences of gender, gonadectomy, and estrous cycle on GABA/BZ receptors and benzodiazepine response in rats. *Brain Res Bull.* 1992;29:165–172.
34. Spiegel E, Wycis H. Anticonvulsant effects of steroids. *J Lab Clin Med.* 1945;30:947–953.
35. Rogawski MA, Reddy DS, Neurosteroids: endogenous modulators of seizure susceptibility. In: Rho JM, Sankar R, Cavazos JE, eds. *Epilepsy: Scientific Foundations of Clinical Practice.* New York: Marcel Dekker; 2004:319–355.
36. Reddy DS, Castaneda DC, O'Malley BW, et al. Anticonvulsant activity of progesterone and neurosteroids in progesterone receptor knockout mice. *J Pharmacol Exp Ther.* 2004;310:230–239.
37. Selye H. Antagonism between anesthetic steroid hormones and pentamethylenetetrazol (Metrazol). *J Lab Clin Med.* 1942;27:1051–1053.
38. Frye CA, Rhodes ME, Walf A, et al. Progesterone reduces pentylenetetrazol-induced ictal activity of wild-type mice but not those deficient in type I 5α-reductase. *Epilepsia.* 2002;43(suppl 5):14–17.
39. Lonsdale D, Burnham WM, The anticonvulsant effects of progesterone and 5α-dihydroprogesterone on amygdala-kindled seizures in rats. *Epilepsia.* 2003;44:1494–1499.
40. Kokate TG, Banks MK, Magee T, et al. Finasteride, a 5α-reductase inhibitor, blocks the anticonvulsant activity of progesterone in mice. *J Pharmacol Exp Ther.* 1999;288:679–684.
41. Reddy DS, Rogawski MA. Neurosteroid replacement therapy for catamenial epilepsy. *Neurotherapeutics.* 2009;6(2):392–401.
42. Lambert JJ, Belelli D, Peden DR, et al. Neurosteroid modulation of GABAA receptors. *Prog Neurobiol.* 2003;71:67–80.
43. Akk G, Shu HJ, Wang C, et al., Neurosteroid access to the GABAA receptor. *J Neurosci.* 2005;25:11605–11613.
44. Meldrum BS, Rogawski MA. Molecular targets for antiepileptic drug development. *Neurotherapeutics.* 2007;4:18–61.
45. Glykys J, Mody I. Activation of GABAA receptors: views from outside the synaptic cleft. *Neuron.* 2007;56:763–770.
46. Hosie AM, Wilkins ME, Smart TG. Neurosteroid binding sites on GABAA receptors. *Pharmacol Ther.* 2007;116:7–19.
47. Smith SS, Shen H, Gong QH, et al. Neurosteroid regulation of GABAA receptors: focus on the α4 and δ subunits. *Pharmacol Ther.* 2007;116:58–76.
48. Gulinello M, Gong QH, Li X, et al. Short-term exposure to a neuroactive steroid increases α4 GABAA receptor subunit levels in association with increased anxiety in the female rat. *Brain Res.* 2001;910:55–66.
49. Kaminski RM, Livingood MR, Rogawski MA. Allopregnanolone analogs that positively modulate GABA receptors protect against partial seizures induced by 6-Hz electrical stimulation in mice. *Epilepsia.* 2004;45:864–867.
50. van Luijtelaar G, Budziszewska B, Jaworska-Feil L, et al. The ovarian hormones and absence epilepsy: a long-term EEG study and pharmacological effects in a genetic absence epilepsy model. *Epilepsy Res.* 2001;46:225–239.
51. Stoffel-Wagner B. Neurosteroid biosynthesis in the human brain and its clinical implications. *Ann NY Acad Sci.* 2003;1007:64–78.
52. Reddy DS. Anticonvulsant activity of the testosterone-derived neurosteroid 3α-androstanediol. *Neuroreport.* 2004;15(3):515–518.
53. Edwards HE, Burnham WM, Mendonca A, et al. Steroid hormones affect limbic after discharge thresholds and kindling rates in adult female rats. *Brain Res.* 1999;838:136–150.
54. Pouliot WA, Handa RJ, Beck SG. Androgen modulates N-methyl-D-aspartate-mediated depolarization in CA1 hippocampal pyramidal cells. *Synapse.* 1996;23:10–19.
55. Frye CA, Rhodes ME, Walf AA, et al. Testosterone reduces pentylenetrazole-induced ictal activity of wildtype mice but not those deficient in type I 5alpha-reductase. *Brain Res.* 2001;918:182–186.
56. Kaminski RM, Marini H, Kim W, et al. Anticonvulsant activity of androsterone and etiocholanolone. *Epilepsia.* 2005;46(6):819–827.
57. Reddy DS. Testosterone modulation of seizure susceptibility is mediated by neurosteroids 3-α-androstanediol and 17β-estradiol. *Neuroscience.* 2004;129(1):195–207.
58. Pfaff DW, Keiner M. Atlas of estradiol-concentrating cells in the central nervous system of the female rat. *J Comp Neurol.* 1973;151:121–158.
59. Simerly RB, Chang C, Muramatsu M, et al. Distribution of androgen and estrogen receptor mRNA-containing cells in the rat brain: an in situ hybridization study. *J Comp Neurol.* 1990;294:76–95.
60. Morrow L, Pace JR, Purdy RH, et al. Characterization of steroid interactions with gamma-aminobutyric acid receptor-gated chloride ion channels: evidence for multiple steroid recognition sites. *Mol Pharmacol.* 1989;37:263–270.
61. Sheridan PJ. The nucleus interstitialis striae terminalis and the nucleus amygdaloideus medialis: prime targets for androgen in the rat forebrain. *Endocrinology.* 1979;104:130–136.

62. Michael RP, Bonsall RW, Rees HD. The uptake of (3H) testosterone and its metabolites by the brain and pituitary gland of the fetal macaque. *Endocrinology.* 1989;124:1319–1326.

63. Sar M, Stumpf WE. Distribution of androgen-concentrating neurons in rat brain. In: Stumpf WE, Grant LD, eds. Anatomical neuroendocrinology. Basel, Switzerland: Karger; 1975:120–133.

64. Sarrieau A, Mitchell JB, Lal S, et al. Androgen binding sites in human temporal cortex. *Neuroendocrinology.* 1990;51:713–716.

65. Weiland NG, Orchinik M, Brooks PJ, et al. Allopregnanolone mimics the action of progesterone on glutamate decarboxylase gene expression in the hippocampus. *Neuroscience.* 1993;19:1191.

66. Stumpf WE, Sar M, Keefer DA. Atlas of estrogen target cells in rat brain. In: Stumpf WE, Grant LD, eds. *Anatomical Neuroendocrinology.* Basel, Switzerland: Kanger; 1975:104–119.

67. Dornan WA, Malsbury CW. Neuropeptides and male sexual behavior. *Neurosci Biobehav Rev.* 1989;13:1–15.

68. Bridges RS, DiBiase R, Loundes DD, et al. Prolactin stimulation of maternal behavior in female rats. *Science.* 1985;227:782–784.

69. Boyd AE, Reichlin S. Neural control of prolactin secretion in men. *Psychoneuroendocrinology.* 1978;3:113–130.

70. Pritchard PB, Wannamaker BB, Sagel J, et al. Endocrine function following complex partial seizures. *Ann Neurol.* 1983;14:27–32.

71. Sperling MR, Pritchard PB, Engel J, et al. Prolactin in partial epilepsy: an indicator of limbic seizures. *Ann Neurol.* 1986;20:716–722.

72. Molaie M, Culebras A, Miller M. Nocturnal plasma prolactin and cortisol levels in epileptics with complex partial seizures and primary generalized seizures. *Arch Neurol.* 1984;44:699–702.

73. Dana-Haeri J, Trimble MR, Oxley J. Prolactin and gonadotrophin changes following generalized and partial seizures. *J Neurol Neurosurg Psychiatry.* 1983;46:331–335.

74. Pritchard PB. Hyposexuality: a complication of complex partial epilepsy. *Trans Am Neurol Assoc.* 1980;105:193–195.

75. Martin JB, Reichlin S. *Clinical Neuroendocrinology.* 2nd ed. Philadelphia, PA: FA Davis; 1987.

76. Gloor P. Physiology of the limbic system. In: Penry JK, Daly DD, eds. *Complex Partial Seizures and Their Treatment, Vol. II: Advances in Neurology.* New York: Raven Press; 1975:27–55.

77. Merchenthaler I, Setalo G, Csontos C, et al. Combined retrograde tracing and immunocytochemical identification of luteinizing hormone-releasing hormone- and somatostatin-containing neurons projecting to the median eminence of the rat. *Endocrinology.* 1989;125:2812–2821.

78. Brann DW, Hendry LB, Mahesh VB. Emerging diversities in the mechanism of action of steroid hormones. *J Steroid Biochem Mol Biol.* 1995; 52:113–133.

79. Amado D, Cavalheiro EA, Bentivoglio M. Epilepsy and hormonal regulation: the patterns of GnRH and galanin immunoreactivity in the hypothalamus of epileptic female rats. *Epilepsy Res.* 1993;14(2):149–159.

80. Friedman MN, Geula C, Holmes GL, Herzog AG. GnRH-immunoreactive fiber changes with unilateral amygdala-kindled seizures. *Epilepsy Res.* 2002;52(2):73–77.

81. Meo R, Bilo L, Nappi C, et al. Derangement of the hypothalamic GnRH pulse generator in women with epilepsy. *Seizure.* 1993;2:241–252.

82. Herzog AG, Drislane FW, Schomer DL, et al. Abnormal pulsatile secretion of luteinizing hormone in men with epilepsy: relationship to laterality and nature of paroxysmal discharges. *Neurology.* 1990;40:1557–1561.

83. Drislane FW, Coleman AE, Schomer DL, et al. Altered pulsatile secretion of luteinizing hormone in women with epilepsy. *Neurology.* 1994;44: 306–310.

84. Quigg M, Kiely JM, Shneker B, et al. Interictal and postictal alterations of pulsatile secretions of luteinizing hormone in temporal lobe epilepsy in men. *Ann Neurol.* 2002;51:559–566.

85. Morell MJ, Sauer M, Guidice L. Pituitary gonadotropin function in women with epilepsy. *Epilepsia.* 2000;41(suppl 7):247.

86. Morell MJ. Reproductive and metabolic disorders in women with epilepsy. *Epilepsia.* 2003;44(suppl 4):11–20.

87. Morrell MJ, Giudice L, Flynn KL, et al. Predictors of ovulatory failure in women with epilepsy. *Ann Neurol.* 2002;52:704–711.

88. Quigg M, Kiely JM, Johnson ML, et al. Interictal and postictal circadian and ultradian luteinizing hormone secretion in men with temporal lobe epilepsy. *Epilepsia.* 2006;47(9):1452–1459.

89. Scharfman HE, Kim M, Hintz TM, et al. Seizures and reproductive function: insights from female rats with epilepsy. *Ann Neurol.* 2008;64(6): 687–697.

90. Bauer J, Isojärvi JIT, Herzog AG, et al. Reproductive dysfunction in women with epilepsy: Recommendations for evaluation and management. *J Neurol Neurosurg Psychiatry.* 2002;73:121–125.

91. Beastall GH, Cowan RA, Gray JM, et al. Hormone binding globulins and anticonvulsant therapy. *Scott Med J.* 1985;30:101–105.

92. Murialdo G, Galimberti CA, Gianelli MV, et al. Effects of valproate, phenobarbital and carbamazepine on sex steroid setup in women with epilepsy. *Clin Neuropharmacol.* 1988;21:52–58.

93. Stoffel-Wagner B, Bauer J, Flügel D, et al. Serum sex hormones are altered in patients with chronic temporal lobe epilepsy receiving anticonvulsant medication. *Epilepsia.* 1998;39:1164–1173.

94. Victor A, Lundberg PO, Johansson ED. Induction of sex hormone binding globulin by phenytoin. *Br Med J.* 1977;2(6092):934–935.

95. Isojärvi JIT, Löfgren E, Juntunen KST, et al. Effect of epilepsy and antiepileptic drugs on male reproductive health. *Neurology.* 2004;62: 247–253.

96. Herzog AG, Drislane FW, Schomer DL, et al. Differential effects of antiepileptic drugs on sexual function and reproductive hormones in men with epilepsy. *Neurology.* 2005;65:1016–1020.

97. Bauer J, Blumenthal S, Reuber M, et al. Epilepsy syndrome, focus localization, and treatment choice affect testicular function in men with epilepsy. *Neurology.* 2004;62:243–246.

98. Lossius MI, Taubøll E, Mowinckel P, et al. Reversible effects of antiepileptic drugs on reproductive endocrine function in men and women with epilepsy—a prospective randomized double-blind withdrawal study. *Epilepsia.* 2007;48(10):1875–1882.

99. Löfgren E, Tapanainen JS, Koivunen R, et al. Effects of carbamazepine and oxcarbazepine on the reproductive endocrine function in women with epilepsy. *Epilepsia.* 2006;47(9):1441–1446.

100. Stephen LJ, Sills GJ, Leach JP, et al. Sodium valproate versus lamotrigine: a randomised comparison of efficacy, tolerability and effects on circulating androgenic hormones in newly diagnosed epilepsy. *Epilepsy Res.* 2007;75(2–3):122–129.

101. Killer N, Hock M, Gehlhaus M, et al. Modulation of androgen and estrogen receptor expression by antiepileptic drugs and steroids in hippocampus of patients with temporal lobe epilepsy. *Epilepsia.* 2009;50(8): 1875–1890. [Epub ahead of print]

102. Tempkin O. *The Falling Sickness: A History of Epilepsy from the Greeks to the Beginnings of Modern Neurology.* Baltimore, MD: Johns Hopkins Press; 1945.

103. Locock C. Discussion. In: Sieveking EH, ed. Analysis of fifty-two cases of epilepsy observed by the author. *Med Times Gaz.* 1857;14:524–526.

104. Sherman BM, Korenman SG. Measurement of serum LH, FSH, estradiol and progesterone in disorders of the human menstrual cycle: the inadequate luteal phase. *J Clin Endocrinol Metab.* 1974;39:145–149.

105. Jones GS. The luteal phase defect. *Fertil Steril.* 1976;27:351–356.

106. Kawakami M, Sawyer CH. Neuroendocrine correlates of changes in brain activity thresholds by sex steroids and pituitary hormones. *Endocrinology.* 1959;65:652–668.

107. Wooley DE, Timiras PS. Gonad-brain relationship: effects of castration and testosterone on convulsions in the rat. *Endocrinology.* 1962;71: 609–617.

108. Finn DA, Ostrom R, Gee KW. Estrus cycle and sensitivity to convulsants and the anticonvulsant effect of 3 α-hydroxy-5α-pregnan-20-one(3α,5α-P). *Neuroscience.* 1993;19:1539.

109. Finn DA, Gee KW. The estrous cycle, sensitivity to convulsants and the anticonvulsant effect of a neuroactive steroid. *J Pharmacol Exp Ther.* 1994;271:164–170.

110. Teyler TJ, Vardaris RM, Lewis D, et al. Gonadal steroids: effects on excitability of hippocampal pyramidal cells. *Science.* 1980;209:1017–,1029.

111. Morrell MJ, Hamdy SF, Seale CG, et al. Self-reported reproductive history in women with epilepsy: puberty onset and effects of menarche and menstrual cycle on seizures. *Neurology.* 1998;50:448.

112. Marques-Assis L. Influencia da menstruação sobre as epilepsias. *Arq Neuropsiquiatr.* 1981;39:390–395.

113. Duncan S, Read CL, Brodie MJ. How common is catamenial epilepsy? *Epilepsia.* 1993;34:827–831.

114. Herzog AG, Klein P, Ransil BJ. Three patterns of catamenial epilepsy. *Epilepsia.* 1997;38:1082–1088.

115. El-Khayat HA, Soliman NA, Tomoum HY, et al. Reproductive hormonal changes and catamenial pattern in adolescent females with epilepsy. *Epilepsia.* 2008;49(9):1619–1626.

116. Hussain Z, Qureshi MA, Hasan KZ, et al. Influence of steroid hormones in women with mild catamenial epilepsy. *J Ayub Med Coll Abbottabad.* 2006;18(3):17–20.

117. Murialdo G, Magri F, Tamagno G, et al. Seizure frequency and sex steroids in women with partial epilepsy on antiepileptic therapy. *Epilepsia.* 2009;50(8):1920–1926. [Epub ahead of print]

118. Quigg M, Fowler KM, Herzog AG, NIH Progesterone Trial Study Group. Circalunar and ultralunar periodicities in women with partial seizures. *Epilepsia.* 2008;49(6):1081–1085.

119. Kumar N, Behari M, Aruja GK, et al. Phenytoin levels in catamenial epilepsy. *Epilepsia.* 1988;29:155–158.

120. Rosciszewska D, Buntner B, Guz I, et al. Ovarian hormones, anticonvulsant drugs, and seizures during the menstrual cycle in women with epilepsy. *J Neurol Neurosurg Psychiatry.* 1986;49:A47–A51.

121. Bäckström T, Jorpes P. Serum phenytoin, phenobarbital, carbamazepine, albumin; and plasma estradiol, progesterone concentrations during the menstrual cycle in women with epilepsy. *Acta Neurol Scand.* 1979; 59(2–3):63–71.

122. Galimberti CA, Magri F, Copello F, et al. Changes in sex steroid levels in women with epilepsy on treatment: relationship with antiepileptic therapies and seizure frequency. *Epilepsia.* 2009;50(suppl 1):28–32.

123. Alexander W. The surgical treatment of some forms of epilepsy. *Lancet.* 1911;2:932.

124. McQuarrie I, Peeler DB. The effects of sustained pituitary antidiuresis and forced water drinking in epileptic children. A diagnostic and etiologic study. *J Clin Invest.* 1931;10:915–940.

125. Stubbe Teglbjaerg HP. Investigations on epilepsy and water metabolism. *Acta Psychiat Neurol.* 1936;(suppl IX):44–165.

126. Ansell B, Clarke E. Epilepsy and menstruation. The role of water retention. *Lancet.* 1956;2:1232–1235.

127. Poser CM. Modification of therapy for exacerbation of seizures during menstruation. *J Pediatr.* 1974;84:779–780.

128. Ansell B, Clarke E. Acetazolamide in treatment of epilepsy. *Br Med J.* 1956;1:650–661.

129. Feely M, Calvert R, Gibson J. Clobazam in catamenial epilepsy: a model for evaluating anticonvulsants. *Lancet.* 1982;2:71–73.

130. Zimmerman AW, Holden KR, Reiter EO, et al. Medroxyprogesterone acetate in the treatment of seizures associated with menstruation. *J Pediatr.* 1973;83:959–963.

131. Mattson RH, Cramer JA, Caldwell BV, et al. Treatment of seizures with medroxyprogesterone acetate: preliminary report. *Neurology.* 1984;34:1255–1258.

132. Herzog AG. Intermittent progesterone therapy of partial complex seizures in women with menstrual disorders. *Neurology.* 1986;36:1607–1610.

133. Herzog AG. Progesterone therapy in women with complex partial and secondary generalized seizures. *Neurology.* 1995;45:1660–1662.

134. Herzog A. Progesterone therapy in women with epilepsy: a 3-year follow-up. *Neurology.* 1999;52:1917–1918.

135. Jesperson B, Nielson H. Sexual dysfunction in male and female patients with epilepsy: a study of 86 outpatients. *Arch Sex Behav.* 1990;19:1–14.

136. Herzog AG, Seibel MM, Schomer DL, et al. Reproductive endocrine disorders in men with partial seizures of temporal lobe origin. *Arch Neurol.* 1986;43:347–350.

137. Blumer D, Walker AE. Sexual behavior in temporal lobe epilepsy. *Arch Neurol.* 1967;16:37–43.

138. Hierons R, Saunders M. Impotence in patients with temporal lobe lesions. *Lancet.* 1966;2:761–764.

139. Taylor DC. Sexual behavior and temporal lobe epilepsy. *Arch Neurol.* 1969;21:510–516.

140. Demerdash A, Shaalon M, Midori A, et al. Sexual behavior of a sample of females with epilepsy. *Epilepsia.* 1991;32:82–85.

141. Troisi A. Sexual disorders in the context of Darwinian psychiatry. *Endocrinol Invest.* 2003;26(suppl 3):54–57.

142. Basson R, Berman J, Burnett A, et al. Report of the international consensus development conference on female sexual dysfunction: definitions and classifications. *J Urol.* 2000;163:888–897.

143. Dennerstein L, Hayes RD. Confronting the challenges: epidemiological study of female sexual dysfunction and the menopause. *J Sex Med.* 2005;2(suppl 3):118–132.

144. McMahon CG, Abdo C, Incrocci L, et al. Disorders of orgasm and ejaculation in men. *J Sex Med.* 2004;1:58–65.

145. Morales A, Buvat J, Gooren LJ, et al. Endocrine aspects of sexual dysfunction in men. *J Sex Med.* 2004;1:69–81.

146. Isidori AM, Gianetta E, Gianfrilli D, et al. Effects of testosterone on sexual function in men: results of a meta-analysis. *Clin Endocrinol.* 2005;63:381–394.

147. Baird AD, Wilson SJ, Bladin PF, et al. The amygdala and sexual drive: insights from temporal lobe epilepsy surgery. *Ann Neurol.* 2004;55:87–96.

148. Baird AD, Wilson SJ, Bladin PF, et al. Sexual outcome after epilepsy surgery. *Epilepsy Behav.* 2003;4:268–278.

149. Herzog AG, Coleman AE, Jacobs AR, et al. Relationship of sexual dysfunction to epilepsy lateralization and reproductive hormone levels in women. *Epilepsy Behav.* 2003;4:407–413.

150. Morrell MJ, Sperling MR, Stecker M, et al. Sexual dysfunction in partial epilepsy: a deficit in physiologic sexual arousal. *Neurology.* 1994;44:243–247.

151. Baker GA, Nashef L, Van Hout BA. Current issues in the management of epilepsy: the impact of frequent seizures on cost of illness, quality of life, and mortality. *Epilepsia.* 1997;38(suppl 1):S1–S8.

152. Morrell MJ. Sexuality in epilepsy. In: Engel J, Pedley TA, eds. *Epilepsy: A Comprehensive Textbook.* New York: Lippincott-Raven; 1997:2021–2026.

153. Jensen SB. Sexuality and chronic illness: biopsychosocial approach. *Semin Neurol.* 1992;12:135–140.

154. Fawley JA, Pouliot WA, Dudek FE. Epilepsy and reproductive disorders: the role of the gonadotropin-releasing hormone network. *Epilepsy Behav.* 2006;8(3):477–482.

155. Herzog AG, Seibel MM, Schomer DL, et al. Reproductive endocrine disorders in women with partial seizures of temporal lobe origin. *Arch Neurol.* 1986;43:341–346.

156. Rodin E, Subramanian MG, Gilroy J. Investigation of sex hormones in male epileptic patients. *Epilepsia.* 1984;25:690–694.

157. Spark RF, Willis CA, Royal H. Hypogonadism, hyperprolactinemia and temporal lobe epilepsy in hyposexual men. *Lancet.* 1984;1:413–417.

158. Sakuma Y. Brain control of female sexual behavior. In: Yokoyama A, ed. *Brain Control of the Reproductive System.* Tokyo: Japan Scientific Societies Press; 1992:141–155.

159. Bergen D, Daugherty S, Eckenfels E. Reduction of sexual activities in females taking antepileptic drugs. *Psychopathology.* 1992;25:1–4.

160. Jensen P, Jensen SB, Sorensen PS, et al. Sexual dysfunction in male and female patients with epilepsy: a study of 86 outpatients. *Arch Sex Behav.* 1990;19:1–14.

161. Duncan S, Blacklaw J, Beastall GH, et al. Sexual function in women with epilepsy. *Epilepsia.* 1997;38:1074–1081.

162. Morrell MJ, Flynn KL, Done S, et al. Sexual dysfunction, sex steroid hormone abnormalities, and depression in women with epilepsy treated with antiepileptic drugs. *Epilepsy Behav.* 2005;6:360–365.

163. Morrell MJ, Guldner GT. Self-reported sexual function and sexual arousability in women with epilepsy. *Epilepsia.* 1996;37:1204–1210.

164. Maes M, Calabrese JR. Mechanisms of action of valproate in affective disorders. In: Joffe RT, Calabrese JR, eds. *Anticonvulsants in Mood Disorders.* New York: Marcel Dekker; 1994:100–101.

165. Grant AC, Oh H. Gabapentin-induced anorgasmia in women [letter]. *Am J Psychiatry.* 2002;159:1247.

166. Mattson RH, Cramer JA, Collins JF, et al. Comparison of carbamazepine, phenobarbital, phenytoin, and primidone in partial and secondarily generalized tonic-clonic seizures. *N Engl J Med.* 1985;313:145–151.

167. Gil-Nagel A, Lopez-Munoz F, Serratosa JM, et al. Effect of lamotrigine on sexual function in patients with epilepsy. *Seizure.* 2006;15:142–149.

168. El-Khayat HA, Shatla HM, Ali GK, et al. Physical and hormonal profile of male sexual development in epilepsy. *Epilepsia.* 2003;44:447–452.

169. Luef G, Krämer G, Stefan H. Oxcarbazepine treatment in male epilepsy patients improves pre-existing sexual dysfunction. *Acta Neurol Scand.* 2009;119(2):94–99.

170. Talbot JA, Sheldrick R, Caswell H, et al. Sexual function in men with epilepsy: how important is testosterone? *Neurology.* 2008;70(16):1346–1352.

171. Clinckers R, Smolders I, Meurs A, et al. Hippocampal dopamine and serotonin elevations as pharmacodynamic markers for the anticonvulsant efficacy of oxcarbazepine and 10,11-dihydro-10-hydroxycarbamazepine. *Neurosci Lett (Ireland).* 2005;390(1):48–53.

172. Daniele A, Azzoni A, Bizza A, et al. Sexual behavior and hemispheric laterality of the focus in the patients with temporal lobe epilepsy. *Biol Psychiatry.* 1997;42:617–624.

173. Ozkara C, Ozdemir S, Yilmaz A, et al. Orgasm-induced seizures: a study of six patients. *Epilepsia.* 2006;47(12):2193–2197.

174. Gerendai I, Halasz B. Asymmetry of the neuroendocrine system. *News Physiol Sci.* 2001;16:92–95.

175. Hum KM, Megna S, McIntyre Burnham W. The effects of right and left amygdala kindling on the female reproductive system in rats. *Epilepsia.* 2009;50(4):880–886.

176. Bartlik BD, Rosenfeld S, Beaton C. Assessment of sexual functioning: sexual history taking for health care practitioners. *Epilepsy Behav.* 2005;7(suppl 2):S15–S21.

177. McGahuey CA, Gelenberg AJ, Laukes CA, et al. The Arizona Sexual Experience Scale (ASEX): reliability and validity. *J Sex Marital Ther.* 2000;26(1):25–40.

178. Harden C, MacLusky NJ. Aromatase inhibitors as add-on treatment for men with epilepsy. *Exp Rev Neurother.* 2005;5(1):123–127.

179. Schwenkhagen A, Studd J. Role of testosterone in the treatment of hypoactive sexual desire disorder. *Maturitas.* 2009;63(2):152–159.

180. Klein P, Serje A, Pezzullo JC. Premature ovarian failure in women with epilepsy. *Epilepsia.* 2001;42:1584–1589.

181. Harden CL, Koppel BS, Herzog AG, et al. Seizure frequency is associated with age of menopause in women with epilepsy. *Neurology.* 2003;61:451–455.

182. Harden CL, Pulver MC, Jacobs AR. The effect of menopause and perimenopause on the course of epilepsy. *Epilepsia.* 1999;40:1402–1407.

183. Burger HG, Dudley EC, Robertson DM, et al. Hormonal changes in the menopause transition. *Recent Prog Horm Res.* 2002;57:257–275.

184. Harden CL, Herzog AG, Nikolov BG, et al. Hormone replacement therapy in women with epilepsy: a randomized, double-blind, placebo-controlled study. *Epilepsia.* 2006;47(9):1447–1451.

185. Harden CL, Leppik I. Optimizing therapy of seizures in women who use oral contraceptives. *Neurology.* 2006;67(12 suppl 4):S56–S58.

186. Kalkbrenner KA, Standley CA. Estrogen modulation of NMDA-induced seizures in ovariectomized and non-ovariectomized rats. *Brain Res.* 2003;964(2):244–249.

187. Galanopoulou AS, Alm EM, Velísková J. Estradiol reduces seizure-induced hippocampal injury in ovariectomized female but not in male rats. *Neurosci Lett.* 2003;342(3):201–205.

188. Ciriza I, Carrero P, Frye CA, et al. Reduced metabolites mediate neuroprotective effects of progesterone in the adult rat hippocampus. The synthetic progestin medroxyprogesterone acetate (Provera) is not neuroprotective. *J Neurobiol.* 2006;66:916–928.

189. Rosario ER, Ramsden M, Pike CJ. Progestins inhibit the neuroprotective effects of estrogen in rat hippocampus. *Brain Res.* 2006;1099(1):206–210.

190. Peebles CT, McAuley JW, Moore JL, et al. Hormone replacement therapy in a postmenopausal woman with epilepsy. *Ann Pharmacother.* 2000;34(9):1028–1031.

191. Azziz R, Carmina E, Dewailly D, et al. Task Force on the Phenotype of the Polycystic Ovary Syndrome of the Androgen Excess and PCOS Society. The Androgen Excess and PCOS Society criteria for the polycystic ovary syndrome: the complete task force report. *Fertil Steril.* 2009;91(2):456–488.

192. Nisenblat V, Norman RJ. Androgens and polycystic ovary syndrome. *Curr Opin Endocrinol Diabetes Obes.* 2009;16(3):224–231.
193. Rasgon N. The relationship between polycystic ovary syndrome and antiepileptic drugs. *J Clin Psychopharmacol.* 2004;24(3):322–334.
194. Azziz R, Woods KS, Reyna R, et al. The prevalence and features of the polycystic ovarian syndrome in an unselected population. *J Clin Endocrinol Metab.* 2004;89(6):2745–2749.
195. Bauer J, Jarre A, Klingmuller M, et al. Polycystic ovary syndrome in patient with focal epilepsy: a study in 93 women. *Epilepsy Res.* 2000; 41(2):163–167.
196. Isojarvi JIT, Laatikainen TJ, Pakarinen AJ, et al. Polycystic ovaries and hyperandrogenism in women taking valproate for epilepsy. *N Eng J Med.* 1993;329:1383–1388.
197. Nelson-De Grave VL, Wickenheisser JK, Cockrell JE, et al., Valproate potentiates androgen biosyntheses in human ovarian theca cells. *Endocrinology.* 2004;145(2):799–808.

198. Tauboll E, Gregoaszczuk EL, Kolodziej A, et al. Valproate inhibits the conversion of testosterone to estradiol and acts as an apoptotic agent in growing porcine ovarian follicular cells. *Epilepsia.* 2003;44(8):1014–1021.
199. Pylvänen V, Pakarinen A, Knip M, et al. Characterization of insulin secretion in Valproate-treated patients with epilepsy. *Epilepsia.* 2006;47(9): 1460–1464.
200. Artama M, Isojärvi JI, Raitanen J, et al. Birth rate among patients with epilepsy: a nationwide population-based cohort study in Finland. *Am J Epidemiol.* 2004;159(11):1057–1063.
201. Löfgren E, Pouta A, von Wendt L, et al. Epilepsy in the northern Finland birth cohort 1966 with special reference to fertility. *Epilepsy Behav.* 2009;14(1):102–107.
202. Scharfman HE, Malthankar-Phatak GH, Friedman D, et al. A rat model of epilepsy in women: a tool to study physiological interactions between endocrine systems and seizures. *Endocrinology.* 2009;150(9):4437–4442 [Epub ahead of print].

CHAPTER 45 ■ TREATMENT OF EPILEPSY DURING PREGNANCY

PAGE B. PENNELL

Treatment during pregnancy in women with epilepsy involves a precarious balancing act between the teratogenic risks of antiepileptic drugs (AEDs) and maintaining maternal seizure control. However, pregnancy registries and other prospective studies have given us invaluable information on how to optimize treatment regimens for the safety of the mother and for the developing fetus, as well as information about safety of breast-feeding. These detailed data should be a key consideration when counseling and treating women with epilepsy.

Epilepsy is the most common neurologic disorder that requires continuous treatment during pregnancy, and AEDs are one of the most frequent chronic teratogen exposures (1,2). Over 1 million women with epilepsy in the United States are in their active reproductive years and give birth to over 24,000 infants each year (3). However, it is estimated that the total number of children in the United States exposed in utero to AEDs is nearly two times that amount with the emergence of AED use for other illnesses including headache, chronic pain, and mood disorders. Although some of the other disorders may allow for discontinuation of the AED prior to a planned pregnancy, most women with epilepsy do not have the luxury of discontinuing AEDs without re-emergence or worsening of seizures.

The vast majority of women with epilepsy will have a normal pregnancy with a favorable outcome, but there are increased maternal and fetal risks compared to the general population (3). Careful planning and management of any pregnancy in a woman with epilepsy is essential to minimize these risks. The reduction of these risks begins with preconceptional planning. The initial visit between the physician and a woman with epilepsy of childbearing age should include a discussion about family planning. Topics should include effective birth control, the importance of planned pregnancies with AED optimization, and folic acid supplementation beginning prior to conception, obstetrical complications, and teratogenicity of AEDs versus the risks of seizures during pregnancy. The goal is effective control of maternal seizures with the least risk to the fetus.

BIRTH CONTROL FOR WOMEN ON ANTIEPILEPTIC DRUGS

Several AEDs induce the hepatic cytochrome P450 system, the primary metabolic pathway of the sex steroid hormones. This leads to rapid clearance of steroid hormones and may allow ovulation in women taking oral contraceptives or other hormonal forms of birth control (4–6). The 1998 guidelines by the American Academy of Neurology recommend use of an

TABLE 45.1

AED EFFECTS ON HORMONAL CONTRACEPTIVE AGENTS

Lowers hormone levels	No significant effects
Phenobarbital	Ethosuximide
Phenytoin	Valproate
Carbamazepine	Gabapentin
Primidone	Lamotrigine
Topiramate	Tiagabine
Oxcarbazepine	Levetiracetam
	Zonisamide

estradiol dose of 50 μg or its equivalent for 21 days of each cycle when using oral contraceptive agents with the enzyme-inducing AEDs (7), although no studies have addressed whether this improves contraceptive efficacy (8,9). Some experts state that it is the progestin component that is more important than the estrogen to prevent ovulation, but the combined oral contraceptive pills with a higher estradiol dose usually also have higher progestin content. Since this may still not be adequate protection against pregnancy, a backup barrier method is recommended. Table 45.1 lists effects of the individual AEDs on hormonal contraceptive agents (4,5,10,11). The transdermal patch and vaginal ring formulations also have higher failure rates with these AEDs since they also rely on serum hormonal levels. Intramuscular medroxyprogesterone provides higher dosages of progestin but still may require dosing at 8- to 10-week intervals rather than 12-week intervals. The effects of intrauterine devices (IUDs) are based on action at the local level of the endometrium, and thus AEDs do not reduce their high protective rates against unplanned pregnancies.

THE FETAL ANTICONVULSANT SYNDROME

Offspring of women with epilepsy on AEDs are at an increased risk for minor anomalies, major congenital malformations, cognitive dysfunction, small for gestational age birthweight, and low APGAR scores at birth (3,12–14). The term "fetal anticonvulsant syndrome" is used to include various combinations of these findings and has been described with virtually all of the AEDs.

Minor Anomalies

Minor anomalies are defined as structural deviations from the norm that do not constitute a threat to health. Minor anomalies affect 6% to 20% of infants born to women with epilepsy, an approximately 2.5-fold increased rate compared to the general population (15). Minor anomalies seen in infants of mothers on AEDs include distal digital and nail hypoplasia, low hairline, posteriorly rotated low-set ears, and the midline craniofacial anomalies (broad nasal bridge, ocular hypertelorism, epicanthal folds, short upturned nose, long philtrum, and altered lips). Many of the craniofacial anomalies are outgrown by age 5 years, but the digital and nail hypoplasias are more likely to persist.

Major Malformations

Major congenital malformations (MCMs) are defined as an abnormality of an essential anatomical structure present at birth that interferes significantly with function and/or requires major intervention. The reported MCM rates in the general population vary between 1.6% and 3.2% (16), and women with a history of epilepsy but of no AEDs show similar MCM rates (17,18). The average MCM rates among all AED exposures vary between 3.1% and 9%, or approximately 1.7- to 4-fold higher than the general population (12,13,19). Reported MCM rates in monotherapy exposures as a single group are 2.3% to 7.8%, while AED polytherapy exposures as a group carry an average MCM rate of 6.5% to 18.8% (13,19).

MCMs (Table 45.2) most commonly associated with AED exposure include congenital heart disease, cleft lip/palate, urogenital defects, and neural tube defects (NTDs) (13,15,19). The congenital heart defects include atrial septal defect, ventricular septal defect, patent ductus arteriosus, pulmonary stenosis, coarctation of the aorta, and tetralogy of Fallot. Urogenital defects commonly involve glandular hypospadias. NTDs are malformations of the central nervous system and its membranes due to faulty neuralation or abnormal development of the neural tube. The NTDs associated with AEDs tend to be the severe open defect spina bifida aperta, frequently complicated by hydrocephaly and other midline defects (12,20). The evidence is most convincing for valproate (VPA) exposure in utero contributing to NTDs as well as facial clefts and hypospadias (12,21). The abnormal neural tube closure usually occurs between the third and fourth weeks of gestation. By the time most women realize they are pregnant,

TABLE 45.2

MAJOR CONGENITAL MALFORMATIONS IN INFANTS OF WOMEN WITH EPILEPSY

Malformations	General population (%)	Infants of women with epilepsy (%)
Congenital heart	0.5	1.5–2
Cleft lip/palate	0.15	1.4
Neural tube defect	0.06	1–3.8 (VPA)
Urogenital defects	0.7	1.7

TABLE 45.3

RELATIVE TIMING AND DEVELOPMENTAL PATHOLOGY OF CERTAIN MALFORMATIONS (116)

Tissues	Malformations	Postconceptional age
CNS	Neural tube defect	28 days
Heart	Ventricular septal defect	42 days
Face	Cleft lip	36 days
	Cleft maxillary palate	47–70 days

it is too late to make medication adjustments to avoid malformations (Table 45.3).

AED Polytherapy During Pregnancy

The risk for MCMs is consistently higher across studies for women on AED polytherapy regimens compared to women on AED monotherapy regimens (12,13,19). The UK Epilepsy and Pregnancy Register collected prospective, full outcome data on 3607 cases (21). MCMs detected within the first 3 months of life were included. The overall MCM rate for all AED exposures was 4.2% (95% CI: 3.6% to 5.0%). The MCM rate was higher for polytherapy than monotherapy (6.0% vs. 3.7%; crude odds ratio [OR] = 1.63 [$P = 0.010$], adjusted OR = 1.83 [$P = 0.002$]). The MCM rate for the monotherapy group did not differ substantially from the group of women with epilepsy on no AEDs during pregnancy, 3.5% (95% CI: 1.8% to 6.8%). In another study, the rate of major malformations increased to 25% for those women on four or more AEDs (20). A study in Japan reported on 172 deliveries; the infants exposed to AED monotherapy had a malformation rate of 6.5%, whereas the infants exposed to polytherapy had a malformation rate of 15.6% ($P = 0.01$) (22). A prospective study in southeast France also reported that the rate of malformations was higher in infants exposed to polytherapy (15%) than in those exposed to monotherapy (5%) ($P < 0.01$) (23). These consistent results have led to the recommendation that AED monotherapy is preferred to polytherapy during pregnancy and should be achieved during the preconception planning phase (12).

Individual AEDs and MCM During Pregnancy

Although features of the fetal anticonvulsant syndrome have been described in association with virtually all of the AEDs, there are some notable differences in the likelihood of occurrence of any MCM and of specific malformations with the different AEDs (13,19).

Valproate

The UK Epilepsy and Pregnancy Register reported that polytherapy combinations containing valproate carried a higher risk of MCM than combinations not containing valproate (OR = 2.49 [95% CI: 1.31 to 4.70]) (21). Additionally, comparisons between monotherapy regimens did reveal a statistically significant increased MCM rate for pregnancies exposed to valproate (6.2% [95% CI: 4.6% to 8.2%]) compared to those exposed to carbamazepine (CBZ) (2.2% [1.4% to 3.4%], [adjusted OR = 2.97 (P < 0.001)]). Although a lower MCM rate was identified for pregnancies exposed to lamotrigine (LTG) (3.2% [95% CI: 2.1% to 4.9%]), the adjusted OR = 0.59 compared to the valproate group was not statistically significant (P = 0.064). The positive dose trend for VPA did not reach statistical significance (9.1% for doses > 1000 mg/day vs. 5.1% for doses ≤ 1000 mg/day).

Artama et al. (24) reported that the risk for MCMs was higher specifically in offspring of women taking VPA as monotherapy (OR 4.18 [2.31 to 7.57]) or as polytherapy (OR 3.54 [1.42 to 8.11]) compared to untreated WWE. The risk did not appear elevated in offspring of women on CBZ, oxcarbazepine (OXC), or PHT, but the number of women on these specific AEDs could have limited the positive findings.

Prospective data from the North American AED Pregnancy Registry (25) reported that with first-trimester VPA monotherapy exposures (n = 149), major birth defects occurred in 10.7% (6.3 to 16.9) of infants, as compared with 2.8% in infants exposed to other AED monotherapies and 1.6% in external control infants (RR 7.3 [4.4 to 12.2]). Perhaps more helpful to the clinician choosing between AEDs, the RR was 4.0 (2.1 to 7.4) compared to the internal comparison group, which were offspring of women on other AED monotherapies. The Australian Pregnancy Registry also demonstrated a higher percentage of births with MCMs with VPA in comparison to the other monotherapies combined (16.0% vs. 2.4%) (40). Additionally, a significant dose–effect was demonstrated; the incidence of MCMs with VPA doses >1100 mg was 30.2% versus 3.2% with doses <1100 mg. Meador et al. (26) replicated the findings of increased risk of VPA exposure compared to other monotherapies as a combined group (CBZ, LTG, PHT) with an RR of 4.59 (2.07 to 10.18). These significant differences were maintained when individually compared to each of the AED monotherapies, and the effect for VPA was dose-dependent. A study examining the Swedish Medical Birth Registry directly compared VPA and CBZ-exposed pregnancies; the authors reported that exposure to VPA monotherapy compared with CBZ monotherapy provided an OR of 2.51 (1.43 to 4.68) for a diagnosis of MCMs (27).

Other studies have supported a dose relationship for VPA, with an increased risk for MCMs with VPA doses above approximately 1000 mg/day or with levels above 70 mcg/mL (24,28–31).

Several studies have reported an increased risk of NTDs with VPA (21,28,32,33). One analysis pooling data from five prospective studies suggested that the absolute risk with VPA monotherapy may be as high as 3.8% for NTDs (34). Increased risks for hypospadias and facial clefts have also been reported (21,28,32).

The consistent findings of these large prospective pregnancy registries scattered across different regions of the world reveal a consistent pattern of amplified risk for the development of MCM in pregnancies exposed to VPA.

Carbamazepine

In an analysis by Samrén et al. (34) of the European prospective studies, the RR for a MCM in children exposed to CBZ monotherapy was 4.9 (95% CI 1.3 to 18.0). For NTDs, Rosa (35) reported that 1% of CBZ-exposed infants had spina bifida. Data from an ongoing case-control study in the United States and Canada compared data on 1242 infants with NTDs with data from a control group of infants with malformations not related to vitamin supplementation. They reported that the adjusted odds ratio of NTDs related to exposure to CBZ was 6.9 (95% CI 1.9 to 25.7) (36). A recent review pooled data from prospective studies and analyzed 1255 cases of exposure to CBZ (37). Among the CBZ-exposed children, 85 (6.7%) were described as having major congenital anomalies compared with 88 (2.34%) of 3756 control children (P < 0.05; OR = 3.02; 95% CI 2.56 to 4.56). The risk for major congenital anomalies was highest when CBZ was used in polytherapy combinations, with a rate of 18.8% (n = 99) versus 5.28% for those exposed to CBZ monotherapy. In this study, the MCMs most commonly reported were NTDs, cardiovascular and urinary tract anomalies, and cleft palate. However, in other studies the most convincing association for CBZ is an increased risk of oral clefts. An analysis of the dataset of the population-based Hungarian Case-Control Surveillance of Congenital Abnormalities, 1980 to 1996, reported an increased risk for posterior cleft palate (38). Holmes et al. recently reported on findings with CBZ monotherapy from the North American AED Pregnancy Registry (39). An increased risk for cleft lip or cleft palate was noted, occurring in 0.57% of the newborns, with an RR of 24 (95% CI 7.9 to 74.4). The overall rate of MCM was 2.5% (95% CI 1.6% to 3.7%) in 873 infants, with an RR of 1.6 (95% CI 0.9 to 2.8) compared to the external comparison group. Therefore, the possible specific risk of oral clefts with CBZ use during pregnancy should be considered in light of the relatively small risk for all MCMs combined together; the UK Pregnancy Register study suggested no increased risk for MCMs for CBZ (n = 927 outcomes) (RR 0.63 [0.28 to 1.41]) and CBZ was associated with the lowest risk of MCM for all monotherapy exposures (21).

Phenytoin

Pregnancy registries and other prospective studies have reported on relatively small number of outcomes for phenytoin (PHT). MCM rates vary between 3.4% and 10.7% (17,21,26,28,40). The finding of an increased risk for the specific MCM of cleft palate was also reported for PHT by the Hungarian Case-Control Surveillance of Congenital Abnormalities (38).

Phenobarbital

Prospective data from the North American AED Pregnancy Registry is available for phenobarbital. Of 77 women who received PB monotherapy, five of the infants had confirmed MCMs (6.5%; 95% CI 2.1% to 14.5%). When compared to the background rate for MCMs in this hospital-based pregnancy registry (1.62%), the RR is 4.2, with a 95% CI of 1.5 to 9.4 (41). Major malformations in exposed infants included one cleft lip and palate and four heart defects. Two other studies reported an increased risk of cardiac malformations associated with PB (32,29).

Lamotrigine

For first-trimester exposure to LTG monotherapy in the North American AED Pregnancy Registry, the rate of MCM reported was 2.3% (95% CI 1.3% to 3.8%) in 684 infants, with an RR of 1.4 (95% CI 0.9 to 2.3) compared to the external comparison group, which was not statistically significant (42). However, increased risk for cleft lip or cleft palate was noted, occurring in 0.73% of the newborns, with an RR of 10.4 (95% CI 4.3 to 24.9) in comparison to the unexposed group. Review of five other pregnancy registries revealed that of 1623 infants exposed to LTG as monotherapy, prevalence for oral clefts was 2.5/1000 (RR: 3.8, 95% CI: 1.4 to 10.0). The UK Pregnancy Register did not see an increase in oral clefts (43). A population-based case-control study based on EUROCAT congenital anomaly registers included a large number of births from 19 registries in the years 1995 to 2005 but a relatively small number of LTG exposures. This study found no evidence for a specific increased risk of isolated orofacial clefts relative to other malformations due to LTG monotherapy (44).

The UK Pregnancy Register reported in 2006 that the MCM rate for pregnancies exposed to LTG was 3.2% (2.1 to 4.9); the adjusted OR 0.59 compared to the VPA group did not quite reach statistical significance ($P = 0.064$). A positive dose response for MCMs was found for LTG ($P = 0.006$), with reports of an MCM rate for doses >200 mg/day of 5.4% (3.3 to 8.7) (21). The investigators more recently refined their findings with a larger number of pregnancies and reported that the increased risk appeared above 400 mg/day during the first trimester (platform presentation at 2007 AES Annual Meeting, Pregnancy Outcomes SIG).

Data from the International Lamotrigine Pregnancy Registry were analyzed to examine the effect of maximal first-trimester maternal dose of LTG monotherapy on the risk of MCMs (45). Among 802 exposures, the frequency of MCMs was 2.7% (95% CI 1.8% to 4.2%). The distribution of dose did not differ between infants with and those without MCMs (mean 248.3 mg/day and 278.9 mg/day, respectively; median 200 mg/day for both groups). A logistic regression analysis showed no difference in the risk of MCMs as a continuous function of dose (summary OR per 100 mg increase = 0.999, 95% CI 0.996 to 1.001). There was also no effect of dose up to 400 mg/day on the frequency of MCMs.

Other studies also support a low overall rate of MCMs, including the Neurodevelopmental Effect of Antiepileptic Drugs (NEAD) study (26). Serious adverse outcomes, defined as fetal death and/or MCM, occurred in only 1.0% of LTG pregnancies, compared to 8.2% of CBZ, 10.7% of PHT, and 20.3% of VPA pregnancies. The UK Pregnancy Register recently updated their outcome data for 1151 live births exposed to LTG as monotherapy in utero, reporting an even lower MCM rate of 2.4% (95% CI 1.7% to 3.5%) (43).

Levetiracetam

The UK Epilepsy and Pregnancy Register recently reported outcomes for 117 pregnancies exposed to levetiracetam (LEV) (46). Three had MCMs (2.7%; 95% CI 0.9% to 7.7%), but all three of these were exposed to AED polytherapy. Updated numbers from the UK Epilepsy and Pregnancy Register are available (personal communication, Stephen Hunt, UK Pregnancy Register). As of the end of November 2008, of 132 first-trimester exposures collected prospectively, there were 123 live births, 1 stillbirth, 1 induced abortion, 7 spontaneous abortions, and no major congenital malformations, MCM rate 0% (95% CI 0% to 3.0%).

The Keppra (Levetiracetam) Pregnancy Registry, sponsored by UCB, reported on 237 prospectively enrolled pregnancies with 238 known outcomes (47). Of these, 214 had a first-trimester exposure. Among the prospectively enrolled cases, birth defects were reported in nine live births, and four of these were with LEV monotherapy first-trimester exposure. Of the nine prospective and two retrospective birth defect cases, four had cardiac defects consisting of ventricular septal defects. This particular finding is being monitored closely as more cases are enrolled.

Other AEDs

The newest generation of AEDs consists of a large number of structurally diverse compounds, most of which have demonstrated teratogenic effects in preclinical animal experiments. With the exception of LTG and possibly LEV, none have sufficient human pregnancy experience to assess their safety or teratogenicity. Human birth defects have been reported with oxcarbazepine (OXC), topiramate (TPM), gabapentin (GBP), tiagabine (TGB), zonisamide (ZNS), pregabalin, and lacosamide, but accurate denominators are not available to calculate rates. Preliminary reports of experience with some of these agents during pregnancy are reported below, but prospective population-based studies in postmarketing evaluation with larger numbers of outcomes are essential to establish safety in human pregnancies.

A series of gabapentin exposures during pregnancy evaluated prospective and retrospective outcomes for 51 fetuses of women with epilepsy and other disorders, with 44 live births. No malformations were seen in the 11 patients on GBP monotherapy. Two newborns had MCMs with polytherapy exposure (VPA, PB) and one had minor anomalies (LTG) (48). However, the number of outcomes is too small to make any definitive conclusions.

The UK Epilepsy and Pregnancy Register also reported on findings with topiramate (49) use in 203 pregnancies resulting in 178 live births. Of these cases, 70 were monotherapy use, with 3 MCMs (4.8%; 95% CI 1.7% to 13.3%). The MCM rate for polytherapy exposures that included TPM was 11.2% (95% CI 6.7% to 18.2%). They also noted a particularly higher rate of oral clefts (2.2%; 95% CI 0.9% to 5.6%), approximately 11 times their background rate, and a high rate of hypospadias (5.1%; 95% CI 0.2% to 10.1%) among the 78 live male births, 2 of which were classified as MCMs.

A case series from Argentina included 35 women on OXC monotherapy and all infants were healthy; of the 20 infants exposed to polytherapy with OXC, 1 had a cardiac malformation (50). The prospective study from Denmark (51) included 37 women on OXC, and 2 (5%) had infants with major malformations, both VSD. One of the mothers was on OXC monotherapy and one on OXC with low-dose LTG.

One case series reported on 26 pregnancies with zonisamide exposure (52). Two of the 26 fetuses (7.7%) had major malformations, although one of these was exposed to PHT also and the other to PHT and VPA.

Prenatal Screening

Women on AEDs during pregnancy should be encouraged to undergo adequate prenatal screening to detect any fetal major malformations (3). Although only a fraction of women may consider therapeutic abortions, the prenatal diagnosis of a cardiac malformation or NTD allows the appropriate specialist to establish any special plans for labor, delivery, and neonatal care. Surgical interventions are often indicated immediately after birth and prenatal interventions are becoming more plausible for some of the cardiac defects.

Transvaginal ultrasonography can be performed early to detect the most severe defects (53). NTDs should be screened for with a combination of maternal serum alpha-fetoprotein at 15 to 22 weeks and expert, targeted Level II (structural) ultrasound at 16 to 20 weeks (54). The latter ideally should be performed by a perinatologist. These tests can identify over 95% of fetuses with open NTDs (3,55–57). Amniocentesis (with measurements of amniotic fluid alpha-fetoprotein and acetylcholinesterase) is not performed routinely but should be offered if these tests are equivocal, increasing the sensitivity for detection of NTDs to greater than 99%. Detailed sonographic imaging of the fetal heart can be performed at 18 to 20 weeks gestation, and may be followed by fetal echocardiography if visualization is suboptimal or any concerns arise. However, some experts now recommend fetal echocardiography for all pregnancies in a higher risk category. One retrospective audit of a cardiac database in South Australia reported that fetal echocardiography had 95.2% sensitivity, 99.5% specificity, 99.0% positive predictive value, and 97.6% negative predictive value for congenital heart defects, and that outflow tract lesions were most commonly missed by routine obstetric ultrasounds (58). Careful imaging of the fetal face for cleft lip and palate can also be performed at 18 to 20 weeks gestational age, but the sensitivity is often greater if repeated at 24 to 28 weeks. The accuracy of prenatal diagnosis is less established (56). If the patient's weight gain and fundal growth do not appear appropriate, serial sonography should be performed to assess fetal size and amniotic fluid (59).

NEURODEVELOPMENTAL OUTCOME

Studies investigating cognitive outcome in children of women with epilepsy report an increased risk of mental deficiency, affecting 1.4% to 6% of children of women with epilepsy, compared to 1% of controls (13,60). Verbal scores on neuropsychometric measures may be selectively more involved (61). A variety of factors contribute to the cognitive problems of children of mothers with epilepsy, but AEDs appear to play a major role. For example, children of mothers with epilepsy have an increased risk of developmental delay but not children of fathers with epilepsy. Furthermore, two studies reported that children of women with epilepsy on no AEDs during pregnancy demonstrate no differences in IQ compared to control children (62,63).

Exposure during the last trimester may actually be the most detrimental (64). Factors other than specific AED use have been associated with cognitive impairment, including

seizures (65), a high number of minor anomalies, major malformations, decreased maternal education, impaired maternal–child relations, and maternal partial seizure disorder (66). It is possible that these risk factors are not only additive but potentially synergistic.

A retrospective survey in the United Kingdom suggested an especially high risk of VPA for the neurodevelopment of children exposed in utero (67). Compared to children of women with epilepsy on no AEDs, the odds ratios for additional educational needs were 1.49 for all children exposed to AEDs in utero and 3.4 for children exposed to VPA monotherapy.

A prospective study conducted in Finland tested 182 preschool or school-age children that had prenatal exposure to AEDs and compared them to 141 control children. Eighty-six children were exposed to CBZ monotherapy and 13 to VPA. The CBZ group actually demonstrated no differences from controls in their mean verbal and nonverbal IQ scores. Significantly reduced verbal IQ scores were found in the polytherapy group and in the VPA monotherapy group (62). The positive finding of reduced cognitive outcomes in children exposed to AED polytherapy in utero has been reported in other studies (68,69). Other studies have replicated lack of reduced cognitive outcomes in children exposed to CBZ in utero (70,71).

A follow-up study from the same UK group performed a battery of neuropsychological tests on mother–child pairs on 249 children ages 6 to 16 years old. Children with in utero exposure to VPA had a significant reduction in verbal IQ (10 to 14 points) when compared to children exposed to other AED monotherapies or the general population (71,72). Other significant predictors of verbal IQ were the mother's IQ and the number of convulsive seizures (72). Greater than five convulsive seizures during pregnancy had a negative effect on verbal IQ (71).

One group analyzed two cohorts of adult men exposed in utero to PB and reported reduced cognitive abilities compared to normative populations (reduced IQ by 0.5 standard deviation [SD]) (64). Reports of outcomes from PHT exposure in utero demonstrated an increased risk for poor cognitive outcomes compared to unexposed controls (70,73,74).

The multicenter, observational study NEAD is an ongoing prospective study that spans 25 epilepsy centers in the United States and the United Kingdom. The primary aim of the study is a comparison of neurodevelopmental outcomes at age 6 years to determine whether outcomes are different among four different monotherapy exposures in utero (LTG, CBZ, VPA, and PHT). Findings of an interim analysis of cognitive outcomes at age 3 years in 309 children were recently released (75). Children exposed in utero to VPA had significantly lower IQ at age 3 than those exposed to other AEDs. Mean IQs (adjusted for maternal IQ, age, AED dose, gestational age at birth, and maternal folic acid supplementation) were: LTG = 101, PHT = 99, CBZ = 98, VPA = 92. The mean IQ differences between each of the three AED groups and VPA were all significant ($P < 0.05$), and the association between VPA and IQ was dose-dependent.

The findings of increased risk for neurodevelopmental consequences with exposure to AED polytherapy or to VPA, and possibly with exposure to PHT, PB, or frequent convulsive seizures should be considered by the prescribing physician and included in the discussion with women with epilepsy.

Mortality

Fetal death (fetal loss at greater than 20 weeks gestational age) may be another increased risk for women with epilepsy (3), although reports from various groups are conflicting. Reported stillbirth rates may vary between 1.3% and 14.0% compared to rates of 1.2% to 7.8% for women without epilepsy (60). Perinatal death rates may also be up to twofold higher for women with epilepsy (1.3% to 7.8%) compared to controls (1.0% to 3.9%). Spontaneous abortions (<20 weeks gestational age) may also occur more frequently, although figures from different studies vary considerably (3,76). The lack of consistent findings is not surprising given the overall low occurrence rates and lack of consistent reporting systems.

Other Neonatal Risks

One population-based study in Finland from 1989 to 2000 included 179 singleton pregnancies of women with epilepsy and 24,778 singleton pregnancies of unaffected controls (77). The rate of small-for-gestational-age (SGA) infants was significantly higher, and the head circumference was significantly smaller in the children born to the WWE. Compared to controls, APGAR scores at 1 min were lower in children of WWE, and the need for care in the neonatal ward and neonatal intensive care was increased. Another study reported a similar twofold risk of SGA for neonates of WWE taking AEDs compared to the expected rate (14).

POTENTIAL MECHANISMS

The causes of the "anticonvulsant embryopathy" are likely multifactorial. However, recent studies have supported that the AEDs are the most significant offending factor, more so than actual traits carried by mothers with epilepsy, environmental factors, or seizures during pregnancy. Teratogenecity by AEDs is likely mediated by several mechanisms, including antifolate effects and reactive intermediates of AEDs (13). Phenytoin, carbamazepine, phenobarbital, and primodone are associated with folic acid deficiency, and valproic acid and lamotrigine interfere with folic acid metabolism (78,79). One treatment paradigm that is generally accepted as being important is the use of supplemental folic acid prior to conception and during pregnancy in women on AEDs (54,80). However, the established benefits of supplemental folic acid are based on studies of women without epilepsy in the general population (81,82) or women at high risk for NTDs, with a positive family history. Studies specifically investigating effects of fetal AED exposure have failed to show a protective effect against major malformations with folic acid administration. These findings either could be due to folic acid's inability to impact AED teratogenic mechanisms or, possibly, to the prescription of inadequate dosage levels of folic acid. The North American AED Pregnancy Registry reported that among the 505 infants born to the study participants, 34 (6.7%) had a major malformation; maternal use of folic acid at the time of conception was not associated with a statistically significant reduction in risk of having an infant with a major malformation (83). The study did not discuss the dose of folic acid, and perhaps folic acid supplementation at higher doses will be more preventive in this special population of women with epilepsy taking AEDs. Some experts, including the American and Canadian Obstetricians and Gynecologists organizations, recommend at least 4 to 5 mg/day of supplemental folic acid, especially if the woman is on VPA (84). However, given the lack of evidence for benefits of folic acid in women on AEDs at any particular dose, the AAN Practice Parameter Update only recommends a minimum of 0.4 mg daily of folic acid (12).

For all women of childbearing age, the maximal benefit of folic acid is achieved only with folic acid supplementation beginning prior to and continuing after conception. Because of this as well as the high rates of unplanned pregnancies and of late contact with a physician, all women with epilepsy of childbearing potential should be placed on folic acid supplementation of at least 0.4 mg/day.

Reactive intermediates of AEDs include free radicals (via peroxidation reactions) and oxidative metabolites, both of which may contribute to AED teratogenesis (85). AED polytherapy may especially promote epoxide production and inhibit epoxide metabolism via epoxide hydrolase. Fetuses may benefit from AEDs which lack epoxide intermediates (such as oxcarbazepine, gabapentin) and avoidance of polytherapy.

SEIZURES DURING PREGNANCY

The effect of pregnancy on seizure frequency is variable. Approximately 20% to 33% of patients will have an increase in their seizures, 7% to 25% a decrease in seizures, and 50% to 83% will experience no significant change (86,87).

The physiologic changes and psychosocial adjustments that accompany pregnancy can alter seizure frequency, including changes in sex hormone concentrations, changes in AED metabolism, sleep deprivation, and new stresses. Noncompliance with medications is common during pregnancy and is in large part due to the strong message that any drugs during pregnancy are harmful to the fetus. Teratogenic effects of AEDs are well described, but risks to the fetus are often exaggerated or misrepresented. Proper education about the risks of AEDs versus the risks of seizures can be very helpful in assuring compliance during pregnancy.

The risk of seizures to the fetus should be discussed thoroughly with the patient and other family members. Generalized tonic–clonic seizures (GTCS) can cause maternal and fetal hypoxia and acidosis (3,88). After a single GTCS, fetal intracranial hemorrhages (85), miscarriages, and stillbirths have been reported (89). A single brief tonic–clonic seizure has been shown to cause depression of fetal heart rate for more than 20 min (90), and longer or repetitive tonic–clonic seizures are incrementally more hazardous to the fetus as well as the mother. Status epilepticus is an uncommon complication of pregnancy, but when it does occur it carries a high maternal and fetal mortality rate.

It is not as clear what the effects of nonconvulsive seizures are on the developing fetus. One case report described that during labor a complex partial seizure was associated with a strong, prolonged uterine contraction with fetal heart rate deceleration for 3.5 minutes (91). Many types of seizures can cause trauma, which can result in ruptured fetal membranes with an increased risk of infection, premature labor, and

TABLE 45.4

ALTERATIONS OF AED CLEARANCE AND/OR CONCENTRATIONS DURING PREGNANCY: SUMMARY OF CLASS I, II, AND III STUDIES[a] (94)

AED	Reported increases in clearance	Reported decreases in total concentrations	Reported changes in free AED or metabolites
PHT	19–150%	60–70%	Free PHT clearance increased in TM3 by 25%; free PHT concentration decreased by 16–40% in TM3
CBZ	−11 to +27%	0–12%	No change
PB	60%		
	55%	Decrease in free PB concentration by 50%	
PRM	Inconsistent	Inconsistent	Decrease in derived PB concentrations, with lower PB/PRM ratios
VPA	Increased by TM2 and TM3		No change in clearance of free VPA; free fraction increased by TM2 and TM3
ESX	Inconsistent	Inconsistent	
LTG	65–230%, substantial interindividual variability		89% increase in clearance of free LTG
OXC		MHD and active moiety decreased by 36–61%	
LEV	243%	60% by TM3	

AED, antiepileptic drug; TM, trimester; PHT, phenytoin; CBZ, carbamazepine; PRM, primidone; PB, phenobarbital; VPA, valproic acid; ESX, ethosuximide; LTG, lamotrigine; OXC, oxcarbazepine; MHD, monohydroxy derivative of oxcarbazepine; LEV, levetiracetam.
[a]From Pennell PB, Hovinga CA. Antiepileptic drug therapy in pregnancy I: gestation-induced effects on AED pharmacokinetics. *Int Rev Neurobiol.* 2008;83:227–240, with permission.

even fetal death (92). Abruptio placenta occurs after 1% to 5% of minor and 20% to 50% of major blunt injuries (93). Restrictions from driving and climbing heights should be reinforced with each patient with special emphasis on the risk to the fetus of what could otherwise seem to be a trivial injury. In addition to the physical risks of seizures to the developing fetus, re-emergence of seizures in a woman who had previously experienced seizure control can be devastating. Besides the immediate risk to herself and the fetus, the loss of the ability to drive legally can have remarkable psychosocial effects.

ANTIEPILEPTIC DRUG MANAGEMENT AND SEIZURE CONTROL

Management of AEDs during pregnancy can be complex. Clearance of most of the AEDs increases during pregnancy, resulting in a decrease in serum concentrations (Table 45.4) (8,95). Several physiologic factors contribute to the decline in AED levels during pregnancy (Table 45.5). Important mechanisms include decreased albumin concentration and induction of the hepatic microsomal enzymes by the increased sex steroid hormones.

Observations on seizure control and treatment were reported from the international EURAP Epilepsy Pregnancy Registry (86). Data was obtained from 1956 pregnancies in 1882 women with epilepsy. Seizure control during the second and third trimesters was compared to the first trimester. The

majority of women (58.3%) were seizure-free throughout pregnancy. Seizure frequency remained unchanged throughout pregnancy in 63.6%, was increased in 17.3%, and decreased in 15.9%. Factors that were associated with an increased risk for occurrence of all seizures were localization-related epilepsy (OR: 2.5; 1.7 to 3.9) and polytherapy (OR: 9.0; 5.6 to 14.8).

TABLE 45.5

PHYSIOLOGIC CHANGES DURING PREGNANCY: EFFECTS ON DRUG DISPOSITION (94)

Parameter	Consequences
↑ Total body water, extracellular fluid	Altered drug distribution
↑ Fat stores	↓ Elimination of lipid soluble drugs
↑ Cardiac output	↑ Hepatic blood flow leading to ↑ elimination
↑ Renal blood flow and glomerular flow rate	↑ Renal clearance of unchanged drug
Altered cytochrome P450 activity and UGT activity	Altered systemic absorption and hepatic elimination
↓ Maternal albumin	Altered free fraction; increased availability of drug for hepatic extraction

[a]From Pennell PB, Hovinga CA. Antiepileptic drug therapy in pregnancy I: gestation-induced effects on AED pharmacokinetics. *Int Rev Neurobiol.* 2008;83:227–240, with permission.

OXC monotherapy was associated with a greater risk for occurrence of convulsive seizures (OR: 5.4; 1.6 to 17.1). The number or dosage of AEDs were more often increased in pregnancies with seizures (OR: 3.6; 2.8 to 4.7) or pregnancies treated with OXC monotherapy (OR: 3.7; 1.1 to 12.9) or LTG monotherapy (OR: 3.8; 2.1 to 6.9). This international, observational study did not dictate a protocol to monitor serum levels or make dosage adjustments. The apparently higher risk of convulsive seizures among women treated with OXC and the need to increase dose or other meds with OXC or LTG monotherapy is consistent with similar major routes of elimination via glucuronidation.

Lamotrigine

The magnitude of alterations in LTG concentrations exceeds that described for many of the older AEDs, which are primarily eliminated via the cytochrome P450 system (64–96). Approximately 90% of LTG undergoes hepatic glucuronidation, catalyzed by UGT1A4, an isozyme of the UGT family of enzymes. This elimination pathway appears particularly susceptible to activation during pregnancy, most likely as a result of direct effects of rising sex steroid hormone levels.

An early retrospective study reported an approximately 150% increase in LTG Cl in the second and third trimesters of pregnancy ($n = 11$) (97), associated with seizure worsening in 45% of the pregnancies and specifically occurring in women that had >60% change in level/dose ratio. Other studies also noted up to 75% of women experienced seizure worsening during pregnancies on LTG or complications of convulsive seizures, status epilepticus, and even fetal loss (96,98,99).

Two Class II studies showed an increase in the LTG clearance (95,96). A more recent Class I study by Pennell et al. (100) of 53 pregnancies in 53 women, using 305 samples throughout preconception baseline, pregnancy, and postpartum reported that both free LTG and total clearance were increased during all three trimesters, with peaks of 94% (total) and 89% (free) in the third trimester. Clearance of free LTG was significantly higher in white patients as compared to black patients. These studies noted substantial interindividual variability, which may be related to UGT polymorphism variants. This study also examined therapeutic drug monitoring and seizure frequency, and changes in LTG dosing to avoid postpartum toxicity. The authors reported that seizure frequency significantly increased when the LTG level decreased to 65% of the preconceptional individualized target LTG concentration. This finding supports the recommendation to monitor levels of LTG and possibly other AEDs for which the levels decrease during pregnancy.

Previous studies on LTG noted a rapid decrease in LTG Cl during the early postpartum period with reports of symptomatic toxicity (96,98). Pennell et al. (100) also examined the effectiveness of using an empiric postpartum taper schedule for LTG, with steady decreases in dosing at postpartum days 3, 7, and 10, with return to preconception dose or preconception dose plus 50 mg to help counteract the effects of sleep deprivation. Patients were assessed for symptoms of LTG toxicity (dizziness, imbalance, and blurred or double vision). Nonadherence to the standard taper schedule was associated with significantly higher risk of experiencing postpartum toxicity ($P = 0.040$).

Oxcarbazepine

The discovery that glucuronidation can be activated by hormonal shifts may apply to other AEDs. Metabolism of VPA is 30% to 50% by glucuronidation, and 50% to 60% of the clearance of OXC is via glucuronidation. Two Class III studies have examined OXC concentrations during pregnancy. Christensen et al. (101) reported retrospectively on nine pregnancies in seven women. The mean dose-corrected concentration of MHD was decreased during pregnancy ($P = 0.0016$), being 72% (SD = 13%) in the first trimester, 74% (SD = 17%) in the second trimester, 64% (SD = 6%) in the third trimester, and 108% (SD = 18%) after pregnancy versus dose-corrected concentration before pregnancy. Mazzucchelli et al. (102) reported on five pregnancies, with measurements of OXC, its active R-($-$)- and S-($+$)-monohydroxy derivatives (MHD), and the metabolite carbamazepine-10,11-trans-dihydrodiol (DHD) at regular intervals. The active moiety was defined as the molar sum of OXC, R-($-$)-MHD, and S-($+$)-MHD. Alterations were significant for R-($-$)-MHD ($P < 0.02$) and borderline for the active moiety ($P = 0.086$). The mean concentration per 100 mg dose was 45% lower in the second trimester compared to the puerperium.

Levetiracetam

Levetiracetam (LEV) is primarily eliminated via renal excretion (66%), with the remainder via extrahepatic hydrolysis. One Class II study prospectively examined LEV trough concentrations in 15 pregnancies in 14 women every trimester and at least 1 month postpartum (103). Tomson et al. reported that in the seven women without dosage changes, plasma LEV concentrations during the third trimester were only 40% of baseline concentrations outside pregnancy ($P < 0.001$). For all 12 pregnancies, clearance of LEV was significantly higher during the third trimester with an increase from mean ($\pm$SD) 124.7 $\pm$ 57.9 L/day at baseline to 427.3 $\pm$ 211.3 ($P < 0.0001$), an increase of 243%.

Carbamazepine

A prospective study by Tomson et al. (104) was fairly large with 50 pregnancies including 35 on CBZ monotherapy without a change in dosage. Total CBZ concentration decreased in TM2 by 9% and TM3 by 12%; free CBZ concentrations and total and free CBZ-epoxide concentrations were unchanged. Other studies have supported that changes occur, but of relatively small magnitude (105). CBZ binds to both albumin and α_1-acid glycoprotein (AGP), which may work together to resist changes in protein binding during pregnancy.

Phenobarbital

Studies of PB during pregnancy are limited, but they do suggest an increase in clearance throughout pregnancy (94). Yerby et al. (106) reported that the mean concentrations of total PB declined by 55% as pregnancy progressed ($P < 0.005$), with the sharpest decline during the first trimester. Free concentration decreases of PB were statistically significant ($P < 0.005$), with a decrease of 50%. Despite prospectively studying only seven women on phenobarbital monthly during pregnancy, Lander et al. reported that the mean ratio of PB plasma clearance in the third trimester to clearance in the pre- or postpregnancy state was 1.6:1 ($P < 0.001$) (107).

Phenytoin

Previous studies of PHT suggest that apparent clearance increases during pregnancy by 20% to 150% and is often associated with increased seizures (94). PHT clearance decreases again to pregestational levels over the first 12 weeks postpartum. Although the ratio of free PHT to total plasma drug concentration increases during pregnancy, most studies have reported that the actual free-drug concentration still declines significantly. Tomson et al. (104) performed a population-based prospective study of 93 pregnancies in 70 women with epilepsy. The vast majority were on AED monotherapy, with 29 patients on PHT monotherapy and seven on polytherapy. Dosages were kept constant unless poor seizure control occurred. Total PHT levels decreased steadily throughout pregnancy and by 61% at the end, but free levels only dropped by 16% compared to baseline. Yerby et al. (106) reported that the mean concentration of PHT declined by 56% ($P \leq 0.005$), with the sharpest decline occurring during the first trimester. Although the free concentrations did not change as dramatically, the free concentrations of PHT during all three trimesters were significantly different from baseline ($P < 0.05$), with an overall decrease in free concentration of 31%.

In summary, many of the AEDs studied are characterized by significant increases in clearance during the course of pregnancy. The evidence is most convincing for gestational-induced increases in the clearance of LTG, PHT, and CBZ (albeit to a small amount that is of questionable clinical importance). Evidence is fairly convincing for OXC, LEV, and PB. Evidence is less robust or contradictory for VPA, ESX, and PRM (80,94). However, even for the AEDs well studied, details of individual predictability of magnitude of alterations and time course of alterations are lacking. Since there is evidence that decreased AED levels during pregnancy are associated with seizure worsening, monitoring of concentrations should be considered for LTG, free PHT, total and free CBZ, and possibly for OXC (MHD), LEV, and free PB (80). However, because of the myriad of factors that can contribute to the decrease in all AED concentrations during pregnancy (including noncompliance, enhanced metabolism, and excretion) and large intraindividual and interindividual variability, some authors have recommended at least monthly monitoring of all AED concentrations, with obtaining free (unbound) measurements for those medications that are highly protein bound (60,94). For each individual patient, the ideal AED (free) level should be established prior to conception, and should be the level at which seizure control is the best possible for that patient without debilitating side effects. Future studies with formal pharmacokinetic modeling of each of the AEDs during pregnancy in women with epilepsy could be very helpful in achieving an optimal balance between minimizing neonatal exposure to the deleterious influences of both AEDs and seizures.

OBSTETRICAL COMPLICATIONS

Many reports in the literature have raised the concern that women with epilepsy may have an increased risk of certain obstetrical complications, including vaginal bleeding, hyperemesis gravidarum, anemia, eclampsia, abruptio placentae, preterm delivery, and the need for induced labor, interventions during labor, and/or cesarean section (3). However, a recent rigorous review of the literature found good evidence that there is probably no substantially increased risk (greater than two times expected) of Cesarean delivery, of late-pregnancy bleeding, of premature contractions or premature labor and delivery (108). There is possibly a substantially increased risk of premature contractions and premature labor and delivery during pregnancy for the women with epilepsy who continue to smoke during pregnancy.

NEONATAL VITAMIN K DEFICIENCY

Previous reports raised the concern that many of the AEDs may inhibit vitamin K transport across the placenta (109,110), including CBZ, PHT, PB, PRM. The reports included changes in prothrombin and PIVKA-II levels in umbilical cord blood in the newborns exposed to these AEDs in utero (110). Due to the potential seriousness of a hemorrhagic disorder in a newborn with high neonatal mortality, the 1998 guidelines recommend prophylactic treatment with vitamin K_1 administered orally as 10 mg to the mother during the last month of pregnancy and 1 mg administered intramuscularly or intravenously to the newborn at birth (7). All newborns in the United States are supposed to receive 1 mg intramuscularly or intravenously at birth. However, the need for oral supplemental vitamin K in the mother's preterm was reconsidered in the Practice Parameter Updates for Management Issues for Women with Epilepsy during Pregnancy (80). An analysis of the studies that actually looked at neonatal hemorrhagic complications in newborns of WWE taking AEDs, excluding studies that looked solely at surrogate markers, determined that there is inadequate evidence to determine if the newborns of WWE taking AEDs have a substantially increased risk of hemorrhagic complications.

Labor and Delivery

The majority of women with epilepsy will not experience seizures during labor and delivery. One research group reported that in their epilepsy population only 1% to 2% of women had generalized tonic–clonic seizures during labor, and an additional 1% to 2% had seizures during the first 24 hours after delivery (111). However, seizures during labor and delivery may be more likely to occur in women with primary generalized epilepsy, with one study reporting an occurrence rate in 12.5% compared to 0% of women with partial epilepsy (112). Sleep deprivation may provoke seizures and obstetric anesthesia may be used to allow for some rest prior to delivery if sleep deprivation has been prolonged. The specific analgesic meperidine should be avoided because of its potential to lower seizure threshold.

During a prolonged labor, oral absorption of AEDs may be erratic and any emesis will confound the problem. Phenobarbital, (fos)phenytoin, levetiracetam, and valproic acid can be given intravenously at the same maintenance dosage. Convulsive seizures and repeated seizures during labor should be treated promptly with parenteral lorazepam or valium. Benzodiazepines can cause neonatal respiratory depression, decreased heart rate, and maternal apnea if given in large doses, and these potential side effects need to be monitored closely. If convulsive seizures occur, oxygen should be administered to the patient and she should be placed on her left side to increase uterine blood flow and decrease the risk of maternal aspiration (59). Prompt cesarean section may need to be performed when repeated GTCS cannot be controlled during labor or when the mother is unable to cooperate during labor because of impaired awareness during repetitive absence or complex partial seizures; however this occurs very rarely (111).

POSTPARTUM CARE

Most of the antiepileptic drug levels gradually increase after delivery and plateau by 10 weeks postpartum. AED levels should be followed closely during this postpartum period. LTG levels, however, increase immediately and plateau within 2 to 3 weeks postpartum. Adjustments in LTG doses may need to be made on an anticipatory basis beginning within the first few days after delivery (100).

Perinatal lethargy, irritability, and feeding difficulties have been attributed to intrauterine exposure to benzodiazepines and barbiturates, and breast-feeding on these medications may prolong sedation and feeding problems. However, most infants of women with epilepsy can successfully breast-feed without complications. The concentrations of the different AEDs in breast milk are considerably less than those in maternal serum (Table 45.6). The infant's serum concentration is determined by this factor as well as the AED elimination half-life in neonates, which is usually more prolonged than that in adults (113,114). A detailed study of excretion of LTG into breast milk, infant serum concentrations, and infant laboratory studies supports breast-feeding (115). The benefits of breast-feeding are believed to outweigh the small risk of adverse effects of AEDs. The parents should be advised to watch for signs of increased lethargy to a degree that interferes with normal growth and development.

TABLE 45.6

ANTIEPILEPTIC DRUG EXPOSURE THROUGH BREAST MILK (114)

AEDs	Breast milk/maternal concentration	Adult half-life	Neonate half-life
CBZ	0.36–0.41	8–25	8–36
PHT	0.06–0.19	12–15	15–105
PB	0.36–0.46	75–125	100–500
ESX	0.86–1.36	32–60	32–38
PRM	0.72	4–12	7–60
VPA	0.01–0.1	6–20	30–60
LTG	0.5–0.77	30	—
ZNS	0.41–0.93	63	61–109
TPM	0.86	21	24
GBP	0.7–1.3	7–9	14
OXC	0.5–0.65	19.3	17–22
LEV	0.8–1.3	6–8	16–18

AED, antiepileptic drug; CBZ, carbamazepine; PHT, phenytoin; PB, phenobarbital; ESX, ethosuximide; PRM, primidone; VPA, valproic acid; LTG, lamotrigine; TPM, topiramate; ZNS, zonisamide; OXC, oxcarbazepine; LEV, levetiracetam.

The puerperium and its inevitable sleep disruption are often a time of seizure worsening and may even provoke seizure recurrence for women with previously controlled seizures. Extra precautions should be taken during this time. Appropriate individualized safety issues must consider the mother's ictal semiology. If she is likely to drop objects she is holding but remain upright, such as with myoclonic seizures or many complex partial seizures, then she should use a harness when carrying the baby. If she is likely to fall, then a stroller within the house is an even better option. Changing diapers and clothes are best performed on the floor rather than on an elevated changing table. Bathing should never be performed alone, as a brief lapse in attention can result in a fatal drowning. The important role that sleep deprivation plays in exacerbation of seizures needs to be emphasized. Especially if the mother is breast-feeding, sleep deprivation may be unavoidable. The possibility of other adults sharing the burden of night-time feedings through the use of formula or harvested breast milk should be considered, and the mother should attempt to make up any missed sleep during the infant's daytime naps.

SUMMARY

Improving maternal and fetal outcomes for women with epilepsy involves effective preconceptional counseling and preparation. The importance of planned pregnancies with effective birth control should be emphasized, with consideration of the effects of the enzyme-inducing AEDs on lowering efficacy of hormonal contraceptive medications.

Before pregnancy occurs, the patient's diagnosis and treatment regimen should be reassessed. Once the diagnosis of epilepsy is confirmed, it is important to verify whether that individual patient continues to need medications and whether she is on the most appropriate AED to balance control of her seizures against teratogenic risks. For most women with epilepsy, withdrawal of all AEDs prior to pregnancy is not a realistic option. In the vast majority of cases requiring continued AED therapy, monotherapy at the lowest effective dose should be employed. If large daily doses are needed, then frequent smaller doses or extended-release formulations may be helpful to avoid high peak levels. Some of the newest information about differential risks between AEDs must be considered. The consistent findings of increased risk for MCMs and neurodevelopmental delay with VPA use during pregnancy should enter into the physician's daily treatment decisions. Given that 50% of pregnancies are unplanned in the United States, prescribing AEDs to females during their reproductive years should be performed with the constant consideration of pregnancy, planned or unplanned. AED monotherapy is the goal, possibly at the lowest effective dose for seizure control. With the now recurring signals of concern for VPA, other medication trials in an individual patient are not only strongly recommended but necessary to decrease the risk of fetal consequences. For women who fail other AEDs and require VPA, the dose should be limited if possible. Folic acid supplementation should be encouraged in all women of childbearing age on any AED and for any indication. Dosing recommendations vary between 0.4 mg and 5 mg daily. The woman's AED regimen should be optimized and folic acid supplementation should begin prior to pregnancy.

If a woman with epilepsy presents after conception on a single AED that is effective, her medication should usually not be changed. Exposing the fetus to a second agent during a crossover period of AEDs only increases the teratogenic risk, and seizures are more likely to occur with any abrupt medication changes. If a woman is on polytherapy, it may be possible to safely switch to monotherapy. Maintaining seizure control during pregnancy is important, and monitoring of serum AED levels can help achieve that goal.

Prenatal screening can detect major malformations in the first and second trimesters. Although women on AEDs for epilepsy, or for other indications, do have increased risks for maternal and fetal complications, these risks can be considerably reduced with effective preconceptional planning and careful multidisciplinary management during pregnancy and the postpartum period.

References

1. Holmes LB. The teratogenicity of anticonvulsant drugs: a progress report. *J Med Genet.* 2002;39:245–247.
2. Fairgrieve SD, Jackson M, Jonas P, et al. Population based, prospective study of the care of women with epilepsy in pregnancy. *Br Med J.* 2000; 321:674–675.
3. Kaplan PW, Norwitz ER, Ben-Menachem E, et al. Obstetric risks for women with epilepsy during pregnancy. *Epilepsy Behav.* 2007;11:283–291.
4. Dutton C, Foldvary-Schaefer N. Contraception in women with epilepsy: pharmacokinetic interactions, contraceptive options, and management. *Int Rev Neurobiol.* 2008;83:113–134.
5. Guberman A. Hormonal contraception and epilepsy. *Neurology.* 1999; 53:S38–S40.
6. Janz D, Schmidt D. Anti-epileptic drugs and failure of oral contraceptives. *Lancet.* 1974;1:113.
7. Report of the quality of standards subcommittee of the American Academy of Neurology. Practice parameter: a guideline for discontinuing antiepileptic drugs in seizure-free patients—summary statement. *Neurology.* 1996;47:600–602.
8. Pennell PB, Gidal BE, Sabers A, et al. Pharmacology of antiepileptic drugs during pregnancy and lactation. *Epilepsy Behav.* 2007;11:263–269.
9. Davis AR, Pack AM, Kritzer J, et al. Reproductive history, sexual behavior and use of contraception in women with epilepsy. *Contraception.* 2008;77:405–409.
10. Krauss GL, Brandt J, Campbell M, et al. Antiepileptic medication and oral contraceptive interactions: a national survey of neurologists and obstetricians. *Neurology.* 1996;46:1534–1539.
11. Rosenfeld WE, Doose DR, Walker SA, et al. Effect of topiramate on the pharmacokinetics of an oral contraceptive containing norethindrone and ethinyl estradiol in patients with epilepsy. *Epilepsia.* 1997;38:317–323.
12. Harden CL, Meador KJ, Pennell PB, et al., American Academy of Neurology; American Epilepsy Society. Practice parameter update: management issues for women with epilepsy-focus on pregnancy (an evidence-based review): teratogenesis and perinatal outcomes. *Neurology.* 2009; 73(2):133–141.
13. Meador KJ, Pennell PB, Harden CL, et al. Pregnancy registries in epilepsy: a consensus statement on health outcomes. *Neurology.* 2008;71: 1109–1117.
14. Hvas CL, Henriksen TB, Ostergaard JR, et al. Epilepsy and pregnancy: effect of antiepileptic drugs and lifestyle on birthweight. *Br J Obstet Gynecol.* 2000;107:896–902.
15. Morrell MJ. Guidelines for the care of women with epilepsy. *Neurology.* 1998;51:S21–S27.
16. Honein MA, Paulozzi LJ, Cragan JD, et al. Evaluation of selected characteristics of pregnancy drug registries. *Teratology.* 1999;60:356–364.
17. Holmes LB, Harvey EA, Coull BA, et al. The teratogenicity of anticonvulsant drugs. *N Engl J Med.* 2001;344:1132–1138.
18. Pennell PB. Using current evidence in selecting antiepileptic drugs for use during pregnancy. *Epilepsy Curr.* 2005;5:45–51.
19. Pennell PB. Antiepileptic drugs during pregnancy: what is known and which AEDs seem to be safest? *Epilepsia.* 2008;49(suppl 9):43–55.
20. Lindhout D, Meinardi H, Meijer JWA, et al. Antiepileptic drugs and teratogenesis in two consecutive cohorts: changes in prescription policy paralleled by changes in pattern of malformations. *Neurology.* 1992; 42:94–110.
21. Morrow J, Russell A, Guthrie E, et al. Malformation risks of antiepileptic drugs in pregnancy: a prospective study from the UK Epilepsy and Pregnancy Register. *J Neurol Neurosurg Psychiatry.* 2006;77:193–198.
22. Kaneko S, Otani K, Fukushima Y, et al. Teratogenicity of antiepileptic drugs: analysis of possible risk factors. *Epilepsia.* 1988;29:459–467.
23. Dravet C, Julian C, Legras C, et al. Epilepsy, antiepileptic drugs, and malformations in children of women with epilepsy: a French prospective cohort study. *Neurology.* 1992;42:75–82.
24. Artama M, Auvinen A, Raudaskoski T, et al. Antiepileptic drug use of women with epilepsy and congenital malformations in offspring. *Neurology.* 2005;64:1874–1878.
25. Wyszynski DF, Nambisan M, Surve T, et al. Increased rate of major malformations in offspring exposed to valproate during pregnancy. *Neurology.* 2005;64:961–965.
26. Meador KJ, Baker GA, Finnell RH, et al. In utero antiepileptic drug exposure: fetal death and malformations. *Neurology.* 2006;67:407–412.
27. Wide K, Winbladh B, Kallen B. Major malformations in infants exposed to antiepileptic drugs in utero, with emphasis on carbamazepine and valproic acid: a nation-wide, population-based register study. *Acta Paediatrica.* 2004;93:174–176.
28. Samren EB, van Duijn CM, Christiaens GC, et al. Antiepileptic drug regimens and major congenital abnormalities in the offspring. *Ann Neurol.* 1999;46:739–746.
29. Canger R, Battino D, Canerini MP, et al. Malformations in offspring of women with epilepsy: a prospective study. *Epilepsia.* 1999;40:1231–1236.
30. Mawer G, Clayton-Smith J, Coyle H, et al. Outcome of pregnancy in women attending an outpatient epilepsy clinic: adverse features associated with higher doses of sodium valproate. *Seizure.* 2002;11:512–518.
31. Omtzigt JG, Los FJ, Grobbee DE, et al. The risk of spina bifida aperta after first-trimester exposure to valproate in a prenatal cohort. *Neurology.* 1992;42:119–125.
32. Arpino C, Brescianini S, Robert E, et al. Teratogenic effects of antiepileptic drugs: use of an international database on malformations and drug exposure (MADRE). *Epilepsia.* 2000;41:1436–1443.
33. Bertollini R, Mastroiacovo P, Segni G. Maternal epilepsy and birth defects: a case-control study in the Italian Multicentric Registry of Birth Defects (IPIMC). *Eur J Epidemiol.* 1985;1:67–72.
34. Samren EB, van Duijn CM, Koch S, et al. Maternal use of antiepileptic drugs and the risk of major congenital malformations: a joint European prospective study of human teratogenesis associated with maternal epilepsy. *Epilepsia.* 1997;38:981–990.
35. Rosa FW. Spina bifida in infants of women treated with carbamazepine during pregnancy. *N Engl J Med.* 1991;324:674–677.
36. Hernandez-Diaz S, Werler MM, Walker AM, et al. Neural tube defects in relation to use of folic acid antagonists during pregnancy. *Am J Epidemiol.* 2001;153:961–968.
37. Matalon S, Schechtman S, Goldzweig G, et al. The teratogenic effect of carbamazepine: a meta-analysis of 1255 exposures. *Reprod Toxicol.* 2002;16:9–17.
38. Puho EH, Szunyogh M, Metneki J, et al. Drug treatment during pregnancy and isolated orofacial clefts in Hungary. *Cleft Palate Craniofac J.* 2007;44:194–202.
39. Hernandez-Diaz S, Smith CR, Wyszynski DF, et al. Risk of major malformations among infants exposed to carbamazepine during pregnancy. *Birth Defects Res A.* 2007;79:357.
40. Vajda F, Lander C, O'Brien T, et al. Australian pregnancy registry of women taking antiepileptic drugs. *Epilepsia.* 2004;45:1466.
41. Holmes LB, Wyszynski DF. North American antiepileptic drug pregnancy registry. *Epilepsia.* 2004;45:1465.
42. Holmes LB, Baldwin EJ, Smith CR, et al. Increased frequency of isolated cleft palate in infants exposed to lamotrigine during pregnancy. *Neurology.* 2008;70:2152–2158.
43. Hunt SJ, Craig JJ, Morrow JI. Increased frequency of isolated cleft palate in infants exposed to lamotrigine during pregnancy. *Neurology.* 2009;72:1108; author reply 1108–1109.
44. Dolk H, Jentink J, Loane M, et al. Does lamotrigine use in pregnancy increase orofacial cleft risk relative to other malformations? *Neurology.* 2008;71:714–722.
45. Cunnington M, Ferber S, Quartey G. Effect of dose on the frequency of major birth defects following fetal exposure to lamotrigine monotherapy in an international observational study. *Epilepsia.* 2007;48:1207–1210.
46. Hunt S, Craig J, Russell A, et al. Levetiracetam in pregnancy: preliminary experience from the UK Epilepsy and Pregnancy Register. *Neurology.* 2006;67:1876–1879.
47. Bronstein KAS,; Leppik I, Montouris G, et al. Keppra (Levetiracetam) pregnancy registry. *Epilepsia.* 2008;49:85.
48. Montouris G. Gabapentin exposure in human pregnancy: results from the Gabapentin Pregnancy Registry. *Epilepsy Behav.* 2003;4:310–317.
49. Hunt S, Russell A, Smithson WH, et al. Topiramate in pregnancy: preliminary experience from the UK Epilepsy and Pregnancy Register. *Neurology.* 2008;71:272–276.
50. Meischenguiser R, D'Giano CH, Ferraro SM. Oxcarbazepine in pregnancy: clinical experience in Argentina. *Epilepsy Behav.* 2004;5:163–167.
51. Sabers A, Dam M, Rogvi-Hansen B, et al. Epilepsy and pregnancy: lamotrigine as main drug used. *Acta Neurol Scand.* 2004;109:9–13.
52. Kondo T, Kaneko S, Amano Y, et al. Preliminary report on teratogenic effects of zonisamide in the offspring of treated women with epilepsy. *Epilepsia.* 2004;37:1242–1244.

53. Timor-Tritsch IE, Fuchs KM, Monteagudo A, et al. Performing a fetal anatomy scan at the time of first-trimester screening. *Obstet Gynecol.* 2009;113:402–407.

54. Report of the Quality Standards Subcommittee of the American Academy of Neurology. Practice parameter: management issues for women with epilepsy (summary statement). *Neurology.* 1998;51:944–948.

55. Cameron M, Moran P. Prenatal screening and diagnosis of neural tube defects. *Prenat Diagn.* 2009;29:402–411.

56. Malone FD, D'Alton ME. Drugs in pregnancy: Anticonvulsants. *Semin Perinatol.* 1997;21:114–123.

57. Pschirrer ER, Monga M. Seizure disorders in pregnancy. *Obstetr Gynecol Clin.* 2001;28:601–611.

58. Khoo NS, Van Essen P, Richardson M, et al. Effectiveness of prenatal diagnosis of congenital heart defects in South Australia: a population analysis 1999–2003. *Aust N Z J Obstet Gynaecol.* 2008;48:559–563.

59. Committee on Educational Bulletins of the American College of O, Gynecologists. Seizure disorders in pregnancy. *Int J Gynecol Obstet.* 1997;56:279–286.

60. Yerby MS. Quality of life, epilepsy advances, and the evolving role of anticonvulsants in women with epilepsy. *Neurology.* 2000;55:21–31.

61. Meador KJ, Zupanc ML. Neurodevelopmental outcomes of children born to mothers with epilepsy. *Cleve Clin J Med.* 2004;71:S38–S40.

62. Gaily E, Kantola-Sorsa E, Hiilesmaa V, et al. Normal intelligence in children with prenatal exposure to carbamazepine. *Neurology.* 2004;62: 28–32.

63. Holmes LB, Rosenberger PB, Harvey EA, et al. Intelligence and physical features of children of women with epilepsy. *Teratology.* 2000;61:196–202.

64. Reinisch JM, Sanders SA, Mortensen EL, et al. In utero exposure to phenobarbital and intelligence deficits in adult men. *J Am Med Assoc.* 1995; 724:1518–1525.

65. Leonard G, Andermann E, Ptito A. Cognitive effects of antiepileptic drug therapy during pregnancy on school-age offspring [abstract]. *Epilepsia.* 1997;38:170.

66. Meador KJ. Neurodevelopmental effects of antiepileptic drugs. *Curr Neurol Neurosci Rep.* 2002;2:373–378.

67. Adab N, Jacoby A, Smith D, et al. Additional educational needs in children born to mothers with epilepsy. *J Neurol Neurosurg Psychiatry.* 2001; 70:15–21.

68. Koch S, Titze K, Zimmermann RB, et al. Long-term neuropsychological consequences of maternal epilepsy and anticonvulsant treatment during pregnancy for school-age children and adolescents. *Epilepsia.* 1999;40: 1237–1243.

69. Losche G, Steinhausen HC, Koch S, et al. The psychological development of children of epileptic parents. II. The differential impact of intrauterine exposure to anticonvulsant drugs and further influential factors. *Acta Paediatr.* 1994;83:961–966.

70. Scolnik D, Nulman I, Rovet J, et al. Neurodevelopment of children exposed in utero to phenytoin and carbamazepine monotherapy. *J Am Med Assoc.* 1994;271:767–770.

71. Adab N, Kini U, Vinten J, et al. The longer term outcome of children born to mothers with epilepsy. *J Neurol Neurosurg Psychiatry.* 2004;75: 1575–1583.

72. Vinten J, Adab N, Kini U, et al. Neuropsychological effects of exposure to anticonvulsant medication in utero. *Neurology.* 2005;64:949–954.

73. Vanoverloop D, Schnell RR, Harvey EA, et al. The effects of prenatal exposure to phenytoin and other anticonvulsants on intellectual function at 4 to 8 years of age. *Neurotoxicol Teratol.* 1992;14:329–335.

74. Wide K, Henning E, Tomson T, et al. Psychomotor development in preschool children exposed to antiepileptic drugs in utero. *Acta Paediatr.* 2002;91:409–414.

75. Meador KJ, Baker GA, Browning N, et al, NEAD study group. Fetal antiepileptic drug exposure and cognitive function at age 3. *N Engl J Med.* 2009;360:1597–1605.

76. Yerby MS, Cawthon ML. Fetal death, malformations and infant mortality in infants of mothers with epilepsy. *Epilepsia.* 1996;37:98.

77. Viinikainen K, Heinonen S, Eriksson K, et al. Community-based, prospective, controlled study of obstetric and neonatal outcome of 179 pregnancies in women with epilepsy. *Epilepsia.* 2006;47:186–192.

78. Dansky L, Rosenblatt D, Andermann E. Mechanisms of teratogenesis: folic acid and antiepileptic therapy. *Neurology.* 1992;42:32–42.

79. Wegner C, Nau H. Alteration of embryonic folate metabolism by valproic acid during organogenesis: implications for mechanisms of teratogenesis. *Neurology.* 1992;42:17–24.

80. Harden CL, Pennell PB, Koppel BS, et al. Practice parameter update: management issues for women with epilepsy-focus on pregnancy (an evidence-based review): vitamin K, folic acid, blood levels, and breastfeeding. *Neurology.* 2009;73:142–149.

81. Honein MA, Paulozzi LJ, Mathews TJ, et al. Impact of folic acid fortification of the US food supply on the occurrence of neural tube defects. *J Am Med Assoc.* 2001;285:2981–2986.

82. De Wals P, Tairou F, Van Allen MI, et al. Spina bifida before and after folic acid fortification in Canada. *Birth Defects Res A Clin Mol Teratol.* 2008;82:622–626.

83. Nambisan M, Wyszynski DF, Holmes LB. No evidence of a protective effect due to periconceptional folic acid (PCFA) intake on risk for congenital anomalies in the offspring of mothers exposed to antiepileptic drugs (AEDs). *Birth Defects Res.* 2003;67:5.

84. Evans JA. Pre-conceptional vitamin/folic acid supplementation 2007. *J Obstet Gynaecol Can.* 2008;30:656–657; author reply 658.

85. Buehler BA, Rao V, Finnell RH. Biochemical and molecular teratology of fetal hydantoin syndrome. *Pediatr Neurogenet.* 1994;12:741–748.

86. Seizure control and treatment in pregnancy: observations from the EURAP epilepsy pregnancy registry. *Neurology.* 2006;66:354–360.

87. Pennell PB. EURAP Outcomes for seizure control during pregnancy: useful and encouraging data. *Epilepsy Curr.* 2006;6:186–188.

88. Stumpf D, Frost M. Seizures, anticonvulsants, and pregnancy. *Am J Dis Child.* 1978;132:746–748.

89. Minkoff H, Schaffer RM, Delke I, et al. Diagnosis of intracranial hemorrhage in utero after a maternal seizure. *Obstet Gynecol.* 1985;65:22S–24S.

90. Teramo K, Hiilesmaa VK, Bardy A, et al. Fetal heart rate during a maternal grand mal epileptic seizure. *J Perinat Med.* 1979;7:3–5.

91. Nei M, Daly S, Liporace J. A maternal complex partial seizure in labor can affect fetal heart rate. *Neurology.* 1998;51:904–906.

92. Yerby MS, Devinsky O, Feldmann E, et al. Epilepsy and pregnancy. In: *Advances in Neurology: Neurological Complications of Pregnancy.* New York: Raven Press; 1994:45–63.

93. Pearlman MD, Tintinalli JE, Lorenz RP. Blunt trauma during pregnancy. *N Engl J Med.* 1990;323:1609–1613.

94. Pennell PB, Hovinga CA. Antiepileptic drug therapy in pregnancy I: gestation-induced effects on AED pharmacokinetics. *Int Rev Neurobiol.* 2008;83:227–240.

95. Pennell PB, Newport DJ, Stowe ZN, et al. The impact of pregnancy and childbirth on the metabolism of lamotrigine. *Neurology.* 2004;62: 292–295.

96. Tran TA, Leppik IE, Blesi K, Sathanandan ST, et al. Lamotrigine clearance during pregnancy. *Neurology.* 2002;59:251–255.

97. Petrenaite V, Sabers A, Hansen-Schwartz J. Individual changes in lamotrigine plasma concentrations during pregnancy. *Epilepsy Res.* 2005; 65:185–188.

98. de Haan GJ, Edelbroek P, Segers J, et al. Gestation-induced changes in lamotrigine pharmacokinetics: a monotherapy study. *Neurology.* 2004; 63:571–573.

99. Vajda FJ, Hitchcock A, Graham J, et al. Foetal malformations and seizure control: 52 months data of the Australian Pregnancy Registry. *Eur J Neurol.* 2006;13:645–654.

100. Pennell PB, Peng L, Newport DJ, et al. Lamotrigine in pregnancy: clearance, therapeutic drug monitoring, and seizure frequency. *Neurology.* 2008;70:2130–2136.

101. Christensen J, Sabers A, Sidenius P. Oxcarbazepine concentrations during pregnancy: a retrospective study in patients with epilepsy. *Neurology.* 2006;67:1497–1499.

102. Mazzucchelli I, Onat FY, Ozkara C, et al. Changes in the disposition of oxcarbazepine and its metabolites during pregnancy and the puerperium. *Epilepsia.* 2006;47:504–509.

103. Tomson T, Battino D. Pharmacokinetics and therapeutic drug monitoring of newer antiepileptic drugs during pregnancy and the puerperium. *Clin Pharmacokinet.* 2007;46:209–219.

104. Tomson T, Lindbom U, Ekqvist B, et al. Disposition of carbamazepine and phenytoin in pregnancy. *Epilepsia.* 1994;35:131–135.

105. Battino D, Binelli S, Bossi L, et al. Plasma concentrations of carbamazepine and carbamazepine 10,11-epoxide during pregnancy and after delivery. *Clin Pharmacokinet.* 1985;10:279–284.

106. Yerby MS, Friel PN, McCormick K, et al. Pharmacokinetics of anticonvulsants in pregnancy: alterations in plasma protein binding. *Epilepsy Res.* 1990;5:223–228.

107. Lander CM, Livingstone I, Tyrer JH, et al. The clearance of anticonvulsant drugs in pregnancy. *Clin Exp Neurol.* 1981;17:71–78.

108. Harden CL,. MKJ, Hauser WA, Wiebe S, et al. Practice parameter update: management issues for women with epilepsy—focus on pregnancy (an evidence-based review): obstetrical complications and change in seizure frequency. *Neurology.* 2009;73:126–132.

109. Srinivasan G, Seeler RA, Tiruvury A, et al. Maternal anticonvulsant therapy and hemorrhagic disease of the newborn. *Obstet Gynecol.* 1982; 59:250–252.

110. Howe AM, Oakes DJ, Woodman PDC, et al. Prothrombin and PIVKA-II levels in cord blood from newborn exposed to anticonvulsants during pregnancy. *Epilepsia.* 1999;40:980–984.

111. Delgado-Escueta A, Janz D. Consensus guidelines: preconception counseling, management, and care of the pregnant woman with epilepsy. *Neurology.* 1992;42:149–160.

112. Katz JM, Devinsky O. Primary generalized epilepsy: a risk factor for seizures in labor and delivery? *Seizure.* 2003;12:217–219.

113. Pennell PB. Is breast milk the best for babies of mothers on levetiracetam? *Epilepsy Curr.* 2006;6:22–24.

114. Hovinga CA, Pennell PB. Antiepileptic drug therapy in pregnancy II: fetal and neonatal exposure. *Int Rev Neurobiol.* 2008;83:241–258.

115. Newport DJ, Pennell PB, Calamaras MR, et al. Lamotrigine in breast milk and nursing infants: determination of exposure. *Pediatrics.* 2008;122:e223–e231.

116. Moore KL. *The Developing Human: Clinically Oriented Embryology.* Philadelphia, PA: WB Saunders; 1988.

CHAPTER 46 ■ BONE HEALTH AND FRACTURES IN EPILEPSY

RAJ D. SHETH AND ALISON PACK

INTRODUCTION

Impaired bone health results in diminished bone strength. The ultimate consequence of diminished bone strength is fractures. Fractures are between two and six times more common in persons with epilepsy than in the general population, with current overall fracture rates in the United States being 2205 per 100,000 person-years (1,2). Although the fracture rate in epilepsy remains to be clearly defined, the rate is estimated to be similar to patients taking steroids (3).

Generally, four main situations predispose persons with epilepsy to fracture: (i) fractures may be caused by seizures themselves or result from seizure-precipitated falls, (ii) fractures may occur as a general risk associated with trauma, or (iii) fractures may be pathologic, occurring in the context of osteopathy: osteoporosis and osteomalacia. (iv) Incoordination associated with either a coexisting comorbid condition or antiepileptic drug (AED)–induced ataxia (4,5) may also increase the persons' likelihood of a fall and a consequent fracture. Vestergaard and colleagues (6) reported that, in persons with epilepsy, seizure-related forces accounted for 33.9% of all fractures suggesting that although seizures account for some of the increase in fractures, there are other influencing factors. Thus, fractures result from the interplay between accidental trauma, seizure-related falls and bone strength (7). Health care costs and societal burden associated with this increased vulnerability to fractures is considerable. For example, in the United States, the direct cost associated with low bone mineral density (BMD) fractures exceeded $11.9 billion in 1989 and is expected to increase significantly as the population ages (8).

BONE ACROSS THE AGE SPECTRUM

Childhood and adolescence are critical periods of skeletal mineralization (7). At birth there is very little mineralization, bone mass peaks between the second and the third decade of life (9). Peak BMD achieved by the end of adolescence determines the risk for later pathologic fractures and osteoporosis (10). Starting in the sixth decade of life, involutional changes result in physiologic reductions of BMD. Chronic disease and medications that interfere with bone mineralization or adversely affect bone health can have significant long-term implications for bone health.

OSTEOPOROSIS

Osteoporosis is the most common pathologic process in bone and increases one's risk of fracture. Persons with epilepsy treated with AEDs may be at even greater risk. As the Surgeon General states (11) in his first ever report on bone and mineral health:

> Osteoporosis is a silent condition that affects millions of Americans. Ten million Americans over age 50 have osteoporosis, the most common bone disease. Another 34 million Americans have low bone mass. If we do not take immediate action, by 2020, half of all Americans over age 50 will have weak bones from osteoporosis and low bone mass.

Osteopenia and osteoporosis are gradations of the same pathology; osteoporosis being more severe. They are clinically defined by reduced BMD secondary to increased bone resorption. Bone resorption and bone formation are integral to the normal accumulation and maintenance of bone. Osteoclasts are the cells responsible for bone resorption whereas osteoblasts are the cells that form bone. An uncoupling of these functions results in either low bone turnover or high bone turnover. In childhood these pathologic turnover processes affect bone accumulation, whereas bone loss occurs in the adult years, potentially resulting in osteoporosis (7).

Diagnosis and Definition of Osteoporosis

Osteoporosis is currently diagnosed using BMD measurements as determined by dual-energy X-ray absorptiometry (DXA). DXA assesses bone mass at central sites, specifically the hip and spine. The obtained BMD measurement in g/cm^2 is compared with large databases maintained by the manufacturers of the DXA devices. This comparison yields two standard deviation scores: T-score and Z-score. The T-score compares the obtained BMD measurement to a sex- and race-matched population at peak BMD, whereas the Z-score compares the BMD measurement to a sex-, race-, and age-matched population. In postmenopausal women and older men, the WHO uses the T-score to define osteopenia (T-score between -1.0 and 2.5) and osteoporosis (T-score less than -2.5) (12). Low BMD is defined in younger women and men using the Z-score (less than -2.0) (13) to avoid falsely diagnosing low BMD if they have not yet obtained peak BMD.

Classification of Osteoporosis

Osteoporosis is classified as either primary or secondary. Primary osteoporosis is defined as bone loss in the perimenopausal years and in older men and women. Secondary osteoporosis may develop because of lifestyle and nutrition factors, underlying medical conditions (e.g., thyroid disease, renal disease) or medications. AED exposure can result in secondary bone loss. Integral to diagnosing primary and secondary osteoporosis is the identification of risk factors (e.g., Asian or Caucasian race, small frame, family history of osteoporosis, tobacco use, excessive alcohol use). Having more risk factors is associated with a higher risk of osteoporosis and fracture (14). For instance, a postmenopausal woman with multiple risk factors has an increased risk of hip fracture when compared to a woman with fewer risk factors (15).

Epilepsy and Osteoporosis

Multiple studies report high percentages of low BMD or osteoporosis in children and adults with epilepsy treated with AEDs. BMD measurements of persons with epilepsy treated with AEDs reveal low BMD or osteoporosis in 38% to 60% (16–18). Pediatric studies find lower BMD in children treated with AEDs when compared to matched controls, suggesting poor bone accrual (7). In adults, low BMD has been described in institutionalized and ambulatory populations at multiple sites including the total hip, femoral neck, and lumbar spine (19). However, the interpretation and generalization of these studies is limited secondary to small samples, cross-sectional design, and lack of controls. One study controlled for genetics by using a female sibling/twin pair cohort (20). Subjects were discordant for epilepsy and treatment with AEDs. BMD measurements revealed significant reduction in siblings treated with AEDs, with the most significant differences being among those treated with AEDs for greater than 2 years, women treated with enzyme-inducing AEDs, and subjects older than age 40. Prospective studies in men and women find significant bone loss in persons treated with AEDs when compared to controls. For instance, young men (ages 24 to 44 years) with epilepsy treated with AEDs had significantly more annual BMD loss at the femoral neck of the hip when compared to a control population (16). Similarly, a cohort of postmenopausal women treated continuously with AEDs had significant bone loss in comparison to nonusers (21). The authors of this study concluded that AED use in postmenopausal women increased the risk of hip fracture by 29%. Over a single year, young women with epilepsy treated with phenytoin in one study sustained significant bone loss at the femoral neck of the hip (22). Women treated with carbamazepine, valproate, and lamotrigine did not have significant bone loss. In contrast, another study of older men found significant bone loss in men treated with non-enzyme-inducing AEDs when compared to nonusers and men treated with enzyme-inducing AEDs (23). Indications for AED use, however, were not specified, and the majority (83%) who were prescribed non-enzyme-inducing AEDs were taking gabapentin, an AED used for epilepsy and other indications including pain. In summary, pediatric and adult studies find high percentages of low BMD and osteoporosis, particularly in association with enzyme-inducing AEDs.

Duration of Epilepsy and Osteoporosis

BMD deficits acquired during childhood have the potential to increase the risk of developing osteoporotic fractures later in life (9). Epilepsy and its treatment have been shown to adversely affect accrual of BMD in childhood (24). Examination of the interaction between duration of epilepsy and BMD to determine the timing of the bone deficit indicates that children treated for epilepsy sustain significant BMD deficit compared to controls during the initial 1 to 5 years of treatment, which progressively worsens thereafter (25). This progressive BMD deficit may be a contributing factor to the increased fracture risk observed in patients with epilepsy and may accelerate aging-related osteoporosis.

Type of Epilepsy and Osteoporosis

Persons with severe physical disabilities and cerebral palsy have reduced BMD and a consequent increase in low-impact fractures (26). However, it is not clear if normally ambulatory persons with epilepsy are similarly vulnerable. Accordingly, Sheth and colleagues compared BMD in normally ambulatory patients with symptomatic epilepsy to those with idiopathic epilepsy and to controls (27). Persons with symptomatic epilepsy had lower BMD compared to those with idiopathic epilepsy and to controls. Furthermore, as the duration of epilepsy increased there were reductions in BMD Z-scores for symptomatic but not for idiopathic epilepsy. In addition, persons with partial seizures and control subjects had similar BMD, whereas persons with generalized seizures had lower BMD. In summary, persons with symptomatic epilepsy had lower BMD Z-scores when compared to those with idiopathic epilepsy and controls, and persons with generalized seizures had lower BMD Z-scores compared to those with partial epilepsy. These findings suggest a negative impact of both symptomatic epilepsy and generalized seizures on BMD.

EPILEPSY AND BONE QUALITY

Bone strength is increasingly recognized as an important determinant of bone health. Both bone quality and BMD contribute to bone strength, and effects on bone quality can increase the risk of bone disease and fracture. Bone quality describes structural and material properties of bone as well as biochemical strength. Osteomalacia, which literally means softening of bone, and rickets are pathologic processes of bone quality. Rickets occurs in children and involves the growth plate. Drug-induced osteomalacia and rickets result because of either insufficient availability of calcium, phosphate, and active vitamin D or interference with the deposition of calcium and phosphate in bone. Osteomalacic biopsy specimens exhibit abnormally thick osteoid (unmineralized bone) seams, a prolonged mineralization lag time, and a decrease in the adjusted apposition rate. Early biopsy studies of adults and children with epilepsy found evidence of osteomalacia and rickets (28–30). However, subjects in these studies were primarily institutionalized and treated with phenytoin, primidone, and phenobarbital. Recent biopsy studies of ambulatory persons have found no evidence of osteomalacia. These studies have reported normal osteoid seam width and normal or increased mineralization rates. (31,32). There may however be more subtle changes in bone quality.

Interestingly, a meta-analysis of studies on fracture and BMD in persons with epilepsy suggests that current available BMD findings do not fully explain reported increased fracture risk in persons with epilepsy (33). Other potential influencing factors including effects on bone quality may explain the increased fracture risk. For example, effects on bone quality were described in one animal study. Bone specimens in rats treated with levetiracetam, phenytoin, and valproate had evidence of changes in bone quality (34). Biochemical competence was affected in those rats treated with low-dose levetiracetam. Further study needs to more definitively assess bone quality in association with epilepsy and AED treatment.

Epilepsy, AEDs, and Fractures

As previously discussed, fractures in persons with epilepsy are often secondary to multiple factors including seizures, falls, and negative effects of AEDs on bone health. In a case-control study evaluating fractures in persons with epilepsy taking AEDs, risk factors for fracture were prolonged seizures, long-term AED use (either enzyme-inducing AEDs or non-enzyme-inducing AEDs), AED polypharmacy, and female gender (35). Therefore, seizure control is of clear importance in preventing fracture in persons with epilepsy. However, since emerging evidence indicates an adverse effect of AEDs on bone metabolism, in particular the enzyme-inducing AEDs, the choice of an AED to prevent seizures and to protect bone health is important as well.

Persons with epilepsy frequently experience injuries resulting from seizure-related falls (6), or trauma occurring in the context of seizure-related impairment of consciousness (36–38). Interestingly, in one study traumatic fractures were more likely to occur in men (55%), whereas pathologic fractures were more common in women (57%) (38). Vestergaard and colleagues (6) reported that seizure-related fractures accounted for 33.9% of all fractures (95% CI: 25.3% to 43.5%) in persons with epilepsy. Fractures of the spine, forearms, femurs, lower legs, and feet and toes were significantly increased after the diagnosis of epilepsy.

AED exposure and in particular enzyme-inducing AEDs may influence the risk of fracture in persons with epilepsy. Phenytoin use was associated with increased fracture risk in one study (6). Souverein and collaborators did not, however, find a difference in fracture risk between hepatic enzyme-inducing and non-enzyme-inducing AEDs (35). This finding is in agreement with a recent Danish case-control study including 124,655 fracture cases, which concluded that liver-inducing potential per se was not responsible for the increased fracture risk (39). Also, no difference in BMD was found between users of inducing and non-inducing AEDs in a case-control study in Scotland among men and women aged 47 years and older (40). Another study found that valproate, a non-enzyme-inducing AED drug, can also affect bone metabolism (41). Therefore, hepatic enzyme-inducing properties of AEDs are likely to account for just a part of the association between AED use and effects on bone health including increased fracture risk.

Individual AEDs and Bone

AEDs have a wide range of somatic metabolic effects including an effect on bone (42). Although most studies do not determine the unique effect of specific AEDs on bone health, individual AEDs likely have differential effects. The AEDs most commonly associated with altered bone metabolism and decreased bone density are inducers of the cytochrome P450 enzyme system, including phenytoin, primidone, and phenobarbital (19). Available data is less consistent for carbamazepine (19). Increased markers of bone turnover have been reported, however, in persons with epilepsy treated with carbamazepine (43,44). Valproate, a cytochrome P450 enzyme inhibitor, is also associated with an increased risk of alterations in bone and mineral metabolism and decreased BMD (19). Polytherapy may independently result in increased abnormalities of bone metabolism (45,46). There is limited data regarding potential effects of new generation AEDs on bone.

Phenytoin, Phenobarbital, Primidone

Multiple studies report decreased BMD in association with phenytoin, phenobarbital, and primidone treatment, and longitudinal studies find significant BMD reductions in phenytoin-treated postmenopausal (21) and premenopausal women (22). Reported alterations in bone and mineral metabolism although not seen consistently include reduced calcium, reduced phosphate, reduced 25-hydroxyvitamin D levels, and elevated markers of bone formation and resorption. These abnormalities support the most commonly identified potential mechanism suggesting that induction of the cytochrome P450 enzyme system leads to increased catabolism of vitamin D to inactive metabolites, decreased gastrointestinal absorption of calcium, hypocalcemia, a rise in circulating parathyroid hormone (PTH), and subsequent increase in mobilization of calcium stores, bone turnover, and bone loss.

In vitro studies support cytochrome P450 enzyme induction leading to increased catabolism of vitamin D. As xenobiotics, phenobarbital, phenytoin, and carbamazepine activate a nuclear receptor known as either the steroid and xenobiotic receptor (SXR) or pregnane X receptor (PXR) (47,48). One in vitro study found that xenobiotics upregulate 25-hydroxyvitamin D_3–24-hydroxylase (CYP24) in the kidney through activation of PXR (47), which then catalyzes the conversion of 25-hydroxyvitamin D to an inactive metabolite. Another in vitro study found that xenobiotic activation of PXR increased expression of the isoenzyme, CYP3A4, in the liver and small intestine (48), generating more polar inactive vitamin D metabolites.

As some studies do not find significant reductions in calcium or vitamin D metabolites, other mechanisms including an indirect effect through changes in reproductive hormones or direct toxicity on bone may explain the reported abnormalities of these AEDs on bone.

Carbamazepine

Studies report conflicting results when evaluating the effect of carbamazepine on BMD and bone and mineral metabolism. Adults treated with carbamazepine in one study did not have significantly decreased BMD as determined by DXA (49), whereas BMD was decreased in another study of men and women treated with enzyme-inducing AEDs including carbamazepine (17). Decreased cortical bone mass as measured by quantitative ultrasound of the phalanges has been described in carbamazepine-treated subjects (50,51). Similarly, inconsistent reports of hypocalcemia, hypophosphatemia, decreased vitamin D metabolites, and elevated markers of bone turnover exist. For instance, a study of male subjects without epilepsy treated with carbamazepine for 10 weeks did not have significant elevations on markers of bone formation and resorption (52), while other studies report elevated markers of bone formation and resorption in carbamazepine-treated subjects (43,44). Interestingly, elevated risk of fracture was observed in persons treated with carbamazepine (39).

A 2-year longitudinal study performed by Verrotti and colleagues in 60 adolescents taking carbamazepine compared serum markers of bone formation and resorption after starting carbamazepine in normal subjects with epilepsy (44). Subjects achieved typical serum concentrations of carbamazepine. They were age and gender matched with controls and divided by developmental status into three groups: prepuberty, puberty, and postpuberty. Following 2 years of carbamazepine treatment, they found a significant increase in several serum markers of collagen and bone turnover. Urinary cross-linked N-telopeptides of type 1 collagen excretion, a marker of osteoclastic activity, was increased 10-fold. Interestingly, this effect occurred despite a normal calcium intake and in the face of similar PTH and vitamin D serum concentrations. Furthermore, pubertal stage did not influence the association. These findings suggest that increased bone turnover occurred despite normal vitamin D levels.

In summary, the conflicting results suggest that persons treated with carbamazepine should be monitored for potential bone disease, but the effects of carbamazepine monotherapy on BMD and bone and mineral metabolism need to be further elucidated.

Valproate

Early reports evaluating indices of bone and mineral metabolism in patients on valproate found no significant abnormalities (46,53,54). In contrast, recent studies find significant effects on BMD and markers of bone and mineral metabolism. For example, long-term valproate monotherapy treatment in 40 adults resulted in decreased BMD and increased serum concentrations of calcium, low vitamin D metabolites, increased markers of bone resorption and formation (18). The increased calcium was postulated to reflect increased bone resorption. Similarly, children treated with valproate had decreased BMD and elevated markers of bone turnover when compared to children not treated with AEDs (24,25) or treated with carbamazepine (24). Specifically, children treated with valproate have a 10% or greater reduction in BMD compared with controls (24). Considering that a 7% reduction of BMD in healthy adults is associated with a 50% increase in osteoporotic fractures (55,56), valproate use in children might be expected to increase the risk of future fractures. Interestingly, valproate was associated with a higher risk of fracture in a population-based epidemiologic study (39). In summary, recent studies suggest a potential effect of valproate on BMD and indices of bone and mineral metabolism but as with carbamazepine, further study is needed to clarify these effects.

The pathogenesis of valproate-associated reduction in BMD remains undefined. Valproate has been associated with reversible Fanconi syndrome (57,58), suggesting that valproate may cause renal tubular dysfunction with increased urinary loss of calcium and phosphorus. Sato et al. found that 23% of patients taking valproate for more than 1 year had a reduction in BMD in the osteoporotic range (18). This effect was present despite increased weight, which is typically associated with a protective effect on bone mineralization.

Newer AEDs

Few studies have evaluated the effect of the new generation AEDs (gabapentin, lamotrigine, oxcarbazepine, levetiracetam, topiramate, and zonisamide) on BMD and bone and mineral metabolism. A recent prospective study in older men (23) identified non-inducing AEDs, mainly gabapentin, as being associated with bone loss. Prescription indication may have influenced the findings as gabapentin is commonly used for indications other than epilepsy including pain. Lamotrigine monotherapy treatment in young women with epilepsy was not associated with bone loss (22) or significant findings in calcium or markers of bone resorption and bone formation (59). Adults treated with oxcarbazepine had reduced vitamin D metabolites and elevated PTH that was most significant at higher doses (60). Limited data also exists on levetiracetam's effects on bone. A limited preliminary clinical study found no effects (61), but a rat study suggests there may be changes in bone quality secondary to low-dose levetiracetam administration (34). Topiramate and zonisamide therapy may have potential effects. As carbonic anhydrase inhibitors, they can promote a renal acidosis resulting in among other things secondary abnormalities in bone. Interestingly though, carbonic anhydrase also potentiates the action of osteoclasts and inhibitors may have a bone-sparing effect. This hypothesis is supported by findings in women with glaucoma treated with acetazolamide, another carbonic anhydrase inhibitor (62). Finally, a double-blind randomized preliminary study of topiramate as treatment for obesity did not find significant changes in bone turnover markers compared to placebo controls (63).

Of the newer AEDs used in the treatment of pediatric epilepsy, only lamotrigine has been evaluated regarding BMD. Guo and collaborators examined the effect of lamotrigine (16 children), valproate (28 children), or a combination of the two (4 children) in children aged 3 to 17 with epilepsy (54). They found that treatment with valproate or lamotrigine for more than 2 years was associated with short stature, low bone mass, and reduced bone formation. The major predictor of lowered bone mass was physical inactivity. However, only total BMD was measured. This study design may account for the differences noted from other studies that used a more standardized approach of measuring BMD in the distal third of the radius, the lumbar spine, and the femoral neck. The authors reasonably suggest that calcium homeostasis would be expected to be more generally linked with whole bone mineralization rather than site-specific changes. Separating the differential effects of medication from the authors' proposed mechanism of reduced physical activity was not possible. Limitations of this study are the presence of a lower range of body height (below the 10th percentile) in 43% of the patients. This raises the interesting issue of the role of growth in bone mineralization. The authors suggest that lower physical activity in their cohort accounted for most of the observed reductions in BMD.

Total BMD was measured in 13 normally ambulatory children with epilepsy treated with lamotrigine monotherapy who had never been exposed to other medications and compared with 36 controls and 40 patients exposed to polytherapy (64). All subjects were ambulatory and had similar physical activity and calcium intake. BMD Z-scores for lamotrigine and controls were similar and higher than in those receiving polytherapy for 1 to 5 years and ≥6 years. Increasing duration of epilepsy was associated with lower BMD for 1 to 5 years polytherapy and ≥6 years polytherapy but not for those treated with lamotrigine. These data suggest that lamotrigine may not interfere with bone accrual (64). Larger studies of single AED exposure for long durations are needed to confirm these results.

Growth stature and pubertal stage were studied in girls receiving oxcarbazepine and carbamazepine (65). The authors did not study bone mineralization directly but looked at body height as an indirect measure of bone growth. The drugs appeared not to affect linear growth or pubertal development.

Screening and Treatment

Screening of persons with epilepsy treated with AEDs for bone disease and treatment of those who have evidence of bone disease have received limited study. Screening tools including DXA scanning and serologic 25-hydroxyvitamin D testing are available. Multiple therapies approved for bone loss are available and may be useful for persons with epilepsy treated with AEDs. Bone health screening guidelines for persons with epilepsy treated with AEDs do not yet exist. Nonetheless, given the current available evidence, routine screening of calcium and vitamin D metabolites for all persons treated with enzyme-inducing AEDs is recommended. DXA scan testing will identify osteoporosis and low BMD and is recommended for persons at risk. As discussed, data suggest that persons treated with enzyme-inducing AEDs and valproate are at risk particularly if they have other risk factors for bone disease.

Individuals with evidence of vitamin D insufficiency (<30 ng/mL) require vitamin D supplementation. Vitamin D supplementation was evaluated in one study of institutionalized and noninstitutionalized subjects receiving AEDs who had low 25-hydroxyvitamin D levels (66). Almost all of the subjects achieved normal levels over a period of 12 months. The doses of vitamin D required ranged from 400 to 4000 IU/day. Given the variability of the vitamin D supplementation, it is difficult to apply these results to clinical practice. A recent randomized double-blind trial over 1 year compared low-dose (400 IU/day for adults and children) and high-dose (4000 IU/day for adults and 2000 IU/day for children) vitamin D supplementation (67). In the adults, the baseline BMD was reduced at all sites when compared to age- and gender-matched controls. After 1 year, there were significant increases in BMD at all sites in those receiving high dose but not low dose vitamin D. The children had normal BMD when compared to age- and gender-matched controls and had significant and comparable increases in BMD in both treatment groups. This study suggests that persons with epilepsy treated with AEDs should be counseled about adequate vitamin D intake. There are currently no definitive evidence-based guidelines for calcium and vitamin D supplementation for persons with epilepsy. It is, however, recommended that all persons receive at least the recommended daily allowance (Table 46.1). For those taking enzyme-inducing AEDs, higher doses of vitamin D_3 (>800 IU per day) than currently recommended are suggested. Higher doses are also recommended for persons with osteoporosis or osteomalacia (68) (see Table 46.1). All persons should have 25-hydroxyvitamin D levels greater than

---

TABLE 46.1

CALCIUM AND VITAMIN D RECOMMENDATIONS

Recommended daily allowance of calcium	
• Adolescents/young adults	1200–1500 mg
• Men	
• 25–65 years	1000 mg
• Over 65 years	1500 mg
• Women	
• 25–50 years	1000 mg
• Over 50 years (postmenopausal)	
• Taking estrogens	1000 mg
• Not taking estrogens	1500 mg
• Over 65 years	1500 mg
• Pregnant and nursing	1200–1500 mg
Recommended vitamin D supplementation (68)[a]	
• Prophylaxis[b]	400–2000 IU/day
• Persons with osteoporosis	2000–4000 IU/day
• Persons with osteomalacia	5000–15,000 IU/day for 3–4 weeks

[a]Vitamin D_3 recommended.
[b]Higher for persons receiving enzyme-inducing AEDs.

30 ng/mL. If the concentration is lower, high-dose supplementation is necessary. In general, an extra 100 IU of supplemental vitamin D_3 is needed to increase the 25-hydroxyvitamin D concentration by 1 ng/mL.

If a person has osteoporosis or low BMD and is prescribed either an enzyme-inducing AED or valproate, changing the AED may reduce the risk of ongoing bone loss. Referral to a bone and mineral metabolism specialist is also advised. Because few studies are available in individuals treated with AEDs, treatment recommendations need to follow other guidelines, such as for postmenopausal women. Multiple therapies exist including the antiresorptive agents, bisphosphonates, selective estrogen reuptake modulators, calcitonin, hormone replacement therapy, and the recently approved PTH. Some treatments are recommended in specific clinical situations. For instance hormone replacement therapy may be useful in a menopausal woman with other significant symptoms including hot flashes. However, if the woman has epilepsy she may be at risk for increased seizure activity (69). Bisphosphonates are known to increase BMD and reduce the risk of fracture but are not routinely recommended in premenopausal women particularly as the teratogenic potential is unknown.

AED Evaluation

Persons with epilepsy who have already sustained a low-intensity fracture should have their AED therapy evaluated. The change from an enzyme-inducing agent or valproate to another AED should be considered. This decision is at times difficult especially for persons who have not experienced a seizure for many years or are concerned about the cost of changing AEDs. Once a low-intensity fracture has occurred the chance of further fractures increases. Furthermore, persons with a BMD < 2.5 should have their AED regimen evaluated. The decision to change AED therapy in persons with a BMD in the osteopenic range (BMD of −1 to −2.5) should be discussed with the patient. For persons with BMD in the normal range, no AED change need be considered.

Persons with epilepsy appear to have an increased risk for fracture due to trauma from both seizures and from fall-related fractures that are not seizure-related. Fractures in persons with epilepsy not directly caused by seizures frequently occur in the lower leg, ankles, and feet (70). These are not typical sites of low BMD, and patients report that these fractures were caused by clumsiness, tripping, and falling (70). The increased fracture rates in the legs, feet, and toes are likely contributed by AED neurotoxicity and discoordination. This risk could be minimized by carefully managing AEDs to avoid toxicity, limiting benzodiazepine use, and avoiding AEDs that can precipitously reach toxic levels, in particular phenytoin. Notably, phenytoin use has been identified as a risk factor for fractures (6), which may be explained by its narrow therapeutic window as well as its effect on bone metabolism.

Follow-Up DXA

Patient with BMD T-score of −1 or higher do not routinely require repeat measurements unless there have been changes in the risk factors. Persons with an osteopenic BMD should usually have a BMD remeasured in 2 years time. More frequent BMD measures may mislead treatment decisions. For those with osteoporosis, particularly if he/she has been started on a bisphosphonate, follow-up BMD measures should be obtained to determine efficacy and compliance with treatment (71).

CONCLUSION

Fracture rates in persons with epilepsy, although not clearly defined, are higher than in the general population. Seizure-related falls, trauma, osteopathies, including osteoporosis and osteomalacia, and incoordination secondary to a comorbid condition or AED exposure likely all contribute. Osteoporosis or low BMD is relatively common in adults and children with epilepsy, particularly in association with certain AED exposure including enzyme-inducing AEDs and valproate. Changes in bone quality have also been described in persons with epilepsy treated with AEDs. Screening tools such as DXA scanning and serologic testing of active vitamin D levels are available and should be routinely considered. When a person with epilepsy treated with AEDs has evidence of an osteopathy or pathologic fracture, treatment options are available and changing the AED may be necessary.

References

1. Persson HB, Alberts KA, Farahmand BY, et al. Risk of extremity fractures in adult outpatients with epilepsy. *Epilepsia*. 2002;43(7):768–772.
2. Souverein PC, Webb DJ, Petri H, et al. Incidence of fractures among epilepsy patients: a population-based retrospective cohort study in the General Practice Research Database. *Epilepsia*. 2005;46(2):304–310.
3. Mattson RH, Gidal BE. Fractures, epilepsy, and antiepileptic drugs. *Epilepsy Behav*. 2004;5(suppl 2):S36–S40.
4. Riggs BL, Melton LJ III. Involutional osteoporosis. *N Engl J Med*. 1986; 314(26):1676–1686.
5. Sheth RD. Bone health in epilepsy. *Epilepsia*. 2002;43(12):1453–1454.
6. Vestergaard P, Tigaran S, Rejnmark L, et al. Fracture risk is increased in epilepsy. *Acta Neurol Scand*. 1999;99(5):269–275.
7. Sheth RD. Bone health in pediatric epilepsy. *Epilepsy Behav*. 2004;5(suppl 2): S30–S35.
8. Chrischilles E, Shireman T, Wallace R. Costs and health effects of osteoporotic fractures. *Bone*. 1994;15(4):377–386.
9. Sheth RD, Hobbs GR, Riggs JE, et al. Bone mineral density in geographically diverse adolescent populations. *Pediatrics*. 1996;98(5):948–951.
10. Sheth RD. Adolescent issues in epilepsy. *J Child Neurol*. 2002;17(suppl 2): 2S23–2S27.
11. Bone health and Osteoporosis: A report of the Surgeon General, U.D.o.H.a.H. Services, Editor. 2004.
12. Blake GM, Fogelman I. The role of DXA bone density scans in the diagnosis and treatment of osteoporosis. *Postgrad Med J*. 2007;83(982):509–517.
13. Lewiecki EM, Gordon CM, Baim S, et al. International Society for Clinical Densitometry 2007 Adult and Pediatric Official Positions. *Bone*. 2008; 43(6):1115–1121.
14. Kanis JA, Oden A, Johnell O, et al. The use of clinical risk factors enhances the performance of BMD in the prediction of hip and osteoporotic fractures in men and women. *Osteoporos Int*. 2007;18(8):1033–1046.
15. Cummings SR, Nevitt MC, Browner WS, et al. Risk factors for hip fracture in white women. Study of Osteoporotic Fractures Research Group. *N Engl J Med*. 1995;332(12):767–773.
16. Andress DL, Ozuna J, Tirschwell D, et al. Antiepileptic drug-induced bone loss in young male patients who have seizures. *Arch Neurol*. 2002;59(5): 781–786.
17. Farhat G, Yamout B, Mikati MA, et al. Effect of antiepileptic drugs on bone density in ambulatory patients. *Neurology*. 2002;58(9):1348–1353.
18. Sato Y, Kondo I, Ishida S, et al. Decreased bone mass and increased bone turnover with valproate therapy in adults with epilepsy. *Neurology*. 2001; 57(3):445–449.
19. Pack A. Bone health in people with epilepsy: is it impaired and what are the risk factors? *Seizure*. 2008;17(2):181–186.
20. Petty SJ, Paton LM, O'Brien TJ, et al. Effect of antiepileptic medication on bone mineral measures. *Neurology*. 2005;65(9):1358–1365.
21. Ensrud KE, Walczak TS, Blackwell T, et al. Antiepileptic drug use increases rates of bone loss in older women: a prospective study. *Neurology*. 2004; 62(11):2051–2057.
22. Pack AM, Morrell MJ, Randall A, et al. Bone health in young women with epilepsy after one year of antiepileptic drug monotherapy. *Neurology*. 2008;70(18):1586–1593.

23. Ensrud KE, Walczak TS, Blackwell TL, et al. Antiepileptic drug use and rates of hip bone loss in older men: a prospective study. *Neurology.* 2008; 71(10):723–730.

24. Sheth RD, Wesolowski CA, Jacob JC, et al. Effect of carbamazepine and valproate on bone mineral density. *J Pediatr.* 1995;127(2):256–262.

25. Sheth RD, Binkley N, Hermann BP. Progressive bone deficit in epilepsy. *Neurology.* 2008;70(3):170–176.

26. Bischof F, Basu D, Pettifor JM. Pathological long-bone fractures in residents with cerebral palsy in a long-term care facility in South Africa. *Dev Med Child Neurol.* 2002;44(2):119–122.

27. Sheth RD. Hermann BP. Bone in idiopathic and symptomatic epilepsy. *Epilepsy Res.* 2008;78(1):71–76.

28. Dent CE, Richens A, Rowe DJ, et al. Osteomalacia with long-term anticonvulsant therapy in epilepsy. *Br Med J.* 1970;4(727):69–72.

29. Richens A, Rowe DJ. Disturbance of calcium metabolism by anticonvulsant drugs. *Br Med J.* 1970;4(727):73–76.

30. Hahn TJ, Scharp CR, Halstead LR, et al. Parathyroid hormone status and renal responsiveness in familial hypophosphatemic rickets. *J Clin Endocrinol Metab.* 1975;41(5):926–937.

31. Mosekilde L, Melsen F. Dynamic differences in trabecular bone remodeling between patients after jejunoileal bypass for obesity and epileptic patients receiving anticonvulsant therapy. *Metab Bone Dis Relat Res.* 1980;2: 77–82.

32. Weinstein RS, Bryce GF, Sappington LJ, et al. Decreased serum ionized calcium and normal vitamin D metabolite levels with anticonvulsant drug treatment. *J Clin Endocrinol Metab.* 1984;58(6):1003–1009.

33. Vestergaard P. Epilepsy, osteoporosis and fracture risk—a meta-analysis. *Acta Neurol Scand.* 2005;112(5):277–286.

34. Nissen-Meyer LS, Svalheim S, Taubøll E, et al. Levetiracetam, phenytoin, and valproate act differently on rat bone mass, structure, and metabolism. *Epilepsia.* 2007;48(10):1850–1860.

35. Souverein PC, Webb DJ, Weil JG, et al. Use of antiepileptic drugs and risk of fractures: case-control study among patients with epilepsy. *Neurology.* 2006;66(9):1318–1324.

36. Melton LJ III, Crowson CS, O'Fallon WM. Fracture incidence in Olmsted County, Minnesota: comparison of urban with rural rates and changes in urban rates over time. *Osteoporos Int.* 1999;9(1):29–37.

37. Buck D, Baker GA, Jacoby A, et al. Patients' experiences of injury as a result of epilepsy. *Epilepsia.* 1997;38(4):439–444.

38. Sheth RD, Gidal BE, Hermann BP. Pathological fractures in epilepsy. *Epilepsy Behav.* 2006;9(4):601–605.

39. Vestergaard P, Rejnmark L, Mosekilde L. Fracture risk associated with use of antiepileptic drugs. *Epilepsia.* 2004;45(11):1330–1337.

40. Stephen LJ, McLellan AR, Harrison JH, et al. Bone density and antiepileptic drugs: a case-controlled study. *Seizure.* 1999;8(6):339–342.

41. Boluk A, Guzelipek M, Savli H, et al. The effect of valproate on bone mineral density in adult epileptic patients. *Pharmacol Res.* 2004;50(1): 93–97.

42. Sheth RD. Metabolic concerns associated with antiepileptic medications. *Neurology.* 2004;63(10 suppl 4):S24—S29.

43. Verrotti A, Greco R, Morgese G, et al. Increased bone turnover in epileptic patients treated with carbamazepine. *Ann Neurol.* 2000;47(3):385–388.

44. Verrotti A, Greco R, Latini G, et al. Increased bone turnover in prepubertal, pubertal, and postpubertal patients receiving carbamazepine. *Epilepsia.* 2002;43(12):1488–1492.

45. Bouillon R, Reynaert J, Claes JH, et al. The effect of anticonvulsant therapy on serum levels of 25-hydroxy-vitamin D, calcium, and parathyroid hormone. *J Clin Endocrinol Metab.* 1975;41(06):1130–1135.

46. Gough H, Goggin T, Bissessar A, et al. A comparative study of the relative influence of different anticonvulsant drugs, UV exposure and diet on vitamin D and calcium metabolism in out-patients with epilepsy. *Q J Med.* 1986;59(230):569–577.

47. Pascussi JM, Robert A, Nguyen M, et al. Possible involvement of pregnane X receptor-enhanced CYP24 expression in drug-induced osteomalacia. *J Clin Invest.* 2005;115(1):177–186.

48. Zhou C, Assem M, Tay JC, et al. Steroid and xenobiotic receptor and vitamin D receptor crosstalk mediates CYP24 expression and drug-induced osteomalacia. *J Clin Invest.* 2006;116(6):1703–1712.

49. Valimaki MJ, Tiihonen M, Laitinen K, et al. Bone mineral density measured by dual-energy x-ray absorptiometry and novel markers of bone formation and resorption in patients on antiepileptic drugs. *J Bone Miner Res.* 1994;9(5):631–637.

50. Pluskiewicz W, Nowakowska J. Bone status after long-term anticonvulsant therapy in epileptic patients: evaluation using quantitative ultrasound of calcaneus and phalanges. *Ultrasound Med Biol.* 1997;23(4):553–558.

51. Pedrera JD, Canal ML, Carvajal J, et al. Influence of vitamin D administration on bone ultrasound measurements in patients on anticonvulsant therapy. *Eur J Clin Invest.* 2000;30(10):895–899.

52. Bramswig S, Zittermann A, Berthold HK. Carbamazepine does not alter biochemical parameters of bone turnover in healthy male adults. *Calcif Tissue Int.* 2003;73(4):356–360.

53. Davie MW, Emberson CE, Lawson DE, et al. Low plasma 25-hydroxyvitamin D and serum calcium levels in institutionalized epileptic subjects: associated risk factors, consequences and response to treatment with vitamin D. *Q J Med.* 1983;52(205):79–91.

54. Guo CY, Ronen GM, Atkinson SA. Long-term valproate and lamotrigine treatment may be a marker for reduced growth and bone mass in children with epilepsy. *Epilepsia.* 2001;42(9):1141–1147.

55. Matkovic V, Kostial K, Simonović I, et al. Bone status and fracture rates in two regions of Yugoslavia. *Am J Clin Nutr.* 1979;32(3):540–549.

56. Allen JR, Humphries IR, Waters DL, et al. Decreased bone mineral density in children with phenylketonuria. *Am J Clin Nutr.* 1994;59(2):419–422.

57. Lande MB, Kim MS, Bartlett C, et al. Reversible Fanconi syndrome associated with valproate therapy. *J Pediatr.* 1993;123(2):320–322.

58. Hawkins E, Brewer E. Renal toxicity induced by valproic acid (Depakene). *Pediatr Pathol.* 1993;13(6):863–868.

59. Pack AM, Morrell MJ, Marcus R, et al. Bone mass and turnover in women with epilepsy on antiepileptic drug monotherapy. *Ann Neurol.* 2005;57(2): 252–257.

60. Mintzer S, Boppana P, Toguri J, et al. Vitamin D levels and bone turnover in epilepsy patients taking carbamazepine or oxcarbazepine. *Epilepsia.* 2006;47(3):510–515.

61. Ali I, et al. Measurement of bone mineral density in patients on levetiracetam monotherapy. American Epilepsy Society Abstract, 2006:3.211.

62. Pierce WM Jr, Nardin GF, Fuqua MF, et al. Effect of chronic carbonic anhydrase inhibitor treatment on bone mineral density in white women. *J Bone Miner Res.* 1991;6(4):347–354.

63. Leung A, Ramsay E. Effect of topiramate on bone resorption in adults [abstract]. *Epilepsia.* 2006;47(suppl 4):2.150.

64. Sheth RD, Hermann BP. Bone mineral density with lamotrigine monotherapy for epilepsy. *Pediatr Neurol.* 2007;37(4):250–254.

65. Rattya J, Vainionpää L, Knip M, et al. The effects of valproate, carbamazepine, and oxcarbazepine on growth and sexual maturation in girls with epilepsy. *Pediatrics.* 1999;103(3):588–593.

66. Collins N, Maher J, Cole M, et al. A prospective study to evaluate the dose of vitamin D required to correct low 25-hydroxyvitamin D levels, calcium, and alkaline phosphatase in patients at risk of developing antiepileptic drug-induced osteomalacia. *Q J Med.* 1991;78(286):113–122.

67. Mikati MA, Dib L, Yamout B, et al. Two randomized vitamin D trials in ambulatory patients on anticonvulsants: impact on bone. *Neurology.* 2006;67(11):2005–2014.

68. Drezner MK. Treatment of anticonvulsant drug-induced bone disease. *Epilepsy Behav.* 2004;5(suppl 2):S41–S47.

69. Harden CL, Herzog AG, Nikolov BG, et al. Hormone replacement therapy in women with epilepsy: a randomized, double-blind, placebo-controlled study. *Epilepsia.* 2006;47(9):1447–1451.

70. Koppel BS, Harden CL, Nikolov BG, et al. An analysis of lifetime fractures in women with epilepsy. *Acta Neurol Scand.* 2005;111(4):225–228.

71. Sheth RD, Harden CL. Screening for bone health in epilepsy. *Epilepsia.* 2007;48(suppl 9):39–41.

CHAPTER 47 ■ TREATMENT OF EPILEPSY IN THE SETTING OF RENAL AND LIVER DISEASE

JANE G. BOGGS, ELIZABETH WATERHOUSE, AND ROBERT J. DELORENZO

Management of seizures in the presence of renal and liver disease has become an increasingly common problem during the past several decades. Prolonged survival, achieved largely through advances in dialysis, pharmacology, and transplantation, accounts for a growing population of patients with altered metabolic capacities. The emergence of opportunistic hepatic infections in acquired immune deficiency syndrome and other immunocompromised conditions, as well as the prevalence of viral hepatitis, has increased the population with impaired liver function. Pharmacologically induced renal dysfunction and systemic diseases, such as hypertension and diabetes, continue to occur frequently in patients whom an epileptologist may encounter. Consequently, neurologists must possess a basic understanding of pharmacology and the specific pharmacokinetics of anticonvulsants in liver and renal disease.

Patients with pre-existing liver and renal disease may require transient treatment with anticonvulsants for seizures as a result of electrolyte shifts associated with worsening uremia and dialysis, as well as hepatic insufficiency caused by chronic alcohol abuse. Secondary effects of disease in either of these organs can adversely affect blood pressure and coagulation, resulting in potentially epileptogenic cerebrovascular events. In addition, patients with epilepsy are not immune to the liver and renal diseases that occur in the general population. Antiepileptic drugs (AEDs) themselves may induce such organ dysfunction, complicating or contraindicating their further use.

This chapter reviews the clinical use in liver and renal disease of the commonly prescribed AEDs and the newer anticonvulsant medications that became available between 1993 and 2004. Because the degree of debility and the response to AEDs vary significantly among patients, specific rules cannot be inferred, and practical guidelines only are offered. The general biopharmacologic principles that precede the discussion of specific agents apply not only to current anticonvulsant therapy but also to drugs potentially available in the future.

MEDICATIONS IN RENAL DISEASE: OVERVIEW

The degree to which renal disease alters the pharmacokinetics of specific drugs depends on their primary mode of elimination. Drugs excreted unchanged by the kidneys have a slower rate of elimination and longer half-life in patients with renal disease than in healthy persons, increasing drug accumulation and necessitating lower doses and longer interdose intervals to prevent toxic effects.

Drugs are divided into three classes: (i) type A, which are eliminated completely by renal excretion; (ii) type B, which are eliminated by nonrenal routes; and (iii) type C, which are eliminated by both renal and nonrenal routes (1,2). Because the relationship between half-life and creatinine clearance (Cl_{Cr}) is not linear, dosing predictions based on renal insufficiency are difficult. However, estimates may be determined from the following linear equation that describes the speed of drug elimination as a function of creatinine clearance (3):

$$K = R \times Cl_{Cr} + K_{NR}$$

where K is the elimination rate constant, R the slope of K against Cl_{Cr}, and K_{NR} is the rate constant for drug elimination by nonrenal routes (4).

Nomograms based on computed values of K and K_{NR} will predict new maintenance doses that are reduced proportionately to the reduction in K. However, such linear equations do not take into account the effect of renal insufficiency on drug biotransformation, elimination of metabolites with toxic properties, or decreases in plasma protein binding.

Studies show that some drug oxidations in liver endoplasmic reticulum can be accelerated in uremia (5,6). The mechanism is undefined, but several possibilities have been proposed. Poorly excreted nutritional substances that can induce microsomal drug metabolism may be present in excess quantities in renal patients. Indole-containing cruciferous plants (cabbage, cauliflower, Brussels sprouts) induce these enzymes in rats (7). Drugs with low hepatic extraction and high protein binding will have higher rates of metabolism in uremia as the free fraction increases, which, in turn, increases plasma clearance and the apparent volume of distribution (V_d) (8):

$$V_d = VP + VT \times \frac{FP}{FT}$$

where VP is the plasma volume, VT is the extravascular volume, FP is the fraction of free drug in plasma, and FT is the fraction of free drug in tissue (9).

Protein binding of anionic acidic drugs (such as phenytoin, which is strongly bound by albumin) decreases in patients with renal dysfunction (Table 47.1). Drugs with organic bases have variable protein binding in renal disease, and those that bind primarily to one site have decreased binding, an effect described in the literature since 1938 (10). However, this reduced binding exceeds the amount that can be accounted for by a simple decrease in serum albumin. Two hypotheses relating to uremia have been proposed to resolve this discrepancy: the existence of small molecules that competitively displace drugs from normal binding sites (11) and altered binding sites of albumin molecules (12). Experimental evidence supports

TABLE 47.1

DISPOSITION OF COMMON ANTIEPILEPTIC DRUGS IN RENAL DISEASE

Drug	Protein binding	Total plasma concentration	Plasma half-life	Risk of intoxication	Dosage adjustment	Removal by dialysis
Phenytoin	↓	↓	↓	Low	Unnecessary	Negligible
Valproic acid	↓	↓	—	Low	Unnecessary	Negligible
Phenobarbital	—	—	— or ↑	High	Slight reduction	Significant
Primidone	—	—	—	High	Slight reduction	Unknown
Carbamazepine	—	—	—	Low	Unnecessary	Unknown
Ethosuximide	NA	—	—	Low	Unnecessary	Unknown
Benzodiazepines	↓	↓	—	Low	Unnecessary	Unknown
Gabapentin	—	↑	↑	Low	Reduction	Significant
Lamotrigine	Unknown	? ↑	↑	Unknown	Unknown	Moderate
Felbamate[a]	Unknown	? ↑	Unknown	Unknown	Reduce by one-half	Moderate
Topiramate	Unknown	↑	↑	Considerable	Reduction	Significant
Tiagabine[b]	—	—	—	Unknown	Unnecessary	Negligible
Zonisamide	Unknown	? ↑	Unknown	Unknown	Reduction	Unknown
Oxcarbazepine[c,d]	Unknown	↑	↑	Considerable	Reduction	Unknown
Levetiracetam[e]	—	↑	Unknown	Unknown	Reduction	50%
Clobazam	↑	—	—	Low	Reduction	Unknown
Lacosamide	Unknown	↑	↑	Unknown	Reduction if ESRD[f]	Significant
Rufinamide	43%	? ↑	↑	Unknown	Slight reduction	Moderate

↓, Reduction; —, unchanged; ↑, increased; NA, not applicable; ESRD, end-stage renal disease.
[a]Package insert.
[b]Cato et al. (111).
[c]Package insert.
[d]Rouan et al. (100).
[e]Patsalos (116).
[f]Package insert.
Adapted from Asconape JJ, Penry JK. Use of antiepileptic drugs in the presence of liver and kidney disease: a review. *Epilepsia.* 1982;23(suppl 1): 565–579.

both mechanisms, and each probably is involved to some extent in individual patients (13). Although drug metabolism may be accelerated in uremic humans, the same drugs may exhibit slowed metabolism in uremic animals, complicating the extrapolation from experimental data (14).

Although dialysis ameliorates renal insufficiency, it alters the response to medications. The removal of drugs from serum by hemodialysis depends on numerous variables, including molecular weight, protein binding, plasma concentration, blood flow, and hematocrit, as well as on the inherent clearance characteristics of the dialyzer. Dialysis also can profoundly affect drug activity through changes in pH level, protein concentration, osmolality, electrolytes, and glucose and urea levels. Peritoneal dialysis, unlike hemodialysis, is influenced by vascular disease because the blood supply presented to the dialysate passes through arterioles. Drug additives are used more frequently in peritoneal dialysis than in hemodialysis solutions, creating a small potential for drug interactions (15). Following hemodialysis, albumin binding of such medications as phenytoin and phenobarbital is decreased, perhaps because of increased levels of nonesterified fatty acids, which bind strongly to albumin (16). This effect has been proposed for heparin, administered systemically during dialysis, with resultant activation of lipoprotein lipase (17).

MEDICATIONS IN LIVER DISEASE: OVERVIEW

Because the liver is a primary site of drug metabolism in humans, hepatic insufficiency can significantly alter biotransformation and disposition, although pathophysiologic changes will vary according to the disease or its stages. Hepatic blood inflow by the portal vein, hepatocellular mass, and functional capacity primarily determine the effects of liver disease on drug handling. Table 47.2 illustrates the major changes found in cirrhosis, acute viral hepatitis, and alcoholic hepatitis (18).

At least five categories of liver disease affect drug disposition: (i) chronic liver disease; (ii) acute hepatitis; (iii) drug-induced hepatotoxicity; (iv) cholestasis; and (v) hepatic infiltrative/neoplastic disease. In addition, medications must be classified not only by protein binding but also by the capacity of the liver to extract drug as blood flows through the organ: flow limited, capacity limited with high protein binding, and capacity limited with low protein binding (19).

Flow-limited drugs have high extraction rates, and clearance is limited primarily by blood flow. Their rate of metabolism depends on the amount of drug presented to the liver,

TABLE 47.2

PATHOPHYSIOLOGIC CHANGES IN VARIOUS TYPES OF LIVER DISEASE

Disease	Total hepatic blood flow	Hepatocellular mass	Hepatocyte function
Cirrhosis			
Moderate	↓	—/↑	—
Severe	↓	↓	↓
Acute/inflammatory			
Liver disease			
Viral hepatitis	—/↑	—/↑	↓
Alcoholic hepatitis	—/↑	—/↑/↓	↓

↓, Decreased; —, unchanged; ↑, increased.
From Blaschke TF, Meffin PJ, Melmon KL, et al. Influence of acute viral hepatitis on phenytoin kinetics and protein binding. *Clin Pharmacol Ther.* 1975;17:685–691, with permission.

which is proportional to blood flow. Most anticonvulsants are capacity-limited drugs, as their extraction ratios are low (<0.2). Table 47.3 lists the extraction ratios of major antiepileptic compounds (18,20–23). The rate of metabolism of capacity-limited drugs depends on the concentration of free drug at hepatic enzyme receptor sites and thus on the extent of protein binding. Capacity-limited, binding-sensitive drugs, such as phenytoin, valproic acid, and carbamazepine, are greater than 85% bound to plasma proteins at therapeutic concentrations; therefore, alterations in plasma protein concentration and binding characteristics can significantly alter their hepatic clearance (23,24). Capacity-limited, binding-insensitive drugs, such as ethosuximide, have a low affinity for plasma protein (usually less than 30% at therapeutic concentrations), and clearance is only minimally affected by changes in protein binding.

The following model, combining the principles of intrinsic metabolic capacity and blood flow, has been proposed (25):

$$Cl_h = \frac{Q \times F_b \times Cl_{int}}{Q + F_b \times Cl_{int}}$$

where Cl_h is the volume of blood cleared by the liver per unit time, Q is total hepatic blood flow, F_b is the fraction of drug bound to protein and cells, and Cl_{int} is the intrinsic metabolic clearance (23,24,26).

The latter term, defined as the volume of liver water cleared of drug per unit time, varies directly with the Michaelis con-

stant. The extraction ratio (E) may be derived by dividing hepatic blood flow into total hepatic clearance (27):

$$\frac{Cl}{Q} = E$$

When combined hepatic and renal clearance occurs, clearances are additive.

Although hypoalbuminemia is frequently a feature of liver disease, drug binding to plasma proteins may be decreased even without measurable changes in albumin concentration (Table 47.4). Mechanisms similar to those causing decreased protein binding in renal insufficiency have been suggested (28,29). Because intrinsic clearance varies with the type and duration of liver disease, the effects of changes in protein binding in capacity-limited, binding-sensitive drugs are complex. If hepatic disease lowers binding without changing intrinsic clearance, total drug concentration will ultimately fall because the rate of metabolism of these drugs depends on the free fraction. If liver disease reduces intrinsic clearance, total drug concentration may remain the same or increase as the free concentration increases. This can result in enhanced response or toxic effects at lower than expected drug levels and may explain the increased incidence of adverse reactions to medications such as valproic acid in liver disease (30).

Capacity-limited, binding-insensitive drugs can be considered relatively pure indicators of intrinsic clearance. However, tissue binding to substances such as ligandin may contribute

TABLE 47.3

EXTRACTION RATIOS OF MAJOR ANTIEPILEPTIC COMPOUNDS

Extraction rates	Extraction ratios	% Bound	Source
Phenytoin	0.03	90	Blaschke et al. (18)
Valproic acid	<0.05		Evans et al. (137)
Carbamazepine	<0.002		Evans et al. (137)
Benzodiazepines (diazepam)	0.03	98	Klotz et al. (21)
Hexobarbitone	0.16		Breimer et al. (20)
Amylobarbitone	0.03	61	Mawer et al. (22)

TABLE 47.4

DISPOSITION OF COMMON ANTIEPILEPTIC DRUGS IN HEPATIC DISEASE

Drug	Protein binding	Total plasma concentration	Plasma half-life	Risk of intoxication	Dosage adjustment
Phenytoin	↓	—	—	Considerable	Unnecessary or slight reduction
Valproic acid	↓	↓	↑	Considerable	Unnecessary or slight reduction
Phenobarbital	Unknown	—	↑	Considerable	Unnecessary or slight reduction
Primidone	Unknown	—	Unknown	Unknown	Unknown
Carbamazepine	↓	—	Unknown	Considerable?	Unknown
Benzodiazepines[a]	↓	—	↑	High	Reduction
Gabapentin	—	—	—	Low	Unnecessary
Lamotrigine	?↓	?↑	?↑	Unknown	Reduction
Clobazam	↑	↑	↑	High	Reduction
Felbamate	?↓	?↑	?↑	Contraindicated	Contraindicated
Tiagabine	↓	↑	↑	Considerable	Reduction
Lacosamide	Unknown	↑	Unknown	Unknown	Reduction/Contraindicated[b]
Rufinamide	34%	—	—	Unknown	Reduction

↓, Reduced; —, unchanged; ↑, increased.
[a]Not applicable to oxazepam.
[b]Reduction with mild or moderate hepatic impairment, not recommended for use with severe hepatic impairment.
Adapted from Asconape JJ, Penry JK. Use of antiepileptic drugs in the presence of liver and kidney disease: a review. *Epilepsia.* 1982;23(suppl 1): 565–579.

to the volume of distribution of drugs and thus to their half-life. The effect of liver disease on the content and function of such binding proteins is poorly understood. Tissue binding can be affected by secondary pathologic changes of liver disease, such as alterations in tissue and plasma pH level (24,31–33) or by ascites (34,35).

Because of various types of drugs and stages of liver disease, as well as interindividual variation, predicting changes in drug kinetics in patients with hepatic insufficiency remains difficult. Studies have identified additional discrepancies between observed changes and those suggested by pharmacokinetic predictions (12,23,36). Another variable is the potential for autoinduction of microsomal enzymes after long-term drug administration. Phenobarbital and carbamazepine and their active metabolites have this potential, with resultant temporal variability in drug levels and efficacy, increased complexity of drug interactions, and the potential increased risk of liver dysfunction.

SPECIFIC DRUGS

Phenytoin

Phenytoin (5,5-diphenylhydantoin) has a dissociation constant (pK_a) of about 8.3 and is approximately 90% bound to plasma proteins, mainly albumin (37). A larger proportion remains free in neonates and in patients with hypoalbuminemia and uremia (38). Apparent volume of distribution is approximately 64% of body weight, as fractional binding in tissues is similar to that in plasma. Elimination occurs nearly exclusively by hepatic microsomal biotransformation, with less than 5% excreted unchanged in urine (39). The primary metabolite, 5-parahydroxyphenyl-5-phenylhydantoin, is inactive and is excreted initially in bile and subsequently in urine, mostly as glucuronide. The corresponding microsomal enzymes are saturable at usual clinical doses. For concentrations less than 10 mg/L, elimination is exponential; at high levels, it is dose dependent (40).

Effects of Renal Disease

Phenytoin is the most extensively studied anticonvulsant in renal dysfunction. Uremic plasma has lower binding capacity for phenytoin than plasma in healthy subjects, with unbound fractions as high as 30%, compared with the usual 10% to 15% (28,41–43). The degree of binding impairment has been correlated with levels of albumin, blood urea nitrogen, serum creatinine, creatinine clearance, and the patient's physical disability (43,44). However, decreased binding is noted frequently in uremic patients with normal albumin levels (45), suggesting the accumulation of competitive or noncompetitive inhibiting substances (11) or altered albumin-binding sites (12). Most consistently, the free fraction of phenytoin directly reflects the degree of renal failure, which can be roughly estimated by serum creatinine values. Reidenberg and Affrime (45) calculated the total phenytoin values that produce free phenytoin levels of 0.7 to 1.4 mg/L (Fig. 47.1). Decreased protein binding results in a proportionate increase in the apparent volume of distribution higher than the usual 0.6 L/kg. In chronic renal failure, this situation results in lower total plasma concentrations, reducing therapeutic ranges from 10 to 20 mg/L to as low as 5 to 10 mg/L (6,46,47).

The half-life of phenytoin is decreased in patients with uremia. Increased hepatic clearance of phenytoin observed in uremic rabbits suggests that heightened drug metabolism may account for more rapid elimination (48). However, additional

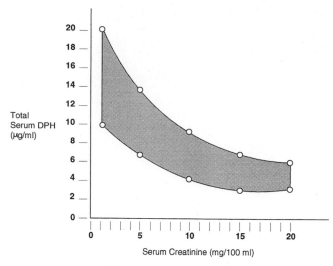

FIGURE 47.1 Calculated values of total serum phenytoin (diphenylhydantoin [DPH]) concentration that will produce a concentration in plasma water of 0.7 to 1.4 μg/mL. (Adapted from Rowland M, Blaschke TF, Meffin PJ, et al. Pharmacokinetics in disease states modifying hepatic and metabolic function. In: Benet LZ, ed. *Effect of Disease States on Drug Pharmacokinetics.* Washington, DC: American Pharmaceutical Association; 1976:53–74.)

studies have not demonstrated enhanced microsomal enzyme activity (49,50). Because 95% of a phenytoin dose is biotransformed, little parent drug accumulates, even in severe renal failure. Nevertheless, accumulation of the glucuronide metabolite, which is primarily excreted by the kidney, does occur in renal failure (5,51). This metabolite has no known anticonvulsant or toxic properties. Some studies suggest that it may inhibit phenytoin biotransformation (52), whereas others report no such effect (27,53).

Dialysis affects phenytoin primarily by altering protein binding. Various studies have suggested either a decrease (3) or an increase (54) in binding capacity following hemodialysis. This apparent contradiction may result from fluctuations in the free fraction of phenytoin during and after hemodialysis, leading to unexpected clinical intoxication (54). Martin and colleagues (55) reported that only 2% to 4% of intravenous phenytoin appeared in the dialysate of seven uremic patients. With a dialyzer of 4.5% efficiency, no postdialysis supplementation was necessary (55).

Finally, certain assays may give incorrect results in renally impaired patients. The enzyme-multiplied immunoassay may falsely elevate total plasma phenytoin levels in patients with severe renal insufficiency (56), tripling values obtained by gas–liquid chromatography. The cause of this discrepancy is unknown, but gas–liquid or high-performance liquid chromatography appears to be a more predictable and clinically useful method in patients with advanced renal disease (57).

Effects of Liver Disease

Plasma from patients with hepatic insufficiency also has reduced binding capacity for phenytoin (28,44,45). The degree of impairment correlates with levels of serum albumin (18,58) or total bilirubin (53), or both (29,44). It has been suggested that the total number of binding sites is reduced as a result of lower albumin concentration in competition with bilirubin

(44). However, studies in alcoholic cirrhosis and acute viral hepatitis indicate that the degree of impairment is unlikely to be significant (18,25). Nevertheless, neonates with hyperbilirubinemia have substantially decreased phenytoin binding and require a reduced dose to prevent toxic effects (29).

Decreased biotransformation capacity in patients with liver disease results in accumulation of drug and increased potential for toxicity. Studies by Kutt and colleagues (14) found that in patients receiving phenytoin or phenobarbital, drug accumulated as hepatic dysfunction increased. Decreased renal excretion of metabolites was also noted.

Clinical Recommendations

Based on the shortened half-life noted in uremia, phenytoin usually should be administered no less frequently than every 8 hours. Lower loading doses may be necessary if protein binding is expected to be markedly decreased, as a high free fraction can be anticipated. Bound and free phenytoin levels should be determined for a stable level of renal function, and maintenance levels adjusted accordingly. The therapeutic range for free phenytoin remains between 1 and 2 mg/L, even in renal disease. Salivary levels closely correlate with free levels. No supplementation should be given after hemodialysis or peritoneal dialysis. Microsomal enzyme induction from long-term phenytoin administration may increase metabolism of 25-hydroxycalciferol, worsening the osteomalacia of uremia (59). Although phenytoin accumulation may accompany severe liver disease, nonlinear kinetics and difficulty in estimating hepatic metabolic capacity limit the clinician's ability to predict dose adjustments. Therefore, frequent serum determinations and gradual dose regulation are necessary.

Phenobarbital

Phenobarbital (5-ethyl-5-phenylbarbituric acid) is a weak acid with a pK_a of 7.2 that is 40% to 60% bound to plasma proteins. Its volume of distribution is approximately 0.9 L/kg (33). Up to 25% of the drug dose is eliminated by renal mechanisms, whereas the remainder is metabolized by the hepatic mixed-function oxidase system. The major metabolites, parahydroxyphenobarbital and N-hydroxyphenobarbital, are inactive and are excreted by the kidneys. Phenobarbital is a potent inducer of the microsomal enzyme system (40).

Effects of Renal Disease

Although the half-life of phenobarbital has been reported to be unchanged in uremic patients (38), some accumulation should be expected, as elimination of long-acting barbiturates depends more on renal excretion than on biotransformation. Because of this, hemodialysis and peritoneal dialysis remove a proportion of phenobarbital from the serum, thereby reducing serum levels. In impaired renal function, severe central nervous system and cardiovascular depression may result from barbiturate accumulation, further worsening the renal condition.

Effects of Liver Disease

Because a significant amount is excreted unchanged by the kidneys, phenobarbital has been promoted as a useful agent in patients with liver disease. Nevertheless, some studies have found a prolonged half-life in certain hepatic illnesses. Animal models with carbon tetrachloride-induced liver damage showed a slight reduction in plasma clearance (60). In cirrhotic patients, phenobarbital half-life was prolonged compared with that in controls (130 ± 15 hours and 86 ± 3 hours, respectively), and reduced amounts of conjugated hydroxyphenobarbital appeared in the urine (61). However, in patients with acute viral hepatitis, no statistically significant prolongation of half-life or change in metabolic excretion clearly occurred, although only one dose of phenobarbital was administered (61). In a previous study, two cirrhotic patients who chronically received phenobarbital appeared to have drug accumulation when the daily dosage exceeded 60 mg. However, this study lacked controls and was complicated by concomitant administration of other drugs (14). Biliary excretion of phenobarbital is minimal, and cholestasis does not change serum levels (61).

Clinical Recommendations

Although no short-term dosage adjustment appears necessary, lower maintenance doses of phenobarbital must be recommended. Supplementation after dialysis is probably necessary (62). The effect of liver disease on patients receiving prolonged phenobarbital therapy varies with the individual as well as with the type of liver damage. Frequent measurement of plasma concentrations will help establish dose modifications; free levels offer little additional information.

Primidone

Primidone (2-deoxyphenobarbital), structurally related to phenobarbital, is not significantly bound to plasma proteins. It is partially converted by the liver to the active forms phenobarbital and phenylethylmalonamide. Approximately 20% of a primidone dose is excreted unchanged in the urine (9).

Effects of Renal Disease

Although little information is available on the use of primidone in renal disease, accumulation with resultant toxicity has been reported, presumably from delayed renal excretion and prolongation of the phenylethylmalonamide half-life. In one report (63), phenylethylmalonamide levels were proportionately higher than those of primidone or phenobarbital and thus were hypothesized to be responsible for clinical toxicity. Another patient showed evidence of intoxication, with high phenylethylmalonamide levels and moderate elevation of phenobarbital in association with renal failure (64).

Effects of Liver Disease

As primidone is metabolized to active compounds by the liver, little difference can be anticipated in a short course of therapy in liver disease. With long-term administration, changes similar to those seen with phenobarbital may be expected. No results from experimental investigation of primidone in liver disease are available.

Clinical Recommendations

Because primidone is metabolized to three active compounds, determination of plasma concentrations may help in assessing intoxications. With very low protein binding, free levels offer little information. Although it is unclear whether primidone may be removed by dialysis, its metabolite phenobarbital certainly will be. Supplementation following dialysis may be necessary and can best be established by measuring levels of primidone, phenobarbital, and phenylethylmalonamide.

Valproic Acid

Valproic acid (2-propylpentanoic acid) is a carboxylic acid with a pK_a of 4.9. The drug is 90% bound to plasma proteins, with a resultant volume of distribution of only 0.1 to 0.4 L/kg. At higher serum concentrations, protein binding decreases (13). Elimination is mostly by hepatic biotransformation, with only 1% to 3% of the dose excreted unchanged in urine. More than 70% is present as metabolites, primarily the glucuronide of 2-propylglutaric acid. This drug has no known enzyme-inducing properties. Its metabolites show anticonvulsant activity in animal studies, particularly 3-oxovalproic acid, which has activity comparable to that of valproic acid in mice. No data on this compound's activity in humans are available (65).

Effects of Renal Disease

As with phenytoin, protein binding of valproic acid decreases in uremia (66,67). The decrease correlates with levels of blood urea nitrogen, creatinine, uric acid, and creatinine clearance but appears to have little relation to albumin and total protein levels (68). Hypoalbuminemia exerts a more significant effect in patients with a nephrotic syndrome than in healthy individuals. Hemodialysis decreased protein binding in 3 of 4 patients in one study (67). Reduced protein binding, with increased apparent volume of distribution, lowers total steady-state concentrations and unchanged free levels. As valproic acid is eliminated primarily by the liver, little accumulation in renal failure should be expected. However, its metabolites may have a prolonged effect because of delayed elimination. A single case report of valproic acid-related hepatobiliary dysfunction and reversible renal failure described decreased renal clearance of total conjugated valproic acid. In vivo production of rearranged valproic acid glucuronide was detected. It is unclear whether the accumulation of these altered substances is related to hepatobiliary or renal dysfunction, or both, and whether these substances are clinically active in humans (69).

Effects of Liver Disease

Valproic acid disposition studies in patients with alcoholic cirrhosis and those recovering from acute viral hepatitis (70) noted variably decreased protein binding (from 88.7% to 70.3% and 78.1%, respectively), with consequent increase in the apparent volume of distribution. Plasma half-life increased from 12.2 ± 3.7 hours in controls to 18.9 ± 5.1 hours in patients with cirrhosis and to 17 ± 3.7 hours in those with hepatitis. Total drug plasma clearance remained unimpaired in both groups, but free drug clearance decreased in cirrhotic patients. Reduced protein binding also increased the entrance of free valproic acid into blood cells and lowered metabolism by limiting substrate concentration. The investigators noted no changes in urinary excretion of valproic acid. Therefore, liver diseases studied appeared to result in reduced metabolic capacity for valproic acid that was compensated for by decreased protein binding. However, another study (68) of patients in acute stages of viral hepatitis showed increased half-life of valproic acid from 14.9 to 25.1 hours, with total drug clearance reduced from 8.6 to 3.8 mL/min.

Altered metabolic profiles of valproic acid have been described primarily in case reports of severe hepatic failure. A case resembling Reye syndrome in a 7-year-old reported significantly increased formation of three monounsaturated and four double-unsaturated metabolites in plasma (58% to 71% of valproic acid compounds compared with a maximum of 15% in controls) and in urine (34% to 61% compared with a maximum of 10% in controls) (71). β-Oxidation, in particular, appeared suppressed, whereas omega-oxidation was increased (1). Serum-free carnitine, as well as the main β-oxidation metabolite 3-ketovalproic acid, decreased despite serum valproic acid concentration at the upper limit of the therapeutic range in a 3-year-old with valproic acid–induced Reye syndrome (72). Autopsy of a set of twins with a progressive hepatic encephalopathy revealed hepatic necrosis only in the sibling who had received valproic acid, indicating that the drug may have aggravated pre-existing hepatic pathology (73).

Rarely, valproic acid precipitates severe hepatotoxicity (74). This idiosyncratic reaction usually occurs during the first 6 months of treatment, and most cases have been reported in children. Other suggested associated risk factors for this condition include developmental delay and polytherapy. Histologic changes are variable, including cholestasis, centrilobular necrosis, and fatty changes. Clinical symptoms, such as nausea, vomiting, malaise, and breakthrough seizures, often appear before liver function tests become abnormal (75). Valproic acid causes metabolic changes because of the inhibition of enzymes involved in intermediary cell metabolism. Moderate elevations of blood ammonia are common in patients receiving valproic acid and usually do not require treatment in the absence of clinical symptoms (76).

Clinical Recommendations

Reduction of valproic acid dose generally is unnecessary in renal disease. However, decreased protein binding will lower the therapeutic range in uremic patients in proportion to the degree of renal failure. No estimated relationship has been established as it has for phenytoin, but free levels can be determined and dose adjustments should be based on clinical grounds and on the increase in free level greater than 10%. No clear evidence indicates that valproic acid must be supplemented following dialysis. Extreme caution should be exercised in the use of valproic acid in liver disease. Significant accumulation may occur as a result of increased half-life and may worsen hepatic function to a precipitous degree. The literature has little information on such cases, as valproic acid was discontinued promptly in all reported patients.

Carbamazepine

Carbamazepine (5-*H*-dibenz[*b,f*]azepine-5-carboxamide) is a neutral iminostilbene that is structurally related to imipramine. Plasma protein binding reaches 70% to 80%, and elimination depends almost entirely on hepatic biotransformation by epoxidation and hydroxylation. The most significant product is 10,11-carbamazepine epoxide, which has pharmacologic activity in animals (77). Carbamazepine can induce its own metabolism, shortening the half-life proportionately to the duration of treatment (40).

Effects of Renal Disease

Hooper and associates (78) found no evidence of reduced protein binding in patients with renal disease. Because only 1% of carbamazepine is eliminated unchanged in urine, accumulation of parent drug or the epoxide metabolite is unlikely. No studies are available on the effects of dialysis on the drug or its metabolites.

Effects of Liver Disease

Significant reduction in the percentage of carbamazepine bound to protein occurred in patients with mild liver disease (78). No clear correlation between any laboratory parameter and the degree of impairment could be determined.

Clinical Recommendations

Dose adjustment is not needed in either renal disease or dialysis. However, close monitoring of serum levels of carbamazepine and the 10,11-epoxide should be maintained, especially with long-term administration in patients with liver dysfunction.

Ethosuximide

Ethosuximide (2-ethyl-2-methylsuccinimide), a weak acid with a pK_a of 9.3, is not bound to plasma proteins. It is metabolized in the liver by hydroxylation at C-2 of the ethyl and methyl side chains with subsequent glucuronidation. Only 10% to 20% is eliminated unchanged in urine, and half-life is age dependent, increasing from approximately 30 hours in children to 60 hours in adults (40). No information is available on the pharmacokinetics of ethosuximide in renal or hepatic disease. Accumulation in renal failure is unlikely because of the small amount excreted. Significant removal during dialysis is probable, owing to the low volume of distribution and negligible protein binding. Supplementation based on serum levels following dialysis is recommended (62).

Benzodiazepines

The most commonly used benzodiazepines in epilepsy are diazepam, clonazepam, chlordiazepoxide, clorazepate, and nitrazepam. All undergo primarily hepatic biotransformation; minimal amounts appear unchanged in urine. Various metabolites such as desmethyldiazepam and oxazepam are clinically active and eliminated by the kidney in the free and glucuronidated forms. Protein binding varies among drugs (40).

Effects of Renal Disease

Although protein binding of diazepam and desmethyldiazepam declines with worsening uremia, the clinical significance of this effect remains unclear (78–80). Levels of chlordiazepoxide and diazepam have not been found to decrease following dialysis (81).

Effects of Liver Disease

Liver disease significantly alters the disposition of most benzodiazepines. Prolonged half-life of diazepam and chlordiazepoxide has been found in cirrhosis and acute viral hepatitis (82–84). Notably, oxazepam shows no evidence of altered disposition in various liver diseases (84,85). Hepatic disease reduces protein binding in all benzodiazepines studied except oxazepam (86).

Clinical Recommendations

Because renal disease has little impact on the elimination of benzodiazepines, no postdialysis supplementation or dose adjustment in uremia should be necessary. In liver disease, however, doses of diazepam, chlordiazepoxide, and probably clorazepate and clonazepam warrant reduction (87). Oxazepam appears to be an exception, as it is eliminated after glucuronidation without significant oxidative metabolism (8).

Lamotrigine

Lamotrigine [6-(2,3-dichlorophenyl)-1,2,4-triazine-3,5-diamine] is a phenyltriazine, chemically unrelated to other AEDs. Plasma protein binding is approximately 55% at therapeutic levels. Lamotrigine is metabolized predominantly by glucuronidation, and then it is eliminated renally. It may induce its own metabolism to a modest degree when multiple doses are administered (88). When it is taken with hepatic enzyme-inducing AEDs (phenytoin, carbamazepine, phenobarbital, primidone), it is eliminated more rapidly. However, lamotrigine clearance is decreased by about 50% in the presence of valproate.

Effects of Renal Disease

Clinical experience in patients with renal dysfunction is limited. In a study of a small number of patients with renal impairment, Fillastre and colleagues (89) found that the elimination half-life of unchanged lamotrigine is prolonged in comparison with that in patients with normal renal function. Twelve volunteers with chronic renal failure and six individuals undergoing hemodialysis were given a single 100-mg dose. The mean plasma half-lives shown were 42.9 hours (chronic renal failure), 13.0 hours (during hemodialysis), and 57.4 hours (between hemodialysis treatments), compared with 26.2 hours in healthy volunteers. Approximately 20% of the amount of lamotrigine present in the body was eliminated during 4 hours of hemodialysis.

Effects of Liver Disease

The disposition of lamotrigine in patients with hepatic dysfunction has not been extensively evaluated. Posner and colleagues (90) evaluated the pharmacokinetics of a single dose of lamotrigine in seven patients with Gilbert syndrome, a benign condition associated with a deficiency in the enzyme bilirubin uridine diphosphate glucuronyltransferase. Although the clearance of lamotrigine was lower and its half-life longer in these patients than in controls, it was felt that these differences were unlikely to be clinically significant. The clearance of lamotrigine is increased in the setting of hepatic impairment, and the package insert states that the mean half-life of lamotrigine in patients with liver impairment that was mild, moderate, severe without ascites, and severe with ascites, was 46 ± 20, 72 ± 44, 67 ± 11, and 100 ± 47 hours respectively, compared with 33 ± 7 hours in healthy controls.

Clinical Recommendations

Lamotrigine should be used with caution in patients with renal or hepatic dysfunction. Initial doses depend upon concomitant AEDs. Maintenance dose reduction is appropriate for patients with severe renal impairment, and close monitoring is warranted. For patients with hepatic impairment, the package insert recommends no dose adjustment for those with mild liver disease, and a 25% reduction in initial, escalation, and maintenance doses in those with moderate liver disease or with severe disease but no ascites. In the setting of severe liver impairment and ascites, lamotrigine doses should be reduced by 50%.

Felbamate

Felbamate (2-phenyl-1,3-propanediol dicarbamate) is a dicarbamate that is structurally similar to meprobamate. It is between 22% and 25% protein bound. Almost half of the dose is eliminated unchanged in the urine; the rest is metabolized by the liver to 2-hydroxy, *p*-hydroxy, and monocarbamate metabolites, none of which demonstrates significant antiepileptic activity (91). There is no autoinduction.

Effects of Renal Disease

Few data are available regarding the use of felbamate in patients with renal dysfunction.

Effects of Liver Disease

As of September 1999, there were 19 reported cases of hepatotoxicity associated with felbamate administration and 5 fatalities. The risk of fatal liver damage associated with felbamate is estimated to be 1 in 24,000 to 32,000 patients (92).

A detailed review of the reported cases of hepatic failure in patients treated with felbamate reveals confounding factors in up to 50% (93). Concomitant medications (valproic acid, carbamazepine, and phenytoin) or the presence of status epilepticus, acetaminophen toxicity, hepatitis, or shock liver may have played a significant role. Although no definitive diagnostic indicator has been established in unconfounded cases, research has identified a potential reactive aldehyde metabolite. Until further data are forthcoming, the clinician should consider potential risks for aplastic anemia and hepatic failure before initiating treatment with this drug.

Clinical Recommendations

Felbamate should not be prescribed for patients with a history of hepatic dysfunction. A patient who develops abnormal liver function values should be immediately withdrawn from the drug. Because felbamate is metabolized by the kidneys as well as the liver, either renal or hepatic dysfunction could decrease drug clearance. Because of the risk of aplastic anemia or hepatic failure, felbamate should not be used as a first-line AED and its use always requires careful hematologic and biochemical monitoring.

Gabapentin

Gabapentin [1-(aminomethyl)cyclohexane acetic acid] was synthesized as a γ-aminobutyric acid (GABA) analogue, although it does not act through direct GABA mechanisms. Gabapentin is not metabolized and does not inhibit or induce AED-metabolizing hepatic enzymes. It does not bind to plasma proteins and does not affect steady-state concentrations of other anticonvulsant drugs (94). It is excreted renally.

Effects of Renal Disease

Because gabapentin is excreted by the kidneys entirely, its elimination depends on renal function. Impairment of renal function decreases gabapentin clearance and increases plasma concentration in proportion to the degree of dysfunction. In 11 anuric patients given a single 400-mg oral dose of gabapentin, the half-life was 132 hours on days when hemodialysis was not performed and 3.8 hours during dialysis (95).

Effects of Liver Disease

Because of its low protein binding and renal elimination, gabapentin is theoretically a good anticonvulsant choice in patients with partial seizures and hepatic dysfunction. However, currently few data are available regarding the use of gabapentin in this population.

Clinical Recommendations

Gabapentin dosage should be decreased or the dosing interval increased in patients with renal dysfunction. The manufacturer recommends the following dosages, based on the patient's creatinine clearance: 400 mg three times a day, more than 60 mL/min; 300 mg twice a day, 30 to 60 mL/min; 300 mg once a day, 15 to 30 mL/min; and 300 mg every other day, less than 15 mL/min. A maintenance dose of 200 to 300 mg is recommended following each 4-hour session of hemodialysis, with no need for further supplementation until the next dialysis.

Oxcarbazepine

Oxcarbazepine (10,11-dihydro-10-oxocarbamazepine) is the keto analogue of carbamazepine. This compound was developed in an attempt to improve the tolerability profile of carbamazepine by elimination of metabolic production of carbamazepine 10,11-epoxide. Oxcarbazepine is rapidly and almost completely absorbed from the gastrointestinal tract after ingestion and is rapidly and nearly completely converted to the active metabolite, 10,11-dihydro-10-hydroxy-*5H*-dibenzo(*b*,*f*)azepine-5-carboxamide (MHD) (96). As MHD is the main compound active in the blood, pharmacokinetic data on oxcarbazepine are based on data for MHD. MHD is highly lipophilic and readily crosses the blood–brain barrier. Approximately 38% of MHD is protein bound in plasma, and its volume of distribution is approximately 0.3 to 0.8 L/kg (97–99). The half-life of MHD in plasma is approximately 8 to 10 hours. More than 95% of MHD is excreted by the kidneys. Oxcarbazepine also shows considerable placental transfer.

Effects of Renal and Liver Disease

Few studies are currently available on the effect of renal disease on oxcarbazepine levels. However, because the active, dominant metabolite is excreted by the kidneys, renal disease significantly impacts the half-life and blood levels of oxcarbazepine, and dose reductions as well as increased dosing intervals are recommended to prevent dose-dependent toxicity (100).

Little is known about the effect of liver disease on oxcarbazepine in humans.

Clinical Recommendations

Patients with renal disease or those receiving dialysis will not eliminate oxcarbazepine as quickly as normal individuals, as noted above. Patients with liver failure may tolerate oxcar-

bazepine, and it may be used cautiously in this group of patients, even though no clinical studies are available at this time to guide usage. Because approximately 40% of the MHD metabolite of oxcarbazepine is protein bound, the effect of renal and liver disease on protein plasma binding may result in increased free levels of MHD.

Topiramate

Topiramate, a sulfamate-substituted monosaccharide [2,3:4,5-bis-O-(1-methylethylidine)-β-D-fructopyranose], is structurally distinct from other anticonvulsant drugs. It is approximately 15% protein bound and not extensively metabolized. Only 20% of a single dose is metabolized by healthy adults; up to 50% of multiple doses is metabolized by patients taking other anticonvulsants. No clinically active metabolites have been identified. The drug is eliminated renally, and about 50% to 80% appears unchanged in the urine (4).

Effects of Renal and Liver Disease

As topiramate is excreted primarily via the kidneys, impaired creatinine clearance may delay elimination. In preclinical studies, topiramate was associated with a 1.5% risk of calcium renal stone formation, but this rate was not greater than that seen in placebo-treated patients (101). No increased incidence of adverse effects has been noted in patients with pre-existing renal or hepatic disease.

Clinical Recommendations

Topiramate has not been associated with hepatic disease. Renal disease is not a contraindication to the use of topiramate, although doses should be decreased and dosing intervals lengthened in patients with impaired renal function. Topiramate should be used with caution in patients with a history of probable kidney stones.

Zonisamide

Zonisamide (1,2-benzisoxazole-3-methanesulfonamide) is an anticonvulsant that is not readily soluble in water at neutral pH, but becomes more soluble as the pH increases to greater than 8. The majority of pharmacokinetic data on zonisamide has been obtained in animals, although some human data are available. In both animal and human studies, zonisamide was rapidly and essentially completely distributed throughout the body, including the brain. The metabolism of zonisamide is extensive, and it is excreted primarily in the urine. Protein binding is 50% to 60% in human sera (102–104) and is not significantly affected by usual therapeutic levels of phenytoin or phenobarbital (103). The major route of metabolism is direct acetyl or glucuronyl conjugation.

Effects of Liver and Renal Disease

There are no data on the effect of liver disease on the metabolism of zonisamide in humans. Because zonisamide is primarily excreted via the kidneys and metabolized extensively by the liver, both renal and liver disease may alter the pharmacokinetics of this drug. High doses of zonisamide have been associated with hepatic impairment in dogs treated with zonisamide doses that are above the maximum recommended human dose. The significance of these findings for humans is not known.

Renal clearance of zonisamide decreases with decreasing renal function. Marked renal impairment $CL_{CR} < 20$ mL/min) is associated with an increase in zonisamide AUC of 35%. Zonisamide has been associated with a statistically significant 8% mean increase in baseline serum creatinine and BUN compared with placebo. This increase has been attributed to a nonprogressive decrease in glomerular filtration rate (GFR), occurring during the first 4 weeks of treatment. GFR returned to baseline within 2 to 3 weeks of drug discontinuation in a 30-day study.

Clinical Recommendations

Because zonisamide is metabolized hepatically and excreted renally, it should be used cautiously in patients with hepatic or renal disease, with slower titration and frequent monitoring. Zonisamide should be discontinued in patients who develop acute renal failure or a significantly increased creatinine/BUN concentration. Zonisamide should not be used in nondialysis patients with renal failure ($Cl_{Cr} < 50$ mL/min), due to insufficient experience regarding drug dosing and toxicity. Like topiramate, zonisamide has been associated with the occurrence of kidney stones, and should be used with caution, if at all, with these patients.

A study of zonisamide in four patients undergoing hemodialysis found that its concentration was reduced by about 50% during one 4.5-hour hemodialysis session. It has been suggested that patients undergoing hemodialysis every 2 to 3 days dose their zonisamide once daily in the evening, and that if seizures occur after hemodialysis, a supplemental dose be given (105).

Tiagabine

Tiagabine [(−)-(R)-1-[4,4-bis(3-methyl-2-thienyl)-3-butenyl]-3-piperidinecarboxylic acid hydrochloride] increases the amount of GABA available in the extracellular space, presumably by preventing GABA uptake into presynaptic neurons. The pharmacokinetics of tiagabine had been studied in healthy individuals and patients with epilepsy, but few studies have been performed on patients with liver or renal disease. Tiagabine is rapidly absorbed and reaches maximal plasma concentrations in less than 2 hours after oral dosing (106,107). The mean elimination half-life ranges from 4 to 9 hours, and little of the drug accumulates in the plasma during multiple dosing (106,107). Hepatic metabolism is extensive, and only approximately 1% of the drug is excreted unchanged in the urine. Tiagabine does not appear to induce or inhibit hepatic microsomal enzyme systems and does not change the clearance of antipyrine, even after 14 days of administration (108,109). Initial studies suggest that tiagabine is greater than 95% protein bound.

Effects of Liver and Renal Disease

A study of 13 patients with mild or moderate impairment of hepatic function found that they had higher and more prolonged plasma concentrations of both total and unbound tiagabine after administration of tiagabine for 5 days. Hepatically impaired patients also had more neurologic side effects. Therefore, tiagabine should be used cautiously in epilepsy patients with hepatic impairment. Reduced dosages

and/or longer dosing intervals may be needed, and patients should be observed closely for neurologic side effects (110). A study of 25 subjects with various degrees of renal function (ranging from normal to requiring hemodialysis) demonstrated that the pharmacokinetics of tiagabine were similar in all subjects, suggesting that dosage adjustment may be unnecessary for epilepsy patients with renal impairment (111).

Vigabatrin

Vigabatrin (γ-vinyl-GABA: (±)-4-amino-hex-5-enoic acid) is a racemate with only the $S(+)$ enantiomer possessing clinical efficacy. It is an irreversible inhibitor of GABA transaminase, is not protein bound, and does not induce liver enzymes. Elimination occurs principally through urinary excretion, with biotransformation accounting for less than 20% (112). Approximately 50% of the $S(+)$ enantiomer and 65% of the $R(−)$ enantiomer are excreted in the urine, and the clearance of both correlates well with creatinine clearance.

Effects of Renal Disease

Because vigabatrin is excreted renally, impaired creatinine clearance may delay elimination. Hemodialysis is expected to remove a high proportion of vigabatrin. Bachmann and coworkers reported that 60% of vigabatrin was removed from the blood pool during hemodialysis (113).

Effects of Liver Disease

Vigabatrin has not been systematically studied in patients with liver disease. Reports of use in patients with hepatic cirrhosis document reductions in plasma alanine aminotransferase (ALT) activity to normal levels after initiation of vigabatrin (114). Use of vigabatrin in patients with porphyria failed to demonstrate a desferoxamine-dependent increase in messenger RNA for 5-aminolevulinate (ALA) synthetase, the rate-limiting enzyme in porphyrin synthesis (115).

Clinical Recommendations

As plasma concentrations are likely to be elevated in patients with renal disease, a decrease in dose or increase in dosing interval may be necessary. To maintain serum concentrations and stable clinical efficacy, single doses administered only every 3 days were necessary in one case (113). As vigabatrin may reduce levels of ALT in patients with pre-existing liver disease, this liver function test may not be a useful index of liver cell damage in some cases.

Levetiracetam

Levetiracetam (S-α-ethyl-2-oxo-1-pyrolidine acetamide) is a racemically pure pyrrolidine derivative. It has rapid and nearly complete absorption, unaffected by food, with peak plasma levels reached within 1 hour of administration and steady-state plasma levels reached within 2 days of initiation. Protein binding is less than 10%, and volume of distribution is 0.7 L/kg. Levetiracetam is excreted primarily via the kidneys, with 66% of the drug appearing unchanged in the urine and the remainder metabolized to an inactive compound formed by hydrolysis of the acetamide group. Levetiracetam's half-life is 7.2 ± 1.1 hours in young, healthy subjects (116).

Effects of Renal Disease

As the major route of excretion of levetiracetam is renal, impaired creatinine clearance will delay elimination and result in accumulation of the drug. The half-life is typically 6 to 8 hours in patients under 16, but increases to 10.2 to 10.4 hours in subjects over 65, presumably because of impaired creatinine clearance (117). When the disposition of levetiracetam was studied in patients with impaired renal function, total body clearance of levetiracetam was reduced in patients with impaired renal function, as follows: 40% in the mild group (Cl_{Cr} = 50 to 80 mL/min), 50% in the moderate group (Cl_{Cr} = 30 to 50 mL/min), and 60% in the severe renal impairment group (Cl_{Cr} < 30 mL/min). In anuric patients, the total body clearance decreased 70% compared with that of normal subjects. Approximately 50% of the pool of levetiracetam in the body is removed during a standard 4-hour hemodialysis procedure (see UCB Pharma package insert for Keppra levetiracetam).

Effects of Liver Disease

The lack of significant hepatic metabolism implies that primary liver disease will not impact metabolism of levetiracetam. Study of potential effects in 11 different drug-metabolizing enzymes using human liver microsomes failed to identify any pharmacokinetic interactions, even in doses exceeding expected therapeutic levels (118).

Clinical Recommendations

Levetiracetam should be used with caution in patients with pre-existing renal disease, and patients should be observed closely for signs of developing toxicity. Decreased doses or increased dosing intervals should be used in patients with impaired creatinine clearance. The package insert recommends the following: Cl_{Cr} > 80: 500 to 1500 mg every 12 hours; Cl_{Cr} = 50 to 80: 500 to 1000 mg every 12 hours; Cl_{Cr} = 30 to 50: 250 to 750 mg every 12 hours; Cl_{Cr} < 30: 250 to 500 mg every 12 hours; end-stage renal disease patients using dialysis: 500 to 1000 mg every 24 hours with a 250- to 500-mg supplemental dose following dialysis.

Clobazam (Frisium)

Clobazam (7-chloro-1-methyl-5-phenyl-1,5-benzodiazepine-2,4(3H)-dione) is a 1,5-benzodiazepine. Oral absorption of clobazam is rapid and complete. After oral ingestion, peak blood levels are achieved in 15 minutes to 4 hours. The drug is highly lipophilic and distributes rapidly in fat and in the brain. Clobazam is approximately 85% to 90% bound to plasma proteins. Over 90% of the clobazam is excreted in the urine as metabolites after oral dosing. Clobazam is markedly metabolized and is not excreted as clobazam, but as metabolites. Clobazam is primarily metabolized in the liver, undergoing dealkylation and hydroxylation before conjugation. The major metabolites produced are N-desmethyl clobazam and 4-hydroxyclobazam with 4-hydroxy-N-desmethyl clobazam being observed to a lesser extent. N-desmethyl clobazam is an active metabolite and reaches maximum plasma concentrations 24 to 72 hours after ingestion of clobazam. The mean half-life of clobazam is 18 hours with a range of 10 to 30 hours. N-desmethyl clobazam has a much longer half-life than clobazam (mean 42 hours, range 36 to 46 hours) (119). In addition, the half-life of clobazam significantly increases with age and aging also produces a reduced clearance after oral ingestion. The distribution volume is increased and the terminal half-life is prolonged in the elderly. The active metabolite also behaves in the same manner. Thus, use of clobazam in the elderly, especially in the debilitated elderly with organic brain dysfunction, can cause significant central nervous system depressant effects even at low doses.

Effects of Renal Disease

Slightly lower dosages may be required if the patient has a history of chronic renal failure. The drug is mainly inactivated by metabolism in the liver, but renal failure can affect the excretion of the metabolites. It has been indicated that renal impairment can lower the plasma concentrations of clobazam primarily due to the impaired absorption of the drug. The terminal half-life of clobazam is mainly independent of renal function. Care should be taken when using clobazam in renal disease.

Effects of Hepatic Disease

Clobazam is primarily metabolized in the liver and is contraindicated in patients with hepatic disease. Hepatic disease can alter both the metabolism and protein binding of clobazam and thus can significantly affect plasma levels. Clobazam has been used in less severe hepatic disease, but care needs to be taken to use low initial doses and very gradual increases in doses with careful observation. In patient with very severe liver disease, the distribution volume of clobazam can be significantly increased and the terminal half-life of the drug is prolonged. Clobazam is contraindicated in patients with severe impairment of liver function and the use of this drug in the setting of hepatic disease can lead to encephalopathy (120).

Rufinamide

Rufinamide (1-[(2,6-difluorophenyl)methyl]-1/+1,2,3-triazole-4-carboxamide) is a triazole derivative that is chemically distinct from any currently marketed AEDs. Oral absorption is relatively slow, and the extent of absorption declines with increasing doses. Pharmacokinetics, however, do not appear altered after multiple doses. Peak plasma concentrations occur between 4 and 6 hours after oral administration. Because food increases absorption, it is recommended that patients be dosed with food. This medication reaches at least 85% absorption after oral administration of a single 600-mg dose in the fed state. Protein binding is relatively low at 34%, predominantly to albumin. The apparent volume of distribution varies with dose and body surface area, and is approximately 50 L at a total daily dose of 3200 mg.

Rufinamide is primarily eliminated through the kidneys with a plasma elimination half-life of 6 to 10 hours. It is extensively metabolized, but with no known active metabolites. It is primarily metabolized by carboxylesterase-mediated hydrolysis of the carboxylamide group to the acid CGP 47292, which, is then metabolized by acyl-glucuronidation. Eighty-five percent of a dose is excreted in the urine, with two thirds of the excretory product appearing as the acid CGP 47292, and only 2% as the parent drug. Rufinamide is not metabolized by cytochrome p450 (CYP). It is, however, a weak inhibitor of CYP 2E1 and a weak inducer of CYP 3A4 isozymes (121,122).

Effects of Renal Disease

As the major route of excretion of rufinamide is renal, impaired creatinine clearance will delay elimination and can result in accumulation of the drug. No significant differences have been identified in age-related pharmacokinetics of this medication. Pharmacokinetic evaluation of nine patients with severe renal impairment (Cl_{Cr} <30 mL/min) also showed no differences from normal subjects. Dialysis within 3 hours of rufinamide dosing reduced AUC by 29% and C_{max} by 16%, indicating that upward dose adjustment may be needed to offset drug removal by dialysis. Administration of postdialysis supplemental dose may be considered (123).

Effects of Liver Disease

There are no studies specifically studying the effect of hepatic disease on rufinamide use. There are no reports in the literature of worsened liver function. As with any drug undergoing some metabolism through the liver, cautious dosing in the setting of liver disease is reasonable. Concomitant use of drugs that are substrates of CYP 2E1 may have increased levels in the presence of rufinamide; conversely, rufinamide may result in decreased effect of drugs that are substrates of CYP 3A4. Small, but potentially significant interactions between rufinamide and other AEDs should be anticipated (123,124).

Clinical Recommendations

As with all drugs with extensive renal elimination, lower doses are needed to achieve clinical effect when creatinine clearance is reduced. Similarly, adverse effects may be encountered at lower doses in patients with hepatic impairment. The metabolism of rufinamide is less extensive than that of older generation AEDs, but still warrants careful dose monitoring, and perhaps dose reduction in patients with liver disease.

Lacosamide

Lacosamide [(R)-2-acetamido-N-benzyl-3-methoxypropionamide] is one of a group of functionalized amino acids screened for anticonvulsant properties. It selectively enhances the slow inactivation of neuronal sodium channels, without affecting fast inactivation. It binds to collapsin-response mediator protein 2 (CRMP-2), a phosphoprotein involved in neuronal differentiation and control of axonal outgrowth (125). Lacosamide is rapidly and completely absorbed, with minimal first-pass effect. Peak plasma levels occur 1 to 4 hours after an oral dose, and the elimination half-life is about 13 hours (126). Lacosamide is less than 15% bound to plasma proteins. A small proportion of lacosamide is demethylated to an inactive O-desmethyl metabolite (127) with an elimination half-life of 15 to 23 hours.

Lacosamide and its metabolite are eliminated from the systemic circulation primarily by renal excretion. After oral and intravenous administration of radiolabeled lacosamide, 95% was recovered in the urine, and less than 0.5% in the feces. The excreted compounds consisted of unchanged lacosamide

(about 40% of the dose), the O-desmethyl metabolite (about 30%), and a structurally unknown polar fraction (about 20%). The plasma exposure of O-desmethyl lacosamide is about 10% that of lacosamide (128).

Effects of Renal Disease

Because lacosamide is metabolized by the liver and excreted by the kidneys, both renal and hepatic dysfunction alter its pharmacokinetics. Impaired renal function does not affect the maximum concentration (C_{max}) of lacosamide. However, compared to subjects with normal renal function, the area under the concentration versus time curve (AUC) of lacosamide is increased by 25% in the setting of mild renal impairment (Cl_{cr} 50 to 80 mL/min) or moderate renal impairment (30 to 50 mL/min), and by 60% in severe renal impairment ($Cl_{cr} \leq$ 30 mL/min) (128).

Effects of Liver Disease

Lacosamide undergoes hepatic metabolism. While lacosamide does not induce cytochrome P-450 isoenzymes, at concentrations many times higher than therapeutic plasma levels, it inhibits CYP 2C19 in vitro. No studies have evaluated its effects in patients with severe hepatic impairment, and lacosamide is not recommended for these patients. Patients with moderate hepatic impairment showed higher plasma concentrations of lacosamide (approximately 50 to 60% higher AUC) compared to healthy subjects (128).

Clinical Recommendations

No dose adjustment of lacosamide is necessary for patients with mild to moderate renal impairment. For patients with severe renal impairment ($Cl_{cr} \leq$ 30 mL/min) or with end-stage renal disease, the maximum recommended dose of lacosamide is 300 mg daily. It is effectively removed from plasma by hemodialysis, with a 4-hour dialysis treatment reducing the AUC of lacosamide by 50%. Following dialysis, a supplemental dose of 50% of the daily dose should be considered (128). In all renally impaired patients, the dose titration should be performed with caution.

Patients with severe hepatic impairment should not use lacosamide. In those with mild to moderate impairment, dose titration should be cautious, with close monitoring, and the maximum dose should not exceed 300 mg daily. Patients with coexisting hepatic and renal impairment should be monitored closely during dose titration.

MEDICATIONS IN LIVER AND RENAL TRANSPLANTATION

Use of AEDs in patients who are being evaluated for renal or liver transplantation is similar to that previously described for patients with renal or liver disease. Care should be taken to avoid further diminishing organ function while a patient waits for availability of a donor organ. However, this interval prior to transplantation may be the optimal time to re-evaluate the diagnosis of epilepsy by video electroencephalographic monitoring or to consider revising AED therapy to reduce the likelihood of interactions with immunosuppressants and antibiotics following transplantation.

Liver transplantation is considered in patients with irreversible and progressive liver dysfunction for which no alternative therapy is available. It is rarely performed in patients older than age 70 years or in patients with coexistent active alcohol or drug abuse. Epilepsy is not a specific contraindication. Allograft donors are matched for ABO blood compatibility and liver size and should test negative for the human immunodeficiency virus (HIV) and hepatitis B and C. Immunosuppression is usually accomplished by combinations of tacrolimus or cyclosporine, steroids, azathioprine, or OKT3 (ornithine ketoacid transaminase, monoclonal antithymocyte globulin). Other immunosuppressants are under investigation. Posttransplantation complications include liver dysfunction from primary nonfunction, acute or chronic rejection, ischemia, hepatic artery thrombosis, and biliary obstruction or leak. Bacterial, viral, fungal, and other opportunistic infections may occur, as well as renal and psychiatric disorders (129).

Renal transplantation is the treatment of choice for most patients with end-stage renal disease. Graft survival is best in living-related transplants, intermediate in living-unrelated transplants, and least in cadaveric transplants. Renal transplantation is contraindicated in patients with active glomerulonephritis, infection, malignancy, HIV, or hepatitis B, and in those with severe comorbid disease. Relative contraindications include age older than 70 years, severe psychiatric disease, moderate comorbidity, and some primary renal diseases (multiple myeloma, amyloidosis, oxalosis). Again, epilepsy is not a specific contraindication. Immunosuppression usually consists of a two- or three-drug regimen, with each drug targeted at a different stage in the immune response. Cyclosporine and prednisone are frequently used together for the first few years after successful grafting. Azathioprine or mycophenolate mofetil is commonly used as the third drug. Tacrolimus is used less commonly in renal than in liver transplantation, but it is used in patients with subacute or chronic rejection. Other immunosuppressive agents are under investigation. Infection is the most common complication of renal transplantation, and ganciclovir or cytomegalovirus (CMV)-immune globulin may be used prophylactically. Risk of fungal and *Pneumocystis carinii* infection increases substantially as prednisone is tapered (130).

In addition to the obvious concerns about using AEDs associated with liver or renal toxicities to treat patients with donated organs, the primary management concerns of the epileptologist are (i) AED interactions with immunosuppressants; (ii) AED interactions with prophylactic antibiotics; and (iii) the appropriate diagnostic and therapeutic approach to new-onset seizures following transplantation.

Antiepileptic Drug Use with Immunosuppressants

It is well documented in the literature that cyclosporine may result in neurotoxic effects, including seizures. Such effects are more frequently seen with high cyclosporine levels, but levels may be within the usual therapeutic range. Dose reduction or withdrawal of cyclosporine usually results in improvement of clinical symptoms (131). Results of animal studies suggest that cyclosporine lowers seizure threshold by inhibiting GABAergic neural activity and binding properties of the GABA receptor (132). Neoral, a newer formulation of cyclosporine, appears to reduce the potential for seizures in liver transplant recipients (133). All formulations of cyclosporine are highly protein bound, with potential for increased blood levels of unbound AEDs. Enzyme-inducing AEDs may lead to increased elimination of cyclosporine because of induction of hepatic microsomal enzymes. This interaction may precipitate or exacerbate graft-versus-host disease and lead to rejection. For this reason, AEDs with low protein binding and minimal metabolism should be considered first in patients taking cyclosporine.

Tacrolimus (FK506) has been less frequently associated with seizures than has cyclosporine (134). After reversing neurologic findings by discontinuation of cyclosporine, substitution with tacrolimus did not result in neurotoxicity (135). Like cyclosporine, however, tacrolimus is highly protein bound and is metabolized by the cytochrome P450 enzymes, with similar potential AED interactions.

Prednisone and other corticosteroids may be used before transplantation as well as chronically in combination with other immunosuppressants following transplantation. The action of corticosteroids may be blunted by enzyme-inducing AEDs, resulting in increased clearance from the circulation and prompting a need for higher steroid doses. Azathioprine is rarely associated with increased risk for seizures and has minimal potential for interaction with AEDs.

Seizures and Infections After Transplantation

Liver and renal transplant recipients are at significantly increased risk for central nervous system and systemic infections or neoplasms, both of which can significantly lower the threshold for seizures. In transplantation patients with new-onset seizures, a diligent search for localized neurologic infection or neoplasia must be conducted, especially if seizures have focal symptoms. A minimal diagnostic evaluation of such patients should include magnetic resonance imaging using fluid attenuated inversion recovery (FLAIR) sequences, usually precontrast and postcontrast, as well as carefully performed electroencephalography with appropriately selected activation procedures.

A review of interactions of AEDs with all possible antibiotic agents is beyond the scope of this chapter. However, it should be mentioned that many antibiotics, especially the β-lactam agents, lower the threshold for seizures and that consideration of this potential is important in selecting antibiotics to treat transplant recipients, who already have a lowered threshold for seizures in comparison with that of the general population. Among the most commonly used posttransplantation prophylactic antibiotics are the antivirals, especially ganciclovir. This agent has minimal protein binding and metabolism, with clearance rate directly related to kidney function. Additive toxicity may be seen (e.g., generalized seizures in patients receiving ganciclovir with imipenem–cilastatin, neutropenia in patients receiving ganciclovir with carbamazepine) and should be a consideration when selecting AEDs. Prophylactic fluconazole is sometimes used after transplantation, resulting in decreased risk for fungal colonization but higher serum cyclosporine levels and thus more potential neurotoxicity (136).

References

1. Kuhara T, Inoue Y, Matsumoto M, et al. Altered metabolic profiles of valproic acid in a patient with Reye's syndrome. *Clin Chim Acta.* 1985;145:135–142.

2. Kunin CM. A guide to use of antibiotics in patients with renal disease. *Ann Intern Med.* 1967;67:151–158.

3. Adler DS, Martin E, Gambertoglio JG, et al. Hemodialysis of phenytoin in a uremic patient. *Clin Pharmacol Ther.* 1975;18:65–69.

4. Dettli L, Spring P, Ryter S. Multiple dose kinetics and drug dosage in patients with kidney disease. *Acta Pharmacol Toxicol (Copenh).* 1971;29(suppl 3):211–224.

5. Letteri JM, Mellk H, Louis S, et al. Diphenylhydantoin metabolism in uremia. *N Engl J Med.* 1971;285:648–652.

6. Odar-Cederlof I, Borga O. Kinetics of diphenylhydantoin in uremia patients: consequences of decreased plasma protein binding. *Eur J Clin Pharmacol.* 1974;7:31.

7. Loub WD, Wattenberg LW, Davis DW. Aryl hydrocarbon hydroxylase induction in rat tissues by naturally occurring indoles of cruciferous plants. *J Natl Cancer Inst.* 1975;54:985.

8. Affrime MB, Lowenthal DT. Analgesics, sedatives, and sedative-hypnotics. In: Anderson RJ, Schrier RW, eds. *Clinical Use of Drugs in Patients with Kidney and Liver Disease.* Philadelphia, PA: WB Saunders; 1981:199–210.

9. Gillette JR. Factors affecting drug metabolism. *Ann N Y Acad Sci.* 1971;179:43.

10. Bennhold H. Die Vekikelfunction der Bluteiweisskorper. In: Bennhold H, Kylin E, Rusznyak S, eds. *Die Eiweisskorper des Blutplasmas.* Leipzig, Germany: Steinkopf; 1938:220–303.

11. Sjoholm I, Kober A, Odar-Cederlof I, et al. Protein binding of drugs in uremia and normal serum: the role of endogenous binding inhibitors. *Biochem Pharmacol.* 1976;25:1205.

12. Shoeman DW, Azarnoff DL. The alterations of plasma proteins in uremia as reflected in their ability to bind digitoxin and diphenylhydantoin. *Pharmacology.* 1972;7:169.

13. Reidenberg MM. The biotransformation of drugs in renal failure. *Am J Med.* 1977;62:482.

14. Kutt H, Winters W, Scherman R, et al. Diphenylhydantoin and phenobarbital toxicity: the role of liver disease. *Arch Neurol.* 1964;11:649–656.

15. Maher JF. Principles of dialysis and dialysis of drugs. *Am J Med.* 1977;62:475.

16. Dromgoole SH. The effect of hemodialysis on the binding capacity of albumin. *Clin Chim Acta.* 1973;46:469.

17. Dromgoole SH. The binding capacity of albumin and renal disease. *J Pharmacol Exp Ther.* 1974;191:318–323.

18. Blaschke TF, Meffin PJ, Melmon KL, et al. Influence of acute viral hepatitis on phenytoin kinetics and protein binding. *Clin Pharmacol Ther.* 1975;17:685–691.

19. Blaschke TF. Protein binding and kinetics of drugs in liver diseases. *Clin Pharmacokinet.* 1977;2:32–44.

20. Breimer DD, Zilly W, Richter E. Pharmacokinetics of hexobarbital in acute hepatitis and after apparent recovery. *Clin Pharmacol Ther.* 1975;18:433–440.

21. Klotz U, Avant GR, Hoyumpa A, et al. The effects of age and liver disease on the disposition and elimination of diazepam in adult man. *J Clin Invest.* 1975;55:347–359.

22. Mawer GE, Miller NE, Turnberg LA. Metabolism of amylobarbitone in patients with chronic liver disease. *Br J Pharmacol.* 1972;44:549–560.

23. Wilkinson GR, Shand DG. A physiological approach to hepatic drug clearance. *Clin Pharmacol Ther.* 1975;18:377–390.

24. Rowland M, Blaschke TF, Meffin PJ, et al. Pharmacokinetics in disease states modifying hepatic and metabolic function. In: Benet LZ, ed. *Effect of Disease States on Drug Pharmacokinetics.* Washington, DC: American Pharmaceutical Association; 1976:53–74.

25. Affrime M, Reidenberg MM. The protein binding of some drugs in plasma from patients with alcoholic liver disease. *Eur J Clin Pharmacol.* 1975;8:267–269.

26. Rowland M, Benet LZ, Graham GG. Clearance concepts in pharmacokinetics. *J Pharmacokinet Biopharm.* 1973;1:123–136.

27. Albert K, Hallmark M, Sakmar E, et al. Plasma concentrations of diphenylhydantoin, its parahydroxylated metabolite, and corresponding glucuronide in man. *Res Commun Chem Pathol Pharmacol.* 1974;9:463–469.

28. Hooper WD, Bochner F, Endre MJ, et al. Plasma protein binding of diphenylhydantoin: effects of sex hormones, renal and hepatic disease. *Clin Pharmacol Ther.* 1974;15:276–282.

29. Rane A, Lunde PKM, Jalling B, et al. Plasma protein binding of diphenylhydantoin in normal and hyperbilirubinemic infants. *J Pediatr.* 1971;78:877–882.

30. Greenblatt DJ, Koch-Weser J. Clinical toxicity of chlordiazepoxide and diazepam in relation to serum albumin concentration: a report from the Boston Collaborative Drug Surveillance Program. *Eur J Clin Pharmacol.* 1974;7:259–262.

31. Brodie BB, Mark LC, Papper EM, et al. The fate of thiopental in man and a method for its estimation in biological material. *J Pharmacol Exp Ther.* 1950;98:85–96.

32. Garrett ER, Bres J, Schnelle K, et al. Pharmacokinetics of saturably metabolized amobarbital. *J Pharmacokinet Biopharm.* 1974;2:43–103.

33. Waddell WJ, Butler TC. The distribution of phenobarbital. *J Clin Invest.* 1957;36:1217–1226.

34. Branch RA, James J, Read EA. A study of factors influencing drug disposition in chronic liver disease, using the model drug (+)propranolol. *Br J Clin Pharmacol.* 1976;3:243–249.

35. Lewis JP, Jusko WJ. Pharmacokinetics of ampicillin in cirrhosis. *Clin Pharmacol Ther.* 1975;18:475–484.

36. Wilkinson GR, Schenker S. Drug disposition and liver disease. *Drug Metab Rev.* 1975;4:139–175.

37. Booker HE, Darcey B. Serum concentrations of free diphenylhydantoin and their relationship to clinical intoxication. *Epilepsia.* 1973;14:177–184.

38. Reidenberg MM, Drayer DE. Effects of renal disease upon drug disposition. *Drug Metab Rev.* 1978;8:293–302.

39. Butler TC. The metabolic conversion of 5,5-diphenylhydantoin to 5-(p-hydroxyphenyl)-5-phenylhydantoin. *J Pharmacol Exp Ther.* 1957;119:111.

40. Gilman AG, Goodman LS, Rall TW, et al., eds. *Goodman & Gilman's the Pharmacological Basis of Therapeutics.* 7th ed. Elmsford, NY: Pergamon; 1985:446–472.

41. Leber HW, Schutterle G. Oxidative drug metabolism in liver microsomes from uremic rats. *Kidney Int.* 1972;2:152.

42. Odar-Cederlof I, Lunde P, Sjoqvist F. Abnormal pharmacokinetics of phenytoin in a patient with uraemia. *Lancet.* 1970;2:831.

43. Reidenberg MM. *Renal Function and Drug Action.* Philadelphia, PA: WB Saunders; 1971.

44. Olsen GD, Bennett WM, Porter GA. Morphine and phenytoin binding to plasma proteins in renal and hepatic failure. *Clin Pharmacol Ther.* 1975;17:677–684.

45. Reidenberg MM, Affrime M. Influence of disease on binding of drugs to plasma proteins. *Ann N Y Acad Sci.* 1973;226:115–126.

46. Ehrnebo M, Odar-Cederlof I. Binding of amobarbital, pentobarbital and diphenylhydantoin to blood cells and plasma proteins in healthy volunteers and uraemic patients. *Eur J Clin Pharmacol.* 1975;8:445–453.

47. Van Peer AP, Belpaire FM, Rosseel MT, et al. Distribution of antipyrine, phenylbutazone and phenytoin in experimental renal failure. *Pharmacology.* 1981;22:139–145.

48. Van Peer AP, Belpaire FM, Bogaert MG. Pharmacokinetics of drugs in rabbits with experimental acute renal failure. *Pharmacology.* 1978;17:307–314.

49. Van Peer AP, Belpaire FM, Bogaert MG. In vitro hepatic oxidative metabolism of antipyrine, phenytoin and phenylbutazone in rabbits with experimental renal failure. *Arch Int Pharmacodyn Ther.* 1978;234:346–347.

50. Van Peer AP, Belpaire FM, Bogaert MG. *In vitro* hepatic oxidative metabolism of antipyrine, phenytoin and phenylbutazone in uraemic rabbits. *J Pharm Pharmacol.* 1980;32:135–136.

51. Borga O, Hoppel C, Odar-Cederlof I, et al. Plasma levels and renal excretion of phenytoin and its metabolites in patients with renal failure. *Clin Pharmacol Ther.* 1979;26:306–314.

52. Borondy P, Chang T, Glazko AJ. Inhibition of diphenylhydantoin (DPH) hydroxylation by 5-(p-hydroxyphenyl)-5-phenylhydantoin (pHPPH) [abstract]. *Fed Proc.* 1972;31:582.

53. Perucca E, Makki K, Richens A. Is phenytoin metabolism dose dependent by enzyme saturation or by feedback inhibition? *Clin Pharmacol Ther.* 1978;22:46–51.

54. Steele WH, Lawrence JR, Elliott HL, et al. Alterations of phenytoin protein binding with in vivo haemodialysis in dialysis encephalopathy. *Eur J Clin Pharmacol.* 1979;15:69–71.

55. Martin E, Gambertoglio JG, Adler DS, et al. Removal of phenytoin by hemodialysis in uremic patients. *JAMA.* 1977;238:1750–1753.

56. Nandedkar A, Williamson R, Kutt H, et al. A comparison of plasma phenytoin level determinations by EMIT and gas-liquid chromatography in patients with renal insufficiency. *Ther Drug Monit.* 1980;2:427–430.

57. Burgess ED, Friel PN, Blair AD, et al. Serum phenytoin concentrations in uremia. *Ann Intern Med.* 1981;94:59–60.

58. Lunde PKM, Rane A, Yaffe SJ, et al. Plasma protein binding of diphenylhydantoin in man: interaction with other drugs and the effect of temperature and plasma dilution. *Clin Pharmacol Ther.* 1970;11:846–855.

59. Richens A. Clinical pharmacokinetics of phenytoin. *Clin Pharmacokinet.* 1979;4:153–169.

60. Breen KJ, Shaw J, Alvin J, et al. Effect of experimental hepatic injury on the clearance of phenobarbital and paraldehyde. *Gastroenterology.* 1973;64:992–1004.

61. Alvin J, McHorse T, Hoyumpa A, et al. The effect of liver disease in man on the disposition of phenobarbital. *J Pharmacol Exp Ther.* 1975;192:224–235.

62. Gambertoglio JG, Lauer RM. Use of neuropsychiatric drugs. In: Anderson RJ, Schrier RW, eds. *Clinical Use of Drugs in Patients with Kidney and Liver Disease.* Philadelphia, PA: WB Saunders; 1981:276–295.

63. Heipertz R, Guthoff A, Bernhardt W. Primidone metabolism in renal insufficiency and acute intoxication. *J Neurol.* 1979;221:101–104.

64. Stern EL. Possible phenylethylmalondiamide (PEMA) intoxication. *Ann Neurol.* 1977;2:356–357.

65. Gugler R, von Unruh GE. Clinical pharmacokinetics of valproic acid. *Clin Pharmacokinet.* 1980;5:67–83.

66. Brewster D, Muir NC. Valproate plasma protein binding in the uremic condition. *Clin Pharmacol Ther.* 1980;27:76–82.

67. Bruni J, Wang LH, Marbury TC, et al. Protein binding of valproic acid in uremic patients. *Neurology.* 1980;30:557–559.

68. Gugler R, Mueller G. Plasma protein binding of valproic acid in healthy subjects and in patients with renal disease. *Br J Clin Pharmacol.* 1978;5:441–446.

69. Dickinson RG, Kluck RM, Hooper WD, et al. Rearrangement of valproate glucuronide in a patient with drug associated hepatobiliary and renal dysfunction. *Epilepsia.* 1985;26:589–593.

70. Klotz U, Rapp T, Mueller WA. Disposition of valproic acid in patients with liver disease. *Eur J Clin Pharmacol.* 1978;13:55–60.

71. Kochen W, Schneider A, Ritz A. Abnormal metabolism of valproic acid in fatal hepatic failure. *Eur J Pediatr.* 1983;141:30–35.

72. Bohles H, Richter K, Wagner-Thiessen E, et al. Decreased serum carnitine in valproate induced Reye's syndrome. *Eur J Pediatr.* 1982;139:185–186.

73. Lenn NJ, Ellis WG, Washburner RB. Fatal hepatocerebral syndrome in siblings discordant for exposure to valproate. *Epilepsia.* 1990;31:578–583.

74. Zafrani BS, Berthelot P. Sodium valproate in the induction of unusual hepatoxicity. *Hepatology.* 1982;2:648–649.

75. Dreifuss FE, Langer WH, Moline KA, et al. Valproic acid and hepatic fatalities, II. US experience since 1984. *Neurology.* 1989;39:201–207.

76. Zaret BS, Beckner RR, Marini AM, et al. Sodium valproate induced hyperammonemia without clinical hepatic dysfunction. *Neurology.* 1982;32:206–208.

77. Faigle JW, Brechbuhler S, Feldman KF, et al. The biotransformation of carbamazepine. In: Birkmayer W, ed. *Epileptic Seizures–Behavior and Pain.* Vienna: Hans Huber; 1975:127–140.

78. Hooper WD, Dubetz DK, Bochner F, et al. Plasma protein binding of carbamazepine. *Clin Pharmacol Ther.* 1975;17:433–440.

79. Kangas L, Kanto J, Forsstrom J, et al. The protein binding of diazepam and *N*-desmethyldiazepam in patients with poor renal function. *Clin Nephrol.* 1976;5:114–118.

80. Kober A, Sjoholm I, Borga O, et al. Protein binding of diazepam and digitoxin in uremic and normal serum. *Biochem Pharmacol.* 1979;28:1037–1042.

81. Garella S, Lorch JA. Use of dialysis and hemoperfusion in drug overdose: an overview. In: Anderson RJ, Schrier RW, eds. *Clinical Use of Drugs in Patients with Kidney and Liver Disease.* Philadelphia, PA: WB Saunders; 1981:269–309.

82. Andreasen PB, Hendel J, Greisen G, et al. Pharmacokinetics of diazepam in disordered liver function. *Eur J Clin Pharmacol.* 1976;10:115–120.

83. Sellers EM, Greenblatt DJ, Giles HG, et al. Chlordiazepoxide and oxazepam disposition in cirrhosis. *Clin Pharmacol Ther.* 1979;26:240–246.

84. Wilkinson GR. The effects of liver disease and aging on the disposition of diazepam, chlordiazepoxide, oxazepam and lorazepam in man. *Acta Psychiatr Scand.* 1978;(suppl 274):56–74.

85. Shull HJ, Wilkinson GR, Johnson R, et al. Normal disposition of oxazepam in acute viral hepatitis and cirrhosis. *Ann Intern Med.* 1976;84:420–425.

86. Patwardhan RV, Schenker S. Drug use in patients with liver disease: an overview. In: Anderson RJ, Schrier RW, eds. *Clinical Use of Drugs in Patients with Kidney and Liver Disease.* Philadelphia, PA: WB Saunders; 1981:166–181.

87. Asconape JJ, Penry JK. Use of antiepileptic drugs in the presence of liver and kidney disease: a review. *Epilepsia.* 1982;23(suppl 1):565–579.

88. Yau MK, Adams MA, Wargin WA, et al. A single-dose and steady-state pharmacokinetic study of lamotrigine in healthy male volunteers. Presented at the Third International Cleveland Clinic–Bethel Epilepsy Symposium; June 16–20, 1992; Cleveland, OH.

89. Fillastre JP, Taburet AM, Fialaire A, et al. Pharmacokinetics of lamotrigine in patients with renal impairment: influence of hemodialysis. *Drugs Exp Clin Res.* 1993;19:25–32.

90. Posner J, Cohen AF, Land G, et al. The pharmacokinetics of lamotrigine (BW 430C) in healthy subjects with unconjugated hyperbilirubinemia (Gilbert's syndrome). *Br J Clin Pharmacol.* 1989;28:117–120.

91. Palmer KJ, McTavisk D. Felbamate. A review of its pharmacodynamic and pharmacokinetic properties, and therapeutic efficacy in epilepsy. *Drugs.* 1993;45:1041–1065.

92. Brodie MJ, Pellock JM. Taming the brain storms: felbamate updated. *Lancet.* 1995;346:918–919.

93. Pellock JM. Felbamate in epilepsy therapy: evaluating the risks. *Drug Saf.* 1999;21:225–239.

94. Data on file. Ann Arbor, MI: Parke-Davis; 1995.

95. Halstenson CE, Keane WF, Tuerck D, et al. Disposition of gabapentin (GAB) in hemodialysis (HD) patients [abstract]. *J Clin Pharmacol.* 1992;32:751.

96. Schutz H, Feldmann KF, Faigle JW, et al. The metabolism of 14C-oxcarbazepine in man. *Xenobiotica.* 1986;16:769–778.

97. Feldmann KF, Brechbuhler S, Faigle JW, et al. Pharmacokinetics and metabolism of GP47779, the main human metabolite of oxcarbazepine (GP47680) in animals and healthy volunteers. In: Dam M, Gram L, Penry JK, eds. *Advances in Epileptology. XIIth Epilepsy International Symposium.* New York: Raven Press; 1981:89–96.

98. Kristensen O, Klitgaard NA, Jonsson B, et al. Pharmacokinetics of 10-*OH*-carbazepine, the main metabolite of the antiepileptic oxcarbazepine, from serum and saliva concentrations. *Acta Neurol Scand.* 1983;68:145–150.

99. Theisohn M, Heimann G. Disposition of the antiepileptic oxcarbazepine and its metabolites in healthy volunteers. *Eur J Clin Pharmacol.* 1982;22:545–551.

100. Rouan MC, Lecaillon JB, Godbillon J, et al. The effect of renal impairment on the pharmacokinetics of oxcarbazepine and its metabolites. *Eur J Clin Pharmacol.* 1994;47:161–167.

101. Data on file. Philadelphia, PA: Ortho-McNeil; 1995.

102. Kimura M, Tanaka N, Kimura Y, et al. Pharmacokinetic interaction of zonisamide in rats: effect of other antiepileptics on zonisamide. *J Pharmacobiodyn.* 1992;15:631–639.

103. Matsumoto K, Miyazaki H, Fujii T, et al. Absorption, distribution and excretion of 3-(sulfamoyl[^{14}C]methyl)-1,2-benzisoxazole (AD-810) in rats, dogs and monkeys and of AD-810 in men. *Arzneimittelforschung.* 1983;33:961–968.

104. Nishiguchi K, Ohniski N, Iwakawa S, et al. Pharmacokinetics of zonisamide: saturable distribution into human and rat erythrocytes and into rat brain. *J Pharmacobiodyn.* 1992;15:409–415.

105. Ijiri Y, Inoue T, Fukuda F, et al. Dialyzability of the antiepileptic drug zonisamide in patients undergoing hemodialysis. *Epilepsia.* 2004;45:924–927.

106. Gustavson LE, Mengel HB. Pharmacokinetics of tiagabine, a gamma-aminobutyric acid-uptake inhibitor, in healthy subjects after single and multiple doses. *Epilepsia.* 1995;36:605–611.

107. Gustavson LE, Mengel HB, Pierce MW, et al. Tiagabine, a new gamma-aminobutyric acid uptake inhibitor antiepileptic drug: pharmacokinetics after single oral doses in man. *Epilepsia.* 1990;31:642.

108. Mengel HB. Tiagabine. *Epilepsia.* 1994;35(suppl 5):S81–S84.

109. Mengel HB, Pierce M, Mant T, et al. Tiagabine, a GABA-uptake inhibitor: safety and tolerance of multiple dosing in normal subjects. *Acta Neurol Scand.* 1990;82(suppl 133):35.

110. Lau AH, Gustavson LE, Sperelakis R, et al. Pharmacokinetics and safety of tiagabine in subjects with various degrees of hepatic function. *Epilepsia.* 1997;38:445–451.

111. Cato A, Gustavson LE, Qian J, et al. Effect of renal impairment on the pharmacokinetics and tolerability of tiagabine. *Epilepsia.* 1998;39:43–47.

112. Richens A. Pharmacology and clinical pharmacology of vigabatrin. *J Child Neurol.* 1991;6(suppl 2):S7–S10.

113. Bachmann D, Ritz R, Wad N, et al. Vigabatrin dosing during haemodialysis. *Seizure.* 1996;5:239–242.

114. Williams A, Sekaninova S, Coakly J. Suppression of elevated alanine aminotransferase activity in liver diseases by vigabatrin. *J Pediatr Child Health.* 1998;34:395–397.

115. Hahn M, Gildemeister OS, Krauss GL, et al. Effects of new anticonvulsant medications on porphyrin synthesis in cultured liver cells: potential implications for patients with acute porphyria. *Neurology.* 1997;49:97–106.

116. Patsalos PN. Pharmacokinetic profile of levetiracetam: toward ideal characteristics. *Pharmacol Ther.* 2000;85:77–85.

117. Bialer M, Johannessen SI, Kupferberg, et al. Progress report on new antiepileptic drugs: a summary of the fourth Eilat conference (EILAT IV). *Epilepsy Res.* 1999;34:1–41.

118. Nicolas JM, Collart P, Gerin B, et al. In vitro evaluation of potential drug interactions with levetiracetam, a new antiepileptic agent. *Drug Metab Dispos.* 1999;27:250–254.

119. Rupp W, Badian M, Christ O, et al. Pharmacokinetics of single and multiple doses of clobazam in humans. *Br J Clin Pharmacol.* 1979;7:51S–57S.

120. Barzaghi F, Fournex R, Mantegazza P. Pharmacological and toxicological properties of clobazam, a new psychotherapeutic agent. *Arzneim Forsch (Drug Res).* 1973;23:683–686.

121. Perucca E, Cloyd J, Critchley D, et al. Rufinamide: clinical pharmacokinetics and concentration-response relationships in patients with epilepsy. *Epilepsia.* 2008;49(7):1123–1141.

122. Cheng-Hakimian A, Anderson GD, Miller JW. Rufinamide: pharmacology, clinical trials, and role in clinical practice. *Int J Clin Pract.* 2006;60(11):1497–1501.

123. Banzel™ (rufinamide) Tablets, package insert. Eisai, 2008.

124. Glauser T, Kluger G, Sachdeo R, et al. Rufinamide for generalized seizures associated with Lennox–Gastaut syndrome. *Neurology.* 2008;70(21):1950–1958.

125. Beyreuther BK, Freitag J, Heers C, et al. Lacosamide: a review of preclinical properties. *CNS Drug Rev.* 2007;13:21–42.

126. Hovinga CA. SPM-927 (Schwarz Pharma). *Idrugs.* 2003;6:479–485.

127. Doty P, Rudd GD, Stoehr T, et al. Lacosamide. *Neurotherapeutics*. 2007; 4:145–148.

128. VIMPAT® [package insert]. Smyrna, GA: UCB; 2008.

129. Dienstag J. Liver transplantation. In: Fauci AS, Braunwald E, Isselbacher K, et al., eds. *Harrison's Principles of Internal Medicine*. 14th ed. New York: McGraw-Hill; 1998:1721–1725.

130. Carpenter CB, Lazarus JM. Dialysis and transplantation in the treatment of renal failure. In: Fauci AS, Braunwald E, Isselbacher K, et al., eds. *Harrison's Principles of Internal Medicine*. 14th ed. New York: McGraw-Hill; 1988:1520–1529.

131. Gitjenbeck JM, van den Bent MJ, Vecht CJ. Cyclosporine neurotoxicity review. *J Neurol*. 1999;246:339–346.

132. Shuto H, Kataoka Y, Fujisaki K, et al. Inhibition of GABA system involved in cyclosporine-induced convulsions. *Life Sci*. 1999;65:879–887.

133. Wijdicks EF, Dahlke LJ, Wiesner RH. Oral cyclosporine decreases severity of neurotoxicity in liver transplant recipients. *Neurology*. 1999;12:1708–1710.

134. Neu AM, Furth SL, Case BW, et al. Evaluation of neurotoxicity in pediatric renal transplant recipients treated with tacrolimus (FK506). *Clin Transplant*. 1997;11(Pt 1):412–414.

135. Wijdicks EF, Wiesner RH, Krom RA. Neurotoxicity in liver transplant recipients with cyclosporine immunosuppression. *Neurology*. 1995; 45:1962–1964.

136. Winston DJ, Pakrasi A, Busuttil RW. Prophylactic fluconazole in liver transplant recipients: a randomized, double blind, placebo-controlled trial. *Ann Intern Med*. 1999;131:729–737.

137. Evans WE, Schentag JJ, Jusko JW, eds. *Applied Pharmacokinetics*. 3rd ed. Spokane, WA: Applied Therapeutics; 1986:542–544.

CHAPTER 48 ■ MONITORING FOR ADVERSE EFFECTS OF ANTIEPILEPTIC DRUGS

L. JAMES WILLMORE, JOHN M. PELLOCK, AND ANDREW PICKENS IV

Treatment of patients with epilepsy strives for complete seizure control without intolerable drug side effects (1). Independent of blood drug levels, toxic effects allow titration to efficacy. However, allergic reactions, metabolically or genetically determined drug-induced illnesses, and idiosyncratic effects of drugs, while rare, may be life-threatening.

Monitoring is an attempt to detect serious systemic toxic reactions of antiepileptic drugs (AEDs) in time to intervene and protect patients. The process begins with the disclosure to patients and family members of all information required for an informed decision delivered within the framework of risks and benefits. Regularly scheduled accumulation of hematologic data, routine serum chemistry values, and results of urinalysis creates an archive (2). A rational basis for this approach was thought to reside in the *Physicians' Desk Reference* (PDR) (3) and the Canadian *Compendium of Pharmaceuticals and Specialties* (4). Although these sources appear to define the standard of practice for many clinicians, they actually preserve observations about specific and well-defined groups of patients under close scrutiny during drug trials. Contrary to some clinical practices and these publications, evidence-based scientific criteria fail to support routine monitoring, and the resulting archival data rarely predict serious drug reactions. For example, two prospective studies (5,6) investigated the efficacy of routine blood and urine testing in patients receiving long-term AED treatment. One study (5) of 199 children evaluated liver, blood, and renal function at initiation of therapy and at 1, 3, and 6 months. Screening studies repeated every 6 months disclosed no serious clinical reactions from phenobarbital, phenytoin, carbamazepine, or valproate. Abnormal but clinically insignificant results prompted retesting in 12 children (6%), and therapy was discontinued unnecessarily in 2 children. The authors concluded that routine monitoring provided no useful information and sometimes prompted unwarranted action. A second study (6) of 662 adults treated with carbamazepine, phenytoin, phenobarbital, or primidone failed to detect significant laboratory abnormalities during 6 months of monitoring and led to the conclusion that routine screening was neither cost-effective nor valuable for asymptomatic patients. Treatment of 480 patients with either carbamazepine or valproic acid in a double-blind, controlled trial also demonstrated the lack of usefulness of routine laboratory monitoring (7).

Although habits vary in the United States and elsewhere, it is good medical practice to measure biochemical function and structural circulating elements in blood at baseline before starting treatment with a new drug (2).

Efficacy and adverse effects of drugs are the foundation for treatment decisions by physicians; however, some adverse events have led to legal actions that also have affected treatment, monitoring, and the need to document patient care. Publication of such cases occurs in several circumstances. In general, a case heard in state court will be published in the official reporters for that state only if an appellate court has produced a decision marked for publication. The same is true for some trial-level decisions made by federal courts. Publication occurs when the issues determined are deemed important or significant. For example, classic cases involving AEDs have centered on medical negligence in dosage, selection of treatment, and questions about informed consent.

The approval process for drugs used in the United States is codified in the federal Food, Drug, and Cosmetic Act of 1938, as amended in 21 USC §301 et seq (2001) and the 1962 Kefauver-Harris amendment to the Food, Drug, and Cosmetic Act; both were updated with the Food, Drug, and Cosmetic Modernization Act of 1997. The U.S. Food and Drug Administration (FDA) does not regulate drug use by physicians, who may use any licensed drug to treat patients. An attempt to restrain physicians in that respect failed (*United States v. Evers*, 453 F Supp 1141 [ND Ala 1978]). At this time, legislative and judicial actions are being considered regarding control of drugs and devices.

U.S. standards of care are derived from expert opinion, source publications, or referred articles that underlie evidence-based medicine. Other sources are textbooks and published practice guidelines, such as those from the American Academy of Neurology and the Office of Quality Assurance and Medical Review of the American Medical Association.

In medical malpractice or negligence cases, determining the standard of care for a particular treatment is of utmost importance. The standard-of-care concept extends also to the methods used to obtain informed consent and a trial is usually established by testimony from experts citing source documents or articles from referred publications. One such reference source is the PDR (8) (Table 48.1).

As with any area of law over which a state has authority, the process for determining the standard of care can differ from state to state, particularly as regards the evidentiary force of the medication package insert and information in the PDR. Historically, states tend to use these materials in one of three ways. Although the differences among these approaches are not absolute, the categorization has educational and discussion value. In the first group are states that consider the PDR and package insert as establishing the standard of care (*Haught v. Maceluch*, 681 F2d 291, *reh'ing denied*, 685 F2d

TABLE 48.1

LEGAL ACTION REGARDING ADVERSE EFFECTS OF ANTIEPILEPTIC DRUGS

Year	Case	Drug	Issue	Outcome
2004	*Dubois v. Haykal*	Tegretol	Failure to warn BCP failure	Reversed lower court decision granting summary judgment in favor of physician
2002	*Serigne v. Ivker*	Dilantin (phenytoin)	Informed consent: teratogenicity	Malformation causation not connected: informed consent was established
2002	*Spano v. Bertocci*	Depakote (valproic acid)	Informed consent	Patient had prior knowledge of pregnancy and effect of valproate: informed consent was established
1988	*Guevara v. Dorsey Laboratories*	Bellargal-S (phenobarbital)	Failure to warn physicians	Community knowledge and PDR adequate warning
1987	*Shinn v. St. James Mercy Hospital*	Phenytoin	Informed consent: SJS	Only required to disclose common adverse effects
1984	*Menefee v. Guerhing*	Phenobarbital	Informed consent: SJS	General warning adequate
1983	*Harbeson v. Parke-Davis*	Phenytoin	Informed consent: teratogenicity	Patient not warned: malformed children: award for plaintiff
1967	*Fritz v. Parke Davis & Co*	Phenytoin	Informed consent: hepatotoxicity	Documented serious illness and skilled care: in favor of physician
1987	*Hendricks v. Charity Hospital of New Orleans*	Phenytoin	Malpractice: dose error	Found for plaintiff
1998	*Martin v. Life Care Centers of America Inc.*	Phenytoin	Malpractice: failure to act on elevated plasma levels: patient death	Found for plaintiff
1992	*Pester v. Graduate Hospital*	Valproate	Malpractice: failure to diagnose pancreatitis	Found for plaintiff

1385 [5th Cir 1985]). In the second group, the package insert and PDR are considered evidence of standard of care and may establish a prima facie case for negligence if a physician does not follow the prescribed directions. Generally, however, a physician may present evidence for using a medication outside the description in the PDR and package insert (*Mulder* rule and echo of *Mulder*; see below) (*Thompson v. Carter*, 518 So2d 609, 613 [Miss 1987]). *Mulder v. Parke-Davis*, 181 NW2d 882 (Minn 1970), required a physician to explain the reason for deviating from the use of a drug as specified in the PDR. Such an explanation is best included in the patient's chart. In the third group of states, the PDR and package insert are given little credence and in some jurisdictions are inadmissible without supporting expert testimony. This is known as the echo of the *Mulder* rule (*Spensieri v. Lasky*, 723 NE2d 544 [NY 1999]) (8).

These discrepancies in the handling of medical malpractice issues illustrate why it is critical for the physician to know local, regional, and national standards of practice and the idiosyncrasies of applicable law in their jurisdiction, as well as why a physician must diligently document the rationale for action in a patient's medical record.

Issues of informed consent have also required adjudication. In *Serigne v. Ivker* (808 So2d 783 [La App 4th Cir 2002]), the plaintiff alleged that informed consent had not been obtained because teratogenicity had not been disclosed. The court found (i) that the plaintiff had failed to establish a connection between malformations and phenytoin and (ii) that informed consent did exist. In *Spano v. Bertocci*, a plaintiff claimed lack of informed consent based on nondisclosure of the teratogenic effects of valproic acid. At the trial and appellate court levels, informed consent was deemed to have been obtained because of the plaintiff's previous knowledge of the danger of valproate use during pregnancy.

The landmark decision of *Harbeson v. Parke-Davis* (656 P.2d 483 [1983]) illustrates the diligence required in providing information for patients with childbearing potential. A woman who delivered children with fetal hydantoin syndrome claimed failure of informed consent causing wrongful birth and wrongful life. The court stated that a physician had a duty to "exercise reasonable care in disclosing 'grave risks' of (any) treatment" advocated. The physician had failed to search the literature, which would have uncovered the dangers of using phenytoin during pregnancy and would have allowed the physician to inform the patient of the risks.

Interactions with other drugs also have been the basis of malpractice claims. In *Dubois v. Haykal* (165 S.W.3d 634 [2004]), the appellate court reversed a decision by the trial court granting summary judgment in favor of the physician. The trial court originally had granted summary judgment finding that the plaintiff had not established causation between the defendant prescribing Tegretol and an unexpected pregnancy while the plaintiff was on oral contraceptives. The plaintiff had presented evidence, including expert testimony, that Tegretol reduced the efficacy of oral contraceptives and asserted that the physician did not warn about the possible interaction.

Serious skin reactions, including Stevens–Johnson syndrome, have also raised issues of informed consent. *Shinn v. St. James Mercy Hospital* (675 F Supp 94 [WDNY 1987])

centered on the claim that serious skin reactions to phenytoin had not been disclosed. The court decided that all adverse effects need not be disclosed to a patient, only the most common. In addition, given the patient's medical circumstance, treatment would not reasonably have been declined even if adverse effects had been delineated. Similarly, another court found that warnings in the PDR and package insert diminished the "danger-in-fact" of the medication: ". . . no reasonable trier of fact could conclude that this . . . medicine is unreasonably dangerous per se" (*Williams v. Ciba-Geigy*, 686 F Supp 573 [WD La 1988]).

Documentation can be critical. A patient treated with phenytoin suffered hepatotoxic reactions, and the court originally found for the plaintiff. That decision was overturned on appeal, the appellate court stating, "Viewing the record . . . the skill and care exhibited by defendant's physicians' diagnosis and treatment were marked by devoted diligence and attention and were wholly consistent with the professional skill . . . employed by other physicians in treating and controlling . . . the complex disease of epilepsy" (*Fritz v. Parke-Davis*, 152 NW2d 129 [1967]).

Errors in the use of AEDs that amount to negligence have resulted in legal action. When a patient who was to take Dilantin 500 mg per day received a prescription for 500 mg three times a day, judgment was for the plaintiff (*Hendricks v. Charity Hospital of New Orleans* [La App 1987]). In *Martin v. Life Care Centers of America* (No. 95-4124-B, 117th Judicial Dist Ct, Nueces County, TX [April 1998]), high plasma levels of Dilantin were associated with a patient's death, resulting in judgment for the plaintiff. One court found for the plaintiff in a case of failure to diagnose pancreatitis from the use of valproate (*Pester v. Graduate Hospital*, No. 87-05-00357, Court of Common Pleas, Philadelphia, PA, Oct 1992).

Serious idiosyncratic drug reactions do not depend on dose and by their nature are unpredictable (9). All organs are affected, the skin most commonly (Table 48.2). Established AEDs, used in millions of patients, are known to cause agranulocytosis, aplastic anemia, blistering skin rash, hepatic necrosis, allergic dermatitis, serum sickness, and pancreatitis. Newly available drugs, used in many fewer patients, have caused allergic dermatitis and serious skin reactions (Table 48.2). With the exception of reactions to felbamate,

other serious reactions have yet to be reported with any alarming frequency.

AT-RISK PROFILES

One way to minimize the risk of serious adverse effects is to identify high-risk patients by constructing clinical profiles from reports of idiopathic drug reactions (9). For example, the risk of hepatotoxic reactions from valproic acid is too nonspecific to be of much practical help; however, at-risk patients are younger than 2 years of age, being treated with several AEDs, and have known metabolic disease with developmental delay (10–12). Patients fitting this profile need detailed laboratory screening for the presence of metabolic disorders, including measurement of serum lactate, serum pyruvate, serum carnitine, and urinary organic acid levels, as well as routine hematologic and chemical tests (2). Prothrombin time, partial thromboplastin time, and determination of arterial blood gas and ammonia levels are also useful tests.

Risk of hypersensitivity, including Stevens–Johnson syndrome and toxic epidermal necrolysis has been identified a markedly increased in those with the HLA-B*1502 allele of the human leukocyte antigen (13). This allele occurs predominantly in those of Han Chinese, Filipino, Malayasian, South Asian Indian, and Thai descent (13). Physicians have been advised by the FDA to screen Asian patients for this allele prior to prescribing carbamazepine and to consider the risk in using phenytoin or fosphenytoin in these patients (13). Cross-reactivity and sensitivity between carbamazepine, phenytoin, phenobarbital, lamotrigine, and oxcarbazepine does occur (14).

After a drug is selected, the physician must review its relative benefits and risks, documenting this discussion in the patient's record. This process forms the basis for informal informed consent. Patients should be told the criteria for success and reminded of the trial and error of drug selection and the methods for changing drugs. Because dose-related side effects aid management but interfere with treatment, negotiation defines this process. The patient must know the nature of side effects, what must be tolerated, and how side effects will influence titration. Serious, life-threatening, idiosyncratic effects must be explained clearly, but within the context of rarity. Although the

TABLE 48.2

IDIOSYNCRATIC REACTIONS TO ANTIEPILEPTIC DRUGS

Reaction	CBZ	ETH	FBM	GBP	LEV	LTG	PB	PHT	TPM	TGB	OXC	ZNS	VPA
Agranulocytosis	X	X	X				X	X					X
Stevens–Johnson syndrome	X	X				X	X	X					X
Aplastic anemia	X	X	X					X					X
Hepatic failure	X		X				X	X					X
Allergic dermatitis	X	X	X	X		X	X	X	X	X	X	X	X
Serum sickness	X	X					X	X					X
Pancreatitis	X												
Nephrolithiasis									X			X	

CBZ, carbamazepine; ETH, ethosuximide; FBM, felbamate; GBP, gabapentin; LEV, levetiracetam; LTG, lamotrigine; PB, phenobarbital; PHT, phenytoin; TPM, topiramate.

TABLE 48.3

ASSESSMENT FOR HIGH-RISK PATIENTS TREATED WITH VALPROATE

At risk	Younger than 2 years of age
	Treated with multiple drugs
	Known metabolic disease
	Delayed development
Specific screening studies	Serum lactate and pyruvate
	Plasma carnitine
	Urinary metabolic screen with organic acids
	Ammonia and arterial blood gases

patient must be ready to report symptoms, the physician must identify patients who lack advocates or who have impaired ability to communicate. Unlike most patients with epilepsy, these individuals may require a monitoring strategy. A screening program may be useful in some high-risk patients (Table 48.3).

CLINICAL MONITORING

Although routine monitoring of hepatic function revealed elevated values in 5% to 15% of patients treated with carbamazepine, fewer than 20 with significant hepatic complications were reported in the United States from 1978 to 1989 (15). Cases of pancreatitis were even rarer (16). Transient leukopenia occurs in up to 12% of adults and children treated with carbamazepine (17,18), and aplastic anemia or agranulocytosis, unrelated to benign leukopenia, occurs in 2 per 575,000, with an annual mortality rate of approximately 1 in 575,000 patients (15). Only 4 of 65 cases of agranulocytosis or aplastic anemia occurred in children.

Hematologic abnormalities in patients developing exfoliative dermatitis, alone or as part of systemic hypersensitivity, were not found until clinical symptoms appeared. Neither benign leukopenia nor transient elevations in hepatic enzyme predicted life-threatening reactions. Routine monitoring does not allow anticipation of life-threatening effects of carbamazepine; data for phenytoin and phenobarbital are similar.

Women of childbearing potential must be warned about contraceptive failure; impact on reproductive health, such as development of polycystic ovaries; and the possible effect of maternal drug treatment on a developing fetus (19,20). Use of AEDs that induce cytochrome P450 enzymes by women taking oral contraceptives increases the risk that contraception will fail (19,21). Gynecologists must be informed of the AED being used and of the need that the contraceptive contain an adequate amount of estrogen (19).

Some AEDs are thought to have direct reproductive consequences for women. Whether temporal lobe epilepsy or a specific drug causes polycystic ovary syndrome has generated continued discussion (22). Either anovulatory cycles with serologic evidence or physical changes of androgen excess can define this syndrome; documentation of polycystic ovaries is not required for diagnosis. Although polycystic ovaries and hyperandrogenism are associated with valproate, high percentages of ovarian changes have been reported in women with localization-related epilepsy (23).

Pregnancy increases the number of seizures in approximately one third of patients. Although changes in drug metabolism, drug absorption, or induction of metabolism may be operative, medication compliance is a major concern (19).

Women treated with AEDs have an increased risk of delivering infants with major malformations. Established drugs are associated with cleft lip and palate and serious cardiac defects (24–26). Reports from the North American Antiepileptic Drug Pregnancy Registry (26) identify phenobarbital as posing the greatest risk (a 12% rate of malformation) followed by valproate (an 8.8% rate of malformation). Carbamazepine has a 0.5% to 1.0% incidence of neural tube defects, including anencephaly and spina bifida (27). The total number of drugs used to treat a mother with epilepsy is also important. When all malformations were considered, incidence was 20.6% with one drug and 28% with two or more drugs (26). Administration of folate to women treated with AEDs is recommended in that low folate levels have been observed in women delivering malformed infants (27).

As new drugs become available, physicians have an obligation to review source documents for those medications and devise a strategy of treatment and for monitoring. Because data tend to be limited, a new drug should be initiated cautiously and patients should be given as much information as possible. Although industry-produced materials may be useful, a better alternative is for physicians to provide copies of package inserts coupled with their own material describing how the drug is to be used and any monitoring strategy planned. Parsimony may be the guiding principle in monitoring when established drugs are being used, but such is not necessarily the case with a newly introduced drug (Table 48.4). Baseline data should be obtained, the patient must be prepared

TABLE 48.4

RECOMMENDATIONS FOR MONITORING

1. Obtain screening laboratory studies before initiation of antiepileptic drug treatment. Baseline studies provide a benchmark and could identify patients with special risk factors that could influence drug selection.
2. Blood and urine monitoring in otherwise healthy and asymptomatic patients is unnecessary.
3. Identify high-risk patients before treatment.
   a. Presumptive biochemical disorders
   b. Altered systemic health
   c. Neurodegenerative disease
   d. History of significant adverse drug reactions
   e. Patients without an advocate
      i. Those unable to communicate require a different strategy
      ii. Patients with multiple handicaps who are institutionalized
4. For newly introduced drugs, follow recommended guidelines for blood monitoring until the numbers of patients treated in this country increase and data become available.

Adapted from Willmore LJ. Clinical risk patterns: summary and recommendations. In: Levy RH, Penry JK, eds. *Idiosyncratic Reactions to Valproate: Clinical Risk Patterns and Mechanisms of Toxicity.* New York: Raven Press; 1991:163–165.

TABLE 48.5

SCREENING LABORATORY TESTS TO
DETECT ADVERSE DRUG REACTIONS
TO ANTIEPILEPTIC DRUGS

Antiepileptic drug	Laboratory tests
Phenytoin	CBC, liver enzymes
Phenobarbital	CBC, liver enzymes
Carbamazepine	CBC, liver enzyme
Valproate	CBC, liver enzymes, hepatic panel, serum amylase and lipase (pancreatitis), ammonia, plasma, and urine carnitine assay
Oxcarbazepine	Serum sodium
Topiramate	Urine for microscopic hematuria and renal ultrasound (renal stones), intraocular pressure (glaucoma)
Zonisamide	Urine for microscopic hematuria and renal ultrasound (renal stones)
Felbamate	CBC, reticulocyte count, liver enzymes, hepatic panel
Ethosuximide	CBC, reticulocyte count

CBC, complete blood count with platelet count.

to get in touch with the physician, and the physician must
facilitate that communication. Chemical and hematologic
monitoring may be recommended in the materials developed
by the manufacturer in concert with the FDA. It may be wise
to follow those guidelines until broader clinical experience is
available. Table 48.5 summarizes screening laboratory tests
that may aid in detection of adverse effects of AEDs. Further,
the FDA has issued an alert regarding AEDs and sucidality.
Patients and care givers must be alerted to this problem and
behavior monitored (28).

SPECIFIC DRUGS

Carbamazepine

When carbamazepine is catalyzed by the hepatic monooxyge-
nases, an epoxide is formed at the 10,11-double bond of the
azepine ring (CBZ-10,11-epoxide); this compound is associated with toxic symptoms (29). Hydration of the epoxide
occurs through microsomal epoxide hydrolase. Inhibition of
that enzyme, as with concomitant administration of valproic
acid, increases the quantity of the epoxide (30).

Severe reactions to carbamazepine can cause hematopoietic,
skin, hepatic, and cardiovascular changes (17). Rash occurs
in 5% to 8% of patients, and in rare cases, may progress
to exfoliative dermatitis or to a bullous reaction, such as
Stevens–Johnson syndrome especially in patients of oriental
descent (13). Transient leukopenia is observed in 10% to 12%
of patients; however, fatal reactions such as aplastic anemia are
rare. Patients and parents must be reassured that frequent monitoring of blood counts and liver values is unnecessary (2).

Presymptomatic blood test abnormalities have not been
reported in patients who develop systemic hypersensitivity

reactions to carbamazepine. Genetic susceptibility among
those patients who are oriental means pretreatment screening
is critically important for patient care (13,31).

Ethosuximide

Ethosuximide causes nausea, gastric distress, and abdominal
pain unless given with meals. Rash, severe headaches, and, on
rare occasions, leukopenia, pancytopenia, and aplastic anemia
have occurred. Neurologic effects include lethargy, agitation,
aggressiveness, depression, and memory problems. Psychiatric
disorders have occurred and drug-induced lupus has been
reported in children (32).

Felbamate

Felbamate, a dicarbamate compound related to meprobamate,
involves vigorous drug interactions that may cause clinically
significant toxic reactions or exacerbate seizures (33). Serious
idiosyncratic reactions to felbamate, including aplastic anemia, have occurred, and clinical risk profiles for felbamate
suggest the need for a screening strategy. Although some features such as white race, female sex, and adult status are not
specific, a previous AED allergic reaction, cytopenia, an
immune disorder, especially lupus erythematosus, and less
than 1 year of treatment are more worrisome. Before felbamate is prescribed, manufacturer recommendations should be
reviewed (34). Hepatotoxic effects of felbamate seem less
clearly associated with risk factors.

Guidelines now emphasize that felbamate should be used
for severe epilepsy refractory to other therapy. Treatment
should be preceded by a careful history to uncover indications
of hematologic, hepatotoxic, and autoimmune diseases.
Women with autoimmune disease account for the largest proportion of those who developed aplastic anemia. Routine
hematologic and liver function tests should be performed at
baseline, and patients and their families must be fully
informed of the potential risks; in the United States written
consent is recommended. The frequency of clinical monitoring
and a specific schedule of blood tests should follow the manufacturer's recommendations, and patients should be educated
about symptoms that may signify either hematologic change
or hepatotoxicity.

Gabapentin

Gabapentin, 1-(aminomethyl)cyclohexane acetic acid, is structurally related to γ-aminobutyric acid (GABA). Adverse events
were typically neurotoxic, but withdrawal from studies was
infrequent. Use in mentally retarded children was accompanied by an increased incidence of hyperactivity and aggressive
behavior (35).

Lamotrigine

Central nervous system side effects included lethargy, fatigue,
and mental confusion (36–38). Serious rash appears to be correlated with the rate of dose increase and may be more
common in children. Current U.S. guidelines require discontinuation if a rash develops.

TABLE 48.6

GUIDELINES FOR USE OF LAMOTRIGINE

	Weeks 1 and 2	Weeks 3 and 4	To achieve maintenance
Information for patients and parents about rash			
For adult patients receiving inducing drugs such as phenytoin, carbamazepine, or barbiturates (but not valproate)	50 mg each day	100 mg each day (in divided doses)	Add 50–100 mg every 1–2 weeks to 200–400 mg each day
For patients treated with valproic acid	25 mg every other day	25 mg each day	Add 25–50 mg every 1–2 weeks to 100–200 mg each day

Adapted from Willmore LJ. General principles. Safety monitoring of antiepileptic drugs. In: Levy RH, Mattson RH, Meldrum BS, et al., eds. *Antiepileptic Drugs.* Philadelphia, PA: Lippincott Williams & Wilkins; 2002:112–118.

Morbilliform erythematous rash, urticaria, or a maculopapular pattern are most common (39–44); however, erythema multiforme and blistering reactions like Stevens–Johnson syndrome or toxic epidermal necrolysis can occur. Simple rashes require careful assessment to rule out a hypersensitivity syndrome. Such sensitivity reactions often include fever, lymphadenopathy, elevated liver enzyme values, and altered numbers of circulating cellular elements of blood (42).

In U.S. drug trials, rash affected approximately 10% of patients; 3.8% had to discontinue the drug and 0.3% were hospitalized (42). Most serious rashes developed within 6 weeks of the start of treatment. In drug trials involving children, rash occurred in 12.9% and was serious in 1.1%, with half of that group having Stevens–Johnson syndrome (42). More than 80% of patients who experienced a serious rash were being treated with valproate or had been given higher-than-recommended doses (42). Rash was suspected to be a drug interaction with valproate, which inhibits the metabolism of lamotrigine, causing diminished clearance and resultant high blood levels (43). When treatment guidelines are followed, the incidence of serious rash may be reduced (42,44,45). In the United States, discontinuation is advised if rash develops. Table 48.6 lists the suggested plan for initiation of lamotrigine treatment.

Levetiracetam

Treatment-emergent side effects typical for a CNS-active drug have been reported from the clinical trials, including somnolence, asthenia, and dizziness (46). Behavioral changes reported in children include aggression, emotional lability, oppositional behavior, and psychosis (47). Exacerbation, a pre-existing tendency has been suggested as a mechanism (48), but behavioral changes consistent with all of the newer drugs have been reported as well (49).

Oxcarbazepine

Oxcarbazepine is a keto analogue of carbamazepine that is rapidly converted to a 10-monohydroxy active metabolite by cytosol arylketone reductase. Renal clearance of the metabolite correlates with measured creatinine clearance. Dizziness, sedation, and fatigue, possibly dose related, were reported in pivotal trials (50–52). Hyponatremia also has occurred (53).

Oxcarbazepine was associated with malformations in a small cohort of a study that failed to identify phenytoin as causing malformations (27). Cross-reactivity in patients allergic to carbamazepine has been reported.

Phenobarbital

Idiosyncratic reactions to phenobarbital include allergic dermatitis, Stevens–Johnson syndrome, serum sickness, hepatic failure, agranulocytosis, and aplastic anemia. Folate deficiency in patients treated with AEDs is claimed to be associated with behavioral changes (54).

Long-term treatment may cause connective tissue changes, with coarsened facial features, Dupuytren contracture, Ledderhose syndrome (plantar fibromas), and frozen shoulder (55). Sedative effects may exacerbate absence, atonic, and myoclonic seizures. Sudden withholding of doses of short-acting barbiturates may precipitate drug-withdrawal seizures or even status epilepticus. Phenobarbital's slow rate of clearance makes such acute seizures less of a problem, but dose tapering is recommended if discontinuation is planned. Some patients may experience mild withdrawal symptoms of tremor, sweating, restlessness, irritability, weight loss, disturbed sleep, and even psychiatric manifestations. Infants of mothers treated with phenobarbital may have irritability, hypotonia, and vomiting for several days after delivery (56).

Phenytoin

Phenytoin is a weak organic acid, poorly soluble in water, and available as free acid and a sodium salt. Because of the drug's saturation kinetics, small changes in the maintenance dose produce large changes in total serum concentration (57); thus, the half-life increases with higher plasma concentrations. Doses must be changed carefully. The steady state of phenytoin is altered by interaction with other drugs (58). Dose-related effects of phenytoin include nystagmus, ataxia, altered coordination, cognitive changes, and dyskinesia. Facial features may coarsen, and body hair may change texture and darken. Acne may develop and gingival hypertrophy is common. Osteoporosis and lymphadenopathy occur with long-term use. Folate deficiency may be severe enough to cause megaloblastic anemia; a transient encephalopathy is said to occur by a similar mechanism (54). Prolonged exposure to high levels of plasma phenytoin has been linked to cerebellar atrophy. Allergic dermatitis, hepatotoxicity, serum sickness, and aplastic anemia may be fatal (59). Drug-induced lupus erythematosus reactions have been observed (60).

Topiramate

Topiramate has a monosaccharide-type structure. The drug appears to influence sodium and a portion of chloride channels, blocks non–N-methyl-D-aspartate glutamate receptors, and inhibits carbonic anhydrase. Nephrolithiasis and dose-related weight loss require discussion with patients. Many side effects in studies were caused by forced titration to high doses. Adverse cognitive effects occur at high doses in adults; however, slowing the pace of dose increases reduces the impact on cognitive function (61,62). Serious rashes have occurred. Reports of acute secondary angle-closure glaucoma mandate cautioning patients to report ocular pain or altered visual acuity immediately (63–65). Children should be monitored for oligohydrosis with hyperthermia, especially in hot weather (66). An encephalopathy has been reported in patients treated with toprimate combined with valproate (67).

Valproate

Children younger than age 2 years who are being treated with several AEDs are at the highest risk for hepatotoxic reactions from treatment with valproate. Additional risk factors are presumed metabolic disorders or severe epilepsy complicating mental retardation and organic brain disease (10,11,68,69). Most clinicians, however, consider this pattern of incidence too restrictive or insufficiently detailed to allow identification of patients at highest risk (70). Moreover, routine laboratory monitoring does not predict fulminant and irreversible hepatic failure (71). Some patients who progressed to fatal hepatotoxic reactions never exhibited abnormalities on specific hepatic function tests. Conversely, abnormal levels of serum ammonia, carnitine, and fibrinogen, as well as hepatic function anomalies have been reported without clinically significant hepatotoxic reactions (45,72). Therefore, reporting of clinical symptoms and identification of highest-risk patients are more reliable means of monitoring (73). Vomiting is an initial symptom in serious cases (72,74). Nausea, vomiting, and anorexia with lethargy, drowsiness, and coma are critical symptoms and must be evaluated immediately. Although early drug discontinuation may reverse hepatotoxic reactions in some patients, fatalities still result (75). No biochemical markers differentiate survivors and those who die. Patients with hepatic failure have been rescued by administration of carnitine (76). Measurement of urinary organic acid and a metabolic evaluation are recommended in high-risk patients or in any patient without an established reason for mental retardation and seizures (70).

Dreifuss and colleagues described high-risk patients (10,11). Most fatalities occurred in the first 6 months of treatment, but some were noted up to 2 years after initiation. Children younger than age 2 years receiving polytherapy had a 1 in 500 to 800 chance of a fatal hepatotoxic event. Patients at negligible risk were those older than age 10 years who were treated with valproate alone and who were free of underlying metabolic or neurologic disorders. Intermediate-risk factors

were use of monotherapy between ages 2 and 10 years and need for polytherapy at any age.

Most cases of fatal liver failure involved mental retardation, encephalopathy, and decline of neurologic function. Two of four reported patients older than age 21 years had degenerative disease of the nervous system. Nine of 16 hepatic fatalities in one report (77), and all members of the 11- to 20-year-old age group in another series were neurologically abnormal. Only 7 of 26 adults with fatal hepatic failure were considered neurologically normal (78).

Specific biochemical disorders associated with valproate-induced hepatotoxic events include urea cycle defects, organic acidurias, multiple carboxylase deficiency, mitochondrial or respiratory chain dysfunction, cytochrome aa_3 deficiency in muscle, pyruvate carboxylase deficiency, and hepatic pyruvate dehydrogenase complex deficiency (brain) (70,79). Clinical disorders include GM_1 gangliosidosis type 2, spinocerebellar degeneration, Friedreich ataxia, Lafora body disease, Alpers disease, and mitochondrial encephalomyelopathy with ragged red fibers (MERRF) (80).

Tremor with sustension and at rest is dose related (81). Weight gain affects from 20% to 54% of patients (82) who report appetite stimulation. Excessive weight change may require drug discontinuation. Hair loss is transient. Hair appears to be fragile, and regrowth results in a curlier shaft (83). Supplementation with zinc-containing multivitamins may be protective. Thrombocytopenia appears to be dose related. Platelet counts vary without dose changes and are asymptomatic. Petechial hemorrhage and ecchymoses necessitate decreases in dose or even discontinuation (84).

Sedation and encephalopathy are less frequently encountered (85). Acute encephalopathy and even coma may develop on initial exposure to valproic acid (86); these patients may be severely acidotic and have elevated excretion of urinary organic acids. Because valproic acid is known to sequester coenzyme A (87), such patients are suspected of having a partially compensated defect in mitochondrial β-oxidation enzymes (85,88). Dermatologic abnormalities, although unusual, may be severe (89).

Acute hemorrhagic pancreatitis may be fatal in younger patients. Abdominal pain should lead to measurement of lipase and amylase levels (16).

Hyperammonemia may occur in the absence of hepatic dysfunction (90,91), possibly caused by inhibition of either nitrogen elimination or urea synthesis (92,93). In rare instances, an insufficiency of urea cycle enzymes such as ornithine transcarbamylase deficiency may be present (94).

Vigabatrin

Vigabatrin, also known as γ-vinyl GABA, increases tissue concentrations of GABA by irreversible inhibition of GABA-transaminase, the enzyme that degrades GABA. Severe changes in behavior with agitation, hallucinations, and altered thinking are thought to be dose related. Depression is a potential problem in all patients. Loss of peripheral retinal function is of concern (95). Up to 40% of adults in one series treated with vigabatrin had concentrically constricted visual fields (95). These visual effects appear not to reverse after the drug is discontinued (95). Use of this drug should be restricted to those children with severe and intractable seizures related to tuberous sclerosis and to patients with severely refractory seizures where risk of visual loss is outweighed by the need for treatment of seizures.

Zonisamide

Zonisamide is a sulfonamide that may cross-react in patients known to be allergic to sulfa-containing compounds (96). Serious skin reactions, drowsiness, and altered thinking have occurred. Patients with a history of renal stones should be informed of the risk of nephrolithiasis and advised to remain adequately hydrated. Children should be monitored for hyperthermia with oligohydrosis, especially during hot weather (97).

LEGAL AND MEDICAL DISCLAIMER

This brief review constitutes an introduction to a topic and has been prepared and provided for educational and informational purposes only; it is not intended to convey, nor should it be considered to convey, legal or medical advice. Legal and/or medical advice requires expert consultation and an in-depth knowledge of your specific situation. Although every effort has been made to provide accurate information herein, laws and precedent are always changing and will vary from state to state and jurisdiction to jurisdiction. As such, the material provided herein is not comprehensive for all legal and medical developments and may contain errors or omissions. For information regarding your particular circumstances, you should contact an attorney to confirm the current laws and how they may apply to your particular situation without delay, in that any delay may result in loss of some or all of your rights. It is hoped that this review helps you understand the need for thorough knowledge and careful documentation.

References

1. Pellock JM. Efficacy and adverse effects of antiepileptic drugs. *Pediatr Clin North Am.* 1989;36:345–348.
2. Pellock JM, Willmore LJ. A rational guide to routine blood monitoring in patients receiving antiepileptic drugs. *Neurology.* 1991;41:961–964.
3. Physicians' Desk Reference. 63rd ed. Montvale, NJ: Thomson Reuters; 2009.
4. CPHA. *Compendium of Pharmaceuticals and Specialities.* 44 ed. Ottawa, Canada: Canadian Pharmaceutical Association; 2009.
5. Camfield C, Camfield P, Smith E, et al. Asymptomatic children with epilepsy: little benefit from screening for anticonvulsant-induced liver, blood or renal damage. *Neurology.* 1986;36:838–841.
6. Mattson RH, Cramer JA, Collins JF, et al. Comparison of carbamazepine, phenobarbital, phenytoin, and primidone in partial and secondarily generalized tonic-clonic seizures. *N Engl J Med.* 1985;313:145–151.
7. Mattson RH, Cramer JA, Collins JF, Department of Veterans Affairs Epilepsy Cooperative Study, No. 264 Group. A comparison of valproate with carbamazepine for the treatment of complex partial seizures and secondarily generalized tonic-clonic seizures in adults. *N Engl J Med.* 1992; 327:765–771.
8. Bradford GE, Elben CC. The drug package insert and the PDR as establishing the standard of care in prescription drug liability cases. *J Mo Bar.* 2001;57:233–242.
9. Glauser TA. Idiosyncratic reactions: new methods of identifying high-risk patients. *Epilepsia.* 2000;41(suppl 8):S16–S29.
10. Dreifuss FE, Santilli N, Langer DH, et al. Valproic acid hepatic fatalities: a retrospective review. *Neurology.* 1987;37:379–385.
11. Dreifuss FE, Langer DH, Moline KA, et al. Valproic acid hepatic fatalities. II. US experience since 1984. *Neurology.* 1989;39:201–207.
12. Bryant AE III, Dreifuss FE. Valproic acid hepatic fatalities. III. U.S. experience since 1986. *Neurology.* 1996;46(2):465–469.
13. Ferrell PB, McLeod HL. Carbamazepine, HLA-B*1502 and risk of Stevens–Johnson syndrome and toxic epidermal necrolysis: US FDA recommendations. *Pharmacogenomics.* 2008;9:1543–1546.
14. Arif H, Buchsbaum R, Weintraub D, et al. Comparison and predictors of rash associated with 15 antiepileptic drugs. *Neurolgy.* 2007;68:1701–1709.
15. Seetharam MN, Pellock JM. Risk-benefit assessment of carbamazepine in children. *Drug Saf.* 1991;6:148–158.
16. Gerstner T, Busing D, Bell N, et al. Valproic acid-induced pancreatitis: 16 new cases and a review of the literature. *J Gastroenterol.* 2007;42: 39–48.
17. Pellock JM. Carbamazepine side effects in children and adults. *Epilepsia.* 1987;28:S64–S70.
18. Hart RG, Easton JD. Carbamazepine and hematological monitoring. *Ann Neurol.* 1982;11:309–312.
19. Pennell PB. Antiepileptic drugs during pregnancy: what is known and which AEDs seem to be safest? *Epilepsia.* 2008;49(suppl 9):43–55.
20. Uziel D, Rozental R. Neurologic birth defects after prenatal exposure to antiepileptic drugs. *Epilepsia.* 2008;49(suppl 9):35–42.
21. Mattson RH, Cramer JA, Darney PD, et al. Use of oral contraceptives by women with epilepsy. *JAMA.* 1986;256:238–240.
22. Morrell MJ. Reproductive and metabolic disorders in women with epilepsy. *Epilepsia.* 2003;44(suppl 4):11–20.
23. Morrell MJ, Giudice L, Flynn KL, et al. Predictors of ovulatory failure in women with epilepsy. *Ann Neurol.* 2002;52:704–711.
24. Annegers JF, Hauser WA, Elveback LR. Congenital malformations and seizure disorders in the offspring of parents with epilepsy. *Int J Epidemiol.* 1978;7:241–247.
25. Friis ML. Facial clefts and congenital heart defects in children of parents with epilepsy: genetic and environmental etiologic factors. *Acta Neurol Scand.* 1989;79:433–459.
26. Holmes LB, Harvey EA, Coull BA, et al. The teratogenicity of anticonvulsant drugs. *N Engl J Med.* 2001;344:1132–1138.
27. Kaaja E, Kaaja R, Hiilesmaa V. Major malformations in offspring of women with epilepsy. *Neurology.* 2003;60:575–579.
28. Shneker BF, Cios JS, Elliott JO. Suicidality, depression screening, and antiepileptic drugs. *Neurology.* 2009;72:987–991.
29. Riley RJ, Kitteringham NR, Park BK. Structural requirements for bioactivation of anticonvulsants to cytotoxic metabolites in vitro. *Br J Clin Pharmacol.* 1989;28:482–487.
30. Pisani F, Caputo M, Fazio A, et al. Interaction of carbamazepine-10,11-epoxide, an active metabolite of carbamazepine, with valproate: a pharmacokinetic study. *Epilepsia.* 1990;31:339–342.
31. Franciotta D, Kwan P, Perucca E. Genetic basis for idiosyncratic reactions to antiepileptic drugs. *Curr Opin Neurol.* 2009;22(2):144–149.
32. Jacobs JC. Systemic lupus erythematosus in childhood. Report of 35 cases, with discussion of seven apparently induced by anticonvulsant medication and the prognosis and treatment. *Pediatrics.* 1963;32:257.
33. Theodore WH, Raubertas RF, Porter RJ, et al. Felbamate: a clinical trial for complex partial seizures. *Epilepsia.* 1991;32:392–397.
34. Thompson CD, Gulden PH, Macdonald TL. Identification of modified atropaldehyde mercapturic acids in rat and human urine after felbamate administration. *Chem Res Toxicol.* 1997;10:457–462.
35. Pellock JM. Utilization of new antiepileptic drugs in children. *Epilepsia.* 1996;37(suppl 1):S66–S73.
36. Binnie CD, Debets RM, Engelsman M, et al. Double-blind crossover trial of lamotrigine (Lamictal) as add-on therapy in intractable epilepsy. *Epilepsy Res.* 1989;4:222–229.
37. Matsuo F, Bergen D, Faught E, et al. Placebo-controlled study of the efficacy and safety of lamotrigine in patients with partial seizures. *Neurology.* 1993;43:2284–2291.
38. Messenheimer JA, Ramsay RA, Willmore LJ, et al. Lamotrigine therapy for partial seizures: a multicenter placebo-controlled, double-blind, crossover trial. *Epilepsia.* 1994;35:113–121.
39. Schlienger RG, Shapiro LE, Shear NH. Lamotrigine-induced severe cutaneous adverse reactions. *Epilepsia.* 1998;39:S22–S26.
40. Pellock JM. Managing pediatric epilepsy syndromes with new antiepileptic drugs. *Pediatrics.* 1999;104:1106–1116.
41. Pellock JM. Overview of lamotrigine and the new antiepileptic drugs: the challenge. *J Child Neurol.* 1997;12:S48–S52.
42. Guberman AH, Besag FMC, Brodie MJ, et al. Lamotrigine-associated rash: risk/benefit considerations in adults and children. *Epilepsia.* 1999;40: 985–991.
43. Willmore LJ, Messenheimer JA. Adult experience with lamotrigine. *J Child Neurol.* 1997;12(suppl 1):S16–S18.
44. Messenheimer JA, Mullens EJ, Giorgi L, et al. Safety review of adult clinical trial experience with lamotrigine. *Drug Saf.* 1998;18:281–296.
45. Motte J, Trevathan E, Arvidsson JFV, et al. Lamotrigine for generalized seizures associated with the Lennox–Gastaut syndrome. *N Engl J Med.* 1994;337:1807–1812.
46. Harden C. Safety profile of levetiracetam. *Epilepsia.* 2001;42:36–39.
47. Glauser TA, Ayala R, Elterman RD, et al. Double-blind placebo-controlled trial of adjunctive levetiracetam in pediatric partial seizures. *Neurology.* 2006;66:1654–1660.
48. Kossoff EH, Bergey GK, Freeman JM, et al. Levetiracetam psychosis in children with epilepsy. *Epilepsia.* 2001;42(12):1611–1613.
49. Glauser TA. Behavioral and psychiatric adverse events associated with antiepileptic drugs commonly used in pediatric patients. *J Child Neurol.* 2004;19(suppl 1):25–38.

50. Schachter SC, Vasquez B, Fisher RS, et al. Oxcarbazepine: a double-blind, placebo-controlled, monotherapy trial for partial seizures. *Neurology.* 1999;52:732–737.
51. Bill PA, Vigonius U, Pohlmann H, et al. A double-blind controlled clinical trial of oxcarbazepine versus phenytoin in adults with previously untreated epilepsy. *Epilepsy Res.* 1997;27:195–204.
52. Christe W, Kramer G, Vigonius U, et al. A double-blind controlled clinical trial: oxcarbazepine versus sodium valproate in adults with newly diagnosed epilepsy. *Epilepsy Res.* 1997;26:451–460.
53. Sachdeo RC, Wasserstein A, Mesenbrink PJ, et al. Effects of oxcarbazepine on sodium concentration and water handling. *Ann Neurol.* 2002;51: 613–620.
54. Reynolds EH, Chanarin I, Milner G, et al. Anticonvulsant therapy, folic acid and vitamin B12 metabolism and mental symptoms. *Epilepsia.* 1966; 7:261–270.
55. Mattson RH, Cramer JA, McCutchen CB. Barbiturate related connective tissue disorders. *Arch Intern Med.* 1989;149:911–914.
56. Morselli PL, Franco-Morselli R, Bossi L. Clinical pharmacokinetics in newborns and infants: age related differences and therapeutic implications. *Clin Pharmacokinet.* 1980;5:485–527.
57. Bender AD, Post A, Meier JP, et al. Plasma protein binding of drugs as a function of age in adult human subjects. *J Pharmaceut Sci.* 1975;64:1711–1713.
58. Kutt H. Interactions between anticonvulsants and other commonly prescribed drugs. *Epilepsia.* 1984;25(suppl 2):S118–S131.
59. Haruda F. Phenytoin hypersensitivity: 38 cases. *Neurology.* 1979;29: 1480–1485.
60. Gleichmann H. Systemic lupus erythematosus triggered by diphenylhydantoin. *Arthritis Rheum.* 1982;25:1387.
61. Ben-Menachem E, Henricksen O, Dam M, et al. Double-blind, placebo-controlled trial of Topiramate as add-on therapy in patients with refractory partial seizures. *Epilepsia.* 1996;37:539–543.
62. Privitera M, Fincham R, Penry JK, et al. Topiramate placebo-controlled dose-ranging trial in refractory partial epilepsy using 600-, 800-, and 1,000-mg daily dosages. *Neurology.* 1996;46:1678–1683.
63. Congdon NG, Friedman DS. Angle-closure glaucoma: impact, etiology, diagnosis and treatment. *Curr Opin Ophthalmol.* 2003;14:70–73.
64. Sankar PS, Pasquale LR, Grosskreutz CL. Uveal effusion and secondary angle-closure glaucoma associated with topiramate use. *Arch Ophthalmol.* 2001;119:2110–2111.
65. Thambi L, Kapcala LP, Chambers W, et al. Topiramate-associated secondary angle-closure glaucoma: a case series. *Arch Ophthalmol.* 2002; 120:1108.
66. Ben-Zeev B, Watemberg N, Augarten A, et al. Oligohydrosis and hyperthermia: pilot study of a novel topiramate adverse effect. *J Child Neurol.* 2003;18:254–257.
67. Cheung E, Wong V, Fung C-W. Topiramate-valproate-induced hyperammonemic encephalopathy syndrome. *J Child Neurol.* 2005;20:157–160.
68. Willmore LJ. Clinical manifestations of valproate hepatotoxicity. In: Levy RH, Penry JK, eds. *Idiosyncratic Reactions to Valproate: Clinical Risk Patterns and Mechanisms of Toxicity.* New York: Raven Press; 1991:3–7.
69. Willmore LJ. Clinical risk patterns: summary and recommendations. In: Levy RH, Penry JK, eds. *Idiosyncratic Reactions to Valproate: Clinical Risk Patterns and Mechanisms of Toxicity.* New York: Raven Press; 1991: 163–165.
70. Willmore LJ, Triggs WJ, Pellock JM. Valproate toxicity: risk-screening strategies. *J Child Neurol.* 1991;6:3–6.
71. Willmore LJ, Wilder BJ, Bruni J, et al. Effect of valproic acid on hepatic function. *Neurology.* 1978;28:961–964.
72. Hamer HM, Knake S, Schomburg U, et al. Valproate-induced hyperammonemic encephalopathy in the presence of topiramate. *Neurology.* 2000;54:230–232.
73. Navarro VJ, Senior JR. Drug-related hepatotoxicity. *N Engl J Med.* 2006;354:731–739.
74. Kifune A, Kubota F, Shibata N, et al. Valproic acid-induced hyperammonemic encephalopathy with triphasic waves. *Epilepsia.* 2000;41:909–912.
75. Koenig SA, Beusing D, Longin E, et al. Valproic acid-induced hepatopathy: nine new fatilities in Germany from 1994 to 2003. *Epilepsia.* 2006;47: 2027–2031.
76. Bohan TP, Helton E, McDonald I, et al. Effect of L-carnitine treatment for valproate-induced hepatotoxicity. *Neurology.* 2001;56:1405–1409.
77. Scheffner D, Konig St, Rauterberg-Ruland I, et al. Fatal liver failure in 16 children with valproate therapy. *Epilepsia.* 1988;29:530–542.
78. Konig SA, Schenk M, Sick C, et al. Fatal liver failure associated with valproate therapy in a patient with Friedreich's disease: review of valproate hepatotoxicity in adults. *Epilepsia.* 1999;40:1036–1040.
79. Jellinger K, Seitelberger F. Spongy encephalopathies in infancy: spong degeneration of CNS and progressive infantile poliodystrophy. In: Goldensohn ES, Appel SA, eds. *Scientific Approaches to Clinical Neurology.* Philadelphia, PA: Lea & Febiger; 1977:363.
80. van Egmond H, Degomme P, de Simpel H, et al. A suspected case of late-onset sodium valproate-induced hepatic failure. *Neuropediatrics.* 1987; 18:96–98.
81. Hyuman NM, Dennis PD, Sinclar KG. Tremor due to sodium valproate. *Neurology.* 1979;29:1177–1180.
82. Dinesen H, Gram L, Andersen T, et al. Weight gain during treatment with valproate. *Acta Neurol Scand.* 1984;70:65–69.
83. Jeavons PM, Clark JE, Hirdme GA. Valproate and curly hair. *Lancet.* 1977;1:359.
84. Loiseau P. Sodium valproate, platelet dysfunction and bleeding. *Epilepsia.* 1981;22:141–146.
85. Triggs WJ, Bohan TP, Lin S-N, et al. Valproate induced coma with ketosis and carnitine insufficiency. *Arch Neurol.* 1990;47:1131–1133.
86. Sackellares JC, Lee SI, Dreifuss FE. Stupor following administration of valproic acid to patients receiving other antiepileptic drugs. *Epilepsia.* 1979; 20:697–703.
87. Millington DS, Bohan TP, Roe CR, et al. Valproylcarnitine: a novel drug metabolite identified by fast atom bombardment and thermospray liquid chromatography-mass spectrometry. *Clin Chim Acta.* 1985;145:69–76.
88. Triggs WJ, Roe CR, Rhead WJ, et al. Neuropsychiatric manifestations of defect in mitochondrial beta oxidation response to riboflavin. *J Neurol Neurosurg Psychiatry.* 1992;55:209–211.
89. Roujeau JC, Stern RS. Severe adverse cutaneous reactions to drugs. *N Engl J Med.* 1994;331:1272–1285.
90. Thom H, Carter PE, Cole GF, et al. Ammonia and cartinine concentrations in children treated with sodium valproate compared with other anticonvulsant drugs. *Dev Med Child Neurol.* 1991;33:795–802.
91. Zaret B, Beckner RR, Marini AM, et al. Sodium valproate-induced hyperammonemia without clinical hepatic dysfunction. *Neurology.* 1982; 32:206–208.
92. Hjelm M, Oberholzer V, Seakins J, et al. Valproate-induced inhibition of urea synthesis and hyperammonemia in healthy subjects. *Lancet.* 1986; 2:859.
93. Hjelm M, de Silva LKV, Seakins JWT, et al. Evidence of inherited urea cycle defect in a case of fatal valproate toxicity. *Br Med J.* 1986;292:23–24.
94. Volzke E, Doose H. Dipropylacetate (Depakine, Ergenyl) in the treatment of epilepsy. *Epilepsia.* 1973;14:185–193.
95. Willmore LJ, Abelson MB, Ben-Menachem E, et al. Vigabatrin: 2008 Update. *Epilepsia.* 2009;50(2):163–173.
96. Leppik IE, Willmore LJ, Homan RW, et al. Efficacy and safety of zonsiamede: results of a multicenter study. *Epilepsy Res.* 1993;14:165–173.
97. Knudsen JF, Thambi LR, Kapcala LP, et al. Oligohydrosis and fever in pediatric patients treated with zonisamide. *Pediatr Neurol.* 2003;28:184–189.

CHAPTER 49 ■ PHARMACOGENETICS OF ANTIEPILEPTIC MEDICATIONS

TOBIAS LODDENKEMPER, TRACY A. GLAUSER, AND DIEGO A. MORITA

Marked interindividual variation in efficacy and adverse effects, a characteristic of antiepileptic drug (AED) therapy, represents the result of a delicate balance between a drug's pharmacokinetic features and its pharmacodynamic effects. As the study of "how the body affects the drug," pharmacokinetics describes the relationship of dose, concentration, and time (1). Pharmacodynamics is the study of how the drug affects the body acting on a biochemical or physiologic system (2,3).

Both genetic and nonheritable factors affect pharmacokinetic and pharmacodynamic profiles, thereby contributing to the variability in clinical response to an AED. The impact of nongenetic factors (age, weight, concomitant medications, and concurrent hepatic or renal disease) is well recognized (Fig. 49.1) (2–5).

The study of the genetic contribution to therapeutic response was first called pharmacogenetics in 1959 (6). Pharmacogenomics, a more recent term, is often used interchangeably (7) with pharmacogenetics, but it refers to the systematic study of drug effects on the entire genome. To date, pharmacogenetic research has focused on the effect of genetic polymorphisms (genotype) on a patient's clinical response to a drug (phenotype). A polymorphism is clinically relevant if two or more phenotypes occur in at least 1% of a defined population (8). These variations in DNA sequences can be single-nucleotide polymorphisms (SNPs), deletions or insertions of at least one DNA base (often hundreds or thousands), or deletions or insertions of repetitive DNA (7). Most polymorphisms are present in noncoding regions, but more than 500,000 reside in exons and can potentially change amino acids to a clinically relevant degree (8).

Genetic variation can affect a drug's pharmacokinetic and pharmacodynamic profile through alterations in any of the classic pharmacokinetic phases—absorption, distribution,

metabolism, and excretion (2,5)—in drug receptor site(s), or drug transporters (Fig. 49.2). The metabolism phase exhibits the greatest potential for variability, and polymorphisms in drug-metabolizing enzyme (DME) genes are responsible for most of the well-described pharmacogenetic differences (7,9). Polymorphisms in the DME receptor and drug-transporter genes account for most of the rest (7,9). A molecular explanation for some of the observed pharmacogenetic differences is not yet available.

To describe the current state of AED pharmacogenetics, this chapter is divided into three sections. The first section identifies AED-specific polymorphic candidate genes that encode AED-specific absorption and distribution, target receptors, metabolizing enzymes, and efflux transporters thereby providing insights into AED efficacy and dosing. The second section reviews clinical data based on a phenotypical approach illustrating the impact of these genetic variations on AED safety in several important adverse effects. The third section describes ongoing and future approaches to clarify the contribution of genetic variation to interindividual variation in AED response.

CANDIDATE GENES FROM ABSORPTION TO ELIMINATION

Absorption and Distribution

Knowledge about AED carriers that mediate drug absorption is limited. Gabapentin and pregabalin are in part absorbed and transported via the large neutral amino acid carrier (system L) (10), but it is unclear whether mutations in this carrier affect absorption (11).

Transporters may also influence drug absorption and distribution by secreting AEDs. Several drug-efflux transporter proteins, in particular, members of the superfamily adenosine triphosphatase (ATPase)-binding cassette (ABC) subfamilies B and C (including ABCB1, ABCC1, and ABCC2) play an important role in the absorption, tissue targeting, and elimination of drugs, thus affecting the pharmacokinetic profile and pharmacodynamic effects of AEDs. The therapeutic effectiveness of AEDs could be limited by the activity of ABCB1, ABCC1, and ABCC2, which have been found to be overexpressed in the blood–brain barrier, glia, or neurons of human epileptogenic tissue (12).

MDR1 (ABCB1, PGY1)

ABCB1, also called P-glycoprotein ("P" for permeability) is an ATPase-dependent membrane transporter efflux pump, coded for by the multidrug-resistance gene 1 (MDR1 or ABCB1 or

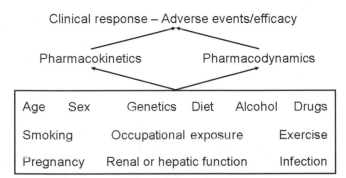

FIGURE 49.1 Interaction among clinical response, drug pharmacokinetics, drug pharmacodynamics, and genetic and noninheritable variables.

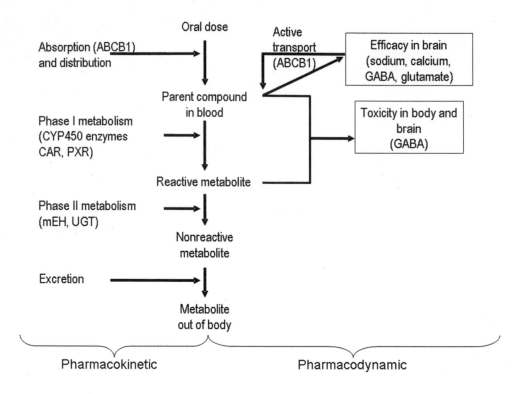

FIGURE 49.2 Sites of potential genetic contribution to the pharmacokinetic and pharmacodynamic profile of an antiepileptic drug.

PGY1), and identified in the intestine and other human tissues as well as the blood–brain barrier (13,14). The MDR1 gene is located on chromosome 7q21.1, encompasses 29 exons, and encodes for ABCB1, a protein with an approximate length of 1280 amino acid residues (15,16). In the intestine, ABCB1 promotes the excretion of drugs in the lumen and could theoretically affect bioavailability of orally administered AEDs (17). More important, lipophilic molecules (such as the AEDs) are good substrates for the ABCB1 efflux transport system at the blood–brain barrier (Fig. 49.3).

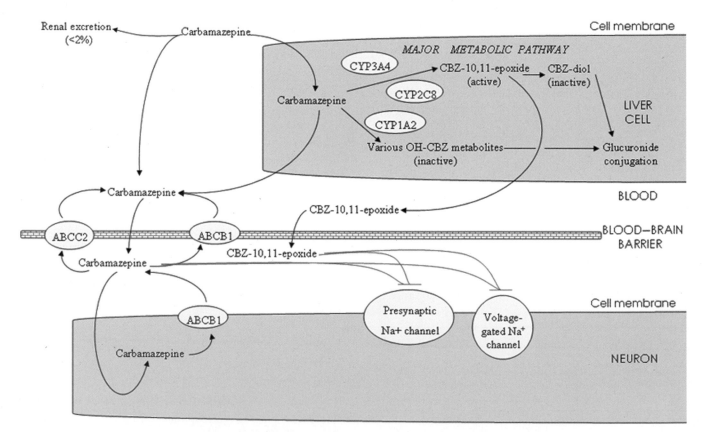

FIGURE 49.3 Carbamazepine pathway demonstrates all known sites for potential genetic contribution to the drug's pharmacokinetics and pharmacodynamics. (Courtesy of Brian Alldredge, PharmD.)

Overexpression of P-glycoprotein may limit drug distribution (18,19). Several studies suggest that increased expression of P-glycoprotein may be associated with subtherapeutic plasma levels of phenytoin (PHT), carbamazepine (CBZ), and valproic acid (20,21). P-glycoprotein expression increase has been well described in epileptic human and animal tissue (18,22). In line with these findings, a study (23) of 19 patients undergoing surgery for treatment-resistant epilepsy demonstrated in 58% (11 of 19) of brain specimens ABCB1 messenger RNA (mRNA) levels more than 10 times higher as compared to normal control brain tissue. A P-glycoprotein inhibitor, tariquidar, has been shown to counteract the decrease of AEDs in epileptic brain regions in animal models (24–26). Several AEDs are substrates of P-glycoprotein encoded by ABCB1 indicating that variations in the gene may affect pharmacokinetics and pharmacodynamics of these drugs (18,19). ABCB1 mRNA was found to be inversely correlated with an active metabolite of oxcarbazepine in patients with epilepsy refractory to oxcarbazepine (27). One study indicated that intestinal P-glycoprotein expression and PHT and CBZ dosing were related to polymorphisms in position 3435 and 2677 of the ABCB1 gene (28).

ABCB1 Polymorphisms. Siddiqui et al. published one of the first studies that suggested an association with 3435C > T polymorphism in the ABCB1 gene and resistance to AED treatment in patients with epilepsy. In 200 patients with drug-resistant epilepsy, the incidence of the ABCB1 C3435T polymorphism was compared to 115 patients with drug-responsive epilepsy, and 200 control subjects without epilepsy (29). The drug-resistant epilepsy group was significantly more likely to have the CC genotype at ABCB1 3435 than the TT genotype (odds ratio, 2.66; 95% CI, 1.32 to 5.38; $P = 0.006$). Despite the statistical association, the authors cautioned that this polymorphism may not be causal. The warning is appropriate for many reasons including, but not limited to, the fact that the polymorphism itself does not alter the amino acid sequence (30) and is within an extensive block of linkage dysequilibrium that spans most of the gene (i.e., it may be linked to the causal polymorphism) (29–32). Loscher et al. (11) reviewed 15 subsequent association studies on ABCB1 polymorphisms in different ethnic populations, with different AEDs and epilepsy types, as well as different definitions of drug resistance and found 8 positive (29,31,33–38) and 7 negative (32,39–44) association studies. Other polymorphisms that may also play a role are 2677G > T and 1236C > T and some association studies analyzed these together with the 3435C > T haplotype (31,35,37,41,42).

Ethnicity and ABCB1 Polymorphism. In a number of ethnic groups, many SNPs have been identified in the genes coding for these transporter proteins (14). Among all ABCB1 variants, the C3435T polymorphism has been found in all ethnic groups studied to date, with the following frequencies: 43% to 54% in whites, 84% in African Americans, 37% to 61% in Asians, 49% to 63% in Oceanians, 73% to 83% in Africans, and 55% in Middle Easterners (14). This polymorphism consists of a C → T transversion at position 3435 in exon 26; it is silent, not altering the amino acid sequence (14). In two positive association studies in non-Caucasian patients, however, patients with intractable epilepsy were more likely to have the

TT genotype (11,37,38) and this adds a layer of complexity to the interpretation of results.

"Silent" ABCB1 polymorphism may alter protein conformation. Furthermore, Kimchi-Sarfaty et al. demonstrated that this "silent" C3435T SNP polymorphism in exon 27, although not related to amino acid changes, results in different substrate specificity (45) and this was ascribed to altered conformations with similar mRNA and protein levels. This study demonstrated that even "silent" SNPs can lead to a similar protein and amino acid chain but with different properties and therefore should be considered in the individual pharmacogenomic approach (45,46).

Imaging, Pathology, and CSF Findings in ABCB1 Polymorphisms. In order to monitor drug distribution in the human brain, PET studies with the P-polyglycan substrate ^{11}C-Verapamil did not show differences in brain distribution (47,48). Postmortem pathological studies indicated a trend to higher P-polyglycan expression in the 3435CC genotype (49). Additionally, 14 patients with dysembryoplastic neuroepithelial tumors had higher P-polyglycan expression in the epileptic tissue, and it was highest in a patient with 3435CC genotype (50). In a prospective study investigating plasma and CSF phenobarbital levels in 60 patients with idiopathic generalized epilepsy on phenobarbital monotherapy, the 3435CC genotype had a lower CSF/plasma ratio and higher overall seizure frequency indicating an association between ABCB1 genotype and response to treatment (51).

MRP1 (ABCC1)

ABCC1, also called multidrug resistance-associated protein 1 (MRP1), is coded for by the MRP1 gene located on chromosome 16p13.1. ABCC1 contains 31 exons, and the encoded protein has 1522 amino acids (52). ABCC1 is ubiquitous and as it occurs with the other MRPs its substrate specificity is partially shared with that of ABCB1 (53). A Japanese study (54) identified 81 SNPs in the ABCC1 gene and 41 SNPs in the ABCC2 gene; no clinical associations have been recognized.

MRP2 (ABCC2)

ABCC2, or MRP2, is encoded by the MRP2 gene, which contains 32 exons and is located on chromosome 10q24. ABCC2 is found primarily in the liver, kidney, and gut (53); it also has been identified in isolated capillaries from rat and pig brains (55). ABCB1 and ABCC1 were overexpressed in reactive astrocytes in resected epileptogenic tissue from patients with dysembryoplastic neuroepithelial tumors, focal cortical dysplasia, and hippocampal sclerosis, all common causes of refractory epilepsy (56). ABCB1 and ABCC1 were also expressed in microvascular endothelial cells in human tissue after resection for mesial temporal sclerosis (57). Similarly, high levels of expression were found in brain tissues resected from a 4-month-old female with tuberous sclerosis and treatment-resistant epilepsy (58) and in a postmortem examination of a patient who died in status epilepticus (59).

Evidence exists that carbamazepine, felbamate, gabapentin, lamotrigine, phenobarbital, phenytoin, topiramate, and valproic acid are substrates for multidrug transporters in the brain (11, 12, 53).

Target Drug Receptors

Two potential types of drug receptors could help to clarify the pharmacogenetics of AEDs: the neuronal AED ion channel receptors (e.g., sodium, calcium channels) and the family of nuclear receptors that regulate induction of AED-specific DME.

SCN1A, SCN2A, SCN3A, and SCN8A

Polymorphisms in genes coding for sodium channels have been the focus of research into the genetic causes of epilepsy (60–67). The sodium channel is composed of a large α subunit with auxiliary β subunits. The α subunit is the pharmacogenetic focus because the β subunits only modulate properties of the channel and are not required for its functioning.

The α subunit isoforms have slightly different electrophysiologic properties and amino acid sequences and are encoded by a family of highly conserved genes denoted by the symbols SCN1A-11A (68). SCN1A, SCN2A1, SCN3A, and SCN8A are expressed in the brain and represent potential candidate genes for pharmacogenetic studies; they map, respectively, to chromosomes 2q23-q24.3, 2q24, and 2q24, whereas SCN8A maps to chromosome 12q13.

The α subunits all have four homologous domains (I to IV), each containing six transmembrane segments (S1 to S6) (69). Site-directed mutagenesis of S6 in domains III and IV (using the *SCN2A* gene) demonstrated that these regions are important for anticonvulsant and antiarrhythmic binding (70,71). When alanine was substituted for certain amino acids in these transmembrane regions, the affinity of phenytoin and lamotrigine decreased two- to eightfold (69,70). This work clearly identified potential candidate genes for further study. Subsequently, a small human tissue electrophysiologic study suggested that sodium channels may exhibit different properties in patients with pharmacoresistant epilepsy as evidenced by different response to carbamazepine (72).

Few published human studies have since examined the relationship between response to therapy and presence of polymorphisms in these genes. Particularly a functional polymorphism in the SCN1A gene (IVS5N+5 G > A, rs3812718) was suggested to influence the dosage requirements for the AEDs carbamazepine and phenytoin in epilepsy patients. This SNP in a 5-splice donor site was shown to influence the alternative splicing of exon 5 which codes for one of the functionally important voltage sensors of the channel (73,74). This SNP (rs3812718) determines whether a neonatal or adult version of exon 5 is included in the final channel (73) and this is under tight control of the protein Nova-2 (74). Results could not be confirmed by the same researchers in a smaller study in Chinese patients (75). However, this study revealed a marginal effect on phenytoin pharmacodynamics and was therefore interpreted as a potential confirmation by the authors (75). A third association study was also negative (76).

Furthermore, determination of genotype and candidate SNPs of SCN1A, 2A, and 3A in 471 Chinese epilepsy patients (272 drug responsive and 199 drug resistant) suggested an association between SCN2A IVS7-32A > G and AED responsiveness (77).

CACNA1G, CACNA1H, and CACNA1I

In a manner analogous to the neuronal sodium channels (and the genes that code for them) the α_1G, α_1H, and α_1I subunits of the T-type calcium channels are the sites of drug action against absence seizures. Voltage-dependent calcium channels in the human brain are multimeric complexes of α_1, β, and $\alpha_2\delta$ subunits (78,79); the γ subunit is expressed only in skeletal muscle. The α_1 subunit, which forms the ion-conducting pore and the channel's voltage sensor to initiate opening, is considered the most likely pharmacologic target (78,79). Its 10 members (α_1A to α_1I and α_1S) encode six functionally distinct calcium channels (types P, Q, L, N, T, and R). Only the genes for the α_1G, α_1H, and α_1I subunits encode the T-type calcium channel, supporting the belief that these three subunits are the pharmacologic targets of AEDs active against T-type calcium channels (80).

The genes that code the α_1G, α_1H, and α_1I subunits of the T-type calcium channel are designated CACNA1G, CACNA1H, and CACNA1I, respectively. CACNA1G has been mapped to 17q22, CACNA1H to 16p13.3, and CACNA1I to chromosome 22q13.1. Significant homology is seen in the membrane-spanning segments coded for by each of these genes. CACNA1H contains at least 27 exons and CACNA1I contains at least 36 exons. No polymorphisms (either naturally occurring or by site-specific mutagenesis) that alter drug binding have been described.

NR1I2 and NR1I3 (Nuclear Receptor Subfamily 1, Group I, Members 2 and 3)

Polymorphisms in DMEs that alter enzyme activity and affect drug pharmacokinetics represent the most intensively studied area of pharmacogenetics; however, interindividual variability may exist in the extent of induction of these cytochrome P450 (CYP) enzymes. The constitutive androstane receptor (CAR) and the pregnane X receptor (PXR), two orphan members of the nuclear receptor superfamily, mediate the induction of CYP2 and CYP3 enzymes, which are involved in the metabolism of many AEDs (Table 49.1) (81–83). The induction begins with exposure to an enzyme-inducing drug like phenobarbital; thereafter, CAR translocates to the nucleus, forms a dimer with the retinoid X receptor, and activates a phenobarbital-responsive enhancer module. An analogous mechanism occurs with PXR (84).

The genes that code CAR and PXR are labeled NR1I3 and NR1I2, respectively. NR1I2 has been mapped to 3q13-q21 and contains nine exons. Research is under way to identify polymorphisms in humans in these and other nuclear receptors that could affect the induction of P450 enzymes that metabolize AEDs.

Metabolism and Excretion

Metabolism of AEDs is divided into two phases (85). Phase I reactions can be oxidative (mediated by CYP enzymes) or reductive (mediated by aldoketoreductases) (85,86). Phase II reactions increase the water solubility of a drug or its phase I metabolite to improve the body's ability to excrete the compound; these reactions conjugate a drug with moieties such as glucuronic acid. Microsomal epoxide hydrolase and uridine diphosphate (UDP)-glucuronosyltransferases (UGTs) are examples of phase II enzymes (85,86). Phase I reactions are considered bioactivating; phase II reactions are considered a form of detoxification (85).

Genetic variability in phase I metabolizing enzymes can alter pharmacokinetic profiles and subsequently drug toxicity.

TABLE 49.1

CYTOCHROME P450 ENZYMES INVOLVED IN THE METABOLISM OF ANTICONVULSANT MEDICATIONS

CYP	CBZ	CZP	DZP	ESM	FBM	MDZ	PB	PHT	TGB	VPA	ZNS
1A2	X										
2A6										X	
2B6			X[a]			X				X	
2C8	X		X					X			
2C9			X				X[a]	X[a]		X	
2C18								X			
2C19			X[a]				X	X		X	X
2E1					X		X				
3A4	X[a]	X	X[a]	X	X	X[a]		X	X		X[a]
3A5			X[a]			X		X			X
3A7						X		X			
4B1						X					

CBZ, carbamazepine; CYP, cytochrome P450; CZP, clonazepam; DZP, diazepam; ESM, ethosuximide; FBM, felbamate; MDZ, midazolam; PB, phenobarbital; PHT, phenytoin; TGB, tiagabine; VPA, valproic acid; ZNS, zonisamide.
[a]Major P450 enzyme involved in metabolism.
Data from Cloyd JC, Remmel RP. Antiepileptic drug pharmacokinetics and interactions: impact on treatment of epilepsy. *Pharmacotherapy.* 2000;20:139S–151S; Rendic S. Summary of information on human CYP enzymes: human P450 metabolism data. *Drug Metab Rev.* 2002;34:83–448; and Glauser TA. Advancing the medical management of epilepsy: disease modification and pharmacogenetics. *J Child Neurol.* 2002;17(suppl 1): S85–S93.

The hepatic microsomal CYP enzymes, the best-studied examples, are coded by a superfamily of CYP genes and play a key role in the metabolism of phenytoin, phenobarbital, carbamazepine, diazepam, ethosuximide, zonisamide, felbamate, and tiagabine (Table 49.1) (87,88). Not all AEDs are metabolized by this enzyme system. Some either do not undergo metabolism (gabapentin, levetiracetam) or are metabolized through alternative non-CYP pathways (lamotrigine by glucuronidation, valproic acid by β-oxidation and glucuronidation, and oxcarbazepine by aldoketoreductases).

Cytochrome P450 Genes

The CYP enzymes metabolize compounds by catalyzing the insertion of an oxygen atom from O_2 into an aromatic or aliphatic molecule to form a hydroxyl group. CYP enzymes are heme-thiolate proteins found in all living organisms (89). In mammals, for example, they are membrane bound and concentrated in the liver. The term *P450* comes from the observation that a broadband peak occurs at a wave length of 450 nm when a difference spectrum is plotted between reduced CYP treated with nitrogen and reduced CYP treated with carbon monoxide placed in the path of a double-beam spectrometer (90).

Sequence similarities have been used to devise a standardized nomenclature for categorizing the P450 proteins into families and subfamilies (89,91). P450 proteins are in the same family if they exhibit more than 40% similarity in protein sequence; within the same family, proteins that have more than 55% sequence homology are in the same subfamily (91). Families are given a unique Arabic number; subfamilies noted by a letter after the family number and individual genes in the subfamily are denoted by a second Arabic number after the subfamily letter, for example, CYP2C9 (7,89,91,92). The website http://www.imm.ki.se/cypalleles is the most informative source for data about CYP allelic variants.

CYP2C9, CYP2C19, and CYP3A4 are particularly important to AED interactions; CYP2C9 and CYP2C19 display noteworthy pharmacogenetic polymorphisms (93–95). The CYP2C subfamily accounts for approximately 18% of the hepatic CYP content in humans (96).

CYP2C9 and CYP2C19

CYP2C9 is the principal CYP2C isoenzyme in the human liver (97). The CYP2C9 gene, mapped to chromosome 10q24.2, encompasses 9 exons and codes for a protein of 490 amino acids (96,98). Of the 34 CYP2C9 alleles identified, CYP2C9*1, the most common, is considered the wild-type allele (96,98). Individuals homozygous for this allele are called extensive metabolizers. Multiple variant alleles have been associated with significant reductions in the metabolism of CYP2C9 substrates, compared with the wild-type allele (99–103). Individuals with at least one variant allele are called poor metabolizers.

Mapped to chromosome 10q24.1-q24.3, the CYP2C19 gene consists of 9 exons encoding a protein of 490 amino acids (93). There are 26 alleles, including the wild-type CYP2C19*1 (104). The first seven variants (CYP2C19*2 to CYP2C19*8) are inactive mutations responsible for the poor-metabolizer phenotype.

Most individuals in all populations studied have the CYP2C19 extensive-metabolizer phenotype involving the wild-type allele. CYP2C19 poor metabolizers are much more numerous among Asians (13% to 23%) than among whites and African Americans (1% to 6%) (93). The CYP2C19*2 and CYP2C19*3 mutations are responsible for the majority of CYP2C19 poor metabolizers. The main defective allele, CYP2C19*2 occurs in 30% of Chinese, approximately 15% of whites, and approximately 17% of African Americans. CYP2C19*3 affects approximately 5% of the Chinese and is almost nonexistent in Caucasians (105). Both alleles together can explain all Asian and approximately 80% of whites poor metabolizers (106).

CYP2C9/CYP2C19 and Phenytoin. Phenytoin's nonlinear metabolism accounts for its considerable interindividual pharmacokinetic variability. In humans, 4'-hydroxylation forms 5-(4'-hydroxyphenyl)-5-phenylhydantoin (4'-HPPH), which is responsible for approximately 80% of the drug's elimination. This reaction is mediated by CYP2C9 and to a lesser extent by CYP2C19 (107,108). Nonlinear pharmacokinetics, a narrow therapeutic index, and a concentration-related toxicity profile mean that small changes in CYP2C9 activity may be clinically significant for phenytoin. Studies in different populations have demonstrated that the CYP2C9*2, CYP2C9*3, CYP2C9*4, and CYP2C9*6 alleles are important in vivo determinants of the drug's disposition (100,101,109–115). Individuals with at least one of these variant alleles are poor metabolizers, exhibiting a reduced ability to metabolize phenytoin and requiring lower-than-average doses to decrease the incidence of concentration-dependent adverse effects (113,116).

Odani and coworkers (109) observed a decrease of approximately 30% in the maximal rate of phenytoin elimination in Japanese heterozygous for CYP2C9*3, compared with those homozygous for the wild-type allele. In another study (116), the mean maintenance dose of phenytoin leading to a therapeutic serum concentration was significantly lower in patients with CYP2C9 allelic variants (199 ± 42.5 mg/day) than in those with the wild type (314 ± 61.2 mg/day; $P < 0.01$). A case report (114) concerning a heterozygous CYP2C9*3 allele carrier described a toxic concentration of phenytoin (32.6 µg/mL) despite a modest dose (187.5 mg/day); the patient showed signs of central nervous system intoxication, ataxia, and diplopia. In an African American woman with signs of neurotoxic phenytoin reactions, clearance was 17% of that in normal patients. She was homozygous for the CYP2C9*6 null polymorphism and did not carry any other known CYP2C9 or CYP2C19 allelic variants.

The activity of the CYP2C9 enzyme alone does not fully explain the large interindividual variability in phenytoin's clinical pharmacokinetics and its reported drug interactions (117). Bajpai and coworkers (118) noted that the contribution of CYP2C19 to the metabolism of phenytoin increases with an increase in drug concentration, suggesting that CYP2C19 might be important when CYP2C9 is saturated. With reported differences in K_m (Michaelis constant) values for CYP2C9-catalyzed and CYP2C19-catalyzed phenytoin hydroxylation (5.5 µmol/L vs. 71.4 µmol/L), CYP2C9 is likely to become saturated at phenytoin "therapeutic concentrations" of 10 to 20 µg/mL (40 to 80 µmol/L) (117). This mechanism explains the increased risk of phenytoin toxic reactions with the coadministration of CYP2C19 inhibitors like ticlopidine or isoniazid. From 1% to 2% of whites are poor metabolizers for both CYP2C9 and CYP2C19, making them particularly susceptible to adverse effects of phenytoin (93).

A Japanese study (109) examining the effect of CYP2C19 polymorphisms on the pharmacokinetics of phenytoin noted an approximately 14% decrease in the maximum metabolic rate in patients with CYP2C19 variants compared with that in extensive metabolizers. In another Japanese study (110), predicted plasma concentrations with a phenytoin dose of 5 mg/kg/day were 18.7, 22.8, and 28.8 µg/mL in CYP2C19

homozygous extensive metabolizers, heterozygous extensive metabolizers, and poor metabolizers.

Following a single 300 mg dose of phenytoin, 96 healthy Turkish volunteers underwent genotyping and analyses of plasma levels of phenytoin and its metabolites (111). The ABCB1 C3435T polymorphism had no statistically significant effect on phenytoin plasma levels ($P = 0.064$). The ABCB1*TT genotype affected the metabolic ratio of p-HPPH versus phenytoin ($P = 0.026$), and the ABCB1*CC genotype was associated with low phenytoin levels ($P \leq 0.001$). On multiple regression analysis, the number of mutant CYP2C9 alleles explained 14.1% of the intrapatient variability in phenytoin plasma levels. The number of ABCB1*T alleles provided some additional explanation (1.3%), and CYP2C19*2 was not a contributory variable. Overall, the combination of CYP2C9 and ABCB1 genotyping accounted for 15.4% of the variability in phenytoin data ($r^2 = 0.154$, $P = 0.0002$). When the findings from the volunteers were applied to 35 patients with epilepsy being treated with phenytoin, the analysis of CYP2C9 and ABCB1 genotypes had "some predictive value not only in the controlled settings of a clinical trial, but also in the daily clinical practice." Conversely, Rosemary et al. did not find a significant difference between the various genotypes (119), but this study included only 27 patients of variable ethnic background.

Tate et al. (73) found a relationship between the CYP2C9*3 genotype and phenytoin dose. Carriers of one or two alleles required a 13% and 30% lower dose of phenytoin, respectively (73).

CYP2C9/CYP2C19 and Phenobarbital. Approximately 20% to 30% of a dose is metabolized to p-hydroxyphenobarbital by CYP2C9 and CYP2C19 (88,120–122). Attempts to clarify the metabolism of phenobarbital in two clinical studies from the same Japanese group reported inconsistent results (123,124). The first study (123) used a population pharmacokinetic approach to analyze the effect of CYP2C19 polymorphisms on 144 serum phenobarbital concentrations from 74 patients being treated with phenobarbital and phenytoin, but not valproic acid (123). All patients were genotyped for CYP2C19. Poor metabolizers (*2/*2 and *2/*3) had lower phenobarbital clearance values (18%; 95% CI, 10.6% to 27.0%) than heterozygous (*1/*2 and *1/*3) and homozygous (*1/*1) extensive metabolizers. One year later, this group administered phenobarbital 30 mg daily for 14 days to 10 healthy volunteers: 5 extensive metabolizers (*1/*1) and 5 poor metabolizers (*2/*2 and *3/*3) (125). Cosegregation of the p-hydroxylation pathway of phenobarbital with the CYP2C19 metabolic polymorphism was confirmed, as the formation clearance (29.8 vs. 21.1 mL/h) and urinary excretion (12.5% vs. 7.7%) of p-hydroxyphenobarbital were significantly lower ($P < 0.05$) in the poor metabolizers than in the extensive metabolizers of CYP2C19. In contrast to the early study, however, the kinetic parameters of phenobarbital did not differ significantly in extensive and poor metabolizers, suggesting that CYP2C19 is not the main enzyme in the drug's metabolism. The authors proposed that the discrepancy may have been related to the concomitant use of phenytoin in the first study, and an interaction of these two drugs with regard to the CYP2C polymorphisms could not be ruled out.

CYP2C19 and Benzodiazepines. At low concentrations, CYP2C19 is responsible for approximately 33% of the

N-demethylation of diazepam to desmethyldiazepam (nordiazepam) and 9% of the 3-hydroxylation of diazepam to temazepam (126). CYP2C19 polymorphisms influence the rate of N-demethylation in Caucasian and Asian populations (127–130). One study in Chinese participants (129) noted a gene dosage effect of CYP2C19 polymorphisms on the metabolism of diazepam and desmethyldiazepam (129). In a separate study of 21 healthy Chinese males (131), serial blood samples were obtained up to 24 days after a single 5-mg oral dose of diazepam. Plasma elimination half-lives of the drug and its metabolite were significantly longer (both $P < 0.05$) and the clearance of diazepam was significantly lower ($P < 0.05$) in the 4 poor metabolizers than in the 17 extensive metabolizers.

CYP3A4 and CYP3A5

CYP3A4 and CYP3A5 appear to metabolize many of the same drugs, and an exclusive substrate for either has yet to be identified. The most abundant form of CYP in the human liver, CYP3A isoenzymes account for approximately 30% of the total CYP protein (132) and metabolize about half of all prescribed drugs (133). The CYP3A locus is found on 7q22.1 and consists of four members; CYP3A4 and CYP3A5 are the main isoenzymes in the liver (132,134). Each CYP3A gene contains 13 exons and encodes a 503-amino acid protein (135).

Most of the 40 CYP3A4 variants consist of SNPs (104,136); large interethnic differences characterize the distribution of these alleles. CYP3A4*1B, which is not associated with altered catalytic activity, is present in 9% of whites and 53% of Africans and is absent in the Taiwanese population (137). CYP3A4*2 occurs in 2.7% of the Finnish population but is absent in whites from Middle and Western Europe, the Chinese, and blacks (138,139). In vitro, this variant showed a lower intrinsic clearance for nifedipine than the wild type but was not significantly different for testosterone 6β-hydroxylation. CYP3A4*3 was first identified in a single Chinese individual and later found in Dutch whites with a frequency of 2.2% (138,140). The allelic variants CYP3A4*4, CYP3A4*5, and CYP3A4*6 were found in the Chinese at a frequencies of 3%, 2%, and 1%, respectively (141). Measurement of the ratio of morning spot urinary 6β-hydroxycortisol to free cortisol in persons with these mutations suggests that these alleles may have a decreased activity compared with the wild type. The CYP3A4*7 through CYP3A4*13 allelic variants have been described in Middle and Western Europeans; CYP3A4*12 showed altered catalytic activity for testosterone and midazolam (139).

CYP3A4*14, CYP3A4*15, and CYP3A4*16 have been described in a study of nine different ethnic populations (136): CYP3A4*14 in a single person of unknown ancestry, CYP3A4*15 in 2% of African Americans, and CYP3A4*16 in 5% of Mexicans and Japanese. The CYP3A4*17 variant occurred in 27% of whites, whereas the CYP3A4*18 and CYP3A4*19 mutations were observed in Asians at allelic frequencies of 2% (142). In vitro assessments of the catalytic activity of CYP3A4 using testosterone and the insecticide chlorpyrifos demonstrated decreased activity for CYP3A4*17 and increased activity for CYP3A4*18. Overall, the heterozygous frequency of at least one nonsynonymous CYP3A4 mutant allele was 14% in whites, 10% in Japanese, and 15% in African Americans and Mexicans (136).

CYP3A5 is one of the two most important CYP3A proteins in the liver (143). Expression is variable, with reported rates in 10% to 29% of livers to at least trace presence in all liver samples, depending on the detection method used (144–147). CYP3A5 is more frequently expressed in hepatic samples of African Americans than in those from whites (60% versus 33%) (134).

Twenty-three variants of CYP3A5 have been described to date (104); however, only individuals with the wild-type CYP3A5*1 allele produce high levels of full-length CYP3A5 mRNA and express the CYP3A5 protein (134). CYP3A5*1 occurs at the following frequencies: 15% in whites and Japanese, 25% in Mexicans and Southeast Asians, 33% in Pacific Islanders, 35% in Chinese, 45% in African Americans, and 60% in Southwestern American Indians (134). The CYP3A5*2 variant was described in two of five whites with no CYP3A5 protein (148) but was not found in the Chinese or African American populations (143,149). The presence of CYP3A5*3 is the most common cause of the absence of the CYP3A5 isoenzyme, which results from alternate splicing and truncation of the protein (134). The frequency of this mutation varies from 27% in African Americans to 75% in Asians and 95% in whites (135,150). CYP3A5*4 and CYP3A5*5 were each found in 1.8% of Chinese persons (149). CYP3A5*6 was identified in 15% of African Americans and was associated with either normal or decreased enzyme activity (134). Ten percent of African Americans had the CYP3A5*7 mutation; correlation with enzymatic activity was unclear (143). The CYP3A5*8 variant occurs in African populations with a frequency of 4%. CYP3A5*9 is present in 2% of Asians, and CYP3A5*10 is found in 2% of whites (150). These three mutations exhibited decreased enzymatic activity for testosterone clearance and nifedipine oxidation, compared with the wild-type allele (150).

EPHX1

Human microsomal epoxide hydrolase (mEH), coded by the EPHX1 gene, is a major phase II enzyme involved in the detoxification of aromatic AED metabolites. This enzyme catalyzes the conversion of epoxides to less toxic trans-dihydrodiols that can subsequently be conjugated with glucuronic acid or glutathione and excreted. This detoxification is critical during the metabolism of phenytoin and phenobarbital (that both form arene oxide intermediates) and carbamazepine (that forms a 10,11-carbamazepine epoxide). mEH occurs abundantly in the liver, intestine, brain, kidney, lung, and adrenal gland, as well as in mononuclear leukocytes (151–153).

The EPHX1 gene is located on chromosome 1q42.1 and contains nine exons separated by eight introns (154). Two SNPs have been described in the gene's coding region. One SNP in exon 3, at amino acid position 113, changes tyrosine to histidine (His-113); the other SNP, in exon 4 at amino acid position 139, changes histidine residue to arginine (Arg-139) (154–156). Despite initial suggestions that these SNPs may alter enzyme function (155), research conducted with human liver microsomal preparations indicates "only modest impact on the enzyme's specific activity in vivo" (157).

UGT1 and UGT2

Glucuronidation by UDP-UGT enzymes is the major phase II reaction, which increases the polarity of target compounds by adding a glucuronic acid group to the substrate, thereby enhancing their excretion in bile or urine (158,159). UGT enzymes are membrane-bound proteins, located primarily in the liver but also found in other organs (160). The nomenclature, as recommended by Mackenzie and coworkers (161), comprises the root UGT followed by an Arabic number representing the family, followed by a letter designating the subfamily and another Arabic number denoting the individual gene.

In humans, more than 26 genes, or complementary DNAs (cDNAs), have been identified, 18 of which correspond to functional proteins. The UGT1 and UGT2 families exhibit 41% sequence homology and are further divided into three subfamilies: UGT1A, UGT2A, and UGT2B. Nine isoenzymes correspond to the UGT1 family (UGT1A1 and UGT1A3 through UGT1A10) and are encoded in a single gene locus, composed of 17 exons, on chromosome 2q37 (162). In contrast, the UGT2B subfamily members (UGT2B4, 7, 10, 11, 15, 17, and 28) are encoded by several independent genes, encompassing six exons, located on chromosome 4q13 (163). The two isoenzymes of the UGT2A subfamily (UGT2A1 and UGT2A2) also reside on chromosome 4q13 (163).

Some of the polymorphisms for UGT enzymes demonstrate altered enzymatic activity compared with the normal or wild-type allele. Of the UGT isoenzymes expressed in human liver, UGT1A1 has more than 60 identified mutations (159). UGT1A1*28, the most common mutation, is associated with Gilbert syndrome, a mild form of inherited unconjugated hyperbilirubinemia (164). It has a frequency of approximately 30% to 40% in whites, African Americans, and Hispanics, and up to 15% in Asians (159). Individuals with this polymorphism have an approximately 30% decrease in UGT1A1 protein expression and may exhibit altered lorazepam clearance compared with those with the wild-type allele (159,165). Six UGT1A3 allelic variants with different levels of enzyme activity have been identified in the Japanese population at frequencies of 5% to 12% (166). Four alleles, including the wild type, are known for UGT1A6. UGT1A6*2 has 27% to 75% lower activity toward different substrates compared with the wild type and has been recognized in 30% of American whites and 22% of Asian Americans (159,167). UGT2B15*2, an allelic variant of UGT2B15, has been identified in 50% to 55% of whites and 38% of African Americans; it exhibits increased catalytic activity for some substrates (159).

OCTN1

Gabapentin is cleared by renal filtration, and additionally by secretion of the organic cation transporter OCTN1. Genetic variation of OCTN1 (L503F) leads to lower renal clearance of gabapentin than in the wild type (168).

PHENOTYPICAL APPROACH TO AED ADVERSE EVENTS

Immune-Mediated Hypersensitivity

Immune-mediated hypersensitivity reactions against AEDs frequently present with cutaneous manifestations ranging from a mild rash to Stevens–Johnson syndrome. AED-related rash occurs in up to 10% of patients (11), and up to 1 in 10,000 develops severe cutaneous reactions (169). Aromatic anticonvulsants like carbamazepine, phenytoin, lamotrigine, and phenobarbital give rise to an array of severe idiosyncratic adverse events, including the anticonvulsant hypersensitivity syndrome (86,170,171). Prediction of cutaneous reaction based on predisposing genetic variants could assist in AED selection (169). Several studies have demonstrated an association between carbamazepine-induced Stevens–Johnson syndrome and HLA-B*1502 in subjects of Asian ethnicity (172–175). Ethnicity is important, as carbamazepine-induced Stevens–Johnson syndrome was not seen in Caucasians (174). These findings led to an FDA recommendation to test patients of Asian decent for the HLA-B*1502 allele prior to initiation of carbamazepine (176).

In lamotrigine-induced idiosyncratic drug reactions T-cell receptor polymorphisms may play a similar role, but no polymorphisms have been described to date (11). In phenytoin, an association between rash and a CYP2C9*3 polymorphism was described in a small subset of patients (177).

The effect of EPHX1 polymorphisms on the occurrence of carbamazepine-related severe adverse reactions has also been the focus of pharmacogenetic research. A series of in vitro experiments demonstrated that inherited deficiencies in mEH detoxification of arene oxides significantly increase a patient's susceptibility to severe idiosyncratic reaction from an aromatic AED (178–181). Subsequently, a single report (182) compared EPHX1 gene polymorphisms in 10 patients with carbamazepine hypersensitivity (including toxic epidermal necrolysis, Stevens–Johnson syndrome, and hepatitis) and 10 healthy volunteers. The gene's nine exons were screened, and new mutations were sequenced. The patients showed more frequent polymorphisms, but no consistent single polymorphism or pattern was detected. In an earlier similar study (183), no EPHX1 polymorphisms were noted in patients with adverse reactions to phenytoin, phenobarbital, or carbamazepine compared with a control group. These data suggest that a single EPHX1 polymorphism "cannot be the sole determinant of the predisposition to carbamazepine hypersensitivity" (182).

Vigabatrin-Associated Visual Field Defects

Visual field constriction occurs in up to 40% of patients taking Vigabatrin. No risk factors for visual field loss and no definite genetic predictors have been identified. A study investigating GABA transporters, GABA transaminase, and the rho subunit of the GABA$_c$ receptor at two centers only revealed weak effect sizes in the selected candidate genes (184). Effectiveness of vigabatrin in infantile spasms and recent FDA approval of vigabatrin in selected patients rekindled the need for pharmacokinetic risk assessment prior to treatment.

Hepatotoxicity

Liver damage due to valproate toxicity has been linked to CYP-metabolized valproic acid metabolites. It is unclear whether not yet described CYP2C9 polymorphisms may play a role (11). An association study also indicated a connection between GSTM1 and GSTT1 gene polymorphisms and γ-GT elevation, but a causal mechanism could not be shown (185). Among multidrug treatment and age under 2 years, mitochondrial disease is a known risk factor for valproic acid induced hepatotoxicity, and may be ruled out by mitochondrial genome screening and/or POLG1 testing in selected patients (169).

Teratogenicity

Neural tube defects in children after maternal valproic acid treatment may be related to genetic and environmental influences. Genetic influences are supported by occurrence of neural tube defects in siblings, even despite folate supplementation, and conception of a healthy child after valproic acid discontinuation in one of these mothers (186–190). Studies investigating polymorphisms in the folate metabolism, such as 5′-10′-methylenetetrafolatereductase (MTHFR) have been inconclusive regarding neural tube defects, possibly indicating a trend toward the MTHFR 677TT genotype as a risk factor (191,192). However, mothers with mutations in the MTHFR gene were more likely to have infants with fetal anticonvulsant syndrome (192).

Fetal hydantoin syndrome presented with low mEH on amniocentesis (193). mEH is encoded by the EPHX1 gene and plays an important role in eliminating oxidative metabolites. Results could not be reproduced using chorionic villi sampling due to local enzyme variability (194).

Hyperhomocysteinemia

Several studies suggested that hyperhomocysteinemia, a risk factor for stroke and cardiovascular disease, may be related to 677C > T and 1298A > C polymorphisms in the MTHFR gene in epilepsy patients (195,196). However, this could not be confirmed in children on AED monotherapy who were tested for the 677C > T polymorphism (197).

Other Future Research Directions

Among many others, cognitive and psychiatric side effects, bone health, and AED-induced weight change may be few of many additional adverse events that may be of interest for AED selection and future targets of pharmacogenetic research (169).

CONCLUSION

Despite their persistent use, high frequency of dose-dependent and long-term toxic reactions, and large pharmacokinetic and pharmacodynamic interindividual variability, AEDs, surprisingly, have not been the subject of intensive pharmacogenetic research. Understanding the genetic contribution to AED response is an opportunity to improve the drugs' efficacy, tolerability, safety, and, ultimately, the patient's quality of life.

Pharmacogenetic association studies traditionally have assessed the effect of one gene's polymorphic variation on the overall phenotype. In a few cases, the impact of allelic variations in one gene is large enough to alter a phenotype in an easily recognizable fashion (e.g., the relationship between HLA-B*1502 and related severe idiosyncratic drug reaction in patients of Asian and Chinese ethnicity). Generally, however, the genetic contribution to drug response is a summary of contributions from all factors that affect a drug's pharmacokinetic and pharmacodynamic profile and is best investi-

gated through a global pathway approach that simultaneously considers polymorphic variations in all relevant genes (see Fig. 49.3). Once the phenotype of drug response is defined, a multivariate analysis can identify which polymorphisms contribute most to the interindividual variation in AED therapy. In many phenotypic correlation studies, a single polymorphism may not be easily detectable because of possible interactions with other polymorphisms that may also influence the risk (198).

To date, pharmacogenetic research has emphasized unidirectional effects (i.e., the effect of genetic polymorphisms on response to a drug); however, the interaction is actually bidirectional. Yet to be examined is the role of potential molecular factors, such as a direct AED effect on the expression of receptors, transporters, and DMEs either alone or in combination with polymorphisms in the genes encoding them and possibly regulatory polymorphisms that affect gene expression and mRNA. Improvement in DNA microarray techniques and genomewide association studies now offer additional ways to simultaneously measure the expression levels of thousands of genes and expand research in directions previously not considered.

Our understanding of the genetic contribution to the interindividual variation in AED response will grow as more AEDs are studied and complementary methodologies are used both to generate new hypotheses and clarify systemic mechanisms underlying drug response. Additional research is needed into the cost-effectiveness of pharmacogenetic testing and the educational needs of clinicians who must incorporate these test results into actual practice. The FDA has already started to implement first recommendations. Additionally, pharmacogenetic and pharmacogenomic characterization of risk profiles and medical intractability may also offer additional treatment approaches, that is, as seen in P-polyglycan inhibitors that may reduce pharmacologic intractability (199).

References

1. Dodson WE. Pharmacokinetic principles of antiepileptic therapy in children. In: Dodson W, Pellock J, eds. *Pediatric Epilepsy: Diagnosis and Therapy*. New York: Demos; 1993:231–240.
2. Rowland M, Tozer T. *Clinical Pharmacokinetics: Concepts and Applications*. Philadelphia, PA: Lippincott, Williams & Wilkins; 1995.
3. Shargel L, Yu A. *Applied Biopharmaceutics and Pharmacokinetics*. New York: Appleton; 1999.
4. Dodson WE. Pharmacokinetic principles of antiepileptic therapy in children. In: Pellock JM, Dodson WE, Bourgeois BFD, eds. *Pediatric Epilepsy: Diagnosis and Therapy*. New York: Demos; 2001:317–327.
5. Eadie MJ. Pharmacokinetic principles of drug treatment. In: Shorvon S, Dreifuss F, Fish D, et al., eds. *The Treatment of Epilepsy*. London: Blackwell; 1996:138–151.
6. Kalow W. *Pharmacogenetics: Heredity and Response to Drugs*. Philadelphia, PA: WB Saunders; 1962.
7. Nebert DW. Pharmacogenetics and pharmacogenomics: why is this relevant to the clinical geneticist? *Clin Genet*. 1999;56(4):247–258.
8. Clancy CE, Kass RS. Pharmacogenomics in the treatment of epilepsy. *Pharmacogenomics*. 2003;4(6):747–751.
9. Vesell ES. Advances in pharmacogenetics and pharmacogenomics. *J Clin Pharmacol*. 2000;40(9):930–938.
10. Su TZ, Feng MR, Weber ML. Mediation of highly concentrative uptake of pregabalin by L-type amino acid transport in Chinese hamster ovary and Caco-2 cells. *J Pharmacol Exp Ther*. 2005;313(3):1406–1415.
11. Loscher W, Klotz U, Zimprich F, et al. The clinical impact of pharmacogenetics on the treatment of epilepsy. *Epilepsia*. 2009;50(1):1–23.
12. Loscher W, Potschka H. Role of multidrug transporters in pharmacoresistance to antiepileptic drugs. *J Pharmacol Exp Ther*. 2002;301(1):7–14.
13. Schinkel AH. P-Glycoprotein, a gatekeeper in the blood-brain barrier. *Adv Drug Deliv Rev*. 1999;36(2–3):179–194.
14. Ieiri I, Takane H, Otsubo K. The MDR1 (ABCB1) gene polymorphism and its clinical implications. *Clin Pharmacokinet*. 2004;43(9):553–576.

15. Callen DF, Baker E, Simmers RN, et al. Localization of the human multiple drug resistance gene, MDR1, to 7q21.1. *Hum Genet.* 1987;77(2): 142–144.

16. Gottesman MM, Hrycyna CA, Schoenlein PV, et al. Genetic analysis of the multidrug transporter. *Annu Rev Genet.* 1995;29:607–649.

17. Fromm MF. Importance of P-glycoprotein for drug disposition in humans. *Eur J Clin Invest.* 2003;33(suppl 2):6–9.

18. Loscher W, Potschka H. Drug resistance in brain diseases and the role of drug efflux transporters. *Nat Rev Neurosci.* 2005;6(8):591–602.

19. Loscher W, Potschka H. Role of drug efflux transporters in the brain for drug disposition and treatment of brain diseases. *Prog Neurobiol.* 2005; 76(1):22–76.

20. Lazarowski A, Czornyj L, Lubienieki F, et al. ABC transporters during epilepsy and mechanisms underlying multidrug resistance in refractory epilepsy. *Epilepsia.* 2007;48(suppl 5):140–149.

21. Lazarowski A, Massaro M, Schteinschnaider A, et al. Neuronal MDR-1 gene expression and persistent low levels of anticonvulsants in a child with refractory epilepsy. *Ther Drug Monit.* 2004;26(1):44–46.

22. Kwan P, Brodie MJ. Potential role of drug transporters in the pathogenesis of medically intractable epilepsy. *Epilepsia.* 2005;46(2):224–235.

23. Tishler DM, Weinberg KI, Hinton DR, et al. MDR1 gene expression in brain of patients with medically intractable epilepsy. *Epilepsia.* 1995;36(1): 1–6.

24. Cucullo L, Hossain M, Rapp E, et al. Development of a humanized in vitro blood-brain barrier model to screen for brain penetration of antiepileptic drugs. *Epilepsia.* 2007;48(3):505–516.

25. Brandt C, Bethmann K, Gastens AM, et al. The multidrug transporter hypothesis of drug resistance in epilepsy: proof-of-principle in a rat model of temporal lobe epilepsy. *Neurobiol Dis.* 2006;24(1):202–211.

26. van Vliet EA, van Schaik R, Edelbroek PM, et al. Region-specific overexpression of P-glycoprotein at the blood-brain barrier affects brain uptake of phenytoin in epileptic rats. *J Pharmacol Exp Ther.* 2007;322(1): 141–147.

27. Marchi N, Guiso G, Rizzi M, et al. A pilot study on brain-to-plasma partition of 10,11-dyhydro-10-hydroxy-5H-dibenzo(b,f)azepine-5-carboxamide and MDR1 brain expression in epilepsy patients not responding to oxcarbazepine. *Epilepsia.* 2005;46(10):1613–1619.

28. Simon C, Stieger B, Kullak-Ublick GA, et al. Intestinal expression of cytochrome P450 enzymes and ABC transporters and carbamazepine and phenytoin disposition. *Acta Neurol Scand.* 2007;115(4):232–242.

29. Siddiqui A, Kerb R, Weale ME, et al. Association of multidrug resistance in epilepsy with a polymorphism in the drug-transporter gene ABCB1. *N Engl J Med.* 2003;348(15):1442–1448.

30. Pedley TA, Hirano M. Is refractory epilepsy due to genetically determined resistance to antiepileptic drugs? *N Engl J Med.* 2003;348(15):1480–1482.

31. Zimprich F, Sunder-Plassmann R, Stogmann E, et al. Association of an ABCB1 gene haplotype with pharmacoresistance in temporal lobe epilepsy. *Neurology.* 2004;63(6):1087–1089.

32. Tan NC, Heron SE, Scheffer IE, et al. Failure to confirm association of a polymorphism in ABCB1 with multidrug-resistant epilepsy. *Neurology.* 2004;63(6):1090–1092.

33. Ebid AH, Ahmed MM, Mohammed SA. Therapeutic drug monitoring and clinical outcomes in epileptic Egyptian patients: a gene polymorphism perspective study. *Ther Drug Monit.* 2007;29(3):305–312.

34. Soranzo N, Cavalleri GL, Weale ME, et al. Identifying candidate causal variants responsible for altered activity of the ABCB1 multidrug resistance gene. *Genome Res.* 2004;14(7):1333–1344.

35. Hung CC, Tai JJ, Lin CJ, et al. Complex haplotypic effects of the ABCB1 gene on epilepsy treatment response. *Pharmacogenomics.* 2005;6(4): 411–417.

36. Hung CC, Jen TJ, Kao PJ, et al. Association of polymorphisms in NR1I2 and ABCB1 genes with epilepsy treatment responses. *Pharmacogenomics.* 2007;8(9):1151–1158.

37. Seo T, Ishitsu T, Ueda N, et al. ABCB1 polymorphisms influence the response to antiepileptic drugs in Japanese epilepsy patients. *Pharmacogenomics.* 2006;7(4):551–561.

38. Kwan P, Baum L, Wong V, et al. Association between ABCB1 C3435T polymorphism and drug-resistant epilepsy in Han Chinese. *Epilepsy Behav.* 2007;11(1):112–117.

39. Sills GJ, Mohanraj R, Butler E, et al. Lack of association between the C3435T polymorphism in the human multidrug resistance (MDR1) gene and response to antiepileptic drug treatment. *Epilepsia.* 2005;46(5): 643–647.

40. Kim DW, Kim M, Lee SK, et al. Lack of association between C3435T nucleotide MDR1 genetic polymorphism and multidrug-resistant epilepsy. *Seizure.* 2006;15(5):344–347.

41. Kim YO, Kim MK, Woo YJ, et al. Single nucleotide polymorphisms in the multidrug resistance 1 gene in Korean epileptics. *Seizure.* 2006;15(1): 67–72.

42. Leschziner G, Jorgensen AL, Andrew T, et al. Clinical factors and ABCB1 polymorphisms in prediction of antiepileptic drug response: a prospective cohort study. *Lancet Neurol.* 2006;5(8):668–676.

43. Ozgon GO, Bebek N, Gul G, et al. Association of MDR1 (C3435T) polymorphism and resistance to carbamazepine in epileptic patients from Turkey. *Eur Neurol.* 2008;59(1–2):67–70.

44. Shahwan A, Murphy K, Doherty C, et al. The controversial association of ABCB1 polymorphisms in refractory epilepsy: an analysis of multiple SNPs in an Irish population. *Epilepsy Res.* 2007;73(2):192–198.

45. Kimchi-Sarfaty C, Oh JM, Kim IW, et al. A "silent" polymorphism in the MDR1 gene changes substrate specificity. *Science.* 2007;315(5811): 525–528.

46. Komar AA. Silent SNPs: impact on gene function and phenotype. *Pharmacogenomics.* 2007;8(8):1075–1080.

47. Brunner M, Langer O, Sunder-Plassmann R, et al. Influence of functional haplotypes in the drug transporter gene ABCB1 on central nervous system drug distribution in humans. *Clin Pharmacol Ther.* 2005;78(2):182–190.

48. Takano A, Kusuhara H, Suhara T, et al. Evaluation of in vivo P-glycoprotein function at the blood-brain barrier among MDR1 gene polymorphisms by using 11C-verapamil. *J Nucl Med.* 2006;47(9):1427–1433.

49. Vogelgesang S, Cascorbi I, Schroeder E, et al. Deposition of Alzheimer's beta-amyloid is inversely correlated with P-glycoprotein expression in the brains of elderly non-demented humans. *Pharmacogenetics.* 2002;12(7): 535–541.

50. Vogelgesang S, Kunert-Keil C, Cascorbi I, et al. Expression of multidrug transporters in dysembryoplastic neuroepithelial tumors causing intractable epilepsy. *Clin Neuropathol.* 2004;23(5):223–231.

51. Basic S, Hajnsek S, Bozina N, et al. The influence of C3435T polymorphism of ABCB1 gene on penetration of phenobarbital across the blood–brain barrier in patients with generalized epilepsy. *Seizure.* 2008; 17(6):524–530.

52. Cole SP, Bhardwaj G, Gerlach JH, et al. Overexpression of a transporter gene in a multidrug-resistant human lung cancer cell line. *Science.* 1992; 258(5088):1650–1654.

53. Borst P, Evers R, Kool M, et al. A family of drug transporters: the multidrug resistance-associated proteins. *J Natl Cancer Inst.* 2000;92(16): 1295–1302.

54. Saito S, Iida A, Sekine A, et al. Identification of 779 genetic variations in eight genes encoding members of the ATP-binding cassette, subfamily C (ABCC/MRP/CFTR. *J Hum Genet.* 2002;47(4):147–171.

55. Miller DS, Nobmann SN, Gutmann H, et al. Xenobiotic transport across isolated brain microvessels studied by confocal microscopy. *Mol Pharmacol.* 2000;58(6):1357–1367.

56. Sisodiya SM, Lin WR, Harding BN, et al. Drug resistance in epilepsy: expression of drug resistance proteins in common causes of refractory epilepsy. *Brain.* 2002;125(Pt 1):22–31.

57. Kubota H, Ishihara H, Langmann T, et al. Distribution and functional activity of P-glycoprotein and multidrug resistance-associated proteins in human brain microvascular endothelial cells in hippocampal sclerosis. *Epilepsy Res.* 2006;68(3):213–228.

58. Lazarowski A, Sevlever G, Taratuto A, et al. Tuberous sclerosis associated with MDR1 gene expression and drug-resistant epilepsy. *Pediatr Neurol.* 1999;21(4):731–734.

59. Sisodiya SM, Thom M. Widespread upregulation of drug-resistance proteins in fatal human status epilepticus. *Epilepsia.* 2003;44(2):261–264.

60. Claes L, Del Favero J, Ceulemans B, et al. De novo mutations in the sodium-channel gene SCN1A cause severe myoclonic epilepsy of infancy. *Am J Hum Genet.* 2001;68(6):1327–1332.

61. Escayg A, Heils A, MacDonald BT, et al. A novel SCN1A mutation associated with generalized epilepsy with febrile seizures plus and prevalence of variants in patients with epilepsy. *Am J Hum Genet.* 2001;68(4):866–873.

62. Kamiya K, Kaneda M, Sugawara T, et al. A nonsense mutation of the sodium channel gene SCN2A in a patient with intractable epilepsy and mental decline. *J Neurosci.* 2004;24(11):2690–2698.

63. Sugawara T, Mazaki-Miyazaki E, Fukushima K, et al. Frequent mutations of SCN1A in severe myoclonic epilepsy in infancy. *Neurology.* 2002;58(7):1122–1124.

64. Wallace R. Mutations in GABA-receptor genes cause human epilepsy. *Lancet Neurol.* 2002;1(4):212.

65. Wallace RH, Scheffer IE, Parasivam G, et al. Generalized epilepsy with febrile seizures plus: mutation of the sodium channel subunit SCN1B. *Neurology.* 2002;58(9):1426–1429.

66. Sander T, Toliat MR, Heils A, et al. Failure to replicate an allelic association between an exon 8 polymorphism of the human alpha(1A) calcium channel gene and common syndromes of idiopathic generalized epilepsy. *Epilepsy Res.* 2002;49(2):173–177.

67. Feucht M, Fuchs K, Pichlbauer E, et al. Possible association between childhood absence epilepsy and the gene encoding GABRB3. *Biol Psychiatry.* 1999;46(7):997–1002.

68. Goldin AL, Barchi RL, Caldwell JH, et al. Nomenclature of voltage-gated sodium channels. *Neuron.* 2000;28(2):365–368.

69. Catterall WA. From ionic currents to molecular mechanisms: the structure and function of voltage-gated sodium channels. *Neuron.* 2000;26(1): 13–25.

70. Ragsdale DS, McPhee JC, Scheuer T, et al. Common molecular determinants of local anesthetic, antiarrhythmic, and anticonvulsant block of voltage-gated Na+ channels. *Proc Natl Acad Sci U S A.* 1996;93(17): 9270–9275.

71. Yarov-Yarovoy V, Brown J, Sharp EM, et al. Molecular determinants of voltage-dependent gating and binding of pore-blocking drugs in

transmembrane segment IIIS6 of the Na(+) channel alpha subunit. *J Biol Chem.* 2001;276(1):20–27.

72. Remy S, Gabriel S, Urban BW, et al. A novel mechanism underlying drug resistance in chronic epilepsy. *Ann Neurol.* 2003;53(4):469–479.
73. Tate SK, Depondt C, Sisodiya SM, et al. Genetic predictors of the maximum doses patients receive during clinical use of the anti-epileptic drugs carbamazepine and phenytoin. *Proc Natl Acad Sci U S A.* 2005;102(15):5507–5512.
74. Heinzen EL, Yoon W, Tate SK, et al. Nova2 interacts with a cis-acting polymorphism to influence the proportions of drug-responsive splice variants of SCN1A. *Am J Hum Genet.* 2007;80(5):876–883.
75. Tate SK, Singh R, Hung CC, et al. A common polymorphism in the SCN1A gene associates with phenytoin serum levels at maintenance dose. *Pharmacogenet Genomics.* 2006;16(10):721–726.
76. Zimprich F, Stogmann E, Bonelli S, et al. A functional polymorphism in the SCN1A gene is not associated with carbamazepine dosages in Austrian patients with epilepsy. *Epilepsia.* 2008;49(6):1108–1109.
77. Kwan P, Poon WS, Ng HK, et al. Multidrug resistance in epilepsy and polymorphisms in the voltage-gated sodium channel genes SCN1A, SCN2A, and SCN3A: correlation among phenotype, genotype, and mRNA expression. *Pharmacogenet Genomics.* 2008;18(11):989–998.
78. Heady TN, Gomora JC, Macdonald TL, et al. Molecular pharmacology of T-type Ca^{2+} channels. *Jpn J Pharmacol.* 2001;85(4):339–350.
79. Felix R. Channelopathies: ion channel defects linked to heritable clinical disorders. *J Med Genet.* 2000;37(10):729–740.
80. Sohal VS, Huguenard JR. It takes T to tango. *Neuron.* 2001;31(1):3–4.
81. Fuhr U. Induction of drug metabolising enzymes: pharmacokinetic and toxicological consequences in humans. *Clin Pharmacokinet.* 2000;38(6):493–504.
82. Goodwin B, Moore LB, Stoltz CM, et al. Regulation of the human CYP2B6 gene by the nuclear pregnane X receptor. *Mol Pharmacol.* 2001;60(3):427–431.
83. Quattrochi LC, Guzelian PS. Cyp3A regulation: from pharmacology to nuclear receptors. *Drug Metab Dispos.* 2001;29(5):615–622.
84. Sueyoshi T, Negishi M. Phenobarbital response elements of cytochrome P450 genes and nuclear receptors. *Annu Rev Pharmacol Toxicol.* 2001;41:123–143.
85. Pirmohamed M, Kitteringham NR, Park BK. The role of active metabolites in drug toxicity. *Drug Saf.* 1994;11(2):114–144.
86. Shapiro LE, Shear NH. Mechanisms of drug reactions: the metabolic track. *Semin Cutan Med Surg.* 1996;15(4):217–227.
87. Cloyd JC, Remmel RP. Antiepileptic drug pharmacokinetics and interactions: impact on treatment of epilepsy. *Pharmacotherapy.* 2000;20(8 Pt 2):139S–151S.
88. Rendic S. Summary of information on human CYP enzymes: human P450 metabolism data. *Drug Metab Rev.* 2002;34(1–2):83–448.
89. Omiecinski CJ, Remmel RP, Hosagrahara VP. Concise review of the cytochrome P450s and their roles in toxicology. *Toxicol Sci.* 1999;48(2):151–156.
90. Evans D. Genetic factors in drug therapy: clinical and molecular pharmacogenetics. In: Evans D, ed. *Cytochrome P450—General Features.* New York: Cambridge University Press; 1993:9–18.
91. Nelson DR, Koymans L, Kamataki T, et al. P450 superfamily: update on new sequences, gene mapping, accession numbers and nomenclature. *Pharmacogenetics.* 1996;6(1):1–42.
92. van der WJ, Steijns LS. Cytochrome P450 enzyme system: genetic polymorphisms and impact on clinical pharmacology. *Ann Clin Biochem.* 1999;36(Pt 6):722–729.
93. Desta Z, Zhao X, Shin JG, et al. Clinical significance of the cytochrome P450 2C19 genetic polymorphism. *Clin Pharmacokinet.* 2002;41(12):913–958.
94. Ingelman-Sundberg M. Pharmacogenetics of cytochrome P450 and its applications in drug therapy: the past, present and future. *Trends Pharmacol Sci.* 2004;25(4):193–200.
95. Gardiner SJ, Begg EJ. Pharmacogenetic testing for drug metabolizing enzymes: is it happening in practice? *Pharmacogenet Genomics.* 2005;15(5):365–369.
96. Lee CR, Goldstein JA, Pieper JA. Cytochrome P450 2C9 polymorphisms: a comprehensive review of the in-vitro and human data. *Pharmacogenetics.* 2002;12(3):251–263.
97. Goldstein JA, de Morais SM. Biochemistry and molecular biology of the human CYP2C subfamily. *Pharmacogenetics.* 1994;4(6):285–299.
98. Schwarz UI. Clinical relevance of genetic polymorphisms in the human CYP2C9 gene. *Eur J Clin Invest.* 2003;33(suppl 2):23–30.
99. Rettie AE, Wienkers LC, Gonzalez FJ, et al. Impaired (S)-warfarin metabolism catalysed by the R144C allelic variant of CYP2C9. *Pharmacogenetics.* 1994;4(1):39–42.
100. Kidd RS, Straughn AB, Meyer MC, et al. Pharmacokinetics of chlorpheniramine, phenytoin, glipizide and nifedipine in an individual homozygous for the CYP2C9*3 allele. *Pharmacogenetics.* 1999;9(1):71–80.
101. Ieiri I, Tainaka H, Morita T, et al. Catalytic activity of three variants (Ile, Leu, and Thr) at amino acid residue 359 in human CYP2C9 gene and simultaneous detection using single-strand conformation polymorphism analysis. *Ther Drug Monit.* 2000;22(3):237–244.
102. Dickmann LJ, Rettie AE, Kneller MB, et al. Identification and functional characterization of a new CYP2C9 variant (CYP2C9*5) expressed among African Americans. *Mol Pharmacol.* 2001;60(2):382–387.
103. Allabi AC, Gala JL, Horsmans Y. CYP2C9, CYP2C19, ABCB1 (MDR1) genetic polymorphisms and phenytoin metabolism in a Black Beninese population. *Pharmacogenet Genomics.* 2005;15(11):779–786.
104. Human Cytochrome P450 (CYP) Allele Nomenclature Committee, 2004. 10-30-2009. Internet Communication: http://www.cypalleles.ki.se/
105. Xie HG, Kim RB, Wood AJ, et al. Molecular basis of ethnic differences in drug disposition and response. *Annu Rev Pharmacol Toxicol.* 2001;41:815–850.
106. Wormhoudt LW, Commandeur JN, Vermeulen NP. Genetic polymorphisms of human N-acetyltransferase, cytochrome P450, glutathione-S-transferase, and epoxide hydrolase enzymes: relevance to xenobiotic metabolism and toxicity. *Crit Rev Toxicol.* 1999;29(1):59–124.
107. Dickinson RG, Hooper WD, Patterson M, et al. Extent of urinary excretion of p-hydroxyphenytoin in healthy subjects given phenytoin. *Ther Drug Monit.* 1985;7(3):283–289.
108. Yasumori T, Chen LS, Li QH, et al. Human CYP2C-mediated stereoselective phenytoin hydroxylation in Japanese: difference in chiral preference of CYP2C9 and CYP2C19. *Biochem Pharmacol.* 1999;57(11):1297–1303.
109. Odani A, Hashimoto Y, Otsuki Y, et al. Genetic polymorphism of the CYP2C subfamily and its effect on the pharmacokinetics of phenytoin in Japanese patients with epilepsy. *Clin Pharmacol Ther.* 1997;62(3):287–292.
110. Mamiya K, Ieiri I, Shimamoto J, et al. The effects of genetic polymorphisms of CYP2C9 and CYP2C19 on phenytoin metabolism in Japanese adult patients with epilepsy: studies in stereoselective hydroxylation and population pharmacokinetics. *Epilepsia.* 1998;39(12):1317–1323.
111. Aynacioglu AS, Brockmoller J, Bauer S, et al. Frequency of cytochrome P450 CYP2C9 variants in a Turkish population and functional relevance for phenytoin. *Br J Clin Pharmacol.* 1999;48(3):409–415.
112. Caraco Y, Muszkat M, Wood AJ. Phenytoin metabolic ratio: a putative marker of CYP2C9 activity in vivo. *Pharmacogenetics.* 2001;11(7):587–596.
113. van der WJ, Steijns LS, van Weelden MJ, et al. The effect of genetic polymorphism of cytochrome P450 CYP2C9 on phenytoin dose requirement. *Pharmacogenetics.* 2001;11(4):287–291.
114. Ninomiya H, Mamiya K, Matsuo S, et al. Genetic polymorphism of the CYP2C subfamily and excessive serum phenytoin concentration with central nervous system intoxication. *Ther Drug Monit.* 2000;22(2):230–232.
115. Brandolese R, Scordo MG, Spina E, et al. Severe phenytoin intoxication in a subject homozygous for CYP2C9*3. *Clin Pharmacol Ther.* 2001;70(4):391–394.
116. Goldstein JA. Clinical relevance of genetic polymorphisms in the human CYP2C subfamily. *Br J Clin Pharmacol.* 2001;52(4):349–355.
117. Levy RH. Cytochrome P450 isozymes and antiepileptic drug interactions. *Epilepsia.* 1995;36(suppl 5):S8–S13.
118. Bajpai M, Roskos LK, Shen DD, et al. Roles of cytochrome P4502C9 and cytochrome P4502C19 in the stereoselective metabolism of phenytoin to its major metabolite. *Drug Metab Dispos.* 1996;24(12):1401–1403.
119. Rosemary J, Surendiran A, Rajan S, et al. Influence of the CYP2C9 AND CYP2C19 polymorphisms on phenytoin hydroxylation in healthy individuals from south India. *Indian J Med Res.* 2006;123(5):665–670.
120. Whyte MP, Dekaban AS. Metabolic fate of phenobarbital. A quantitative study of p-hydroxyphenobarbital elimination in man. *Drug Metab Dispos.* 1977;5(1):63–70.
121. Gidal BE, Zupanc ML. Potential pharmacokinetic interaction between felbamate and phenobarbital. *Ann Pharmacother.* 1994;28(4):455–458.
122. Reidenberg P, Glue P, Banfield CR, et al. Effects of felbamate on the pharmacokinetics of phenobarbital. *Clin Pharmacol Ther.* 1995;58(3):279–287.
123. Mamiya K, Hadama A, Yukawa E, et al. CYP2C19 polymorphism effect on phenobarbitone. Pharmacokinetics in Japanese patients with epilepsy: analysis by population pharmacokinetics. *Eur J Clin Pharmacol.* 2000;55(11–12):821–825.
124. Hadama A, Ieiri I, Morita T, et al. P-hydroxylation of phenobarbital: relationship to (S)-mephenytoin hydroxylation (CYP2C19) polymorphism. *Ther Drug Monit.* 2001;23(2):115–118.
125. Bertilsson L, Henthorn TK, Sanz E, et al. Importance of genetic factors in the regulation of diazepam metabolism: relationship to S-mephenytoin, but not debrisoquin, hydroxylation phenotype. *Clin Pharmacol Ther.* 1989;45(4):348–355.
126. Jung F, Richardson TH, Raucy JL, et al. Diazepam metabolism by cDNA-expressed human 2C P450s: identification of P4502C18 and P4502C19 as low K(M) diazepam N-demethylases. *Drug Metab Dispos.* 1997;25(2):133–139.
127. Andersson T, Cederberg C, Edvardsson G, et al. Effect of omeprazole treatment on diazepam plasma levels in slow versus normal rapid metabolizers of omeprazole. *Clin Pharmacol Ther.* 1990;47(1):79–85.
128. Sohn DR, Kusaka M, Ishizaki T, et al. Incidence of S-mephenytoin hydroxylation deficiency in a Korean population and the interphenotypic differences in diazepam pharmacokinetics. *Clin Pharmacol Ther.* 1992;52(2):160–169.

129. Qin XP, Xie HG, Wang W, et al. Effect of the gene dosage of CgammaP2C19 on diazepam metabolism in Chinese subjects. *Clin Pharmacol Ther.* 1999;66(6):642–646.

130. Klotz U. The role of pharmacogenetics in the metabolism of antiepileptic drugs: pharmacokinetic and therapeutic implications. *Clin Pharmacokinet.* 2007;46(4):271–279.

131. Wan J, Xia H, He N, et al. The elimination of diazepam in Chinese subjects is dependent on the mephenytoin oxidation phenotype. *Br J Clin Pharmacol.* 1996;42(4):471–474.

132. Shimada T, Yamazaki H, Mimura M, et al. Interindividual variations in human liver cytochrome P-450 enzymes involved in the oxidation of drugs, carcinogens and toxic chemicals: studies with liver microsomes of 30 Japanese and 30 Caucasians. *J Pharmacol Exp Ther.* 1994;270(1): 414–423.

133. Wrighton SA, VandenBranden M, Ring BJ. The human drug metabolizing cytochromes P450. *J Pharmacokinet Biopharm.* 1996;24(5):461–473.

134. Kuehl P, Zhang J, Lin Y, et al. Sequence diversity in CYP3A promoters and characterization of the genetic basis of polymorphic CYP3A5 expression. *Nat Genet.* 2001;27(4):383–391.

135. Wojnowski L. Genetics of the variable expression of CYP3A in humans. *Ther Drug Monit.* 2004;26(2):192–199.

136. Lamba JK, Lin YS, Thummel K, et al. Common allelic variants of cytochrome P4503A4 and their prevalence in different populations. *Pharmacogenetics.* 2002;12(2):121–132.

137. Walker AH, Jaffe JM, Gunasegaram S, et al. Characterization of an allelic variant in the nifedipine-specific element of CYP3A4: ethnic distribution and implications for prostate cancer risk. Mutations in brief no. 191. Online. *Hum Mutat.* 1998;12(4):289.

138. Sata F, Sapone A, Elizondo G, et al. CYP3A4 allelic variants with amino acid substitutions in exons 7 and 12: evidence for an allelic variant with altered catalytic activity. *Clin Pharmacol Ther.* 2000;67(1):48–56.

139. Eiselt R, Domanski TL, Zibat A, et al. Identification and functional characterization of eight CYP3A4 protein variants. *Pharmacogenetics.* 2001;11(5):447–458.

140. van Schaik RH, de Wildt SN, Brosens R, et al. The CYP3A4*3 allele: is it really rare? *Clin Chem.* 2001;47(6):1104–1106.

141. Hsieh KP, Lin YY, Cheng CL, et al. Novel mutations of CYP3A4 in Chinese. *Drug Metab Dispos.* 2001;29(3):268–273.

142. Dai D, Tang J, Rose R, et al. Identification of variants of CYP3A4 and characterization of their abilities to metabolize testosterone and chlorpyrifos. *J Pharmacol Exp Ther.* 2001;299(3):825–831.

143. Hustert E, Haberl M, Burk O, et al. The genetic determinants of the CYP3A5 polymorphism. *Pharmacogenetics.* 2001;11(9):773–779.

144. Aoyama T, Yamano S, Waxman DJ, et al. Cytochrome P-450 hPCN3, a novel cytochrome P-450 IIIA gene product that is differentially expressed in adult human liver. cDNA and deduced amino acid sequence and distinct specificities of cDNA-expressed hPCN1 and hPCN3 for the metabolism of steroid hormones and cyclosporine. *J Biol Chem.* 1989;264(18): 10388–10395.

145. Wrighton SA, Brian WR, Sari MA, et al. Studies on the expression and metabolic capabilities of human liver cytochrome P450IIIA5 (HLp3). *Mol Pharmacol.* 1990;38(2):207–213.

146. Boobis AR, Edwards RJ, Adams DA, et al. Dissecting the function of cytochrome P450. *Br J Clin Pharmacol.* 1996;42(1):81–89.

147. Paulussen A, Lavrijsen K, Bohets H, et al. Two linked mutations in transcriptional regulatory elements of the CYP3A5 gene constitute the major genetic determinant of polymorphic activity in humans. *Pharmacogenetics.* 2000;10(5):415–424.

148. Jounaidi Y, Hyrailles V, Gervot L, et al. Detection of CYP3A5 allelic variant: a candidate for the polymorphic expression of the protein? *Biochem Biophys Res Commun.* 1996;221(2):466–470.

149. Chou FC, Tzeng SJ, Huang JD. Genetic polymorphism of cytochrome P450 3A5 in Chinese. *Drug Metab Dispos.* 2001;29(9):1205–1209.

150. Lee SJ, Usmani KA, Chanas B, et al. Genetic findings and functional studies of human CYP3A5 single nucleotide polymorphisms in different ethnic groups. *Pharmacogenetics.* 2003;13(8):461–472.

151. Farin FM, Omiecinski CJ. Regiospecific expression of cytochrome P-450s and microsomal epoxide hydrolase in human brain tissue. *J Toxicol Environ Health.* 1993;40(2–3):317–335.

152. de W, I, Cugnenc PH, Yang CS, et al. Cytochrome P 450 isoenzymes, epoxide hydrolase and glutathione transferases in rat and human hepatic and extrahepatic tissues. *J Pharmacol Exp Ther.* 1990;253(1):387–394.

153. Seidegard J, Ekstrom G. The role of human glutathione transferases and epoxide hydrolases in the metabolism of xenobiotics. *Environ Health Perspect.* 1997;105(suppl 4):791–799.

154. Hassett C, Robinson KB, Beck NB, et al. The human microsomal epoxide hydrolase gene (EPHX1): complete nucleotide sequence and structural characterization. *Genomics.* 1994;23(2):433–442.

155. Hassett C, Aicher L, Sidhu JS, et al. Human microsomal epoxide hydrolase: genetic polymorphism and functional expression in vitro of amino acid variants. *Hum Mol Genet.* 1994;3(3):421–428.

156. Hassett C, Lin J, Carty CL, et al. Human hepatic microsomal epoxide hydrolase: comparative analysis of polymorphic expression. *Arch Biochem Biophys.* 1997;337(2):275–283.

157. Omiecinski CJ, Hassett C, Hosagrahara V. Epoxide hydrolase—polymorphism and role in toxicology. *Toxicol Lett.* 2000;112–113:365–370.

158. Evans WE, Relling MV. Pharmacogenomics: translating functional genomics into rational therapeutics. *Science.* 1999;286(5439):487–491.

159. Guillemette C. Pharmacogenomics of human UDP-glucuronosyltransferase enzymes. *Pharmacogenomics J.* 2003;3(3):136–158.

160. Tukey RH, Strassburg CP. Human UDP-glucuronosyltransferases: metabolism, expression, and disease. *Annu Rev Pharmacol Toxicol.* 2000;40: 581–616.

161. Mackenzie PI, Miners JO, McKinnon RA. Polymorphisms in UDP glucuronosyltransferase genes: functional consequences and clinical relevance. *Clin Chem Lab Med.* 2000;38(9):889–892.

162. Gong QH, Cho JW, Huang T, et al. Thirteen UDPglucuronosyltransferase genes are encoded at the human UGT1 gene complex locus. *Pharmacogenetics.* 2001;11(4):357–368.

163. Wells PG, Mackenzie PI, Chowdhury JR, et al. Glucuronidation and the UDP-glucuronosyltransferases in health and disease. *Drug Metab Dispos.* 2004;32(3):281–290.

164. Monaghan G, Ryan M, Seddon R, et al. Genetic variation in bilirubin UPD-glucuronosyltransferase gene promoter and Gilbert's syndrome. *Lancet.* 1996;347(9001):578–581.

165. Herman RJ, Chaudhary A, Szakacs CB. Disposition of lorazepam in Gilbert's syndrome: effects of fasting, feeding, and enterohepatic circulation. *J Clin Pharmacol.* 1994;34(10):978–984.

166. Iwai M, Maruo Y, Ito M, et al. Six novel UDP-glucuronosyltransferase (UGT1A3) polymorphisms with varying activity. *J Hum Genet.* 2004; 49(3):123–128.

167. Ciotti M, Marrone A, Potter C, et al. Genetic polymorphism in the human UGT1A6 (planar phenol) UDP-glucuronosyltransferase: pharmacological implications. *Pharmacogenetics.* 1997;7(6):485–495.

168. Urban TJ, Brown C, Castro RA, et al. Effects of genetic variation in the novel organic cation transporter, OCTN1, on the renal clearance of gabapentin. *Clin Pharmacol Ther.* 2008;83(3):416–421.

169. Kasperaviciute D, Sisodiya SM. Epilepsy pharmacogenetics. *Pharmacogenomics.* 2009;10(5):817–836.

170. Dreifuss FE, Langer DH. Hepatic considerations in the use of antiepileptic drugs. *Epilepsia.* 1987;28(suppl 2):S23–S29.

171. Arif H, Buchsbaum R, Weintraub D, et al. Comparison and predictors of rash associated with 15 antiepileptic drugs. *Neurology.* 2007;68(20): 1701–1709.

172. Chung WH, Hung SI, Hong HS, et al. Medical genetics: a marker for Stevens–Johnson syndrome. *Nature.* 2004;428(6982):486.

173. Hung SI, Chung WH, Jee SH, et al. Genetic susceptibility to carbamazepine-induced cutaneous adverse drug reactions. *Pharmacogenet Genomics.* 2006;16(4):297–306.

174. Lonjou C, Thomas L, Borot N, et al. A marker for Stevens–Johnson syndrome. . .: ethnicity matters. *Pharmacogenomics J.* 2006;6(4):265–268.

175. Man CB, Kwan P, Baum L, et al. Association between HLA-B*1502 allele and antiepileptic drug-induced cutaneous reactions in Han Chinese. *Epilepsia.* 2007;48(5):1015–1018.

176. FDA Alert. 12-12-2007. Ref Type: Internet Communication: http://www.fda.gov/Drugs/DrugSafety/PostmarketDrugSafetyInformationforPatients andProviders/ucm107834.htm./

177. Lee AY, Kim MJ, Chey WY, et al. Genetic polymorphism of cytochrome P450 2C9 in diphenylhydantoin-induced cutaneous adverse drug reactions. *Eur J Clin Pharmacol.* 2004;60(3):155–159.

178. Spielberg SP. In vitro analysis of idiosyncratic drug reactions. *Clin Biochem.* 1986;19(2):142–144.

179. Park BK, Pirmohamed M, Kitteringham NR. Idiosyncratic drug reactions: a mechanistic evaluation of risk factors. *Br J Clin Pharmacol.* 1992;34(5): 377–395.

180. Spielberg SP. In vitro assessment of pharmacogenetic susceptibility to toxic drug metabolites in humans. *Fed Proc.* 1984;43(8):2308–2313.

181. Gibaldi M. Adverse drug effect-reactive metabolites and idiosyncratic drug reactions: part I. *Ann Pharmacother.* 1992;26(3):416–421.

182. Green VJ, Pirmohamed M, Kitteringham NR, et al. Genetic analysis of microsomal epoxide hydrolase in patients with carbamazepine hypersensitivity. *Biochem Pharmacol.* 1995;50(9):1353–1359.

183. Gaedigk A, Spielberg SP, Grant DM. Characterization of the microsomal epoxide hydrolase gene in patients with anticonvulsant adverse drug reactions. *Pharmacogenetics.* 1994;4(3):142–153.

184. Kinirons P, Cavalleri GL, Singh R, et al. A pharmacogenetic exploration of vigabatrin-induced visual field constriction. *Epilepsy Res.* 2006;70(2–3):144–152.

185. Fukushima Y, Seo T, Hashimoto N, et al. Glutathione-S-transferase (GST) M1 null genotype and combined GSTM1 and GSTT1 null genotypes are risk factors for increased serum gamma-glutamyltransferase in valproic acid-treated patients. *Clin Chim Acta.* 2008;389(1–2):98–102.

186. Kozma C. Valproic acid embryopathy: report of two siblings with further expansion of the phenotypic abnormalities and a review of the literature. *Am J Med Genet.* 2001;98(2):168–175.

187. Malm H, Kajantie E, Kivirikko S, et al. Valproate embryopathy in three sets of siblings: further proof of hereditary susceptibility. *Neurology.* 2002;59(4):630–633.

188. Omtzigt JG, Los FJ, Hagenaars AM, et al. Prenatal diagnosis of spina bifida aperta after first-trimester valproate exposure. *Prenat Diagn.* 1992;12(11):893–897.

189. Omtzigt JG, Los FJ, Grobbee DE, et al. The risk of spina bifida aperta after first-trimester exposure to valproate in a prenatal cohort. *Neurology.* 1992;42(4 suppl 5):119–125.

190. Duncan S, Mercho S, Lopes-Cendes I, et al. Repeated neural tube defects and valproate monotherapy suggest a pharmacogenetic abnormality. *Epilepsia.* 2001;42(6):750–753.

191. Kini U, Lee R, Jones A, et al. Influence of the MTHFR genotype on the rate of malformations following exposure to antiepileptic drugs in utero. *Eur J Med Genet.* 2007;50(6):411–420.

192. Dean J, Robertson Z, Reid V, et al. Fetal anticonvulsant syndromes and polymorphisms in MTHFR, MTR, and MTRR. *Am J Med Genet A.* 2007;143A(19):2303–2311.

193. Buehler BA, Delimont D, van Waes M, et al. Prenatal prediction of risk of the fetal hydantoin syndrome. *N Engl J Med.* 1990;322(22):1567–1572.

194. Buehler BA, Bick D, Delimont D. Prenatal prediction of risk of the fetal hydantoin syndrome. *N Engl J Med.* 1993;329(22):1660–1661.

195. Vilaseca MA, Monros E, Artuch R, et al. Anti-epileptic drug treatment in children: hyperhomocysteinaemia, B-vitamins and the 677C→T mutation of the methylenetetrahydrofolate reductase gene. *Eur J Paediatr Neurol.* 2000;4(6):269–277.

196. Belcastro V, Gaetano G, Italiano D, et al. Antiepileptic drugs and MTHFR polymorphisms influence hyper-homocysteincmia recurrence in epileptic patients. *Epilepsia.* 2007;48(10):1990–1994.

197. Vurucu S, Demirkaya E, Kul M, et al. Evaluation of the relationship between C677T variants of methylenetetrahydrofolate reductase gene and hyperhomocysteinemia in children receiving antiepileptic drug therapy. *Prog Neuropsychopharmacol Biol Psychiatry.* 2008;32(3):844–848.

198. Sankar R. Teratogenicity of antiepileptic drugs: role of drug metabolism and pharmacogenomics. *Acta Neurol Scand.* 2007;116(1):65–71.

199. Iannetti P, Spalice A, Parisi P. Calcium-channel blocker verapamil administration in prolonged and refractory status epilepticus. *Epilepsia.* 2005;46(6):967–969.

CHAPTER 50 ■ CARBAMAZEPINE AND OXCARBAZEPINE

CARLOS A. M. GUERREIRO AND MARILISA M. GUERREIRO

Carbamazepine (CBZ) is one of the most often prescribed drugs worldwide for the treatment of neurologic disorders. CBZ is considered an efficacious agent for the treatment of partial and secondarily generalized seizures in children and adults, with an excellent side-effect profile (1).

Oxcarbazepine (OXC), the 10-keto analogue of CBZ, has been used largely as an alternative for CBZ because of its more favorable pharmacologic and adverse-event profiles.

CHEMISTRY AND MECHANISM OF ACTION OF CARBAMAZEPINE AND OXCARBAZEPINE

CBZ is an iminodibenzyl derivative. Both CBZ and OXC are tricyclic anticonvulsant agents that are structurally similar to antidepressants. However, unlike the tricyclic antidepressants, CBZ and OXC are neutral substances because of their carbamoyl side chains (Fig. 50.1).

OXC as a prodrug is rapidly and completely metabolized to the monohydroxy derivative (MHD). CBZ and OXC (and also their active metabolites—CBZ epoxide and MHD) share many known actions of antiepileptic drugs (AEDs). They produce blockade of voltage-dependent ionic membrane conductance (especially sodium, potassium, and calcium), resulting in stabilization of hyperexcited neural membranes and synaptic actions of such neurotransmitters as γ-aminobutyric acid (GABA), glutamate, purine, monoamine, N-methyl-D-aspartate and acetylcholine receptors; the effect is diminution of propagation of synaptic impulses (2). There are subtle differences in the mechanisms of action of CBZ and OXC. For instance, MHD blocks N-type calcium channels, whereas CBZ blocks L-type (3).

CARBAMAZEPINE

Absorption and Distribution

CBZ is absorbed from the gastrointestinal tract slowly, with an estimated bioavailability of about 80% to 90%. The bioavailability of the agent is similar for all formulations—that is, tablets, solution, oral suspension, chewable tablets, and extended-release tablets/capsules. However, some studies have demonstrated the advantages in reducing serum level fluctuation with controlled-release forms of CBZ. Peak plasma concentration with chronic dosing is 3 to 4 hours. CBZ is a lipophilic compound that crosses the blood–brain barrier readily and is rapidly distributed to various organs, including fetal tissues and amniotic fluid as well as breast milk (4). Pharmacokinetic parameters are shown in Table 50.1 (5–7).

Metabolism

CBZ clearance is accomplished almost entirely via hepatic metabolism. The major pathways of CBZ biotransformation, consecutively or as parallel reactions, are the epoxide-diol pathway, aromatic hydroxylation, and conjugation. Metabolites from these major routes account for 80% to 90% of total

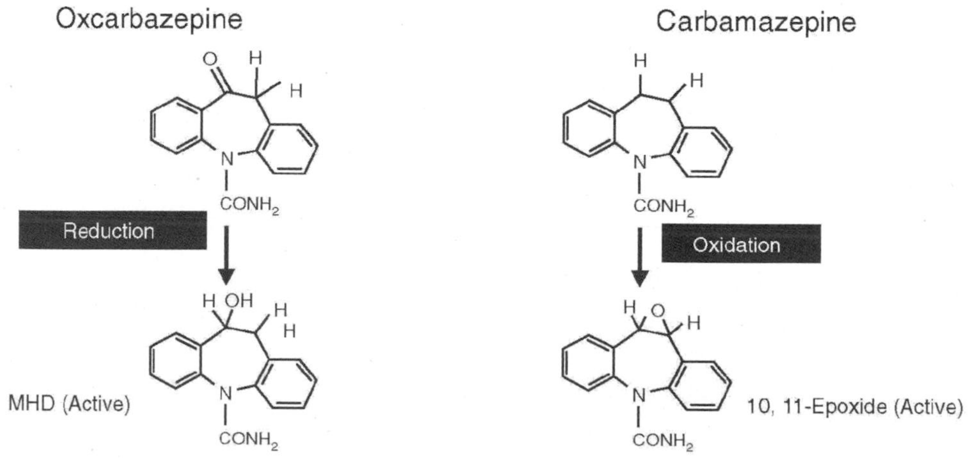

FIGURE 50.1 Chemical structure and main first-step metabolic pathways of oxcarbazepine and carbamazepine, and their active metabolites, MHD and CBZ-10,11-epoxide (CBZ-E).

TABLE 50.1

PHARMACOKINETIC PARAMETERS OF CBZ, OXC, AND MHD (5–7)

	F (%)	T_{max} (h)	V_d (L/kg)	Protein binding (%)	$t_{1/2}$ (h)	T_{ss} (d)	Therapeutic range (µg/L)	Dose (mg/kg/d)
CBZ	75–85	4–12	0.8–1.9	70–80	5–20	20–30	3–12	10–30
OXC	>95	1–2	—	—	2	—	—	10–50
MHD	—	3–5	0.75	40	8–15	2	8–20	—

CBZ, carbamazepine; OXC, oxcarbazepine; MHD, monohydroxy derivative; F, bioavailability; T_{max}, time interval between ingestion and maximum serum concentration; V_d, volume of distribution; protein binding, fraction to serum protein; $t_{1/2}$, elimination half-life; T_{ss}, steady state; therapeutic range, therapeutic range of serum concentration.

urinary radioactivity. The main metabolites found in urine are due 40% to oxidation of the 10,11 double bond of the azepine rings, 25% to hydroxylation of the six-membered aromatic rings, 15% to direct N-glucuronidation at the carbamoyl side chain, and 5% to substitution of the six-membered rings with sulfur-containing groups. CBZ is oxidized by the cytochrome P450 system (CYP3A4 and CYP2C8 isoforms) to CBZ-10,11-epoxide (CBZ-E), which is considered the most important product of CBZ metabolism (see Fig. 50.1). CBZ-E is an active metabolite that may contribute to rash and other side effects associated with CBZ use. CBZ induces the activity of CYP3A4, with the metabolic clearance of CBZ-E nearly doubled in induced patients (4).

CBZ leads to autoinduction, which increases clearance (double in monotherapy), shortens serum half-life, and decreases serum concentrations. This process takes approximately 2 to 6 weeks to occur (4).

CBZ-E is hydrolyzed primarily to trans-10,11-dihydroxy-10,11-dihydrocarbamazepine (trans-CBZ-diol). The diol is excreted in the urine and accounts for 35% of a CBZ dose. Another, somewhat less important metabolic pathway of CBZ is the hydroxylation at different positions of the six-membered aromatic rings. The third most important step in CBZ biotransformation is conjugation reactions. CBZ may be directly conjugated with glucuronic acid. Direct N-glucuronidation of CBZ and its metabolites depends on microsomal uridine diphosphate glucuronosyltransferase (UDPGT). Additionally, CBZ and its phenolic metabolites can be conjugated with sulfuric acid (4).

Drug Interactions

CBZ has a narrow therapeutic range, and plasma concentrations are often maximized to the upper limit of tolerance. As a low-clearance drug, CBZ is sensitive to enzyme induction or inhibition, especially by the large number of agents that induce or inhibit CYP3A4 isoenzymes. CBZ as well as its metabolites induce CYP3A4, CYP2C9, CYP2C19, and CYP1A2. As a result, the metabolism of other agents, including AEDs, is increased, which accounts for the decrease in blood levels (8).

The effectiveness of hormonal contraceptives, independent of preparation (oral, subcutaneous, intrauterine, implant, or injectable), can be reduced by CBZ administration. Oral contraceptives should contain ≥50 µg of estrogen. Midcycle spotting or bleeding is a sign that ovulation has not been suppressed (8). On the other hand, agents that interfere with the production of these isoenzymes can have a great effect on plasma levels of CBZ, leading to toxicity. Drugs that inhibit CYP3A4 increase plasma concentrations of CBZ. Polytherapy that associates CBZ with inducing and inhibiting other AEDs leads to unpredictable blood levels. Pharmacokinetic interactions among CBZ, OXC, and AEDs are shown in Table 50.2 (5,9).

Efficacy

The efficacy of CBZ in patients with epilepsy was first demonstrated in the early 1960s (10). The agent continues to be a first-line treatment for patients with focal-onset seizures.

Randomized, Monotherapy, Controlled Trials: CBZ versus Other Agents

Most studies have demonstrated no difference in efficacy between CBZ and phenytoin (PHT) as monotherapy for adults and children with epilepsy (10). No difference in efficacy was reported in trials comparing CBZ and phenobarbital (PB) in children. The second Veterans Administration (VA) Cooperative Study, a multicenter, randomized, double-blind,

TABLE 50.2

PHARMACOKINETIC INTERACTIONS AMONG CBZ, OXC, AND OTHER AEDs (5,9)

On levels of	Effects of the addition of						
	CBZ	PHT	PB	PRM	VPA	OXC	ZNS
CBZ	↓	↓	↓	↓	↑E	↑E	↑E
OXC	↓	↓	↓	↓			

CBZ, carbamazepine; OXC, oxcarbazepine; PHT, phenytoin; PB, phenobarbital; PRM, primidone; VPA, valproate; ZNS, zonisamide; E, CBZ epoxide.
Note: Ethosuximide, felbamate, lamotrigine, gabapentin, tiagabine, pregabalin, levetiracetam and vigabatrin addition do not affect level of OXC.

parallel-group trial, compared CBZ with valproate (VPA) for the treatment of 480 adults with complex partial ($n = 206$) or secondarily generalized ($n = 274$) seizures. The patient population comprised recently diagnosed, AED-naïve patients with epilepsy, as well as those who were being suboptimally treated. In patients with tonic–clonic seizures, there was no difference in efficacy between the two agents. However, CBZ appeared more efficacious than VPA for the treatment of patients with partial seizures, according to several outcome measures: number of seizures, seizure rate, seizure score, and time to first seizure [11]. Other studies did not reveal any significant differences between CBZ and VPA in adults or children [10].

Large Trials Comparing Several AEDs with CBZ

The first VA study was a double-blind, comparative study of monotherapy with PB, PHT, primidone (PRM), and CBZ in 622 adults with partial and secondarily generalized tonic–clonic seizures [12]. CBZ was found to be similarly as effective as PB, PHT, and PRM in controlling secondarily generalized tonic–clonic seizures. However, CBZ was more effective than barbiturates for the treatment of partial seizures, whether simple or complex. No difference was found between CBZ and PHT.

Other studies in the United Kingdom [10] did not demonstrate any difference between CBZ and PB, PHT, or VPA. However, the patients from the United Kingdom had been recently diagnosed with epilepsy, whereas half of the patients in the VA trials had been previously treated. Nevertheless, the large number of patients with complex partial seizures in the VA studies may provide the power to detect statistically significant differences. Because of the above-mentioned data, CBZ has been considered a first-line AED for the treatment of partial and secondarily generalized tonic–clonic seizures, and is used as an active control in trials of all new compounds.

A multicentric class I study of 593 elderly subjects with newly diagnosed seizures, comparing gabapentin (GBP), lamotrigine (LTG), and CBZ concluded that there were no significant differences in the seizure-free rate at 12 months, but the main limiting factor in patient retention was adverse drug reactions. Patients taking LTG or GBP did better than those taking CBZ. Seizure control was similar among the groups. Based on the findings, the authors proposed that LTG and GBP should be considered as initial therapy for older patients with newly diagnosed seizures [13].

CBZ has been tested against almost all new AEDs in monotherapy trials. The majority of these studies have shown no difference in efficacy between CBZ and LTG in adults, adolescents, and children, OXC [10], or topiramate (TPM) in children and adults [14]. CBZ was significantly more efficacious than vigabatrin (VGB) [15], remacemide [16], and probably GBP [17]. Some studies have suggested that GBP, LTG, VGB, and OXC are better tolerated than CBZ.

There are several methodologic limitations in many trials, with some satisfying regulatory agencies but not necessarily guaranteeing clinical use. Most studies are either undertaken with insufficient numbers of patients to demonstrate significant differences or the follow-up is relatively short, considering the seizure-free period, for a true improvement in quality of life to be realized.

A recent study comparing CBZ and levetiracetam did not show differences in the efficacy and effectiveness between these AEDs [18].

The available data suggest that CBZ is as effective as any of the other AEDs that have been investigated. More studies that assess the economic impact of epilepsy treatment are warranted to compare several therapies.

According to the evidence-based analysis of the AED efficacy and effectiveness as initial monotherapy for adults with partial-onset seizures, CBZ was considered a level A recommendation [19]. Based on the same guidelines, CBZ is not a level A, but a level C recommendation for elderly patients with partial-onset epilepsy.

Adverse Events

Accurate determination of adverse events has been a limitation in several AED trials. Systematic active questioning of patients has revealed a completely different picture of a spontaneously self-reporting adverse event. The perception of the adverse-event profile can influence a patient's current health status [20]. Although up to 50% of patients treated with CBZ experience adverse events, only 5% to 10% need to discontinue therapy [21,22].

Neurotoxicity

Most adverse events associated with CBZ use involve the central nervous system (CNS) and are mild, transient, and dose related; severe idiosyncratic reactions occur rarely. The most common adverse events are nausea, gastrointestinal discomfort, headache, dizziness, incoordination, vertigo, sedation, diplopia or blurred vision, nystagmus, tremor, and ataxia. Adverse events are similar in children and more common in elderly patients [21,22].

As with most AEDs, CBZ may cause several psychic disturbances, including asthenia, restlessness, insomnia, agitation, anxiety, and psychotic reactions. Neuropsychological adverse events associated with nontoxic, chronic CBZ use are generally minimal. Some investigators believe that the use of a sustained-release preparation may be advantageous in both children and adults [22].

Movement disorders, including dystonia, choreoathetosis, and tics, are associated with the use of CBZ, possibly with toxic plasma levels of the agent.

Hypersensitivity Reactions

The incidence of rash with CBZ use is approximately 10% [12,23]. CBZ causes the anticonvulsant hypersensitivity syndrome (AHS), characterized by fever, skin rash, and internal organ involvement [23,24]. AHS is associated with the aromatic AEDs—that is, PHT, PB, PRM, CBZ, and LTG. AHS begins within 2 to 8 weeks after AED therapy initiation; the reaction usually starts with low- or high-grade fever, and over the next 1 or 2 days a cutaneous reaction, lymphadenopathy, and pharyngitis may develop. Involvement of various internal organs may occur, resulting in hepatic, hematologic, renal, or pulmonary impairment. The most prominent manifestations are hepatitis, eosinophilia, blood dyscrasias, and nephritis. The most common cutaneous manifestation is an exanthema with or without pruritus. Rarely, severe skin reactions may occur, such as erythema multiforme, Stevens–Johnson syndrome, and toxic epidermal necrolysis [23]. It is important for the management of the patient to be aware of acute cross-reactivity, which may be as high as 70% to 80% among CBZ, PHT, and PB (22,24). VPA is considered a safe, acute alternative for the treatment of patients with AHS. Systemic corticosteroids are usually required for full recovery (24).

Systemic lupus erythematosus may be induced by CBZ. Symptoms generally appear 6 to 12 months after initiation of therapy. Discontinuation of CBZ usually leads to disappearance of the symptoms. Hair loss associated with CBZ use has been reported. Myocarditis has been described as a manifestation of CBZ hypersensitivity (22).

Hematologic Effects

Transient leukopenia occurs within the first 3 months of treatment in 10% to 20% of patients taking CBZ. Persistent leukopenia, which is seen in 2% of patients, reverses with discontinuation of CBZ treatment (22). In the VA study, only one patient had a transient, clinically significant neutropenia (<1000 cells/mm^3) associated with CBZ use, and the treatment was not discontinued (22). Isolated thrombocytopenia associated with CBZ treatment has been described at a rate of 0.9 per 100,000. The risk for aplastic anemia in the general population is about 2 to 2.5 per million. Aplastic anemia occurs with CBZ exposure in 5.1 per million (1/200,000) (21,25).

Endocrinologic Effects

Hyponatremia is an adverse event provoked by CBZ treatment. The risk for hyponatremia increases in proportion to the dose CBZ and age of the patient; it is unusual in children (22).

Although thyroid function tests may be abnormal due to CBZ use, treated patients remain clinically euthyroid. Because of the induction effect of CBZ on the metabolism of thyroid hormones, hypothyroid patients may require higher doses of T$_4$ to maintain euthyroid states (22).

The effect of CBZ on metabolism of testosterone, pituitary responsiveness to gonadotrophin-releasing hormones, prolactin, follicle-stimulating hormone, and luteinizing hormone have been studied, although the clinical relevance of the findings has not been thoroughly elucidated (22,26).

Teratogenic Effects

As with other established AEDs, CBZ exhibits teratogenic effects. CBZ exposure has also been associated with neural tube defects (27) and major congenital malformations in monotherapy: 2.2 to 4.0 (28). Polytherapy with two or more agents significantly elevates the teratogenic risk. Despite uncertainty about the efficacy of periconceptual folate supplementation in women with epilepsy, most authors recommend its use at the same dosage as that recommended for the general population: 0.4 to 0.6 mg/day. Women taking CBZ should have prenatal diagnostic ultrasonography to detect any congenital malformations (27). The overall risk for CBZ causing major congenital malformation appears relatively low. Breast-feeding is considered safe for women being treated with CBZ.

Miscellaneous Adverse Events

Weight gain is a common side effect associated with the use of AEDs, including CBZ, although it is not as pronounced as with VPA use (22).

Hepatic enzymes may be elevated in patients receiving CBZ treatment—mostly mild elevations with no clinical significance. Rarely, CBZ hepatotoxicity can be a serious adverse event that leads to death. Cases in pediatric patients are probably less common than in adults (21). Cardiac arrhythmias have also been associated with CBZ use (22).

Over the past several years, bone health impairment and increased risk of fractures have been associated with epilepsy and AEDs, including CBZ, both in children and in adults. Many authors recommend vitamin D and calcium supplementation. Nevertheless, there is no evidence-based guidance about the efficacy of dietary supplements or the appropriate amount to be used (29,30).

Clinical Use

CBZ is one of the agents of choice for the treatment of cryptogenic and symptomatic localization-related epilepsies, as well as for generalized tonic–clonic seizures. Doses must be adjusted individually because of great variability in different epileptic syndromes and intra- and interindividual responses. When clinical condition permits, CBZ treatment should be initiated with 100 to 200 mg/day in adults and children >12 years of age (>40 kg). Increments up to an initial target dose of 600 to 800 mg (10 mg/kg) in adults (60 to 80 kg) (10,11) and changes at weekly intervals is preferred, whenever possible. Risk for AHS or rash is higher with rapid titration. Newly diagnosed patients usually require lower doses (mean dose, 7.5 mg/kg) than those with chronic epilepsy (mean dose, 10.3 mg/kg). The mean effective dose in children is probably 20 mg/kg in those <5 years of age and 10 mg/kg in those >5 years of age. If seizures cannot be controlled, doses should be gradually increased by 100- or 200-mg increments until either control is achieved or unacceptable adverse events appear. Control doses range from 600 to >1600 mg in adults and 10 to >40 mg/kg/day in children. It is not possible to define any absolute therapeutic range for CBZ. Although plasma level monitoring is a useful tool for the clinician, it has no definite value. It is necessary to push the CBZ dose to the maximum clinically tolerated dose, independent of plasma level, in uncontrolled patients. Plasma level monitoring may be useful in patients receiving polytherapy, with usual concentrations in the range of 4 to 12 mg/L (10).

The dosage interval depends both on the severity of the epilepsy and on the difficulty with control. Most responsive patients, such as those newly diagnosed, need modest doses twice daily. If higher doses are necessary, however, toxicity may be avoided by taking CBZ three times per day. Two or three times per day provides similar levels, with fluctuations of 57% ± 20% and 56% ± 29%, respectively. In children, the interdose variation was 21% for patients receiving CBZ sustained-release and 41% for those treated with standard CBZ preparation. Children metabolize CBZ faster than do adults and thus may need higher doses. Elderly patients retain their sensitivity to dose-dependent autoinduction and heteroinduction by CBZ, but their metabolism rates remain considerably lower than those observed in matched controls. As a result, elderly individuals will require a lower dosage to achieve serum concentrations comparable to those found in nonelderly adults (10). In patients receiving doses that approximate the maximal tolerated doses, the use of sustained-release formulations of

CBZ twice daily minimizes dose fluctuations and may help to adequately control seizures (31).

Precautions and Contraindications

CBZ should not be used in patients with a known hypersensitivity to any tricyclic antidepressant or to OXC. Use of CBZ can worsen some epileptic conditions by aggravating preexisting seizures or by leading to new seizure types, particularly absence and myoclonic seizures. An increase in the number of generalized seizures has been documented in children (10).

Serious allergic cutaneous reactions caused by CBZ therapy are significantly more common in patients with a particular human leukocyte antigen (HLA) allele: HLA-B* 1502. This allele occurs almost exclusively in patients with Asian ancestry. A recent FDA alert recommends that patients with ancestry of an at-risk population be screened for the HLA-B* 1502 allele prior to starting CBZ and that positive patients not be exposed to it (32).

OXCARBAZEPINE

Absorption, Distribution, and Metabolism

Orally administered OXC is rapidly and almost completely absorbed, with absorption being largely unaffected by food. As discussed earlier, the pharmacologic effect of OXC in humans is exerted predominantly through its main metabolite, MHD (monohydroxy derivative), which accounts for its unique pharmacokinetic and pharmacodynamic profile (33,34) (see Fig. 50.1). OXC undergoes rapid and extensive metabolism to MHD. The half-life of OXC is 1 to 3.7 hours and the half-life of MHD is 8 to 10 hours. As a lipophilic compound, MHD is widely distributed throughout the body and easily crosses the blood–brain barrier (35). The plasma protein binding of MHD is approximately 40%, which is less than that of CBZ (70% to 90%). Steady state is achieved after three to four doses. At steady state, the pharmacokinetics of OXC is linear over the dose range of 300 to 2400 mg/day (7). After oral administration of ^{14}C-labeled MHD, most of the dose is excreted in the urine within 6 days after dosing, <1% as unchanged drug (34). As with most AEDs, placental transfer of OXC appears to occur.

Drug Interactions

OXC exhibits no enzyme autoinduction and has a limited potential for heteroinduction. Induction of the cytochrome P450 system is much less pronounced with OXC than with CBZ (34). Therefore, polytherapy is much simpler with OXC. Levels of the MHD are not significantly modified by CBZ, felbamate, LTG, PB, PHT, or VPA (36).

Whereas CBZ induces many cytochrome P450 isoenzymes (CYP1A2, CYP2C9, CYP2C19, and CYP3A4), OXC is a weak inhibitor of CYP2C19 and a weak inducer of CYP3A4. Since CYP2C19 is involved in PHT metabolism, OXC may increase plasma levels of PHT. As the CYP3A subfamily is responsible for the metabolism of estrogens, oral contraceptive levels may be lower in patients receiving OXC therapy

(36). The same precautions used with CBZ therapy apply to OXC therapy, relative to coadministration with hormonal contraceptives.

Efficacy

Monotherapy

Most studies found OXC to be efficacious as monotherapy for patients with partial and generalized tonic–clonic seizures. OXC has a similar efficacy to CBZ, but with a more favorable tolerability profile (37).

In two large, similarly designed trials of previously untreated patients with recently diagnosed epilepsy, OXC was as effective as PHT (38) and VPA (39). A total of 287 adult patients with either partial or generalized tonic–clonic seizures, were randomized in a double-blind, parallel-group comparison of OXC and PHT (38). In the efficacy analyses, no statistically significant differences were found between the treatment groups. Seventy patients (59.3%) in the OXC group and 69 (58%) in the PHT group were seizure-free during the 48-week maintenance period (35). In the comparison of OXC and VPA (39), 249 adult patients with either partial or generalized seizures were randomized. As with OXC and PHT, no statistically significant differences were found between the treatment groups in the efficacy analyses. Sixty patients (56.6%) in the OXC group and 57 (53.8%) in the VPA group were seizure-free during the 48 weeks of maintenance treatment (39).

A multicenter, double-blind, randomized, parallel-group trial compared the efficacy of two different doses of OXC as monotherapy in a refractory epilepsy patient population. In the intent-to-treat analysis, 12% of patients in the higher-dose (2400 mg/day) OXC group were seizure-free, compared with 0% in the lower-dose (300 mg/day) OXC group (40).

A multicenter, double-blind, randomized, parallel-group, dose-controlled monotherapy trial compared OXC 2400 mg/day with OXC 300 mg/day in patients with uncontrolled partial-onset seizures previously receiving CBZ monotherapy. The trial demonstrated that OXC 2400 mg/day is efficacious when administered as monotherapy in patients with uncontrolled partial-onset seizures (41).

In another monotherapy trial, OXC was compared with placebo in a double-blind, randomized, two-arm, parallel-group design in hospitalized patients with refractory partial and secondarily generalized seizures. Both primary and secondary efficacy variables showed a statistically significant effect in favor of OXC (42).

A double-blind, controlled clinical trial of OXC versus PHT in children and adolescents with newly diagnosed epilepsy showed that OXC was comparable to PHT in terms of efficacy, but had significant advantages over PHT in terms of tolerability and treatment retention (43). A total of 193 patients 5 to 18 years of age with either partial or generalized tonic–clonic seizures were enrolled. In the efficacy analyses, no statistically significant differences were found between the treatment groups. Forty-nine patients (61%) in the OXC group and 46 (60%) in the PHT group were seizure-free during the 48-week maintenance period (43).

A long-term extension phase of two multicenter, randomized, double-blind, controlled trials (38,43) showed that the estimated seizure-free rate after 52 weeks on open follow-up was 67.2% with OXC and 62.2% with PHT. This 2-year study revealed that the majority of patients were seizure-free, suggesting an improvement in seizure control during the second year of OXC monotherapy.

Adjunctive Therapy

Several adjunctive studies have shown that patients treated with OXC experienced a significantly greater reduction in partial seizure frequency than those treated with placebo (7).

Adverse Events

Monotherapy

The main adverse events associated with OXC treatment are CNS-related effects, gastrointestinal symptoms, and idiosyncratic reactions (37–40,42–44). The most common adverse events are somnolence, headache, dizziness, diplopia, fatigue, nausea, vomiting, ataxia, abnormal vision, abdominal pain, tremor, dyspepsia, abnormal gait, and rash.

When OXC was compared with placebo (42), most adverse events with OXC were mild or moderate in intensity and similar to those with placebo. Adverse events reported at some time during the trial by ≥5% of all treated patients were headache, nausea, dizziness, pruritus, somnolence, diplopia, vomiting, fatigue, constipation, dyspepsia, and insomnia. Each of these adverse events occurred with greater frequency in the OXC treatment group. Three patients in the OXC group discontinued treatment prematurely—one for a transient rash, one for postictal psychosis, and one for an administrative reason. Two patients discontinued prematurely from the placebo group, both for administrative reasons.

The trial that compared OXC with PHT (38) showed that the number of premature discontinuations due to adverse experiences with OXC was significantly lower than that with PHT. Five of 143 patients in the OXC group discontinued treatment because of tolerability reasons—rash in one case, pregnancy in one case, an astrocytoma not previously diagnosed in one case, a suicide attempt with OXC intoxication in one case, and gastrointestinal discomfort combined with depression/anxiety in one case. Sixteen of 144 patients in the PHT group discontinued treatment because of tolerability reasons—rash in 10 cases, hirsutism/gum hypertrophy in 5 cases, and cerebellar symptoms/sedation in the last case. Somnolence, headache, dizziness, nausea, and rash occurred in ≥10% of the patients in both groups. Gum hyperplasia, tremor, diplopia, acne, nervousness, and nystagmus occurred in <10% of the patients in both groups (38). When differences in the incidence of adverse events were apparent between the groups, these were nearly all in favor of OXC therapy.

The comparison of OXC and VPA in 249 adults revealed no statistically significant difference between treatment groups with respect to the total number of premature discontinuations or those due to adverse events. The most frequent reason for withdrawal due to adverse events in the OXC group was allergic reaction with skin symptoms (six patients); in the VPA group, it was hair loss (four patients). The most common adverse events considered to have a causal relationship to the trial treatment were somnolence, weight increase, fatigue, headache, alopecia, dizziness, nausea, tremor, abdominal pain, impaired concentration, increased appetite, and diarrhea. When differences in incidence existed between the groups, these generally favored OXC treatment. Abnormally low plasma sodium levels were reported in two OXC-treated patients. Both patients were asymptomatic with respect to their low plasma sodium levels, and neither discontinued treatment prematurely (39).

The study that compared two different doses of OXC (2400 mg/day vs. 300 mg/day) concluded that OXC was well tolerated, with fatigue, dizziness, somnolence, nausea, ataxia, and headache the most common adverse events (41). Most of the adverse events were transient and rated as mild to moderate in intensity (40).

The trial that compared the efficacy and safety of OXC with that of PHT in 193 children and adolescents (43) found that 2 patients in the OXC group and 14 patients in the PHT group discontinued treatment prematurely for tolerability reasons. The number of premature discontinuations due to adverse events was statistically significantly lower in the OXC group than in the PHT group. Moreover, the odds of an individual discontinuing prematurely were almost twice as high in the PHT group. Based on the findings of this trial, the authors concluded that OXC has significant advantages over PHT in terms of tolerability and treatment retention.

OXC therapy in elderly patients (≥65 years of age) seems as safe as treatment in younger adults. The four most common adverse events experienced by elderly patients were vomiting (19%), dizziness (17%), nausea (17%), and somnolence (15%). Three of 52 patients developed an asymptomatic hyponatremia, with at least one patient's serum sodium level <125 mEq/L (44).

Adjunctive Therapy

The study that evaluated the safety of a broad OXC dosage as adjunctive therapy in patients with uncontrolled partial seizures (44) found that the most common adverse events were related to the nervous and digestive systems. Rapid and fixed titration to high doses was associated with an increased risk for adverse events, which could potentially be reduced by adjusting concomitant AEDs and using a slower, flexible OXC titration schedule.

The trial that compared the safety of OXC with placebo as adjunctive therapy in children with inadequately controlled partial seizures (44) found that 91% of the OXC group and 82% of the placebo group reported at least one adverse event. Vomiting, somnolence, dizziness, and nausea occurred more frequently in the OXC-treated group. The majority of these adverse events were mild to moderate in severity. The incidence of rash was 4% in the OXC group and 5% in the placebo group. Fourteen patients (10%) in the OXC group and four patients (3%) in the placebo group discontinued treatment prematurely because of adverse events. The most common reasons for discontinuation in the OXC group were adverse events involving the digestive system (primarily nausea and vomiting), which occurred in five patients, and rash (maculopapular and erythematous), which occurred in four patients.

Hyponatremia

Hyponatremia is usually defined as a serum sodium level <135 mEq/L. Clinically significant hyponatremia (sodium level <125 mEq/L) has been observed in 2.5% of OXC-treated patients in 14 controlled trials (7). Acute symptoms of hyponatremia include headache, nausea, vomiting, tremors, delirium, seizures, and decerebrate posturing, whereas chronic symptoms include anorexia, cramps, personality changes, gait disturbance, stupor, nausea, and vomiting (7). The 14 trials that evaluated 1966 patients showed that hyponatremia increased with age, from 0% at <6 years and 0.5% at <18 years to 3.4% between 18 and 64 years and 7.3% at >65 years (7,44,45). OXC-induced hyponatremia has not been attributable to the syndrome of inappropriate secretion of antidiuretic hormone. Possible mechanisms include a direct effect of OXC on the renal collecting tubules or an enhancement of their responsiveness to circulating antidiuretic hormone. Although hyponatremia has been reported, it is only rarely accompanied by clinical symptomatology and rarely leads to OXC discontinuation. The degree of hyponatremia seems to be related to the dose of OXC. Rapid titration may be another risk factor (45).

Other Potential Adverse Events

An analysis of 29 trials involving 2191 patients treated with OXC for up to 11.5 months showed no clinically significant weight changes in the OXC group compared with the placebo group (46). However, the authors have seen patients with weight gain that reversed with OXC substitution. This information is also described in very few other clinical trials (7).

OXC in monotherapy or combination therapy has no effect on blood pressure and electrocardiograms (7).

The teratogenic potential of OXC is unknown (27). Major malformations in offspring of mothers with epilepsy are associated with the use of AEDs, including OXC, during early pregnancy (47).

OXC does not appear to affect cognitive function in healthy volunteers or adults with newly diagnosed epilepsy. The cognitive effects of the agent in children and adolescents have not been systematically studied (48).

OXC, like CBZ, has been reported to aggravate some seizures in children (49). Clinical and EEG monitoring may be important, especially in patients who do not show adequate response to OXC.

Clinical Use

OXC is indicated for use as monotherapy or adjunctive therapy in the treatment of partial seizures, with or without secondary generalized seizures, and primary generalized tonic–clonic seizures in adults and children with epilepsy. OXC is available as 150-mg, 300-mg, and 600-mg film-coated tablets for oral administration. OXC is also available as a 300-mg/5 mL (60 mg/mL) oral suspension (7). It can be taken with or without food.

In adults, treatment with OXC monotherapy should be initiated at a dose of 300 to 600 mg/day. Increases at weekly intervals are advisable and titration should be planned according to the clinical condition of the patient, since slow and gradual initiation of therapy minimizes side effects. In the case of frequent seizures, the interval may be shortened (e.g., every second day). The recommended monotherapy dosage is 600 to 1200 mg/day in two divided doses. OXC dosages range from 600 to 3000 mg/day. As adjunctive therapy, treatment with OXC should be initiated at a dose of 600 mg/day, administered as a twice-daily regimen. The recommended dosage for adjunctive therapy is 1200 mg/day or higher, if needed, which may be increased at weekly intervals (7).

In children, treatment should be initiated at a daily dose of 8 to 10 mg/kg, generally not to exceed 600 mg/day, administered as a twice-daily regimen. The target maintenance dose of OXC should be between 30 and 50 mg/kg/day. The pharmacokinetics of OXC are similar in older children (>8 years of age) and adults. However, younger children (<8 years of age) have an increased clearance compared with older children and adults; therefore, they should receive the highest maintenance doses (7).

A multicentric study has shown improvement in the quality of life in patients with partial seizures after conversion to OXC monotherapy (50).

Therapeutic drug monitoring is claimed to be of little or no value with OXC because of the linear pharmacokinetics of the agent, although measuring drug levels is undoubtedly useful for individualization of treatment in selected cases in a particular clinical setting. The plasma concentrations associated with antiepileptic effect was reported to be 5 to 50 mg/L (34).

It is believed that there is no need to monitor sodium levels regularly in asymptomatic patients, unless there are special risks, such as in patients taking high doses or diuretics and in the elderly individuals. OXC is not a drug of first choice for the elderly patients (45).

CARBAMAZEPINE VERSUS OXCARBAZEPINE

CBZ and OXC are among the most efficacious AEDs available. The literature suggests that CBZ and OXC do not differ in terms of seizure control efficacy. However, OXC has a better safety profile, including its association with fewer severe adverse events, such as idiosyncratic reactions, aplastic anemia, and agranulocytosis. Except for sodium monitoring under special circumstances with OXC treatment, laboratory monitoring of drug levels is not necessary. The OXC pharmacokinetic profile is also better than that of CBZ, with lack of autoinduction, low protein binding, linear pharmacokinetics, and minimal drug interactions, except with contraceptive use. OXC does not appear to change endogenous hormonal levels. In conclusion, OXC should be considered one of the first-line treatment options for patients with partial-onset seizures.

In some cases, a decision may be made to switch a patient from CBZ to OXC. This can either be done gradually or with a more abrupt changeover. Typically, the conversion ratio for similar efficacy is on the order of 1:1.5.

According to the ILAE guidelines, OXC was considered a level A recommendation for efficacy and effectiveness as initial monotherapy for children with partial-onset seizures (19).

References

1. Brodie MJ, Ditcher MA. Antiepileptic drugs. *N Engl J Med.* 1996;334: 168–175.
2. Macdonald RL. Carbamazepine. Mechanism of action. In: Levy RH, Mattson RH, Meldrum BS, et al., eds. *Antiepileptic Drugs.* 5th ed. Philadelphia, PA: Lippincott Williams & Wilkins; 2002:227–235.
3. McLean MJ. Oxcarbazepine. Mechanism of action. In: Levy RH, Mattson RH, Meldrum BS, et al., eds. *Antiepileptic Drugs.* 5th ed. Philadelphia, PA: Lippincott Williams & Wilkins; 2002:451–458.
4. Spina E. Carbamazepine. Chemistry, biotransformation, and pharmacokinetics. In: Levy RH, Mattson RH, Meldrum BS, et al., eds. *Antiepileptic Drugs.* 5th ed. Philadelphia, PA: Lippincott Williams & Wilkins; 2002: 236–246.

5. Bourgeois BFD. Pharmacokinetic properties of current antiepileptic drugs: what improvements are needed? *Neurology.* 2000;55(suppl 3):S11–S16.
6. Bourgeois BFD. Pharmacokinetics and pharmacodynamics of antiepileptic drugs. In: Wyllie E, ed. *The Treatment of Epilepsy: Principles and Practice.* 3rd ed. Philadelphia, PA: Lippincott Williams & Wilkins; 2001:729–739.
7. Novartis Pharmaceutical Corporation. Trileptal (oxcarbazepine) prescription information [online]. 2009. Available at: http://www.pharma.us.novartis.com/product/pi/pdf/trileptal.pdf. Accessed January 24, 2009.
8. Wurden CJ, Levy RH. Carbamazepine: interactions with other drugs. In: Levy RH, Mattson RH, Meldrum BS, et al., eds. *Antiepileptic Drugs.* 5th ed. Philadelphia, PA: Lippincott Williams & Wilkins; 2002:247–261.
9. Bourgeois BFD. Important pharmacokinetic properties of antiepileptic drugs. *Epilepsia.* 1995;36(suppl 5):S1–S7.
10. Loiseau P. Carbamazepine. Clinical efficacy and use in epilepsy. In: Levy RH, Mattson RH, Meldrum BS, et al., eds. *Antiepileptic Drugs,* 5th ed. Philadelphia, PA: Lippincott Williams & Wilkins; 2002:262–272.
11. Mattson RH, Cramer JA, Collins JF. A comparison of valproate with carbamazepine for the treatment of complex partial seizures and secondarily generalized tonic-clonic seizures. *N Engl J Med.* 1992;327:765–771.
12. Mattson RH, Cramer JA, Collins JK, et al. Comparison of carbamazepine, phenobarbital, phenytoin, and primidone in partial and secondarily generalized tonic-clonic seizures. *N Engl J Med.* 1985;313:145–151.
13. Rowan AJ, Ramsay RE, Collins JF, et al. New onset geriatric epilepsy: a randomized study of gabapentin, lamotrigine, and carbamazepine. *Neurology.* 2005;64(11):1868–1873.
14. Privitera MD, Brodie MJ, Mattson RH, et al. Topiramate, carbamazepine and valproate monotherapy: double-blind comparison in newly diagnosed epilepsy. *Acta Neurol Scand.* 2003;107:165–175.
15. Kälviäinen R, Aikia M, Saukkonen AM, et al. Viagabatrin versus carbamazepine monotherapy in patients with newly diagnosed epilepsy: a randomized controlled study. *Arch Neurol.* 1995;52:989–996.
16. Brodie MJ, Wroe SJ, Dean AD, et al. Efficacy and safety of remacemide versus carbamazepine in newly diagnosed epilepsy: comparison by sequential analysis. *Epilepsy Behav.* 2002;3:140–146.
17. Chadwick DW, Anhut H, Greiner MJ, et al. A double-blind trial of gabapentin monotherapy for newly diagnosed partial seizures. *Neurology.* 1998;51:1282–1288.
18. Brodie MJ, Perucca E, Ryvlin P, et al. Comparison of levetiracetam and controlled-release carbamazepine in newly diagnosed epilepsy. *Neurology.* 2007;68(6):402–408.
19. Glauser T, Ben-Menachem E, Bourgeois B, et al. ILAE treatment guidelines: evidence-based analysis of antiepileptic drug efficacy and effectiveness as initial monotherapy for epileptic seizures and syndromes. *Epilepsia.* 2006; 47(7):1094–1120.
20. Gilliam F. Optimizing health outcomes in active epilepsy. *Neurology.* 2002; 58(suppl 5):S9–S20.
21. Pellock JM. Carbamazepine side effects in children and adults. *Epilepsia.* 1987;28 (suppl 3):S64–S70.
22. Holmes GL. Carbamazepine. Adverse effects. In: Levy RH, Mattson RH, Meldrum BS, et al., eds. *Antiepileptic Drugs.* 5th ed. Philadelphia, PA: Lippincott Williams & Wilkins; 2002:285–297.
23. Schlienger RG, Shear NH. Antiepileptic drug hypersensitivity syndrome. *Epilepsia.* 1998;39(suppl 7):S3–S7.
24. Bohan KH, Mansuri TF, Wilson NM. Anticonvulsivant hypersensitivity syndrome: implications for pharmaceutical care. *Pharmacotherapy.* 2007;27(10):1425–1439.
25. Blackburn SC, Oliart AD, Garcia Rodriguez LA, et al. Antiepileptics and blood dyscrasias: a cohort study. *Pharmacotherapy.* 1998;18:1277–1283.
26. Herman S. Sex hormones and epilepsy: no longer just for women. *Epilepsy Curr.* 2008;8(1):6–8.
27. Yerby MS. Clinical care of pregnant women with epilepsy: neural tube defects and folic acid supplementation. *Epilepsia.* 2003;44(suppl 3):S33–S40.
28. Meador K. Effects of in utero antiepileptic drug exposure. *Epilepsy Curr.* 2008;8(6):143–147.
29. Bergen DC. Maintaining strong bones: strong opinions, little evidence. *Epilepsy Curr.* 2007;7(5):123–124.
30. Abou-Khalil BW. When should clinicians worry about bone density for patients with epilepsy? *Epilepsy Curr.* 2008;8(6):148–149.
31. The Tegretol OROS Osmotic Release Delivery System Study Group. Double-blind crossover comparison of Tegretol-XR and Tegretol in patients with epilepsy. *Neurology.* 1995;45:1703–1707.
32. Information for healthcare professionals. Carbamazepine (market as Carbatrol, Equetro, Tegretol and generics). FDA Alert 12/12/07, updated 1/31/08. Available at: http:www.fda.gov/cder/drug/InfoSheet/HCP/carbamazepineHCP.htm. Accessed January 10, 2009.
33. Faigle JW, Menge GP. Metabolic characteristics of oxcarbazepine and their beneficial implications for enzyme induction and drug interactions. *Behav Neurol.* 1990;3:21–30.
34. Bialer M. Oxcarbazepine: chemistry, biotransformation, and pharmacokinetics. In: Levy RH, Mattson RH, Meldrum BS, et al., eds. *Antiepileptic Drugs.* 5th ed. Philadelphia, PA: Lippincott Williams & Wilkins; 2002: 459–465.
35. Gram L. Oxcarbazepine. In: Engel J Jr, Pedley TA, eds. *Epilepsy: A Comprehensive Textbook.* Philadelphia, PA: Lippincott-Raven Publishers; 1997:1541–1546.
36. Patsalos PN, Perucca E. Clinically important drug interactions in epilepsy: general features and interactions between antiepileptic drugs. *Lancet Neurol.* 2003;2:347–356.
37. Dam M, Ekberg R, Loyning Y, et al. A double-blind study comparing oxcarbazepine and carbamazepine in patients with newly diagnosed, previously untreated epilepsy. *Epilepsy Res.* 1989;3:70–76.
38. Bill PA, Vigonius U, Pohlmann H, et al. A double-blind controlled clinical trial of oxcarbazepine versus phenytoin in adults with previously untreated epilepsy. *Epilepsy Res.* 1997;27:195–204.
39. Christe W, Krämer G, Vigonius U, et al. A double-blind controlled clinical trial: oxcarbazepine versus sodium valproate in adults with newly diagnosed epilepsy. *Epilepsy Res.* 1997;26:451–460.
40. Beydoun A, Sachdeo RC, Rosenfeld WE, et al. Oxcarbazepine monotherapy for partial-onset seizures: a multicenter, double-blind, clinical trial. *Neurology.* 2000;54:2245–2251.
41. Sachdeo R, Beydoun A, Schachter S, et al. Oxcarbazepine (Trileptal) as monotherapy in patients with partial seizures. *Neurology.* 2001;57: 864–871.
42. Schachter SC, Vazquez B, Fisher RS, et al. Oxcarbazepine: double-blind, randomized, placebo-control, monotherapy trial for partial seizures. *Neurology.* 1999;52:732–737.
43. Guerreiro MM, Vigonius U, Pohlmann H, et al. A double-blind controlled clinical trial of oxcarbazepine versus phenytoin in children and adolescents with epilepsy. *Epilepsy Res.* 1997;27:205–213.
44. Beydoun A, Nasreddine WM, Albini F. Oxcarbazepine. In: Engel J Jr, Pedley TA, eds. *Epilepsy: A Comprehensive Textbook.* 2nd ed. Philadelphia, PA: Lippincott Williams & Wilkins; 2008:1593–1598.
45. Krämer G. Oxcarbazepine: adverse effects. In: Levy RH, Mattson RH, Meldrum BS, et al., eds. *Antiepileptic Drugs.* 5th ed. Philadelphia, PA: Lippincott Williams & Wilkins; 2002:479–486.
46. Pedersen B, D'Souza J. Oxcarbazepine (Trileptal) therapy results in no clinically significant changes in weight. *Epilepsia.* 2002;43(suppl 8):149. Abstract.
47. Pennell PB. Using current evidence in selecting antiepileptic drugs for use during pregnancy. *Epilepsy Curr.* 2005;5(2):45–51.
48. Aldenkamp AP, Krom MD, Reijs R. Newer antiepileptic drugs and cognitive issues. *Epilepsia.* 2003;44:21–29.
49. Vendrame M, Khurana DS, Cruz M, et al. Aggravation of seizures and/or EEG features in children treated with oxcarbazepine monotherapy. *Epilepsia.* 2007;48(11):2116–2120.
50. Sachdeo RC, Gates JR, Bazil CW, et al. Improved quality of life in patients with partial seizures after conversion to oxcarbazepine monotherapy. *Epilepsy and Behavior.* 2006;(9):457–463.

CHAPTER 51 ■ VALPROATE

ANGELA K. BIRNBAUM, SUSAN E. MARINO, AND BLAISE F. D. BOURGEOIS

HISTORICAL BACKGROUND

The anticonvulsant effect of valproic acid, or valproate (VPA), was discovered serendipitously when the agent was used as a solvent for compounds tested in an animal model of seizures (1). VPA has been used in the treatment of epilepsy for more than 40 years (2), and was approved in the United States in 1978. Since then, it has been regarded as one of the major antiepileptic drugs (AEDs), distinguished from previous agents by its broad spectrum of activity against many seizure types in both children and adults (3,4) as well as by its relatively low sedative effect. In addition to being the first agent to be highly effective against several primarily generalized seizure types, such as absence, myoclonic, and tonic–clonic seizures, VPA was found to be effective in the treatment of partial seizures, Lennox–Gastaut syndrome, infantile spasms, neonatal seizures, and febrile seizures (5,6). Although VPA is also used in the treatment of migraine headaches (7,8), affective disorders (9,10), neuropathic pain (11,12), and Sydenham chorea (13), these indications will not be included in the present discussion.

CHEMISTRY AND MECHANISM OF ACTION

Valproate (MW 144.21; Fig. 51.1), a short-chain, branched fatty acid, is a colorless liquid with low solubility in water. Other forms include: (i) sodium valproate (MW 166.19), a highly water-soluble, hygroscopic white, crystalline powder and (ii) divalproex sodium, a complex composed of equal parts of VPA and sodium valproate (Fig. 51.1). The antiepileptic activity of VPA, demonstrated in several animal models (14,15), includes protection against maximal electroshock-induced seizures; seizures induced chemically by pentylenetetrazol, bicuculline, glutamic acid, kainic acid, strychnine, ouabain, nicotine, and intramuscular penicillin; and seizures induced by kindling (16). This broad spectrum of efficacy of VPA in animal models suggests that the agent is effective in both preventing the spread and lowering the threshold of seizures. Although several effects of VPA have been demonstrated at the cellular level, the precise mechanism underlying its antiepileptic effect has not been fully elucidated. Identified mechanisms include potentiation of γ-aminobutyric acid (GABA)ergic function, inhibition of γ-hydroxybutyric acid formation (17), inhibition of voltage-sensitive sodium channels (18), antagonism of NMDA receptor–mediated neural excitation (5,19) and its more recently discovered activity as a broad acting, histone deacetylase (HDAC) inhibitor (20) that may act to induce the GABA synthetic enzyme, glutamate decarboxylase (21,22). It is not known to what extent any of these actions contributes to clinical seizure protection by VPA.

ABSORPTION, DISTRIBUTION, AND METABOLISM

The main pharmacokinetic parameters of VPA are summarized in Chapter 42, Table 42.1. Different preparations of VPA are available, although not all are available in any given

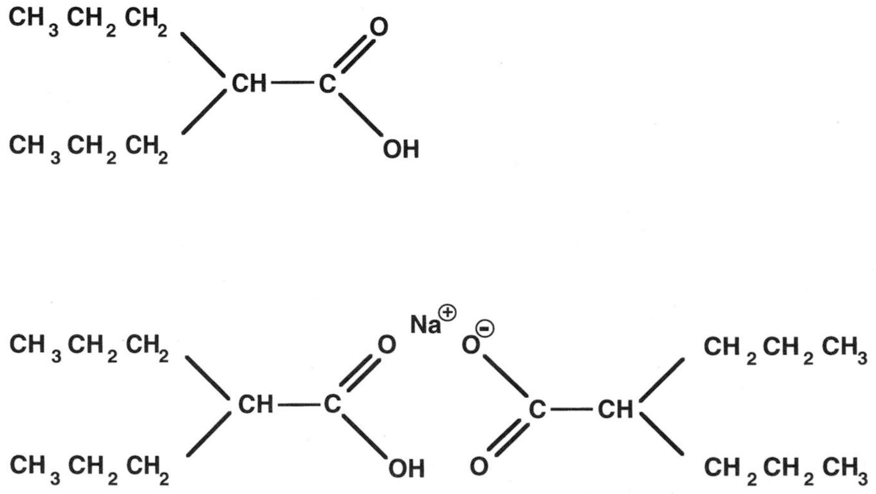

FIGURE 51.1 Structural formulas for valproic acid (N-dipropylacetic acid) and sodium hydrogen divalproate (divalproex sodium).

country. Oral preparations of VPA include VPA capsules, tablets, and syrup (immediate-release); enteric-coated tablets of sodium valproate or sodium hydrogen divalproate (divalproex sodium); divalproex sodium enteric-coated sprinkles; slow-release oral preparations; and valpromide (the amide of VPA). A parenteral formulation of sodium valproate for intravenous (IV) use is also available.

The bioavailability of oral preparations of VPA is virtually complete compared with that of the IV route (23). The purpose of the enteric coating of tablets is to prevent gastric irritation associated with release of VPA in the stomach. The rate of absorption of VPA after oral administration is variable, depending on the formulation. Administration of syrup or uncoated regular tablets or capsules is followed by rapid absorption and peak levels within 2 hours. Absorption from enteric-coated tablets is delayed but rapid. The onset of absorption varies as a function of the state of gastric emptying at the time of ingestion, and peak levels may be reached only 3 to 8 hours after oral ingestion of enteric-coated tablets (24–26) (Chapter 45, Fig. 45.1). Therefore, in patients treated chronically with enteric-coated VPA, the true trough level may occur in the late morning or early afternoon (27). The bioavailability of enteric-coated sprinkles of divalproex sodium was compared with that of VPA syrup in 12 children, with no difference noted between the two formulations (28). However, the average time to maximal VPA concentrations was longer for sprinkles (4.2 hours) than for syrup (0.9 hours). Diurnal variation in VPA concentrations of particular VPA formulations have been observed with the enteric-coated tablets resulting in nighttime drug concentrations of 30% to 40% of daytime values (29–35). The recently approved extended-release divalproex formulation does not seem to exhibit this variation after administration to healthy volunteers (36). With the IV formulation, peak VPA serum levels are reached at the end of the recommended infusion time of 60 minutes. Compared with oral syrup, the relative bioavailability of VPA suppositories was found to be 80% in volunteers (37,38). Suppositories are not available commercially. Rectal preparations from the syrup and capsule formulations can be prepared and have been given to patients (39,40).

The volume of distribution of VPA is relatively small (0.13 to 0.19 L/kg in adults and 0.20 to 0.30 L/kg in children). VPA is highly bound to serum proteins; this binding appears to be saturable at therapeutic concentrations, with the free fraction of VPA increasing as the total concentration increases (41): 7% at 50 mg/L, 9% at 75 mg/L, 15% at 100 mg/L, 22% at 125 mg/L, and 30% at 150 mg/L. On the basis of these values, with an only threefold increase in the total concentration of VPA, from 50 to 150 mg/L, the free level of VPA would increase more than 10 times, from 3.5 to 45 mg/L. Accordingly, there is a curvilinear relationship between VPA maintenance dose and total steady-state concentrations, with relatively smaller increases in concentrations at higher doses (42). VPA unbound fraction decreases from 15% at maximum concentration to 9% at 45mg/L when rapid infusion (infusions of VPA administered in less than 60 minutes) of intravenous VPA is given (43). Several factors including induction status, albumin concentration, and infusion rate can significantly affect VPA pharmacokinetics. Infusion of VPA at a rate up to 3 mg/kg/min produces predictable total VPA concentrations when hepatic induction status and albumin levels are considered. Unpredictable protein binding can also be seen in critically ill patients and after rapid administration of VPA.

Four children receiving doses (8.3 to 15.4 mg/kg) in less than 15 minutes had a fraction unbound of 45% (44). Monitoring of unbound drug concentration may be useful when protein-binding alterations are suspected.

The elimination half-life of VPA varies as a function of comedication. In the absence of inducing drugs, the half-life in adults is 13 to 16 hours (24,45), whereas in adults receiving polytherapy with inducing drugs, the average half-life is 9 hours (23). In children, the half-life is slightly shorter. Cloyd and colleagues (35) reported an average half-life of 11.6 hours in children receiving monotherapy and 7.0 hours in those receiving polytherapy. Newborns eliminate VPA slowly; the half-life in this population is longer than 20 hours (33). In vitro studies from human liver microsomes show no difference in the rates of valproate-glucuronide formation in microsomes from young versus elderly (>65 years of age) livers (46). Approximately 55% of elderly nursing home residents are maintained at total VPA concentrations below the adult therapeutic range for epilepsy of 50 to 100 mg/mL regardless of indication (37,47). The population clearance from a study of 146 (405 VPA concentrations) elderly nursing home residents (average age 78.5 years ± 8.0 (SD)) was 0.843 L/hr (48). Apparent oral clearances in elderly nursing residents are reported to be 27% lower in female residents, even after adjusting for weight, and 25% greater in residents using the nonsyrup formulation (48). Approximately 20% of elderly nursing home residents take VPA syrup (37). The lower clearances seen with the syrup formulation may be a function of the patient's pathophysiology rather than a difference in the bioavailability of the syrup formulation.

Several enzymes (UDP-glucuronosyltransferases: UGTs, β-oxidation, and cytochrome P450: CYP) are predominantly involved in the metabolism of VPA. The most abundant metabolites of VPA are glucuronide and 3-oxo-VPA, which represent about 40% and 33%, respectively, of the urinary excretion of a VPA dose (32). Several UGTs—UGT1A3, UGT1A4, UGT1A6, UGT1A8, UGT1A9, and UGT1A10—have been identified in vitro to be involved in forming the acyl glucuronide conjugate (46,49–51). Two desaturated metabolites of VPA, 2-ene-VPA and 4-ene-VPA, have anticonvulsant activity that is similar in potency to that of VPA itself (31). Because there is delayed but significant accumulation of 2-ene-VPA in the brain and because it is cleared more slowly than VPA (30), the formation of 2-ene-VPA provides a possible explanation for the discrepancy between the time courses of VPA concentrations and antiepileptic activity (29). It appears that 2-ene-VPA does not have the pronounced embryotoxicity (52) and hepatotoxicity (53) of 4-ene-VPA. Both are produced by the action of cytochrome P450 enzymes, which are induced by certain other AEDs (32,54). This may explain the increased risk for hepatotoxicity in patients receiving VPA concomitantly with these agents (55). However, elevation of 4-ene-VPA levels has not yet been found in patients with VPA hepatotoxicity, short-term adverse effects, or hyperammonemia (56). Cytochrome CYP2C9*1 is the predominant catalyst in the formation of 4-ene-VPA, 4-OH-VPA, and 5-OH-VPA metabolites (75% to 80%) with CYP2A6 and CYP2B6 being responsible for the remainder of these reactions. CYP2A6 is involved in approximately 50% of the formation of 3-OH-VPA (57). Population pharmacokinetic studies indicate that knowledge of a patient's CYP2C9 and CYP2C19 genotype may aid in predicting a patient's response to VPA (58).

DRUG INTERACTIONS

Pharmacokinetic interactions with VPA fall into three categories, based on the following features: (i) the metabolism of VPA is sensitive to enzymatic induction; (ii) VPA itself can inhibit the metabolism of other agents; and (iii) VPA has a high affinity for serum proteins and can displace other agents or be displaced from proteins (59–61). Concomitant administration of enzyme-inducing drugs has been repeatedly shown to lower VPA levels relative to the dose (62). Carbamazepine (63–65) and phenytoin (65) lower VPA levels by one third to one half, or even more, in children (66–68). When children receiving polytherapy discontinued treatment with other agents, VPA levels increased 122% after withdrawal of phenytoin, 67% after withdrawal of phenobarbital, and 50% after withdrawal of carbamazepine (69). In elderly nursing home residents VPA clearance is increased 41% in residents who are also taking phenytoin or carbamazepine (48). In contrast, levels of VPA are increased by coadministration of felbamate: 28% with felbamate 1200 mg/day and 54% with felbamate 2400 mg/day (70,71). According to one study, clobazam may significantly reduce the clearance of VPA (72).

VPA affects the kinetics of other drugs either by enzymatic inhibition or by displacement from serum proteins. Phenobarbital levels have been found to increase by 57% (73) to 81% (74) after the addition of VPA. Levels of ethosuximide can also be raised by the addition of VPA, mostly in the presence of additional AEDs (75). Although VPA does not increase levels of carbamazepine itself, levels of the active metabolite carbamazepine-10,11-epoxide may double (76,77). Elimination of lamotrigine is markedly inhibited by VPA, resulting in a two- to threefold prolongation of the lamotrigine half-life (78). Although this is a competitive interaction that is likely to be rapidly reversible upon discontinuation of VPA, the inhibition seems to persist even at low VPA concentrations (79,80). A pharmacokinetic interaction occurs between VPA and phenytoin, partly because both agents have a high affinity for serum proteins. Displacement of one highly protein bound drug by a second highly protein bound drug can cause a reduction in total but not unbound drug concentrations (34). However, VPA also interferes with the metabolism of phenytoin resulting in a decrease in total and an increase in unbound phenytoin concentrations (i.e., VPA increases the free fraction of phenytoin) (81,82). Thus, in the presence of VPA, total phenytoin concentrations in the usual therapeutic range may be associated with clinical toxicity. In contrast to inducing AEDs, VPA is not associated with oral contraceptive failure (83); however, oral contraceptives may decrease VPA levels in women taking both compounds (84).

EFFICACY

VPA is a highly effective first-line agent for the treatment of primarily generalized idiopathic seizures, such as absence generalized tonic–clonic and myoclonic seizures (85). The indication for VPA when it was first released in North America in 1978 was for treatment of absence seizures. In patients with typical and atypical absence seizures, a reduction of spike-and-wave discharges was demonstrated (86–89). In two studies, comparison of VPA and ethosuximide for the treatment of absence seizures showed equal efficacy for the two agents (90,91). It appears that absence seizures are more likely to be fully controlled when they occur alone than when they are mixed with another seizure type (69,92). Overall, VPA appears to be somewhat less effective against atypical or "complex" absences than against simple absences (93,94). VPA can also be used effectively in patients with recurrent absence status (95).

VPA was found to be effective in the treatment of certain generalized convulsive seizures (96–99). Among 42 patients with intractable seizures, generalized tonic–clonic seizures were fully controlled in 14 patients by add-on VPA therapy (69). VPA was compared with phenytoin in 61 previously untreated patients with generalized tonic–clonic, clonic, or tonic seizures, and seizures were controlled in 82% of VPA-treated patients versus 76% of those treated with phenytoin (100). In another randomized comparison of VPA and phenytoin in patients with previously untreated tonic–clonic seizures, a 2-year remission was achieved in 27 of 37 patients receiving VPA and in 22 of 39 patients receiving phenytoin (99). Monotherapy with VPA was assessed in two studies of patients with primary (or idiopathic) generalized epilepsies (92,101). Among patients who had generalized tonic–clonic seizures only, complete seizure control was achieved in 51 of 70 patients (101) and in 39 of 44 patients (92), respectively. VPA monotherapy in children with generalized tonic–clonic seizures was also found to be highly effective (102).

Currently, VPA is often a first choice for most myoclonic seizures, particularly for those occurring in patients with primary or idiopathic generalized epilepsies (92,93,101). In a group of patients with primary generalized epilepsy given VPA monotherapy, 22 patients had myoclonic seizures and 20 of them experienced at least one other seizure type, either absence or tonic–clonic. The myoclonic seizures were controlled by VPA monotherapy in 18 of the 22 patients (92). Patients with juvenile myoclonic epilepsy have an excellent response to VPA (103), which remains an agent of first choice for this condition. Benign myoclonic epilepsy of infancy also responds well to treatment with VPA (102). Some success has been achieved with VPA in patients with postanoxic intention myoclonus (104,105). A combination of VPA and clonazepam is often used to treat the myoclonic and tonic–clonic seizures associated with severe progressive myoclonus epilepsy (106).

Like all other AEDs, VPA is less effective in the treatment of generalized encephalopathic epilepsies of infancy and childhood, such as infantile spasms and Lennox–Gastaut syndrome. In a series of 38 patients with myoclonic astatic epilepsy, seven patients became and remained seizure free with VPA therapy and 50% to 80% improvement was achieved in one third of patients (93).

Reports on the use of VPA for the treatment of infantile spasms include small numbers of patients (107–109), or patients receiving corticotropin and VPA simultaneously. Overall, there was a trend toward a better response with corticotropin, but the incidence and severity of side effects was lower with VPA. A retrospective study of VPA monotherapy in 30 patients with simple partial and complex partial seizures in whom previous drugs had failed showed a remarkable response (110). Seizure control was achieved in 12 patients, a greater than 50% seizure reduction occurred in 10 patients, and only 9 patients showed no improvement. Comparison of VPA with carbamazepine or phenytoin showed little difference (111,112).

Mattson and colleagues (113) reported the most comprehensive controlled comparison of VPA and carbamazepine monotherapy for the treatment of partial and secondarily generalized seizures. Several seizure indicators, as well as neurotoxicity and systemic neurotoxicity, were assessed quantitatively. Four of five efficacy indicators for partial seizures were significantly in favor of carbamazepine, and a combined composite score for efficacy and toxicity was higher for carbamazepine than for VPA at 12 months, but not at 24 months. Outcomes for secondarily generalized seizures did not differ between the two agents. Two studies—one comparing VPA and carbamazepine (114) and the other comparing VPA, carbamazepine, phenytoin, and phenobarbital (115)—were conducted in children. Equal efficacy against generalized and partial seizures was reported with all agents. Unacceptable side effects necessitating withdrawal occurred in patients receiving phenobarbital, which was prematurely eliminated from the study. VPA was also evaluated in 143 adult patients with poorly controlled partial epilepsy randomized to VPA monotherapy at low plasma levels (25 to 50 mg/L) or high plasma levels (80 to 150 mg/L) (116). The reduction in frequency of both complex partial and secondarily generalized tonic–clonic seizures was significantly higher among patients in the high-level group.

Several studies have demonstrated the efficacy of VPA in the prevention of febrile seizures (117–123). Based on risk–benefit ratio considerations, VPA cannot be recommended for this indication. A small group of newborns with seizures have also been treated with VPA administered rectally (124) or orally (33). Results were favorable overall. In newborns treated with VPA, a long elimination half-life (26.4 hours) and high levels of ammonia were reported (33).

ADVERSE EFFECTS

Neurologic Effects

A dose-related tremor is relatively common in patients treated with VPA. If it does not improve sufficiently with dosage reduction, propranolol may be tried (125). Drowsiness, lethargy, and confusional states are uncommon with VPA, but may occur in some patients, usually at levels >100 mg/L. There have also been case reports of reversible dementia and pseudoatrophy of the brain (126–128). Treatment with VPA has been associated with a somewhat specific and unique adverse effect, characterized by an acute mental change that can progress to stupor or coma (129,130). It is usually associated with generalized delta slowing in the electroencephalographic tracing. The mechanism is not known with certainty, but it is probably not caused by hyperammonemia or carnitine deficiency. This encephalopathic picture is more likely to occur when VPA is added to another AED, and it is usually reversible within 2 to 3 days upon discontinuation of VPA or the other AED. In addition, Meador et al. recently reported that, when compared with other AEDs, VPA can significantly lower, in a dose-related fashion, the IQ of children 3 years of age who have been exposed to VPA in utero (131).

Gastrointestinal Effects

The most common gastrointestinal (GI) adverse effects associated with VPA use are nausea, vomiting, GI distress, and anorexia. These effects may be due, in part, to direct gastric irritation by VPA; the incidence is lower with enteric-coated tablets. Excessive weight gain is another common problem (132,133). This is not entirely attributable to increased appetite, and decreased β-oxidation of fatty acids has been postulated as a mechanism (134). Excessive weight gain seems to be less of a problem in children, and a recent report suggests that VPA is not associated with greater weight gain, compared with carbamazepine, in children (94).

Fatal hepatotoxicity remains the most feared adverse effect of VPA (30,135–138). Two main risk factors have been clearly identified: young age and polytherapy (135). The risk for fatal hepatotoxicity in patients receiving VPA polytherapy is approximately 1:600 at younger than 3 years of age, 1:8,000 from 3 to 10 years, 1:10,000 from 11 to 20 years, 1:31,000 from 21 to 40 years, and 1:107,000 at older than 41 years of age. The risk is much lower in patients receiving monotherapy; it varies between 1:16,000 (3 to 10 years of age) and 1:230,000 (21 to 40 years of age) (135). No fatalities in patients receiving VPA monotherapy have been reported in certain age groups (0 to 2 years, 11 to 20 years, and older than 40 years of age) (135). Because a benign elevation of liver enzymes is common during VPA therapy and because severe hepatotoxicity is not preceded by a progressive elevation of liver enzymes, laboratory monitoring is of little value despite the fact that it is often performed routinely. The diagnosis of VPA-associated hepatotoxicity depends mostly on recognition of the clinical features, which include nausea, vomiting, anorexia, lethargy, and, at times, loss of seizure control, jaundice, or edema. One study indicates a possible protective effect of L-carnitine administration in cases of established VPA-induced hepatotoxicity (139). Among 92 patients with severe, symptomatic VPA-induced hepatotoxicity, 48% of the 42 patients treated with L-carnitine survived, as opposed to 10% of the 50 patients receiving similar supportive treatment without L-carnitine. The results suggested better survival with IV, rather than enteral, L-carnitine (139).

Another serious complication of VPA treatment is the development of acute hemorrhagic pancreatitis (140–144). Suspicion should be raised by the occurrence of vomiting and abdominal pain. Serum amylase and lipase are the most helpful diagnostic tests, and abdominal ultrasonography may also be considered.

Hematologic Effects

Hematologic alterations are relatively common with VPA therapy, but they seldom lead to discontinuation of treatment (145,146). Thrombocytopenia (145,147) can fluctuate and tends to improve with dosage reduction. In conjunction with altered platelet function (148,149) and other VPA-mediated disturbances of hemostasis (150,151), it may cause excessive bleeding. Therefore, the common practice of withdrawing VPA before elective surgery may be recommended despite the fact that several reports found no objective evidence of excessive operative bleeding in patients maintained on VPA therapy (152–154).

Hyperammonemia

Mild hyperammonemia is a very common finding in asymptomatic patients receiving chronic VPA therapy, particularly in those taking VPA along with an enzyme-inducing AED

(155,156), and routine monitoring of ammonium levels is not warranted. Although hyperammonemia can be reduced with L-carnitine supplementation (157), there is no documentation that this is necessary or clinically beneficial (158). Chronic treatment with VPA, especially in polytherapy, tends to lower carnitine levels (159,160); however, a role for carnitine deficiency in the development of severe adverse effects of VPA has not been established. A beneficial effect of L-carnitine supplementation in acute VPA overdoses has been suggested (161,162), and a panel of pediatric neurologists has made recommendations for routine supplementation with L-carnitine in a subgroup of pediatric patients being treated with VPA (163).

Reproductive Issues

In women, VPA has been reported to cause menstrual irregularities, hormonal changes such as hyperandrogenism and hyperinsulinism, polycystic ovaries, and pubertal arrest (164–168). An additional concern has been the possible association of VPA therapy, polycystic ovaries, and elevated testosterone levels (164–166,169). In a comparison of women treated with VPA, 21 with phenobarbital, 23 with carbamazepine, and 20 healthy untreated women, polycystic ovary prevalence, ovary volumes, and hirsutism scores did not differ among the groups (170). Epilepsy itself, other AEDs, and additional factors may be involved in the development of polycystic ovary syndrome (171,172). Treatment with VPA during the first trimester of pregnancy has been found to be associated with an estimated 1% to 2% risk of neural tube defect (170,173,174); a pharmacogenetic susceptibility has been suggested (175). Folate supplementation appears to reduce the risk (176), and a daily dose of at least 1 mg should be considered in all female patients of childbearing age who are taking VPA. However, the finding that by age 3, children who have been exposed to VPA in utero are cognitively impaired compared to children who had fetal exposure to other AEDs supports the recommendation by Meador et al. that, "VPA not be used as a first-choice drug in women of childbearing potential"(131).

Miscellaneous Effects

Excessive hair loss may be seen during treatment with VPA, and although the hair tends to grow back, it may become different in texture (177) or color (178). Facial and limb edema can occur in the absence of VPA-induced hepatic injury (179). Children may develop secondary nocturnal enuresis after initiation of VPA therapy (111,133,180–182). Hyponatremia (183) has been reported in one patient. The occurrence of rash with VPA therapy is very rare (184).

CLINICAL USE

An initial VPA dosage of approximately 15 mg/kg/day is recommended, with subsequent increases, as necessary and tolerated, of 5 to 10 mg/kg/day at weekly intervals. The optimal VPA dose or concentration may vary according to a patient's seizure type (185). Daily doses between 10 and 20 mg/kg are often sufficient for VPA monotherapy in patients with primary generalized epilepsies (69,92,100,101); children may require higher doses (74,93) whereas elderly nursing home residents may require lower doses (37). Dosages of 30 to 60 mg/kg/day (in children, >100 mg/kg/day) may be necessary to achieve adequate VPA levels in patients being treated concomitantly with enzyme-inducing agents. If therapeutic levels of VPA are to be achieved rapidly or if patients are unable to take VPA orally, the agent can be administered intravenously (186). This route has also been suggested for the treatment of patients with status epilepticus, with an initial dose of 15 mg/kg (at 20 mg/min) followed by 1 mg/kg/hr (187). A more rapid loading with an initial dose of 20 mg/kg has also been advocated, given at a rate of 33.3 to 555 mg/min (188) or ≤6 mg/kg/min (189). Rapid IV VPA loading seems to be well tolerated (190).

Because of the short half-life of VPA, it is common to divide the total daily dose into two or three doses. However, the pharmacodynamic profile of VPA may explain why equally good results have been achieved with a single daily dose (93,191,192). In addition, the availability of an extended-release divalproex formulation makes once a day dosing even more appealing. The value of monitoring serum levels of VPA is limited. First, there is a considerable fluctuation in VPA levels because of the short half-life and variable absorption rate of the agent. Second, there seems to be a poor correlation between VPA serum levels and clinical effect, and the pharmacodynamic effect of VPA may lag behind its blood concentrations (92,193–196). Although the usual therapeutic range for VPA serum levels is 50 to 100 mg/L (350 to 700 μmol/L), levels up to 150 mg/L may be both necessary and well tolerated. In selected cases, and particularly during combination therapy with enzyme-inducing agents, VPA serum levels can be valuable, but a single measurement must be interpreted cautiously (197). Routine monitoring of liver enzymes and complete blood count with platelets is a common practice, but may be of little value. It may be more useful to perform these tests if unusual bruising or bleeding occurs or if there are any symptoms or signs of liver failure.

ACKNOWLEDGMENT

Results presented in this chapter were funded in part by NIH NINDS K01 NS050309 and P50 NS16308.

References

1. Meunier H, Carraz G, Neunier Y, et al. Pharmacodynamic properties of N-dipropylacetic acid. *Therapie.* 1963;18:435–438.
2. Carraz G, Fau R, Chateau R, et al. Communication concerning 1st clinical tests of the anticonvulsive activity of N-dipropylacetic acid (sodium salt). *Ann Med Psychol.* 1964;122:577–585.
3. Sarisjulis N, Dulac P. Valproate in the treatment of epilepsies in children. In: Loscher W, ed. *Valproate.* Basel: Birkhauser; 1999:131–152.
4. Davis R, Peters DH, McTavish D. Valproic acid. A reappraisal of its pharmacological properties and clinical efficacy in epilepsy. *Drugs.* 1994; 47(2):332–372.
5. Löscher W. Basic pharmacology of valproate: a review after 35 years of clinical use for the treatment of epilepsy. *CNS Drugs.* 2002;16(10): 669–694.
6. Bourgeois BFD. Clinical efficacy and use in epilepsy. In: Levy RH, Mattson RH, Meldrum BS, et al., eds. *Antiepileptic Drugs.* Philadelphia, PA: Lippincott Williams & Wilkins; 2002:808–817.
7. Silberstein SD, Lipton RB, Goadsby PJ. *Headache in Clinical Practice.* Oxford: Isis Medical Media; 1998.
8. Silberstein SD, Saper JR, Freitag F. Migraine: diagnosis and treatment. In: Silberstein SD, Lipton RB, Dalessio DJ. eds. *Wolff's Headache and Other Head Pain.* New York: Oxford University Press; 2001.

9. Emrich HM, Dose M, von Zerssen D. The use of sodium valproate, carbamazepine and oxcarbazepine in patients with affective disorders. *J Affect Disord.* 1985;8(3):243–250.

10. Swann AC. Valproic acid: Clinical efficacy and use in psychiatric disorders. In: Levy RH, Maattson RH, Meldrum BS, et al., eds. *Antiepileptic Drugs.* Philadelphia, PA: Lippincott Williams & Wilkins; 2002: 828–835.

11. Hardy JR, Rees EA, J. Gwilliam B, et al. A phase II study to establish the efficacy and toxicity of sodium valproate in patients with cancer-related neuropathic pain. *J Pain Symptom Manage.* 2001;21(3):204–209.

12. Johannessen Landmark C. Antiepileptic drugs in non-epilepsy disorders: relations between mechanisms of action and clinical efficacy. *CNS Drugs.* 2008;22(1):27–47.

13. Daoud AS, Zaki M, Shakir R, et al. Effectiveness of sodium valproate in the treatment of Sydenham's chorea. *Neurology.* 1990;40:1140–1141.

14. Frey HH, Löscher W, Reiche R, et al. Anticonvulsant potency of common antiepileptic drugs in the gerbil. *Pharmacology.* 1983;27:330–335.

15. Pellegrini A, Gloor P, Sherwin AL. Effect of valproate sodium on generalized penicillin epilepsy in the cat. *Epilepsia.* 1978;19:351–360.

16. Leviel V, Naquet R. A study of the action of valproic acid on the kindling effect. *Epilepsia.* 1977;18:229–234.

17. Löscher W. Valproic acid: mechanisms of action. In: Levy RH, Mattson RH, Meldrum BS, et al., eds. *Antiepileptic Drugs.* Philadelphia, PA: Lippincott Williams & Wilkins; 2002:767–779.

18. Large CH, Kalinichev M, Lucas A, et al. The relationship between sodium channel inhibition and anticonvulsant activity in a model of generalised seizure in the rat. *Epilepsy Res.* 2009;85(1):96–106.

19. Zeise ML, Kasparow S, Zieglgansberger W. Valproate suppresses N-methyl-D-aspartate-evoked, transient depolarizations in the rat neocortex in vitro. *Brain Res.* 1991;5442:345–348.

20. Gottlicher M, Minucci S, Zhu P, et al. Valproic acid defines a novel class of HDAC inhibitors inducing differentiation of transformed cells. *EMBO J.* 2001;20(24):6969–6978.

21. Tremolizzo L, Carboni G, Ruzicka WB, et al. An epigenetic mouse model for molecular and behavioral neuropathologies related to schizophrenia vulnerability. *Proc Natl Acad Sci U S A.* 2002;99(26):17095–17100.

22. Nalivaeva, NN, Belyaev, ND, & Turner, AJ, Sodium valproate: an old drug with new roles. *Trends Pharmacol Sci.* 2009;30(10):509–514.

23. Perucca E, Gatti G, Frigo GM, et al. Disposition of sodium valproate in epileptic patients. *Br J Clin Pharmacol.* 1978;5:495–499.

24. Gugler R, Schell A, Eichelbaum M, et al. Disposition of valproic acid in man. *Eur J Clin Pharmacol.* 1977;12:125–132.

25. Klotz U, Antonin KH. Pharmacokinetics and bioavailability of sodium valproate. *Clin Pharmacol Ther.* 1977;21:736–743.

26. Levy RH, Conraud B, Loiseau P, et al. Meal-dependent absorption of enteric-coated sodium valproate. *Epilepsia.* 1980;21:273–280.

27. Issakainen J, Bourgeois BFD. Bioavailability of sodium valproate suppositories during repeated administration at steady state in epileptic children. *Eur J Pediatr.* 1987;146:404–407.

28. Cloyd J, Kriel R, Jones-Saete C, et al. Comparison of sprinkle versus syrup formulations of valproate for bioavailability, tolerance, and preference. *J Pediatr.* 1992;120:634–638.

29. Nau H, Löscher W. Valproic acid: brain and plasma levels of the drug and its metabolites, anticonvulsant effects and gamma-aminobutyric acid (GABA) metabolism in the mouse. *J Pharmacol Exp Ther.* 1982;220: 654–659.

30. Pollack GM, McHugh WB, Gengo FM, et al. Accumulation and washout kinetics of valproic acid and its active metabolites. *J Clin Pharmacol.* 1986;26:668–676.

31. Löscher W, Nau H. Pharmacological evaluation of various metabolites and analogues of valproic acid. *Neuropharmacology.* 1985;24:427–435.

32. Levy RH, Rettenmeier AW, Anderson GD. Effects of polytherapy with phenytoin, carbamazepine, and stiripentol on formation of 4-ene-valproate, a hepatotoxic metabolite of valproic acid. *Clin Pharmacol Ther.* 1990;48:225–235.

33. Gal P, Oles KS, Gilman JT, et al. Valproic acid efficacy, toxicity, and pharmacokinetics in neonates with intractable seizures. *Neurology.* 1988;38:467–471.

34. Cloyd J. Pharmacokinetic pitfalls of present antiepileptic medications. *Epilepsia.* 1991;32(suppl 5):S53–S65.

35. Cloyd JC, Fischer JH, Kriel RL, et al. Valproic acid pharmacokinetics in children. IV. Effects of age and antiepileptic drugs on protein binding and intrinsic clearance. *Clin Pharmacol Ther.* 1993;53:22–29.

36. Dutta S, Reed RC, Cavanaugh JH. Pharmacokinetics and safety of extended-release divalproex sodium tablets: morning versus evening administration. *Am J Health Syst Pharm.* 2004;61(21):2280–2283.

37. Birnbaum AK, Hardie NA, Conway JM, et al. Valproic acid doses, concentrations, and clearances in elderly nursing home residents. *Epilepsy Res.* 2004;62(2–3):157–162.

38. Holmes GB, Rosenfeld WE, Graves NM, et al. Absorption of valproic acid suppositories in human volunteers. *Arch Neurol.* 1989;46: 906–909.

39. Conway JM, Kriel RL, Birnbaum AK. Antiepileptic drug therapy in children. In: *Pediatric Neurology: Principles and Practice.* Philadelphia, PA: Elsevier; 2006.

40. Cloyd JC, Kriel RL. Bioavailability of rectally administered valproic acid syrup. *Neurology.* 1981;31(10):1348–1352.

41. Cramer JA, Mattson RH, Bennett DM, et al. Variable free and total valproic acid concentrations in sole-and multi-drug therapy. *Ther Drug Monit.* 1986;8:411–415.

42. Gram L, Flachs H, Wurtz-Jorgensen A, et al. Sodium valproate, serum level and clinical effect in epilepsy: a controlled study. *Epilepsia.* 1979;20:303–312.

43. Cloyd JC, Dutta S, Cao G, et al. Valproate unbound fraction and distribution volume following rapid infusions in patients with epilepsy. *Epilepsy Res.* 2003;53(1–2):19–27.

44. Birnbaum AK, Kriel RL, Norberg SK, et al. Rapid infusion of sodium valproate in acutely ill children. *Pediatr Neurol.* 2003;28(4):300–303.

45. Perucca E, Grimaldi R, Gatti G, et al. Pharmacokinetics of valproic acid in the elderly. *Br J Clin Pharmacol.* 1984;17:665–669.

46. Argikar UA, Remmel RP. Effect of aging on glucuronidation of valproic acid in human liver microsomes and the role of UDP-glucuronosyltransferase UGT1A4, UGT1A8, and UGT1A10. *Drug Metab Dispos.* 2009; 37(1):229–236.

47. Schachter SC, Cramer GW, Thompson GD, et al. An evaluation of antiepileptic drug therapy in nursing facilities. *J Am Geriatr Soc.* 1998; 46(9):1137–1141.

48. Birnbaum AK, Hardie NA, Conway JM, et al. Population pharmacokinetics of valproic acid concentrations in elderly nursing home residents. *Ther Drug Monit.* 2007;29(5):571–575.

49. Ethell BT, Anderson GD, Burchell B. The effect of valproic acid on drug and steroid glucuronidation by expressed human UDP-glucuronosyltransferases. *Biochem Pharmacol.* 2003;65(9):1441–1449.

50. Green MD, King CD, Mojarrabi B, et al. Glucuronidation of amines and other xenobiotics catalyzed by expressed human UDP-glucuronosyltransferase 1A3. *Drug Metab Dispos.* 1998;26(6):507–512.

51. Green MD, Tephly TR. Glucuronidation of amines and hydroxylated xenobiotics and endobiotics catalyzed by expressed human UGT1.4 protein. *Drug Metab Dispos.* 1996;24(3):356–363.

52. Nau H, Hauck RA, Ehlers K. Valproic acid-induce neural tube defects in mouse and human: aspects of chirality, alternative drug development, pharmacokinetics, and possible mechanisms. *Pharmacol Toxicol.* 1991; 69:310–321.

53. Kesterson JW, Granneman GR, Machinist JM. The hepatotoxicity of valproic acid and its metabolites in rats. I. Toxicologic, biochemical and histopathologic studies. *Hepatology.* 1984;4:1143–1152.

54. Rettie AE, Rettenmeier AW, Howald WN, et al. Cytochrome P-450—catalyzed formation of delta 4-VPA, a toxic metabolite of valproic acid. *Science.* 1987;235:890–893.

55. Dreifuss FE, Langer DH, Moline KA, et al. Valproic acid hepatic fatalities. II. US experience since 1984. *Neurology.* 1984;39:201–207.

56. Paganini M, Zaccara G, Moroni F, et al. Lack of relationship between sodium valproate-induced adverse effects and the plasma concentration of its metabolite 2-propylpenten-4-oic acid. *Eur J Clin Pharmacol.* 1987;32:219–222.

57. Kiang TK, Ho PC, Anari MR, et al. Contribution of CYP2C9, CYP2A6, and CYP2B6 to valproic acid metabolism in hepatic microsomes from individuals with the CYP2C9*1/*1 genotype. *Toxicol Sci.* 2006;94(2):261–271.

58. Jiang D, Bai X, Zhang Q, Lu W, Wang Y, Li L, Müller M. Effects of CYP2C19 and CYP2C9 genotypes on pharmacokinetic variability of valproic acid in Chinese epileptic patients: nonlinear mixed-effect modeling. *Eur J Clin Pharmacol.* 2009;65(12):1187–1193.

59. Bourgeois BFD. Pharmacologic interactions between valproate and other drugs. *Am J Med.* 1988;84:29–33.

60. Levy RH, Koch KM. Drug interactions with valproic acid. *Drugs.* 1982; 24:543–556.

61. Scheyer RD, Mattson RH. Valproic acid: interactions with other drugs. In: Levy R, Mattson R, Meldrum B. eds. *Antiepileptic Drugs.* New York: Raven Press; 1995:621–631.

62. May T, Rambeck B. Serum concentrations of valproic acid: influence of dose and comedication. *Ther Drug Monit.* 1985;7:387–390.

63. Bowdle TA, Levy RH, Cutler RE. Effect of carbamazepine on valproic acid kinetics in normal subjects. *Clin Pharmacol Ther.* 1979;26:629–634.

64. Hoffmann F, von Unruh GE, Jancik BC. Valproic acid disposition in epileptic patients during combined antiepileptic maintenance therapy. *Eur J Clin Pharmacol.* 1981;19:383–385.

65. Reunanen MI, Luoma P, Myllyla V, et al. Low serum valproic acid concentrations in epileptic patients on combination therapy. *Curr Ther Res.* 1980;28:456–462.

66. Cloyd JC, Kriel RL, Fischer JH. Valproic acid pharmacokinetics in children. II. Discontinuation of concomitant antiepileptic drug therapy. *Neurology.* 1985;35:1623–1627.

67. de Wolff FA, Peters ACB, van Kempen GMJ. Serum concentrations and enzyme induction in epileptic children treated with phenytoin and valproate. *Neuropediatrics.* 1982;13:10–13.

68. Sackellares JC, Sato S, Dreifuss FE, et al. Reduction of steady-state valproate levels by other antiepileptic drugs. *Epilepsia.* 1981;22:437–441.

69. Henriksen O, Johannessen SI. Clinical and pharmacokinetic observations on sodium valproate: a 5-year follow-up study in 100 children with epilepsy. *Acta Neurol Scand.* 1982;65:504–523.

70. Hooper WD, Franklin ME. Glue P, et al. Effect of felbamate on valproic acid disposition in healthy volunteers: inhibition of beta-oxidation. *Epilepsia.* 1996;37:91–97.

71. Wagner ML, Graves NM, Leppik IE, et al. The effect of felbamate on valproate disposition. *Epilepsia.* 1991;32:15.

72. Theis JG, Koren G, Daneman R, et al. Interactions of clobazam with conventional antiepileptics in children. *J Child Neurol.* 1997;12:208–213.

73. Suganuma T, Ishizaki T, Chiba K, et al. The effect of concurrent administration of valproate sodium on phenobarbital plasma concentration/dosage ratio in pediatric patients. *J Pediatr.* 1981;99:314–317.

74. Redenbaugh JE, Sato S, Penry JK, et al. Sodium valproate: pharmacokinetics and effectiveness in treating intractable seizures. *Neurology.* 1980;30:1–6.

75. Mattson RH, Cramer JA. Valproic acid and ethosuximide interaction. *Ann Neurol.* 1980;7:583–584.

76. Levy RH, Moreland TA, Morselli PL, et al. Carbamazepine/valproic acid interaction in man and rhesus monkey. *Epilepsia.* 1984;25:338–345.

77. Pisani F, Fazio A, Oteri G, et al. Sodium valproate and valpromide: differential interactions with carbamazepine in epileptics patients. *Epilepsia.* 1986;27:548–552.

78. Yuen AWC, Land G, Weatherly BC, et al. Sodium valproate acutely inhibits lamotrigine metabolism. *Br J Clin Pharmacol.* 1992;33:511–513.

79. Kanner AM, Frey M. Adding valproate to lamotrigine: a study of their pharmacokinetic interaction. *Neurology.* 2000;55:588–591.

80. Gidal BE, Anderson GD, Rutecki PR, et al. Lack of an effect of valproate concentration on lamotrigine pharmacokinetics in developmentally disabled patients with epilepsy. *Epilepsy Res.* 2000;42:23–31.

81. Pisani FD, Perri RGD. Intravenous valproate: effects on plasma and saliva phenytoin levels. *Neurology.* 1981;31:467–470.

82. Rodin EA, Sousa GD, Haidukewych D, et al. Dissociation between free and bound phenytoin levels in presence of valproate sodium. *Arch Neurol.* 1981;38:240–242.

83. Mattson RH, Cramer JA, Darney PD, et al. Use of oral contraceptives by women with epilepsy. *JAMA.* 1986;256:238–240.

84. Herzog AG, Blum AS, Farina EL, et al. Valproate and lamotrigine level variation with menstrual cycle phase and oral contraceptive use. *Neurology.* 2009;72(10):911–914.

85. Jeavons PM, Clark JE, Maheshwari MC. Treatment of generalized epilepsies of childhood and adolescence with sodium valproate ("Epilim"). *Dev Med Child Neurol.* 1977;19:9–25.

86. Adams DJ, Lüders H, Pippenger CE. Sodium valproate in the treatment of intractable seizure disorders: a clinical and electroencephalographic study. *Neurology.* 1978;28:152–157.

87. Maheshwari MC, Jeavons PM. Proceedings: The effect of sodium valproate (Epilim) on the EEG. *Electroencephalogr Clin Neurophysiol.* 1975;39:429.

88. Braathen G, Theorell K, Persson A, et al. Valproate in the treatment of absence epilepsy in children. *Epilepsia.* 1988;29:548–552.

89. Mattson RH, Cramer JA, Williamson PD, et al. Valproic acid in epilepsy: clinical and pharmacological effects. *Ann Neurol.* 1978;3:20–25.

90. Callaghan N, O'Hare J, O'Driscoll, D, et al. Comparative study of ethosuximide and sodium valproate in the treatment of typical absence seizures (petit mal). *Dev Med Child Neurol.* 1982;24:830–836.

91. Sato S, White BG, Penry JK, et al. Valproic acid versus ethosuximide in the treatment of absence seizures. *Neurology.* 1982;32:157–163.

92. Bourgeois B, Beaumanoir A, Blajev B, et al. Monotherapy with valproate in primary generalized epilepsies. *Epilepsia.* 1987;28:S8–S11.

93. Covanis A, Gupta AK, Jeavons PM. Sodium valproate: monotherapy and polytherapy. *Epilepsia.* 1982;23:693–720.

94. Erenberg G, Rothner AD, Henry CE, et al. Valproic acid in the treatment of intractable absence seizures in children: a single-blind clinical and quantitative EEG study. *Am J Dis Child.* 1982;136:526–529.

95. Berkovic SF, Andermann F, Guberman A, et al. Valproate prevents the recurrence of absence status. *Neurology.* 1989;39:1294–1297.

96. Dulac O, Steru D, Rey E, et al. Sodium valproate (Na VPa) monotherapy in childhood epilepsy. *Arch Fr Pediatr.* 1982;39:347–352.

97. Ramsay RE, Wilder BJ, Murphy JV, et al. Efficacy and safety of valproic acid versus phenytoin as sole therapy for newly diagnosed primary generalized tonic–clonic seizures. *J Epilepsy.* 1992;5:55–60.

98. Spitz MC, Deasy DN. Conversion to valproate monotherapy in nonretarded adults with primary generalized tonic–clonic seizures. *J Epilepsy.* 1991;4:33–38.

99. Turnbull DM, Howel D, Rawlins MD, et al. Which drug for the adult epileptic patient: phenytoin or valproate? *Br Med J.* 1985;290:816–819.

100. Wilder BJ, Ramsay RE, Murphy JV, et al. Comparison of valproic acid and phenytoin in newly diagnosed tonic–clonic seizures. *Neurology.* 1983;33:1474–1476.

101. Feuerstein J. A long-term study of monotherapy with sodium valproate in primary generalized epilepsy. *Br J Clin Pract.* 1983;27:17–23.

102. Dulac O, Steru D, Rey E, et al. Sodium valproate monotherapy in childhood epilepsy. *Brain Dev.* 1986;8:47–52.

103. Delgado-Escueta AV, Enrile-Bacsal F. Juvenile myoclonic epilepsy of Janz. *Neurology.* 1984;34:285–294.

104. Fahn S. Post-anoxic action myoclonus: improvement with valproic acid. *N Engl J Med.* 1978;299:313–314.

105. Rollinson RD, Gilligan BS. Postanoxic action myoclonus (Lance–Adams syndrome) responding to valproate. *Arch Neurol.* 1979;36:44–45.

106. Iivanainen M, Himberg JJ. Valproate and clonazepam in the treatment of severe progressive myoclonus epilepsy. *Arch Neurol.* 1982;39:236–238.

107. Barnes SE, Bower BD. Sodium valproate in the treatment of intractable childhood epilepsy. *Dev Med Child Neurol.* 1975;17:175–181.

108. Olive D, Tridon P, Weber M. Effect of sodium dipropylacetate on certain varieties of epileptogenic encephalopathies in infants. *Schweiz Med Wochenschr.* 1969;99:87–92.

109. Rohmann E, Arndt, R. Effectiveness of ergenyl (dipropylacetate) in hypsarrhythmia. *Kinderarztl Prax.* 1976;44:109–113.

110. Dean JC, Penry JK. Valproate monotherapy in 30 patients with partial seizures. *Epilepsia.* 1988;29:140–144.

111. Loiseau P, Cohadon S, Jogeix M, et al. Efficacy of sodium valproate in partial epilepsy. Crossed study of valproate and carbamazepine. *Rev Neurol.* 1984;140:434–437.

112. Callaghan N, Kenny RA, O'Neill B, et al. A prospective study between carbamazepine, phenytoin and sodium valproate as monotherapy in previously untreated and recently diagnosed patients with epilepsy. *J Neurol Neurosurg Psychiatry.* 1985;48:639–644.

113. Mattson RH, Cramer JA, Collins JF. A comparison of valproate with carbamazepine for the treatment of complex partial seizures and secondarily generalized tonic–clonic seizures in adults. *N Engl J Med.* 1992;327:765–771.

114. Verity CM, Hosking G, Easter DJ. A multicentre comparative trial of sodium valproate and carabamazepine in paediatric epilepsy. The Paediatric EPITEG Collaborative Group. *Dev Med Child Neurol.* 1995;37:97–108.

115. DeSilva M, MacArdle B, McGowan M, et al. Randomized comparative monotherapy trial of phenobarbitone, phenytoin, carbamazepine, or sodium valproate for newly diagnosed childhood epilepsy. *Lancet.* 1996;347:709–713.

116. Beydoun A, Sackellares JC, Shu V. Safety and efficacy of divalproex sodium monotherapy in partial epilepsy: a double-blind, concentration-response design clinical trial. Depakote Monotherapy for Partial Seizures Study Group. *Neurology.* 1997;48:182–188.

117. Cavazzutti GB. Prevention of febrile convulsions with dipropylacetate (Depakine). *Epilepsia.* 1975;16:647–648.

118. Herranz JL, Armijo JA, Arteaga R. Effectiveness and toxicity of phenobarbital, primidone and sodium valproate in the prevention of febrile convulsions, controlled by plasma levels. *Epilepsia.* 1984;25:89–95.

119. Lee K, Melchior JC. Sodium valproate versus phenobarbital in the prophylactic treatment of febrile convulsions in childhood. *Eur J Pediatr.* 1981;137:151–153.

120. Mamelle N, Mamelle JC, Plasse JC, et al. Prevention of recurrent febrile convulsions—a randomized therapeutic assay: sodium valproate, phenobarbital and placebo. *Neuropediatrics.* 1984;15:37–42.

121. Minagawa K, Miura H. Phenobarbital, primidone and sodium valproate in the prophylaxis of febrile convulsions. *Brain Dev.* 1981;3:385–393.

122. Ngwane E, Bower B. Continuous sodium valproate or phenobarbitone in the prevention of simple febrile convulsions. Comparison by a double-blind trial. *Arch Dis Child.* 1980;55:171–174.

123. Rantala H, Tarkka R, Uhari M. A meta-analytic review of the preventive treatment of recurrences of febrile seizures. *J Pediatr.* 1997;131:922–925.

124. Steinberg A, Shaley RS, Amir N. Valproic acid in neonatal status convulsion. *Brain Dev.* 1986;8:278–279.

125. Karas BJ, Wilder BJ, Hammond EJ, et al. Treatment of valproate tremors. *Neurology.* 1983;33:1380–1382.

126. McLachlan RS. Pseudoatrophy of the brain with valproic acid monotherapy. *Can J Neurol Sci.* 1987;14:294–296.

127. Papazian O, Canizales E, Alfonso I, et al. Reversible dementia and apparent brain atrophy during valproate therapy. *Ann Neurol.* 1995;38:687–691.

128. Shin C, Gray L, Armond C. Reversible cerebral atrophy: radiologic correlate of valproate-induced parkinson-dementia syndrome. *Neurology.* 1992;42:277.

129. Marescaux C, Warter JM, Micheletti G, et al. Stuporous episodes during treatment with sodium valproate: report of seven cases. *Epilepsia.* 1982;23:297–305.

130. Sackellares JC, Lee SI, Dreifuss FE. Stupor following administration of valproic acid to patients receiving other antiepileptic drugs. *Epilepsia.* 1979;20:697–703.

131. Meador KJ, Baker GA, Browning N, et al. Cognitive function at 3 years of age after fetal exposure to antiepileptic drugs. *N Engl J Med.* 2009;360(16):1597–1605.

132. Dean JC, Penry JK. Weight gain patterns in patients with epilepsy: comparison of antiepileptic drugs. *Epilepsia.* 1995;36:72.

133. Dinesen H, Gram L, Andersen, T, et al. Weight gain during treatment with valproate. *Acta Neurol Scand.* 1984;70:65–69.

134. Breum L, Astrup A, Gram L, et al. Metabolic changes during treatment with valproate in humans: implications for weight gain. *Metabolism.* 1992;41:666–670.

135. Bryant AEI, Dreifuss FE. Valproic acid hepatic fatalities. III. U.S. experience since 1986. *Neurology.* 1996;46:465–469.
136. Dreifuss FE, Santilli N, Langer DH, et al. Valproic acid hepatic fatalities: a retrospective view. *Neurology.* 1987;37:379–385.
137. König SA, Siemes H, Blaker F, et al. Severe hepatotoxicity during valproate therapy: an update and report of eight new fatalities. *Epilepsia.* 1994;35:1005–1015.
138. Scheffner D, König S, Rauterberg-Ruland I, et al. Fatal liver failure in 16 children with valproate therapy. *Epilepsia.* 1988;29:530–542.
139. Bohan TP, Helton E, McDonald I, et al. Effect of L-carnitine treatment for valproate-induced hepatotoxicity. *Neurology.* 2001;56:1405–1409.
140. Asconape JJ, Penry JK, Dreifuss FE, et al. Valproate-associated pancreatitis. *Epilepsia.* 1993;34:177–183.
141. Camfield PR. Pancreatitis due to valproic acid. *Lancet.* 1979;1:1198–1199.
142. Coulter DL, Allen RJ. Pancreatitis associated with valproic acid therapy for epilepsy. *Ann Neurol.* 1980;7:693–720.
143. Williams LHP, Reynolds RP, Emery JL. Pancreatitis during sodium valproate treatment. *Arch Dis Child.* 1983;58:543–544.
144. Wyllie E, Wyllie R, Cruse RP, et al. Pancreatitis associated with valproic acid therapy. *Am J Dis Child.* 1984;138:912–914.
145. Hauser E, Seidl R, Freilinger M, et al. Hematologic manifestations and impaired liver synthetic function during valproate monotherapy. *Brain Dev.* 1996;18:105–109.
146. May RB, Sunder TR. Hematologic manifestations of long-term valproate therapy. *Epilepsia.* 1993;34:1098–1101.
147. Neophytides AN, Nutt JG, Lodish JR. Thrombocytopenia associated with sodium valproate treatment. *Ann Neurol.* 1978;5:389–390.
148. Kis B, Szupera Z, Mezei Z, et al. Influence of valproate monotherapy on platelet activation and hematologic values. *Epilepsia.* 1999;40:186–189.
149. Zeller JA, Schlesinger S, Runge U, et al. Influence of valproate monotherapy on platelet activation and hematologic values. *Epilepsia.* 1999;40(2):186–189.
150. Gidal B, Spencer N, Maly M, et al. Valproate-mediated disturbances of hemostasis: relationship to dose and plasma concentration. *Neurology.* 1994;44:1418–1422.
151. Kreuz W, Linde M, Funk R, et al. Valproate therapy induces von Willebrand disease type I. *Epilepsia.* 1991;33:178–184.
152. Anderson GD, Lin YX, Berge C, et al. Absence of bleeding complications in patients undergoing cortical surgery while receiving valproate treatment. *J Neurosurg.* 1997;87:252–256.
153. Ward MM, Barbaro NM, Laxer KD, et al. Preoperative valproate administration does not increase blood loss during temporal lobectomy. *Epilepsia.* 1996;37:98–101.
154. Winter SL, Kriel RL, Novacheck TF, et al. Perioperative blood loss: the effect of valproate. *Pediatr Neurol.* 1996;15:19–22.
155. Haidukewych D, John G, Zielinski JJ, et al. Chronic valproic acid therapy and incidence of increases in venous plasma ammonia. *Ther Drug Monit.* 1985;7:290–294.
156. Zaccara G, Paganini M, Campostrini R, et al. Effect of associated antiepileptic treatment on valproate-induced hyperammonemia. *Ther Drug Monit.* 1985;7:185–190.
157. Gidal BE, Inglese CM, Meyer JF, et al. Diet- and valproate-induced transient hyperammonemia: effect of L-carnitine. *Pediatr Neurol.* 1997;16:301–305.
158. Bohles H, Sewell AC, Wenzel D. The effect of carnitine supplementation in valproate-induced hyperammonaemia. *Acta Paediatr.* 1996;85:446–449.
159. Coulter DL. Carnitine deficiency in epilepsy: risk factors and treatment. *J Child Neurol.* 1995;10:S32–S39.
160. Laub MC, Paetake-Brunner I, Jaeger G. Serum carnitine during valproate acid therapy. *Epilepsia.* 1986;27:559–562.
161. Ishikura H, Matsuo N, Matsubara M, et al. Valproic acid overdose and L-carnitine therapy. *J Anal Toxicol.* 1996;20:55–58.
162. Murakami K, Sugimoto T, Woo M, et al. Effect of L-carnitine supplementation on acute valproate intoxication. *Epilepsia.* 1996;37:687–689.
163. Vivo DD, Bohan T, Coulter DL, et al. L-carnitine supplementation in childhood epilepsy: current perspectives. *Epilepsia.* 1998;39:1216–1225.
164. Isojärvi JI, Laatikainen TJ, Knip M, et al. Obesity and endocrine disorders in women taking valproate for epilepsy. *Ann Neurol.* 1996;39:579–584.
165. Isojärvi JI, Laatikainen TJ, Pakarinen AJ, et al. Polycystic ovaries and hyperandrogenism in women taking valproate for epilepsy. *N Engl J Med.* 1993;19:1383–1388.
166. Isojärvi JI, Rattya J, Myllyla VV, et al. Valproate, lamotrigine, and insulin-mediated risks in women with epilepsy. *Ann Neurol.* 1998;43:446–451.
167. Margraf JW, Dreifuss FE. Amenorrhea following initiation of therapy with valproic acid. *Neurology.* 1981;31:159.
168. Luef G, Abraham I, Trinka E, et al. Hyperandrogenism, postprandial hyperinsulinism and the risk of PCOS in a cross sectional study of women with epilepsy treated with valproate. *Epilepsy Res.* 2002;48:295–304.
169. Sharma S, Jacobs HS. Polycystic ovary syndrome associated with treatment with the anticonvulsant sodium valproate. *Curr Opin Obstet Gynecol.* 1997;9:391–392.
170. Bjerkedal T, Czeizel A, Goujard J, et al. Valproic acid and spina bifida. *Lancet.* 1982;2:1096.
171. Genton P, Bauer J, Duncan S, et al. On the association of valproate and polycystic ovaries. *Epilepsia.* 2001;42:295–304.
172. Isojärvi JI, Tauboll E, Tapanainen JS, et al. On the association between valproate and polycystic ovary syndrome: a response and an alternative view. *Epilepsia.* 2001;42:305–310.
173. Lindhout D, Meinardi H. Spina bifida and in-utero exposure to valproate. *Lancet.* 1984;2:396.
174. Omtzigt JGC, Los FJ, Grobbee DE, et al. The risk of spina bifida aperta after first-trimester exposure to valproate in a prenatal cohort. *Neurology.* 1992;42(4 suppl 5):119–125.
175. Duncan S, Mercho S, Lopes-Cendes I, et al. Repeated neural tube defects and valproate monotherapy suggest a pharmacogenetic abnormality. *Epilepsia.* 2001;42:750–753.
176. Wegner C, Nau H. Alteration of embryonic folate metabolism by valproic acid during organogenesis. *Neurology.* 1992;42:17–24.
177. Jeavons PM, Clark JE, Harding GFA. Valproate and curly hair. *Lancet.* 1977;1:359.
178. Herranz JL, Arteaga R, Armijo JA. Change in hair colour induced by valproic acid. *Dev Med Child Neurol.* 1987;23:386–387.
179. Ettinger A, Moshe S, Shinnar S. Edema associated with long-term valproate therapy. *Epilepsia.* 1990;31:211–213.
180. Choonra IA. Sodium valproate and enuresis. *Lancet.* 1985;1:1276.
181. Herranz JL, Arteaga R, Armijo JA. Side effects of sodium valproate in monotherapy controlled by plasma levels: a study in 88 pediatric patients. *Epilepsia.* 1982;23:203–214.
182. Panayiotopoulos CP. Nocturnal enuresis associated with sodium valproate. *Lancet.* 1985;1:980–981.
183. Branten AJ, Wetzels JF, Weber AM, et al. Hyponatremia due to sodium valproate. *Ann Neurol.* 1998;43:265–267.
184. Hyson C, Sadler M. Cross sensitivity of skin rashes with antiepileptic drugs. *Can J Neurol Sci.* 1997;24:245–249.
185. Lundberg B, Nergardh A, Boreus LO. Plasma concentrations of valproate during maintenance therapy in epileptic children. *J Neurol.* 1982;228:133–141.
186. Devinsky O, Leppik I, Willmore LJ, et al. Safety of intravenous valproate. *Ann Neurol.* 1995;38:670–674.
187. Giroud M, Gras D, Escousse A, et al. Use of injectable valproic acid in status epilepticus: a pilot study. *Drug Invest.* 1993;5:154–159.
188. Limdi NA, Faught E. The safety of rapid valproic acid infusion. *Epilepsia.* 2000;41:1342–1345.
189. Wheless J, Venkataraman V. Safety of high intravenous valproate loading doses in epilepsy patients. *J Epilepsy.* 1998;11:319–324.
190. Venkataraman V, Wheless J. Safety of rapid intravenous infusion of valproate loading doses in epilepsy patients. *Epilepsy Res.* 1999;35:147–153.
191. Gjerloff I, Arentsen J, Alving J, et al. Monodose versus 3 daily doses of sodium valproate: a controlled trial. *Acta Neurol Scand.* 1984;69:120–124.
192. Stefan H, Burr W, Fichel H, et al. Intensive follow-up monitoring in patients with once daily evening administration of sodium valproate. *Epilepsia.* 1974;25:152–160.
193. Brachet-Liermain A, Demarquez JL. Pharmacokinetics of dipropylacetate in infants and young children. *Pharm Weekbl.* 1977;112:293–297.
194. Bruni J, Wilder BJ. Valproic acid. Review of a new antiepileptic drug. *Arch Neurol.* 1979;36:393–398.
195. Burr W, Fröscher W, Hoffmann F, et al. Lack of significant correlation between circadian profiles of valproic acid serum levels and epileptiform electroencephalographic activity. *Ther Drug Monit.* 1984;6:179–181.
196. Rowan AJ, Binnie CD, Warfield CA, et al. The delayed effect of sodium valproate on the photoconvulsive response in man. *Epilepsia.* 1979;20:61–68.
197. Chadwick DW. Concentration-effect relationships of valproic acid. *Clin Pharmacokinet.* 1985;10:155–163.

CHAPTER 52 ■ PHENYTOIN AND FOSPHENYTOIN

DIEGO A. MORITA AND TRACY A. GLAUSER

HISTORICAL BACKGROUND

Phenytoin

From the second half of the 19th century until 1938, the antiepileptic effect of commonly used medications (bromides and phenobarbital) was attributed to their sedative effects (1). The landmark work of Merritt and Putnam in 1937 and 1938 (2,3) demonstrated that the antiepileptic potential of drugs could be tested in animals, the anticonvulsant effect and sedative effects could be separated, and anticonvulsant activity could be achieved without sedation. Phenytoin (compared with bromides and phenobarbital) showed the greatest anticonvulsant potency with the least hypnotic activity in the cat model they devised, which compared a drug's ability to change the seizure threshold with its sedative effects.

In a subsequent series of articles, Merritt and Putnam demonstrated that phenytoin was effective in humans; the first clinical trial of phenytoin in epilepsy (4) documented freedom from seizures in 50% of 142 patients with refractory disease. This trial showed, for the first time, that a drug effective against seizures in experimental animals could be successfully used in humans. In fact, Merritt and Putnam's electroconvulsive test in animals remains the most reliable experimental indicator of antiepileptic drug (AED) efficacy in tonic–clonic and partial seizures in humans. A follow-up study described effectiveness in complex partial seizures, with or without secondarily generalized tonic–clonic seizures, but not in absence seizures (5). Today, phenytoin is one of the world's most widely prescribed AEDs (6).

Fosphenytoin

Because phenytoin is poorly soluble in water, parenteral phenytoin sodium has been formulated as an aqueous vehicle containing propylene glycol, ethanol, and sodium hydroxide, adjusted to a pH of 12 (7,8). Unfortunately, parenteral phenytoin sodium is associated with cardiovascular complications and phlebitis (9,10). First synthesized in 1973, fosphenytoin was developed as a water-soluble phenytoin prodrug that might reduce the risks of the cardiovascular complications and phlebitis from parenteral phenytoin administration (11).

CHEMISTRY AND MECHANISM OF ACTION

Phenytoin

Phenytoin is commercially available as the free acid and the sodium salt. The molecular weight is 252.26 for the free acid

and 274.25 for the sodium salt. A weak organic acid, phenytoin is poorly soluble in water. The apparent dissociation constant (pK_a) ranges from 8.1 to 9.2 and requires an alkaline solution to achieve solubility in high concentrations. As a result, parenteral phenytoin sodium must be formulated as an aqueous vehicle containing 40% propylene glycol and 10% ethanol in water for injection, adjusted to a pH of 12 with sodium hydroxide (7,8,11).

Phenytoin affects ion conductance, sodium–potassium adenosine triphosphatase activity, various enzyme systems, synaptic transmission, posttetanic potentiation, neurotransmitter release, and cyclic nucleotide metabolism (12). Despite these numerous sites of action, the major anticonvulsant mechanism of action is believed to be the drug's effect on the sodium channel. Phenytoin blocks membrane channels through which sodium moves from the outside to the inside of the neuron during depolarization, suppressing the sustained repetitive firing that results from presynaptic stimulation (12–14).

Fosphenytoin

Fosphenytoin, a phenytoin prodrug, is the disodium phosphate ester of 3-hydroxymethyl-5,5-diphenylhydantoin (molecular weight 406.24) (Fig. 52.1). Following conversion, 1.5 mg of fosphenytoin yields 1 mg of phenytoin. To avoid confusion, fosphenytoin (Cerebyx) is packaged as milligram phenytoin equivalents (mg PE). Thus, 100 mg of parenteral phenytoin (Dilantin) and 100 mg PE of parenteral fosphenytoin (Cerebyx) have equal molar amounts of phenytoin.

Fosphenytoin's phosphate ester group on the basic phenytoin molecule significantly increases solubility. The water solubility of fosphenytoin at 37°C is 75,000 µg/mL, compared with 20.5 µg/mL for phenytoin (11). Thus, fosphenytoin is freely soluble in aqueous solutions and can be formulated without organic solvents (15). Fosphenytoin is formulated as a ready-mix solution of 50 mg PE/mL in water for injection, USP, and tromethamine, USP (Tris) buffer adjusted to pH 8.6 to 9.0 with either hydrochloric acid, NF, or sodium hydroxide,

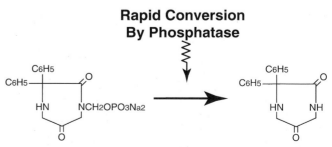

FIGURE 52.1. Structural formulas of fosphenytoin (*left*) and phenytoin (*right*).

NF (16). Fosphenytoin itself has no known anticonvulsant activity and derives its utility from its rapid and total conversion to phenytoin (15,16).

ABSORPTION, DISTRIBUTION, METABOLISM, AND EXCRETION

Phenytoin

Absorption

Phenytoin is available in various formulations for both oral and parenteral use (Table 52.1). Both the rate and extent of absorption may differ among the formulations, leading to clinically significant alterations in serum concentrations when switching among products.

The rate and extent of absorption of phenytoin from its site of entrance depends on pK_a and lipid solubility, the pH of the medium in which it is dissolved, solubility in the medium, and concentration. These factors are frequently altered by the presence of foods or drugs in the intestinal tract and by the formulations. Little phenytoin is absorbed in the stomach because the drug is insoluble in the acidic pH of gastric juice (about 2.0), even though it is in its nonionized form in the stomach. Absorption occurs primarily in the duodenum, where the higher pH increases the solubility of phenytoin. Absorption from the jejunum and ileum is slower than from the duodenum and is poor from the colon (17,18).

In humans, the rate of absorption is variable and prolonged (19,20), and significantly influenced by the rate of elimination (21). Because dissolution is the rate-limiting process in the absorption of phenytoin, any factor that affects dissolution or solubility will affect absorption. After oral administration of a single dose, peak blood drug levels are generally reached between 4 and 8 hours later (range, 3 to 12 hours) (22,23). In patients ingesting massive amounts of phenytoin, absorption may continue for as long as 60 hours (24). Relative bioavailability increases with age, suggesting an age-dependent effect on drug absorption (25). In newborns and infants up to 3 months old, phenytoin is absorbed slowly and incompletely after both oral and intramuscular administration (26); absorption in older infants and children is similar to that in adults. Stable isotope tracer doses have been used to assess the bioavailability of phenytoin (27,28).

After intramuscular administration, phenytoin is absorbed slowly, as poor water solubility leads to precipitation of drug at the injection site, forming almost a depot repository (20). This prolonged absorption and pain on administration mandate use of the intravenous route if parenteral administration is required.

The reported bioavailability of rectally administered phenytoin sodium is approximately 25% (29).

Absorption of Generic Preparations

Several generic phenytoin preparations have been approved by the Food and Drug Administration (FDA) and are available in the United States; however, they are not equivalent owing to differences in their rate of absorption. Most of the generic products are not rated as bioequivalent to brand name Dilantin because of their rapid ("prompt") absorption profile. Steady-state concentrations of the prompt formulation have been found to be either higher than those of the brand extended-release form (30), lower (31,32), or not different (33). Thus, when stable concentrations are desirable, an extended-release profile is preferred. In 1998, a 100-mg generic extended-release product (manufactured by Mylan Pharmaceuticals) was approved as bioequivalent to Dilantin Kapseals 100 mg.

In contrast, the generic prompt-release formulation is useful when rapid serum concentrations are desired, such as with an oral loading dose. Prompt-release phenytoin administered in three divided doses of 6 mg/kg every 3 hours reaches maximal concentrations almost 4 hours sooner than does the brand name extended-release form given according to the same regimen (34).

Distribution

Protein Binding. Phenytoin is approximately 90% bound to plasma proteins, primarily albumin, in most healthy, ambulatory patients. Only the unbound (free) portion is pharmacologically active because protein-bound drug cannot cross the

TABLE 52.1

FORMULATIONS OF PHENYTOIN AND FOSPHENYTOIN

Formulation	Preparation	Strength	Acid or salt	Amount of drug	Prompt or extended
Dilantin Kapseals	Capsule	30 mg	Sodium salt	27.6 mg	Extended
Dilantin Kapseals	Capsule	100 mg	Sodium salt	92 mg	Extended
Dilantin Infatabs	Chewable tablet	50 mg	Free acid	50 mg	Prompt
Dilantin-125 suspension	Suspension	125 mg/5 mL	Free acid	125 mg/mL	Prompt
Phenytek	Capsule	200 mg	Sodium salt	184 mg	Extended
Phenytek	Capsule	300 mg	Sodium salt	276 mg	Extended
Phenytoin (generic)	Capsule	30 mg	Sodium salt	27.6 mg	Prompt and extended
Phenytoin (generic)[a]	Capsule	100 mg	Sodium salt	92 mg	Prompt and extended
Phenytoin (generic)	Suspension	125 mg/5 mL	Free acid	125 mg/mL	Prompt
Phenytoin (generic)	Injectable solution	50 mg/mL	Sodium salt	46 mg/mL	
Fosphenytoin	Injectable solution	50 mg PE/mL	Disodium salt	50 mg PE/mL	

[a]The prompt-release generic phenytoin 100-mg capsules are not bioequivalent to Dilantin 100-mg Kapseals. The extended-release generic phenytoin 100-mg capsules are considered bioequivalent. The prescriber should be cautious when writing prescriptions.

blood–brain barrier. Because unbound phenytoin distributes passively between plasma and cerebrospinal fluid, concentrations are the same in both sites (35), and the unbound plasma concentration can be used to estimate the cerebrospinal fluid concentration (18).

The generally established therapeutic range for phenytoin of 10 to 20 μg/mL includes both bound and unbound drugs. As 10% is normally unbound, the equivalent unbound therapeutic range is 1 to 2 μg/mL. The extent of protein binding varies little with phenytoin plasma concentration.

The percentage of binding (70% to 95%) depends on albumin concentration and coexisting medications or illnesses. Low serum albumin, renal failure, or concomitant medications that displace phenytoin from protein-binding sites increase the risk for changes in protein binding. Both exogenous (other highly protein-bound medications) and endogenous (increased bilirubin) substances can compete for binding sites and increase unbound phenytoin concentrations. Valproic acid significantly alters phenytoin binding to serum albumin, whereas phenobarbital, ethosuximide, diazepam, carbamazepine, and folic acid do not (36). Binding is decreased in uremia (84.2%), hepatic disease, and acquired immunodeficiency syndrome (18); in renal dysfunction, it is most apparent at creatinine clearances below 25 mL/min (37). In patients with uremia who undergo renal transplantation, binding returns to normal when renal function recovers (38).

Total phenytoin concentrations that are below the normal range can be associated with unbound phenytoin concentrations in the therapeutic range. For example, if a patient has a subtherapeutic total phenytoin concentration of 5 μg/mL but an unbound fraction of 20%, the equivalent unbound phenytoin concentration is 1 μg/mL, which is in the "therapeutic" range. Thus patients at high risk for altered protein binding may respond to clinically subtherapeutic total concentrations and may not tolerate total serum concentrations within the therapeutic range. If such patients experience toxic reactions despite therapeutic concentrations, measurement of unbound concentrations may be warranted. Total phenytoin concentrations may be a misleading test in developing countries, where hypoalbuminemia is highly prevalent (39).

Among the methods that predict total phenytoin concentrations in the face of reduced albumin levels, the best documented is the Sheiner-Tozer method (40,41):

$$C_n = C_o/(0.2 \times \text{Alb} + 0.1)$$

where C_o is the measured total phenytoin concentration (milligrams/liter), Alb is albumin concentration (grams/deciliter), and C_n is the total phenytoin concentration that would have been observed with normal albumin concentrations.

Volume of Distribution. Phenytoin is distributed freely in the body with an average volume of distribution in humans of 0.78 L/kg (18). The volume of distribution after single intravenous doses (9.4 to 21.3 mg/kg) in children declines with age and range from 1 to 1.5 L/kg below the age of 5 years and from 0.6 to 0.8 L/kg above the age of 8 years (42). At the pH of plasma, phenytoin exists predominantly in the nonionized form, thus allowing rapid movement across cell membranes by nonionic diffusion. The volume of distribution, which correlates with body weight (43), is larger in morbidly obese patients, who may require large loading doses to achieve therapeutic concentrations (44,45).

Metabolism

In humans, the major pathway of phenytoin elimination (approximately 80%) is 4′-hydroxylation to form 5-(4′-hydroxyphenyl)-5-phenylhydantoin (4′-HPPH). This reaction is mediated mainly by the cytochrome P450 (CYP) enzyme CYP2C9, and to a lesser extent by CYP2C19 (46,47). Approximately 10% of phenytoin is eliminated to a dihydrodiol, and another 10% is metabolized to 5-(3-hydroxyphenyl)-5-phenylhydantoin (3′,4′-diHPPH) (7,46,48). An arene oxide, which precedes the formation of these compounds, has been implicated in the toxicity and teratogenicity of phenytoin; however, its transient presence in patients with normally functioning arene oxide detoxification systems is unlikely to account for many of the toxic reactions (49,50).

Because phenytoin has nonlinear pharmacokinetics, a narrow therapeutic index, and a concentration-related toxicity profile, small changes in CYP2C9 activity may be clinically significant. Of the more than 30 CYP2C9 alleles identified to date, the most common, designated as CYP2C9*1, is considered the wild-type allele (51,52). Individuals homozygous for the wild-type allele are called extensive metabolizers. Studies in various populations demonstrated that the CYP2C9*2, CYP2C9*3, CYP2C9*4, and CYP2C9*6 alleles are important in vivo determinants of phenytoin disposition (53–62). Individuals with at least one of these variant alleles are called poor metabolizers and have a reduced ability to metabolize phenytoin. They may require lower-than-average phenytoin doses to decrease the incidence of concentration-dependent adverse effects (57,63).

While two thirds of Caucasians possess the wild-type allele, one third are heterozygous for the CYP2C9*2 or CYP2C9*3 allele (51). These two variant alleles are much less prevalent in African Americans and Asians, with more than 95% of these groups expressing the wild-type genotype (51). The CYP2C9*4, CYP2C9*5, and CYP2C9*6 allelic variants have been identified in the Japanese (CYP2C9*4) and African American (CYP2C9*5 and CYP2C9*6) populations (62,64,65). The CYP2C9*7 through CYP2C9*12 alleles have been discovered by resequencing CYP2C9 DNA from Caucasians, Asians, and Africans (African Americans and African Pygmies) (66). A study in a Black Beninese population, demonstrated that CYP2C9 alleles *5, *6, *8, and *11 were associated with a decreased phenytoin metabolism (67). The allele CYP2C9*13 was identified in the Chinese population, and found to be associated with reduced plasma clearance of drugs that are substrates for CYP2C9 (68). A clear association between the newer discovered alleles and an altered phenytoin metabolism has not yet been demonstrated. The allelic variants CYP2C9*14 to CYP2C9*20 were found in a recent study of Southeast Asians (Chinese and Indians) (69). The alleles CYP2C9*21 to CYP2C9*23 were described in European Americans (70). CYP2C19*24 was described in a patient on warfarin therapy (71). The alleles CYP2C19*25 to CYP2C19*30 were recently reported in the Japanese population (72). Two recently discovered allelic variants, CYP2C9*31 and CYP2C9*32, were described in the African population (73).

Odani and coworkers observed a decrease of approximately 30% in the maximal rate of phenytoin elimination in Japanese heterozygous for CYP2C9*3 compared with those homozygous for the wild-type allele (53). Moreover, the mean phenytoin maintenance dose leading to a therapeutic serum concentration was significantly lower in patients with CYP2C9 allelic variants (199 ± 42.5 mg/day) than in those with the wild-type allele (314 ± 61.2 mg/day; $P < 0.01$) (57). A case report of a heterozygous CYP2C9*3 allele carrier described excessive phenytoin concentrations relative to the doses taken; a toxic level (32.6 μg/mL) was reached despite a modest dose (187.5 mg/day). The patient showed signs of central nervous system intoxication, ataxia, and diplopia (58).

The activity of CYP2C9 alone, however, does not fully explain the large interindividual variability in the clinical pharmacokinetics and reported drug interactions of phenytoin (74). More than 20 CYP2C19 alleles have been described to date (52). The first seven, CYP2C19*2 to CYP2C19*8, are inactive and are responsible for the poor-metabolizer phenotype. The allelic variants CYP2C19*9 to CYP2C19*15 are potentially defective, although none have yet been studied in vivo (75). The CYP2C19*17 variant has been associated with ultrarapid drug metabolisms for two of its substrates, omeprazole and escitalopram, which might imply increased risk of therapeutic failure (76,77).

The majority of all populations studied have the CYP2C19 extensive-metabolizer phenotype involving the wild-type CYP2C19*1 allele. The frequency of CYP2C19 poor metabolizers is much higher in Asians (13% to 23%) than in Caucasians and African Americans (1% to 6%) (78). The CYP2C19*2 and CYP2C19*3 mutations are responsible for most of the CYP2C19 poor metabolizers. CYP2C19*2, the main defective allele, occurs with a frequency of 30% in the Chinese population, approximately 15% in Caucasians, and approximately 17% in African Americans. The CYP2C19*3 variant affects approximately 5% of Chinese, and is almost nonexistent in Caucasians (79). Together, the CYP2C19*2 and CYP2C19*3 alleles can explain all Asian and approximately 80% of Caucasian poor metabolizers (80).

Because the contribution of CYP2C19 to the metabolism of phenytoin increases with an increase in drug concentration, CYP2C19 may be important when CYP2C9 is saturated. The reported differences in K_m values for CYP2C9-catalyzed and CYP2C19-catalyzed phenytoin hydroxylation (5.5 μmol/L vs. 71.4 μmol/L) suggest that CYP2C9 is likely to become saturated at phenytoin therapeutic concentrations of 10 to 20 μg/mL (40 to 80 μmol/L) (81). This mechanism explains the increased risk of toxic reactions with the coadministration of CYP2C19 inhibitors such as ticlopidine or isoniazid. The 1% to 2% of Caucasian poor metabolizers for both CYP2C9 and CYP2C19 are particularly susceptible to phenytoin's adverse effects (78). Dosage adjustments based on the CYP2C9 and CYP2C19 genotypes may decrease the risk of concentration-dependent adverse effects in allelic variant carriers, particularly at the beginning of therapy.

A Japanese epilepsy study (53) noted an approximate decrease of 14% in the maximum metabolic rate in patients with CYP2C19 variants compared with those with the extensive-metabolizer phenotype. In another Japanese study (54), the predicted plasma concentrations with a phenytoin dose of 5 mg/kg/day were 18.7, 22.8, and 28.8 μg/mL in CYP2C19 homozygous extensive metabolizers, heterozygous extensive metabolizers, and poor metabolizers, respectively. Although the effect of CYP2C polymorphisms on the pharmacokinetic parameters has been reported, caution is advised when estimating the usefulness of genotyping the CYP2C subfamily for the determination of phenytoin dosage regimens. There are

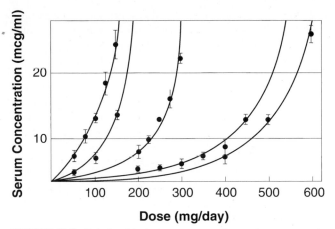

FIGURE 52.2. Relationship between serum phenytoin concentration and daily dose in five patients. Each point represents the mean (±SD) of three to eight measurements at steady state. The curves were fitted by computer through use of the Michaelis–Menten equation. (From Richens A, Dunlop A. Serum phenytoin levels in the management of epilepsy. *Lancet.* 1975;2:247–248, with permission.)

other factors, such as concurrent drug treatment and many environmental factors, that may overwhelm the significance of genotyping in clinical practice (82,83).

Enzyme saturation kinetics lead to phenytoin plasma concentrations increasing nonproportionally with changes in dose (Fig. 52.2) (84). The relationship between dose and concentration can be expressed by the Michaelis–Menten equation:

$$\text{Dose (mg/day)} = \frac{V_{max} C_{ss}}{K_m + C_{ss}}$$

where V_{max} is the maximal rate of drug metabolism, C_{ss} the steady-state serum concentration, and K_m the concentration at which V_{max} is half-maximal. The mean apparent phenytoin K_m in adults 20 to 39 years old is 5.7 μg/mL (range, 1.5 to 20.7 μg/mL); the mean V_{max} is 7.5 mg/kg/day (85). In most patients, phenytoin exhibits nonlinear pharmacokinetics because the usual therapeutic plasma concentrations exceed the usual K_m. Concomitant illnesses (86) or medications, pregnancy (87,88), genetic makeup (89–91), and age can significantly affect V_{max} or K_m (or both). Children have higher V_{max} values, but similar K_m values, compared with adults (92–94); elderly individuals have lower V_{max} values (mean, 6.0 mg/kg/day) (85).

Excretion

Up to 95% of phenytoin is excreted in urine and feces as metabolites, with 5% or less of unchanged phenytoin excreted in urine. Phenytoin is also excreted in breast milk (95). Some investigators have suggested that phenytoin enhances its own elimination through enzyme induction (96).

Fosphenytoin

Absorption and Bioavailability

Fosphenytoin can be administered either intravenously or intramuscularly. The values for the area under the plasma total phenytoin and free phenytoin concentration versus time curves, after either intravenous or intramuscular administration of fosphenytoin, are almost identical to that for intravenous phenytoin sodium, indicating complete bioavailability by either route (11). These findings are based on studies involving single-dose intravenous and intramuscular administration to drug-free volunteers and single-dose intravenous administration to patients with therapeutic plasma phenytoin concentrations (11,97,98).

The total and complete conversion to phenytoin presents a potential clinical problem. A milligram for mg PE conversion from oral phenytoin (Dilantin) capsules to parenteral fosphenytoin (Cerebyx) solution represents a 9% increase in total dosage, because 100-mg Dilantin capsules actually contain only 92 mg of phenytoin. Dosage adjustment is not usually necessary when Cerebyx is used for up to 1 week, although a phenytoin plasma concentration should be checked after longer periods of administration.

Distribution

Protein Binding. Like phenytoin, fosphenytoin is highly bound (95% to 99%) to serum albumin in a nonlinear fashion (11). This protein binding is not affected by prior diazepam administration (99). However, in the presence of fosphenytoin, phenytoin is displaced from binding sites, rapidly increasing unbound phenytoin concentrations as a function of plasma fosphenytoin concentration. This displacement is accentuated by fosphenytoin doses of at least 15 mg PE/kg delivered at rates of 50 to 150 mg PE/min. As plasma fosphenytoin concentrations decline, phenytoin protein binding returns to normal. There is little displacement of phenytoin after intramuscular administration of fosphenytoin (11).

Volume of Distribution. Fosphenytoin's volume of distribution is reported to be 0.13 L/kg in patients receiving 1200 mg PE fosphenytoin at 150 mg PE/min. At lower doses and slower infusion rates, the volume of distribution is lower, 2.6 L, or approximately 0.04 L/kg for a 70-kg human (11,97,100). Fosphenytoin, a very polar molecule, achieves a rapid equilibrium between plasma and associated tissues (100).

Metabolism

After intravenous or intramuscular administration, the phosphate group of fosphenytoin is cleaved by ubiquitous nonspecific phosphatases to produce active phenytoin. The half-life of this conversion is approximately 8 to 18 minutes, is complete in a little more than an hour, and is independent of age, dose, or infusion rate (11,16,101–103). The tissue phosphatases responsible for this conversion are present at all ages; age, plasma phenytoin or fosphenytoin concentrations, and other medications do not alter their activity. The conversion of fosphenytoin to phenytoin is slightly faster in patients with hepatic or renal disease, consistent with decreased binding of fosphenytoin to plasma proteins and increased fraction of unbound fosphenytoin resulting from hypoproteinemia in these diseases (101). In addition, fosphenytoin's phosphate load of 0.0037 mmol phosphate/mg PE fosphenytoin should be considered in patients with severe renal impairment (16).

A pharmacokinetic meta-analysis of plasma total and free phenytoin concentration from seven clinical trials involving neurosurgical patients, patients with status epilepticus, patients with stroke, and healthy volunteers demonstrated that fosphenytoin loading doses of 15 to 20 mg PE/kg administered either intravenously or intramuscularly consistently

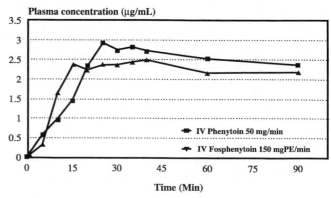

FIGURE 52.3. Free phenytoin concentration achieved in patients receiving an equivalent intravenous phenytoin-loading dose (20 mg/kg) at 50 mg/min and an equivalent intravenous fosphenytoin loading dose at 150 mg PE/min. (From Eldon M, Loewen G, Voightman R, et al. Pharmacokinetics and tolerance of fosphenytoin and phenytoin administration intravenously to healthy subjects. *Can J Neurol Sci.* 1993;20:5810, with permission.)

resulted in total phenytoin plasma concentrations of 10 μg/mL or more and free phenytoin concentrations of 1 μg/mL or more. These therapeutic plasma phenytoin concentrations were reached in most subjects within 10 minutes, if rapid intravenous fosphenytoin dosing (≥100 mg PE/min) was used, or within 30 minutes, if slower intravenous (<100 mg PE/min) or intramuscular fosphenytoin dosing was used (104).

In one study, after administration of 1200 mg of phenytoin at 50 mg/min, peak unbound phenytoin concentrations of approximately 3 μg/mL were achieved within 0.5 hour; administration of the equivalent fosphenytoin dose, infused at a rate of 150 mg PE/min, produced similar peak unbound phenytoin concentrations (Fig. 52.3) (105). This rapid infusion rate was well tolerated (see below). Therefore, when rapid achievement of therapeutic phenytoin concentrations is critical, as in the treatment of status epilepticus, fosphenytoin should be administered at a rate of 150 mg PE/min. Slower infusion rates (50 to 100 mg PE/min) may be acceptable in nonemergencies (105).

Excretion

A clinically insignificant amount of fosphenytoin (0% to 4% of a dose) is excreted renally (103).

PLASMA DRUG CONCENTRATIONS

Phenytoin

Most laboratories and textbooks assume a therapeutic range for phenytoin of 10 to 20 μg/mL, which clinical experience and literature have called into question. Seizures have been controlled with concentrations lower than 10 μg/mL (106), although at times, more than 20 μg/mL is needed (107). This variability in seizure control may be due to the underlying disorder, the seizure type, or genetic determinants (107). In one study (108), 51% of patients achieved complete control at concentrations either below or above that range. No significant association was evident between the serum phenytoin concentration and any measures of efficacy or toxicity.

Fosphenytoin

Measurement of fosphenytoin levels does not provide clinically useful information for patient care but rather has been utilized only in clinical research settings. Fosphenytoin may interfere with the ability of common laboratory immunoanalytic techniques, such as TDx/TDxFLx (fluorescence polarization) and Emit 2000 (enzyme multiplication), to measure phenytoin levels, because of cross-reactivity resulting in an artifactually elevated phenytoin concentration value. Waiting until all of the fosphenytoin to phenytoin conversion has occurred (approximately 2 hours after intravenous fosphenytoin administration or 4 hours after intramuscular fosphenytoin administration) before attempting to measure a patient's phenytoin concentrations is recommended (11).

DRUG INTERACTIONS

Phenytoin

Phenytoin can affect, and be affected by, a number of medications (Tables 52.2 and 52.3) (109). Although these drug interactions do not preclude concomitant administration, they signal the need for more frequent determination of serum concentrations, increased monitoring for the appearance of side effects, and, if appropriate, changes in dose. Patient-specific factors, such as genetic makeup, previous exposure to other compounds, and susceptibility to the clinical outcomes of the interaction, govern the extent and clinical significance of any drug interaction. In addition, a drug may act as an inhibitor in one patient and an inducer in another (e.g., phenobarbital's effect on phenytoin).

Interactions can affect any of the four primary pharmacokinetic phases. A drug that affects absorption most likely will decrease phenytoin serum concentration. For example, administration of phenytoin with a continuous high-calorie, nitrogen liquid complete-nutrition formula through nasogastric tube feedings causes a decrease in phenytoin serum concentrations from a mean of 9.8 μg/mL to 2.72 μg/mL at the same dose (110).

Drugs that affect protein binding increase the percentage of unbound phenytoin, usually with no change in the unbound concentration and with a decrease in the total concentration. Valproic acid displaces phenytoin from protein-binding sites. When valproic acid is added to a phenytoin regimen, total phenytoin concentrations decrease, free fraction increases, and free concentrations either stay the same or increase slightly. The following equation may be used to measure unbound phenytoin concentration in a patient receiving this combination (111,112):

$$\text{Free PHT} = [0.095 + 0.001(\text{VPA})]\text{PHT}$$

where PHT is phenytoin and VPA is valproic acid. Metabolic interactions usually cause either enzyme induction or inhibition. Addition of an inducer decreases phenytoin concentrations; addition of an inhibitor increases them. The order of addition

---

TABLE 52.2

BIDIRECTIONAL INTERACTIONS BETWEEN PHENYTOIN AND OTHER ANTIEPILEPTIC DRUGS

Specific drug	Effect of AED on phenytoin concentration	Mechanism of AED effect	Effect of phenytoin on AED concentration	Mechanism of phenytoin effect
Carbamazepine	↑↓	CYP2C19 induction	↓↓	CYP3A4 induction
Ethosuximide	«		↓↓	CYP3A4 induction
Felbamate	↑↑	CYP2C19 inhibition	↓↓	CYP3A4 induction
Fosphenytoin	↑ Free phenytoin	Protein-binding displacement	«	
Gabapentin	«		«	
Lacosamide	«		«	
Lamotrigine	«		↓↓	UDPGT induction
Levetiracetam	«		«	
Oxcarbazepine	↑	CYP2C19 inhibition	↓ MHD	Unknown
Phenobarbital	↑↓	CYP2C9 and CYP2C19 induction	↑	Unclear
Pregabalin	«		«	
Rufinamide	↑	Unknown	↓	Unknown
Stiripentol	↑	CYP2C9 and 2C19 inhibition	↓	Unclear
Topiramate	↑	CYP2C19 inhibition	↓↓	Unknown
Tiagabine	«		↓↓	CYP3A4 induction
Valproic acid	↓/?↑ Free phenytoin	Protein-binding displacement and CYP2C9 inhibition	↓↓	CYP2C9 and CYP2C19 induction
Vigabatrin	↓	Unknown	«	
Zonisamide	«		↓↓	CYP3A4 induction

↑↓, Variable; ↑, minor increase; ↓, minor decrease; ↑↑, important increase; ↓↓, important decrease; «, no change; MHD, monohydroxy derivative.

TABLE 52.3

BIDIRECTIONAL INTERACTIONS BETWEEN PHENYTOIN AND OTHER DRUGS

Drug	Effect on phenytoin concentration	Mechanism of effect	Effect of phenytoin on drug concentration	Mechanism of effect
Antimicrobials				
Albendazole			↓	CYP3A4 induction
Isoniazid	↑	CYP2C9 inhibition		
Rifampicin	↓	CYP2C9 and CYP2C19 induction	↓	CYP3A4 induction
Sulfaphenazole	↑	CYP2C9 inhibition		
Miconazole	↑	CYP2C9 inhibition		
Fluconazole	↑	CYP2C9 inhibition		
Itraconazole	↑	CYP2C9 inhibition	↓	CYP3A4 induction
Nevirapine			↓	CYP3A4 induction
Efavirenz			↓	CYP2B6 induction
Delavirdine			↓	CYP3A4 induction
Indinavir			↓	CYP3A4 induction
Ritonavir			↓	CYP3A4 induction
Saquinavir			↓	CYP3A4 induction
Antineoplastic drugs				
Cyclophosphamide			↓	CYP2B6 and CYP2C19 induction
Ifosfamide			↓	CYP2B6 induction
Teniposide			↓	CYP3A4 and CYP2C19 induction
Etoposide			↓	CYP3A4 induction
Paclitaxel			↓	CYP3A4 induction
Methotrexate	↓	↓ Absorption		
Fluorouracil	↑	CYP2C9 inhibition		
Carmustine	↓	↓ Absorption		
Vinblastine	↓	↓ Absorption		
Vincristine	↓	↓ Absorption		
Bleomycin	↓	↓ Absorption		
Cardiovascular drugs				
Quinidine			↓	CYP3A4 induction
Amiodarone	↑	CYP2C9 inhibition	↓	CYP3A4 induction
Propranolol			↓	CYP1A2 and CYP2C19 induction
Nifedipine			↓	CYP3A4 induction
Felodipine			↓	CYP3A4 induction
Nisolpidine			↓	CYP3A4 induction
Verapamil (oral)			↓	CYP3A4 induction
Losartan			↓ Active metabolite	CYP2C9 inhibition
Ticlopidine	↑	CYP2C19 inhibition		
Digoxin			↓	CYP3A4 induction
Atorvastatin			↓	CYP3A4 induction
Lovastatin			↓	CYP3A4 induction
Simvastatin			↓	CYP3A4 induction
Fluvastatin			↓	CYP2C9 induction
Warfarin			↑ Free warfarin (initially), then ↓	CYP2C9 induction
Ticlopidine	↑	CYP2C19 inhibition		
Gastrointestinal drugs				
Antacids	↓	↓ Absorption		

(continued)

TABLE 52.3

BIDIRECTIONAL INTERACTIONS BETWEEN PHENYTOIN AND OTHER DRUGS (*continued*)

Drug	Effect on phenytoin concentration	Mechanism of effect	Effect of phenytoin on drug concentration	Mechanism of effect
Sucralfate	↓	↓ Absorption		
Cimetidine	↑	CYP2C9 and CYP2C19 inhibition		
Omeprazole	↑	CYP2C19 inhibition		
Immunosuppressant drugs				
Cyclosporin			↓	CYP3A4 induction
Tacrolimus	↑	Protein-binding displacement	↓	CYP3A4 induction
Sirolimus			↓	CYP3A4 induction
Psychotropic drugs				
Amitriptyline	↑	CYP2C19 inhibition	↓	CYP2C19 and CYP3A4 induction
Imipramine	↑	CYP2C19 inhibition	↓	CYP1A2 and CYP2C19 induction
Clomipramine			↓	CYP1A2 and CYP2C19 induction
Mianserin			↓	CYP3A4 induction
Bupropion			↓	CYP2B6 induction
Citalopram			↓	CYP3A4 and CYP2C19 induction
Paroxetine	↑	CYP2C19 and CYP2C9 inhibition		
Fluoxetine	↑	CYP2C19 inhibition		
Fluvoxamine	↑	CYP2C19 inhibition		
Sertraline	↑	CYP2C9 inhibition		
Haloperidol			↓	CYP3A4 induction
Chlorpromazine			↓	CYP3A4 induction
Clozapine			↓	CYP1A2 induction
Quetiapine			↓	CYP3A4 induction
Trazodone	↑	CYP2C19 inhibition		
Diazepam			↓	CYP3A4 and CYP2C19 induction
Alprazolam			↓	CYP3A4 induction
Midazolam			↓	CYP3A4 induction
Steroids				
Hydrocortisone			↓	CYP3A4 induction
Dexamethasone			↓	CYP3A4 induction
Prednisone			↓	CYP3A4 induction
Steroidal oral contraceptives			↓	CYP3A4 induction
Miscellaneous				
Theophylline			↓	CYP3A4 induction
Fentanyl			↓	CYP3A4 induction
Methadone			↓	CYP3A4 and CYP2B6 induction
Tolbutamide	↑ Free phenytoin	Protein-binding displacement		

↑, increase; ↓, decrease.

or deletion is important. An inducer added to another compound may lead to decrease in the serum concentration of the preexisting drug; however, if that same drug is added to the inducer, the interaction would have a less noticeable clinical significance because nothing has changed—the added drug would simply require a higher dose. When an enzyme-inhibiting drug is removed from a regimen, the concentration of the remaining compound is likely to increase (113).

Fosphenytoin

As described above, in the presence of fosphenytoin, phenytoin is displaced from binding sites, rapidly increasing unbound phenytoin concentrations as a function of plasma fosphenytoin concentration (11).

EFFICACY

Phenytoin

Phenytoin is effective in the abortive treatment of acute seizures (including acute repetitive seizures and status epilepticus) or as chronic maintenance therapy to prevent seizure recurrence. As maintenance therapy, phenytoin is effective against partial-onset seizures and generalized tonic–clonic seizures but has limited efficacy in absence, clonic, myoclonic, tonic, or atonic seizures. In juvenile myoclonic epilepsy, it may be effective if tonic–clonic seizures are the sole or major seizure type. Similarly, in Lennox–Gastaut syndrome, efficacy appears limited to the tonic–clonic component (114,115).

Acute Seizures (Acute Repetitive Seizures and Status Epilepticus)

Multiple open-label series have indicated that patients with acute repetitive seizures or status epilepticus respond promptly to intravenous administration of phenytoin (114). In 60% to 80% of patients, a response was noted within 20 minutes after the initiation of an infusion (116,117). In one pediatric study (118), loading doses produced a complete or partial effect in 30 of 35 patients. The youngest children had lower concentrations and responded less favorably than did the older children.

A double-blind, randomized trial compared the efficacy of four treatments for generalized convulsive status epilepticus: diazepam (0.15 mg/kg) + phenytoin (18 mg/kg), lorazepam (0.1 mg/kg), phenobarbital (15 mg/kg), and phenytoin (18 mg/kg) (119). Success was defined as complete cessation of motor and electroencephalographic seizure activity within 20 minutes after the drug infusion began, without return of seizure activity during the next 40 minutes. Analyses were performed both on an intent-to-treat basis and including only patients with a verified diagnosis of generalized convulsive status epilepticus. Among the 384 patients with verified overt generalized convulsive status epilepticus, lorazepam was the most successful treatment (64.9%, $P = 0.02$ for the overall comparison), followed by phenobarbital (58.2%), diazepam + phenytoin (55.8%), and phenytoin alone (43.6%). Lorazepam was superior to phenytoin in a direct pairwise comparison ($P = 0.002$). However, the four groups did not differ significantly either for the subgroup of verified subtle generalized convulsive status epilepticus or in the intent-to-treat analysis. The authors concluded that lorazepam is more effective than phenytoin for the treatment of overt generalized convulsive status epilepticus (119).

Controlled studies have shown that phenytoin does not prevent nonepileptic alcohol-related seizures (120,121). Ninety alcoholic patients were enrolled prospectively in a randomized, double-blind trial within 6 hours of an initial alcohol-related seizure during a withdrawal episode and assigned to receive either 1000 mg of intravenous phenytoin or placebo. None of the patients had a history of seizures not related to alcohol withdrawal, and 71 patients had seizures during prior withdrawals. Six of 45 patients in the phenytoin group and 6 of 45 in the placebo group had at least one recurrent seizure during the postinfusion observation period. Phenytoin serum concentrations were similar in patients with and without subsequent seizures. Response rates in the two arms did not differ significantly ($P > 0.05$) (120).

Another identically designed trial (121) assigned 55 patients with alcohol withdrawal seizures and without other previous seizures to intravenous phenytoin or placebo. Of 28 patients treated with phenytoin, 6 (21%) had a seizure recurrence, compared with 5 (19%) of 27 patients given placebo. Again, response rates in the two groups did not differ significantly ($P > 0.05$) (121).

Partial-Onset and Generalized Tonic–Clonic Seizures

Multiple studies have compared the efficacy and tolerability of phenytoin with those of other AEDs (including carbamazepine, phenobarbital, primidone, valproic acid, lamotrigine, and oxcarbazepine) in the treatment of partial-onset and generalized tonic–clonic seizures. Overall, phenytoin has consistently demonstrated equal or superior efficacy compared with all other AEDs against these seizure types (122).

In the first Veterans Administration (VA) Cooperative Study (122), 622 adults were randomly assigned to treatment with phenytoin, carbamazepine, phenobarbital, or primidone and remained on therapy unless unacceptable toxic reactions or lack of efficacy was evident. Carbamazepine and phenytoin were more effective and had greater tolerability over time compared with primidone and phenobarbital in the treatment of complex partial seizures. All four AEDs were equally effective as monotherapy for generalized tonic–clonic seizures. Carbamazepine and phenytoin produced the highest rates of success, as defined by retention in the study (Fig. 52.4), and were recommended as "drugs of first-choice for single-drug therapy of adults with partial or generalized tonic–clonic seizures or with both."

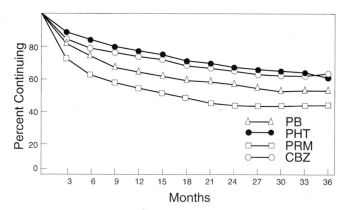

FIGURE 52.4. Cumulative percentage of patients remaining in the study during 36 months of follow-up. There were 275 patients at 12 months, 164 at 24 months, and 97 at 36 months. (From Mattson RH, Cramer JA, Collins JF, et al. Comparison of carbamazepine, phenobarbital, phenytoin, and primidone in partial and secondarily generalized tonic–clonic seizures. *N Engl J Med.* 1985;313:145–151, with permission.)

In several other comparative trials, phenytoin was as effective as carbamazepine and valproic acid, with similar potential to cause major side effects (123–126). In a comparison with phenobarbital, carbamazepine, and valproic acid in 243 adults with new-onset partial or generalized tonic–clonic seizures, 27% of the patients remained seizure free and 75% had entered 1 year of remission by 3 years of follow-up. No significant differences in efficacy were found among the four drugs at 1, 2, or 3 years of follow-up. The incidence of unacceptable side effects necessitating withdrawal from treatment was 10% (127).

Two studies compared the efficacy and tolerability of oxcarbazepine and phenytoin monotherapy in patients with recent-onset partial seizures or generalized tonic–clonic seizures (128,129). Each study was a randomized (1:1 oxcarbazepine:phenytoin), double-blind, parallel-group trial consisting of a 14-day screening phase followed by a 56-week double-blind period (8-week flexible titration phase followed by a 48-week maintenance phase). One study (128) involving 287 adults and adolescents, ages 15 to 91 years, demonstrated no difference in the proportion of seizure-free patients during the 48 weeks of maintenance between the oxcarbazepine group (59%) and the phenytoin group (58%). The second trial (129), in 193 children and adolescents, ages 5 to 17 years, also showed no difference in the proportion of seizure-free patients during the 48-week maintenance period between the oxcarbazepine group (61%) and the phenytoin group (60%).

Lamotrigine and phenytoin monotherapy were compared in a double-blind, parallel-group study of patients with newly diagnosed untreated partial-onset seizures or generalized tonic–clonic seizures (130). After randomization to either lamotrigine ($n = 86$) or phenytoin ($n = 95$), patients entered a 6-week flexible titration phase, followed by a 48-week maintenance phase. No between-treatment difference in efficacy was detected on the basis of percentages of patients remaining on each treatment arm, those remaining seizure free during the last 24 and 40 weeks of the study, and times to first seizure after the initial 6 weeks of treatment (dose-titration period).

No monotherapy trials have compared phenytoin with felbamate, gabapentin, topiramate, tiagabine, zonisamide, or levetiracetam in the treatment of partial-onset or generalized tonic–clonic seizures.

One study compared the efficacy and toxicity of phenytoin, phenobarbital, carbamazepine, and valproate as monotherapy in children with newly diagnosed epilepsy (131). In this study, 167 children, ages 3 to 16 years (median 10.3 years) were stratified by seizure type (generalized tonic–clonic seizures or partial seizures with or without secondary generalization) and the presence or absence of additional handicaps. These children were randomized in an open-labeled fashion to one of the four AEDs as monotherapy, and were followed-up for a median duration of 44 months (range, 3 to 88). Comparative efficacy was assessed by analysis of time to first seizure recurrence after the initiation of therapy, and by time to achieve a 1-year of seizure freedom. The likelihood ratio comparing the four drugs showed no difference between the drugs for either measure of efficacy at 1, 2, or 3 years of follow-up. Nine percent of the children had adverse effects requiring withdrawal. Patients on phenobarbital were more likely to withdraw because of intolerable side effects, compared to those on the other drugs. There was no significant difference in the rate of withdrawal between the other drugs (131).

Neonatal Seizures

Phenytoin and phenobarbital monotherapy were compared in a randomized trial of 59 neonates with seizures confirmed by electroencephalography (132). Seizures were controlled in 43% of the phenobarbital group and in 45% of the phenytoin group. Monotherapy or subsequent duotherapy controlled seizures in 59% of the neonates. The authors concluded that both drugs were "equally but incompletely effective as anticonvulsants in neonates."

In a sample of practice in major US pediatric hospitals, 6099 infants with neonatal seizures were identified over 62 months. As expected, the most common treatment for neonatal seizures was phenobarbital, which was given to 76% of all infants in the study (range, 56% to 89%, $P < 0.001$), and 97% of the infants who received a nonbenzodiazepine AED (range, 92% to 100%). Overall, 80% of the neonates treated with phenobarbital did not receive any other nonbenzodiazepine AEDs. Phenytoin was the second most commonly used nonbenzodiazepine AED but it was usually used in combination with another AED. It was used to treat 16% of all neonates diagnosed with neonatal seizures (range, 8% to 36%, $P < 0.001$), and 20% of the neonates who received a nonbenzodiazepine AED (range, 12% to 42%, $P < 0.001$). Phenytoin was used without phenobarbital in only 11% of these neonates and was used without any other nonbenzodiazepine AEDs in only 83 infants overall (8%). Phenytoin was started at least 1 day after phenobarbital 46% of the time, started on the same day as phenobarbital 32% of the time, and started at least 1 day before phenobarbital 11% of the time (133).

Evidence as Initial Monotherapy

The International League Against Epilepsy elaborated an evidence-based guideline for AED efficacy and effectiveness as initial monotherapy for different epileptic seizures and syndromes (134). The guideline concluded that based on available efficacy and effectiveness evidence alone, phenytoin and carbamazepine were efficacious or effective as initial monotherapy for adults with newly diagnosed or untreated partial-onset seizures (with the highest level of evidence, Level A). The findings in children was not that robust, and therefore, based on available efficacy and effectiveness evidence alone, phenytoin, carbamazepine, phenobarbital, topiramate, and valproate were possibly efficacious or effective as initial monotherapy for children with newly diagnosed or untreated partial-onset seizures (Level C). Similarly, phenytoin, carbamazepine, phenobarbital, oxcarbazepine, lamotrigine, topiramate, and valproate were found to be possibly efficacious or effective as initial monotherapy for adults with generalized tonic–clonic seizures (Level C). In children with generalized tonic–clonic seizures, phenytoin, carbamazepine, phenobarbital, topiramate, and valproate were possibly efficacious or effective (Level C) (134).

Other Seizure Types

Phenytoin is considered effective for primary generalized tonic–clonic seizures (115,125); however, there is no convincing evidence that it is effective against absence, clonic, myoclonic, tonic, or atonic seizures. Phenytoin is not recommended for infantile spasms, Lennox–Gastaut syndrome, or primary generalized epilepsy syndromes such as childhood absence or juvenile myoclonic epilepsy.

Prophylaxis

For seizure prophylaxis in pregnancy-induced hypertension, phenytoin has similar (135) or inferior (136,137) efficacy to magnesium sulfate. Patients receiving phenytoin had more rapid cervical dilation, a smaller decrease in hematocrit after delivery, and a lower incidence of hot flushes (138). In addition, phenytoin did not confound the computer analysis of fetal heart rate (139).

Phenytoin is often used following neurosurgical procedures and cerebrovascular accidents. A randomized, double-blind trial compared the efficacy, tolerability, and impact on quality of life and cognitive functioning of anticonvulsant prophylaxis with phenytoin versus valproate in 100 patients following craniotomy (140). Fourteen patients (seven in each group) experienced postoperative seizures. No major between-treatment differences emerged in efficacy, tolerability, impact on quality of life, or cognitive functioning (140). A double-blind comparison of phenytoin or carbamazepine with no treatment after supratentorial craniotomy noted no significant differences but a higher incidence of side effects in the treated group (141). Thus, prophylactic anticonvulsants cannot be recommended routinely after this type of procedure.

The efficacy of phenytoin in the prevention of posttraumatic seizures was studied in a randomized, double-blind trial of 404 patients with serious head trauma (142). Patients received a phenytoin-loading dose within 24 hours of injury; free phenytoin serum levels were maintained in a range from 0.75 to 1.5 μg/mL. From the time of drug loading to day 7, significantly fewer seizures occurred in the phenytoin group than in the placebo group (3.6% vs. 14.2%, $P < 0.001$). No benefit was seen in the phenytoin group after day 8, however, leading to the conclusion that phenytoin had an early suppressive effect, but not a true prophylactic effect, on seizures, and that it reduced the incidence of seizures only during the first week after injury. In a secondary analysis of this study (143), no significant difference in mortality was found between patients assigned to phenytoin and those assigned to placebo (143). In a randomized, double-blind, placebo-controlled trial in children with moderate to severe blunt head injury, phenytoin did not prevent posttraumatic seizures within 48 hours of the trauma (144).

Nonepileptic Disorders

Phenytoin has been shown to be useful in neuropathic pain (145), motion sickness (146,147), cardiac arrhythmias, continuous muscle fiber activity syndrome, myotonic muscular dystrophy, and myotonia congenita (148). It may also have a role in the treatment of recessive dystrophic epidermolysis bullosa, intermittent explosive disorder, and anxiety disorder (148), and as topical therapy for burns, refractory skin ulcers (148,149), and wound healing (150).

Fosphenytoin

Fosphenytoin itself has no known anticonvulsant activity; it derives its utility from its rapid and total conversion to phenytoin (15,16).

ADVERSE EFFECTS

Phenytoin

Concentration-Dependent Effects

The most common concentration-dependent phenytoin side effects are related to the central nervous system and consist of nystagmus, ataxia, incoordination (151,152), diplopia (vestibulo-oculo-cerebellar syndrome), and drowsiness. Some patients may experience prominent side effects at concentrations in the lower end of the therapeutic range, while others may be free of complaints despite elevated drug concentrations. These effects are reversible with appropriate adjustments in dose. Although small decreases may completely alleviate complaints, significant dose alterations may dramatically decrease serum concentrations, leading to a recurrence of seizures. Nausea, vomiting, and epigastric pain are often improved by dividing the dose or taking it with meals (or both).

Symptoms noted at serum phenytoin concentrations higher than 30 μg/mL include dysarthria, far-lateral nystagmus, movement disorders (usually choreoathetosis and orofacial dyskinesia), exacerbation of seizures, external ophthalmoplegia, or encephalopathy (including lethargy, delirium, "psychosis," stupor, and coma) (103,152–157).

Reports of the effect of phenytoin on cognitive function vary, depending on the type of patients, presence or absence of concomitant AEDs, measurement instruments, and comparative drugs. In general, however, effects appear modest when serum concentrations are kept within standard therapeutic ranges and polypharmacy is avoided (158,159). Unfortunately, patients taking phenytoin may suffer from cognitive side effects even when these guidelines are followed (160).

Compared with carbamazepine, no difference (159, 161–165) or more changes (160,166,167) in cognition with phenytoin have been noted. In one study, phenytoin appeared to be associated with more cognitive effects than carbamazepine, although reanalysis excluding patients with elevated phenytoin concentrations showed no difference (161,168). When used as prophylaxis against seizures following head trauma, phenytoin demonstrated negative cognitive effects compared with placebo (169). No clinically significant difference in cognitive effects between phenytoin and valproate was detected in either healthy adults (170) or patients following craniotomy (140).

In one study of elderly patients, phenytoin and valproic acid had similar effects (171), whereas a second study reported no cognitive impairment resulting from modest increases in serum phenytoin concentrations (between 11 μg/mL and 16 μg/mL) (172). Motor disturbances are common in children taking phenytoin (173). In children withdrawn from AEDs, cognitive function remains unchanged, whereas psychomotor speed improves (174). Fluctuations in phenytoin serum concentrations by as much as 50% had no or an immeasurably small effect in children with well-controlled seizures receiving monotherapy with low therapeutic dosages (175). Removal of chronic phenytoin in patients receiving polypharmacy resulted in significant improvement in one test of concentration and two tests of psychomotor function (162).

Idiosyncratic Reactions

Phenytoin's idiosyncratic reactions are proposed to result from the formation of a reactive metabolite (an arene oxide) that either directly (owing to deficiencies in detoxification resulting from inadequate epoxide hydrolase activity) or indirectly (through an immune response or free radical–mediated injury) causes cell, tissue, or organ injury and, at times, death (176).

The most common idiosyncratic reaction is rash, which may occur in up to 8.5% of patients, particularly children and adolescents (177–179). The in vivo and in vitro cross-reactivity between phenytoin, phenobarbital, and carbamazepine is as high as 70% to 80% (180). A recent study on cross-sensitivity of skin rashes among commonly used AEDs ($n = 1875$), found evidence of specific cross-sensitivity between carbamazepine and phenytoin (181). The phenytoin rash rate in patients who also had a rash to carbamazepine ($n = 59$) was 57.6%, which was significantly higher compared to the phenytoin rash rate in patients with rashes to any other AEDs (38.8%; $P < 0.0016$) (181). The rate of cross-sensitivity between phenytoin and other AEDs (phenobarbital, lamotrigine, oxcarbazepine, and zonisamide) was not as high as with carbamazepine (181). A more severe dermatologic idiosyncratic reaction is the "hypersensitivity syndrome" (180). In a series of 38 affected patients, the most common manifestations were rash, fever, lymphadenopathy, eosinophilia, abnormal liver function test results, blood dyscrasias, serum sickness, renal failure, and polymyositis. Symptoms usually occur within the first 3 months of therapy (182).

Other reported idiosyncratic reactions include Stevens–Johnson syndrome (SJS), toxic epidermal necrolysis, aplastic anemia, hepatitis, pseudolymphoma, and a lupus-like reaction (152). Recent data suggests a possible association between HLA-B*1052 and phenytoin-induced SJS (183,184). The human leukocyte antigen allele, HLA-B*1502, occurs almost exclusively in patients with ancestry across broad areas of Asia, including Han Chinese, Filipinos, Malaysians, South Asian Indians, and Thais. A study from Hong Kong reported that HLA-B*1052 was associated with SJS in a patient who started phenytoin within 8 weeks prior to the development of the cutaneous reaction, and in whom no other causes for the reaction were found (183). More recently, a Thai study reported a significant association between HLA-B*1052 and SJS in four patients on phenytoin ($P = 0.005$). One of the four patients who developed phenytoin-induced SJS, was tolerant to carbamazepine. The authors concluded that while HLA-B*1052 may be necessary, it is not sufficient to cause SJS from phenytoin in the Thai population (184).

Adverse Effects with Long-Term Therapy

Long-term administration of phenytoin has been associated with gingival hyperplasia (185,186), hirsutism, acne, and rash. The exact incidence of gingival hyperplasia attributable to phenytoin is not known (186); reports range from 13% of patients attending general medical practices (187) to about 40% of patients taking phenytoin long term in a community-based cross-sectional study in Ferrara, Northern Italy (188). In the latter report, younger age and poorer oral hygiene seemed to predispose to the severest level of gingival involvement (188). Hyperplasia regresses after discontinuation of phenytoin (189,190).

Cerebellar atrophy has been reported after long-term (191,192) and acute use (193) of high doses, although whether the true etiologic agent was phenytoin or the seizures is unclear (194,195); single-photon-emission computed tomography scans may be a means for early detection (194).

Among other effects of long-term phenytoin therapy are alterations in laboratory values, including reduction in bone mineral density (196), low folate levels (103), macrocytosis (103), and decreases in levels of carnitine (197), low-density lipoprotein cholesterol, and apolipoprotein B (198). Levels of prolactin (199) and apolipoprotein A and A1 (198) increase, as does high-density lipoprotein cholesterol, although at doses of 100 mg/day this lipid fraction was unchanged (200). Phenytoin may decrease levels of free testosterone and enhance its conversion to estradiol (201).

Changes in thyroid hormones have been reported (202). The thyroxine (T_4) and free T_4 index, total T_4 and triiodothyronine (T_3), free T_4, and free T_3 all decrease. Increases in serum levels of thyroid-stimulating hormone (203,204) may involve protein-binding displacement and induction of cellular metabolism (205). Phenytoin therapy may suppress immunoglobulin (Ig) production, leading to decreases in IgG (206,207) and IgA (206,208). Panhypoglobulinemia was reported in one patient infected with the human immunodeficiency virus (209). It is unclear whether these changes are a direct result of phenytoin or epilepsy (206) or if they occur with any drug with arene oxide intermediates (206,210).

Teratogenicity

"Fetal hydantoin syndrome" was described in 1975 and consisted of growth retardation, microcephaly, mental retardation, and numerous "minor" congenital anomalies (179,211). However, "fetal anticonvulsant syndrome" has replaced this term because the malformations are seen in children of mothers taking a wide variety of AEDs. Although there is agreement that anticonvulsant polypharmacy and folic acid deficiency increase the risk of malformation (212), the absolute and relative teratogenicity of phenytoin is not completely known. One study showed an increased risk for cleft palate in the offspring with phenytoin use during pregnancy (213).

Two recent studies described the pregnancy outcomes of women with epilepsy taking AEDs; one focused on fetal malformations (214) and the other one on the neurocognitive outcome for AED exposure in utero (215). The Australian Pregnancy Registry of AEDs, an ongoing, observational prospective study, monitored 1002 pregnancies, 875 of which were exposed to AEDs. Of the 31 pregnancies exposed to phenytoin as monotherapy, at least in the first trimester, 3.23% (1 of 31) had birth defects. This finding was not significant compared with the 3.61% (3 of 83) malformation rate in women with epilepsy who were not taking an AED in the first trimester (214). The Neurodevelopmental Effect of Antiepileptic Drugs (NEAD) study is an ongoing prospective observational study that recently reported on the cognitive outcome at age 3 years, in 309 children born to mothers who were taking a single AED during pregnancy. On average, the IQ of children exposed to phenytoin ($n = 48$) was 7 points better than the ones exposed to valproate (95% CI, 0.2 to 14.0; $P = 0.04$) but not different than the ones exposed to carbamazepine or lamotrigine ($P = 0.68$) (215). Three earlier studies showed that the use of phenytoin carries a higher risk of poor cognitive outcome compared to unexposed controls (216–218).

Intravenous Administration

Administration of parenteral phenytoin solution is associated with local reactions, including pain and burning at the infusion site, phlebitis, and vessel cording (8,9,219). Extravasation can lead to phlebitis, chemical cellulitis, or frank necrosis (10). A unique effect of unknown etiology, purple glove syndrome (220,221), begins with discoloration and progresses to a petechial rash; severe cases may require surgical intervention. In one report (222), 9 of 152 patients (5.9%) receiving intravenous phenytoin developed purple glove syndrome.

Intravenously administered phenytoin can also lead to cardiovascular complications, such as hypotension, atrial and ventricular conduction depression, and ventricular fibrillation (9). The major risk factors for these complications include preexisting disease, advanced age, and rapid infusion (9,219). In patients without cardiovascular disease, phenytoin can be administered at 40 to 50 mg/min (223). Rates should not exceed 25 mg/min in patients with arteriosclerotic cardiovascular disease (224).

Fosphenytoin

Concentration-Dependent Effects

Intravenous fosphenytoin infusion has a favorable side-effect profile (8,105,225). The local reactions associated with administration of parenteral phenytoin solution (infusion-site pain, phlebitis, and vessel cording) occur significantly less often with fosphenytoin (8). Pain at the site of fosphenytoin infusion is rare, but 48.9% of patients reported pruritus or tingling (without rash) in the perianal region, elsewhere on the trunk, or on the back of the head (225). Pruritus or tingling appears soon after an infusion starts, abates rapidly when the infusion stops, and can be reduced or abolished by slowing the infusion. Decreases in systolic and diastolic blood pressure have been observed, but the changes were judged to be clinically insignificant and did not require cessation of the infusion (226). Cardiac arrhythmias have not been noted (226). Dizziness, somnolence, and ataxia were observed with a frequency similar to that after phenytoin infusion (226).

Adverse effects have been even less notable after intramuscular fosphenytoin injection (227–229). Mild local irritation occurred in only 5% of 60 patients who received intramuscular loading doses, even though the volume of injected solution was usually 15 to 20 mL (mean, 17.8 mg/PE/kg or 1359.8 mg PE total) (228).

Idiosyncratic Reactions, Long-Term Adverse Reactions, Teratogenicity

No idiosyncratic reactions are associated specifically with fosphenytoin. As fosphenytoin is used only on a short-term basis, data about long-term adverse reactions are lacking. There are also no data on possible teratogenic effects with fosphenytoin.

CLINICAL USE

Phenytoin

For rapid increase in drug concentration, phenytoin doses of 15 to 20 mg/kg are used (119,230). Doses of 18 mg/kg increase phenytoin serum concentrations by approximately 23 μg/mL in adults being treated for acute seizures (231); in children with status epilepticus, similar or higher doses have been administered (118). The intravenous route is used during status epilepticus. In less acute situations, oral administration is appropriate, but the loading dose is divided into three or four doses, given 2 to 3 hours apart to improve bioavailability and rate of absorption (232–234).

When given intravenously to adults, phenytoin should be diluted in normal saline (not in dextrose 5% in water); the infusion should not exceed 50 mg/min and should be injected directly into a large vein through a large-gauge needle or intravenous catheter. The intramuscular route is not recommended owing to the drug's slow and erratic absorption, as well as painful local reactions likely associated with crystallization at the injection site. If, however, no other routes of administration are available, intramuscular doses 50% higher than oral doses may be needed to maintain plasma concentrations (235–237). Adjustments in dosage and monitoring of serum levels may be necessary on switching from one route to another. Therapeutic levels of phenytoin administered rectally have not been maintained in patients with seizures (238).

For maintenance therapy, the nonlinear pharmacokinetics and wide interindividual variability in metabolism and absorption necessitate individualized regimens. The typical initial dose of 300 mg/day results in concentrations between 10 and 20 μg/mL in fewer than 30% of patients, and more than 57% will achieve concentrations below 10 μg/mL (41). Doses of 6 to 8 mg/kg will produce concentrations between 10 and 20 μg/mL in approximately 45% of otherwise healthy patients, less than 10 μg/mL in 35%, and more than 20 μg/mL in 20% (41). Thereafter, adjustments should be based on clinical response, increasing dosage for lack of seizure control or lowering dosage for concentration-dependent toxic reactions.

Privitera (239) proposed the following guidelines based on initial plasma concentration: increase dosage by 100 mg/day for an initial plasma concentration of less than 7 μg/mL; increase by 50 mg/day for concentrations from 7 to 12 μg/mL; increase by 30 mg/day for concentrations greater than 12 μg/mL. This formula was tested in 129 dosage increases of 50 or 100 mg in 77 patients. All 53 increases that were within the guidelines produced plasma concentrations less than 25 μg/mL, whereas 36% of the increases that exceeded the guidelines produced plasma concentrations greater than 25 μg/mL (239).

Accurate predictions of phenytoin plasma concentrations cannot be accomplished with the Michaelis–Menten equation unless patient-specific values for V_{max} and K_m are obtainable, which is rarely possible in clinical situations. When at least some clinical data are available, numerous methods can assist in estimating an individual patient's dose (240–243) to achieve predetermined serum concentrations (244,245). The nonlinear pharmacokinetics of phenytoin not only lead to nonproportional changes in serum concentration with changes in dose but also increase the apparent elimination half-life with higher concentrations. Thus, patients with "high" concentrations exhibit smaller peak–trough variability and require a longer time to achieve steady state. For most patients whose concentrations are within the therapeutic range, the peak–trough remains relatively unaffected, and steady state is reached in approximately 1 to 2 weeks. Thus, any changes in dose will require 1 to 2 weeks to achieve maximum effect.

Patients receiving prompt-release phenytoin products and those with low serum concentrations and rapid phenytoin metabolism (e.g., children or patients with relatively high dose requirements) are at high risk for large peak–trough variability and often need multiple daily doses to prevent wide fluctuations in clinical response.

Children require higher milligrams per kilogram daily doses, whereas the elderly should be started on 2 to 3 mg/kg/day and doses increased carefully. Concomitant illnesses can alter phenytoin pharmacokinetics and, consequently, dosage requirements. Critically ill patients may require plasmapheresis, continuous ambulatory peritoneal dialysis, or hemofiltration. Plasmapheresis does not appear to remove a significant amount of phenytoin (246); continuous ambulatory peritoneal dialysis may not either (247). In contrast, continuous hemofiltration at a high ultrafiltration rate may remove significant amounts of phenytoin in patients with renal failure with significant protein-binding changes (248). Pregnancy may necessitate an increase in phenytoin dose, especially during the third trimester (87,88).

Formulation switches to generics has recently become a common cost containment strategy for the management of health care resources. In the case of phenytoin, a drug with narrow therapeutic index and nonlinear pharmacokinetics, generic substitution may present a problem (249). Both increases and decreases in phenytoin serum concentrations with generic substitution have been reported, with associated increase in side effects and loss of seizure control (30,250).

Fosphenytoin

The three main situations in which fosphenytoin is used are during status epilepticus, as a temporary substitute for oral phenytoin, and in a nonemergency hospital situation, such as in a patient undergoing a neurosurgical procedure. Fosphenytoin can be diluted in a variety of vehicles, such as dextrose 5% and 10%, lactated Ringer's solution, and mannitol 20% (251).

Allen and colleagues (252) reported preliminary results of an open-label, single-dose study of intravenous fosphenytoin for treatment of status epilepticus in 54 patients. With a mean fosphenytoin dose of 967 mg PE (16.4 mg PE/kg) infused at a mean rate of 120 mg PE/min, total and free phenytoin concentrations at or above 10 µg/mL and 1 µg/mL, respectively, were achieved within 10 to 20 minutes. No patients had cardiac arrhythmias or clinically significant hypotension. Three percent of patients reported tenderness at the infusion site 24 hours later, but no inflammation or phlebitis was observed. Seizures were controlled in 50 of the 53 patients who received an adequate dose.

Fosphenytoin (rather than phenytoin) has become part of the standard-of-care treatment protocols for convulsive status epilepticus in adults and children in many US hospitals. It is preferred to phenytoin because of better tolerability at the infusion site, lack of cardiovascular complications, and overall ease of administration (253). For the treatment of convulsive status epilepticus, a fosphenytoin "loading dose" of 15 to 20 mg PE/kg can be given intravenously, with an infusion rate of at least 100 mg PE/min and up to 150 mg PE/min. The dose should be adjusted in patients who have hepatic impairment or hypoalbuminemia.

Fosphenytoin (given either intravenously or intramuscularly) is useful as a temporary substitute for oral phenytoin when the patient is unable to take oral medications. In this situation, the fosphenytoin dose and frequency would be the same as the patient's oral phenytoin dose and frequency.

Fosphenytoin can be useful in the prophylaxis of seizures in neurosurgical patients. A single nonemergency loading dose is given either intravenously or intramuscularly. The dose is usually 10 to 20 mg PE/kg, with an intravenous infusion rate of up to 150 mg PE/min.

Fosphenytoin is significantly more expensive than phenytoin (254). A number of studies and editorials have reported pharmacoeconomic comparisons between fosphenytoin and intravenous phenytoin (233,254–256). The overall cost of patient care with intravenous fosphenytoin was less than with intravenous phenytoin in an emergency department setting (256). Substitution of intravenous fosphenytoin for intravenous phenytoin was associated with reduced "adverse events at a reasonable increase in total hospital costs" in a second study (255). An editorial suggested that pharmacoeconomic decisions should be based on outcome cost, not acquisition costs (254). Overall, in terms of cost effectiveness, studies in the past decade showed that despite higher acquisition cost, use of intravenous fosphenytoin appeared to be at least equivalent to, if not better than, intravenous phenytoin. However, two recent studies (233,257) have challenged this impression. The administration of intravenous fosphenytoin to adults in an emergency department did not significantly decrease the incidence of drug-related adverse effects or decrease the length of stay in the emergency department compared with the use of intravenous phenytoin. This result suggests that intravenous fosphenytoin may not be more cost effective than intravenous phenytoin.

References

1. Friedlander WJ. Putnam, Merritt, and the discovery of Dilantin. *Epilepsia*. 1986;27(suppl 3):S1–S20.
2. Putnam T, Merritt H. Experimental determination of the anticonvulsant properties of some phenyl derivatives. *Science*. 1937;85:525–526.
3. Merritt H, Putnam T. A new series of anticonvulsant drugs tested by experiments in animals. *Arch Neurol Psychiatry*. 1938;39:1003–1015.
4. Merritt H, Putnam T. Sodium diphenyl hydantoinate in the treatment of convulsive disorders. *JAMA*. 1938;111:1068–1073.
5. Merritt H, Putnam T. Further experience with the use of sodium diphenyl hydantoinate in the treatment of convulsive disorders. *Am J Psychiatry*. 1940;96:1023–1027.
6. Leppik I. Antiepileptic drug selection: a view from the United States. *Epilepsia*. 1995;36:S90.
7. Browne T, LeDuc B. Phenytoin: chemistry and biotransformation. In: Levy R, Mattson R, Meldrum B, eds. *Antiepileptic Drugs*. 4th ed. New York: Raven Press; 1995:283–300.
8. Jamerson BD, Dukes GE, Brouwer KL, et al. Venous irritation related to intravenous administration of phenytoin versus fosphenytoin. *Pharmacotherapy*. 1994;14(1):47–52.
9. Mattson RH. Parenteral antiepileptic/anticonvulsant drugs. *Neurology*. 1996;46(6 suppl 1):S8–S13.
10. Hayes A, Chesney T. Necrosis of the hand after extravasation of intravenously administered phenytoin. *J Am Acad Dermatol*. 1993;28: 360–363.
11. Browne TR, Kugler AR, Eldon MA. Pharmacology and pharmacokinetics of fosphenytoin. *Neurology*. 1996;46(6 suppl 1):S3–S7.
12. DeLorenzo R. Phenytoin mechanisms of action. In: Levy R, Mattson R, Meldrum B, eds. *Antiepileptic Drugs*. New York: Raven Press; 1995: 271–282.
13. Esplin D. Effects of diphenylhydantoin on synaptic transmission in cat spinal cord and stallate ganglion. *J Pharmacol Exp Ther*. 1957;120: 301–323.
14. Francis J, Burnham W. (3H) Phenytoin identifies a novel anticonvulsant-binding domain on voltage-dependent sodium channels. *Mol Pharmacol*. 1992;42:1097–1103.

15. Knapp LE, Kugler AR. Clinical experience with fosphenytoin in adults: pharmacokinetics, safety, and efficacy. *J Child Neurol.* 1998;13(suppl 1): S15–S18.

16. Boucher BA. Fosphenytoin: a novel phenytoin prodrug. *Pharmacotherapy.* 1996;16(5):777–791.

17. Meinardi H, Kleijn E, Meijer Jvd, et al. Absorption and distribution of antiepileptic drugs. *Epilepsia.* 1975;16:353–365.

18. Treiman DM, Woodbury DM. Phenytoin: absorption, distribution, and excretion. In: Levy RH, Mattson RH, Meldrum BS, eds. *Antiepileptic Drugs.* New York: Raven Press; 1995:301–314.

19. Davis A, Begg E, Kennedy M, et al. Application of a simplified method to determine bioavailability of an oral dose of phenytoin. *J Pharmacokinet Biopharm.* 1993;21:195–208.

20. Jusko W. Bioavailability and disposition kinetics of phenytoin in man. In: Kellaway P, Petersen I, eds. *Quantitative Analytic Studies in Epilepsy.* New York: Raven Press; 1976:115–36.

21. Irvin J, Notari R. Computer-aided dosage form design, III: feasibility assessment for an oral prolonged-release phenytoin product. *Pharm Res.* 1991;8:232–237.

22. Dill W, Kazenko A, wolff L, et al. Studies on 5, 5-diphenylhydantoin (Dilantin) in animals and man. *J Pharmacol Exp Ther.* 1956;118: 270–279.

23. O'Malley W, Denckla M, O'Doherty D. Oral absorption of diphenylhydantoin as measured by gas liquid chromatography. *Trans Am Neurol Assoc.* 1969;94:318–319.

24. Wilder B, Ramsay R. Correlation of acute diphenylhydantoin intoxication with plasma levels and metabolite excretion. *Neurology* 1976;23: 1329–32.

25. Matsukura M, Ikeda T, Higashi A, et al. Relative bioavailability of two different phenytoin preparations. Evidence for an age dependency. *Dev Pharmacol Ther.* 1984;7(3):160–168.

26. Jalling B, Boreus L, Rane A, et al. Plasma concentrations of diphenylhydantoin in young infants. *Pharmacol Clin (Berlin).* 1970;2:200–202.

27. Browne T, Szabo G, Schumacher G, et al. Bioavailability studies of drugs with nonlinear pharmacokinetics, I: tracer dose AUC varies directly with serum concentration. *J Clin Pharmacol.* 1992;32:1141–1145.

28. Kasuya Y, Mamada K, Baba S, et al. Stable-isotope methodology for the bioavailability study of phenytoin during multiple-dosing regimens. *J Pharm Sci.* 1985;74:503–507.

29. Chang S, da Silva JH, Kuhl DR. Absorption of rectally administered phenytoin: a pilot study. *Ann Pharmacother.* 1999;33(7–8):781–786.

30. Mikati M, Bassett N, Schachter E. Double-blind randomized study comparing brand-name and generic phenytoin monotherapy (published erratum appears in *Epilepsia.* 1992;33(6):1156). *Epilepsia.* 1992;33:359–365.

31. Rosenbaum D, Rowan A, Tuchman L, et al. Comparative bioavailability of a generic phenytoin and Dilantin. *Epilepsia.* 1994;35:656–660.

32. Tsai JJ, Lai ML, Yang YH, et al. Comparison on bioequivalence of four phenytoin preparations in patients with multiple-dose treatment. *J Clin Pharmacol.* 1992;32(3):272–276.

33. Petker M, Morton D. Comparison of the effectiveness of two oral phenytoin products and chronopharmacokinetics of phenytoin. *J Clin Pharm Ther.* 1993;18:213–217.

34. Goff D, spunt A, Jung D, et al. Absorption characteristics of three phenytoin sodium products after administration of oral loading doses. *Clin Pharm.* 1984;3:634–638.

35. Woodbury D. Pharmacology of anticonvulsant drugs in CSF. In: Woods J, ed. *Neurobiology of Cerebrospinal Fluid.* New York: Plenum Press; 1983:615–628.

36. Pospisil J, Perlik F. Binding parameters of phenytoin during monotherapy and polytherapy. *Int J Clin Pharmacol Ther Toxicol.* 1992;30:24–28.

37. Liponi D, Winter M, Tozer T. Renal function and therapeutic concentrations of phenytoin. *Neurology.* 1984;34:395–397.

38. Kang H, Leppik I. Phenytoin binding and renal transplantation. *Neurology.* 1984;34:83–86.

39. Fedler C, Stewart MJ. Plasma total phenytoin: a possibly misleading test in developing countries. *Ther Drug Monit.* 1999;21(2):155–160.

40. Dager W, Inciardi J, Howe T. Estimating phenytoin concentrations by the Sheiner-Tozer method in adults with pronounced hypoalbuminemia. *Ann Pharmacother.* 1995;29:667–670.

41. Tozer TN, Winter ME. Phenytoin. In: Evans WE, Schentag JJ, Jusko WJ, eds. *Applied Pharmacokinetics Principles of Therapeutic Drug Monitoring.* 3rd ed. Vancouver, Washington: Applied Therapeutics Inc.; 1992: 25-1–25.44.

42. Koren G, Brand N, Halkin H, et al. Kinetics of intravenous phenytoin in children. *Pediatr Pharmacol (New York).* 1984;4(1):31–38.

43. Vozeh S, Uematsu T, Aarons L, et al. Intravenous phenytoin loading in patients after neurosurgery and in status epilepticus. A population pharmacokinetic study. *Clin Pharmacokinet.* 1988;14(2):122–128.

44. Abernethy D, Greenblatt D. Phenytoin disposition in obesity. Determination of loading dose. *Arch Neurol.* 1985;42:468–471.

45. Oca G, Gums J, Robinson J. Phenytoin dosing in obese patients: two case reports. *Drug Intell Clin Pharm.* 1988;22:708–710.

46. Dickinson R, Hooper W, Patterson M, et al. Extent of urinary excretion of *p*-hydroxyphenytoin in healthy subjects given phenytoin. *Ther Drug Monit.* 1985;7:283–289.

47. Yasumori T, Chen LS, Li QH, et al. Human CYP2C-mediated stereoselective phenytoin hydroxylation in Japanese: difference in chiral preference of CYP2C9 and CYP2C19. *Biochem Pharmacol.* 1999;57(11): 1297–1303.

48. Komatsu T, Yamazaki H, Asahi S, et al. Formation of a dihydroxy metabolite of phenytoin in human liver microsomes/cytosol: roles of cytochromes P450 2C9, 2C19, and 3A4. *Drug Metab Dispos.* 2000; 28(11):1361–1368.

49. Spielberg S, Gordon G, Blake D, et al. Anticonvulsant toxicity in vitro: possible role of arene oxides. *J Pharmacol Exp Ther.* 1981;217:386–389.

50. Strickler S, Dansky L, Miller M, et al. Genetic predisposition to phenytoin induced birth defects. *Lancet.* 1985;1:746–749.

51. Lee CR, Goldstein JA, Pieper JA. Cytochrome P450 2C9 polymorphisms: a comprehensive review of the in-vitro and human data. *Pharmacogenetics.* 2002;12(3):251–263.

52. Human Cytochrome P450 (CYP) Allele Nomenclature Committee. 2008. Last accessed at http://www.cypalleles.ki.se/ on 07/04/2009.

53. Odani A, Hashimoto Y, Otsuki Y, et al. Genetic polymorphism of the CYP2C subfamily and its effect on the pharmacokinetics of phenytoin in Japanese patients with epilepsy. *Clin Pharmacol Ther.* 1997;62(3): 287–292.

54. Mamiya K, Ieiri I, Shimamoto J, et al. The effects of genetic polymorphisms of CYP2C9 and CYP2C19 on phenytoin metabolism in Japanese adult patients with epilepsy: studies in stereoselective hydroxylation and population pharmacokinetics. *Epilepsia.* 1998;39(12):1317–1323.

55. Aynacioglu AS, Brockmoller J, Bauer S, et al. Frequency of cytochrome P450 CYP2C9 variants in a Turkish population and functional relevance for phenytoin. *Br J Clin Pharmacol.* 1999;48(3):409–415.

56. Caraco Y, Muszkat M, Wood AJ. Phenytoin metabolic ratio: a putative marker of CYP2C9 activity in vivo. *Pharmacogenetics.* 2001;11(7): 587–596.

57. van der Weide J, Steijns LS, van Weelden MJ, et al. The effect of genetic polymorphism of cytochrome P450 CYP2C9 on phenytoin dose requirement. *Pharmacogenetics.* 2001;11(4):287–291.

58. Ninomiya H, Mamiya K, Matsuo S, et al. Genetic polymorphism of the CYP2C subfamily and excessive serum phenytoin concentration with central nervous system intoxication. *Ther Drug Monit.* 2000;22(2):230–232.

59. Kidd RS, Straughn AB, Meyer MC, et al. Pharmacokinetics of chlorpheniramine, phenytoin, glipizide and nifedipine in an individual homozygous for the CYP2C9*3 allele. *Pharmacogenetics* 1999;9(1):71–80.

60. Brandolese R, Scordo MG, Spina E, et al. Severe phenytoin intoxication in a subject homozygous for CYP2C9*3. *Clin Pharmacol Ther.* 2001; 70(4):391–394.

61. Ieiri I, Tainaka H, Morita T, et al. Catalytic activity of three variants (Ile, Leu, and Thr) at amino acid residue 359 in human CYP2C9 gene and simultaneous detection using single-strand conformation polymorphism analysis. *Ther Drug Monit.* 2000;22(3):237–244.

62. Kidd RS, Curry TB, Gallagher S, et al. Identification of a null allele of CYP2C9 in an African-American exhibiting toxicity to phenytoin. *Pharmacogenetics.* 2001;11(9):803–808.

63. Goldstein JA. Clinical relevance of genetic polymorphisms in the human CYP2C subfamily. *Br J Clin Pharmacol.* 2001;52(4):349–355.

64. Imai J, Ieiri I, Mamiya K, et al. Polymorphism of the cytochrome P450 (CYP) 2C9 gene in Japanese epileptic patients: genetic analysis of the CYP2C9 locus. *Pharmacogenetics.* 2000;10(1):85–89.

65. Dickmann LJ, Rettie AE, Kneller MB, et al. Identification and functional characterization of a new CYP2C9 variant (CYP2C9*5) expressed among African Americans. *Mol Pharmacol.* 2001;60(2):382–387.

66. Goldstein J. Polymorphism in the human CYP2C subfamily. *Drug Metab Rev.* 2002;34(suppl 1):5.

67. Allabi AC, Gala JL, Horsmans Y. CYP2C9, CYP2C19, ABCB1 (MDR1) genetic polymorphisms and phenytoin metabolism in a Black Beninese population. *Pharmacogenet Genomics.* 2005;15(11):779–786.

68. Si D, Guo Y, Zhang Y, et al. Identification of a novel variant CYP2C9 allele in Chinese. *Pharmacogenetics.* 2004;14(7):465–469.

69. Zhao F, Loke C, Rankin SC, et al. Novel CYP2C9 genetic variants in Asian subjects and their influence on maintenance warfarin dose. *Clin Pharmacol Ther.* 2004;76(3):210–219.

70. Veenstra DL, Blough DK, Higashi MK, et al. CYP2C9 haplotype structure in European American warfarin patients and association with clinical outcomes. *Clin Pharmacol Ther.* 2005;77(5):353–364.

71. Herman D, Peternel P, Stegnar M, et al. A novel sequence variant in exon 7 of CYP2C9 gene (CYP2C9*24) in a patient on warfarin therapy. *Thromb Haemost.* 2006;95(1):192–194.

72. Maekawa K, Fukushima-Uesaka H, Tohkin M, et al. Four novel defective alleles and comprehensive haplotype analysis of CYP2C9 in Japanese. *Pharmacogenet Genomics.* 2006;16(7):497–514.

73. Matimba A, Del-Favero J, Van Broeckhoven C, et al. Novel variants of major drug-metabolising enzyme genes in diverse African populations and their predicted functional effects. *Hum Genomics.* 2009;3(2):169–190.

74. Levy RH. Cytochrome P450 isozymes and antiepileptic drug interactions. *Epilepsia.* 1995;36(suppl 5):S8–S13.

75. Blaisdell J, Mohrenweiser H, Jackson J, et al. Identification and functional characterization of new potentially defective alleles of human CYP2C19. *Pharmacogenetics.* 2002;12(9):703–711.

76. Sim SC, Risinger C, Dahl ML, et al. A common novel CYP2C19 gene variant causes ultrarapid drug metabolism relevant for the drug response to proton pump inhibitors and antidepressants. *Clin Pharmacol Ther.* 2006;79(1):103–113.

77. Rudberg I, Mohebi B, Hermann M, et al. Impact of the ultrarapid CYP2C19*17 allele on serum concentration of escitalopram in psychiatric patients. *Clin Pharmacol Ther.* 2008;83(2):322–327.

78. Desta Z, Zhao X, Shin JG, et al. Clinical significance of the cytochrome P450 2C19 genetic polymorphism. *Clin Pharmacokinet.* 2002;41(12):913–958.

79. Xie HG, Kim RB, Wood AJ, et al. Molecular basis of ethnic differences in drug disposition and response. *Annu Rev Pharmacol Toxicol.* 2001;41:815–850.

80. Wormhoudt LW, Commandeur JN, Vermeulen NP. Genetic polymorphisms of human N-acetyltransferase, cytochrome P450, glutathione-S-transferase, and epoxide hydrolase enzymes: relevance to xenobiotic metabolism and toxicity. *Crit Rev Toxicol.* 1999;29(1):59–124.

81. Bajpai M, Roskos LK, Shen DD, et al. Roles of cytochrome P4502C9 and cytochrome P4502C19 in the stereoselective metabolism of phenytoin to its major metabolite. *Drug Metab Dispos.* 1996;24(12):1401–1403.

82. Taguchi M, Hongou K, Yagi S, et al. Evaluation of phenytoin dosage regimens based on genotyping of CYP2C subfamily in routinely treated Japanese patients. *Drug Metab Pharmacokinet.* 2005;20(2):107–112.

83. Lee SY, Lee ST, Kim JW. Contributions of CYP2C9/CYP2C19 genotypes and drug interaction to the phenytoin treatment in the Korean epileptic patients in the clinical setting. *J Biochem Mol Biol.* 2007;40(3):448–452.

84. Richens A, Dunlop A. Serum phenytoin levels in the management of epilepsy. *Lancet.* 1975;2:247–248.

85. Bauer L, Blouin R. Age and phenytoin kinetics in adult epileptics. *Clin Pharmacol Ther.* 1982;31:301–304.

86. Adithan C, Srinivas B, Indhiresan J, et al. Influence of type I and type II diabetes mellitus on phenytoin steady-state levels. *Int J Clin Pharmacol Ther Toxicol.* 1991;29:310–313.

87. Lander C, Smith M, Chalk J, et al. Bioavailability and pharmacokinetics of phenytoin during pregnancy. *Eur J Clin Pharmacol.* 1984;27:105–110.

88. Tomson T, Lindbom U, Ekqvist B, et al. Disposition of carbamazepine and phenytoin in pregnancy. *Epilepsia.* 1994;35(1):131–135.

89. Grasela T, Sheiner L, Rambeck B, et al. Steady state pharmacokinetics of phenytoin from routinely collected patient data. *Clin Pharmacokinet.* 1983;8:355–364.

90. Yukawa E, Higuchi S, Aoyama T. Population pharmacokinetics of phenytoin from routine clinical data in Japan. *J Clin Pharm Ther.* 1989;14(1):71–77.

91. Yukawa E, Higachi S, Aoyama T. Population pharmacokinetics of phenytoin from routine clinical data in Japan: an update. *Chem Pharm Bull.* 1990;38:1973–1976.

92. Bauer L, Blouin R. Phenytoin Michaelis–Menten pharmacokinetics in Caucasian paediatric patients. *Clin Pharmacokinet.* 1983;8:545–549.

93. Koren G, Brand N, MacLeod S. Influence of bioavailability on the calculated Michaelis–Menten parameters of phenytoin in children. *Ther Drug Monit.* 1984;6:11–14.

94. Suzuki Y, Mimaki T, Cox S, et al. Phenytoin age-dose-concentration relationship in children. *Ther Drug Monit.* 1994;16:145–150.

95. Chaplin SS, G; Smith, J. Drug excretion in human breast milk. *Adv Drug React Toxicol Rev.* 1982;1:255–287.

96. Chetty M, Miller R, Seymour MA. Phenytoin auto-induction. *Ther Drug Monit.* 1998;20(1):60–62.

97. Jamerson BD, Donn KH, Dukes GE, et al. Absolute bioavailability of phenytoin after 3-phosphoryloxymethyl phenytoin disodium (ACC-9653) administration to humans. *Epilepsia.* 1990;31(5):592–597.

98. Browne TR, Davoudi H, Donn KH, et al. Bioavailability of ACC-9653 (phenytoin prodrug). *Epilepsia.* 1989;30(suppl 2):S15–S21.

99. Hussey EK, Dukes GE, Messenheimer JA, et al. Evaluation of the pharmacokinetic interaction between diazepam and ACC-9653 (a phenytoin prodrug) in healthy male volunteers. *Pharm Res.* 1990;7(11):1172–1176.

100. Leppik IE, Boucher BA, Wilder BJ, et al. Pharmacokinetics and safety of a phenytoin prodrug given i.v. or i.m. in patients. *Neurology.* 1990;40(3 Pt 1):456–460.

101. Aweeka FT, Gottwald MD, Gambertoglio JG, et al. Pharmacokinetics of fosphenytoin in patients with hepatic or renal disease. *Epilepsia.* 1999;40(6):777–782.

102. Morton LD. Clinical experience with fosphenytoin in children. *J Child Neurol.* 1998;13(suppl 1):S19–S22.

103. Browne TR. Phenytoin and other hydantoins. In: Engel J Jr, Pedley TE, eds. *Epilepsy: A Comprehensive Textbook.* Philadelphia, PA: Lippincott-Raven Publishers; 1998:1557–1579.

104. Kugler AR, Knapp LE, Eldon MA. Rapid attainment of therapeutic phenytoin concentrations following administration of loading doses of fosphenytoin: a metaanalysis. *Neurology.* 1996;46(2):A176.

105. Eldon M, Loewen G, Voightman R, et al. Pharmacokinetics and tolerance of fosphenytoin and phenytoin administration intravenously to healthy subjects. *Can J Neurol Sci.* 1993;20:5810.

106. Hayes G, Kootsikas M. Reassessing the lower end of the phenytoin therapeutic range: a review of the literature. *Ann Pharmacother.* 1993;27:1389–1392.

107. Patsalos PN, Berry DJ, Bourgeois BF, et al. Antiepileptic drugs—best practice guidelines for therapeutic drug monitoring: a position paper by the subcommission on therapeutic drug monitoring, ILAE Commission on Therapeutic Strategies. *Epilepsia.* 2008;49(7):1239–1276.

108. Schmidt D, Haenel F. Therapeutic plasma levels of phenytoin, phenobarbital, and carbamazepine: individual variation in relation to seizure frequency and type. *Neurology.* 1984;34:1252–1255.

109. Tatro D. Drug facts and comparisons. In: *Facts & Comparisons.* St. Louis, MO: Facts and Comparisons; 1996.

110. Bauer L. Interference of oral phenytoin absorption by continuous nasogastric feedings. *Neurology.* 1982;32:570–572.

111. Haidukewych D, Rodin E, Zielinski J. Derivation and evaluation of an equation for prediction of free phenytoin concentration in patients comedicated with valproic acid. *Ther Drug Monit.* 1989;11:134–139.

112. Kerrick J, Wolff D, Graves N. Predicting unbound phenytoin concentrations in patients receiving valproic acid: a comparison of two prediction methods. *Ann Pharmacother.* 1995;29:470–474.

113. Duncan JS, Patsalos PN, Shorvon SD. Effects of discontinuation of phenytoin, carbamazepine, and valproate on concomitant antiepileptic medication. *Epilepsia.* 1991;32(1):101–115.

114. Wilder B. Phenytoin: clinical use. In: Levy R, Mattson R, Meldrum B, eds. *Antiepileptic Drugs.* New York: Raven Press; 1995:339–344.

115. Mattson RH. Efficacy and adverse effects of established and new antiepileptic drugs. *Epilepsia.* 1995;36(suppl 2):S13–S26.

116. Leppik I, Patrick B, Crawford R. Treatment of acute seizures and status epilepticus with intravenous phenytoin. In: Delgado-Escueta A, Wasterlain C, Treiman D, et al., eds. *Status Epilepticus: Mechanisms of Brain Damage and Treatment.* New York: Raven Press; 1983:447–451.

117. Wilder B. Efficacy of phenytoin in the treatment of status epilepticus. In: Delgado-Escueta A, Wasterlain C, Treiman D, et al., eds. *Status Epilepticus: Mechanisms of Brain Damage and Treatment.* New York: Raven Press; 1983:441–446.

118. Richard M, Chiron C, d'Athis P, et al. Phenytoin monitoring in status epilepticus in infants and children. *Epilepsia.* 1993;34:144–150.

119. Treiman DM, Meyers PD, Walton NY, et al. A comparison of four treatments for generalized convulsive status epilepticus. Veterans Affairs Status Epilepticus Cooperative Study Group. *N Engl J Med.* 1998;339(12):792–798.

120. Alldredge BK, Lowenstein DH, Simon RP. Placebo-controlled trial of intravenous diphenylhydantoin for short-term treatment of alcohol withdrawal seizures. *Am J Med.* 1989;87(6):645–648.

121. Chance J. Emergency department treatment of alcohol withdrawal seizures with phenytoin. *Ann Emerg Med.* 1991;20:520–522.

122. Mattson RH, Cramer JA, Collins JF, et al. Comparison of carbamazepine, phenobarbital, phenytoin, and primidone in partial and secondarily generalized tonic–clonic seizures. *N Engl J Med.* 1985;313(3):145–151.

123. Callaghan N, Kenny R, O'Neill B, et al. A prospective study between carbamazepine, phenytoin, and sodium valproate as monotherapy in previously untreated and recently diagnosed patients with epilepsy. *J Neurol Neurosurg Psychiatry.* 1985;48:639–644.

124. Ramsay RE, Wilder BJ, Berger JR, et al. A double-blind study comparing carbamazepine with phenytoin as initial seizure therapy in adults. *Neurology.* 1983;33(7):904–910.

125. Wilder B, Ramsay R, Willmore L, et al. Comparison of valproic acid and phenytoin in newly diagnosed tonic–clonic seizures. *Neurology.* 1983;33:1474–1476.

126. Turnbull DM, Howel D, Rawlins MD, et al. Which drug for the adult epileptic patient: phenytoin or valproate? *Br Med J (Clin Res Ed).* 1985;290(6471):815–819.

127. Heller AJ, Chesterman P, Elwes RDC, et al. Phenobarbitone, phenytoin, carbamazepine or sodium valproate for newly diagnosed adult epilepsy: a randomised comparative monotherapy trial. *J Neurol Neurosurg Psychiatry.* 1995;58:44–50.

128. Bill PA, Vigonius U, Pohlmann H, et al. A double-blind controlled clinical trial of oxcarbazepine versus phenytoin in adults with previously untreated epilepsy. *Epilepsy Res.* 1997;27(3):195–204.

129. Guerreiro MM, Vigonius U, Pohlmann H, et al. A double-blind controlled clinical trial of oxcarbazepine versus phenytoin in children and adolescents with epilepsy. *Epilepsy Res.* 1997;27(3):205–213.

130. Steiner TJ, Dellaportas CI, Findley LJ, et al. Lamotrigine monotherapy in newly diagnosed untreated epilepsy: a double-blind comparison with phenytoin. *Epilepsia.* 1999;40(5):601–607.

131. de Silva M, MacArdle B, McGowan M, et al. Randomised comparative monotherapy trial of phenobarbitone, phenytoin, carbamazepine, or sodium valproate for newly diagnosed childhood epilepsy. *Lancet.* 1996;347(9003):709–713.

132. Painter MJ, Scher MS, Stein AD, et al. Phenobarbital compared with phenytoin for the treatment of neonatal seizures. *N Engl J Med.* 1999;341(7):485–489.

133. Blume HK, Garrison MM, Christakis DA. Neonatal seizures: treatment and treatment variability in 31 United States pediatric hospitals. *J Child Neurol.* 2009;24(2):148–154.

134. Glauser T, Ben-Menachem E, Bourgeois B, et al. ILAE treatment guidelines: evidence-based analysis of antiepileptic drug efficacy and effectiveness as initial monotherapy for epileptic seizures and syndromes. *Epilepsia.* 2006;47(7):1094–1120.

135. Appleton M, Kuehl T, Raebel M, et al. Magnesium sulfate versus phenytoin for seizure prophylaxis in pregnancy-induced hypertension. *Am J Obstet Gynecol.* 1991;165:907–913.

136. Anonymous. Which anticonvulsant for women with eclampsia? Evidence from the Collaborative Eclampsia Trial. *Lancet.* 1995;345:1455–1463.

137. Lucas M, Leveno K, Cunningham F. A comparison of magnesium sulfate with phenytoin for the prevention of eclampsia. *N Engl J Med.* 1995;333:201–205.

138. Friedman S, Lim K, Baker C, et al. Phenytoin versus magnesium sulfate in preeclampsia: a pilot study. *Am J Perinatol.* 1993;10:233–238.

139. Guzman E, Conley M, Stewart R, et al. Phenytoin and magnesium sulfate effects on fetal heart rate tracings assessed by computer analysis. *Obstet Gynecol.* 1993;82:375–379.

140. Beenen LF, Lindeboom J, Trenit DG, et al. Comparative double blind clinical trial of phenytoin and sodium valproate as anticonvulsant prophylaxis after craniotomy: efficacy, tolerability, and cognitive effects. *J Neurol Neurosurg Psychiatry.* 1999;67(4):474–480.

141. Foy P, Chadwick D, Rajgopala N, et al. Do prophylactic anticonvulsant drugs alter the pattern of seizures after craniotomy? *J Neurol Neurosurg Psychiatry.* 1992;55:753–757.

142. Temkin N, Dikmen S, Wilensky A, et al. A randomized, double-blind study of phenytoin for the prevention of post-traumatic seizures. *N Engl J Med.* 1990;323:497–502.

143. Haltiner AM, Newell DW, Temkin NR, et al. Side effects and mortality associated with use of phenytoin for early posttraumatic seizure prophylaxis. *J Neurosurg.* 1999; 91(4):588–592.

144. Young KD, Okada PJ, Sokolove PE, et al. A randomized, double-blinded, placebo-controlled trial of phenytoin for the prevention of early posttraumatic seizures in children with moderate to severe blunt head injury. *Ann Emerg Med.* 2004;43(4):435–446.

145. McCleane G. Intravenous infusion of phenytoin relieves neuropathic pain: a randomized, double-blind, placebo controlled, crossover study. *Anesth Analg.* 1999;89(4):985–988.

146. Knox G, Woodard D, Chelen W, et al. Phenytoin for motion sickness: clinical evaluation. *Laryngoscope.* 1994;104(8 pt 1):935–939.

147. Woodard D, Knox G, Myers K, et al. Phenytoin as a countermeasure for motion sickness in NASA maritime operations. *Aviat Space Environ Med.* 1993;64:363–366.

148. Finkel M. Phenytoin revisited. *Clin Ther.* 1984;6:577–591.

149. Pendse A, Sharma A, Sodani A, et al. Topical phenytoin in wound healing. *Int J Dermatol.* 1993;32:214–217.

150. Modaghegh S, Salehian B, Tavassoli M, et al. Use of phenytoin in healing of war and non-war wounds. A pilot study of 25 cases. *Int J Dermatol.* 1989;28(5):347–350.

151. Wilder B, Bruni J. Medical management of seizure disorders. In: *Seizure Disorders: A Pharmacological Approach to Treatment.* New York: Raven Press; 1981:35–39.

152. Bruni J. Phenytoin: Toxicity. In: Levy R, Mattson R, Meldrum B, eds. *Antiepileptic Drugs.* New York: Raven Press; 1995:345–350.

153. Harrison MB, Lyons GR, Landow ER. Phenytoin and dyskinesias: a report of two cases and review of the literature. *Mov Disord.* 1993;8(1):19–27.

154. Howrie D, Crumrine P. Phenytoin-induced movement disorder associated with intravenous administration for status epilepticus. *Clin Pediatr.* 1985;24:467–469.

155. Micheli F, Lehkuniec E, Gatto M, et al. Hemiballism in a patient with partial motor status epilepticus treated with phenytoin. *Funct Neurol.* 1993;8:103–107.

156. Moss W, Ojukwu C, Chiriboga C. Phenytoin-induced movement disorder. Unilateral presentation in a child and response to diphenhydramine. *Clin Pediatr.* 1994;33:634–638.

157. Stilman N, Masdeu J. Incidence of seizures with phenytoin toxicity. *Neurology.* 1985;35:1769–1772.

158. Drane DL, Meador KJ. Epilepsy, anticonvulsant drugs and cognition. *Baillieres Clin Neurol.* 1996;5(4):877–885.

159. Devinsky O. Cognitive and behavioral effects of antiepileptic drugs. *Epilepsia.* 1995;36(suppl 2):S46–S65.

160. Aldenkamp AP, Alpherts WC, Diepman L, et al. Cognitive side-effects of phenytoin compared with carbamazepine in patients with localization-related epilepsy. *Epilepsy Res.* 1994;19(1):37–43.

161. Dodrill CB, Troupin AS. Neuropsychological effects of carbamazepine and phenytoin: a reanalysis. *Neurology.* 1991;41(1):141–143.

162. May TW, Bulmahn A, Wohlhuter M, et al. Effects of withdrawal of phenytoin on cognitive and psychomotor functions in hospitalized epileptic patients on polytherapy. *Acta Neurol Scand.* 1992;86(2):165–170.

163. Meador KJ, Loring DW, Allen ME, et al. Comparative cognitive effects of carbamazepine and phenytoin in healthy adults. *Neurology.* 1991;41(10):1537–1540.

164. Smith KR, Jr., Goulding PM, Wilderman D, et al. Neurobehavioral effects of phenytoin and carbamazepine in patients recovering from brain trauma: a comparative study. *Arch Neurol.* 1994;51(7):653–660.

165. Aldenkamp AP, Vermeulen J. Phenytoin and carbamazepine: differential effects on cognitive function. *Seizure.* 1995;4(2):95–104.

166. Pulliainen V, Jokelainen M. Effects of phenytoin and carbamazepine on cognitive functions in newly diagnosed epileptic patients. *Acta Neurol Scand.* 1994;89(2):81–86.

167. Pulliainen V, Jokelainen M. Comparing the cognitive effects of phenytoin and carbamazepine in long-term monotherapy: a two-year follow-up. *Epilepsia.* 1995;36(12):1195–1202.

168. Dodrill CB, Troupin AS. Psychotropic effects of carbamazepine in epilepsy: a double-blind comparison with phenytoin. *Neurology.* 1977; 27(11):1023–1028.

169. Dikmen SS, Temkin NR, Miller B, et al. Neurobehavioral effects of phenytoin prophylaxis of posttraumatic seizures. *JAMA.* 1991;265(10):1271–1277.

170. Meador KJ, Loring DW, Moore EE, et al. Comparative cognitive effects of phenobarbital, phenytoin, and valproate in healthy adults. *Neurology.* 1995;45(8):1494–1499.

171. Craig T, Tallis R. Impact of valproate and phenytoin on cognitive function in elderly patients: results of a single-blind randomized comparative study. *Epilepsia.* 1994;35(2):381–390.

172. Read CL, Stephen LJ, Stolarek IH, et al. Cognitive effects of anticonvulsant monotherapy in elderly patients: a placebo-controlled study. *Seizure.* 1998;7(2):159–162.

173. Wallace SJ. A comparative review of the adverse effects of anticonvulsants in children with epilepsy. *Drug Saf.* 1996;15(6):378–393.

174. Aldenkamp AP, Alpherts WC, Blennow G, et al. Withdrawal of antiepileptic medication in children—effects on cognitive function: The Multicenter Holmfrid Study. *Neurology.* 1993;43(1):41–50.

175. Aman MG, Werry JS, Paxton JW, et al. Effects of phenytoin on cognitive-motor performance in children as a function of drug concentration, seizure type, and time of medication. *Epilepsia.* 1994;35(1):172–180.

176. Leeder JS. Mechanisms of idiosyncratic hypersensitivity reactions to antiepileptic drugs. *Epilepsia.* 1998;39(suppl 7):S8–S16.

177. Chadwick D, Shaw M, Foy P, et al. Serum anticonvulsant concentrations and the risk of drug induced skin eruptions. *J Neurol Neurosurg Psychiatry.* 1984;47:642–644.

178. Leppik I, Lapora J, Loewenson R. Seasonal incidence of phenytoin allergy unrelated to plasma levels. *Arch Neurol.* 1985;42:120–122.

179. Leppik IE. Phenytoin. In: Resor SR, Kutt H, eds. *The Medical Treatment of Epilepsy.* New York, Basel, Hong Kong: Marcel Dekker, Inc.; 1992:279–291.

180. Schlienger RG, Shear NH. Antiepileptic drug hypersensitivity syndrome. *Epilepsia.* 1998;39(suppl 7):S3–S7.

181. Hirsch LJ, Arif H, Nahm EA, et al. Cross-sensitivity of skin rashes with antiepileptic drug use. *Neurology.* 2008;71(19):1527–1534.

182. Haruda F. Phenytoin hypersensitivity: 38 cases. *Neurology.* 1979; 29(11):1480–1485.

183. Man CB, Kwan P, Baum L, et al. Association between HLA-B*1502 allele and antiepileptic drug-induced cutaneous reactions in Han Chinese. *Epilepsia.* 2007;48(5):1015–1018.

184. Locharernkul C, Loplumlert J, Limotai C, et al. Carbamazepine and phenytoin induced Stevens–Johnson syndrome is associated with HLA-B*1502 allele in Thai population. *Epilepsia.* 2008;49(12):2087–2091.

185. Dahllof G, Preber H, Eliasson S, et al. Peridontal condition of epileptic adults treated long-term with phenytoin or carbamazepine. *Epilepsia.* 1993;34:960–964.

186. Hassell T, Hefti A. Drug-induced gingival overgrowth: old problem, new problem. *Crit Rev Oral Biol Med.* 1991;2:103–137.

187. Thomason J, Seymour R, Rawlins M. Incidence and severity of phenytoin-induced gingival overgrowth in epileptic patients in general medical practice. *Community Dent Oral Epidemiol.* 1992;20:288–291.

188. Casetta I, Granieri E, Desideri M, et al. Phenytoin-induced gingival overgrowth: a community-based cross-sectional study in Ferrara, Italy. *Neuroepidemiology.* 1997;16(6):296–303.

189. Brunsvold M, Tomasovic J, Ruemping D. The measured effect of phenytoin withdrawal on gingival hyperlasia. *ASDC J Dent Child* 1985;52:417–421.

190. Dahllof G, Axio E, Modeer T. Regression of phenytoin-induced gingival overgrowth after withdrawal of medication. *Swed Dent J.* 1991;15:139–143.

191. Baier W, Beck U, Doose H, et al. Cerebellar atrophy following diphenylhydantoin intoxication. *Neuropediatrics.* 1984;15:76–81.

192. Baier W, Beck U, Hirsch W. CT findings following diphenylhydantoin intoxication. *Pediatr Radiol.* 1985;15:220–221.

193. Lindvall O, Nilsson R. Cerebellar atrophy following phenytoin intoxication. *Ann Neurol.* 1984;16:258–260.

194. Jibiki I, Kido H, Matsuda H, et al. Probable cerebellar abnormality of 123I-IMP SPECT scans in epileptic patients with long-term high-dose phenytoin therapy. Based on observation of multiple cases. *Acta Neurol.* 1993;15:16–24.

195. Ney G, Lantos G, Barr W, et al. Cerebellar atrophy in patients with long-term phenytoin exposure and epilepsy. *Arch Neurol.* 1994;51:767–771.

196. Kubota F, Kifune A, Shibata N, et al. Bone mineral density of epileptic patients on long-term antiepileptic drug therapy: a quantitative digital radiography study. *Epilepsy Res.* 1999;33(2–3):93–97.

197. Hug G, McGraw CA, Bates SR, et al. Reduction of serum carnitine concentrations during anticonvulsant therapy with phenobarbital, valproic acid, phenytoin, and carbamazepine in children. *J Pediatr.* 1991;119(5):799–802.

198. Calandre E, Porta BS, Calzada DGdl. The effect of chronic phenytoin treatment on serum lipid profile in adult epileptic patients. *Epilepsia.* 1992;33:154–157.

199. Elwes R, Dellaportas C, Reynolds E, et al. Prolactin and growth hormone dynamics in epileptic patients receiving phenytoin. *Clin Endocrinol.* 1985;23:263–270.
200. McKenney J, Petrizzi K, Briggs G, et al. The effect of low-dose phenytoin on high-density lipoprotein cholesterol. *Pharmacotherapy.* 1992;12:183–188.
201. Hcroz A, Levesque L, Drislane F, et al. Phenytoin-induced elevation of serum estradiol and reproductive dysfunction in men with epilepsy. *Epilepsia.* 1991;32:550–553.
202. Smith P, Surks M. Multiple effects of 5,5'-diphenylhydatoin on the thyroid hormone system. *Endocr Rev.* 1984;5:514–524.
203. Frey B, Frey F. Phenytoin modulates the pharmacokinetics of prednisolone and the pharmacodynamics of prednisolone as assessed by the inhibition of the mixed lymphocyte reaction in humans. *Eur J Clin Invest.* 1984;1 4:1–6.
204. Hegedus L, Hansen J, Luhdorf K, et al. Increased frequency of goitre in epileptic patients on long-term phenytoin or carbamazepine treatment. *Clin Endocrinol.* 1985;23:423–429.
205. Franklyn J, Sheppard M, Ramsden D. Measurement of free thyroid hormones in patients on long-term phenytoin therapy. *Eur J Clin Pharmacol.* 1984;26:633–634.
206. Basaran N, Hincal F, Kansu E, et al. Humoral and cellular immune parameters in untreated and phenytoin- or carbamazepine-treated epileptic patients. *Int J Immunopharmacol.* 1994;16:1071–1077.
207. Ishizaka A, Nakaniski M, Kasahara E, et al. Phenytoin-induced IgG2 and IgG4 deficiencies in a patient with epilepsy. *Acta Paediatr.* 1992;81:646–648.
208. Kondo N, Takao A, Tomatsu S, et al. Suppression of IgA production by lymphocytes induced by diphenylhydantoin. *J Invest Allergol Clin Immunol.* 1994;4:255–257.
209. Britigan B. Diphenylhydantoin-induced hypogammaglobulinemia in a patient infected with human immunodeficiency virus. *Am J Med.* 1991;90:524–527.
210. Lazoglu A, Boglioli L, Dorsett B, et al. Phenytoin-related immunodeficiency associated with Loeffler's syndrome. *Ann Allergy Asthma Immunol.* 1995;74:479–482.
211. Hanson JW, Smith DW. The fetal hydantoin syndrome. *J Pediatr.* 1975;87(2):285–290.
212. Kaneko S, Battino D, Andermann E, et al. Congenital malformations due to antiepileptic drugs. *Epilepsy Res.* 1999;33(2–3):145–158.
213. Puho EH, Szunyogh M, Metneki J, et al. Drug treatment during pregnancy and isolated orofacial clefts in Hungary. *Cleft Palate Craniofac J.* 2007;44(2):194–202.
214. Vajda FJ, Hitchcock A, Graham J, et al. The Australian Register of Antiepileptic Drugs in Pregnancy: the first 1002 pregnancies. *Aust N Z J Obstet Gynaecol.* 2007;47(6):468–474.
215. Meador KJ, Baker GA, Browning N, et al. Cognitive function at 3 years of age after fetal exposure to antiepileptic drugs. *N Engl J Med.* 2009;360(16):1597–1605.
216. Vanoverloop D, Schnell RR, Harvey EA, et al. The effects of prenatal exposure to phenytoin and other anticonvulsants on intellectual function at 4 to 8 years of age. *Neurotoxicol Teratol.* 1992;14(5):329–335.
217. Scolnik D, Nulman I, Rovet J, et al. Neurodevelopment of children exposed in utero to phenytoin and carbamazepine monotherapy [published erratum appears in *JAMA.* 1994;Jun 8;271(22):1745] [see comments]. *JAMA.* 1994;271(10):767–770.
218. Wide K, Henning E, Tomson T, et al. Psychomotor development in preschool children exposed to antiepileptic drugs in utero. *Acta Paediatr.* 2002;91(4):409–414.
219. Earnest MP, Marx JA, Drury LR. Complications of intravenous phenytoin for acute treatment of seizures. Recommendations for usage. *JAMA.* 1983;249(6):762–765.
220. Hanna DR. Purple glove syndrome: a complication of intravenous phenytoin. *J Neurosci Nurs.* 1992;24(6):340–345.
221. Helfaer MA, Ware C. Purple glove syndrome. *J Neurosurg Anesthesiol.* 1994;6(1):48–49.
222. O'Brien TJ, Cascino GD, So EL, et al. Incidence and clinical consequence of the purple glove syndrome in patients receiving intravenous phenytoin. *Neurology.* 1998;51(4):1034–1039.
223. Carducci B, Hedges J, Beal J, et al. Emergency phenytoin loading by constant intravenous infusion. *Ann Emerg med.* 1984;13:1027–1059.
224. Donovan P, Cline D. Phenytoin administration by constant intravenous infusion: selective rates of administration. *Ann Emerg Med.* 1991;20:139–142.
225. Ramsay R, Philbrook B, Martinez D, et al. A double-blind, randomized safety comparison of rapidly infused intravenous loading doses of fosphenytoin vs. phenytoin. *Epilepsia.* 1995;36(suppl 4):90.
226. Ramsay RE, DeToledo J. Intravenous administration of fosphenytoin: options for the management of seizures. *Neurology.* 1996;46(suppl 1):S17–S19.
227. Dean J, Smith K, Boucher B, et al. Safety, tolerance and pharmacokinetics of intramuscular (IM) fosphenytoin, a phenytoin prodrug, in neurosurgery patients. *Epilepsia.* 1993;34(suppl 6):111.
228. Ramsay R, Barkley D, Garnett W, et al. Safety and tolerance of intramuscular fosphenytoin (Cerebyx) in patients requiring a loading dose of phenytoin. *Neurology.* 1995;45(suppl 4):A249.
229. Wilder B, Ramsay R, Marriot J, et al. Safety and tolerance on intramuscular administration of fosphenytoin, a phenytoin prodrug, for 5 days in patients with epilepsy. *Neurology.* 1994;43(suppl 2):A308.
230. Lowenstein DH, Alldredge BK. Status epilepticus. *N Engl J Med.* 1998;338(14):970–976.
231. Cranford R, Leppik I, Patrick B, et al. Intravenous phenytoin: clinical and pharmacokinetic aspects. *Neurology.* 1978;28:874–880.
232. Jung D, Powell J, Walson P, et al. Effect of dose on phenytoin absorption. *Clin Pharmacol Ther.* 1980;28:479–485.
233. Rudis MI, Touchette DR, Swadron SP, et al. Cost-effectiveness of oral phenytoin, intravenous phenytoin, and intravenous fosphenytoin in the emergency department. *Ann Emerg Med.* 2004;43(3):386–397.
234. Swadron SP, Rudis MI, Azimian K, et al. A comparison of phenytoin-loading techniques in the emergency department. *Acad Emerg Med.* 2004;11(3):244–252.
235. Hvidberg EF, Dam M. Clinical pharmacokinetics of anticonvulsants. [Review] [175 refs]. *Clinical Pharmacokinetics.* 1976;1(3):161–188.
236. Serrano EE, Roye DB, Hammer RH, et al. Plasma diphenylhydantoin values after oral and intramuscular administration of diphenylhydantoin. *Neurology.* 1973;23(3):311–317.
237. Wilensky AJ, Lowden JA. Inadequate serum levels after intramuscular administration of diphenylhydantoin. *Neurology.* 1973;23(3):318–324.
238. Fuerst RH, Graves NM, Kriel RL, et al. Absorption and safety of rectally administered phenytoin. *Eur J Drug Metab Pharmacokinet.* 1988;13(4):257–260.
239. Privitera MD. Clinical rules for phenytoin dosing. [see comments]. *Ann Pharmacother.* 1993;27(10):1169–1173.
240. Armijo J, Cavada F. Graphic estimation of phenytoin dose in adults and children. *Ther Drug Monit.* 1991;13:507–510.
241. Bachmann K, Schwartz J, Forney R Jr, et al. Single dose phenytoin clearance during erythromycin treatment. *Res Commun Chem Pathol Pharmacol.* 1984;46:207–217.
242. Cai W, Chu X, Chen G. A Bayesian graphic method for predicting individual phenytoin dosage schedule. *Acta Pharmacol Sin.* 1991;12:141–144.
243. Flint N, Lopez L, Robinson J, et al. Comparison of eight phenytoin dosing methods in institutionalized patients. *Ther Drug Moni.* 1985;7:74–80.
244. Nakashima E, Matsushita R, Kido H, et al. Systematic approach to a dosage regimen for phenytoin based on one-point, steady-state plasma concentration. *Ther Drug Monit.* 1995;17:12–18.
245. Pryka R, Rodvold K, Erdman S. An updated comparison of drug dosing methods, part I: phenytoin. *Clin Pharmacokinet.* 1991;20:209–217.
246. Tobias J, Baker D, Hurwitz C. Removal of phenytoin by plasmapheresis in a patient with thrombotic thrombocytopenia purpura. *Clin Pediatr.* 1992;31:105–108.
247. Hays DP, Primack WA, Abroms IF. Phenytoin clearance by continuous ambulatory peritoneal dialysis. *Drug Intell Clin Pharm.* 1985;19(6):429–431.
248. Lau A, Kronfol N. Effect of continuous hemofiltration of phenytoin elimination. *Ther Drug Monit.* 1994;16:53–57.
249. Kramer G, Biraben A, Carreno M, et al. Current approaches to the use of generic antiepileptic drugs. *Epilepsy Behav.* 2007;11(1):46–52.
250. Burkhardt RT, Leppik IE, Blesi K, et al. Lower phenytoin serum levels in persons switched from brand to generic phenytoin. *Neurology.* 2004;63(8):1494–1496.
251. Fischer JH, Cwik MJ, Luer MS, et al. Stability of fosphenytoin sodium with intravenous solutions in glass bottles, polyvinyl chloride bags, and polypropylene syringes. *Ann Pharmacother.* 1997;31(5):553–559.
252. Allen F, Runge J, Legarda S. Safety, tolerance, and pharmacokinetics of intravenous fosphenytoin (Cerebyx) in status epilepticus. *Epilepsia.* 1995;36(suppl 4):90.
253. Wheless JW. Pediatric use of intravenous and intramuscular phenytoin: lessons learned. *J Child Neurol.* 1998;13(suppl 1):S11–S14.
254. Browne TR. Intravenous phenytoin: cheap but not necessarily a bargain. *Neurology.* 1998;51(4):942–943.
255. Armstrong EP, Sauer KA, Downey MJ. Phenytoin and fosphenytoin: a model of cost and clinical outcomes. *Pharmacotherapy.* 1999;19(7):844–853.
256. Marchetti A, Magar R, Fischer J, et al. A pharmacoeconomic evaluation of intravenous fosphenytoin (Cerebyx) versus intravenous phenytoin (Dilantin) in hospital emergency departments. *Am J Health Syst Pharm.* 1996;53(19):2249.
257. Coplin WM, Rhoney DH, Rebuck JA, et al. Randomized evaluation of adverse events and length-of-stay with routine emergency department use of phenytoin or fosphenytoin. *Neurol Res.* 2002;24(8):842–848.

CHAPTER 53 ■ PHENOBARBITAL AND PRIMIDONE

BLAISE F. D. BOURGEOIS

HISTORICAL BACKGROUND

Although its use has been decreasing, phenobarbital (PB) is still a major antiepileptic drug (AED). PB has been prescribed for the treatment of epilepsy since 1912, with only bromide having been used longer. Although PB is associated with more sedative and behavioral side effects than most other AEDs, it has relatively low systemic toxicity and a conveniently long half-life, can be administered intravenously and intramuscularly, is effective in patients with status epilepticus and in neonates, and is inexpensive.

Primidone (PRM) has been in clinical use since its synthesis in 1952 (1). Often referred to as a barbiturate, PRM does not strictly belong in this class; its pyrimidine ring contains only two carbonyl groups, compared with the three groups of barbituric acid (Fig. 53.1), but the remainder of the structure is identical to that of PB. Therapeutically, however, PRM is appropriately considered a barbiturate, as its effect can be attributed predominantly to the derived PB. This hepatic biotransformation has heretofore made it impossible to establish whether therapy with PRM differs clinically from that with PB or whether PRM is a PB prodrug. Complicating this issue is the experimental demonstration of independent antiepileptic activity for the other main metabolite of PRM, phenylethylmalonamide (PEMA) (see Fig. 53.1).

CHEMISTRY AND MECHANISM OF ACTION

Chemically, PB is 5-ethyl-5-phenylbarbituric acid (see Fig. 53.1). The molecular weight is 232.23 and the conversion factor from milligrams to micromoles is 4.31 (1 mg/L = 4.31 μmol/L). The sodium salt of PB is water soluble. PB in its free acid form is a white crystalline powder soluble in organic solvents, but with limited water and lipid solubility; it is a weak acid with a pK_a of 7.3. Many actions of PB at the cellular level have been described. Although it is not certain which are responsible for seizure protection, the available evidence seems to favor enhancement of γ-aminobutyric acid (GABA) inhibition (2). In animal models, PB protects against electroshock-induced seizures and, unlike phenytoin, carbamazepine, and PRM, against seizures induced by chemical convulsants, such as pentylenetetrazol. In normal animals, PB raises the threshold and shortens the duration of afterdischarges elicited by electrical stimulation (3). Like other barbiturates, PB enhances postsynaptic $GABA_A$ receptor-mediated chloride (Cl^-) currents by prolonging the opening of the Cl^- ionophore (4). Increased flow of Cl^- into the cell decreases excitability. Presynaptically, PB can cause a concentration-dependent reduction of calcium (Ca^{2+})-dependent action potentials (5), which may contribute to seizure protection at

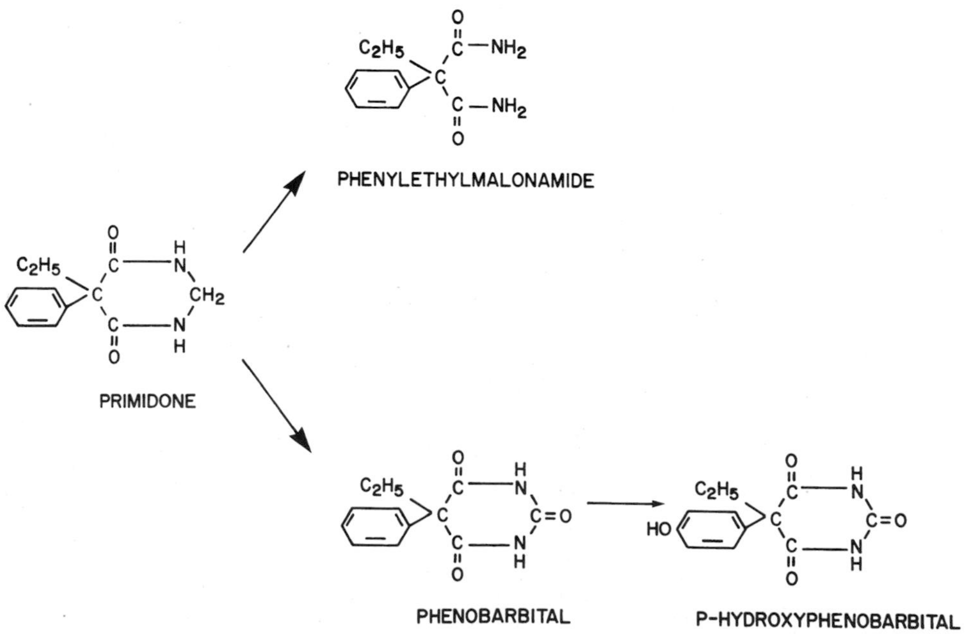

FIGURE 53.1 Structural formulas of primidone and its main metabolites.

higher therapeutic levels and, especially, to sedative and anesthetic effects.

Chemically, PRM is 5-ethyldihydro-5-phenyl-4,6(1-*H*,5*H*) pyrimidinedione. The molecular weight is 218.264 and the conversion factor from milligrams to micromoles is 4.59 (1 mg/L = 4.59 μmol/L). PRM is very poorly soluble in water, somewhat soluble in ethanol, and virtually insoluble in organic solvents.

The basic pharmacologic mechanism of action of PRM has received relatively little attention, not least because it was uncertain for some time whether the agent itself has independent antiepileptic activity. The basic anticonvulsant action of PRM has been studied in mouse neurons in cell culture (6). PRM was compared with PB for its effect on amino acid responses and on sustained, high-frequency firing. In contrast to PB, PRM had no effect on postsynaptic GABA and glutamate responses at concentrations up to 50 μg/mL. However, both agents limited sustained, high-frequency, repetitive firing at relatively high concentrations (>50 μg/mL). Together, PRM and PB limited sustained high-frequency, repetitive firing at clinically relevant concentrations (12 μg/mL and 20 μg/mL, respectively). The authors concluded that PRM and PB may act synergistically to reduce sustained, high-frequency, repetitive firing. These in vitro findings are in accordance with observations made in whole animals.

All the evidence regarding the individual antiepileptic properties of PRM, PB, and PEMA is derived from experiments in animals whose seizures were provoked. Because the metabolites accumulate a few hours after administration of the first dose, a possible long-term protection by PRM alone against spontaneously occurring seizures cannot be assessed in humans. In addition, PEMA may be involved in the overall pharmacodynamic effect of PRM. The first evidence of the independent anticonvulsant activity of PRM came from dogs that were protected against experimental seizures at a lower concentration of PB when PRM was also present than when PB alone was present (7). Rats were similarly protected against induced seizures after a single dose of PRM before the active metabolites could be detected (8), as were mice pretreated with a metabolic blocker that delayed the biotransformation of PRM (9,10). The anticonvulsant potency of PRM against maximal electroshock-induced seizures is similar to that of PB, but unlike PB, PRM was ineffective against chemically induced seizures caused by pentylenetetrazol or biculline (9). Thus, the experimental anticonvulsant spectrum of PRM differs from that of PB and is similar to that of carbamazepine and phenytoin; therefore, PRM and PB may be two different AEDs with different mechanisms of action.

On the basis of brain concentrations in mice, PRM appears to be 2.5 times less neurotoxic than PB, with a superior therapeutic index (9). When PB and PRM were administered together in single-dose experiments in mice (11), their anticonvulsant activity was supra-additive (potentiated) and their neurotoxic effect was infra-additive. A PB–PRM brain concentration ratio of 1:1 provided the best therapeutic index. This ratio is not usually seen in patients, especially those taking PRM combined with enzyme-inducing drugs such as phenytoin or carbamazepine. If PRM is different from or even better than PB for the treatment of epilepsy, its different effect would be likely only when the PRM concentration equals or exceeds the PB concentration. Such a ratio is achieved only rarely with PRM monotherapy and almost never when PRM

is added to phenytoin or carbamazepine, or combined with PB. The results of pharmacodynamic interactions between PRM and PB in mice were confirmed by experiments in amygdala-kindled rats. After single doses, the anticonvulsant effect of PB was potentiated by PRM, whereas side effects of PB, such as ataxia and muscle relaxation, were not increased by combined treatment with PRM (12).

In rats (13) and mice (9,10), PEMA had relatively weak anticonvulsant activity of its own. On the basis of brain concentrations in mice (9), PEMA was 16 times less potent than PB in seizure protection and 8 times less potent in neurotoxic effects, but it potentiated the anticonvulsant (11,13) and neurotoxic effects (11) of PB. Nevertheless, a quantitative analysis of these experimental results, together with the blood levels encountered in clinical practice, suggests that PEMA does not significantly add to the antiepileptic effect or neurotoxicity of PRM therapy.

ABSORPTION, DISTRIBUTION, AND METABOLISM

Phenobarbital

Most formulations of PB contain sodium salt because of good aqueous solubility. The absolute bioavailability of oral preparations of PB is usually greater than 90% (14). Absorption of PB following intramuscular (IM) administration was found to be as complete as that following administration of oral tablets, compared with intravenous (IV) administration (15). Accumulation half-life for the IM route (0.73 hours) was not shorter than for the oral route (0.64 hours). Time to peak concentration is usually 2 to 4 hours. In newborns, however, peak PB plasma levels after oral administration may be reached later than after IM administration (16). A parenteral solution of PB administered rectally has a bioavailability of 89%, compared with that of IM administration (17); average time to peak concentration was 4.4 hours.

PB is not highly bound to serum proteins (45%). Protein binding of PB is lower during pregnancy and in newborns, with a bound fraction between 30% and 40% in pregnant women and their offspring (18). Reported values for the volume of distribution vary. Following IV administration, average values were 0.54 L/kg in adult volunteers and 0.61 L/kg in adult patients with epilepsy (15), both well within the reported range. The volume of distribution of PB approached 1.0 L/kg in newborns (19).

PB is eliminated mostly via renal excretion of the unchanged drug, and via hepatic metabolism and renal excretion of the metabolites. An average of 20% to 25% of PB is eliminated unchanged by the kidneys in adults, with large interindividual variability (20,21). The main metabolite of PB is *p*-hydroxyphenobarbital (Fig. 53.1). At steady state, approximately 20% to 30% of the PB dose is transformed into this metabolite, approximately 50% of which is conjugated to glucuronic acid (20,21). Nitrogen glucosidation, another relevant pathway of PB metabolism, accounts for 25% to 30% of total PB disposition (22). Other identified metabolites of PB represent a very low percentage of the total elimination.

The elimination of PB from serum follows first-order, or linear, kinetics. The half-life of PB is age dependent. It is usually well above 100 hours in newborns (23) and averages 148 hours in asphyxiated newborns (24). During the neonatal period, PB elimination accelerates markedly; thereafter, half-lives are very short, with average values of 63 hours during the first year of life and 69 hours between the ages of 1 and 5 years (25). Half-lives in adults range between 80 and 100 hours, and no evidence of autoinduction of PB metabolism has been demonstrated (15).

Primidone

PRM is supplied as 250-mg and 50-mg tablets and as syrup (1 mL = 50 mg); extremely low solubility precludes parenteral administration. After oral ingestion of tablets, the time to peak serum concentrations in adult patients with epilepsy was 2.7 (26) and 3.2 hours (27), respectively, and 4 to 6 hours after single-dose administration in children (28). In the same study, an average of 92% of the dose (range, 72% to 123%) was excreted in the urine as unchanged PRM and metabolites, probably indicating complete oral bioavailability. Concomitant administration of acetazolamide reduced the oral absorption of PRM (29). One generic preparation was found to have a lower bioavailability than the trademark product (30).

The volume of distribution of PRM ranged from 0.54 L/kg following acute intoxication (31) to 0.86 L/kg (32). The volume of distribution of PEMA after its oral administration was 0.69 L/kg (33). In human plasma, protein binding of both PRM and PEMA was less than 10% (13,27,33). Brain concentrations of PRM were found to be lower than simultaneous plasma concentrations in mice (9,10) and in rats (8). In patients undergoing surgery for intractable epilepsy, one group of investigators found an average brain-to-plasma ratio of 87% (34). In another report (10) of six patients whose mean plasma PRM concentration was 6.3 µg/mL, brain concentrations ranged between nondetectable and 2.2 µg/g. Brain concentrations of PEMA in mice were 93% (10) and 77% (9) of the plasma levels. In humans, the cerebrospinal fluid–plasma ratio for PRM ranged from 0.8 to 1.13 (27,34,35), which is similar to human saliva-to-plasma ratios (36) and which is consistent with the high free fraction of plasma PRM.

The elimination half-life of PRM varies, mainly because of enzymatic induction by comedication. In adults receiving long-term PRM monotherapy, the elimination half-life ranged from 10 to 15 hours (37–39). Therapy with additional AEDs was associated with values of 6.5 and 8.3 hours (26,27,38,39). In 12 children (4 treated with PRM monotherapy, 8 treated with PRM and phenytoin), half-lives ranged from 4.5 to 11 hours (mean, 8.7 hours) (28). In newborns, however, the average PRM half-life was 23 hours (range, 8 to 80 hours) (40), which was associated with a limited biotransformation to the metabolites (41).

After oral ingestion of PEMA itself, the half-life of PRM was 15.7 hours (33). The elimination rate of PEMA cannot be determined accurately in patients taking PRM because the liver produces PEMA as long as PRM is measurable in the blood.

Because two metabolites of PRM accumulate after repeated administration of the agent and because both have independent anticonvulsant activity, an understanding of the qualitative and quantitative aspects of PRM metabolism is needed before any rational clinical use of this drug can be undertaken. Ideally, before prescribing the agent, the physician should know the relative antiepileptic potency, relative toxicity, and expected relative blood levels of PRM and its two active metabolites. Unfortunately, this information is only partially available. Although relative efficacy and relative toxicity of PRM and its metabolites have been studied acutely in animals (9,11), similar investigations are virtually impossible in humans because the three compounds are always present simultaneously during long-term therapy.

Figure 53.1 shows the relevant metabolic pathways for PRM. The first metabolite of PRM to be identified, PEMA, was found initially in rats (42) and thereafter in every species studied. PB and p-hydroxyphenobarbital were discovered only 4 years later, in 1956 (43), and toxic reactions attributed to the derived PB were first reported in 1958 (44). Other metabolites of PRM, with either negligible or nondetectable blood levels during long-term therapy, have no practical significance. Numerous clinical studies have discussed the quantitative aspects of the biotransformation of PRM to PB and PEMA. A comparison of the ratios of PB serum levels to dose during long-term PB therapy and during long-term PRM therapy in the same patients demonstrated that 24.5% of the PRM dose is converted to PB (45). This is in accordance with the report that average PRM doses (in mg/kg/day) required to maintain a given PB level are about five times higher than the equivalent PB doses (46). The extent of PRM biotransformation and the ratios of the blood levels of PRM and its metabolites are very sensitive to interactions with other AEDs and are discussed separately.

INTERACTIONS WITH OTHER AGENTS

Most of the interactions of PB reflect its status as an enzymatic inducer that accelerates the biotransformation of some AEDs, as well as other agents. No clinically significant interaction with PB has been reported that involves absorption. Moreover, because PB is only 55% protein bound in serum, significant interactions involving displacement from serum proteins do not occur. Clinically, the most significant interaction affecting PB levels is the inhibition of PB elimination by valproate (47). Seen in the majority of patients, the extent of this interaction is variable, although the increase in PB concentration can reach 100%, often necessitating dosage adjustments. The concentrations of PB derived from PRM are equally affected by valproate.

In the great majority of interactions, PB affects levels of other agents. Levels of valproate (48) and carbamazepine (49) are often reduced by the addition of PB. Levels of the active metabolite of carbamazepine, the 10,11-epoxide, are less affected or may even increase, and the epoxide–carbamazepine ratio is usually higher in the presence of PB. Relative to the metabolism of phenytoin, PB appears to cause both enzymatic induction and competitive inhibition. The two effects tend to balance out in patients, and dosage adjustments of phenytoin are seldom necessary (50). PB significantly increases the clearance of lamotrigine (51), as well as that of ethosuximide, felbamate, topiramate, zonisamide, tiagabine (52), and rufinamide (53).

PB induces the metabolism of many agents besides AEDs. Among the relevant interactions, clearance and dosage requirements of theophylline (54) increase following the addition of

PB. Induction of the metabolism of coumarin anticoagulants, such as warfarin (55), can cause problems when PB is introduced or discontinued. In both cases, the anticoagulant dose may require adjustment to avoid excessively long prothrombin times or loss of the desired prothrombin time prolongation. Finally, PB can accelerate the metabolism of steroids, including those contained in oral contraceptives, leading to breakthrough bleeding and contraceptive failure (56). Medium- or high-dose oral contraceptive preparations are recommended in women taking PB (57).

PRM is the cause, as well as the object, of numerous pharmacokinetic interactions (58). Because PB is invariably present during long-term PRM treatment, all of the effects of PB on other agents, described above, can be expected with PRM. The degree of enzymatic induction by other AEDs causes the extent of PRM biotransformation to vary among patients. Most reports describe enzymatic induction of the conversion of PRM to PB; some note inhibition. These interactions change not only the blood levels of PRM, PB, and PEMA relative to the PRM dose, but also the ratios among the three substances. Phenytoin, a known potent inducer (38,59–61), causes the most extensive acceleration of PRM conversion, leading to a decrease in the PRM–PB serum concentration ratio. The rate of PRM biotransformation is slower with carbamazepine (38,58), which may also inhibit the conversion of PRM to PB, causing an increase in the PRM–PB serum concentration ratio (62). Table 53.1 summarizes the effect of comedication with phenytoin, carbamazepine, or both on the concentration-to-dose ratios and on the relative concentration ratios of PRM, PB, and PEMA (63). Compared with PRM monotherapy, the morning trough levels of PRM were reduced by about 50% at the same daily dose. Inversely, PB levels were increased by a factor of approximately 1.6. Thus, when patients receive concomitant phenytoin or carbamazepine, the average PRM dose required to maintain a given PB level is about 1.6 times lower than that with PRM monotherapy. Because derived PB is the product of enzymatic conversion and not the substrate, this difference is the opposite of what is usually seen with inducing interaction, namely, that the drug dose must be increased to maintain the same drug level. With PRM, such an increase often yields PB levels associated with toxic reactions.

Table 53.1 also shows that the PB–PRM concentration ratio in a morning predose blood sample was more than three times higher in patients taking phenytoin or carbamazepine in addition to PRM (5.83 vs. 1.65, respectively). This means that at a PRM level of 10 mg/L, the corresponding average PB level would be 16.5 mg/L in a patient receiving PRM monotherapy, but 58.3 mg/L in a patient also taking phenytoin or carbamazepine.

Different effects of valproate on PRM kinetics have been described. In one study (64), transient elevations of PRM levels were observed after the addition of valproate; PB levels were not included in this analysis. Other investigators (58) found no consistent changes in PRM or PB levels after the addition of valproate to PRM therapy.

In all patients receiving long-term PRM therapy, the PB level is almost always higher than the PRM level. Attempts have been made to elevate the PRM level in relation to the PB level to obtain a greater therapeutic effect from PRM itself. Adding nicotinamide to the drug regimen (62) could achieve such a change in ratio, but the necessary doses may cause gastrointestinal side effects and hepatotoxic reactions. The antituberculosis drug isoniazid also markedly inhibits PRM biotransformation, producing relatively high PRM levels relative to PB levels (65).

EFFICACY

PB can show at least some degree of efficacy against every seizure type, except absence seizures, but is used mainly for the treatment of generalized convulsive seizures and partial seizures. It is an agent of first choice only in neonates with seizures. In a large-scale, controlled comparison of 622 adults with partial and secondarily generalized tonic–clonic seizures (66), phenytoin, carbamazepine, PB, and PRM were equally effective in achieving complete control. PB and PRM controlled partial seizures in a lower percentage of patients than did carbamazepine; the difference in overall success rate

---

TABLE 53.1

SERUM CONCENTRATION: PRM DOSE RATIOS AND SERUM CONCENTRATION RATIOS OF PRIMIDONE, PHENOBARBITAL, AND PHENYLETHYLMALONAMIDE AT STEADY STATE[a]

	No. of patients	Serum concentration: PRM dose[b]			Serum concentration ratio[b]	
		PRM	PB	PEMA	PB/PRM	PEMA/PRM
Monotherapy	10	0.78 ±0.25	1.47 ±0.53	0.64 ±0.39	1.65 ±0.74	0.70 ±0.36
Comedications[c]	53	0.40 ±0.15	2.40 ±0.98	0.75A ±0.42	5.83 ±2.62	1.71 ±0.75

PB, phenobarbital; PEMA, phenylethylmalonamide; PRM, primidone.
[a]All blood samples were drawn before the first morning dose in hospitalized patients.
[b]Mean ± standard deviation (SD), PRM dose in mg/kg/day, serum levels in mg/L.
[c]Combination therapy included phenytoin or carbamazepine, or both.
From Bourgeois BFD. Primidone. In: Resor SR, Kutt H, eds. *Medical Treatment of Epilepsy.* New York: Marcel Dekker; 1992:371–378, with permission.

between the agents was based mainly on their side-effect profiles. Evidence-based comparison of PB with phenytoin (67) and with carbamazepine (68) revealed no overall difference in seizure control, but PB was more likely to be withdrawn than the other two agents, presumably because of side effects. In children, PB was as effective as carbamazepine for up to 1 year in the treatment of partial seizures (36). In a randomized study of previously untreated children, PB, phenytoin, carbamazepine, and valproate were compared (69). After 6 of the first 10 children randomized to PB discontinued treatment mainly because of behavioral side effects, PB was eliminated from the study for ethical reasons. Generalized myoclonic seizures and, in particular, juvenile myoclonic epilepsy (70) also respond to PB, although it is not an agent of first choice. A major agent in the treatment of patients with convulsive status epilepticus, PB is usually given if seizures persist following administration of a benzodiazepine and phenytoin (71). The main disadvantages associated with its use are respiratory depression and pronounced sedation. In patients with status epilepticus, PB was as effective as a combination of diazepam and phenytoin (72). Very high doses of PB have been recommended for the treatment of refractory status epilepticus in children (73,74). This approach controlled seizures when no limits were imposed relative to maximum dose, and serum levels of 70 to 344 mg/L were achieved (73). In this series, most patients were initially intubated but recovered good spontaneous respiration despite persistently high PB levels; hypotension was uncommon. PB is the agent of first choice in newborns with any type of seizure, with control achieved in about one third of the infants (19,75,76). An efficacy rate of 85% against various neonatal seizures was noted with loading doses of up to 40 mg/kg (77); however, this high response rate cannot be explained solely on the basis of increased doses. In a recent study, newborns with seizures were randomized to initial treatment with PB or phenytoin (78). There was no difference in the percentage of neonates in whom seizure control was achieved with PB (43%) and with phenytoin (45%).

PB has been the most widely used agent for chronic prophylaxis of febrile seizures, with efficacy demonstrated at levels higher than 15 mg/L (79,80). Failure of prophylaxis was often due to noncompliance with the regimen and subtherapeutic levels at the time of seizure recurrence. However, such treatment is now rarely considered, for several reasons: improved understanding of the benign nature of simple febrile seizures; the efficacy of intermittent short-term use of rectal or oral diazepam therapy (81–83); and reservations about the possible detrimental effect on cognitive function (84,85).

Neurologic side effects have prevented PRM from becoming an agent of first choice for the treatment of any seizure type. Indications are similar to those for PB, except for the treatment of status epilepticus and neonatal seizures (PRM is not available in a parenteral formulation), and the prophylaxis of febrile seizures. PRM is effective against generalized tonic–clonic seizures and, when used as a primary agent, juvenile myoclonic epilepsy (86,87). However, because of its greater efficacy and lower toxicity, valproate is now preferred for the latter condition. The clinical efficacy of PRM and PB has been compared in various studies. Several demonstrated no superiority of PRM, but neither was the drug less effective (45,88,89). In one crossover study (90), the efficacy of PRM and PB was compared sequentially in the same patients. Similar PB levels were maintained during both therapies, and

PRM was found to be slightly more effective than PB against generalized tonic–clonic seizures.

In partial and secondarily generalized seizures, PRM use was associated with the same degree of seizure control as phenytoin or carbamazepine (89,91). The aforementioned study by Mattson and colleagues (66), which is the most comprehensive and systematic controlled comparison of carbamazepine, phenytoin, PB, and PRM in these seizure types, showed little difference in efficacy among the agents; however, the percentage of treatment failures was highest with PRM because of an increased incidence of side effects early on. Carbamazepine and phenytoin were associated with the lowest percentage of failures. The choice between PB and PRM may depend on individual factors. After PB has failed, PRM may still be tried. However, selecting PRM before PB may save one therapeutic step, based on the assumption that PB is unlikely to be effective if maximal tolerated doses of PRM have not controlled seizures. PRM is rarely indicated against any type of seizure other than partial and secondarily generalized seizures. In particular, the agent has little or no place in the treatment of generalized epilepsies encountered in childhood, such as absence epilepsy and Lennox–Gastaut syndrome. Although some potential use has been demonstrated in the treatment of neonatal seizures (41), PRM is rarely used for this indication. PRM is contraindicated in any patient with a previous allergic or severe idiosyncratic reaction to PRM or to PB. Like PB, PRM is also contraindicated in patients with hepatic porphyria.

ADVERSE EFFECTS

Among AEDs, PB and PRM are more likely to cause dose-related neurotoxic reactions, although serious systemic side effects are rare. These agents invariably produce sedation and drowsiness at high doses in adults, whereas children often become hyperactive and irritable even at levels in the therapeutic range. Sedation, usually present at relatively low levels during the first few days of treatment, subsides thereafter as tolerance to this effect develops. Sedation or somnolence reappears only at high therapeutic or supratherapeutic levels, usually >30 mg/L. As dose levels increase further, neurologic toxicity appears, characterized by dysarthria, ataxia, incoordination, and nystagmus. In children, sedation from PB is much less common than behavioral side effects, mainly hyperactivity, aggressiveness, and insomnia, which may be seen in almost half of all children receiving PB and can appear at levels <15 mg/L (80). Depression has been attributed to PB (92,93) as well as to PRM therapy (94). Although its effect may have been overemphasized, double-blind, controlled studies have confirmed that PB affects cognitive abilities even at levels in the therapeutic range. Children treated with PB had lower memory and concentration scores than those receiving placebo, and these differences correlated significantly with plasma levels (95). Double-blind comparisons of PB-treated children versus untreated children (96,84) or valproate-treated children (97) demonstrated subtle but significantly lower intelligence quotient (IQ) scores in the PB groups. In an intention-to-treat analysis comparing children treated with PB or placebo for febrile seizures, the average IQ score was 8.4 points lower with PB (84) and remained 5.2 points lower 6 months after discontinuation of PB. Some differences persisted 3 to 5 years later (85). Movement disorders, such as dyskinesia, may be induced by PB, but they are rare (98). Like other AEDs, PB can exacerbate seizures or induce de novo seizures (99).

Allergic rashes and hypersensitivity reactions are relatively rare with PB and PRM treatment (100). In one study of crosssensitivity, among patients who developed a rash on carbamazepine and phenytoin, 26.7% and 19.5%, respectively, also subsequently had a rash on PB (101). Inversely, among patients who developed a rash on PB, 66.7% had a rash on carbamzepine and 53.3% had a rash on phenytoin. Hematologic toxicity is quite rare with PB or with PRM (102,103). Like phenytoin and carbamazepine, PB can exacerbate acute intermittent porphyria (104) and cause osteoporosis, decreased bone mineral density, and increased risk of fracture, presumably through accelerated vitamin D metabolism (105–107). Vitamin K-deficient hemorrhagic disease in newborns of mothers treated with PB (108) can be prevented by administration of vitamin K to the mother before delivery. Connective tissue disorders associated with long-term PB therapy are well-known (109) and have recently received renewed attention. These include Dupuytren contractures, plantar fibromatosis, heel and knuckle pads, frozen shoulder, and diffuse joint pain (110). Connective tissue disorders are an unusual side effect in children.

Like every AED, PB has been known to increase the risk for minor and major malformations in the offspring of mothers who were chronically exposed during pregnancy. Assessment of the specific risk for a given agent in clinical studies has been complicated by polytherapy and the underlying risk for malformation due to maternal epilepsy. No evidence suggests that PB is more teratogenic than other AEDs or that it causes a specific spectrum of malformations (111). Folic acid supplementation taken at 5 to 12 weeks of amenorrhea may decrease the risk of anomalies (112). Like valproate and phenytoin, PB may be associated with reduced cognitive outcome in the child (113). Evidence that PB increases the risk for any type of tumor development in humans is lacking (114).

Acute and chronic toxic PRM reactions can be distinguished clearly from one another, but long-term PRM side effects are difficult to separate from those associated with derived PB. Because the ratio of PRM to PB varies, toxic side effects may occur at different PRM concentrations. Moreover, reliable evidence that long-term PRM side effects differ from those with comparable PB therapy is lacking. This is also true for potential teratogenic effects. Ventriculoseptal defects, microcephaly, and poor somatic development (115) have been described in the offspring of women taking PRM, although no specific teratogenic pattern has been attributed to the agent.

The acute initial toxicity clearly differentiates PRM from PB. Even after a low initial dose of PRM, some patients experience transient side effects—usually drowsiness, dizziness, ataxia, nausea, and vomiting (66)—that are so debilitating they may be reluctant to take a second dose. Because this acute toxic reaction occurs before PB or PEMA is detected in the blood, it must be associated with PRM itself. That much larger doses of PRM are later tolerated by the same patients during long-term therapy argues for the development of tolerance to PRM probably within hours to days. The ratio of clinical toxicity score to serum PRM levels, determined in a group of patients receiving their first PRM dose (116), decreased significantly as early as 6 hours after the ingestion of drug. PB probably produces a crosstolerance to this acute PRM toxicity, because patients on long-term PB therapy are less likely to experience the same degree of toxicity on first exposure to PRM (116,117). Crosstolerance to PRM following PB exposure can be demonstrated in experimental animals. To achieve the same degree of seizure protection and the same level of neurotoxicity, higher brain concentrations of PRM were necessary in mice that had received PB daily for 2 weeks than in mice without any drug exposure (118).

CLINICAL USE

On the basis of its relative efficacy and toxicity profile, PB is no longer an agent of first choice for the treatment of any seizure type, except for neonates with seizures and for long-term prophylaxis of febrile seizures, if indicated. PB remains an agent of second or third choice for the treatment of generalized convulsive seizures and partial seizures at any age, and is prescribed widely for infants because it is easier to use and is associated with less systemic toxicity than several other AEDs.

In adults, the daily maintenance dose of PB, between 1.5 and 4 mg/kg, achieves steady-state levels within the recommended therapeutic range of 15 to 40 mg/L. Because of its long elimination half-life and slow accumulation, the full maintenance dose can be administered on the first treatment day, although steady-state plasma levels will be reached only after 2 to 3 weeks. The daily maintenance dose of PB in children varies between 2 and 8 mg/kg; doses >8 mg/kg may be necessary in some infants to achieve high therapeutic levels. The dose is roughly inversely proportional to the child's age: 2 months to 1 year, 4 to 11 mg/kg/day; 1 to 3 years, 3 to 7 mg/kg/day; and 3 to 6 years, 2 to 5 mg/kg/day (119). Given the long half-life of PB, dividing the daily dose of the agent into two or more doses appears unnecessary, even in children (120). Close monitoring of plasma levels and dosage reductions may be necessary in patients with advanced renal disease (121) and cirrhosis (122).

The IV loading dose of PB for the treatment of status epilepticus varies between 10 and 30 mg/kg; 15 to 20 mg/kg is most common. The rate of administration should not exceed 100 mg/min (2 mg/kg/min in children weighing less than 40 kg). PB penetrates the brain relatively slowly; however, although full equilibrium is not reached for as long as 1 hour, therapeutic brain concentrations are reached within 3 minutes (123). The initial loading dose of 15 to 20 mg/kg in newborns is similar to the dose in children and adults, and will achieve a plasma level of about 20 mg/L. This level can usually be maintained in newborns with a dose of 3 to 4 mg/kg/day (124). Loading doses up to 40 mg/kg have been used (77).

PRM should be used alone or in combination with a noninducing drug, such as gabapentin, lamotrigine, topiramate, tiagabine, zonisamide, levetiracetam, vigabatrin, or a benzodiazepine. An inducing drug will shift the PRM–PB ratio to such an extent that one might just as well prescribe PB instead of PRM. For the same reason, prescribing PRM and PB simultaneously for the same patient makes no sense. Valproate may also increase PB levels, on the basis of its demonstrated inhibition of PB elimination. A low starting dose is more important with PRM than with most other AEDs because of the occurrence of transient, but severe, neurotoxic reactions. A first dose of one-half tablet (125 mg) at bedtime is often well-tolerated, but some patients initially need as little as one-quarter tablet (62.5 mg) or less. The dose can then be increased every 3 days as tolerated, to a final daily maintenance dose of 10 to 20 mg/kg. Maintenance doses are 15 to 25 mg/kg/day in newborns, 10 to 25 mg/kg/day in infants, and 10 to 20 mg/kg/day in children.

A schedule that allows rapid advancement to the full maintenance dose of PRM was devised (125) on the basis of observations in humans (116) and experimental animals (118) that PB produces crosstolerance to the effects of PRM. After initial administration of PB, the dose is titrated as rapidly as tolerated to achieve a serum level up to 20 mg/L; abrupt switch to the full maintenance dose of PRM follows. Experimentation with various PB titration schedules revealed that most patients tolerate the following increases with minimal or no sedation: 5 mg/L after 24 hours; 10 mg/L after 48 hours; 15 mg/L after 72 hours; and 20 mg/L after 96 hours (end of day 4). These levels can be achieved in adults by administering 3 mg/kg of PB orally on day 1 (two doses of 1.5 mg/kg each, 12 hours apart); 3.5 mg/kg on day 2; 4 mg/kg on day 3; and 5 mg/kg on day 4 (Fig. 53.2). On day 5, the patient can receive a full PRM maintenance dose of 12.5 to 20 mg/kg, with no significant new toxicity. This beneficial effect of PB pretreatment on initial PRM toxicity has been confirmed in a more recent study (126).

PRM monotherapy at a daily dose of 20 mg/kg will achieve, on average, PB levels of 30 mg/L (see Table 53.1); however, steady-state PB levels will be reached only after 2 to 3 weeks at the same PRM dose. In patients comedicated with carbamazepine or phenytoin, the same PB level will be achieved with an average PRM dose of 10 to 15 mg/kg/day. As with most AEDs, average dosage requirements may be higher in children and lower in the elderly. Because of the relatively short half-life of PRM, usual recommendations call for dividing the daily dose into three doses, although the need to do so has never been documented. If blood levels are used to adjust the PRM dose, then PB rather than PRM levels are preferred, because at the usual concentration ratios the side effects from a high PB level are more likely to limit further dosage increases. Although a therapeutic range of 3 to 12 mg/L has

been suggested for PRM (127), monitoring PRM levels is of little help in clinical practice. This is true for PEMA as well, which probably has no significant pharmacologic effect at levels measured in patients.

After long-term administration, PB and PRM should always be discontinued gradually over several weeks. Barbiturates and benzodiazepines are the AEDs most commonly associated with withdrawal seizures on rapid discontinuation. This phenomenon is due to pharmacodynamic mechanisms that cause a state of rebound hyperexcitability when the amount of the drug decreases in the brain, resulting in a lower seizure threshold, and predisposing the patient to more severe than usual seizures or even to status epilepticus. The phenomenon is unrelated to pharmacokinetics, and the fact that PB has a long elimination half-life does not protect the patient or preclude the need for very gradual withdrawal over weeks or months. Since patients treated with PRM are also chronically exposed to PB, the same caution should be exercised when discontinuing PRM therapy. Unless there is a specific reason to proceed faster, it is appropriate to taper the PB or PRM dose linearly over 3 to 6 months, with reductions each month.

References

1. Bogue JY, Carrington HC. The evaluation of "mysoline," a new anticonvulsant drug. *Br J Pharmacol.* 1953;8:230–236.
2. Olson RW. Phenobarbital and other barbiturates: mechanism of action. In: Levy RH, Mattson RH, Meldrum BS, et al., eds. *Antiepileptic Drugs.* 5th ed. Philadelphia, PA: Lippincott Williams & Wilkins; 2002:489–495.
3. Straw R, Mitchell C. Effect of phenobarbital on cortical after-discharge and overt seizure patterns in the rat. *Int J Neuropharmacol.* 1966;5:323–330.
4. MacDonald R, Twyman R. Kinetic properties and regulation of GABA receptor channels. In: Narahashi R, ed. *Ion Channels.* New York: Plenum; 1992:315–343.
5. Heyer E, Macdonald R. Barbiturate reduction of calcium-dependent action potentials: correlation with anesthetic action. *Brain Res.* 1982;236:157–171.
6. MacDonald R, McLean M. Anticonvulsant drugs: mechanisms of action. *Adv Neurol.* 1986;44:713–736.
7. Frey HH, Hahn I. Research on the significance of phenobarbital, produced by biotransformation, for the anticonvulsant action of pyrimidone [German]. *Arch Int Pharmacodyn Ther.* 1960;128:281–290.
8. Baumel IP, Gallagher BB, DiMicco D, et al. Metabolism and anticonvulsant properties of primidone in the rat. *J Pharmacol Exp Ther.* 1973;186:305–314.
9. Bourgeois BFD, Dodson WE, Ferrendelli JA. Primidone, phenobarbital, and PEMA: I. Seizure protection, neurotoxicity, and therapeutic index of individual compounds in mice. *Neurology.* 1983;33:283–290.
10. Leal KW, Rapport RL, Wilensky AJ, et al. Single-dose pharmacokinetics and anticonvulsant efficacy of primidone in mice. *Ann Neurol.* 1979;5:470–474.
11. Bourgeois BFD, Dodson WE, Ferrendelli JA. Primidone, phenobarbital, and PEMA: II. Seizure protection, neurotoxicity, and therapeutic index of varying combinations in mice. *Neurology.* 1983;33:291–295.
12. Loscher W, Honack D. Comparison of the anticonvulsant efficacy of primidone and phenobarbital during chronic treatment of amygdala-kindled rats. *Eur J Pharmacol.* 1989;162:309–322.
13. Baumel IP, Gallagher BB, Mattson RH. Phenylethylmalonamide (PEMA). An important metabolite of primidone. *Arch Neurol.* 1972;27:34–41.
14. Nelson E, Powell J, Conrad K, et al. Phenobarbital pharmacokinetics and bioavailability in adults. *J Clin Pharmacol.* 1982;18:31–42.
15. Wilensky A, Friel P, Levy R, et al. Kinetics of phenobarbital in normal subjects and epileptic patients. *Eur J Clin Pharmacol.* 1982;23:87–92.
16. Jalling B. Plasma concentrations of phenobarbital in the treatment of seizures in the newborn. *Acta Paediatr Scand.* 1975;64:514–524.
17. Graves NM, Holmes GB, Kriel RL, et al. Relative bioavailability of rectally administered phenobarbital sodium parenteral solution. *DICP.* 1989;23:565–568.
18. Kuhnz W, Koch S, Helge H, et al. Primidone and phenobarbital during lactation period in epileptic women: total and free drug serum levels in the nursed infants and their effects on neonatal behavior. *Dev Pharmacol Ther* 1988;1:147–154.
19. Painter MJ, Pippenger C, Wasterlain C, et al. Phenobarbital and phenytoin in neonatal seizures: metabolism and tissue distribution. *Neurology.* 1981;31:1107–1112.

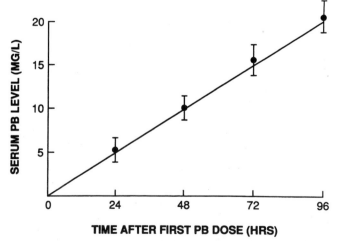

FIGURE 53.2 Phenobarbital (PB) loading dose over 4 days for rapid introduction of primidone. The PB values represent the average of 11 patients with standard deviation *(vertical bars).* The *solid straight line* connects the corresponding predicted values (5, 10, 15, and 20 mg/L). (Courtesy of Bourgeois BFD, unpublished data, 1991.)

20. Kapetanovic I, Kupferberg H, Porter R, et al. Mechanism of valproate-phenobarbital interaction in epileptic patients. *Clin Pharmacol Ther.* 1981;29:480–486.
21. Whyte M, Dekaban A. Metabolic fate of phenobarbital. A quantitative study of p-hydroxyphenobarbital elimination in man. *Drug Metab Dispos.* 1977;5:63–70.
22. Tang B, Kalow W, Grey AA. Metabolic fate of phenobarbital in man. N-glucoside formation. *Drug Metab Dispos.* 1979;7:315–318.
23. Pitlick W, Painter M, Pippenger C. Phenobarbital pharmacokinetics in neonates. *Clin Pharmacol Ther.* 1978;23:346–350.
24. Gal P, Toback J, Erkan N, et al. The influence of asphyxia on phenobarbital dosing requirements in neonates. *Dev Pharmacol Ther.* 1984;7:145–152.
25. Heimann G, Gladtke E. Pharmacokinetics of phenobarbital in childhood. *Eur J Clin Pharmacol.* 1977;12:305–310.
26. Gallagher BB, Baumel IP, Mattson RH. Metabolic disposition of primidone and its metabolites in epileptic subjects after single and repeated administration. *Neurology.* 1972;22:1186–1192.
27. Gallagher BB, Baumel IP. Primidone. Absorption, distribution and excretion. In: Woodbury DM, Penry JK, Schmidt RP, eds. *Antiepileptic Drugs.* New York: Raven Press; 1972:357–359.
28. Kauffman RE, Habersang R, Lansky J. Kinetics of primidone metabolism and excretion in children. *Clin Pharmacol Ther.* 1977;22:200–205.
29. Syverson GB, Morgan JP, Weintraub M, et al. Acetazolamide-induced interference with primidone absorption. *Arch Neurol.* 1977;34:80–84.
30. Wyllie E, Pippenger CE, Rothner AD. Increased seizure frequency with generic primidone. *JAMA.* 1987;258:1216–1217.
31. Matzke GR, Cloyd JC, Sawchuk RJ. Acute phenytoin and primidone intoxication. A pharmacokinetic analysis. *J Clin Pharmacol.* 1981;21:92–99.
32. Pisani F, Perucca E, Primerano G, et al. Single-dose kinetics of primidone in acute viral hepatitis. *Eur J Clin Pharmacol.* 1984;27:465–469.
33. Pisani F, Richens A. Pharmacokinetics of phenylethylmalonamide (PEMA) after oral and intravenous administration. *Clin Pharmacol.* 1983;8:272–276.
34. Houghton GW, Richens A, Toseland PA, et al. Brain concentrations of phenytoin, phenobarbital and primidone in epileptic patients. *Eur J Clin Pharmacol.* 1975;9:73–78.
35. Monaco F, Piredda S, Mastropaolo C, et al. Diphenylhydantoin and primidone in tears. *Epilepsia.* 1981;22:185–188.
36. Mitchell W, Chavez J. Carbamazepine versus phenobarbital for partial onset seizures in children. *Epilepsia.* 1987;28:56–60.
37. Booker HE, Hosokowa K, Burdette RD, et al. A clinical study of serum primidone levels. *Epilepsia.* 1970;11:395–402.
38. Cloyd JC, Miller KW, Leppik IE. Primidone kinetics: effects of concurrent drugs and duration of therapy. *Clin Pharmacol Ther.* 1981;29:402–407.
39. Zavadil P, Gallagher BB. Metabolism and excretion of ^{14}C-primidone in epileptic patients. In: Janz D, ed. *Epileptology.* Stuttgart, Germany: Thieme; 1976:129–139.
40. Nau H, Rating D, Hauser I, et al. Placental transfer and pharmacokinetics of primidone and its metabolites phenobarbital, PEMA and hydroxyphenobarbital in neonates and infants of epileptic mothers. *Eur J Clin Pharmacol.* 1980;18:31–42.
41. Powell C, Painter MJ, Pippenger CC. Primidone therapy in refractory neonatal seizures. *J Pediatr.* 1984;105:651–654.
42. Bogue JY, Carrington HC. Personal communication, 1952, cited by Goodman LS, Swinyard EA, Brown WC, et al. Anticonvulsant properties of 5-phenyl-5-ethyl hexahydropyrimidine-4,6-dione (Mysoline), a new antiepileptic. *J Pharmacol Exp Ther.* 1953;108:428–436.
43. Butler TC, Waddell WJ. Metabolic conversion of primidone (mysoline) to phenobarbital. *Proc Soc Exp Biol Med.* 1956;93:544–546.
44. Plaa GL, Fujimoto JM, Hine CH. Intoxication from primidone due to its biotransformation to phenobarbital. *JAMA.* 1958;168:1769–1770.
45. Oleson OV, Dam M. The metabolic conversion of primidone to phenobarbitone in patients under long-term treatment. *Acta Neurol Scand.* 1967;43:348–356.
46. Bogan J, Smith H. The relation between primidone and phenobarbitone blood levels. *J Pharm Pharmacol.* 1968;20:64–67.
47. De Gatta M, Gonzales A, Sanches M, et al. Effect of sodium valproate on phenobarbital serum levels in children and adults. *Ther Drug Monit.* 1986;8:416–420.
48. May T, Rambeck B. Serum concentrations of valproic acid: influence of dose and comedication. *Ther Drug Monit.* 1985;7:387–390.
49. Riva R, Contin M, Albani F, et al. Free concentration of carbamazepine and carbamazepine-10,11-epoxide in children and adults. Influence of age and phenobarbitone co-medication. *Clin Pharmacokinet.* 1985;10:524–531.
50. Browne T, Szabo G, Evan J, et al. Phenobarbital does not alter phenytoin steady-state concentration or pharmacokinetics. *Neurology.* 1988;38:639–642.
51. Eriksson A, Hoppu K, Nergardh A, et al. Pharmacokinetic interactions between lamotrigine and other antiepileptic drugs in children with intractable epilepsy. *Epilepsia.* 1996;37:769–773.
52. Riva R, Albani F, Contin M, et al. Pharmacokinetic interactions between antiepileptic drugs: clinical considerations. *Clin Pharmacokinet.* 1996;31:470–493.
53. Perucca E, Cloyd J, Critchley D, et al. Rufinamide: clinical pharmacokinetics and concentration-response relationship in patients with epilepsy. *Epilepsia.* 2008;49:1123–1141.
54. Jonkman J, Upton R. Pharmacokinetic drug interactions with theophylline. *Clin Pharmacokinet.* 1984;9:309–334.
55. MacDonald M, Robinson D. Clinical observations of possible barbiturate interference with anticoagulation. *JAMA.* 1968;204:97–100.
56. Hempel E, Klinger W. Drug stimulated biotransformation of hormonal steroid contraceptives: clinical implications. *Drugs.* 1976;12:442–448.
57. Mattson R, Cramer J. Epilepsy, sex hormones and antiepileptic drugs. *Epilepsia.* 1985;26(suppl):S40–S55.
58. Fincham RW, Schottelius DD. Primidone: interactions with other drugs. In: Levy RH, Dreifuss F, Mattson RH, et al., eds. *Antiepileptic Drugs.* New York: Raven Press; 1989:413–422.
59. Battino D, Avanzini G, Bossi L, et al. Plasma levels of primidone and its metabolite phenobarbital: effect of age and associated therapy. *Ther Drug Monit.* 1983;5:73–79.
60. Fincham RW, Schottelius DD, Sahs AL. The influence of diphenylhydantoin on primidone metabolism. *Arch Neurol.* 1974;30:259–262.
61. Reynolds EH, Fenton G, Fenwick P, et al. Interaction of phenytoin and primidone. *Br Med J.* 1975;2:594–595.
62. Bourgeois BFD, Dodson WE, Ferrendelli JA. Interactions between primidone, carbamazepine, and nicotinamide. *Neurology.* 1982;32:1122–1126.
63. Bourgeois BFD. Primidone. In: Resor SR, Kutt H, eds. *Medical Treatment of Epilepsy.* New York: Marcel Dekker; 1992:371–378.
64. Windorfer A, Sauer W, Gadeke R. Elevation of diphenylhydantoin and PRIMIDONE serum concentrations by addition of dipropylacetate, a new anticonvulsant drug. *Acta Paediatr.* 1975;64:771–772.
65. Sutton G, Kupferberg HJ. Isoniazid as an inhibitor of primidone metabolism. *Neurology.* 1975;25:1179–1181.
66. Mattson RH, Cramer JA, Collins JF, et al. Comparison of carbamazepine, phenobarbital, phenytoin and primidone in partial and secondarily generalized tonic–clonic seizures. *N Engl J Med.* 1985;313:145–151.
67. Taylor S, Tudur SC, Williamson PR, et al. Phenobarbitone versus phenytoin monotherapy for partial onset seizures and generalized onset tonic-clonic seizures. *Cochrane Database Syst Rev.* 2001;4:CD002217.
68. Tudur SC, Marson AG, Williamson PR. Carbamazepine versus phenobarbitone monotherapy for epilepsy. *Cochrane Database Syst Rev.* 2003;1:CD001904.
69. de Silva M, MacArdle B, McGowan M, et al. Randomised comparative monotherapy trial of phenobarbitone, phenytoin, carbamazepine, or sodium valproate for newly diagnosed childhood epilepsy. *Lancet.* 1996;347:709–713.
70. Resor SR, Resor LD. The neuropharmacology of juvenile myoclonic epilepsy. *Clin Neuropharmacol.* 1990;6:465–491.
71. Miller LC, Drislane FW. Treatment of status epilepticus. *Expert Rev Neurother.* 2008;8:1817–1827.
72. Shaner MD, McCurdy S, Herring M, et al. Treatment of status epilepticus: a prospective comparison of diazepam and phenytoin versus phenobarbital and optional phenytoin. *Neurology.* 1988;38:202–207.
73. Crawford TO, Mitchell WG, Fishman LS, et al. Very-high-dose phenobarbital for refractory status epilepticus in children. *Neurology.* 1988;38:1035–1040.
74. Tiamkao S, Mayurasakorn N, Suko P, et al. Very high dose phenobarbital for refractory status epilepticus. *J Med Assoc Thai.* 2007;90:2597–2600.
75. Lockman L, Kriel R, Zaske D. Phenobarbital dosage for control of neonatal seizures. *Neurology.* 1979;29:1445–1449.
76. Van Orman C, Darwish HZ. Efficacy of phenobarbital in neonatal seizures. *Can J Neurol Sci.* 1985;12:95–99.
77. Gal P, Toback J, Boer H, et al. Efficacy of phenobarbital monotherapy in treatment of neonatal seizures—relationship to blood vessels. *Neurology.* 1982;32:1401–1404.
78. Painter MJ, Scher MS, Stein AD, et al. Phenobarbital compared with phenytoin for the treatment of neonatal seizures. *N Engl J Med.* 1999;341:485–489.
79. Faero O, Kastrup K, Nielsen E, et al. Successful prophylaxis of febrile convulsions with phenobarbital. *Epilepsia.* 1972;13:279–285.
80. Wolf SM, Forsythe A. Behavior disturbance, phenobarbital, and febrile seizures. *Pediatrics.* 1978;61:728–731.
81. Knudsen FU. Effective short-term diazepam prophylaxis in febrile convulsions. *J Pediatr.* 1985;106:487–490.
82. Rosman NP, Colton T, Labazzo J, et al. A controlled trial of diazepam administered during febrile illnesses to prevent recurrence of febrile seizures. *N Engl J Med.* 1993;329:79–84.
83. Baumann RJ, Duffner PK. Treatment of children with simple febrile seizures: the AAP practice parameter. *Pediatr Neurol.* 2000;23:11–17.
84. Farwell JR, Lee YJ, Hirtz DG, et al. Phenobarbital for febrile seizures—effects on intelligence and on seizure recurrence. *N Engl J Med.* 1990;322:364–369.
85. Sulzbacher S, Farwell JR, Temkin N, et al. Late cognitive effects of early treatment with phenobarbital. *Clin Pediatrics.* 1999;38:387–394.
86. Delgado-Escueta AV, Enrile-Bascal F. Juvenile myoclonic epilepsy of Janz. *Neurology.* 1984;34:285–294.
87. Janz D. Epilepsy with impulsive petit mal (juvenile myoclonic epilepsy). *Acta Neurol Scand.* 1985;72:449–459.

88. Gruber CM Jr, Brock JT, Dyken M. Comparison of the effectiveness of phenobarbital, mephobarbital, primidone, diphenylhydantoin, ethotoin, metharbital, and methylphenylethylhydantoin in motor seizures. *Clin Pharmacol Ther.* 1962;3:23–28.

89. White PT, Pott D, Norton J. Relative anticonvulsant potency of primidone. A double-blind comparison. *Arch Neurol.* 1966;14:31–35.

90. Oxley J, Hebdige S, Laidlaw J, et al. A comparative study of phenobarbitone and primidone in the treatment of epilepsy. In: Johannessen SI, Morselli PL, Pippenger CE, et al., eds. *Antiepileptic Therapy. Advances in Drug Monitoring.* New York: Raven Press; 1980:237–245.

91. Rodin EA, Rim CS, Kitano H, et al. A comparison of the effectiveness of primidone versus carbamazepine in epileptic outpatients. *J Nerv Ment Dis.* 1976;163:41–46.

92. Brent D, Crumrine P, Varma R, et al. Phenobarbital treatment and major depressive disorder in children with epilepsy: a naturalistic follow-up. *Pediatrics.* 1987;80:909–917.

93. Miller JM, Kustra RP, Vuong A, et al. Depressive symptoms in epilepsy: prevalence, impact, aetiology, biological correlates and effect of treatment with antiepileptic drugs. *Drugs.* 2008;68:1493–1509.

94. Lopez-Gomez M, Ramirez-Bermudez J, Campillo C, et al. Primidone is associated with interictal depression in patients with epilepsy. *Epilepsy Behav.* 2005;6:413–416.

95. Camfield PR. Pancreatitis due to valproic acid. *Lancet.* 1979;1:1198–1199.

96. Calandre EP, Dominguez-Granados R, Gomez-Rubio M, et al. Cognitive effects of long-term treatment with phenobarbital and valproic acid in school children. *Acta Neurol Scand.* 1990;81:504–506.

97. Vining EP, Mellitis ED, Dorsen MM, et al. Psychologic and behavioral effects of antiepileptic drugs in children: a double-blind comparison between phenobarbital and valproic acid. *Pediatrics.* 1987;80:165–174.

98. Wiznitzer M, Younkin D. Phenobarbital-induced dyskinesia in a neurologically-impaired child. *Neurology.* 1984;34:1600–1601.

99. Hamano S, Mochizuki M, Morikawa T. Phenobarbital-induced absence seizure in benign childhood epilepsy with centrotemporal spikes. *Seizure.* 2002;11:201–204.

100. Arif H, Buchsbaum R, Weintraub D, et al. Comparison and predictors of rash associated with 15 antiepileptic drugs. *Neurology.* 2007;68:1701–1709.

101. Hirsch LJ, Arif H, Nahm EA, et al. Cross-sensitivity of skin rashes with antiepileptic drug use. *Neurology.* 2008;71:1527–1534.

102. Hawkins C, Meynell M. Macrocytosis and macrocytic anemia caused by anticonvulsant drugs. *Am J Med.* 1958;27:45–63.

103. Focosi D, Kast RE, Benedetti E, et al. Phenobarbital-associated bone marrow aplasia: a case report and review of the literature. *Acta Haematol.* 2008;119:18–21.

104. Magnussen C, Doherthy J, Hess R, et al. Grand mal seizures and acute intermittent porphyria: the problem of differential diagnosis and treatment. *Neurology.* 1975;25:1121–1125.

105. Christiansen C, Rodbro P, Lund M. Incidence of anticonvulsant osteomalacia and effect of vitamin D: controlled therapeutic trial. *Br Med J.* 1973;4:695–701.

106. Farhat G, Yamout B, Mikati MA, et al. Effect of antiepileptic drugs on bone density in ambulatory patients. *Neurology.* 2002;58:1348–1353.

107. Vestergaard P, Rejnmark L, Mosekilde L. Fracture risk associated with use of antiepileptic drugs. *Epilepsia.* 2004;45:1330–1337.

108. Deblay MF, Vert P, Andre M, et al. Transplacental vitamin K prevents hemorrhagic disease of infants of epileptic mothers. *Lancet.* 1982;1:1247.

109. Baulac M, Cramer JA, Mattson RH. Phenobarbital and other barbiturates: adverse effects. In: Levy RH, Mattson RH, Meldrum BS, et al., eds. *Antiepileptic Drugs.* 5th ed. Philadelphia, PA: Lippincott Williams & Wilkins; 2002:528–540.

110. Strzelczyk A, Vogt H, Hamer HM, et al. Continuous phenobarbital treatment leads to recurrent plantar fibromatosis. *Epilepsia.* 2008 May 29. [Epub ahead of print]

111. Meador KJ. Effects of in utero antiepileptic drug exposure. *Epilepsy Curr.* 2008;8:143–147.

112. Kjaer D, Horvath-Puhó E, Christensen J, et al. Antiepileptic drug use, folic acid supplementation, and congenital abnormalities: a population-based case-control study. *BJOG.* 2008;115:98–103.

113. Pennell PB. Antiepileptic drugs during pregnancy: what is known and which AEDs seem to be safest? *Epilepsia.* 2008;49(suppl 9):43–55.

114. Olsen H, Boice J, Jensen J, et al. Cancer among epileptic patients exposed to anticonvulsant drugs. *J Natl Cancer Inst.* 1989;81:803–808.

115. Rating D, Nau H, Jager-Roman E, et al. Teratogenic and pharmacokinetic studies of primidone during pregnancy and in the offspring of epileptic women. *Acta Paediatr Scand.* 1982;71:301–311.

116. Leppik IE, Cloyd JC, Miller K. Development of tolerance to the side effects of primidone. *Ther Drug Monit.* 1984;6:189–191.

117. Gallagher BB, Baumel IP, Mattson RH, et al. Primidone, diphenylhydantoin and phenobarbital. Aspects of acute and chronic toxicity. *Neurology.* 1973;23:145–149.

118. Bourgeois B. Individual and crossed tolerance to the anticonvulsant effect and neurotoxicity of phenobarbital and primidone in mice. In: Frey H, Froscher W, Koella WP, et al., eds. *Tolerance to Beneficial and Adverse Effects of Antiepileptic Drugs.* New York: Raven Press; 1986:17–24.

119. Rossi L. Correlation between age and plasma level/dosage for phenobarbital in infants and children. *Acta Paediat Scand.* 1979;68:431–434.

120. Davis A, Mutchie K, Thompson J, et al. Once-daily dosing with phenobarbital in children with seizure disorders. *Pediatrics.* 1981;68:824–827.

121. Asconape J, Penry J. Use of antiepileptic drugs in the presence of liver and kidney disease: a review. *Epilepsia.* 1982;23(suppl 1):S65–S79.

122. Alvin J, McHorse T, Hoyumpa A, et al. The effect of liver disease in man on the disposition of phenobarbital. *J Pharmacol Exp Ther.* 1975;192:224–235.

123. Ramsay RE, Hammond EJ, Perchalski RJ, et al. Brain uptake of phenytoin, phenobarbital, and diazepam. *Arch Neurol.* 1979;36:535–539.

124. Painter MJ, Pippenger C, MacDonald H, et al. Phenobarbital and phenytoin blood levels in neonates. *Pediatrics.* 1977;92:315–319.

125. Bourgeois BFD, Luders H, Morris H, et al. Rapid introduction of primidone using phenobarbital loading: acute primidone toxicity avoided. *Epilepsia.* 1989;30:667.

126. Kanner AM, Parra J, Frey M. The "forgotten" cross-tolerance between phenobarbital and primidone: it can prevent acute primidone-related toxicity. *Epilepsia.* 2000;41:1310–1314.

127. Schottelius DD, Fincham RW. Clinical application of serum primidone levels. In: Pippenger CE, Penry JK, Kutt H, eds. *Antiepileptic Drugs: Quantitative Analysis and Interpretation.* New York: Raven Press; 1978:273–282.

CHAPTER 54 ■ ETHOSUXIMIDE

ANDRES M. KANNER, TRACY A. GLAUSER, AND DIEGO A. MORITA

Ethosuximide (ETS) is one of the first generation antiepileptic drugs (AEDs) which, despite the advent of several new AEDs, continues to maintain its position as a first-line treatment of absence seizures. Its narrow therapeutic profile has limited its use to the treatment of childhood absence epilepsy. Some studies have also suggested a potential therapeutic effect in epileptic negative myoclonus (1). In addition, data from several experimental animal models of pain suggest that ETS may have potential analgesic properties. Despite its 52-year existence in the market, additional research continues to further elucidate the mechanisms of action of this AED. The purpose of this chapter is to review the latest experimental and clinical data of ETS.

HISTORICAL BACKGROUND

The development of ETS was a response to the need in the 1950s to develop a more effective, safer, and better- tolerated anticonvulsant for the treatment of absence seizures (2). Introduced in the 1940s, trimethadione and its analogue paramethadione were the first anticonvulsants to demonstrate efficacy against absence seizures, but they were associated with significant toxicity (3–6). These toxicity issues spurred the discovery and testing in the 1950s of the succinimide family of anticonvulsants (ETS, methsuximide, and phensuximide) (6). Of the succinimides, ETS had the greatest efficacy and least toxicity when used against absence seizures (6). Because of this combination of efficacy and safety, ETS has been considered as first-line therapy for absence seizures since its introduction in 1958 (7,8).

CHEMISTRY

ETS (2-ethyl-2-methylsuccinimide), with a molecular mass of 141.2, is a chiral compound containing a five-member ring, with two negatively charged carbonyl oxygen atoms with a ring nitrogen between them and one asymmetric carbon atom (9,10) (Fig. 54.1). Its chemical characteristics include a melting point of 64°C to 65°C, a weakly acidic pK_a of 9.3, and a partition coefficient of 9 (chloroform-to-water; pH 7) (10). ETS is freely soluble in ethanol and water (solubility, 190 mg/5 mL) (10). A white crystalline material, ETS is used clinically as a racemate and is commercially available in 250-mg capsules or 250 mg/5 mL of syrup (7,9).

MECHANISM OF ACTION

As stated above, in addition to its antiepileptic effect, ETS appears to have an analgesic effect.

Antiepileptic Effects

The presumed mechanism of action against absence seizures is reduction of low-threshold T-type calcium currents in thalamic neurons (11,12). The spontaneous pacemaker oscillatory activity of thalamocortical neurons involves low-threshold T-type calcium currents (13). These oscillatory currents are considered to be the generators of the 3-Hz spike-and-wave rhythms in patients with absence epilepsy (13). Voltage-dependent blockade of the low-threshold, T-type calcium current was demonstrated at clinically relevant ETS concentrations in thalamic neurons isolated from rats and guinea pigs (11,12,14). ETS does not alter gating of these T-type Ca^{2+} channels (6,12). Combining these findings, it is proposed that ETS's effect on low-threshold, T-type calcium currents in thalamocortical neurons prevents the "synchronized firing associated with spike-wave discharges" (11).

In addition to the effects on voltage-dependent Ca^{2+} currents of the thalamus, studies have investigated the impact of ETS on GABA, on persistent Na^+ and sustained K^+ currents in cortical and thalamic neurons, and more recently on G protein-activated inwardly rectifying K^+ channels. Here are some of the data.

The genetic absence epilepsy rats from Strasbourg (GAERS) have been identified as one of the ideal animal models of absence epilepsy (15). In this animal model, the frequency of spike-and-wave discharges is high with one third of recorded EEG presenting as seizure activity. The use of ETS has been effective in stopping such epileptic activity (16). The impact of ETS on GABA was investigated in this animal model by various investigators all of who recognize a pivotal pathogenic role of excess GABA in absence epilepsy (17). In one study, ETS was shown to reduce GABA concentration in primary motor cortex of GAERS (18), confirming the findings from a previous study (16).

Using a different animal model of absence epilepsy (WAG/Rij rats), investigators have demonstrated the initiation of epileptic activity in somatosensory cortex (19). Furthermore, the effect of infusion of ETS into thalamic nuclei (ventrobasal and reticular nuclei) was significantly lower than that seen with its infusion in somatosensory cortex. The potential effect of ETS on GABA was also suggested in a study using a mouse with a mutation in the gamma2 subunit of the GABA receptor. Such mutation has been identified in childhood absence epilepsy and febrile seizures. Tan et al. developed a mouse model with a gamma2-subunit point mutation (R43Q) in a large Australian family. ETS blocked the 6- to 7-HZ spike-and-wave discharges and clinical events consisting of behavioral arrest recorded in mice heterogeneous for the mutation (20).

In cortical tissue, at concentrations significantly greater than those used for anticonvulsant effect, ETS inhibits Na^+, K^+-adenosine triphosphatase (Na^+, K^+-ATPase) activity

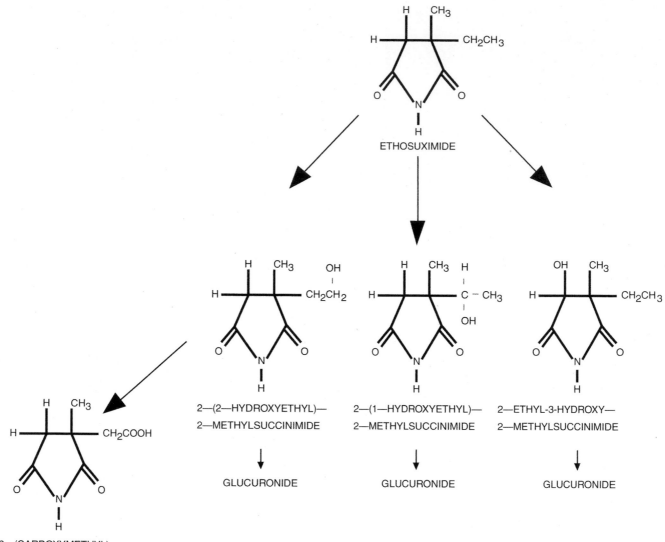

FIGURE 54.1 Structure and biotransformation pathways of ethosuximide. (From Pisani F, Meir B. Ethosuximide: chemistry biotransformation. In: Levy R, Mattson R, Meldrum B, eds. *Antiepileptic Drugs.* 4th ed. New York: Raven Press; 1995:655–658, with permission.)

(21–25). Yet, one in vitro study suggested that ETS lowers the persistent Na^+- and Ca^{2+}-activated K^+ currents of layer V cortical pyramidal and thalamic relay neurons of rats and cats, but has no effect on the transient Na^+ current (26).

G protein-activated inwardly rectifying K^+ channels (GIRK) have been found to play an important role in the regulation of neuronal excitability (27). Using the Xenopus oocyte expression assay, Kobayashi et al. demonstrated that ETS inhibited GIRK at clinically relevant concentrations and in a concentration and time-dependent manner but such inhibition was voltage independent during each voltage pulse (27).

Analgesic Effects

T-type Ca^{2+} channels appear to be important targets for treating persistent pain syndromes. Accordingly, various animal models of pain have suggested a potential analgesic effect of ETS (see section Efficacy).

PHARMACOKINETICS

Implications of Racemic Mixture

ETS has always been used clinically as a racemate. It is theoretically possible that the two enantiomers could demonstrate different pharmacokinetic parameters or anticonvulsant effects. In rats, ETS's disposition is nonstereoselective (10). Chiral gas chromatographic analysis of enantiomer concentrations in plasma samples obtained for routine monitoring, 33 patients demonstrated that the enantiomer ratio was close to unity, and there was little interindividual variability (28). This implies that the disposition of ETS in humans is nonstereoselective and that measurement of total ETS for therapeutic monitoring is reasonable and appropriate (10,29). A small study (three pregnancies in two women taking ETS) demonstrated that the nonstereoselective disposition was unaffected by pregnancy, placental transfer, or passage into breast milk (29).

ABSORPTION

In rats, dogs, and monkeys, absorption is rapid, with nearly complete oral bioavailability in dogs (88% to 95%) and monkeys (93% to 97.5%) (30–35). In children and adults, absorption is considered to be rapid and nearly complete (90% to 95%), even though no intravenous formulation can be used as a reference standard to determine absolute bioavailability in humans (2,34,36,37). Absorption is reported to remain efficient over multiple administrations (34). In two single-dose capsule administration studies three volunteers given a single 1-g oral dose and four healthy adults given a 0.5-g oral dose, peak ETS plasma concentrations were reached between 1 and 4 hours after administration (35,37,38). A separate study with five institutionalized children that compared capsules and syrup demonstrated peak plasma concentrations within 3 to 7 hours with either formulation (8,34–36,39). The syrup had a faster absorption rate than the capsules, but the two formulations were bioequivalent (7,8,34–36,39).

DISTRIBUTION

Tissue Distribution

In rats, ETS distributes evenly to brain, plasma, and other tissues, except for adipose tissue (in which steady-state concentrations are approximately one third of those reached in plasma) (34). ETS crosses the placenta in rats (35,40), and in dog and rat studies readily passed through the blood–brain barrier (30,35). In dogs, the plasma to cerebrospinal fluid (CSF) ratio was 1.01 ± 0.15, with an estimated half-life of entry into the CSF at about 4 to 5 minutes (30,34,35,41). In one study in rats, the whole brain to plasma ETS concentrations ratio was near unity, whereas a second study in rats found uniform distribution in four discrete brain areas (cerebral cortex, cerebellum, midbrain, and pons medulla) (33,35). However, a third study in rats receiving a single intraperitoneal (i.p.) dose of 50 mg/kg found a decrease in brain to plasma concentrations over time, suggesting that ETS may be actively transported out of the rat brain (34,42).

In humans, ETS homogeneously distributes throughout the body (7). Saliva, tears, and CSF concentrations are similar to plasma concentrations (34,35,43–48). In three studies (involving 6, 15, and 19 patients), the respective correlations between saliva and serum concentrations were $R = 0.99$, $R = 0.99$, and $R = 0.74$ (46–48). A fourth study, which examined concentrations in paired parotid saliva and plasma samples from 10 patients, showed the average saliva to plasma ratio to be 1.04, which appeared constant over the measured time intervals (45). In light of these results, multiple studies have concluded that saliva can be used in lieu of plasma for therapeutic monitoring of ETS (35,43,45–48).

ETS crosses the placenta in humans and has been detected in cord serum and amniotic fluid at concentrations of 104% and 111% of maternal serum concentrations, respectively (7,50). In two separate reports, ETS was detected in either the urine or plasma of a newborn of a woman receiving long-term therapy (35,51,52). The serum concentration in the newborn was similar to that in the mother (34,52). ETS is excreted in the breast milk of mothers receiving long-term therapy (34). In multiple studies, the average breast milk to maternal serum concentration ratio ranged from 0.8 to 0.94 (34,52–55). The ETS serum concentration of breast-feeding infants of mothers given long-term therapy was 30% to 50% of their mothers' serum concentration (34,54,55). The American Academy of Pediatrics, however, considers ETS to be usually compatible with breast-feeding (56).

Volume of Distribution and Protein Building

The apparent volume of distribution in rats, dogs, and rhesus monkeys ranges from 0.7 to 0.8 L/kg (30,31,34,57). In humans, ETS's apparent volume of distribution is 0.62 to 0.65 L/kg in adults and 0.69 L/kg in children, implying distribution through total body water (7,34,36,37,44).

ETS protein binding is 0% to 10% in humans, dogs, and rats (28,34,36,39,43,58).

METABOLISM AND EXCRETION

Animals

Metabolism is the main method of ETS elimination in animals. In rhesus monkeys and rats, the drug and its metabolites are excreted predominantly by the kidney, with only a small proportion recovered in the feces (34,40). Unchanged ETS accounts for only 12% of urinary recovery in rats (59).

In rats, biotransformation is catalyzed predominantly by hepatic cytochrome P450 (CYP)3A isoenzymes, with possible minor contributions by CYP2E, CYP2B, and CYP2C isoenzymes (10,34,57,60,61). These CYP enzymes are inducible, and autoinduction has been reported in rats (34,57). The major metabolite in rats and monkeys is 2-(1-hydroxyethyl)-2-methylsuccinimide, and the two minor metabolites are 2-ethyl-3-hydroxy-2-methyl-succinimide and 2-(2-hydroxyethyl)-2-methylsuccinimide (34,63). ETS provided complete protection against pentylenetetrazol-induced clonic seizures in mice at a dose of 125 mg/kg; in contrast, the major metabolite demonstrated "no significant anticonvulsant activity" (63).

Elimination appears to follow first-order kinetics in animals, except in dogs, in which Michaelis–Menten kinetics may apply (30,34,63). Studies of single- and multiple-dose ETS administration in monkeys have demonstrated comparable elimination half-life and total body clearance (7,31,32). In animals, elimination half-lives range from 1 hour in mice to 9 to 26 hours in rats and 11 to 25 hours in dogs (30,34,63). Steady-state plasma concentrations are significantly higher in the morning than in the evening in rhesus monkeys receiving intravenous ETS at a constant rate. These fluctuations may result from circadian changes in ETS metabolizing enzymes (34,63,64).

Humans

As in animals, metabolism is the main method of ETS elimination in humans. ETS undergoes extensive hepatic oxidative biotransformation (80% to 90%) to pharmacologically inactive metabolites. Although most of the remaining drug is excreted unchanged in the urine, small amounts of unchanged ETS can be recovered from bile and feces (65). ETS oxidation is catalyzed mainly by enzymes of the CYP3A subfamily (7). In vitro studies with humanized heterologous CYP microsomal systems showed that ETS is primarily oxidized by CYP3A4, with CYP2E1 playing a minor role in its metabolism (66).

The major metabolite recovered from human urine in patients receiving ETS is 2-(1-hydroxyethyl)-2-methylsuccinimide, of which at least 40% is excreted as a glucuronide conjugate (10,66). Two other metabolites recovered (often as a glucuronide conjugate) from human urine, are 2-ethyl-3-hydroxy-2-methylsuccinimide and 2-(2-hydroxyethyl)-2-methylsuccinimide. The latter metabolite can undergo subsequent metabolism by the hepatic mixed-function oxidase system to form the fourth major metabolite, 2-carboxymethyl-2-methylsuccinimide (10,63,66) (Fig. 54.1).

In humans, ETS's elimination follows first-order kinetics. Total body clearance in adults averages 0.01 L/kg/h (37) and in two children was 0.016 and 0.013 L/kg/h (36). This is significantly lower than hepatic plasma flow (0.9 L/kg/h) implying that ETS does not undergo a significant first-pass effect, and that drug clearance is not blood flow limited (34,35). Total body clearance has been reported to decrease slightly after repeated dosing (34). ETS does not induce hepatic microsomal CYP enzymes or the uridine diphosphate glucuronosyltransferase (UDPGT) system (58,67,68). In humans, in contrast to rats, autoinduction does not occur (68,69).

In general, ETS has a long elimination half-life that varies with age. Its mean half-life in adults reportedly ranges from 40 to 60 hours, compared with 30 to 40 hours in children (36–38,44,63,69–72). Large variations have been observed in pediatric studies, with half-lives ranging from 15 to 68 hours (35,63,70). In neonates, half-lives ranging from 32 to 41 hours have been reported (52,54). The time to reach steady-state concentration after a dosage change is 6 to 7 days for children and 12 days for adults (7,73). ETS clearance is reported to be lower in women than men (74). Dose size and repeated dosing do not affect the elimination half-life (44,70).

The effects of liver and renal disease on ETS elimination have not been formally studied (34). It would seem that liver disease would impair ETS elimination because of the drug's substantial hepatic oxidative metabolism, whereas renal disease would have much less impact on ETS elimination (34). Hemodialysis can readily remove ETS. One report estimated that approximately 50% of the body's ETS was removed over a 6-hour dialysis interval and that the drug's half-life dropped to 3 to 4 hours during dialysis (34,75). In a separate case report, peritoneal dialysis decreased ETS concentrations in a child taking ETS and phenobarbital (76).

DRUG INTERACTIONS

Interactions with Other Antiepileptic Drugs

ETS's lack of effect on either the hepatic microsomal CYP enzymes or the UDPGT system, along with negligible protein binding, indicates a low potential for drug interactions (58,73). Most investigators conclude that ETS therapy does not have a clinically significant effect on the pharmacokinetics of phenytoin, phenobarbital, or carbamazepine, despite scattered reports of some changes in phenytoin or phenobarbital concentrations when ETS is used in combination with phenytoin or primidone (7,77–84). There is no alteration in the plasma protein binding of carbamazepine or phenytoin when ETS is used concomitantly, nor is there a change in the formation of phenobarbital from primidone (85). One study reported a significant decrease in valproic acid serum concentration after the addition of ETS (120.0 ± 20.1 µg/mL before ETS vs. 87.0 ± 13.1 µg/mL during cotherapy with ETS; $P < 0.01$). After cessation of ETS, valproic acid levels rose 36.7%. The mechanism underlying this observed effect is unknown (86).

In contrast, because of ETS's extensive hepatic oxidative metabolism by CYP isoenzymes, concomitant therapy with enzyme-inducing AEDs would be predicted to increase ETS's total clearance (84). ETS's clearance is significantly accelerated (leading to a drop in the serum concentration) when the drug is used concurrently with phenobarbital, phenytoin, or carbamazepine (58,84,87–90). In one study, discontinuation of concomitant carbamazepine therapy increased ETS plasma concentrations by 48% (91). The magnitude of this effect may vary considerably among patients (87).

The effect of concomitant therapy with valproic acid (VPA) on the pharmacokinetics of ETS is variable, with studies showing increases, decreases, or no change in ETS clearance (58,69,72,81,92–94). Some investigators postulate that valproic acid may inhibit the metabolism of ETS leading to an increase in the plasma ETS concentration (95).

Whenever an AED–ETS interaction could occur, serum concentration and clinical response of both AEDs should be monitored. No formal pharmacokinetic interaction studies have examined potential ETS interactions with felbamate, gabapentin, lamotrigine (LTG), tiagabine, topiramate, oxcarbazepine, levetiracetam, or zonisamide.

Interactions with Nonantiepileptic Drugs

The clearance of ETS is substantially increased when it is used in combination with rifampin, an inducer of CYP3A isoenzymes (89). In contrast, concomitant use with isoniazid, a potent inhibitor of CYP isoenzymes, resulted in increased ETS serum concentrations and psychotic behaviors (96).

EFFICACY

Antiepileptic Effects

Animal Models

ETS exhibits very different efficacy profiles in the two major traditional animal models of epilepsy, the maximal electroshock test (MES) and the pentylenetetrazol seizure test. The MES is used to identify agents able to prevent the spread of seizures, and has been hypothesized to identify agents effective against partial-onset and generalized tonic–clonic seizures (6,97). ETS was ineffective against MES-induced tonic seizures, except at anesthetic doses (6,97–99), but ETS blocked clonic seizures produced by subcutaneously administered pentylenetetrazol or bicuculline (6,97,99,100). These chemically induced seizure models are hypothesized to identify agents that raise the seizure threshold and may be effective against absence seizures. ETS's activity profile suggests that the drug exerts its anticonvulsant effects by raising the seizure threshold rather than by blocking the spread of seizures, and it predicts efficacy against absence rather than partial-onset or generalized tonic–clonic seizures.

ETS demonstrated activity against spontaneously occurring absence seizures in three other animal models (mutant tottering mice, Wistar rats, and spontaneously epileptic rats) (101–103), as well as activity against spike-wave seizures induced by systemic administration of α-hydroxybutyrate (97,104–105).

Humans

ETS is an effective first-line monotherapy against typical absence seizures. A recent multicenter, double-blind, controlled study has been completed comparing the efficacy of ETS to that of VPA and LTG given as monotherapy for the treatment of childhood absence epilepsy. The results of this study revealed that ETS and VPA were found to be more effective than LTG in the treatment of childhood absence epilepsy, but ETS was associated with fewer adverse attentional effects (106). Prior to that study, two studies conducted in the 1970s strongly suggest the efficacy of ETS in childhood absence epilepsy (107,108). Efficacy against typical partial seizures was examined in a study with a well-constructed method for patient selection and assessment. Each patient's absence seizures were required to meet a predetermined clinical definition and be witnessed by the principal investigator. Seizure frequency was then assessed by five separate measures: the ward's staff observation; trained observer's observation; mother's observation; physician's observation (including during patient hyperventilation); and standardized video-electroencephalographic (video-EEG) recording. These measures were combined into a "seizure index" (107). Thirty-seven patients were enrolled. By the eighth week of treatment, 19% (7 of 37 patients) were seizure free, with a 100% reduction in seizure index. Overall, during ETS therapy, 49% (18 of 37) of patients demonstrated at least a 90% reduction in seizures, and 95% (35 of 37) had a 50% or more reduction. The full antiabsence effect occurred within a week for any given ETS dose. Plasma ETS concentrations ranged from 16.6 to 104.0 μg/mL (doses of 6.5 to 36.7 mg/kg) and, on the basis of the seizure index, the investigators suggest that the optimal ETS plasma concentrations in this study were 40 to 100 μg/mL (107).

The second major study was a prospective, longitudinal, open-label investigation that used therapeutic drug monitoring to maximize clinical response (108). Seventy patients were enrolled; 54% (38 of 70) were female, with ages ranging from 4 to 28 years (median, 12 years). Thirty-eight patients (54%) had only absence seizures. The remaining patients had either absence seizures with tonic–clonic seizures (30%) or absence seizures, and one or more other generalized seizure type (16%). Approximately 50% of the patients were taking other AEDs in addition to ETS. Patients received between 9.4 and 73.5 mg/kg/day of ETS and were evaluated at 6-month intervals. Introduction of ETS therapy completely controlled seizures in 47% (33 of 70) of the patients. None of these patients had plasma ETS concentrations below 30 μg/mL; only 9% were below 40 μg/mL (108).

During the next 2.5 years, attempts were made to achieve plasma ETS concentrations above 40 μg/mL in the remaining 53% (37 of 70) of patients with uncontrolled absence seizures. Improved compliance and higher dosages led to significantly higher ETS plasma concentrations in 19 patients, 10 of whom became seizure free. At the 2.5-year follow-up, 61% (43 of 70) of the group was seizure free. In these patients, ETS's effectiveness persisted over the next 2.5 years of follow-up (total, 5 years). In contrast, ETS was not able to control absence seizures in patients with both absence seizures and tonic–clonic seizures who were receiving combination AED therapy (108).

Three randomized, controlled, prospective trials have compared ETS and valproic acid as monotherapy for absence seizures (109–111), and a recent Cochrane review reexamined the results (112). A parallel, open study enrolled 28 drug-naive patients, between 4 and 15 years of age, who had typical absence seizures, and followed them up for a mean of 3 years (range, 18 months to 4 years) (109). The relative risk (RR) estimate with 95% confidence interval (CI) for seizure freedom (RR < 1 favors ETS) was 0.70 (95% CI, 0.32 to 1.51); the RR estimate for 50% or more reduction in seizure frequency was 1.02 (95% CI, 0.70 to 1.48). The outcomes were confirmed by 6-hour telemetry and clinical observation. Although no difference was apparent for either outcome, the CIs were wide; the possibility of important differences could not be excluded, and equivalence of ETS and valproic acid could not be inferred (109,112).

Another trial of similar design enrolled 20 patients between 5 and 8 years of age whose simple absence seizures had begun less than 6 months before (110). Follow-up lasted for 1 to 2 years and outcomes were confirmed by clinical observation and EEG. Again, wide CIs and the possibility of important differences precluded confirmation of equivalence of ETS and valproic acid. All patients achieved at least a 50% reduction in seizure frequency (110,112).

A double-blind, crossover study used a complex response-conditional design and recruited 45 patients between 4 and 18 years of age (111). The enrollment included both treatment-naive patients and those with drug-resistant disease. Some had only absence seizures; others had other seizure types as well. In the first phase of this trial, patients were assigned to receive either ETS with placebo valproic acid or valproic acid with placebo ETS for 6 weeks. Responders continued with the randomized drug for a further 6 weeks. This group included treatment-naive patients who became seizure free, and previously treated patients who had an 80% or more reduction in seizure frequency. Nonresponders and those with adverse effects were crossed over to the alternative treatment and followed up for another 6 weeks. No differences emerged between therapies, but the CIs were wide and equivalence could not be inferred. The reduction in seizure frequency, determined by a 12-hour video-EEG telemetry, was 100% for the drug-naive group and 80% for the drug-resistant group (111,112).

No studies have compared initial monotherapy with ETS against either placebo or LTG monotherapy. Controlled trials of ETS's long-term efficacy or effectiveness are also lacking.

Combination therapy with ETS and valproic acid for absence seizures resistant to either drug alone was reported in one open-label study of five patients (113), and many investigators subsequently recommended this combination for patients with absence seizures resistant to monotherapy

(8,39,73,114). Similarly, ETS in patients with both absence and tonic–clonic seizures should be combined with another AED effective against tonic–clonic seizures, such as valproic acid, carbamazepine, or phenytoin (8,73,114). Despite being reported as "highly effective" against atypical absence seizures (73,114), ETS is almost always used as part of combination therapy for patients with atypical absence seizures because of the high incidence of coexisting seizure types (8).

ETS is useful in the prevention and treatment of absence status epilepticus at serum concentrations greater than 120 µg/mL (115,116), and there are reports of effectiveness in severe myoclonic epilepsy in infancy (117), childhood epileptic encephalopathy (Lennox–Gastaut syndrome) (5,118), juvenile myoclonic epilepsy (119,120), epilepsy with myoclonic absences (120), eyelid myoclonia with absences (120), epilepsy with continuous spike-and-wave during slow-wave sleep (121), photosensitive seizures (122), and gelastic seizures (39,123). No controlled studies have investigated ETS's effectiveness against simple partial, complex partial, or partial secondarily generalized tonic–clonic seizures.

Epileptic negative myoclonus consists of an interruption of tonic muscle activity, which is time-locked to an epileptic EEG abnormality, without evidence of an antecedent positive myoclonia in the agonist–antagonist muscles (1). It can be identified in various types of seizure disorders, including idiopathic, cryptogenic, and symptomatic epileptic disorders. ETS has been shown to be effective in epileptic negative myoclonus associated with childhood idiopathic partial epilepsy. Capovilla et al. reported a remission of the motor disorder in nine patients after the addition of ETS to other AEDs (124). Furthermore, Oguni et al. reported total remission of epileptic negative myoclonus in 6 of 10 patients with the use of ETS (125).

Analgesic Effects

Animal Models

Barton et al. investigated the effect of ETS in acute and persistent nociceptive tests in the rat (126). Intraperitoneal administration of ETS reversed capsaicin-induced mechanical hyperalgesia in a dose-dependent manner. In addition, ETS produced antinociceptive effects in the rat tail-flick reflex test and displayed significant analgesic effects in both early and late phase formalin-induced behaviors. Similar findings were reported by Shannon et al. (127). Of note, in this study ETS increased the doses of pentylenetetrazol required to produce both first twitch and clonic seizures, thus showing that the analgesic effects can be obtained at doses that yield an anticonvulsant effect.

Todorovic et al. injected ETS intradermally into peripheral receptive fields of sensory neurons in the hind paws of adult rats, and studied pain perception using the model of acute thermal nociception; ETS induced dose-dependent analgesia in the injected paw, but not in the contralateral (noninjected) paw (128). These findings suggest an analgesic effect mediated at peripheral nerve endings of rat sensory neurons.

Flatters and Bennett demonstrated the analgesic properties of ETS in an animal model using male Sprague–Dawley rats, to which four i.p. injections of 2 mg/kg paclitaxel were administered on alternate days (129). Paclitaxel is a chemotherapeutic agent known to produce neuropathic pain and sensory abnormalities in patients treated with this agent both during therapy and after its discontinuation. The development of

mechanical and cold allodynia/hyperalgesia was demonstrated with behavioral assessment using von Frey filaments and acetone. ETS administered by i.p. route at doses of 450 mg/kg yielded a near complete remission of mechanical allodynia/hyperalgesia. No tolerance of the analgesic effect was found following repetitive dosing with i.p. ETS at doses of 100 or 300 mg/kg daily for 3 days. Furthermore, i.p. administration of ETS at doses of 300 mg/kg also reversed paclitaxel-induced cold allodynia and vincristine-induced mechanical allodynia/hyperalgesia. Of note, paclitaxel-induced pain was resistant to opioid therapy.

Finally, Wang and Thompson demonstrated an analgesic effect of ETS in an animal model of central pain syndrome (130). These investigators created unilateral electrolytic or demyelinating lesions in the spinothalamic tract of the spinal cord of rats resulting in thermal hyperalgesia and mechanical allodynia in all four paws that were attenuated significantly with the administration of ETS. Clearly, ETS appears to have analgesic properties in various animal models of pain.

Human Studies

There have been no open or controlled studies that have investigated the analgesic efficacy of ETS in humans.

ADVERSE EFFECTS

Effects That Depend on Concentration

The incidence of adverse effects due to ETS in initial published reports in 1952, 1958, and 1961 was very low, ranging from 1% to 9%; subsequent studies have indicated an incidence ranging from 31% to 44% (107,131–137). Most adverse effects depend on concentration and are related to the primary and secondary pharmacologic effects of the drug. These reactions are usually predictable, dose dependent, and host independent; they resolve with dose reduction (138,139).

The most common ETS concentration-dependent adverse effects involve the gastrointestinal system and include nausea (the most common), abdominal discomfort, anorexia, vomiting, and diarrhea (2,8,39,131,132,140). Between 20% and 33% of children experience these symptoms, usually at the onset of therapy (39,140). Symptoms are considered mild and respond promptly to dose reduction (39,131,132,140). Techniques to reduce the symptoms include dividing the total daily dose and administering the smaller doses at mealtime (7).

Central nervous system (CNS)-related adverse events (e.g., drowsiness) are the second most common form of ETS concentration-dependent adverse events. Drowsiness usually occurs at the onset of therapy and responds promptly to dose reduction (7,131,132,140). Other CNS-related adverse events include insomnia, nervousness (12% of children), dizziness, hiccups, lethargy, fatigue, ataxia, and behavior changes (e.g., aggression, euphoria, irritability, hyperactivity) (8,140). A direct relationship between ETS therapy and these reported behavioral changes is not certain, because poor methodology (e.g., lack of reliable methods for objectively measuring behavior changes, confounding variable of polypharmacy, and lack of serum AED measurements) makes analysis of existing reports difficult at best (131,132).

Few trials have examined the potential cognitive effects of ETS in a controlled fashion, accounting for confounding variables such as plasma concentrations, underlying mental retardation, concomitant AEDs, or seizure type. In one early report, psychometric testing of 25 children receiving ETS for various seizure types revealed memory, speech, and emotional disturbances (141). However, no plasma concentrations were measured; all the patients were also taking barbiturates; 60% of the cohort had intelligence quotient (IQ) scores below 83; and no matched control group was used (141). In a cohort of children without epilepsy but with learning disorders, and 14- and 6-Hz positive spikes on EEG recording, administration of ETS significantly improved verbal and full-scale IQ scores, without changing motor performance or personality test scores (142).

In a well-designed study, psychometric performance improved significantly over 8 weeks of ETS therapy in 17 (46%) of 37 children with absence seizures (107). This improvement was significantly greater than that of a control group tested in the same fashion over the same interval (107). Only 25% of the study group had IQ scores below 83, and only 32% were receiving other AEDs (107).

Dreifuss (131,132) reported a probable dose-dependent, ETS-related granulocytopenia that often resolves with dose reduction without the need to terminate therapy. Distinction between this probable adverse event and ETS-associated idiosyncratic bone marrow depression (see section Idiosyncratic Reactions) is critical. Careful clinical and laboratory monitoring are essential in making this decision.

Effects That Do Not Depend on Concentration

Some ETS adverse effects do not appear to be concentration dependent, but are also not idiosyncratic reactions in the usual sense. Headaches, reported in 14% of children, may not respond to dose reduction and may persist (7,131,132,140,143).

Episodes of psychotic behavior (i.e., anxiety, depression, visual hallucinations, auditory hallucinations, and intermittent impairment of consciousness) have been noted with ETS (131,144–147) and are most likely in young adults with a history of mental disorders (7,131). The acute psychotic episodes appeared after ETS-induced seizure control with associated EEG improvement, and they resolved when ETS was stopped and seizures returned, illustrating the phenomenon of *forced normalization* (7,131). Psychotic symptoms have recurred when ETS was restarted in patients with previous ETS-related psychotic episodes (131). This forced normalization reaction is not dose dependent and, among all antiabsence AEDs, occurs with highest frequency with ETS (7,148).

Most studies find no evidence of ETS-associated seizure exacerbation (107,131,135,149,150); however, scattered reports describe exacerbation of myoclonic and absence seizures and transformation of absence into "grand mal" seizures in patients receiving ETS (131,133,151). Dreifuss considered this exacerbation effect to be a consequence of the high incidence of generalized tonic–clonic seizures in patients with absences seizures, coupled with ETS's lack of efficacy against generalized tonic–clonic seizures (131).

Idiosyncratic Reactions

Idiosyncratic drug reactions are unpredictable, dose-independent, host-dependent reactions that are not associated with the known pharmacologic effects of the drug; they can be serious and life-threatening. Preclinical animal toxicologic testing may not detect these reactions, and often they cannot be reproduced in animal models (138,139). In general, the skin is the most commonly affected site, followed by the formed elements of the blood and liver and, to a lesser extent, the nervous system and kidneys (138,152). These reactions may be organ specific or may manifest with generalized nonspecific symptoms, such as lymphadenopathy, arthralgias, eosinophilia, and fever (138,153). Idiosyncratic reactions are believed to result from toxic metabolites that cause injury directly or indirectly (i.e., through an immunologic response or free radical-mediated process) (154).

ETS has been associated to various degrees with a wide array of idiosyncratic reactions (131,132,140,155), including allergic dermatitis, rash, erythema multiforme, Stevens–Johnson syndrome (156), systemic lupus erythematosus (157–159), lupus–scleroderma syndrome (160), a lupus-like syndrome (161), blood dyscrasias (aplastic anemia, agranulocytosis) (107,137,149,162–169), dyskinesia (170,171), akathisia (170), autoimmune thyroiditis (172), and diminished renal allograft survival (173).

Mild cutaneous reactions, including allergic dermatitis and rash, are the most common ETS-associated idiosyncratic reactions. They frequently resolve with withdrawal of the drug, but some patients may require steroid therapy. Patients who develop Stevens–Johnson syndrome, a potentially life-threatening condition, require more aggressive in-hospital therapy.

The symptoms of the lupus-like syndrome are described as fever, malar rash, arthritis, lymphadenopathy, and, on occasion, pleural effusions, myocarditis, and pericarditis (131). After discontinuation of ETS, these patients usually fully recover, but the recovery may be prolonged (131).

The manifestations of ETS-associated blood dyscrasias range from thrombocytopenia to pancytopenia and aplastic anemia (107,137,149,162–167). Between 1958 and 1994, only eight cases of ETS-associated aplastic anemia were reported, with onsets of 6 weeks to 8 months after initiation of therapy (166). Six patients were receiving polypharmacy; five were taking phenytoin or ethotoin in combination with ETS (166). Despite therapy, five of the eight patients died (107,137,149,162–167).

Long-Term Effects

Adverse effects resulting from long-term therapy are related to the cumulative dose (138,139). Severe bradykinesia and parkinsonian syndrome have been reported after several years of ETS treatment (136,174).

Delayed Effects

In mice, ETS exhibits considerably less teratogenic effect than carbamazepine, phenytoin, phenobarbital, or primidone (175). In humans, because ETS is predominantly indicated for absence seizures, which frequently remit before childbearing years, little is known about the risks that maternal use poses to the fetus (131). Not enough data are available to accurately assess the teratogenic effect of ETS in humans.

CLINICAL USE

Indications

ETS, like valproic acid, is regarded as effective first-line monotherapy against typical absence seizures. ETS may be the first choice in children younger than 10 years old with absence epilepsy, but as adolescence approaches and the risk of generalized tonic–clonic seizures increases, valproic acid clearly becomes the drug of choice (176). ETS as adjunctive therapy may be beneficial for patients whose absence seizures are not controlled by valproic acid monotherapy, patients with both absence and tonic–clonic seizures, and patients with atypical absence seizures (8,39,73,114,176). No evidence supports a role for ETS as monotherapy or adjunctive therapy in patients with only simple partial, complex partial, or partial secondarily generalized tonic–clonic seizures.

Starting and Stopping

A common starting dosage for children is 10 to 15 mg/kg/day with subsequent titration to clinical response (7,8). Maintenance dosages frequently range from 15 to 40 mg/kg/day (73). In older children and adults, therapy can begin at 250 mg/day and increase by 250-mg increments until the desired clinical response is reached. The interval between dosage changes for older children and adults varies from 3 days (8) to every 12 to 15 days (7). Common maintenance doses for older children and adults are 750 to 1500 mg/day (7,8). In elderly patients, titration should involve smaller increments with longer intervals between changes (8). After a dosage change, steady-state concentration is reached in 6 to 7 days in children and 12 days in adults (7,73). ETS can be administered once, twice, or even thrice daily (with meals) for maximum seizure control with minimum adverse effects (7,8).

If intolerable side effects without seizure control or 2 or more years' freedom from absence seizures occur, discontinuation may be warranted, with gradual reduction over 4 to 8 weeks (7,8). If necessary, abrupt discontinuation is probably safe because of ETS's long half-life (8).

Monitoring

ETS should always be titrated to maximal seizure control with minimal side effects. The generally accepted therapeutic range is 40 to 100 µg/mL (7,8); some patients with refractory seizures or absence status may need serum concentrations up to 150 µg/mL (8). Monitoring ETS's serum concentration may help to identify noncompliance and aid in maximizing seizure control (108).

There is no evidence that monitoring of blood count values during therapy anticipates the drug's idiosyncratic hematologic reactions. Patients must alert their physicians immedi-

ately if fever, sore throat, and cutaneous or other hemorrhages occur (131). However, one recommendation for monitoring is that "periodic blood counts be performed at no greater than monthly intervals for the duration of treatment with ETS, and that the dosage be reduced or the drug discontinued should the total white blood cell count fall below 3500 or the proportion of granulocytes below 25% of the total white blood cell count" (131).

References

1. Rubboli G, Tassinari CA. Negative myoclonus. An overview of its clinical features, pathophysiological mechanisms and management. *Clin Neurophysiol.* 2006;35:337–343.
2. Brodie M, Dichter M. Established antiepileptic drugs. *Seizure.* 1997;6:159–174.
3. Lennox W. The petit mal epilepsies: their treatment with tridione. *JAMA.* 1945;129:1069–1074.
4. Lennox W. Tridione in the treatment of epilepsy. *JAMA.* 1947;134:138–143.
5. Mattson RH. Efficacy and adverse effects of established and new antiepileptic drugs. *Epilepsia.* 1995;36:S13–S26.
6. Rogawski M, Porter R. Antiepileptic drugs: pharmacological mechanisms and clinical efficacy with consideration of promising developmental state compounds. *Pharmacol Rev.* 1990;42:223–286.
7. Sabers A, Dam M. Ethosuximide and methsuximide. In: Shorvon S, Dreifuss F, Fish D, et al., eds. *The Treatment of Epilepsy.* London: Blackwell Science; 1996:414–420.
8. Bromfield E. Ethosuximide and other succinimides. In: Engel J, Pedley T, eds. *Epilepsy: A Comprehensive Textbook.* Philadelphia, PA: Lippincott-Raven; 1997:1503–1508.
9. Millership JS, Mifsud J, Collier PS. The metabolism of ethosuximide. *Eur J Drug Metab Pharmacokinet.* 1993;18:349–353.
10. Pisani F, Meir B. Ethosuximide: chemistry and biotransformation. In: Levy R, Mattson R, Meldrum B, eds. *Antiepileptic Drugs.* 4th ed. New York: Raven Press, 1995:655–658.
11. White HS. Comparative anticonvulsant and mechanistic profile of the established and newer antiepileptic drugs. *Epilepsia.* 1999;40:S2–S10.
12. Macdonald RL, Kelly KM. Antiepileptic drug mechanisms of action. *Epilepsia.* 1993;34:S1–S8.
13. Davies JA. Mechanisms of action of antiepileptic drugs. *Seizure.* 1995; 4:267–271.
14. Coulter C, Huguenard J, Price D. Characterization of ethosuximide reduction of low-threshold calcium current in thalamic neurons. *Ann Neurol.* 1989;25:582–593.
15. Marescaux C, Vergnes M, Depaulis A. Genetic absence epilepsy in rats from Strasbourg: a review. *J NeuralTransm Suppl.* 1992;35:37–69.
16. Manning J-PA, Richards DA, Leresche N, et al. Cortical-area specific block of genetically determined absence seizures by ethosuximide. *Neuroscience.* 2004;123:5–9.
17. Goren MZ, Onat F. Ethosuximide: from bench to bedside. *CNS Drug Rev.* 2007;13:224–239.
18. Terzioglu B, Aypak C, Onat F, et al. The effects of ethosuximide on amino acids in genetic absence epilepsy rat model. *J Pharmacol Sci.* 2006;100:227–233.
19. Richards DA, Manning J-PA, Barnes D. Targeting thalamic nuclei is not sufficient for the full anti-absence action of ethosuximide in a rat model of absence epilepsy. *Epilepsy Res.* 2003;54:97–107.
20. Tan HO, Reid CA, Single FN, et al. Reduced cortical inhibition in a mouse model of familial childhood absence epilepsy. *Proc Natl Acad Sci U S A.* 2007;104:17536–17541.
21. Ferrendelli J, Holland K. Ethosuximide, mechanisms of action. In: Levy R, Mattson R, Meldrum B, et al., eds. *Antiepileptic drugs.* 3rd ed. New York: Raven Press; 1989:653–661.
22. Lin-Mitchell E, Chweh A. Effects of ethosuximide alone and in combination with gamma-aminobutyric acid receptor antagonists on brain gamma-aminobutyric acid concentration, anticonvulsant activity, and neurotoxicity in mice. *J Pharmacol Exp Ther.* 1986;237:486–489.
23. Gilbert J, Buchan P, Scott A. Effects of anticonvulsant drug on monosaccharide transport and membrane ATPase activities of cerebral cortex. In: Harris P, Mawdsley C, eds. *Epilepsy.* Edinburgh: Churchill Livingstone; 1974:98–104.
24. Gilbert J, Scott A, Wyllie M. Effects of ethosuximide on adenosine triphosphate activities of some subcellular fractions prepared from rat cerebral cortex. *Br J Pharmacol.* 1974;50:452P–453P.
25. Gilbert J, Wyllie M. The effects of the anticonvulsant ethosuximide on adenosine triphosphatase activities of synaptosomes prepared from rat cerebral cortex. *Br J Pharmacol.* 1974;52:139P–140P.
26. Crunelli V, Leresche N. Childhood absence epilepsy: genes, channels, neurons and networks. *Nat RevNeurosci.* 2002;3:371–382.

27. Kobayashi T, Ikedaq K. G protein-activated inwardly rectifying potassium channels as potential therapeutic targets. *Curr Pharm Des.* 2006;12:4513–4523.
28. Villen T, Bertilsson L, Sjoqvist F. Nonstereoselective disposition of ethosuximide in humans. *Ther Drug Monit.* 1990;12:514–516.
29. Tomson T, Villen T. Ethosuximide enantiomers in pregnancy and lactation. *Ther Drug Monit.* 1994;16:621–623.
30. El-Sayed M, Loscher W, Frey H. Pharmacokinetics of ethosuximide in the dog. *Arch Int Pharmacodyn Ther.* 1978;234:180–192.
31. Patel I, Levy R, Bauer T. Pharmacokinetic properties of ethosuximide in monkeys. Single dose intravenous and oral administration. *Epilepsia.* 1975;16:705–716.
32. Patel I, Levy R. Pharmacokinetic properties of ethosuximide in monkeys, II: chronic intravenous and oral administration. *Epilepsia.* 1975;16:717–730.
33. Patel I, Levy R, Rapport R. Distribution characteristics of ethosuximide in discrete areas of rat brain. *Epilepsia.* 1977;18:533–541.
34. Bialer M, Ziadong S, Perucca E. Ethosuximide: absorption, distribution, excretion. In: Levy R, Mattson R, Meldrum B, eds. *Antiepileptic Drugs.* 4th ed. New York: Raven Press; 1995:659–665.
35. Chang T. Ethosuximide: absorption, distribution, and excretion. In: Levy R, Mattson R, Meldrum B, et al., eds. *Antiepileptic Drugs.* 3rd ed. New York: Raven Press; 1989:671–678.
36. Buchanan R, Fernandez L, Kinkel A. Absorption and elimination of ethosuximide in children. *J Clin Pharmacol.* 1969;7:213–218.
37. Eadie M, Tyrer J, Smith J, et al. Pharmacokinetics of drugs used for petit mal absence epilepsy. *Clin Exp Neurol.* 1977;14:172–183.
38. Alvarez N, Besag F, Iivanainen M. Use of antiepileptic drugs in the treatment of epilepsy in people with intellectual disability. *J Intellect Disabil Res.* 1998;42:1–15.
39. Wallace SJ. Use of ethosuximide and valproate in the treatment of epilepsy. *Neurol Clin.* 1986;4:601–616.
40. Chang T, Dill W, Glazko A. Ethosuximide: absorption, distribution and excretion. In: Woodbury D, Penry J, Schmidt R, eds. *Antiepileptic Drugs.* New York: Raven Press; 1972:417–423.
41. Loscher W, Frey H. Kinetics of penetration of common anticonvulsant drugs in serum of dog and man. *Epilepsia.* 1984;25:346–352.
42. Aguilar-Veiga E, Sierra-Paredes G, Galan-Valiente J, et al. Correlations between ethosuximide brain levels measured by high performance liquid chromatography and its antiepileptic potential. *Res Comm Chem Pathol Pharmacol.* 1991;7:351–364.
43. Liu H, Delgado MR. Therapeutic drug concentration monitoring using saliva samples. Focus on anticonvulsants. *Clin Pharmacokinet.* 1999;36:453–470.
44. Buchanan R, Kinkel A, Smith T. The absorption and excretion of ethosuximide. *Int J Clin Pharmacol.* 1973;7:213–218.
45. Horning M, Brown L, Nowlin J, et al. Use of saliva in therapeutic drug monitoring. *Clin Chem.* 1977;23:157–164.
46. Piredda S, Monaco F. Ethosuximide in tears, saliva and cerebral fluid. *Ther Drug Monit.* 1981;3:321–323.
47. McAuliffe J, Sherwin A, Leppik I, et al. Salivary levels of anticonvulsants: a practical approach to drug monitoring. *Neurology.* 1977;27:409–413.
48. Van H. Comparative study of the levels of anticonvulsants and their free fraction in venous blood, saliva and capillary blood in man. *J Pharmacol.* 1984;15:27–35.
49. Bachmann K, Schwartz J, Sullivan T, et al. Single sample estimate of ethosuximide clearance. *Int J Clin Pharmacol Ther Toxicol.* 1986;24:546–550.
50. Meyer F, Quednow B, Potrafki A, et al. Pharmacokinetics of anticonvulsants in the perinatal period. *Zentralbe Gynakol.* 1988;110:1195–1205.
51. Horning M, Stratton C, Nowlin J, et al. Metabolism of 2-ethyl-2-methyl-succinimide in the rat and human. *Drug Metab Dispos.* 1973;1:569–576.
52. Koup J, Rose J, Cohen M. Ethosuximide pharmacokinetics in a pregnant patient and her newborn. *Epilepsia.* 1978;19:535–539.
53. Kaneko S, Sato T, Suzuki K. The levels of anticonvulsants in breast milk. *Br J Clin Pharmacol.* 1979;7:624–627.
54. Kuhnz W, Koch S, Hartmann A, et al. Ethosuximide in epileptic women during pregnancy and lactation period. Placental transfer, serum concentrations in nursed infants and clinical status. *Br J Clin Pharmacol.* 1984;18:671–677.
55. Hancock E, Osborne J, Milner P. Treatment of infantile spasms. *Cochrane Database Syst Rev.* 2003:CD001770.
56. American Academy of Pediatrics Committee on Drugs. Transfer of drugs and other chemicals into human milk. *Pediatrics.* 2001;108:776–789.
57. Bachmann K, Jahn D, Yang C, et al. Ethosuximide disposition kinetics in rats. *Xenobiotica.* 1988;18:373–380.
58. Tanaka E. Clinically significant pharmacokinetic drug interactions between antiepileptic drugs. *J Clin Pharmacol Ther.* 1999;24:87–92.
59. Burkett A, Chang T, Glazko A. A hydroxylated metabolite of ethosuximide (Zarontin) in rat urine. *Fed Proc.* 1971;30:391.
60. Bachmann K. The use of single sample clearance estimates to probe hepatic drug metabolism in rats, IV: a model for possible application to phenotyping xenobiotic influences on human drug metabolism. *Xenobiotica.* 1989;19:1449–1459.
61. Bachmann K, Madhira M, Rankin G. The effects of cobalt chloride, SKF-525A and N-(3,5-dichlorophenyl) succinimide on in vivo hepatic mixed function oxidase activity as determined by single-sample plasma clearances. *Xenobiotica.* 1992;22:27–31.
62. Bachmann K, Chu C, Greear V. In vivo evidence that ethosuximide is a substrate for cytochrome P450IIIA. *Pharmacology.* 1992;45:121–128.
63. Chang T. Ethosuximide. Biotransformation. In: Levy R, Mattson R, Meldrum B, et al., eds. *Antiepileptic Drugs.* 3rd ed. New York: Raven Press; 1989:679–683.
64. Patel I, Levy R, Bauer T. Time dependent kinetics, II: diurnal oscillations in steady state plasma ethosuximide levels in rhesus monkeys. *J Pharm Sci.* 1977;66:650–653.
65. Eadie MJ. Formation of active metabolites of anticonvulsant drugs. A review of their pharmacokinetic and therapeutic significance. *Biomed Chromatogr.* 1991;5:212–215.
66. Bachmann K, He Y, Sarver JG, et al. Characterization of the cytochrome P450 enzymes involved in the in vitro metabolism of ethosuximide by human hepatic microsomal enzymes. *Xenobiotica.* 2003;33:265–276.
67. Gilbert J, Scott A, Galloway D, et al. Ethosuximide: liver enzyme induction and D-glucaric acid excretion. *Br J Clin Pharmacol.* 1974;1:249–252.
68. Glazko A. Antiepileptic drugs: biotransformation, metabolism, and serum half-life. *Epilepsia.* 1975;16:376–391.
69. Bauer L, Harris C, Wilensky A, et al. Ethosuximide kinetics: possible interaction with valproic acid. *Clin Pharmacol Ther.* 1982;31:741–745.
70. Buchanan R, Kinkel A, Turner J, et al. Ethosuximide dosage regimens. *Clin Pharmacol Ther.* 1976;19:143–147.
71. Dill W, Peterson L, Chang T, et al. Physiologic disposition of alpha-methyl-alpha-ethyl succinimide (ethosuximide; Zarontin) in animals and in man. Presented at the 149th National Meeting of the American Chemical Society; 1965; Detroit, MI.
72. Pisani P, Narbone M, Trunfio C. Valproic acid-ethosuximide interaction: a pharmacokinetic study. *Epilepsia.* 1984;25:229–233.
73. Sherwin A. Ethosuximide: clinical use. In: Levy R, Mattson R, Meldrum B, eds. *Antiepileptic Drugs.* 4th ed. New York: Raven Press; 1995:667–673.
74. Bachmann KA, Schwartz J, Jauregui L, et al. Use of three probes to assess the influence of sex on hepatic drug metabolism. *Pharmacology.* 1987;35:88–93.
75. Marbury T, Lee C, Perchalski R. Hemodialysis clearance of ethosuximide in patients with chronic renal failure. *Am J Hosp Pharm.* 1981;38:1757–1760.
76. Marquardt E, Ishisaka D, Batra K, et al. Removal of ethosuximide and phenobarbital by peritoneal dialysis in a child. *Clin Pharm.* 1992;11:1030–1031.
77. Browne T, Feldman R, Buchanan R. Methsuximide for complex seizures: efficacy, toxicity, clinical pharmacology, and drug interactions. *Neurology.* 1983;33:414–418.
78. Dawson G, Brown H, Clark B. Serum phenytoin after ethosuximide. *Ann Neurol.* 1978;4:583–584.
79. Frantzen E, Hansen J, Hansen O, et al. Phenytoin (Dilantin) intoxication. *Acta Neurol Scand.* 1967;43:440–446.
80. Rambeck B. Pharmacological interactions of methsuximide with phenobarbital and phenytoin in hospitalized epileptic patients. *Epilepsia.* 1979;20:147–156.
81. Smith G, McKauge L, Dubetz D, et al. Factors influencing plasma concentrations of ethosuximide. *Clin Pharmacokinet.* 1979;4:38–52.
82. Schmidt D. The effect of phenytoin and ethosuximide on primidone metabolism in patients with epilepsy. *J Neurol.* 1975;209:115–123.
83. Battino D, Avanzini G, Bossi L. Plasma levels of primidone and its metabolite phenobarbital: effect of age and associated therapy. *Ther Drug Monit.* 1983;5:73–79.
84. Riva R, Albani F, Contin M, et al. Pharmacokinetic interactions between antiepileptic drugs. Clinical considerations. *Clin Pharmacokinet.* 1996;31:470–493.
85. Eadie M, Tyrer J. In: Eadie M, Tyrer J, eds. *Anticonvulsant Therapy. Pharmacological Basis and Practice.* 2nd ed. Edinburgh: Churchill Livingstone; 1980:211–223.
86. Salke-Kellermann R, May T, Boenigk H. Influence of ethosuximide on valproic acid serum concentrations. *Epilepsy Res.* 1997;26:345–349.
87. Warren JJ, Benmaman J, Wannamaker B, et al. Kinetics of a carbamazepine-ethosuximide interaction. *Clin Pharmacol.* 1980;28:646–651.
88. Battino D, Cusi C, Franceschetti S, et al. Ethosuximide plasma concentrations: influence of age and associated concomitant therapy. *Clin Pharmacokinet.* 1982;7:176–180.
89. Bachmann K, Jauregui L. Use of single sample clearance estimates of cytochrome P450 substrates to characterize human hepatic CYP status in vivo. *Xenobiotica.* 1993;23:307–315.
90. Giaconne M, Bartoli A, Gatti G, et al. Effect of enzyme inducing anticonvulsants on ethosuximide pharmacokinetics in epileptic patients. *Br J Clin Pharmacol.* 1996;41:575–579.
91. Duncan JS, Patsalos PN, Shorvon SD. Effects of discontinuation of phenytoin, carbamazepine, and valproate on concomitant antiepileptic medication. *Epilepsia.* 1991;32:101–115.
92. Bourgeois B. Pharmacologic interactions between valproate and other drugs. *Am J Med.* 1988;84:28–33.
93. Gram L, Wulff K, Rasmussen K, et al. Valproate sodium: a controlled clinical trial including monitoring of drug levels. *Epilepsia.* 1977;18:141–148.
94. Mattson R, Cramer J. Valproic acid and ethosuximide interaction. *Ann Neurol.* 1980;7:583–584.
95. Levy R, Koch K. Drug interactions with valproic acid. *Drugs.* 1982;24:543–556.

96. van Wieringen A, Vrijlandt C. Ethosuximide intoxication caused by interaction with isoniazid. *Neurology.* 1983;33:1227–1228.

97. White HS. Clinical significance of animal seizure models and mechanism of action studies of potential antiepileptic drugs. *Epilepsia.* 1997;38: S9–S17.

98. Reinhard J, Reinhard J. Experimental evaluation of anticonvulsants. In: Vida J, ed. *Anticonvulsants.* New York: Academic Press; 1977:57–111.

99. Woodbury D. Applications to drug evaluations. In: Purpura P, Penry J, Tower D, et al., eds. *Experimental Models of Epilepsy: A Manual for The Laboratory Worker.* New York: Raven Press; 1972:557–583.

100. Swinyard E, Woodhead J, White H, et al. General principles. Experimental selection, quantification and evaluation of anticonvulsants. In: Levy R, Mattson R, Meldrum B, et al., eds. *Antiepileptic Drugs.* 3rd ed. New York: Raven Press; 1989:85–102.

101. Heller A, Dichter M, Sidman R. Anticonvulsant sensitivity of absence seizures in the tottering mutant mouse. *Epilepsia.* 1983;25:25–34.

102. Marescaux C, Micheletti G, Vergnes M, et al. A model of chronic spontaneous petit mal-like seizures in the rat: comparison with pentylenetetrazol-induced seizures. *Epilepsia.* 1984;25:326–331.

103. Sasa M, Ohno Y, Ujihara H. Effects of antiepileptic drugs on absence-like and tonic seizures in the spontaneously epileptic rat, a double mutant rat. *Epilepsia.* 1988;29:505–513.

104. Godschalk M, Dzoljic M, Bonta I. Antagonism of gamma-hydroxybutyrate-induced hypersynchronization in the ECoG of the rat by anti-petit mal drugs. *Neurosci Lett.* 1976;3:145–150.

105. Snead OI. Gamma-hydroxybutyrate in the monkey, II: effect of chronic oral anticonvulsant drugs. *Neurology.* 1978;28:643–648.

106. Glauser TA, Cnaan A, Shinnar S, Hirtz DG, Dlugos D, Masur D, Clark PO, Capparelli EV, Adamson PC; Childhood Absence Epilepsy Study Group. Ethosuximide, valproic acid, and lamotrigine in childhood absence epilepsy. *N Engl J Med.* 2010 Mar 4;362(9):790–9.

107. Browne TR, Dreifuss FE, Dyken PR, et al. Ethosuximide in the treatment of absence (petit mal) seizures. *Neurology.* 1975;25:515–524.

108. Sherwin A, Robb P, Lechter M. Improved control of epilepsy by monitoring plasma ethosuximide. *Arch Neurol.* 1973;28:178–181.

109. Callaghan N, O'Hara J, O'Driscoll D, et al. Comparative study of ethosuximide and sodium valproate in the treatment of typical absence seizures (petit mal). *Dev Med Child Neurol.* 1982;24:830–836.

110. Martinovic Z. Comparison of ethosuximide with sodium valproate. In: Parsonage M, Grant R, Craig AW Jr, eds. *Advances in Epileptology. XIVth Epilepsy International Symposium.* New York: Raven Press; 1983:301–305.

111. Sato S, White BG, Penry JK, et al. Valproic acid versus ethosuximide in the treatment of absence seizures. *Neurology.* 1982;32:157–163.

112. Posner EB, Mohamed K, Marson AG. Ethosuximide, sodium valproate or lamotrigine for absence seizures in children and adolescents. *Cochrane Database Syst Rev.* 2003:CD003032.

113. Rowan A, Meijer J, deBeer-Pawlikowski N, et al. Valproate-ethosuximide combination therapy for refractory absence seizures. *Arch Neurol.* 1983; 40:797–802.

114. Sherwin A. Ethosuximide: clinical use. In: Levy R, Dreifuss F, Mattson R, et al., eds. *Antiepileptic Drugs.* 3rd ed. New York: Raven Press; 1989: 685–698.

115. Guberman A, Cantu-Reyna G, Stuss D, et al. Nonconvulsive generalized status epilepticus: clinical features, neuropsychological testing, and long-term follow-up. *Neurology.* 1986;36:1284–1291.

116. Browne TR, Dreifuss FE, Penry JK, et al. Clinical and EEG estimates of absence seizure frequency. *Arch Neurol.* 1983;40:469–472.

117. Roger J, Genton P, Bureau M, et al. Less common epileptic syndromes. In: Wyllie E, ed. *The Treatment of Epilepsy: Principles and Practice.* Philadelphia, PA: Lea & Febiger; 1993:624–635.

118. Farrell K. Secondary generalized epilepsy and Lennox-Gastaut syndrome. In: Wyllie E, ed. *The Treatment of Epilepsy: Principles and Practice.* Philadelphia, PA: Lea & Febiger; 1993:604–613.

119. Serratosa J, Delgado-Escueta A. Juvenile myoclonic epilepsy. In: Wyllie E, ed. *The Treatment of Epilepsy: Principles and Practice.* Philadelphia, PA: Lea & Febiger; 1993:552–570.

120. Wallace S. Myoclonus and epilepsy in childhood: a review of treatment with valproate, ethosuximide, lamotrigine and zonisamide. *Epilepsy Res.* 1998;29:147–154.

121. Yasuhara A, Yoshida H, Hatanaka T, et al. Epilepsy with continuous spike-waves during slow sleep and its treatment. *Epilepsia.* 1991;32:59–62.

122. Zifkin B, Andermann F. Epilepsy with reflex seizures. In: Wyllie E, ed. *The Treatment of Epilepsy: Principles and Practice.* Philadelphia, PA: Lea & Febiger; 1993:614–623.

123. Ames F, Enderstein O. Ictal laughter: a case report with clinical, cinefilm, and EEG observations. *J Neurol Neurosurg Psychiatry.* 1975;38:11–17.

124. Capovilla G, Beccaria F, Veggoiotti P, et al. Ethosuximide is effective in the treatment of epileptic negative myoclonus in childhood partial epilepsy. *J Child Neurol.* 1999;14:395–400.

125. Oguni H, Uehara T, Tanaka T, et al. Dramatic effect of ethosuximide on epileptic negative myoclonus: implications for the neurophysiological mechanism. *Neuropediatrics.* 1998;29:29–34.

126. Barton ME, Eberle EL, Shannon HE. The antihyperalgesic effects of the T-type calcium channel blockers ethosuximide, trimethadione, and mibefradil. *Eur J Pharmacol.* 2005;521:79–85.

127. Shannon HE, Eberle EL, Peters SC. Comparison of the effects of anticonvulsant drugs with diverse mechanism of action in the formalin test in rats. *Neuropharmacology.* 2005;48:1012–1020.

128. Todorovic SM, Rastogi AJ, Jevtovic-Todorovic V. Potent analgesic effects of anticonvulsants on peripheral thermal nociception in rats. *Br J Pharmacol.* 2003;140(2):255–260.

129. Flatters SJ, Bennett GJ. Ethosuximide reverses paclitaxel- and vincristine-induced painful peripheral neuropathy. *Pain.* 2004;109:150–161.

130. Wang G, Thompson SM. Maladaptive homeostatic plasticity in a rodent model of central pain syndrome: thalamic hyperexcitability after spinothalamic tract lesions. *J Neurosci.* 2008;12(28):11959–11969.

131. Dreifuss F. Ethosuximide: toxicity. In: Levy R, Mattson R, Meldrum B, eds. *Antiepileptic Drugs.* 4th ed. New York: Raven Press; 1995:675–679.

132. Dreifuss F. Ethosuximide: toxicity. In: Levy R, Mattson R, Meldrum B, et al., eds. *Antiepileptic Drugs.* 3rd ed. New York: Raven Press; 1989: 699–705.

133. Gordon N. Treatment of epilepsy with *O*-ethyl-*o*-methylsuccinimide (P.M. 671). *Neurology.* 1961;11:266–268.

134. Livingston S, Pauli L, Najimabadi A. Ethosuximide in the treatment of epilepsy. *JAMA.* 1952;180:104–107.

135. Zimmerman F, Bergemeister B. A new drug for petit mal epilepsy. *Neurology.* 1958;8:769–776.

136. Goldensohn E, Hardie J, Borea E. Ethosuximide in the treatment of epilepsy. *JAMA.* 1962;180:840–842.

137. Weinstein A, Allen R. Ethosuximide treatment of petit mal seizures. A study of 87 pediatric patients. *Am J Dis Child.* 1966;111:63–67.

138. Park BK, Pirmohamed M, Kitteringham NR. Idiosyncratic drug reactions: a mechanistic evaluation of risk factors. *Br J Clin Pharmacol.* 1992;34: 377–395.

139. Pirmohamed M, Kitteringham NR, Park BK. The role of active metabolites in drug toxicity. *Drug Saf.* 1994;11:114–144.

140. Wallace SJ. A comparative review of the adverse effects of anticonvulsants in children with epilepsy. *Drug Saf.* 1996;15:378–393.

141. Guey J, Charles C, Coquery C, et al. Study of psychological effects of ethosuximide (Zarontin) on 25 children suffering from petit mal epilepsy. *Epilepsia.* 1967;8:129–141.

142. Smith L, Phillips M, Guard H. Psychometric study of children with learning problems and 14-6 positive spike EEG patterns, treated with ethosuximide (Zarontin) and placebo. *Arch Dis Child.* 1968;43:616–619.

143. Abu-Arafeh I, Wallace S. Unwanted effects of antiepileptic drugs. *Dev Med Child Neurol.* 1988;30:117–121.

144. Fischer M, Korskjaer G, Pedersen E. Psychotic episodes in Zarontin treatment. Effects and side-effects in 105 patients. *Epilepsia.* 1965;6:325–334.

145. Cohadon F, Loiseau P, Cohadon S. Results of treatment of certain forms of epilepsy of the petit mal type by ethosuximide. *Rev Neurol.* 1964; 110:201–207.

146. Lairy C. Psychotic signs in epileptics during treatment with ethosuximide. *Rev Neurol.* 1964;110:225–226.

147. Sato T, Kondo Y, Matsuo T, et al. Clinical experiences of ethosuximide (Zarontin) in therapy-resistant epileptics. *Brain Nerve (Tokyo).* 1965;17: 958–964.

148. Wolf P, Inoue Y. Therapeutic response of absence seizures in patients of an epilepsy clinic for adolescents and adults. *J Neurol.* 1984;231:225–229.

149. Buchanan R. Ethosuximide: toxicity. In: Woodbury D, Penry J, Schmidt R, eds. *Antiepileptic Drugs.* New York: Raven Press; 1972:449–454.

150. Heathfield K, Jewesbury E. Treatment of petit mal with ethosuximide. *Br Med J.* 1961;2:565.

151. Todorov A, Lenn N, Gabor A. Exacerbation of generalized non-convulsive seizures with ethosuximide therapy. *Arch Neurol.* 1978;35: 389–391.

152. Uetrecht JP. The role of leukocyte-generated reactive metabolites in the pathogenesis of idiosyncratic drug reactions. *Drug Metab Rev.* 1992;24: 299–366.

153. Gibaldi M. Adverse drug effect—reactive metabolites and idiosyncratic drug reactions: part I. *Ann Pharmacother.* 1992;26:416–421.

154. Glauser TA. Idiosyncratic reactions: new methods of identifying high-risk patients. *Epilepsia.* 2000;41:S16–S29.

155. Pellock JM. Standard approach to antiepileptic drug treatment in the United States. *Epilepsia.* 1994;35:S11–S18.

156. Taafe A, O'Brien C. A case of Stevens-Johnson syndrome associated with the anticonvulsants sulthiame and ethosuximide. *Br Dent J.* 1975;138:172–174.

157. Dabbous IA, Idriss HM. Occurrence of systemic lupus erythematosus in association with ethosuccimide therapy. Case report. *J Pediatr.* 1970;76: 617–620.

158. Alter BP. Systemic lupus erythematosus and ethosuccimide. *J Pediatr.* 1970;77:1093–1095.

159. Livingston S, Rodriguez H, Greene CA, et al. Systemic lupus erythematosus. Occurrence in association with ethosuximide therapy. *JAMA.* 1968;203: 731–732.

160. Teoh PC, Chan HL. Lupus-scleroderma syndrome induced by ethosuximide. *Arch Dis Child.* 1975;50:658–661.

161. Singsen B, Fishman L, Hanson V. Antinuclear antibodies and lupus-like syndromes in children receiving anticonvulsants. *Pediatrics.* 1976;57:529–534.

162. Cohn R. A neuropathological study of a case of petit mal epilepsy. *Electroencephalogr Clin Neurophysiol.* 1968;24:282.

163. Kiorboe E, Paludan J, Trolle E, et al. Zarontin (ethosuximide) in the treatment of petit mal and related disorders. *Epilepsia.* 1964;5:83–89.

164. Kousoulieris E. Granulopenia and thrombocytopenia after ethosuximide. *Lancet.* 1967;2:310–311.

165. Spittler J. Agranulocytosis due to ethosuximide with a fatal outcome. *Klin Paediatr.* 1974;186:364–366.

166. Massey GV, Dunn NL, Heckel JL, et al. Aplastic anemia following therapy for absence seizures with ethosuximide [review]. *Pediatr Neurol.* 1994;11:59–61.

167. Mann L, Habenicht H. Fatal bone marrow aplasia associated with administration of ethosuximide (Zarontin) for petit mal epilepsy. *Bull Los Angeles Neurol Soc.* 1962;27:173–176.

168. Seip M. Aplastic anemia during ethosuximide medication. Treatment with bolus-methylprednisolone. *Acta Paediatr Scand.* 1983;72:927–929.

169. Imai T, Okada H, Nanba M, et al. Ethosuximide induced agranulocytosis. *Brain Dev.* 2003;25:522–524.

170. Ehyai A, Kilroy A, Fenicheal G. Dyskinesia and akathisia induced by ethosuximide. *Am J Dis Child.* 1978;132:527–528.

171. Kirschberg G. Dyskinesia—an unusual reaction to ethosuximide. *Arch Neurol.* 1975;32:137–138.

172. Nishiyama J, Matsukura M, Fugimoto S, et al. Reports of 2 cases of autoimmune thyroiditis while receiving anticonvulsant therapy. *Eur J Pediatr.* 1983;140:116–117.

173. Wassner S, Pennisi A, Malekzadeh M, et al. The adverse effect of anticonvulsant therapy on renal allograft survival. A preliminary report. *J Pediatr.* 1976;88:134–137.

174. Porter R, Penry J, Dreifuss F. Responsiveness at the onset of spike-wave bursts. *Electroencephalogr Clin Neurophysiol.* 1973;34:239–245.

175. Sullivan F, McElhatton P. A comparison of the teratogenic activity of the antiepileptic drugs carbamazepine, clonazepam, ethosuximide, phenobarbital, phenytoin, and primidone in mice. *Toxicol Appl Pharmacol.* 1977;40:365–378.

176. Bourgeois BF. Important pharmacokinetic properties of antiepileptic drugs. *Epilepsia.* 1995;36:S1–S7.

CHAPTER 55 ■ BENZODIAZEPINES

LAZAR JOHN GREENFIELD, JR., HOWARD C. ROSENBERG, AND ELIZABETH I. TIETZ

Benzodiazepines (BZs) were initially developed in 1933 from a class of heterocyclic compounds known since 1891 (1). Chlordiazepoxide was introduced as an anxiolytic agent in 1960, followed by diazepam (2) and nitrazepam (3), and the BZs soon became the most widely prescribed drugs in the United States. In 1965, diazepam was first used to treat status epilepticus (SE) in humans (4,5). Clonazepam was introduced in the 1970s primarily as an antiepileptic drug (AED) (6), and clobazam, a 1,5-BZ, was later developed as an AED with reduced sedative effect (7,8). However, at the turn of the 21st century, only a few BZs have been approved for acute or chronic use as AEDs in the United States.

The mechanism of action of the BZs remained obscure until the discovery of high affinity, saturable BZ binding to a CNS receptor (9,10). The BZs were also shown to enhance inhibitory neurotransmission mediated by GABA (γ-aminobutyric acid), the major inhibitory neurotransmitter of the mammalian brain (11). Subsequent studies confirmed that the brain BZ receptor was in fact a binding site on the $GABA_A$ receptor, where the BZs act as positive allosteric modulators (12).

CHEMISTRY AND MECHANISM OF ACTION

The basic BZ structure is shown in Figure 55.1. The term BZ refers most often to the 5-aryl-1,4-BZs, however, clobazam is a 1,5-BZ with antiepileptic properties but less sedative effect

(7,8,13). Some agents (e.g., midazolam and flumazenil) have fused R1 and R2 substituents, creating further ring complexity.

BZ potency correlates with binding affinity at BZ sites on neuronal $GABA_A$ receptors (Table 55.1) (14,15). An electron-withdrawing group at position 7 increases receptor binding affinity (16) and potency, and all useful anticonvulsant BZs have such a group. A methyl group on the position 1 nitrogen (as in diazepam and clobazam) increases binding affinity and potency, as does a halogen at the 2' position. A hydroxyl group at position 3 (as in lorazepam) decreases potency and binding affinity.

BZ activity at the $GABA_A$ receptor is a function of the drug's affinity for the BZ-binding site and its intrinsic allosteric effect on the $GABA_A$ receptor. The efficacy of individual compounds varies widely. Most BZ AEDs are full agonists that maximally enhance $GABA_A$ receptor activity. Competitive antagonists bind to the BZ site but do not affect $GABA_A$ receptor function. The BZ antagonist, flumazenil, is used to reverse sedation induced by BZs in anesthesia (18,19), and to treat BZ overdose (20). Several "partial agonists" at the BZ-binding site have been characterized, including abecarnil (21), imidazenil (22), and bretazenil (23). Although less effective than full agonists like diazepam, these agents have demonstrated anticonvulsant efficacy in animal models and appear less prone to the development of tolerance (24,25). Still other compounds behave as "inverse agonists" at the BZ site, and inhibit GABA-binding or GABA-evoked currents (26). These agents, which can induce convulsive seizures or anxiety (26,27), have no known clinical utility.

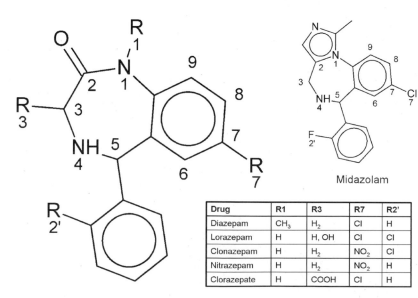

Drug	R1	R3	R7	R2'
Diazepam	CH₃	H₂	Cl	H
Lorazepam	H	H, OH	Cl	Cl
Clonazepam	H	H₂	NO₂	Cl
Nitrazepam	H	H₂	NO₂	H
Clorazepate	H	COOH	Cl	H

Midazolam

FIGURE 55.1 Structure of the 1,4-benzodiazepines. Substituents at the named sites are given in the table for diazepam, lorazepam, clonazepam, nitrazepam, and clorazepate. Midazolam with its fused R1 ring is shown separately.

TABLE 55.1

ANTICONVULSANT ACTIVITY, MOTOR IMPAIRMENT, AND RECEPTOR BINDING OF SOME BZS

BZ	ED_{50} to suppress clonus in kindled rats (mg/kg)[a]	ED_{50} for ataxia (mg/kg)[a]	IC_{50} to inhibit [^{3}H]flunitrazepam specific binding (nM)[b]
Clobazam	2.8	13.2	870
Diazepam	0.4	1.5	78
Clonazepam	0.09	0.9	16
7-Amino-clonazepam	>40	—	195

[a]Dose required to inhibit forelimb clonus or to cause ataxia in 50% of amygdala-kindled rats (data from Ref. 17, except 7-amino-clonazepam data, which has been taken from HC Rosenberg, EI Tietz, and TH Chiu, unpublished data, 1987).
[b]Concentration required to displace 50% of 2 nM [^{3}II]flunitrazepam specifically bound to rat cerebral cortical membranes (EI Tietz, TH Chiu, and HC Rosenberg, unpublished data, 1990).

Anticonvulsant Activity

BZs are effective against virtually every experimental seizure type, but there are large quantitative differences between individual drugs in their potency and efficacy in specific seizure models and their other clinical effects (28). BZs are particularly effective against seizures induced by the convulsant, pentylenetetrazol (29), but are less effective against tonic seizures induced by "maximal electroshock" (30). The dose ratio between clinical efficacy and adverse effects varies among specific agents. For example, the diazepam dose for blocking pentylenetetrazol seizures is 1% of that necessary to abolish the righting response; for clonazepam, the ratio is less than 0.02%, suggesting a greater therapeutic window. BZs have also been shown to slow the development of amygdaloid kindling (31).

BZ Actions at the GABA$_A$ Receptor

In 1977, a high affinity, saturable-binding site for BZs was discovered on CNS neuronal membranes (9,10,14). BZ receptor binding was "coupled" to GABA binding (32), which led to the idea of a "GABA$_A$ receptor complex" incorporating binding sites for GABA, the BZs and barbiturates, and a ligand-gated chloride channel. Only later it was clear that BZs and GABA bind to sites on a single pentomeric channel. This fit well with electrophysiologic studies which demonstrated that BZs increased the amplitude of GABA-mediated inhibitory postsynaptic potentials (IPSPs) (11) by increasing the opening frequency of the GABA-gated chloride channel (33); this was later confirmed with single channel studies (34).

In whole-cell patch-clamp recordings of CNS neurons, BZs produce a leftward shift of the concentration–response curve for GABA (35), which is due to an increase in the affinity for GABA at its binding site, with no change in the kinetics of channel gating (34). The BZs thus increase the current produced by low GABA concentrations, but not by high synaptic concentrations at which receptor binding is saturated. Thus, BZs do not increase the amplitude of miniature inhibitory postsynaptic currents (mIPSCs) from individual synapses, but instead prolong the mIPSC decay phase (36,37) by slowing the dissociation of GABA from the receptor (38,39). Prolongation

of the mIPSC increases the likelihood of temporal and spatial summation of multiple synaptic inputs, which in turn increases the amplitude of stimulus-evoked polysynaptic IPSCs. The BZs thus increase the inhibitory "tone" of GABAergic synapses, which reduces the hypersynchronous firing of neuron populations that underlies seizure activity (40).

Molecular Biology of GABA$_A$ Receptors

GABA$_A$ receptors are pharmacologically complex, with binding sites for BZs, barbiturates, neurosteroids, general anesthetics, the novel anticonvulsant, loreclezole, and the convulsant toxins, picrotoxin and bicuculline. Protein subunits from seven different subunit families (41) assemble to form pentameric (42) transmembrane chloride channels (Fig. 55.2). In mammals, 16 subunit subtypes have been cloned, including six α, three β, and three γ subtypes, as well as δ, π (43), ε (44), and θ (45) and alternatively spliced variants of the β2 and γ2 subtypes. Though thousands of subunit compositions are possible, expression is regulated by region and cell type (46), and also developmentally regulated (47,48), reducing the number of possible isoforms in specific brain regions and individual neurons. The most common GABA receptor has a presumed stoichiometry of two α1, two β2, and a single γ2 subunit; the δ subunit may in some cases substitute for γ, particularly when receptors are expressed extrasynaptically. The subunits are arranged around a central water-filled pore, which can open to conduct Cl$^-$ ions when GABA is bound (see Fig. 55.2). Studies of recombinant receptors have shown that individual subunit subtypes confer different sensitivities to GABA$_A$ receptor modulators including BZs (49,50), loreclezole (51), and zinc ions (52).

GABA$_A$ Receptor Subunits and BZ Pharmacology

BZ augmentation of GABA$_A$ receptor currents requires a γ subunit, and the selectivity of BZ responsiveness is determined by which α subunits are present (41,53). The α1 subunit results in a receptor with high affinity for the hypnotic, zolpidem, defining the "BZ-1" (or Ω-1) receptor type (54,55). The α2 and α3 subunits result in receptors with moderate zolpidem affinity, termed BZ-2 receptors. GABA$_A$ receptors with the α5 subunit and/or the γ3 subunit are sensitive to diazepam, but not to zolpidem, and are termed BZ-3 receptors.

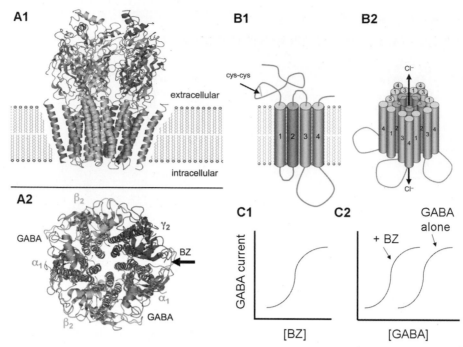

FIGURE 55.2 Model of a GABA$_A$ receptor in the plasma membrane. A space-filling model of the pentomer in side view (**A1**) and top view (**A2**) based on the high sequence homology with the nicotinic acetylcholine receptor. There are with two binding sites for GABA, between α and β subunits, and one for BZs between α and γ subunits *(arrow)*. A schematic view shows the topology of each subunit with a large extracellular loop containing a cysteine loop (**B1**) and four transmembrane domains from which the second forms the lining of the chloride ion channel (**B2**). Binding of GABA allows the channel to open and conduct Cl$^-$ ions, resulting in the fast inhibitory post-synaptic potential (IPSP). (Derived from the published structure: RCSB PDB Database·PDB ID: 2BG9 from Unwin, N. Refined structure of the nicotinic acetylcholine receptor at 4A resolution. *J Mol. Biol.* 2005;346:967.) Images modified from those found at en.wikipedia.org/wiki/GABA$_A$ receptor, with permission (public domain). **C1:** BZ binding enhances the affinity for GABA, resulting in prolonged IPSCs and BZ concentration-dependent increases in GABA currents. **C2:** With a single BZ concentration, currents are generated by lower GABA concentrations resulting in a left shift of the GABA concentration response curve, but no increase in maximal current. The BZs have no effect in the absence of GABA.

GABA$_A$ receptors with the α4 or α6 subunits are insensitive to most BZs. Given the dependence of BZ binding and action on α and γ subunits, it is not surprising that the BZ-binding site is located in a cleft between the extracellular amino termini of these two subunits (56).

GABA$_A$ receptors with particular subunit compositions are associated with specific BZ clinical actions. In particular, BZ binding at receptors that contain the α1 subunit is responsible for sedative, amnestic, and anticonvulsant actions (57,58). Unfortunately, these findings underscore the association between sedative and anticonvulsant efficacy for the BZs at α1-containing GABA$_A$ receptors. The anxiolytic (59) and myorelaxant (60) properties of BZs appear to derive from α2- and (at higher BZ concentrations) α3-containing GABA$_A$ receptors, and more recent studies have implicated the α5 subunit as critical for amnestic effects (61). BZs may also have a true analgesic effect independent of their sedative and anxiolytic actions effect, associated with the α2 and α3 more than α5 subunits (62).

The role of individual subunits in GABA$_A$ receptor function is further underscored by studies in which antisense oligodeoxynucleotides (ASO) were used to selectively reduce the expression of specific subunits. Progesterone withdrawal (which occurs naturally at the end of the menstrual cycle) results in anxiety and increased seizure susceptibility associated with an increase in expression of the α4 subunit (63), which is BZ insensitive. Pretreating rats with an ASO against the α4 subunit prevented the increase in seizure susceptibility (64); this finding may have significance for catamenial epilepsy. Treatment with an ASO for the γ2 subunit produced the expected decrease in BZ binding, but no change in GABA binding to the GABA receptor site (65–67). Similarly, mice lacking the γ2 subunit expressed GABA$_A$ receptors with almost no BZ recognition sites, and only a minor reduction in GABA-binding sites (68).

GABA$_A$ Receptors and Epilepsy

The anticonvulsant properties of BZs are likely related to the prominent role of GABA$_A$ receptors in epilepsy. The evidence linking epilepsy with dysfunction of GABAergic inhibition is substantial (40). GABA$_A$ receptors are the target not only of the BZs, but other AEDs including the barbiturates and, indirectly, two newer agents that increase GABA concentration at the synapse, tiagabine and vigabatrin (40). Several animal models of epilepsy have altered GABA$_A$ receptor number or function (40,69–71). Moreover, changes in the composition or structure of the transmembrane protein subunits that make up GABA$_A$ receptors can result in epilepsy. GABA$_A$ receptor subunit expression is altered in the hippocampi of experimental animals with recurrent seizures (72) and in patients with temporal lobe epilepsy (73,74). Reduction of the GABA$_A$R γ2 subunit expression using an antisense oligodeoxynucleotide in rats (to block translation of endogenous mRNA for that subunit) led to spontaneous electrographic seizures that evolved into limbic SE (75). In humans, Angelman syndrome, a neurodevelopmental disorder associated with severe mental retardation and epilepsy, is linked to a deletion mutation on chromosome 15q11-13 (76) in a region encoding the GABA$_A$ receptor β3 subunit (77). In addition, two mutations in the γ2 subunit that impair GABA$_A$ receptor function (78), K289M (79) and R43Q (71), have been linked to a human syndrome of childhood absence epilepsy and febrile seizures, and a loss-of-function mutation in the α1 subunit was found in a family with autosomal dominant juvenile myoclonic epilepsy (80). The R43Q mutation in the γ2 subunit reduces BZ sensitivity (81) by altering GABA$_A$ receptor assembly (82–84) and trapping the receptor in the endoplasmic reticulum (85).

Other BZ Actions

With a few caveats (27), the BZs appear to derive their anticonvulsant properties from their specific interaction with GABA$_A$ receptors. At doses used to treat SE, BZs can also inhibit voltage-gated sodium (86) and calcium channels (87), and can increase GABA levels in cerebrospinal fluid (88). However, it should be noted that the BZs have no interaction with the G-protein–linked GABA$_B$ receptor, which can either suppress voltage-gated Ca^{2+} channels or activate inward rectifying K$^+$ channels (89).

The BZs also bind to the "peripheral BZ receptor" (PBR) (90,91), an 18-kDa protein in the outer mitochondrial membrane that functions as part of the mitochondrial permeability transition pore involved in cholesterol transport (91), apoptosis, and regulation of mitochondrial function (92). Although the PBR is widely expressed throughout the body, its expression in the CNS is restricted to ependymal cells and glia (90), hence it is unlikely that the PBR is involved in the clinical properties of the BZs.

Excitatory GABA$_A$ Currents

BZ enhancement of GABA$_A$ receptor function may not always be anticonvulsant, or even inhibitory. Early in CNS development, neurons express the Na$^+$/K$^+$/Cl$^-$ cotransporter, NKCC1, rather than the K$^+$/Cl$^-$ cotransporter, KCC2, which is expressed in adult neurons. NKCC1 increases intracellular Cl$^-$ resulting in a depolarizing Cl$^-$ reversal potential, while KCC2 exports Cl$^-$ yielding the hyperpolarizing Cl$^-$ reversal potential found in adult neurons (93). As a result, activation of GABA$_A$ receptor channels can be excitatory during early development (94) and play a trophic role in neuronal migration and connectivity (95,96), but this may also contribute to epileptogenesis (97,98). In fact, endogenous GABA appears to be proconvulsant in early postnatal rat hippocampal slices, as GABA$_A$ antagonists

blocked epileptiform activity induced by depolarization with high external [K$^+$] (99). However, BZ anticonvulsant efficacy appears to be intact, likely because persistent opening of GABA channels (in the presence of BZs) may reduce the depolarizing chloride reversal potential, resulting in "shunt" inhibition, or alternatively, subthreshold GABA-evoked depolarization may inactivate sodium channels and prevent action potential firing (100,101). The current through GABA$_A$ receptor channels can also be altered by changes in intracellular bicarbonate (93,102), which, like Cl$^-$, can flow through the channel (103). Changes in bicarbonate may underlie reduced synaptic GABA currents during development of BZ tolerance (104,105). Depolarizing GABA$_A$ currents may also be a source of interictal spike activity, as observed in epileptic subiculum neurons in hippocampal brain slices removed from patients with temporal lobe epilepsy (106). Changes in the GABA current reversal potential might also explain why diazepam can be less effective in children with epileptic encephalopathies (107), and rarely can cause SE in patients with the Lennox–Gastaut syndrome (108,109).

ABSORPTION, DISTRIBUTION, AND METABOLISM

The major anticonvulsant role of the BZs is in the treatment of SE and seizure clusters, for which they represent first-line therapy. The IV route of administration is preferred (110). In very young children, this may be difficult or impossible, necessitating administration via rectal (111–116), intraosseous (117), buccal (118,119), or nasal (120–122) routes. With IV administration, the main factor in a drug's effectiveness is the rate at which it crosses the blood–brain barrier (BBB). The BZs are highly lipophilic and cross the BBB rapidly (123), though this varies more than 50-fold between agents (124) and is fastest for the most lipophilic agents. Protein binding also correlates with lipophilicity and is high for most BZs, up to nearly 99% for diazepam. The BZs are fully absorbed after oral ingestion.

Despite generally long plasma half-lives, most BZs are relatively "short-acting" after administration of a single dose due to rapid distribution from the brain and vascular compartments to peripheral tissues (125,126). BZ pharmacokinetics are best fit by a two-compartment model: high levels occur rapidly in the brain and other well-perfused organs, then decline rapidly with an initial brief half life due to distribution into peripheral tissues and lipid stores, followed by a much slower elimination half-life related to enzymatic metabolism and excretion. For example, the elimination half-life of diazepam ranges from 20 to 54 hours (127), but the duration of action after a single IV injection is only 1 hour, with peak brain concentrations present for only 20 to 30 minutes (128).

The BZs are metabolized in the liver by cytochrome P450 enzymes, particularly CYP3A4 and CYP2C19, with relatively little enzyme induction. The presence of biologically active metabolites (e.g., nordazepam as a metabolite of diazepam) can significantly prolong the biologic half-lives of some BZs. Elimination may be prolonged by enterohepatic circulation, particularly in the elderly. Most BZs cross the placenta and are secreted into breast milk. A schematic of BZ metabolic pathways is shown in Figure 55.3. The biotransformation and pharmacokinetics of the BZs have been extensively reviewed

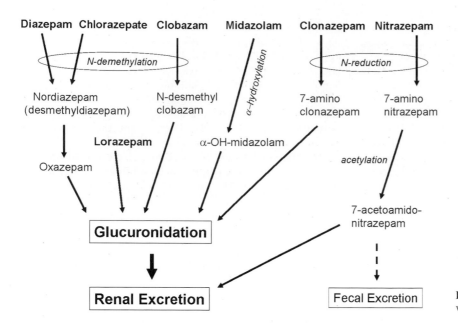

FIGURE 55.3 Hepatic metabolism of the anticonvulsant BZs.

(129–134) and will be presented in more detail for the individual agents below.

DRUG INTERACTIONS

BZs interact with other drugs more prominently through pharmacodynamic than pharmacokinetic mechanisms. They do not significantly affect plasma protein binding or metabolism of other drugs. CNS depression is increased when BZs are given in conjunction with other CNS-depressant drugs (124,135). Pharmacokinetic interactions with other anticonvulsants are infrequent and inconsistent, with the exception of phenobarbital. Diazepam enhances phenobarbital elimination (136), and phenobarbital increases the clearance (137) and lowers plasma levels of clonazepam (138). Clobazam increases the 10,11-epoxide metabolite of carbamazepine (139). Valproate reduces diazepam protein binding, increasing free drug levels (140), and enhances diazepam's effects in the CNS (138). Other AEDs may augment metabolism and clearance of N-desmethyl-diazepam (DMD) derived from clorazepate (141). Inhibitors of CYP3A4, including erythromycin, clarithromycin, ritonavir, itraconazol, ketaconazole, nefazodone, and grapefruit juice, can slow BZ metabolism (142). Cimetidine decreases the clearance of diazepam (143,144) and nitrazepam (145). Rifampin increases the clearance and shortens the half-life of nitrazepam (146). Lorazepam half-life is markedly increased by probenecid (147).

EFFICACY AS ANTIEPILEPTIC AGENTS

Status Epilepticus

SE is associated with significant morbidity and mortality (148,149), and requires emergent medical treatment to avoid neuronal damage and its neurologic consequences (150–152). The BZs have become agents of choice for initial therapy due to their rapid onset, proven efficacy (153), and lower risk of cardiotoxicity or respiratory depression compared to the barbiturates (154). The role of BZs in SE has been confirmed in several well-controlled clinical trials, including the multicenter, double-blind Veterans Affairs (VA) Cooperative SE Trial (155).

Lorazepam and diazepam were compared for treatment of SE in a double-blind study of 78 adults with epilepsy (153). Intravenous lorazepam (4 mg) stopped SE in 78% of patients and diazepam (10 mg) in 58% after the first injection; both had similar efficacy (89% and 76%, respectively) after the second injection. An open-label, prospective, randomized trial compared lorazepam (0.05 to 0.1 mg/kg) and diazepam (0.3 to 0.4 mg/kg) in children with acute convulsions, including convulsive SE (156). Lorazepam was more effective ($P < 0.01$) after the first dose and apparently safer than diazepam. A meta-analysis of 11 randomized controlled trials with 2017 participants found that lorazepam was better than both diazepam and phenytoin alone for reducing risk of seizure continuation (157). A population-based study of 182 children with convulsive SE showed that IV lorazepam was 3.7 times more likely than rectal diazepam to terminate seizures (158). Lorazepam's superiority may be due to its longer duration of action, based on a longer distribution half-life (see below).

Lorazepam has largely replaced diazepam as the agent of choice for prehospital treatment of SE. A prehospital trial of lorazepam and diazepam found that SE had terminated by arrival at the emergency department in 59.1% of patients treated with lorazepam (2 mg), compared to 42.6% of patients treated with diazepam (5 mg) and 21.1% of patients given placebo (159). Rates of circulatory or ventilatory complications for lorazepam and diazepam were similar (10.6% and 10.3%, respectively) and lower than that of placebo (22.5%), confirming the safety and efficacy of BZ treatment of SE in this setting.

Early treatment of SE increases the probability of seizure termination (159), likely because prolonged seizures alter GABA$_A$ receptor susceptibility to BZs (160). Reduction in

GABA$_A$ receptor BZ sensitivity can occur within minutes in SE (161,162) and may be responsible in part for both the persistent epileptic state and its refractoriness to treatment. Refractoriness to BZs may be mediated by N-methyl-D aspartate (NMDA) receptor mechanisms, as NMDA antagonists improve the response to diazepam in late pilocarpine-induced SE (163). These findings suggest a possible strategy for treatment of late, BZ-refractory SE with combinations of a BZ and an NMDA receptor antagonist such as the dissociative general anesthetic, ketamine. Efficacy of combined diazepam and ketamine has been demonstrated in a rat model of SE (164), and a recent trial of oral ketamine for refractory nonconvulsive SE in children showed efficacy in five of five cases (165). Treatment protocols involving NMDA antagonists have been suggested (166,167), but such approaches will require validation in controlled clinical trials.

Both lorazepam and diazepam have been approved by the United States Food and Drug Administration (U.S. FDA) for treatment of SE in adults; diazepam has also been approved in children older than 30 days. Parenteral preparations of other BZs, including midazolam, flunitrazepam, and clonazepam, expand the possibilities for BZ treatment of SE. However, parenteral clonazepam is currently available only in Germany and the United Kingdom, and flunitrazepam is not available in the United States. Alternative routes of administration, including intramuscular (IM) injection and intranasal (121,122), buccal (119), endotracheal (168,169), or rectal (117,170,171) instillation, have also rapidly produced therapeutic levels and demonstrated efficacy against SE or seizure clusters.

Acute Repetitive Seizures

The availability of alternative methods of BZ administration increases the therapeutic options for treatment of acute repetitive seizures. Individual agents can be selected for specific clinical situations. For example, repeated seizures in a patient rapidly tapered off anticonvulsants for inpatient epilepsy monitoring could be treated with diazepam (rather than lorazepam) since its shorter peak duration of action may be less likely to suppress seizure activity needed later for localization of seizure onset. In the case of serial seizures, the need for immediate high drug levels is less urgent, and ease of administration by family or allied health workers becomes important. Diazepam rectal gel is effective in preventing subsequent seizures during seizure clusters (170–172) and can reduce the frequency of emergency department visits (113). Buccal (173,174) and intranasal (175) routes may be equally effective and more acceptable (176). Table 55.2 compares the clinical and pharmacologic properties of the BZs used for acute seizures.

Chronic Treatment of Epilepsy

Although the use of BZs in chronic treatment of epilepsy is limited by sedation and the development of tolerance, BZs may have specific therapeutic indications, such as adjunctive treatment of myoclonic and other generalized seizure types, or in conjunction with comorbid anxiety disorders. For example, lorazepam improved control of seizures associated with psychological stressors (177). Intermittent use of BZs when seizure thresholds are transiently reduced may be the ideal strategy for these AEDs. Not only are they suited pharmacokinetically for such applications, but short-term use may avoid the development of tolerance. For example, catamenial seizures improved with intermittent administration of clobazam (178). AED efficacy for specific indications will be discussed with the individual agents below.

TABLE 55.2

CLINICAL PHARMACOLOGY OF BZs USED FOR ACUTE SEIZURES

| Characteristic | Diazepam | | Lorazepam | | Midazolam | | Clonazepam |
	IV	Rectal	IV[a]	Buccal[a]	IV[a]	IM[a]	IV[b]
Bolus dose (mg)	10–20	0.5–1/kg	4	2–4	0.125–0.15/kg	0.2/kg	0.01–0.09/kg
Infusion rate	8 mg/h	—	—	—	0.15–0.2 mg/kg/h	—	—
Minimum effective concentration	500 ng/mL	NA	30 ng/mL	NA	NA	NA	30 ng/mL
Onset of effect (min)	<1	2–6	<2	NA	<2	2–30	<1
Peak effect (min)	3–15	10–120	30	NA	10–50	25 ± 23	NA
Duration of effect	<20 min	NA	>360 min	NA	<50 min	20–120 min	24 h
Protein bound (%)	96–97	96–97	85–93	85–93	95 ± 2	95 ± 2	86 ± 5
Volume of distribution (L/kg)	133	133	12	12	NA	NA	NA
Distribution half-life	0.96–2.2 h	NA	2–3 h	NA	5.7 ± 2.4 min	NA	NA
Elimination half-life (h)	36 ± 4.9	36 ± 4.9	14.1	14.1	1.9 ± 0.6	1.9 ± 0.6	20–80

NA, not available.
[a]Not approved by the U.S. Food and Drug Administration for seizures.
[b]Not available in the United States.

TOLERANCE AND DEPENDENCE

BZ Tolerance

Chronic BZ treatment is associated with tolerance, a decrease in sedative or anticonvulsant properties, and dependence, the need for continued drug to prevent a withdrawal syndrome (179). The development of tolerance is a significant clinical problem, requiring escalation of drug doses and increasing the risk of withdrawal seizures. Chronic treatment with BZs can also reduce their subsequent effectiveness in acute conditions (180), rendering them less useful for treatment of SE. In animal studies, tolerance develops proportionally to agonist efficacy. BZ partial agonists develop much less tolerance than full agonists, and the antagonist flumazenil causes no tolerance-related changes in receptor number or function (24). Tolerance to one BZ with a particular regimen may not induce tolerance to a different BZ, suggesting drug-specific interactions at their receptors (181). The duration of tolerance also varies between BZs (182). Several studies of tolerance have noted changes in $GABA_A$ receptor subunit expression (183–189) as well as functional changes (190–193); however, such changes are dependent not only on the drug and dosage, but also on the duration and method of drug administration, all of which contribute to chronic BZ receptor occupancy that predisposes to tolerance. Measurements of tolerance also depend on the animal seizure model and the behavioral tests used to assess BZ clinical properties (194).

Physical Dependence

Abrupt cessation of prolonged BZ therapy can result in withdrawal symptoms, including restlessness and agitation, anxiety, loss of appetite, nausea, lethargy, dizziness, headache, palpitations, irritability, confusion, and in some cases, seizures. The short-acting antagonist, flumazenil, precipitated a withdrawal syndrome in subjects given chronic low-dose diazepam (mean dose 11.2 mg/day) for an average of 4.6 years (195). Four of 13 patients developed panic attacks. A short-lived withdrawal syndrome was elicited by IV flumazenil following 7, 14, or 28 days of oral diazepam (15 mg/70 kg) administration to healthy volunteers (196). There is debate whether withdrawal symptoms, such as heightened anxiety, might represent rebound of existing symptoms to a level greater than that before treatment, and whether withdrawal anxiety can result in relapse to the previous state of anxiety (197). BZ prescription misuse has been ascribed to patients' efforts to alleviate withdrawal symptoms, which can lead to a drug dependence syndrome (198,199). BZ self-administration is enhanced in long-term therapeutic users suddenly switched to placebo relative to those whose dose was tapered gradually (200).

Changes in $GABA_A$ receptors related to tolerance might be assumed to underlie withdrawal symptoms and physical dependence (201,202). Yet, evidence from animal models suggests that enhancement of excitatory systems in a variety of brain regions (203,204) may underlie anxiety behavior (205–207) and increased seizure activity (207). Enhanced glutamatergic neurotransmission involves a selective increase in GluR1-containing α-amino-3-hydroxy-5-methyl-4-isoxazole propionic acid (AMPA) receptors (142,207,208), which correlates with increased anxiety-like behavior (205,209). Such plastic changes in the hippocampus are similar to those found with long-term potentiation (LTP) (210). LTP depends on AMPA receptor-mediated depolarization and subsequent relief of the Mg^{2+} block from NMDA receptors, allowing Ca^{2+} entry, which in turn activates kinases resulting in persistent enhancement of GluR1 AMPA receptors. In contrast, for BZ withdrawal, the calcium signal that mediates enhancement of GluR1 AMPA receptors enters through voltage-gated Ca^{2+} channels (VGCCs) (205,206). In fact, VGCC currents double during chronic BZ treatment and withdrawal, and anxiety can be alleviated by prior administration of the VGCC antagonist, nimodipine (206). The increased anxiety and other symptoms abate over time, associated with downregulation of NMDA receptors (205,211,212), which may serve as a natural brake on withdrawal symptoms.

ADVERSE EVENTS

With acute treatment of SE, the primary toxicity issue is respiratory and cardiovascular depression (153,213). For IV infusions, the propylene glycol solvent contributes to toxicity (214,215). Other toxic effects such as sedation and amnesia are of relatively little consequence in this setting, and difficult to distinguish from the effects of SE itself. However, sedation after termination of convulsive SE often necessitates EEG evaluation to ensure that convulsive seizures have not been converted to nonconvulsive SE. When BZs have been administered in conjunction with other CNS-active drugs, such as phenobarbital, respiratory, and cardiovascular toxicity may be enhanced (135). Rarely, parenterally administered BZs can induce tonic SE in patients with Lennox–Gastaut syndrome (109,216). Thrombophlebitis may occur (217,218), and intra-arterial injection may produce tissue necrosis (219).

With chronic use, all of the BZs induce similar untoward effects including sedation and drowsiness, lightheadedness, ataxia, cognitive slowing and confusion, and anterograde amnesia. Other effects include weakness, headache, blurred vision, vertigo, nausea and vomiting, GI distress and diarrhea. Joint aches, chest pains, and incontinence occur more rarely (124). The risk of tolerance, dependence and abuse is significant, but low in patients prescribed with these agents for appropriate indications (126,220). Abrupt withdrawal of the BZs has been associated with convulsions, worsening of insomnia, psychosis, and delirium tremens in nonepileptic individuals using diazepam, clonazepam, clorazepate, or nitrazepam (221–223). The incidence of allergic, hepatotoxic, or hematologic reactions to the BZs is extremely low. The BZs can sometimes increase the frequency of seizures in epileptic patients. Specific adverse effects will be discussed with the individual agents below.

INDIVIDUAL BZs

We will initially discuss agents with predominantly short-term uses: diazepam, lorazepam, and midazolam, and subsequently present the BZs used more commonly in chronic epilepsy treatment: clonazepam, clorazepate, clobazam, and nitrazepam.

Diazepam

Diazepam, the first BZ used in the treatment of epilepsy (4), became a standard initial therapy for SE in adults and children (153), though its primary role has been usurped by lorazepam (155,159). Diazepam is available in both oral and parenteral preparations. The classification of rectal diazepam as an orphan drug in 1993 allowed the development of rectal diazepam gel (Diastat).

Diazepam and other BZs induce an increase in β-frequency activity and slowing of the background on EEG, which can be quantified by spectral analysis (224). The pattern of EEG changes may be of prognostic value in seizure control; 88% of patients (29/33) whose EEG responded to diazepam with loss of abnormal activity or emergence of fast (β frequency) activity had a good prognosis (seizure-free or 50% seizure reduction) (225).

Absorption, Distribution, and Metabolism

Diazepam is highly lipophilic, which allows rapid entry into the brain but also results in rapid subsequent redistribution into peripheral tissues. It is extensively bound to plasma proteins (90% to 99%) (226). The volume of distribution is 1.1 L/kg. Plasma concentration declines rapidly during the distribution phase with an initial half-life ($t_{1/2\alpha}$) of 1 hour (227). Diazepam undergoes demethylation to desmethyldiazepam (DMD, nordiazepam), a metabolite with anticonvulsant activity and a long half-life (>20 hours), followed by slow hydroxylation to oxazepam, which is also active (see Fig. 55.3) (228). Small amounts of temazepam are also formed by 3-hydroxylation of diazepam. The hydroxylated metabolites are conjugated with glucuronic acid in the liver (229) followed by renal excretion (230) with an elimination half-life ($t_{1/2\beta}$) of 24 to 48 hours (136,227). Diazepam treatment causes modest induction of cytochrome P450 type 2B (CYP2B) (230). There is little evidence of enterohepatic circulation (231,232), but diazepam may be secreted in the gastric juices resulting in enterogastric circulation (233). Like most BZs, diazepam crosses the placenta and is excreted to some extent in breast milk (124,227).

Adverse Effects and Drug Interactions

Diazepam can produce respiratory depression (234), which may be exacerbated by postictal CNS depression and necessitate ventilatory support (235). Sedative effects, including inattention and drowsiness, occur at plasma levels of about 200 ng/mL (236,237), the same level needed to suppress spikes (238) and maintain control of SE in acute studies (136). Drowsiness, fatigue, amnesia, ataxia, and falls are more prominent in the elderly. Intravenous diazepam can cause thrombophlebitis and lactic acidosis (due to the propylene glycol vehicle) (217,218). Rare paradoxical responses include increased seizure frequency, muscle spasms, or SE (239). An idiosyncratic allergic interstitial nephritis has also been reported (240). Other rare adverse events include cardiac arrhythmias, hepatotoxicity, gynecomastia, blurred vision and diplopia, neutropenia or thrombocytopenia, rash

and urticaria, and anaphylaxis (241). There is potential for abuse, though it is rare in patients prescribed diazepam for appropriate indications (126). The teratogenicity of diazepam is uncertain, but diazepam taken during the first trimester has been associated with oral clefts (242). Diazepam may also amplify the teratogenic potential of valproic acid (243).

Diazepam enhances the elimination of phenobarbital (136), likely due to induction of cytochrome P450 (230). Valproic acid displaces diazepam bound to plasma proteins, leading to increased free diazepam and associated increased sedation (140).

Clinical Applications

Status Epilepticus. Diazepam is effective initial therapy in both convulsive and nonconvulsive SE (155). It may be particularly effective in generalized absence SE, with 93% of patients initially controlled (244). In the same early study, diazepam also controlled 89% of generalized convulsions, 88% of simple motor seizures, and 75% of complex partial SE. These numbers are higher than those observed in the VA Cooperative SE Trial (155), possibly due to differences in patient populations.

Diazepam is typically administered initially as a single IV bolus of 10 to 20 mg (136). A 20 mg bolus given at a rate of 2 mg/min stopped convulsions in 33% of patients within 3 minutes and in 80% within 5 minutes (245), but a single injection often does not produce lasting control, due to its short duration of action, and may be less effective when status results from acute CNS disease or structural brain lesions (130). Strategies to avoid this problem have included giving subsequent 5 to 10 mg IV doses every few hours, following diazepam with a longer lasting anticonvulsant (e.g., phenytoin (155)), or continuous IV diazepam. Repeated dosing results in a decrease in apparent volume of distribution and clearance, hence subsequent doses should be tapered to prevent toxicity (246). Diazepam (100 mg in 500 mL of 5% dextrose in water) infused at 40 mL/hr delivers 20 mg/hr (110) and may be suitable to obtain a serum level in the range of 200 to 800 ng/mL; 500 ng/mL appears to be effective for termination of status (136,247). Complete suppression of 3-Hz spike-and-wave required 600 to 2000 ng/mL (248). Continuous infusion has been used in patients hypersensitive to anticonvulsants (249). Diazepam is absorbed onto PVC bags, with a reduction in bioavailability of 50% after 8 hours (250), which should be taken into account if a chronic infusion of diazepam for SE is contemplated. As noted above, the efficacy of BZs decreases with duration of SE (160), hence higher levels or alternative treatments may be necessary if seizures are refractory.

Pediatric Status Epilepticus. The initial recommended IV diazepam dose in children is 0.1 to 0.3 mg/kg IV by slow bolus (<5 mg/min) repeating every 15 minutes for 2 doses, with a maximum of 5 mg in infants and 15 mg in older children (251,252). If IV administration is not possible, a diazepam solution (0.5 to 1 mg/kg), placed 3 to 6 cm into the rectum, has been effective (113). Continuous IV infusion of diazepam has also been used effectively in pediatric SE. Continuous diazepam infusion (0.01 to 0.03 mg/kg/min) controlled seizures in 86% of patients (49/57) within an average of 40 minutes (253). Hypotension occurred in one patient

(2%), respiratory depression in six patients (12%), and death in seven patients (14%). A meta-analysis of 111 pediatric patients (1 month to 18 years) with refractory generalized convulsive SE, treated with diazepam, midazolam, thiopental, pentobarbital, or isoflurane, suggested that diazepam was less effective as continuous therapy than the other agents (86% vs. 100%) after stratifying for etiology of SE (254). However, all of the patients receiving diazepam were from one region (India), and none received continuous EEG monitoring, suggesting that differences in location or details of care may have been contributory. Mortality was 20% in symptomatic cases and 4% in idiopathic cases, and was less frequent in midazolam-treated patients.

Although IV administration is preferable, rectal administration of diazepam rapidly produces effective drug levels (255) and safely aborts SE in pediatric patients (111,115). In children found to be in electrographic SE during EEG monitoring, rectal diazepam resulted in cessation of paroxysmal activity in 58% of cases (256). Rectal diazepam was particularly effective in patients with electrical SE during sleep, and less effective in patients with hypsarrhythmia. Intraosseous injection is a viable alternative in children of suitable age when IV access is not available (117).

Febrile Convulsions. Rectal diazepam is effective in aborting febrile and nonfebrile seizures in the home setting (112). While the concept of chronic prophylaxis for childhood febrile convulsions has long been in disrepute, it has not been clear whether there was benefit to short-term seizure prophylaxis during fever. A prospective trial randomized 289 children in Denmark to intermittent prophylaxis (diazepam at fever) or no prophylaxis (diazepam at seizure), and assessed neurologic outcome, motor, cognitive and scholastic achievement and likelihood of future seizures 12 years later (257). There were no differences in these measures, suggesting that short-term prophylaxis is probably not necessary. Moreover, the incidence of respiratory depression in children treated with IV and/or rectal diazepam is fairly high, with 9% showing decreased respiratory rate or oxygen saturation in one study (235).

Acute Repetitive Seizures. In a large-scale multicenter open-label trial of rectal diazepam gel (Diastat) in 149 patients older than 2 years, 77% of diazepam administrations resulted in seizure freedom for the ensuing 12 hours (171). There was no loss of effectiveness with more frequent (>8) doses, suggesting that tolerance did not reduce the effectiveness of diazepam under these conditions. Sedation occurred in 17% of patients. Diazepam rectal gel was also useful against serial seizures in adult patients with refractory epilepsy (116,170), with 0.5 mg/kg found to be an effective dose (114). Intramuscular diazepam injection may also be suitable for prophylaxis of serial seizures, but absorption is not rapid enough to be effective against SE. Intranasal diazepam administration is another alternative in this setting. In healthy human volunteers, peak serum concentrations of diazepam (2 mg) after intranasal administration occurred after 18 ± 11 minutes with bioavailability of about 50% (120). A pharmacodynamic effect was seen after 5 minutes.

Chronic Epilepsies. Periodic courses of diazepam have been proposed as therapy for several chronic conditions, including West syndrome, Lennox–Gastaut syndrome, Landau–Kleffner syndrome, and electrical SE during sleep (258). Oral diazepam (0.5 to 0.75 mg/kg/day) administered in cycles of 3-weeks duration were beneficial in interrupting electrical SE, and improved neuropsychological function in some cases.

Lorazepam

Lorazepam (see Fig. 55.1) has greater potency and a longer duration of action than diazepam, and has become the agent of choice for initial treatment of SE in adults (149). Lorazepam is also less likely to produce significant respiratory depression (156). It is available in both oral and parenteral preparations.

Pharmacokinetics

Lorazepam is rapidly absorbed but less bioavailable after oral administration due to first-pass biotransformation in the liver (259). Peak plasma levels occur 90 to 120 minutes after oral dosing (260). Lorazepam is about 90% protein bound, with CSF levels approximately equivalent to free serum levels (261). Sleep spindles in EEG recordings were observed within 30 seconds to 4 minutes after IV lorazepam (262), though peak brain concentrations and maximal EEG effect did not occur until 30 minutes (263). The volume of distribution is about 1.8 L/kg (263). After a single IV injection, plasma levels decrease initially due to tissue distribution with a half-life ($t_{1/2\alpha}$) of 2 to 3 hours. The minimal effective plasma concentration for control of SE was 30 ng/mL (264); after IV injection of 5 mg, plasma levels remain above that level for about 18 hours (265). Sedation, amnesia, and anxiolysis occur at plasma levels between 10 and 30 ng/mL (260).

Lorazepam is metabolized in the liver via glucuronidation at the 3-hydroxy group (266) and then excreted by the kidneys (267) (see Fig. 55.3). The half-life for elimination ($t_{1/2\beta}$) is in the 8 to 25 hours range (mean 15 hours), and is the same for oral administration (268).

Adverse Effects and Drug Interactions

Sedation, dizziness, vertigo, weakness, and unsteadiness are relatively common, with disorientation, depression, headache, sleep disturbances, agitation or restlessness, emotional disturbances, hallucinations, and delirium less common (262,269). Psychomotor impairment, dysarthria, and anterograde amnesia have also been observed. Mild respiratory depression sometimes occurs, particularly with the first IV dose (270). Rare adverse events include neutropenia. A paradoxical effect was observed in a patient with Lennox–Gastaut syndrome in which lorazepam precipitated tonic seizures (271). Abuse liability is relatively low. Although lorazepam is in U.S. FDA pregnancy category D, of unknown teratogenic potential, short-term use in treatment of SE may be of life-saving benefit and likely to outweigh the uncertain risks. Sudden discontinuation after chronic use has caused withdrawal seizures (272).

Valproic acid increased plasma concentrations of lorazepam (273), and decreased lorazepam clearance by 40% (274), apparently by inhibiting hepatic glucuronidation, though lorazepam does not affect valproic acid levels (273).

Probenecid increased the half-life of lorazepam by inhibiting glucuronidation, resulting in toxicity in patients on long-term therapy (147).

Clinical Applications

Status Epilepticus. The recommended IV dose of lorazepam for SE is 0.1 mg/kg (up to a maximum of 4 mg) administered at 2 mg/min, with repeat doses after 10 to 15 minutes if necessary (155). Although lorazepam is less lipophilic than diazepam, it crosses the BBB readily. Onset of action occurred within 3 minutes, with control of SE in 89% of episodes within 10 minutes (153). In another early study, all 10 patients with generalized convulsive SE had seizures controlled with IV lorazepam (mean 4 mg), but 9 of 11 patients with complex partial SE experienced problems, including respiratory depression (275). Other studies have shown response rates of 80% (131) and 92% (270). Similar success rates were achieved with simple partial SE (180,270). As noted above, the VA Cooperative Status Epilepticus Trial demonstrated superiority of lorazepam (0.1 mg/kg) over phenytoin (18 mg/kg) in response rate to initial therapy (64.9% vs. 43.6%), with slightly better results for lorazepam than diazepam (0.15 mg/kg) (155). Intravenous lorazepam (4 mg) was effective against post-anoxic myoclonic SE after cardiac arrest in six patients (276). However, continuous EEG monitoring during lorazepam treatment is advisable, as electroclinical dissociation has been observed (electrographic seizures despite cessation of convulsive activity).

Pediatric Status Epilepticus. The usual IV lorazepam dose in pediatric SE is 0.05 mg/kg, repeated twice at intervals of 15 to 20 minutes (156,180). This regimen terminated seizure activity in 81% of 31 children aged 2 to 18 (270). In a prospective randomized trial of 178 children, lorazepam (0.1 mg/kg) had the same efficacy (100%) as diazepam (0.2 mg/kg) plus phenytoin (18 mg/kg), with similar rates of respiratory depression (about 5%) (277). A retrospective study found that lorazepam (0.1 mg/kg in children and 0.07 mg/kg in adolescents) was most effective in partial SE terminating seizures in 90% of cases (180). Prior treatment of SE with phenytoin, phenobarbital, or diazepam did not alter the effectiveness of lorazepam, though chronic BZ treatment with clonazepam or clorazepate significantly reduced the effectiveness of lorazepam in SE (180), indicating tolerance. Respiratory depression, when observed, occurred after the first injection.

Lorazepam was effective in neonatal seizures refractory to phenobarbital and/or phenytoin in several small studies. In seven neonates (gestational ages 30 to 43 weeks) treated with IV lorazepam (0.05 mg/kg), seizures were controlled within 5 minutes in all seven patients, with no recurrence in five, and at least 8 hours of control in the remaining two patients (278). No respiratory depression or other adverse effects were reported. In another small series, SE in six of seven neonates was terminated with lorazepam (0.05 to 0.14 mg/kg) (279).

Pediatric Serial Seizures. Sublingual lorazepam (1 to 4 mg) was effective against serial seizures in 80% (8 of 10) and partially effective in 20% (2 of 10) of children, with onset of clinical effects within 15 minutes in most cases (280).

Alcohol Withdrawal Seizures. Lorazepam (2 mg) administered after a witnessed ethanol withdrawal seizure prevented a second seizure better than placebo (3% vs. 24%), and may be the agent of choice in this setting (281).

Chronic Epilepsy. Lorazepam was effective as adjunctive treatment of complex partial seizures, with an optimal dose of 5 mg/day after slow upward titration from 1 mg twice daily (213). Therapeutic levels were in the range of 20 to 30 ng/mL. However, long-term treatment with lorazepam is likely to result in tolerance, and is not generally recommended.

Midazolam

Midazolam (see Fig. 55.1) is widely used for induction of anesthesia or as a preanesthetic agent. It is three to four times as potent as diazepam. Midazolam has gained popularity in acute treatment of SE by either IV or IM use, though its short duration of action necessitates continuous IV maintenance or subsequent therapy with an additional anticonvulsant. Midazolam (10 mg) IM injection reduced interictal spike frequency in EEG recordings as well as IV diazepam (20 mg) (282), and this route provides a valuable alternative when IV access is unavailable.

Pharmacokinetics

Midazolam is water soluble, but at physiologic pH a conformational change in the BZ ring makes it lipid soluble (283). Serum midazolam levels after IV administration were best fit by a two-compartment model, with an initial tissue distribution phase ($t_{1/2\alpha}$ of 5.7 ± 2.4 minutes) and an elimination phase ($t_{1/2\beta}$ of 66 ± 37 minutes) (227). After IV administration in eight healthy adult volunteers, plasma concentration for a half-maximal increase in β-frequency activity on EEG recording was 276 ± 64 µmol/L (284). With an IM injection, peak serum concentration occurred after 25 ± 23 minutes (285). After oral administration, $44 \pm 17\%$ of the dose was bioavailable (227), while intranasal midazolam bioavailability ranged from 50% (286) to 83% (287). Bioavailability after rectal administration was 52% (288) and 74.5% after buccal administration (118). Midazolam is $95 \pm 2\%$ protein bound, with a volume of distribution of 1.1 ± 0.6 L/kg and a half-life in the range of 1.9 (227,289) to 2.8 hours (285). The clearance rate was 6.6 ± 1.8 mL/min/kg, with $56 \pm 26\%$ urinary excretion. The pharmacokinetics of midazolam were altered in children and critically ill patients. In children aged 1 to 5 years, administration of midazolam (0.2 mg/kg) by intranasal or IV route resulted in a similar elimination half-life, 2.2 hours for intranasal and 2.4 hours for IV administration (290). In critically ill neonates, the elimination half-life after IV administration was 12.0 hours (291). In adult ICU patients, the volume of distribution (3.1 L/kg) and elimination half-life (5.4 hours) were significantly greater than in healthy volunteers (0.9 L/kg and 2.3 hours, respectively) (292) though clearance was not significantly different (6.3 vs. 4.9 mL/min/kg for patients and volunteers, respectively).

Midazolam is metabolized rapidly by α-hydroxylation of the methyl group on the fused imidazo ring (Figs. 55.1 and 55.3) (285). This metabolite is biologically active, but is eliminated with a half-life of about 1 hour after hepatic conjugation with glucuronic acid (293).

Adverse Effects and Drug Interactions

Dose-dependent sedation with midazolam may be prolonged after continuous infusion despite its short half-life (294). Retrograde amnesia, euphoria, confusion, and dysarthria also occur. Midazolam syrup has been associated with respiratory depression and arrest, and should only be given where resuscitative drugs, equipment, and experienced personnel are immediately available. Paradoxical reactions (agitation, tremor, involuntary movements, hyperactivity, and combativeness) occur in about 2%, seizures and nystagmus in about 1%. Nausea and vomiting occur with midazolam syrup in 8% and 4%, respectively, but are far less common with IV administration. Hypotension and decreased cardiac output likely result from peripheral vasodilatation (283). Sudden discontinuation after long-term use can result in withdrawal seizures (295). Midazolam is in U.S. FDA pregnancy risk category D.

Erythromycin prolongs the half-life of midazolam to 10 to 20 hours (296). Phenytoin and carbamazepine reduce the bioavailability of oral midazolam by inducing cytochrome P450, which enhances first-pass hepatic metabolism (297).

Clinical Applications

Status Epilepticus. For refractory SE, IV midazolam 0.2 mg/kg by slow bolus injection followed by 0.75 to 10 µg/kg/min maintenance infusion has been recommended (149,298). Midazolam suppresses respiratory drive, so patients must be entubated and mechanically ventilated. Typically, infusion is maintained for 24 hours and then slowly tapered during continuous EEG monitoring; if seizure activity returns, midazolam infusion is resumed for additional 12 hour periods. Tolerance may develop, and doses up to 2 mg/kg/hr have been required for seizure control (298). Advantages of midazolam over other BZs include rapid onset of action, ease of administration and titration (with the possibility of initial IM injection) (299), good efficacy, and lack of serious adverse effects (298). Continuous IV infusion of midazolam was effective for treatment of refractory SE, terminating seizures within 100 seconds in seven patients who had failed treatment with diazepam, lorazepam, and phenytoin with or without phenobarbital (300). Intramuscular midazolam has been used successfully for SE in several small series, with an effective dose of 0.2 mg/kg (299,301).

Pediatric Status Epilepticus Midazolam is also safe and effective in pediatric SE. In a retrospective study of unprovoked refractory convulsive SE in epileptic children 1 to 15 years old, repeated bolus midazolam (0.1 mg/kg every 5 minutes), controlled 89% of the episodes after three doses, with infrequent adverse events (respiratory depression 13%) (302). In another study, midazolam (0.15 mg/kg bolus followed by 1 to 5 µg/kg/min infusion), either alone or with concomitant phenytoin or phenobarbital, controlled SE in 19 of 20 children (mean age 4 years) (303). In a series of eight pediatric patients (age 17 days to 16 years) with refractory SE treated with prolonged (>48 hours) midazolam coma, the average dose for seizure cessation was 14 µg/kg/min and mean duration of therapy was 192 hours; one patient could not be successfully weaned and died after 4 weeks (304). In a similar series of 20 children (mean age 4 years), midazolam was well tolerated and stopped seizures in 95% of patients (305). Intravenous

midazolam was safe and effective as first-line therapy in 15 of 16 episodes of SE in 10 children (20 months to 16 years), using a loading dose of 0.1 to 0.3 mg/kg followed by average infusion of 2.7 µg/kg/min for 12 hours to 6 days (306). It was also effective as a second-, third-, or fourth-line drug, with seizure control in 34 of 38 SE episodes. In neonates (1 to 9 days, 30 to 41 weeks gestational age) midazolam (0.1 to 0.4 mg/kg/hr) controlled overt seizures refractory to high-dose phenobarbital in six patients within 1 hour (307); electrographic seizures continued in two of the six for another 12 hours. Midazolam was tolerated well by neonates, with no change in pulse or blood pressure and no adverse reactions.

Febrile Seizures. In a prospective, randomized study of 47 children, intranasal midazolam was as effective as IV diazepam for controlling prolonged febrile convulsions, with shorter mean time to starting treatment and shorter time for controlling seizures (3.5 vs. 5.5 minutes) (122).

Pediatric Acute Repetitive Seizures. A study comparing IM midazolam to IV diazepam in children with seizures lasting longer than 10 minutes found similar efficacy between these agents, though patients in the midazolam group received medication sooner and seizures ended sooner (308). Intranasal midazolam was rapidly effective (175,309), and parents preferred it over rectal diazepam due to faster action and the ability to give it in public (175). In a prospective randomized trial comparing rectal diazepam (0.3 mg/kg) to intranasal midazolam (0.2 mg/kg), mean time from drug administration to cessation of seizure was less in the midazolam group, and mean respiratory rate and oxygen saturation were lower in the diazepam group (176). A randomized trial in children (aged 5 to 19 years) with the Lennox–Gastaut syndrome or other symptomatic generalized epilepsies showed that midazolam (10 mg in 2 mL) administered to the buccal mucosa stopped 75% of seizures, compared to 59% of seizures stopped by rectal diazepam (10 mg) (119). The time to end of seizure was not different between groups, and no cardiorespiratory adverse events occurred. Intrabuccal and intranasal midazolam are thus viable routes of administration in this patient population.

Clonazepam

Clonazepam (see Fig. 55.1) is unique among the BZs in that it is used primarily as an anticonvulsant and may be administered for treatment of both acute seizures and chronic epilepsy. It is effective in several types of SE (310), but in the United States, clonazepam is available only as an oral preparation.

Pharmacokinetics

The initial distribution half-life after IV injection has not been studied. Clonazepam is 81% to 98% absorbed after oral administration, with peak plasma levels occurring in 1 to 4 hours (6). It is highly lipid soluble with somewhat lower plasma protein binding (86%) than diazepam (124). The volume of distribution is 1.5 to 4.4 L/kg (6), greater than that of diazepam or lorazepam. Clonazepam is primarily metabolized to an inactive product, 7-amino-clonazepam, which is conjugated to glucuronide and excreted by the kidneys (6). Plasma half-lives were similar in single and multiple-dose studies, with ranges of 18.7 to 39 hours and 31 to 42 hours, respectively, suggesting relatively little hepatic enzyme induction (6).

Adverse Effects and Drug Interactions

Drowsiness and lethargy occur in about 50% of adult patients initially, but tolerance to these symptoms develops with continued administration (311). Drowsiness was seen in up to 85% of children treated with clonazepam and, along with other side effects, necessitated termination of the drug in 27% of patients (6). Respiratory and cardiovascular depression can occur with IV use. Nystagmus is fairly common; incoordination, ataxia, hypotonia, dysarthria, and dizziness are less frequent. Behavior disturbances including aggression, hyperactivity, and paranoia can be seen in up to 12% of children (312). Seizure frequency is sometimes increased by clonazepam, and seizures (313) or SE (314) can occur upon abrupt withdrawal. Increased salivary and bronchial secretions, anorexia, or hyperphagia can also occur. A "burning mouth syndrome" with painful oral dysesthesias has been described (315).

Clinical Applications

Status Epilepticus. Intravenous injection of 0.01 to 0.09 mg/kg terminates SE in most cases (6). A single 1-mg dose controlled various types of SE in 80% of adult patients (316). Both IV and oral clonazepam were effective treatments for SE in children (310,317). The minimum effective plasma level of clonazepam for control of convulsive SE was 30 ng/mL (130). In children and adults with absence SE, clonazepam (1 to 4 mg) was effective in 83.3% (318). Dissolving clonazepam into a droplet of propylene glycol followed by buccal administration achieved therapeutic levels in 10 to 15 minutes, and might be a strategy for treating serial seizures (319). An open-label study comparing clonazepam and lorazepam for SE in 50 adults with various epilepsies found similar effectiveness (68% and 69%) (320). However, neither diazepam nor clonazepam were found to be effective for SE in another study of 55 patients with symptomatic generalized epilepsy, primarily Lennox–Gastaut syndrome (316).

Pediatric Status Epilepticus. An IV 0.25-mg bolus of clonazepam, repeated as needed up to 0.75 mg, terminated SE in all 17 children (2 weeks to 15 years old) (310). Doses ranged from 0.01 to 0.09 mg/kg; the mean clonazepam levels were 185 ng/mL at 10 minutes after seizure termination, and 43 ng/mL at 30 minutes.

Chronic Epilepsy. The dose for chronic therapy in children is 0.01 to 0.02 mg/kg/day; in adults, it may range up to 8 mg/day in two to three divided doses. Good control of absence seizures was obtained at plasma levels of 13 to 72 ng/mL (317). However, correlation between plasma clonazepam levels and efficacy is relatively poor (6,321) due to the development of tolerance to antiseizure effects (322). Children require relatively higher doses than adults due to a higher clearance rate. Because of rapid absorption and elimination, children should receive the total daily amount divided into three equal doses (6). Clonazepam can be safely discontinued with dosage reduction of 0.04 mg/kg per week (323).

Severe Childhood Epilepsies. Although clonazepam is effective against a wide variety of seizure types, side effects limit its use to the most difficult epileptic conditions. Clonazepam pro-

duced lasting improvement in 5 of 24 patients with infantile spasms and in 3 of 13 patients with Lennox–Gastaut syndrome at doses of 0.1 to 0.3 mg/kg/day (324). Similarly, complete seizure control was achieved in about one-third of 42 cases of infantile spasms and 37 cases of Lennox–Gastaut syndrome (325).

Myoclonic Seizures. Clonazepam is effective in various myoclonic seizure disorders including myoclonic atonic seizures (326), myoclonic seizures (327), Unverricht–Lundborg myoclonic epilepsy (328), and intention myoclonus (329). Other conditions reported to respond to clonazepam include hyperekplexia (330), acute intermittent porphyria (331), epilepsy with continuous spike-and-wave during slow-wave sleep (332), and neonatal seizures (333).

Clorazepate

Clorazepate (see Fig. 55.1) is used in adjunctive treatment of seizure disorders, anxiety, and alcohol withdrawal. Its role in epilepsy is limited to adjunctive therapy of refractory generalized or partial seizure disorders, particularly in the setting of comorbid anxiety disorders.

Pharmacokinetics

Clorazepate is a prodrug for nordiazepam (N-desmethyldiazepam, DMD), the major active metabolite of diazepam (see Fig. 55.3). Nonenzymatic decarboxylation at position 3 occurs at gastric pH, with 90% of clorazepate converted to DMD in less than 10 minutes. Decarboxylation of absorbed clorazepate continues more slowly in the blood. DMD is responsible for most of clorazepate's anticonvulsant effect. Clorazepate is 100% bioavailable by the IM route (334) and 91% (as DMD) by oral ingestion (335). Clorazepate and DMD are 97% to 98% protein bound. The time to peak DMD concentration is 0.7 to 1.5 hours, with peak response in 1 to 2.5 hours (336). Volume of distribution ranged from 0.9 to 1.5 L/kg, and was greater in the elderly and in obese subjects (337). The elimination half-life of clorazepate is 2.3 hours, but the half-life of DMD is about 46 hours (338), longer in elderly males and neonates (339). DMD is then hydroxylated to oxazepam (see Fig. 55.3), which is then conjugated to glucuronic acid in the liver (229) and excreted by the kidneys with an elimination half-life of 1 to 2 days (136). As with diazepam, drugs and conditions that alter hepatic metabolism can dramatically affect the metabolism and clearance of clorazepate, DMD, and oxazepam.

Adverse Effects and Drug Interactions

Clorazepate is reportedly less sedating than other BZ anticonvulsants, although sedation is still its most common side effect (340). Dizziness, ataxia, nervousness, and confusion are less commonly seen. Memory problems, difficulty in concentration, irritability, and depression also occur, particularly in association with primidone (341). Paradoxical akathisia has been reported in two patients with history of head trauma and seizure disorders (342). Personality changes with aggressive behavior, irritability, rage, or depression have been described (343), though some have attributed these changes to the underlying temporal lobe epilepsy (344). Hepatotoxicity (345) and transient skin rashes have also been reported. Withdrawal symptoms after chronic use include nervousness, insomnia, irritability, diarrhea, muscle aches, and memory impairment. Clorazepate is in U.S. FDA pregnancy category D; major malformations were reported in one infant born to a mother who took clorazepate during the first trimester (346).

Clinical Applications

The recommended initial dose for adjunctive treatment is 7.5 mg three times daily (0.3 mg/kg/day), with slow increases as required, to a maximal daily dose of 90 mg (about 1 mg/kg/day) in adults and up to 3 mg/kg/day in children (340). Rapid absorption and conversion to DMD requires divided dosing to avoid toxicity, despite the long elimination half-life (141). A sustained release preparation delivers 22.5 mg in a single daily dose (Tranxene-SD). Plasma DMD levels of 0.5 to 1.9 mg/mL may represent the therapeutic range (227).

Clorazepate has been used primarily as add-on therapy. Clorazepate was ineffective as monotherapy, but improved seizure control as adjunctive therapy in 59 patients with various seizure disorders (347). Other studies have found limited effectiveness (348), or drowsiness at effective doses (349). Clorazepate was no more effective than phenobarbital as an adjunct to phenytoin treatment, but patients preferred clorazepate (350). Clorazepate controlled refractory generalized seizures in 11 children (age 3 to 17 years), though seizures recurred in 3, likely due to tolerance (351). However, a recent review suggested that clorazepate's long half-life, slow release formulation, and slow induction of tolerance may make it more useful than some other BZ's for chronic treatment of epilepsy (352).

Clobazam

Clobazam (8-chloro-5-methyl-1-phenyl-1,5-benzodiazepine-2,4-dione) has become the most widely used BZ for the long-term treatment of epilepsy because of effectiveness and relatively low tendency to produce sedation (353), despite a trend for the development of tolerance. In post-temporal lobectomy patients, clobazam is the third most common anticonvulsant employed after carbamazepine and phenytoin (354). Clobazam has primarily been used as add-on therapy, but the Canadian Study Group for Childhood Epilepsy (355) has found it effective as monotherapy in children. It is not available in the United States.

Pharmacokinetics

Clobazam is the only 1,5-BZ in clinical use as an anticonvulsant. Clobazam has a relatively low binding affinity and a correspondingly low potency (see Table 55.1). It is well absorbed, with peak concentrations in 1 to 4 hours, is highly lipid soluble, and is 85% protein bound. N-desmethylclobazam, the major metabolite, is the primary anticonvulsant component in patients undergoing long-term therapy. The mean elimination half-life is 18 hours for clobazam and 42 hours for N-desmethylclobazam. Clobazam induces hepatic enzymes, leading to more rapid conversion to N-desmethylclobazam with long-term treatment (356). Plasma levels of clobazam and N-desmethylclobazam correlated with both therapeutic effect and toxicity, but therapeutic levels have not been established, likely due to presence of the active metabolite or the development of tolerance (357).

Adverse Effects and Drug Interactions

Clobazam may have fewer or milder side effects than other BZs at equipotent doses (7,358,359). Levels of the metabolite, N-desmethylclobazam correlated with side effects (360). In epileptic patients, the predominant side effects of clobazam are drowsiness and fatigue (356). Of 23 open-label studies of clobazam, ataxia was described in 4, dizziness in 19, and vertigo in 2 (356). Memory disturbance, aggressiveness, dysphoria, and illusional and psychotic symptoms occur relatively infrequently. Clobazam has been associated with blurred vision. Negative myoclonus has been observed when clobazam was added to carbamazepine (361). Tolerance occurs with clobazam as with the 1,4-BZs (362). Increased seizure activity can occur with discontinuation of the drug (363).

Clinical Applications

Clobazam doses range from 10 to 50 mg/day, with most studies using 10 to 30 mg/day in one or two doses. In the Canadian Clobazam Cooperative trial of 877 patients, the average dose in adults was 30.8 mg, while the average dose for children was 0.86 mg/kg (364).

Clobazam is effective against all seizure types (365), but the benefits may be short-lived. In the Canadian Clobazam Cooperative Study, more than 40% of patients with a single seizure type had a 50% or greater reduction in seizure frequency, and 60% of patients with multiple seizure types had improvement in at least one type of seizure (364). About a third developed drowsiness as a side effect, but this was severe enough to cause discontinuation in only 11%. About 9% discontinued due to recurrence of seizures, which was thought to represent tolerance. In a randomized, double-blind study of clobazam as adjunctive therapy for drop seizures in Lennox–Gastaut syndrome, clobazam provided a significant, dose-related reduction in drop seizure rates, with non-drop seizures also reduced; adverse effects were rare and mild (366). Clobazam may be particularly effective in the Lennox–Gastaut syndrome (353), but tolerance prevents it from being the drug of first choice for most epilepsies (356). In a large prospective U.S. study of 251 refractory patients prescribed adjunctive clobazam (5 to 60 mg/day, mean 23.9 mg/day), 7 patients (11.3%) became seizure-free for at least 6 months after introduction of clobazam, and the 1-year retention rate was 61% (367). Clobazam was effective when used intermittently in catamenial epilepsy, as tolerance to the anticonvulsant effect was apparently avoided (177). Clobazam has also been shown safe and effective in the treatment of epileptic encephalopathies of childhood (368) though its ability to suppress EEG spike-and-wave activity has caused confusion in the diagnosis of electrical SE during sleep (369).

Despite reports of rapid development of tolerance, the Canadian Clobazam Cooperative Study (364) reported that 40% to 50% of patients remained on clobazam for 4 years or longer. Patients who had a seizure reduction exceeding 75% when clobazam was added were likely to sustain this response if their epilepsy was not longstanding and had a known cause (370).

Nitrazepam

Nitrazepam (see Fig. 55.1) has been used as a hypnotic and anticonvulsant, with benefit against infantile spasms and as adjunctive therapy for severe generalized epilepsies of childhood. Nitrazepam may be particularly effective against myoclonic seizures.

Pharmacokinetics

Oral bioavailability is about 78% (371), with peak concentration occurring in 1.4 hours (372). Nitrazepam is 85% to 88% protein bound (373) and has a volume of distribution of 2.4 L/kg in healthy young adults, higher in the elderly and in women (371). Nitrazepam is metabolized in the liver to an inactive product (see Fig. 55.3) (374). It does not induce its own metabolism. A portion is apparently bound in tissues for prolonged periods (375). Metabolism is slowed in patients with hypothyroidism (376) and obesity (377).

Adverse Effects and Drug Interactions

Like other BZs, nitrazepam can produce disorientation, confusion, and drowsiness, particularly in elderly patients (373). Vivid nightmares have occurred at the onset of therapy (378). Drooling and aspiration have occurred in children (379,380), apparently caused by impaired swallowing (380) though this did not occur at doses less than 0.8 mg/kg/day (380). Respiratory depression has occurred in elderly patients (381). Increased seizure frequency and new seizure types are sometimes seen (382). Tolerance can develop with chronic use, and withdrawal symptoms have occurred (221,383,384).

Nitrazepam is in U.S. FDA pregnancy category C. Infants born to mothers on nitrazepam late in pregnancy have been somnolent, floppy, poorly responsive, and required tube feeding, but recovered in several days (385). Like other BZs, nitrazepam is associated with increased teratogenic risk, particularly oral clefts (242).

Nitrazepam therapy increased the risk of death in young patients with intractable epilepsy. In a retrospective analysis of 302 patients treated with nitrazepam, 21 patients died, 14 of whom were taking nitrazepam at time of death (386). In patients younger than 3.4 years, the death rate was 3.98 per 100 pt × years, compared with 0.26 deaths per 100 pt × years in patients not taking nitrazepam. Nitrazepam had a slight protective effect in patients older than 3.4 years. It should therefore be used with extreme caution if at all in children younger than 4 years.

Clinical Applications

Nitrazepam is not available for clinical use in the United States. The usual daily dose is 1 mg/kg for children and 0.5 mg/kg for adults. Initial doses of 1 to 6 mg daily, with gradual increases up to 60 mg daily, have been used in treatment of pediatric seizure disorders (387–389). In children, satisfactory seizure control was associated with a mean plasma concentration of 114 ng/mL (373); levels above 220 ng/mL were more likely to be toxic. Nitrazepam (0.25 to 0.5 mg/kg/day, in t.i.d. dosing during fever) was effective in prophylaxis of febrile convulsions (390).

Nitrazepam was particularly effective for infantile spasms, myoclonic seizures, and the Lennox–Gastaut syndrome (387,389,391). In 52 patients (1 to 24 months) with infantile spasms and hypsarrhythmia on EEG, nitrazepam (0.2 to 0.4 mg/kg/day in two divided doses) and adrenocorticotrophic hormone (ACTH, 40 U IM daily) were similar in efficacy and incidence of adverse effects (392). Both regimens resulted in 75% to 100% reduction in seizure frequency in 50% to 60% of patients. Twenty children (4 to 28 months) with infantile spasms or early Lennox–Gastaut syndrome were treated with nitrazepam (median dose 1.5 mg/kg/day); of these, five had complete cessation of seizures, seven had greater than 50% seizure reduction, and eight had no response (393). Twelve children experienced pooling of oral secretions and six developed sedation, but no serious side effects were reported.

Flumazenil: Potential Uses in Epilepsy

The BZ antagonist, flumazenil has been used primarily to reverse BZ-induced sedation (18,19), but may also have benefit in reversing hepatic coma (394,395) in patients who had no prior exposure to BZs. Ammonia and manganese activate mitochondrial BZ receptors leading to increased production of neuroactive steroids, some of which (e.g., allopregnanolone, THDOC) enhance inhibitory neurotransmission via allosteric modulation of the $GABA_A$ receptor (396,397). The reversal of hepatic coma has bolstered arguments for an endogenous BZ ligand or "endozapine," which could be displaced by flumazenil (398,399). An endogenous "diazepam-binding inhibitor" peptide has been characterized (400), though its role in inhibitory neurotransmission remains unclear.

Flumazenil may be of use in epilepsy by reversing tolerance, but may also have intrinsic antiepileptic effects. Brief exposure to flumazenil can reverse tolerance-related changes in $GABA_A$ receptor function (401,402) and subunit expression (403). Flumazenil has been used with modest success to treat BZ dependence (404). The concept of using intermittent low doses of flumazenil to reverse BZ anticonvulsant tolerance has been explored in humans (405). Three patients with daily seizures who had become tolerant to clonazepam (1 mg b.i.d.) were treated with a single IV dose of flumazenil (1.5 mg, corresponding to 55% receptor occupancy), resulting in a mild withdrawal syndrome (shivering) lasting 30 minutes, followed by seizure freedom for 6 to 21 days (mean 13 days). Refinement of this approach may allow more extensive use of the BZs in the chronic treatment of epilepsy. Curiously, flumazenil itself has shown anticonvulsant efficacy in some animal models, possibly due to partial agonism at high doses (406–408) or antagonism of an endogenous proconvulsant (405). Flumazenil also reduced epileptiform discharges in hippocampal slices (409) and slowed the development of kindling (410). Flumazenil (0.75 to 15 mg) suppressed focal epileptiform activity in six patients with partial (temporal lobe) seizures, but had no effect on generalized spike-and-wave activity in six patients with generalized seizures (411). Several small studies have suggested possible benefit as an AED in humans (411,412). In 9 of 11 previously untreated patients with epilepsy, oral flumazenil (10 mg once to three times daily) caused a 50% to 75% reduction in seizure frequency, and 9 of 16 patients experienced 50% to 75% reduction in seizure frequency when flumazenil was added as an adjunctive anticonvulsant (413). Flumazenil's ability to prevent interictal epileptiform discharges on EEG was similar to that of diazepam (405,414).

Flumazenil can precipitate seizures, particularly in the setting of hepatic encephalopathy, in BZ-dependent patients, or in patients who have ingested multiple agents in overdose (e.g., tricyclic antidepressants) (415). The ability of flumazenil to induce seizures in patients previously treated with BZs has been used to precipitate partial seizures during inpatient epilepsy monitoring to localize seizure onset (416). In addition, [^{11}C]flumazenil has been used diagnostically in positron emission tomography (PET) studies to demonstrate regions of neuronal loss associated with epilepsy (417–419), and may be useful in localizing the seizure focus in patients with dual pathology (420).

FUTURE DIRECTIONS: NEW STRATEGIES FOR THE BZS

Partial BZ agonists (abecarnil, bretazenil, imidazenil) may retain anticonvulsant efficacy but be less prone to the development of tolerance. The utility of these agents in human epilepsy has not been adequately explored. Combination therapy using a full agonist with a partial agonist or antagonist (flumazenil), or intermittent use during periods of higher seizure risk (e.g., catamenial epilepsy), might prevent the development of tolerance and provide new strategies for BZ use. Novel routes of administration via the nasal, buccal, or rectal mucosa provide less invasive means to use BZs acutely in the outpatient setting. Another novel approach involves using BZs in a device capable of detecting seizure discharges and injecting the drug at the onset of seizure activity, either locally onto the epileptic focus, into the cerebral ventricles, or systemically. A model for this type of device in rats showed a decrease in seizure frequency and duration when diazepam rather than vehicle was injected onto a bicuculline-created seizure focus (421). Such approaches may increase the future role of BZs in the treatment of SE, serial seizures, and epilepsy.

References

1. Sternbach LH. Chemistry of the 1,4-benzodiazepines and some aspects of the structure-activity relationship. In: Garattini S, Mussini R, Randall LO, eds. *The Benzodiazepines*. New York: Raven Press; 1973:1–26.
2. Sternbach LH, Reeder E. Quinazolines and 1,4-benzodiazepines, IV: transformations of 7-chloro-2-methylamino-5-phenyl-^{3}H-1,4-benzodiazepine-4-oxide. *J Org Chem*. 1961;26:4936–4941.
3. Sternbach LH, Fryer RI, Keller O, et al. Quinazolines and 1,4-benzodiazepines, X: nitro-substituted 5-phenyl-1,4-benzodiazepine derivatives. *J Med Chem*. 1963;6:261–265.
4. Gastaut H, Naquet R, Poire R, et al. Treatment of status epilepticus with diazepam (Valium). *EPA*. 1965;6:167–182.
5. Naquet R, Soulayrol R, Dolce G, et al. First attempt at treatment of experimental status epilepticus in animals and spontaneous status epilepticus in man with diazepam (Valium). *Electroencephalogr Clin Neurophysiol*. 1965;18:4–27.
6. Sato S. Benzodiazepines, clonazepam. In: Levy RH, Mattson RH, Meldrum BS, eds. *Antiepileptic Drugs*. 4th ed. New York: Raven Press; 1995:725–734.
7. Chapman AG, Horton RW, Meldrum BS. Anticonvulsant action of a 1,5-benzodiazepine, clobazam, in reflex epilepsy. *EPA*. 1978;19:293–299.
8. Robertson MM. Current status of the 1,4- and 1,5-benzodiazepines in the treatment of epilepsy: the place of clobazam. *EPA*. 1986;(27 suppl 1):S27–S41.
9. Braestrup C, Squires RF. Specific benzodiazepine receptors in rat brain characterized by high-affinity [^{3}H]diazepam binding. *Proc Natl Acad Sci U S A*. 1977;74:3805–3809.
10. Mohler H, Okada T. Benzodiazepine receptor: demonstration in the central nervous system. *Science*. 1977;198:849–851.
11. Macdonald R, Barker JL. Benzodiazepines specifically modulate GABA-mediated postsynaptic inhibition in cultured mammalian neurones. *Nature*. 1978;271:563–564.
12. Macdonald RL, Olsen RW. GABA$_A$ receptor channels. *Annu Rev Neurosci*. 1994;17:569–602.
13. Gastaut H, Low MD. Antiepileptic properties of clobazam, a 1,5 benzodiazepine, in man. *EPA*. 1979;20:437–446.
14. Braestrup C, Squires RF. Pharmacological characterization of benzodiazepine receptors in the brain. *Eur J Pharmacol*. 1978;48:263–270.
15. Mohler H, Okada T, Heitz P, et al. Biochemical identification of the site of action of benzodiazepines in human brain by ^{3}H-diazepam binding. *Life Sci*. 1978;22:985–995.
16. Sieghart W, Schuster A. Affinity of various ligands for benzodiazepine receptors in rat cerebellum and hippocampus. *Biochem Pharmacol*. 1984;33:4033–4038.
17. Tietz EI, Rosenberg HC, Chiu TH. A comparison of the anticonvulsant effects of 1,4- and 1,5-benzodiazepines in the amygdala-kindled rat and their effects on motor function. *Epilepsy Res*. 1989;3:31–40.
18. Gross JB, Blouin RT, Zandsberg S. Effect of flumazenil on ventilatory drive during sedation with midazolam and alfentanil. *Anesthesiology*. 1996;85:713–720.
19. Shannon M, Albers G, Burkhardt K. Safety and efficacy of flumazenil in the reversal of benzodiazepine-induced conscious sedation. *J Pediatr*. 1997;131:582–586.
20. Mullins ME. First-degree atrioventricular block in alprazolam overdose reversed by flumazenil. *J Pharm Pharmacol*. 1999;51:367–370.
21. Turski L, Stephens DN, Jensen LH, et al. Anticonvulsant action of the beta-carboline abecarnil: studies in rodents and baboon, *Papio papio*. *J Pharmacol Exp Ther*. 1990;253:344–352.
22. Zanotti A, Mariot R, Contarino A, et al. Lack of anticonvulsant tolerance and benzodiazepine receptor downregulation with imidazenil in rats. *Br J Pharmacol*. 1996;117:647–652.
23. Rundfeldt C, Wlaz P, Honack D, et al. Anticonvulsant tolerance and withdrawal characteristics of benzodiazepine receptor ligands in different seizure models in mice. Comparison of diazepam, bretazenil and abecarnil. *J Pharmacol Exp Ther*. 1995;275:693–702.
24. Natolino F, Zanotti A, Contarino A, et al. Abecarnil, a beta-carboline derivative, does not exhibit anticonvulsant tolerance or withdrawal effects in mice. *Naunyn Schmiedebergs Arch Pharmacol*. 1996;354: 612–617.
25. Hernandez TD, Heninger C, Wilson MA, et al. Relationship of agonist efficacy to changes in GABA sensitivity and anticonvulsant tolerance following chronic benzodiazepine ligand exposure. *Eur J Pharmacol*. 1989; 170:145–155.
26. Haefely W, Kyburz E, Gerecke M, et al. Recent advances in the molecular pharmacology of benzodiazepine receptors and in the structure-activity relationships of their agonists and antagonists. *Adv Drug Res*. 1985;14: 165–322.
27. Polc P. Electrophysiology of benzodiazepine receptor ligands: multiple mechanisms and sites of action. *Prog Neurobiol*. 1988;31:349–423.
28. Randall LO, Kappell B. Pharmacological activity of some benzodiazepines and their metabolites. In: Garattini S, Mussini E, Randall LO, eds. *The Benzodiazepines*. New York: Raven Press; 1973:27–51.
29. Rogawski MA, Porter RJ. Antiepileptic drugs: pharmacological mechanisms and clinical efficacy with consideration of promising developmental stage compounds. *Pharmacol Rev*. 1990;42(3):223–286.
30. Swinyard EA, Castellion AW. Anticonvulsant properties of some benzodiazepines. *J Pharmacol Exp Ther*. 1966;151:369–375.
31. Albertson TE, Stark LG, Derlet RW. Modification of amygdaloid kindling by diazepam in juvenile rats. *Brain Res Dev Brain Res*. 1990;51:249–252.
32. Karobath M, Sperk G. Stimulation of benzodiazepine receptor binding by γ-aminobutyric acid. *Proc Natl Acad Sci U S A*. 1979;76:1004–1006.
33. Study RE, Barker JL. Diazepam and (−)-pentobarbital: fluctuation analysis reveals different mechanisms for potentiation of γ-aminobutyric acid responses in cultured central neurons. *Proc Natl Acad Sci U S A*. 1981;78:7180–7184.
34. Rogers CJ, Twyman RE, Macdonald RL. Benzodiazepine and beta-carboline regulation of single GABA$_A$ receptor channels of mouse spinal neurones in culture. *J Physiol (Lond)*. 1994;475:69–82.
35. Twyman RE, Rogers CJ, Macdonald RL. Differential regulation of γ-aminobutyric acid receptor channels by diazepam and phenobarbital. *Ann Neurol*. 1989;25:213–220.
36. Edwards FA, Konnerth A, Sakmann B. Quantal analysis of inhibitory synaptic transmission in the dentate gyrus of rat hippocampal slices: a patch-clamp study. *J Physiol (Lond)*. 1990;430:213–249.
37. Puia G, Costa E, Vicini S. Functional diversity of GABA-activated Cl$^−$ currents in purkinje versus granule neurons in rat cerebellar slices. *Neuron*. 1994;12:117–126.
38. Otis TS, Mody I. Modulation of decay kinetics and frequency of GABA$_A$ receptor-mediated spontaneous inhibitory post-synaptic currents in hippocampal neurons. *Proc Natl Acad Sci U S A*. 1992;78:7180–7184.
39. Mody I, De Doninck Y, Otis TS, et al. Bridging the cleft at GABA synapses in the brain. *Trends Neurosci*. 1994;17:517–525.

40. Treiman DM. GABAergic mechanisms in epilepsy. *EPA*. 2001;42(3): 8–12.

41. Macdonald RL, Olsen RW. GABA_A receptor channels. *Annu Rev Neurosci*. 1994;17:569–602.

42. Nayeem N, Green TP, Martin IL, et al. Quaternary structure of the native GABA_A receptor determined by electron microscopic image analysis. *J Neurochem*. 1994;62:815–818.

43. Hedblom E, Kirkness EF. A novel class of GABA_A receptor subunit in tissues of the reproductive system. *J Biol Chem*. 1997;272:15346–15350.

44. Davies PA, Hanna MC, Hales TG et al. Insensitivity to anesthetic agents conferred by a class of GABA_A receptor subunit. *Nature*. 1997;385: 820–823.

45. Bonnert TP, McKernan RM, Le Bourdelles B, et al. Θ, a novel γ-aminobutyric acid type A subunit. *Proc Natl Acad Sci U S A*. 1999;96:9891–9896.

46. Wisden W, Laurie DJ, Monyer H, et al. The distribution of 13 GABA_A receptor subunit mRNAs in the rat brain. I. Telencephalon, diencephalon, mesencephalon. *J Neurosci*. 1992;12:1040–1062.

47. Brooks-Kayal AR, Pritchett DB. Developmental changes in human γ-aminobutyric acid_A receptor subunit composition. *Ann Neurol*. 1993;34: 687–693.

48. Brooks-Kayal AR, Jin H, Price M, et al. Developmental expression of GABA_A receptor subunit mRNAs in individual hippocampal neurons in vitro and in vivo. *J Neurochem*. 1998;70:1017–1028.

49. Pritchett DB, Sontheimer H, Shivers BD, et al. Importance of a novel GABA_A subunit for benzodiazepine pharmacology. *Nature*. 1989;338: 582–585.

50. Wieland HA, Luddens H, Seeburg PH. A single histidine in GABA_A receptors is essential for benzodiazepine agonist binding. *J Biol Chem*. 1992; 267:1426–1429.

51. Wingrove PB, Wafford KA, Bain C, et al. The modulatory action of loreclezole at the γ-aminobutyric acid type A receptor is determined by a single amino acid in the β_2 and β_3 subunit. *Proc Natl Acad Sci U S A*. 1994;91:4569–4573.

52. Draguhn A, Verdorn TA, Ewert M, et al. Functional and molecular distinction between recombinant rat GABA_A receptor subtypes by Zn^{2+}. *Neuron*. 1990;5:781–788.

53. Verdoorn TA, Draguhn A, Ymer S, et al. Functional properties of recombinant rat GABA_A receptors depend upon subunit composition. *Neuron*. 1990;4:919–928.

54. Lüddens H, Korpi ER, Seeburg P. GABA_A/benzodiazepine receptor heterogeneity: neurophysiological implications. *NPH*. 1995;34:245–254.

55. Doble A, Martin IL. Multiple benzodiazepine receptors—no reason for anxiety. *Trends Pharmacol Sci*. 1992;13:76–81.

56. Smith GB, Olsen RW. Functional domains of GABA_A receptors. *Trends Pharmacol Sci*. 1995;16:162–168.

57. Rudolph U, Crestani F, Benke D, et al. Benzodiazepine actions mediated by specific γ-aminobutyric acid_A receptor subtypes. *Nature*. 2000;401: 796–800.

58. McKernan RM, Rosahl TW, Reynolds DS, et al. Sedative but not anxiolytic properties of benzodiazepines are mediated by the GABA_A receptor α1 subunit. *Nat Neurosci*. 2000;3:529–530.

59. Low K, Crestani F, Keist R, et al. Molecular and neuronal substrate for the selective attenuation of anxiety. *Science*. 2000;290:131–134.

60. Crestani F, Low K, Keist R, et al. Molecular targets for the myorelaxant action of diazepam. *Mol Pharmacol*. 2001;59:442–445.

61. Crestani F, Keist R, Fritschy JM, et al. Trace fear conditioning involves hippocampal alpha5 GABA(A) receptors. *Proc Natl Acad Sci U S A*. 2002;99:8980–8985.

62. Knabl J, Zeilhofer UB, Crestani F, et al. Genuine antihyperalgesia by systemic diazepam revealed by experiments in GABA_A receptor point-mutated mice. *Pain*. 2009;141:233–238.

63. Smith SS, Gong QH, Li X, et al. Withdrawal from 3alpha-OH-5alpha-pregnan-20-One using a pseudopregnancy model alters the kinetics of hippocampal GABAA-gated current and increases the GABAA receptor alpha4 subunit in association with increased anxiety. *J Neurosci*. 1998;18:5275–5284.

64. Smith SS, Gong QH, Hsu FC, et al. GABA(A) receptor alpha4 subunit suppression prevents withdrawal properties of an endogenous steroid. *Nature*. 1998;392:926–930.

65. Karle J, Witt MR, Nielsen M. Diazepam protects against rat hippocampal neuronal cell death induced by antisense oligodeoxynucleotide to GABA(A) receptor gamma2 subunit. *Brain Res*. 1997;765:21–29.

66. Karle J, Witt MR, Nielsen M. The use of in vivo antisense oligonucleotide technology for the investigation of brain GABA receptors. *Neurochem Int*. 1997;31:437–446.

67. Zhao TJ, Li M, Chiu TH, et al. Decreased benzodiazepine binding with little effect on gamma-aminobutyric acid binding in rat brain after treatment with antisense oligodeoxynucleotide to the gamma-aminobutyric acid A receptor gamma-2 subunit. *J Pharmacol Exp Ther*. 1998;287: 752–759.

68. Gunther U, Benson J, Benke D, et al. Benzodiazepine-insensitive mice generated by targeted disruption of the gamma 2 subunit gene of gamma-aminobutyric acid type A receptors. *Proc Natl Acad Sci U S A*. 1995; 92:7749–7753.

69. Jones-Davis DM, Macdonald RL. GABA(A) receptor function and pharmacology in epilepsy and status epilepticus. *Curr Opin Pharmacol*. 2003;3:12–18.

70. Olsen RW, DeLorey TM, Gordey M, et al. GABA receptor function and epilepsy. *Adv Neurol*. 1999;79:499–510.

71. Wallace RH, Marini C, Petrou S, et al. Mutant GABA(A) receptor gamma2-subunit in childhood absence epilepsy and febrile seizures. *Nat Genet*. 2001;28:49–52.

72. Kokaia M, Pratt GD, Elmer E, et al. Biphasic differential changes of GABA_A receptor subunit mRNA levels in denate gyrus granule cells following recurrent kindling-induced seizures. *Mol Brain Res*. 1994;23:323–332.

73. Brooks-Kayal AR, Shumate MD, Jin H, et al. Selective changes in single cell GABA_A receptor subunit expression and function in temporal lobe epilepsy. *Nat Med*. 1998;4:1166–1172.

74. Loup F, Weiser HG, Yonekawa Y, et al. Selective alterations in GABA_A receptor subtypes in human temporal lobe epilepsy. *J Neurosci*. 2000;20:5401–5419.

75. Karle J, Woldbye DP, Elster L, et al. Antisense oligonucleotide to GABA(A) receptor gamma2 subunit induces limbic status epilepticus. *J Neurosci Res*. 1998;54:863–869.

76. Matsumoto A, Kumagai T, Miura K, et al. Epilepsy in Angelman syndrome associated with chromosome 15q deletion. *EPA*. 1992;33:1083–1090.

77. DeLorey TM, Handforth A, Anagnostaras SG, et al. Mice lacking the beta3 subunit of the GABAA receptor have the epilepsy phenotype and many of the behavioral characteristics of Angelman syndrome. *J Neurosci*. 1998;18:8505–8514.

78. Bianchi MT, Song L, Zhang H, et al. Two different mechanisms of disinhibition produced by GABA_A receptor mutations linked to epilepsy in humans. *J Neurosci*. 2002;22:5321–5327.

79. Baulac S, Huberfeld G, Gourfinkel-An I, et al. First genetic evidence of GABA_A receptor dysfunction in epilepsy: a mutation in the γ2-subunit gene. *Nat Genet*. 2001;28:46–48.

80. Cossette P, Liu L, Brisebois K, et al. Mutation of GABRA1 in an autosomal dominant form of juvenile myoclonic epilepsy. *Nat Genet*. 2002;31:184–189.

81. Bowser DN, Wagner DA, Czajkowski C, et al. Altered kinetics and benzodiazepine sensitivity of a GABAA receptor subunit mutation [gamma 2(R43Q)] found in human epilepsy. *Proc Natl Acad Sci U S A*. 2002;99:15170–15175.

82. Frugier G, Coussen F, Giraud MF, et al. A gamma 2(R43Q) mutation, linked to epilepsy in humans, alters GABAA receptor assembly and modifies subunit composition on the cell surface. *J Biol Chem*. 2007; 282:3819–3828.

83. Hales TG, Tang H, Bollan KA, et al. The epilepsy mutation, gamma2(R43Q) disrupts a highly conserved inter-subunit contact site, perturbing the biogenesis of GABAA receptors. *Mol Cell Neurosci*. 2005;29:120–127.

84. Sancar F, Czajkowski C. A GABAA receptor mutation linked to human epilepsy (gamma2R43Q) impairs cell surface expression of alpha-betagamma receptors. *J Biol Chem*. 2004;279:47034–47039.

85. Kang JQ, Macdonald RL. The GABAA receptor gamma2 subunit R43Q mutation linked to childhood absence epilepsy and febrile seizures causes retention of alpha1beta2gamma2S receptors in the endoplasmic reticulum. *J Neurosci*. 2004;24:8672–8677.

86. McLean MJ, Macdonald RL. Benzodiazepines, but not beta carbolines, limit high frequency repetitive firing of action potentials of spinal cord neurons in cell culture. *J Pharmacol Exp Ther*. 1988;244:789–795.

87. Reuveny E, Twombly DA, Narahashi T. Chlordiazepoxide block of two types of calcium channels in neuroblastoma cells. *J Pharmacol Exp Ther*. 1993;264:22–28.

88. Löscher W, Schmidt D. Diazepam increases gamma-aminobutyric acid in human cerebrospinal fluid. *J Neurochem*. 1987;49:152–157.

89. Ong J, Kerr DI. Recent advances in GABAB receptors: from pharmacology to molecular biology. *Acta Pharmacol Sin*. 2000;21:111–123.

90. Casellas P, Galiegue S, Basile AS. Peripheral benzodiazepine receptors and mitochondrial function. *Neurochem Int*. 2002;40:475–486.

91. Papadopoulo V. Peripheral benzodiazepine receptor: structure and function in health and disease. *Ann Pharm Fr*. 2003;61:30–50.

92. Galiegue S, Tinel N, Casellas P. The peripheral benzodiazepine receptor: a promising therapeutic drug target. *Curr Med Chem*. 2003;10: 1563–1572.

93. Staley KJ, Soldo BL, Proctor WR. Ionic mechanisms of neuronal excitation by inhibitory GABA_A receptors. *Science*. 1995;269:977–981.

94. Brumback AC, Staley KJ. Thermodynamic regulation of NKCC1-mediated Cl-cotransport underlies plasticity of GABA(A) signaling in neonatal neurons. *J Neurosci*. 2008;28:1301–1312.

95. Ben-Ari Y. Developing networks play a similar melody. *Trends Neurosci*. 2001;24:353–360.

96. Kriegstein AR, Owens DF. GABA may act as a self-limiting trophic factor at developing synapses. *Sci STKE*. 2001;2001:E1.

97. Kahle KT, Staley KJ. The bumetanide-sensitive Na-K-2Cl cotransporter NKCC1 as a potential target of a novel mechanism-based treatment strategy for neonatal seizures. *Neurosurg Focus*. 2008;25:E22.

98. Dzhala VI, Talos DM, Sdrulla DA, et al. NKCC1 transporter facilitates seizures in the developing brain. *Nat Med*. 2005;11:1205–1213.

99. Dzhala VI, Staley KJ. Excitatory actions of endogenously released GABA contribute to initiation of ictal epileptiform activity in the developing hippocampus. *J Neurosci.* 2003;23:1840–1846.

100. Thompson SM, Deisz RA, Prince DA. Relative contributions of passive equilibrium and active transport to the distribution of chloride in mammalian cortical neurons. *J Neurophysiol.* 1988;60:105–124.

101. Zhang SJ, Jackson MB. GABAA receptor activation and the excitability of nerve terminals in the rat posterior pituitary. *J Physiol.* 1995;483 (Pt 3):583–595.

102. Staley K. Enhancement of the excitatory actions of GABA by barbiturates and benzodiazepines. *Neurosci Lett.* 1992;146:105–107.

103. Bormann J, Hamill OP, Sakmann B. Mechanism of anion permeation through channels gated by glycine and gamma-aminobutyric acid in mouse cultured spinal neurones. *J Physiol (Lond).* 1987;385:243–286.

104. Zeng X, Tietz EI. Depression of early and late monosynaptic inhibitory postsynaptic potentials in hippocampal CA1 neurons following chronic benzodiazepine administration: role of a reduction in Cl-driving force. *Synapse.* 1997;25:125–136.

105. Zeng XJ, Tietz EI. Role of bicarbonate ion in mediating decreased synaptic conductance in benzodiazepine tolerant hippocampal CA1 pyramidal neurons. *Brain Res.* 2000;868:202–214.

106. Cohen I, Navarro V, Clemenceau S, et al. On the origin of interictal activity in human temporal lobe epilepsy in vitro. *Science.* 2002;298:1418–1421.

107. Shorvon SD. *Status Epilepticus. Its Clinical Features and Treatment in Children and Adults.* New York: Cambridge University Press; 1994.

108. Tassinari CA, Dravet C, Roger J, et al. Tonic status epilepticus precipitated by intravenous benzodiazepine in five patients with Lennox–Gastaut syndrome. *EPA.* 1972;13:421–435.

109. Bittencourt PRM, Richens A. Anticonvulsant-induced status epilepticus in Lennox–Gastaut syndrome. *EPA.* 1981;22:129–134.

110. Delgado-Escueta AV, Wasterlain C, Treiman DM, et al. Current concepts in neurology: management of status epilepticus. *N Engl J Med.* 1982;306:1337–1340.

111. Albano A, Reisdorff EJ, Wiegenstein JG. Rectal diazepam in pediatric status epilepticus. *Am J Emerg Med.* 1989;7:168–172.

112. Camfield CS, Camfield PR, Smith E, et al. Home use of rectal diazepam to prevent status epilepticus in children with convulsive disorders. *J Child Neurol.* 1989;4:125–126.

113. Kriel RL, Cloyd JC, Hadsall RS, et al. Home use of rectal diazepam for cluster and prolonged seizures: efficacy, adverse reactions, quality of life, and cost analysis. *Pediatr Neurol.* 1991;7:13–17.

114. Remy C, Jourdil N, Villemain D, et al. Intrarectal diazepam in epileptic adults. *EPA.* 1992;33:353–358.

115. Dieckmann RA. Rectal diazepam for prehospital pediatric status epilepticus. *Ann Emerg Med.* 1994;23:216–224.

116. Dreifuss FE, Rossman NP, Cloyd JC. A comparison of rectal diazepam gel and placebo for acute repetitive seizures. *N Engl J Med.* 1998;338:1869–1875.

117. McNamara RM, Spivey WH, Unger HD, et al. Emergency applications of intraosseous infusion. *J Emerg Med.* 1987;5:97–101.

118. Schwagmeier R, Alincic S, Striebel HW. Midazolam pharmacokinetics following intravenous and buccal administration. *Br J Clin Pharmacol.* 1998;46:203–206.

119. Scott RC, Besag FM, Neville BG. Buccal midazolam and rectal diazepam for treatment of prolonged seizures in childhood and adolescence: a randomized trial. *Lancet.* 1999;353:623–626.

120. Gizurarson S, Gudbrandsson FK, Jonsson H, et al. Intranasal administration of diazepam aiming at the treatment of acute seizures: clinical trials in healthy volunteers. *Biol Pharm Bull.* 1999;22:425–427.

121. Kendall JL, Reynolds M, Goldberg R. Intranasal midazolam in patients with status epilepticus. *Ann Emerg Med.* 1997;29:415–417.

122. Lahat E, Goldman M, Barr J, et al. Comparison of intranasal midazolam with intravenous diazepam for treating febrile seizures in children: prospective randomized study. *Br Med J.* 2000;321:83–86.

123. Borea PA, Bonora D. Brain receptor binding and the lipophilic character of benzodiazepines. *Biochem Pharmacol.* 1983;32:603–607.

124. Charney DS, Mihic SJ, Harris RA. Hypnotics and sedatives. In: Hardman JG, Limbird LE, eds. *Goodman and Gilman's The Pharmacological Basis of Therapeutics.* 10th ed. New York: McGraw Hill; 2001:399–427.

125. Greenblatt DJ, Divoll M, Abernathy DR. Clinical pharmacokinetics of the newer benzodiazepines. *Clin Pharmacokinet.* 1983;8:233–252.

126. Greenblatt DJ, Shader RI, Abernethy DR. Current status of benzodiazepines (first of two parts). *N Engl J Med.* 1983;309:354–358.

127. Ochs HR, Greenblatt DJ, Divoll M. Diazepam kinetics in relation to age and sex. *Pharmacology.* 1981;23:24–30.

128. Arendt RM, Greenblatt DJ, deJong RH, et al. In vitro correlates of benzodiazepine cerebrospinal fluid uptake, pharmacodynamic action and peripheral distribution. *J Pharmacol Exp Ther.* 1993;277:98–106.

129. Hoogerkamp A, Arends RH, Bomers AM, et al. Pharmacokinetic/pharmacodynamic relationship of benzodiazepines in the direct cortical stimulation model of anticonvulsant effect. *J Pharmacol Exp Ther.* 1996;279:803–812.

130. Treiman DM. Pharmacokinetics and clinical use of benzodiazepines in the management of status epilepticus. *EPA.* 1989;30(2):S4–S10.

131. Greenblatt DJ. Benzodiazepine hypnotics: sorting the pharmacokinetic facts. *J Clin Psychiatry.* 1991;52:4–10.

132. Greenblatt DJ. Pharmacology of benzodiazepine hypnotics. *J Clin Psychiatry.* 1992;53:7–13.

133. Laurijssens BE, Greenblatt DJ. Pharmacokinetic-pharmacodynamic relationships for benzodiazepines. *Clin Pharmacokinet.* 1996;30:52–76.

134. Rey E, Treluyer JM, Pons G. Pharmacokinetic optimization of benzodiazepine therapy for acute seizures. Focus on delivery routes. *Clin Pharmacokinet.* 1999;36:409–424.

135. Prensky AL, Raff MC, Moore MS, et al. Intravenous diazepam in the treatment of prolonged seizure activity. *N Engl J Med.* 1967;276:779–786.

136. Schmidt D. Benzodiazepines, diazepam. In: Levy RH, Dreifuss FE, Mattson RH, et al., eds. *Antiepileptic Drugs.* 3rd ed. New York: Raven Press; 1989:735–764.

137. Bekersky I, Maggio AC, Mattaliano V Jr., et al. Influence of phenobarbital on the disposition of clonazepam and antipyrine in the dog. *J Pharmacokinet Biopharm.* 1977;5:507–512.

138. Nanda RN, Johnson RH, Keogh HJ, et al. Treatment of epilepsy with clonazepam and its effect on other anticonvulsants. *J Neurol Neurosurg Psychiatry.* 1977;40:538–543.

139. Munoz JJ, De Salamanca RE, Diaz-Obregon C, et al. The effect of clobazam on steady state plasma concentrations of carbamazepine and its metabolites. *Br J Clin Pharmacol.* 1990;29:763–765.

140. Dhillon S, Richens A. Valproic acid and diazepam interaction in vivo. *Br J Clin Pharmacol.* 1982;13:553–560.

141. Wilensky AJ, Levy RH, Troupin AS, et al. Clorazepate kinetics in treated epileptics. *Clin Pharmacol Ther.* 1978;24:22–30.

142. Das P, Lilly SM, Zerda R, et al. Increased AMPA receptor GluR1 subunit incorporation in rat hippocampal CA1 synapses during benzodiazepine withdrawal. *J Comp Neurol.* 2008;511:832–846.

143. Klotz U, Reimann I. Elevation of steady-state diazepam levels by cimetidine. *Clin Pharmacol Ther.* 1981;30:513–517.

144. Klotz U, Reimann I. Delayed clearance of diazepam due to cimetidine. *N Engl J Med.* 1980;302:1012–1014.

145. Ochs HR, Greenblatt DJ, Gugler R, et al. Cimetidine impairs nitrazepam clearance. *Clin Pharmacol Ther.* 1983;34:227–230.

146. Brockmeyer NH, Mertins L, Klimek K, et al. Comparative effects of rifampin and/or probenecid on the pharmacokinetics of temazepam and nitrazepam. *Int J Clin Pharmacol Ther Toxicol.* 1990;28:387–393.

147. Abernethy DR, Greenblatt DJ, Ameer B, et al. Probenecid impairment of acetaminophen and lorazepam clearance: direct inhibition of ether glucuronide formation. *J Pharmacol Exp Ther.* 1985;234:345–349.

148. Towne AR, Pellock JM, Ko D, et al. Determinants of mortality in status epilepticus. *EPA.* 1994;35:27–34.

149. Lowenstein DH, Alldredge BK. Status epilepticus. *N Engl J Med.* 1998;338:970–976.

150. DeLorenzo RJ, Sun DA. Basic mechanisms in status epilepticus: role of calcium in neuronal injury and the induction of epileptogenesis. *Adv Neurol.* 2006;97:187–197.

151. Fujikawa DG. Prolonged seizures and cellular injury: understanding the connection. *Epilepsy Behav.* 2005;7(suppl 3):S3–S11.

152. Holmes GL. Seizure-induced neuronal injury: animal data. *Neurology.* 2002;59:S3–S6.

153. Leppik IE, Derivan AT, Homan RW, et al. Double-blind study of lorazepam and diazepam in status epilepticus. *JAMA.* 1983;249:1452–1454.

154. Treiman DM. The role of benzodiazepines in the management of status epilepticus. *Neurology.* 1990;40:32–42.

155. Treiman DM, Meyers PD, Walton NY, et al. A comparison of four treatments for generalized convulsive status epilepticus. Veterans Affairs Status Epilepticus Cooperative Study Group. *N Engl J Med.* 1998;339:792–798.

156. Appleton R, Sweeney A, Choonara I, et al. Lorazepam versus diazepam in the acute treatment of epileptic seizures and status epilepticus. *Dev Med Child Neurol.* 1995;37:682–688.

157. Prasad K, Krishnan PR, Al-Roomi K, et al. Anticonvulsant therapy for status epilepticus. *Br J Clin Pharmacol.* 2007;63:640–647.

158. Chin RF, Neville BG, Peckham C, et al. Treatment of community-onset, childhood convulsive status epilepticus: a prospective, population-based study. *Lancet Neurol.* 2008;7:696–703.

159. Alldredge BK, Gelb AM, Isaacs SM, et al. A comparison of lorazepam, diazepam, and placebo for the treatment of out-of-hospital status epilepticus. *N Engl J Med.* 2001;345:631–637.

160. Walton NY, Treiman DM. Response of status epilepticus induced by lithium and pilocarpine to treatment with diazepam. *Exp Neurol.* 1988;101:267–275.

161. Kapur J, Macdonald RL. Rapid seizure-induced reduction of benzodiazepine and Zn^{2+} sensitivity of hippocampal dentate granule cell GABAA receptors. *J Neurosci.* 1999;17:7532–7540.

162. Mazarati AM, Baldwin RA, Sankar R, et al. Time-dependent decrease in the effectiveness of antiepileptic drugs during the course of self-sustaining status epilepticus. *Brain Res.* 1998;814:179–185.

163. Rice AC, DeLorenzo RJ. N-methyl-D-aspartate receptor activation regulates refractoriness of status epilepticus to diazepam. *Neurosciences.* 1999;93:117–123.

164. Martin BS, Kapur J. A combination of ketamine and diazepam synergistically controls refractory status epilepticus induced by cholinergic stimulation. *EPA.* 2008;49:248–255.

165. Mewasingh LD, Sekhara T, Aeby A, et al. Oral ketamine in paediatric non-convulsive status epilepticus. *Seizure.* 2003;12:483–489.

166. Abend NS, Dlugos DJ. Treatment of refractory status epilepticus: literature review and a proposed protocol. *Pediatr Neurol.* 2008;38: 377–390.

167. Wasterlain CG, Chen JW. Mechanistic and pharmacologic aspects of status epilepticus and its treatment with new antiepileptic drugs. *EPA.* 2008;49(9):63–73.

168. Pasternak SJ, Heller MB. Endotracheal diazepam in status epilepticus. *Ann Emerg Med.* 1985;14:485.

169. Rusli M, Spivey WH, Bonner H. Endotracheal diazepam: absorption and pulmonary pathologic effects. *Ann Emerg Med.* 1987;16:314.

170. Kriel RL, Cloyd JC, Pellock JM, et al. Rectal diazepam gel for treatment of acute repetitive seizures. The North American Diastat Study Group. *Pediatr Neurol.* 1999;20:282–288.

171. Mitchell WG, Conry JA, Crumrine PK, et al. An open-label study of repeated use of diazepam rectal gel (Diastat) for episodes of acute breakthrough seizures and clusters: safety, efficacy and tolerance. North American Diastat Group. *EPA.* 1999;40:1610–1617.

172. Fakhoury T, Chumley A, Bensalem-Owen M. Effectiveness of diazepam rectal gel in adults with acute repetitive seizures and prolonged seizures: a single-center experience. *Epilepsy Behav.* 2007;11:357–360.

173. Talukdar B, Chakrabarty B. Efficacy of buccal midazolam compared to intravenous diazepam in controlling convulsions in children: a randomized controlled trial. *Brain Dev.* 2009;31:744–749.

174. Mpimbaza A, Ndeezi G, Staedke S, et al. Comparison of buccal midazolam with rectal diazepam in the treatment of prolonged seizures in Ugandan children: a randomized clinical trial. *Pediatrics.* 2008;121:e58–e64.

175. Kyrkou M, Harbord M, Kyrkou N, et al. Community use of intranasal midazolam for managing prolonged seizures. *J Intellect Dev Disabil.* 2006;31:131–138.

176. Bhattacharyya M, Kalra V, Gulati S. Intranasal midazolam vs rectal diazepam in acute childhood seizures. *Pediatr Neurol.* 2006;34: 355–359.

177. Moffett A, Scott DF. Stress and epilepsy: the value of a benzodiazepine–lorazepam. *J Neurol Neurosurg Psychiatry.* 1984;47:165–167.

178. Feely M, Gibson J. Intermittent clobazam for catamenial epilepsy: tolerance avoided. *J Neurol Neurosurg Psychiatry.* 1984;47:1279–1282.

179. Lader M. Withdrawal reactions after stopping hypnotics in patients with insomnia. *CNS Drugs.* 1998;10:425–440.

180. Crawford TO, Mitchell WG, Snodgrass SR. Lorazepam in childhood status epilepticus and serial seizures: effectiveness and tachyphylaxis. *Neurology.* 1987;37:190–195.

181. Ramsey-Williams VA, Wu Y, Rosenberg HC. Comparison of anticonvulsant tolerance, crosstolerance, and benzodiazepine receptor binding following chronic treatment with diazepam or midazolam. *Pharmacol Biochem Behav.* 1994;48:765–772.

182. Rosenberg HC. Differential expression of benzodiazepine anticonvulsant cross-tolerance according to time following flurazepam or diazepam treatment. *Pharmacol Biochem Behav.* 1995;51:363–368.

183. Heninger C, Saito N, Tallman JF, et al. Effects of continuous diazepam administration on GABA$_A$ subunit mRNA in rat brain. *Mol Neurosci.* 1990;2:101–107.

184. Kang I, Miller LG. Decreased GABA$_A$ receptor mRNA concentrations following chronic lorazepam administration. *Br J Pharmacol.* 1991;103: 1285–1287.

185. O'Donovan MC, Buckland PR, Spurlock G, et al. Bi-directional changes in the levels of messsenger RNA's encoding γ-aminobutyric acid$_A$ receptor α subunits after flurazepam treatment. *Eur J Pharmacol.* 1992;226: 335–341.

186. Zhao TJ, Chiu TH, Rosenberg HC. Reduced expression of γ-aminobutyric acid type A benzodiazepine receptor γ2 and α5 subunit mRNAs in brain regions of flurazepam-treated rats. *Mol Pharmacol.* 1994;45:657–663.

187. Tietz EI, Huang X, Weng X, et al. Expression of α1, α5, and γ2 GABA$_A$ receptor subunit mRNA's measured *in situ* in rat hippocampus and cortex following chronic flurazepam administration. *J Mol Neurosci.* 1994;4: 277–292.

188. Tietz EI, Huang X, Chen S, et al. Temporal and regional regulation of α1, β2 and β3, but not α2, α4, α6, β1, or γ2 GABA$_A$ receptor subunit messenger RNAs following one week oral flurazepam administration. *Neurosciences.* 1999;91:327–341.

189. Li M, Szabo A, Rosenberg HC. Downregulation of benzodiazepine binding to α5 subunit-containing GABA$_A$ receptors in tolerant rat brain indicates particular involvement of the hippocampal CA1 region. *J Pharmacol Exp Ther.* 2000;295:689–696.

190. Tietz EI, Rosenberg HC. Behavioral measurement of benzodiazepine tolerance and GABAergic subsensitivity in the substantia nigra pars reticulata. *Brain Res.* 1988;438:41–51.

191. Xie XH, Tietz EI. Chronic benzodiazepine treatment of rats induces reduction of paired pulse inhibition in CA1 region of in vitro hippocampal slices. *Brain Res.* 1991;561:69–76.

192. Zeng X, Xie XH, Tietz EI. Impairment of feedforward inhibition in CA1 region of hippocampus after chronic benzodiazepine treatment. *Neurosci Lett.* 1994;173:40–44.

193. Zeng XJ, Tietz EI. Benzodiazepine tolerance at GABAergic synapses on hippocampal CA1 pyramidal cells. *Synapse.* 1999;31:263–277.

194. Loscher W, Rundfeldt C, Honack D, et al. Long-term studies on anticonvulsant tolerance and withdrawal characteristics of benzodiazepine receptor ligands in different seizure models in mice. I. Comparison of diazepam, clonazepam, clobazam and abecarnil. *J Pharmacol Exp Ther.* 1996;279:561–572.

195. Mintzer MZ, Stoller KB, Griffiths RR. A controlled study of flumazenil-precipitated withdrawal in chronic low-dose benzodiazepine users. *Psychopharmacology (Berl).* 1999;147:200–209.

196. Mintzer MZ, Griffiths RR. Flumazenil-precipitated withdrawal in healthy volunteers following repeated diazepam exposure. *Psychopharmacology (Berl).* 2005;178:259–267.

197. Schweizer E, Rickels K. Benzodiazepine dependence and withdrawal: a review of the syndrome and its clinical management. *Acta Psychiatr Scand Suppl.* 1998;393:95–101.

198. Higgitt A, Fonagy P. Benzodiazepine dependence syndromes and syndromes of withdrawal. In: Hallström C, ed. *Benzodiazepine Dependence.* Oxford: Oxford University Press; 1993:58–70.

199. Griffiths RR, Weerts EM. Benzodiazepine self-administration in humans and laboratory animals—implications for problems of long-term use and abuse. *Psychopharmacology (Berl).* 1997;134:1–37.

200. Cappell H, Busto U, Kay G, et al. Drug deprivation and reinforcement by diazepam in a dependent population. *Psychopharmacology (Berl).* 1987;91:154–160.

201. Bateson AN. Basic pharmacologic mechanisms involved in benzodiazepine tolerance and withdrawal. *Curr Pharm Des.* 2002;8:5–21.

202. Wafford KA. GABAA receptor subtypes: any clues to the mechanism of benzodiazepine dependence? *Curr Opin Pharmacol.* 2005;5:47–52.

203. Allison C, Pratt JA. Neuroadaptive processes in GABAergic and glutamatergic systems in benzodiazepine dependence. *Pharmacol Ther.* 2003;98:171–195.

204. Costa E, Auta J, Grayson DR, et al. GABAA receptors and benzodiazepines: a role for dendritic resident subunit mRNAs. *NPH.* 2002;43:925–937.

205. Van Sickle BJ, Xiang K, Tietz EI. Transient plasticity of hippocampal CA1 neuron glutamate receptors contributes to benzodiazepine withdrawal-anxiety. *Neuropsychopharmacology.* 2004;29:1994–2006.

206. Xiang K, Tietz EI. Benzodiazepine-induced hippocampal CA1 neuron alpha-amino-3-hydroxy-5-methylisoxasole-4-propionic acid (AMPA) receptor plasticity linked to severity of withdrawal anxiety: differential role of voltage-gated calcium channels and N-methyl-D-aspartic acid receptors. *Behav Pharmacol.* 2007;18:447–460.

207. Izzo E, Auta J, Impagnatiello F, et al. Glutamic acid decarboxylase and glutamate receptor changes during tolerance and dependence to benzodiazepines. *Proc Natl Acad Sci U S A.* 2001;98:3483–3488.

208. Song J, Shen G, Greenfield LJ Jr., et al. Benzodiazepine withdrawal-induced glutamatergic plasticity involves up-regulation of GluR1-containing alpha-amino-3-hydroxy-5-methylisoxasole-4-propionic acid receptors in Hippocampal CA1 neurons. *J Pharmacol Exp Ther.* 2007;322: 569–581.

209. Shen G, Van Sickle BJ, Tietz EI. Calcium/Calmodulin-Dependent Protein Kinase II Mediates Hippocampal Glutamatergic Plasticity During Benzodiazepine Withdrawal. *Neuropsychopharmacology.* 2010 May 5. [Epub ahead of print], in press.

210. Liao D, Hessler NA, Malinow R. Activation of postsynaptically silent synapses during pairing-induced LTP in CA1 region of hippocampal slice. *Nature.* 1995;375:400–404.

211. Van Sickle BJ, Cox AS, Schak K, et al. Chronic benzodiazepine administration alters hippocampal CA1 neuron excitability: NMDA receptor function and expression(1). *NPH.* 2002;43:595–606.

212. Xiang K, Earl DE, Davis KM, et al. Chronic benzodiazepine administration potentiates high voltage-activated calcium currents in hippocampal CA1 neurons. *J Pharmacol Exp Ther.* 2008;327:872–883.

213. Walker JE, Homan RW, Crawford IL. Lorazepam: a controlled trial in patients with intractable partial complex seizures. *EPA.* 1984;25: 464–466.

214. Lolin Y, Francis DA, Flanagan RJ, et al. Cerebral depression due to propylene glycol in a patient with chronic epilepsy—the value of the plasma osmolal gap in diagnosis. *Postgrad Med J.* 1988;64:610–613.

215. Arbour RB. Propylene glycol toxicity related to high-dose lorazepam infusion: case report and discussion. *Am J Crit Care.* 1999;8:499–506.

216. Waltregny A, Dargent J. Preliminary study of parenteral lorazepam in status epilepticus. *Acta Neurol Belg.* 1975;75:219–229.

217. Graham CW, Pagano RR, Conner JT. Pain and clinical thrombophlebitis following intravenous diazepam and lorazepam. *Anaesthesia* 1978;33: 188–191.

218. Parkes RB, Blanton PL, Thrash WJ. Incidence of thrombophlebitis in humans with the diazepam vehicle. *Anesth Prog.* 1982;29:168–169.

219. Gould JD, Lingam S. Hazards of intra-arterial diazepam. *Br Med J.* 1977;2:298–299.
220. Greenblatt DJ, Shader RI, Abernethy DR. Current status of benzodiazepines (second of two parts). *N Engl J Med.* 1983;309:410–416.
221. Busto U, Sellers EM, Naranjo CA, et al. Withdrawal reaction after long-term therapeutic use of benzodiazepines. *N Engl J Med.* 1986;315:854–859.
222. Salzman C. The benzodiazepine controversy: therapeutic effects versus dependence, withdrawal, and toxicity. *Harv Rev Psychiatry.* 1997;4:279–282.
223. Schweitzer E, Rickels K. Benzodiazepine dependence and withdrawal: a review of the syndrome and its clinical management. *Acta Psychiatr Scand.* 1998;98(393):95–101.
224. Huang ZC, Shen DL. Studies of quantitative beta activity in EEG background changes produced by intravenous diazepam. *Clin Electroencephalogr.* 1997;28:172–178.
225. Huang ZC, Shen DL. The prognostic significance of diazepam-induced EEG changes in epilepsy: a follow-up study. *Clin Electroencephalogr.* 1993;24:179–187.
226. Greenblatt DJ, Divoll M. Diazepam vs. lorazepam: relationship of drug distribution to duration of clinical action. In: Delgado-Escueta AV, Wasterlain C, Treiman DM, et al., eds. *Status Epilepticus: Mechanism of Brain Damage and Treatment.* New York: Raven Press; 1983:487–490.
227. Hardman JG, Limbird LE, Gilman AG. Appendix II. In: Hardman JG, Limbird LE, Gilman AG, eds. *Goodman and Gilman's The Pharmacological Basis of Therapeutics.* 10th ed. New York: McGraw Hill; 2001.
228. Schwartz MA, Koechlin BA, Postma E, et al. Metabolism of diazepam in rat, dog and man. *J Pharmacol Exp Ther.* 1965;149:423–435.
229. Klotz U, Antonin KH, Brügel H, et al. Disposition of diazepam and its major metabolite desmethyldiazepam in patients with liver disease. *Clin Pharmacol Ther.* 1977;21:430–436.
230. Nims RW, Prough RA, Jones CR, et al. In vivo induction and in vitro inhibition of hepatic cytochrome P450 activity by the benzodiazepine anticonvulsants clonazepam and diazepam. *Drug Metab Dispos.* 1997;25:750–756.
231. Eustace PW, Hailey DM, Cox AG, et al. Biliary excretion of diazepam in man. *Br J Anaesth.* 1975;47:983–985.
232. Mahon WA, Inaba T, Umeda T, et al. Biliary elimination of diazepam in man. *Clin Pharmacol Ther.* 1976;19:443–450.
233. Ma YM, Sun RY. Second peak of plasma diazepam concentration and enterogastric circulation. *Zhongguo Yao Li Xue Bao.* 1993;14:218–221.
234. Nichol CF, Tutton IC, Smith BH. Parenteral diazepam in status epilepticus. *Neurology.* 1969;19:332–343.
235. Norris E, Marzouk O, Nunn A, et al. Respiratory depression in children receiving diazepam for acute seizures: a prospective study. *Dev Med Child Neurol.* 1999;41:340–343.
236. Korttila K, Linnoila M. Absorption and sedative effects of diazepam after oral administration and intramuscular administration into the vastus lateralis muscle and the deltoid muscle. *Br J Anaesth.* 1975;47:857–862.
237. Korttila K, Linnoila M. Psychomotor skills related to driving after intramuscular administration of diazepam and meperidine. *Anesthesiology.* 1975;42:685–691.
238. Milligan N, Dhillon S, Oxley J, et al. Absorption of diazepam from the rectum and its effect on interictal spikes in the EEG. *EPA.* 1982;23:323–331.
239. Al Tahan A. Paradoxic response to diazepam in complex partial status epilepticus. *Arch Med Res.* 2000;31:101–104.
240. Sadjadi SA, McLaughlin K, Shah RM. Allergic interstitial nephritis due to diazepam. *Arch Intern Med.* 1987;147:579.
241. Haley CJ, Haun WM, Lin S, et al. *Diazepam.* In: DRUGDEX® System [Internet database]. Greenwood Village, Colorado: Thomson Reuters (Healthcare) Inc. Updated periodically. 2001.
242. Saxén I, Saxén L. Association between maternal intake of diazepam and oral clefts. *Lancet.* 1975;2:498.
243. Laegreid L, Kyllerman M, Headner R, et al. Benzodiazepine amplification of valproate teratogenic effects in children of mothers with absence epilepsy. *Neuropediatrics.* 1993;24:88–92.
244. Browne TR, Penry JK. Benzodiazepines in the treatment of epilepsy. A review. *EPA.* 1973;14:277–310.
245. Delgado-Escueta AV, Enrile-Bacsal F. Combination therapy for status epilepticus: intravenous diazepam and phenytoin. *Adv Neurol.* 1983;34:477–485.
246. Walker MC, Tong X, Brown S, et al. Comparison of single- and repeated-dose pharmacokinetics of diazepam. *EPA.* 1998;39:283–289.
247. Ferngren HG. Diazepam treatment for acute convulsions in children. *EPA.* 1974;15:27–37.
248. Booker HE, Celesia GG. Serum concentrations of diazepam in subjects with epilepsy. *Arch Neurol.* 1973;29:191–194.
249. Bertz RJ, Howrie DL. Diazepam by continuous intravenous infusion for status epilepticus in anticonvulsant hypersensitivity syndrome. *Ann Pharmacother.* 1993;27:298–301.
250. Mahomed K, Nyamurera T, Tarumbwa A. PVC bags considerably reduce availability of diazepam. *Cent Afr J Med.* 1998;44:172–173.
251. Phelps SJ, Cochran EB. Diazepam. In: American Society of Hospital Pharmacists, ed. *Guidelines for Administration of Intravenous Medications to Pediatric Patients.* 4th ed. Bethesda, MD: Intelligence Publications; 1993.
252. Agurell S, Berlin A, Ferngren H, et al. Plasma levels of diazepam after parenteral and rectal administration. *EPA.* 1975;16:277–283.
253. Singhi S, Banerjee S, Singhi P. Refractory status epilepticus in children: role of continuous diazepam infusion. *J Child Neurol.* 1998;13:23–26.
254. Gilbert DL, Gartside PS, Glauser T. Efficacy and mortality in treatment of refractory generalized convulsive status epilepticus. *J Child Neurol.* 1999;14:602–609.
255. Meberg A, Langslet A, Bredesen JE, et al. Plasma concentration of diazepam and N-desmethyldiazepam in children after a single rectal or intramuscular dose. *Eur J Clin Pharmacol.* 1978;14:273–276.
256. De Negri M, Baglietto MG, Battaglia FM, et al. Treatment of electrical status epilepticus by short diazepam (DZP) cycles after DZP rectal bolus test. *Brain Dev.* 1995;17:330–333.
257. Knudsen FU, Paerregaard A, Andersen R, et al. Long term outcome of prophylaxis for febrile convulsions. *Arch Dis Child.* 1996;74:13–18.
258. De Negri M, Baglietto MG, Biancheri R. Electrical status epilepticus in childhood: treatment with short cycles of high dosage benzodiazepine (preliminary note). *Brain Dev.* 1993;15:311–312.
259. Herman RJ, Van Pham JD, Szakacs CB. Disposition of lorazepam in human beings: enterohepatic recirculation and first-pass effect. *Clin Pharmacol Ther.* 1989;46:18–25.
260. Bradshaw EG, Ali AA, Mulley BA, et al. Plasma concentrations and clinical effects of lorazepam after oral administration. *Br J Anaesth.* 1981;53:517–521.
261. Ochs HR, Busse J, Greenblatt DJ, et al. Entry of lorazepam into cerebrospinal fluid. *Br J Clin Pharmacol.* 1980;10:405–406.
262. Greenblatt DJ, Joyce KA, Comer WH, et al. Clinical pharmacokinetics of lorazepam: III Intravenous injection. Preliminary results. *J Clin Pharmacol.* 1977;17:490–494.
263. Greenblatt DJ, Ehrenberg BL, Gunderman J, et al. Kinetic and dynamic study of intravenous lorazepam: comparison with intravenous diazepam. *J Pharmacol Exp Ther.* 1989;250:134–140.
264. Walker JE, Homan RW, Vasko MR, et al. Lorazepam in status epilepticus. *Ann Neurol.* 1979;6:207–213.
265. Homan RW, Treiman DM. Lorazepam. In: Levy RH, Meldrum BS, eds. *Antiepileptic Drugs.* 4th ed. New York: Raven Press; 1995:779–790.
266. Ochs HR, Greenblatt DJ, Eichelkraut W, et al. Contribution of the gastrointestinal tract to lorazepam conjugation and clonazepam nitroreduction. *Pharmacology.* 1991;42:36–48.
267. Greenblatt DJ, Schillings RT, Kyriakopoulos AA, et al. Clinical pharmacokinetics of lorazepam: absorption and disposition of oral ¹⁴C-lorazepam. *Clin Pharmacol Ther.* 1976;21:222–230.
268. Greenblatt DJ, Shader RI, Franke K, et al. Pharmacokinetics and bioavailability of intravenous, intramuscular, and oral lorazepam in humans. *J Pharm Sci.* 1979;68:57–63.
269. Ameer B, Greenblatt DJ. Lorazepam: a review of its clinical pharmacological properties and therapeutic uses. *Drugs.* 1981;21:162–200.
270. Lacey DJ, Singer WD, Horwitz SJ, et al. Lorazepam therapy of status epilepticus in children and adolescents. *J Pediatr.* 1986;108:771–774.
271. DiMario FJ Jr., Clancy RR. Paradoxical precipitation of tonic seizures by lorazepam in a child with atypical absence seizures. *Pediatr Neurol.* 1988;4:249–251.
272. Kahan BB, Haskett RF. Lorazepam withdrawal and seizures. *Am J Psychiatry.* 1984;141:1011–1012.
273. Samara EE, Granneman RG, Witt GF, et al. Effect of valproate on the pharmacokinetics and pharmacodynamics of lorazepam. *J Clin Pharmacol.* 1997;37:442–450.
274. Anderson GD, Gidal BE, Kantor ED, et al. Lorazepam–valproate interaction: studies in normal subjects and isolated perfused rat liver. *EPA.* 1994;35:221–225.
275. Levy RJ, Krall RL. Treatment of status epilepticus with lorazepam. *Arch Neurol.* 1984;41:605–611.
276. Vincent FM, Vincent T. Lorazepam in myoclonic seizures after cardiac arrest [letter]. *Ann Intern Med.* 1986;104:586.
277. Sreenath TG, Gupta P, Sharma KK, et al. Lorazepam versus diazepam–phenytoin combination in the treatment of convulsive status epilepticus in children: a randomized controlled trial. *Eur J Paediatr Neurol.* 2010;14:162–168.
278. Deshmukh A, Wittert W, Schnitzler E, et al. Lorazepam in the treatment of refractory neonatal seizures. A pilot study. *Am J Dis Child.* 1986;140:1042–1044.
279. Maytal J, Novak GP, King KC. Lorazepam in the treatment of refractory neonatal seizures. *J Child Neurol.* 1991;6:319–323.
280. Yager JY, Seshia SS. Sublingual lorazepam in childhood serial seizures. *Am J Dis Child.* 1988;142:931–932.
281. D'Onofrio G, Rathlev NK, Ulrich AS, et al. Lorazepam for the prevention of recurrent seizures related to alcohol. *N Engl J Med.* 1999;340:915–919.
282. Jawad S, Oxley J, Wilson J, et al. A pharmacodynamic evaluation of midazolam as an antiepileptic compound. *J Neurol Neurosurg Psychiatry.* 1986;49:1050–1054.

283. Dundee JW, Halliday NJ, Harper KW, et al. Midazolam. A review of its pharmacological properties and therapeutic use. *Drugs.* 1984;28: 519–543.

284. Breimer LT, Burm AG, Danhof M, et al. Pharmacokinetic–pharmacodynamic modelling of the interaction between flumazenil and midazolam in volunteers by aperiodic EEG analysis. *Clin Pharmacokinet.* 1991;20: 497–508.

285. Bell DM, Richards G, Dhillon S, et al. A comparative pharmacokinetic study of intravenous and intramuscular midazolam in patients with epilepsy. *Epilepsy Res.* 1991;10:183–190.

286. Burstein AH, Modica R, Hatton M, et al. Pharmacokinetics and pharmacodynamics of midazolam after intranasal administration. *J Clin Pharmacol.* 1997;37:711–718.

287. Bjorkman S, Rigemar G, Idvall J. Pharmacokinetics of midazolam given as an intranasal spray to adult surgical patients. *Br J Anaesth.* 1997; 79:575–580.

288. Clausen TG, Wolff J, Hansen PB, et al. Pharmacokinetics of midazolam and α-hydroxy-midazolam following rectal and intravenous administration. *Br J Clin Pharmacol.* 1988;25:457–463.

289. Thummel KE, O'Shea D, Paine MF, et al. Oral first-pass elimination of midazolam involves both gastrointestinal and hepatic CYP3A-mediated metabolism. *Clin Pharmacol Ther.* 1996;59:491–502.

290. Rey E, Delaunay L, Pons G, et al. Pharmacokinetics of midazolam in children: comparative study of intranasal and intravenous administration. *Eur J Clin Pharmacol.* 1991;41:355–357.

291. Jacqz-Aigrain E, Oxley J, Wilson J, et al. Pharmacokinetics of midazolam during continuous infusion in critically ill neonates. *Eur J Clin Pharmacol.* 1992;42:329–332.

292. Malacrida R, Fritz ME, Suter PM, et al. Pharmacokinetics of midazolam administered by continuous intravenous infusion to intensive care patients. *Crit Care Med.* 1992;20:1123–1126.

293. Oldenhof H, de Jong M, Steenhoek A, et al. Clinical pharmacokinetics of midazolam in intensive care patients, a wide interpatient variability? *Clin Pharmacol Ther.* 1988;43:263–269.

294. Caldwell CB, Gross JB. Physostigmine reversal of midazolam-induced sedation. *Anesthesiology.* 1982;57:125–127.

295. Hantson P, Clemessy JL, Baud FJ. Withdrawal syndrome following midazolam infusion. *Intensive Care Med.* 1995;21:190–194.

296. Olkkola KT, Aranko K, Luurila H, et al. A potentially hazardous interaction between erythromycin and midazolam. *Clin Pharmacol Ther.* 1993;53:298–305.

297. Backman JT, Olkkola KT, Ojala M, et al. Concentrations and effects of oral midazolam are greatly reduced in patients treated with carbamazepine or phenytoin. *EPA.* 1996;37:253–257.

298. Hanley FD, Kross JF. Use of midazolam in the treatment of refractory status epilepticus. *Clin Ther.* 1998;20:1093–1105.

299. Towne AR, DeLorenzo RJ. Use of intramuscular midazolam for status epilepticus. *J Emerg Med.* 1999;17:323–328.

300. Kumar A, Bleck TP. Intravenous midazolam for the treatment of refractory status epilepticus. *Crit Care Med.* 1992;20:483–488.

301. Wroblewski BA, Joseph AB. The use of intramuscular midazolam for acute seizure cessation of behavioral emergencies in patients with traumatic brain injury. *Clin Neuropharmacol.* 1992;15:44–49.

302. Papavasiliou AS, Kotsalis C, Paraskevoulakos E, et al. Intravenous midazolam in convulsive status epilepticus in children with pharmacoresistant epilepsy. *Epilepsy Behav.* 2009;14:661–664.

303. Lal KR, Raj AG, Chacko A, et al. Continous midazolam infusion as treatment of status epilepticus. *Arch Dis Child.* 1997;76:445–448.

304. Igartua J, Silver P, Maytal J, et al. Midazolam for refractory status epilepticus in children. *Crit Care Med.* 1999;27:1982–1985.

305. Koul RL, Raj AG, Chacko A, et al. Continuous midazolam infusion as treatment of status epilepticus. *Arch Dis Child.* 1997;76:445–448.

306. Yoshikawa H, Yamazaki S, Abe T, et al. Midazolam as a first-line agent for status epilepticus in children. *Brain Dev.* 2000;22:239–242.

307. Sheth RD, Buckley DJ, Gingold M, et al. Midazolam in the treatment of refractory neonatal seizures. *Clin Neuropharmacol.* 1996;19:165–170.

308. Chamberlain JM, Altieri MA, Futterman C, et al. A prospective, randomized study comparing intramuscular midazolam with intravenous diazepam for the treatment of seizures in children. *Pediatr Emerg Care.* 1997;13:92–94.

309. Jeannet PY, Roulet E, Maeder-Ingvar M, et al. Home and hospital treatment of acute seizures in children with nasal midazolam. *Eur J Paediatr Neurol.* 1999;3:73–77.

310. Congdon PJ, Forsythe WI. Intravenous clonazepam in the treatment of status epilepticus in children. *EPA.* 1980;21:97–102.

311. Edwards VE. Side effects of clonazepam therapy. *Proc Aust Assoc Neurol.* 1974;11:199–202.

312. Rothschild AJ, Shindul R, Viguera A, et al. Comparison of the frequency of behavioral disinhibition on alprazolam, clonazepam, or no benzodiazepine in hospitalized psychiatric patients. *J Clin Psychopharmacol.* 2000;20:7–11.

313. Buchanan N, Sharpe C. Clonazepam withdrawal in 13 patients with active epilepsy and drug side effects. *Seizure.* 1994;3:271–275.

314. Sechi GP, Zoroddu G, Rosati G. Failure of carbamazepine to prevent clonazepam withdrawal status epilepticus. *Ital J Neurol Sci.* 1984;5:285–287.

315. Culhane NS, Hodle AD. Burning mouth syndrome after taking clonazepam. *Ann Pharmacother.* 2001;35:874–876.

316. Tassinari CA, Daniele O, Michelucci R, et al. Benzodiazepines: efficacy in status epilepticus. *Adv Neurol.* 1983;34:465–475.

317. Dreifuss FE, Penry JK, Rose SW, et al. Serum clonazepam concentrations in children with absence seizures. *Neurology.* 1975;25:255–258.

318. Ketz E, Bernoulli C, Siegfried J. Clinical and electroencephalographic trial with clonazepam (Ro 5-4023) with special regard to status epilepticus. *Acta Neurol Scand Suppl.* 1973;53:47–53.

319. Sakata O, Onishi H, Machida Y. Clonazepam oral droplets for the treatment of acute epileptic seizures. *Drug Dev Ind Pharm.* 2008;34: 1376–1380.

320. Sorel L, Mechler L, Harmant J. Comparative trial of intravenous lorazepam and clonazepam im status epilepticus. *Clin Ther.* 1981;4:326–336.

321. Naito H, Wachi M, Nishida M. Clinical effects and plasma concentrations of long-term clonazepam monotherapy in previously untreated epileptics. *Acta Neurol Scand.* 1987;76:58–63.

322. McNamara JO. Drugs effective in the therapy of the epilepsies. In: Hardman JG, Limbird LE, Gilman AG, eds. *Goodman and Gilman's The Pharmacological Basis of Therapeutics.* 10th ed. New York: McGraw Hill; 2001:521–548.

323. Sugai K. Seizures with clonazepam: discontinuation and suggestions for safe discontinuation rates in children. *EPA.* 1993;34:1089–1097.

324. Vassella F, Pavlincova E, Schneider HJ, et al. Treatment of infantile spasms and Lennox–Gastaut syndrome with clonazepam (Rivotril). *EPA.* 1973; 14:165–175.

325. Dumermuth G, Kovacs E. The effect of clonazepam (Ro 5-4023) in the syndrome of infantile spasms with hypsarrhythmia and in petit mal variant of Lennox syndrome. Preliminary report. *Acta Neurol Scand Suppl.* 1973;53:26–28.

326. Mikkelsen B, Birket-Smith E, Bradt S, et al. Clonazepam in the treatment of epilepsy. A controlled clinical trial in simple absences, bilateral massive epileptic myoclonus, and atonic seizures. *Arch Neurol.* 1976;33: 322–325.

327. Hanson RA, Menkes JH. A new anticonvulsant in the management of minor motor seizures. *Dev Med Child Neurol.* 1972;14:3–14.

328. Laitinen L, Toivakka E. Clonazepam (Ro 5-4023) in the treatment of myoclonus epilepsy. Four case reports. *Acta Neurol Scand Suppl.* 1973;53:72–76.

329. Goldberg MA, Dorman JD. Intention myoclonus: successful treatment with clonazepam. *Neurology.* 1976;26:24–26.

330. Ryan SG, Sherman SL, Terry JC, et al. Startle disease, or hyperekplexia: response to clonazepam and assignment of the gene (STHE) to chromosome 5q by linkage analysis. *Ann Neurol.* 1992;31:663–668.

331. Suzuki A, Aso K, Ariyoshi C, et al. Acute intermittent porphyria and epilepsy: safety of clonazepam. *EPA.* 1992;33:108–111.

332. Yasuhara A, Yoshida H, Hatanaka T, et al. Epilepsy with continuous spike-waves during slow sleep and its treatment. *EPA.* 1991;32: 59–62.

333. Andre M, Boutroy MJ, Bianchetti G, et al. Clonazepam in neonatal seizures: dose regimens and therapeutic efficacy. *Eur J Clin Pharmacol.* 1991;40:193–195.

334. Bertler A, Lindgren S, Magnusson J-O, et al. Intramuscular bioavailability of clorazepate as compared to diazepam. *Eur J Clin Pharmacol.* 1985;28:229–230.

335. Greenblatt DJ, Divoll MK, Soong MH, et al. Desmethyldiazepam pharmacokinetics: studies following intravenous and oral desmethyldiazepam, oral clorazepate, and intravenous diazepam. *J Clin Pharmacol.* 1988;28:853–859.

336. Greenblatt DJ, Shader RI, Harmatz JS, et al. Self-rated sedation and plasma concentrations of desmethyldiazepam following single doses of clorazepate. *Psychopharmacology (Berl).* 1979;66:289–290.

337. Abernethy DR, Greenblatt DJ, Divoll M, et al. Prolongation of drug half-life due to obesity: studies of desmethyldiazepam (clorazepate). *J Pharm Sci.* 1982;71:942–944.

338. Bertler A, Lindgren S, Magnusson J-O, et al. Pharmacokinetics of clorazepate after intravenous and intramuscular administration. *Psychopharmacology.* 1983;80:236–239.

339. Shader RI, Greenblatt DJ, Ciraulo DA, et al. Effect of age and sex on disposition of desmethyldiazepam formed from its precursor clorazepate. *Psychopharmacology.* 1981;75:193–197.

340. Wilensky AJ, Friel PW. Benzodiazepines, clorazepate. In: Levy RH, Mattson RH, Meldrum BS, eds. *Antiepileptic Drugs.* 4th ed. New York: Raven Press; 1995:751–762.

341. Vining EP. Use of barbiturates and benzodiazepines in treatment of epilepsy. *Neurol Clin.* 1986;4:617–632.

342. Joseph AB, Wroblewski BA. Paradoxical akathesia caused by clonazepam, clorazepate and lorazepam in patients with traumatic encephalopathy and seizure disorder: a subtype of benzodiazepine-induced disinhibition. *Behav Neurol.* 1993;6:221–223.

343. Karch FE. Rage reaction associated with clorazepate dipotassium. *Ann Intern Med.* 1979;91:61–62.

344. Livingston S, Pauli LL. Clorazepate in epilepsy. *JAMA.* 1977;237:1561.

345. Parker JL. Potassium clorazepate (Tranxene)-induced jaundice. *Postgrad Med J.* 1979;55:908–910.

346. Patel DA, Patel AR. Clorazepate and congenital malformations. *JAMA.* 1980;244:135–136.

347. Booker HE. Clorazepate dipotassium in the treatment of intractable epilepsy. *JAMA.* 1974;299:552–555.

348. Berchou RC, Odin EA, Russell ME. Clorazepate therapy for refractory seizures. *Neurology.* 1981;31:1483–1485.

349. Fujii T, Okuno T, Go T, et al. Clorazepate therapy for intractable epilepsy. *Brain Dev.* 1987;9:288–291.

350. Wilensky AJ, Ojemann LM, Temkin NR, et al. Clorazepate and pheno-barbital as antiepileptic drugs: a double-blind study. *Neurology.* 1981;31:1271–1276.

351. Naidu S, Gruener G, Brazis P. Excellent results with clorazepate in recalcitrant childhood epilepsies. *Pediatr Neurol.* 1986;2:18–22.

352. Riss J, Cloyd J, Gates J, et al. Benzodiazepines in epilepsy: pharmacology and pharmacokinetics. *Acta Neurol Scand.* 2008;118:69–86.

353. Shorvon SD. The use of clobazam, midazolam and nitrazepam in epilepsy. *EPA.* 1998;39(1):S15–S23.

354. Maher J, McLachlan RS. Antiepileptic drug treatment following temporal lobectomy. *Neurology.* 1998;51:305–307.

355. Canadian Study Group for Childhood Epilepsy. Clobazam has equivalent efficacy to carbamazepine and phenytoin as monotherapy for childhood epilepsy. *EPA.* 1998;39:952–959.

356. Shorvon S. Benzodiazepines, clobazam. In: Levy RH, Mattson RH, Meldrum BS, eds. *Antiepileptic Drugs.* 4th ed. New York: Raven Press; 1995:763–777.

357. Guberman A, Couture M, Blaschuk K, et al. Add-on trial of clobazam in intractable adult epilepsy with plasma level correlations. *Can J Neurol Sci.* 1990;17:311–316.

358. Hanks GW. Clobazam: pharmacological and therapeutic profile. *Br J Clin Pharmacol.* 1979;7(1):151S–155S.

359. Hindmarch I. Some aspects of the effects of clobazam on human psychomotor performance. *Br J Clin Pharmacol.* 1979;7(1):77S–82S.

360. Bardy AH, Seppala T, Salokorpi T, et al. Monitoring of concentrations of clobazam and norclobazam in serum and saliva of children with epilepsy. *Brain Dev.* 1991;13:174–179.

361. Genton P, Nguyen VH, Mesdjian E. Carbamazepine intoxication with negative myoclonus after the addition of clobazam. *EPA.* 1998;39:1115–1118.

362. Rosenberg HC, Tietz EI, Chiu TH. Tolerance to anticonvulsant effects of diazepam, clonazepam, and clobazam in amygdala-kindled rats. *EPA.* 1989;30:276–285.

363. Allen JW, Oxley J, Robertson MM, et al. Clobazam as adjunctive treatment in refractory epilepsy. *Br Med J (Clin Res Ed).* 1983;286:1246–1247.

364. Canadian Clobazam Cooperative Group. Clobazam in treatment of refractory epilepsy: the Canadian experience. A retrospective study. *EPA.* 1991;32:407–416.

365. Koeppen D, Baruzzi A, Capozza M, et al. Clobazam in therapy-resistant patients with partial epilepsy: a double-blind placebo-controlled crossover study. *EPA.* 1987;28:495–506.

366. Conry JA, Ng YT, Paolicchi JM, et al. Clobazam in the treatment of Lennox–Gastaut syndrome. *EPA.* 2009;50:1158–1166.

367. Montenegro MA, Arif H, Nahm EA, et al. Efficacy of clobazam as add-on therapy for refractory epilepsy: experience at a US epilepsy center. *Clin Neuropharmacol.* 2008;31:333–338.

368. Silva RC, Montenegro MA, Guerreiro CA, et al. Clobazam as add-on therapy in children with epileptic encephalopathy. *Can J Neurol Sci.* 2006;33:209–213.

369. Bahi-Buisson N, Savini R, Eisermann M, et al. Misleading effects of clonazepam in symptomatic electrical status epilepticus during sleep syndrome. *Pediatr Neurol.* 2006;34:146–150.

370. Singh A, Guberman AH, Boisvert D. Clobazam in long-term epilepsy treatment: sustained responders versus those developing tolerance. *EPA.* 1995;36:798–803.

371. Rieder J. Plasma levels and derived pharmacokinetic characteristics of unchanged nitrazepam in man. *Arzneimittelforschung.* 1973;23:212–218.

372. Nicholson AN. Hypnotics: their place in therapeutics. *Drugs.* 1986;31:164–176.

373. Kangas L, Iisalo E, Kanto J, et al. Human pharmacokinetics of nitrazepam: effect of age and diseases. *Eur J Clin Pharmacol.* 1979;15:163–170.

374. Breimer DD. Pharmacokinetics and metabolism of various benzodiazepines used as hypnotics. *Br J Clin Pharmacol.* 1979;8:7S–13S.

375. Baruzzi A, Michelucci R, Tassinari CA. Benzodiazepines, nitrazepam. In: Levy RH, Dreifus FE, Mattson RH, et al., eds. *Antiepileptic Drugs.* New York: Raven Press; 1989:785–804.

376. Kenny RA, Kafetz K, Cox M, et al. Impaired nitrazepam metabolism in hypothyroidism. *Postgrad Med.* 1984;60:296–297.

377. Abernethy DR, Greenblatt DJ, Lockniskar A, et al. Obesity effects on nitrazepam disposition. *Br J Clin Pharmacol.* 1986;22:551–557.

378. Taylor F. Nitrazepam and the elderly. *Br Med J.* 1973;1:113–114.

379. Hagberg B. The chlordiazepoxide HCl (Librium®) analogue nitrazepam (Mogadon®) in the treatment of epilepsy in children. *Dev Med Child Neurol.* 1968;10:302–308.

380. Wyllie E, Wyllie R, Cruse RP, et al. The mechanism of nitrazepam-induced drooling and aspiration. *N Engl J Med.* 1986;314:35–38.

381. Clark TJH, Collins JV, Tong D. Respiratory depression caused by nitrazepam in patients with respiratory failure. *Lancet.* 1971;2:737–738.

382. Gibbs FA, Anderson EM. Treatment of hypsarrhythmia and infantile spasms with a Librium analogue. *Neurology.* 1965;15:1173–1176.

383. Darcy L. Delirium tremens following withdrawal from nitrazepam. *Med J Aust.* 1972;2:450.

384. Speirs CJ, Navey FL, Brooks DJ, et al. Opisthotonos and benzodiazepine withdrawal in the elderly. *Lancet.* 1986;2:1101.

385. Speight AN. Floppy infant syndrome and maternal diazepam and/or nitrazepam. *Lancet.* 1977;2:878.

386. Rintahaka PJ, Shewmon DA, Kyyronen P, et al. Incidence of death in patients with intractable epilepsy during nitrazepam treatment. *EPA.* 1999;40:492–496.

387. Baldwin R, Kenny TJ, Segal J. The effectiveness of nitrazepam in a refractory epileptic population. *Curr Ther Res.* 1969;11:413–416.

388. Peterson WG. Clinical study of Mogadon®, a new anticonvulsant. *Neurology.* 1967;17:878–880.

389. Millichap JG, Ortiz WR. Nitrazepam in myoclonic epilepsies. *Am J Dis Child.* 1966;112:242–248.

390. Vanasse M, Masson P, Geoffroy G, et al. Intermittent treatment of febrile convulsions with nitrazepam. *Can J Neurol Sci.* 1984;11:377–379.

391. Snyder CH. Myoclonic epilepsy in children: short-term comparative study of two benzodiazepine derivatives in treatment. *South Med J.* 1968;61:17–20.

392. Dreifus FE, Farwell J, Holmes GL, et al. Infantile spasms: comparative trial of nitrazepam and corticotropin. *Arch Neurol.* 1986;43:1107–1110.

393. Chamberlain MC. Nitrazepam for refractory infantile spasms and the Lennox–Gastaut syndrome. *J Child Neurol.* 1996;11:31–34.

394. Grimm G, Ferenci P, Katzenschlager R, et al. Improvement of hepatic encepalopathy treated with flumazenil. *Lancet.* 1988;2:1392–1394.

395. Pomierlayrargues G, Giguere JF, Lavoie J, et al. Flumazenil in cirrhotic patients in hepatic coma—a randomized double-blind placebo-controlled crossover trial. *Hepatology.* 1994;19:32–37.

396. Norenberg MD, Itzhak Y, Bender AS. The peripheral benzodiazepine receptor and neurosteroids in hepatic encephalopathy. *Adv Exp Med Biol.* 1997;420:95–111.

397. Butterworth RF. Pathophysiology of hepatic encephalopathy: the concept of synergism. *Hepatol Res.* 2008;38:S116–S121.

398. Grimm G, Katzenschlager R, Holzner F, et al. Effect of flumazenil in hepatic encephalopathy. *Eur J Anaesthesiol Suppl.* 1988;2:147–149.

399. Sand P, Kavvadias D, Feineis D, et al. Naturally occurring benzodiazepines: current status of research and clinical implications. *Eur Arch Psychiatry Clin Neurosci.* 2000;250:194–202.

400. Alho H, Costa E, Ferrero P, et al. Diazepam-binding inhibitor: a neuropeptide located in selected neuronal populations of rat brain. *Science.* 1985;229:182.

401. Gonsalves SF, Gallager DW. Persistent reversal of tolerance to anticonvulsant effects and GABAergic subsensitivity by a single exposure to benzodiazepine antagonist during chronic benzodiazepine administration. *J Pharmacol Exp Ther.* 1987;244:79–83.

402. Gonsalves SF, Gallager DW. Spontaneous and RO15-1788-induced reversal of subsensitivity to GABA following chronic benzodiazepines. *Eur J Pharmacol.* 1985;110:163–170.

403. Tietz EI, Zeng X, Chen S, et al. Antagonist-induced reversal of functional and structural measures of hippocampal benzodiazepine tolerance. *J Pharmacol Exp Ther.* 1999;291:932–942.

404. Hood S, O'Neil G, Hulse G. The role of flumazenil in the treatment of benzodiazepine dependence: physiological and psychological profiles. *J Psychopharmacology.* 2009;23:401–409.

405. Savic I, Widen L, Stone-Elander S. Feasibility of reversing benzodiazepine tolerance with flumazenil. *Lancet.* 1991;337:133–137.

406. Nutt DJ, Cowan PJ, Little HJ. Unusual interactions of benzodiazepine receptor antagonists. *Nature.* 1982;295:436–438.

407. Vellucci SV, Webster RA. Is RO15-1788 a partial agonist at benzodiazepine receptors? *Eur J Pharmacol.* 1983;90:263–268.

408. Polc P, Jahromi SS, Facciponte G, et al. Benzodiazepine antagonist flumazenil reduces hippocampal epileptiform activity. *Neuroreport.* 1995;6:1549–1552.

409. Polc P, Jahromi SS, Facciponte G, et al. Benzodiazepine antagonists reduce epileptiform discharges in rat hippocampal slices. *EPA.* 1996;37:1007–1014.

410. Robertson HA, Riives ML. A benzodiazepine antagonist is an anticonvulsant in an animal model for limbic epilepsy. *Brain Res.* 1983;270:380–382.

411. Sharief MK, Sander JWAS, Shorvon S. The effects of oral flumazenil on interictal epileptic activity: results of a double-blind, placebo-controlled study. *Epilepsy Res.* 1993;15:53–60.

412. Scollo-Lavizzari G. The anticonvulsant effect of the benzodiazepine antagonist, Ro15-1788: an EEG study of 4 cases. *Eur Neurol.* 1984;23:1–6.

413. Scollo-Lavizzari G. The clinical anticonvulsant effects of flumazenil, a benzodiazepine antagonist. *Eur J Anaesthesiol.* 1988;129–138.

414. Hart YM, Meinardi H, Sander JW, et al. The effect of intravenous flumazenil on interictal electroencephalographic epileptic activity: results of a placebo-controlled study. *J Neurol Neurosurg Psychiatry.* 1991;54:305–309.

415. Spivey WH. Flumazenil and seizures: analysis of 43 cases. *Clin Ther.* 1992;14:292–305.

416. Schulze-Bonhage A, Elger CE. Induction of partial epileptic seizures by flumazenil. *EPA.* 2000;41:186–192.

417. Henry TR. Functional neuroimaging with positron emission tomography. *EPA.* 1996;37:1141–1154.

418. Lamusuo S, Pitkanen A, Jutila L, et al. [11C]Flumazenil binding in the medial temporal lobe in patients with temporal lobe epilepsy: correlation with hippocampal MR volumetry, T2 relaxometry and neuropathology. *Neurol Res.* 2000;17:190–192.

419. Padma MV, Simkins R, White P, et al. Clinical utility of 11C-flumazenil positron emission tomography in intractable temporal lobe epilepsy. *Neurol India.* 2004;52:457–462.

420. Juhasz C, Nagy F, Muzik O, et al. [11C]Flumazenil PET in patients with epilepsy with dual pathology. *EPA.* 1999;40:566–574.

421. Stein AG, Eder HG, Blum DE, et al. An automated drug delivery system for focal epilepsy. *Epilepsy Res.* 2000;39:103–114.

CHAPTER 56 ■ GABAPENTIN AND PREGABALIN

MICHAEL J. MCLEAN AND BARRY E. GIDAL

Gabapentin (1-[aminomethyl]cyclohexaneacetic acid or 3-cyclohexyl α-aminobutyric acid) and pregabalin (3-[aminomethyl]-5-methyl-,[3S]-hexanoic acid, or 3-isobutyl-GABA) are 3-substituted derivatives of GABA (γ-amino butyric acid) (Fig. 56.1). They are currently the only two clinically used compounds from a group of GABA analogs known as gabapentinoids.

The precise cellular mechanism(s) of action of gabapentinoids is unclear and remains a topic of intense research. Multiple, similar actions of gabapentin and pregabalin have been reported in animal and cell models (1–4). Activity in a variety of animal seizure models suggests a mechanism(s) of gabapentinoids that differs from other antiepileptic drugs (AEDs) (5). The weight of evidence suggests that binding to the $\alpha_2\delta$ modulatory subunit of voltage-sensitive calcium channels, unique to gabapentinoids, may account for much of the clinical effects of both drugs (6–8). The affinity of pregabalin for the binding site is greater than that of gabapentin. Binding is thought to result in decreased release of neurotransmitters (9). A mutation (R217A) in the extracellular domain of the $\alpha_2\delta$ subunit markedly reduced pregabalin binding and effects on neurotransmission (6). Intracellular binding sites also may be involved in altering presynaptic calcium channel traffic and intracellular signaling of both drugs (10). Greater potency and bioavailability of pregabalin go far in explaining differences from gabapentin in the laboratory and in the clinic.

GABAPENTIN

Indications and Dosing

Although initially intended to be a spasmolytic agent, gabapentin was developed to treat epilepsy (11–13). Initially, gabapentin was approved by the U.S. Food and Drug Administration (FDA) at the end of 1993 as an adjunctive agent for the treatment of partial seizures with or without secondary generalization in patients over 12 years of age. It was approved for children 3 to 12 years of age in 2001. It has been approved as initial monotherapy for seizures in about 40 countries outside the United States. In 2002, gabapentin was also approved for the treatment of postherpetic neuralgia in the United States.

In the U.S. Prescribing Information (14) based on three pivotal trials (see below), the effective dose of gabapentin (Neurontin) for patients with epilepsy over the age of 12 is given as 900 to 1800 mg/day in three doses. Doses up to 2400 mg/day are included as having been well tolerated in long-term clinical studies. Doses of 3600 mg/day are mentioned as having been administered to a small number of patients for a relatively short duration; these doses were well tolerated. In clinical studies of postherpetic neuralgia, efficacy was demonstrated for doses from 1800 to 3600 mg/day in divided doses (two or three times daily) with comparable effects across the dose range. Doses greater than 1800 mg/day were not shown to provide greater efficacy in the randomized parallel group trials.

Some patients received higher doses in the course of optimization of benefit on an individual basis. Evidence is summarized below controlled and open studies published in the peer-reviewed medical literature for safety, tolerability, and efficacy of doses of gabapentin greater than 1800 mg/day.

Chemistry

Gabapentin is an amorphous crystalline substance with a molecular weight of 171.24. It is freely soluble in water (11,15). Gabapentin is a zwitterion, ionized at both the amino and carboxyl groups of the GABA spine, at physiologic pH (11,15). It is actively transported between body compartments by the L-system amino acid transporter. This same transporter recognizes naturally occurring, bulky, neutral amino acids such as

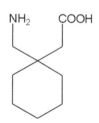

Gabapentin
(CI-945)
1-(aminomethyl)
cyclohexaneacetic acid

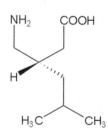

Pregabalin
(CI-1008)
S-(+)-3-isobutyl-GABA
active enantiomer

Pregabalin
(PD 14450)
R-(-)-isobutyl-GABA
inactive enantiomer

FIGURE 56.1 Chemical structure of gabapentin and pregabalin.

L-leucine, L-isoleucine, L-valine, and L-phenylalanine. This transporter is presumed to mediate transport across the gut wall, the blood–brain barrier, and cell membranes Z (16,17). Gabapentin concentrations can be measured in protein-free plasma samples by high-performance liquid chromatography (18,19) and gas chromatography (20). Blood level assays are commercially available. Gabapentin degrades slowly to a lactam in solution as a function of pH, temperature, and buffer concentration (21). The lactam has both proconvulsant (22) and neuroprotective (23) properties in laboratory models. Proprietary synthetic methods result in a low-lactam product (24).

Pharmacokinetics

Absorption

Gabapentin is absorbed primarily in the small intestine where the L-amino acid transporter is concentrated (25). Absorption from the colon is poor in animals and humans (26,27).

Bioavailability of gabapentin by the oral route is limited and dose dependent. The plasma level after a single 300-mg oral dose was about 60% of the level reached by intravenous (IV) administration of 300 mg (28). On a multidose regimen of 1600 mg t.i.d., bioavailability decreased to about 35% (29).

In phase 1 pharmacokinetic studies, plasma concentrations of gabapentin increased in proportion to the dose, that is, linearly, up to 1800 mg/day. At doses between 1800 and 4800 mg/day (600 to 1600 mg q8h), plasma levels continued to rise, but less than expected (30). A nonlinear increase in plasma levels was also noted in the data from some clinical trials (31,32). This was likely the result of saturable absorption of gabapentin from the intestine (16).

Pharmacokinetic studies including gabapentin doses of 2700 to 6000 mg/day have demonstrated substantial interindividual variability in absorption (33–35). While apparent absorption can vary substantially between individuals, less variability is noted within subjects (35).

Administration with food or enteral nutritional formulations did not impair absorption of gabapentin (29,35,36). Mean plasma levels increased by 36% and the area under the curve (AUC) by 12% after high-protein meals and meals rich in neutral amino acids (37,38). The physiologic basis for this effect has not been determined. Enhanced amino acid transport (costimulation) or increased paracellular absorption could contribute. Other investigators confirmed the lack of impairment in gabapentin absorption following a high-protein meal, but they did not demonstrate significantly increased oral absorption (36).

Gabapentin is usually prescribed in three divided doses per day. Four divided doses may be necessary at high doses (39). In a study of 36 healthy volunteers, age did not influence C_{max} or time to maximal serum concentration (T_{max}) age (40).

Distribution

Gabapentinoids do not bind significantly to plasma proteins (1,41,42). Pooled data yield a mean volume of distribution (V_d) of 60.9 L, or 0.65 to 1.04 L/kg (29,42).

Gabapentin crosses the human blood–brain barrier and is distributed throughout the central nervous system (CNS). Ratios of cerebrospinal fluid (CSF) to plasma concentration were 0.1 at 6 hours and 0.2 at 24 hours after a single 1200-mg oral dose of gabapentin (43–45). After 3 months of treatment with gabapentin 900 or 1200 mg/day, concentrations in CSF varied from 6% to 34% of those in plasma (43–45). Two clearance mechanisms—passive diffusion and active transport—appear to limit accumulation (46–49).

The CNS to plasma partition ratio was 0.8:1.0 between 1 and 8 hours after a single IV dose of gabapentin (46,50). Assuming a partition ratio of 0.8 and C_{max} ranging from 2 to 25 μg/mL at steady state, brain tissue concentrations of 1.6 to 20 μg/g may be reached.

Elimination

The absorbed fraction of gabapentin is excreted unchanged in the urine (11,29). Gabapentin is metabolized little, if at all, in humans (11,29). Repeated dosing does not appear to affect the elimination of gabapentin (41,42).

The elimination half-life ($t_{1/2}$) of gabapentin was originally estimated to be 7 to 9 hours (42,48); however, more recent data indicate a broader range of elimination $t_{1/2}$s from 4 to 22 hours (50). Renal clearance of gabapentin is linearly related to creatinine clearance (ClCr) and glomerular filtration rate in adults and children (29,51–53). Clearance of gabapentin is similar between genders (40). On a mg/kg basis, younger children appear to require doses approximately 33% larger than those of older children because of greater variability of gabapentin clearance in children under 5 years of age (53).

Age- and disease-related decreases in renal function substantially reduce elimination (35,40,48,50). Longer elimination $t_{1/2}$s and higher relative steady-state plasma concentrations occur in elderly patients. Dosage guidelines based on renal function have been generated from pharmacokinetic studies (14,48,50).

Drug–Drug Interactions

Gabapentin did not induce or inhibit hepatic microsomal enzymes involved in the metabolism of other drugs (42). It did not alter the metabolism of carbamazepine or its epoxide, phenobarbital, phenytoin, or valproate (30). Coadministration of gabapentin was associated with a 50% prolongation of the elimination $t_{1/2}$ of felbamate in 11 patients, presumably due to interaction at a renal site (54). Liver-metabolized AEDs did not affect the pharmacokinetics of gabapentin. Similarly, no clinically significant interactions were noted with antacids Z (55), oral contraceptives (56), or lithium (57).

Concentration–Effect Relationship

The therapeutic range of gabapentin concentrations in plasma is not completely characterized. Plasma levels ≥2 μg/mL were associated with significant clinical improvement in controlled studies (58,59). Improved clinical response was observed in a group of patients with refractory partial seizures and gabapentin serum concentrations ranging between 6 and 20 μg/mL (34). Well-tolerated, early-morning trough plasma levels exceeded 20 μg/mL in some patients receiving 4800 mg/day (52). Other studies have been unable to establish a significant concentration–effect relationship (60).

Some important pharmacokinetic properties of gabapentin are summarized in Table 56.1.

TABLE 56.1

PHARMACOKINETIC PROFILES OF GABAPENTIN AND PREGABALIN, WITH SIGNIFICANT DIFFERENCES LIMITED TO ABSORPTION

Absorption	Mediated by L-amino acid transporter
	Gabapentin: Dose-limiting bioavailability
	Pregabalin: >90% bioavailability
Distribution	Water soluble
	Not extensively bound to plasma proteins
Metabolism	Not metabolized by liver
	No induction of hepatic enzymes
	No autoinduction
	No inhibition of hepatic enzymes
Elimination	Excreted intact in urine
	Excretion proportional to creatinine clearance
	Gabapentin: $t_{1/2}$ 4–22 hours; average, 5–7 hours
	Pregabalin: $t_{1/2}$ 5–7 hours
Interactions	No effect on other AEDs or oral contraceptives
	No effect of gabapentin on levels of other AEDs
	None with hepatic enzymes
	None with protein-binding sites

AEDs, antiepileptic drugs; $t_{1/2}$, half-life.

Clinical Studies

Adjunctive Therapy: Placebo-Controlled Studies

Three parallel-group, placebo-controlled, double-blind, add-on trials were the basis for approval of gabapentin for the treatment of refractory partial epilepsy, with or without secondarily generalized tonic–clonic seizures (61–63) (Tables 56.2 and 56.3). These trials extended findings from two smaller dose-ranging studies that demonstrated the antiepileptic efficacy of the agent (58,59).

Adjunctive Therapy: Open-Label Studies

Company-sponsored, open-label studies were conducted in France (64), Canada (65), the United States (66,67), and Australia (68) to obtain additional information in the office setting about the safety, tolerability, and efficacy of gabapentin at doses higher than 1800 mg/day. These studies were catalyzed, in large part, by investigators during continuation phases of the controlled trials and by prescribers in the postmarketing period who found higher doses useful for some patients. More than 2500 patients were involved in these studies that incorporated methods of dosing AEDs in the clinical setting, namely dose optimization on an individual basis rather than forced titration characteristic of the pivotal controlled trials. Useful lessons were learned might have been tested in additional controlled trials. Data in Table 56.2 reveal increased, dose-dependent efficacy without altering the safety profile of gabapentin at doses up to 4800 mg/day. Gabapentin was the first add-on for most patients in the Canadian study,

TABLE 56.2

PIVOTAL TRIALS OF GABAPENTIN (GBP) AS ADD-ON THERAPY FOR PATIENTS WITH REFRACTORY PARTIAL AND SECONDARILY GENERALIZED TONIC–CLONIC SEIZURES

Study	Number of subjects	Doses	Mean RRatio[a]	Responder rate (%) (P Value)[a]
UK Gabapentin Study Group (1990)	127	GBP 1200 mg/day vs. placebo	GBP: −0.192 Placebo: −0.060 ($P = 0.0056$)	GBP: 23% Placebo: 9% ($P = 0.049$)
U.S. Gabapentin Study Group No. 5 (1993)	306	GBP 600, 1200, and 1800 mg/day vs. placebo	1800 mg/day: −0.233 ($P < 0.001$) 1200 mg/day: −0.118 ($P < 0.023$) 600 mg/day: −0.151 ($P < 0.007$) Placebo: −0.025	1800 mg/day: 26.4% ($P < 0.007$) 1200 mg/day: 17.6% ($P < 0.080$) 600 mg/day: 18.4% ($P < 0.138$) Placebo: 8.4%
International Gabapentin Study Group (Anhut et al., 1994)	272	GBP 900 and 1200 mg/day vs. placebo	1200 mg/day: −0.157 ($P = 0.0055$) 900 mg/day: −0.136 ($P = 0.0046$) Placebo: −0.025	1200 mg/day: 28.0% ($P = 0.008$) 900 mg/day: 22.9% ($P = 0.0046$) Placebo: 10.1%

The three parallel-group studies were 12 weeks in duration, multicenter, randomized, double-blind, and placebo controlled. Study medications were given in three divided doses. Significance is expressed as *P* values versus placebo.
[a]Definitions: RRatio, response ratio, a measure of the percent change in seizure frequency from baseline to the end of the masked treatment period (3 months), distributed normally between ±100%; amenable to analysis with parametric statistics. A 50% reduction in seizures corresponds to an RRatio of 0.33; responder rates, a secondary efficacy measure, representing the percentage of patients with a 50% reduction or more in the seizures. From Refs. 61–63.

TABLE 56.3

OPEN-LABEL STUDIES OF GABAPENTIN AS ADD-ON THERAPY FOR PATIENTS WITH PARTIAL AND SECONDARILY GENERALIZED TONIC–CLONIC SEIZURES

Study (in order of publication)	Design	Duration	Subjects	Efficacy	Tolerability (AEs)	Dropouts
The French Gabapentin Collaborative Group (Baulac et al., 1998)	• GBP as add-on at doses of 1200–2400 mg/day (mean dose 1739 mg/day at 6 months) • Two or more concomitant AEDs	6 months	610	• Overall responder rate 33.9% • 13% seizure free at end of study; 1.5% seizure free at baseline	• 62% reported AEs • – Somnolence and asthenia most common • 7.4% serious AEs (hypersomnolence, personality change, falls, surgery) • Dose-related weight gain, average 5.4 kg in 8.8%	9.3%
NEON (Bruni et al., 1998)	• GBP as first add-on • GBP doses of 300–3200 (median 1600) mg/day	20 weeks	114/119 evaluable	• 71% responder rate • –46% seizure free at completion • 52% seizure free at 1 year follow-up	• 16% somnolence • 9% dizziness • 6% asthenia	~11% due to mild-moderate AEs; no increase in dropouts at higher doses
STEPS (McLean et al., 1999; Morrell et al., 2000)	• GBP as add-on up to 3600 mg/day • GBP dose optimization • One to two concomitant AEDs	16 weeks	1639/2216 = 74% completers	• Dose-dependent efficacy • 46% of completers (23% by ITT) were seizure free in the last month on GBP doses of 2400–3600 mg/day • No long-term follow-up (Morrell et al., 2000)	More AEs occurred at <1800 mg/day; comparable incidence of somnolence de novo at doses above and below 1800 mg/day (McLean et al., 1999)	~11% for AEs; six serious AEs: one each of sudden death, infection, overdose, ataxia, new generalized tonic–clonic seizures, and hostility
AUS-STEPS (Beran et al., 2001)	• GBP as add-on up to 4800 mg/day • GBP dose optimization • One to three concomitant AEDs	6 months	174/176 evaluable	• 53% responder rate • Dose-dependent response 27% (N = 82) responders at 2400–3600 mg/day • 30% (N = 10) responders at 3600–4800 mg/day	• 94% reported AEs at some point • 31% dizziness, 29% fatigue, 27% somnolence, 21% headache, 20% ataxia • Incidence of AEs comparable at high and low doses	~10% for AEs; one suicide thought unrelated to GBP

the study with the most formal follow-up period (65). The chance of becoming seizure free when gabapentin was added early was nearly 50% (65). Complete seizure control persisted at this rate for a year after completion of one study (65). Side effects were common, but few were serious; 9% to 11% of patients dropped out of the studies prematurely because of adverse events.

Retrospective chart reviews of add-on use of gabapentin in office practice at doses of 900 to 6400 mg/day (average,

2688 mg/day) for 2 to 18 months in patients with refractory partial seizures with or without secondary generalization were presented in abstract form (69–74). The reports corroborated what was seen in the studies mentioned above: efficacy was dose-related and increased at higher doses of gabapentin than were used in the controlled trials. Gabapentin monotherapy was achieved in 2% to 17% of individuals. A greater than 75% reduction in seizure frequency was observed in 28% of patients, and a 50% or more reduction was noted in 44%. No change was seen in 30%, and 26% of patients worsened (a greater than 50% increase in seizures). Side effects were reported in 4% to 43% of patients but were infrequent causes of discontinuation. Dysphoria (aggression, irritability) and weight gain were more evident in these patients than among those in the controlled trials.

Long-term follow-up studies demonstrated sustained efficacy of gabapentin (75–80). Seizure freedom was achieved for some patients by adding gabapentin, particularly if they had failed less than three AEDs before the addition of gabapentin. Tolerability was generally good, with the majority of side effects occurring at doses ≤1800 mg/day (66), often being self-limited and mild to moderate in intensity. Weight gain appeared to be dose- and time-dependent. Withdrawal rates for adverse effects ranged from 9% to 17%. In most instances, gabapentin was administered in three or four doses per day. Some patients benefitted from twice-daily dosing (81).

Monotherapy Trials

Gabapentin does not have an indication for use in monotherapy in the United States. Several controlled trials support this use, however. Reduction to monotherapy with gabapentin involved 275 outpatients with refractory partial and generalized tonic–clonic seizures (31). After an 8-week baseline, gabapentin was titrated to 600, 1200, or 2400 mg/day, and other medications were discontinued over 8 weeks. The patients were then followed on gabapentin monotherapy for 16 weeks. Although 15% to 26% converted successfully to monotherapy, there was no significant difference among the three doses. In the open-label extension, some patients taking ≥4800 mg/day were able to remain on monotherapy with gabapentin (82). Gabapentin therapy was associated with improved cognitive function, mood, and psychosocial adjustment in this dose-controlled study without a placebo group (82,86).

A randomized, placebo-controlled monotherapy study lasting 8 days compared gabapentin 300 mg/day with gabapentin 3600 mg/day in 82 hospitalized patients whose other medications had been stopped during video monitoring for diagnostic purposes or presurgical evaluation (32). Gabapentin was titrated to the target dose within 24 hours. Rapid titration to 3600 mg/day was well tolerated and no patient discontinued because of side effects. Seventeen percent of the group randomized to 300 mg/day and 53% of those randomized to 3600 mg/day completed the 8-day study ($P = 0.002$). Brief inpatient trials lend insight into the short-term tolerability and efficacy of a medication, but they do not provide evidence for long-term effectiveness.

Two European studies evaluated gabapentin as initial monotherapy. In the first trial, Chadwick and associates randomized 292 patients with newly diagnosed and previously untreated partial epilepsy to monotherapy with gabapentin (300, 900, or 1800 mg/day; blinded arms) or carbamazepine (600 mg/day; open-label treatment) for 6 months (83). Roughly equal percentages of patients taking gabapentin 900 or 1800 mg/day and carbamazepine 600 mg/day remained in the study at 6 months. Time to exit based on worsening seizures was significantly longer in patients receiving gabapentin 900 or 1800 mg/day, compared with those receiving gabapentin 300 mg/day. Study withdrawal rates because of adverse events were higher for patients receiving

carbamazepine. These results suggest a role for gabapentin monotherapy in the newly diagnosed patient with infrequent seizures.

In the second double-blind, randomized, comparative trial, Brodie and colleagues (84) evaluated gabapentin and lamotrigine in a group of newly diagnosed patients with partial and/or generalized tonic–clonic seizures ($N = 309$). Patients were titrated to gabapentin doses between 1800 and 3600 mg/day, or lamotrigine up to 300 mg/day. By study end (30 weeks), there was no significant difference in time to exit, proportion of patients that were seizure free, or time to first seizure, indicating that gabapentin was comparable to lamotrigine in this population. The majority of patients randomized to the gabapentin arm who completed the study were receiving 1800 mg/day (74.3%), versus 22% receiving doses between 1800 and 3600 mg/day and 3.7% receiving 3600 mg/day. Similar proportions of patients in both study arms withdrew as result of adverse events. The most common adverse events reported in this study were dizziness, asthenia, and headache.

Three AEDs were compared as initial monotherapy for the treatment of newly diagnosed partial epilepsy in elderly patients (≥65 years of age; $N = 593$) in a Veterans Affairs Cooperative Study (85). Patients were randomized to receive monotherapy with lamotrigine ($N = 200$, target dose = 150 mg/day); gabapentin ($N = 195$, target dose = 1500 mg/day, highest dose 3600 mg/day); or carbamazepine ($N = 198$, target dose = 600 mg/day). Doses could be optimized on the basis of clinical response. Significantly more patients receiving lamotrigine (57.9%) or gabapentin (49.2%) remained in the study for 12 months, compared with those receiving carbamazepine (37%; $P = 0.010$ for gabapentin and 0.00003 for lamotrigine vs. carbamazepine). The difference between lamotrigine and gabapentin for this endpoint did not reach statistical significance. Although carbamazepine was the most efficacious agent, discontinuation rates were significantly higher in carbamazepine-treated versus gabapentin-treated patients. Adverse effects were the main reason for study withdrawal.

Patients with porphyria have been seizure free or nearly so with gabapentin monotherapy (86–88). In one study, refractory generalized tonic–clonic, but not absence or myoclonic, seizures responded to gabapentin, but the results were not statistically significant compared with the placebo group (89).

Pediatric Trials

A study of benign rolandic epilepsy with centrotemporal spikes demonstrated the efficacy of gabapentin over placebo (90). Gabapentin has been studied as add-on therapy for refractory partial seizures (91–94). Appleton and colleagues (92) conducted a large, 12-week, double-blind, placebo-controlled trial of gabapentin (25 to 35 mg/kg/day) as adjunctive treatment for 247 patients aged 3 to 12 years with refractory partial seizures. The median frequency of seizures was reduced by 35% for complex partial seizures and by 28% for secondarily generalized seizures. Gabapentin was well tolerated. Somnolence was the most common CNS-related adverse event (8%). Five percent of gabapentin-treated patients withdrew from the study because of adverse events. The safety and tolerability of 24 and 70 mg/kg/day of gabapentin were also noted in a smaller study involving 52 children (2 to 17 years of age) with refractory partial seizures (93).

Gabapentin also was both effective and well tolerated in children aged 3 to 12 years in an open-label, multicenter study of gabapentin as add-on therapy for refractory partial seizures in 237 children over a 6-month period (94). All children received gabapentin 24 to 70 mg/kg/day. The overall responder rate was 34%. Approximately 5% of the children withdrew due to adverse events.

In a placebo-controlled study evaluating the efficacy of gabapentin for the treatment of childhood absence seizures (ages 4 to 16 years; $N = 33$), Trudeau and associates (95) reported no difference between gabapentin and placebo in either efficacy or adverse event rates. Absence seizures did not worsen. Given the small sample size, it is difficult to draw firm conclusions from this study, however.

Behavioral side effects were noted, along with increased seizures, in some children with pre-existing behavioral disorders and mental retardation (96–99). Atypical absence and myoclonic seizures were reported to increase in a child with Lennox–Gastaut syndrome (100).

Long-Term Retention

More patients appear to continue on topiramate (30%) at 3 years compared with lamotrigine (29%) or gabapentin at a mean dose of 1440 mg/day (retention <10%; dose range 180 to 3600 mg/day), despite the fact that topiramate had the highest incidence of adverse events (101). Depondt et al. (102) found 65% patients continued levetiracetam at 2 years. In a review of 500 long-term open-label studies, seizure freedom for 6 months or longer was less for gabapentin (1350 to 2400 mg/day) than levetiracetam, topiramate, and lamotrigine (103); no data was available for oxcarbazepine, pregabalin, tiagabine, or zonisamide. Withdrawal due to side effects showed levetiracetam and lamotrigine to be better tolerated than gabapentin; topiramate was least tolerable (103).

In a review of retention of new AEDs in adults with refractory epilepsy and learning disability, Simister et al. (104) found drug continuation at 2 years to be 85% for oxcarbazepine, 57% for lamotrigine, 56% for levetiracetam, 45% for topiramate, 24% for tiagabine, and 15% for gabapentin (doses tried ranged from 800 to 5400, mean 2687 mg/day). Three-year retention rates of new AEDs in order of frequency of use in institutionalized patients with intellectual disability were lamotrigine 70% (used for 68% of patients); levetiracetam 52% (for 58%); topiramate 51% (for 28%); and gabapentin 33% (for 8%; average dose of 1890 mg/day calculated) (105).

It would appear that long-term continuation of therapy with gabapentin is less than that with some other newer AEDs. The finding is quite consistent. However, variable methodology and the impact of a number of factors have not been analyzed uniformly. These include the number of previous AEDs, which AEDs failed in a given patient before gabapentin was tried, the number and identification of concomitant AEDs, seizure type(s), age, and etiology of mental disability. Also, these were retrospective, nonrandomized studies. Further examination of long-term retention of the new AEDs with additional criteria seems to be warranted.

Safety

Gabapentin has not been associated with specific organ toxicities. Status epilepticus and sudden deaths occurring in clinical trials were similar in frequency to those in the general epileptic population (106). Rare deaths have occurred because of hypersensitivity (Stevens–Johnson syndrome) in patients taking gabapentin along with other AEDs known to cause such hypersensitivity (106). In addition, abrupt discontinuation of the agent has been accomplished safely, with no reports of status epilepticus or significant increases in seizure frequency (106).

Deliberate overdoses in suicide attempts have also been reported. One individual took 49 g of gabapentin without life-threatening complications or sequelae (107). Another patient attempting suicide took 91 g of gabapentin, 54 g of valproate, and had a serum ethanol level of 136 mg/dL (108). Drowsiness, dizziness, and slurred speech lasted 9 to 11 hours, without sequelae.

After review of 199 clinical trials of 11 AEDs, including gabapentin, the FDA issued on January 31, 2008 (update February 16, 2008) an alert stating that patients randomized to receive any one of the drugs in mono- or adjunctive therapy for epilepsy or any other disorder had almost twice the risk of suicidal behavior and ideation (0.43%) as patients who received placebo (0.24%) (109). The risk increased as early as 1 week after initiation of treatment and remained elevated throughout the period of observation in the studies. The risk associated with AEDs was higher than that of psychiatric and other drugs and appeared to be a class effect of AEDs. The AEDs considered included drugs with a variety of mechanisms of action: carbamazepine (marketed as Carbatrol, Equetro, Tegretol, Tegretol XR); divalproex sodium (marketed as Depakote, Depakote ER); felbamate (marketed as Felbatol); gabapentin (marketed as Neurontin); lamotrigine (marketed as Lamictal); levetiracetam (marketed as Keppra); oxcarbazepine (marketed as Trileptal); pregabalin (marketed as Lyrica); tiagabine (marketed as Gabitril); topiramate (marketed as Topamax); and zonisamide (marketed as Zonegran). A statistical review and evaluation of all these AEDs is available online (110). A letter was sent to manufacturers directing changes to the labeling (111). In the alert, the FDA recommended that all patients taking or about to start taking AEDs should be informed of this risk and monitored for changes of behavior indicative of worsening depression or suicidal ideation.

Adverse Effects

Adverse effects of gabapentin and pregabalin are similar (Table 56.4). In controlled trials, side effects of gabapentin typically involved the CNS, began within the first few days of therapy, and lasted approximately 2 weeks, without discontinuation of therapy (107). Similar adverse effects were reported in the various studies described above. The dropout rate due to side effects was less than 15%. The most common adverse effects encountered in the add-on and monotherapy trials were somnolence and dizziness. Modest weight gain has been reported to be dose related (64,112–114). Abnormal movements also can occur with gabapentin therapy (115–117). Irritability and behavioral adverse effects have been noted (e.g., aggression, anger, oppositional behavior), particularly in developmentally disabled patients and those with comorbid attention-deficit hyperactivity disorder (96–99,117,118). Leg edema with or

SOME COMMONLY OCCURRING ADVERSE EVENTS ENCOUNTERED IN CLINICAL TRIALS OF GABAPENTIN AND PREGABALIN, AND THEIR RESPECTIVE PLACEBO GROUPS

	U.S. Gabapentin Study Group No. 5 (1993)			Kugler et al. (2002) (136)		
	GBP (N = 208)	PBO (N = 99)	GBP/PBO	PGB (N = 758)	PBO (N = 294)	PGB/PBO
Somnolence	24.5	12.5	1.96	20.8	10.9	1.91
Dizziness	23.1	9.2	2.51	28.9	10.5	2.75
Ataxia	20.2	11.2	1.80	13.2	4.1	3.22
Fatigue/asthenia	11.5	7.1	1.62	11.2	8.2	1.36
Headache	14.4	12.2	1.18	9.1	11.6	0.78
Weight gain	5–15%[a]	—	—	10.4	1.4	7.43
AE-related withdrawal rate	3	1	—	15.3	6.1	

Incidence is expressed as percentage; relative incidence is expressed as the ratio of percentages in AED-treated and placebo groups.
Doses studied: GBP as 900, 1200, and 1800 mg/day in three doses per day; PGB as 50, 150, and 300 mg/day in three doses per day and 600 mg/day in two and three doses per day.
AE, adverse event; AED, antiepileptic drug; GBP, gabapentin; PBO, placebo; PGB, pregabalin.
[a]Not given in USGBP No. 5, 1993; from Baulac et al. (1998) (64).

without discoloration of the skin was reported during clinical trials and in open use (107,119). The edema resolves with discontinuation of gabapentin. Rash is relatively uncommon with gabapentin, and there are no clinical data suggesting a cross-reactivity between gabapentin and other medications. The occurrence of adverse effects with gabapentin is not strictly dose related (66,107). Some individuals do not tolerate even small doses of gabapentin.

Pregnancy and Teratogenicity

Animal studies conducted by the manufacturer revealed that gabapentin was fetotoxic in rodents (120). Gabapentin was not mutagenic in vitro or in vivo in standard assays. As a result, gabapentin has been assigned to pregnancy category C (14).

There is little published experience, including that in pregnancy registries, about the use of gabapentin in pregnant women (121). In general, polytherapy carries a greater risk of fetal malformations (121–123).

Carcinogenicity

Increased incidence of noninvasive, nonmetastasizing pancreatic acinar carcinomas in male Wistar rats taking high doses of gabapentin led to a temporary suspension of controlled trials (124). Increased incidence was not observed in female rats, in mice of either gender, or in monkeys. Survival was not significantly affected. Human pancreatic cancers tend to be ductal rather than acinar. In addition, Ki-ras mutations found in human pancreatic carcinomas were not observed in gabapentin-induced pancreatic tumors in rats (125). This species- and gender-specific effects have no clear relationship to human carcinogenic potential.

Male rat-specific α_{2u} globulin nephropathy is associated with many xenobiotics and increased nephrocarcinogenesis. The incidence of nephropathy increased in male rats fed with high doses of gabapentin and reversed upon cessation, without significant increase in carcinomas (126).

PREGABALIN

Indications

The new drug application (NDA) containing data supporting indications for use of pregabalin to treat generalized anxiety disorder, painful diabetic neuropathy, postherpetic neuralgia, and partial seizures was submitted to the FDA in November 2003. Pregabalin was approved for use as add-on therapy for patients with refractory partial and secondarily generalized seizures, for pain associated with diabetic neuropathy, and for postherpetic neuralgia in mid-2004 and for fibromyalgia in June of 2007. Development for anxiety continues. Dose-dependent efficacy was shown in the course of clinical trials for each indication. Dosage recommendations were based on the data from those studies. Doses up to 600 mg daily (as 200 mg three times daily or 300 mg twice daily) were recommended for treatment of partial epilepsy and postherpetic neuralgia. For painful diabetic neuropathy, 100 mg three times daily was recommended. For fibromyalgia, 300 to 450 mg/day in two or three doses was recommended. For painful diabetic neuropathy and fibromyalgia, 600 mg/day was also studied. This dose was not recommended because it was less tolerable and provided no additional efficacy.

Pregabalin was approved by the Committee for Medicinal Products for Human Use of the European Medicines Evaluation Agency for treatment of partial seizures in the add-on role and peripheral neuropathic pain in July 2004 and for generalized anxiety disorder in 2006.

Chemistry

Pregabalin is a water-soluble compound with a molecular weight of 159.23. It is several times more potent than gabapentin on a mg/kg basis in various animal seizure models (1). Bioavailability is 90% or more, suggesting that the L-system amino acid transporter concentrated in the duodenum is not saturated by useful doses of pregabalin (1). Additional uptake mechanisms for pregabalin may exist but have not been elucidated. Serum concentrations have been determined with high-performance liquid chromatography–ultraviolet methods (127). Plasma levels of pregabalin are commercially available.

Pharmacokinetics

Absorption

The absorption of pregabalin was linearly related to the dose in studies of single and multiple oral doses in patients (128). T_{max} was about 1 hour with oral bioavailability 90% or more (128), compared with the limited, dose-dependent uptake of gabapentin. This suggests that pregabalin absorption is not limited by a saturable process and may involve different or multiple absorption mechanisms. Pregabalin uptake was sodium dependent and involved multiple amino acid carriers ($b^{0,+}$, B^0, and $B^{0,+}$) in brush-border membrane vesicles prepared from duodenum, jejunum, and ileum of rats and rabbits (129). In the same model, gabapentin absorption was mediated by a sodium-independent transporter ($b^{0,+}$) and was greatest in the duodenum and ileum (129). Other mechanisms for pregabalin absorption have not been ruled out, but the short elimination $t_{1/2}$ suggests that absorption does not take place throughout the intestine.

Distribution

Gabapentinoids do not bind significantly to plasma proteins (1,41,42). Pooled data from several studies of gabapentin yield a mean volume of distribution (V_d) of 60.9 L, or 0.65 to 1.04 L/kg (29,42).

Pregabalin is not metabolized significantly in humans (<2% is recovered in urine as metabolites), is not bound significantly to plasma proteins, and enters the brain readily (1). As in the case of gabapentin, anticonvulsant efficacy appeared with a delay after entry of pregabalin into the brain, as measured by microdialysis, and persisted to some extent as interstitial brain concentrations fell (49). Efficacy was not strictly proportional to the concentration of pregabalin in the brain, and could have been caused by delayed (e.g., biochemical) action of the agent (49).

Metabolism

Pregabalin is not metabolized significantly in humans (1). Less than 2% of pregabalin can be recovered in the urine as metabolites. There are no known active metabolites.

Elimination

Pregabalin is excreted intact in the urine in proportion to ClCr (130). The elimination $t_{1/2}$ was approximately 9 hours for ClCr >60 mL/min, 25 hours for ClCr 15 to 30 mL/min, and 55 hours for hemodialysis patients (130). Renal function was the only factor that altered pregabalin pharmacokinetics; age was not an independent factor (131).

Drug–Drug Interactions

Steady-state plasma levels of pregabalin were not affected significantly by carbamazepine, lamotrigine, phenobarbital, phenytoin, tiagabine, topiramate, or valproate (132). The addition of pregabalin had no effect on trough plasma levels, C_{max}, AUC, or $t_{1/2}$ of carbamazepine, lamotrigine, phenytoin, or valproate administered as monotherapy in patients with partial epilepsy (132,133). In one study (134), comedication with drug-inducing AEDs was associated with unexpected 20% to 30% reduction of serum pregabalin levels. Further investigation is needed to try to duplicate and explain this reduction.

Dose and Concentration–Effect Relationships

Efficacy was proportional to oral dose up to 600 mg/day (in two or three divided doses) in three clinical trials (135). The concentration–effect relationship was also linear (134).

Clinical Studies of Efficacy and Safety

Adjunctive Therapy: Placebo-Controlled Studies

Data from three pivotal, parallel-groups, placebo-controlled, double-blind, add-on trials of pregabalin for the treatment of refractory partial seizures were used to support the new drug application and the results have been published in peer-reviewed journals (136–139) (Table 56.5). The study by French et al. (137) involved 453 patients with a median baseline seizure frequency of 10 seizures per month while taking one to three concomitant AEDs. There was a dose–response relationship when pregabalin was added at doses of 50, 150, 300, or 600 mg/day (65). Arroyo et al. (138) found 150 and 600 mg of pregabalin daily to be superior to placebo; 600 mg/day was superior to 150 mg/day. Beydoun et al. (139) found 300 mg twice daily to be equivalent to 200 mg three times daily. Analysis of data from all three trials supported a dose–response relationship in three of four patients and indicated that treatment with pregabalin 186 mg/day should be expected to result in a 50% reduction in seizures from baseline (140). A significant reduction in seizures among patients taking pregabalin 150 to 600 mg/day was evident by study at day 2 (141). Twelve percent of patients were seizure free for 6 months or more by one estimate (142). Methodology can affect estimates of seizure freedom in clinical trials. Using the last-observation-carried-forward (LOCF) method to treat data from patients who exit trials prematurely, the seizure free percentage for those taking pregabalin was 3.7% to 7.9%; 1.3% to 1.4% of those who completed the trials were seizure free (143).

A fourth controlled trial in Europe showed significant reduction of seizures by two regimens of pregabalin, either a fixed dose of 300 mg twice daily or flexible dosing (150 to 600 mg/day) adjusted for optimal benefit and tolerability (144). Patients treated with both pregabalin regimens experienced significantly greater reduction of seizure frequency compared with placebo treatment (35.4% reduction for flexible dosing dose [$P = 0.0091$] and 49.3% reduction for the fixed-dose regimen [$P = 0.0001$] versus 10.6% for placebo). Seizure reduction in fixed-dose group was superior to that in the flexible-dose group ($P = 0.0337$). Most adverse events were mild or moderate. Discontinuation rates due to adverse events were 6.8% for those receiving placebo, 12.2% for those on the flexible-dose pregabalin regimen, and 32.8% for those on the fixed-dose pregabalin regimen.

Post-hoc analysis of data from the three U.S. studies showed 600 mg/day of pregabalin to be effective in reducing

TABLE 56.5

PIVOTAL TRIALS OF PREGABALIN (PGB) AS ADD-ON THERAPY FOR PATIENTS WITH REFRACTORY PARTIAL AND SECONDARILY GENERALIZED TONIC–CLONIC SEIZURES

Study	Number of subjects	Doses	Mean RRatio		Responder rate (%)[a]: (P value)	
1008-009 Beydoun et al. (2005)	312	PGB 600 mg/day as b.i.d. or t.i.d. vs. placebo	b.i.d. t.i.d. Placebo	−28 (P ≤ 0.001) −36 (P ≤ 0.001) −0.6	b.i.d. t.i.d. Placebo	43% (P ≤ 0.001) 48% (P ≤ 0.001) 10%
1008-011 Arroyo et al. (2004)	287	PGB 150 or 600 mg/day as t.i.d. vs. placebo	150 mg/day 600 mg/day Placebo	−12 (P ≤ 0.0007) −31 (P ≤ 0.0001) 0.9	150 mg/day 600 mg/day Placebo	14% (NS) 43% (P ≤ 0.001) 6%
1008-034 French et al. (2003)	453	PGB 50, 150, 300, 600 mg/day as b.i.d. vs. placebo	50 mg/day 150 mg/day 300 mg/day 600 mg/day	−6 (NS) −21 (P ≤ 0.001) −28 (P ≤ 0.001) −37 (P ≤ 0.001)	50 mg/day 150 mg/day 300 mg/day 600 mg/day	14% (NS) 15% (P ≤ 0.006) 40% (P ≤ 0.001) 50% (P ≤ 0.001)

Studies were 12 weeks in duration, multicenter (United States, Canada, Europe, Australia), randomized, double-blind, and placebo-controlled. Clinically significant efficacy was present in the first week in all three studies (Pfizer Global Research and Development, Data on file).

RRatio, response ratio; b.i.d., twice daily; t.i.d., three times a day; NS, not significant.

[a]Estimated from graph on poster handout by Kugler et al. (2002) (136).

the frequency of secondarily generalized tonic–clonic seizures along with partial seizures, but not solely based on blocking seizure spread from the focus, as would have been indicated by constant frequency of partial seizures while tonic–clonic seizures were significantly reduced (145). Meta-analysis of the four U.S. and European controlled trials revealed significantly higher responder rates while taking pregabalin 150 to 600 mg/day compared to placebo (Mantel–Haenszel odds ratio 5.93 [95% CIs 1.24, 2.35]) (146). Withdrawal for any reason was about the same for those taking pregabalin or placebo (0.9% to 2.8% of patients taking different doses of pregabalin, 2.3% of patients taking placebo; Mantel–Haenszel odds ratio 1.71 [95% CIs 1.24, 2.35] (146). These results compare favorably with other new AEDs and vagus nerve stimulation evaluated in previous meta-analyses (147).

Pregabalin, Adjunctive Therapy: Open-Label Studies

Eighty-three percent of study patients elected to enter long-term, open-label extensions of the placebo-controlled trials (136). Interim analysis indicates sustained benefit of pregabalin 225 to 600 mg/day administered in two or three doses per day. Responder rates at different doses were in the range of 35% to 61% at 1 to 2 years. About 12% of patients withdrew because of treatment-related adverse effects.

Retrospective analysis of the effects of adding pregabalin to medications of seven mentally challenged patients with multiple seizure types showed that an average dose of 293 mg/day (range: 150 to 350 mg/day) led to a significant reduction of seizures (P = 0.018 vs. historical baseline) with 71% responder rate; side effects included weight gain, myoclonus, and sedation (148).

The cost effectiveness of adding 300 mg/day of pregabalin was found to be comparable to adding other AEDs (149).

Pregabalin, Monotherapy Trials

There are no peer-reviewed publications with results of studies of pregabalin as monotherapy.

Pregabalin, Pediatric Trials

There are no peer-reviewed publications with results of studies of pregabalin for the treatment of pediatric epilepsies.

Pregabalin Effects on Sleep in Epilepsy

Acute effects of pregabalin on the sleep of adult rats differed from those of a benzodiazepine (150). Pregabalin increased non-REM sleep (increased duration of NREM episodes; decreased number of NREM episodes), decreased REM sleep, and increased EEG power density in the delta range. Triazolam increased non-REM sleep, had no effect on REM sleep, and reduced low frequency power density on EEG.

Twenty-four normal adult volunteers underwent a randomized, double-blind three-way crossover study with 1 week washout between treatments (151). Pregabalin 150 mg, alprazolam 1 mg, or placebo were given three times daily in identical capsules for 3 days with polysomnograms recorded nightly. Compared to control, the effects of treatment with pregabalin were different from those of the benzodiazepine. Pregabalin decreased the latency of sleep onset; increased slow-wave sleep (SWS; NREM) as a proportion of both total sleep and duration of stage 4; decreased REM time as a proportion of total sleep without affecting REM latency; and decreased the number of awakenings. Alprazolam decreased the latency to sleep onset; decreased the proportion of SWS; increased REM latency; and decreased REM time. Ease of getting to sleep and quality of sleep were perceived to be improved by both pregabalin and alprazolam. Effects of both drugs were diminished after oral administration was stopped.

In a double-blind placebo-controlled exploratory trial, seizure-free patients with partial epilepsy and disturbed sleep over the past 6 months were randomized in double-blind fashion to receive 300 mg of pregabalin ($N = 8$) or placebo ($N = 7$) daily for 1 month (152). Polysomnography was performed at baseline and after 1 month of treatment. Pregabalin treatment was associated with a significant reduction of awakenings ($P < 0.02$ vs. placebo) and significant improvement in the sleep quantity and sleep disturbance subscales of the Medical Outcome Studies Sleep Scale. The authors interpreted this as an indication of improvement of sleep continuity by pregabalin (152).

In another study, 12 patients, 8 of whom had >50% reduction of seizures, underwent polysomnography before and after 3 months of treatment with pregabalin. Compared to baseline, there was an increase in sleepiness and in REM sleep independent of seizure frequency. The authors felt this could be due to direct effects on sleep generators and secondary to clinical efficacy; they also stressed the potential significance of anticonvulsant effects of increased REM (153).

Safety and Toxicity

Safety

The highest overdose during the clinical trials of pregabalin was 8000 mg, and there were no significant clinical consequences or sequelae (135). In open-label continuation phases of the clinical trials, some patients took as much as 2400 mg/day with no significant difference in the type or severity of adverse reactions compared to those experienced by patients exposed to 600 mg/day in the blinded phases of the clinical trials (135).

Pregabalin was included in the FDA alert of January 31, 2008 as 1 of 11 AEDs associated with increased risk of suicidal behavior and ideation (109–111) (see section on gabapentin safety). In a suicide attempt described in a peer-reviewed publication, a 29-year-old man ingested 32 g of lamotrigine and 11.5 g of pregabalin (154). He was initially unresponsive with facial grimacing and hemiballism that responded to benzodiazepines. EEG showed no seizures. EKG showed no conduction abnormalities. The pregabalin level in serum fell from 45 to 0 μg/mL over 12 days and the lamotrigine level fell from 60 to 0 over 4.5 days with supportive care. The 16-day stay in the intensive care unit was complicated by aspiration pneumonia. Glascow Coma Scale scores ranged from 9 to 12. Renal and hepatic functions remained normal throughout the course; hematologic parameters fell transiently without complications. Recurrence of seizures was controlled by addition of phenytoin, then carbamazepine. The patient was discharged home without sequelae after 28 days.

Adverse Effects

Adverse effects of pregabalin in pivotal trials were similar to those of gabapentin, with dizziness (29%), somnolence (21%), ataxia (13%), and weight gain (10%) (136). The intensity was generally mild to moderate, with withdrawal rates because of adverse effects ranging from 1.2% to 25%, depending on the dose. No deaths were reported, and the occurrence of serious adverse effects was infrequent (136). The occurrence of adverse effects of pregabalin in 257 patients followed for 6 months to 2 years during open-label continuation studies was somewhat different (1,142). The most common adverse effects were weight gain (27%), followed by dizziness (22%) and somnolence (20%); leg edema was not among the 11 most common adverse effects. About 12% of patients withdrew because of treatment-related adverse effects. Myoclonus has been reported in about 1% of those treated with pregabalin overall (155). Huppertz et al. (156) reported myoclonus in 4 or 19 subjects of one study. Two patients treated with pregabalin for chronic pain developed myoclonic status epilepticus (157) and another developed asterixis after the first dose of pregabalin (158). Erectile dysfunction due to pregabalin has been reported in a small series (159). Mild, transient elevations in liver enzymes occurred in nonepileptic healthy volunteers taking pregabalin 900 mg/day during multidose pharmacokinetic studies (160). Pregabalin had minimal effects on cognitive and psychomotor functions as compared to alprazolam (161).

In a meta-analysis of double-blind, add-on, randomized, placebo-controlled trials of new AEDs, pregabalin was significantly associated with somnolence, dizziness, ataxia, and fatigue (162). Meta-analysis of the four double-blind, randomized, add-on, placebo-controlled trials of pregabalin demonstrated that the most common adverse effects were dizziness and somnolence (146). These symptoms were most pronounced in the first week then waned. Dose-dependent weight gain was reported by 5.4% to 17.1% of subjects, but it was infrequently a cause for premature withdrawal from the studies (0.74%).

Pregnancy and Teratogenicity

Pregabalin is listed as pregnancy category C due to detection of increased incidences of fetal structural abnormalities and other manifestations of developmental toxicity (e.g., lethality, growth retardation, skeletal malformations, abnormal ossification, and functional impairment of nervous and reproductive systems) in the offspring of rats and rabbits given exposed to pregabalin at doses equivalent to more than five times the maximum recommended dose of 600 mg/day during pregnancy throughout the period of organogenesis (135).

Pregnancies registries have begun to log information about births to women who received pregabalin in pregnancy, but there are no publications about this in the peer-reviewed literature so far. The package insert recommends that pregabalin should be prescribed during pregnancy only if the potential benefit outweighs the potential risk to the fetus (135).

Carcinogenicity

An unexpectedly high, dose-dependent increase in incidence of malignant hemangiosarcomas was found in two strains of mice, but not in rats, during standard preclinical lifetime carcinogenicity studies (135,163). This delayed submission of the NDA (164). After required additional toxicology studies were completed, the NDA was submitted in November 2003. The clinical significance of this finding is unknown. No reports associating pregabalin treatment with increased incidence of cancers, specifically hemangiosarcomas, were found in the course of online literature searches.

Potential for Drug Abuse and Dependence

During the pivotal trials of over 5500 patients, 4% of patients treated with pregabalin and 1% of those who received placebo-reported euphoria. This and some preclinical observations led to review by the Drug Enforcement Agency.

Pregabalin does not appear to work through opioid pathways (164,165) commonly linked to drugs of abuse. Abrupt or rapid discontinuation of pregabalin resulted in reports by some patients of symptoms suggestive of physical dependence (135). A group of 15 recreational drug user (sedative/hypnotic drugs, e.g., alcohol) reported that a single 450-mg pregabalin dose produced subjective feelings comparable to a single 30 mg dose of diazepam (135). These findings led to the classification of pregabalin (Lyrica) as a Schedule V controlled substance (135). Prescribers should inform patients about and observe signs of drug abuse at follow-up visits.

Other Precautions

The U.S. package insert warns of several additional issues (135): angioedema, including life-threatening angioedema with respiratory compromise, has been reported in the postmarketing period. A history of angioedema in response to other drugs or taking other agents known to cause angioedema (such as angiotensin converting-enzyme inhibitors) should raise concern. Occurrence of angioedema should lead to immediate discontinuation of pregabalin.

Blurred vision was reported in 7% of patients taking pregabalin and 2% of patients taking placebo in controlled trials and 1% withdrew because of this. The blurriness resolved during continued dosing in most instances. In prospective studies of more than 3600 individuals, there were slightly more patients taking pregabalin than placebo with reduced visual acuity (7% vs. 5%), visual field changes (13% vs. 12%), and funduscopic changes (2% vs. 2%). Patients with treatment-emergent visual changes should be instructed to notify their physicians and appropriate investigation should ensue.

Three patients in controlled trials had rhabdomyolysis. Threefold or greater elevations of creatine kinase above normal were observed in 1.5% of pregabalin subjects and 0.7% of placebo subjects in the trials. Patients should be instructed to report new muscle-related problems promptly.

Decreased numbers of platelets were detected at higher incidence in pregabalin-exposed patients in clinical trials. There was one case of thrombocytopenia <20,000. There was no increase in incidence of bleeding diathesis due to exposure to pregabalin in the course of the pivotal trials.

Pregabalin doses >300 mg/day were associated with 3 to 6 msec prolongation of the PR interval. No clinically significant prolongations or arrhythmias were reported during the pivotal trials.

GABAPENTIN AND PREGABALIN: SUMMARY

In summary, the main advantages of gabapentinoids include lack of organ toxicity, lack of significant drug–drug interactions, and lack of protein binding. Both gabapentin and pregabalin are generally safe, but both carry a low risk of increased suicidal ideation or suicide attempts.

Both drugs are generally tolerable, but side effects of pregabalin tend to be dose dependent. The principal disadvantage of gabapentin seems to be interindividual variability in absorption because of saturation kinetics. Mixed results in monotherapy trials may have resulted from failure to incorporate strategies to compensate for variable absorption in the study designs. This led to extensive examination of doses higher than those tested in pivotal trials in the postmarketing period. Anecdotally, some physicians have used plasma levels as an index of the ability of

an individual patient to absorb gabapentin or of when to discontinue it as the drug was titrated. Optimization of dosing on an individual basis has been important in determining the potential benefits of gabapentin.

Pregabalin is more potent than gabapentin and it is absorbed linearly throughout the range of recommended doses. Both agents have short $t_{1/2}$s. However, pregabalin can be administered twice daily with good clinical efficacy. Gabapentin is generally given three to four times daily. When the results of pivotal trials of similar design were compared, patients treated with pregabalin (600 mg/day) achieved a greater reduction in seizures than did those treated with gabapentin at the highest dose tested (1800 mg/day). Greater potency and reliable oral bioavailability are significant advantages of pregabalin over gabapentin. Patients with a limited capacity to absorb gabapentin may benefit from treatment with pregabalin.

Both gabapentin and pregabalin are approved for adjunctive use in the treatment of partial epilepsy. Though neither drug is approved for these uses in the United States, both drugs have anxiolytic effects and positively affect sleep architecture. These actions could help to prevent seizure exacerbations due to anxiety and insomnia. Neither drug has been approved to use as monotherapy to treat epilepsy in the United States. Gabapentin was approved for use as monotherapy in 40 countries around the world. Testing of pregabalin for use in monotherapy is in progress. Gabapentin is approved for use in children. Pregabalin is not; trials in childhood epilepsy are in progress.

References

1. Ben-Menachem E, Kugler AR. Drugs in development: pregabalin. In: Levy RH, Mattson RH, Meldrum BS, Perucca E, eds. *Antiepileptic Drugs*. 5th ed. New York: Raven Press; 2002:901–905.
2. Taylor CP, Gee NS, Su TZ, et al. A summary of mechanistic hypotheses of gabapentin pharmacology. *Epilepsy Res*. 1998;29:233–249.
3. Taylor CP. Gabapentin: mechanisms of action. In: Levy RH, Mattson RH, Meldrum BS, Perucca E, eds. *Antiepileptic Drugs*. 5th ed. New York: Raven Press; 2002:321–334.
4. Kavoussi R. Pregabalin: From molecule to medicine. *Eur Neuropsychopharmacol*. 2006;16:S128–S133.
5. Vartanian MG, Radulovic LL, Kinsora JJ, et al. Activity profile of pregabalin in rodent models of epilepsy and ataxia. *Epilepsy Res*. 2006;68: 189–205.
6. Bian F, Li Z, Offord J, et al. Calcium channel alpha2-delta type 1 subunit is the major binding protein for pregabalin in neocortex, hippocampus, amygdala, and spinal cord: an ex vivo autoradiographic study in alpha2-delta type 1 genetically modified mice. *Brain Res*. 2006;1075:68–80.
7. Taylor CP, Angelotti T, Eric Fauman E. Pharmacology and mechanism of action of pregabalin: The calcium channel $\alpha_2\delta$ (alpha2-delta) subunit as a target for antiepileptic drug discovery. *Epilepsy Res*. 2007;73:137–150.
8. Sills GJ. The mechanisms of action of gabapentin and pregabalin. *Curr Opin Pharmacol*. 2006;6:108–113.
9. Joshi I, Taylor CP. Pregabalin action at a model synapse: binding to presynaptic calcium channel α_2-δ subunit reduces neurotransmission in mice. *Eur J Pharmacol*. 2006;553:82–88.
10. Taylor, CP. Mechanisms of analgesia by gabapentin and pregabalin—calcium channel $\alpha_2\delta$ [Ca$_v$ α_2-δ] ligands. *Pain*. 2009;142:13–16
11. Schmidt B. Potential antiepileptic drugs: gabapentin. In: Levy R, Mattson R, Meldrum BS, Penry JK, Dreifuss FE, eds. *Antiepileptic Drugs*. 3rd ed. New York: Raven Press; 1989:925–935.
12. Taylor CP. Mechanisms of action of new antiepileptic drugs. In: Chadwick D, ed. *New Trends in Epilepsy Management: The Role of Gabapentin*. London: Royal Society of Medicine Services; 1993:13–40.
13. Satzinger G. Antiepileptics from gamma-aminobutyric acid. *Arzneimittelforschung*. 1994;44:261–266.
14. US Prescribing Information for Gabapentin (Neurontin). Available at http://professionals.epilepsy.com/medications/p_neurontin_pi.html.
15. Bartoszyk GD, Meyerson N, Reimann W, et al. Gabapentin. In: Meldrum BS, Porter RJ, eds. *New Anticonvulsant Drugs*. London: John Libbey; 1986:147–463.

16. Stewart BH, Kugler AR, Thompson PR, et al. A saturable transport mechanism in the intestinal absorption of gabapentin is the underlying cause of lack of proportionality between increasing dose and drug levels in plasma. *Pharm Res.* 1993;10:276–281.

17. Su TZ, Lunney E, Campbell G, et al. Transport of gabapentin, a gamma-amino acid drug, by system L alpha-amino acid transporters: a comparative study in astrocytes, synaptosomes and CHO cells. *J Neurochem.* 1995;64:2125–2131.

18. Hengy H, Kölle EU. Determination of gabapentin in plasma and urine by high-performance liquid chromatography and pre-column labelling for ultraviolet detection. *J Chromatogr.* 1985;341:473–478.

19. Lensmeyer GL, Kempf T, Gidal BE, et al. Optimized method for determination of gabapentin in serum by high-performance liquid chromatography. *Ther Drug Monit.* 1995;17:251–258.

20. Wolf CE, Saady JJ, Poklis A. Determination of gabapentin in serum using solid-phase extraction and gas-liquid chromatography. *J Analyt Toxicol.* 1996;20:498–501.

21. Zour E, Lodhi SA, Nesbitt RU, et al. Stability studies of gabapentin in aqueous solutions. *Pharm Res.* 1992;9:595–600.

22. Potschka H, Feuerstein TJ, Löscher W. Gabapentin-lactam, a close analogue of the anticonvulsant gabapentin, exerts convulsant activity in amygdale kindled rats. *Naunyn Schmiedebergs Archiv Pharmacol.* 2000;361:200–205.

23. Jehle T, Lagreze WA, Blauth E, et al. Gabapentin-lactam (8-aza-spiro[5,4]decan-9-on; GBP-L) inhibits oxygen glucose deprivation-induced [^{3}H]glutamate release and is a neuroprotective agent in a model of acute retinal ischemia. *Naunyn Schmiedebergs Archiv Pharmacol.* 2000;362:74–81.

24. United States Patent 6,054,482, entitled Lactam-free Amino Acids. Inventors: Augart, et al. Assignee: Gödecke Aktiengesellschaft, issued April 25, 2000.

25. Maurer HH, Rump AFE. Intestinal absorption of gabapentin in rats. *Arzneimittelforschung.* 1991;41:104–106.

26. Stevenson CM, Kim JS, Fleisher D. Colonic absorption of anticpileptic agents. *Epilepsia.* 1997;38:63–67.

27. Kriel RL, Birnbaum AK, Cloyd JC, et al. Failure of absorption of gabapentin after rectal administration. *Epilepsia.* 1997;38:1242–1244.

28. Vollmer KO, Anhut H, Thomann P, et al. Pharmacokinetic model and absolute bioavailability of the new anticonvulsant gabapentin. *Adv Epileptol.* 1987;17:209–211.

29. Richens A. Clinical pharmacokinetics of gabapentin. In: Chadwick D, ed. *New Trends in Epilepsy Management: The Role of Gabapentin.* London: Royal Society of Medicine Services; 1993:41–46.

30. McLean MJ. Gabapentin. *Epilepsia.* 1995;36(suppl 2):S73–S76.

31. Beydoun A, Fischer J, Labar DR, et al. Gabapentin monotherapy: II. A 26-week, double-blind, dose-controlled, multicenter study of conversion from polytherapy in outpatients with refractory complex partial or secondarily generalized seizures. The US Gabapentin Study Group 82/83. *Neurology.* 1997;49:746–752.

32. Bergey GK, Morris HH, Rosenfeld W, et al. Gabapentin monotherapy: I. An 8-day, double-blind, dose-controlled, multicenter study in hospitalized patients with refractory complex partial or secondarily generalized seizures. The US Gabapentin Study Group 88/89. *Neurology.* 1997;49:739–745.

33. Beydoun A, Fakhoury T, Nasreddine W, et al. Conversion to high-dose gabapentin monotherapy in patients with medically refractory partial epilepsy. *Epilepsia.* 1998;39:188–193.

34. Wilson EA, Sills GJ, Forrest G, et al. High-dose gabapentin in refractory epilepsy: clinical observations in 50 patients. *Epilepsy Res.* 1998;29:161–166.

35. Gidal BE, Radulovic LL, Kruger S, et al. Inter- and intra-subject variability in gabapentin absorption and absolute bioavailability. *Epilepsy Res.* 2000;40:123–127.

36. Benetello P, Furlanut M, Fortunato M, et al. Oral gabapentin disposition in patients with epilepsy after a high-protein meal. *Epilepsia.* 1997;38:1140–1142.

37. Gidal BE, Maly MM, Kowalski JW, et al. Gabapentin absorption: effect of mixing with foods of varying macronutrient composition. *Ann Pharmacother.* 1998;32:405–408.

38. Gidal BE, Maly MM, Budde J, et al. Effect of a high-protein meal on gabapentin pharmacokinetics. *Epilepsy Res.* 1996;23:71–76.

39. Gidal BE, DeCerce J, Bockbrader HN, et al. Gabapentin bioavailability: effect of dose and frequency of administration in adult patients with epilepsy. *Epilepsy Res.* 1998;31:91–99.

40. Boyd RA, Türck D, Sedman AJ, et al. Effect of age and gender on the single dose pharmacokinetics of gabapentin. *Epilepsia.* 1999;40:474–479.

41. Vollmer KO, von Hodenberg A, Kölle EU. Pharmacokinetics and metabolism of gabapentin in rat, dog and man. *Arzneimittelforschung.* 1986;36:830–839.

42. Bockbrader HN. Clinical pharmacokinetics of gabapentin. *Drugs of Today.* 1995;31:19–25.

43. Ben-Menachem E, Hedner T, Persson LI. Seizure frequency and CSF gabapentin, GABA, and monoamine metabolite concentrations after 3 months' treatment with 900 mg or 1,200 mg gabapentin daily in patients with intractable complex partial seizures. *Neurology.* 1990;40(suppl 1):158.

44. Ben-Menachem E, Persson LI, Hedner T. Selected CSF biochemistry and gabapentin concentrations in the CSF and plasma in patients with partial seizures after a single oral dose of gabapentin. *Epilepsy Res.* 1990;11:45–49.

45. Ben-Menachem E, Sodefelt B, Hamberger A, et al. Seizure frequency and CSF parameters in a double-blind, placebo-controlled trial of gabapentin in patients with intractable complex partial seizures. *Epilepsy Res.* 1995;21:231–236.

46. Wang Y, Welty DF. The simultaneous estimation of the influx and efflux blood–brain barrier permeabilities of gabapentin using a microdialysis-pharmacokinetic approach. *Pharm Res.* 1996;13:398–403.

47. Radulovic LL, Türck D, Hodenberg AV, et al. Disposition of gabapentin (Neurontin) in mice, rats, dogs, and monkeys. *Drug Metab Disp.* 1995;23:441–448.

48. Vollmer KO, Türck D, Bockbrader HN, et al. Summary of Neurontin (gabapentin) clinical pharmacokinetics. *Epilepsia.* 1992;33(suppl 3):77.

49. Feng MR, Turluck D, Burleigh J, et al. Brain microdialysis and PK/PD correlation of pregabalin in rats. *Eur J Drug Metab Pharmacokin.* 2001;26:123–128.

50. Ojemann LM, Friel PN, Ojemann GA. Gabapentin concentrations in human brain. *Epilepsia.* 1988;29:694.

51. Blum RA, Comstock TJ, Sica DA, et al. Pharmacokinetics of gabapentin in subjects with various degrees of renal function. *Clin Pharmacol Ther.* 1994;56:154–159.

52. Callerame KJ, Toledo C, Martinez OA, et al. Gabapentin serum levels in patients on doses greater than 1,800 mg/day. *Epilepsia.* 1995;36(suppl 4):70.

53. Ouellet D, Bockbrader HN, Wesche DL, et al. Population pharmacokinetics of gabapentin in infants and children. *Epilepsy Res.* 2001;47:229–241.

54. Hussein G, Troupin AS, Montouris G. Gabapentin interaction with felbamate. *Neurology.* 1996;47:1106.

55. Busch JA, Radulovic LL, Bockbrader HN, et al. Effect of Maalox TC on single-dose pharmacokinetics of gabapentin capsules in healthy subjects. *Pharm Res.* 1992;9(suppl):S315.

56. Eldon MA, Underwood BA, Randinitis EJ, et al. Gabapentin does not interact with a contraceptive regimen of norethindrone acetate and ethinyl estradiol. *Neurology.* 1998;50:1146–1148.

57. Frye MA, Kimbrell TA, Dunn RT, et al. Gabapentin does not alter single-dose lithium pharmacokinetics. *J Clin Psychopharmacol.* 1998;18:461–464.

58. Crawford P, Ghadualis E, Lane R, et al. Gabapentin as an antiepileptic drug in man. *J Neurol Neurosurg Psychiatry.* 1987;50:682–686.

59. Sivenius J, Kalviainen R, Ylinen A, et al. Double-blind study of gabapentin in the treatment of partial seizures. *Epilepsia.* 1991;32:539–542.

60. Lindberger M, Luhr O, Johannessen S, et al. Serum concentrations and effects of gabapentin and vigabatrin: observations from a dose titration study. *Ther Drug Monit.* 2003;25:457–462.

61. UK Gabapentin Study Group. Gabapentin in partial epilepsy. *Lancet.* 1990;335:1114–1117.

62. US Gabapentin Study Group, No 5. Gabapentin as add-on therapy in refractory partial epilepsy: a double-blind, placebo-controlled, parallel-group study. *Neurology.* 1993;43:2292–2298.

63. Anhut H, Ashman P, Feuerstein TJ, et al. Gabapentin (Neurontin) as add-on therapy in patients with partial seizures: a double-blind, placebo-controlled study. The International Gabapentin Study Group. *Epilepsia.* 1994;35:795–801.

64. Baulac M, Cavalcanti D, Semah F, et al. Gabapentin add-on therapy with adaptable dosages in 610 patients with partial epilepsy: an open, observational study. *Seizure.* 1998;7:55–62.

65. Bruni J. Outcome evaluation of gabapentin as add-on therapy for partial seizures. "NEON" Study Investigators Group. Neurontin Evaluation of Outcomes in Neurological Practice. *Can J Neurol Sci.* 1998;25:134–140.

66. McLean MJ, Morrell MJ, Willmore LJ, et al. Safety and tolerability of gabapentin as adjunctive therapy in a large multicenter study. *Epilepsia.* 1999;40:965–972.

67. Morrell MJ, McLean MJ, Willmore LJ, et al. Efficacy of gabapentin as adjunctive therapy in a large multicenter study. *Seizure.* 2000;9:241–248.

68. Beran R, Berkovic S, Black A, et al. AUStralian study of titration to effect profile of safety (AUS-STEPS): high-dose gabapentin (Neurontin) in partial seizures. *Epilepsia.* 2001;42:1335–1339.

69. Agomuoh TC, Barkley GL. Clinical experience with gabapentin in a tertiary referral center. *Epilepsia.* 1995;36(suppl 4):70.

70. Anderson BL, Haessly SM, Weatherford KJ, et al. An observational study of efficacy and tolerance of gabapentin. *Epilepsia.* 1995;36(suppl 4):S70.

71. Doherty KP, Gates JR, Penovich PE, et al. Gabapentin in a medically refractory epilepsy population. Seizure response and unusual side effects. *Epilepsia.* 1995;36(suppl 4):S71.

72. Hosain S, Labar DR, Nikolov B, et al. Gabapentin use in the general epileptic population. *Epilepsia.* 1995;36(suppl 4):S70.

73. Kelly KM, Kothary SP, Beydoun A. Safety and efficacy of extended gabapentin therapy for patients with complex partial or secondarily generalized seizures. *Epilepsia.* 1995;36(suppl 4):S69.

74. Piña-Garza JE, Bukhari AA, Laowattana S, et al. Treatment of patients with refractory partial epilepsies with gabapentin: a retrospective analysis. *Epilepsia.* 1995;36(suppl 4):S69.

75. Perry JR, Sawka C. Add-on gabapentin for refractory seizures in patients with brain tumours. *Can J Neurol Sci.* 1996;23:128–131.
76. Ojemann LM, Wilensky AJ, Temkin NR, et al. Long-term treatment with gabapentin for partial epilepsy. *Epilepsy Res.* 1992;13:159–165.
77. US Gabapentin Study Group. The long-term safety and efficacy of gabapentin (Neurontin) as add-on therapy in drug-resistant partial epilepsy. *Epilepsy Res.* 1994;18:67–73.
78. Leidermann DB, Koto EM, LaMoreaux LK, et al. Long-term therapy with gabapentin (GBP; Neurontin): 5-year experience from a US open-label trial. US Gabapentin Study Group 13. *Epilepsia.* 1995;36(suppl 4):S68.
79. Handforth A, Treiman DM. Efficacy and tolerance of long-term, high-dose gabapentin: additional observations. *Epilepsia.* 1994;35:1032–1037.
80. Sivenius J, Ylinen A, Kalviainen R, et al. Long-term study with gabapentin in patients with drug-resistant epileptic seizures. *Arch Neurol.* 1994;51:1047–1050.
81. Muscas GC, Chiroli S, Luceri F, et al. Conversion from thrice daily to twice daily administration of gabapentin (GBP) in partial epilepsy: analysis of clinical efficacy and plasma levels. *Seizure.* 2000;9:47–50.
82. Leach JP, Girvan J, Paul A, et al. Gabapentin and cognition: a double-blind, dose-ranging, placebo-controlled study in refractory epilepsy. *J Neurol Neurosurg Psychiatry.* 1997;62:372–376.
83. Chadwick D, Anhut H, Murray G, et al. Gabapentin (GBP; Neurontin) monotherapy in patients with newly diagnosed epilepsy: results of a double-blind fixed-dose study comparing three dosages of gabapentin and open-label carbamazepine. *Epilepsia.* 1997;38:34.
84. Brodie MJ, Chadwick DW, Anhut H, et al. Gabapentin versus lamotrigine monotherapy: a double-blind comparison in newly diagnosed epilepsy. *Epilepsia.* 2002;43:993–1000.
85. Rowan AJ, Ramsay RE. Outcome of VA Coop Study #428: treatment of seizures in the elderly population. International Geriatric Epilepsy Symposium; September 12–14, 2003; Coral Gables, FL.
86. Tatum WO, Zachariah SB. Gabapentin treatment of seizures in acute intermittent porphyria. *Neurology.* 1995;45:1216–1217.
87. Yandel ML, Watters MR. Treatment of complex partial epilepticus unmasking acute intermittent porphyria in a patient with resected anaplastic glioma. *Clin Neurol Neurosurg.* 1995;97:261–263.
88. Krauss GL, Simmons-O'Brien E, Campbell M. Successful treatment of seizures and porphyria with gabapentin. *Neurology.* 1995;45:594–595.
89. Chadwick D, Leiderman DB, Sauerman W, et al. Gabapentin in generalized seizures. *Epilepsy Res.* 1996;25:191–197.
90. Bourgeois B, Brown L, Pellock J, et al. Gabapentin (Neurontin) monotherapy in children with benign childhood epilepsy with centrotemporal spikes (BECTS): a 36-week, double-blind, placebo-controlled study. *Epilepsia.* 1998;39(suppl 6):163.
91. Khurana DS, Riviello J, Helmers S, et al. Efficacy of gabapentin therapy in children with refractory partial seizures. *J Pediatr.* 1996;128:829–833.
92. Appleton R, Fichtner K, LaMoreaux L, et al. Gabapentin as add-on therapy in children with refractory partial seizures: a 12-week, multicentre, double-blind, placebo-controlled study. Gabapentin Paediatric Study Group. *Epilepsia.* 1999;40:1147–1154.
93. Korn-Merker E, Boursiak P, Boenigk HE. Gabapentin in childhood epilepsy: a prospective evaluation of efficacy and safety. *Epilepsy Res.* 2000;38:2732.
94. Appleton R, Fichtner K, LaMoreaux L, et al. Gabapentin as add-on therapy in children with refractory partial seizures: a 24-week, multicentre, open-label study. *Dev Med Child Neurol.* 2001;43:269–273.
95. Trudeau V, Myers S, LaMoreaux L, et al. Gabapentin in naive childhood absence epilepsy: results from two double-blind, placebo-controlled, multicenter studies. *J Child Neurol.* 1996;11:470–475.
96. Litzinger MJ, Wiscombe N, Hanny A, et al. Increased seizures and aggression seen in persons with mental retardation and epilepsy treated with Neurontin. *Epilepsia.* 1995;36(suppl 4):S71.
97. Zupanc ML, Schroeder VM. Behavioral changes in children on gabapentin. *Epilepsia.* 1995;36(suppl 4):S73.
98. Wolf SM, Shinnar S, Kang H, et al. Gabapentin toxicity in children manifesting as behavioral changes. *Epilepsia.* 1996;36:1203–1205.
99. Lee DO, Steingard RJ, Cesena M, et al. Behavioral side effects of gabapentin in children. *Epilepsia.* 1996;37:87–90.
100. Vossler DG. Exacerbation of seizures in Lennox–Gastaut syndrome by gabapentin. *Neurology.* 1996;46:852–853.
101. Lhatoo SD, Wong CK, Polizzi G, et al. Long-term retention rates of lamotrigine, gabapentin and topiramate in chronic epilepsy. *Epilepsia.* 2000;41:1592–1596.
102. Depondt C, Yuen AWC, Bell GS, et al. The long term retention of levetiracetam in a large cohort of patients with epilepsy. *J Neurol Neurosurg Psychiatr.* 2006;77:101–103.
103. Zaccara G, Messori A, Cincotta M, et al. Comparison of the efficacy and tolerability of new antiepileptic drugs: what can we learn from long-term studies? *Acta Neurol Scand.* 2006;114:157–168.
104. Simister RJ, Sander JW, Koepp MJ. Long-term retention rates of new antiepileptic drugs in adults with chronic epilepsy and learning disability. *Epilepsy Behav.* 2007;10:336–339.
105. Carpay JA, Aalbers K, Graveland GA, et al. Retention of new AEDs institutionalized intellectually disabled patients. *Seizure.* 2009;18:119–123.
106. New drug application for gabapentin. Morris Plains, NJ: Parke-Davis, Division of Warner-Lambert Company.
107. Fischer JH, Barr AN, Rogers SL, et al. Lack of serious toxicity following gabapentin overdose. *Neurology.* 1994;44:982–983.
108. Fernandez MC, Walter FG, Petersen LR, et al. Gabapentin, valproic acid, and ethanol intoxication: elevated blood levels with mild clinical effects. *Clin Toxicol.* 1996;34:437–439.
109. FDA ALERT [1/31/2008, updated: 12/16/2008]: Information for Healthcare Professionals Suicidal Behavior and Ideation and Antiepileptic Drugs. Available at http://www.fda.gov/CDER/drug/InfoSheets/HCP/antiepilepticsHCP.htm.
110. FDA statistical review and evaluation, antiepileptic drugs and suicide. Available at http://www.fda.gov/ohrms/dockets/ac/08/briefing/2008-4372b1-01-FDA.pdf.
111. FDA Sponsor Letter, Antiepileptic Drugs and Suicide. Available at http://www.fda.gov/CDER/drug/InfoSheets/HCP/antiepilepticsHCP.htm.
112. Asconape J, Collins T. Weight gain associated with the use of gabapentin. *Epilepsia.* 1995;36(suppl 4):S72.
113. Gidal BE, Maly MM, Nemire RE, et al. Weight gain and gabapentin therapy. *Ann Pharmacother.* 1995;29:1048.
114. De Toledo JC, Toledo C, DeCerce J, et al. Changes in body weight with chronic, high-dose gabapentin therapy. *Ther Drug Monit.* 1997;19:394–396.
115. Buetefisch CM, Gutierrez A, Gutmann L. Choreoathetotic movements: a possible side effect of gabapentin. *Neurology.* 1996;46:851–852.
116. Chudnow RS, Dewey RB, Lawson CR. Choreoathetosis as a side effect of gabapentin therapy in severely neurologically impaired patients. *Arch Neurol.* 1997;54:910–912.
117. Reeves AL, So EL, Sharbrough FW, et al. Movement disorders associated with the use of gabapentin. *Epilepsia.* 1996;37:988–990.
118. Tallian KB, Nahata MC, Lo, W, et al. Gabapentin associated with aggressive behavior in pediatric patients with seizures. *Epilepsia.* 1996;37:501–502.
119. Rowbotham M, Harden N, Stacey B, et al. Gabapentin for the treatment of postherpetic neuralgia: a randomized controlled trial. *JAMA.* 1998;280:1837–1842.
120. Data on file. Parke-Davis, Division of Warner-Lambert Company, now Pfizer Inc.
121. Pennell PB. Antiepileptic drugs during pregnancy: what is known, and which AEDs seem to be safest? *Epilepsia.* 2008;49(suppl 9):43–55.
122. Tomson T, Battino D. Teratogenic effects of antiepileptic drugs. *Seizure.* 2008;17:166–171.
123. Meador KJ, Pennell PB, Harden CL, et al. Pregnancy registries in epilepsy. A consensus statement on health outcomes. *Neurology.* 2008;71:1109–1117.
124. Sigler RE, Gough AW, de la Iglesia FA. Pancreatic acinar cell neoplasia in male Wistar rats following 2 years of gabapentin exposure. *Toxicology.* 1995;98:73–92.
125. Fowler ML, Sigler RE, de la Iglesia FA, et al. Absence of Ki-ras mutations in exocrine pancreatic tumors from male rats chronically exposed to gabapentin. *Mutat Res.* 1995;327:151–160.
126. Dominick MA, Robertson DG, Bleavins MR, et al. Alpha 2u-globulin nephropathy without nephrocarcinogenesis in male Wistar rats administered 1-(aminomethyl)cyclohexaneacetic acid. *Toxicol Appl Pharmacol.* 1991;111:375–387.
127. Bockbrader HN, Burger PJ, Kugler AR, et al. The oral clearance (CL/F) of commonly prescribed antiepileptic drugs (AEDs) is unaffected by concomitant administration of pregabalin in adult patients with refractory partial seizures. *Neurology.* 2000;54(suppl 3):421.
128. Bockbrader HN, Hunt T, Strand J, et al. Pregabalin pharmacokinetics and safety in healthy volunteers: results from two phase I studies. *Neurology.* 2000;54(suppl 3):A421.
129. Piyapolrungroj N, Li C, Bockbrader H, et al. Mucosal uptake of gabapentin vs. pregabalin in the small intestine. *Pharm Res.* 2001;18:1126–1130.
130. Randinitis EJ, Posvar EL, Alvey CW, et al. Pharmacokinetics of pregabalin in subjects with various degrees of renal function. *J Clin Pharmacol.* 2003;43:277–283.
131. Corrigan BW, Bockbrader H, Burger PJ, et al. Pregabalin population pharmacokinetics in patients with refractory seizures. Presented at the 5th European Congress on Epileptology; October 9, 2002; Madrid, Spain.
132. Wilson E, Brodie MJ, Bockbrader HN, et al. Pregabalin drug interaction studies in patients with epilepsy maintained on either valproate (VPA), lamotrigine (LTG), phenytoin (PHY), or carbamazepine (CBZ). Presented at the 5th European Congress on Epileptology; October 9, 2002; Madrid, Spain.
133. Brodie MJ, Wilson EA, Wesche DL, et al. Pregabalin drug interaction studies: lack of effect on the pharmacokinetics of carbamazepine, phenytoin, lamotrigne, and valproate in patients with partial epilepsy. *Epilepsia.* 2005;46(9):1407–1413.
134. May TW, Rambeck B, Neb R, et al. Serum concentrations of pregabalin in patients with epilepsy: the influence of dose, age, and comedication. *Ther Drug Monit.* 2007;29(6):789–794.
135. US Full Prescribing Information for Pregabalin (Lyrica). Available at http://media.pfizer.com/files/products/uspi_lyrica.pdf.
136. Kugler AR, Robbins JL, Strand JC, et al. Pregabalin overview: a novel CNS-active compound with anticonvulsant activity. Presented at the 56th Annual Meeting of the American Epilepsy Society; December 11, 2002; Seattle, Washington.

137. French JA, Kugler AR, Robbins JL, et al. Dose-response trial of pregabalin adjunctive therapy in patients with partial seizures. *Neurology.* 2003;60: 1631–1637.

138. Arroyo S, Anhut H, Kugler AR et al. Pregabalin add-on treatment: a randomized, double-blind, placebo-controlled, dose-response study in adults with partial seizures. *Epilepsia.* 2004;45:20–27.

139. Beydoun A, Uthman BM, Kugler AR et al. Safety and efficacy of two pregabalin regimens for add-on treatment of partial epilepsy. *Neurology.* 2005;64:475–480.

140. Miller R, Frame B, Corrigan B, et al. Exposure-response analysis of pregabalin add-on treatment of patients with refractory partial seizures. *Clin Pharmacol Ther.* 2003;73:491–505.

141. Perucca E, Ramsay RE, Robbins JL, et al. Pregabalin demonstrates anticonvulsants activity onset by the second day. Presented at the 56th Annual Meeting of the American Epilepsy Society; December 11, 2002; Seattle, Washington.

142. Uthman BM, Beydoun A, Kugler AR, et al. Long-term efficacy and tolerability of pregabalin in patients with partial seizures. Presented at the 56th Annual Meeting of the American Epilepsy Society; December 11, 2002; Seattle, Washington.

143. Gazzola DM, Balcer LJ, French JA. Seizure-free outcome in randomized add-on trials of the new antiepileptic drugs. *Epilepsia.* 2007;48(7): 1303–1307.

144. Elger CE, Brodie MJ, Anhut H, et al. Pregabalin add-on treatment in patients with partial seizures: a novel evaluation of flexible-dose and fixed-dose treatment in a double-blind, placebo-controlled study. *Epilepsia.* 2005;46:1926–1936.

145. Briggs DE, Lee CM, Spiegel K, et al. Reduction of secondarily generalized tonic–clonic (SGTC) seizures with pregabalin. *Epilepsy Res.* 2008;82: 86–92.

146. Gil-Nagel A, Zaccara G, Baldinetti F, et al. Add-on treatment with pregabalin for partial seizures with or without generalization: pooled data analysis of four randomized placebo-controlled trials. *Seizure.* 2009;18:184–192.

147. Otoul C, Arrigo C, van Rijckevorsel K, et al. Meta-analysis and indirect comparisons of levetiracetam with other second-generation antiepileptic drugs in partial epilepsy. *Clin Neuropharmacol.* 2005;28:72–78.

148. Modur PN, Milteer WE. Adjunctive pregabalin therapy in mentally retarded, developmentally delayed patients with epilepsy. *Epilepsy Behav.* 2008;13:554–556.

149. Vera-Llonch M, Brandenburg NA, Oster G. Cost-effectiveness of add-on therapy with pregabalin in patients with refractory partial epilepsy. *Epilepsia.* 2008;49(3):431–437.

150. Kubota T, Fang J, Meltzer LT, et al. Pregabalin enhances nonrapid eye movement sleep. *J Pharmacol Exp Therap I.* 2001;299:1095–1105.

151. Hindmarch I, Dawson J, Stanley N. A double-blind study in healthy volunteers to assess the effects of on sleep of pregabalin compared to alprazolam and placebo. *Sleep.* 2005;28:187–193.

152. de Haas S, Otte A, deWeerd A, et al. Exploratory polysomnographic evaluation of pregablin on sleep disturbance in patients with epilepsy. *J Clin Sleep Med.* 2007;3:473–478.

153. Romigi A, Izzi F, Marciani MG, et al. Pregabalin as add-on therapy induces REM sleep enhancement in partial epilepsy: a polysomonographic study. *Eur J Neurol.* 2009;16:70–75.

154. Braga AJ, Chidley K. Self-poisoning with lamotrigine and pregabalin. *Anaesthesia.* 2007;62:524–527.

155. Brigell MG, Carter CM, Smith F, et al. Prospective evaluation of the ophthalmologic safety of pregabalin shows no evidence of toxicity. Presented at the 56th Annual Meeting of the American Epilepsy Society; December 11, 2002; Seattle, Washington.

156. Huppertz H-J, Feuerstein TJ, Schulze-Bonhage A. Myoclonus in epilepsy patients with anticonvulsive add-on therapy with pregabalin. *Epilepsia.* 2001;42:790–792.

157. Knake S, Klein KM, Hattemer K, et al. Pregabalin-induced generalized myoclonic status epilepticus in patients with chronic pain. *Epilepsy Behav.* 2007;11:471–473.

158. Hellwig S, Amtage F. Letter to the Editor. Pregabalin-induced cortical negative myoclonus in a patient with neuropathic pain. *Epilepsy Behav.* 2008;13:418–420.

159. Hitiris N, Barrett JA, Brodie MJ. Erectile dysfunction associated with pregabalin add-on treatment in patients with partial seizures: five case reports. *Epilepsy Behav.* 2006;8:418–421.

160. Hindmarch I, Dawson J, Stanley N. Evaluation of cognitive and psychomotor profile of pregabalin compared to alprazolam in normal volunteers. Presented at the 56th Annual Meeting of the American Epilepsy Society; December 11, 2002; Seattle, Washington.

161. Zaccara G, Gangemi PF, Cincotta M. Central nervous system adverse effects of new antiepileptic drugs. A meta-analysis of placebo-controlled studies. *Seizure.* 2008;17:405–421.

162. www.pfizerpro.com.

163. *Datamonitor,* a publication of Pfizer Inc. August 20, 2001.

164. Field MJ, Oles RJ, Lewis AS, et al. Gabapentin (Neurontin) and S-(+)-3-isobutylgaba represent a novel class of selective antihyperalgesic agents. *Br J Pharmacol.* 1997;121:1513–1522.

165. Field MJ, Coz PJ, Stott E et al. Identification of the α2-δ-1 subunit of voltage-dependent calcium channels as a molecular target for pain mediating the analgesic actions of pregabalin. *Proc Natl Acad Sci.* 2004;103: 17537–17542.

CHAPTER 57 ■ LAMOTRIGINE

FRANK GILLIAM AND BARRY E. GIDAL

CHEMISTRY AND MECHANISM OF ACTION

Lamotrigine is a phenyltriazine, tertiary amine derivative (3,5-diamino-6-(2,3-dichlorophenyl)-1,2,4-trizine, MW = 256.09) which is poorly soluble in water or alcohol. A primary cellular mechanism of action for lamotrigine is blockade of neuronal sodium channels that is both voltage and use-dependent (greater blockade during repetitive activation) (1–7). Lamotrigine blockade of sodium channels activated from depolarized membrane potentials occurs at lower concentrations than those required to elicit blockade from hyperpolarized membrane, and occurs at clinically achievable concentrations (6). Lamotrigine appears to stabilize the inactivated state of the Na^+ channel. Recently, a potential binding site within the Na^+ channel pore has been identified (8). In addition to sodium channels, lamotrigine produces dose-dependent inhibition of high voltage-activated Ca^{++} currents, possibly through inhibition of presynaptic N- and P/Q-type Ca^{++} channels (9,10). Despite its apparent clinical activity in human absence seizures, lamotrigine does not appear to inhibit low-voltage currents mediated by T-type Ca^{++} channels. Although these actions are mechanistically similar to those of phenytoin, important differences do exist between these agents. Veratrine-evoked release of both glutamate and GABA are inhibited by phenytoin. At similar concentrations, however, lamotrigine is twice as effective in inhibiting the release of glutamate as compared to GABA (11). Release of excitatory amino acid neurotransmitters such as glutamate and aspartate is blocked during sustained repetitive firing. Animal models also suggest that lamotrigine inhibits ischemia-induced release of excitatory neurotransmitters (12–15). Inhibition of nitric oxide release (16) and serotonin uptake (17) may also modestly contribute to lamotrigine's action in both epilepsy and affective disorders. Lamotrigine appears to display only modest inhibition of potassium channels. Similarly, lamotrigine is only a weak inhibitor of 5_HT uptake in humans or rodents (17). Lamotrigine is not an N-methyl-D-aspartate (NMDA) receptor antagonist (18), nor does it displace other ligands for this receptor complex (CNQX, CGS, TCHP). Further, lamotrigine does not appear to alter either plasma or brain GABA concentrations in humans (19,20). Most likely, the antiepileptic actions and clinical spectrum of lamotrigine can be predominantly explained by the combination of both Na^+ and Ca^{++}(N, P/Q) channel inhibition.

Lamotrigine is effective in preventing maximal electroshock seizures in mice with potency and duration being similar to phenytoin and carbamazepine (21). Lamotrigine does not prevent pentylenetetrazole-induced clonus, a model of absence seizures (21). Lamotrigine is active in suppressing photically evoked afterdischarges and photoconvulsive responses (22), and has demonstrated activity in the genetic epilepsy-prone rat (23). Lamotrigine has also demonstrated efficacy in the electrically induced electroencephalogram after discharge model (24). While lamotrigine does not prevent the development of cortical kindling in rats, it does attenuate kindled seizures in a dose-dependent manner (24–26).

ABSORPTION, DISTRIBUTION, AND METABOLISM

Lamotrigine is an orally administered drug, and is available in a variety of dosage strengths, including dispersible tables. Bioequivalence has been established between these various product formulations. Lamotrigine is completely absorbed, with a bioavailability of 98% (27,28). Peak serum concentrations are achieved within 1 to 3 hours following oral administration (29–31). Lamotrigine displays linear oral absorption, with proportionality observed following doses up to 700 mg (32–34). A secondary peak in serum concentration may occur between 4 to 6 hours following either oral or parenteral administration, suggesting enterohepatic recycling. Food does not significantly affect drug absorption (35).

Recently, an extended release formulation of lamotrigine has been marketed (Lamictal XR). This dosage formulation is enteric coated and has a modified release core. A small aperture is drilled through the coating, allowing for a gradual dissolution rate over approximately 12 to 15 hours. Pharmacokinetic studies in patients with epilepsy (36) have demonstrated that this new extended-release formulation is bioequivalent to the immediate-release brand product, when patients are converted from twice-daily branded lamotrigine (Lamictal), to once-daily Lamictal XR. In this study, peak-to-trough fluctuations were minimized (as compared to immediate-release Lamictal) following conversion to once-daily administration, particularly in those patients receiving a concomitant enzyme-inducing antiepileptic drug (AED).

Lamotrigine is also systemically absorbed following rectal administration, although mean AUC are approximately 50% of corresponding oral administration values (37,38).

Lamotrigine is only moderately bound to plasma proteins (approximately 56%) and is constant over a concentration range of at least 1 to 10 μg/mL (32). In vitro studies have demonstrated that lamotrigine protein binding is unaffected by phenytoin, phenobarbital, carbamazepine, or valproate (32).

Lamotrigine volume of distribution is independent of dose and ranges between 0.9 to 1.2 L/kg in healthy volunteers (14,39). Data derived from rodents as well as human ex vivo placental perfusion studies suggest that lamotrigine easily and rapidly crosses the placenta (39) and that lamotrigine is present in maternal milk at potentially clinically significant levels (40). In humans, lamotrigine is extensively hepatically metabolized by UDP-glucuronyltransferase (UGT 1A4) (41). Glucuronide conjugation can occur at both heterocyclic nitrogen atoms to form a quaternary amine glucuronide (42). In healthy volunteers, 70% of a single dose was recovered in the urine (32), with the 5-N and 2-N-glucuronide metabolite accounting for 90% of the recovered dose. This glucuronide metabolite is pharmacologically inactive. Renal elimination of unchanged drug accounts for a minor fraction of administered dose (<10%).

When given as monotherapy in adults, lamotrigine elimination half-life is approximately 24 to 29 hours. Oral clearance average 0.35 to 0.59 mL/min/kg (43). Lamotrigine clearance is higher in children, and lower in the elderly as compared to young adults. The concentration/dose ratio of lamotrigine was approximately 30% to 50% lower in young children (3 to 6 years) versus that seen in older children (7 to 15 years) or young adults (44). Mean lamotrigine oral clearance and elimination half-life were 0.64 mL/kg/min and 32 hours, respectively in 12 children (4 to 11 years) receiving monotherapy (45). Advancing age has modest effects upon lamotrigine clearance and half-life. In a group of elderly volunteers, age 65 to 76 years, lamotrigine clearance was 37% lower when compared to a group of young adults (26 to 38 years) (31).

There is evidence demonstrating that lamotrigine undergoes autoinduction. Population analysis of sparse data obtained retrospectively from 163 monotherapy patients demonstrated a 17% increase in clearance over a 48-week period (46). As lamotrigine initiation usually involves gradual dose escalation, this modest degree of autoinduction is not clinically meaningful.

Hepatic disease, depending upon severity, can influence lamotrigine pharmacokinetics, and patients with Child–Pugh scores of 5 to 6 (B) or 7 to 9 (C) requiring dosage reductions of 50% to 75%, respectively (47). No significant differences in the plasma clearance of lamotrigine have been noted in patients with chronic renal failure (48). Approximately 17% of a lamotrigine dose may be removed by hemodialysis, with a corresponding reduction in half-life to about 13 hours (49).

The apparent oral clearance of lamotrigine does not appear to significantly differ between men and women (46). Importantly, recent data suggest that lamotrigine oral clearance may be markedly (>65%) increased during pregnancy, with changes being most evident during the second and third trimester. Lamotrigine clearance appears to return to prepregnancy values during the postpartum period (50). The magnitude of alterations in lamotrigine concentrations exceeds that described for many of the older AEDs, perhaps due to sex-hormone mediated activation of UDP-glucuronyltransferase (51,52).

Lamotrigine apparent oral clearance may increase by as much as 150% during the second and third trimesters, and there are indications that women treated with this agent may experience increased seizure frequency. Data from Pennell et al. (53) suggested that lamotrigine total and unbound oral clearance were increased during all three trimesters, with peaks of 94% (total) and 89% (unbound) in the third trimester. In this study, it was noted that seizure frequency significantly increased when the LTG level decreased to 65% of the preconceptional individualized target lamotrigine serum concentration. Lamotrigine oral clearance appears to return to baseline values during the early postpartum period, which will likely necessitate further dose modifications. These observations clearly support the notion of monitoring lamotrigine serum concentrations both during pregnancy as well as postpartum.

A well-defined serum concentration–effect range for lamotrigine has yet to be conclusively established (54) and individual patients may respond to a wide range of plasma concentrations. A target range of 4 to 14 µg/mL has been suggested by some investigators however for patients with epilepsy (55,56). Use of serum concentration data may aid in the interpretation of drug interactions and compliance issues. Given ongoing concerns regarding the interchangeability of various generic formulations of this drug (57,58), additional monitoring of serum concentrations both before, and following generic substitution would also seem prudent.

DRUG INTERACTIONS

Effect of Other Drugs on Lamotrigine

Comedication with Inducing AEDs

Lamotrigine displays substantial interpatient variability in plasma clearance; a phenomenon that can largely be explained by the presence or absence of concomitant drug therapy (59,60). Lamotrigine elimination half life is reduced by approximately 50% ($t_{1/2}$ about 12 to 15 hours) in the presence of UGT-inducing drugs, such as carbamazepine, phenobarbital, primidone, and phenytoin (22). While the effect of adding an enzyme inducer to a regimen containing lamotrigine is well recognized, an important clinical question involves the time course of *deinduction*, following the removal of a concomitant inducer such as phenytoin or carbamazepine. In a recent pharmacokinetic analysis of lamotrigine serum concentration data derived from the pivotal conversion to monotherapy trial (61), Anderson et al. found that mean lamotrigine plasma concentrations approximately doubled following the withdrawal of concomitant phenytoin treatment, increases of only 50% to 75% occurred following the withdrawal of carbamazepine cotherapy. Interestingly these data suggested that lamotrigine concentrations did not significantly change (increase) until the concomitant enzyme-inducing drug was completely removed, and concentrations of either phenytoin or carbamazepine approached zero (62).

There do not appear to be any significant interactions between lamotrigine and newer AEDs such as topiramate, felbamate, gabapentin, pregabalin, zonisamide, vigabatrin or levetiracetam. Similarly, pharmacokinetic interactions between lacosamide and lamotrigine would not be expected. Modest reductions (~30%) in lamotrigine serum concentrations have been noted in patients receiving concomitant oxcarbazepine (63–66).

Comedication with Valproate

As lamotrigine does not undergo cytochrome P450-dependent metabolism, only drugs that inhibit UGTs, such as valproate, will decrease lamotrigine clearance and result in increased plasma concentrations. Valproate can markedly reduce lamotrigine clearance and prolong elimination half-life ($t_{1/2}$ about 60 hours) (67). Recent pharmacokinetic studies in adult volunteers have suggested that the maximal theoretical inhibition of lamotrigine clearance by valproate is approximately 65%, with 50% of maximal inhibition occurring at valproate plasma concentrations of approximately 5 to 6 µg/mL. Maximal theoretical inhibition appears to occur at valproate concentrations of approximately 50 µg/mL. These data suggest that valproate-mediated inhibition of lamotrigine begins at very low valproate doses (e.g., 125 to 250 mg/day), with maximal inhibition occurring at valproate doses of approximately 500 mg/day (68).

While earlier studies suggested that concurrent treatment with lamotrigine may result in modestly decreased valproate serum concentrations, this is unlikely to be of clinical significance (69,70).

Effect of Lamotrigine upon Other Drugs

Lamotrigine does not induce or inhibit the mixed-function oxidase system (cytochrome P450 isozymes). In addition, lamotrigine is not extensively bound to plasma proteins. These properties would predict lamotrigine to have a low incidence of *causing* pharmacokinetic interactions. Addition of lamotrigine does not alter serum concentrations of either phenytoin, phenobarbital, primidone, carbamazepine, or carbamazepine epoxide (43,49,71,72). Lamotrigine does not appear to significantly alter hormone concentrations in female volunteers taking oral contraceptives (OCPs) (73).

Effect of Non-AEDs on Lamotrigine

Daily doses of acetaminophen, a drug that is 55% eliminated by glucuronide conjugation, but not an inducer of UGT, unexpectedly increased lamotrigine clearance. Occasional use of acetaminophen would not be expected to alter lamotrigine pharmacokinetics (74). One anecdotal report has suggested a potential interaction between the serotonin-selective reuptake inhibitor sertraline and lamotrigine, with lamotrigine serum concentrations increasing following the addition of the antidepressant (75).

While lamotrigine does not alter the pharmacokinetics of oral contraceptive medications, recent clinical reports have suggested that concomitant treatment with combined OCPs may decrease lamotrigine serum concentrations, possibly due to induction of UGT by ethinyl estradiol (76,77). The addition of an OCP containing ethinyl estradiol may decrease lamotrigine serum concentrations by as much as 50%. Importantly, this interaction dissipates quite rapidly during the pill-free week, and within 1 week following discontinuation of OCP.

EFFICACY

Lamotrigine is indicated as adjunctive therapy for the following seizure types in patients ≥2 years of age:

- partial seizures.
- primary generalized tonic–clonic seizures.
- generalized seizures of Lennox–Gastaut syndrome.

The newer extended-release formulation is currently only FDA approved as adjunctive treatment for partial seizures (with or without secondary generalization) in patients greater than 13 years of age.

In addition, lamotrigine is indicated for conversion to monotherapy in adults (≥16 years of age) with partial seizures who are receiving treatment with carbamazepine, phenytoin, phenobarbital, primidone, or valproate as the single background AED. To date, although data from several U.S. and European clinical trials suggest utility, lamotrigine has not yet received FDA approval as initial monotherapy.

Adjunctive Therapy for Partial Seizures

Seven premarketing multicenter, double-blind, placebo-controlled add-on trials supported the efficacy of lamotrigine as adjunctive treatment for partial seizures in adults (78). The study with the highest dose (500 mg) (79) demonstrated a mean reduction in seizure frequency of 36% compared to baseline. Seizure frequency was reduced by greater than 50% in about one quarter of these patients. The placebo group had an 8% reduction in seizure frequency relative to baseline. These studies supported the initial approval for the indication of lamotrigine as adjunctive therapy for partial seizures in persons 16 years and older. A subsequent pediatric trial demonstrated efficacy over placebo in 201 children from 40 sites in the United States and France, and supported an FDA indication for children up to age 2 years (80).

Naritoku and colleagues (81) have recently confirmed that once-daily, extended-release lamotrigine was effective as adjunctive treatment in patients (13 years and older) with partial seizures, many of whom had failed multiple other AEDs. In this study, the percentage of patients with at least a 50% reduction in seizure frequency was significantly greater than placebo (42% vs. 24%, $P = 0.0037$).

Monotherapy for Partial Seizures

Efficacy as monotherapy in partial seizures was shown by a multicenter, double-blind, randomized trial comparing 500 mg of lamotrigine to an active control of 1000 mg of valproate (61). The primary endpoint was proportion of patients completing the trial by not meeting the exit criteria of a doubling of greatest 2-day or 1-month seizure rates observed in the baseline period; in the protocol analysis, 56% of patients taking lamotrigine completed compared to 20% receiving low-dose valproate. Lamotrigine has been shown to have equivalent efficacy to immediate-release carbamazepine (82) and phenytoin (83) in double-blind, randomized clinical studies of recent onset epilepsy in adults. Similarly, lamotrigine was shown to have comparable effectiveness when compared to controlled-release carbamazepine in newly diagnosed elderly patients with epilepsy (84).

The recently published SANAD trial (85), an unblinded randomized effectiveness trial conducted in the United Kingdom, suggested that lamotrigine was at least as effective as carbamazepine in patients with newly diagnosed partial seizures. Patients treated with lamotrigine were found to have a significantly longer time to treatment failure than either gabapentin or topiramate.

Lennox–Gastaut Syndrome in Children

A large ($n = 169$) multicenter, double-blind, randomized add-on trial of lamotrigine demonstrated efficacy of lamotrigine for the treatment major motor seizures in children and young adults with Lennox–Gastaut syndrome (86). The age range for the study was 2 to 25 years. The target dose of lamotrigine was 15 mg/kg for patients not taking valproate and 5 mg/kg for those taking valproate. Major motor seizures, defined as atonic, tonic, major myoclonic, and tonic–clinic, were reduced by 32% compared to baseline. Only a 9% reduction in major motor seizures was observed in the placebo group. This study supported the FDA indication for major motor seizures in

Lennox–Gastaut syndrome in adults and children. Other studies have supported the efficacy of lamotrigine in Lennox–Gastaut syndrome (87–89).

Idiopathic Generalized Epilepsies

Although lamotrigine has not received FDA approval for the indication of treatment of idiopathic generalized epilepsy in the United States due to the small number of patients in randomized controlled trials, several studies have suggested effectiveness for childhood absence epilepsy and juvenile myoclonic epilepsy (90–94). A double-blind, randomized, placebo-controlled, "responder-enriched" study of recently diagnosed typical absence seizures that confirmed seizure frequency by 24-hour EEG and hyperventilation EEG found that 62% of patients were seizure-free compared to 21% in the placebo group (94). Glauser and colleagues however have recently reported that in children with newly diagnosed childhood absence, treatment with either valproate or ethosuximide appeared to be more efficacious when compared to treatment with lamotrigine (95). Another double-blind, placebo-controlled add-on crossover study of treatment-resistant generalized epilepsy demonstrated that lamotrigine significantly reduced seizures that had not been controlled by other AEDs; 25% of the sample became seizure-free (90). A small case series suggested that myoclonus may worsen with lamotrigine treatment in some patients with idiopathic generalized epilepsy (96).

Data from Biton and colleagues (97) suggest that lamotrigine is effective as adjunctive therapy for primary generalized tonic–clonic (PGTC) seizures. In a double-blind, placebo-controlled trial where lamotrigine was added to patients with recurrent PGTC seizures and concurrently receiving one or two background AEDs, seizure frequency was reduced by approximately 66% (vs. 34% in the placebo arm). Seventy-two percent of patients treated with lamotrigine (vs. 49% of placebo) experienced a 50% reduction in seizures. Importantly, no serious adverse events, nor aggravation of other seizure types was noted.

In an unblinded, randomized effectiveness trial, Marson and colleagues (98) found that in patients with idiopathic generalized seizures, initial treatment with valproate was significantly better with respect to time to 12-month remission than with lamotrigine; however, no significant differences were seen for time to treatment failure between these two treatments. While these data are certainly useful, the decision as to which agent should be considered drug of first choice will likely still depend on patient-specific characteristics (e.g., gender, pregnancy, weight gain, etc.).

TOLERABILITY

Similar to efficacy, the safety profile of lamotrigine has been defined by numerous clinical studies. Of the side effects reported with lamotrigine, rash has received the most attention (99,100). The pathologic mechanism is not known, but may have a genetic basis (101). There appears to be crossreactivity for rash with other antiepileptic medications, especially carbamazepine and phenytoin (102).

The incidence of serious rash associated with hospitalization and discontinuation of lamotrigine in the pediatric population was assessed in a prospectively followed cohort of pediatric patients (2 to 16 years of age) with epilepsy receiving adjunctive therapy. In these patients, the incidence of serious rash was approximately 0.8%. In the adult population, serious rash associated with lamotrigine occurred in 0.3%. Interestingly, in clinical trials in patients with bipolar disorders was 0.08% in adult patients receiving lamotrigine as initial monotherapy and 0.13% in those who received the drug as adjunctive therapy.

In general, risk for serious rash appears to be increased when lamotrigine is either initiated at too high a starting dose, or when dosage is rapidly escalated (100). Attention and adherence to FDA-approved dosage and titration schedules are clearly prudent. There is also evidence that the combination of valproate and lamotrigine may increase the risk of serious rash in both pediatric and adult patients.

With regard to comparison with other AEDs, prior monotherapy studies of new onset epilepsy found no difference in rash rates between lamotrigine and carbamazepine (82) or phenytoin (83).

The most common central nervous system and systemic side effects reported with lamotrigine conversion and monotherapy are shown in Table 57.1. Some adverse events

TABLE 57.1

MOST COMMON ADVERSE EVENTS IN PIVOTAL TRIAL ($N = 156$) OF LAMOTRIGINE (500 MG/DAY) AS MONOTHERAPY COMPARED TO ACTIVE-CONTROL VALPROATE (1000 MG/DAY) (83)

	Transition phase		Monotherapy phase	
	Lamotrigine (500 mg)	Low-dose valproate	Lamotrigine	Low-dose valproate
Dizziness	20%	23%	7%	0%
Nausea	16%	19%	7%	2%
Headache	13%	13%	7%	14%
Asthenia	12%	13%	2%	0%
Coordination abnormality	12%	0%	7%	0%
Vomiting	11%	9%	9%	0%
Rash	11%	8%	2%	2%
Somnolence	8%	14%	0%	2%
Tremor	7%	10%	5%	7%
Dyspepsia	0%	14%	7%	2%

are related to pharmacodynamic interactions, most commonly with carbamazepine. Several double-blind, randomized monotherapy studies indicate that lamotrigine causes significantly less sedation than most other AEDs (61,82,83). Steiner et al. (83) reported that 28% of patients reported sleepiness while taking phenytoin, compared to 7% ($P < 0.05$) with lamotrigine. Brodie et al. (82) also found less sedation compared to carbamazepine (12% vs. 22%, $P < 0.05$), and more patients withdrew from the study due to adverse events on carbamazepine (15% vs. 27%).

Some prior studies suggest that lamotrigine has a favorable psychotropic profile, and may improve mood in some patients (103–105). This observation is potentially confounded by decreased sedations and improved concentration after converting from less well-tolerated antiepileptic medications (106), but available evidence supports that lamotrigine can improve mood or even protect against adverse mood effects of other medications. For example, Mula and colleagues reported that concomitant treatment with lamotrigine was associated with reduced rates of adverse psychiatric reactions to levetiracetam (107) or topiramate (108).

References

1. Lang DG, Wang CM, Cooper BR. Lamotrigine, phenytoin and carbamazepine interactions on the sodium current present in N4TG1 mouse neuroblastoma cells. *J Pharmacol Exp Ther.* 1993;266:829–835.
2. Errington AC, Stohr T, Heers C, et al. The investigational anticonvulsant lacosamide selectively enhances slow inactivation of voltage-gated sodium channels. *Mol Pharmacol.* 2008;73:157–169.
3. Song JH, Nagata K, Huang CS, et al. Differential block of two types of sodium channels by anticonvulsants. *Neuroreport.* 1996;7:3031–3036.
4. Kuo CC. A common anticonvulsant binding site for phenytoin, carbamazepine, and lamotrigine in neuronal Na$^+$ channels. *Mol Pharmacol.* 1998;54:712–721.
5. Macdonald RL, Kelly KM. Antiepileptic drug mechanisms of action. *Epilepsia.* 1995;36(suppl 2):S2–S12.
6. Coulter DA. Antiepileptic drug cellular mechanisms of action: Where does lamotrigine fit in? *J Child Neurol.* 1997;12(suppl 1):S2–S9.
7. Lees G, Leach MJ. Studies on the mechanism of action of the novel anticonvulsant lamotrigine (Lamictal) using primary neurological cultures from rat cortex. *Brain Res.* 1993;612:190–199.
8. Yarov-Yarovoy V, Brown J, Sharp EM, et al. Molecular determinants of voltage-dependent gating and binding of pore-blocking drugs in transmembrane segment IIIS6 of the Na$^+$ channel alpha subunit. *J Biol Chem.* 2001;276:20–27.
9. Stefani A, Spadoni F, Siniscalchi A, et al. Lamotrigine inhibits Ca^{2+} currents in cortical neurons: functional implications. *Eur J Pharmacol.* 1996;307:113–116.
10. Stefani A, Spadoni F, Bernardi G. Voltage-activated calcium channels: targets of antiepileptic drug therapy? *Epilepsia.* 1997;38:959–965.
11. Leach MJ, Marden CM, Miller AA. Pharmacological studies on lamotrigine, a novel potential antiepileptic drug: II. Neurochemical studies on the mechanism of action. *Epilepsia.* 1986;27:490–497.
12. Conroy BP, Black D, Lin CY, et al. Lamotrigine attenuates cortical glutamate release during global cerebral ischemia in pigs on cardiopulmonary bypass. *Anesthesiology.* 1999;90:844–854.
13. Koinig H, Morimoto Y, Zornow MH. The combination of lamotrigine and mild hypothermia prevents ischemia-induced increase in hippocampal glutamate. *J Neurosurg Anesthesiol.* 2001;13:106–112.
14. Bacher A, Zornow MH. Lamotrigine inhibits extracellular glutamate accumulation during transient global cerebral ischemia in rabbits. *Anesthesiology.* 1997;86:459–463.
15. Shuaib A, Mahmood RH, Wishart T, et al. Neuroprotective effects of lamotrigine in global ischemia in gerbils. A histological, in vivo microdialysis and behavioral study. *Brain Res.* 1995;702:199–206.
16. Lizasoain I, Knowles RG, Moncada S. Inhibition by lamotrigine of the generation of nitric oxide in rat forebrain slices. *J Neurochem.* 1995;64:636–642.
17. Southam E, Kirkby D, Higgins GA, et al. Lamotrigine inhibits monoamine uptake in vitro and modulates 5-hydroxytryptamine uptake in rats. *Eur J Pharmacol.* 1998;358:19–24.
18. McGeer EG, Zhu SG. Lamotrigine protects against kainate but not ibotenate lesions in rat striatum. *Neurosci Lett.* 1990;112:348–351.
19. Shiah I, Yatham LN, Gau Y, et al. Effect of lamotrigine on plasma GABA levels in healthy humans. *Prog Neuropsychopharmacol Biol Psychiatry.* 2003;27:419–423.
20. Kuznicky R, Ho S, Pan J, et al. Modulation of cerebral GABA by topiramate, lamotrigine, and gabapentin in healthy adults. *Neurology.* 2002;58:368–372.
21. Miller AA, Wheatley P, Sawyer DA, et al. Pharmacological studies on lamotrigine, a novel potential antiepileptic drug: I. Anticonvulsant profile in mice and rats. *Epilepsia.* 1986;27:483–489.
22. Binnie CD, van Emde Boas W, Kasteleijn-Nolste-Trenite DG, et al. Acute effects of lamotrigine (BW430C) in persons with epilepsy. *Epilepsia.* 1986;27:248–254.
23. Smith SE, al-Zubaidy ZA, Chapman AG, et al. Excitatory amino acid antagonists, lamotrigine and BW 1003C87 as anticonvulsants in the genetically epilepsy-prone rat. *Epilepsy Res.* 1993;15:101–111.
24. Wheatley PL, Miller AA. Effects of lamotrigine on electrically induced afterdischarge duration in anaesthetised rat, dog, and marmoset. *Epilepsia.* 1989;30:34–40.
25. O'Donnell RA, Miller AA. The effect of lamotrigine upon development of cortical kindled seizures in the rat. *Neuropharmacology.* 1991;30:253–258.
26. Otsuki K, Morimoto K, Sato K, et al. Effects of lamotrigine and conventional antiepileptic drugs on amygdala- and hippocampal-kindled seizures in rats. *Epilepsy Res.* 1998;31:101–112.
27. Fitton A, Goa KL. Lamotrigine. An update of its pharmacology and therapeutic use in epilepsy. *Drugs.* 1995;50:691–713.
28. Goa KL, Ross SR, Chrisp P. Lamotrigine. A review of its pharmacological properties and clinical efficacy in epilepsy. *Drugs.* 1993;46:152–176.
29. Garnett WR. Lamotrigine: Pharmacokinetics. *J Child Neurol.* 1997;12(suppl 1):S10–S15.
30. Biton V. Pharmacokinetics, toxicology and safety of lamotrigine in epilepsy. *Expert Opin Drug Metab Toxicol.* 2006;2:1009–1018.
31. Posner J, Cohen AF, Land G, et al. The pharmacokinetics of lamotrigine (BW430C) in healthy subjects with unconjugated hyperbilirubinaemia (Gilbert's syndrome). *Br J Clin Pharmacol.* 1989;28:117–120.
32. Cohen AF, Land GS, Breimer DD, et al. Lamotrigine, a new anticonvulsant: pharmacokinetics in normal humans. *Clin Pharmacol Ther.* 1987;42:535–541.
33. Rambeck B, Wolf P. Lamotrigine clinical pharmacokinetics. *Clin Pharmacokinet.* 1993;25:433–443.
34. Peck AW. Clinical pharmacology of lamotrigine. *Epilepsia.* 1991;32(suppl 2):S9–S12.
35. Ramsay RE, Pellock JM, Garnett WR, et al. Pharmacokinetics and safety of lamotrigine (Lamictal) in patients with epilepsy. *Epilepsy Res.* 1991;10:191–200.
36. Tompson DJ, Oliver-Willwong R, et al. Steady-state pharmacokinetics of lamotrigine when converting from twice-daily immediate-release to once-daily extended-release formulation in subjects with epilepsy (The COMPASS study). *Epilepsia.* 2008;49:410–417.
37. Birnbaum AK, Kriel RL, Burkhardt RT, et al. Rectal absorption of lamotrigine compressed tablets. *Epilepsia.* 2000;41:850–853.
38. Birnbaum AK, Kriel RL, Im Y, et al. Relative bioavailability of lamotrigine chewable dispersible tablets administered rectally. *Pharmacotherapy.* 2001;21:158–162.
39. Myllynen PK, Pienimaki PK, Vahakangas KH. Transplacental passage of lamotrigine in a human placental perfusion system in vitro and in maternal and cord blood in vivo. *Eur J Clin Pharmacol.* 2003;58:677–682.
40. Ohman I, Vitols S, Tomson T. Lamotrigine in pregnancy: Pharmacokinetics during delivery, in the neonate, and during lactation. *Epilepsia.* 2000;41:709–713.
41. Magdalou J, Herber R, Bidault R, et al. In vitro N-glucuronidation of a novel antiepileptic drug, lamotrigine, by human liver microsomes. *J Pharmacol Exp Ther.* 1992;260:1166–1173.
42. Hawes EM. N$^+$-glucuronidation, a common pathway in human metabolism of drugs with a tertiary amine group. *Drug Metab Dispos.* 1998;26:830–837.
43. Jawad S, Yuen WC, Peck AW, et al. Lamotrigine: single-dose pharmacokinetics and initial 1 week experience in refractory epilepsy. *Epilepsy Res.* 1987;1:194–201.
44. Provinciali L, Bartolini M, Mari F, et al. Influence of vigabatrin on cognitive performances and behaviour in patients with drug-resistant epilepsy. *Acta Neurol Scand.* 1996;94:12–18.
45. Chen C, Casale EJ, Duncan B, et al. Pharmacokinetics of lamotrigine in children in the absence of other antiepileptic drugs. *Pharmacotherapy.* 1999;19:437–441.
46. Hussein Z, Posner J. Population pharmacokinetics of lamotrigine monotherapy in patients with epilepsy: retrospective analysis of routine monitoring data. *Br J Clin Pharmacol.* 1997;43:457–465.
47. Bialer M, Johannessen SI, Kupferberg HJ, et al. Progress report on new antiepileptic drugs: a summary of the fourth Eilat conference (EILAT IV). *Epilepsy Res.* 1999;34:1–41.
48. Wootton R, Soul-Lawton J, Rolan PE, et al. Comparison of the pharmacokinetics of lamotrigine in patients with chronic renal failure and healthy volunteers. *Br J Clin Pharmacol* 1997;43:23–27.

49. Fillastre JP, Taburet AM, Fialaire A, et al. Pharmacokinetics of lamotrigine in patients with renal impairment: influence of haemodialysis. *Drugs Exp Clin Res.* 1993;19:25–32.
50. Tran TA, Leppik IE, Blesi K, et al. Lamotrigine clearance during pregnancy. *Neurology.* 2002;59:251–255.
51. Pennell PB, Hovinga CA. Antiepileptic drug therapy in pregnancy I: gestation-induced effects on AED pharmacokinetics. *Int Rev Neurobiol.* 2008;83:227–240.
52. Pennell PB, Newport DJ, Stowe ZN, et al. The impact of pregnancy and childbirth on the metabolism of lamotrigine. *Neurology.* 2004;62:292–295
53. Pennell PB, Peng L, Newport DJ, et al. Lamotrigine in pregnancy: clearance, therapeutic drug monitoring, and seizure frequency. *Neurology.* 2008;70:2130–2136.
54. Kilpatrick ES, Forrest G, Brodie MJ. Concentration–effect and concentration–toxicity relations with lamotrigine: a prospective study. *Epilepsia.* 1996;37:534–538.
55. Morris RG, Black AB, Harris AL, et al. Lamotrigine and therapeutic drug monitoring: retrospective survey following the introduction of a routine service. *Br J Clin Pharmacol.* 1998;46:547–551.
56. Froscher W, Keller F, Vogt H, et al. Prospective study on concentration-efficacy and concentration-toxicity: correlations with lamotrigine serum levels. *Epileptic Disord.* 2002;4:49–56.
57. LeLorier J, Duh MS, Paradis PE, et al. Clinical consequences of generic substitution of lamotrigine for patients with epilepsy. *Neurology.* 2008;70(22 Pt 2):2179–2186.
58. Andermann F, Duh MS, Gosselin A, . Compulsory generic switching of antiepileptic drugs: high switchback rates to branded compounds compared with other drug classes. *Epilepsia.* 2007;48:464–469.
59. Battino D, Croci D, Granata T, et al. Lamotrigine plasma concentrations in children and adults: influence of age and associated therapy. *Ther Drug Monit.* 1997;19:620–627.
60. Vauzelle-Kervroedan F, Rey E, Cieuta C, et al. Influence of concurrent antiepileptic medication on the pharmacokinetics of lamotrigine as add-on therapy in epileptic children. *Br J Clin Pharmacol.* 1996;41:325–330.
61. Gilliam F, Vazquez B, Sackellares JC, et al. An active-control trial of lamotrigine monotherapy for partial seizures [see comments]. *Neurology.* 1998;51:1018–1025.
62. Anderson GD, Gidal BE, Messenheimer JA, Gilliam FG. Time course of lamotrigine de induction: impact of step-wise withdrawal of carbamazepine or phenytoin. *Epilepsy Res.* 2002;49:211–217.
63. Perucca E, Gidal BE, Baltes E. Effects of antiepileptic comedication on levetiracetam pharmacokinetics: a pooled analysis of data from randomized adjunctive therapy trials. *Epilepsy Res.* 2003;53:47–56.
64. Gidal BE, Kanner A, Maly M, et al. Lamotrigine pharmacokinetics in patients receiving felbamate. *Epilepsy Res.* 1997;27:1–5.
65. Berry DJ, Besag FMC, Pool F, et al. Lack of an effect of topiramate on lamotrigine serum concentrations. *Epilepsia.* 2002;43:818–823.
66. May TW, Rambeck B, Jurgens U. Influence of oxcarbazepine and methsuximide on lamotrigine concentrations in epileptic patients with and without valproic acid comedication: Results of a retrospective study. *Ther Drug Monit.* 1999;21:175–181.
67. Yuen AW, Land G, Weatherley BC, et al. Sodium valproate acutely inhibits lamotrigine metabolism. *Br J Clin Pharmacol.* 1992;33:511–513.
68. Gidal BE, Sheth R, Parnell J, et al. Evaluation of VPA dose and concentration effects on lamotrigine pharmacokinetics: implications for conversion to lamotrigine monotherapy. *Epilepsy Res.* 2003;57(2–3):85–93.
69. Anderson GD, Yau MK, Gidal BE, et al. Bidirectional interaction of valproate and lamotrigine in healthy subjects. *Clin Pharmacol Ther.* 1996;60:145–56.
70. Mataringa MI, May TW, Rambeck B. Does lamotrigine influence valproate concentrations? *Ther Drug Monit.* 2002;24:631–636.
71. Gidal BE, Rutecki P, Shaw R, et al. Effect of lamotrigine on carbamazepine epoxide/carbamazepine serum concentration ratios in adult patients with epilepsy. *Epilepsy Res.* 1997;28:207–211.
72. Pisani F, Xiao B, Fazio A, et al. Single dose pharmacokinetics of carbamazepine-10,11-epoxide in patients on lamotrigine monotherapy. *Epilepsy Res.* 1994;19:245–248.
73. Sidhu J, Job S, Singh S, et al. The pharmacokinetic and pharmacodynamic consequences of the co-administration of lamotrigine and a combined oral contraceptive in healthy female subjects. *Br J Clin Pharmacol.* 2006;61: 191–199.
74. Depot M, Powell JR, Messenheimer JA, Jr, et al. Kinetic effects of multiple oral doses of acetaminophen on a single oral dose of lamotrigine. *Clin Pharmacol Ther.* 1990;48:346–355.
75. Kaufman KR, Gerner R. Lamotrigine toxicity secondary to sertraline. *Seizure.* 1998;7:163–165.
76. Sabers A, Ohman I, Christensen J, et al. Oral contraceptives reduce lamotrigine plasma levels. *Neurology.* 2003;61:570–571.
77. Christensen J, Petrenaite V, Atterman J, et al. Oral contraceptives induce lamotrigine metabolism: evidence from double-blind placebo controlled trial. *Epilepsia.* 2007;48:484–489.
78. French JA, Kanner AM, Bautista J, et al. Efficacy and tolerability of the new antiepileptic drugs II: treatment of refractory epilepsy. report of the therapeutics and technology assessment subcommittee and quality standards subcommittee of the American academy of neurology and the American epilepsy society. *Neurology.* 2004;62:1261–1273.
79. Matsuo F, Bergen D, Faught E, et al. Placebo-controlled study of the efficacy and safety of lamotrigine in patients with partial seizures. *Neurology.* 1993;43:2284.
80. Duchowny M, Pellock JM, Graf WD, et al. A placebo-controlled trial of lamotrigine add-on therapy for partial seizures in children. Lamictal Pediatric Partial Seizure Study Group. *Neurology.* 1999;53:1724–1731.
81. Naritoku DK, Warnock CR, Messenheimer JA, et al. Lamotrigine extended-release as adjunctive therapy for partial seizures. *Neurology.* 2007;69:1610–1618.
82. Brodie MJ, Richens A, Yuen AW. Double-blind comparison of lamotrigine and carbamazepine in newly diagnosed epilepsy. UK Lamotrigine/Carbamazepine Monotherapy Trial Group [published erratum appears in Lancet 1995 Mar 11;345(8950):662] [see comments]. *Lancet.* 1995;345: 476–479.
83. Steiner TJ, Dellaportas CI, Findley LJ, et al. Lamotrigine monotherapy in newly diagnosed untreated epilepsy: a double-blind comparison with phenytoin. *Epilepsia.* 1999;40:601–607.
84. Saetre E, Perucca E, Isojarvi J, et al. LAM 40089 Study Group. An international multicenter randomized double-blind controlled trial of lamotrigine and sustained-release carbamazepine in the treatment of newly diagnosed epilepsy in the elderly. *Epilepsia.* 2007;48: 1292–1302.
85. Marson AG, Al-Kharusi AM, Alwaidh M, et al. The SANAD study of effectiveness of carbamazepine, gabapentin, lamotrigine, oxcarbazepine, or topiramate for treatment of partial epilepsy: an unblinded randomised controlled trial. *Lancet.* 2007;369:1000–1015.
86. Motte J, Trevathan E, Arvidsson JF, et al. Lamotrigine for generalized seizures associated with the Lennox–Gastaut syndrome. Lamictal Lennox–Gastaut Study Group. *N Engl J Med.* 1997;337:1807–1812.
87. Donaldson JA, Glauser TA, Olberding LS. Lamotrigine adjunctive therapy in childhood epileptic encephalopathy (the Lennox–Gastaut syndrome). *Epilepsia.* 1997;38:68–73.
88. Schlumberger E, Chavez F, Palacios L, et al. Lamotrigine in treatment of 120 children with epilepsy. *Epilepsia.* 1994;35:359–367.
89. Timmings PL, Richens A. Lamotrigine as an add-on drug in the management of Lennox-Gastaut syndrome. *Eur Neurol.* 1992;32:305–307.
90. Beran RG, Berkovic SF, Dunagan FM, et al. Double-blind, placebo-controlled, crossover study of lamotrigine in treatment-resistant generalised epilepsy [see comments]. *Epilepsia.* 1998;39:1329–1333.
91. Buchanan N. The use of lamotrigine in juvenile myoclonic epilepsy. *Seizure.* 1996;5:149–151.
92. Buoni S, Grosso S, Fois A. Lamotrigine in typical absence epilepsy. *Brain Dev.* 1999;21:303–306.
93. Ferrie CD, Robinson RO, Knott C, et al. Lamotrigine as an add-on drug in typical absence seizures. *Acta Neurol Scand.* 1995;91:200–202.
94. Frank LM, Enlow T, Holmes GL, et al. Lamictal (lamotrigine) monotherapy for typical absence seizures in children. *Epilepsia.* 1999; 40:973–979.
95. Glauser TA, Cnaan A, Shinnar S, et al. Ethosuximide, valproic acid and lamotrigine in childhood absence epilepsy. *N Engle J Med.* 2010;362: 790–799.
96. Crespel A, Genton P, Berramdane M, et al. Lamotrigine associated with exacerbation or de novo myoclonus in idiopathic generalized epilepsies. *Neurology.* 2005;65:762–764.
97. Biton V, Sackellares JC, Vuong A, et al. Double-blind, placebo-controlled study of lamotrigine in primary generalized tonic-clonic seizures. *Neurology.* 2005;65(11):1737–1743.
98. Marson AG, Al-Kharusi AM, Alwaidh M, et al. The SANAD study of effectiveness of valproate, lamotrigine, or topiramate for generalized and unclassifiable epilepsy: an unblinded randomized controlled trial. *Lancet.* 2007;369:1016–1026.
99. Dooley J, Camfield P, Gordon K, et al. Lamotrigine-induced rash in children. *Neurology.* 1996;46:240–242.
100. Guberman AH, Besag FM, Brodie MJ, et al. Lamotrigine-associated rash: risk/benefit considerations in adults and children [see comments]. *Epilepsia.* 1999;40:985–991.
101. Kazeem GR, Cox C, Aponte J, et al. High-resolution HLA genotyping and severe cutaneous adverse reactions in lamotrigine-treated patients. *Pharmacogenet Genomics.* 2009;19:661–665.
102. Hirsch LJ, Arif H, Nahm EA, et al. Cross-sensitivity of skin rashes with antiepileptic drug use. *Neurology.* 2008;71:1527–1534.
103. Ettinger AB, Kustra RP, Hammer AE. Effect of lamotrigine on depressive symptoms in adult patients with epilepsy. *Epilepsy Behav.* 2007;10: 148–154.
104. Fakhoury TA, Barry JJ, Mitchell Miller J, et al. Lamotrigine in patients with epilepsy and comorbid depressive symptoms. *Epilepsy Behav.* 2007; 10:155–162.
105. Rogawski MA, Loscher W. The neurobiology of antiepileptic drugs for the treatment of nonepileptic conditions. *Nat Med.* 2004;10: 685–692.
106. Gilliam FG, Barry JJ, Hermann BP, et al. Rapid detection of major depression in epilepsy: a multicentre study. *Lancet Neurol.* 2006;5:399–405.
107. Mula M, Trimble MR, Yuen A, et al. Psychiatric adverse events during levetiracetam therapy. *Neurology.* 2003;61:704–706.
108. Mula M, Trimble MR, Lhatoo SD, et al. Topiramate and psychiatric adverse events in patients with epilepsy. *Epilepsia.* 2003;44:659–663.

CHAPTER 58 ■ TOPIRAMATE

WILLIAM E. ROSENFELD

HISTORICAL BACKGROUND

Topiramate (TPM) is a highly oxygenated sulfamate-substituted monosaccharide that is structurally distinct from other anticonvulsant medications. Available in the United States as Topamax (Ortho-McNeil Pharmaceutical), it is a broad-spectrum agent that has been extensively studied in double-blind, randomized, controlled trials in adults and children. Initially approved for use as adjunctive therapy in adults with partial-onset seizures. Subsequently, TPM was approved in children and adults with partial-onset seizures, primary generalized tonic–clonic seizures, and multiple seizure types associated with Lennox–Gastaut syndrome.

TPM is now also approved in the United States for monotherapy in adults and children 10 years of age and older. The drug was originally discovered in a screening protocol using the standard maximal electroshock seizure (MES) test. Anticonvulsant effects were similar to phenytoin and carbamazepine (1). Most of the known benefits and side effects were noted for this medication from the first couple of 1000 patients (except narrow angle glaucoma which is a much rarer phenomena). Efficacy was seen early (in blinded studies family and friends often noted so much improvement they were often referring other friends). Side effects were also noted early due to not yet knowing the most effective dosages without side effects. Too high and too rapid titration often occurred and the most common side effects noted were word finding, mathematical difficulties, paresthesias, weight loss, and kidney stones. A 1.5% incidence of kidney stones was seen early and remained the same even despite millions of patients being on such (not necessarily dose or titration related).

CHEMISTRY

TPM (2,3:4,5-di-O-isopropylidene-β-D-fructopyranose sulfamate; Fig. 58.1) is a white crystalline powder, which is freely soluble in acetone, chloroform, dimethylsulfoxide, and ethanol. TPM is supplied as 25-, 50-, 100-, and 200-mg tablets and as 15- and 25-mg sprinkle capsules that can be opened and sprinkled onto soft food for children and for patients who may have difficulty swallowing tablets.

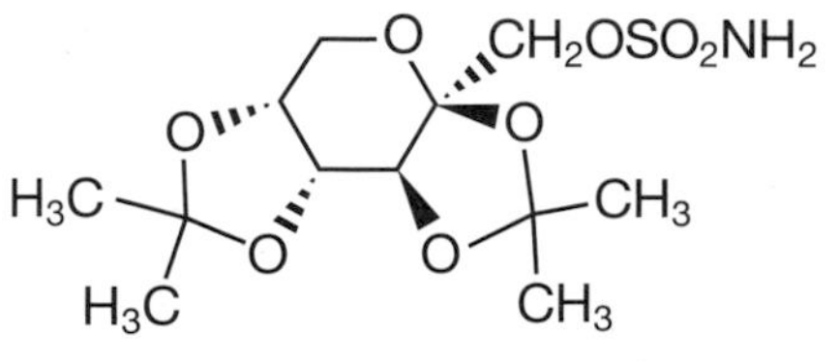

FIGURE 58.1. Topiramate (2,3:4,5-Di-O-isopropylidene-β-D-fructopyranose sulfamate).

MECHANISMS OF ACTION

TPM has a unique combination of activities at various receptor sites and ion channels, which may account for its broad-spectrum profile in epilepsy and other neurologic disorders. It blocks the kainate/AMPA (α-amino-3-hydroxy-5-methylisoxazole-4-propionic acid) subtype of the glutamate receptor (2–5), with no direct effect on NMDA (N-methyl-D-aspartate) receptor activity; blocks voltage-activated sodium channels to limit sustained repetitive firing (6–10); enhances α-aminobutyric acid (GABA)-mediated chloride flux at GABA$_A$ receptors (11,12); reduces the amplitude of high-voltage–activated calcium currents (13,14); and activates potassium conductance (15,16). It has been hypothesized that effects of TPM on voltage-activated sodium channels, high-voltage–activated calcium channels, GABA$_A$ receptors, and AMPA/kainate receptors reflect a common modulator involving protein phosphorylation (17). TPM is also a weak inhibitor of carbonic anhydrase isoenzymes (CA II and CA IV), which may modulate pH-dependent activation of voltage- and receptor-gated ion channels (18); its inhibitory effect is less than acetazolamide.

ANIMAL MODELS

The anticonvulsant properties of TPM have been demonstrated in several animal models of epilepsy. TPM exhibited potent and long-lasting anticonvulsant activity when evaluated using the MES test in rodents with a median effective dose of 47.6 mg/kg in the mouse and 15.8 mg/kg in the rat (19). TPM inhibited chronic motor seizures and absence-like seizures when administered intraperitoneally (17). TPM blocked sound-induced clonic and tonic–clonic seizures (20). TPM effectively inhibited tonic, clonic, and wild running seizures in a postischemia model of epilepsy in rats, and its potency was similar to that of phenytoin for all three seizure types (21). TPM also produced a dose-related inhibition of amygdala-kindled seizures in rats (22). Experimental studies have shown that TPM reduced seizure-induced hippocampal neuronal injury (23) and prevented spontaneous seizures following status epilepticus (24). In an experimental model of neonatal hypoxia/ischemia, TPM suppressed acute seizures and reduced subsequent susceptibility to neuronal injury and seizures induced by a second insult (kainate) (25).

TABLE 58.1

PHARMACOKINETIC CHARACTERISTICS OF TOPIRAMATE

Characteristic	Value
Elimination half-life (hr)	19–23
Peak plasma concentration (mg/L)	1.7 (100-mg single dose)
	7.7 (400-mg single dose)
	28.7 (1200-mg single dose)
Time to maximum concentration (hr)	1.8–4.3
Fraction of systemically available drug excreted	
Unchanged into the urine (%)	70–97
Apparent oral clearance (mL/min)	22–36
Apparent volume of distribution (L/kg)	0.6–0.8
Unbound fraction of drug in plasma (%)	Predominantly unbound

Adapted with permission from Bialer (26) and Rosenfeld (27).

PHARMACOKINETICS

Renal elimination, low protein binding, and a long half-life make TPM relatively easy to manage from a pharmacokinetic perspective (Table 58.1) (26,27).

Absorption

TPM is rapidly absorbed with peak plasma concentrations occurring in 1 to 4 hours with TPM doses of 100 to 400 mg. Absorption is nearly complete with less than 80% of a 100-mg dose recovered in urine. Coadministration with food slightly delays absorption but does not decrease bioavailability (28). TPM exhibits linear kinetics; plasma concentrations increase in proportion to dose increases (29).

Distribution and Protein Binding

The apparent volume of distribution for TPM is 38.5 to 58 L (0.6 to 0.8 L/kg, weight normalized), consistent with distribution to total body water. Binding to plasma proteins is minimal (13% to 17%) and is not considered to be a major factor in dosing and drug interactions (29).

Metabolism and Excretion

In the absence of hepatic enzyme induction, approximately 20% of a TPM dose is metabolized. When TPM is coadministered with enzyme-inducing antiepileptic drugs (AEDs), up to 50% of the TPM dose may be metabolized. Hepatic metabolism appears to involve hydroxylation, hydrolysis, and glucuronidation; none of the metabolites constitutes >5% of an administered dose, and they are quickly cleared (29).

Elimination of TPM is primarily via renal excretion, with 50% to 80% being eliminated in the urine unchanged. The half-life of TPM in adults is 20 to 30 hours in the absence of enzyme induction, allowing steady-state plasma concentrations to be reached in 4 to 8 days. In the presence of enzyme induction, the TPM half-life in adults is 12 to 15 hours (29). In children 4 to 17 years of age, clearance is approximately 50% higher than in adults (30). Steady-state concentrations for the same mg/kg dose were correspondingly lower in children than in adults. Consistent with the higher clearance, the calculated half-life of TPM in children is approximately 15 hours without enzyme induction and 7.5 hours with enzyme induction. In young children (younger than 4 years old), clearance rates were the same or slightly higher than in older children (31). In elderly patients (65 to 85 years of age), clearance decreases only to the extent that renal function itself is reduced by age; age alone does not alter clearance in adults (32).

TPM clearance is reduced by 40% to 50% in patients with moderate (creatinine clearance 30 to 69 mL/min) or severe (creatinine clearance, <30 mL/min) renal impairment compared with subjects with normal renal function (creatinine clearance, >70 mL/min) (29). One half of the usual TPM dose is recommended in patients with moderate or severe renal impairment. TPM plasma concentrations fell by an average of 50.1% during hemodialysis. The mean hemodialysis plasma clearance of TPM has been reported to be approximately nine times higher than that found in subjects not receiving hemodialysis (33). Modest decreases in TPM clearance have been reported when comparing age- and sex-matched healthy controls to individuals with moderate to severe hepatic impairment; mean clearance was decreased 26% (31.8 vs. 23.5 mL/min) and half-life increased 36% (25 vs. 34 hours), with parallel increases in plasma concentrations (29).

THERAPEUTIC DRUG MONITORING

Drug monitoring is of relatively little importance in initial titration of TPM. It is most important for compliance and also if utilizing higher dose therapy. Steady-state plasma concentrations of TPM are generally linear, with dose-proportional increases in plasma concentration (29). Mean plasma concentrations achieved during maintenance in randomized, controlled trials of TPM monotherapy were: 50 mg/day, 1.6 and 1.9 µg/mL; 97 mg/day, 3.8 µg/mL; 189 mg/day, 6.4 µg/mL; 313 mg/day, 11.7 µg/mL; 367 mg/day, 12.4 µg/mL (34). Studies of TPM as monotherapy have provided the opportunity to examine the relationship between TPM plasma levels and clinical response. In a study comparing 50 and 500 mg/day TPM as monotherapy, plasma concentrations >9.91 µg/mL were associated with better seizure control compared with plasma concentrations of 1.77 to 9.91 µg/mL and ≤1.76 µg/mL (35). However, because of the intraindividual variations in blood levels associated with seizure control and side effects, a traditional "therapeutic range" cannot be identified. As expected, plasma concentrations are higher when TPM is administered as monotherapy (6.4 to 12.4 µg/mL with ~200 to 400 mg/day) versus its use as add-on to enzyme-inducing AEDs (1.4 to 5.3 µg/mL with ~200 to 400 mg/day). Despite the substantially higher plasma concentration with monotherapy, the incidence of central nervous system (CNS)-related adverse events, particularly cognitive effects, was substantially lower with TPM monotherapy than with adjunctive therapy. This finding underscores the contribution of pharmacodynamic interactions to the occurrence of adverse events during TPM polytherapy and the limited benefit of therapeutic drug monitoring in TPM-treated patients.

The relationship between TPM dose and plasma level was examined in children in whom TPM was titrated to clinical response or side effects (36). Among 21 children aged 6 to 12 years, TPM plasma levels were predictably related to dose (1:1 ratio). With monotherapy, a mean dose of 9.7 mg/kg/day (range, 5.5 to 16.5 mg/kg/day) resulted in a mean plasma level of 9.8 µg/mL (range, 3.4 to 16.6 µg/mL). For 20 younger children (younger than 6 years of age), however, higher monotherapy doses were needed (mean, 22.5 mg/kg/day; range, 11 to 35 mg/kg/day) to achieve seizure control; mean plasma level was 14.8 µg/mL (range, 6.1 to 23.7 µg/mL). When TPM was administered with an enzyme-inducing drug, the TPM dosage in younger children (mean, 14.2 mg/kg/day) was double than that in older children (7.0 mg/kg/day) (36).

Patients with levels close to 25 µg/mL or more rarely obtained additional benefit at higher dosages and side effects increased. Therapeutic ranges are often quoted in the 2 to 25 µg/mL range. It is this author's opinion that there are two ranges. Monotherapy patients who are relatively easy to control can often be controlled in the 2 to 6 µg/mL range and those who are more intractable may need higher doses.

DRUG INTERACTIONS

Interaction studies were performed with the three leading AEDs carbamazepine, phenytoin, and valproic acid and also later with lamotrigine. Similar study designs were utilized.

Topiramate and Carbamazepine

The steady-state pharmacokinetics of carbamazepine and TPM as adjunctive therapy and monotherapy were determined in 12 adults whose epilepsy was stabilized with carbamazepine 300 to 800 mg t.i.d. (37). No significant differences were observed in the pharmacokinetics of total or unbound carbamazepine or carbamazepine epoxide in the absence of TPM or with TPM 100 to 400 mg b.i.d. TPM AUC, C_{max}, average concentration, and minimum concentration levels were approximately 40% lower in the presence of carbamazepine than with TPM monotherapy (27).

Topiramate and Phenytoin

The steady-state pharmacokinetics of phenytoin and TPM were determined in 12 adults with partial epilepsy who were stabilized on phenytoin (38). During concomitant phenytoin therapy, TPM pharmacokinetics were proportional for dosages ranging from 100 to 400 mg. During TPM adjunctive therapy with phenytoin, TPM concentrations were reduced by approximately 50%. The investigators hypothesized that the increase in TPM clearance during concomitant phenytoin therapy was due to enzyme induction by phenytoin. In half the patients, TPM had no measurable effect on the pharmacokinetics of phenytoin; in the other patients, however, particularly those taking phenytoin twice a day, phenytoin concentrations were approximately 25% higher. No patients required adjustment of phenytoin or discontinued the trial. In clinical practice, patients receiving dosages in the higher therapeutic ranges of phenytoin should be observed carefully, because they may be more likely to require a downward adjustment of phenytoin dosage (27).

Topiramate and Valproic Acid

The steady-state pharmacokinetics of valproic acid and TPM were determined in 12 patients whose partial epilepsy was treated with valproic acid (39). TPM plasma concentrations were approximately 14% lower during adjunctive therapy with valproic acid. Valproic acid concentrations decrease by 11% when TPM 400 mg b.i.d. was added. The clinical significance of these changes is probably minimal (27).

Topiramate and Lamotrigine

An open-label, sequential, single group, dose escalating, PK study was performed in 13 patients with epilepsy. No PK interactions were noted between TPM and lamotrigine at observed doses of 100 to 400 mg/day TPM (40).

Topiramate and Oral Contraceptives

Interaction studies evaluating the effect of TPM on combination oral contraceptives showed that TPM has no effect on the progestin (norethindrone 1.0 mg) component (41,42). At doses of ≤200 mg/day, TPM has no significant effect on estrogen (ethinyl estradiol 35 µg) concentrations (41,42). Initial studies showed the mean serum estradiol to be reduced by 18% at 200 mg/day but repeat testing at the same 200 mg dosage showed only an 11% decrease. At higher doses (400 and 800 mg/day), TPM was associated with 21% and 30% reductions, respectively, in ethinyl estradiol concentrations, suggesting a modest induction of estrogen clearance (42). The level of induction is substantially less than that associated with potent enzyme-inducing agents such as carbamazepine (42% reduction in estrogen concentration) (41). The dose-related effect of TPM on estrogen clearance is consistent with the concentration-dependent induction of cytochrome P450 (CYP450) CYP3A4 activity measured in vitro (43). TPM-induced CYP3A4 enzymes only at concentrations >50 µM, a concentration that is unlikely to be achieved with dosages up to 400 mg/day; enzyme induction was still less than that associated with known inducers (phenobarbital and rifampicin) used in this study.

Predominantly renal elimination and low protein binding minimize the potential for drug interactions. Pharmacokinetic interactions between TPM and other AEDs are limited primarily to the effects of enzyme-inducing drugs on TPM. TPM plasma levels are approximately 50% lower when TPM is given with an enzyme-inducing AED (37–45) compared to TPM use alone or in combination with nonenzyme-inducing drugs (39,37–45). The addition of TPM does not significantly affect plasma concentrations of carbamazepine (37), valproate (39), phenobarbital/primidone (44), or lamotrigine (40). However, phenytoin plasma levels may be increased as much as 25% in some patients, particularly those in whom phenytoin metabolism may be at or near saturation (45). Studies of TPM in models designed to predict drug interactions related to the CYP450 enzyme system have shown inhibition of only the CYP2C19 isozyme, which may account for the potential interaction with phenytoin (46). Although pharmacokinetic interactions between TPM and other AEDs are limited, the lower incidence of adverse effects with TPM monotherapy (35,47,48) suggests that pharmacodynamic interactions may affect tolerability when TPM is added to existing therapy.

A slight decrease in digoxin clearance has been observed with the addition of TPM (49), but generally does not require dosage adjustments. Changes in metformin pharmacokinetics suggest that diabetic control should be monitored when TPM is added or withdrawn (50).

EFFICACY

Adjunctive Therapy

Partial-Onset Seizures

The effectiveness of TPM as adjunctive therapy across a wide range of doses (200 to 1000 mg/day) in adults with refractory partial-onset seizures has been well documented in randomized, double-blind, placebo-controlled trials (51–59). Similarity of trial design and patient populations allowed pooled analysis of data from six of these trials (51–56). Among 743 adults (median baseline frequency, 12 seizures per month), median seizure reduction was 44% with TPM treatment versus 2% with placebo ($P \leq 0.001$); 43% of TPM-related patients (placebo, 12%; $P \leq 0.001$) achieved at least 50% seizure reduction (60). During 11 to 19 weeks of double-blind treatment, 5% of patients in the TPM group were seizure free, while no patients in the placebo group were seizure free ($P \leq 0.001$) (60). Initially it was felt that dosages of 200 mg/day would be placebo-like and therefore 79% of the original patients were at dosages of 400 to 1000 mg/day. On initial review of the data, it appeared that there was a flattening of the efficacy curve at higher dosages. However, one must remember that this was intent to treat data. If a patient due to side effects did not make it to his assigned upper dosage (even if seizure free or significantly reduced in seizure frequency), the patient was considered as not succeeding at that dosage. Therefore, from an efficacy point of view, there was a dose–response curve. Although dosages as high as 1000 mg/day were evaluated, the most clinically useful adjunctive therapy dosages appear to be 200 to 400 mg/day. In a 12-week,

double-blind trial to further evaluate the lower end of the presumed dosing range (59), 200 mg/day TPM was added to carbamazepine. Median seizure reduction in TPM-treated patients ($N = 168$) was 44% (vs. 20% with placebo, $N = 91$; $P < 0.001$); 45% of TPM-treated patients (placebo, 24%; $P = 0.001$) achieved at least 50% seizure reduction. After 2 weeks, median seizure reduction in patients receiving TPM 100 mg/day ($N = 84$) was 60% (placebo, 17%; $P < 0.001$), which suggests that 100 mg/day may be a target dose at which seizure control should be initially evaluated.

The initial overestimation of TPM dosage needs is evident from prospective, in-practice studies in which adults with refractory partial-onset seizures achieved good seizure control with 264 mg/day (48% of patients had 50% or more seizure reduction rate; 9% were seizure free) (61) and 323 mg/day (68% of patients had a 50% or more seizure reduction rate) (62). When titrating to response, patients with fewer baseline seizures (less than four per month) required lower TPM dosages (303 mg/day) than those with higher baseline seizure frequency (341 mg/day in patients with four or more seizures per month) (62). In a prospective study, 17% of refractory patients had at least 50% seizure reduction and 8% were seizure free with TPM dosages of 100 or less mg per day (63).

In treatment-resistant epilepsy patients treated at a tertiary epilepsy center, estimated long-term retention rates among 393 TPM-treated patients were 52% after 1 year, 42% at 2 years, 30% at 3 years, and 28% at 5 years (64,65). Although these rates were higher than those with another new-generation agent (lamotrigine), the low retention rate at 5 years reflects the limitations of medical therapy in patients with refractory epilepsy.

TPM was evaluated as adjunctive therapy in 86 children (2 to 16 years of age) with refractory partial-onset seizures (66). With a mean daily dose of 6 mg/kg (target dose, 5 to 9 mg/kg/day), median seizure reduction was 33% (placebo, 11%; $P = 0.03$). More TPM-treated children had at least 50% reduction in seizures (39% vs. 20% with placebo; $P = 0.08$); 5% of children receiving TPM had no seizures, while no placebo-treated children were seizure free.

All 83 children completing the double-blind phase entered the long-term, open-label extension in which the dosages of TPM and concomitant AEDs could be adjusted according to clinical response (67). Mean treatment duration was 15 months, with some children being treated as long as 2.5 years; the mean TPM dosage was 9 mg/kg/day (range, 4 to 22 mg/kg/day). Among children treated for at least 6 months, 64% had at least a 50% reduction in seizures; 14% were seizure free for a minimum of 6 months. During open-label in-practice studies in children with refractory partial-onset seizures (68–71), 4% to 20% of TPM-treated children were seizure free during treatment periods as long as 33 months.

Lennox–Gastaut Syndrome

TPM was evaluated as adjunctive therapy in 98 patients with Lennox–Gastaut syndrome confirmed by an electroencephalographic (EEG) pattern of slow spike-and-wave, multiple seizure types, including drop attacks, and a history of atypical absence episodes (72). At a maximum dose of 6 mg/kg/day, median reduction for drop attacks was 15% compared with a 5% increase with placebo; 28% of TPM-treated patients were responders (placebo 14%). A combined measure of drop attacks and tonic–clonic seizures showed a 26% reduction with TPM and a 5% increase with placebo ($P = 0.015$); respective responder rates were 33% and 8% ($P = 0.002$). These outcomes compared favorably with those reported for lamotrigine in this population (73). The placebo-adjusted responder rate for drop attacks was 14% for TPM and 15% for lamotrigine; respective rates for major motor seizures were 25% and 17% (72,73).

During the long-term, open-label extension in which the dosages of TPM and concomitant AEDs could be adjusted according to clinical response (74), 55% of the 82 children treated with TPM for more than 6 months had at least a 50% reduction in drop attacks during the last 6 months of treatment; 15% experienced no drop attacks. Two patients were free of all seizures. The mean duration of TPM treatment was 18 months, with treatment periods as long as 3.4 years. The mean TPM dosage was 10 mg/kg/day (range, 1 to 29 mg/kg/day). Among patients treated as long as 8 years, 21% to 40% of patients had at least 50% seizure reduction, with major motor seizures being the most responsive (75,76).

Generalized Tonic–Clonic Seizures of Nonfocal Origin

Two double-blind, placebo-controlled trials (77,78) evaluated TPM in the treatment of generalized, nonfocal tonic–clonic seizures (i.e., primary generalized tonic–clonic seizures). Inclusion criteria specified tonic–clonic seizures with or without other generalized seizure types and EEG or CCTV/EEG patterns consistent with generalized epilepsy (generalized, symmetric, synchronous spike-wave discharges, and normal background activity); patients with Lennox–Gastaut syndrome or partial-onset seizures were excluded. In the two trials, more than 70% of patients had primary generalized tonic–clonic seizures plus at least one other type of generalized seizure (i.e., absence, myoclonic, or tonic).

TPM was initiated as adjunctive therapy in adults and children (at least 4 years of age) with refractory generalized tonic–clonic seizures despite treatment with one or two AEDs. The target dose was 5 to 9 mg/kg/day and the maximum daily dose was 400 mg. In one trial (77), baseline seizure frequency in the TPM-treated group ($N = 39$) was five generalized tonic–clonic seizures per month (placebo 4.5 generalized tonic–clonic seizures per month; $N = 41$). Median seizure reduction was 57% (placebo 9%; $P < 0.02$) for tonic–clonic seizures and 42% (placebo, 1%; $P = 0.003$) for all generalized seizures. Among TPM-treated patients, generalized tonic–clonic seizures and all generalized seizures were reduced at least 50% in 56% and 46%, respectively (respective placebo values: 20%, $P = 0.001$; 17%, $P = 0.003$). No generalized tonic–clonic seizures occurred during the 20-week study in 13% of TPM-treated patients (placebo 5%); 5% had no generalized seizures of any type (placebo 0% of patients).

Because the two trials were identically designed, data were pooled and analyzed. As had been observed in the single trial, TPM reduced the frequency of generalized tonic–clonic and all generalized seizures, with significantly more patients achieving 50% or greater reduction in generalized tonic–clonic (55% vs. 28% with placebo; $P \leq 0.001$) and all generalized seizures (43% vs. 19% with placebo; $P = 0.001$). Although small sample sizes limited analysis, TPM was also more effective than placebo in reducing the frequency of tonic and myoclonic seizures and did not exacerbate absence seizures.

All 131 patients who completed the double-blind phase entered an open-label extension phase (79). During the last 6 months of treatment, 16% had no generalized tonic–clonic seizures and 7% were seizure free for at least 6 months. TPM was also effective against other generalized seizure types; during the last 6 months of treatment, 10% of patients with absence seizures, 33% of patients with myoclonic seizures, and 21% of patients with tonic seizures were seizure free for at least 6 months.

In a study evaluating EEG changes and seizure control in TPM-treated patients with primary generalized epilepsies (80), more than half of patients showed reductions in epileptiform spike-wave activity, although TPM was less likely to suppress activity in patients with very high discharge frequencies at baseline. As with other broad-spectrum AEDs, seizure reduction (36% seizure free) did not correlate with EEG response, and no correlation was observed between clinical or EEG response and TPM blood levels.

Juvenile Myoclonic Epilepsy (JME)

In a pilot study, 15 patients who had previously failed valproic acid (one wanted off strictly due to weight gain and 5 wished to get off due to weight issues) were switched from valproic acid to TPM. Myoclonic seizures stopped in 60% of patients, 49% of generalized tonic–clonic seizure patients became seizure free of that type of seizure and 25% of absence seizure patients stopped having this type of seizure (81).

A small subset of patients with JME was included in the controlled trials evaluating TPM in primary generalized tonic–clonic seizures (77,78). Among 11 patients with JME receiving TPM, primary generalized tonic–clonic seizures were reduced at least 50% in 73% (vs. 18% of patients receiving placebo, $N = 11$; $P = 0.03$) (82). In addition, the frequency of myoclonic seizures was reduced and the number of weeks without absence seizures was increased in TPM-treated patients. In a randomized, open-label study in patients with JME (83), TPM and valproate were similarly effective (seizure-free rates following 12 weeks' treatment: 47% and 33%, respectively). The treatment groups were similar in neurotoxicity scores; however, TPM was associated with less systemic toxicity than valproate.

West Syndrome

Eleven children with refractory West syndrome participated in a pilot study of TPM (84). At a maximum daily dose of 24 mg/kg, the frequency of infantile spasms was reduced by at least 50% in nine children, including five (45%) who were completely controlled. Ancillary seizures responded in four of six children. After 18 months of TPM (mean dosage, 29 mg/kg/day), eight children (73%) continued on medication; four (50%) children were free of spasms, and seven (88%) children had spasms reduced by at least one half (85).

Childhood Absence Epilepsy

Five children 4 to 11 years of age with EEG-documented absence seizures and childhood absence epilepsy were treated with open-label TPM (maximum dose, 12 mg/kg/day) (86). Three children experienced a minimum reduction of 50% at daily dosages of 5 to 6 mg/kg; two children were seizure free. Frequency was unchanged in the remaining two children, even at the maximum dosage.

Severe Myoclonic Epilepsy in Infancy

During a prospective, multicenter, open-label study in 18 patients with severe myoclonic epilepsy in infancy and refractory seizures of different types, three patients became seizure free, six patients had greater than 75% seizure reduction, and four patients had greater than 50% seizure reduction with TPM treatment (87). Seizure frequency was unchanged in five patients; no patients experienced seizure worsening. Mean treatment duration was 12 months (range, 2 to 24 months); mean TPM dose was 5.4 mg/kg/day (range, 2.8 to 10 mg/kg/day).

Patients with Mental Retardation, Learning Disabilities, and/or Developmental Disabilities

Among 64 patients (16 to 65 years of age) with refractory epilepsy and learning disability treated with TPM in an open-label study, 16 patients became seizure free and 29 patients had at least a 50% seizure reduction (88). Many patients, including 63% of those who were seizure free and 66% of treatment responders, were receiving TPM dosages of ≤200 mg/day. In a study evaluating the effect of TPM in 20 adults (21 to 57 years of age) with intractable mixed seizures, mental retardation, and development disabilities, two patients became seizure free and 11 patients had at least a 50% seizure reduction with TPM treatment (89). In addition, the duration and/or severity of seizures were reduced in 44% of patients. The mean duration of treatment was 42 weeks (range, 20 to 54 weeks); the mean TPM dose was 189 mg/day (range, 50 to 350 mg/day).

Refractory Status Epilepticus

In six cases of refractory status epilepticus unresponsive to sequential trials of multiple agents, including one patient who had been in a prolonged pentobarbital coma, TPM (300 to 1600 mg/day) administered via nasogastric tube successfully terminated refractory status epilepticus (90). TPM was effective against both generalized convulsive and nonconvulsive status epilepticus. All patients were subsequently discharged from the hospital.

Monotherapy

The 1990s ushered in a new era—at least in the United States—for clinical studies in newly diagnosed, previously untreated epilepsy. The use of traditional AEDs (carbamazepine, phenytoin, valproate) as first-line monotherapy is largely based on landmark Veterans' Administration Cooperative trials (91,92) and similar open-label trials in the United Kingdom (93,94). However, the U.S. Food and Drug Administration (FDA) began requiring randomized, double-blind trials demonstrating a statistically significant difference between treatments as evidence of efficacy, generating considerable debate as to how to safely and ethically accomplish this goal. One such approach is an active-control conversion-to-monotherapy design in which patients are randomized to study drug or a minimally effective active-control and pre-existing AED therapy is gradually withdrawn (95). Such a design parallels the technique clinicians use to switch patients to a second trial of AED monotherapy when the first agent has failed because of ineffective seizure control or intolerable side effects. Such a design was used as a proof-of-principle trial for TPM monotherapy (96).

Monotherapy trial design becomes particularly complex when evaluating new AEDs in patients with newly or recently diagnosed epilepsy. The use of a placebo control in untreated epilepsy patients remains controversial, and only one such trial has been conducted (97). Unlike their European counterparts, regulatory authorities in the United States are unwilling to accept monotherapy equivalence trials for AEDs already approved as adjunctive therapy (95). The argument is that a trial showing equivalence of two treatments could be interpreted as meaning that both treatments were equally ineffective or that the trial simply failed to detect existing differences (95,98). Given the responsiveness of patients with newly diagnosed epilepsy, some have doubted the possibility of demonstrating a treatment effect with active-control or dose-control trials. These trial types are also controversial in relation to ethical equipoise (99).

TPM has been evaluated as first-line monotherapy in adults and children with newly or recently diagnosed epilepsy in three multicenter, randomized, double-blind trials. Two trials were dose-controlled trials (35,48), and one trial used a novel trial design to simultaneously compare TPM with two standard AEDs (i.e., carbamazepine and valproate) (47).

In the first dose-controlled trial (35), 252 adults and children who had been diagnosed with epilepsy within 3 years of study entry and who had one to six partial-onset seizures during a 3-month retrospective baseline were randomized to 50 mg/day or 500 mg/day TPM (patients weighing ≤50 kg were randomized to 25 mg/day or 200 mg/day). Patients were untreated or had been treated for more than 1 month with one AED. The primary efficacy outcome was time to exit, which was time to second seizure in 96% of patients. Time to exit was longer in patients receiving TPM 200/500 mg/day (median 422 days vs. 293 days in patients receiving 25/50 mg/day), although the difference was not significant. When time to exit was analyzed using time to first seizure as a covariate, the difference between treatment groups was significant ($P = 0.01$). This finding reflected the higher seizure-free rate in patients receiving TPM 200/500 mg/day (54% vs. 39% with 25/50 mg/day; $P = 0.02$) as well as the longer interval before the first seizure (median 317 days vs. 108 days with 25/50 mg/day; $P = 0.06$). In this study, seizure-free rates with 50 mg/day (39%) and TPM 400 mg/day (54%) were at the lower and upper ends for the range of seizure-free rates (36% to 43%) reported with therapeutic dosages of other AEDs in double-blind studies (100,101). The mean dosage among patients randomized to TPM 500 mg/day was 366 mg/day. A significant difference between treatment groups was observed for patients with one or two seizures in the 3-month baseline, but not for patients with three or more seizures in the 3-month baseline. This finding suggested that higher seizure frequency may serve as an indicator of more treatment-resistant seizures in patients with untreated epilepsy and is consistent with other reports linking higher seizure frequency before initial treatment with refractory epilepsy (102).

Results from the first dose-controlled study (35) suggested that TPM 50 mg/day was an effective dose in some patients responsive to anticonvulsant therapy and could serve as an active control to treatment with TPM 400 mg/day. Moreover, patients with one or two seizures in a 3-month baseline may represent the population of patients with newly diagnosed epilepsy who are most likely to benefit from monotherapy and not require polytherapy because of drug-resistant epilepsy. In the second dose-controlled study (48), 470 adults and children (weighing at least 25 kg) were eligible if they had untreated epilepsy diagnosed within 3 months of study entry, or if epilepsy had relapsed while they were not receiving anticonvulsant therapy. Patients could have only one or two partial-onset or generalized tonic–clonic seizures during the 3-month retrospective baseline. The primary efficacy end point was time to first seizure; seizure-free rates at 6 months and 1 year were secondary efficacy measures. Kaplan–Meier survival analyses for time to first seizure showed a significantly greater treatment effect with the 400 mg/day group versus the 50 mg/day group ($P = 0.0002$). The probability of being seizure free was 83% with the 400 mg/day group and 71% with the 50 mg/day group ($P = 0.005$) after 6 months treatment and 76% and 59% ($P = 0.001$) after 12 months. A difference between dose groups emerged within the first week after randomization when patients were receiving 25 mg/day or 50 mg/day; the between-group difference was significant after 2 weeks when patients were receiving 25 mg/day or 100 mg/day. The mean dosage achieved for each of these groups was 46 mg/day (in the so-called 50 mg/day group) and 275 mg/day (in the so-called 400 mg group). The reason that the numbers were less than 50 and 400 mg/day was that for example for the higher dosage patients, they had to be increased to at least 150 mg/day but not necessarily to 400 mg/day. Approximately half of the patients were not fully titrated to 400 mg/day and approximately half were titrated up to 400 mg/day (investigator discretion). Similarly one could stop at 25 mg/day for the low dosage group and did not have to increase to 50 mg/day.

The effectiveness of TPM 100 mg/day as initial monotherapy in patients with newly diagnosed epilepsy was established further with a randomized, double-blind trial comparing TPM, carbamazepine, and valproate in adults and children ($N = 613$) with newly diagnosed epilepsy (47). No seizure types/epilepsy syndromes were excluded. During this trial, investigators selected carbamazepine (600 mg/day) or valproate (1250 mg/day) as the preferred therapy according to each patient's clinical presentation. Patients were then assigned to the carbamazepine or valproate treatment branch. Within each branch, patients were randomized to double-blind treatment with the investigator's choice of traditional AED (carbamazepine or valproate), TPM 100 mg/day, or TPM 200 mg/day. Patients continued double-blind treatment until exiting the study or until 6 months after the last patient was randomized.

The initial efficacy analysis compared time to first seizure for the two TPM dosages (100 and 200 mg/day). If TPM 200 mg/day was significantly more effective than TPM 100 mg/day, then 200 mg/day was to be compared with carbamazepine and valproate. If 200 mg/day was not significantly more effective, the protocol required TPM dosage groups to be pooled within each branch and compared with traditional therapy. For the comparison between TPM and traditional therapy, the primary efficacy measure was time to exit; secondary efficacy end points were time to first seizure and proportion of patients seizure free during the last 6 months of double-blind treatment.

No difference was observed for the initial efficacy analysis comparing the two TPM dosages groups. Therefore, the combined TPM groups were compared with carbamazepine and valproate treatment. In both the carbamazepine and valproate branches, time to exit did not differ between the combined TPM treatment groups and traditional therapy. Because the branches were homogeneous, pooled data across branches were used to calculate 95% confidence intervals (CIs) for treatment differences. Although retention rates were higher among patients receiving TPM compared with those receiving carbamazepine or valproate, 95% CIs included zero, which indicated that between-group differences were not statistically significant. Similar results were observed for time to first seizure. The proportion of patients with no seizures during the last 6 months of double-blind treatment was 49% among patients receiving TPM 100 mg/day and 44% in each of the other three treatment groups (i.e., TPM 200 mg/day, carbamazepine, and valproate). The 95% CIs were narrow and included zero, indicating no difference among the four treatment groups.

Results from two trials showing that TPM 100 mg/day is effective in adults and children with newly diagnosed epilepsy support clinical findings suggesting that only low to moderate dosages of AEDs are required in patients with new-onset epilepsy that is responsive to treatment (103).

Other Clinical Uses

Studies suggest that TPM may prevent migraine attacks. Two randomized, double-blind, placebo-controlled trials evaluated the efficacy of TPM treatment (50, 100, and 200 mg/day) in 970 patients with migraine (104,105). The primary efficacy measure was change in mean monthly migraine frequency from baseline during double-blind treatment. Compared with placebo, significant reductions in monthly migraine frequency were reported with TPM dosages of 100 and 200 mg/day; migraine frequency was also reduced with 50 mg/day, although the difference from placebo was not statistically significant. The proportion of treatment responders with a 50% or more reduction in monthly migraine frequency was significantly greater in TPM-treated patients (36% to 54% vs. 23% with placebo) (104,105). TPM may also have favorable effects in patients with cluster headache; in a case series, cluster remission occurred in nine of 10 patients (106).

TPM may have a potential role in movement disorder treatment. In a double-blind, placebo-controlled, crossover trial in 62 patients with essential tremor, TPM was associated with significant improvements in tremor severity, motor task performance, and functional disability (107), findings that were consistent with those in an earlier pilot study (108). In a retrospective chart review, TPM seemed to be effective in reducing tics in children and adolescents with Tourette syndrome (109); 59% (19/32) of patients had at least 50% reduction in tic severity scores.

Several studies suggest that TPM may be effective in various impulse control disorders. In a randomized, double-blind, placebo-controlled trial in 150 patients with alcohol dependence, TPM-treated patients had significantly fewer drinks per day, drinks per drinking per day, and heavy drinking days and significantly more abstinent days compared with placebo (110). Plasma α-glutamyl transferase, an objective index of alcohol consumption, was also significantly lower in TPM-treated patients. Among 61 obese patients with binge-eating disorder who were participating in a randomized, double-blind, placebo-controlled trial, TPM treatment was associated with significantly greater reductions in binge frequency, binge per day frequency, body mass index (BMI), body weight, and obsessive–compulsive scores (111). Open-label treatment with TPM has been reported to improve behavior, mood, weight control, compulsive eating problems, and self-mutilating behavior (notably skin picking) associated with Prader–Willi syndrome (112,113).

The observation that TPM is associated with weight loss and expected improvement in metabolic parameters (e.g., lipids, blood pressure, glucose levels) (114), led to studies of TPM (64 to 384 mg/day) in obese patients (115). After 6 months, mean percent decrease in baseline body weight was significantly greater among TPM-treated patients (range, 4.8% to 6.3% depending on TPM dose; 2.6% with placebo). A similar pattern of weight loss was observed in patients with diabetes who participated in three double-blind, placebo-controlled trials evaluating the efficacy of TPM in painful diabetic neuropathy (116). Moreover, in these trials diabetic control, measured as HbA1c levels, improved significantly compared with placebo, with reductions in HbA1c occurring independent of weight loss. These findings are supported by data from an animal model of diabetes, in which TPM demonstrated dose-dependent decreases in blood glucose and plasma triglycerides without significant body weight changes (117).

In view of the role of glutamate and AMPA in the pathobiology of neuronal injury, attention has been focused on TPM because of its activity as an AMPA antagonist. Potential neuroprotective and disease-modifying effects of TPM have been observed in models of seizure-related neuronal injury (23), focal cerebral ischemia (118), and glutamate excitotoxicity (119). Preliminary data in patients with diabetic neuropathy suggest that TPM may improve or restore nerve function through preservation/regeneration of C-fibers, with associated improvement in functional parameters (120). Studies using a cerebral microdialysis technique in patients with traumatic brain injury showed that TPM reduced glutamate levels compared with historical controls (121). In a double-blind, placebo-controlled trial, high-dose TPM (800 mg/day) did not provide beneficial effects in patients with amyotrophic lateral sclerosis (ALS) and may have accelerated the loss of arm muscle strength. In this study, TPM treatment was associated with an increased risk of side effects (122). These findings are useful for advancing our understanding of potential therapeutic targets.

Use in Pregnancy

TPM carries a category C classification (42). According to the PDR 2009, a category C rating indicates "adequate, well controlled human studies are lacking and animal studies have shown a risk to the fetus or are lacking as well. There is a chance of fetal harm if the drug is administered during pregnancy, but the potential benefits may outweigh the potential risks" (123). In animal studies, fetal abnormalities were similar to those observed with other carbonic anhydrase inhibitors such as acetazolamide, whose use has not been linked to teratogenic effects in humans. The effects of TPM in humans are unknown. One company sponsored study with 75 pregnancies with 29 monotherapy exposures revealed two malformations. The other 46 pregnancies in

that study were exposed to at least one other AED; 7 infants had a malformation (124). Preliminary experience from the UK Epilepsy and Pregnancy Registry which is a prospective observational registry and follow-up study revealed 203 pregnancies with 173 live births. There were 16 major congenital malformations (MCM) (9%). Of these 16 patients, 3 cases were on monotherapy (out of 70 monotherapy cases) (4.8%) and 13 were on polypharmacy (11.2%). Four MCMs were oral clefts (2.2%). There were four cases of hypospadias among 78 live male births. Two of these cases were classified as major malformations (125). Caution is advised due to sample size and wide CIs. Of additional note, approximately half of these patients were migraine patients and not all were epilepsy patients. In addition much of the data was in polypharmacy. These are the first data we have had on TPM in pregnancy and while these findings are of potential concern, until we have more research from other pregnancy registries, they cannot be interpreted as definitive (126). Pregnancy registries in the United States and Europe are collecting information about the use of TPM and other AEDs during pregnancy. A recent progress report from the North American Antiepileptic Drug Registry showed 8 total malformations out of 197 enrolled monotherapy pregnancies with TPM (prevalence 4.1%) (95% CIs 1.9 to 7.6%) (127). Identified malformations were eight separate, common birth defects and did not show an increase for any specific abnormality. (Data preliminary since predictions would be much more certain with a larger sample size—preferably greater than 600 pregnancies.)

TPM is extensively excreted in human breast milk and nursing infants are exposed to TPM (plasma concentrations in infants are 10% to 20% of maternal concentrations); the significance of this exposure is unknown (128).

ADVERSE EFFECTS

Central Nervous System

As expected with anticonvulsants, CNS effects were the most commonly reported side effects in randomized, controlled trials with TPM. Their relatively high incidence in early double-blind, placebo-controlled trials were attributable in part to high starting doses, rapid dose escalation, and high drug load when supratherapeutic dosages of TPM were added to maximum tolerated dosages of one or more AEDs (60). Various studies showed that the incidence and severity of CNS effects, as well as premature discontinuations because of side effects, could be reduced with more gradual dose escalation, lower target doses, and reductions in the dosages of concomitant AEDs as TPM was titrated to effect (62,129,130).

Although many of the CNS effects were nonspecific complaints seen with all AEDs (e.g., somnolence, fatigue, dizziness, ataxia, confusion), the early studies were characterized by a relatively high incidence of adverse events coded to the term "abnormal thinking" per WHOART (World Health Organization Adverse Reporting Terminology) (51,52). Subsequently, neurobehavioral adverse events were coded with an expanded adverse-event term list that included psychomotor slowing, memory difficulty, concentration/attention difficulty, speech problems, language problems, and mood problems, among others. A double-blind study comparing

TPM with carbamazepine and valproate as monotherapy in newly diagnosed epilepsy was the first in which the adverse events occurring with other AEDs were coded with the dictionary that is unique to TPM trials (47). The incidence of neurobehavioral side effects was low with all three medications. TPM 100 mg/day and carbamazepine 600 mg/day were indistinguishable in terms of most neurobehavioral side effects (concentration and attention difficulty, 4% in each group; psychomotor slowing, 4%; confusion, 3%; speech disorders, 2%), which occurred less frequently in patients receiving valproate 1250 mg/day (concentration and attention difficulty, 1%; psychomotor slowing, 1%; no reports of confusion or speech problems). Cognitive problems not otherwise specified, as well as memory difficulty, were slightly more common with TPM than with the other agents (cognitive problems not otherwise specified: TPM, 3%; carbamazepine and valproate, 1%; memory difficulty: TPM, 8%; valproate, 6%; carbamazepine, 5%), while language problems were somewhat more common with carbamazepine (carbamazepine, 6%; valproate, 4%; TPM, 3%).

Although TPM and carbamazepine have not been compared in terms of their effects on objective measures of cognitive function, two studies have compared TPM and valproate added to carbamazepine in patients with uncontrolled partial-onset seizures (131,132). In a double-blind study in which patients were followed for 20 weeks, 1 of 17 neuropsychometric variables (short-term verbal memory) showed a statistically significant difference between treatments (worsening of scores with TPM and improvement with valproate). Although the study did not include measures of language function, it used the titration schedule most commonly used in clinical practice when adding TPM to other AEDs (i.e., 25 mg/day starting dose increased weekly in 25-mg increments to a target dose of 200 to 400 mg/day). In a double-blind study using a more rapid escalation schedule (50 mg/day starting dose increased weekly in 50-mg increments to a target dose of 400 mg/day) to add TPM to carbamazepine, cognitive performance was significantly worse from baseline in seven of 24 variables at the end of the 8-week titration period but in only 2 of 24 variables (controlled oral word association and symbol digit modalities) after an additional 3 months of treatment (132). Compared with valproate added to carbamazepine, TPM scores during neuropsychometric testing were slightly worse overall. In this study, it appeared that a subset of patients was more sensitive to TPM and accounted for much of the worsening in cognitive function scores. Because pharmacodynamic interactions are a major factor in the neurobehavioral adverse events that have been reported with TPM polytherapy, neuropsychometric testing during TPM monotherapy would be a better indicator of the effects of TPM on cognitive function. However, no such study in patients with epilepsy has been published. A short-term study in healthy volunteers showed that a high starting dose (100 mg/day) and escalation to 400 mg/day in 4 weeks was associated with significant decreases from baseline on measures of attention and word fluency (133). However, the results of this study have little clinical relevance since the 400 mg/day dosage was four times higher than the recommended target dose of 100 mg/day in newly diagnosed epilepsy.

Although the comparative study of TPM, carbamazepine, and valproate as monotherapy showed that language and speech disorders were actually no more common with TPM, at least as monotherapy, than with carbamazepine, the occurrence of word-finding difficulty during TPM therapy has generated considerable interest, as evidenced by the studies using comprehensive neuropsychometric test batteries. In addition, investigators have sought potential risk factors for adverse cognitive effects with TPM. In a prospective study from a tertiary epilepsy center, left temporal lobe epilepsy and simple partial seizures were most strongly associated with the occurrence of word-finding difficulty in the 31 of 431 patients (7%) who developed word-finding difficulty during TPM therapy (134). As in the double-blind cognitive function study (132), it appeared that the word-finding difficulty in a small subset of patients reflected a biologic vulnerability.

The original double-masked placebo-controlled studies were all forced-titration studies that increased each patient's dosage to a target dose, usually at weekly increments of 100 to 200 mg/day. The recommended titration rate (weekly increments of 50 mg/day or less) is slower and has clearly been associated with improved tolerability (27). TPM may be increased at 25 to 50 mg/week increments and it is this author's opinion that 2-week intervals may be best. If TPM is titrated too quickly, patients may complain of agitation, anxiety, or nervousness as well as word-finding difficulties. This can often be ameliorated by slowing the rate of titration. Keeping TPM total dosage per day at no greater than 200 mg by 6 to 8 weeks is often best. Reduction in the dose of concomitant AEDs can further decrease side effects. Particularly in patients with high valproic acid levels reduction of the dose of valproate can improve cognitive side effects. Patients with thrombocytopenia while taking valproate may have a futher reduction in platelet count with the addition of TPM (39). Platelet counts increase when the valproate dose is reduced. In most cases, side effects are manageable and do not require discontinuation of the drug (27).

Carbonic Anhydrase Inhibition

Side effects that can be linked to TPM inhibition of carbonic anhydrase isozymes (CA II and CA IV) are paresthesia, renal stones, and decreased serum bicarbonate. Paresthesias are often transient, resolve with continuing treatment, and rarely lead to drug discontinuation. Paresthesias are more common with TPM monotherapy (35,47,48) than as add-on treatment (60), which is likely caused by higher TPM plasma levels in the absence of hepatic enzyme-inducing AEDs.

As in the general population, renal stone formation in TPM clinical trials was more common in men. Other risk factors for renal stone formation include personal or family history of renal stones, chronic metabolic acidosis, and coadministration of other carbonic anhydrase inhibitors or the ketogenic diet. Although chronic metabolic acidosis may increase the risk of renal stone formation, serum bicarbonate levels are not reliable predictors of renal stone formation. Patients should maintain adequate hydration to increase urinary output and lower the concentration of stone-forming substances.

In some patients, carbonic anhydrase inhibition is associated with laboratory findings of reduced serum bicarbonate levels. In clinical trials, the mean serum bicarbonate reduction was 4 mEq/L. Although reductions in serum bicarbonate levels are usually asymptomatic, nonspecific symptoms may include fatigue, anorexia, nausea, and vomiting; no correlation between these symptoms and serum bicarbonate levels was observed in TPM-treated patients. Cases of metabolic acidosis marked by hyperventilation and acute changes in mental status have been reported in patients receiving TPM, primarily children (135–137), although most cases have been asymptomatic (138–140). Reductions in serum bicarbonate levels generally occur early in treatment and tend to stabilize without progression during continued treatment (nevertheless, more pronounced at higher doses). Conditions that increase bicarbonate loss (e.g., renal disease, diarrhea, other carbonic anhydrase inhibitors), interfere with carbon dioxide regulation via the lungs (e.g., severe respiratory disorders, surgery, status epilepticus), or alter acid–base balance (ketogenic diet) may have additive effects. It is prudent to monitor serum bicarbonate in patients with any of these potentially exacerbating conditions.

Due to the potential for untreated hyperchloremic normal anion gap, metabolic acidosis the potential for osteomalacia (rickets) with reduced growth rates in children has been raised as a hypothetical concern. The effect of these metabolic abnormalities on adult bone remain speculative.

Adverse Effects in Children

During controlled clinical trials with TPM adjunctive therapy, the incidence of CNS effects in children, including cognitive effects, was generally lower than that in adults, perhaps reflecting a more gradual dose-escalation schedule (60,66,72,77,78). The most common CNS effects in children were somnolence and decreased appetite. TPM did not negatively affect measures of mental status as evaluated by parents and guardians during double-blind treatment (66), although a formal study with neuropsychological testing has not been performed in children. Temporary slowing of weight gain or minor weight loss occurred with TPM treatment; however, weight gain resumed in most children with continued therapy (141). TPM does not adversely affect growth, measured as height, in children (142).

Pooled data from three randomized, double-blind trials (35,47,48) in which 245 children/adolescents as young as 3 years of age with newly or recently diagnosed epilepsy received 50 to 500 mg/day TPM as first-line monotherapy showed that the incidence of CNS effects, including neurobehavioral effects, was lower than with adjunctive therapy, even though the treatment periods were longer (median 8 months; treatment periods as long as 2.2 years) (143). The most common CNS effects were headache, decreased appetite, and somnolence. In most children, body weight increased or did not change; among 13 patients who lost 10% or more of baseline body weight, 12 were adolescents (12 to 15 years old). No child/adolescent discontinued TPM monotherapy because of weight loss. As noted above, metabolic acidosis may be more likely to be symptomatic in children receiving TPM compared with adults.

Idiosyncratic Toxicity

No clinically significant abnormalities in hematologic or hepatic function were reported during clinical trials (60), and laboratory test values remained generally unchanged other than expected reductions in serum bicarbonate levels and increased chloride levels.

TPM has been associated with a rare ocular syndrome consisting of acute myopia with increased intraocular pressure (144). The syndrome occurs bilaterally and at any age, in contrast to primary narrow angle closure, which is rarely bilateral and rare in individuals younger than 40 years of age. Symptoms occur early in TPM therapy (within the first month) and include acute (usually quite apparent) onset of blurred vision and/or ocular pain and/or red eyes. Ophthalmologic findings were bilateral and could include severe myopia, conjunctival hyperemia, shallowing of the anterior chambers, and increased intraocular pressure. Mydriasis was an inconsistent finding. Symptoms resolve upon prompt discontinuation of TPM treatment.

Decreased sweating (oligohidrosis) and an elevation in body temperature have been reported in association with TPM use; the majority of reports were in children. Most cases occurred after exposure to hot weather (145).

Weight Loss

Weight loss of 1.6 to 6.5 kg was reported in patients during the clinical trials. Patients who weighed most (>100 kg) before TPM therapy experienced the greatest weight loss (mean weight loss, 9.6 kg) compared with those who weighed least (<60 kg) before TPM treatment (mean weight loss, 1.3 kg). For patients receiving long-term TPM therapy, body-weight reductions were most commonly noted during the first 3 months of treatment and peaked at 12 to 18 months. This was partially reversed in some patients who gained weight starting with the second year of therapy (27).

Pooled data from double-blind, placebo-controlled trials and open-label studies showed that 85% of 1319 adults with epilepsy receiving TPM as monotherapy or as adjunctive therapy lost weight; mean body weight change was 3.8 kg loss (4.6% of baseline body weight) (146). Weight loss was a function of baseline body weight, with greater losses occurring in patients with higher pretreatment weight. Weight loss was gradual, typically began during the initial 3 months of therapy, and peaked at 12 to 18 months. Weight loss was accompanied by positive changes in lipid profile, glycemic control, and blood pressure. In a prospective study evaluating weight changes associated with TPM treatment (114), more than 80% of adults lost weight without changes in diet or exercise; obese patients (BMI $\geq$ 30 kg/m^2) had the greatest degree of weight loss. Reduction of body fat mass represented 60% to 70% of the absolute weight loss. In these patients, weight loss was associated with improvements in glucose, insulin, and total cholesterol levels.

Weight loss has been observed in patients receiving TPM for conditions other than epilepsy. During two double-blind, placebo-controlled trials in patients with migraine (104,105), dose-related decreases in body weight were observed; the mean percent change in body weight compared with placebo was significantly greater in patients receiving TPM. During three double-blind, placebo-controlled trials in patients with diabetic neuropathy, 18% to 40% had clinically significant weight loss (5% or more of baseline body weight) with TPM treatment (116). The observed improvement in diabetic control, measured as reduction in HbA1c levels, did not seem to correlate with TPM-induced weight loss.

CLINICAL USE

The initial randomized, controlled trials with TPM as adjunctive therapy identified TPM 200 to 400 mg/day as an appropriate target dose in adults with refractory epilepsy; subsequent studies have shown that many patients respond to TPM dosages of ≤200 mg/day. While gradual introduction improves tolerability, TPM can be added rapidly, if needed. Reducing the dose of concomitant AEDs as TPM is added also improves tolerability. In children receiving TPM as adjunctive therapy, the recommended daily dose is 5 to 9 mg/kg; the starting dose of 1 to 3 mg/kg/day can be increased in 1- to 3-mg/kg increments every 1 to 2 weeks.

As first-line monotherapy in adults with newly or recently diagnosed epilepsy, 100 mg/day is an appropriate target dose to initially assess patient response. It appears the optimal starting dose in adults is 25 to 50 mg/day, with weekly or biweekly increases of 25 to 50 mg/day. As initial monotherapy in children, the recommended dose is 3 to 6 mg/kg/day, using a starting dose of 0.5 to 1 mg/kg/day and incremental increases of 0.5 to 1 mg/kg at 1- or 2-week intervals.

ACKNOWLEDGMENTS

I would like to thank Michael D. Privitera, MD, Professor and Vice-Chair Neurology, Director, Cincinnati Epilepsy Center, Medical Director, UC Physicians—University of Cincinnati Medical Center, for his earlier excellent contributions to a previous edition chapter. I would like to thank my wife, Susan M. Lippmann, MD, my partner in epilepsy and life for assisting with this publication. I would like to thank Caren Hein for her excellent administrative assistance.

References

1. Patsalos PN, Sander JWAS. Newer antiepileptic drugs. Towards an improved risk-benefit ration. *Drug Saf.* 1994;11:37–67.
2. Gibbs JW, Sombati S, DeLorenzo RJ, et al. Cellular actions of topiramate blockade of kainate-evoked inward currents in cultured hippocampal neurons. *Epilepsia.* 2000;41(suppl 1):S10–S16.
3. Skradski S, White HS. Topiramate blocks kainate-evoked cobalt influx into cultured neurons. *Epilepsia.* 2000;41(suppl 1):S45–S47.
4. Coulter DA, Sombati S, DeLorenzo RJ. Topiramate effects on excitatory amino acid-mediated responses in cultured hippocampal neurons: selective blockade of kainate currents [abstract]. *Epilepsia.* 1995;36(suppl 3):S40.
5. Rogawski MA, Gryder D, Castaneda D, et al. GluR5 kainate receptors, seizures, and the amygdala. *Ann N Y Acad Sci.* 2003;985:150–162.
6. DeLorenzo RJ, Sombati S, Coulter DA. Effects of topiramate on sustained repetitive firing and spontaneous recurrent seizure discharge in cultured hippocampal neurons. *Epilepsia.* 2000;41(suppl 1):S40–S44.
7. McLean MJ, Bukhari AA, Wamil AW. Effects of topiramate on sodium-dependent action-potential firing by mouse spinal cord neurons in cell culture. *Epilepsia.* 2000;41(suppl 1):S21–S24.
8. Taverna S, Sancini G, Mantegazza M, et al. Inhibition of transient and persistent Na+ current fractions by the new anticonvulsant topiramate. *J Pharmacol Exp Ther.* 1999;288:960–968.
9. Zona C, Ciotti MT, Avoli M. Topiramate attenuates voltage-gated sodium currents in rat cerebellar granule cells. *Neurosci Lett.* 1997;231:123–126.
10. Wu SP, Tsai JJ, Gean PW. Frequency-dependent inhibition of neuronal activity by topiramate in rat hippocampal slices. *Br J Pharmacol.* 1998;125:826–832.
11. White HS, Brown SD, Woodhead JH, et al. Topiramate modulates GABA-evoked currents in murine cortical neurons by a nonbenzodiazepine mechanism. *Epilepsia.* 2000;41(suppl 1):S17–S20.
12. White HS, Brown SD, Woodhead JH, et al. Topiramate enhances GABA-mediated chloride flux and GABA-evoked chloride currents in murine brain neurons and increases seizure threshold. *Epilepsy Res.* 1997;28:167–179.
13. Zhang X-l, Velumian AA, Jones OT, et al. Modulation of high-voltage-activated calcium channels in dentate granule cells by topiramate. *Epilepsia.* 2000;41(suppl 1):S52–S60.
14. Ängehagen M, Ben-Menachem E, Rönnbäck L, et al. Topiramate protects against glutamate- and kainate-induced neurotoxicity in primary neuronal-astroglial cultures. *Epilepsy Res.* 2003;54:63–71.
15. Herrero AI, Del Olmo N, Gonzalez-Escalada JR, et al. Two new actions of topiramate: inhibition of depolarizing GABA (A)-mediated responses and activation of a potassium conductance. *Neuropharmacology.* 2002;42:210–220.
16. Russo E, Constanti A. Topiramate hyperpolarizes and modulates the slow post stimulus AHP of rat olfactory cortical neurones in vitro. *Br J Pharmacol.* 2004;141:285–301.
17. Shank RP, Gardocki JF, Streeter AJ, et al. An overview of the preclinical aspects of topiramate: pharmacology, pharmacokinetics, and mechanism of action. *Epilepsia.* 2000;41(suppl 1):S3–S9.
18. Dodgson SJ, Shank RP, Maryanoff BE. Topiramate as an inhibitor of carbonic anhydrase isoenzymes. *Epilepsia.* 2000;41(suppl 1):S35–S39.
19. Shank RP, Gardocki JF, Vaught JL, et al. Topiramate: preclinical evaluation of a structurally novel anticonvulsant. *Epilepsia.* 1994;35:450–460.
20. Nakamura J, Tamura S, Kanda T, et al. Inhibition by topiramate of seizures in spontaneously epileptic rats and DBA/2 mice. *Eur J Pharmacol.* 1994;254:83–89.
21. Edmonds HL Jr, Jiang YD, Zhang PY, et al. Anticonvulsant activity of topiramate and phenytoin in a rat model of ischemia-induced epilepsy. *Life Sci.* 1996;59:PL127–PL131.
22. Wauquier A, Zhou S. Topiramate: a potent anticonvulsant in the amygala-kindled rat. *Epilepsy Res.* 1996;24:73–77.
23. Niebauer M, Gruenthal M. Topiramate reduces neuronal injury after experimental status epilepticus. *Brain Res.* 1999;837:263–269.
24. DeLorenzo RJ, Morris TA, Blair RE, et al. Topiramate is both neuroprotective and antiepileptogenic in the pilocarpine model of status epilepticus [abstract]. *Epilepsia.* 2002;43(suppl 7):15.
25. Koh S, Jensen FE. Topiramate blocks perinatal hypoxia-induced seizures in rat pups. *Ann Neurol.* 2001;50:366–372.
26. Bialer M. Comparative pharmacokinetics of the newer antiepileptic drugs. *Clin Pharmacokinet.* 1993;24:441–452.
27. Rosenfeld, WE. Topiramate: a review of preclinical, pharmacokinetic, and clinical data. *Clin Ther.* 1997;19(6):1294–1308.
28. Doose DR, Walker SA, Gisclon LG, et al. Single-dose pharmacokinetics and effect of food on the bioavailability of topiramate, a novel antiepileptic drug. *J Clin Pharmacol.* 1996;36:884–891.
29. Garnett WR. Clinical pharmacology of topiramate: a review. *Epilepsia.* 2002;41(suppl 1):S61–S65.
30. Rosenfeld WE, Doose DR, Walker SA, et al. A study of topiramate pharmacokinetics and tolerability in children with epilepsy. *Pediatr Neurol.* 1999;20:339–344.
31. Glauser TA, Miles MV, Tang P, et al. Topiramate pharmacokinetics in infants. *Epilepsia.* 1999;40:788–791.
32. Doose DR, Larson KL, Natarajan J, et al. Comparative single-dose pharmacokinetics of topiramate in elderly versus young men and women [abstract]. *Epilepsia.* 1998;39(suppl 6):56.
33. Gisclon LG, Curtin CR, Sica DA, et al. The pharmacokinetics (PK) of topiramate (TPM) in subjects with end-stage renal disease undergoing hemodialysis. *Clin Pharmacol Ther.* 1994;55:196. [Abstract PIII-56].
34. Faught E, Squires L, Wang S, et al. Tolerability and safety of topiramate as first-line monotherapy in 1,000+ epilepsy patients [abstract]. *Epilepsia.* 2003;44(suppl 9):100.
35. Gilliam FG, Veloso F, Bomhof MAM, et al. A dose-comparison trial of topiramate as monotherapy in recently diagnosed partial epilepsy. *Neurology.* 2003;60:196–202.
36. Schwabe MJ, Wheless JW. Clinical experience with topiramate dosing and serum levels in children 12 years or under with epilepsy. *J Child Neurol.* 2001;16:806–808.
37. Sachdeo RC, Sachdeo SK, Walker SA, et al. Steady-state pharmacokinetics of topiramate and carbamazepine in patients with epilepsy during monotherapy and concomitant therapy. *Epilepsia.* 1996;37:774–780.
38. Gisclon LG, Curtin CR, Kramer LD. The steady-state pharmacokinetics of phenytoin (Dilantin Kapseals brand) and of Topamax (topiramate) in male and female epileptic patients on monotherapy, and during combination therapy. *Epilepsia.* 1994;35(suppl 8):54. [Abstract].
39. Rosenfeld WE, Liao S, Kramer LD, et al. Comparison of the steady-state pharmacokinetics of topiramate and valproate in patients with epilepsy during monotherapy and concomitant therapy. *Epilepsia.* 1997;38:324–333.
40. Doose DR, Brodie ME, Wilson EA, et al. Topiramate and lamotrigine pharmacokinetics during repetitive monotherapy and combination therapy in epilepsy patients. *Epilepsia.* 2003;44:917–922.
41. Doose DR, Wang S-S, Padmanabhan M, et al. Effect of topiramate or carbamazepine on the pharmacokinetics of an oral contraceptive containing norethindrone and ethinyl estradiol in healthy obese and nonobese female subjects. *Epilepsia.* 2003;44:540–549.
42. Rosenfeld WE, Doose DR, Walker SA, et al. Effect of topiramate on the pharmacokinetics of an oral contraceptive containing norethindrone and ethinyl estradiol in patients with epilepsy. *Epilepsia.* 1997;38:317–323.

43. Nallani SC, Glauser TA, Hariparsad N, et al. Dose-dependent induction of cytochrome P450(CYP)3A4 and activation of pregnane X receptor by topiramate. *Epilepsia.* 2003;44:1521–1528.
44. Doose DR, Walker SA, Pledger G, et al. Evaluation of phenobarbital and primidone/phenobarbital (primidone's active metabolite) plasma concentrations during administration of add-on topiramate therapy in five multicenter, double-blind, placebo-controlled trials in outpatients with partial seizures [abstract]. *Epilepsia.* 1995;36(suppl 3):S158.
45. Sachdeo RC, Sachdeo SK, Levy RH, et al. Topiramate and phenytoin pharmacokinetics during repetitive monotherapy and combination therapy to epileptic patients. *Epilepsia.* 2002;43:691–696.
46. Levy RH, Bishop F, Streeter AJ, et al. Explanation and prediction of drug interactions with topiramate using a CYP450 inhibition spectrum [abstract]. *Epilepsia.* 1995;36(suppl 4):S47.
47. Privitera MD, Brodie MJ, Mattson RH, et al. Topiramate, carbamazepine and valproate monotherapy: double-blind comparison in newly diagnosed epilepsy. *Acta Neurol Scand.* 2003;107:165–175.
48. Arroyo S, Squires L, Wang S, et al. Topiramate: effective as monotherapy in dose-response study in newly diagnosed epilepsy [abstract]. *Epilepsia.* 2002;43(suppl 7):241.
49. Liao S, Palmer M. Digoxin and topiramate drug interaction study in male volunteers [abstract]. *Pharm Res.* 1993;10(suppl):S405.
50 Topamax® (topiramate) tablets/(topiramate capsules) Sprinkle Capsules package insert. Raritan, NJ: Ortho-McNeil Pharmaceutical, Inc., December 2003.
51. Faught E, Wilder BJ, Ramsay RE, et al. Topiramate placebo-controlled dose-ranging trial in refractory partial epilepsy using 200-, 400-, and 600-mg daily dosages. *Neurology.* 1996;46:1684–1690.
52. Privitera M, Fincham R, Penry J, et al. Topiramate placebo-controlled dose-ranging trial in refractory partial epilepsy using 600-, 800-, and 1000-mg daily dosages. *Neurology.* 1996;46:1678–1683.
53. Sharief M, Viteri C, Ben-Menachem E, et al. Double-blind, placebo-controlled study of topiramate in patients with refractory partial epilepsy. *Epilepsia Res.* 1996;25:217–224.
54. Tassinari CA, Michelucci R, Chauvel P, et al. Double-blind, placebo-controlled trial of topiramate (600 mg daily) for the treatment of refractory partial epilepsy. *Epilepsia.* 1996;37:763–768.
55 Ben-Menachem E, Henriksen O, Dam M, et al. Double-blind, placebo-controlled trial of topiramate as add-on therapy in patients with refractory partial seizures. *Epilepsia.* 1996;37:539–543.
56. Rosenfeld W, Abou-Khalil B, Reife R, et al. Placebo-controlled trial of topiramate as adjunctive therapy to carbamazepine or phenytoin for partial-onset epilepsy [abstract]. *Epilepsia.* 1996;37(suppl 5):153.
57. Korean Topiramate Study Group. Topiramate in medically intractable partial epilepsies: double-blind placebo-controlled randomized parallel group trial. *Epilepsia.* 1999;40:1767–1774.
58. Yen D-J, Yu H-Y, Guo Y-C, et al. A double-blind, placebo-controlled study of topiramate in adult patients with refractory partial epilepsy. *Epilepsia.* 2000;41:1162–1166.
59. Guberman A, Neto W, Gassmann-Mayer C, et al. Low-dose topiramate in adults with treatment-resistant partial-onset seizures. *Acta Neurol Scand.* 2002;106:183–189.
60. Reife R, Pledger G, Wu S. Topiramate as add-on therapy: pooled analysis of randomized controlled trials in adults. *Epilepsia.* 2000;41(suppl 1): S66–S71.
61. Korean Topiramate Study Group. Low dose and slow titration of topiramate as adjunctive therapy in refractory partial epilepsies: a multicentre open clinical trial. *Seizure.* 2002;11:255–260.
62. Dodson WE, Kamin M, Kraut L, et al. Topiramate titration to response: analysis of individualized therapy study (TRAITS). *Ann Pharmacother.* 2003;37:615–620.
63. Stephen LJ, Sills GJ, Brodie MJ. Topiramate in refractory epilepsy: a prospective observational study. *Epilepsia.* 2000;41:977–980.
64. Lhatoo SD, Wong ICK, Polizzi G, et al. Long-term retention rates of lamotrigine, gabapentin, and topiramate in chronic epilepsy. *Epilepsia.* 2000; 41:1592–1596.
65. Lhatoo SD, Wong ICK, Sander JWAS. Prognostic factors affecting long-term retention of topiramate in patients with chronic epilepsy. *Epilepsia.* 2000;41:338–341.
66. Elterman RD, Glauser TA, Wyllie E, et al. A double-blind, randomized trial of topiramate as adjunctive therapy for partial-onset seizures in children. *Neurology.* 1999;52:1338–1344.
67. Ritter FJ, Glauser TA, Elterman R, et al. Effectiveness, tolerability and safety of topiramate in children with partial-onset seizures. *Epilepsia.* 2000;41(suppl 1):S82–S85.
68. Mikaeloff Y, de Saint-Martin A, Mancini J, et al. Topiramate: efficacy and tolerability in children according to epilepsy syndromes. *Epilepsy Res.* 2003;53:225–232.
69. Coppola G, Caliendo G, Terracciano MM, et al. Topiramate in refractory partial-onset seizures in children, adolescents, and young adults: a multicentric open trial. *Epilepsy Res.* 2001;43:255–260.
70. Mohamed K, Appleton R, Rosenbloom L. Efficacy and tolerability of topiramate in childhood and adolescent epilepsy: a clinical experience. *Seizure.* 2000;9:137–141.
71. Guerreiro MM, Squires L, Mohandoss E. Topiramate as adjunctive therapy: a prospective study of 500+ children/adolescents with refractory epilepsy [abstract]. *Epilepsia.* 2002;43(suppl 7):58.
72. Sachdeo RC, Glauser TA, Ritter F, et al. A double-blind, randomized trial of topiramate in Lennox–Gastaut syndrome. *Neurology.* 1999;52: 1882–1887.
73. Motte J, Trevathan E, Arvidsson JFV, et al. Lamotrigine for generalized seizures associated with the Lennox–Gastaut syndrome. *N Engl J Med.* 1997;337:1807–1812.
74. Glauser TA, Levisohn P, Ritter F, et al. Topiramate in Lennox–Gastaut syndrome: open-label treatment of patients completing a randomized controlled trial. *Epilepsia.* 2000;41(suppl 1): S86–S90.
75. Guerreiro MM, Manreza MLG, Scotoni AE, et al. A pilot study of topiramate in children with Lennox–Gastaut syndrome. *Arq Neuropsiquiatr.* 1999;57:167–175.
76. Coppola G, Caliendo G, Veggiotti P, et al. Topiramate as add-on drug in children, adolescents and young adults with Lennox–Gastaut syndrome: an Italian multicentric study. *Epilepsy Res.* 2002;51:147–153.
77. Biton V, Montouris GD, Ritter F, et al. A randomized, placebo-controlled study of topiramate in primary generalized tonic–clonic seizures. *Neurology.* 1999;52:1330–1337.
78. Ben-Menachem E, Topiramate YTC-E Study Group. A double-blind trial of topiramate in patients with generalised tonic–clonic seizures of non-focal origin [abstract]. *Epilepsia.* 1997;38(suppl 3):60.
79. Montouris G, Biton V, Rosenfeld WE, et al. Non-focal generalized tonic–clonic seizures: response during long-term topiramate treatment. *Epilepsia.* 2000;41(suppl 1):S77–S81.
80. Ting TY, Herman S, Herman JA, et al. Seizure control and EEG response in primary generalized epilepsy patients treated with topiramate [abstract]. *Epilepsia.* 2002;41(suppl 7):202.
81. Rosenfeld WE. Topiramate, a broad spectrum agent, in patients with juvenile myoclonic epilepsy. *Epilepsia.* 1994;40 (suppl 2):226.
82. Biton V, Rosenfeld WE, Twyman R, et al. Topiramate (TPM) in juvenile myoclonic epilepsy (JME): observations from randomized controlled trials in primary generalized tonic–clonic seizures (PGTCS) [abstract]. *Epilepsia.* 1999;40(suppl 7):218.
83. Levisohn PM, Holland KD, Hulihan JF, et al. Topiramate versus valproate in patients with juvenile myoclonic epilepsy [abstract]. *Epilepsia.* 2003;44(suppl 9):267–268.
84. Glauser TA, Clark PO, Strawsburg R. A pilot study of topiramate in the treatment of infantile spasms. *Epilepsia.* 1998;39:1324–1328.
85. Glauser TA, Clark PO, McGee K. Long-term response to topiramate in patients with West syndrome. *Epilepsia.* 2000;41(suppl 1):S91–S94.
86. Cross JH. Topiramate monotherapy for childhood absence seizures: an open-label pilot study. *Seizure.* 2002;11:406–410.
87. Coppola G, Capovilla G, Montagnini A, et al. Topiramate as add-on drug in severe myoclonic epilepsy in infancy: an Italian multicenter open trial. *Epilepsy Res.* 2002;49:45–48.
88. Kelly K, Stephen LJ, Sills GJ, et al. Topiramate in patients with learning disability and refractory epilepsy. *Epilepsia.* 2002;43:399–402.
89. Singh BK, White-Scott S. Role of topiramate in adults with intractable epilepsy, mental retardation, and developmental disabilities. *Seizure.* 2002;11:47–50.
90. Towne AR, Garnett LK, Waterhouse EJ, et al. The use of topiramate in refractory status epilepticus. *Neurology.* 2003;60:332–334.
91. Mattson RH, Cramer JA, Collins JF, et al. Comparison of carbamazepine, phenobarbital, phenytoin, and primidone in partial and secondarily generalized tonic–clonic seizures. *N Engl J Med.* 1985;313:145–151.
92. Mattson RH, Cramaer JA, Collins JF, et al. A comparison of valproate with carbamazepine for the treatment of complex partial seizures and secondarily generalized tonic–clonic seizures in adults. *N Engl J Med.* 1992; 327:765–771.
93. Heller AJ, Chesterman P, Elwes RDC, et al. Phenobarbitone, phenytoin, carbamazepine, or sodium valproate for newly diagnosed adult epilepsy: a randomised comparative monotherapy trial. *J Neurol Neurosurg Psychiatry.* 1995;58:44–50.
94. de Silva M, MacArdle B, McGowan M, et al. Randomised comparative monotherapy trial of phenobarbitone, phenytoin, carbamazepine, or sodium valproate for newly diagnosed childhood epilepsy. *Lancet.* 1996; 347:709–713.
95. Pledger GW, Kramer LD. Clinical trials of investigational antiepileptic drugs: monotherapy designs. *Epilepsia.* 1991;32:716–721.
96. Sachdeo RC, Reife RA, Lim P, et al. Topiramate monotherapy for partial onset seizures. *Epilepsia.* 1997;38:294–300.
97. Sachdeo RC, Edwards K, Hasegawa H, et al. Safety and efficacy of oxcarbazepine 1200 mg per day in patients with recent-onset partial epilepsy [abstract]. *Neurology.* 1999;52(suppl 2):A391.
98. Leber P. Hazards of inference: the active control investigation. *Epilepsia.* 1989;30(suppl 1):S57–S63.
99. Chadwick D, Privitera M. Placebo-controlled trials in neurology: where do they stop? *Neurology.* 1999;52:682–685.
100. Brodie MJ, Richens A, Yuen AWC, et al. Double-blind comparison of lamotrigine and carbamazepine in newly diagnosed epilepsy. *Lancet.* 1995; 345:476–479.

101. Steiner TJ, Dellaportas CI, Findley LJ, et al. Lamotrigine monotherapy in newly diagnosed untreated epilepsy: a double-blind comparison with phenytoin. *Epilepsia.* 1999;40:601–607.

102. Kwan P, Brodie MJ. Early identification of refractory epilepsy. *N Engl J Med.* 2000;342:314–319.

103. Kwan P, Brodie MJ. Effectiveness of first antiepileptic drug. *Epilepsia.* 2001;42:1255–1260.

104. Brandes JL, Saper JR, Diamond M, et al. Topiramate for migraine prevention: a randomized controlled trial. *JAMA.* 2004;291:965–973.

105. Dodick DW, Neto W, Schmitt J, et al. Topiramate in migraine prevention (MIGR-001): additional efficacy measures from a randomized, double-blind, placebo-controlled trial. *Neurology.* 2003;60(suppl 1): A237–A238.

106. Wheeler SD, Carrazana EJ. Topiramate-treated cluster headache. *Neurology.* 1999;53:274–276.

107. Hulihan J, Connor GS, Wu S-C, et al. Topiramate in essential tremor: pooled data from a double-blind, placebo-controlled, crossover trial [abstract]. *Neurology.* 2003;60(suppl 1):A291.

108. Connor GS. A double-blind placebo-controlled trial of topiramate treatment for essential tremor. *Neurology.* 2002;59:132–134.

109. Nelson TY, Lesser PS, Bost MT. Topiramate in children and adolescents with Tourette's syndrome [abstract]. *Ann Neurol.* 2002;52(suppl 1): S128.

110. Johnson BA, Ait-Daoud N, Bowden CL, et al. Oral topiramate for treatment of alcohol dependence: a randomized controlled trial. *Lancet.* 2003; 36:1677–1685.

111. McElroy SL, Arnold LM, Shapira NA, et al. Topiramate in the treatment of binge-eating disorder associated with obesity: a randomized, placebo-controlled trial. *Am J Psychiatry.* 2003;160:255–261.

112. Nigro MA, Smathers SA. An open-label trial on the efficacy of topiramate in the treatment of behavior, mood, and compulsive eating disorder of Prader–Willi syndrome [abstract]. *Neurology.* 2001;56(suppl 3):A42.

113. Shapira NA, Lessig MC, Murphy TK, et al. Topiramate attenuates self-injurious behavior in Prader–Willi syndrome. *Int J Neuropsychopharmacol.* 2002;5:141–145.

114. Ben-Menachem E, Axelsen M, Johanson EH, et al. Predictors of weight loss in adults with topiramate-treated epilepsy. *Obes Res.* 2003;11:556–562.

115. Bray GA, Hollander P, Klein S, et al. A 6-month randomized, placebo-controlled, dose-ranging trial of topiramate for weight loss in obesity. *Obes Res.* 2003;11:722–733.

116. Thienel U, Neto W, Goldstein H. Effect of topiramate on diabetic control and weight in diabetic patients [abstract]. *Epilepsia.* 2002;43(suppl 7): 221–222.

117. Demarest K, Conway B, Osborne M, et al. Topiramate improves glucose tolerance and may improve insulin sensitivity in animal models of type 2 diabetes [abstract]. *Diabetes.* 2001;50(suppl 2):A302.

118. Yang Y, Shuaib A, Li Q, et al. Neuroprotection by delayed administration of topiramate in a rat model of middle cerebral artery embolization. *Brain Res.* 1998;804:169–176.

119. Angehagen M, Hansson E, Ronnback L, et al. Does topiramate (TPM) have protective effects on astroglia cells and neurons in primary cortical cultures [abstract] *Epilepsia.* 1998;39(suppl 6):44.

120. Vinik AI, Pittenger GL, Anderson SA, et al. Topiramate improves C-fiber neuropathy and features of the dysmetabolic syndrome in type 2 diabetes. Presented at the American Diabetes Association 63rd Scientific Sessions; June 13, 2002; New Orleans, Louisiana.

121. Alves OL, Doyle AJ, Clausen T, et al. Evaluation of topiramate neuroprotective effect in severe TBI using microdialysis. *Ann N Y Acad Sci.* 2003;993:25–34.

122. Cudkowicz ME, Shefner JM, Schoenfeld DA, et al. for the Northeast ALS Consortium. A randomized, placebo-controlled trial of topiramate in amyotrophic lateral sclerosis. *Neurology.* 2003;61:456–464.

123. PDR, 63 Edition 2009. Thomson Reuters.

124. *Medscape Medical News* 2008, July 23, 2008.

125. Hunt S, Russell A, Smithson WH, et al. Topiramate in pregnancy: preliminary experience from the UK Epilepsy and Pregnancy Register. *Neurology.* 2008;71:272–276.

126. *Medscape Medical News* 2008, Quotation from Kim Meador, M.D., July 23, 2008.

127. The North American Anti-Epileptic Drug Pregnancy Registry, Winter 2009 Newsletter.

128. Öhman I, Vitols S, Luef G, et al. Topiramate kinetics during delivery, lactation, and in the neonate: preliminary observations. *Epilepsia.* 2002;43: 1157–1160.

129. Biton V, Edwards KR, Montouris GD, et al. Topiramate titration and tolerability. *Ann Pharmacother.* 2001;35:173–179.

130. Naritoku DK, Hulihan J, Karim R, et al. Reduction of antiepileptic drug (AED) co-therapy improves tolerability of add-on therapy with topiramate a novel randomized study [abstract]. *Epilepsia.* 2001;42(suppl 7):258.

131. Aldenkamp AP, Baker G, Mulder OG, et al. A multicenter, randomized clinical study to evaluate the effect on cognitive function of topiramate compared with valproate as add-on therapy to carbamazepine in patients with partial-onset seizures. *Epilepsia.* 2000;41:1167–1178.

132. Meador KJ, Loring DW, Hulihan JF, et al. Differential cognitive and behavioral effects of topiramate and valproate. *Neurology.* 2003;60:1483–1488.

133. Martin R, Kuzniecky R, Ho S, et al. Cognitive effects of topiramate gabapentin, and lamotrigine in healthy young adults. *Neurology.* 1999; 52:321–327.

134. Mula M, Trimble MR, Thompson P, et al. Topiramate and word-finding difficulties in patients withepilepsy. *Neurology.* 2003;60:1104–1107

135. Stowe CD, Bolliger T, James LP, et al. Acute mental status changes and hyperchloremic metabolic acidosis with long-term topiramate therapy. *Pharmacotherapy.* 2000;20:105–109.

136. Ko C-h, Kong C-k. Topiramate-induced metabolic acidosis: report of two cases. *Dev Med Child Neurol.* 2001;43:701–704.

137. Philippi H, Boor R, Reitter B. Topiramate and metabolic acidosis in infants and toddlers. *Epilepsia.* 2002;43:744–747.

138. Wilner A, Raymond K, Pollard R. Topiramate and metabolic acidosis. *Epilepsia.* 1999;40:792–795.

139. Takeoka M, Holmes GL, Thiele E, et al. Topiramate and metabolic acidosis in pediatric epilepsy. *Epilepsia.* 2001;42:387–392.

140. Takeoka M, Riviello JJ, Pfeifer H, et al. Concomitant treatment with topiramate and ketogenic diet in pediatric epilepsy. *Epilepsia.* 2002;43:1072–1075.

141. Riviello JJ, Wheless J, Wu SC, et al. Body weight (BW) changes during topiramate (TPM) therapy in children with epilepsy [abstract]. *Epilepsia.* 1999;40(suppl 7):127.

142. Morita DA, Glauser TA, Guo SS. Effect of topiramate on linear growth in children with refractory complex partial seizures [abstract]. *Neurology.* 2000;54(suppl 3):A193.

143. Dlugos DJ, Squires L, Wang S. Topiramate as first-line therapy: tolerability and safety in children and adolescents [abstract]. *Neurology.* 2003; 60(suppl 1):A474–A475.

144. Keates E, Clark T. Acute myopia and secondary angle closure glaucoma: a rare ocular syndrome in topiramate-treated patients [abstract]. *Neurology.* 2002;58:A422.

145. Ben-Zeev B, Watemberg N, Augarten A, et al. Oligohydrosis and hyperthermia: pilot study of a novel topiramate adverse effect. *J Child Neurol.* 2003;18:254–257.

146. Rosenfeld WE, Slater J. Characterization of topiramate-associated weight changes in adults with epilepsy. *Epilepsia.* 2002;43(suppl 7):220–221.

CHAPTER 59 ■ ZONISAMIDE

TIMOTHY E. WELTY

Zonisamide was first synthesized in 1974 in Japan. In the early 1980s, clinical trials of zonisamide were initiated in the United States. Due to an increased risk of nephrolithiasis in patients receiving active drug, further development in the United States was halted. Development of zonisamide continued in Japan, and the drug was approved for marketing in Japan in 1989. Additional studies in Europe and the United States were initiated with approval for marketing granted in the United States in 2000. Zonisamide is an antiepileptic drug (AED) that appears to have broad activity in various seizure types and epilepsy syndromes.

CHEMISTRY

Zonisamide is classified as a sulfonamide AED that is a 1, 2-benzisoxazole derivative and is the first compound from this group of chemicals to be developed as an AED. It is unrelated chemically to other AEDs (Fig. 59.1). It is moderately soluble in water (0.8 mg/mL) and has a pK_a of 10.2. Zonisamide is a white powder and has a molecular weight of 212.23.

MECHANISM OF ACTION

There are several pharmacologic effects of zonisamide that may be responsible for its activity as an AED. Results from several studies demonstrate the most likely mechanism of action for zonisamide to be through blockade of T-type calcium channels, inhibition of slow sodium channels, and possibly through inhibition of glutamate release (1–5). However, zonisamide differs from ethosuximide in that zonisamide does not inhibit G protein-activated inwardly rectifying K^+ channels (6). Zonisamide does have activity as a carbonic anhydrase inhibitor, but this is not responsible for its antiepileptic activity (7). In animal models, zonisamide demonstrates broad spectrum as an AED (8–11). Beside its antiepileptic activity, zonisamide has some effect as a neuroprotective agent in ischemia (12,13). Additionally, other pharmacologic activities may make zonisamide useful in the treatment of Parkinson disease and essential tremor (14,15).

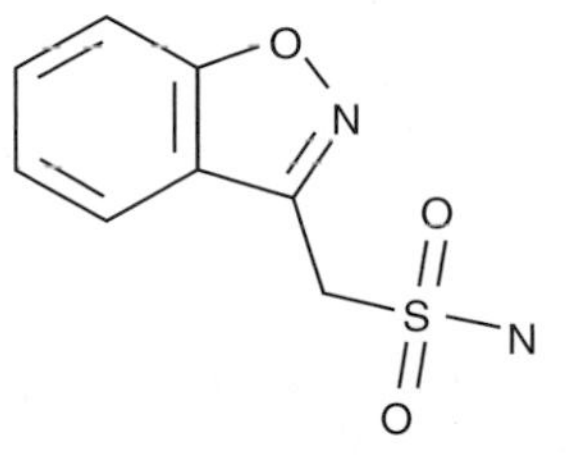

FIGURE 59.1. Zonisamide.

PHARMACOKINETICS

Absorption

Zonisamide is rapidly absorbed following oral administration with maximum concentrations achieved within 2 to 5 hours (16). The absolute bioavailability in humans is unknown, due to the lack of a parenteral product. Nagatomi et al. measured the absolute bioavailability of orally administered zonisamide at 81% in rats (17). In the same study, the bioavailability of zonisamide in a rectal preparation was 96%. Zonisamide is metabolized by cytochrome P450 3A4 (CYP 3A4) (18). Intestinal CYP 3A4 may account for decreased bioavailability of the oral preparation.

Distribution and Protein Binding

Like many sulfonamide drugs, zonisamide has a dose-dependent decrease in volume of distribution (V_d/F) (19). The volume of distribution for a 200-mg dose is 1.8 L/kg and for an 800-mg dose is 1.2 L/kg. Saturable binding to erythrocytes, especially to intracellular carbonic anhydrase, is the most likely explanation for this phenomenon (20–22). Additionally, 40% to 60% of zonisamide is bound to plasma proteins, especially albumin (22,23).

Therefore, zonisamide is concentrated in the erythrocytes compared to plasma. With saturable binding to erythrocytes, the whole blood zonisamide concentration is nonlinear as the dosage increases. However, the plasma zonisamide concentration is linear with increased doses (16). Care must be taken in laboratory analysis and interpretation of zonisamide concentrations. Results should be identified as coming from whole blood or plasma.

Metabolism and Clearance

Following oral administration the half-life ($t_{1/2}$) of zonisamide is estimated at 50 to 69 hours (16,24). Apparent oral clearance (Cl/F) following single and repeated oral doses is 0.6 to 0.71 L/hr (24). Less than 30% of zonisamide is eliminated unchanged in the urine and most of the drug undergoes extensive hepatic metabolism (25). The relatively long $t_{1/2}$ and slow clearance allow for once-daily dosing of zonisamide.

Early studies of the pharmacokinetics of zonisamide suggested that concentrations increased in a nonlinear relationship to doses (19,26). Following an 800-mg dose, zonisamide clearance was 22% lower than clearance estimates following 200-mg and 400-mg doses. Clearance estimates at steady state with doses ranging from 400 to 1200 mg daily were 40% lower than those seen following a single 400-mg dose (16,27). A study by Wilensky et al. showed steady-state zonisamide concentrations to be higher than predicted from single-dose data, but steady-state plasma concentrations did increase in a linear relationship to daily dose (28). These observations were considered to be related to the saturable, preferential binding of zonisamide to erythrocytes. However, an analysis of zonisamide doses and concentrations in children using a nonlinear mixed effects model and population pharmacokinetic methodology demonstrated dose-dependent, Michaelis–Menten, pharmacokinetics of zonisamide with a mean V_{max} of 27.6 mg/day/kg and K_m of 45.9 µg/mL (29). Because the V_{max} is well above the typical range of daily zonisamide doses, it is unlikely that the nonlinear nature of zonisamide clearance will profoundly impact clinical practice.

The major metabolite of zonisamide is 2-sulfamoy-lacetylphenol (SMAP), formed under anaerobic conditions by liver microsomal enzymes (18,30,31). The formation of SMAP appears to be primarily through cytochrome P 450 3A4 (CYP 3A4) (18,30). In these studies, metabolism of zonisamide to SMAP was inhibited by cimetidine and ketoconazole, known CYP 3A4 inhibitors. Zonisamide is metabolized to a much lesser extent by CYP 2C19 and CYP 3A5 (32). Studies of the effect of genetic polymorphisms on zonisamide metabolism have shown a 16% to 30% reduction in clearance in individuals who were CYP 2C19 heterozygous extensive metabolizers or homozygous poor metabolizers compared to homozygous extensive metabolizers (33). The clinical implications of this observation are unclear.

Serum Concentrations and Doses

The manufacturer's recommended dose for adults is 300 to 400 mg daily, but doses of 600 mg daily have been used in clinical trials (34). Doses above 400 mg have not consistently been associated with increased efficacy. The recommended doses of zonisamide are typically associated with steady-state plasma concentrations of 10 to 38 µg/mL (24,29,35). However, a relationship between concentration and response has not been established. Other investigators have suggested that concentrations >30 µg/mL are associated with increased adverse effects (19,28). Therefore, it may be advisable to maintain zonisamide concentrations <30 to 40 µg/mL. The pharmacokinetics and dosing of zonisamide are summarized in Table 59.1.

Special Populations

Pediatrics

No formal pharmacokinetic studies have been done in children. In a study of zonisamide for infantile spasms by Suzuki and colleagues, daily doses of 4 to 5 mg/kg yielded plasma concentrations of 5.2 to 16.3 µg/mL (36). Additional work by this group substantiated these findings with zonisamide doses of 4 to 12 mg/kg/day producing plasma concentrations of 5.2 to 30 µg/mL (37). Table 59.2 summarizes typical mean plasma concentrations related to dose and age. A comparison

TABLE 59.1

SUMMARY OF ZONISAMIDE PHARMACOKINETICS AND DOSING

Parameter	Value
Oral bioavailability	81%[a]
Volume of distribution (V_d/F)	1.2–1.8 L/kg[b]
Protein binding	40–60%[c]
Half-life	50–69 hours
Clearance (Cl/F)	0.6–0.71 L/hr
Usual plasma concentrations	10–30 µg/mL[d]
Recommended dose	200–400 mg/day[e]

[a]Based upon animal data.
[b]Volume of distribution is inversely related to dose, due to saturable binding to erythrocytes.
[c]Additionally, zonisamide is highly and preferentially bound to erythrocytes.
[d]These are typical concentrations observed with usual doses. A relationship between concentrations and response has not been established.
[e]Higher doses have been used in clinical trials.

TABLE 59.2

MEAN ZONISAMIDE PLASMA CONCENTRATIONS RELATED TO AGE AND DAILY DOSE (38)

Age (years)	Mean daily dose (mg/kg)	Mean plasma concentration (µg/mL)
>16	5.9	20.0
7–15	7.1	20.7
2–6	8.8	19.9
≤1	8.6	19.6

of pharmacokinetic parameters derived from population data in children and adults shows a similar volume of distribution, but more rapid clearance of zonisamide in children (29,39). Thus, children appear to require larger doses of zonisamide, based on body weight, to achieve plasma concentration similar to those seen in adults (40).

Three case reports have provided some documentation regarding transfer of zonisamide across the placenta and into breast milk. Kawada and colleagues measured zonisamide concentrations in umbilical cord blood, infant blood, and maternal blood of two infants born to mothers taking zonisamide for epilepsy (41). In these infants, zonisamide concentrations were 92% of that in maternal blood. Kawada also measured zonisamide concentrations in the breast milk of these mothers, showing these concentrations to be 41% to 57% of maternal plasma concentrations. In a separate case, evaluating zonisamide concentrations in breast milk to 30 days postpartum, Shimoyama observed breast milk concentrations to range from 81% to 100% of maternal plasma concentrations (42). It appears that zonisamide readily crosses the placenta. Zonisamide also appears in breast milk at concentrations similar to maternal plasma concentrations. No clinically important adverse effects related to zonisamide were documented in these case reports.

Pregnancy

Case reports suggest that clearance of zonisamide may increase toward the end of the second trimester, requiring an increase in dose (43).

Renal Failure

A single-dose study of zonisamide in individuals with moderate renal failure (creatinine clearance >0.6 L/hr) did not demonstrate any difference in pharmacokinetic parameters compared to normal individuals (44). Studies in severe renal dysfunction and multiple-dose studies in renal failure have not been reported.

DRUG INTERACTIONS

Because zonisamide is primarily metabolized through CYP 3A4 and to a lesser extent by CYP 2C19, it is potentially prone to drug–drug interactions involving these enzyme systems. Several interactions have been studied in animals and in humans (Table 59.3). However, the exact clinical implications of these interactions are poorly documented.

Influence of Other Drugs on Zonisamide

Using in vitro studies of the CYP 3A system, Nakasa and colleagues showed that cyclosporine A, ketoconazole, dihydroergotamine, and triazolam profoundly inhibit zonisamide metabolism (32). These drugs reduced zonisamide metabolism by 85% to 95% compared to control. Other known inhibitors of CYP 3A, diazepam, terfenadine, erythromycin, and lidocaine did not produce a marked reduction in metabolism. The percent reduction in metabolism with these agents ranged from 35% to 45%. Clinical correlates to these findings have not been documented, so recommendations for dosage adjustments in patient care are not available. However, patients receiving known inhibitors of CYP 3A may require lower doses of zonisamide to reduce the risk of adverse events.

Inducers of CYP 3A have been shown to increase the metabolism of zonisamide (32). Phenytoin and carbamazepine have been shown to induce zonisamide metabolism, with phenytoin possibly having a greater influence than carbamazepine (45,46). In a study of 12 patients receiving phenytoin

or carbamazepine concomitantly with zonisamide, the mean oral clearance (Cl/F) of zonisamide was 33.9 mL/hr/kg with phenytoin and 20.6 mL/hr/kg with carbamazepine (45). However, some researchers have observed inhibition of zonisamide metabolism by carbamazepine (32). Other known inducers of hepatic metabolism, especially phenobarbital and primidone, can also increase the metabolism of zonisamide (16). When zonisamide is used in combination with known CYP 3A inducers, doses of zonisamide may need to be increased to achieve seizure control. In the case of carbamazepine, care must be taken to determine if induction or inhibition is predominant in a given patient and zonisamide doses adjusted accordingly.

Zonisamide Influence on Other Drugs

Studies with zonisamide have shown that it does not induce or inhibit hepatic enzymes (47,48). A study of zonisamide's effects on ethinyl estradiol–norethindrone oral contraceptives demonstrated no alteration of hormonal effect or loss of contraceptive efficacy (49). A survey of interactions between zonisamide and cancer chemotherapy agents demonstrated no known interactions (50). It appears that zonisamide does not cause clinically significant alteration of the pharmacokinetic disposition of other drugs.

Drug–Food Interactions with Zonisamide

As a substrate for CYP 3A4, zonisamide is a candidate for drug–food interactions. Within the intestinal wall, are high concentrations of CYP 3A4 that can metabolize drugs before they are absorbed into systemic circulation. Several foods, especially grapefruit juice, lime juice, and Seville orange juice, contain substances that inhibit the activity of intestinal CYP 3A4. When these foods are eaten with drugs that are metabolized by CYP 3A4, there is increased absorption of the drug and a potential for adverse effects. Although this potential interaction with zonisamide has not been documented, it should be of concern. In a study of rectal administration, (a route that bypasses intestinal CYP 3A4), of zonisamide, Nagatomi and colleagues consistently demonstrated increased bioavailability and absorption of zonisamide (17).

CLINICAL TRIALS

Clinical studies of zonisamide have evaluated its use in several different types of epilepsy and epilepsy syndromes. Additionally, zonisamide has been used extensively in Japan and has gained increasing use in the remainder of the world. Despite this history, there have been no direct comparisons of zonisamide to other AEDs in specific seizure types. The best published comparison has been in two meta-analyses of clinical trials of other newer AEDs, including zonisamide (51,52). In the first study, Marson and colleagues evaluated the odds ratio of zonisamide producing a ≥50% reduction in seizure

TABLE 59.3

DRUG INTERACTIONS WITH ZONISAMIDE

Reduce zonisamide metabolism	Increase zonisamide metabolism	Variable effect on zonisamide metabolism
Cyclosporine A	Phenytoin	Carbamazepine
Ketoconazole	Phenobarbital	
Dihydroergotamine	Primidone	
Triazolam		
Diazepam		
Erythromycin		

frequency compared to placebo (51). Combining data from two clinical trials, zonisamide was shown to be significantly better than placebo in controlling seizures. Additionally, significantly more patients receiving zonisamide stopped taking the drug compared to patients taking placebo. A comparison of zonisamide to gabapentin, lamotrigine, tiagabine, topiramate, and vigabatrin failed to demonstrate any statistically significant differences between these drugs. In a second meta-analysis, Marson did not include any additional studies from his first report, but was able to identify from these the five most common adverse effects patients on zonisamide experienced (52). This type of analysis shows that zonisamide is equally effective to the other new AEDs in treating seizures. However, it is not extremely helpful in determining the specific place in therapy for zonisamide.

Focal-Onset Epilepsies/Partial Seizures

Clinical studies of zonisamide have evaluated its use in several different types of epilepsy and epilepsy syndromes. However, there have been no direct comparisons of zonisamide to other AEDs in specific seizure types. The best published comparisons are in meta-analyses of clinical trials of other newer AEDs, including zonisamide (51–53). In the first study, Marson and colleagues evaluated the odds ratio of zonisamide producing a ≥50% reduction in seizure frequency compared to placebo (51). Combining data from two clinical trials, zonisamide was shown to be significantly better than placebo in controlling seizures. Additionally, significantly more patients receiving zonisamide stopped taking the drug compared to patients taking placebo. A comparison of zonisamide to gabapentin, lamotrigine, tiagabine, topiramate, and vigabatrin failed to demonstrate any statistically significant differences between these drugs. In a second meta-analysis, Marson did not include any additional studies from his first report, but was able to identify from these the five most common adverse effects patients on zonisamide experienced (52). In a study designed to compare intention to treat to last observation carried forward methodology, zonisamide had a 3% seizure-free rate compared to 0.8%, 2.6%, 7.1%, and 1.4% for lamotrigine, oxcarbazepine, levetiracetam, and pregabalin, respectively (53). This type of analysis shows that zonisamide is at least equally effective to the other new AEDs in treating seizures.

Several clinical trials of zonisamide for partial seizures have been published. In an open trial of zonisamide in 10 patients with refractory partial epilepsy, all but 1 patient had a ≥50% reduction in seizure frequency (27). A second pilot study by Wilensky and colleagues was conducted in eight patients with refractory epilepsy (28). Zonisamide doses ranged from 400 to 1200 mg daily with a mean of 475 mg/day.

A multicenter, placebo-controlled, double-blind, parallel-group, add-on study showed zonisamide to be more effective than placebo (54). Zonisamide was increased over 4 weeks to a dose of 6 mg/kg/day in 139 patients. The mean reduction at the end of the study in all seizures was 16% and in complex partial seizures was 16.4%. Mean doses of zonisamide were 7.0 mg/kg at the end of the trial and did not differ between responders and nonresponders. Nearly 30% of patients on zonisamide had ≥50% reduction in seizure frequency compared to 9.4% of patients receiving placebo.

Another similar study evaluated zonisamide efficacy in 167 adults over 3 months (55). Zonisamide doses were titrated upward based upon individual tolerance and ranged from 50 to 1100 mg daily with a median dose of 500 mg/day. The median percent reduction in seizure frequency at the end of the study was 51.8%. Forty-one percent of study participants had ≥50% reduction in seizure frequency and six became seizure-free on zonisamide. When complex partial seizures were independently evaluated, the median reduction was 40.6% overall and 43.2% of the participants had ≥50% reduction in seizure frequency. Generalized tonic–clonic seizures were also reduced significantly during zonisamide therapy. At the end of this study, patients were able to continue in a long-term safety study. One hundred thirteen individuals chose to continue zonisamide. Of these, only 16 patients discontinued zonisamide due to perceived lack of efficacy. Two thirds of the patients choosing to continue zonisamide remained on the drug 1 year after initiation. This study demonstrates that zonisamide has good efficacy in refractory partial epilepsy and may have prolonged benefit to patients.

A third multicenter, double-blind study employed a different approach to zonisamide dosing (56). In this study, patients in the placebo group were crossed over to zonisamide following 12 weeks of placebo treatment. Individuals who were randomized to receive zonisamide were divided between a slow and rapid initial titration of the active drug. All patients receiving zonisamide were ultimately increased to 400 mg/day. The median reduction in seizures for all patients initially started on zonisamide was 32.3% compared to 5.6% for placebo. Significantly more individuals on zonisamide had a ≥50% or ≥75% reduction in seizure frequency. Among those who were in the placebo group and crossed over to zonisamide, the median reduction in the frequency of all seizures was 40.1% and for complex partial seizures was 55% compared to the placebo seizure frequency. The slow titration schedule in one of the zonisamide groups allowed for evaluation of efficacy at 100 mg/day and 200 mg/day. At these doses, the median reduction in the frequency of all seizures and responder rate was statistically significant in favor of zonisamide.

Another study of adjunctive zonisamide therapy compared to placebo showed significant reductions in all seizures types and partial seizures (57). The 50% responder rate was only significant for complex partial seizures at a median dose of 500 mg/day or 6.4 mg/kg/day. In a dose-ranging study, Brodie and colleagues demonstrated a dose–response relationship with doses ranging from 300 to 500 mg/day (58). For adults, it appears that a reduction in seizures can occur with doses ranging from 100 to 500 mg/day, and that increasing doses in this range increases the number of patients who respond.

A summary of Japanese studies using zonisamide in pediatric patients with partial seizures estimated that 34% of children responded to zonisamide (39). Otherwise, there are few published reports on the use of zonisamide specifically for partial seizures. Kluger reported a prospective open-label study of zonisamide in childhood-onset seizures that included pediatric patients (59). In this report 75% of the patients had focal seizures, and 58.3% of all patients had a ≥50% reduction in seizure frequency. In a safety study of zonisamide use in 109 pediatric patients, there was a significant reduction in all seizure types and partial seizures with 7 patients discontinuing therapy due to serious adverse events (60). Limited data on pediatric use of zonisamide for partial seizures appear to indicate that it is effective and safe.

Generalized Epilepsies

Formal studies of zonisamide in adults with primary generalized epilepsies are lacking. A small clinical trial suggested that zonisamide decreases cortical excitability in patients with idiopathic generalize epilepsies (61). Henry and colleagues report two cases of progressive myoclonic epilepsy where zonisamide use was associated with reduced seizure frequency and improved functioning (62). A case series of patients with juvenile myoclonic epilepsy indicated that zonisamide was well tolerated and associated with reduced seizures compared to valproate (63). A similar retrospective study of juvenile myoclonic epilepsy indicated that zonisamide was easily titrated and had a rapid onset of action (64).

More extensive evaluation of zonisamide in primary generalized epilepsies has been done in children. Several studies using zonisamide for West syndrome have been published. In children with newly diagnosed infantile spasms, Suzuki et al. used 3 to 10 mg/kg/day of zonisamide in an open-label trial (36). A total of 11 infants from 11 hospitals were enrolled in this study. Of these children who started on zonisamide, four had complete seizure control and cessation of hypsarrhythmia with doses of 4 to 5 mg/kg/day. Kishi and colleagues reported their experience with zonisamide in children with hypsarrhythmia (65). In this group of three patients, zonisamide resulted in elimination of hypsarrhythmia and seizures. A larger study in 54 patients, newly diagnosed with West syndrome, was done (37). Zonisamide doses ranged from 4 to 14 mg/kg/day with a mean dose and serum concentration of 7.2 mg/kg/day and 15.3 µg/mL, respectively. Eleven infants had complete elimination of seizures and hypsarrhythmia, seven children had >50% reduction in seizure frequency, and 14 with cryptogenic West syndrome responded. Of those who the authors categorized as not responding, four were seizure-free transiently, six had a <50% reduction in seizure frequency, and 33 had no change in seizure frequency. The 11 individuals in this study who had elimination of seizures and hypsarrhythmia were entered into a long-term follow-up study, evaluating their response out to 79 months (mean duration of 53 months) (66). Seven of the infants who had an initial cessation of seizures continued to be seizure-free. Presence of epileptiform activity on the EEG at the end of 3 weeks was predictive of recurrence of seizures. Yanagaki and colleagues studied the use of zonisamide starting at 10 mg/kg/day, demonstrating this scheme was well tolerated in children with West syndrome (67).

Although case series reports and open-label studies suggest that zonisamide may be effective in patients with generalized epilepsies, it has not been well studied in this patient population. The most extensive information on zonisamide use in generalized epilepsies is in children with West syndrome. These data suggest that zonisamide may be a useful alternative for infants with this disorder. For other types of generalized epilepsies, zonisamide may prove to be a useful alternative.

Monotherapy

Few clinical trials have evaluated the use of zonisamide in monotherapy for the treatment of epilepsy. The most exten-

sive studies have been in children with West syndrome (36,66). Additionally, Kumagai and colleagues studied zonisamide as a single agent in 44 children with epilepsy (68). In this open-label trial, 30 children with various seizure types became seizure-free and 6 children had to discontinue the drug due to adverse effects.

There are much less data available in adults with epilepsy. The only published study of zonisamide monotherapy was done by Wilensky and colleagues (28). In this study, eight adults with partial seizures and receiving phenytoin were randomized to carbamazepine or zonisamide and then crossed over in an open-label design. Two subjects had improved seizure control with zonisamide compared to carbamazepine and a third individual had a similar response, but had to discontinue zonisamide due to the development of Stevens–Johnson syndrome.

The limited available data on zonisamide monotherapy treatment indicate that zonisamide may be effective as a single agent for epilepsy. However, larger, double-blind clinical trials must be done before zonisamide monotherapy can be recommended.

Nonepilepsy Indications

Preliminary clinical trials of zonisamide in disorders other than epilepsy indicate it may be useful for other indications. One study of zonisamide in patients with mania and acute psychotic conditions indicated that 71% responded at least moderately to treatment (69). In an open-label trial of zonisamide in 35 patients with neuropathic pain, mean pain scores showed little or no improvement after 8 weeks of therapy (70). A trial in nine patients with Parkinson disease demonstrated that seven of the nine patients had improvement in their symptoms, especially wearing-off phenomenon, when zonisamide was added to their other medications (71). Preliminary data suggest that zonisamide is at least as effective as propranolol in patients with head tremor or essential tremor (14,72).

ADVERSE EFFECTS

Common Adverse Effects

In the initial and major clinical trials of zonisamide as adjunctive therapy, several adverse effects were commonly reported (Table 59.4) (27,28,54–56). Schmidt et al. reported the statistical evaluation of adverse events reported in their trial (54). Dizziness, somnolence, anorexia, abnormal thinking, ataxia, and confusion were more common with zonisamide compared to placebo. A meta-analysis, which calculated the odds ratios of adverse events reported in clinical trials, showed that patients on zonisamide were more likely to experience anorexia, ataxia, dizziness, and fatigue compared to patients receiving placebo (52). These adverse events and their frequency are similar to those reported with other new AEDs.

Adverse events in children appear to be similar to those in adults. The adverse events that are reported in >10% of children on zonisamide in combination with other AEDs are somnolence, anorexia, ataxia, fatigue, dizziness, cognitive impairment, irritability, and exanthema (39). Monotherapy of

TABLE 59.4

MOST FREQUENTLY REPORTED ADVERSE EFFECTS
IN CLINICAL TRIALS

Adverse event	Percent reporting range
Fatigue	3.3–22.5%
Ataxia	3.3–11.3%
Nausea/Vomiting	4.2–15%
Headache	5–15.9%
Somnolence	5.2–18.3%
Rhinitis	5.2–14.4%
Confusion	5.6–10.6%
Anorexia	6.7–15%
Dizziness	6.9–16.9%
Nervousness	8.8–9.9%
Thinking abnormal	9.7–11.3%

zonisamide in pediatrics has been more extensively studied than in adults. When zonisamide is used by itself in children, the only adverse effect that occurs in >10% of individuals is somnolence (39). Thus, common adverse events, especially in children, may be limited by decreasing or eliminating other AEDs.

Anorexia was a commonly observed adverse event in the clinical trials. In some of these studies, this translated into a definite weight loss for many of the patients. A post hoc analysis of data from the major clinical trials demonstrated that significantly more patients on zonisamide (21.6%) lost >5 pounds compared to patients on placebo (56). A retrospective analysis of patients from European and American clinical trials (54–56) showed that 28.9% of individuals receiving zonisamide lost >5 pounds compared to 8.4% receiving placebo, a significant difference (73). The mean weight loss for all patients on zonisamide was 4.3 pounds. As a follow-up to the weight-loss effects, a double-blind, placebo-controlled study of 60 obese nonepileptic patients demonstrated a mean weight loss of 9.2 kg with zonisamide compared to a mean weight loss of 1.5 kg in those receiving placebo (74). A second study compared diet alone to diet and zonisamide in obese women (75). Women who took zonisamide had an additional 5 pounds weight loss compared to those only on a diet.

Zonisamide appears to produce a mild to moderate weight loss. Patients who are obese or have experienced weight gain associated with the use of other AEDs may benefit from the addition of zonisamide to their regimen.

Rare Adverse Effects

Early in the clinical trials of zonisamide, the formation of renal calculi was observed in some patients (55). Four patients of the 113 enrolled in this study had kidney stones form during the study. Kubota reported three cases of nephrolithiasis in patients receiving zonisamide (76) and Miyamoto reported the case of a 10-year-old girl with a kidney stone after starting zonisamide (77). The precise mechanism for this adverse effect has not been determined. Some have speculated that renal calculi formation is related to inhibition of carbonic anhydrase by zonisamide. However, zonisamide is an extremely weak carbonic anhydrase inhibitor (76). It is important to note that all published reports of renal calculi with zonisamide are in individuals who were taking other AEDs. Zonisamide is not contraindicated with patients with a history of kidney stones, but care should be taken when using zonisamide in these patients. Prudent management of patients on zonisamide should include adequate hydration to maintain good urine flow.

Allergic reactions to zonisamide are rare, but did occur in the clinical trials. Rash was the predominant allergic type reaction reported, with at least four individuals (one with Stevens–Johnson syndrome) in these studies being discontinued due to dermatologic reactions. A mild, relative neutropenia was also observed in several individuals. A study by Hirsch and colleagues demonstrates that there is no cross-reactivity with other AEDs (78). Because zonisamide is chemically related to sulfonamide drugs, caution should be taken when using zonisamide in patients who note a prior allergic reaction to these agents. The exact cross-reactivity in patients known to be allergic to sulfonamides has not been determined.

Oligohidrosis can occur with zonisamide, and is marked by decreased sweating and hyperthermia. Postmarketing surveillance indicates that oligohidrosis occurs primarily in children, with all reported cases in individuals ≤18 years of age. The estimated rate of incidence is approximately 12 cases per 10,000 patient-years (79). When zonisamide is used in children, parents should be instructed to carefully monitor for decreased sweating and increased body temperature. Children on zonisamide should not be exposed for prolonged periods of time to extreme heat.

As with other AEDs that possess carbonic anhydrase inhibition activity, zonisamide can produce a metabolic acidosis. Individuals with impaired pulmonary or renal function are especially at risk for this side effect, and serum electrolytes should be monitored.

Cognitive and behavioral effects of AEDs have received increasing attention. The cognitive effects of zonisamide were studied early in its development. Berent and colleagues studied 11 patients who were on stable regimens of two to three other AEDs (80). Zonisamide doses were calculated to maintain plasma concentrations of 15 to 40 μg/mL, and a battery of neuropsychological tests were administered prior to starting and after 12 weeks of zonisamide therapy. When plasma concentrations of zonisamide exceeded 30 μg/mL the acquisition and consolidation of new information, especially verbal learning, were impaired. Miyamoto et al. reviewed 74 reported cases of psychosis associated with zonisamide use, and only 14 of these cases exhibited symptoms of true psychosis (81). There were significantly more men than women with psychosis, and this group was younger than the general population of patients with epilepsy. Hirai and colleagues reported on 27 children in a prospective clinical trial of zonisamide monotherapy and two displayed behavioral disturbances (82). One child presented with selective mutism and the other child developed obsessive–compulsive disorder. As with other AEDs, zonisamide may alter cognition and behavior in some individuals. It is difficult to truly assess the incidence of these effects, because none of the reports accounted for the number of individuals taking zonisamide. Additionally, most of the reports of cognitive or behavioral problems were in patients taking multiple AEDs.

Few data are available on the teratogenic effects of zonisamide. Kondo surveyed 381 hospitals in Japan during June 1989 regarding pregnancies in women using AEDs (83). Only two women exposed to zonisamide during pregnancy bore children with major malformations. In both of these cases, multiple AEDs were taken by the mothers. The authors conclude that zonisamide is associated with no greater risk of teratogenicity than other AEDs.

SUMMARY

Clinical studies have proven the effectiveness of zonisamide as adjunctive therapy for partial seizures. Zonisamide has been used in a variety of age groups, seizure types, and as monotherapy. However, clinical study data outside of the primary indication are lacking. Current evidence suggests that zonisamide has broad utility as an AED in children and adults. The adverse effect and pharmacokinetic profile of zonisamide is favorable with few severe adverse effects reported and a long half-life that allows once-daily dosing.

Zonisamide should be considered an alternative adjunctive agent when typical AEDs have failed in treating partial seizures. It may also be useful in patients with other seizure types and in monotherapy. Individuals who are concerned about weight gain or desire to lose weight may benefit from zonisamide therapy. Care should be exercised when using zonisamide in patients with a history of renal calculi and true sulfa allergies. However, these items do not constitute absolute contraindications to zonisamide use. Zonisamide has been used safely and effectively in pediatrics, but children need to be monitored carefully for oligohidrosis.

References

1. Suzuki S, Kawakami K, Nishimura S, et al. Zonisamide blocks T-type calcium channel in cultured neurons of rat cerebral cortex. *Epilepsy Res.* 1992;12(1):21–27.
2. Rock DM, Macdonald RL, Taylor CP. Blockade of sustained repetitive action potentials in cultured spinal cord neurons by zonisamide (AD 810, CI 912), a novel anticonvulsant. *Epilepsy Res.* 1989;3(2):138–143.
3. Schauf CL. Zonisamide enhances slow sodium inactivation in Myxicola. *Brain Res.* 1987;413(1):185–188.
4. Okada M, et al. Interaction between Ca^{2+}, K^+, carbamazepine and zonisamide on hippocampal extracellular glutamate monitored with a microdialysis electrode. *Br J Pharmacol.* 1998;124(6):1277–1285.
5. Fromm GH, Shibuya T, Terrence CF. Effect of zonisamide (CI-912) on a synaptic system model. *Epilepsia.* 1987;28(6):673–679.
6. Kobayashi M, Hirai H, Iino M, et al. Inhibitory effects of the antiepileptic drug ethosuximide on G protein-activated inwardly rectifying K^+ channels. *Neuropharmacology.* 2008;56:8.
7. Thone J, et al. Antiepileptic activity of zonisamide on hippocampal CA3 neurons do not depend on carbonic anhydrase inhibition. *Epilepsy Res.* 2008;79(2–3):105–11.
8. Wada Y, Hasegawa H, Yamaguchi N, Effect of a novel anticonvulsant, zonisamide (AD-810, CI-912), in an experimental model of photosensitive epilepsy. *Epilepsy Res.* 1990;7(2):117–120.
9. Hamada K, Ishida S, Yagi K, et al. Anticonvulsant effects of zonisamide on amygdaloid kindling in rats. *Neurosciences.* 1990;16:407–412.
10. Takano K, et al. Zonisamide: electrophysiological and metabolic changes in kainic acid-induced limbic seizures in rats. *Epilepsia.* 1995;36(7): 644–648.
11. Akaike K, et al. Regional accumulation of 14C-zonisamide in rat brain during kainic acid-induced limbic seizures. *Can J Neurol Sci.* 2001;28(4):341–345.
12. Minato H, et al. Protective effect of zonisamide, an antiepileptic drug, against transient focal cerebral ischemia with middle cerebral artery occlusion-reperfusion in rats. *Epilepsia.* 1997;38(9):975–980.
13. Tokumaru J, et al. In vivo evaluation of hippocampal anti-oxidant ability of zonisamide in rats. *Neurochem Res.* 2000;25(8):1107–1111.
14. Ondo WG. Zonisamide for essential tremor. *Clin Neuropharmacol.* 2007; 30(6):345–349.
15. Okada M, et al. Effects of zonisamide on dopaminergic system. *Epilepsy Res.* 1995;22(3):193–205.
16. Perucca E, Bialer M. The clinical pharmacokinetics of the newer antiepileptic drugs. Focus on topiramate, zonisamide and tiagabine. *Clin Pharmacokinet.* 1996;31(1):29–46.
17. Nagatomi A, et al. Utility of a rectal suppository containing the antiepileptic drug zonisamide. *Biol Pharm Bull.* 1997;20(8):892–896.
18. Nakasa H, et al. Rat liver microsomal cytochrome P-450 responsible for reductive metabolism of zonisamide. *Drug Metab Dispos.* 1993;21(5): 777–781.
19. Taylor CP, McLean JR, Bockrader HN, et al. Zonisamide. In: Meldrum BS, Porter RJ, eds. *New Anticonvulsant Drugs.* London: John Libbey; 1986: 277–294.
20. Nishiguchi K, et al. Pharmacokinetics of zonisamide; saturable distribution into human and rat erythrocytes and into rat brain. *J Pharmacobiodyn.* 1992;15(8):409–415.
21. Matsumoto K, et al. Binding of sulfonamides to erythrocyte proteins and possible drug-drug interaction. *Chem Pharm Bull (Tokyo).* 1989;37(10): 2807–2810.
22. Matsumoto K, et al. Binding of sulfonamides to erythrocytes and their components. *Chem Pharm Bull (Tokyo).* 1989;37(7):1913–1915.
23. Kimura M, et al. Factors influencing serum concentration of zonisamide in epileptic patients. *Chem Pharm Bull (Tokyo).* 1992;40(1):193–195.
24. Kochak GM, et al. Steady-state pharmacokinetics of zonisamide, an antiepileptic agent for treatment of refractory complex partial seizures. *J Clin Pharmacol.* 1998;38(2):166–171.
25. Walker MC, Patsalos PN. Clinical pharmacokinetics of new antiepileptic drugs. *Pharmacol Ther.* 1995;67(3):351–384.
26. Wagner JG, Sackellares JC, Donofrio PD, et al. Nonlinear pharmacokinetics of CI-912 in adult epileptic patients. *Ther Drug Monit.* 1984;6:277–283.
27. Sackellares JC, et al. Pilot study of zonisamide (1,2-benzisoxazole-3-methanesulfonamide) in patients with refractory partial seizures. *Epilepsia.* 1985;26(3):206–211.
28. Wilensky AJ, et al. Zonisamide in epilepsy: a pilot study. *Epilepsia.* 1985;26(3):212–220.
29. Hashimoto Y, et al. Population analysis of the dose-dependent pharmacokinetics of zonisamide in epileptic patients. *Biol Pharm Bull.* 1994;17(2): 323–326.
30. Nakasa H, Komiya M, Ohmori S, et al. Characterization of human liver microsomal cytochrome P450 involved in the reductive metabolism of zonisamide. *Mol Pharmacol.* 1993;44:216–221.
31. Stiff DD, Robicheau T, Zemaitis MA. Reductive metabolism of the anticonvulsant agent zonisamide, a 1,2-benzisoxazole Derivative. *Xenobiotica.* 1992;22(1):1–11.
32. Nakasa H, et al. Prediction of drug-drug interactions of zonisamide metabolism in humans from in vitro data. *Eur J Clin Pharmacol.* 1998;54(2): 177–183.
33. Okada Y, et al. Population estimation regarding the effects of cytochrome P450 2C19 and 3A5 polymorphisms on zonisamide clearance. *Ther Drug Monit.* 2008;30(4):540–543.
34. *Zonegran.* 2004 [cited 2009 March 31]. Available at: http://www.eisai.com/package_inserts/ZonegranPI-12-2004.pdf.
35. Johannessen SI, Tomson T. Pharmacokinetic variability of newer antiepileptic drugs: when is monitoring needed? *Clin Pharmacokinet.* 2006;45(11):1061–1075.
36. Suzuki Y, et al. Zonisamide monotherapy in newly diagnosed infantile spasms. *Epilepsia.* 1997;38(9):1035–1038.
37. Suzuki Y, Zonisamide in West syndrome. *Brain Dev.* 2001;23(7):658–661.
38. Yagi K, Seino M. Methodological requirements for clinical trials in refractory epilepsies: our experience with zonisamide. In: *Symposium on Advances in Basic Research and Treatment of Refractory Epilepsy.* Kyoto: Dainippon Pharmaceutical Company Limited; 1990.
39. Odani A, Hashimoto Y, Takayanagi K, et al. Population pharmacokinetics of phenytoin in Japanese patients with epilepsy: analysis with a dose-dependent clearance model. *Biol Pharm Bull.* 1996;19(3):444–448.
40. Glauser TA, Pellock JM. Zonisamide in pediatric epilepsy: review of the Japanese experience. *J Child Neurol.* 2002;17(2):87–96.
41. Kawada K, et al. Pharmacokinetics of zonisamide in perinatal period. *Brain Dev.* 2002;24(2):95–97.
42. Shimoyama R, Ohkubo T, Sugawara K. Monitoring of zonisamide in human breast milk and maternal plasma by solid-phase extraction HPLC method. *Biomed Chromatogr.* 1999;13(5):370–372.
43. Oles KS, Bell WL, Zonisamide concentrations during pregnancy. *Ann Pharmacother.* 2008;42(7):1139–1141.
44. Schentag JJ, Gengo FM, Wilton JH, et al. Influence of phenobarbital, cimetidine, and renal disease on zonisamide kinetics. *Pharm Res.* 1987; (suppl):S79.
45. Ojemann LM, et al. Comparative pharmacokinetics of zonisamide (CI-912) in epileptic patients on carbamazepine or phenytoin monotherapy. *Ther Drug Monit.* 1986;8(3):293–296.
46. Shinoda M, et al. The necessity of adjusting the dosage of zonisamide when coadministered with other anti-epileptic drugs. *Biol Pharm Bull.* 1996;19(8):1090–1092.
47. Mather G, Carlson S, Trager EF, et al. Prediction of zonisamide interactions based on metabolic enzymes. *Epilepsia.* 1997;38(suppl 8):108.

48. Hachad H, Ragueneau-Majlessi I, Levy RH. New antiepileptic drugs: review on drug interactions. *Ther Drug Monit.* 2002;24(1):91–103.

49. Griffith SG, Dai, Y. Effect of zonisamide on the pharmacokinetics and pharmacodynamics of a combination ethinyl estradiol-norethindrone oral contraceptive in healthy women. *Clin Ther.* 2004;26(12): 2056–2065.

50. Yap KY, Chui WK, Chan A. Drug interactions between chemotherapeutic regimens and antiepileptics. *Clin Ther.* 2008;30(8):1385–1407.

51. Marson AG, Kadir ZA, Chadwick DW. New antiepileptic drugs: a systematic review of their efficacy and tolerability. *BMJ.* 1996;313(7066): 1169–1174.

52. Marson AG, et al. The new antiepileptic drugs: a systematic review of their efficacy and tolerability. *Epilepsia.* 1997;38(8):859–880.

53. Gazzola DM, Balcer LJ, French JA, Seizure-free outcome in randomized add-on trials of the new antiepileptic drugs. *Epilepsia.* 2007;48(7):1303–1307.

54. Schmidt D, et al. Zonisamide for add-on treatment of refractory partial epilepsy: a European double-blind trial. *Epilepsy Res.* 1993;15(1):67–73.

55. Leppik IE, et al. Efficacy and safety of zonisamide: results of a multicenter study. *Epilepsy Res.* 1993;14(2):165–173.

56. Faught E, et al. Randomized controlled trial of zonisamide for the treatment of refractory partial-onset seizures. *Neurology.* 2001;57(10): 1774–1779.

57. Sackellares JC, et al. Randomized, controlled clinical trial of zonisamide as adjunctive treatment for refractory partial seizures. *Epilepsia.* 2004;45(6): 610–617.

58. Brodie MJ, et al. Dose-dependent safety and efficacy of zonisamide: a randomized, double-blind, placebo-controlled study in patients with refractory partial seizures. *Epilepsia.* 2005;46(1):31–41.

59. Kluger G, Zsoter A, Holthausen H. Long-term use of zonisamide in refractory childhood-onset epilepsy. *Eur J Paediatr Neurol.* 2008;12(1):19–23.

60. Shinnar S, Pellock JM, Conry JA. Open-label, long-term safety study of zonisamide administered to children and adolescents with epilepsy. *Eur J Paediatr Neurol.* 2009;13(1):3–9.

61. Joo EY, et al. Zonisamide decreases cortical excitability in patients with idiopathic generalized epilepsy. *Clin Neurophysiol.* 2008;119(6):1385–1392.

62. Henry TR, et al. Progressive myoclonus epilepsy treated with zonisamide. *Neurology.* 1988;38(6):928–931.

63. Welty T, Kuzniecky R, Faught, E. Outcomes of using new AED in juvenile myoclonic epilepsy. *Neurology.* 2003.

64. Kothare SV, et al. Efficacy and tolerability of zonisamide in juvenile myoclonic epilepsy. *Epileptic Disord.* 2004;6(4):267–270.

65. Kishi T, et al. Successful zonisamide treatment for infants with hypsarrhythmia. *Pediatr Neurol.* 2000;23(3):274–277.

66. Suzuki Y, et al. Long-term response to zonisamide in patients with West syndrome. *Neurology.* 2002;58(10):1556–1559.

67. Yanagaki S, et al. Zonisamide for West syndrome: a comparison of clinical responses among different titration rate. *Brain Dev.* 2005;27(4):286–290.

68. Kumagai N, et al. Monotherapy for childhood epilepsies with zonisamide. *Jpn J Psychiatry Neurol.* 1991;45(2):357–359.

69. Kanba S, Yagi G, Kamijima K, et al. The first open study of zonisamide, a novel anticonvulsant, shows efficacy in mania. *Prog Neuro-Psychopharmacol Biol Psychiatry.* 1994;18:707–715.

70. Backonja MM. Use of anticonvulsants for treatment of neuropathic pain. *Neurology* 2002;59(5 suppl 2):S14–S17.

71. Murata M, Horiuchi E, Kanazawa I. Zonisamide has beneficial effects on Parkinson's disease patients. *Neurosci Res.* 2001;41(4):397–399.

72. Song IU, et al. Effects of zonisamide on isolated head tremor. *Eur J Neurol.* 2008;15(11):1212–1215.

73. Welty TE, Kuzniecky RI, Limdi N, et al. Weight loss associated with use of zonisamide in European and US clinical trials. *Epilepsia.* 2001;42 (abstract) page 262.

74. Gadde KM, et al. Zonisamide for weight loss in obese adults: a randomized controlled trial. *JAMA.* 2003;289(14):1820–1825.

75. Kim, C.S., Zonisamide effective for weight loss in women. *J Fam Pract.* 2003;52(8):600-1.

76. Kubota M, et al. Zonisamide-induced urinary lithiasis in patients with intractable epilepsy. *Brain Dev.* 2000;22(4):230–233.

77. Miyamoto A, Sugai R, Okamoto T, et al. Urine stone formation during treatment with zonisamide. *Brain Dev.* 2000;22:460.

78. Hirsch LJ, et al. Cross-sensitivity of skin rashes with antiepileptic drug use. *Neurology.* 2008;71(19):1527–1534.

79. O'Brien C. Important drug warning. In: Professionals H, ed. Elan Pharmaceuticals; 2002.

80. Berent S, et al. Zonisamide (CI-912) and cognition: results from preliminary study. *Epilepsia.* 1987;28(1):61–67.

81. Miyamoto T, Kohsaka M, Koyama T. Psychotic episodes during zonisamide treatment. *Seizure.* 2000;9(1):65–70.

82. Hirai K, et al. Selective mutism and obsessive compulsive disorders associated with zonisamide. *Seizure.* 2002;11(7):468–470.

83. Kondo T, et al. Preliminary report on teratogenic effects of zonisamide in the offspring of treated women with epilepsy. *Epilepsia.* 1996;37(12): 1242–1244.

CHAPTER 60 ■ LEVETIRACETAM

JOSEPH I. SIRVEN AND JOSEPH F. DRAZKOWSKI

Levetiracetam (LEV) is a novel antiepileptic drug (AED) approved in 2000 by the U.S. Food and Drug Administration as adjunctive therapy for patients with partial epilepsy. The compound was developed as a derivative of the nosotropic agent piracetam, with a wide spectrum of anticonvulsant effects in animal models of various types of epileptic seizures (1). It is chemically unrelated to existing AEDs. In addition to its unique chemical structure, LEV has a distinct mechanism of action and a favorable pharmacokinetic and safety profile, making it an attractive therapy for seizure management.

CHEMISTRY

LEV is a single enantiomer (−)-(S)-α-ethyl-2-oxo-1-pyrrolidine acetamide with a molecular weight of 170.21 (1,2). The structural formula of the agent is shown in Figure 60.1. The drug is a white to off-white crystalline powder with a faint odor and bitter taste. It is very soluble in water (104.0 g/100 mL), freely soluble in chloroform and in methanol, and soluble in ethanol. It is much less soluble to insoluble in acetonitrile and n-hexane.[1] LEV tablets contain LEV and the inactive ingredients silicon dioxide, cornstarch, methylcellulose, magnesium stearate, polyethylene glycol 4000, and coloring agents. LEV is supplied as 250-mg (blue), 500-mg (yellow), and 750-mg (orange) tablets, a 10% oral solution at 100 mg/mL, a 500-mg extended-release tablet, and a 500 mg/5 mL vial intravenous solution (2).

MECHANISM OF ACTION

Prior to undergoing standardized AED testing by the National Institutes of Health, LEV was found to have antiepileptic properties. In contrast to all approved AEDs, LEV lacked conventional modulation of the acute seizure model (maximum electroshock seizure [MES] test and pentylenetetrazol [PTZ]), suggesting a novel mechanism of action (3–5). Moreover, LEV displays unique potent protection against kindled seizures in both mice and rats during kindling models (3,4). In comparative tests with established AEDs in a number of animal models of epileptic seizures, LEV displays potent protection in a broad range of animal models of chronic epilepsy, including partial and primary generalized seizures (5).

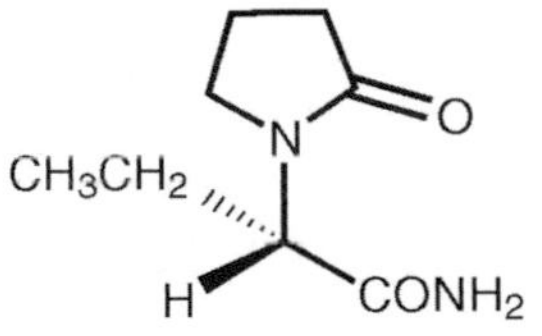

The precise mechanism by which LEV exerts its AED effect is unknown. It does not appear to derive its function from known mechanisms involved in inhibitory and excitatory neurotransmission, but it may be active at a brain-specific binding site (6). A stereoselective binding site for LEV has been shown to exist exclusively in membranes from cells in the central nervous system (CNS), but not in peripheral tissue (3,6). The central binding site is now known and is a presynaptic protein (SVA2) located on synaptic vesicles (7). The function of the protein is unknown but is believed to be a modulator of the vesicle fusion process (7). LEV binds to this protein, but how this interaction results in antiseizure activity is not known. There is no significant displacement (≤10 mm) of ligands specific for 55 different binding sites. Established AEDs, such as carbamazepine, phenytoin, valproate, phenobarbital, and clonazepam, do not possess an affinity for this binding site (6). LEV does not modulate any of the conventional mechanisms relevant to the action of other AEDs.

In studies performed to demonstrate the cellular pharmacodynamics of LEV, the agent reduces calcium current through neuron-specific, high-voltage–activated N-type calcium channels, thus reducing seizure potential (8). It does not modulate neuronal voltage-gated sodium, T-type calcium currents, or glutamate receptor-mediated neurotransmission in the spinal cord, nor does it have any conventional effects at the gamma-aminobutyric acid (GABA) A receptors (8). However, LEV does promote inhibitory neurotransmission by reducing negative allosteric effects of zinc and the beta-carbolines on GABA A and glycine receptors (9). In vitro and in vivo recordings of epileptiform activity from the hippocampus have shown that LEV inhibits burst firing without affecting normal neuronal excitability, suggesting selective suppression of hypersynchronization of epileptiform burst firing and propagation of seizure activity (10). The only certainty regarding the mechanism of action is that further investigation is warranted to elucidate the ways in which LEV exerts its selective effects.

ABSORPTION, DISTRIBUTION, AND METABOLISM

Overview

LEV is rapidly and almost completely absorbed following oral administration. The pharmacokinetics is linear and time invariant, with low individual variability (11). LEV is not protein bound (less than 10%), and its volume of distribution is close to the volume of intracellular and extracellular water (11,12). Sixty-six percent of the dose is unchanged as it is

FIGURE 60.1 The chemical structure of levetiracetam.

[1]Keppra is a registered trademark of UCB Pharma, Inc.

excreted renally (11). The major metabolic profile of LEV is an enzymatic hydrolysis of the acetamide group (11,12). LEV is not liver cytochrome P450–dependent (11). Its metabolites have no known pharmacologic activity and are renally excreted. The plasma half-life of LEV across studies is approximately 6 to 8 hours. The effects of the agent are increased in the elderly (primarily due to impaired renal clearance) and in patients with renal impairment (11,12).

Absorption and Distribution

Absorption of LEV is rapid, with peak plasma concentrations occurring about 1 hour following oral administration. Oral bioavailability is 100%, with no effect from ingestion of food. Linear pharmacokinetics characterizes LEV over a dose range of 500 to 5000 mg. Steady state is achieved after 2 days of multiple twice-daily dosing. LEV is less than 10% bound to plasma proteins; clinically significant interactions with other drugs through competition for protein-binding sites are unlikely (11,12).

Metabolism and Elimination

LEV is not extensively metabolized in humans with the major metabolic pathway of enzymatic hydrolysis of the acetamide group, which produces the pharmacologically inactive carboxylic acid metabolite. There is no dependency on P450 cytochrome liver metabolism (11,12).

LEV is eliminated by renal excretion as unchanged drug, which represents 66% of the administered dose (11). The total body clearance is 0.96 mL/min/kg and the renal clearance is 0.6 mL/min/kg (11,12). The mechanism of excretion is glomerular filtration with subsequent partial tubular reabsorption. Elimination is correlated with creatinine clearance (CrCl) (11).

Special Populations

Pediatrics

The pharmacokinetics of LEV has been evaluated in children 6 to 12 years of age following single 20-mg/kg doses. The apparent clearance of LEV was approximately 40% higher in children than in adults. The half-life in children is 4 to 8 hours, compared with approximately 7 hours in adults. The maximum concentration of drug (C_{max}) and area under the curve (AUC) values are comparable to those in adults. There is no correlation between age and clearance among pediatric patients (12).

Elderly

In older adults, total body clearance decreased by 38%, and the half-life was 2.5 hours longer compared with healthy adults (11).

Renal Impairment

Total body clearance of LEV is reduced in patients with impaired renal function by 40% in those with mild renal impairment (CrCl 50 to 80 mL/min), 50% in those with moderate impairment (CrCl 30 to 50 mL/min), and 60% in those with severe renal impairment (CrCl < 30 mL/min). In patients

with end-stage renal disease, total body clearance decreased by 70% compared with those with normal renal function. About 50% of LEV is removed during a standard 4-hour hemodialysis procedure. Thus, dosage should be reduced in patients with impaired renal function and supplemental doses should be given after hemodialysis (11).

Hepatic Impairment

The pharmacokinetics of LEV is unchanged in individuals with hepatic impairment. No dose adjustment is needed in patients with hepatic impairment (11).

DRUG INTERACTIONS

In vitro data on metabolic interactions indicate that LEV is unlikely to produce or be affected by pharmacokinetic interactions. Minimal plasma protein binding makes interactions due to competition for protein-binding sites unlikely (13). Potential pharmacokinetic interactions were assessed, but none were reported in clinical pharmacokinetic studies with phenytoin, warfarin, digoxin, and oral contraceptives (14–17). Analysis of Phase 3 studies also revealed no pharmacokinetic interactions with other AEDs, such as phenytoin, carbamazepine, valproic acid, and phenobarbital (14,18).

EFFICACY

Partial-Onset Seizures

There have been several trials investigating LEV for a number of varied seizure conditions (2,19–41). The effectiveness of LEV as adjunctive therapy in adults was established in three multicenter, randomized, double-blind, placebo-controlled clinical trials in patients with refractory partial-onset seizures with or without secondary generalization (19–21). Patients (N = 904) were randomized to one of four treatment arms: placebo, LEV 1000 mg, LEV 2000 mg, or LEV 3000 mg/day. Responder rates (50% or more reduction in seizure frequency compared with baseline) of 37.1% and 20.8%, respectively, were reported for 1000-mg/day doses for studies 1 and 2. At 2000 mg/day, a responder rate of 35.2% was reported; responder rates of 39.6% and 39.4%, respectively, were noted for 3000 mg/day (19–21). All of the response rates were statistically significant when all three LEV treatment arms were compared with placebo. Complete seizure freedom was reported to be 2% at 1000 mg and 6.7% at 3000 mg/day (19–21).

An interesting finding in study 1 was the rapid onset of efficacy of LEV (19). A significant reduction in weekly seizure frequency compared with that of the baseline period was observed during the first 2 weeks of the titration period, indicating that the agent has a rapid clinical effect at an initial dose (19,41). Open-label community trials confirmed the results noted in the pivotal trials, with efficacy achieved in patients at a dose of only 500 mg b.i.d. (22).

Four published studies have demonstrated the sustained efficacy of LEV as add-on epilepsy therapy for a period of at least 12 months and for as long as 54 months. The long-term tolerability of the agent is similar to that seen in the short-term, placebo-controlled trials (23–28).

Myoclonic Seizures in JME

The effectiveness of LEV as adjunctive therapy in patients 12 years of age or older with juvenile myoclonic epilepsy (JME) experiencing myoclonic seizures was established after one multicenter, randomized, double-blind, placebo-controlled study conducted at 37 sites in 14 countries. One hundred and thirteen patients were randomized to either placebo or LEV at a target dose of 3000 mg/day; 60.4% of the LEV group responded (>50% reduction from baseline in myoclonic seizure days per week) (29).

Primary Generalized Tonic–Clonic Seizures

LEV was evaluated for efficacy as adjunctive therapy in patients with idiopathic generalized epilepsy experiencing primary generalized tonic–clonic seizures by one randomized controlled trial conducted at 50 sites in 8 countries. Patients were randomized to either placebo or a target dose of 3000 mg/day or 60 mg/kg/day for children. Patients randomized to the LEV group showed a 77.6% reduction in seizures as compared to baseline. The LEV group also had a responder rate of 72.2% (29).

Monotherapy

Individuals with refractory partial epilepsy who completed a multicenter, double-blind, placebo-controlled, parallel-group with LEV 3000 mg/day were eligible for a monotherapy trial (21). Forty-nine patients entered the monotherapy arm. The median percent reduction in partial seizures was 73.8%, with a 50% responder rate of 59.2%. Nine patients (18.4%) remained seizure-free on monotherapy (21).

In a multicenter, noninferiority comparison trial conducted in newly diagnosed patients with epilepsy, LEV was compared to controlled-release carbamazepine as initial treatment. At 1 year, seizure outcomes were similar, with 56.6% of patients randomized to LEV ($N = 288$) and 58.5% of patients receiving controlled-release carbamazepine ($N = 291$) were seizure-free. Withdrawal rates due to treatment-emergent adverse events were 14.4% with LEV and 19.2% for those treated with controlled-release carbamazepine (30). LEV is not currently FDA approved as initial monotherapy.

Pediatrics

LEV has been evaluated in partial-onset seizures in children with epilepsy. One randomized, double-blind, placebo-controlled study was performed in North America with 60 sites and 198 pediatric patients between the ages of 4 to 16 years of age (39). Patients were randomized to placebo or to a dose of 20 mg/kg/day in two divided doses to a target dose of 60 mg/kg/day. The results showed a responder rate of 44.6% and a 26.8% reduction in weekly partial-onset seizures. A comparative trial was recently performed comparing LEV versus carbamazepine monotherapy for partial epilepsy in children less than 16 years of age. LEV was shown to have equal efficacy to carbamazepine (31).

Two open-label trials have been conducted to assess the efficacy and safety of LEV in children with partial seizures (12,32). Twenty-three children 6 to 12 years of age with treatment-resistant partial-onset seizures who were receiving one standard AED were eligible (32). Seizure frequency in these children was evaluated and compared with a 4-week baseline seizure frequency, using a 6-week titration to a target dose of 40 mg/kg/day. Twelve children (52%) responded (50% seizure reduction), with two patients remaining seizure-free during the entire study period (32).

A 10% oral grape-flavored solution (100 mg/mL) with an indication as an alternative formulation for adults and children with partial-onset epilepsy who have difficulty swallowing tablets is available. This will likely have utility both in the pediatric population and in patients who require feeding tubes (29).

ADVERSE EVENTS

Central Nervous System

Three main types of CNS adverse effects are associated with LEV use: fatigue, coordination difficulties, and behavioral problems (19–21,32). In the three pivotal clinical trials, 14.7% of patients reported fatigue, whereas 3.4% had coordination problems. Coordination difficulties included ataxia, abnormal gait, and incoordination. Dose reduction improved these symptoms. Fatigue and coordination problems occurred most frequently within the first 4 weeks of treatment. Of patients treated with LEV, 13% reported such behavioral symptoms as agitation, hostility, anxiety, apathy, emotional lability, depersonalization, and depression (Table 60.1). Most of these symptoms occurred within 4 weeks of drug initiation (19–21). Dose reduction was associated with improvement in these behavioral problems, with only 0.8% of treated patients requiring hospitalization. In the open-label trial of children, there were no differences between adverse events reported in this population and those reported in adults (33).

Other Systemic Adverse Events

Table 60.2 illustrates systemic adverse effects that have been reported in clinical trials with LEV. The most frequently reported adverse events included asthenia, somnolence, and dizziness, which occurred predominantly during the first

TABLE 60.1

NEUROLOGIC AND PSYCHIATRIC ADVERSE EFFECTS OF LEVETIRACETAM

Neurologic effect	Reported incidence in placebo-controlled trials in adults
Somnolence	14.8%
Vertigo	3%
Agitation	6% (pediatric trials)
Nervousness	4%
Depression	6.7%
Irritability	7%
Suicidal ideation	0.5%
Anxiety	2%

ADVERSE EFFECTS OF LEVETIRACETAM: SYSTEMIC

Body system	Adverse effects
Cardiac	No effect
Dermatologic	Minimal rash potential
Gastrointestinal	No significant effect
Hematologic	Minor decreases in hemoglobin, red blood cell count, and white blood cell (WBC) count
	No patients required treatment discontinuation because of these effects
Hepatic	No meaningful changes in liver function tests
Infectious	Pharyngitis, rhinitis with no relationship to WBC count
Pulmonary	No effect

4 weeks of treatment. In 15% of patients treated with LEV, somnolence was most often associated with discontinuation or dose reduction, followed by breakthrough seizures or dizziness (19–21).

Pregnancy

LEV is a pregnancy Category C drug, meaning that animal studies have produced evidence of developmental anomalies at doses similar to or greater than those used in humans (2). However, there are no adequate controlled studies of LEV in pregnant women. The effect of this drug on labor and delivery in humans is unknown. It is unclear whether LEV is excreted in human milk. Moreover, there is no impairment in male or female fertility (2,19–21).

CLINICAL USE

The recommended dosage of LEV is between 1000 and 3000 mg/day in two divided doses (2,11–39). Although in some studies there was a tendency toward greater response with higher doses, a consistent increase in response with increased dose has not been reported. Indeed, some older adults may respond to a dose as low as 500 mg/day (41). Dosage should guide titration to clinical response.

LEV should be introduced gradually at 250 mg b.i.d., in order to reduce the potential for side effects and to identify the minimum effective dose. Increases of 250 mg/day at 1- to 2-week intervals are recommended. If behavioral symptoms occur, reducing the dose may be beneficial. Although LEV has a rapid onset of effect, dose escalation that is too rapid could lead to adverse effects. A therapeutic dose range, in terms of concentration, has not been established for LEV. Dosage should be guided by clinical response. LEV may be ideally suited for individuals with seizures who are hepatically compromised or are taking multiple medications.

There are no clear guidelines established for dosing in patients younger than 16 years of age. However, open-label, postmarketing trials are attempting to fill this knowledge gap.

Data from these trials suggest for partial-onset seizures and primary generalized seizures, children from age 4 to 16 years should be initiated with a daily dose of 20 mg/kg in two divided doses. The daily dose can be increased every 2 weeks by increments of 20 mg/kg to a target dose of 60 mg/kg/day. In children with myoclonic seizures from JME and are 12 years of age or older, treatment should be initiated with a dose of 1000 mg/day given as b.i.d. doses. The target maximum dose is 3000 mg/day (29–35).

OTHER PREPARATIONS

Extended-Release Formulation

Keppra XR is an extended-release preparation of oral LEV based on matrix pill technology. The bioavailability of Keppra XR tablets is similar to that of immediate-release LEV. Similarly no differences exist between extended-release formulations and immediate-release LEV with regard to metabolism or renal excretion. Keppra XR is different than immediate-release LEV in that the time to peak plasma concentrations is about 3 hours longer with extended-release LEV than with immediate-release LEV. Single administration of two 500-mg Keppra XR tablets once a day produces comparable maximal plasma concentration and AUC plots as one 500-mg immediate-release LEV taken twice daily. There are no tablet skeletons/shells seen in the stool.

Keppra XR was evaluated for efficacy as adjunctive therapy in one multicenter, double-blind, randomized, placebo-controlled study in patients with refractory partial seizures (36). Patients were randomized to placebo versus two 500-mg tables of extended-release LEV. When compared to placebo, median reduction in seizure frequency for the extended-release group was 46.1% versus 33.4% ($P = 0.038$) for placebo during the 12-week treatment period. Patients did not have any different adverse effects than that reported for immediate-release LEV. There were no study withdrawals due to either excess sedation nor irritability. The manufacturer suggests that treatment should be initiated as adjunctive therapy for partial seizures with a dose of 1000 mg once daily with dosage adjusted in increments of 1000 mg every 2 weeks to a maximum recommended dose of 3000 mg/day. There are no data for the use of extended-release LEV in myoclonic seizures, primary generalized epilepsy, and children. This new formulation can be taken with or without food, but must be swallowed whole and should not be crushed or chewed. While generic formulations of immediate-release LEV have been FDA approved and marketed, currently there is no generic formulation of Keppra XR.

Intravenous Preparation

A new intravenous formulation of LEV is now available for adult patients 16 years and older when oral administration is temporarily not feasible (37–39). This preparation does not have an indication for seizure emergencies (29). Intravenous LEV and oral LEV result in equivalent pharmacokinetic parameters when IV LEV is administered as a 15-minute infusion. Its distribution, metabolism, and elimination are no different than oral LEV. In fact, intravenous LEV is almost interchangeable with oral LEV. In switching from oral LEV to intravenous LEV, the total daily dosage of medication should be equivalent. The manufacturer suggests that the total daily dose of LEV be administered as a 15-minute infusion following dilution in 100 mL of a compatible diluent. There is no evidence to suggest that a loading dose is necessary. Compatible diluents include: sodium chloride (0.9%), lactated Ringer's solution, and dextrose (5%). There is no randomized, controlled trial showing efficacy of intravenous LEV for acute seizures or status epilepticus.

CONCLUSION

LEV is a highly efficacious broad spectrum agent that can be used for a number of seizure types including partial seizures, myoclonic seizures of JME, and generalized tonic–clonic seizures of primary generalized epilepsy in both adults and children. LEV has linear and predictable pharmacokinetics, renal metabolism with few drug interactions, and multiple dosing preparations. These pharmacologic characteristics reduce the need for frequent serum therapeutic monitoring and allow the agent to be utilized in a variety of clinical settings. Although LEV has few adverse effects, its main drawback is concerns relating to its behavioral side effects. These effects can be mitigated by patient education and avoiding the drug in patients with ongoing psychiatric comorbid conditions.

References

1. Genton P, Van Vleyman BV. Piracetam and levetiracetam: close structural similarities but different pharmacological and clinical profiles. *Epileptic Disord.* 2000;2:99–105.
2. Keppra. In: *Physician's Desk Reference®.* 62nd ed. Montvale, NJ: Medical Economics; 2008.
3. Klitgaard H, Matagne A, Gobert J, et al. Evidence for a unique profile of levetiracetam in rodent models of seizures and epilepsy. *Eur J Pharmacol.* 1998;353:191–206.
4. Loscher W, Honack D. Profile of ucb L059, a novel anticonvulsant drug, in models of partial and generalized epilepsy in mice and rats. *Eur J Pharmacol.* 1993;232:147–158.
5. Gower AJ, Hirsch E, Boehrer A, et al. Effects of levetiracetam, a novel antiepileptic drug, on convulsant activity in two genetic rat models of epilepsy. *Epilepsy Res.* 1995;22:207–213.
6. Noyer M, Gillard M, Matagne A, et al. The novel antiepileptic drug levetiracetam (ucb L059) appears to act via a specific binding site in CNS membranes. *Eur J Pharmacol.* 1995;286:137–146.
7. Lynch BA, Lamberg N, Nocka K, et al. The synpatic vesicle protein SVA2 is the binding site for the antiepileptic drug LEV. *Proc Natl Acad Sci.* 2004;101(26):9861–9866.
8. Lukyanetz EA, Shkryl VM, Kostyuk PG. Selective blockade of N-type calcium channels by levetiracetam. *Epilepsia.* 2002;43:9–18.
9. Rigo JM, Hans G, Nguyen L, et al. The anti-epileptic drug levetiracetam reverses the inhibition by negative allosteric modulators of neuronal GABA- and glycine-gated currents. *Br J Pharmacol.* 2002;136:659–672.
10. Niespodziany I, Klitgaard H, Margineanu DG. Levetiracetam inhibits the high-voltage-activated Ca (2+) current in pyramidal neurones of rat hippocampal slices. *Neurosci Lett.* 2001;306:5–8.
11. Patsalos PN. Pharmacokinetic profile of levetiracetam: toward ideal characteristics. *Pharmacol Ther.* 2000;85:77–85.
12. Pellock JM, Glauser TA, Bebin EM, et al. Pharmacokinetic study of levetiracetam in children. *Epilepsia.* 2001;42:1574–1579.
13. Nicolas JM, Collart P, Gerin B, et al. In vitro evaluation of potential drug interactions with levetiracetam, a new antiepileptic agent. *Drug Metab Dispos.* 1999;27:250–254.
14. Perucca E, Gidal BE, Baltes E. Effects of antiepileptic comedication on levetiracetam pharmacokinetics: a pooled analysis of data from randomized adjunctive therapy trials. *Epilepsy Res.* 2003;53:47–56.
15. Ragueneau-Majlessi I, Levy RH, Janik F. Levetiracetam does not alter the pharmacokinetics of an oral contraceptive in healthy women. *Epilepsia.* 2002;43:697–702.
16. Levy RH, Ragueneau-Majlessi I, Baltes E. Repeated administration of the novel antiepileptic agent levetiracetam does not alter digoxin pharmacokinetics and pharmacodynamics in healthy volunteers. *Epilepsy Res.* 2001; 46:93–99.
17. Ragueneau-Majlessi I, Levy RH, Meyerhoff C. Lack of effect of repeated administration of levetiracetam on the pharmacodynamic and pharmacokinetic profiles of warfarin. *Epilepsy Res.* 2001;47:55–63.
18. Gidal BE, Baltes E, Otoul C, et al. Effect of levetiracetam on the pharmacokinetics of adjunctive antiepileptic drugs: a pooled analysis of data from randomized clinical trials. *Epilepsy Research.* 2005;64(1–2):1–11.
19. Cereghino JJ, Biton V, Abou-Khalil B, et al. Levetiracetam for partial seizures: results of a double-blind, randomized clinical trial. *Neurology.* 2000;55:236–242.
20. Shorvon SD, Lowenthal A, Janz D, et al. Multicenter double-blind, randomized, placebo-controlled trial of levetiracetam as add-on therapy in patients with refractory partial seizures. *Epilepsia.* 2000;4:1179–1186.
21. Ben-Menachem E, Falter U. Efficacy and tolerability of levetiracetam 3000 mg/d in patients with refractory partial seizures; a multicenter, double-blind, responder-selected study evaluating monotherapy. *Epilepsia.* 2000; 41:1276–1283.
22. Abou-Khalil B, Hemdal P, Privitera M. An open-label study of levetiracetam at individualised doses between 1000 and 3000 mg day (−1) in adult patients with refractory epilepsy. *Seizure.* 2003;12:141–149.
23. Krakow K, Walker M, Otoul C, et al. Long-term continuation of levetiracetam in patients with refractory epilepsy. *Neurology.* 2001;56:1772–1774.
24. Ben-Menachem E, Gilland E. Efficacy and tolerability of levetiracetam during 1-year follow-up in patients with refractory epilepsy. *Seizure.* 2003;12: 131–135.
25. Betts T, Waegemans T, Crawford P. A multicentre, double-blind, randomized parallel group study to evaluate the tolerability and efficacy of two oral doses of levetiracetam, 2000 mg daily and 4000 mg daily, without titration in patients with refractory epilepsy. *Seizure.* 2000;9:80–87.
26. Grant R, Shorvon SD. Efficacy and tolerability of 1000–4000 mg per day of levetiracetam as add-on therapy in patients with refractory epilepsy. *Epilepsy Res.* 2000;42:89–95.
27. Ben-Menachem E, Edrich P, Van Vleyman B, et al. Evidence for sustained efficacy of levetiracetam as add-on epilepsy therapy. *Epilepsy Res.* 2003; 53:57–64.
28. Betts T, Yarrow H, Greenhill L, et al. Clinical experience of marketed levetiracetam in an epilepsy clinic—a one year follow up study. *Seizure.* 2003;12:136–140.
29. Levetiracetam. Available at: http://www.accessdata.fda.gov/Scripts/cder/ DrugsatFDA/index.cfm?fuseaction=Search.Label_ApprovalHistory. Accessed January 24, 2009.
30. Brodie MJ, Perucca E, Ryvlin P, et al. Comparison of levetiracetam and controlled-release carbamazepine in newly diagnosed epilepsy. *Neurology.* 2007;68:402–408.
31. Perry S, Holt P, Benatar M. Levetiracetam versus carbamazepine monotherapy for partial epilepsy in children less than 16 years of age. *J Child Neurol.* 2008;23:515–519.
32. Glauser TA, Pellock JM, Bebin EM, et al. Efficacy and safety of levetiracetam in children with partial seizures: an open-label trial. *Epilepsia.* 2002; 43:518–524.
33. Harden C. Safety profile of levetiracetam. *Epilepsia.* 2001;42(suppl 4): 36–39.
34. Frost MD, Gustafson MC, Ritter FJ. Use of levetiracetam in children younger than 2 years [abstract]. *Epilepsia.* 2002;43(suppl 7):57.
35. Peltola J, Coetzee C, Jimenez J, et al. Once daily extended release levetiracetam as adjunctive treatment of partial-onset seizures in patients with epilepsy; a double blind, randomized, placebo-controlled trial. *Epilepsia.* 2009;50:406–414.
36. Baulac M, Brodie MJ, Elger CE, et al. Levetiracetam intravenous infusion as alternative to oral dosing in patients with partial-onset seizures. *Epilepsia.* 2007;48:589–592.
37. Ramael S, Daoust A, Otoul C, et al. Levetiracetam intravenous infusion: a randomized, placebo-controlled safety and pharmacokinetic study. *Epilepsia.* 2006;47:1128–1135.
38. Ramael S, De Smedt F, Toublanc N, et al. Single dose bioavailability of levetiracetam intravenous infusion relative to oral tablets and multiple dose pharmacokinetics and tolerability of levetiracetam intravenous infusion compared with placebo in healthy subjects. *Clin Ther.* 2006;28:734–744.
39. Glauser TA, Ayala R, Elterman RD, et al. Double-blind placebo-controlled trial of adjunctive levetiracetam in pediatric partial seizures. *Neurology.* 2006;66:1654–1660.
40. Ferrendelli JA, French J, Leppik I, et al. Use of levetiracetam in a population of patients aged 65 years and older: a subset analysis of the KEEPER trial. *Epilepsy Behav.* 2003;4:702–709.
41. French J, Arrigo C. Rapid onset of action of levetiracetam in refractory epilepsy patients. *Epilepsia.* 2005;46:324–326.

CHAPTER 61 ■ TIAGABINE

DANA EKSTEIN AND STEVEN C. SCHACHTER

HISTORICAL BACKGROUND AND CHEMISTRY

Tiagabine (−)-(R)-1-[4,4-bis(3-methyl-2-thienyl)-3-butenyl] nipecotic acid hydrochloride (TGB; Gabitril) received regulatory clearance from the U.S. Food and Drug Administration (FDA) for the adjunctive treatment of partial seizures in adults and children 12 years and older in October 1997. TGB was synthesized by using an aliphatic chain to link nipecotic acid to a lipophilic anchor (Fig. 61.1). Nipecotic acid is effective against seizures in animal models only when injected into the cerebral ventricles, because it does not cross the blood–brain barrier (BBB) (1). The lipophilic anchor allows the attached nipecotic acid to readily cross the BBB.

MECHANISM OF ACTION

TGB blocks the neuronal and glial reuptake of gamma-aminobutyric acid (GABA) after its release from postsynaptic GABA receptors, thereby enhancing GABA-mediated inhibition at central nervous system (CNS) sites (2,3). Accordingly, TGB suppresses hyperexcitability in the dentate gyrus and CA3 area in epileptic E1 mice (4). In electrophysiologic experiments in hippocampal slices in culture, TGB prolonged the inhibitory postsynaptic potentials (IPSP) and inhibitory postsynaptic currents (IPSC) in CA1 and CA3 areas produced by the addition of exogenous GABA; while in vivo microdialysis showed that TGB also increases extracellular GABA overflow in a dose-dependent manner (5). TGB does not reduce the frequency of spontaneous bursting in brain slices from rats with kainite-induced chronic epilepsy, but does reduce their duration and area under the curve of the bursts, at low concentrations (6).

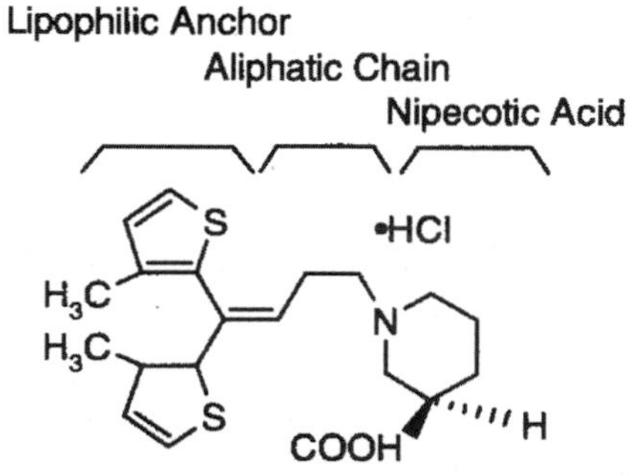

FIGURE 61.1 Chemical structure of tiagabine. (From Schachter SC. Tiagabine: current status and potential clinical applications. *Exp Opin Invest Drugs* 1996;5:1377–1387, with permission.)

TGB binds to the GABA uptake carrier GAT-1 in animals (5,7) and postmortem human brain tissue (8,9), but not to any other neurotransmitter uptake sites or receptors. TGB has no significant effect on sodium or calcium channels (5,10).

Animal Seizure Models

TGB reduces the severity and duration of convulsions in amygdala-kindled rats (5) and significantly retards kindling (11). In addition, TGB reduces maximal electroshock-induced seizures and bicuculline (BIC)-induced seizures in rats (5), and picrotoxin-induced convulsions in mice (12). The agent partially protects against photically induced myoclonus in photosensitive baboons (5) and blocks audiogenic convulsions in genetically epilepsy-prone rats (GEPR) in a dose-dependent manner (13). TGB is a potent anticonvulsant agent against methyl-6,7-dimethyoxy-4-ethyl-B-carboline-3-carboxylate (DMCM)-induced clonic convulsions, subcutaneous pentylenetetrazol (PTZ)-induced tonic convulsions, and GEPRs. TGB is partially efficacious against subcutaneous PTZ-induced clonic convulsions. However, TGB is weakly efficacious in the intravenous PTZ seizure threshold and the maximal electroshock seizure (MES) tests and produces only partial protection against BIC-induced convulsions in rats (5).

Efficacy for TGB has also been described in animal models of pain (14), depression (15), ethanol (16), cocaine and food (17) addictions, panic disorder (18), experimental Huntington disease (19), dystonia, (20) and experimental cerebral ischemia (21–24).

PHARMACOKINETICS

Absorption and Distribution

TGB is rapidly and almost completely absorbed (25). Oral bioavailability is approximately 90%, and the absorption of TGB is linear over the therapeutic dosage range. Maximum serum concentrations are attained within 45 to 90 minutes in the fasting state and after a mean of 2.6 hours when taken with food (10). The extent of TGB absorption is not affected by food. Binding to serum proteins is up to 96%.

In animal studies, TGB was found to have rapid CSF and brain penetration, with linear kinetics. However, CSF concentrations did not reflect free drug concentrations in serum, and its elimination from the brain greatly outlasted that seen in blood. It distributed evenly in brain cerebral cortex and hippocampus (26).

Metabolism and Elimination

Extensive oxidation of TGB occurs in the liver via isoform 3A of the cytochrome P450 (CYP450) family of enzymes (27). Only 2% of the administered dose is excreted as parent drug. The E- and Z-5-oxo-tiagabine isomers are the prominent metabolites in plasma and urine. Two major metabolites in human feces remain unidentified. TGB elimination is linear over the therapeutic dosage range (28).

The plasma half-life of TGB is 5 to 8 hours in patients with uninduced liver function (29) and 2 to 3 hours in patients taking hepatic enzyme-inducing antiepileptic drugs (AEDs) (10,28). More frequent dosing does not appear to be necessary to compensate for the shortened half-life, however, possibly due to the different kinetics of the drug inside the CNS. TGB 32 mg/day, as add-on therapy, is equally effective whether administered as a 16-mg dose twice daily or as an 8-mg dose four times per day (30). Similarly, twice-daily and thrice-daily regimens for patients with partial epilepsy were equally effective both during titration to 40 mg/day and a flexible continuation period of 12 weeks at 30 to 70 mg/day. However, during the titration period more adverse events were experienced by the patients who received TGB twice a day (31).

When adjusted for body weight, TGB elimination is two times higher in children than in uninduced adults with epilepsy (32). The pharmacokinetics of TGB are similar in healthy elderly volunteers and healthy young volunteers (33).

TGB pharmacokinetics are unaffected by renal impairment (34). However, the half-life of the agent is increased to 12 to 16 hours in patients with hepatic impairment (35), necessitating dosage reductions and less frequent dosing intervals.

Drug Interactions

Concurrently administered drugs that enhance the activity of CYP3A increase the clearance of TGB and decrease the half-life of the agent. Therefore, TGB serum concentrations may increase if treatment with concomitantly administered enzyme-inducing AEDs is discontinued (36).

Because TGB neither induces nor inhibits most hepatic microsomal enzymes involved in drug metabolism, it minimally affects the serum concentrations of other agents (29). However, since TGB was found to inhibit CYP45019, it might affect the balance between sex hormones (37). Moreover, although TGB is up to 96% protein bound, its serum concentration is too low to cause significant displacement of other protein-bound AEDs from albumin.

The metabolism of oral contraceptives is unaffected by TGB 8 mg/day (38), though it is unknown whether higher doses may have an effect on oral contraceptive metabolism.

EFFICACY

Add-on Studies of Patients with Refractory Partial Seizures

Five multicenter, double-blind, randomized, placebo-controlled studies evaluated TGB for the adjunctive treatment of partial-onset seizures in 951 patients, 675 of whom were randomly assigned to receive TGB (39–42). Three pivotal studies with parallel-group, add-on designs (30,41,42) enrolled patients taking one to three concomitant hepatic enzyme-inducing AEDs. The dose-response study compared the efficacy of three different doses of TGB (16, 32, and 56 mg/day) with that of placebo (43). The thrice-daily dosing study compared the efficacy of TGB 10 mg administered three times per day with that of placebo (44). A meta-analysis of the five placebo-controlled studies found a relative risk of 3.16 for having more than 50% seizures reduction (45). In the dose-response study, the reduction in median seizure rates was statistically significant for both higher dosage groups (32 mg and 56 mg) compared with the placebo group (43). In the thrice-daily dosing study, TGB 10 mg administered three times per day was significantly more effective than placebo in reducing 4-week complex partial seizure (CPS) rates and simple partial seizure rates from baseline (43). A large postmarketing open-label study followed 330 patients with partial-onset seizures for 10 weeks and found a better response to TGB when combined with valproic acid than when added to carbamazepine (46).

TGB was shown to have efficacy similar to topiramate in a small open-label study (47) and to levetiracetam (LEV) in a meta-analysis (48).

Monotherapy Trials

A dose-ranging study determined that the median tolerated dose of TGB as monotherapy for patients whose CPSs were not adequately controlled with one AED was 38.4 mg/day (range, 24 to 54 mg) (49).

The high- versus low-dose study randomized patients with CPS with or without secondarily generalized tonic–clonic seizures to either TGB 6 mg/day or TGB 36 mg/day (36). Median CPS rates decreased significantly in both dosage groups during TGB monotherapy in those patients who completed 12 weeks of fixed-dose treatment ($P < 0.05$). Additionally, nearly twice as many patients in the TGB 36-mg/day group as in the TGB 6-mg/day group experienced a reduction of $\geq 50\%$ in CPS rates (31% vs. 18%, respectively; $P = 0.038$) (49).

Long-Term Efficacy

Approximately 1200 patients received TGB for ≥ 1 year in six trials. CPS rates declined by a median of 28.4% after 3 to 6 months of treatment and by 44% after treatment for ≥ 1 year. Seizure reductions were maintained for up to 24 months (50). More recently, significant proportions of TGB-treated patients with learning disabilities were found to remain on TGB long-term (51).

ADVERSE EFFECTS

Add-On Studies of Patients with Refractory Partial Seizures

In the add-on trials, dizziness, asthenia (fatigue or generalized muscle weakness), nervousness, tremor, abnormal thinking (difficulty concentrating, mental lethargy, or slowness of thought), depression, aphasia (dysarthria, difficulty speaking, or speech arrest), and abdominal pain occurred significantly more often with TGB treatment than with placebo (30,43,44). Severe adverse effects were reported in 9% of the patients who received TGB and 5% of the patients who received placebo. Of patients treated with TGB, 13% withdrew from the study prematurely because of adverse effects, compared with 5% of those treated with placebo. In a meta-analysis of the five placebo-controlled studies, the side effects that occurred significantly more often with TGB than placebo were dizziness, fatigue, nervousness, and tremor (45). There were no significant differences between TGB and placebo for side effects related to mood, cognition, and adjustment. In a different meta-analysis, no difference in withdrawal rates was found between TGB and LEV (48).

Complex or simple partial status epilepticus occurred in 4 of 494 (0.8%) TGB recipients and 2 of 275 (0.7%) placebo recipients. Rash and psychosis occurred with approximately equal frequency in both groups (52). No clinically important effects attributable to TGB treatment were indicated in hematologic and biochemical test results, electrocardiograms, and vital signs. Neuropsychologic testing did not reveal any evidence of worsening in mood or cognitive abilities (53).

Long-Term Studies

No new adverse events occurred in long-term studies, nor were any additional severe adverse effects reported other than those already noted with short-term therapy (54). A review of 53 clinical trials involving nearly 3100 patients treated with TGB found no clinically important effects on laboratory tests, hepatic metabolism, or concomitant AED therapy (55). More recently, no significant difference in cognitive function was seen during 52 weeks of TGB 20 to 30 mg/day as monotherapy when compared to either carbamazepine monotherapy or untreated patients after their first seizure (56). Similarly, TGB-treated patients showed fewer long-term cognitive side effects than patients who received topiramate in a small open-label study (47).

The TGB safety database was scanned for adverse effects suggestive of symptomatic visual field loss. Of the eight patients who had visual symptoms, two had visual field defects from fixed lesions (temporal lobe resection, cortical infarct) and six had transient visual complaints. Physical examination did not reveal any fixed visual defects (57).

CLINICAL USE

Case reports have documented thrombocytopenia (58), convulsive status epilepticus (59), exacerbation of essential tremor (60), athetosis (61), dose-dependent balance disorder (62), and reversible acute dystonic reactions (63) in patients treated with TGB.

Numerous other reports have documented confusional states or nonconvulsive status epilepticus in TBG-treated patients with partial-onset or generalized seizures (64–76); remission has been observed with decreased TGB daily dose or with the addition of clonazepam or lorazepam (67,69,70,72,77). As noted earlier, the incidence of symptoms consistent with nonconvulsive status epilepticus in blinded trials was not higher in patients treated with TGB than in those who received placebo. The relationship of nonconvulsive status epilepticus to rapid dose increase (68,78) and TGB overdose (79) in nonepileptic adults (80,81) and pediatric patients (82,83) remains to be fully explored (26,84).

Add-on TGB therapy has no effect on weight (85) and appears to have similar effects on mood as does add-on carbamazepine and phenytoin (86), more so during the titration period (87). No relationship of TGB to psychosis (87), increased risk of fractures (88) and saccadic eye movements (89) has been demonstrated. The safety and pharmacokinetics of TGB in pregnancy are not known (90).

Open-label case series have shown no evidence of visual field changes with long-term TGB treatment (91–93). A patient with bipolar disease treated with adjunctive TGB was reported to have asymptomatic visual field defects that reversed when the TGB was discontinued (94). Color perception abnormality was seen in 7 of 17 patients and no contrast abnormalities were observed among the same 17 patients (95).

TGB continues to be used largely as an adjunctive agent in patients with partial-onset epilepsy (96). An intriguing report suggests that TGB may have particular efficacy for seizures due to glial tumors, but this awaits confirmation (97).

Based on its mechanism of action, TGB has been proposed for numerous off-label uses. However, it is not more effective than placebo for spasticity (98), anxiety (99), post-traumatic stress disorder (PTSD) (100), alcohol (101) and cocaine (102) abuse, and bipolar disorder (103). Possible benefit for migraine (104), chronic pain (105), and primary insomnia (106,107) need to be confirmed with controlled studies.

TGB is available in the United States as 2-, 4-, 12-, and 16-mg tablets. Dosages should be titrated slowly to 32 to 56 mg daily in two or three divided doses in patients taking concomitant enzyme-inducing AEDs and to 12 to 22 mg/day in uninduced patients. Dosages in children have not been well established; in one pediatric trial, doses ≤0.4 mg/kg were used in children with uninduced hepatic function and doses ≤0.7 mg/kg in children taking enzyme-inducing AEDs.

The clinical utility of TGB serum concentrations is uncertain because of its short half-life in induced patients (108,109) and because the serum level may not reliably reflect the concentration of TGB in the brain (26). Routine monitoring of liver, renal, and bone marrow function does not appear to be necessary.

CONCLUSION

TGB is a potent AED with linear, predictable pharmacokinetics that inhibits GABA reuptake into neurons and glia. TGB has no clinically relevant effects on hepatic metabolism or serum concentrations of other AEDs, nor does it interact with many commonly used non-AEDs. The most common side effects are CNS related, usually mild to moderate in severity, and minimized by slow dosage titration. At doses of 32 to 56 mg/day, TGB has proved effective as add-on treatment in patients with partial seizures. Higher doses are well tolerated and appear to benefit some patients in open studies and in clinical experience. Additional controlled studies are needed to confirm the efficacy of TGB as monotherapy and to determine the effective dosage range.

References

1. Krogsgaard-Larsen P, Falch E, Larsson OM, et al. GABA uptake inhibitors: relevance to antiepileptic drug research. *Epilepsy Res.* 1987;1:77–93.
2. Braestrup C, Nielsen EB, Sonnewald U, et al. (R)-N-[4,4-bis(3-methyl-2-thienyl)but-3-en-1-yl]nipecotic acid binds with high affinity to the brain gamma-aminobutyric acid uptake carrier. *J Neurochem.* 1990;54:639–647.
3. Giardina WJ. Anticonvulsant action of tiagabine, a new GABA-uptake inhibitor. *J Epilepsy.* 1994;7:161–166.
4. Fueta Y, Schwarz W, Ohno K, et al. Selective suppression of hippocampal region hyperexcitability related to seizure susceptibility in epileptic El mice by the GABA-transporter inhibitor tiagabine. *Brain Res.* 2002;947: 212–217.
5. Suzdak PD, Jansen JA. A review of the preclinical pharmacology of tiagabine: a potent and selective anticonvulsant GABA uptake inhibitor. *Epilepsia.* 1995;36(6):612–626.
6. Smith MD, Saunders GW, Clausen RP, et al. Inhibition of the betaine-GABA transporter (mGAT2/BGT-1) modulates spontaneous electrographic bursting in the medial entorhinal cortex (mEC). *Epilepsy Res.* 2008;79(1):6–13.
7. Borden LA, Dhar TGM, Smith KE, et al. Tiagabine, SK&F 89976-A, CI-966, and NNC-711 are selective for the cloned GABA transporter GAT-1. *Eur J Pharmacol.* 1994;269:219–224.
8. Eriksson IS, Allard P, Marcusson J. [3H]Tiagabine binding to GABA uptake sites in human brain. *Brain Res.* 1999;851:183–188.
9. Sundman-Eriksson I, Allard P. [(3)H]Tiagabine binding to GABA transporter-1 (GAT-1) in suicidal depression. *J Affect Disord.* 2002;71:29–33.
10. Brodie MJ. Tiagabine pharmacology in profile. *Epilepsia.* 1995;36(suppl 6):S7–S9.
11. Morimoto K, Sato H, Yamamoto Y, et al. Antiepileptic effects of tiagabine, a selective GABA uptake inhibitor, in the rat kindling model of temporal lobe epilepsy. *Epilepsia.* 1997;38:966–974.
12. Nielsen EB, Suzdak PD, Andersen KE, et al. Characterization of tiagabine (NO-328), a new potent and selective GABA uptake inhibitor. *Eur J Pharmacol.* 1991;196:257–266.
13. Faingold CL, Randall ME, Anderson CA. Blockade of GABA uptake with tiagabine inhibits audiogenic seizures and reduces neuronal firing in the inferior colliculus of the genetically epilepsy-prone rat. *Exp Neurol.* 1994;126:225–232.
14. Ipponi A, Lamberti C, Medica A, et al. Tiagabine antinociception in rodents depends on GABA(B) receptor activation: parallel antinociception testing and medial thalamus GABA microdialysis. *Eur J Pharmacol.* 1999;368:205–211.
15. Pistovcakova J, Dostalek M, Sulcova A, et al. Tiagabine treatment is associated with neurochemical, immune and behavioural alterations in the olfactory bulbectomized rat model of depression. *Pharmacopsychiatry.* 2008;41(2):54–59.
16. Nguyen SA, Deleon CP, Malcolm RJ, et al. Tiagabine reduces ethanol reward in C57BL/6 mice under acute and chronic administration regimens. *Synapse.* 2005;56(3):135–146.
17. Weerts EM, Froestl W, Griffiths RR. Effects of GABAergic modulators on food and cocaine self-administration in baboons. *Drug Alcohol Depend.* 2005;80(3):369–376.
18. Zwanzger P, Rupprecht R. Selective GABAergic treatment for panic? Investigations in experimental panic induction and panic disorder. *J Psychiatry Neurosci.* 2005;30(3):167–175.
19. Dhir A, Akula KK, Kulkarni SK. Tiagabine, a GABA uptake inhibitor, attenuates 3-nitropropionic acid-induced alterations in various behavioral and biochemical parameters in rats. *Prog Neuropsychopharmacol Biol Psychiatry.* 2008;32(3):835–843.
20. Kreil A, Richter A. Antidystonic efficacy of gamma-aminobutyric acid uptake inhibitors in the dtsz mutant. *Eur J Pharmacol.* 2005;521(1–3): 95–98.
21. Yang Y, Li Q, Wang CX, et al. A. Dose-dependent neuroprotection with tiagabine in a focal cerebral ischemia model in rat. *Neuroreport.* 2000;11:2307–2311.
22. Chen Xu W, Yi Y, Qiu L, et al. Neuroprotective activity of tiagabine in a focal embolic model of cerebral ischemia. *Brain Res.* 2000;874:75–77.
23. Iqbal S, Baziany A, Gordon S, et al. Neuroprotective effect of tiagabine in transient forebrain global ischemia: an in vivo microdialysis, behavioral, and histological study. *Brain Res.* 2002;946:162–170.
24. Costa C, Leone G, Saulle E, et al. Coactivation of GABA(A) and GABA(B) receptor results in neuroprotection during in vitro ischemia. *Stroke.* 2004;35(2):596–600.
25. Mengel H. Tiagabine. *Epilepsia.* 1994;35(suppl 5):S81–S84.
26. Wang X, Ratnaraj N, Patsalos PN. The pharmacokinetic inter-relationship of tiagabine in blood, cerebrospinal fluid and brain extracellular fluid (frontal cortex and hippocampus). *Seizure.* 2004;13(8):574–581.
27. Bopp BA, Nequist GE, Rodrigues AD. Role of the cytochrome P450 3A subfamily in the metabolism of [14C] tiagabine by human hepatic microsomes. *Epilepsia.* 1995;36(suppl 3):S159.
28. Samara EE, Gustavson LE, El-Shourbagy T, et al. Population analysis of the pharmacokinetics of tiagabine in patients with epilepsy. *Epilepsia.* 1998;39:868–873.
29. Gustavson LE, Mengel HB. Pharmacokinetics of tiagabine, a gamma-aminobutyric acid-uptake inhibitor, in healthy subjects after single and multiple doses. *Epilepsia.* 1995;36:605–611.
30. Sachdeo RC, Leroy RF, Krauss GL, et al. Tiagabine therapy for complex partial seizures. A dose-frequency study. *Arch Neurol.* 1997;54:595–601.
31. Arroyo S, Boothman BR, Brodie MJ, et al. A randomised open-label study of tiagabine given two or three times daily in refractory epilepsy. *Seizure.* 2005;14(2):81–84.
32. Gustavson LE, Boellner SW, Granneman GR, et al. A single-dose study to define tiagabine pharmacokinetics in pediatric patients with complex partial seizures. *Neurology.* 1997;48:1032–1037.
33. Snel S, Jansen JA, Mengel HB, et al. The pharmacokinetics of tiagabine in healthy elderly volunteers and elderly patients with epilepsy. *J Clin Pharmacol.* 1997;37:1015–1020.
34. Cato A, Gustavson LE, Quian J, et al. Effect of renal impairment on the pharmacokinetics and tolerability of tiagabine. *Epilepsia.* 1998;39:43–47.
35. Lau AH, Gustavson LE, Sperelakis R, et al. Pharmacokinetics and safety of tiagabine in subjects with various degrees of hepatic function. *Epilepsia.* 1997;38:445–451.
36. Schachter SC. Tiagabine monotherapy in the treatment of partial epilepsy. *Epilepsia.* 1995;36(suppl 6):S2–S6.
37. Jacobsen NW, Halling-Sorensen B, Birkved FK. Inhibition of human aromatase complex (CYP19) by antiepileptic drugs. *Toxicol In Vitro.* 2008;22(1):146–153.
38. Mengel HB, Houston A, Back DJ. An evaluation of the interaction between tiagabine and oral contraceptives in female volunteers. *J Pharm Med.* 1994;4:141–150.
39. Ostergaard LH, Gram L, Dam M. Potential antiepileptic drugs. Tiagabine. In: Levy RH, Mattson RH, Meldrum BS, eds. *Antiepileptic drugs.* New York: Raven Press; 1995:1057–1061.
40. Richens A, Chadwick DW, Duncan JS, et al. Adjunctive treatment of partial seizures with tiagabine: a placebo-controlled trial. *Epilepsy Res.* 1995;21:37–42.
41. Lassen LC, Sommerville K, Mengel HB, et al. Summary of five controlled trials with tiagabine as adjunctive treatment of patients with partial seizures. *Epilepsia.* 1995;36(suppl 3):S148.
42. Crawford P, Meinardi H, Brown S, et al. Tiagabine: efficacy and safety in adjunctive treatment of partial seizures. *Epilepsia.* 2001;42:531–538.
43. Uthman BM, Rowan AJ, Ahmann PA, et al. Tiagabine for complex partial seizures: a randomized, add-on, dose-response trial. *Arch Neurol.* 1998;55:56–62.
44. Kalviainen R, Brodie MJ, Duncan J, et al. A double-blind, placebo-controlled trial of tiagabine given three-times daily as add-on therapy for refractory partial seizures. *Epilepsy Res.* 1998;30:31–40.
45. Pereira J, Marson AG, Hutton JL. Tiagabine add-on for drug-resistant partial epilepsy. *Cochrane Database Syst Rev.* 2002;(3):CD001908.
46. Jedrzejczak J. Tiagabine as add-on therapy may be more effective with valproic acid—open label, multicentre study of patients with focal epilepsy. *Eur J Neurol.* 2005;12(3):176–180.
47. Fritz N, Glogau S, Hoffmann J, et al. Efficacy and cognitive side effects of tiagabine and topiramate in patients with epilepsy. *Epilepsy Behav.* 2005;6(3):373–381.
48. Otoul C, Arrigo C, van Rijckevorsel K, et al. Meta-analysis and indirect comparisons of levetiracetam with other second-generation antiepileptic drugs in partial epilepsy. *Clin Neuropharmacol.* 2005;28(2):72–78.
49. Schachter SC, Cahill WT, Wannamaker BB, et al. Open-label dosage and tolerability study of tiagabine monotherapy in patients with refractory complex partial seizures. *J Epilepsy.* 1998;11:248–255.
50. Schachter SC, Deaton R, Sommerville K. Long-term use of tiagabine for partial seizures. *Epilepsia.* 1997;38(suppl 8):S105–S106.
51. Simister RJ, Sander JW, Koepp MJ. Long-term retention rates of new antiepileptic drugs in adults with chronic epilepsy and learning disability. *Epilepsy Behav.* 2007;10(2):336–339.
52. Sackellares JC, Krauss G, Sommerville KW, et al. Occurrence of psychosis in patients with epilepsy randomized to tiagabine or placebo treatment. *Epilepsia.* 2002;43:394–398.
53. Dodrill CB, Arnett JL, Sommerville KW, et al. Cognitive and quality of life effects of differing dosages of tiagabine in epilepsy. *Neurology.* 1997;48:1025–1031.
54. Leppik IE. Tiagabine: the safety landscape. *Epilepsia.* 1995;36(suppl 6):S10–S13.
55. Leppik IE, Gram L, Deaton R, et al. Safety of tiagabine: summary of 53 trials. *Epilepsy Res.* 1999;33:235–246.
56. Aikia M, Jutila L, Salmenpera T, et al. Comparison of the cognitive effects of tiagabine and carbamazepine as monotherapy in newly diagnosed adult patients with partial epilepsy: pooled analysis of two long-term, randomized, follow-up studies. *Epilepsia.* 2006;47(7):1121–1127.
57. Collins SD, Brun S, Kirstein YG, et al. Absence of visual field defects in patients taking tiagabine. *Epilepsia.* 1998;39(suppl 6):S146–S147.
58. Willert C, Englisch S, Schlesinger S, et al. Possible drug-induced thrombocytopenia secondary to tiagabine. *Neurology.* 1999;52:889–891.
59. Ostrovskiy D, Spanaki MV, Morris GL III. Tiagabine overdose can induce convulsive status epilepticus. *Epilepsia.* 2002;43:773–774.
60. Zesiewicz TA, Sullivan KL, Ward CL, et al. Tiagabine and exacerbation of essential tremor. *Mov Disord.* 2007;22(14):2132–2133.

61. Tombini M, Pacifici L, Passarelli F, et al. Transient athetosis induced by tiagabine. *Epilepsia.* 2006;47(4):799–800.

62. Sirven JI, Fife TD, Wingerchuk DM, et al. Second-generation antiepileptic drugs' impact on balance: a meta-analysis. *Mayo Clin Proc.* 2007;82(1):40–47.

63. Wolanczyk T, Grabowska-Grzyb A. Transient dystonias in three patients treated with tiagabine. *Epilepsia.* 2001;42:944–946.

64. Brouns R, Van Paesschen W. Recurrent complex partial status epilepticus associated with tiagabine rechallenge. *Acta Neurol Belg.* 2002;102:19–20.

65. Fitzek S, Hegemann S, Sauner D, et al. Drug-induced nonconvulsive status epilepticus with low dose of tiagabine. *Epileptic Disord.* 2001;3:147–150.

66. Eckardt KM, Steinhoff BJ. Nonconvulsive status epilepticus in two patients receiving tiagabine treatment. *Epilepsia.* 1998;39:671–674.

67. Trinka E, Moroder T, Nagler M, et al. Clinical and EEG findings in complex partial status epilepticus with tiagabine. *Seizure.* 1999;8:41–44.

68. de Borchgrave V, Lienard F, Willemart T, et al. Clinical and EEG findings in six patients with altered mental status receiving tiagabine therapy. *Epilepsy Behav.* 2003;4:326–337.

69. Imperiale D, Pignatta P, Cerrato P, et al. Nonconvulsive status epilepticus due to a de novo contralateral focus during tiagabine adjunctive therapy. *Seizure.* 2003;12:319–322.

70. Kellinghaus C, Dziewas R, Ludemann P. Tiagabine-related non-convulsive status epilepticus in partial epilepsy: three case reports and a review of the literature. *Seizure.* 2002;11:243–249.

71. Ettinger AB, Bernal OG, Andriola MR, et al. Two cases of nonconvulsive status epilepticus in association with tiagabine therapy. *Epilepsia.* 1999;40:1159–1162.

72. Knake S, Hamer HM, Schomburg U, et al. Tiagabine-induced absence status in idiopathic generalized epilepsy. *Seizure.* 1999;8:314–317.

73. Balslev T, Uldall P, Buchholt J. Provocation of non-convulsive status epilepticus by tiagabine in three adolescent patients. *Eur J Paediatr Neurol.* 2000;4:169–170.

74. Skodda S, Kramer I, Spittler JF, et al. Non-convulsive status epilepticus in two patients receiving tiagabine add-on treatment. *J Neurol.* 2001;248:109–112.

75. Koepp MJ, Edwards M, Collins J, et al. Status epilepticus and tiagabine therapy revisited. *Epilepsia.* 2005;46(10):1625–1632.

76. Vinton A, Kornberg AJ, Cowley M, et al. Tiagabine-induced generalised non convulsive status epilepticus in patients with lesional focal epilepsy. *J Clin Neurosci.* 2005;12(2):128–133.

77. Zhu Y, Vaughn BV. Non-convulsive status epilepticus induced by tiagabine in a patient with pseudoseizure. *Seizure.* 2002;11:57–59.

78. Skardoutsou A, Voudris KA, Vagiakou EA. Non-convulsive status epilepticus associated with tiagabine therapy in children. *Seizure.* 2003;12(8):599–601.

79. Spiller HA, Winter ML, Ryan M, et al. Retrospective evaluation of tiagabine overdose. *Clin Toxicol (Phila).* 2005;43(7):855–859.

80. Leikin JB, Benigno J, Dubow JS, et al. Status epilepticus due to tiagabine ingestion. *Am J Ther.* 2008;15(3):290–291.

81. Vollmar C, Noachtar S. Tiagabine-induced myoclonic status epilepticus in a nonepileptic patient. *Neurology.* 2007;68(4):310.

82. Jette N, Cappell J, VanPassel L, et al. Tiagabine-induced nonconvulsive status epilepticus in an adolescent without epilepsy. *Neurology.* 2006;67(8):1514–1515.

83. Kazzi ZN, Jones CC, Morgan BW. Seizures in a pediatric patient with a tiagabine overdose. *J Med Toxicol.* 2006;2(4):160–162.

84. Stein V, Nicoll RA. GABA generates excitement. *Neuron.* 2003;37(3):375–378.

85. Hogan RE, Bertrand ME, Deaton RL, et al. Total percentage body weight changes during add-on therapy with tiagabine, carbamazepine and phenytoin. *Epilepsy Res.* 2000;41:23–28.

86. Dodrill CB, Arnett JL, Deaton R, et al. Tiagabine versus phenytoin and carbamazepine as add-on therapies: effects on abilities, adjustment, and mood. *Epilepsy Res.* 2000;42:123–132.

87. Mula M, Sander JW. Negative effects of antiepileptic drugs on mood in patients with epilepsy. *Drug Saf.* 2007;30(7):555–567.

88. Vestergaard P, Rejnmark L, Mosekilde L. Fracture risk associated with use of antiepileptic drugs. *Epilepsia.* 2004;45(11):1330–1337.

89. Zwanzger P, Schule C, Eser D, et al. Saccadic eye velocity after selective GABAergic treatment with tiagabine in healthy volunteers. *Neuropsychobiology.* 2005;52(3):147–150.

90. Tomson T, Battino D. Pharmacokinetics and therapeutic drug monitoring of newer antiepileptic drugs during pregnancy and the puerperium. *Clin Pharmacokinet.* 2007;46(3):209–219.

91. Krauss GL, Johnson MA, Sheth S, et al. A controlled study comparing visual function in patients treated with vigabatrin and tiagabine. *J Neurol Neurosurg Psychiatry.* 2003;74:339–343.

92. Fakhoury TA, Abou-Khalil B, Lavin P. Lack of visual field defects with long-term use of tiagabine. *Neurology.* 2000;54(suppl 3):A309.

93. Nousiainen I, Mantyjarvi M, Kalviainen R. Visual function in patients treated with the GABAergic anticonvulsant drug tiagabine. *Clin Drug Invest.* 2000;20:393–400.

94. Kaufman KR, Lepore FE, Keyser BJ. Visual fields and tiagabine: a quandary. *Seizure.* 2001;10:525–529.

95. Sorri I, Kalviainen R, Mantyjarvi M. Color vision and contrast sensitivity in epilepsy patients treated with initial tiagabine monotherapy. *Epilepsy Res.* 2005;67(3):101–107.

96. Schmidt D, Gram L, Brodie M, et al. Tiagabine in the treatment of epilepsy—a clinical review with a guide for the prescribing physician. *Epilepsy Res.* 2000;41:245–251.

97. Striano S, Striano P, Boccella P, et al. Tiagabine in glial tumors. *Epilepsy Res.* 2002;49:81–85.

98. Chu ML, Sala DA. The use of tiagabine in pediatric spasticity management. *Dev Med Child Neurol.* 2006;48(6):456–459.

99. Pollack MH, Tiller J, Xie F, et al. Tiagabine in adult patients with generalized anxiety disorder: results from 3 randomized, double-blind, placebo-controlled, parallel-group studies. *J Clin Psychopharmacol.* 2008;28(3):308–316.

100. Davidson JR, Brady K, Mellman TA, et al. The efficacy and tolerability of tiagabine in adult patients with post-traumatic stress disorder. *J Clin Psychopharmacol.* 2007;27(1):85–88.

101. Karila L, Gorelick D, Weinstein A, et al. New treatments for cocaine dependence: a focused review. *Int J Neuropsychopharmacol.* 2008;11(3):425–438.

102. Minozzi S, Amato L, Davoli M, et al. Anticonvulsants for cocaine dependence. *Cochrane Database Syst Rev.* 2008;(2):CD006754.

103. Young AH, Geddes JR, Macritchie K, et al. Tiagabine in the treatment of acute affective episodes in bipolar disorder: efficacy and acceptability. *Cochrane Database Syst Rev.* 2006;3:CD004694.

104. Freitag FG, Diamond S, Diamond ML. Tiagabine in the prophylaxis of migraine. *Neurology.* 1999;52(suppl 2):A208.

105. Todorov AA, Kolchev CB, Todorov AB. Tiagabine and gabapentin for the management of chronic pain. *Clin J Pain.* 2005;21(4):358–361.

106. Roth T, Wright KP, Jr., Walsh J. Effect of tiagabine on sleep in elderly subjects with primary insomnia: a randomized, double-blind, placebo-controlled study. *Sleep.* 2006;29(3):335–341.

107. Walsh JK, Zammit G, Schweitzer PK, et al. Tiagabine enhances slow wave sleep and sleep maintenance in primary insomnia. *Sleep Med.* 2006;7(2):155–161.

108. Perucca E. Is there a role for therapeutic drug monitoring of new anticonvulsants? *Clin Pharmacokinet.* 2000;38:191–204.

109. Johannessen SI, Tomson T. Pharmacokinetic variability of newer antiepileptic drugs: when is monitoring needed? *Clin Pharmacokinet.* 2006;45(11):1061–1075.

CHAPTER 62 ■ FELBAMATE

EDWARD FAUGHT

HISTORICAL BACKGROUND

Felbamate (FBM) is historically significant as the first of the new generation of antiepileptic drugs (AEDs) introduced in the 1990s, after a dormant period of 15 years with no major advances in medical therapy for epilepsy. It was first synthesized in the 1950s as a potential tranquilizer, but unlike the related dicarbamate, meprobamate, it has no tranquilizing nor sedative action. Eventually, it was submitted to the National Institutes of Health (NIH) antiepileptic drug-screening program, and demonstrated encouraging results in animal seizure models (1). Human clinical trials began in 1985 (2–5). Monotherapy trials for partial-onset seizures yielded impressive results (6,7) and FBM was approved for use in the United States in 1993. Dangerous side effects were not anticipated based on the experience of the 2100 patients enrolled in clinical trials, but in 1994, FBM was found to be associated with a high incidence of aplastic anemia (8). FBM remains available for patients with refractory seizures who respond poorly to other medications.

CHEMISTRY AND MECHANISM OF ACTION

Chemistry

FBM (2 phenyl-1,3-propanediol dicarbamate, molecular weight 238.24) differs from meprobamate by having a phenyl group, rather than an aliphatic chain, at the 2-carbon position (Fig. 62.1). It is lipophilic and relatively insoluble in water (9). No parenteral preparation for humans is available, but intravenous administration in mice has been achieved by encapsulating FBM molecules with hydrophobic diketopiperazine microspheres (10).

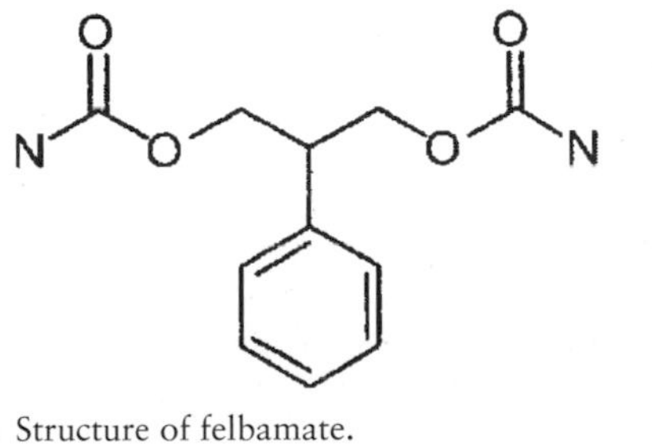

FIGURE 62.1 Structure of felbamate.

Antiepileptic Profile in Animals

FBM displayed high protective indices (toxic $dose_{50}$/effective $dose_{50}$) against both the tonic phase of maximal electroshock seizures (MES) and subcutaneous pentylenetetrazol-induced seizures in rodents (1). It is effective in amygdala-kindled, phenytoin-resistant rats (11). A synergistic effect with levetiracetam was demonstrated in the mouse MES model (12).

Mechanisms of Action

The major antiepileptic mechanism of action of FBM is probably binding to open channels of the N-methyl D-aspartate (NMDA) subtype of glutamate receptor, blocking sodium and calcium excitatory conductances (13). This action is unique among AEDs. FBM binds selectively to some NMDA-receptor subtypes, especially those containing NR2B subunits (14,15). Subtype specificity may account for the lack of serious neurobehavioral complications typical of other NMDA-receptor blockers such as MK-801 (16).

Other mechanisms may be clinically relevant. FBM interferes with voltage-gated sodium channels, resulting in blockade of sustained repetitive neuronal firing and prevention of seizure spread (17). It may have a blocking action on non-NMDA-type glutamatergic receptors (18). An inhibitory effect on high-threshold, voltage-sensitive calcium currents was reported (19).

An antiglutamergic mechanism may underlie neuroprotective effects: FBM reduced neuronal damage in a rat model of hypoxia–ischemia (20), protected CA1 hippocampal neurons from apoptosis in a gerbil ischemia model (21), and exhibited neuroprotective effects in a rat model of status epilepticus (22). FBM and related compounds have potential as treatments for status epilepticus. Fluorofelbamate stopped seizures in the rat self-sustaining status epilepticus model; it also retarded the development of subsequent spontaneous seizures, which suggests an antiepileptogenic effect (23).

ABSORPTION, DISTRIBUTION, AND METABOLISM

FBM is well absorbed; more than 90% of ^{14}C-labeled FBM, or its metabolites, is recovered in urine and feces after oral administration (24), and the rate and extent of absorption are not affected by food or antacids (25). Protein binding in human plasma is low, 22% to 25% (24). Animal studies confirm the basic characteristics of FBM absorption and distribution (26). FBM readily crosses the blood–brain barrier, with brain and cerebrospinal fluid concentrations in humans close to plasma concentrations (27).

Of the absorbed FBM dose, 30% to 50% is excreted in the urine unchanged (24), with renal clearance decreasing to 9% to 22% of the total dose in patients with renal dysfunction (28). The remainder is metabolized by the liver utilizing the cytochrome P450 system, especially CYP2E1 (29). Clearance in children is higher, with mean values 40% higher in children 2 to 12 years old in comparison to adults (30). Pharmacokinetic differences in patients 67 to 78 years of age were minor (31).

FBM exhibits linear first-order pharmacokinetics over a dose range of 1200 to 6000 mg/day in humans (32). Peak plasma concentration is reached 3 hours after an oral dose (24). Monotherapy with FBM 3600 mg/day produced a mean trough plasma level of 78.4 µg/mL (range, 23.7 to 136.6 µg/mL) in one study (6) and a mean (±standard deviation) level of 65(±23) µg/mL after 112 days in another (7).

The terminal elimination half-life of 20 hours (range, 13 to 23 hours) with FBM monotherapy decreases to 13 to 14 hours in the presence of phenytoin or carbamazepine (3). The apparent volume of distribution is 0.8 L/kg (33), and steady-state plasma levels are achieved approximately 4 days following initiation of therapy (34).

EFFICACY

FBM is approved for use in the United States as either adjunctive therapy or monotherapy for patients older than 14 years of age with partial seizures, with or without generalization, and as adjunctive therapy for patients of any age with Lennox–Gastaut syndrome and its component seizure types (33).

Partial-Onset Seizures

The initial clinical studies of FBM employed standard adjunctive trial designs. Adding FBM to carbamazepine (4,5) or to phenytoin (4) produced modest reductions in seizure frequency. In 1988, new monotherapy designs for AED trials were proposed in a workshop sponsored by the NIH (34). Clinical investigators of FBM were the first to use these designs.

In an inpatient, presurgical evaluation trial (35), FBM or placebo was added to the AEDs in use after diagnostic electroencephalogram (EEG)-video monitoring. The primary endpoint was time to occurrence of the fourth seizure or 29 days, whichever came first. Of patients randomized to placebo, 88% had a fourth seizure, compared with 46% taking FBM ($P = 0.03$). In outpatient monotherapy trials (6,7), standard therapy was withdrawn over 28 days, and FBM 3600 mg/day or valproate 15 mg/kg/day was substituted. The valproate dose was a compromise between a placebo control, considered unsafe, and a full-dose active control, which could have reduced the chance of detecting a difference (36). It should be noted that 15 mg/kg/day is the recommended starting dose for valproate. The endpoint, treatment failure, was defined according to predetermined criteria, including a doubling of seizure frequency during any 2 days or 1 month, compared

with pretreatment baseline. Patients taking low-dose valproate met escape criteria more often than FBM-treated patients (86% vs. 14%, respectively, of 42 patients in the single-center study (6); 78% vs. 40%, respectively, of 95 patients in the multicenter study (7)). The "presurgical" design was repeated as a monotherapy trial and further confirmed efficacy (37). Experience with partial-onset seizures in children is limited. Adjunctive open-label use reduced seizure frequency by 53% among 30 children aged 2 to 17 years (38).

Lennox–Gastaut Syndrome

FBM 45 mg/kg/day was used as adjunctive therapy, most often with valproate, in a multicenter, double-blind, controlled trial of 73 patients (39). Atonic seizures (drop attacks) were reduced by 34% and all seizures by 19%, versus a 9% decrease and a 4% increase, respectively, with placebo. No difference in atypical absence frequency could be demonstrated. During a 12-month, open-label follow-up, seizure frequency decreased by 50% in FBM plus standard therapy patients, compared with 15% in the placebo plus standard therapy group (40).

Other Seizure Types

Secondarily generalized tonic–clonic seizures respond to FBM treatment (41). There are reports of efficacy in small, uncontrolled series of patients with infantile spasms (42), primary generalized seizures (4,43), absence seizures (44), atypical absence seizures not part of the Lennox–Gastaut syndrome (45,46). Eight children with myoclonic–astatic seizures responded well to FBM (47).

DRUG INTERACTIONS

Skillful use of FBM requires knowledge of several drug interactions. Clinically significant interactions with phenytoin, carbamazepine, valproate, and phenobarbital have been established (Table 62.1). FBM affects the hepatic cytochrome P450 system by two major mechanisms: induction of CYP3A4 and inhibition of CYP2C19. Most drug interactions are therefore predictable. For example, FBM inhibits phenytoin clearance by inhibiting CYP2C19 (48). FBM is metabolized primarily by CYP2E1 and to a minor extent by CYP3A4 (30). CYP2E1 inhibitors such as chlorzoxazone increase FBM levels, but CYP3A4 inhibitors such as erythromycin have little effect (49). Carbamazepine, phenytoin, and phenobarbital induce CYP3A4 and increase FBM clearance (50).

Effect on Carbamazepine

When FBM is added to carbamazepine (CBZ), levels of CBZ decrease 20% to 30%, but carbamazepine epoxide (CBZ-E) levels increase by 50% to 60% (51). FBM induces CYP3A4-mediated CBZ metabolism, and may also inhibit epoxide hydrolase, which metabolizes CBZ-E. An increase in CBZ-E can cause clinical toxicity, often dizziness, diplopia, or headache.

TABLE 62.1

INTERACTIONS OF FELBAMATE WITH OTHER AEDS

	Effect of felbamate on other AEDs		Effect of other AEDs on felbamate
	AED change in concentration (%)	Recommended dose adjustment (%)	Change in concentration (%)
Phenytoin	↑ (30–50)	↓ (20–33)	↓ (15)
Carbamazepine (total)	↓ (30)	↓ (20–33)	↓ (15)
Carbamazepine (epoxide)	↑ (50–60)	—	—
Valproate	↑ (25–50)	↓ (20–33)	↔ (Variable)
Phenobarbital	↑ (24)	↓ (25)	—

AEDs, antiepileptic drugs.

Effect on Phenytoin

FBM reduces phenytoin (PHT) clearance by a mean of 20% (50). PHT serum levels may increase by 30% to 50%. This effect varies directly with the FBM dose and baseline PHT level because FBM inhibits CYP2C19, a secondary enzyme for the clearance of PHT, which becomes more important at high PHT serum levels. Typical adverse effects of PHT, such as dizziness and ataxia, may occur. This can be confirmed by measurement of serum PHT level and may require reduction in PHT dose.

Effect on Valproate

FBM increases valproate levels by inhibiting its metabolism by beta-oxidation. In 10 patients treated with stable FBM doses, the addition of FBM 600 mg/day increased mean steady-state valproate concentrations from 69.9 to 85.5 mg/L; FBM 1200 mg/day caused an increase to 103.0 mg/L (52).

Effects of Other Agents on Felbamate

Both CBZ and PHT induce the metabolism of FBM, producing levels about 15% lower in the presence of either agent (49). These effects are additive. The addition of valproate may increase the plasma level of FBM slightly (49).

Other Interactions

One patient's warfarin requirement fell by 50% when FBM was added (53). FBM may raise phenobarbital levels by 24% (54). There are no interactions with lamotrigine (55) or oxcarbazepine (56). Interactions with renally excreted drugs such as levetiracetam, gabapentin, pregabalin, and vigabatrin have not been reported and would not be expected.

ADVERSE EFFECTS

Common Adverse Effects

Gastrointestinal disturbances, headache, anorexia, and insomnia are reported frequently (6,7,33).

Headache and anorexia are probably the most troublesome common side effects. The combination of FBM and CBZ may be especially likely to cause headache. Weight loss is most likely over the first year of use, then weight tends to level off in most patients (57). Dizziness, diplopia, and ataxia were common in adjunctive therapy trials (4,5), but may have been related to pharmacokinetic elevations in PHT and CBZ-E levels.

Adverse effects are less common with monotherapy. Among 366 adults receiving monotherapy, 4.1% experienced nausea, 3.6% insomnia, 3% anorexia, 2% to 5% dizziness, and 2% weight loss (41). Administering FBM in three daily doses after meals may reduce stomachache. Giving the largest dose in the morning may help insomnia.

FBM has a stimulant effect in many patients. This is a major advantage in comparison to other AEDs, but it may be associated with insomnia, irritability, and behavioral changes. In one open-label, add-on assessment, behavioral problems were the leading cause of discontinuation (57). At 3% to 4%, the incidence of rash did not differ between FBM and placebo in clinical trials (33). Two children experienced involuntary dyskinetic movements (58).

The overall dropout rate caused by adverse effects in clinical trials was 12% (33). As expected with most drugs, this rate is higher in community practice—21% in one open-label series (57).

Dose-Limiting Effects

Doses in the clinical trials were limited to 3600 mg/day for adults and 45 mg/kg/day for children, with most research patients achieving these targets without dose-limiting toxicities. Higher doses may produce limiting symptoms. Among 50 patients stabilized on FBM 3600 mg or 45 mg/kg/day who received increases to 4200 to 7200 mg/day (mean 5412 mg/day, mean serum concentration 110 mg/L), 32% developed new or increased side effects, but only 15% required dose reductions (59). The most common dose-limiting effects were dizziness, ataxia, and nausea.

Aplastic Anemia

FBM can cause severe or fatal aplastic anemia. In 1994, 33 cases were reported to the Food and Drug Administration

(60,61). Another case was reported in 2000 and a questionable one in 2007 (61). There have been 14 fatalities. However, relatively few patients have been started on FBM since 1994. At present, about 14,000 patients worldwide are receiving FBM (61).

Detailed review of the first 31 cases according to International Agranulocytosis and Aplastic Anemia Study criteria revealed that 23 (74%) met criteria for a diagnosis of aplastic anemia (60). Six others had preexisting blood dyscrasias or systemic lupus erythematosus. Of the 23 confirmed cases, FBM was implicated as the most likely cause in 14; the others had other plausible causes, usually other medications known to cause aplastic anemia.

Based on a 1997 estimate of 110,000 patients exposed, the authors of this review suggested a most probable incidence of 127 per million (1/8000 cases), compared with a population rate of 2 per million per year (60). By comparison, estimates for CBZ range from 5 to 39 per million per year (60). A more conservative estimate is 300 per million (61). All FBM-related aplastic anemia cases were diagnosed within 1 year of starting the drug, two third within 6 months (62). Therefore, the risk drops substantially after 1 year.

Patients developing aplastic anemia were more likely to have histories of blood dyscrasias, especially cytopenia, autoimmune disorders, and rashes or significant toxicities with previous drugs (62). It seems best to avoid FBM use in such patients. Caucasian women were the demographic group most likely to develop aplastic anemia (62). Children may be safer; only one child, a postpubescent 14-year-old reported in 2007, has been affected (61).

Liver Failure

Among patients taking FBM for 25 to 959 days, 18 reported cases of liver failure resulted in 9 fatalities (62). Of these, eight cases could have been caused by other factors—five associated with status epilepticus and one case each of hepatitis A, acetaminophen poisoning, and severe hypotension. Using population exposure estimates (62), this implies a risk of about 1 per 10,000 patient exposures. The authors of a 1997 review concluded that the rate of hepatotoxicity "is within the general range of that seen with valproate and, perhaps, with other AEDs" (63).

Mechanisms of Toxicity

The mechanism by which FBM causes bone marrow and liver toxicity is unknown, but the formation of a toxic metabolite that triggers an immune reaction is suspected. The second step in FBM metabolism is formation of 3-carbamoyl-2-phenylproprionaldehyde (CBMA) (64). CBMA is then metabolized by three competing pathways, one of which leads to the formation of 2-phenylpropenal, also known as atropaldehyde (62). Atropaldehyde is cytotoxic and immunogenic (65), and it may be that individuals who form more of this compound on a genetic basis are more prone to severe idiosyncratic reactions. Since atropaldehyde is detoxified by glutathione, and glutathione stores are depleted by acetaminophen, it seems prudent to advise patients on FBM therapy not to take acetaminophen, although this notion is purely theoretical.

Fluorofelbamate, a potent antiepileptic compound that is not metabolized to atropaldehyde, has been proposed as a safer alternative to FBM (66) and is in early clinical trials. There may be other mechanisms for blood toxicity. Both felbamate and its initial metabolite, 2-phenyl-1,3-propanediol monocarbamate, cause apoptosis of bone marrow progenitor cells in vitro (67).

CLINICAL USE

Patient Selection

Because of the potential for serious blood or liver reactions, FBM should not be used as initial epilepsy therapy or in patients for whom an effective alternative agent can be found. Patients with partial-onset seizures refractory to several previous drugs, especially those who have both severe epilepsy and problems with sedative effects, may be considered for treatment with FBM. A Quality Standards Subcommittee of the American Academy of Neurology and the American Epilepsy Society has formulated practice guidelines for use in specific patient populations (68) (Table 62.2). All patients or their caretakers must be able to report side effects reliably, comply with blood testing, and understand the potential risks and benefits.

Initial Therapy

Both children and adults may be started on FBM 15 mg/kg/day in three divided doses, taken after meals, with increases to 30 mg/kg/day and 45 mg/kg/day at 1- or 2-week intervals (33). FBM is more effective and better tolerated as monotherapy than as an add-on agent, but if a seizure-free state without toxicity is achieved during the polytherapy interim, it is not unreasonable to defer further dose changes.

Maintenance Dosage

The target adult dose is 3600 mg/day; the target pediatric dose is 45 mg/kg/day. Lower doses may be effective, and some patients have tolerated doses as high as 7200 mg (adults) or 100 mg/kg/day (children) (69). Higher relative doses may be necessary for younger children in whom clearance is increased (38). Because FBM is involved in many drug interactions, determination of its serum level in polytherapy may be useful. The average therapeutic range for FBM has been reported to be 50 to 110 mg/L (59,69).

Monitoring for Adverse Effects

Because in patients with aplastic anemia from other causes, symptoms often precede laboratory confirmation (70), the best protection for patients is probably education about early symptoms, especially unusual fatigue, pallor, dyspnea, easy bruising, and bleeding. However, it is not known whether this is also true for FBM-induced cases. Nausea, vomiting, or jaundice may be indicative of hepatic problems.

TABLE 62.2

RECOMMENDATIONS FOR USE OF FELBAMATE

A. Patients for whom risk-to-benefit ratio supports use because there is class I evidence of benefit.
 1. Patients with Lennox–Gastaut syndrome >4 years of age who are unresponsive to primary AEDs.
 2. Intractable partial seizures in patients >18 years of age who have failed standard AEDs at therapeutic levels (monotherapy data indicate a better risk-to-benefit ratio for felbamate used as monotherapy).
 3. Patients taking felbamate >18 months.
B. Patients for whom the current risk-to-benefit assessment does not support the use of felbamate.
 1. New onset epilepsy in adults or children.
 2. Patients who have experienced significant prior hematologic adverse events.
 3. Patients in whom follow-up and compliance will not allow careful monitoring.
 4. Patients unable to discuss risks to benefits (i.e., those with mental retardation, developmental disability) and for whom no parent or legal guardian is available to provide consent.
C. Patients in whom risk-to-benefit ratio is unclear and based on case reports and expert opinion (class III) only, but under certain circumstances, depending on the nature and severity of the patient's seizure disorder, felbamate use may be appropriate.
 1. Children with intractable partial epilepsy.
 2. Patients with other generalized epilepsies unresponsive to primary agents.
 3. Patients who experience unacceptable sedative or cognitive side effects with traditional AEDs.
 4. Patients with Lennox–Gastaut syndrome <4 years of age who are unresponsive to other AEDs.

Adapted from French J, Smith M, Faught E, et al. Practice advisory: the use of felbamate in the treatment of patients with intractable epilepsy. Report of the Quality Standards Subcommittee of the American Academy of Neurology and the American Epilepsy Society. *Neurology*. 1999;52:1540–1546, with permission.

It is important to tell patients that periodic blood testing may not detect adverse events early enough to prevent serious illness or death. Nevertheless, the manufacturer recommends periodic blood counts and liver function tests, but the frequency is not mandated (33). A reasonable schedule is monthly testing for the first 6 months and every 2 months for the next 6 months. Experience has shown that patients comply poorly with more frequent blood tests. The lessening of risk after 1 year of therapy requires less frequent testing, perhaps every 3 months during the second year, then only if symptoms develop thereafter. There is no clinical evidence that higher doses of FBM are more likely to cause aplastic anemia or hepatic failure. Since most serious reactions began 3 to 12 months after initiation of FBM, consideration should be given to withdrawing the drug if no benefit is observed after a few months (62).

Withdrawal from Felbamate

Dramatic increases in seizure frequency and even status epilepticus can occur with rapid withdrawal from FBM (71). Remember that as the dose of FBM is reduced, levels of PHT, phenobarbital, and valproate will also decrease. Surveillance for hematologic and hepatic effects should be continued for 6 months after FBM therapy ends, because damage to bone marrow stem cells may not be manifested immediately in peripheral blood counts.

SUMMARY

FBM is effective for patients with partial-onset seizures, especially as monotherapy, and may work even after failure of several other agents. It is possible that this is because of its unique mechanism of action as a selective antagonist of certain NMDA-type glutamate receptors. Animal studies and experience with Lennox–Gastaut syndrome suggest a broad spectrum of activity against generalized seizures as well. FBM is nonsedating, a very good feature. Nevertheless, it is not easy to use because of the many pharmacokinetic interactions.

Serious toxicities preclude FBM use except in those patients who do not achieve complete seizure control with safer agents. Safety may be improved by avoiding FBM use in patients with autoimmune diseases and previous histories of significant cytopenia or serious drug reactions (62). The combined risk for serious bone marrow or hepatic toxicity with FBM is about 1 in 5000 patients, and for death perhaps 1 in 10,000. These risks are almost certainly less than the risks of continued poor seizure control.

References

1. Swinyard EA, Sofia RD, Kupferberg HJ. Comparative anticonvulsant activity and neurotoxicity of felbamate and four prototype antiepileptic drugs in mice and rats. *Epilepsia*. 1986;27:27–34.
2. Sheridan PH, Ashworth M, Milne K, et al. Open pilot study of felbamate (ADD 03055) in partial seizures. *Epilepsia*. 1986;27:649.
3. Wilensky AJ, Friel PN, Ojemann LM, et al. Pharmacokinetics of W-554 (ADD 03055) in epileptic patients. *Epilepsia*. 1985;26:602–606.
4. Leppik IE, Dreifuss FE, Pledger GW, et al. Felbamate for partial seizures; results of a controlled clinical trial. *Neurology*. 1991;141:1785–1789.
5. Theodore WH, Raubertas RF, Porter RJ, et al. Felbamate: a clinical trial for complex partial seizures. *Epilepsia*. 1991;32:392–397.
6. Sachdeo R, Kramer LD, Rosenberg A, et al. Felbamate monotherapy: controlled trial in patients with partial onset seizures. *Ann Neurol*. 1992;32:386–392.
7. Faught E, Sachdeo R, Remler M, et al. Felbamate monotherapy for partial onset seizures: an active-control trial. *Neurology*. 1993;43:688–692.
8. Nightingale SL. Recommendation to immediately withdraw patients from treatment with felbamate. *JAMA*. 1994;272:995.
9. Kucharczyk N. Felbamate: chemistry and biotransformation. In: Levy RH, Mattson RH, Meldrum BS, eds. *Antiepileptic Drugs*. New York: Raven Press; 1995:795–806.

10. Lian H, Steiner SS, Sofia RD, et al. A self-complementary, self-assembling microsphere system: application for intravenous delivery of the antiepileptic and neuroprotectant compound felbamate. *J Pharm Sci.* 2000;89: 867–875.

11. Ebert U, Reissmuller E, Loscher W. The new antiepileptic drugs lamotrigine and felbamate are effective in phenytoin-resistant kindled rats. *Neuropharmacology.* 2000;39:1893–1903.

12. Luszczki JJ, Andres-Mach MM, Ratnaraj N, et al. Levetiracetam and felbamate interact both pharmacodynamically and pharmacokinetically: an isobolographic analysis in the mouse maximal electroshock model. *Epilepsia.* 2007;48:806–815.

13. Kuo EC, Lin B-J, Chang HR. Use-dependent inhibition of the NMDA currents by felbamate: a gating modifier with selective binding to the desensitized channels. *Mol Pharmacol.* 2004;65:370–380.

14. Kleckner NW, Glazewski JC, Chen CC, et al. Subtype-selective antagonism of *N*-methyl-D-aspartate receptors by felbamate: insights into the mechanism of action. *J Pharmacol Exp Ther.* 1999;289:886–894.

15. Harty TP, Rogawski MA. Felbamate block of recombinant *N*-methyl-D-aspartate receptors: selectivity for the NR2B subunit. *Epilepsy Res.* 2000; 39:47–55.

16. Chang H-R, Kuo C-C. Molecular determinants of the anticonvulsant felbamate binding site in the NMDA receptor. *J Med. Chem.* 2008;51: 1534–1545.

17. White HS, Wolf HH, Swinyard EA, et al. A neuropharmacological evaluation of felbamate as a novel anticonvulsant. *Epilepsia.* 1992;33:564–572.

18. DeSarro G, Ongini E, Bertorelli R, et al. Excitatory amino acid neurotransmission through both NMDA and non-NMDA receptors is involved in the anticonvulsant activity of felbamate in DBA/2 mice. *Eur J Pharmacol.* 1994;262:11–19.

19. Stefani A, Spadoni F, Barnardi E. Voltage-activated calcium channels: targets of antiepileptic drug activity? *Epilepsia.* 1997;38:959–965.

20. Wasterlain CG, Adams LM, Schwartz PH, et al. Posthypoxia treatment with felbamate is neuroprotective in a rat model of hypoxia-ischemia. *Neurology.* 1993;43:2303–2310.

21. Wasterlain CG, Adams LM, Wichmann JK, et al. Felbamate protects CA1 neurons from apoptosis in a gerbil model of global ischemia. *Stroke.* 1996;27:1236–1240.

22. Mazarati AM, Baldwin RA, Sofia RD, et al. Felbamate in experimental model of status epilepticus. *Epilepsia.* 2000;41:123–127.

23. Mazarati AM, Sofia RD, Wasterlain CG. Anticonvulsant and antiepileptogenic effects of fluorofelbamate in experimental status epilepticus. *Seizure.* 2002;11:423–430.

24. Shumaker RC, Fantel C, Kelton E, et al. Evaluation of the elimination of (^{14}C) felbamate in healthy men. *Epilepsia.* 1990;31:642.

25. Gudipati RM, Raymond RH, Ward DL, et al. Effect of food on the absorption of felbamate (Felbatol^{TM}) in healthy male volunteers. *Neurology.* 1992;42:332.

26. Adusumalli VE, Yang JT, Wong KK, et al. Felbamate pharmacokinetics in the rat, rabbit, and dog. *Drug Metab Dispos.* 1991;19:1116–1125.

27. Adusumalli VE, Wichmann JK, Kucharczyk N, et al. Drug concentrations in human brain tissue samples from epileptic patients treated with felbamate. *Drug Metab Dispos.* 1994;22:168–170.

28. Glue P, Sulowicz W, Colucci R, et al. Single-dose pharmacokinetics of felbamate in patients with renal dysfunction. *Br J Clin Pharmacol.* 1997;44: 91–93.

29. Glue P, Banfield CR, Perhach JL, et al. Pharmacokinetic interactions with felbamate. In vitro–in vivo correlation. *Clin Pharmacokinet.* 1997;33: 214–224.

30. Barfield CR, Zhu GR, Jer JF et al. The effect of age on the apparent clearance of felbamate: a retrospective analysis using nonlinear mixed-effects modelling. *Ther Drug Monit.* 1996;18:19–29.

31. Richens A, Banfield CR, Salfi M, et al. Single and multiple dose pharmacokinetics of felbamate in the elderly. *Br J Clin Pharmacol.* 1997;44: 129–134.

32. Sachdeo RC, Narang-Sachdeo SK, Shumaker RC, et al. Tolerability and pharmacokinetics of monotherapy felbamate doses of 1200–6000 mg/day in subjects with epilepsy. *Epilepsia.* 1997;38:887–892.

33. Felbatol package insert; September 2003, MedPointe Healthcare Inc., Somerset, NJ, USA.

34. Pledger GW, Kramer LD. Clinical trials of investigational antiepileptic drugs: monotherapy designs. *Epilepsia.* 1991;32:716–721.

35. Bourgeois BFD, Leppik IE, Sackellares JC, et al. Felbamate double-blind efficacy trial following presurgical monitoring. *Epilepsia.* 1991;32: 481–486.

36. Leber P. Hazards of inference: the active control investigation. *Epilepsia.* 1989;30:S57–S63.

37. Devinsky O, Faught RE, Wilder BJ, et al. Efficacy of felbamate monotherapy in patients undergoing presurgical evaluation of partial seizures. *Epilepsy Res.* 1995;20:241–246.

38. Carmant L, Holmes GL, Sawyer S, et al. Efficacy of felbamate in therapy for partial epilepsy in children. *J Pediatr.* 1994;125:481–486.

39. The Felbamate Study Group in Lennox-Gastaut Syndrome. Efficacy of felbamate in childhood epileptic encephalopathy (Lennox–Gastaut syndrome). *N Engl J Med.* 1993;328:29–33.

40. Dodson WE. Felbamate in the treatment of Lennox–Gastaut syndrome: results of a 12-month open-label study following a randomized clinical trial. *Epilepsia.* 1993;34:S18–S24.

41. Sachdeo RC, Wagner ML. Felbamate in generalized tonic–clonic seizures. *Epilepsia.* 1991;32(suppl 3):54.

42. Hurst DL, Rolan TD. The use of felbamate to treat infantile spasms. *J Child Neurol.* 1995;10:134–136.

43. Leroy RF, Castain T. Pilot study of felbamate in adult medically refractory primary generalized seizure patients. *Epilepsia.* 1991;32:13.

44. Devinsky O, Kothari M, Rubin R, et al. Felbamate for absence seizures. *Epilepsia.* 1992;33:84.

45. Kuzniecky R, Thompson G, Faught E, et al. Felbamate add-on therapy in intractable atypical absence. *Epilepsia.* 1991;32:10.

46. Sachdeo RC, Murphy JV, Kamin M. Felbamate in juvenile myoclonic epilepsy. *Epilepsia.* 1992;33(suppl 3):118.

47. Grosso S, Condelli DM, Coppola G, et al. Efficacy and safety of felbamate in children under 4 years of age: a retrospective chart review. *Eur J Neurol.* 2008;15:940–946.

48. Graves NM, Holmes GB, Fuerst RH, et al. Effect of felbamate on phenytoin and carbamazepine serum concentrations. *Epilepsia.* 1989;30: 225–229.

49. Sachdeo RC, Narang-Sachdeo SK, Montgomery PA, et al. Evaluation of the potential interaction between felbamate and erythromycin in patients with epilepsy. *Clin Pharmacol Ther.* 1998;38:184–190.

50. Wagner ML, Leppik IE, Graves NM, et al. Felbamate serum concentrations: effect of valproate, carbamazepine, phenytoin, and phenobarbital. *Epilepsia.* 1990;31:642.

51. Albani F, Theodore WH, Washington P, et al. Effect of felbamate on plasma levels of carbamazepine and its metabolites. *Epilepsia.* 1991;32: 130–132.

52. Wagner ML, Graves NM, Leppik IE, et al. The effect of felbamate on valproic acid disposition. *Clin Pharmacol Ther.* 1994;56:494–502.

53. Tisdel KA, Israel DS, Kolb KW. Warfarin-felbamate interaction: first report [letter]. *Ann Pharmacother.* 1994;28:805.

54. Reidenberg P, Glue P, Banfield CR, et al. Effects of felbamate on the pharmacokinetics of phenobarbital. *Clin Pharmacol Ther.* 1995;58: 279–287.

55. Gidal BE, Kanner A, Maly M, et al. Lamotrigine pharmacokinetics in patients receiving felbamate. *Epilepsy. Res.* 1997;27:1–5.

56. Hulsman JA, Rentmeester TW, Banfield CR, et al. Effects of felbamate on the pharmacokinetics of the monohydroxy and dihydroxy metabolites of oxcarbazepine. *Clin Pharmacol Ther.* 1995;58:383–389.

57. Li LM, Nashef L, Moriarty J, et al. Felbamate as add-on therapy. *Eur Neurol.* 1996;36:146–148.

58. Kerrick JM, Kelley BJ, Maister BH, et al. Involuntary movement disorders associated with felbamate. *Neurology.* 1995;45:185–187.

59. Faught E, Kuzniecky R, Thompson G. Tolerability of high-dose felbamate. *Epilepsia.* 1994;35:32.

60. Kaufman DW, Kelly JP, Anderson T, et al. Evaluation of case reports of aplastic anemia among patients treated with felbamate. *Epilepsia.* 1997; 38:1265–1269.

61. Gever L. Personal communication, *Meda Pharmaceuticals.* 26 January 2009.

62. Pellock JM. Felbamate in epilepsy therapy: evaluating the risks. *Drug Saf.* 1999;21:225–239.

63. Pellock JM, Brodie MJ. Felbamate: 1997 update. *Epilepsia.* 1997;38: 1261–1264.

64. Thompson CD, Barthen MT, Hopper DW, et al. Quantification in patient urine samples of felbamate and three metabolites: acid carbamate and two mercapturic acids. *Epilepsia.* 1999;40:769–776.

65. Popovic M, Nierkens S, Pieters R, et al. Investigating the role of 2-phenylpropenal in felbamate-induced idiosynncratic drug reactions. *Chem Res Toxicol.* 2004;17:1568–1576.

66. Roecklein BA, Sacks HJ, Mortko H, et al. Fluorofelbamate. *Neurotherapeutics.* 2007;4:97–101.

67. Husain Z, Pinto C, Sofia RD, et al. Felbamate-induced apoptosis of hematopoietic cells is mediated by redox-sensitive and redox-independent pathways. *Epilepsy Res.* 2002;48:57–69.

68. French J, Smith M, Faught E, et al. Practice advisory: the use of felbamate in the treatment of patients with intractable epilepsy. Report of the Quality Standards Subcommittee of the American Academy of Neurology and the American Epilepsy Society. *Neurology.* 1999;52:1540–1546.

69. Leppik IE. Felbamate. *Epilepsia.* 1995;36:S66–S72.

70. Kelly JP, Jurgelon JM, Issargrisil S, et al. An epidemiological study of aplastic anemia: relationship of drug exposures to clinical features and outcome. *Eur J Hematol.* 1996;37:47–52.

71. Welty TE, Privitera M, Shukla R. Increased seizure frequency associated with felbamate withdrawal in adults. *Arch Neurol.* 1998;55:641–645.

CHAPTER 63 ■ VIGABATRIN

ELIZABETH A. THIELE

HISTORICAL BACKGROUND

Vigabatrin (VGB) was initially synthesized in 1977 by Jung and colleagues (1), designed as a specific inhibitor of gamma-aminobutyric acid (GABA)-transaminase (GABA-T), the enzyme responsible for metabolizing GABA at the synapse. It was hypothesized that inhibiting GABA-T would then increase whole brain levels of GABA, making it more available to its receptor site, thus increasing GABAergic inhibition. For decades prior to this, the role of GABA in seizure activity had been proposed by the apparent proconvulsant properties of compounds either inhibiting GABA synthesis or blocking its postsynaptic action, by the ability of drugs enhancing GABA-mediated inhibition to act as anticonvulsants in many animal models, and by the identification of abnormalities in the GABA receptor in certain genetically determined epilepsy animal models. Although several compounds have been developed over the last 30 years that function to modulate GABA-A-mediated inhibition via various mechanisms, VGB is the only drug that does so by specifically inhibiting GABA-T.

VGB was initially approved and marketed in the United Kingdom in 1989, and currently is available in over 50 countries worldwide, including most countries of the European Union, Canada, and Mexico. Although the initial NDA for VGB in the United States was submitted in 1994 for adult patients with complex partial seizures (CPS), the medication was only approved for use in 2009. Since initial approval in 1989, over 1.5 million have been treated with VGB. Multiple clinical studies conducted around the world, including the United States have established the efficacy of VGB in the treatment of refractory complex partial seizures and infantile spasms (IS).

GENERAL CHARACTERISTICS

VGB (4-amino-5-hexenoic acid or gamma-vinyl-GABA) is a structural analogue of GABA that contains a vinyl appendage (Fig. 63.1). It was designed to specifically and irreversibly inhibit GABA-T, and is the only currently available drug with this mechanism of action. It may also stimulate GABA release (2). VGB is highly water soluble, only slightly soluble in ethanol and methanol, and insoluble in hexane and toluene. VGB is a white to off-white crystalline solid, with a molecular mass of 129.16 and a melting point of 171°C to 117°C. It exists as a racemic mixture of R(−) and S(+) isomers, which occur in equal proportions, and has no optical activity. The pharmacologic activity is thought to be associated only with the S(+) enantiomer, and the R(−) enantiomer is thought to be entirely inactive (3,4). The major pharmacologic effects are determined by effects of VGB on GABA-T half-life and activity rather than the drug itself.

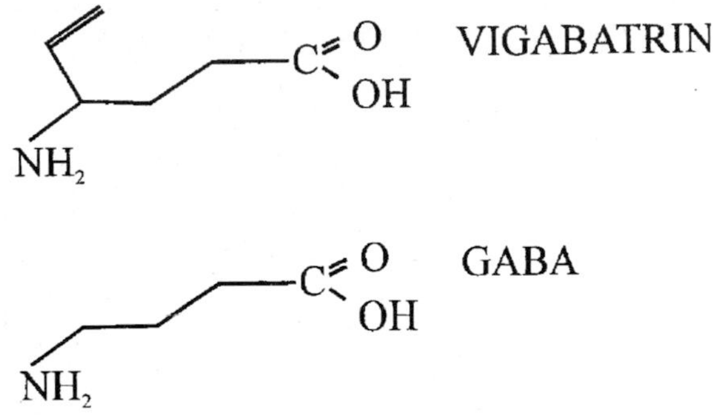

FIGURE 63.1 Chemical structure of vigabatrin.

PHARMACOKINETICS

Administration

Current formulations of VGB include 500-mg tablets, and 500-mg powder packets or sachets. Following oral administration, VGB is almost completely absorbed, with peak VGB concentrations reached within 2 hours of administration of doses ranging from 0.5 to 3 g (3,5,6). VGB can be given at or between meals, as presence or type of food does not have a significant effect on absorption and therefore should not influence clinical response.

Distribution

VGB is widely distributed throughout the body with a volume of distribution at steady state of 1.1 L/kg (7) and a half-life of distribution of 1 to 2 hours. Concentrations of VGB in the CSF are approximately 10% of blood levels (8). VGB has pharmacokinetics that is dose proportional and linear following single and repeated dosing (9,10). VGB does not bind to plasma proteins, and does not cause hepatic induction of hepatic cytochrome P450-dependent enzymes (5,11). Passage of VGB across the human placenta occurs at a low level, comparable to other alpha-amino acids; the maximum amount of VGB that a nursing infant would be exposed to each day is approximately 3.6% of the R(−) and 1% of the S(+) enantiomer of the maternal VGB dose (12).

VGB has been shown to have minimal drug–drug interactions with other AEDs, ethanol, and oral contraceptive agents (13,14). VGB plasma levels are not affected by CBZ, clorazepate, primidone or valproic acid. A modest reduction of about 20% in phenytoin plasma levels has been reported.

Metabolism

VGB is not metabolized, and is eliminated primarily as the parent drug by renal excretion. The half-life of VGB is approximately 5 to 8 hours, although it is thought that plasma levels do not correlate with clinical effect (7). Children have a lower AUC than adults following VGB dosing, although renal clearance is similar. Therefore, children may require higher doses of VGB to achieve the same clinical effect as seen in adults.

SPECIAL POPULATIONS

Age

The renal clearance of VGB in healthy elderly patients (>65 years of age) was 36% less than that observed in healthy younger patients (10). The VGB half-life in elderly patients with reduced creatinine clearance is approximately twice that of normal healthy volunteers.

Gender

No gender-specific differences for the pharmacokinetics parameters of VGB have been observed.

Race

Limited data are available regarding race-specific variability in pharmacokinetics of VGB. A single report compared the pharmacokinetic parameters of Caucasian and Japanese patients; all parameters were similar except for mean renal clearance of VGB, which was slightly higher among the Caucasians.

Renal Impairment

As VGB is renally excreted, its pharmacokinetics is affected in the setting of renal impairment. Mean AUC values were found to increase 32% and 253% and $t_{1/2}$ increase 4.0 hours and 15.3 hours, respectively, in patients with mild to moderate (creatinine clearance of 40 to 79 mL/min) and severe (creatinine clearance of 10 to 39 mL/min) renal impairment (5).

EFFICACY

Now in clinical use for over 20 years, the efficacy of VGB in the treatment of partial onset seizures and IS is well recognized.

Complex Partial Seizures

Numerous single-blind and double-blind studies have shown that VGB is effective in the treatment of intractable partial-onset seizures. A meta-analysis of the first 10 single-blind studies of VGB, which included a total of 352 patients, showed a 55.8% responder rate (patients with a >50% seizure reduction) (8,15–19).

Several European-conducted, double-blind, placebo-controlled, crossover studies also found VGB to be effective in the treatment of refractory partial-onset seizures. With doses ranging from 2 to 3 g/day as add-on treatment, the studies reported responder rates between 33% and 64%, with between 0% and 7% of patients becoming seizure-free. In addition, two U.S. studies showed VGB to be effective as adjunctive treatment for intractable or refractory CPS. Both U.S. studies were placebo controlled and enrolled patients between 18 and 60 years of age; over 50% of patients in both studies were on two or more concomitant anticonvulsant medications at time of enrollment and had on average an over 20-year history of epilepsy, the majority having been treated with over three anticonvulsant medications. The first U.S. study, which included 182 patients, showed a 43% responder rate (compared to 19% placebo responder rate), including 5.4% of VGB-treated patients who became seizure-free (20). The second U.S. study, which enrolled 174 patients, evaluated doses of 1, 3, or 6 g/day of VGB, with significant reductions in seizure frequency seen in the two higher doses with a 51% responder rate in the VGB 3 g/day group and 54% responder rate in the VGB 6 g/day group (21). During the last 8 weeks of the study, 9.3% and 12.2% of patients in the 3 g/day and 6 g/day groups respectively were seizure-free, compared with no patients in the placebo-controlled or the VGB 1 g/day groups. Efficacy was also seen relatively early in the study, with a significant reduction in seizures seen after 14 days of treatment.

Open-label trials of VGB in children with mixed seizure types have shown similar efficacy of VGB in CPS as the adult studies (22,23), myoclonic seizures appeared to be exacerbated.

Infantile Spasms

The efficacy of VGB in the treatment of IS has been appreciated for almost 20 years. The initial report of an uncontrolled study of VGB in 70 patients with IS in 1991 showed a 68% responder rate in infants with refractory IS with 71% of those with IS due to tuberous sclerosis complex (TSC) becoming seizure-free (24). The effectiveness of VGB as a monotherapy treatment for IS was established in three controlled studies, including one conducted in the United States and two outside the United States, one of which was restricted to the treatment of IS due to TSC (25–27). In all three studies, cessation of IS was observed, with onset of efficacy between 2 and 4 weeks. The U.S. study, which was the largest study with 221 infants completing the study, found VGB effective across etiologies of IS, and found that doses of >100 mg/kg/day were more effective than lower doses (25). In addition, several uncontrolled studies have examined the efficacy of VGB in IS, finding between 38% and 76% of infants having cessation of spasms (28–31). The UK Infantile Spasm Study (UKISS) compared the efficacy of VGB to prednisolone and ACTH in IS due to etiologies other than TSC; at 2 weeks of treatment 54% of those on VGB had experienced cessation of spasms compared to 73% receiving hormonal treatment (30). On follow-up analysis at 12 to 14 months, 75% of those treated with VGB continued to be spasm free compared to 76% receiving hormonal treatment (31). An American Academy of Neurology practice parameter published in 2004 found that VGB was possibly effective in the treatment of IS (32). A meta-analysis of 11 randomized controlled trials in IS found VGB to be as effective as other treatments, namely ACTH and steroids, in the treatment of IS (33).

SAFETY

Adverse Events

Overall, VGB is well tolerated, but can be associated with adverse events (AEs). The most frequently noted AEs in clinical trials for complex partial seizures and in clinical use included fatigue and somnolence; dizziness, nystagmus, tremor, headache, weight increase, blurred vision, diarrhea, and irritability can also be seen. Serious AEs were also noted in the controlled trials, and included visual field defects (VFDs) (discussed below), status epilepticus, and psychiatric complaints including most commonly depression, but also confusion, aggression, insomnia, irritability, suicidal ideation, and suicide attempt. In clinical trials for IS, most common AEs included upper respiratory tract infection, otitis media, pyrexia, viral infection, irritability, somnolence, sedation, vomiting, constipation, pneumonia, diarrhea, insomnia, and rash. Serious adverse events also were seen in the IS studies, most commonly status epilepticus and pneumonia.

Chronic Toxicity

Intramyelinic Edema

Studies in animals revealed that treatment with VGB could be associated with intramyelinic edema (IME), or edema occurring within the myelin sheath (34,35). This finding, observed in rats and dogs but not monkeys, is characterized histopathologically by microvacuolation of specific regions of the brain, predominantly within the white matter.

IME was found to develop within several weeks of VGB treatment, stabilize without further progression, and resolve within 12 to 16 weeks after drug discontinuation. No residual histopathology was observed following drug discontinuation in dogs; however, rats retained swollen axons as well as foci of microscopic mineralization in the cerebellum. Further characterization of VGB-related IME identified both evoked potentials as well as MRI as sensitive noninvasive techniques to diagnose IME in rats and dogs. These studies also were used to support the absence of IME in monkeys and humans. Monkeys were treated with VGB at doses up to 300 mg/kg/day, which provided maximal plasma concentrations of 38 μg/mL, for up to 6 years to characterize possible toxicities; evaluation after 16 months of treatment did not yield conclusive evidence of IME. This dosing and plasma levels were consistent with that of infants and young children at a dosing of 50 mg/kg/day (36).

Additional studies to further characterize VGB-related IME in rodents included a juvenile toxicity study to evaluate the effects of VGB treatment on the physical and behavioral development of rats compared to controls (37). Microscopic evaluation of animals revealed mild vacuolar changes within the neuropil in select brain regions following VGB treatment at 50 mg/kg/day. Most affected brain regions included gray matter in the midbrain tegmentum, substantia nigra, dorsal subiculum, deep cerebellar nuclei, posterior thalamus, basal forebrain, and medulla oblongata. Additional although significantly less abundant vacuoles were also seen in some white matter tracks, including the medial longitudinal fasciculus and the medial forebrain bundle. Although it was not possible to determine which cell type was vacuolated, it was felt that the neuronal cell bodies, blood vessel endothelium, and perivascular astrocytic end processes were not affected. The authors felt that although the morphologic appearance was consistent with IME seen in older rodents, the distribution of involvement was different in the younger animals as it was found predominantly in subcortical gray matter. The behavior and development of these animals were evaluated by a variety of observational and standardized testing; there was no evidence of significant adverse developmental effects of these pathologic findings. Reproductive and ocular development were also assessed and not found to be significantly affected by the pathologic changes, however, the VGB-treated animals receiving higher doses of VGB (15 and 50 mg/kg/day) were found to have significant reductions in food intake and growth.

Subsequently, ultrastructural characterizations of these changes were performed using electron microscopy that showed an evolution of vacuoles, which were found to begin as splits of myelin sheaths along the intraperiod line (38). These initial splits in the myelin sheaths then expanded and evolved into large, fluid-filled, membrane-rich vacuoles. Lesions in the cerebellum were found to appear prior to those in the reticular formation and more rostral brain regions. The distribution of changes appeared to vary with age, species, and possibly timing and duration of treatment although the process appeared limited to myelinated nerve fibers or axons. Changes in adult rats were characterized by vacuoles in large white matter regions of the brain; neonatal and juvenile rats instead had lesions in white matter fibers traversing in or near the gray matter.

Following these observations, significant efforts were made to see if VGB treatment-related IME occurred in humans. Studies involved review of data obtained during several VGB clinical trials over a 15-year period of time, including review of effects of VGB treatment on brain MRI and evoked potentials. In addition, surgical brain and autopsy samples of VGB-treated patients were evaluated histopathologically for evidence of IME. In an estimated 350,000 patients' years of VGB exposure (correlating to approximately 175,000 patients treated for 2 years at an average daily dose of 2 g), no definite evidence of VGB-related IME was identified (39).

However, Pearl et al. (40) reported the initial observation of MRI T2 signal abnormalities involving the deep gray nuclei in 3/15 young children treated with VGB. Subsequent reports describe similar findings occurring in 20% to 30% of infants treated with VGB for IS (41–43). The characteristic MRI T2 signal changes seen involve the basal ganglia, thalamus, dentate nucleus, brainstem, and cerebellum. On diffusion weighted imaging (DWI), apparent diffusion coefficient (ADC) maps also suggested restricted diffusion in these regions. These changes appeared to be resolved following drug discontinuation, dosage reduction, and also with continuation of drug. Risk factors for developing these MRI signal changes during VGB therapy are thought to include age (since observed during treatment for IS, but not seen in older children or adults), and VGB dose (since changes more frequently seen in infants on VGB doses of 150 mg/kg/day and higher). There have been no reports of definite clinical sequelae of these signal changes, although this has not been carefully studied. It is unclear how these signal changes relate histopathologically to VGB-related IME well characterized in animal models, but they are thought to likely represent similar mechanisms.

Visual Field Defects

VGB treatment is associated with possible development of a VFD, typically characterized by a bilateral, concentric constriction of the peripheral visual fields. First reported in 1997 (44), this VGB-related VFD has now been well characterized by numerous studies providing understanding regarding the pathophysiology of the VFD as well as incidence, prevalence, and functional impact of the VFD as well as most effective methods to diagnose and monitor the VFD (45–48). The VGB-related VFD has been described as typically a slowly progressive bilateral concentric peripheral constriction of visual fields, which many studies have found to be more marked nasally than temporally. Central vision and color vision are spared.

Pathophysiology. The retina has been identified as the site of injury in VGB-related VFD via nonclinical studies as well as electroretinography (ERG) studies in humans (49). Visual evoked potentials and brain imaging have demonstrated that the optic nerve and central visual pathways are not involved. ERG studies in humans have suggested that the postreceptor cone responses of the inner retina are most affected by VGB treatment, which has been supported by ophthalmoscopic identification of nerve fiber atrophy in some VGB-treated patients and abnormal nerve fiber layer thickness measurements by optical coherence tomography (OCT) (50,51). However, a single postmortem examination of human retina following VGB treatment showed cell loss in all retinal layers (52).

The pathophysiologic mechanisms of these changes and the related VFD are unknown, although several hypotheses have been proposed. One hypothesis suggested that since VGB is more effectively transported into retina than brain that the resulting levels of GABA could contribute to the retinal toxicity (53). Subsequent studies have suggested a possible role for aberrant protein kinase C-alpha activity (PKC-alpha) after identifying VGB dose-related changes in translocation of the enzyme in rod bipolar cells as well as a significant decrease in the number of PKC-alpha labeled rod bipolar cells in VGB-treated animals (54). Most recently, the effects of VGB on taurine levels were investigated given the VFD similarities between VGB treatment and those characterized with taurine deficiency (55). The authors found significant reductions in taurine levels in VGB-treated animals compared to controls as well as in VGB-treated infants. Taurine supplementation led to diminished retinal toxicity in both rats and mice.

Clinical Features. The actual prevalence and incidence of VGB-related VFD are difficult to determine due to limited data sets and study design, however they are thought to be influenced by age of the patient and extent of exposure to VGB (including dose and duration of treatment or cumulative VGB exposure). There is a likely 25% to 50% prevalence of VFD in adults, a 15% prevalence in children, and a range of 15% to 31% prevalence in infants (56). It is believed that the VGB-related VFD most likely occurs with more prolonged drug treatment, although there are limited prospective data. The earliest identification of a VFD in adults is after 9 months of treatment, with a mean time to onset of 4.8 years. The earliest identification of a VFD is after 11 months of treatment, with a mean time of onset of 5.5 years. In infants, the earliest onset of a presumed VGB-related retinal abnormal detected by ERG is 3.1 months. There are rare case reports of VGB-related VFD occurring in adults with less than 6 months of

treatment. The literature also has varying estimates of the severity of the VGB associated VFD, although most agree that it is usually mild and asymptomatic. However, severe visual peripheral field constrictions (defined as <30 degrees of retained temporal field or <60 degrees of binocular field) can occur ("tunnel vision"), and occur in 2% to 40% of patients. Although it is possible that the VFD can progress, it typically remains stable, and may improve although not normalize following drug discontinuation. Progression of the VFD following drug discontinuation cannot be ruled out, but available evidence suggests that it is unlikely for this to occur.

Clinical Assessment. Standard methods for assessing visual fields in adults and older children include Goldmann kinetic perimetry and Humphrey's static automated perimetry. Both are sensitive and specific enough to establish baseline visual field function and to monitor for possible treatment-related effects on peripheral function. Kinetic perimetry is less reliable in children less than 9 years of age and in the neurologically impaired population.

ERG is an electrophysiologic measurement of retinal function that can also be used to assess for possible VFD, especially in infants, young children, and others not able to cooperate with visual perimetry testing. Although typically widely available, testing often requires sedation or anesthesia in infants, young children, and impaired individuals, which dramatically limits access. The 30-Hz flicker response component of the ERG is thought to be the most predictive of the presence and degree of severity of VGB-induced VFD (57,58). Other measures, namely b-cone amplitude, are also thought to be measures of VGB toxicity. However, the exact relationship between these ERG findings in infants and subsequent visual field abnormalities has not firmly been established.

OCT is a recently developed technology that shows great promise for monitoring for possible VGB-induced VFD although further studies are needed to better characterize its sensitivity and specificity.

Teratogenicity

Pregnancy

Limited data are available on the teratogenic effects of VGB therapy in animals, except for a possible increased incidence of cleft palate in rabbits receiving a high dose, and possible mandibular and maxillary hypoplasia, arched palate, cleft palate, limb defects, and exophthalmia in the TO mouse after receiving high doses (300 to 450 mg/kg) (59). Similar to other AEDs, VGB has a class warning against use in pregnancy due to inadequate evidence of possible human teratogenic effects.

CLINICAL USE

Administration

The daily adult dose of VGB used in most clinical trials and reports is between 2 and 3 g/day, with 3 g accepted as an optimal adult dose. Higher doses can improve efficacy, such as the U.S. double-blind study that employed 6 g/day, however higher doses have also been shown to be associated with increased side effects (21). If clinical response is not achieved at a dose of 3 g/day, consideration should be given to discontinuation of the medication, particularly given the risk of VGB-related VFD. In infants and children, dosing of VGB is similar to other medications, and calculated on a mg/kg/day basis. VGB is frequently titrated up to 100 to 150 mg/day in b.i.d. dosing as needed for seizure control. Although higher doses may be effective in some infants being treated for IS, caution should be used given the probable increased risk both of VGB-related VFD as well as VGB-related MRI T2 signal changes.

Titration

In order to minimize side effects, particularly psychiatric or behavioral difficulties, gradual titration of the medication is suggested for both adults and infants and children.

Discontinuation

Efficacy of VGB is usually seen within the first 3 months of treatment. Should the medication not prove effective or tolerated, it should be discontinued. VGB should be tapered slowly to minimize possibility of rebound seizures including status epilepticus, and of significant behavioral abnormalities. Discontinuing VGB over a period of 1 to 2 months is usually well tolerated.

The optimal duration of VGB treatment if effective is not clear, particularly given the possibility that VGB-related VFD increases with cumulative VGB exposure. Typically, infants being treated for IS have continued on the medication for 1 year; currently, the long-term efficacy of shorter duration treatment is being evaluated.

Laboratory Monitoring

Although assays to measure VGB levels in blood and CSF are available, they are not felt to be clinically useful as blood level has not been shown to correlate with clinical effectiveness. Routine blood monitoring of blood counts and hepatic enzyme levels are not recommended as VGB has not been shown to have a significant effect on these values. Due to limited drug–drug interactions with other AEDs, routine AED levels are also not recommended unless clinically indicated.

Clinical Monitoring

Due to the risk of VGB-related VFD, clinical monitoring of visual function is important. In adults, visual field perimetry should ideally be obtained at baseline, and subsequently at regular intervals throughout the duration of treatment. Should abnormalities appear, consideration should be given to discontinue VGB treatment based on a risk–benefit assessment with the patient. In infants, young children, and those who are neurologically impaired and not able to cooperate with perimetry, visual fields should be assessed at baseline by confrontational testing. Repeat confrontational testing should be performed at 3-month intervals for the duration of treatment. Ideally infants should also be followed by experienced pediatric ophthalmologists and by ERG, although access to these services is not always readily available and should not delay treatment.

Should abnormalities appear, consideration of discontinuation of VGB should also be considered, with careful risk–benefit assessment of continued treatment, especially in the context of VGB treatment for IS. FDA approval in the U.S. mandates ophthalmologic evaluation at 3-month intervals throughout the duration of VGB treatment in infants and adults due to the risks of retinal toxicity.

CONCLUSION

VGB has been shown to be an effective AED in a wide variety of seizure types affecting both adults and children, particularly refractory complex partial seizures and IS. It has a unique mechanism of action from other available AEDs, and is generally well tolerated. However, VGB-related VFD is a possible and possibly significant side effect of the medication. Therefore, patients started on VGB should be closely monitored for visual field changes. VGB appears to be particularly effective in the treatment of IS, a catastrophic pediatric epilepsy syndrome with limited effective treatments available. In this setting, the use of VGB should be strongly considered, as the risks of the impact of uncontrolled IS on subsequent neurocognitive development may outweigh the risks of possible VGB-related VFD. The MRI T2 signal changes seen in infants treated with VGB are another possible risk of the medication. However, no significant clinical changes have been seen with these changes, and further studies are needed to understand any possible significance that could affect continuation of VGB treatment.

References

1. Jung MJ, Lippert B, Metcalf BW, et al. Gamma-Vinyl GABA (4-amino-hex-5-enoic acid), a new selective irreversible inhibitor of GABA-T: effects on brain GABA metabolism in mice. *J Neurochem.* 1977;29(5):797–802.
2. Schechter PJ. Vigabatrin. In: Meldrum B, Porter, RJ, eds. *New Anticonvulsant Drugs.* London: John Libbey; 1986:265–275.
3. Haegele KD, Schechter PJ. Kinetics of the enantiomers of vigabatrin after an oral dose of the racemate or the active S-enantiomer. *Clin Pharmacol Ther.* 1986;40(5):581–586.
4. Rey E, Pons G, Richard MO, et al. Pharmacokinetics of the individual enantiomers of vigabatrin (gamma-vinyl GABA) in epileptic children. *Br J Clin Pharmacol.* 1990;30(2):253–257.
5. Haegele KD, Huebert ND, Ebel M, et al. Pharmacokinetics of vigabatrin: implications of creatinine clearance. *Clin Pharmacol Ther.* 1988;44(5):558–565.
6. Saletu B, Grunberger J, Linzmayer L, et al. Psychophysiological and psychometric studies after manipulating the GABA system by vigabatrin, a GABA-transaminase inhibitor. *Int J Psychophysiol.* 1986;4(1):63–80.
7. Rey E, Pons G, Olive G. Vigabatrin. Clinical pharmacokinetics. *Clin Pharmacokinet.* 1992;23(4):267–278.
8. Ben-Menachem E. Pharmacokinetic effects of vigabatrin on cerebrospinal fluid amino acids in humans. *Epilepsia.* 1989;30(suppl 3):S12–S14.
9. Durham SL, Hoke JF, Chen TM. Pharmacokinetics and metabolism of vigabatrin following a single oral dose of [14C]vigabatrin in healthy male volunteers. *Drug Metab Dispos.* 1993;21(3):480–484.
10. Hoke JF, Yuh L, Antony KK, et al. Pharmacokinetics of vigabatrin following single and multiple oral doses in normal volunteers. *J Clin Pharmacol.* 1993;33(5):458–462.
11. Mumford JP. A profile of vigabatrin. *Br J Clin Pract Suppl.* 1988;61:7–9.
12. Tran A, O'Mahoney T, Rey E, et al. Vigabatrin: placental transfer in vivo and excretion into breast milk of the enantiomers. *Br J Clin Pharmacol.* 1998;45(4):409–411.
13. Hachad H, Ragueneau-Majlessi I, Levy RH. New antiepileptic drugs: review on drug interactions. *Ther Drug Monit.* 2002;24(1):91–103.
14. Crawford P. Interactions between antiepileptic drugs and hormonal contraception. *CNS Drugs.* 2002;16(4):263–272.
15. Schechter PJ, Hanke NF, Grove J, et al. Biochemical and clinical effects of gamma-vinyl GABA in patients with epilepsy. *Neurology.* 1984;34(2):182–186.

16. Browne TR, Mattson RH, Penry JK, et al. Vigabatrin for refractory complex partial seizures: multicenter single-blind study with long-term follow-up. *Neurology.* 1987;37(2):184–189.

17. Cocito L, Maffini M, Perfumo P, et al. Vigabatrin in complex partial seizures: a long-term study. *Epilepsy Res.* 1989;3(2):160–166.

18. Mumford JP, Dam M. Meta-analysis of European placebo controlled studies of vigabatrin in drug resistant epilepsy. *Br J Clin Pharmacol.* 1989; 27(suppl 1):101S–107S.

19. Michelucci R, Tassinari CA. Response to vigabatrin in relation to seizure type. *Br J Clin Pharmacol.* 1989;27(suppl 1):119S–124S.

20. French JA, Mosier M, Walker S, et al. A double-blind, placebo-controlled study of vigabatrin three g/day in patients with uncontrolled complex partial seizures. Vigabatrin Protocol 024 Investigative Cohort. *Neurology.* 1996;46(1):54–61.

21. Dean C, Mosier M, Penry K. Dose–response study of Vigabatrin as add-on therapy in patients with uncontrolled complex partial seizures. *Epilepsia.* 1999;40(1):74–82.

22. Livingston JH, Beaumont D, Arzimanoglou A, et al. Vigabatrin in the treatment of epilepsy in children. *Br J Clin Pharmacol.* 1989;27(suppl 1): 109S–112S.

23. Luna D, Dulac O, Pajot N, et al. Vigabatrin in the treatment of childhood epilepsies: a single-blind placebo-controlled study. *Epilepsia.* 1989;30(4): 430–437.

24. Chiron C, Dulac O, Beaumont D, et al. Therapeutic trial of vigabatrin in refractory infantile spasms. *J Child Neurol.* 1991;(suppl 2):S52–S59.

25. Elterman RD, Shields WD, Mansfield KA, et al. Randomized trial of vigabatrin in patients with infantile spasms. *Neurology.* 2001;57(8): 1416–1421.

26. Chiron C, Dumas C, Jambaque I, et al. Randomized trial comparing vigabatrin and hydrocortisone in infantile spasms due to tuberous sclerosis. *Epilepsy Res.* 1997;26(2):389–395.

27. Vigevano F, Cilio MR. Vigabatrin versus ACTH as first-line treatment for infantile spasms: a randomized, prospective study. *Epilepsia.* 1997;38(12): 1270–1274.

28. Siemes H, Brandl U, Spohr HL, et al. Long-term follow-up study of vigabatrin in pretreated children with West syndrome. *Seizure.* 1998;7(4): 293–297.

29. Villeneuve N, Soufflet C, Plouin P, et al. Treatment of infantile spasms with vigabatrin as first-line therapy and in monotherapy: apropos of 70 infants. *Arch Pediatr.* 1998;5(7):731–738.

30. Lux AL, Edwards SW, Hancock E, et al. The United Kingdom Infantile Spasms Study comparing vigabatrin with prednisolone or tetracosactide at 14 days: a multicentre, randomised controlled trial. *Lancet.* 2004;364(9447): 1773–1778.

31. Lux AL, Edwards SW, Hancock E, et al. The United Kingdom Infantile Spasms Study (UKISS) comparing hormone treatment with vigabatrin on developmental and epilepsy outcomes to age 14 months: a multicentre randomised trial. *Lancet Neurol.* 2005;4(11):712–717.

32. Mackay MT, Weiss SK, Adams-Webber T, et al. Practice parameter: medical treatment of infantile spasms: report of the American Academy of Neurology and the Child Neurology Society. *Neurology.* 2004;62(10): 1668–1681.

33. Hancock E, Osborne J, Milner P. Treatment of infantile spasms. *Cochrane Database Syst Rev.* 2003;(3):CD001770.

34. Weiss KL, Schroeder CE, Kastin SJ, et al. MRI monitoring of vigabatrin-induced intramyelinic edema in dogs. *Neurology.* 1994;44(10):1944–1949.

35. Yarrington JT, Gibson JP, Dillberger JE, et al. Sequential neuropathology of dogs treated with vigabatrin, a GABA-transaminase inhibitor. *Toxicol Pathol.* 1993;21(5):480–489.

36. Beaumont D. *Pharmacokinetics of the Enantiomers of Vigabatrin in Infants and Children of the Racemate.* Protocol: Report W-90-0001-C. Ovation Pharmaceuticals.

37. Foss JA. *Oral (Gavage) Repeated-Dose Toxicity Study of Vigabatrin in Rats.* Study No. OV-1007, Report DMQ00001. Ovation Pharmaceuticals.

38. Newcomb DL. *Nine-Week Oral (Gavage) Repeat-Dose Toxicity Study of Vigabatrin in Neonatal Rats.* Study No. OVNC-9004, Report DMQ00012. Ovation Pharmaceuticals; 2007.

39. Cohen JA, Fisher RS, Brigell MG, et al. The potential for vigabatrin-induced intramyelinic edema in humans. *Epilepsia.* 2000;41(2):148–157.

40. Pearl PL, Molloy-Wells E, McClintock WM, et al. MRI abnormalities associated with vigabatrin therapy: higher risk in infants? *Epilepsia.* 2006; 47(s4):14.

41. Milh M, Villeneuve N, Chapon F, et al. Transient brain magnetic resonance imaging hyperintensity in basal ganglia and brain stem of epileptic infants treated with vigabatrin. *J Child Neurol.* 2009;24(3):305–315.

42. Wheless JW, Carmant L, Bebin M, et al. Magnetic resonance imaging abnormalities associated with vigabatrin in patients with epilepsy. *Epilepsia.* 2009;50(2):195–205.

43. Pearl PL, Vezina LG, Saneto RP, et al. Cerebral MRI abnormalities associated with vigabatrin therapy. *Epilepsia.* 2009;50(2):184–194.

44. Eke T, Talbot JF, Lawden MC. Severe persistent visual field constriction associated with vigabatrin. *BMJ.* 1997;314(7075):180–181.

45. Wild JM, Martinez C, Reinshagen G, et al. Characteristics of a unique visual field defect attributed to vigabatrin. *Epilepsia.* 1999;40(12): 1784–1794.

46. Malmgren K, Ben-Menachem E, Frisen L. Vigabatrin visual toxicity: evolution and dose dependence. *Epilepsia.* 2001;42(5):609–615.

47. Kalviainen R, Nousiainen I, Mantyjarvi M, et al. Vigabatrin, a gabaergic antiepileptic drug, causes concentric visual field defects. *Neurology.* 1999;53(5):922–926.

48. Kinirons P, Cavalleri GL, O'Rourke D, et al. Vigabatrin retinopathy in an Irish cohort: lack of correlation with dose. *Epilepsia.* 2006;47(2): 311–317.

49. Krauss GL, Johnson MA, Sheth S, et al. A controlled study comparing visual function in patients treated with vigabatrin and tiagabine. *J Neurol Neurosurg Psychiatry.* 2003;74(3):339–343.

50. Wild JM, Robson CR, Jones AL, et al. Detecting vigabatrin toxicity by imaging of the retinal nerve fiber layer. *Invest Ophthalmol Vis Sci.* 2006;47(3):917–924.

51. Krauss GL, Johnson MA, Miller NR. Vigabatrin-associated retinal cone system dysfunction: electroretinogram and ophthalmologic findings. *Neurology.* 1998;50(3):614–618.

52. Ravindran J, Blumbergs P, Crompton J, et al. Visual field loss associated with vigabatrin: pathological correlations. *J Neurol Neurosurg Psychiatry.* 2001;70(6):787–789.

53. Sills GJ. Pre-clinical studies with the GABAergic compounds vigabatrin and tiagabine. *Epileptic Disord.* 2003;5(1):51–56.

54. Kjellstrom U, Bruun A, Ghosh F, et al. Dose-related changes in retinal function and PKC-alpha expression in rabbits on vigabatrin medication. Effect of vigabatrin in the rabbit eye. *Graefes Arch Clin Exp Ophthalmol.* 2009;247(8):1057–1067.

55. Jammoul F, Wang Q, Nabbout R, et al. Taurine deficiency is a cause of vigabatrin-induced retinal phototoxicity. *Ann Neurol.* 2009;65(1):98–107.

56. Willmore LJ, Abelson MB, Ben-Menachem E, et al. Vigabatrin: 2008 update. *Epilepsia.* 2009;50(2):163–173.

57. Harding GF, Wild JM, Robertson KA, et al. Separating the retinal electrophysiologic effects of vigabatrin: treatment versus field loss. *Neurology.* 2000;55(3):347–352.

58. Harding GF, Wild JM, Robertson KA, et al. Electro-oculography, electroretinography, visual evoked potentials, and multifocal electroretinography in patients with vigabatrin-attributed visual field constriction. *Epilepsia.* 2000;41(11):1420–1431.

59. Abdulrazzaq YM, Bastaki SM, Padmanabhan R. Teratogenic effects of vigabatrin in TO mouse fetuses. *Teratology.* 1997;55(3):165–176.

CHAPTER 64 ■ RUFINAMIDE

GREGORY KRAUSS AND STEFANIE DARNLEY

Rufinamide was identified as a potential antiepileptic drug (AED) by Ciba-Geigy in Europe and was initially developed by Novartis Pharmaceuticals. In 2004, Eisai Pharmaceuticals obtained development rights to rufinamide. In 2008, the company obtained regulatory approval in Europe and the United States for using rufinamide to treat seizures in patients with Lennox–Gastaut syndrome. The drug is marketed in the United States with FDA approval as an orphan drug "Banzel" and in Europe as "Inovelon." It is being evaluated for use in adjunctive treatment of partial-onset seizures.

CHEMISTRY

Rufinamide (1-[2,6-difluorobenzyl]-1H-1,2,3-triazole-4-carboxamide) is a triazole ($C_2H_3N_3$) ring structure, which is structurally dissimilar to other AEDs (lamotrigine has a "triazine" two ring structure) (Fig. 64.1).

Rufinamide is nearly insoluble in water and slightly soluble in methanol and ethanol. This would make it difficult to prepare an intravenous preparation. Solubility in water and gastric fluid is approximately 40 to 70 mg/L at 37°C. Dissolution is the rate-limiting step for absorption. Rufinamide forms a white crystalline powder and is compacted into scored film tabs of 100, 200, and 400 mg tablets.

MECHANISMS OF ACTION

Rufinamide modulates voltage-dependent neuronal sodium channels; however, it also inhibits seizures triggered by GABA antagonists, and its anticonvulsant mechanisms in humans are unknown. The drug interacts with sodium channels in cultured rodent cortical neurons, prolongs inactivation of voltage-dependent sodium channels in spinal cord neurons, and acts to reduce repetitive firing of sodium channel–dependent neurons (1). The drug does not interact, however, with several subtypes of rodent and human voltage-gated sodium channels: rat $Na_v1.2a$, rat $Na_v1.8$, and human $Na_v1.5$ (2). Interactions with sodium channel isoforms, such as human $Na_v1.2$, involved in familial epilepsy syndromes have not been evaluated.

Rufinamide's effects in prolonging inactivation of voltage-dependent sodium channels is consistent with its potent inhi-

bition of maximal electroshock (MES) triggered seizures in rodents (oral ED50 = 4 to 24 mg/kg) (3). Rufinamide's inhibition of MES seizures was additive with other AEDs, but it did not potentiate or reduce the effects of other AEDs (4). Rufinamide also prevents clonic seizures induced by injected (s.c. and i.p.) pentylenetetrazole (PTZ) in mice, but did not prevent seizures caused by oral PTZ treatment. Rufinamide caused behavioral toxicity on the rotorod test only at extremely high doses; consequently, rufinamide's protective indexes for MES and PTZ tests are much higher than traditional AEDs (e.g., phenytoin in MES model; valproic acid in PTZ model) (3).

Rufinamide inhibits seizures induced by the GABA-A antagonists bicuculline and picrotoxin, with less effect on strychnine-induced seizures. Rufinamide does not inhibit seizures in the WAG/Rij rat, however, which is a genetic model of absence epilepsy with GABA-A receptor abnormalities (5). Rufinamide also does not interact directly with GABA receptors or modulators. This suggests rufinamide's influences on cortical inhibition are indirect, possibly mediated by modulation of voltage-dependent sodium channels in cortical interneurons.

Rufinamide has mixed effects on chronic seizure models: it delayed development of electrically kindled after-discharges in the cat, but not in the rat. It markedly reduced recurring motor seizures induced by aluminum hydroxide placed on monkey cortex (6). Overall, these studies suggest that rufinamide modulation of voltage-dependent sodium channels may indirectly influence seizures via effects on cortical inhibition. However, associations between these mechanisms and effects on seizures associated with Lennox–Gastaut syndrome are unknown.

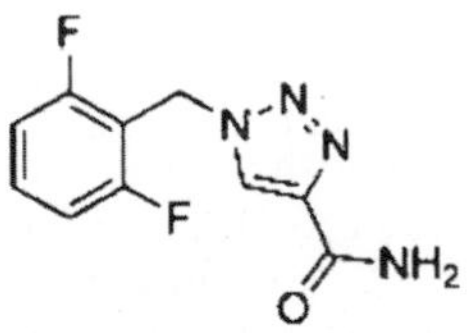

ABSORPTION, METABOLISM, AND DRUG INTERACTIONS

The pharamacologic profile for rufinamide is summarized in Table 64.1.

FIGURE 64.1 Chemical structure of rufinamide.

MW 238.2 ($C_{10}H_8F_2N_4O$)

TABLE 64.1

PHARMACOKINETIC PROPERTIES OF RUFINAMIDE

Half-life	Mean 9.5 hours (range 8–12 hours)
T_{max}	Fed 6 hours; fasted 8 hours
Bioavailability	Fed 70%; fasted 49%
Protein binding	34%
Mean C_{max}	3.03 µg/mL (400 mg dose in healthy adult male volunteers)
V_d	Range: 50–80 L

Rufinamide is well absorbed orally in the fed state (≥85% absorption in healthy volunteers) with a slow rate of absorption; absorption decreases slightly at high doses (7). The relative extent of absorption of rufinamide was lower at a dose of 1600 mg/day compared to 200 to 800 mg/day in a large pharmacokinetic study (8). Bioavailability of single doses of rufinamide are increased by food, however, food effects were not seen with chronic dosing (9). Patients received rufinamide only with food in clinical trials, and it is approved to be dosed with food. Peak rufinamide concentrations occur approximately 6 hours after dosing when taken with food and approximately 8 hours when dosed while fasting (10). Rufinamide has relatively low (34%) protein binding—mostly to albumin—and is distributed in the bloodstream equally between erythrocytes and plasma (7). Rufinamide's apparent volume of distribution (V_d) is approximately 50 L at a 3200 mg/day dose and increases slightly with very high doses and high body surface area (11).

Rufinamide is eliminated via hydrolysis into an inactive carboxylic acid metabolite (CGP 47292), which is renally excreted. Less than 2% of rufinamide is recovered in the urine (4). A small fraction of metabolite is glucuronidated and subsequently excreted. Rufinamide is hydrolyzed by a carboxylesterase, which is concentrated in the liver, but is present in brain and other tissues (7). Rufinamide does not induce carboxylesterase and its metabolism is not dependent on cytochrome p450 (CYP) isozymes thus major drug–drug interactions are unlikely (7). With the exception of a valproic acid interaction in children, the overall pharmacokinetics for rufinamide are similar in children and in adults, including the elderly, with clearance proportionate to dose and body surface area (12).

In clinical studies, rufinamide had only small effects on concentrations of several other AEDs (13): phenytoin clearance was decreased slightly, with plasma concentrations increasing from 7% to 21%; carbamazepine, lamotrigine, and phenobarbital concentrations decreased from 7% to 13%; topiramate and valproate concentrations were unchanged. Patients taking valproic acid, especially children, had increases in rufinamide concentrations (14). Valproic acid caused average increase in rufinamide plasma concentrations of 40% in children and 11% in adults (12). Small children (<30 kg) with very high valproic acid concentrations (e.g., 100 mg/L) had increases in rufinamide concentrations of up to 70%, however, this varied widely across patients (14). Rufinamide doses were not adjusted in clinical trials for patients receiving valproic acid, however, reduced dose reductions of 50% to 60% have been recommended for small children (<30 kg) taking valproic acid (14). European regulators have requested an additional pediatric monitoring study to evaluate this interaction further. Adolescents and adults receiving valproic acid had much small increases in rufinamide concentrations than children: ≤26% increases in adolescents and <16% increases in adults (14). Other AEDs were associated with small, but variable, decreases in rufinamide concentrations: carbamazepine (19% to 26%), phenobarbital (25% to 46%), phenytoin (25% to 46%), and primidone (25% to 46%). Lamotrigine and topiramate did not alter rufinamide concentrations (6).

Rufinamide had a modest interaction with oral contraceptives: repeated administration of 1600 mg/day of rufinamide decreased ethinyl estradiol concentrations by 22% and norethindrone by 14%. It is unclear whether higher doses of rufinamide might produce greater hormonal plasma concentration reductions and subsequent contraceptive failure (15).

Triazolam clearance increased slightly with rufinamide treatment (4). Increased clearance is most likely caused by modest induction of CYP3A4 and is not believed to be clinically relevant (16).

Due to extensive metabolism, rufinamide elimination is not influenced by renal dysfunction and no specific dosage changes are required for patients with renal impairments (11). No marked difference in rufinamide concentrations was found in patients experiencing severe renal impairment as compared to healthy individuals after a single 400 mg dose (14). During dialysis, area under plasma concentration-time curve (AUC) was decreased by approximately 30%. Simulations have indicated that an approximate 12% decrease in total rufinamide exposure (AUC) would result over 1 week including three 3-hour dialysis sessions. These results indicate that no specific dose adjustment is likely to be required for patients with renal failure undergoing hemodialysis (14).

CLINICAL STUDIES

Lennox–Gastaut Syndrome

Rufinamide is approved for adjunctive treatment of Lennox–Gastaut syndrome in the United States and Europe. Patients with Lennox–Gastaut syndrome typically have multiple seizure types along with encephalopathies. Their most characteristic (and serious) seizure types are tonic and tonic/atonic "drop attacks," which cause sudden falls and injuries. Patients also have varying patterns of atypical absence, myoclonic, atonic, tonic–clonic, and complex motor seizures. Most patients have slow spike-and-wave discharges and generalized slowing on EEG. Effects of rufinamide in treating seizures in patients with Lennox–Gastaut were evaluated in a randomized, parallel-design, placebo-controlled study ($N = 138$) (17). Seizures associated with falls (predominantly tonic and tonic/atonic seizures) and total seizures were assessed. Patients were treated with rufinamide 45 mg/kg, up to a maximum of 3200 mg/day, divided BID. Patients receiving rufinamide had a 42.5% median reduction in tonic–atonic seizures compared to a 1.4% increase in seizures for patients receiving placebo treatment (Fig. 64.2A). The patients' total seizure frequency was reduced 32.7% during rufinamide treatment compared to a median of 11.7% for placebo treatment. Seizure responder rates (proportions of patients with >50% seizure reduction) were also significantly higher for patients treated with rufinamide (42.5%) compared to placebo (16.7%) (Fig. 64.2B).

Efficacy was sustained during open-label extension treatment, with decreases in seizure frequency of 43% to 79% during 6 to 36 months of treatment; patients converting from placebo to rufinamide also had substantial reductions in seizures (18). Responder rates for patients, during their most recent 6 months of therapy, were 45.1% for total seizures and 47.9% for tonic/atonic seizures. A total of 9.4% of patients were free of tonic/atonic seizures during their last 6 months of open-label treatment (16).

Most patients with Lennox–Gastaut syndrome tolerated rufinamide well; especially considering that treatment was combined with one to three concomitant AEDs (17). The most common adverse events (AEs) (≥10%) seen in rufinamide-treated patients as compared to those receiving placebo were: somnolence (24.3% vs. 12.5%), vomiting (21.6% vs. 6.3%),

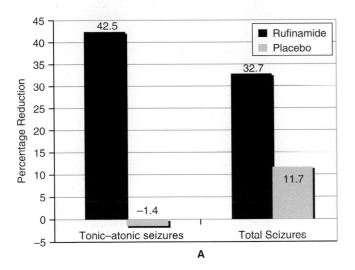

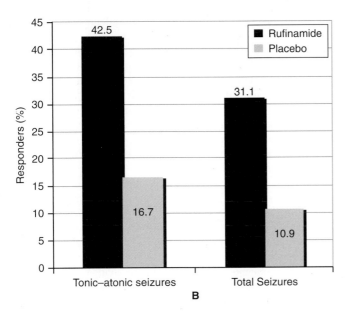

FIGURE 64.2 **A:** Median percentage reduction in total seizure frequency and tonic–atonic seizure frequency. **B:** Percentage of patients (responders) who experienced at least 50% reduction in tonic–atonic seizure frequency.

pyrexia (13.5% vs. 17.2%), and diarrhea (5.4% vs. 10.9%), respectively. Vomiting and somnolence were the only AEs occurring at an incidence of 5% greater than placebo treatment. Of the 124 patients entering open-label extension treatment (median dose 1800 mg/day), 12 subsequently discontinued treatment due to AEs (18). The most commonly reported AEs during the uncontrolled extension treatment phase were vomiting (30.6%), pyrexia (25.8%), upper respiratory tract infection (21.8%), and somnolence (21.0%).

Partial-Onset Seizure Trials

Rufinamide demonstrated variable efficacy for reducing partial-onset seizures in adults in two large randomized, placebo-controlled, multicenter trials. A third pivot trial was completed in 2009. In one large trial of adults ($\geq$16 years, $N = 313$), patients were randomized to receive either rufinamide (3200 mg/day) or placebo during a 13-week double-

blind maintenance treatment phase (19). Rufinamide reduced median seizure frequency by 20.4% compared to a 1.6% increase during placebo treatment. The responder rate (proportion of patients with >50% seizure reduction) was 28.2% with rufinamide treatment compared to 18.6% with placebo treatment ($P = 0.038$).

A second large pivotal trial (20) ($N = 647$) in adults (ages 15 to 65 years) compared treatment with four doses of rufinamide 200, 400, 800, or 1600 mg/day (given b.i.d.) and placebo. There was a significant linear trend in dose–response across patients receiving the four rufinamide doses ($P = 0.003$): 50% responder rates ranged from 9% with placebo to 4.7% with rufinamide 200 mg/day, 16% for 400 mg/day ($P = 0.027$), 12% for 800 mg/day dose ($P = 0.012$), and 14% with a 1600 mg/day dose ($P = 0.016$). Seizure frequencies were not reported, but were significantly reduced for the 400 mg/day ($P < 0.03$), 800 mg/day ($P < 0.02$), and 1600 mg/day ($P < 0.02$) treatment groups compared to placebo.

Monotherapy Treatment for Partial Onset

Two clinical trials evaluated the efficacy of monotherapy treatment in patients >12 years of age. One study (21) included patients ($N = 104$) with uncontrolled partial seizures completing an evaluation for epilepsy surgery. Patients were randomized to rufinamide 3200 mg (divided b.i.d) or placebo with efficacy determined by time required for patients to reach an end point of four seizures. Although rufinamide treatment significantly increased patients' time to having one, two, or three seizures compared to placebo ($P < 0.04$), their times to reaching the primary end point of a fourth seizure was only slightly longer for patients treated with rufinamide ($P = 0.051$). The median times for patients to have second and third seizures, however, were more than twice as long for patients randomized to rufinamide monotherapy than for patients treated with placebo.

An additional outpatient monotherapy study compared patients receiving full doses of rufinamide, 3200 mg/day, versus low doses of 300 mg/day (22). Efficacy end points were defined as proportions of patients reaching several exit criteria of recurring seizures. The number of patients meeting the exit criterion were not significantly different for the high-dose treatment (66.7%) and low-dose (72.5%) groups ($P = 0.44$). The median time to reach the exit criterion slightly favored high-dose rufinamide therapy (56 days) versus low-dose therapy (32 days) ($P = 0.097$).

Partial-Onset Pediatric Trials

A randomized, double-blind, placebo-controlled, adjunctive trial enrolled 269 pediatric patients between the ages of 4 to 15 years of age (23). Seizure frequencies for children treated with rufinamide (45 mg/kg/day) decreased by an average of only 7% compared to a 12.8% reduction with placebo treatment ($P = 0.62$). A number of children with very high seizure frequencies appeared to influence the assessment of seizure frequencies. Children treated with rufinamide had slightly higher responder rates (>50% reduction in seizures) (27.2%) compared to those treated with placebo (18.3%), though, this difference did not reach statistical significance ($P = 0.082$).

Generalized Epilepsy

The safety and efficacy of treating patients ($N = 153$) with inadequately controlled, primary, generalized tonic–clonic seizures was evaluated in a multicenter, double-blind, placebo-controlled study using a relatively low dose of rufinamide (800 mg/day) (24). Patients receiving rufinamide had a greater mean reduction in frequency of generalized tonic–clonic seizures (median reduction, 36.4%) than those receiving placebo (25.6%); however, this difference was not statistically significant ($P = 0.63$) and responses to higher doses have not been explored.

SAFETY AND TOLERABILITY

Rufinamide safety and tolerability were assessed in 11 double-blind, randomized, placebo-controlled studies (25); long-term safety was evaluated in 14 controlled and open-label extension studies. These included all patients receiving ≥1 dose of rufinamide. Overall, 98.2% of all patients with epilepsy received at least one concomitant AED, the most common medications being carbamazepine (52.9%), valproate (31.6%), phenytoin (22.9%), and clonazepam (19.7%).

Short-Term Therapy

Safety and tolerability were evaluated in patients receiving rufinamide treatment ($N = 1240$, with a mean age of 31.7 years) in controlled studies compared to those receiving placebo ($N = 635$, with a mean age of 28.6 years). The mean dose of rufinamide was 1373 mg/day with a median daily dose of 1000 mg/day. Eleven percent of patients receiving rufinamide reported no AEs. The most commonly reported AEs associated with rufinamide treatment (compared to placebo) were headache, dizziness, fatigue, somnolence, and nausea (Table 64.2). Other significant AEs included rash (children 4%, adults <2%), AED hypersensitivity syndrome (three

children), cognitive symptoms (mostly somnolence), psychiatric symptoms, status epilepticus, and convulsions. The percentage of rufinamide-treated patients experiencing serious AEs was slightly greater than for placebo-treated patients.

Long-Term Therapy

Safety and tolerability during long-term rufinamide therapy was evaluated in 1978 patients (mean age of 31.3 years) in controlled and open studies lasting between <1 month and >4 years. The mean daily dose of rufinamide was 1700 mg/day with a median daily dose of 1600 mg/day. The most frequently reported AEs were headache, dizziness, and fatigue. The majority of common AEs appeared during the first 2 weeks of therapy, with few patients developing new AEs during chronic therapy. Although most AEs were mild to moderate in severity, at least one severe AE occurred in 20.8% of patients: 261 patients reported serious AEs during treatment, most commonly convulsions, status epilepticus, and pneumonia.

In extensive cardiac testing, rufinamide shortened QT intervals in ECG up to 20 msec in a large proportion (46%) of patients treated with recommended doses (2400 mg/day to 3200 mg/day) (11). Treatment, however, did not shorten QT intervals to a clinically significant range of <300 msec, which is associated with ventricular arrhythmias. There were no increased risks for sudden cardiac death or other cardiac abnormalities identified in clinical trials.

Pregnancy risks for women treated with rufinamide are unknown. Only 13 women (out of >2000 patients treated) in clinical trials had pregnancies: 6 had healthy babies, 3 had planned terminations, 1 had a spontaneous abortion, and 3 did not have pregnancy outcomes determined. A pregnancy registry has been established in Europe to monitor risks for pregnancy with rufinamide treatment; a U.S. AED registry monitors outcomes for patients treated with all AEDs. Due to a lack of outcome data, women of childbearing age receiving rufinamide are recommended to avoid pregnancies with careful contraceptive use. Patients becoming pregnant will require individual assessments of their risk benefits for continuing rufinamide therapy.

AEs Causing Discontinuation of Treatment

A larger proportion of patients discontinued rufinamide due to AEs ($N = 100$; 8.1%) during double-blind studies than those receiving placebo ($N = 27$; 4.3%). The most common AEs associated with discontinuing treatment were dizziness, fatigue, headache, nausea, and diplopia. The percentage of patients discontinuing treatment due to serious AEs was also slightly increased for patients treated with rufinamide (6.3%) compared to placebo (3.9%)—"convulsions" were most commonly reported. During long-term extension treatment, 259 (13.1%) patients discontinued treatment due to AE's; the most common symptoms were fatigue, headache, dizziness, and nausea.

CLINICAL USE

Rufinamide is approved in the United States and Europe for adjunctive treatment of seizures in children (>4 years) and adults with Lennox–Gastaut syndrome. Based on the

TABLE 64.2

MOST COMMON ADVERSE EVENTS REPORTED BY PATIENTS IN ADJUNCTIVE TRIALS FOR PARTIAL-ONSET EPILEPSY

	Rufinamide-treated patients (%)	Placebo-treated patients (%)
Short-term therapy [$N = 1875$]		
Headache	22.9	18.9
Dizziness	15.5	9.4
Fatigue	13.6	9.0
Somnolence	11.8	9.1
Nausea	11.4	7.6
Serious AEs	6.3	3.9
Long-term therapy [$N = 1978$]		
Headache	29.5	
Dizziness	22.5	
Fatigue	17.7	
Serious AEs	13.2	

Lennox–Gastaut trial, very rapid (1 week) schedules for titrating rufinamide were approved. The approved schedule for treating children with rufinamide is an initial dose of approximately 10 mg/kg/day (divided b.i.d.), followed by an increase of 10 mg/kg every 2 days to a target dose of 45 mg/kg (or a maximum of 3200 mg/day), divided b.i.d. These doses can be achieved using scored 200 and 400 mg tablets; an additional 100 mg tablet is available in Europe. The approved schedule for adults is similar: an initial dose of 400 to 800 mg/day (divided b.i.d.) followed by a 400 to 800 mg/day increase every 2 days to a maximum dose of 3200 mg/day, divided b.i.d. A more gradual 2-week titration schedule is recommended for patients who have difficulty tolerating the drug. Small children (<30 kg) adding rufinamide to valproic acid treatment may begin treatment at one half of these doses.

Clinicians often find that AED titration schedules slower than those used in clinical trials help minimize drug-related side effects. An early open treatment series, for example, showed that gradual rufinamide titration, with increases every 5 to 7 days, along with reductions in ineffective concomitant AEDs, appears to reduce AEs seen during titration in clinical trial, such as somnolence and dizziness (26). Patients with Lennox–Gastaut syndrome have frequent seizures and can also have maximum rufinamide doses determined by their treatment responses—some patients may respond to doses lower than 45 mg/kg. It will be important to explore another possible finding in an early uncontrolled series—that rufinamide may be effective for treating seizures in patients with multifocal seizures and encephalopathies (26), but who do not meet clinical criteria for having Lennox–Gastaut syndrome (27).

SUMMARY

Rufinamide is a unique AED, which prolongs inactivation of voltage-dependent sodium channels in neurons and has a very high protective index in animal seizure models, but also blocks seizures triggered by GABA-A receptor antagonists. Rufinamide was generally well tolerated in clinical trials with CNS-related side effects most common (headache, dizziness, fatigue, etc.). The drug was effective in a well-controlled clinical trial of Lennox–Gastaut syndrome and continues to be investigated as adjunctive treatment of partial-onset seizures.

References

1. Mclean MJ, Schmutz M, Pozza M. The influence of rufinamide on sodium currents and action potential firing in rodent neurons. *Epilepsia*. 2005;46: 296.
2. Vickory RG, Amagasu SM, Chang R, et al. Comparison of the pharmacological properties of rat Nav1.8 with rat NAv1.2a and human Nav1.5 voltage-gated sodium channel subtypes using a membrane potential sensitive dye and FLIPR. *Recept Channels*. 2004;10:11–23.
3. White HS, Franklin MR, Kupferberg HJ, et al. The anticonvulsant profile of rufinamide (CGP 33101) in rodent seizure models. *Epilepsia*. 2008;49(7):1213–1220.
4. Arroyo S. Rufinamide. *Neurotherapeutics*. 2007;4(1):155–162.
5. Rogawski MA. Diverse mechanisms of antiepileptic drugs in the development pipeline. *Epilepsy Res*. 2006;69:273–294.
6. Bialer M, Johannessen SI, Kupferberg HJ, et al. Progress report on new antiepileptic drugs: a summary of the Eighth Eilat Conference (EILAT VIII). *Epilepsy Res*. 1999;34(1):1–41.
7. Waldmeier F. Metabolism of the new anticonvulsant trial drug rufinamide (CGP33101) in healthy male volunteers. *Epilepsia*. 1996;37(suppl 5):167.
8. Brunner LA, Harrigan EP, John VA, et al. Pharmacokinetics of a new anticonvulsany (CGP 33101) in epileptic male patients and healthy male subjects after single ascending oral doses of 400–1200 mg. *Am J Ther*. 1994;1: 215–220.
9. Cardot JM, Lecaillon JB, Czendlik C, et al. The influence of food on the disposition of the antiepileptic rufinamide in healthy volunteers. *Biopharm Drug Dispos*. 1998;19:259–262.
10. Cheng-Hakimian A, Anderson GD, Miller JW. Rufinamide: pharmacology, clinical trials, and role in clinical practice. *Int J Clin Pract*. 2006;60(11): 1497–1501.
11. Banzel[package insert]. Woodcliff Lake, NJ: Eisai Co., Ltd.; 2008. http://www.eisai.com/package_inserts/Banzel%20PI%200109.PDF.
12. Critchley D, Fuseau E, Perdomo C, et al. Pharmacokinetic and pharmacodynamic parameters of adjunctive rufinamide in patients with Lennox-Gastaut syndrome. *Epilepsia*. 2005;46:209.
13. Fuseau E, Critchley D, Perdomo C, et al. Population pharmacokinetic drug-drug interaction analyses of rufinamide studies in patients with epilepsy. *Epilepsia*. 2005;46(suppl 8):210–211. Abstract.
14. Perucca E, Cloyd J, Critchley D, et al. Rufinamide: clinical pharmacokinetics. *Epilepsia*. 2008;49(7):1123–1141.
15. Svendson KD, Choid L, Chen B-L. Single-center, open-label, multiple-dose pharmacokinetic trial investigating the effect of rufinamide administration on Ortho-Novum 1/35 in healthy women. *Epilepsia*. 1998;39(suppl 6):59.
16. Deeks E, Scott LJ. Rufinamide. *CNS Drugs*. 2006;20(9):751–760.
17. Glauser T, Kluger G, Sachdeo R, et al. Rufinamide for generalized seizures associated with Lennox Gastaut syndrome. *Neurology*. 2008;70:1950–1958.
18. Kluger G, Glauser T, Krauss G, et al. Adjunctive rufinamide in Lennox-Gastaut syndrome: a long-term, open-label extension study. *Acta Neurolologica Scandinavica*. 2010;9999.
19. Brodie MJ, Rosenfeld W, Vazquez B, et al. Rufinamide for the adjunctive treatment of partial seizures in adults and adolescents: A randomized placebo-controlled trial. *Epilepsia*. 2009;50:1899–1909.
20. Elger C, Stefan H, Perdomo C, et al. A 24-week multicenter, randomized, double-blind parallel-group, dose-ranging study of rufinamide in adults and adolescents with inadequately controlled partial seizures. *Epilepsy Research*. 2010;88:255–263.
21. Lesser RP, Biton V, Sackelares JC, et al. Efficacy and safety of rufinamide monotherapy for the treatment of patients with refractory partial seizures. *Epilepsia*. 2005;46: 177–178.
22. Todorov A, Biton V, Krauss GL, et al. Efficacy and safety of high- versus low-dose rufinamide monotherapy in patients with inadequately controlled partial seizures. *Epilepsia*. 2005;46(suppl 8):218–219. Abstract.
23. Glauser T, Arzimanoglou A, Litzinger M, et al. Efficacy and safety of rufinamide as adjunctive therapy for inadequately controlled partial seizures in pediatric patients. *Epilepsia*. 2005;46(suppl 8):194–195.
24. Biton V, Sachdeo RC, Rosenfeld W, et al. Efficacy and safety of adjunctive rufinamide in patients with inadequately controlled primary generalized tonic-clonic seizures. *Epilepsia*. 2005;46(suppl 18):206.
25. Krauss GL, Perdomo CA, Arroyo S. Short-term and long-term safety of rufinamide in patients with epilepsy [poster]. In: *7th European Congress on Epileptology (ECE)*; July 2–6, 2006; Helsinki, Finland.
26. Friedo AL, Bohlmann K, Straub HB. First experiences with rufinamide: tolerability and effectiveness in clinical practice. In: *Programs and abstracts of the 8th European Congress on Epileptology*. Berlin, Germany; September 21–25, 2008. Poster E539.
27. Arzimanoglou A, French J, Blume WT, et al. Lennox-Gastaut syndrome: a consensus approach on diagnosis, assessment, management, and trial methodology. *Lancet Neurol*. 2009;8(1):82–93.

CHAPTER 65 ■ LACOSAMIDE

RAJ D. SHETH AND HARRY S. ABRAM

HISTORICAL BACKGROUND

Lacosamide (Vimpat; previously harkoseride) is the *R*-enantiomer of 2-acetamido *N*-benzyl-3-methoxypropionamide (Fig. 65.1). Lacosamide is a new investigational antiepileptic medication approved for use as adjunctive therapy for adults with partial complex seizures. Formulations as a tablet, syrup, and an intravenous injection are available. The drug was initially developed by Harris LLC with preclinical trials conducted by Schwartz Pharma and subsequently acquired by UCB Pharma. Although, it was specifically synthesized as an antiepileptic medication, as with many newer agents, it was found to have additional pharmacologic properties including a role in the alleviation of pain associated with diabetic neuropathy. The indication for pain associated with diabetic neuropathy is under Food and Drug Administration review. Preclinical development suggests neuroprotection in animal models of seizures as well as in status epilepticus models. Most studies have examined activity in the maximal electroshock-induced seizure test used in rodents. Human randomized controlled trials have shown lacosamide to have efficacy as an adjunctive therapy in adults with partial-onset seizures, although, efficacy in other epilepsy syndromes is being investigated.

GENERAL CHARACTERISTICS

Lacosamide belongs to a class of functionalized amino acids that were specifically designed to have potential anticonvulsant properties (see Fig. 65.1). It is a light yellow crystalline powder that is soluble in phosphate-buffered saline (pH of 7.5 at 25°C) and has a chemical formula of $C_{13}H_{18}N_2O_3$.

MECHANISM OF ACTION

Animal Models

Lacosamide has a dual mechanism of action, both of which appear novel and operational across a wide variety of animal seizure models when administered intraperitoneally in a dosage range of 1 to 30 mg/kg (1). Animal models where lacosamide has had antiseizure activity demonstrated include mice with audiogenic seizures and maximal electroshock and *N*-methyl-D-aspartate induced seizures (2).

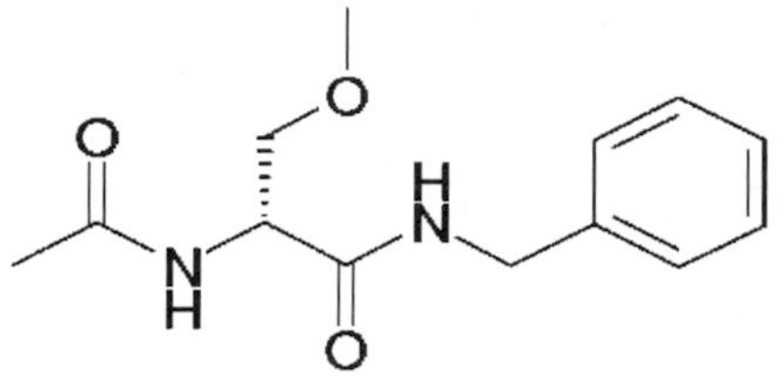

Lacosamide appears to have two main mechanisms of actions. The primary mechanism of action appears to be selective enhancing the slow inactivation of voltage-gated sodium channels without interfering with fast inactivation. Slow inactivation of sodium channels is an endogenous mechanism whereby neurons reduce ectopic hyperactivity, and may represent an effective mechanism to selectively reduce ictal hyperactivity without altering physiologic function (3). Lacosamide, unlike carbamazepine, lamotrigine, and phenytoin, did not produce frequency-dependent facilitation of block of 3-seconds, 10-Hz pulse stimulation train. The slow inactivation voltage curve was shifted in the hyperpolarizing direction and significantly promoted the shift of channels to the slow inactivated state without impairing rate of recovery. Such modulation of neuronal activity may underlie lacosamide's therapeutic activity in the management of pain (2).

A second mechanism of action is lacosamide's interaction with the collapsin response mediator protein 2 (CRMP-2). Brain derived neurotrophic factor and neurotrophin-3 activate a transduction cascade that ultimately results in increased CRMP-2 which enhances neuronal sprouting and axonal outgrowth (Fig. 65.2) (1). Lacosamide inhibits CRMP-2, thereby potentially inhibiting axonal sprouting and outgrowth that may underlie the progression reported in chronic epilepsy. Brandt et al. examined the effect of lacosamide administered in 3, 10, or 30 mg/kg/day over 22 to 23 days during amygdala kindling (4). They found a dose-dependent inhibitory effect on the development of kindling and concluded that lacosamide could retard kindling-induced epileptogenesis. This mechanism may be neuroprotective. While the role of these potential neuroprotective effects may treat seizures and prevent epilepsy progression, they are yet to be evaluated clinically.

Lacosamide in Acute Status Epilepticus

Lacosamide is highly potent in acute status epilepticus models. In rats, it has been shown to have the potential for disease modification that may be CRMP-2 dependent (5). Lacosamide's inhibition of CRMP-2 may render it effective as both a traditional antiepileptogenic agent while also having efficacy in acute seizures. Male rats rendered in self-sustaining EEG, and clinical status epilepticus treated with early (10 minutes) or delayed (40 minutes) lacosamide showed dose-dependent and potent reduction in both the frequency of seizures as well as the cumulative duration of seizures. Early treatment with lacosamide resulted in a dose-dependent reduction of the number of spontaneous recurrent seizures of up to 70%. Late

FIGURE 65.1 Structure of lacosamide ($C_{13}H_{18}N_2O_3$).

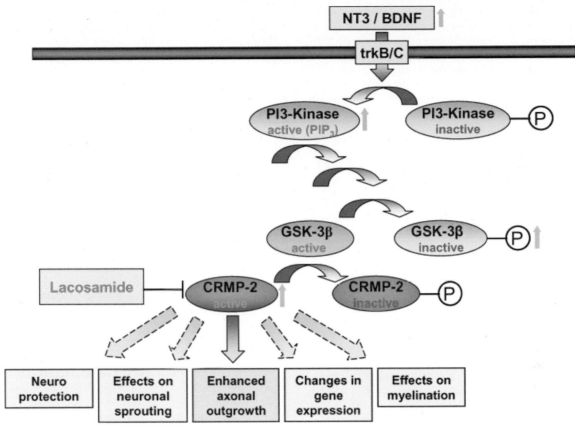

FIGURE 65.2 Schema showing CRMP-2-mediated transduction of neurotrophic signals to neuronal response and the possible interaction of lacosamide. Neurotrophins like NT-3 and BDNF activate their receptors in the plasma membrane, triggering a transduction cascade, which regulates the activity of intracellular protein kinases (e.g., PI3 kinase or GSK-3β) finally resulting in increased levels of active CRMP-2. Active, nonphosphorylated CRMP-2 has been shown to enhance axonal outgrowth, and might also be involved in the induction of other cellular responses. Interaction site of lacosamide is indicated (1).

treatment with lacosamide resulted in a 50% reduction in the frequency of spontaneous recurrence. The number of seizure-free animals increased from 0% in the untreated group to 65% in the highest dose groups. Protection of hippocampal structures within 72 hours following induction of status epilepticus was greatly enhanced.

CLINICAL STUDIES

Lacosamide has been studied in two clinical settings: (i) in adults with partial seizures as an adjunctive agent and (ii) in pain associated with diabetic neuropathy. Dose ranges that were tested in these situations are between 200 and 600 mg/day (Table 65.1), following indications from initial trials of efficacy between 100 and 600 mg/day.

Randomized Controlled Trials in Epilepsy

A total of three randomized controlled trials in adults with partial complex epilepsy where lacosamide was used as an adjunctive have been completed to date. All three used similar randomization with double-blind parallel-group design in a 12-week dose escalation with target 100 mg/day increments followed by a 12-week maintenance period.

TABLE 65.1

CHANGE IN SEIZURE FREQUENCY PER 28 DAYS DURING THE FIRST 2 WEEKS OF LACOSAMIDE EXPOSURE

Randomized treatment group	Reduction over placebo (%)	P-value
First week of exposure to LCM (LCM 100 mg/day)		
LCM 200-mg/day group	17.6	0.031
LCM 400-mg/day group	21.2	0.002
Second week of exposure to LCM (LCM 200 mg/day)		
LCM 200-mg/day group	25.3	0.001
LCM 400-mg/day group	18.3	0.007

Ben-Menachem et al., in a multicenter, international, double-blind, placebo-controlled, randomized, dose–response study, involving 418 adults with refractory partial epilepsy, demonstrated significant efficacy at doses of 400 and 600 mg/day (6,7). At these dosages, compared to placebo, median seizure frequency was reduced 40%, with 49% of patients experiencing a 50% or greater reduction in seizure frequency. A dose-adverse effects relationship was seen with doses of 600 mg/day most consistently associated with the highest adverse event rate. In these studies, adverse effects included common neurologic symptoms, including nausea, headache, ataxia, fatigue, and diplopia. Serious adverse effects resulting in medication withdrawal occurred in less than 1% of all patients. Adverse effects resulting in withdrawal most frequently consisted of exacerbation of convulsive seizures and intolerable dizziness. Lacosamide appeared to be neutral on its effect on body weight. Importantly, there was no change in the serum concentrations of coadministered anticonvulsants.

Dose-Range Study

Dose-finding studies are critically important in the clinical development of a new drug. They help define the no-effect, the mean effective, and the maximal effective doses and determine a potentially optimal therapeutic dose range. In a pooled post hoc review of 1294 patients treated in three placebo-controlled, double-blind, international clinical trials evaluating the efficacy and safety of adjunctive lacosamide (200 to 600 mg/day) in adults ≥16 years with partial-onset seizures with or without secondary generalization, Chung et al. (American Epilepsy Society 2008) found consistent seizure reduction for lacosamide dosages 400 and 600 mg/day. Dosage with 200 mg/day produced a variable effect, although pooled data suggested that 200 mg/day was efficacious compared to placebo. Lacosamide 400 mg/day added to between one and three other antiepileptic medications in 466 patients with intractable epilepsy in Phase II and III double-blind, placebo-controlled studies were examined to understand medication's efficacy (8).

Lacosamide was added to carbamazepine (33%), lamotrigine (33%), levetiracetam (30%), valproate (23%), topiramate (23%), and oxcarbazepine (17%). Median percent reduction over 28 days in seizure frequency from baseline was 36.8% for lacosamide 400 mg/day versus 18.4% for placebo. Lacosamide showed a similar magnitude of reduction versus placebo regardless of which combination of antiepileptic medication regimens it was added to. Importantly, efficacy was demonstrated whether lacosamide was added to a sodium channel blocking AED or to an AED with other mechanisms of action. This suggests an independent additive efficacy in excess of that provided by pre-existing antiepileptic medication to which lacosamide was added.

The time of onset of efficacy is an important consideration in the choice of antiepileptic medication. Lacosamide appears to have an early onset of efficacy against seizures. Secondary analysis of lacosamide in a pooled analysis of three Phase II and Phase III trials demonstrated efficacy in the early weeks after addition (9).

Lacosamide in fixed doses of 200, 400, or 600 mg/day were used in these pooled data. Titration was started at 100 mg/day during the initial week of lacosamide exposure, followed by weekly titration in 100-mg increments to the assigned target dose. After the first week of lacosamide exposure to 100 mg/day, the percent reduction of seizures over placebo was 17.9% ($P < 0.01$) and only slightly improved to 20.4% by the second week when patients were receiving 200 mg/day. Post hoc pooled analysis showed an early onset of efficacy starting at a dose of 100 mg/day in the first week and increasing modestly after that for patients where lacosamide was added to their antiepileptic medication

regimen. Thus, efficacy can be expected in the first week or two following initiation of adjunctive lacosamide. Prospective trials are required to confirm these findings.

Clinical use suggests that lacosamide be initiated as an adjunctive at 50 mg twice daily with subsequent dose increases on a weekly basis to a target dose of 200 to 400 mg/day in adults with partial epilepsy. The availability of a parenteral formulation has the potential to be useful in the management of acute seizures, although, studies in status epilepticus are still to be performed. Studies in other populations, including pediatrics and the elderly, are needed to further define the therapeutic spectrum of lacosamide.

Studies in Diabetic Neuropathy

At least three randomized, placebo-controlled, double-blind trials have been completed to test the efficacy of lacosamide in diabetic neuropathy related pain. Lacosamide appears to be effective in doses up to 400 mg/day. However, doses of 600 mg/day were not associated with further increments in efficacy and were generally less well tolerated (10).

ABSORPTION, DISTRIBUTION, AND METABOLISM

The pharmacokinetic properties of lacosamide include a fast rate of absorption, little metabolism with cytochrome P450 iso-enzymes with about 20% metabolized via CYP2C19, limited effect of age and gender on plasma levels, and low potential for drug–drug interactions (11).

Oral administration of lacosamide results in rapid and near complete absorption with minimal first-pass effects (12). Bioavailability after oral administration approaches 100%, with peak plasma concentration being reached after 30 min to 4 hours following oral administration. Dose to plasma concentrations are linear with low intra- and intersubject variability. Food appears to have no influence on lacosamide's absorption with oral bioavailability reaching 100% (13). Escalating dose administration orally results in near-linear increases in serum concentration. Lacosamide administered in a 300-mg single dose following consumption of a high fat diet did not influence its serum concentration. Lacosamide has an apparent volume of distribution of about 40 to 60 L (0.5 to 0.8 L/kg) and has a low plasma protein binding, with less than 15% of serum lacosamide being bound to plasma protein. Distribution in placenta and breast milk and distribution in children has not been examined.

Metabolism

Almost 40% of lacosamide is excreted unchanged in the urine. A further 30% is metabolized by demethylation to the pharmacologically inactive O-desmethyl metabolite that is excreted in the urine (14). In addition, a polar fraction (~20% of the dose) is also excreted into urine after both oral and intravenous administration. Small amounts of further metabolites representing 0.5% to 2% of the dose are also found in urine. Cytochrome P450 (CYP) 2C19 is involved in the demethylation of lacosamide. The relative contribution of other CYP isoforms to lacosamide metabolism is currently not clear.

Population-based pharmacokinetics of lacosamide examined in adults with partial-onset seizures was characterized in a total of 2370 lacosamide plasma concentrations using nonlinear, mixed-effect modeling in two Phase III, double-blind, multicenter, randomized, parallel-group, placebo-controlled trials where subjects received 200, 400, or 600 mg/day lacosamide in divided doses twice daily (15). As a class, inducer antiepileptic medications increased clearance by approximately 36%. Individually, coadministration of the CYP inducers carbamazepine or phenytoin resulted in an approximate decrease in area under the curve by 20%, and coadministration of phenobarbital yielded an approximate 30% decrease. The observed effect of inducer antiepileptic medications on lacosamide exposure was modest. Accordingly, this finding is unlikely to be clinically significant when adding lacosamide to an existing treatment regimen. Furthermore, no significant change in lacosamide PK was seen in CYP2C19 poor metabolizers or following comedication with omeprazole.

INTERACTIONS WITH OTHER DRUGS

Given the pharmacokinetic properties, the probability of drug–drug interactions with lacosamide treatment is likely to be low (7,16). When used at therapeutic concentrations, lacosamide did not have a significant effect on the cytochrome P450 enzyme system. Human hepatocyte showed no potential to induce cytochrome P450 isoforms including 1A2, 2B6, 2C9, 2C19, and 3A4. At 30 times higher than "therapeutic" human plasma concentrations, lacosamide exerted a 60% inhibition of CYP2C19 function. The dosage at which this inhibition would be expected is unlikely to be routinely achieved in the treatment of human epilepsy.

ADVERSE EFFECTS

Animal Toxicology

Single as well as 3-, 6-, and 12-month repeated dose studies in mice, rats, and dogs did not demonstrate adverse effects that persisted after discontinuation of lacosamide. Signs of dose-related toxicity, typically seen with other antiepileptic medication—including ataxia, tremor, and reduced motility—occurred. At high doses, paradoxical convulsions were observed. This supratherapeutic effect was similar to that described for phenytoin, gabapentin, and carbamazepine.

Clinical Adverse Effects

Adverse events were evaluated in 944 subjects randomized to receive either lacosamide 200 mg/day ($n = 270$), 400 mg/day ($n = 471$), or 600 mg/day ($n = 203$), or placebo ($n = 364$) (17). A dose–adverse-effect relationship was seen for frequently reported nervous system and gastrointestinal adverse effects. All patients were on between 1 and 3 other concomitantly administered AEDs, including carbamazepine (35%), lamotrigine (31%), levetiracetam (29%), valproate (24%), topiramate (22%), oxcarbazepine (18%), and phenytoin (14%).

Frequently reported treatment-emergent adverse events are shown in Table 65.2. Other adverse events including peripheral

TABLE 65.2

MOST COMMON TREATMENT-EMERGENT ADVERSE EFFECTS (≥2%) RESULTING IN EARLY DISCONTINUATION

Adverse effects	Placebo ($n = 364$) (%)	LCM 200 mg/day ($n = 270$) (%)	LCM 400 mg/day ($n = 471$) (%)
Dizziness	0.3	0.4	4.2
Vomiting	0.3	0.4	2.3
Diplopia	0.3	1.5	2.1

edema (1%), weight gain (1%), memory impairment (2%), pancreatitis (0.1%), and psychotic disorders (0.2%) were low and generally similar to placebo. Clinically relevant changes in observed laboratory parameters, ECGs, vital signs, or body weight measurements were not seen, although, there was a small, dose-related increase in PR interval. Generally, lacosamide was well tolerated when combined with up to three concomitant antiepileptic medications. Lacosamide has been FDA approved in the United States as a Class V controlled substance. The teratogenic potential of lacosamide has not been defined.

Intravenous Administration

Intravenous administration of lacosamide was studied in a multicenter, double-blind, double-dummy, randomized, inpatient trial evaluating the safety, tolerability, and pharmacokinetics as replacement for oral lacosamide (18). This study utilized patients from an open-label extension trial of oral lacosamide and randomized to either intravenous lacosamide and oral placebo or intravenous placebo and oral lacosamide. Infusions occurred over either 30- or 60-minute time periods. Treatment-emergent adverse events were mild and included dizziness, headache, back pain, somnolence, and injection site pain and were similar to oral lacosamide. There were no significant cardiac/hemodynamic adverse effects noted and there does not appear to be the need for special monitoring of cardiovascular function. Efficacy of the intravenous formulation in partial complex seizures or status epilepticus has not been studied. There have not been clinical trials evaluating lacosamide for status epilepticus. This is not surprising given the very recent availability of an intravenous formulation. Given lacosamide's pharmacokinetic profile, a 1:1 substitution of intravenous to oral dosage has been approved by the Federal Drug Administration. Optimum effective dosage in adults is 200 to 400 mg/day suggesting similar type dosages for intravenous formulation. Case reports of usage in adults with status epilepticus have reported the use of 200 mg administered intravenously over 30 minutes with a subsequent repeat in 30 minutes. However, such recommendations need to be substantiated by carefully designed clinical studies.

CONCLUSION

Lacosamide is a novel anticonvulsant with a favorable pharmacokinetic profile including low protein binding, a long half-life, and good bioavailability that is not affected by food intake. Furthermore, the lack of induction or inhibition of the hepatocyte CYP family renders a low potential for clinically significant drug–drug interactions. Weight neutrality and absent skin rashes, at least in limited studies, are favorable features. Efficacy from pooled analysis indicates target doses of 200 to 400 mg/day are likely to have optimum effect with an acceptable and low adverse effect rate. Clinical use in adults with partial epilepsy suggest that lacosamide be initiated as an adjunctive at 50 mg twice daily with subsequent dose increases on a weekly basis to a target dose of 200 mg/day. Dizziness is the most common adverse event, followed by gastrointestinal disturbances such as nausea and vomiting. The availability of a parenteral formulation has the potential to be useful in the management of acute seizures, although, studies in status epilepticus are still to be performed. Studies in other populations, including pediatrics and the elderly, are also needed to further define the therapeutic spectrum of lacosamide in these populations.

References

1. Beyreuther BK, et al. Lacosamide: a review of preclinical properties. *CNS Drug Rev.* 2007;13(1):21–42.
2. Errington AC, et al. The investigational anticonvulsant lacosamide selectively enhances slow inactivation of voltage-gated sodium channels. *Mol Pharmacol.* 2008;73(1):157–169.
3. Errington AC, et al. Seeking a mechanism of action for the novel anticonvulsant lacosamide. *Neuropharmacology.* 2006;50(8):1016–1029.
4. Brandt C, et al. Effects of the novel antiepileptic drug lacosamide on the development of amygdala kindling in rats. *Epilepsia.* 2006;47(11):1803–1809.
5. Stoehr T, Wasterlain C. Acute and long-term effects of lacosamide in an animal model of status epilepticus. *Epilepsia.* 2008;49(suppl 7):116–117.
6. Ben-Menachem E. Lacosamide: an investigational drug for adjunctive treatment of partial-onset seizures. *Drugs Today (Barc).* 2008;44(1):35–40.
7. Ben-Menachem E, et al. Efficacy and safety of oral lacosamide as adjunctive therapy in adults with partial-onset seizures. *Epilepsia.* 2007;48(7):1308–1317.
8. Rosenfeld WE, et al. Lacosamide efficacy is independent of concomitant AED treatment. *Epilepsia.* 2008;49(suppl 7):451.
9. Sperling M, et al. Early onset of efficacy in the initial weeks of treatment with lacosamide: a pooled analysis of three phase 2/3 trials. *Epilepsia.* 2008;49(suppl 7):457.
10. Rauck RL, et al. Lacosamide in painful diabetic peripheral neuropathy: a phase 2 double-blind placebo-controlled study. *Clin J Pain.* 2007;23(2):150–158.
11. Biton V. Lacosamide for the treatment of diabetic neuropathic pain. *Expert Rev Neurother.* 2008;8(11):1649–1660.
12. Doty P, et al. Lacosamide. *Neurotherapeutics.* 2007;4(1):145–148.
13. Cawello W, et al. Food does not affect the pharmacokinetics of SPM 927. *Epilepsia.* 2004;45(suppl 7):307.
14. Bialer M, et al. Progress report on new antiepileptic drugs: a summary of the Eighth Eilat Conference (EILAT VIII). *Epilepsy Res.* 2007;73(1):1–52.
15. Brunhild N, et al. Population pharmacokinetics of lacosamide in subjects with partial-onset seizures: results from two phase III trials. *Epilepsia.* 2008;49(suppl 7):337–475.
16. Thomas D, Scharfenecker U, Nickel B, Doty P, et al. Lacosamide has a low potential for drug-drug interaction. *Epilepsia.* 2007;60:227.
17. Rosenfeld W, et al. Lacosamide: an interim evaluation of long-term safety and efficacy as oral adjunctive therapy in subjects with partial-onset seizures. *Epilepsia.* 2007;48(48):318–319.
18. Biton V, et al. Intravenous lacosamide as replacement for oral lacosamide in patients with partial-onset seizures. *Epilepsia.* 2008;49(3):418–424.

CHAPTER 66 ■ ADRENOCORTICOTROPIN AND STEROIDS

CRISTINA Y. GO AND ORLANDO CARTER SNEAD III

HISTORICAL BACKGROUND

In 1950, Klein and Livingston (1) reported on the efficacy of adrenocorticotropin (ACTH) therapy for childhood seizures after observing its benefits in various types of intractable generalized seizures. Eight years later, Sorel and Dusaucy-Bauloye (2) reported control of seizures and an improvement in electroencephalographic (EEG) findings for children with infantile spasms treated with the drug. The benefit of oral steroids in this condition was established soon after that of ACTH (3–7), and since then, both drugs have been used in a number of other epilepsy syndromes, including Ohtahara syndrome, Lennox–Gastaut syndrome, other myoclonic epilepsies, and Landau–Kleffner syndrome.

ACTH and steroid therapy uniquely affect epilepsy syndromes that have an age-related onset during a critical period of brain development that can cause a characteristic regression or plateau of acquired developmental milestones at seizure onset and subsequent long-term cognitive impairment. For some of these patients, ACTH or steroids, or both, can improve the short-term developmental trajectory and the long-term prognosis for language and cognitive development, in addition to the beneficial effects on the convulsive state (8–13).

INFANTILE SPASMS

General Considerations

In 1841, Dr. William West wrote a letter to Lancet in which he described an unusual condition affecting his 4-month-old son, James, as a peculiar form of infantile convulsions (14). He went on to describe a reduction in developmental trajectory in his child that was normal prior to the onset of the event. This letter, now over 160 years old, remains the most eloquent clinical description of what we now know as infantile spasms.

In 1952, Gibbs and Gibbs described the classical interictal EEG pattern associated with this condition, called hypsarrhythmia, which is characterized by high-voltage chaotic slowing with multifocal spikes and marked asynchrony (15). The term West syndrome refers to an age-related triad of epileptic spasms, developmental regression, and hypsarrhythmia on EEG. Although this term has been used synonymously with infantile spasms, the latter should refer strictly to the massive myoclonus because infantile spasms may occur in the absence of either mental retardation or the hypsarrhythmia EEG pattern.

Published studies on the efficacy of ACTH and corticosteroids in infantile spasms display considerable variability in design, complicating the establishment of research-based recommendations for optimal treatment (16–18). A few observations are generally accepted. The cumulative spontaneous remission rate over the first 12 months of seizures is about 25% (19). Seizures are almost always intractable to treatment with traditional anticonvulsant drugs. ACTH or oral steroid therapy should significantly reduce seizures in 50% to 75% of patients, but ACTH protocols, particularly those employing high-dose, long-acting synthetic formulations, are associated with a significantly high rate of side effects (20,21). The best chance for a treatment response is probably between 4 and 12 months of age in children who are neurologically normal when spasms begin that have no demonstrable cause (11,12,20,22–24). The ultimate prognosis is dismal for most patients and depends heavily on the cause of the spasms, preexisting neurologic and developmental status, the presence or absence of other seizures concomitant with the spasms, and the patient's age at seizure onset (8,12,20,25–28).

The controversies surrounding the management of infantile spasms continue to outnumber the areas of agreement. Which is the most effective therapy: ACTH or steroids; other medical treatment including the ketogenic diet; other anticonvulsants such as vigabatrin, valproic acid, benzodiazepines, topiramate, zonisamide, or levetiracetam; pyridoxine; some or all of these in combination? What is the impact of treatment with ACTH compared with steroids, the ketogenic diet, or anticonvulsants on the long-term outcome in recurrence of spasms, evolution into other forms of intractable epilepsy, and cognitive or behavioral function? Does treatment change the outcome for a patient with preexisting mental retardation and a structurally abnormal brain? What is the optimal dosage of these drugs, and how long should the treatment last? Does the ultimate outcome depend on timing of treatment? Does the efficacy of ACTH depend on the formulation (natural vs. synthetic, sustained release vs. short acting)? More than 160 years after this syndrome was described by Dr. West, most of these questions remain unanswered.

Mechanisms of Action

The pathogenesis of infantile spasms and therefore the mechanisms of action of ACTH and steroids in this condition are unknown, principally because of a paucity of valid animal model for this disorder is lacking (29–32). Infantile spasms is an epileptic syndrome that begins in infancy within a narrow range of ages, with initial onset mostly between 3 and 7 months of life in more than 50% of cases. Various abnormalities have been causally linked (symptomatic cases); however, infantile spasms may also occur without apparent cause (idiopathic and cryptogenic cases). The effect of ACTH and corticosteroids is frequently all or nothing and the steroid-induced seizure-free state is often sustainable even after drug withdrawal. These observations support the theory that the developing brain experiences a significant stress response to various etiologies that results in this age-dependent epileptic encephalopathy. Within this very narrow developmental window, ACTH and steroids may be able to reset the deranged homeostatic mechanisms of the brain, thereby reducing the convulsive tendency and improving the developmental trajectory.

The Brain–Adrenal Axis

Evidence suggests that the effects of ACTH on infantile spasms may be independent of steroidogenesis (33,34). Efficacy studies have demonstrated the superiority of ACTH to corticosteroids in treating infantile spasms and its efficacy in adrenal-suppressed patients (35–38). Substantial physiologic and pharmacologic data indicate that ACTH has direct effects on brain function: increasing dendrite outsprouting in immature animals (39); stimulating myelination (40); regulating the synthesis, release, uptake, and metabolism of dopamine, norepinephrine, acetylcholine, serotonin, and γ-aminobutyric acid; regulating the binding at glutamatergic, serotonergic, muscarinic type 1, opiate, and dopaminergic receptors (41,42); and altering neuronal membrane lipid fluidity, permeability, and signal transduction (39). These neurobiologic effects can influence synaptic function and neurotransmission and may reside in fragments of the peptide devoid of corticotropic activity.

Baram and colleagues (37,43,44) proposed the important role of corticotropin-releasing hormone (CRH) in the pathogenesis of infantile spasms as well as its response to ACTH. The hypothesis is that diverse etiologies resulting in infantile spasms cause activation of the brain's stress response, leading to excessive release of CRH. CRH is an excitatory neuromodulator, with potent age-specific convulsant effects demonstrated in animal models. In immature brains, CRH can cause neuronal hyperexcitability, seizures and neuronal death in the amygdala and hippocampus (45,46). High brain CRH levels can decrease ACTH levels due to desensitization of CRH receptors after chronic activation, which then decreases ACTH release. Low ACTH levels have been found in the cerebrospinal fluid of children with infantile spasms (45,47).

ACTH has a down-regulatory effect on CRH by reducing CRH gene expression in specific brain regions, an effect demonstrated in the absence of adrenal steroids and achieved only with the use of only the 4 to 10 fragment of ACTH, which does not release adrenal steroids (37). Melanocortin-receptor antagonists blocked this effect, suggesting that these are the targets of ACTH action (37).

By suppressing CRH expression, possibly through the action of peptide fragments of ACTH on melanocortin receptors, neuronal hyperexcitability may be reduced, ameliorating infantile spasms. Indirect evidence to support this hypothesis was reported recently by Liu et al., who found that genetic variants in the central melanocortin-4-receptor promoter are associated with the development of infantile spasms and

influence treatment response to ACTH in children with infantile spasms (48). Clinical trials of ACTH fragments without activity on adrenals have yielded disappointing results (49,50), but these studies used the 4 to 9 rather than 4 to 10 peptide fragment studied in animal models (37).

Efficacy and Dosage

Table 66.1 lists the different preparations of depot corticotrophin. The biologic activity, expressed in international units (IU), permits a comparison of potency but represents the relative ability of the peptide to stimulate the adrenals and may not reflect its ability to affect brain function. The biologic activity of natural ACTH in the brain may differ from that of synthetic ACTH (12) as a result of ACTH fragments and possibly other pituitary hormones with neurobiologic activity in the brain that are present in the pituitary extracts. These compounds could enhance the therapeutic efficacy of natural ACTH (51). Any differences in the biologic effects of sustained ACTH levels provided by the depot formulations, as opposed to those of the short-acting preparations, are unknown. Given in high doses, however, long-acting depot preparations are associated with an increased incidence of severe side effects, including death from overwhelming infection (21).

Although most efficacy studies of ACTH and steroids are retrospective, an expanding body of prospective data is available (12,27,52–62). Most published literature supports the hypothesis that the natural ACTH 1 to 39 peptide (p-ACTH) is superior to oral steroids. In randomized, controlled trials, spasms ceased in 42% to 87% of children treated with ACTH, compared with 29% to 33% of children treated with prednisone (46–50). In these studies, the relapse rates were 15% to 31% for ACTH and 29% to 33% for prednisone. Based on these and other data, the current American Academy of Neurology Practice Parameter for the medical treatment of infantile spasms has concluded that ACTH is probably an effective agent in the short-term treatment of infantile spasms (16).

TABLE 66.1

PREPARATIONS OF DEPOT CORTICOTROPIN

Preparation	Biologic activity (100 IU)[a] equivalent to	Duration of action (hr)
Short-acting forms		
Corticotropin (ACTH 1–39)—porcine pituitary extract		
Acthar gel, 80 IU/mL	0.72 mg	24–48
ACTH-carboxymethyl-cellulose	Not available	~24
Cosyntropin/tetracosactin (ACTH 1–24)—synthetic		
Cortrosyn	1.0 mg	~24
Long-acting forms		
Cosyntropin/tetracosactin (ACTH 1–24)—synthetic		
Synacthen-zinc	2.5 mg	~72
Cortrosyn-Z	2.5 mg	~72

[a]Commercial preparations are described in international units (IU), based on a potency assay in hypophysectomized rats in which depletion of adrenal ascorbic acid is measured after subcutaneous ACTH injection.

Most institutions have their own treatment protocol for infantile spasms, with a wide variety of dose and duration (63–65). The most effective dose and duration of treatment with p-ACTH for remission of infantile spasms continues to be a controversial issue. Compared to prednisone, no major advantage was demonstrated by low doses of ACTH, whereas high doses were superior (55,56). High-dose p-ACTH at 60 IU/day or 150 IU/m^2/day has produced excellent short-term response rates of 87% to 93% in prospective studies (55,60). In the only randomized, prospective comparison of p-ACTH, however, Hrachovy and associates (57) found no difference between high-dose and low-dose therapy. A prospective study using synthetic ACTH (59) by Yanagaki and associates compared very-low-dose (0.2 IU/kg/day) and low-dose (1 IU/kg/day) ACTH and found equivalent efficacy, with response and relapse rates comparable to those in other studies. Describing a stepwise increase in dosage, Heiskala and colleagues (62) demonstrated that while some patients can be controlled on lower doses of carboxymethyl-cellulose ACTH (3 IU/kg/day), others required high doses (12 IU/kg/day). Spasms were controlled initially in 65% of patients, but the relapse rate was high.

Although there are some data suggesting that a good response to ACTH appears to be associated with better long-term outcome (24), the evidence is not rigorous (16). Similarly, while some evidence supports high-dose ACTH over low-dose ACTH or oral steroids in cognitive outcome (9,11), the data are contradictory and not Class I. Glaze and colleagues (52) found no difference between low-dose p-ACTH (20 to 30 IU/day) and prednisone (2 mg/kg/day). In a comparison of high-dose p-ACTH (110 IU/m^2/day) and steroids, however, Lombroso (12) showed a higher rate of normal cognitive outcome in cryptogenic patients treated with ACTH than in those treated with prednisone alone (55% vs. 17%). In a retrospective comparison of different ACTH dosage regimens (66), Ito and coworkers also noted a positive correlation between dose and developmental outcome.

Although some data support high-dose ACTH as being more effective than low-dose ACTH, the precise dosage and duration are undetermined. The optimal dose may lie between 50 and 200 IU/m^2/day. Doses of 400 IU/m^2/day or higher are contraindicated because of a high incidence of life-threatening side effects (20,21,66).

Adverse Effects

ACTH and steroids, particularly at the high doses recommended for infantile spasms, can produce dangerous side effects. These are more frequent and more pronounced with ACTH. In prospective controlled trials, cushingoid features and extreme irritability were seen frequently; hypertension, while less common, was associated with higher doses (56–59). Vigilance is required for signs of sepsis, pneumonia, glucosuria, metabolic abnormalities involving the electrolytes calcium and phosphorus (67–69), and congestive heart failure (70,71). Of five deaths reported in prospective studies, at least two were directly attributable to ACTH (12,61).

Cerebral ventriculomegaly (56,72–76), which is not always reversible (52), can lead to subdural hematoma (77,78). The cause of the apparent cerebral atrophy is obscure, but its existence emphasizes the importance of diagnostic neuroimaging before initiation of ACTH.

Because hypothalamic–pituitary or adrenocortical dysfunction can result from ACTH therapy (79,80), morning levels of cortisol should be monitored during a taper and any medical stress treated with high-dose steroids (81). Treatment with ACTH or steroids can also be immunosuppressant and associated with infectious complications, perhaps as a result of impaired function of polymorphonuclear leukocytes (82). Both agents are therefore contraindicated in the face of serious bacterial or viral infection such as varicella or cytomegalovirus. Because of the high rate of fatal *Pneumocystis* pneumonia as an infectious complication of ACTH therapy (20,83–85), prophylaxis with trimethoprim–sulfamethoxazole, accompanied by folate supplementation and frequent blood counts, may be prudent in infants older than 2 months of age. In rare cases, ACTH can exacerbate seizures (86,87).

Vigabatrin versus Adrenocorticotropin

The current American Academy of Neurology Practice Parameter for the medical treatment of infantile spasms has concluded that vigabatrin is possibly an effective agent in the short-term treatment of infantile spasms (16). Based on data from randomized controlled trials, from 23% to 65% of children treated with vigabatrin achieve short-term remission of infantile spasms, with relapse rates of 4% to 20% (18,58,88–90).

Although vigabatrin is thought to be particularly effective against infantile spasms associated with tuberous sclerosis (58,91,92) and is frequently advocated as a first-line therapy for this disorder, the data supporting this are retrospective (16). Limiting its use is the characteristic concentric constriction of visual fields. This effect does occur in childhood, and the risk may be cumulative with longer duration of therapy (93–97). The incidence in very young children is not known, and perimetric testing is often impossible in this group. Electrophysiologic studies in infants, although not as sensitive as perimetry, have confirmed vigabatrin-associated abnormalities (96–99). Vigabatrin may have a place as a short-term treatment, although its safety remains uncertain.

Other Agents in Infantile Spasms

Valproate (100,101), nitrazepam (102), pyridoxine (103), felbamate (104), intravenous immunoglobulin (105), topiramate (106), zonisamide (107), ganaxolone (108), levetiracetam (109), and the ketogenic diet (110,111) have been studied in small uncontrolled trials. However, there is insufficient evidence of efficacy and safety to recommend any of these therapies at this time.

Recommended Protocols for Adrenocorticotropin

The optimal dose of ACTH required to enhance short-term response and long-term cognitive outcome is unknown; however, relatively high doses given early in the disease, accompanied by a second course in the event of relapse, appear warranted. The following high-dose ACTH regimen that has been used successfully in more than 500 children (55,60,112) is recommended (Table 66.2). A suggested protocol using synacthen (cosyntropin or tetracosactide) based on the study

TABLE 66.2

PROTOCOL FOR ACTH THERAPY FOR INFANTILE SPASMS

Initial assessment before therapy begins

    History and physical examination including Wood's light

    EEG with pyridoxine injection

    Blood counts, routine blood chemical analysis, urinalysis including glucose, and thyroid
       and adrenal function tests

    Electrocardiogram

    Magnetic resonance imaging of brain

    Family counseling and education for administration and monitoring of side effects

Clinical monitoring during ACTH therapy

    Blood pressure and urine dipstick for glucose: daily first week, then thrice weekly

    Blood counts, routine blood chemical analysis weekly first month, then fortnightly

    EEG once during and after therapy and as indicated

    Provide family with letter describing treatment and prompting urgent assessment in case
      of fever or other signs of infection

High-dose schedule for ACTH[a]

Week 1	150 IU/m^2/day IM, two divided doses
Week 2	75 IU/m^2/day IM, single daily dose
Reassess	If spasms stop and hypsarrhythmia resolves, continue with taper; if no clinical or EEG response, change ACTH lot or select alternative therapy and taper ACTH as appropriate
Week 3	75 IU/m^2/day IM, alternate days
Week 4	60 IU/m^2/day IM, alternate days
Week 5	50 IU/m^2/day IM, alternate days
Week 6	40 IU/m^2/day IM, alternate days
Week 7	30 IU/m^2/day IM, alternate days
Week 8	20 IU/m^2/day IM, alternate days
Week 9	10 IU/m^2/day IM, alternate days
Week 10	5 IU/m^2/day IM, alternate days, then stop ACTH

Lower-dose schedule for ACTH

Weeks 1 and 2	40 IU/day

If response is complete: taper ACTH over 1–4 months

If response is incomplete: increase to 60–80 IU/day over 1–2 weeks

If response remains incomplete: taper ACTH and try other medications

Suggested schedule for Synacthen (cosyntropin) in infantile spasms

Week number	Date of injection	Dose given intramuscularly
Week 1	Day 1	1.9 mg/m^2
	Day 3	1.9 mg/m^2
	Day 5	1.9 mg/m^2
	Day 7	1.9 mg/m^2
Week 2	Day 9	0.94 mg/m^2
	Day 11	0.94 mg/m^2
	Day 13	0.94 mg/m^2

Reassess after 2 weeks; responders will finish protocol on the following taper schedule

Week 3	Day 15	0.94 mg/m^2
	Day 17	0.94 mg/m^2
	Day 19	0.94 mg/m^2
	Day 21	0.94 mg/m^2
Week 4	Day 23	0.94 mg/m^2
	Day 25	0.94 mg/m^2
	Day 27	0.94 mg/m^2

(continued)

TABLE 66.2

PROTOCOL FOR ACTH THERAPY FOR INFANTILE SPASMS (*continued*)

Week number	Date of injection	Dose given intramuscularly
Week 5	Day 29	0.75 mg/m^2
	Day 31	0.75 mg/m^2
	Day 33	0.75 mg/m^2
	Day 35	0.75 mg/m^2
Week 6	Day 37	0.75 mg/m^2
	Day 39	0.75 mg/m^2
	Day 41	0.75 mg/m^2
Week 7	Day 43	0.63 mg/m^2
	Day 45	0.63 mg/m^2
	Day 47	0.63 mg/m^2
	Day 49	0.63 mg/m^2
Week 8	Day 51	0.5 mg/m^2
	Day 53	0.5 mg/m^2
	Day 55	0.5 mg/m^2
Week 9	Day 57	0.38 mg/m^2
	Day 59	0.38 mg/m^2
	Day 61	0.38 mg/m^2
Week 10	Day 63	0.25 mg/m^2
	Day 65	0.25 mg/m^2
	Day 67	0.25 mg/m^2
	Day 69	0.25 mg/m^2
Week 11	Day 71	0.13 mg/m^2
	Day 73	0.13 mg/m^2
	Day 75	0.13 mg/m^2
	Day 77	0.13 mg/m^2
Week 12	Day 79	0.06 mg/m^2
	Day 81	0.06 mg/m^2
	Day 83	0.06 mg/m^2, then stop ACTH

[a]This protocol developed and used at the Hospital for Sick Children, Toronto, Ontario.

done by Snead and colleagues (60) with 0.25 mg of synacthen equivalent to 25 units of corticotropin is also included.

The child is admitted to a daycare unit for initiation therapy. Parents are taught to administer the injection, measure urine glucose three times daily with Chemstix, and recognize spasms so as to keep an accurate seizure calendar. Any diagnostic workup indicated by clinical circumstances is also performed, including screening for occult infections. Before ACTH is started, an endocrine profile, complete blood count, urinalysis, electrolyte panel, baseline renal function tests, and calcium, phosphorus, and serum glucose levels are obtained. Blood pressure is measured and an electrocardiogram performed. The drug is not given if any of these studies show abnormal results. Diagnostic neuroimaging is indicated before initiation of ACTH or steroids because of the association with ventriculomegaly.

The initial dose of ACTH is 150 IU/m^2/day of ACTH gel, 80 IU/mL, intramuscularly in two divided doses for 1 week. In the second week, 75 IU/m^2/day is given, followed by 75 IU/m^2 every other day in the third week. Over the next 6 weeks, the dose is gradually tapered. The lot number of the ACTH gel is carefully recorded. Usually, a response is seen within the first 7 days; if within 2 weeks no response is noted or a steroid effect is evident, the lot is changed.

Blood pressure must be measured daily at home during the first week and three times weekly thereafter. Control of hypertension is attempted with salt restriction and amlodipine therapy rather than discontinuation of ACTH. The patient is monitored in the outpatient clinic weekly for the first month and then biweekly, with appropriate blood work at each visit. Waking and sleeping EEG patterns are obtained during and after the start of ACTH to assess treatment response. Because a response is usually noted within a week or two of initiating ACTH (54,55,57), positive results are suggested when properly trained parents report no seizures in a child whose waking and sleeping EEG patterns are normal.

If relapse occurs, the dose may be increased to the previously effective dose for 2 weeks and another tapering begun. If seizures continue, the dose may be increased to 150 IU/m^2/day and the regimen restarted.

Recommended Protocols for Prednisone

If prednisone is chosen because of its oral formulation and lower incidence of serious side effects, the pretreatment laboratory evaluation described earlier is performed. The initial dose is 3 mg/kg/day in four divided doses for 2 weeks, followed by a 10-week taper (112). A multiple daily dose regimen of high-dose ACTH therapy is recommended to produce sustained elevations of plasma cortisol (54,60).

OTHER SEIZURE DISORDERS

Ohtahara and Lennox–Gastaut syndromes are believed to represent earlier and later manifestations, respectively, of a spectrum of infantile epileptic encephalopathies that include infantile spasms (113–116). These conditions respond poorly to traditional anticonvulsant drug therapies but are sometimes improved by the antiepileptic drugs used in infantile spasms: ACTH, steroids, benzodiazepines, and valproic acid. ACTH of steroids also may be beneficial in Landau–Kleffner syndrome.

Ohtahara Syndrome

Also known as early infantile epileptic encephalopathy, Ohtahara syndrome is characterized by spasms beginning within the first 3 months of life associated with persistent burst suppression on the EEG in all stages of the sleep–wake cycle (113). Despite reports of improvement after ACTH (113,117), vigabatrin (118), and zonisamide (113), the long-term prognosis usually is unchanged by any treatment (113,115) and involves high mortality and severely handicapped survivors. If used, ACTH should be administered as described for infantile spasms.

Lennox–Gastaut Syndrome and Other Myoclonic Disorders

ACTH and steroids have been found useful in younger children with various combinations of severe and intractable seizures, particularly atypical absence, myoclonic, tonic, and atonic seizures (1,38,112,119–124). This group includes patients with Lennox–Gastaut syndrome, a disorder characterized by mental retardation, generalized slow spike-and-wave discharges, intractable atypical absence, myoclonus, and frequent ictal falls. Several uncontrolled, retrospective studies suggest that ACTH is superior to oral steroids against these seizure types (113,119,121,122), and the regimen described in this chapter for ACTH or prednisone is recommended. Nevertheless, ACTH and steroids should be reserved for the most severe and intractable disease. Usually, the best result is temporary relief, because 70% to 90% of patients with multiple seizure types suffer a relapse during the ACTH taper (112).

In another age-dependent disorder first described by Doose (125), myoclonic astatic seizures begin between 7 months and 6 years of age in a previously normal child and are associated with generalized discharges on the EEG (126). This disorder is resistant to most conventional antiepileptic drugs; however, a retrospective study has reported response to the ketogenic diet, ACTH, and ethosuximide (126).

Landau–Kleffner Syndrome and Related Disorders

Described in 1957 (127), Landau–Kleffner syndrome, also known as acquired epileptic aphasia, is characterized by regression in receptive and expressive language associated with epileptic seizures. The usual presentation occurs between the ages of 2 and 8 years. Clinical seizures may precede, be coincident with, or develop after the onset of language deterioration, and up to 25% of patients with language loss and epileptiform EEG patterns never experience clinical seizures (128,129). Behavioral disturbances are frequent, ranging from hyperactivity and aggressiveness to autism and global cognitive deterioration. Some children display sustained agnosia and mutism; others show a waxing and waning course that parallels the EEG changes; still others demonstrate spontaneous resolution (129). The EEG typically shows 1- to 3-Hz high-amplitude spike and slow waves; these may be unilateral, bilateral, unifocal, or multifocal but often include the temporal region, with or without parietal and occipital involvement, and are activated in sleep (130).

Valproate and benzodiazepines may control the syndrome's clinical seizures but have only a partial and transient effect on the EEG abnormalities (10,131). In 1974, McKinney and McGreal described the beneficial effect of ACTH on the characteristic seizures, language regression, and behavioral change (132). Since then, although no controlled prospective trials of ACTH or steroids have been published, case reports and retrospective series have demonstrated improvements in seizure control and language in children treated with varying ACTH or corticosteroid regimens (10,129–131,133–135).

The use of ACTH or corticosteroids in patients with Landau–Kleffner syndrome appears justified; however, further study of dose and duration of therapy is warranted, as is exploration of new anticonvulsants. High-dose ACTH or prednisone, as described in this chapter for infantile spasms, may be useful, with a longer tapering schedule and concomitant use of valproic acid.

References

1. Klein R, Livingston S. The effect of adrencorticotrophic hormone in epilepsy. *J Pediatr.* 1950;37:733–742.
2. Sorel L, Dusaucy-Bauloye A. A propos de cas d'hypsarythmia de Gibbs: son traitement spectulaire par l'ACTH. *Acta Neurol Belg.* 1958;58:130–141.
3. Dumermuth G. Über die Blitz-Nick-Salaam-Krämpfe und ihre Behandlung mit ACTH und Hydrocortison. *Mitt Helv Pediatr Acta.* 1959;14:250–270.
4. Gastaut H, Salfiel J, Raybaud C, et al. A propos du traitement par l'ACTH des encéphalites myoclonique de la première enfance avec majeure (hypsarythmie). *Pediatrie.* 1959;14:35–45.
5. Low N. Infantile spasms with mental retardation, I: treatment with cortisone and adrenocorticotrophin. *Pediatrics.* 1958;22:1165–1169.
6. McQuarrie I, Anderson JA, Ziegler RR. Observations on the antagonistic effects of posterior pituitary and cortico-adrenal hormones in the epileptic subject. *J Clin Endocrinol.* 1942;2:406–410.
7. Stamps FW, Gibbs EL, Rosenthal IM, et al. Treatment of hypsarrhythmia with ACTH. *JAMA.* 1959;171:408–411.
8. Koo B, Hwang P, Logan W. Infantile spasms: outcome and prognostic factors of cryptogenic and symptomatic groups. *Neurology.* 1993;43:2322–2327.
9. Lerman P, Kivity S. The efficacy of corticotropin in primary infantile spasms. *J Pediatr.* 1982;101:294–296.
10. Marescaux C, Hirsch E, Finck S, et al. Landau–Kleffner syndrome: a pharmacologic study of five cases. *Epilepsia.* 1990;31:768–777.
11. Sher PK, Sheikh MR. Therapeutic efficacy of ACTH in symptomatic infantile spasms with hypsarrhythmia. *Pediatr Neurol.* 1993;9:451–456.
12. Lombroso C. A prospective study of infantile spams: clinical and therapeutic correlations. *Epilepsia.* 1983;24:135–158.
13. Kivity S, Lerman P, Ariel R, et al. Long-term cognitive outcomes of a cohort of children with cryptogenic infantile spasms treated with high-dose adrenocorticotropic hormone. *Epilepsia.* 2004;45:255–262.
14. West W. On a peculiar form of infantile convulsions. *Lancet.* 1841;1:724–725.
15. Gibbs FA, Gibbs EL. *Atlas of Electroencephalography, II: Epilepsy.* Cambridge, MA: Addison-Wesley; 1952.

16. MacKay MT, Weiss SK, Adams-Webber T, et al. Practice parameter: medical treatment of infantile spasms: report of the American Academy of Neurology and the Child Neurology Society. *Neurology.* 2004;62:1668–1681.
17. Hancock EC, Osbourne JP, Edwards SW. Treatment of infantile spasms. *Cochrane Database Syst Rev.* 2008;(4):CD001770.
18. Lux AL, Edwards SW, Hancock E, et al. The United Kingdom infantile spasms study comparing Vigabatrin with prednisolone or tetracosactide at 14 days: a multicentre, randomized controlled trial. *Lancet.* 2004;364: 1773–1778.
19. Hrachovy RA, Glaze DG, Frost JD. A retrospective study of spontaneous remission and long-term outcome in patients with infantile spasms. *Epilepsia.* 1991;32:212–214.
20. Riikonen R. A long-term follow-up study of 214 children with the syndrome of infantile spasms. *Neuropediatrics.* 1982;13:14–23.
21. Riikonen R, Donner M. ACTH therapy in infantile spasms: side effects. *Arch Dis Child.* 1980;55:664–672.
22. Chevrie J, Aicardi J. Le prognostic psychique des spasms infantiles traités par l'ACTH ou les cortocoides. Analyse statistique de 78 cas suivis plus d'un an. *J Neurol Sci.* 1971;12:351–368.
23. Jeavons PM, Bower BD, Dimitrakoudi M. Long-term prognosis of 150 cases of "West syndrome." *Epilepsia.* 1973;14:153–164.
24. Riikonen R. Long-term outcome of West syndrome: a study of adults with a history of infantile spasms. *Epilepsia.* 1996;37:367–372.
25. Dulac O, Plouin P, Jambaque I, et al. Benign epileptic infantile spasms. *Rev Electroencephalogr Neurophysiol Clin.* 1986;16:371–382.
26. Favata I, Leuzzi V, Curalto P. Mental outcome in West syndrome: prognostic value of some clinical factors. *J Ment Defic Res.* 1987;31:9–15.
27. Nolte R, Christen HJ, Doerrer J. Preliminary report of a multi-center study on the West syndrome. *Brain Dev.* 1988;10:236–244.
28. Pollack MA, Zion TE, Kellaway PR. Long term prognosis of patients with infantile spasms following ACTH therapy. *Epilepsia.* 1979;20:255–260.
29. Snead OC III. Neuropeptides and infantile spasms: search for an animal model. In: Porter R, ed. *Advances in Epileptology: XVth Epilepsy International Symposium.* New York: Raven Press; 1984:193–196.
30. Lee CL, Frost JD, Swann JW, et al. A new animal model of infantile spasms with unprovoked persistent seizures. *Epilepsia.* 2008;49:298–307.
31. Vilisek L, Jehle K, Asche S, et al. Model of infantile spasms induced by N-methyl-D-aspartic acid in prenatally impaired brain. *Ann Neurol.* 2007; 61:109–119.
32. Cortez MA, Shjen L, Wu Y, et al. Infantile spasms and Down syndrome: a new animal model. *Pediatr Res.* 2009;65:499–503.
33. Bornstein SR, Engeland WC, Erhart-Bornstein M, et al. Dissociation of ACTH and glucocoticoids. *Trends Endocrinol Metab.* 2008;19:175–180.
34. Jaseja H. A plausible explanation for superiority of adrenocorticotrophic hormone (ACTH) over oral corticosteroids in the treatment of infantile spasms (West syndrome). *Med Hypotheses.* 2006;67:721–724.
35. Crosley CJ, Richman RA, Thorpy MJ. Evidence for cortisol-independent anticonvulsant activity of adrenocorticotropic hormone in infantile spasms. *Ann Neurol.* 1980;8:220.
36. Farwell J, Milstein J, Opheim K, et al. Adrenocorticotropic hormone controls infantile spasms independently of cortisol stimulation. *Epilepsia.* 1984;25:605–608.
37. Brunson K, Khan N, Eghbal-Ahmadi M, et al. Corticotropin (ACTH) acts directly on amygdala neurons to down-regulate corticotropin-releasing hormone gene expression. *Ann Neurol.* 2001;49:304–312.
38. Willig RP, Lagenstein I, Iffland E. Cortisoltagesprofile unter ACTH und Dexamethason-Therapie fruhkindlicher Anfalle (BNS- und Lennox-Syndrom). *Monatsschr Kinderheilk.* 1977;126:191–197.
39. Pranzatelli MR. On the molecular mechanism of adrenocorticotrophic hormone in the CNS: neurotransmitters and receptors. *Exp Neurol.* 1994; 125:142–161.
40. Palo J, Savolainen H. The effect of high dose synthetic ACTH on rat brain. *Brain Res.* 1974;70:313–320.
41. Pranzatelli MR. In vivo and in vitro effects of adrenocorticotropic hormone on serotonin receptors in neonatal rat brain. *Dev Pharmacol Ther.* 1989; 12:49–56.
42. Kendall DA, McEwen BS, Enne SJ. The influence of ACTH and corticosterone on ^{3}[H]GABA receptor binding in rat brain. *Brain Res.* 1982;236:365–374.
43. Baram TZ. Pathophysiology of massive infantile spasms: perspective on the putative role of the brain adrenal axis. *Ann Neurol.* 1993;33:231–236.
44. Brunson KL, Avishai-Eliner S, Baram TZ. ACTH treatment of infantile spasms: mechanisms of its effects in modulation of neuronal excitability. *Int Rev Neurobiol.* 2002;49:185–197.
45. Baram TZ, Mitchell WG, Snead OC III, et al. Brain-adrenal axis hormones are altered in CSF of infants with massive infantile spasms. *Neurology.* 1992;42:1171–1175.
46. Baram TZ, Hirsch E, Snead OC III, et al. Corticotropin-releasing hormone-induced seizures in infant rats originate in the amygdala. *Ann Neurol.* 1992;31:488–494.
47. Nagamitsu S, Matsuishi T, Yamashita Y, et al. Decreased cerebrospinal fluid levels of β-endorphin and ACTH in children with infantile spasms. *J Neural Transm.* 2001;108:363–371.
48. Liu ZL, He B, Fang F, et al. Analysis of single nucleotide polymorphisms in the melanocortin-4-receptor promoter in infantile spasms. *Neuropediatrics.* 2007;28:304–309.
49. Pentella K, Bachman DS, Sandman CA. Trial of an ACTH 4-9 analog (ORG 2766) in children with intractable seizures. *Neuropediatrics.* 1982; 13:59–62.
50. Willig RP, Lagenstein I. Use of ACTH fragments in children with intractable seizures. *Neuropediatrics.* 1982;13:55–58.
51. Snead OC III, Chiron C. Medical management. In: Dulac O, Chugani HT, Dalla Bernadina B, eds. *Infantile Spasms and West Syndrome.* London: WB Saunders; 1994:244–256.
52. Glaze DG, Hrachovy RA, Forst JD, et al. Prospective study of outcome of infants with infantile spasms treated during controlled studies of ACTH and prednisone. *J Pediatr.* 1988;112:389–396.
53. Hrachovy RA, Frost JD, Kellaway PR, et al. A controlled study of prednisone therapy in infantile spasms. *Epilepsia.* 1979;20:403–407.
54. Hrachovy RA, Frost JD, Kellaway PR, et al. A controlled study of ACTH therapy in infantile spasms. *Epilepsia.* 1980;21:631–636.
55. Baram TZ, Mitchell WG, Tournay A, et al. High-dose corticotropin (ACTH) versus prednisone for infantile spasms: a prospective, randomized, blinded study. *Pediatrics.* 1996;97:375–379.
56. Hrachovy RA, Forst JD, Kellaway PR, et al. Double-blind study of ACTH vs. prednisone therapy in infantile spasms. *J Pediatr.* 1983;103:641–645.
57. Hrachovy RA, Frost JD, Glaze DG. High dose, long duration vs. low dose, short duration corticotropin therapy in infantile spasms. *J Pediatr.* 1994; 124:803–806.
58. Vivegano F, Cilio MR. Vigabatrin versus ACTH as first-line treatment for infantile spasms: a randomized, prospective study. *Epilepsia.* 1997;38: 1270–1274.
59. Yanagaki S, Oguni H, Hayashi K, et al. A comparative study of high-dose and low-dose ACTH therapy for West syndrome. *Brain Dev.* 1999;21: 461–467.
60. Snead OC III, Benton JW, Hosey LC, et al. Treatment of infantile spasms with high-dose ACTH: efficacy and plasma levels of ACTH and cortisol. *Neurology.* 1989;39:1027–1031.
61. Kusse MC, van Nieuwenhuizen O, van Huffelen AC, et al. The effect of non-depot ACTH (1-24) on infantile spasms. *Dev Med Child Neurol.* 1993;35:1067–1073.
62. Heiskala H, Riikonen R, Santavuori P, et al. West syndrome: individualized ACTH therapy. *Brain Dev.* 1996;18:456–460.
63. Bobele GB, Bedensteiner JB. The treatment of infantile spasms by child neurologists. *J Child Neurol.* 1994;9:432–435.
64. Appleton RE. The treatment of infantile spasms by paediatric neurologists in the UK and Ireland. *Dev Med Child Neurol.* 1996;38:278–279.
65. Ito M, Seki T, Takuma Y. Current therapy for West syndrome in Japan. *J Child Neurol.* 2000;15:424–428.
66. Ito M, Okuno T, Fujii T, et al. ACTH therapy in infantile spasms: relationship between dose of ACTH and initial effect or long-term prognosis. *Pediatr Neurol.* 1990;6:240–244.
67. Hanefeld F, Sperner J, Rating D, et al. Renal and pancreatic calcification during treatment of infantile spasms with ACTH. *Lancet.* 1984;1:901–904.
68. Rausch HP. Medullary nephrocalcinosis and pancreatic calcifications demonstrated by ultrasound and CT in infants after treatment with ACTH. *Radiology.* 1984;153:105–107.
69. Riikonen R, Simell O, Jääskeläinen J, et al. Disturbed calcium and phosphate homeostasis during treatment with ACTH of infantile spasms. *Arch Dis Child.* 1986;61:671–676.
70. Tacke E, Kupferschmid C, Lang D. Hypertrophic cardiomyopathy during ACTH treatment. *Klin Padiatr.* 1983;195:124–128.
71. Alpert BS. Steroid-induced hypertrophic cardiomyopathy in an infant. *Pediatr Cardiol.* 1984;5:117–118.
72. Deona T, Voumard C. Reversible cerebral atrophy and corticotropin. *Lancet.* 1979;2:207–209.
73. Glaze DG, Hrachovy RA, Frost JD, et al. Computed tomography in infantile spasms: effects of hormonal therapy. *Pediatr Neurol.* 1986;2:23–27.
74. Konishi Y, Yasujima M, Kuriyama M, et al. Magnetic resonance imaging in infantile spasms: effects of hormonal therapy. *Epilepsia.* 1992;33:304–309.
75. Lagenstein I, Willig RP, Kuhne D. Cranial computed tomography (CCT) findings in children treated with ACTH and dexamethasone: first results. *Neuropadiatrie.* 1979;10:370–384.
76. Lyen KR, Holland IM, Lyen YC. Reversible cerebral atrophy in infantile spasms caused by corticotropin. *Lancet.* 1979;2:237–238.
77. Hara K, Watanabe K, Miyazaki S, et al. Apparent brain atrophy and subdural hematoma following ACTH therapy. *Brain Dev.* 1981;3:45–49.
78. Okuno T, Ito M, Konishi Y, et al. Cerebral atrophy following ACTH therapy. *J Comput Assist Tomogr.* 1980;4:20–23.
79. Rao JK, Willis J. Hypothalomo-pituitary-adrenal function in infantile spasms: effects of ACTH therapy. *J Child Neurol.* 1987;2:220–223.
80. Ross DL. Suppressed pituitary ACTH response after ACTH treatment of infantile spasms. *J Child Neurol.* 1986;1:34–37.
81. Perheentupa J, Riikonen R, Dunkel L, et al. Adrenocortical hyporesponsiveness after treatment with ACTH of infantile spasms. *Arch Dis Child.* 1986;61:750–753.
82. Colleselli P, Milan M, Drigo P, et al. Impairment of polymorphonuclear leucocyte function during therapy with synthetic ACTH in children affected by epileptic encephalopathies. *Acta Paediatr Scand.* 1986;75:159–169.
83. Goetting MG. Fatal *Pneumocystis* pneumonia from ACTH therapy for infantile spasms. *Ann Neurol.* 1986;19:307–308.

84. Quittell LM, Fisher M, Foley CM. *Pneumocystis carinii* pneumonia in infants given adrenocorticotropic hormone for infantile spasms. *J Pediatr.* 1987;110:901–903.

85. Shamir R, Garty BZ. *Pneumocystis carinii* pneumonia associated with adrenocorticotropic hormone treatment for infantile spasms. *Eur J Pediatr.* 1992;151:867–895.

86. Kanayama M, Ishikawa T, Tauchi A, et al. ACTH-induced seizures in an infant with West syndrome. *Brain Dev.* 1989;11:329–331.

87. Rutledge SL, Snead OC III, Kelly DR, et al. Pyruvate carboxylase deficiency: acute exacerbation after ACTH treatment of infantile spasms. *Pediatr Neurol.* 1989;5:201–206.

88. Appleton RE, Peters ACB, Mumford JP, et al. Randomised, placebo-controlled study of vigabatrin as first-line treatment of infantile spasms. *Epilepsia.* 1999;40:1627–1633.

89. Elterman RD, Shields WD, Mansfield KA, et al. Randomized trial of vigabatrin in patients with infantile spasms. *Neurology.* 2001;57:1416–1421.

90. Lux AL, Edwards SW, Hancock E, et al. The United Kingdom infantile spasms study (UKISS) comparing hormone treatment with Vigabatrin on developmental and epilepsy outcomes to age 14 months: a multicentre randomized trial. *Lancet Neurol.* 2005;4:712–717.

91. Wohlrab G, Boltshauser E, Schmitt B. Vigabatrin as first-line drug in West syndrome: clinical and electroencephalographic outcome. *Neuropediatrics.* 1998;29:133–136.

92. Chiron C, Dumas C, Jambaque I, et al. Randomized trial comparing vigabatrin and hydrocortisone in infantile spasms due to tuberous sclerosis. *Epilepsy Res.* 1997;26:389–395.

93. Wohlrab G, Boltshauser E, Schmitt B, et al. Visual field constriction is not limited to children treated with vigabatrin. *Neuropediatrics.* 1999;30:130–132.

94. Vanhatalo S, Nousiainen I, Eriksson K, et al. Visual field constriction in 91 Finnish children treated with vigabatrin. *Epilepsia.* 2002;43:748–756.

95. Hardus P, Verduin WM, Engelsman M, et al. Visual field loss associated with vigabatrin: quantification and relation to dosage. *Epilepsia.* 2001;42:262–267.

96. Gross-Tsur V, Banin E, Shahar E, et al. Visual impairment in children with epilepsy treated with vigabatrin. *Ann Neurol.* 2000;48:60–64.

97. Koul R, Chacko A, Ganesh A, et al. Vigabatrin associated retinal dysfunction in children with epilepsy. *Arch Dis Child.* 2001;85:469–473.

98. Westall C, Logan WJ, Smith K, et al. The Hospital for Sick Children, Toronto, longitudinal ERG study of children on vigabatrin. *Doc Ophthalmol.* 2002;104:133–149.

99. Camposano SE, Major P, Halpern E, et al. Vigabatrin in the treatment of childhood epilepsy: a retrospective chart review of efficacy and safety profile. *Epilepsia.* 2008;49:1123–1141.

100. Siemes H, Spohr HL, Michael T, et al. Therapy of infantile spasms with valproate: results of a prospective study. *Epilepsia.* 1988;29:553–560.

101. Schlumberger E, Dulac O. A simple, effective and well-tolerated treatment regime for West syndrome. *Dev Med Child Neurol.* 1994;36:863–872.

102. Chamberlain MC. Nitrazepam for refractory infantile spasms and the Lennox-Gastaut syndrome. *J Child Neurol.* 1996;11:31–34.

103. Toribe Y. High-dose vitamin B6 treatment in West syndrome. *Brain Dev.* 2001;23:654–657.

104. Hurst DL, Rolan TD. The use of felbamate to treat infantile spasms. *J Child Neurol.* 1997;10:134–136.

105. Echenne B, Dulac O, Parayre-Chanez MJ, et al. Treatment of infantile spasms with intravenous gamma-globulins. *Brain Dev.* 1991;13:313–319.

106. Glauser T, Clark PO, Strawsburg R. A pilot study of topiramate in the treatment of infantile spasms. *Epilepsia.* 1998;39:1324–1328.

107. Suzuki Y, Imai K, Toribe Y, et al. Long-term response to zonisamide in patients with West syndrome. *Neurology.* 2002;58:1556–1559.

108. Kerrigan JF, Shields WD, Nelson TY, et al. Ganaxolone for treating intractable infantile spasms: a multicentre, open-label, add-on trial. *Epilepsy Res.* 2000;42:133–139.

109. Mikati MA, El Banna D, Sinno D, et al. Response of infantile spasms to levetiracetam. *Neurology.* 2008;70:574–575.

110. Kossoff EH, Pyzik PL, McGrogan JR, et al. Efficacy of the ketogenic diet for infantile spasms. *Pediatrics.* 2002;109:780–783.

111. Kossoff EH, Hedderick EF, Turner Z, et al. A case-control evaluation of the ketogenic diet versus ACTH for new onset infantile spasms. *Epilepsia.* 2008;49:1504–1509.

112. Snead OC III, Benton JW, Myers GJ. ACTH and prednisone in childhood seizure disorders. *Neurology.* 1983;33:966–970.

113. Yamatogi Y, Ohtahara S. Early-infantile epileptic encephalopathy with suppression-bursts, Ohtahara syndrome; its overview referring to our 16 cases. *Brain Dev.* 2002;24:13–23.

114. Yamatogi Y, Ohtahara S. Age dependent epileptic encephalopathy: a longitudinal study. *Folia Psych Neurol Jpn.* 1981;35:321–332.

115. Martinez BA, Roche C, Lopez-Martin V, et al. Early infantile epileptic encephalopathy. *Rev Neurol.* 1995;23:297–300.

116. Donat JF. The age dependent epileptic encephalopathies. *J Child Neurol.* 1992;7:7–21.

117. Campistol J, Garcia-Garcia JJ, Lobera E, et al. The Ohtahara syndrome: a special form of age dependent epilepsy. *Rev Neurol.* 1997;25:212–214.

118. Baxter PS, Gardner-Medwin D, Barwick DD, et al. Vigabatrin monotherapy in resistant neonatal seizures. *Seizure.* 1995;4:57–59.

119. Dobbs JM, Baird HW. The use of corticotropin and a corticosteroid in patients with minor motor seizures. *Am J Dis Child.* 1960;100:584–585.

120. Kurakawa T, Nagahide G, Fukuyama Y, et al. West syndrome and Lennox-Gastaut syndrome: a survey of natural history. *Pediatrics.* 1980;65:81–88.

121. Lagenstein I, Willig RP, Iffland E. Behandlung fruhkindlicher Anfalle mit ACTH und Dexamethasone unter standardisierten Bedingungen, I: klinische Ergebnisse. *Monatsschr Kinderheilk.* 1978;126:492–499.

122. Lagenstein I, Willig RP, Iffland E. Behandlung fruhkindlicher Anfalle mit ACTH und Dexamethasone unter standardisierten Bedingungen, II: elektrocencephalographische Beobachtungen. *Monatsschr Kinderheilk.* 1978;126:500–506.

123. Paul L, O'Neal R, Ybanez M, et al. Minor motor epilepsy. Treatment with corticotropin (ACTH) and steroid therapy. *JAMA.* 1960;172:1408–1412.

124. O'Regan ME, Brown JK. Is ACTH a key to understanding anticonvulsant action? *Dev Med Child Neurol.* 1998;40:82–89.

125. Doose H. Myoclonic-astatic epilepsy. *Epilepsy Res Suppl.* 1992;6:163–168.

126. Oguni H, Tanaka T, Hayashi K, et al. Treatment and long-term prognosis of myoclonic-astatic epilepsy of early childhood. *Neuropediatrics.* 2002;33:122–132.

127. Landau W, Kleffner FR. Syndrome of acquired aphasia with convulsive disorder in children. *Neurology.* 1957;7:523–530.

128. Appleton RE. The Landau-Kleffner syndrome. *Arch Dis Child.* 1995;72:386–387.

129. Robinson RO, Baird G, Robinson G, et al. Landau-Kleffner syndrome: course and correlates with outcome. *Dev Med Child Neurol.* 2001;43:243–247.

130. Lerman P, Lerman-Sagie T, Kivity S. Effects of early corticosteroid therapy for Landau-Kleffner syndrome. *Dev Med Child Neurol.* 1991;33:257–266.

131. Hirsch E, Marescaux C, Finck S, et al. Landau-Kleffner syndrome: a clinical and EEG study of five cases. *Epilepsia.* 1990;31:756–767.

132. McKinney W, McGreal DA. An aphasic syndrome in children. *Can Med Assoc J.* 1974;110:637–639.

133. Kellerman K. Recurrent aphasia with subclinical bioelectric status epilepticus during sleep. *Eur J Pediatr.* 1978;128:207–212.

134. Van der Sandt-Koenderman WME, Smit IAC, Van Dongen HR, et al. A case of acquired aphasia and convulsive disorder. Some linguistic aspects of recovery and breakdown. *Brain Lang.* 1984;21:174–183.

135. Tsuru T, Mori M, Mizuguchi M, et al. Effects of high-dose intravenous corticosteroid therapy in Landau-Kleffner syndrome. *Pediatr Neurol.* 2000;22:145–147.

CHAPTER 67 ■ NEWER ANTIEPILEPTIC DRUGS

DEANA M. GAZZOLA, NORMAN DELANTY, AND JACQUELINE A. FRENCH

Despite advances in epilepsy treatment, there remains a continuing need for the development of new medications (1–4). Among those with epilepsy, 30% to 40% continue to have seizures or experience unacceptable side effects that affect their quality of life (5,6). In a prospective study of 525 patients in a single epilepsy center between 1984 and 1997, only 63% remained seizure-free for more than 1 year, with seizure-free rates being similar regardless of whether a new or an established antiepileptic drug (AED) was used (7). Moreover, the available anticonvulsant drugs neither influence the process of epileptogenesis in humans nor alter the underlying brain dysfunction that expresses itself as epilepsy. Rather, they merely suppress the symptoms of epilepsy, and therefore are not actually antiepileptic or antiepileptogenic. An agent considered to be truly antiepileptogenic or antiepileptic in nature would prevent epilepsy (e.g., after a head injury or stroke), alter the underlying mechanisms of a particular epilepsy, or prevent or ameliorate its progression (8). The ideal AED would provide complete seizure control without significant side effects or idiosyncratic life-threatening reactions; have simple, predictable pharmacokinetics; be unaffected by other drugs or medical conditions; and be nonteratogenic, affordable, and available in a parenteral formulation.

Although multiple new agents have been introduced in recent years, with attendant marketing considerations, many novel compounds with promise as useful AEDs are currently in various stages of development (Tables 67.1 and 67.2). Some of these resulted from the Antiepileptic Drug Development

TABLE 67.1

CHEMISTRY AND POSSIBLE MECHANISMS OF ACTION OF SOME NEW ANTIEPILEPTIC DRUGS

Drug	Chemistry	Possible mechanism of action
Eslicarbazepine acetate	*S-(–)-10-acetoxy-10,11-dihydro-5H-dibenz[b,f]azepine-5-carboxamide*; shares the dibenzazepine nucleus bearing the 5-carboxamide substitute with carbamazepine	Stabilizes the inactivated state of voltage-gated sodium channels
Brivaracetam	Pyrrolidone derivative in the same class as levetiracetam and piracetam	Binds to the synaptic vesicle protein 2A (SV2A) like its parent compound levetiracetam, but with higher affinity; also inhibits sodium channel currents
Propylisopropyl acetate (PID)	Chiral isomer of valpromide	(R) enantiomer is more potent; mechanism of action unknown
Carisbamate	*S-2-O-carbamoyl-1-o-chlorophenyl-ethanol*	Inhibits voltage-gated sodium channels; modest inhibition of high-voltage activated calcium channels
Ganaxolone	*3α-hydroxy-3β-methyl-5α-pregnan-20-one*	Positive allosteric modulator of the GABA(A) receptor
Huperzine A	Sesquiterpene lycopodium alkaloid	N-methyl-D-aspartate receptor and acetylcholinesterase inhibitor
JZP-4	*3-(2,3,5-trichloro-phenyl)-pyrazine-2,6-diamine*; structurally related to lamotrigine	Sodium- and calcium-channel blocker
NAX 5055	Analog of the endogenous neuropeptide galanin	Agonist of galanin receptor subtypes GalR1 and GalR2; this is thought to decrease glutamate release
Retigabine	Carbamacic acid ethyl ester	*Opens inward rectifying K$^+$ channels; GABA potentiation*
Stiripentol	Aromatic allylic alcohol	Inhibits synaptosomal GABA uptake; enhances GABAergic transmission; inhibits hepatic cytochrome P450 enzymes
YKP3089	Unknown	Unknown

TABLE 67.2

IMPORTANT PHARMACOKINETIC PARAMETERS OF NEW ANTIEPILEPTIC
COMPOUNDS IN HUMANS

Drug	T_{max} (hr)	Protein binding (%)	Half-life (hr)	Excretion
Eslicarbazepine acetate	2–3	30	20–24	Renal
Brivaracetam	1–2	Weak	8	Renal
Propylisopropyl acetate (PID)	Unknown	Unknown	Unknown	Unknown
Carisbamate	1–3	44	12	Renal
Ganaxolone	1.5–2	99	35–40	Hepatic
Huperzine A	Unknown	Unknown	Unknown	Unknown
JZP-4	Unknown	Unknown	10	Renal
NAX-5055	Unknown	Unknown	Unknown	Unknown
Retigabine	1–2	Less than 80	8–10	Renal
Stiripentol	1.5	99	Nonlinear pharmacokinetics (Michaelis–Menten)	Unknown
YKP3089	1.5–3.5	Unknown	30–75	Unknown

(ADD) Program sponsored by the U.S. National Institutes of Health (9), which has screened more than 24,000 compounds (provided by industry and academia) for potential anticonvulsant efficacy in traditional animal models (9,10). These models have focused mainly on the maximum electroshock (MES) test and the pentylenetetrazol (PTZ) test, which in the past were believed to predict efficacy against tonic–clonic and absence seizures, respectively, although this has not completely borne out in the clinic. Although this approach has identified drugs such as topiramate, it does not always recognize potentially useful compounds, predict activity in humans, or test antiepileptogenic potential (11). Newer models, such as pilocarpine, kainate, or electrically induced post-status epilepsy models, are aimed at mimicking human disease and may be better suited to identify useful compounds, but are not effective for high-throughput screening of new chemical entities. Research elucidating the molecular mechanisms underlying some specific epilepsy syndromes, such as benign neonatal convulsions (12) and Unverricht–Lundborg progressive myoclonic epilepsy (13), suggests that targeted therapeutic approaches may prove more successful than mass screening techniques for some of the epilepsies. This may also be true for some of the more common forms of epilepsy, such as juvenile myoclonic epilepsy (14). Despite the limitations of screening methods, promising compounds are in development (15–18). Some are at a late stage of development (e.g., brivaracetam, retigabine), while others are at earlier stages of clinical testing (e.g., huperzine A, JZP-4, YKP3089). However, not all of these compounds will be approved for use, which is exemplified by the fact that seven of the compounds discussed in the prior version of this chapter are no longer in development.

In the fourth edition of this textbook, this chapter discussed 11 anticonvulsant drugs (19). Rufinamide and lacosamide (formerly known as harkoseride), both originally discussed in this chapter, are now covered in Chapters 64 and 65, respectively. Information on retigabine, UCB 34714 (now called brivaracetam), and the valproate derivatives has been

updated. Carabersat, DP-VPA, fluorofelbamate, NPS 1776, safinamide, talampanel, and valrocemide will not be discussed in this chapter as the interval development of these agents has been either temporarily stalled for different reasons, or has ceased altogether due to an unfulfilled promise of efficacy. Compounds newly developed as potential AEDs since the writing of the last edition have been added; included are carisbamate, eslicarbazepine, huperzine A, JZP-4, NAX 5055, propylisopropyl acetate (PID), stiripentol, and YKP3089. The chapter has also been reorganized; drugs whose chemical structure are related to pre-existing parent compounds are discussed first under the derivative compound section, followed by a section devoted to compounds that are novel in their chemical structure.

DERIVATIVE COMPOUNDS

Carbamazepine Derivatives: Eslicarbazepine Acetate

Eslicarbazepine acetate (*S*-(−)-10-acetoxy-10,11-dihydro-5H-dibenz/*b,f*/azepine-5-carboxamide, formerly BIA 2-093) is structurally similar to carbamazepine and oxcarbazepine, sharing the dibenzazepine nucleus that bears the 5-carboxamide substitute (20). It most resembles oxcarbazepine, a pro-drug that is metabolized to *S*- and *R*-enantiomers of licarbazepine (also known as *S*- and *R*-MHD). However, eslicarbazepine acetate's unique structure at the 10,11-position results in different metabolism (15). Eslicarbazepine actetate undergoes biotransformation via presystemic first-pass hepatic hydrolysis to the major active metabolite eslicarbazepine (also called *S*-licarbazepine or *S*-MHD). Oxcarbazepine and *R*-licarbazepine are minor active metabolites formed by non-cytochrome P450 (CYP450)-mediated metabolism. Thus, whereas ingestion of oxcarbazepine will result in exposure to oxcarbazepine (briefly, before conversion), as well as *R*- and *S*-licarbazepine, eslicarbazepine acetate ingestion will lead to exposure almost exclusively to eslicarbazepine acetate (before conversion) and *S*-licarbazepine (95% of total exposure). It is unknown to what extent, if at all, the two enantiomers will differ in their clinical properties. While the exact mechanism of action of the drug is unknown, the major active metabolite eslicarbazepine has been found to stabilize the inactivated state of voltage-gated sodium channels, and it also binds more selectively to rapidly firing neurons (21,22). Eslicarbazepine acetate displays linear pharmacokinetics. No food effect on absorption has been appreciated (22). Peak plasma concentration C_{max} occurs 2 to 3 hours post dose. It has an elimination half-life of approximately 20 to 24 hours, reaching steady state after 4 to 5 days (22). Metabolites are primarily renally excreted unchanged and as glucuronide conjugates (16,23); a recent study showed that mild renal impairment in patients affects clearance, thereby requiring a dose adjustment (24). Eslicarbazepine acetate is not highly protein bound (30%). In in vitro studies, it had no impact on the majority of cytochrome P450 isozymes, but moderate inhibition of CYP2C9 and mild activation of UGT1A1-mediated ethinylestradiol glucuronidation were observed. In a clinical study assessing interaction with the Oral contraceptive (OCP), the area under plasma concentration-time curve (AUC) of levonorgestrel and ethinylestradiol decreased by 24% and 32%, respectively. Whereas this is lower than oxcarbazepine, which decreases both levonorgestrel and ethinylestradiol AUC by 47%, an impact of effectiveness of the OCP cannot be ruled out (22). Eslicarbazepine does not appear to significantly affect the plasma concentrations of *R*-warfarin. In preliminary studies, serum concentrations of lamotrigine and topiramate were significantly reduced by b.i.d., but not q.d. administration of ESL (22).

In general eslicarbazepine acetate has been well tolerated. The most common adverse effects reported include nausea, headache, dizziness, somnolence, and circumoral/lips/tongue paresthesias. Phase II and Phase III clinical trials have been completed. Results from three recent multicenter, randomized, double-blind, placebo-controlled Phase III trials were presented at the 8th European Congress on Epileptology in September 2008 (25–27). Patients with refractory partial epilepsy were randomized to receive eslicarbazepine acetate (400, 800, or 1200 mg depending on the study) or placebo for a 12-week maintenance period. Pooled data revealed that at doses of 800 and 1200 mg/day, eslicarbazepine acetate was associated with a statistically significant median relative reduction of seizure frequency (800 mg group 36.4%; 1200 mg group 46.4%) compared to placebo (15%). In addition, the responder rate (defined as equal to or greater than 50% reduction in seizure frequency) was also higher in those patients treated with eslicarbazepine acetate (800 mg: 36%, $P < 0.001$ and 1200 mg: 44%, $P < 0.0001$) compared to placebo (22%) (16,28).

The most common adverse effects reported in clinical trials have been CNS-related (e.g., dizziness, somnolence, nausea). In the Phase III clinical trials, adverse effects were usually mild to moderate in intensity and occurred in the beginning of treatment (16,28). Hyponatremia (reported in 4/1050 patients) and rash (reported in 13/1050 patients) were rare. This may distinguish eslicarbazepine acetate from oxcarbazepine but as of now, the two drugs have not been compared head to head. Another difference is that eslicabazepine acetate was effective when administered once per day in clinical trials.

The above findings suggest that eslicarbazepine acetate, if approved for use, will be a useful addition to the current repertoire of AEDs. Preparation of a New Drug Application to the U.S. Food and Drug Administration (FDA) was underway at the time of writing of this chapter.

Lamotrigine Derivatives: JZP-4

JZP-4 (3-(2,3,5-trichloro-phenyl)-pyrazine-2,6-diamine) is a novel sodium- and calcium-channel blocker, structurally related to lamotrigine. It has effectively inhibited seizures in multiple mouse and rat models suggesting broad-spectrum anticonvulsant activity (15). In addition to its potential use as an AED, JZP-4 may have other applications. JZP-4 might possess antidepressant and antimania properties as evidenced by its activity in the rat forced swim test and the chlordiazepoxide–amphetamine model. In addition, JZP-4 was active in the harmaline-induced tremor model of essential tremor, and prevented hyperalgesia in neuropathic pain models (16).

JZP-4 is rapidly absorbed after oral dosing, is primarily eliminated in the urine, and has a terminal-phase half-life of approximately 10 hours (16). In vitro analysis has demonstrated minimal inhibition of hepatic CYP isoenzymes at high concentrations of drug, and results from testing in isolated human hepatocytes suggest JZP-4 is not a hepatic enzyme inducer (16). Two proof-of-concept studies are currently ongoing to assess the antiepileptic properties of JZP-4.

Levetiracetam Derivatives: Brivaracetam

Brivaracetam (UCB 34714) is a pyrrolidone derivative in the same class as levetiracetam and piracetam. It binds to the synaptic vesicle protein 2A (SV2A) like its parent compound levetiracetam, but with higher affinity. SV2A is a membrane glycoprotein found in all synaptic and endocrine vesicles. There is no settled mechanism by which binding to this site leads to anticonvulsant effect. In contrast to levetiracetam, brivaracetam also inhibits sodium-channel currents as demonstrated in rat cortical neurons in vitro (29). It exhibits superior activity against secondarily generalized motor seizures in corneally kindled mice, and prevents clonic convulsions in audiogenic-susceptible mice (30). Brivaracetam suppresses spike-and-wave discharges in GAERS (Generalized Absence Epilepsy Rat from Strasbourg) rats, and also suppresses both motor seizure severity and after-discharge duration in amygdala-kindled rats (30).

Brivaracetam is rapidly absorbed following oral administration, displays linear pharmacokinetics, binds weakly to plasma proteins, and has an approximately 8 hour half-life (31,32). Its volume of distribution, like levetiracetam, is close to body water. Inactive metabolites that are primarily renally cleared are produced via hydrolysis of the acetamide group and CYP2C8-mediated hydroxylation (32). In contrast to levetiracetam, which does not impact metabolism of concomitantly administered medications, brivaracetam has been demonstrated in vitro to have some impact on metabolizing enzymes. Specifically, it inhibits epoxide hydrolase and to a lesser extent CYP3A4 and 2C19, and is a weak inducer of CYP3A4 (33). Brivaracetam has been shown to slightly reduce carbamazepine concentrations, while slightly increasing levels of carbamazepine-10, 11-epoxide. Brivaracetam has equivocal effects on phenytoin, possibly lowering serum concentrations, and has no effect on the concentrations of lamotrigine, levetiracetam, oxcarbazepine, topiramate, and valproic acid (15,34). Enzyme-inducing AEDs increase brivaracetam clearance, leading to a 30% reduction of AUC (16). There is no change in exposure in elderly and renally impaired patients, indicating that no dose adjustments should be necessary. However, severe hepatic impairment will increase exposure by about 50% (16). High doses of brivaracetam have been shown to moderately reduce the estrogen and progesterone components of oral contraceptives, but this has not been shown to impact ovulation (15,33).

Tolerability of brivaracetam is good overall, with the most common adverse effects being CNS-related, mild to moderate in intensity, and transient. Brivaracetam was administered in a randomized trial in photosensitive epilepsy patients, utilizing the photoparoxysmal response (PPR) paradigm (35). At the lowest dose of 10 mg, brivaracetam abolished or suppressed photoparoxysmal EEG discharges in all patients, and at higher levels abolished discharges completely in all patients for a mean of 60 hours. The latter result not only indicates brivaracetam's antiepileptic potential, but also suggests that the compound's pharmacodynamic half-life likely outlasts its pharmacokinetic half-life. Two Phase IIb dose-ranging clinical studies, conducted in patients with refractory partial epilepsy, also yielded promising efficacy and tolerability data (36,37). In a Phase II study, which had a relatively short (7 week) maintenance period (36), a 50% responder rate was observed in 32.0% (P = NS), 44.2% (P = 0.014), and 55.8% ($P <$ 0.001) of patients receiving brivaracetam doses of 5, 20, and 50 mg/day, respectively, compared to placebo (16.7%). Seizure freedom was attained in 8.0%, 7.7%, and 7.7% of patients receiving 5, 20, and 50 mg/day of drug compared to 1.9% of the placebo group (36). Of note, more patients in the placebo group than in the highest treatment dose arm (50 mg) dropped out due to side effects (2 vs. 0, respectively). In a second study (37), 50% responder rates were 39.6% and 33.3% in those patients receiving 50 and 150 mg/day brivaracetam, respectively, compared to 23.1% in the placebo group. Seizure freedom was achieved in 9.4% and 5.8% of patients on 50 and 150 mg/day of drug, respectively, compared to 1.9% of patients on placebo (P = NS).

Three Phase III clinical trials are currently underway: two double-blind, placebo-controlled studies randomizing patients with refractory partial-onset epilepsy to different doses of brivaracetam for a 12-week period and a third study designed to assess the safety and tolerability of brivaracetam in patients with primary generalized epilepsy. Brivaracetam has also gained orphan drug status for the progressive myoclonic epilepsies, and two studies using the drug in patients with Unverricht–Lundborg disease are in progress.

Of note, a second levetiracetam derivative, seletracetam, has been under development; however, clinical trials have been halted, and it is unclear whether development will continue.

Valproate Derivatives: Propylisopropyl Acetamide (PID)

Interest has centered on the search for clinically effective valproate-like compounds that lack the hepatotoxic or teratogenic potential of the parent drug (38,39), and which do not inhibit the detoxifying enzyme epoxide hydrolase (40). Several compounds have raised interest in the past several years, including but not limited to DP-VPA, NPS 1776, and PID. The latter compound, chosen from a drug-discovery program seeking a nontoxic valproate derivative, has shown the most promise of advancing in development. Of note, the majority of the published literature on PID to date covers the pharmacologic properties of the compound, as well as its pharmacokinetic profile. There is presently an absence of data from clinical trials as they are yet to be performed.

Valpromide is the corresponding pro-drug and amide of valproic acid (41,42). It is a more potent AED than valproic acid, and is also much less teratogenic in animal models (41,43). However, the pro-drug nature of valpromide makes it structurally unstable as it transforms to the more teratogenic and less potent valproic acid, requiring the need to find an alternative compound that is similar in structure and function to valpromide, but chemically stable. PID, a chiral isomer of valpromide, is such a compound (41). The (R)- and (S)-enantiomer forms of PID have demonstrated anticonvulsant activity in various animal models, including the MES and PTZ models (41,42). When compared to the (S)-enantiomer, the (R)-enantiomer is more potent and possesses a longer half-life in mice (44). Preliminary findings regarding teratogenicity are promising. In two separate gestational studies using two different mouse strains sensitive to valproic-acid–induced teratogenicity, single doses of either the racemic form of PID, or one of the (R)- or (S)-PID enantiomers, were administered to pregnant mice. No teratogenic effects were found (43,45).

Future studies to determine the potential clinical efficacy of PID in the treatment of epilepsy are being planned.

STRUCTURALLY NOVEL COMPOUNDS

Carisbamate

Carisbamate (*S*-2-*O*-carbamoyl-1-*o*-chlorophenyl-ethanol, formerly RWJ-333369) is a novel molecule that has exhibited potent and broad activity in rodent seizure models including audiogenic seizure models and seizures induced by MES, PTZ, BIC, and picrotoxin, as well as in corneal-kindled rats (15). Carisbamate also suppressed the duration of spike-and-wave discharges in the GAERS model (46), and has shown efficacy in additional rat models. Approximately 44% of the drug is protein-bound, and primary routes of metabolism include *O*-glucuronidation and carbamate ester hydrolysis followed by oxidation of the aliphatic side chain (47). Unlike felbamate, there is low likelihood of conversion to the reactive metabolite mercapturic acid or its conjugates (48). It has a 12-hour half-life allowing for twice daily dosing, and follows linear pharmacokinetics (49). Maximum concentrations (C_{max}) occur 1 to 3 hours after dosing. Oral (metabolic) clearance is low. It is primarily renally excreted. Carisbamate has minimal impact on CYP450 hepatic enzymes and only slightly increases valproic acid and lamotrigine clearance (48). While carisbamate has no effect on carbamazepine pharmacokinetics, the C_{max} of carisbamate is reduced by approximately 30% when administered with carbamazepine (50). Carisbamate plasma concentration is reduced to a lesser extent when administered with an oral contraceptive (48).

A multicenter proof of principle study was performed using the photosensitivity model (51). Three of the 13 evaluable patients had complete abolition of photosensitivity, and an additional 7 had clinically significant reduction. A dose of 1000 mg was the highest tested and was also most effective. Reduction in photosensitivity was long lasting, up to 32 hours, which is longer than would have been expected from the drug's half-life. Maximum effect, however, seemed to correlate with C_{max}.

A randomized, double-blind, placebo-controlled, dose-ranging Phase IIb study for adjunctive use in partial-onset seizures has recently been completed (52). At carisbamate doses of 300, 800, and 1600 mg/day, patients experienced a reduced seizure frequency of 24% ($P < 0.001$), 21% ($P \leq 0.006$), and 29% ($P < 0.001$), respectively, compared to a 6% reduction in the placebo group. The most common adverse events in patients were CNS-related (headaches, dizziness, somnolence), and led to drug discontinuation in 6%, 12%, and 19% in each of the respective carisbamate-treated groups (vs. 8% in the placebo group). An open-label extension trial is currently ongoing.

Ganaxolone

Ganaxolone (3α-hydroxy-3β-methyl-5α-pregnan-20-one) is the 3-β-methyl analog of the neurosteroid allopregnanolone (16). It is a positive allosteric modulator of the GABA(A) receptor, and is similar to its natural analog allopregnanolone in potency and efficacy (53). Ganaxolone has protective antiepileptic activity in several seizure models, including the PTZ and bicuculline models, the 6-Hz model, and the cocaine-kindling models (53–56). Findings from animal models also suggest that certain neurosteroids may possess antiepileptogenic properties, slowing the development of spontaneous recurrent seizures (57).

Ganaxolone is rapidly absorbed and undergoes metabolism primarily by the CYP3A4/3A5 hepatic enzymes (16). It has a 10-hour effective half-life and a terminal elimination half-life of 35 to 40 hours (16). One issue is its variable absorption pattern in the presence or absence of food; plasma exposure values are 5 to 15 times higher when ganaxolone is taken with food, compared to values when ingested during fasting. To combat this problem, several unique formulations have been created including two solid capsule forms, one immediate-release and the other pH-sensitive delayed-release. Ganaxolone is highly protein-bound (>99%) (16), but in vitro drug–drug interaction studies have thus far failed to show any significant interactions between ganaxolone and other AEDs (58). Phase II trials assessing drug–drug interactions are ongoing.

Three Phase II open-label, adjunctive-therapy studies with ganaxolone have been performed in the pediatric population. The largest of the three enrolled a total of 45 patients with partial or generalized refractory seizures, ages 2 to 15 years. A maximum dose of ganaxolone of 12 mg/kg three times daily was administered for an 8-week maintenance period. Of the original 45 patients, 27 (60%) completed the entire study and 12 patients (27%) experienced a >50% reduction in seizure frequency (58). Therapy has been continued in patients on a compassionate use basis, citing improvement in behavior and seizure frequency as beneficial effects (58). The main adverse event observed in the clinical studies to date is somnolence,

and no serious adverse events have yet been reported. Two additional Phase II clinical trials, one in adults with partial-onset seizures and one in pediatric patients with infantile spasms, are currently ongoing. The efficacy of ganaxolone in the treatment of women with catamenial epilepsy is also being investigated.

Huperzine A

Huperzine A, an N-methyl-D-aspartate receptor and acetylcholinesterase inhibitor, is a sesquiterpene lycopodium alkaloid isolated from the Chinese club moss *Huperzia serrata*, traditionally used in China for swelling, fever and inflammation, blood disorders, and schizophrenia (16,59,60). Huperzine A is approved for use in China for Alzheimer's disease, and is considered a dietary supplement by the U.S. FDA, available in health food stores. While huperzine A has not been shown to protect against seizures in the MES-induced seizure model, it has been found to be protective against subcutaneous PTZ-induced seizures in mice. A maximum protection was observed at three doses of 1, 2, and 4 mg/kg in mice; however, rotarod test impairment was observed in a majority of mice at doses of 2 and 4 mg/kg (61). Currently, a pilot dose-ranging study is planned to evaluate the tolerability and efficacy of adjunctive huperzine A in human patients with medically refractory epilepsy. A trial is underway in patients with Alzheimer's disease using doses of 200 and 400 μg b.i.d.

NAX-5055

NAX-5055 is an analog of the endogenous neuropeptide galanin. Mazarati and colleagues (62–66) have demonstrated that injecting galanin into rat hippocampus decreases the severity of picrotoxin-induced kindled seizures. However, galanin is metabolically unstable and cannot penetrate the blood–brain barrier, thereby necessitating the development of an analog.

NAX-5055 binds and acts as an agonist at galanin receptor subtypes GalR1 and GalR2 (G-protein coupled receptors). This is thought to lead to a decrease in glutamate release, which could theoretically explain the drug's effect on seizures in animal models. NAX-5055 has thus far been effective in multiple rodent seizure models. It is effective at lower doses against PTZ- and MES-induced seizures, but is inactive at substantially higher doses, a property similar to levetiracetam (16). NAX-5055 also inhibits seizures in the 6-Hz seizure model, the corneal-kindled mouse model of partial epilepsy, and the hippocampal-kindled rat. Efficacy in kindling models, particularly the corneal-kindled mouse, suggests that there may be a role for NAX-5055 in the treatment of partial seizures specifically (16,67). Ongoing evaluations are planned, aimed at further defining the drug's therapeutic potential.

Retigabine

Retigabine (N-(2-amino-4-[4-fluorobenzylamino]-phenyl) carbamic acid ethyl ester) acts by opening the Kv7 (formerly KCNQ2/Q3) potassium channel (68,69), which mediates the potassium M-current (16,70), leading to neuronal hyperpolarization. Mutations in potassium channels have been described in benign familial neonatal convulsions (71). Retigabine also potentiates GABA-mediated currents at higher concentrations. Nontoxic doses of retigabine were effective against a broad range of experimental models, including genetic models of epilepsy and the amygdala-kindling model (72–74). The Kv7 site of action of retigabine might ultimately expand the application of the drug. Its use in the treatment of neuropathic pain, as well as neuroprotection in the setting of acute stroke, has been investigated and early findings have been promising (71,75,76). In addition, Kv7 subunits are expressed in bladder and intestinal smooth muscle, as well as in auditory pathways, suggesting a possible role for retigabine in the treatment of urinary incontinence, irritable bowel syndrome, and deafness and tinnitus (77–81).

The bioavailability of retigabine is 60% and although maximum concentration may be slightly higher after a high-fat meal, AUC is not affected. T_{max} is 1.5 hours. Retigabine has a half-life of 8 to 10 hours, and displays linear pharmacokinetics (in doses up to 1200 mg/day) (16,80). Protein binding is <80%, and therefore not likely to produce interactions (16). It is metabolized primarily by glucuronidation and acetylation producing two inactive N-glucuronide metabolites and one N-acetylated metabolite which has minimal pharmacologic activity (16). Retigabine is not metabolized by the CYP450 pathway. The majority of retigabine and its metabolites are renally excreted (16). Retigabine does not appear to alter the metabolism of oral contraceptives, although the agent appears to modestly increase the metabolism of lamotrigine by an unknown mechanism (with trough levels reduced by up to 20% in one Phase III clinical trial); conversely, phenytoin and carbamazepine increase the clearance of retigabine (16). Clearance is reduced by 30% in the elderly, indicating lower doses will be needed (16). Clearance is also reduced by moderate and severe hepatic impairment, by 30% and 50%, respectively, and by mild and severe renal impairment by 25% and 50%, respectively (16).

In Phase II studies, the most common adverse events involved the CNS and appeared to be dose-related (15,16), including astenia, dizziness, and somnolence. No clinically significant changes have been seen in either electrocardiograms or laboratory parameters (15,16). One recent Phase II double-blind, placebo-controlled trial randomized 399 patients with refractory partial epilepsy to placebo or add-on retigabine therapy. Retigabine doses of 600, 900, and 1200 mg/day produced a median percent reduction of 23%, 29%, and 35%, respectively, in monthly total seizures compared to 13% with placebo. In addition, ≥50% seizure reduction was seen in 23%, 32%, and 33% in patients receiving 600, 900, and 1200 mg retigabine, respectively, compared to 16% for those receiving placebo (80,81).

Two large-scale, Phase III trials, RESTORE-1 and RESTORE-2 (Retigabine Efficacy and Safety Trials for Partial-Onset Epilepsy) have been completed (82,83). Both studies enrolled patients with refractory partial-onset seizures. RESTORE-1 randomized subjects to 1200 mg versus placebo. Median percent seizure reduction was 44.3% (1200 mg) versus 17.5% (placebo) ($P < 0.001$). RESTORE-2 randomized subjects to 600 mg, 900 mg, or placebo. Median percent seizure reduction was 39.9% (900 mg), 27.9% (600 mg), and 15.9% (placebo) ($P < 0.001$ for both doses vs. placebo). Dropout rates increased with increasing dose (27% vs. 9% for 1200 mg vs. placebo, 26% vs. 17% vs. 6% for 900 and 600 mg vs.

placebo, respectively). In both studies, side effects leading to discontinuation included dizziness, somnolence, headache and fatigue, as well as confusion and dysarthria at the 1200-mg dose (82,83).

Two pharmaceutical companies are currently collaborating on the drug and are planning to file a New Drug Application with the U.S. FDA.

Stiripentol

Stiripentol [4,4 dimethyl-1-(3,4-methylenedioxyphenyl)-1-penten-3-ol] is a structurally novel molecule belonging to the aromatic allylic alcohol family. It has been used in France and Canada for over 10 years, but only recently began development for use in the United States. Animal studies have shown that stiripentol both inhibits synaptosomal GABA uptake and also enhances GABAergic transmission in CA3 pyramidal neurons of immature rats (84,85). In addition, stiripentol inhibits the hepatic cytochrome P450 enzymes, which likely also contributes to the drug's antiepileptogenic properties when it is combined with other AEDs, as serum concentrations of many concomitant AEDs will rise (86). This feature of stiripentol has made it difficult to study clinically. Patients with refractory epilepsy are often on concomitant AEDs, making it difficult to attribute any observed therapeutic effects purely to stiripentol. Specifically, stiripentol inhibits CYP3A4, CYP2C19, and CYP1A2. The coadministration of stiripentol with carbamazepine significantly increases the ratio of carbamazepine to carbamazepine epoxide. Stiripentol also inhibits the hydroxylation of the active metabolite of clobazam, desmethylclobazam. These interactions underscore the need to reduce the dose of carbamazepine and clobazam when stiripentol is added as adjunctive therapy. Because of its broad inhibition of the CYP system, stiripentol has the propensity to cause many other drug–drug interactions, including the elevation of theophylline and caffeine through CYP1A2 inhibition. Stiripentol is 99% protein-bound, and demonstrates nonlinear pharmacokinetics, decreasing in clearance as drug dose increases (87).

Since 1995 studies in adults have been discontinued due to lack of efficacy; however, results in children have been more promising. The first trial was an open-label adjunctive therapy study, which included children with partial-onset epilepsy, as well as children with Dravet syndrome (severe myoclonic epilepsy in infants) (88). Two thirds of the children with partial epilepsy treated with stiripentol were responders to drug, and 20% became seizure-free. In addition, 10 out of 20 children with Dravet syndrome were responders, and three became seizure-free. Given these findings, two additional small add-on trials were performed, one in France and one in Italy. Children 3 to 18 years of age with Dravet syndrome were enrolled. Stiripentol significantly reduced clonic and tonic–clonic seizure frequency, and led to complete seizure freedom in 9/21 patients and 3/12 patients in the two respective trials (89). Whether these results are purely attributable to stiripentol alone, or to secondary increases in concomitant AEDs, remains to be determined.

Adverse effects of stiripentol are fairly common, but can be minimized by adjusting doses of coadministered drugs. The most frequently observed adverse effects include drowsiness, slowing of mental function, ataxia, diplopia, loss of appetite causing weight loss, nausea, abdominal pain, and occasionally asymptomatic neutropenia (90). Currently, stiripentol is available from some hospitals in France and has been granted orphan drug status by the European Union for use in Dravet syndrome.

YKP3089

YKP3089 is a novel compound in early stages of development. It has been effective in a wide variety of epilepsy and seizure animal models, suggesting its potential use as a broad-spectrum AED (16). Its mechanism of action is currently unknown. Phase I clinical trials have documented linear pharmacokinetics over a single dose range of 5 to 750 mg, and a half-life of 30 to 75 hours (16). Single dose studies have shown the drug to be well tolerated, with a low incidence of CNS-related adverse effects. A proof-of-concept Phase IIa study performed in the photosensitivity model was recently closed, and results are pending.

CONCLUSIONS AND FUTURE DIRECTIONS

As in other areas of therapeutics, the choice of clinically effective novel anticonvulsant compounds will likely expand and help more patients with epilepsy live with fewer seizures and side effects. Continued vigilance will be needed to detect rare idiosyncratic side effects, which should include the use of postmarketing surveillance studies. Interest will also grow in the elucidation of optimal combination therapies using the available and upcoming drugs. Improvements in drug delivery systems and an increased choice of parenteral formulations are other reasonable expectations. The identification of compounds with antiepileptogenic neuroprotective properties should be an immediate priority, with clinical trials enrolling high-risk patients after head injury and stroke. The ability to predict an individual's response to a particular drug in terms of efficacy and side effects may be enhanced by advances in pharmacogenetics.

References

1. Delanty N, French JA. New options in epilepsy pharmacotherapy. *Formulary.* 1998;33:1190–1206.
2. Marson AG, Chadwick DW. New drug treatments for epilepsy. *J Neurol Neurosurg Psychiatry.* 2001;70:143–147.
3. Nguyen DK, Spencer SS. Recent advances in the treatment of epilepsy. *Arch Neurol.* 2003;60:929–935.
4. Sills GJ, Brodie MJ. Update on the mechanisms of action of antiepileptic drugs. *Epileptic Disord.* 2001;3:165–172.
5. Dichter MA, Brodie MJ. New antiepileptic drugs. *N Engl J Med.* 1996; 334:1583–1590.
6. Devinsky O. Patients with refractory epilepsy. *N Engl J Med.* 1999;340: 1565–1570.
7. Kwan P, Brodie MJ. Early identification of refractory epilepsy. *N Engl J Med.* 2000;342:314–319.
8. Tasch E, Cendes F, Li LM, Dubeau F, et al. Neuroimaging evidence of progressive neuronal loss and dysfunction in temporal lobe epilepsy. *Ann Neurol.* 1999;45:568–576.
9. White HS, Wolf HH, Woodhead JH, et al. The National Institutes of Health Anticonvulsant Drug Development Program: screening for efficacy. In: French J, Leppik I, Dichter MA, eds. *Antiepileptic Drug Development.* Philadelphia, PA: Lippincott-Raven; 1998:29–39.
10. White HS. Clinical significance of animal seizure models and mechanism of action studies of potential antiepileptic drugs. *Epilepsia.* 1997;38(suppl 1): S9–S17.
11. Loscher W, Leppik IE. Critical re-evaluation of previous preclinical strategies for the discovery and the development of new antiepileptic drugs. *Epilepsy Res.* 2002;50:17–20.
12. Singh NA, Charlier C, Stauffer D, et al. A novel potassium channel gene, KCNQ2, is mutated in an inherited epilepsy of newborns. *Nat Genet.* 1998;18:25–29.
13. Pennacchio LA, Lehesjoki AE, Stone NE, et al. Mutations in the gene encoding cystatin B in progressive myoclonic epilepsy (EPM1). *Science.* 1996;271:1731–1734.
14. Cossette P, Liu L, Brisebois K, et al. Mutation of GABA1 in an autosomal dominant form of juvenile myoclonic epilepsy. *Nat Genet.* 2002;31: 184–189.
15. Bialer M, Johannessen SI, Kupferberg HJ, et al. Progress report on new antiepileptic drugs: a summary of the Eight Eilat Conference (EILAT VIII). *Epilepsy Res.* 2007;73:1–52.
16. Bialer M, Johannessen SI, Levy RH, et al. Progress report on new antiepileptic drugs: a summary of the Ninth Eilat Conference (EILAT IX). *Epilepsy Res.* 2008;doi:10.1016/j.eplepsyres.2008.09.005.
17. Rogawski MA, Bazil CW. New molecular targets for antiepileptic drugs: $\alpha 2\delta$, SV2A, and Kv7/KCNQ/M potassium channels. *Curr Neurol Neurosci Rep.* 2008;8:345–352.
18. Meldrum BS, Rogawski MA. Molecular targets for antiepileptic drug development. *Neurotherapeutics.* 2007;4:18–61.
19. Delanty N, French JA. Newer antiepileptic drugs. In: Wyllie E, ed. *The Treatment of Epilepsy: Principles and Practice.* 4th ed. Baltimore, MD: Lippincott Williams & Wilkins; 2001:977–983.
20. Benes J, Parada A, Figueiredo AA, et al. Anticonvulsant and sodium channel-blocking properties of novel 10,11-dihydro-5H-dibenz[b,f]azepine-5-carboxamide derivatives. *J Med Chem.* 1999;42:2582–2587.
21. Bonifacio MJ, Sheridan RD, Parada A, et al. Interaction of the novel anticonvulsant, BIA 2-093, with voltage-gated sodium channels: comparison with carabamazepine. *Epilepsia.* 2001;42:600–608.
22. Almcida L, Soares-da-Silva P. Eslicarbazepine acetate (BIA 2-093). *Neurotherapeutics.* 2007;4:88–96.
23. Almeida L, Soares-da-Silva P. Safety, tolerability, and pharmacokinetic profile of BIA 2-093, a novel putative antiepileptic, in a rising multiple-dose study in young healthy humans. *J Clin Pharmacol.* 2004;44:906–918.
24. Maia J, Almeida L, Falcao A, et al. Effect of renal impairment on the pharmacokinetics of eslicarbazepine acetate. *Int J Clin Pharmacol Ther.* 2008; 46:119–130.
25. Elger C, Halasz P, Maia J, et al. Efficacy and safety of eslicarbazepine acetate as add-on treatment in adults with refractory partial-onset seizures: BIA-2093-301 study. Abstract and Oral Communication, Presented at the 8th European Congress on Epileptology; September 21–25, 2008; Berlin, Germany.
26. Hufnagel A, Ben-Menachem E, Gabbai A, et al. Efficacy and safety of eslicarbazepine acetate as add-on treatment in adults with refractory partial-onset seizures: BIA-2093-302 study. Abstract and Oral Communication, Presented at the 8th European Congress on Epileptology; September 21–25, 2008; Berlin, Germany.
27. Lopes-Lima J, Gil-Nagel A, Maia J, et al. Efficacy and safety of eslicarbazepine acetate as add-on treatment in adults with refractory partial-onset seizures: BIA-2093-303 study. Abstract and Oral Communication, Presented at the 8th European Congress on Epileptology; September 21–25, 2008; Berlin, Germany.
28. Elger C, French J, Halasz P, et al. Efficacy and safety of eslicarbazepine acetate as add-on treatment in patients with partial-onset seizures: pooled analysis of three double-blind phase III clinical studies. *Epilepsia.* 2008;3:199. Abstract.
29. Zona C, Pieri M, Klitgaard H, et al. UCB 34714, a new pyrrolidone derivative, inhibits Na+-currents in rat cortical neurons in culture. *Epilepsia.* 2004;45(suppl 7):146.
30. Matagne A, Margineanu DG, Kenda B, et al. Anticonvulsive and antiepileptic properties of brivaracetam (UCB 34714), a high affinity synaptic vesicle protein SV2A ligand. *Br J Pharmacol.* 2008;154:1662–1671.
31. Sargentini-Maier ML, Rolan P, Connell J, et al. The pharmacokinetics, CNS pharmacodynamics and adverse event profile of brivaracetam after single increasing oral doses in healthy males. *Br J Clin Pharmacol.* 2007; 63:680–688.
32. Sargentini-Maier ML, Espié P, Coquette A, et al. Pharmacokinetics and metabolism of 14C-brivaracetam, a novel SV2A ligand, in healthy subjects. *Drug Metab Dispos.* 2008;36:36–45.
33. von Rosenstiel, P. Brivaracetam (UCB 34714). *Neurotherapeutics.* 2007;4: 84–87.
34. Otoul C, von Rosenstiel P, Stockis A. Evaluation of the pharmacokinetic interaction of brivaracetam on other antiepileptic drugs in adults with partial-onset seizures. *Epilepsia.* 2007;48(suppl 6):334.
35. Kasteleijn-Nolst Trenite DG, Genton P, Parain D, et al. Evaluation of brivaracetam, a novel SV2A ligand, in the photosensitivity model. *Neurology.* 2007;69:1027–1034.
36. French JA, von Rosenstiel P on behalf of the Brivaracetam N01193 Study Group. Efficacy and tolerability of 5, 30 and 50 mg/day brivaracetam (UCB 34714) as adjunctive treatment in adults with refractory partial-onset seizures. *Epilepsia.* 2007;48(suppl 6):400.
37. van Paesschen W, von Rosenstiel P on behalf of the Brivaracetam N01114 Study Group. Efficacy and tolerability of 50 and 150 mg/day brivaracetam

(UCB 34714) as adjunctive treatment in adults with refractory partial-onset epilepsy. *Epilepsia.* 2007;48(suppl 6):329.

38. Bialer M, Haj-Yehia A, Badir K, et al. Can we develop improved derivatives of valproic acid? *Pharm World Sci.* 1994;16:2–6.

39. Hadad S, Bialer M. Pharmacokinetic analysis and antiepileptic activity of N-valproyl derivatives of GABA and glycine. *Pharm Res.* 1995;2:905–910.

40. Kerr BM, Levy RH. Inhibition of epoxide hydrolase by anticonvulsants and risk of teratogenicity. *Lancet.* 1989;1:610–611.

41. Bialer M. Clinical pharmacology of valpromide. *Clin Pharmacokinet.* 1991;20:114–122.

42. Spiegelstein O, Yagen B, Levy RH, et al. Stereoselective pharmacokinetics and pharmacodynamics of propylisopropyl acetamide, a CNS-active chiral amide analog of valproic acid. *Pharm Res.* 1999;16:1582–1588.

43. Radatz M, Ehlers K, Yagen B, et al. Valnoctamide, valpromide and valnoctic acid are much less teratogenic in mice than valproic acid. *Epilepsy Res.* 1998;30:41–48.

44. Isoherranen N, Yagen B, Woodhead JH, et al. Characterization of the anticonvulsant profile and enantioselective pharmacokinetics of the chiral valproylamide propylisopropyl acetamide in rodents. *Br J Pharmacol.* 2003;138:602–613.

45. Spiegelstein O, Bialer M, Radatz M, et al. Enantioselective synthesis and teratogenicity of propylisopropyl acetamide, a CNS-active chiral amide analogue of valproic acid. *Chirality.* 1999;11:645–650.

46. Francois J, Boehrer A, Nehlig A. Effects of carisbamate (RWJ-333369) in two models of genetically determined generalized epilepsy, the GAERS and the audiogenic Wistar AS. *Epilepsia.* 2008;49:393–399.

47. Mannens GSJ, Hendricks J, Janssen C, et al. The absorption, metabolism and excretion of the novel neuromodulator RWJ-333369 (1,2-ethanediol, [1-2-chlorophenyl]-, 2-carbamate, [S]-) in humans. *Drug Metab Dispos.* 2007;35(4):554–565.

48. Novak GP, Kelley M, Zannikos P, et al. Carisbamate (RWJ-333369). *Neurotherapeutics.* 2007;4:106–109.

49. Yao C, Chien S, Doose DR, et al. Pharmacokinetics of the new antiepileptic and CNS drug RWJ-333369, following single and multiple dosing to humans. *Epilepsia.* 2006;47:1822–1829.

50. Chien S, Yao C, Solanki B, et al. Pharmacokinetic interaction study between the new antiepileptic and CNS drug RWJ-333369 and carbamazepine in healthy subjects. *Epilepsia.* 2006;47:1830–1840.

51. Dorothée GA, Kasteleijn-Nolst Trenité DGA, French JA, et al. Evaluation of carisbamate, a novel antiepileptic drug, in photosensitive patients: an exploratory, placebo-controlled study. *Epilepsy Res.* 2007;74(2–3):193–200.

52. Faught E, Holmes GL, Rosenfeld WE, et al. Randomized, controlled, dose-ranging trial of carisbamate for partial-onset seizures. *Neurology.* 2008;71:1586–1593.

53. Carter RB, Wood PL, Wieland S, et al. Characterization of the anticonvulsant properties of ganaxolone (CCD1042; 3alpha-hydroxy-3beta-methyl-5alpha-pregnan-20-one), a selective, high-affinity, steroid modulator of the gamma-aminobutyric acid receptor. *J Pharmacol Exp Ther.* 1997;280:1284–1295.

54. Leskiewicz M, Budziszewska B, Jaworska-Feil L, et al. Inhibitory effect of some neuroactive steroids on cocaine-induced kindling in mice. *Polish J Pharmacol.* 2003;55:1131–1136.

55. Kaminski RM, Gasior M, Carter RB, et al. Protective efficacy of neuroactive steroids against cocaine kindled-seizures in mice. *Eur J Pharmacol.* 2003;474:217–222.

56. Kaminski RM, Livingood MR, Rogawski MA. Allopregnanolone analogs that positively modulate GABA receptors protect against partial seizures induced by 6-Hz electrical stimulation in mice. *Epilepsia.* 2004;45:864–867.

57. Biagini G, Baldelli E, Longo D, et al. Endogenous neurosteroids modulate epileptogenesis in a model of temporal lobe epilepsy. *Exp Neurol.* 2006;201:519–524.

58. Nohria V, Giller E. Ganaxolone. *Neurotherapeutics.* 2007;4:102–105.

59. Zangara A. The psychopharmacology of huperzine A: an alkaloid with cognitive enhancing and neuroprotective properties of interest in the treatment of Alzheimer's disease. *Pharmacol. Biochem. Behav.* 2003;75:675–686.

60. Ward J, Caprio V. A radical mediated approach to the core structure of Huperzine A. *Tetrahedron Lett.* 2006;47:553–556.

61. White HS, Schachter S, Lee D, et al. Anticonvulsant activity of Huperzine A, an alkaloid extract of Chinese club moss (*Huperzia serrata*). *Epilepsia.* 2005;46(suppl 8):220.

62. Mazarati A, Lundstrom L, Sollenberg U, et al. Regulation of kindling epileptogenesis by hippocampal galanin type 1 and type 2 receptors: the effects of subtype-selective agonists and the role of G-protein-mediated signalling. *J Pharmacol Exp Ther.* 2006;318:700–708.

63. Mazarati A, Lu X. Regulation of limbic status epilepticus by hippocampal galanin type 1 and type 2 receptors. *Neuropeptides.* 2005;39:277–280.

64. Mazarati A, Langel U, Bartfai T. Galanin: an endogenous anticonvulsant? *Neuroscientist.* 2001;7:506–517.

65. Mazarati AM, Liu H, Soomets U, et al. Galanin modulation of seizures and seizure modulation of hippocampal galanin in animal models of status epilepticus. *J Neurosci.* 1998;18:10070–10077.

66. Mazarati AM, Halaszi E, Telegdy G. Anticonvulsive effects of galanin administered into the central nervous system upon the picrotoxin-kindled seizure syndrome in rats. *Brain Res.* 1992;589:164–166.

67. Matagne A, Klitgaard H. Validation of corneally kindled mice: a sensitive screening model for partial epilepsy in man. *Epilepsy Res.* 1998;31:59–71.

68. Rundfeldt C. The new anticonvulsant retigabine (D-23129) acts as an opener of K+ channels in neuronal cells. *Eur J Pharmacol.* 1997;336:243–249.

69. Rundfeldt C. Characterization of the K+-opening effect of the anticonvulsant retigabine in PC12 cells. *Epilepsy Res.* 1999;35:99–107.

70. Main MJ, Cryan JE, Dupere JRB, et al. Modulation of KCNQ2/3 potassium channels by the novel anticonvulsant retigabine. *Mol Pharmacol.* 2000;58:253–262.

71. Biervert C, Schroeder BC, Kubisch C, et al. A potassium channel mutation in neonatal human epilepsy. *Science.* 1998;279:403–406.

72. Dailey JW, Cheong JH, Ko KH, et al. Anticonvulsant properties of D-20443 in genetically epilepsy prone rats: prediction of clinical response. *Neurosci Lett.* 1995;195:77–80.

73. Tober C, Rundfeldt C, Rostock A, et al. The phenyl carbamic acid ester D-23129 is highly effective in epilepsy models for generalized and focal seizures at nontoxic doses. *Abstr Soc Neurosci.* 1994;20:1641. Abstract.

74. Tober C, Rostock A, Rundfeldt C, et al. D-23129: a potent anticonvulsant in the amygdala kindling model of complex partial seizures. *Eur J Pharmacol.* 1996;303:163–169.

75. Blackburn-Munro G, Jensen BS. The anticonvulsant retigabine attenuates nociceptive behaviours in rat models of persistent and neuropathic pain. *Eur J Pharmacol.* 2003;460:109–116.

76. Dost R, Rostock A, Rundfeldt C. The anti-hyperalgesic activity of retigabine is mediated by KCNQ potassium channel activation. *Naunyn Schmiedebergs Arch Pharmacol.* 2004;369:382–390.

77. Argentieri TM, Sheldon JH, Bowlby MR, inventors; American Home Products Corporation, assignee. Methods for modulating bladder function. US patent 6 348 486. February 19, 2002.

78. Burbridge SA, Clare JJ, Cox B, et al. New uses for potassium channel openers. WO Patent WO1407768. January 11, 2001.

79. Kharkovets T, Hardelin JP, Safieddine S, et al. KCNQ4, a K-channel mutated in a form of dominant deafness, is expressed in the inner ear and the central auditory pathway. *Proc Natl Acad Sci.* 2000;97:4333–4338.

80. Porter RJ, Nohria V, Rundfeldt C. Retigabine. *Neurotherapeutics.* 2007;4:149–154.

81. Porter RJ, Partiot, A, Sachdeo R, et al. Randomized, multicenter, dose-ranging trial of retigabine for partial-onset seizures. *Neurology.* 2007;68:1197–1204.

82. Brodie M, Mansbach H. Retigabine 600 or 900 mg/day as adjunctive therapy in adults with partial-onset seizures. *Epilepsia.* 2008;49(suppl 7):110.

83. French J, Mansbach H. 1200 mg/day retigabine as adjunctive therapy in adults with refractory partial-onset seizures. *Epilepsia.* 2008;49(suppl 7):112–113.

84. Poisson M, Huguet F, Savattier A, et al. A new type of anticonvulsant, stiripentol: pharmacological profile and neurochemical study. *Arzneimittelforschung.* 1984;34:199–204.

85. Quilichini PP, Chiron C, Ben-Ari Y, et al. Stiripentol, a putative antiepileptic drug, enhances the duration of opening of GABAA-receptor channels. *Epilepsia.* 2006;47:704–716.

86. Tran A, Rey E, Pons G, et al. Influence of stiripentol on cytochrome P450-mediated metabolic pathways in humans: in vitro and in vivo comparison and calculation of in vivo inhibition constants. *Clin Pharmacol Ther.* 1997;62:490–504.

87. Levy RH, Loiseau P, Guyot M, et al. Stiripentol kinetics in epilepsy: nonlinearity and interactions. *Clin Pharmacol Ther.* 1984;36:661–669.

88. Perez J, Chiron C, Musial C, et al. Stiripentol: efficacy and tolerability in children with epilepsy. *Epilepsia.* 1999;40:1618–1626.

89. Chiron C, Marchand MC, Tran A, et al. Stiripentol in severe myoclonic epilepsy in infancy: a randomised placebo-controlled syndrome-dedicated trial. STICLO study group. *Lancet.* 2000;356:1638–1642.

90. Chiron C. Stiripentol. *Neurotherapeutics.* 2007;4:123–125.

CHAPTER 68 ■ LESS COMMONLY USED ANTIEPILEPTIC DRUGS

BASIM M. UTHMAN

Despite the availability of a large number of marketed antiepileptic drugs (AEDs), physicians use only a few to treat most patients with epilepsy. The six traditional AEDs used for epileptic seizures include phenytoin, carbamazepine, valproate, primidone, phenobarbital, and ethosuximide. In 1999, phenytoin (Dilantin) had a 42% market share of total AED prescriptions for epilepsy in the United States, proprietary (Tegretol) and generic carbamazepine had a 24% share, and divalproex sodium (Depakote) had captured 17% of the market (1). The remaining 17% of the market was held by all other products and generics. The availability of less-sedating AEDs led to a gradual decline in the use of primidone and phenobarbital in the United States. This prescribing pattern reflects the physician's familiarity with a particular agent, its efficacy, tolerability, pharmacokinetic profile, and cost. Results of comparative trials have led to improved objectivity in the selection of the best agent for specific seizure disorders.

Over the past decade, the introduction of new AEDs—felbamate (Felbatol[1]), gabapentin (Neurontin), lamotrigine (Lamictal), topiramate (Topamax), tiagabine (Gabitril), zonisamide (Zonegran), oxcarbazepine (Trileptal), levetiracetam (Keppra), and pregabalin (Lyrica)—has expanded the range of choices when first-line agents fail to control seizures or produce intolerable adverse events. Felbamate has been of limited use because of toxic reactions affecting the liver and bone marrow. Because of improved tolerability and fewer drug–drug interactions, newer AEDs may replace older ones as first-line agents in the treatment of epilepsy. The availability of new AEDs has reduced the use of older AEDs over the last few years. In June 2003, the market share of Dilantin in the United States dropped to 33.3% of total AED prescriptions.

This chapter discusses less frequently used AEDs: ethotoin, methsuximide, methylphenobarbital, acetazolamide, vitamin B$_6$, and bromides (Table 68.1). Inferior efficacy, poor tolerability, or both have forced withdrawal of several AEDs from the market. The use of vagus nerve stimulation and the ketogenic diet is discussed elsewhere in this volume.

[1]Tegretol and Trileptal are registered trademarks of Novartis Pharmaceuticals; Depakote is a registered trademark of Abbott Laboratories; Felbatol is a registered trademark of Wallace Laboratories; Dilantin, Lyrica, and Neurontin are registered trademarks of Pfizer, Inc.; Lamictal is a registered trademark of GlaxoSmithKline; Topamax is a registered trademark of Ortho-McNeil Pharmaceutical; Gabitril is a registered trademark of Cephalon, Inc.; Zonegran is a registered trademark of Elan Pharmaceuticals; Keppra is a registered trademark of UCB Pharma, Inc.

TABLE 68.1

ANTIEPILEPTIC DRUGS MARKETED IN THE UNITED STATES

Year	Nonproprietary name[a]	Trade name introduced
1912	**Phenobarbital**[b]	Luminal
1935	Mephobarbital	Mebraral
1938	**Phenytoin**	Dilantin
1946	Trimethadione	Tridione
1947	Mephenytoin	Mesantoin
1949	Paramethadione	Paradione
1951	Phenacemide	Phenurone
1952	Metharbital	Gemonil
1953	Phensuximide	Milontin
1954	**Primidone**	Mysoline
1957	Methsuximide	Celontin
1957	Ethotoin	Peganone
1960	**Ethosuximide**	Zarontin
1968	Diazepam	Valium
1974	**Carbamazepine**	Tegretol
1975	Clonazepam	Clonopin
1978	**Valproate**	Depakene
1981	Clorazepate	Tranxene
1992	Felbamate	Felbatol
1994	**Gabapentin**	Neurontin
1995	**Lamotrigine**	Lamictal
1996	**Topiramate**	Topamax
1997	**Tiagabine**	Gabitril
2000	**Oxcarbazepine**	Trileptal
2000	**Zonisamide**	Zonegran
2000	**Levetiracetam**	Keppra
2005	**Pregabalin**	Lyrica

[a]Withdrawn AEDs are not included.
[b]Boldface indicates major AEDs.
Adapted from Levy R, Mattson R, Meldrum B, et al., eds. *Antiepileptic Drugs.* 3rd ed. New York: Raven Press; 1989:24.

ETHOTOIN

Historical Background

Until phenytoin was marketed as an AED in 1938, phenobarbital was well established as the agent of choice in the treatment of seizures. Merritt and Putnam (2,3), searching for

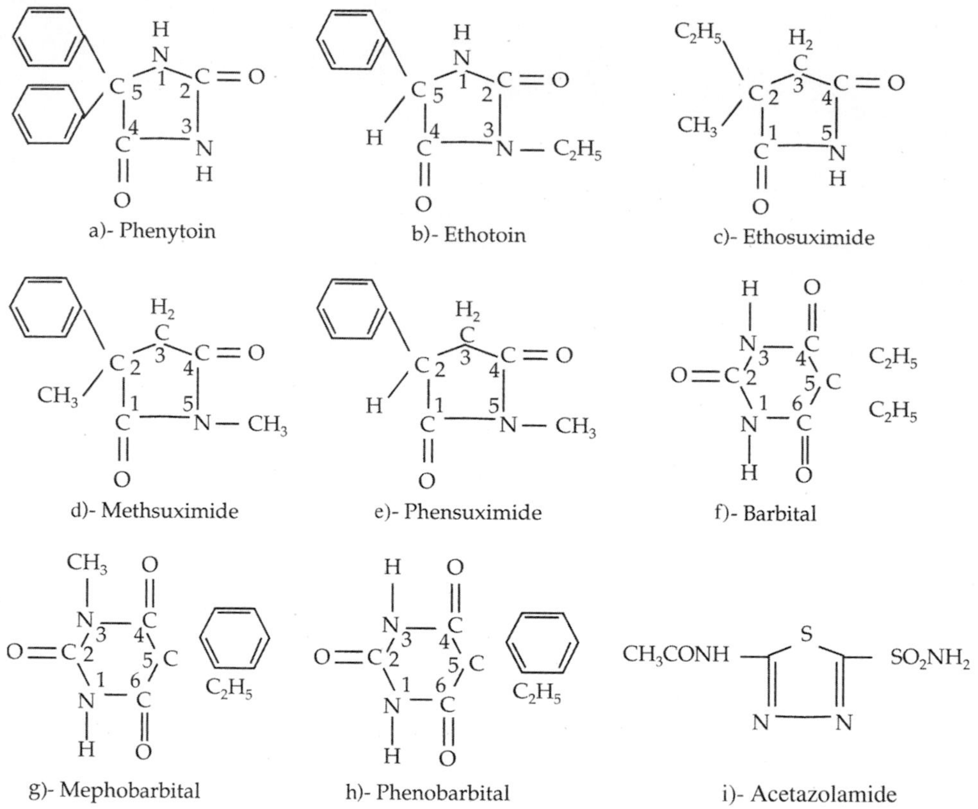

a)- Phenytoin

b)- Ethotoin

c)- Ethosuximide

d)- Methsuximide

e)- Phensuximide

f)- Barbital

g)- Mephobarbital

h)- Phenobarbital

i)- Acetazolamide

FIGURE 68.1. Chemical structures of selected minor and major antiepileptic drugs: **A:** Phenytoin. **B:** Ethotoin. **C–E:** Methsuximide belongs to the succinimide family (ethosuximide and phensuximide), which shares a common heterocyclic ring. **D:** Methsuximide. **F–G:** Mephobarbital is structurally similar to barbital. **H:** Phenobarbital. **I:** Acetazolamide.

AEDs devoid of sedative effects, first reported on the anticonvulsant properties of phenyl derivatives in animal studies. They recommended clinical trials of phenytoin (Dilantin; 5,5-diphenylhydantoin; Fig. 68.1A), and soon demonstrated the superiority of the agent over phenobarbital and its lack of significant hypnotic effects (4). Phenytoin has since become the world's most commonly used agent for the treatment of patients with generalized tonic–clonic and simple and complex partial seizures. Other hydantoins were also tested, but only ethotoin is still in use today.

Chemistry and Mechanism of Action

Ethotoin (Peganone, 3-ethyl-5-phenylhydantoin; Fig. 68.1B) is similar to phenytoin, except for the deletion of one phenyl group from position 5 and the addition of an ethyl group in position 3 of the hydantoin ring. It has a molecular weight of 204.22. Ethotoin has a broad spectrum of activity, and inhibits seizures induced by maximal electroshock and pentylenetetrazol.

Absorption, Distribution, and Metabolism

Ethotoin is slowly absorbed from the gastrointestinal (GI) tract. Absorption is dose-dependent; the time to peak plasma concentration increases with increasing dose. This nonlinear profile may explain the poor correlation between daily dose and steady-state serum levels of ethotoin (5).

Ethotoin is metabolized in the liver by hydroxylation and deethylation of the hydantoin ring. It has a relatively short half-life of 6 to 9 hours.

Efficacy and Clinical Use

The clinical use of ethotoin has been limited by its hypnotic properties and low anticonvulsant potency (6). The lack of gingival hyperplasia and hirsutism, side effects of phenytoin therapy, may make ethotoin an attractive alternative AED; however, it is only one fourth as effective as phenytoin in inhibiting electrically induced convulsions in animals. Few clinical trials of ethotoin are cited in the literature. In one study (7), ethotoin reduced seizure frequency in most of the children ($N = 17$) with uncontrolled seizures treated with dosages of 19 to 49 mg/kg/day. Two hours after ingestion, serum levels ranged from 14 to 34 μg/mL (conversion for ethotoin: μmol/L = μg/mL $\times$ 4.90) (5). In a retrospective study of adults with medically refractory epilepsy, ethotoin as adjunctive therapy reduced overall seizure frequency, especially the frequency of tonic seizures (8). The efficacy of the agent, however, was reduced by one half within 10 months, suggesting relatively rapid onset of tolerance. Ethotoin is ineffective in treating and may exacerbate absence seizures. Because of its short half-life, ethotoin is given in four divided doses of 20 to 40 mg/kg/day. Ethotoin is available in 250- and 500-mg tablets.

Interactions with Other Agents and Adverse Effects

No drug–drug interactions have been documented with ethotoin.

Although the agent is relatively free of the common adverse effects of phenytoin, ataxia, diplopia, dizziness, insomnia, rash, and GI distress may occur during ethotoin use. Isolated cases of lymphadenopathy have been reported. Cleft lip, cleft palate, and other malformations have occurred in infants born to mothers taking ethotoin (9,10).

Ethotoin has been available for more than five decades, but its efficacy and safety have not been adequately established in well-controlled clinical trials, and its use in the treatment of seizures and epilepsy remains limited.

METHSUXIMIDE

Historical Background

Introduced in 1957 for the treatment of refractory absence seizures, methsuximide (Celontin[2]) belongs to the succinimide family (i.e., ethosuximide and phensuximide), which shares a common heterocyclic (succinimide) ring (Fig. 68.1C–E). The diverse effects of these agents in a variety of experimental and clinical seizure types are probably related to the substitution of different chemical groups in the succinimide ring. Since phensuximide is no longer available, only methsuximide is discussed in some detail in this chapter.

Chemistry and Mechanism of Action

The chemical structure of methsuximide (*N*-2-dimethyl-2-phenyl-succinimide) is shown in Figure 68.1D. Phenyl group substitution at the 2C position counteracts experimentally induced maximal electroshock seizures, whereas alkyl group substitution at the 2C position counteracts experimentally induced pentylenetetrazol seizures. Methyl group substitution at the 5N position adds to the antipentylenetetrazol effect and the sedative activity. Alkyl substitution at the 5N and 2C positions and phenyl substitution at the 2C position provide activity against pentylenetetrazol- and maximal-electroshock–induced seizure activity (11).

Methsuximide is a nonpolar chemical compound that is water soluble and slightly lipophilic. Its exact effects on excitable membranes are unknown. Because of its effectiveness against absence and partial seizures, the agent probably has more than one mechanism of action, including effects on transmitter release, calcium uptake into presynaptic endings, and conductance of sodium, potassium, and chloride.

Absorption, Distribution, and Metabolism

Methsuximide is quickly absorbed through the GI tract, with peak plasma levels achieved in 2 to 4 hours. The agent is distributed evenly throughout the body and penetrates brain and fat tissue better than ethosuximide (12). Because of its low protein binding and poor solubility, methsuximide equilibrates with CSF (B. J. Wilder, unpublished data, 1980). It is rapidly metabolized to *N*-desmethyl-methsuximide or 2-methyl-2-phenyl succinimide (12–15) and has a mean half-life of 1.4 hours. Trough plasma concentrations of methsuximide are reportedly undetectable in fasting specimens (16). A major active metabolite of methsuximide, *N*-desmethyl-methsuximide,

achieves high steady-state plasma levels and exerts a major anticonvulsant effect. The mean half-life of this metabolite is 38 hours (range, 37 to 48 hours) (13), although some investigators (16) have reported half-lives of 51.6 to 80.2 hours in patients who received maximal doses of methsuximide. Another methsuximide metabolite, *N*-methyl-2-hydroxy-methyl-2-phenylsuccinimide, was detected by means of gas chromatography and mass spectrometry of the serum of a patient with a fatal overdose of primidone and methsuximide.

Optimal clinical effect may be achieved with a nontrough *N*-desmethyl-methsuximide plasma concentration of 20 to 24 μg/mL (15), near the middle of the therapeutic range of 10 to 40 μg/mL, reported by Strong and colleagues (14). Browne and associates (16) reported a therapeutic range of 10 to 30 μg/mL for fasting *N*-desmethyl-methsuximide plasma concentrations. Steady-state plasma concentration is reached between 8.1 and 16.8 days from onset of maintenance methsuximide dose. The usual dosage increase of 150 or 300 mg/day can be made at biweekly intervals to avoid toxicity. Methsuximide is no longer available in 150-mg tablets; biweekly dosage increments of one tablet (300 mg) every other day may be used (16).

Efficacy and Clinical Use

Methsuximide has a wide spectrum of antiepileptic activity and is effective in patients with complex partial seizures (15–17), generalized tonic–clonic seizures, and absence seizures (18–21). Wilder, Buchanan, and Uthman (15,22) found methsuximide to be an effective adjunctive agent in the management of refractory complex partial seizures. Twenty-one patients taking phenytoin, phenobarbital, primidone, or carbamazepine as monotherapy or in combination were studied. Of these patients, 71% achieved good to excellent control of complex partial seizures, and a dose reduction or discontinuation of one or more AED was possible in 42%. Optimal plasma levels and control of complex partial seizures were associated with daily methsuximide dosages of 9.5 to 11.0 mg/kg, with maximal seizure control observed at *N*-desmethyl-methsuximide plasma levels of 20 to 24 μg/mL (conversion factor for methsuximide: μmol/L = 4.92 × μg/mL). A dose–response relationship was determined after the addition of methsuximide, and seizure frequency progressively decreased as *N*-desmethyl-methsuximide serum levels increased.

Browne and colleagues (16) described the use of adjunctive methsuximide in 26 patients with medically refractory complex partial seizures. The maximal tolerated dose of methsuximide was maintained for 8 weeks. Of the total population, eight patients (31%) had a 50% or more reduction in seizure frequency, and four (15%) became seizure-free. Eight patients withdrew from the study because of adverse events and three because of increased seizure frequency (these patients had a history of severe seizure flurries before and after initiation of methsuximide treatment). Of the eight patients who responded, five continued to have a 50% or more reduction in frequency of complex partial seizures for 3 to 34 months.

Sigler and associates (23) used methsuximide as add-on therapy in children with epilepsy refractory to first- and second-line AEDs. Forty patients (35.7%) had a 50% or more reduction in seizure frequency, and 10 (8.9%) became seizure-free during the short-term phase (mean, 9.1 weeks). Of the 112

---

[2]Celontin is a registered trademark of Pfizer Inc.

patients studied, 22 (19.6%) continued to benefit from the drug (a 50% or more reduction in seizure frequency compared with baseline and absence of intolerable side effects) at long-term follow-up (mean, 3.7 years; range, 18 months to 7.1 years). In patients with good seizure control, fasting plasma levels of N-desmethyl-methsuximide were 25.3 to 44.7 mg/L (mean, 36.0 mg/L); thus, effective plasma concentrations of N-desmethyl-methsuximide in children were found to be higher than previously described. No serious or irreversible side effects were reported. Likewise, Tennison and colleagues (24) used methsuximide as add-on therapy in children with complex partial and "minor motor" seizures refractory to first- and second-line AEDs; 15 patients (60%) had a 50% or more reduction in seizure frequency, and no serious adverse events were reported.

Other reports of methsuximide as adjunctive medical therapy for complex partial seizures showed complete seizure control in 0% to 38% of patients and a 50% or more reduction in seizure frequency in 6% to 100% of patients (17,19,25–28). In one study of previously untreated patients (29), seizures were controlled in 18%, and 27% had a 50% or more reduction in seizure frequency.

Results of early studies of methsuximide showed some efficacy in patients with absence seizures (19–21). In one study (20), methsuximide was used in previously untreated patients; absences were not completely controlled in any patient, and only 20% had a greater than 50% reduction in seizure frequency. Rabe (30) reported that 10 of 16 patients became completely free of absences and another five had seizure frequency reduced by 75%. He suggested two possible explanations for the greater effectiveness of methsuximide in his study compared with earlier work: most of his patients had epilepsy of relatively recent onset, and he used considerably higher doses of methsuximide (1200 to 2100 mg/day) than did previous investigators.

Rabe also reported on the efficacy of methsuximide in four patients with juvenile myoclonic epilepsy (30). Two patients became completely free of myoclonus and two had a reduction in frequency of at least 75%. One case report described methsuximide used with primidone to be very effective in a 17-year-old boy with drawing-induced myoclonic seizures (31). Hurst (32) described five adolescent girls with juvenile myoclonic epilepsy who became seizure-free taking methsuximide; four were maintained on monotherapy.

Tolerance to the anticonvulsant effect of methsuximide develops in approximately 50% of patients treated with maximal doses, and seizure frequency returns to baseline. The low overall efficacy of methsuximide relative to that of first-line AEDs may reflect the selectively more refractory seizures in the patients studied. Failures because of toxic reactions might have occurred when the dose of methsuximide was increased too rapidly. The dose should not be increased more often than every 2 weeks in adults receiving multidrug therapy (16). Methsuximide should be considered in patients who are allergic to or whose disease is refractory to other AEDs.

Interactions with Other Agents and Adverse Effects

Methsuximide interacts with other AEDs, necessitating close monitoring of serum levels and adjustment of concurrent AED

dose, especially in the face of clinical toxicity. Rambeck (33) reported that concurrent administration of methsuximide increased the mean serum concentration of phenobarbital by 37% in patients receiving this agent and by 40% in patients receiving primidone. The mean serum concentration of phenytoin increased by 78%. Patients taking phenobarbital or phenytoin had increased serum levels of N-desmethyl-methsuximide compared with patients taking methsuximide alone. These increases were attributed to competition by the drugs for a common hydroxylating enzyme system.

Conversely, the addition of methsuximide induces the metabolization of other AEDs (34,35). Methsuximide decreased the mean serum concentrations of carbamazepine (16), valproic acid (36,37), lamotrigine (35,38), and topiramate (39) when added to the treatment regimen. Methsuximide mitigated the effect of valproic acid on lamotrigine; the combination of valproic acid and lamotrigine increased the concentration of lamotrigine by 211% compared with lamotrigine monotherapy; however, if methsuximide was added, the increased concentration of lamotrigine dropped to 8% (35).

GI disturbance, lethargy, somnolence, fatigue, and headache may be experienced, but these adverse effects are usually transient and dose-related. Other adverse experiences include hiccups, irritability, ataxia, blurred vision or diplopia, inattention, dysarthria, and psychic changes (16). In some patients, headache, photophobia, and hiccups require withdrawal of methsuximide (15). Transient leukopenia and a movement disorder have been reported (40). Delayed, profound coma following methsuximide overdose has been described (41). Charcoal hemoperfusion was successful in one case of methsuximide overdose (42).

BARBITURATES

Historical Background

Approximately 2500 barbiturate compounds have been synthesized since barbituric acid was first produced in 1864. About 25 (1%) of these compounds are licensed by the U.S. Food and Drug Administration as hypnotics, anesthetics, and anticonvulsants (11). Two barbiturates are currently marketed as AEDs: mephobarbital (Mebaral,[3] methylphenobarbital, methylphenobarbitone) and phenobarbital (Luminal; Fig. 68.1H). Primidone (Mysoline) is a deoxybarbiturate metabolized to phenobarbital and phenylethyl-malonamide. All these compounds are derived from barbital, the first synthetic hypnotic barbiturate.

Phenobarbital was introduced as an AED in 1912 (43) and remains one of the major agents used worldwide for the treatment of generalized tonic–clonic and simple or complex partial seizures. It has a special use in patients with status epilepticus and is widely prescribed for prophylaxis of febrile seizures and alcohol- and drug-withdrawal seizures. Phenobarbital and primidone were reported to be less well tolerated than phenytoin and carbamazepine for the treatment of seizures of partial onset (44). A number of studies have reported on the behavioral and cognitive side effects of phenobarbital (45–49). Phenobarbital and primidone are discussed in detail in other chapters. Mephobarbital is considered here.

---

[3]Mebaral is a registered trademark of Ovation Pharmaceuticals, Inc.

Chemistry and Mechanism of Action

The chemical structure of mephobarbital (5-ethyl-1-methyl-5-phenylbarbituric acid) is similar to the structure of barbital, as illustrated in Figure 68.1F and G. Mephobarbital is similar to phenobarbital except for the methyl group at the 3N position. The molecular mass of mephobarbital is 246.26. The mechanism of anticonvulsant action is probably similar to that of phenobarbital, essentially inhibiting the spread of seizure activity and elevating seizure threshold (50). All the commercially available hypnotic barbiturates exhibit anticonvulsant activity at anesthetic doses and inhibit epileptic seizures induced by electroshock, tetanus, strychnine, or pentylenetetrazol. This anticonvulsant activity is separate from the sedative or anesthetic effects and is not diminished by the concurrent administration of agents that counteract sedation (11).

Absorption, Distribution, and Metabolism

Mephobarbital is highly soluble in lipids, with lipid to water partition ratio of 100. The agent is easily absorbed and readily crosses biologic membranes. A bioavailability of 75% was found in a pharmacokinetic study of mephobarbital in two volunteers (51). It appears to be widely distributed in the body, with higher concentrations in adipose tissue and brain. In rats, brain mephobarbital levels were eight times those simultaneously measured in blood (52). In vitro studies suggest that 58% to 68% of mephobarbital in highly concentrated solution is bound to human serum albumin (53).

Mephobarbital is metabolized to phenobarbital by demethylation in the liver (54,55) and is affected by the cytochrome P450 system (56). A portion is excreted in human urine as a p-hydroxyphenyl glucuronide derivative of the parent drug (57). Phenobarbital is a known liver enzyme inducer, with this effect possibly responsible for the decrease in mephobarbital elimination half-life from approximately 50 hours initially to 12 to 24 hours during long-term therapy.

Efficacy and Clinical Use

In view of mephobarbital's metabolism, the clinical efficacy and safety of the agent could be expected to resemble those of its metabolite, phenobarbital. Use of mephobarbital began in 1932 (58). Although attempts to correlate dose and serum levels with anticonvulsant effect were made, well-controlled studies comparing the efficacy and safety of the agent with those of other AEDs for the treatment of epilepsy are not available. Nevertheless, mephobarbital is reputed to be as effective as phenobarbital in humans and less sedative (59). National Health Service prescriptions for mephobarbital in Australia have remained similar to those for phenobarbital and primidone over several years (59). There is no reason to believe that mephobarbital is more effective or has a wider anticonvulsant spectrum than the less expensive phenobarbital. It is difficult to differentiate the anticonvulsant effect of the parent drug, mephobarbital, and that of its active metabolite, phenobarbital, during long-term treatment in humans.

Because of the slower metabolism of phenobarbital, its steady-state plasma concentrations exceed those of the parent drug. Probably for that reason, the therapeutic range of mephobarbital traditionally has been expressed in terms of plasma phenobarbital concentrations. Some believe that by ignoring plasma mephobarbital levels, a measure of one active anticonvulsant substance present in the body may be overlooked (59). It is argued that because of its apparent high volume of distribution relative to that of phenobarbital and its lipid solubility, mephobarbital probably has substantially higher brain levels than plasma levels compared with phenobarbital. Usual therapeutic plasma levels of phenobarbital range from 10 to 40 μg/mL. Steady-state plasma phenobarbital levels correlate closely with mephobarbital dose.

Mephobarbital dosages of 3 to 4 mg/kg/day produce mean plasma phenobarbital levels of 15 μg/mL; a dosage of 5 mg/kg/day produces mean levels of 20 μg/mL (59). At higher mephobarbital doses and plasma levels, proportionately lower phenobarbital plasma levels are seen. This may suggest a rate-limited metabolism at high plasma mephobarbital concentrations (59). In one small study (60), plasma phenobarbital levels averaged 20 times those of mephobarbital (conversion for mephobarbital: [μmol/L] = 4.06 × [μg/mL]; phenobarbital: [μmol/L] = 4.31 × [μg/mL]).

Interactions with Other Agents and Adverse Effects

Any interaction that is known to occur with phenobarbital (see Chapter 53) probably will also happen with mephobarbital. Subtle adverse effects in the form of intellectual impairment and depression of cognitive abilities are of major concern in patients receiving long-term therapy with mephobarbital or metharbital (61). Other untoward reactions include hypnotic effects, irritability, hyperactivity, and alterations in sleep patterns. Up to 40% of children and probably as many elderly patients taking phenobarbital experience unpleasant side effects (11). Impairment of immediate memory and attention has been demonstrated with long-term phenobarbital use at therapeutic plasma drug levels (62,63). This effect on short-term memory and attention is a significant problem, considering the large number of school-aged children who receive phenobarbital or mephobarbital. Children who take barbiturates may experience irritability and hyperactivity. In one study (64), six of 11 children on maintenance doses of phenobarbital or mephobarbital had clear behavioral changes, including irritability, oppositional attitudes, and overactivity, compared with age-matched controls. Many of our patients reported feeling "dumb" or "mentally dull" when they received barbiturate drugs. In others, already taking barbiturates when referred to us, intellectual impairment became apparent in retrospect after the drug was withdrawn. When other, safer AEDs have failed and phenobarbital or mephobarbital must be used, patients should be treated with the lowest dose that effects adequate seizure control.

Another side effect of phenobarbital that is unintentionally ignored by physicians is impotence or decreased libido. Usually, male patients are reluctant to discuss their sex lives, and physicians tend to ascribe the problem to psychosocial conflict. In a Veterans Administration Cooperative study,

Mattson and colleagues (44) found that 15% of patients complained of decreased potency, decreased libido, or both. Of 56 patients who took phenobarbital for 1 year, 14% reported a transient or continuous decrease in sexual function. The problem usually disappeared when phenytoin or carbamazepine was substituted for phenobarbital, but not when phenobarbital was changed to another barbiturate.

ACETAZOLAMIDE

Historical Background

Carbonic anhydrase activity was first demonstrated in red blood cells in the early 1930s. It catalyzes reaction I:

$$CO_2 + H_2O \leftrightarrow H_2CO_3 \leftrightarrow H^+ + HCO_3^-$$

Carbonic anhydrase has subsequently been found in many tissues, including the pancreas, gastric mucosa, renal cortex, eye, and CNS. Inhibition of carbonic anhydrase activity was observed when sulfanilamide was introduced as a chemotherapeutic agent. A large number of sulfonamides have been synthesized and tested as carbonic anhydrase inhibitors and potential diuretics. Among these, acetazolamide has been the most extensively studied. Acetazolamide was introduced as an AED by Bergstrom and coworkers (65), and later reports confirmed its effectiveness in most seizure types (66–70). Its usefulness, however, is limited by the rapid development of tolerance.

Chemistry and Mechanism of Action

Acetazolamide (Diamox,[4] N-(5-sulfamoyl-1,3,4-thiadiazol-2-yl-)acetamide; Fig. 68.1I) is a weak acid with a molecular mass of 222. In the brain, acetazolamide acts through inhibition of carbonic anhydrase, causing carbon dioxide to accumulate and inducing the anticonvulsant action. Blocking carbonic anhydrase in other tissues, particularly red blood cells, causes even greater retention of carbon dioxide in the brain (71). This results in blockade of anion transport, which prevents spread of seizure activity and elevates seizure threshold. The anticonvulsant effect of acetazolamide, as measured by prevention of maximal electroshock-induced seizures (72,73), correlates with the degree of inhibition of brain carbonic anhydrase. Acetazolamide is one of the most potent carbonic anhydrase (CA) isozymes—that is, CA I and CA II—and the agent exhibited strong anticonvulsant properties in a maximal electroshock test in mice (74). Acetazolamide increases brain levels of GABA; however, increased carbon dioxide levels have also been shown to raise brain GABA levels. The carbonic anhydrase inhibitory effect with subsequent increase in intracellular carbon dioxide is probably responsible for the anticonvulsant properties of acetazolamide (75). Carbonic anhydrase inhibitor sukthiame decreases the intracellular pH of hippocampal CA_3 neurons by 0.17 ± 0.10 within 10 minutes, and action potentials and the frequency of epileptiform bursts 10 to 15 minutes after administration (76).

---

[4]Diamox is a registered trademark of Wyeth.

High doses of acetazolamide may produce a paradoxical effect, resulting in disruption of acid–base homeostasis in the brain (77). The drug also alters choroid plexus function by its effect on carbonic anhydrase, decreasing production of CSF by limiting chloride and bicarbonate transport across the plexus (78). Woodbury (78) showed that the development of tolerance to acetazolamide is attributable to the induction of increased carbonic anhydrase synthesis in glial cells and to glial proliferation.

Absorption, Distribution, and Metabolism

Acetazolamide is rapidly absorbed from the GI tract, and peak plasma levels occur 2 to 4 hours after a single oral dose. Because acetazolamide is a weak acid, most of its absorption takes place in the duodenum and upper jejunum after some amount has been absorbed in the stomach. In humans, the agent is 90% protein-bound; concentrations are lower in CSF than in plasma. The greatest concentration of acetazolamide is in red blood cells. After distribution to various tissues, it binds to carbonic anhydrase and remains in a relatively stable carbonic anhydrase–acetazolamide complex. The plasma half-life of acetazolamide is 2 to 4 days. It is eliminated in the urine unchanged through glomerular filtration, tubular filtration, and tubular secretion. Increasing urinary pH increases excretion. Acetazolamide is also excreted in the bile to be resorbed from the intestinal tract.

Efficacy and Clinical Use

Acetazolamide is effective against various seizure types, particularly absence seizures, when it is used as an adjunct to other AEDs (79). After several weeks of continuous treatment, however, tolerance usually develops. Transient or intermittent use of acetazolamide is beneficial when seizures are temporarily exacerbated. This avoids the development of tolerance and may offer protection beyond that provided by AEDs administered long term. Perhaps the best application of acetazolamide is in catamenial epilepsy. The drug can be started 5 days before the expected onset of menses and continued for 11 to 14 days. With a half-life of 2 to 4 days, steady-state plasma levels occur 5 to 7 days after the initial dose, and adequate levels continue for 3 to 5 days after the agent is discontinued. This regimen can be repeated with each menstrual cycle. In a retrospective study of 20 women with catamenial epilepsy, 40% reported a 50% or greater decrease in seizure frequency; the response rates were similar in generalized versus focal epilepsy and temporal versus extratemporal epilepsy (80). In a retrospective study of 31 patients with juvenile myoclonic epilepsy treated with long-term acetazolamide monotherapy, generalized tonic–clonic seizures were controlled in 45% (81).

Katayama and associates (82) examined the long-term effectiveness and side effects of acetazolamide when used as an adjunct to other AEDs in children with refractory epilepsy. Complete seizure control for more than 3 years was obtained in four (10.8%) of 37 patients, and six patients (16.2%) showed a greater than 50% decrease in seizure frequency for more than 6 months after the introduction of acetazolamide. None of the patients (n = 28) that were examined after long-term acetazolamide therapy, which ranged from 10 months to

14 years, showed evidence of renal calculi. A summary of the pharmacologic and pharmacokinetic properties, efficacy, and safety of acetazolamide in the treatment of epilepsy has been published (83).

The recommended daily dosage is 10 mg/kg given in a single dose or in two or three divided doses. Usual effective therapeutic plasma levels range from 8 to 14 μg/mL (conversion for acetazolamide: μmol/L = 4.5 × μg/mL). Acetazolamide is available in 125-, 250-, and 500-mg scored tablets. Delayed-release 500-mg tablets are also marketed.

Interactions with Other Agents and Adverse Effects

Elimination of acetazolamide may decrease and the half-life of the agent may increase with the concomitant use of probenecid, which blocks renal tubular secretion of acids. The absorption of salicylate may be increased and that of amphetamine may be delayed when these drugs are taken with acetazolamide. Acetazolamide is a relatively benign agent, with only a few adverse effects known. Lethargy, paresthesias, rashes, abdominal distention, and cyanosis have been reported with its use. In up to 90% of patients, acetazolamide can alter taste sensation (84) by eliminating the tingly or prickly sensation of carbonation and giving a false flat taste to carbonated beverages; we have not seen this effect in any of our patients who had been placed on intermittent treatment. Renal calculi have been reported after long-term use (81). Patients who have been taking phenytoin, barbiturates, and/or acetazolamide for 5 years or more show decreased bone mineral density (BMD) compared with healthy controls (85). A 7-year follow-up (total of ≥12 years of use) with these subjects revealed significantly lower BMDs when compared with their previous measurement at 5 years of treatment. In one study (86), standard height and weight scores were significantly reduced in children receiving acetazolamide along with other AEDs. The investigators speculated that acetazolamide-induced metabolic acidosis might have been responsible for this growth suppression. Caution is advised when the agent is used in children. Teratogenic effects have been induced in animals. Although acetazolamide use may be considered if seizures are exacerbated during pregnancy, the drug should be avoided during the first trimester.

PYRIDOXINE

Historical Background

Two types of pyridoxine-related seizures occur in the newborn: those caused by pyridoxine (vitamin B_6) deficiency (87,88) and those caused by pyridoxine dependency (89,90). These rare conditions carry a poor prognosis for mental development if prompt treatment is not rendered. Pyridoxine dependency as a cause of generalized seizures in children was reported about 40 years ago (91). An autosomal recessive disorder (92), it typically manifests in neonates, but onset has been reported up to the age of 19 months (93,94). Vitamin B_6 levels are reduced in pyridoxine deficiency but are normal in pyridoxine-dependent epilepsy. In either case, vitamin B_6 is the only effective treatment; in pyridoxine deficiency, a single dose is sufficient, whereas pyridoxine dependency requires continuous vitamin B_6 administration.

Chemistry and Mechanism of Action

Pyridoxal phosphate, the active metabolite of vitamin B_6, is the coenzyme for glutamic acid decarboxylase (GAD) and GABA transaminase, the enzymes necessary for the production and metabolism of CNS GABA. In the pyridoxine dependency and deficiency states, GABA levels in CSF are significantly reduced (95). Similarly, GABA and GAD concentrations were reduced in the cortex of a patient with pyridoxine-dependent seizures (94). The underlying defect in pyridoxine-dependent epilepsy is unknown, but one theory is that it is caused by faulty GAD, which catalyzes the conversion of glutamic acid to GABA (92,96). However, glutamate and GABA studies in CSF have been contradictory, and recent genetic studies have not found any linkage between the two brain isoforms (97). Another recent hypothesis is that there may be an abnormality of pyridoxine transport, which underlies the pathophysiology of the disorder (98).

Efficacy and Clinical Use

Pyridoxine Dependency

The diagnosis is established by remission of seizures (generalized seizures or status epilepticus) with vitamin B_6 and relapse without this treatment. Given parenterally in pharmacologic amounts (50 to 100 mg), pyridoxine hydrochloride stops the seizures within minutes (89,99–101). In pyridoxine dependency, lifelong supplementation with vitamin B_6 is needed. Withdrawal of pyridoxine even after several years of effective therapy causes seizures to reappear within days or weeks (99,101,102). Untreated patients develop intractable epilepsy, and most die within days or months (102).

Psychomotor retardation and progressive neurologic deterioration result when therapy is delayed; therefore, early diagnosis and treatment are important for stopping the seizures and preventing a chronic encephalopathy. In one study (103), serial magnetic resonance imaging (MRI) scans of the heads of children with neonatal seizures and pyridoxine dependency demonstrated progressive dilation of the ventricular system and atrophy of the cortex and subcortical white matter, which was thought to result from an imbalance of GABA and glutamic acid levels causing chronic excitotoxicity in the cerebrum. Pyridoxine-dependent seizures atypically may involve prolonged seizure-free periods with conventional AEDs before pyridoxine treatment (99,100), need for large doses before an effect is seen (104), and late onset several months after birth (100,105). Bass and coworkers (106) reported other atypical features in a child whose seizures stopped only after repeated trials of pyridoxine. The investigators warned of the possibility of decreased levels of consciousness with intravenous (IV) pyridoxine and of the need to have resuscitative equipment available.

Recommended daily oral maintenance dosages range from 2 to 300 mg, corresponding to doses from 0.2 to 30 mg/kg/day (94,95,99–102,104,105,107), with most patients becoming seizure-free with doses between 20 and 100 mg/day (103). The single report of long-term follow-up suggested that the prognosis for complete seizure control is excellent (102). However, it was found that elevated cerebral glutamic acid concentrations in children with pyridoxine-dependent epilepsy may not normalize after vitamin B_6 doses sufficient to stop the seizures (108). To prevent psychomotor retardation in patients with this condition, adjustments in the vitamin B_6 dosage should be based on seizure control and on normalization of glutamate concentration in the CSF (108).

Pyridoxine-Responsive Epilepsy

The finding that CSF levels of GABA were lower in patients with infantile spasms than in controls (109,110) led to a number of trials of vitamin B_6 for the treatment of this syndrome (111–114). In the first and largest trial (113), children received daily vitamin B_6 doses of 30 to 400 mg; 13% became seizure-free within 2 weeks after initiation of treatment. Vitamin B_6 as monotherapy or in combination with valproic acid was also investigated in 20 children with infantile spasms (112). Treatment began at 10 to 20 mg/kg/day, with a maintenance dose of 20 to 50 mg/kg/day in three doses. Vitamin B_6 monotherapy reduced seizure frequency in 23% of patients, although only one patient remained seizure-free during the 15-month follow-up. No statistically significant difference was identified between patients treated with vitamin B_6 monotherapy and valproate monotherapy (30 to 63 mg/kg/day); however, these agents administered in combination produced significantly better seizure reduction and electroencephalographic effects than did vitamin B_6 alone. Corticotropin was more effective than vitamin B_6 as monotherapy or in combination with valproic acid, having an excellent effect in 86% of patients who did not respond to the combination treatment; many patients, however, had later recurrences of seizures.

Blennow and Starck (111) successfully treated three children with doses ranging between 200 and 400 mg/kg/day. In another study (114), five of 17 children with infantile spasms responded to 300 mg/kg/day of vitamin B_6 within the first week of treatment, with all five becoming seizure-free within 4 weeks. The investigators proposed that treatment begin with high doses for 4 to 6 weeks and be followed by a slow dosage reduction (114). In a randomized, prospective trial (115) of neonates, infants, and children younger than 12 years of age with acute recurrent seizures, adjunctive therapy with IV pyridoxine (30 to 50 mg/kg) infused over 2 to 4 hours was significantly superior to monotherapy with a conventional AED. Of note, Wang and Kuo (116) suggest using pyridoxal phosphate (PLP), the active form of vitamin B_6, instead of pyridoxine in pediatric epilepsy. They reason that PLP is as inexpensive as pyridoxine is and patients with one of the four inborn errors of vitamin B_6 metabolism, pyridoxine phosphate oxidase deficiency, respond to PLP and not to pyridoxine.

Adverse Effects

After IV vitamin B_6 administration, apnea, lethargy, pallor, decreased responsiveness, and hypotonia may occur immediately and persist for several hours (102). These reactions have also followed intramuscular administration (100,117) and the initial oral dose (118). Believed to result from a massive initial release of GABA (118), these symptoms are usually mild, but on rare occasions have necessitated intubation and assisted ventilation (119). Loss of appetite, periods of restlessness and crying, vomiting, and apathy have been reported during therapy for infantile spasms with high doses of vitamin B_6 (114).

Long-term pyridoxine use can cause a peripheral neuropathy, which has been documented in animals (120) and humans (121–123), and produced experimentally in animals (124) and humans (125). The original reports suggested that doses of 2000 to 6000 mg/day were toxic to dorsal root ganglia, with subsequent degeneration of the peripheral sensory nerves. Later reports indicated that daily doses as low as 500 mg (126) and possibly 200 mg (122) could be neurotoxic. Early recognition of the potential toxicity of high pyridoxine doses and the complete reversal of symptoms on withdrawal of supplementation has averted permanent disability in all but two patients who received a single dose of >100 g of parenteral pyridoxine (127). Prospective studies of 70 adult patients taking daily doses of 100 to 150 mg reported no clinical or electrophysiologic evidence of neurotoxicity (128,129).

On the basis of findings in adults, high doses of pyridoxine may be potentially harmful in infants (130). Although no sensory neuropathy was observed in patients with homocystinuria who received 10 to 90 mg/kg/day during the first 10 years of life (131), nor in three children with infantile spasms treated with very high doses of vitamin B_6, prudence dictates (111) use of the minimum effective dosage. One case of sensory neuropathy caused by high-dose, long-term pyridoxine therapy for pyridoxine-dependent epilepsy has been reported (132).

BROMIDES

Historical Background

In 1857, at a time when seizures were linked to hysteria and masturbation, bromides, with putative antiaphrodisiac properties, were introduced for the treatment of epilepsy (133). They remained the principal AED until phenobarbital became available in 1912.

Chemistry and Mechanism of Action

The anticonvulsant mechanism of bromides is unknown, although hyperpolarization of postsynaptic membranes has been proposed. In radioligand studies, halide ions (including bromide and chloride) were found to enhance binding to benzodiazepine receptors, probably at an anion-binding site related to the GABA-gated chloride channels (134). Because bromide has a smaller hydrated diameter than chloride, it crosses cell membranes faster and tends to hyperpolarize the postsynaptic membrane, which is activated by inhibitory neurotransmitters (135).

Absorption, Distribution, and Metabolism

Bromide salts are rapidly absorbed from the GI tract and have nearly complete bioavailability (136). Not bound to plasma proteins, they can freely diffuse across membranes. The volume of distribution of bromides is similar to that of chloride ions. Tissues do not distinguish between these two anions, and their concentration in extracellular fluids depends on their relative intake and excretion. After oral administration, bromides have a half-life of approximately 12 days (136). Excretion by the kidneys occurs slowly and depends on concomitant chloride intake. A high chloride load increases the excretion of bromides and shortens the half-life. Conversely, a salt-deficient diet reduces bromide clearance and prolongs the half-life (135).

Efficacy and Clinical Use

Most reports about the efficacy of bromides include a small number of patients with a variety of seizure types treated with a number of AEDs. Bromides have generally been found to be most effective in treating patients with refractory generalized tonic–clonic seizures and to be considerably less effective in other seizure types (137–141). A retrospective, controlled clinical evaluation (140) of 60 children with medically refractory generalized tonic–clonic seizures found a 50% or more seizure reduction in 58% of patients, with 27% achieving complete control.

Bromides are usually administered as the triple bromide elixir (i.e., combination of sodium, potassium, and ammonium bromide salts) containing 240 mg/mL of bromide salt. The usual dosage in children younger than 6 years of age ranges from 300 mg twice daily to 600 mg three times daily. For children older than 6 years of age, 300 to 1000 mg is administered three times daily (137). The therapeutic plasma concentration (135) ranges from 750 to 1250 µg/mL (10 to 15 mEq/L). Because toxic adverse effects may occur at a concentration of 1500 µg/mL, careful monitoring of serum is required. A steady salt intake should be maintained during treatment. Bromide treatment should be reserved for patients whose disease is refractory to other AEDs and especially for those with refractory generalized tonic–clonic seizures.

Interactions with Other Agents and Adverse Effects

No interactions of bromides with other agents have been described. Sedation is the most frequently encountered side effect of bromides. Although rare cases of acute intoxication with marked nephrotoxicity and ototoxicity have been reported, the more common adverse effects occur as a result of chronic toxicity. Referred to as bromism (142), these effects target the CNS, skin, and GI tract in older individuals or those with compromised renal function. Chronic intoxication is associated with weakness, tiredness, headaches, irritability, confusion, restlessness, psychosis, and sometimes coma. Dermatologic manifestations include rash, nodular or pustular lesions, and ulcerations (135,142). Anorexia, constipation, and GI distress may also occur. Bromism is treated by the administration of a large quantity of sodium chloride and a chloruretic agent. Hemodialysis or peritoneal dialysis can be used to lower bromide levels rapidly (143).

CONCLUSION

Major AEDs may fail because of lack of efficacy or increased toxicity and serious reactions. In these cases, less commonly used AEDs may be efficacious and may help provide better seizure control especially when alternative surgical options are

not choice solutions. Although these drugs are usually administered as adjunctive therapy, the physician should be encouraged to aim for monotherapy with these second-line agents if seizure frequency is reduced. Monotherapy simplifies the drug regimen, reduces cost, decreases toxic reactions, and probably further improves seizure control. Nonpharmacologic therapy, such as intermittent vagus nerve stimulation, may provide another alternative for patients with medically refractory seizures. Other neurostimulation techniques for the purpose of preventing recurrent seizures are under study.

ACKNOWLEDGMENTS

The authors thank Dr. K. A. Abboud of the University of Florida, Department of Chemistry, who prepared Figure 68.1.

References

1. Scott Levin's PPDA, MAT. February 1999.
2. Merritt HH, Putnam TJ. A new series of anticonvulsant drugs tested by experiments on animals. *Arch Neurol Psychiatry.* 1938;39:1003–1015.
3. Putnam TJ, Merritt HH. Experimental determination of anticonvulsant properties of some phenyl derivatives. *Science.* 1937;85:525–526.
4. Merritt HH, Putnam TJ. Sodium diphenylhydantoinate in treatment of convulsive disorders. *J Am Med Assoc.* 1938;111:1068–1073.
5. Kupferberg HJ. Other hydantoins: mephenytoin and ethotoin. In: Levy R, Mattson R, Meldrum B, et al., eds. *Antiepileptic Drugs.* 3rd ed. New York: Raven Press; 1989:257–266.
6. Schwade ED, Richards RK, Everett GM. Peganone, a new anticonvulsant drug. *Dis Nerv Syst.* 1956;17:155–158.
7. Carter CA, Helms RA, Boehm R. Ethotoin in seizures of childhood and adolescence. *Neurology.* 1984;34:791–795.
8. Biton V, Gates JR, Ritter FJ, et al. Adjunctive therapy for intractable epilepsy with ethotoin. *Epilepsia.* 1990;31:433–437.
9. Finnell RH, Dilibert JH. Hydantoin-induced teratogenesis: are arene oxide intermediates really responsible? *Helv Paediatr Acta.* 1983;38: 171–177.
10. Zablen M, Brand N. Cleft lip and palate with the anticonvulsant ethotoin. *N Engl J Med.* 1977;297:1404.
11. Wilder BJ, Bruni J. *Seizure Disorders: A Pharmacological Approach to Treatment.* New York: Raven Press; 1981.
12. Glazko AJ, Dill WA. Other succinimides: methsuximide and phensuximide. In: Woodbury DM, Penry JK, Schmidt RP, eds. *Antiepileptic Drugs.* New York: Raven Press; 1972:455–464.
13. Porter RJ, Penry JK, Lacy IR, et al. Plasma concentrations of phensuximide, methsuximide and their metabolites in relation to clinical efficacy. *Neurology.* 1979;29:1509–1513.
14. Strong JM, Abe R, Gibbs EL, et al. Plasma levels of methsuximide and N-desmethylmethsuximide during methsuximide therapy. *Neurology.* 1974;24:250–255.
15. Wilder BJ, Buchanan RB. Methsuximide for refractory complex partial seizures. *Neurology.* 1981;31:741–744.
16. Browne TR, Feldman RG, Buchanan RA, et al. Methsuximide for complex partial seizures: efficacy, toxicity, clinical pharmacology, and drug interactions. *Neurology.* 1983;33:414–418.
17. Coroba EF, Strobos RRJ. N-methyl-2-methylphenyl-succinimide, in psychomotor epilepsy. *Dis Nerv Syst.* 1956;17:383–385.
18. Aird RB, Woodbury DM. *The Management of Epilepsy.* Springfield, IL: Charles C Thomas; 1974.
19. French EG, Rey-Bellet J, Lennox WG. Methsuximide in psychomotor and petit mal seizures. *N Engl J Med.* 1958;253:892–894.
20. Livingston S, Pauli L. Celontin in the treatment of epilepsy. *Pediatrics.* 1957;19:614–618.
21. Zimmerman FT, Burgemeister BB. Use of N-methyl-a,-a-methylphenylsuccinimide in the treatment of petit mal epilepsy. *Arch Neurol Psychiatry.* 1954;72:720–725.
22. Uthman BM, Wilder BJ. Methsuximide. In: Kutt H, Resor SR, eds. *Medical Treatment of Epilepsy.* New York: Marcel Dekker; 1991: 379–384.
23. Sigler M, Strassburg HM, Boenigk HE. Effective and safe but forgotten: methsuximide in intractable epilepsies in childhood. *Seizure.* 2001;10: 120–124.
24. Tennison MB, Greenwood RS, Miles MV. Methsuximide for intractable childhood seizures. *Pediatrics.* 1991;87:186–189.
25. Carter CH, Maley MC. Use of Celontin in the treatment of mixed epilepsy. *Neurology.* 1957;7:483–484.

26. Dow RW, McFarlane JP, Stevens JR. Celontin in patients with refractory epilepsy. *Neurology.* 1958;8:201–204.
27. Scholl ML, Abbott JA, Schwab RS. Celontin—a new anticonvulsant. *Epilepsia.* 1959;1:105–109.
28. Zimmerman FT. N-methyl-a,a-methylphenylsuccinimide in psychomotor epilepsy treatment. *Arch Neurol Psychiatry.* 1956;76:65–71.
29. Livingston S, Eisner V, Pauli L. Minor motor epilepsy: diagnosis, treatment and prognosis. *Pediatrics.* 1958;21:916–928.
30. Rabe F. Celontin (Petinutin)—a contribution to the differential therapy of epilepsy [German]. *Nervenarzt.* 1960;7:306–312.
31. Brenner RP, Seelinger DF. Drawing-induced seizures. *Arch Neurol.* 1979;36:515–516.
32. Hurst DL. Methsuximide therapy of juvenile myoclonic epilepsy. *Seizure.* 1996;5:47–50.
33. Rambeck B. Pharmacological interactions of methsuximide with phenobarbital and phenytoin in hospitalized epileptic patients. *Epilepsia.* 1979;20:147–156.
34. Eichelbaum M, Kothe KW, Hoffmann F, et al. Kinetics and metabolism of carbamazepine during combined antiepileptic drug therapy. *Clin Pharmacol Ther.* 1979;26:366–371.
35. May T, Rambeck B, Jurgens U. Influence of oxcarbazepine and methsuximide on lamotrigine concentrations in epileptic patients with and without valproic acid comedication: results of a retrospective study. *Ther Drug Monit.* 1999;21:175–181.
36. Besag FM, Berry DJ, Vasey M. Methsuximide reduces valproic acid serum levels. *Ther Drug Monit.* 2001;23:694–697.
37. Mataringa MI, May TW, Rambeck B. Does lamotrigine influence valproate concentrations? *Ther Drug Monit.* 2002;24:631–636.
38. Besag FM. Methsuximide lower lamotrigine blood levels: a pharmacokinetic antiepileptic drug interaction. *Epilepsia.* 2000;41:624–627.
39. May TW, Rambeck B, Jurgens U. Serum concentrations of topiramate in patients with epilepsy: influence of dose, age, and comedication. *Ther Drug Monit.* 2002;24:366–374.
40. Dooley J, Camfield P, Buckley D, et al. Methsuximide-induced movement disorder. *Pediatrics.* 1991;88:1291–1292.
41. Karch SB. Methsuximide overdose: delayed onset of profound coma. *J Am Med Assoc.* 1973;223:1463–1465.
42. Baehler RW, Work J, Smith W, et al. Charcoal hemoperfusion in the therapy for methsuximide and phenytoin overdose. *Arch Intern Med.* 1980;140:1466–1468.
43. Hauptman A. Luminal bei Epilepsie. *Munch Med Wochenschr.* 1912;59:1907–1909.
44. Mattson RH, Cramer JA, Collins JF, et al. Comparison of carbamazepine, phenobarbital, phenytoin, and primidone in partial and secondary generalized tonic-clonic seizures. *N Engl J Med.* 1985;313:145–151.
45. Farwell JR, Lee YJ, Hirtz DG, et al. Phenobarbital for febrile seizures: effects on intelligence and on seizure recurrence. *N Engl J Med.* 1990;322:364–369.
46. Goldberg RN, Moscoso P, Bauer CR, et al. Use of barbiturate therapy in severe perinatal asphyxia: a randomized controlled trial. *J Pediatr.* 1986;109:851–856.
47. Kuban KCK, Krishnamoorthy KS, Littlewood Teele R, et al. Neonatal intracranial hemorrhage and phenobarbital. *Pediatrics.* 1986;77:443–450.
48. Painter MJ. How to use phenobarbital. In: Morselli PL, Pippenger CE, Penry JK, eds. *Antiepileptic Drug Therapy in Pediatrics.* New York: Raven Press; 1983:245–250.
49. Wallin A, Boreus LO. Phenobarbital prophylaxis for hyperbilirubinemia in preterm infants: a controlled study of bilirubin disappearance and infant behavior. *Acta Pediatr Scand.* 1984;73:488–497.
50. Pritchard JW. Phenobarbital mechanisms of action. In: Woodbury D, Penry JK, Pippenger CE, eds. *Antiepileptic Drugs.* 2nd ed. New York: Raven Press; 1982:1332–1335.
51. Hooper WD, Kunze HE, Eadie MJ. Qualitative and quantitative studies of methylphenobarbital metabolism in man. *Drug Metab.* 1981;9:381–385.
52. Craig CR, Shideman FE. Metabolism and anticonvulsant properties of mephobarbital and phenobarbital in rats. *J Pharmacol Exp Ther.* 1971;176:35–41.
53. Buch H, Knabe J, Buzello W, et al. Stereospecificity of anaesthetic activity, distribution, inactivation and protein binding of the optical antipodes of two N-methylated barbiturates. *J Pharmacol Exp Ther.* 1970;176:709–716.
54. Smith JA, Waddell WJ, Butler TC. Demethylation of N-methyl derivatives of barbituric acid, hydantoin and 2,4-oxazolidinedione by rat liver microsomes. *Life Sci.* 1963;7:486–492.
55. Butler TC, Mahaffee D, Mahaffee C. The role of the liver in the metabolic disposition of mephobarbital. *J Pharmacol Exp Ther.* 1952;106:364–369.
56. Kobayashi K, Morita J, Chiba K, et al. Pharmacogenetic roles of CYP2C19 and CYP2B6 in the metabolism of R- and S-mephobarbital in humans. *Pharmacogenetics.* 2004;14(8):549–556.
57. Hooper WD, Kunze HE, Eadie MJ. Pharmacokinetics and bioavailability of methylphenobarbital in man. *Ther Drug Monit.* 1981;3:39–44.
58. Blum E. Die Bekanfung epileptischer Anfalle und iher Folgeer Scheinungen mit Prominal. *Dtsch Med Wochenschr.* 1932;58:230–236.
59. Eadie MJ. Other barbiturates: methyl-phenobarbital and metharbital. In: Levy R, Mattson R, Meldrum B, et al., eds. *Antiepileptic Drugs.* 3rd ed. New York: Raven Press; 1989:357–378.
60. Kupferberg HJ, Longacre-Shaw J. Mephobarbital and phenobarbital plasma concentrations in epileptic patients treated with mephobarbital. *Ther Drug Monit.* 1979;1:117–122.
61. Hutt SJ, Jackson PM, Belsham A, et al. Perceptual-motor behavior in relation to blood phenobarbital level: a preliminary report. *Dev Med Child Neurol.* 1968;10:626–632.
62. Camfield C. *Clinical Trials of Phenobarbital.* Presented at the NIH Consensus Development Conference on Febrile Seizures; May 19–21, 1980; Bethesda, MD.
63. McLeod CM, Dekaban AS, Hunt E. Memory impairment in epileptic patients: selective effects of phenobarbital concentrations. *Science.* 1978; 202:1102–1104.
64. Willis J, Nelson A, Black FW, et al. Barbiturate anticonvulsants: a neuropsychological and quantitative electroencephalographic study. *J Child Neurol.* 1997;12:169–171.
65. Bergstrom WH, Carzoli RF, Lombroso C, et al. Observations on metabolic and clinical effects of carbonic anhydrase inhibitors in epileptics. *Am J Dis Child.* 1952;84:771–772.
66. Ansell B, Clarke E. Acetazolamide in treatment of epilepsy. *Br Med J.* 1956;1:650–661.
67. Forsythe WI, Owens JR, Toothill C. Effectiveness of acetazolamide in the treatment of carbamazepine-resistant epilepsy in children. *Dev Med Child Neurol.* 1981;23:761–769.
68. Golla FL, Sessions HR. Control of petit mal by acetazolamide. *J Ment Sci.* 1957;103:214–217.
69. Lombroso CT, Davidson DT Jr, Gross-Bianchi ML. Further evaluation of acetazolamide (Diamox) in treatment of epilepsy. *J Am Med Assoc.* 1956;160:268–272.
70. Millichap JG. Anticonvulsant action of Diamox in children. *Neurology.* 1956;6:552–559.
71. Maren TH, Mayer E, Wadsworth BC. Carbonic anhydrase inhibition, I: the pharmacology of Diamox (2-acetylamino-1,3,4–thiadiazole-5-sulfonamide). *Bull Johns Hopkins Hosp.* 1954;95:199–243.
72. Millichap JG, Woodbury DM, Goodman LS. Mechanism of the anticonvulsant action of acetazolamide, a carbonic anhydrase inhibitor. *J Pharmacol Exp Ther.* 1955;115:251–258.
73. Velisek L, Moshé SL, Xu SG, et al. Reduced susceptibility to seizures in carbonic anhydrase II deficient mutant mice. *Epilepsy Res.* 1993;14:115–121.
74. Masereel B, Rolin S, Abbate F, et al. Carbonic anhydrase inhibitors: anticonvulsant sulfonamides incorporating valproyl and other lipophilic moieties. *J Med Chem.* 2002;45:312–320.
75. Woodbury DM. Pharmacology and mechanisms of action of antiepileptic drugs. In: Goldensohn ES, Appel SH, eds. *Scientific Approaches to Clinical Neurology.* Philadelphia, PA: Lea & Febiger; 1977:693–726.
76. Leniger T, Wiemann M, Bingmann D, et al. Carbonic anhydrase inhibitor sulthiame reduces intracellular pH and epileptiform activity of hippocampal CA3 neurons. *Epilepsia.* 2002;43:469–474.
77. Woodbury DM, Kemp JW. Basic mechanisms of seizures: neurophysiological and biochemical etiology. In: Shagass C, Gerson S, Friedhoff AJ, eds. *Psychopathology and Brain Dysfunction.* New York: Raven Press; 1977:149–182.
78. Woodbury DM. Antiepileptic drugs: carbonic anhydrase inhibitors. In: Glaser GH, Penry JK, Woodbury DM, eds. *Antiepileptic Drugs: Mechanisms of Action.* New York: Raven Press; 1980:617–634.
79. Panayiotopoulos CP. Treatment of typical absence seizures and related epileptic syndromes. *Paediatr Drugs.* 2001;3:379–403.
80. Lim LL, Foldvary N, Mascha E, Lee J. Acetazolamide in women with catamenial epilepsy. *Epilepsia.* 2001;42:746–749.
81. Resor SR, Jr, Resor LD. Chronic acetazolamide monotherapy in the treatment of juvenile myoclonic epilepsy. *Neurology.* 1990;40:1677–1681.
82. Katayama F, Miura H, Takanashi S. Long-term effectiveness and side effects of acetazolamide as an adjunct to other anticonvulsants in the treatment of refractory epilepsies. *Brain Dev.* 2002;24:150–154.
83. Reiss WG, Oles KS. Acetazolamide in the treatment of epilepsy. *Ann Pharmacother.* 1996;30:514–519.
84. Woodbury DM, Kemp JW. Other antiepileptic drugs: sulfonamides and derivatives. In: Levy R, Mattson R, Meldrum B, et al., eds. *Antiepileptic Drugs.* 3rd ed. New York: Raven Press; 1989:855–876.
85. Kubota F, Kifune A, Shibata N, et al. Bone mineral density of epileptic patients on long-term antiepileptic drug therapy: a quantitative digital radiography study. *Epilepsy Res.* 1999;33:93–97.
86. Futagi Y, Atani K, Abe J. Growth suppression in children receiving acetazolamide with antiepileptic drugs. *Pediatr Neurol.* 1996;15:323–326.
87. Bessey OA, Adam DJD, Hansen AE. Intake of vitamin B-6 and infantile convulsions: a first approximation of requirements of pyridoxine in infants. *Pediatrics.* 1957;10:33–44.
88. Livingston SJ, Hsu M, Petersen DC. Ineffectiveness of pyridoxine (vitamin B-6) in the treatment of epilepsy. *Pediatrics.* 1955;16:250–251.
89. Scriver CR. Vitamin B-6–dependency infantile convulsions. *Pediatrics.* 1960;26:62–74.
90. Scriver CR, Hutchison JH. The vitamin B-6 deficiency syndrome in human infancy: biochemical and clinical observations. *Pediatrics.* 1963;31:240–250.
91. Hunt AD, Stokes J, McCrory WW, et al. Pyridoxine dependency: report of a case of intractable convulsions in an infant controlled by pyridoxine. *Pediatrics.* 1954;13:140–145.

92. Scriver CR, Whelan DT. Glutamic acid decarboxylase (GAD) in mammalian tissue outside the central nervous system, and its possible relevance to hereditary vitamin B-6 dependency with seizures. *Ann N Y Acad Sci.* 1969;166:83–96.

93. Bachmann DS. Late-onset pyridoxine-dependency convulsions. *Ann Neurol.* 1983;14:692–693.

94. Coker SB. Postneonatal vitamin B-6–dependent epilepsy. *Pediatrics.* 1992;90:221–223.

95. Kurleman G, Loscher W, Dominick HC, et al. Disappearance of neonatal seizures and low CSF GABA levels after treatment with vitamin B-6. *Epilepsy Res.* 1987;1:152–154.

96. Yoshida T, Tada K, Arakawa T. Vitamin B 6-dependency of glutamic acid decarboxylase in the kidney from a patient with vitamin B 6 dependent convulsion. *Tohoku J Exp Med.* 1971;104:195–198.

97. Baxter P. Pyridoxine-dependent seizures: a clinical and biochemical conundrum. *Biochim Biophys Acta.* 2003;1647:36–41.

98. Gospe SM. Pyridoxine-dependent seizures: findings from recent studies pose new questions. *Pediatr Neurol.* 2002;26:181–185.

99. Bankier A, Turner M, Hopkins IJ. Pyridoxine dependent seizures: a wider clinical spectrum. *Arch Dis Child.* 1983;58:415–418.

100. Goutieres F, Aicardi J. Atypical presentations of pyridoxine-dependent seizures: a treatable cause of intractable epilepsy in infants. *Ann Neurol.* 1985;17:117–120.

101. Mikati MA, Trevathan E, Krishnamoorthy KS, et al. Pyridoxine-dependent epilepsy: EEG investigations and long-term follow-up. *Electroencephalogr Clin Neurophysiol.* 1991;78:215–221.

102. Haenggeli CA, Girardin E, Paunier L. Pyridoxine-dependent seizures, clinical therapeutic aspects. *Eur J Pediatr.* 1991;150:452–455.

103. Gospe SM, Jr, Hecht ST. Longitudinal MRI findings in pyridoxine-dependent seizures. *Neurology.* 1998;51:74–78.

104. Clarke TA, Saunders BS, Feldman B. Pyridoxine-dependent seizures requiring high doses of pyridoxine for control. *Am J Dis Child.* 1979;133:963–965.

105. Krishnamoorthy KS. Pyridoxine-dependency seizure: report of a rare presentation. *Ann Neurol.* 1983;13:103–104.

106. Bass NE, Wyllie E, Cohen B, et al. Pyridoxine-dependent epilepsy: the need for repeated pyridoxine trials and the risk of severe electrocerebral suppression with intravenous pyridoxine infusion. *J Child Neurol.* 1996;11:422–424.

107. Lott IT, Coulombe T, DiPaolo RV, et al. Vitamin B 6-dependent seizures: pathology chemical findings in brain. *Neurology.* 1978;28:47–54.

108. Friedrich AM, Baumeister MD, Gsell W, et al. Glutamate in pyridoxine-dependent epilepsy: neurotoxic glutamate concentration in the cerebrospinal fluid and its normalization by pyridoxine. *Pediatrics.* 1994; 94:318–321.

109. Ito M, Mikawa M, Tangiguchi T. Cerebrospinal fluid GABA levels in children with infantile spasms. *Neurology.* 1984;34:235–238.

110. Loscher W, Siemes H. Cerebrospinal fluid: aminobutyric acid levels in children with different types of epilepsy: effect of anticonvulsant treatment. *Epilepsia.* 1985;16:314–319.

111. Blennow G, Starck L. High dose B-6 treatment in infantile spasms. *Neuropediatrics.* 1986;17:7–10.

112. Ito M, Okuno T, Hattori H, et al. Vitamin B-6 and valproic acid in treatment of infantile spasms. *Pediatr Neurol.* 1991;7:91–96.

113. Ohtsuka Y, Matsuda M, Kohno C, et al. Pyridoxal phosphate in the treatment of the West syndrome. In: Akimoto H, Seino M, Ward AA, Jr, eds. *Advances in Epileptology. XIIIth Epilepsy International Symposium.* New York: Raven Press; 1982:311–313.

114. Pietz J, Benninger C, Schafer H, et al. Treatment of infantile spasms with high-dosage vitamin B6. *Epilepsia.* 1993;34:757–763.

115. Jiao FY, Takuma Y, Wu S, et al. Randomized, controlled trial of high-dose intravenous pyridoxine in the treatment of recurrent seizures in children. *Pediatr Neurol.* 1997;17:54–57.

116. Wang HS, Kuo MF. Vitamin B6 related epilepsy during childhood. *Chang Gung Med J.* 2007;30(5):396–401.

117. Garty R, Yonis Z, Braham J, et al. Pyridoxine-dependent convulsions in an infant. *Arch Dis Child.* 1962;37:21–24.

118. Kroll J. Pyridoxine for neonatal seizures: an unexpected danger. *Dev Med Child Neurol.* 1985;27:369–382.

119. Heeley A, Puch RJP, Clayton BE, et al. Pyridoxol metabolism in vitamin B-6 responsive convulsions of early infancy. *Arch Dis Child.* 1978;53:794–802.

120. Antopol W, Tarlov IM. Experimental study of the effects produced by large doses of vitamin B-6. *J Neuropathol Exp Neurol.* 1942;1:330–336.

121. Dalton K, Dalton JT. Characteristics of pyridoxine overdose neuropathy syndrome. *Acta Neurol Scand.* 1987;76:8–11.

122. Parry GJ, Bredesen DE. Sensory neuropathy with low-dose pyridoxine. *Neurology.* 1985;35:1466–1468.

123. Schaumburg H, Kaplan J, Windebank A, et al. Sensory neuropathy from pyridoxine abuse: a new megavitamin syndrome. *N Engl J Med.* 1983; 309:445–448.

124. Xu Y, Sladky JT, Brown MJ. Dose-dependent expression of neuronopathy after experimental pyridoxine intoxication. *Neurology.* 1989;39:1077–1083.

125. Berger AR, Schaumburg HH, Schroeder C, et al. Dose response, coasting, and differential fibre vulnerability in human toxic neuropathy: a prospective study of pyridoxine neurotoxicity. *Neurology.* 1992;42:1367–1370.

126. Berger A, Schaumburg HH. More on neuropathy from pyridoxine abuse. *N Engl J Med.* 1984;311:986–987.

127. Albin R, Alpers JW, Greenberg HS, et al. Acute sensory neuropathy-neuronopathy from pyridoxine overdose. *Neurology.* 1987;37:1729–1732.

128. Bernstein AL, Lobitz CS. A clinical and electrophysiologic study of the treatment of painful diabetic neuropathies with pyridoxine. In: Leklem JE, Reynolds RD, eds. *Clinical and Physiological Applications of Vitamin B-6. Current Topics in Nutrition and Disease.* New York: Alan R. Liss; 1988;19:415–423.

129. Del Tredici AM, Bernstein AL, Chinn K. Carpal tunnel syndrome and vitamin B-6 therapy. In: Reynolds RD, Leklem JE, eds. *Vitamin B-6: Its Role in Health and Disease. Current Topics in Nutrition and Disease.* New York: Alan R. Liss; 1985;13:459–462.

130. Reynolds RD. Pyridoxine dependent seizures. *Arch Dis Child.* 1984;59:906–907.

131. Mpofu C, Alani SM, Whitehouse C, et al. No sensory neuropathy during pyridoxine treatment in homocystinuria. *Arch Dis Child.* 1991;66:1081–1082.

132. McLachlan RS, Brown WF. Pyridoxine dependent epilepsy with iatrogenic sensory neuronopathy. *Can J Neurol Sci.* 1995;22:50–51.

133. Locock C. In discussion of Sieveking EH. Analysis of 52 cases of epilepsy observed by author. *Lancet.* 1857;1:527.

134. Palachios JM, Nieholt DL, Kuhar MJ. Ontogeny of GABA and benzodiazepine receptors: effects of Triton X-100, bromide and muscimol. *Brain Res.* 1979;179:390–395.

135. Woodbury DM, Pippenger CE. Bromides. In: Woodbury DM, Penry JK, Pippenger CE, eds. *Antiepileptic Drugs.* 2nd ed. New York: Raven Press; 1986:791–801.

136. Vaiseman N, Koren G, Pencharz P. Pharmacokinetics of oral and intravenous bromide in normal volunteers. *Clin Toxicol.* 1986;24:403–413.

137. Dreifuss FE. Bromides. In: Levy R, Mattson R, Meldrum B, et al., eds. *Antiepileptic Drugs.* 3rd ed. New York: Raven Press; 1989:877–879.

138. Ernst J, Doose H, Baier WK. Bromides were effective in intractable epilepsy with generalized tonic-clonic seizures and onset in early childhood. *Brain Dev.* 1988;10:385–388.

139. Oguni H, Hayashi K, Oguni M, et al. Treatment of severe myoclonic epilepsy in infants with bromide and its borderline variant. *Epilepsia.* 1994;35:1140–1145.

140. Steinhoff BJ, Kruse R. Bromide treatment of pharmaco-resistant epilepsies with generalized tonic-clonic seizures: a clinical study. *Brain Dev.* 1992;14:144–149.

141. Stewart LS. Anticonvulsant medications. *Emerg Med Serv.* 2001;30:56–66.

142. James LP, Farrar HC, Griebel ML, et al. Bromism: intoxication from a rare anticonvulsant therapy. *Pediatr Emerg Care.* 1997;13:268–270.

143. Lichtenberg R, Zeller WP, Gatson R, et al. Bromate poisoning. *J Pediatr.* 1989;114:891–894.

CHAPTER 69 ■ THE KETOGENIC DIET

DOUGLAS R. NORDLI JR AND DARRYL C. DE VIVO

The ketogenic diet is a high-fat, low-carbohydrate, low-protein regimen that has been used for more than 80 years in thousands of patients. It is an effective and safe medical treatment for epilepsy, but it must be judiciously applied and carefully monitored.

HISTORICAL HIGHLIGHTS

There are biblical references to the salutary effects of starvation upon seizure control, but the earliest scientific observations were made by Geyelin at New York Presbyterian Hospital in 1921 (1). Shortly thereafter, Wilder proposed a high-fat diet to mimic the effects of starvation (2). Since this high-fat diet increased the production of ketone bodies, the regimen became known as a "keto," or ketogenic diet. It had previously been discovered that ketone bodies were in the urine of patients with diabetes and that they were produced when fatty acids were oxidized. This led to the notion that ketone bodies were potentially toxic metabolites of fatty acid degradation and that their anticonvulsant effect was caused by a sedative property, similar to the mechanisms of action of the available anticonvulsants of that era—bromides and phenobarbital.

This notion was challenged when Krebs suggested that ketone bodies were fuel for respiration in 1961 (3). In 1967, Owen and colleagues proved that ketone bodies were the major fuel for brain metabolism during starvation (4). Appleton and De Vivo (1974) developed an animal model, which showed that ketone bodies utilization during starvation altered brain metabolites and increased cerebral energy reserves (5). In 1976, Huttenlocher found that the level of ketosis correlated with efficacy (6). Livingston and associates reported extensive (41-year) experience with the ketogenic diet for the treatment of myoclonic seizures of childhood, stating that it completely controlled seizures in 54% of his patients and markedly improved control in another 26% (7). Subsequently, valproate (VPA) and other antiepileptic drugs (AEDs) effective for the control of myoclonic seizures were introduced in the United States. Yet, despite the availability of these agents, the ketogenic diet continues to be used in many centers across the country. The first report of a randomized controlled trial of the ketogenic diet was published in 2008, 87 years after its introduction (8).

PRODUCTION AND UTILIZATION OF KETONE BODIES

The major precursors of ketone bodies are nonesterified fatty acids. During the fasting state, the decrease in blood glucose reduces plasma insulin production, stimulates lipolysis in fatty tissues, and increases the flux of nonesterified fatty acids to the liver. Nonesterified fatty acids can be esterified or metabolized to ketone bodies. The fate of fatty acids in the liver is determined, at least in part, by the carbohydrate status of the host (9). A critical component of this regulation is malonyl-coenzyme A (CoA), an intermediate in the pathway of lipogenesis (10,11). Malonyl-CoA inhibits carnitine acyltransferase I, which is needed to shuttle long-chain fatty acyl-CoA into the mitochondria for oxidation. The production of glucose from glycogen provides the carbon source for lipogenesis and, in particular, malonyl-CoA. If glucose is reduced, so is malonyl-CoA. The reduction in malonyl-CoA decreases the inhibition of (or increases the net activity of) carnitine acyltransferase. This allows more movement of fatty acids into the mitochondria, where fatty acyl-CoA is converted to acetyl-CoA and later to acetoacetate (AcAc). AcAc is in equilibrium with β-hydroxybutyrate, the major ketone body used by the brain.

Passage of ketone bodies into the brain may be the critical factor limiting the rate of brain utilization of these chemicals. Movement of ketone bodies into the brain relies on the monocarboxylic acid transporter-1 system. This is upregulated during fasting in adults and during milk feeding in neonates (12,13). Work in rodents with PET scans has shown a marked increase in transport of ketone bodies during ketogenic diet administration (14). Fasting studies in humans demonstrated that the brain's ability to extract ketone bodies is inversely related to the age of the subject (4). In contrast to glucose, ketone bodies can pass directly into mitochondria without being processed in the cytosol and may be used directly by neurons for metabolism (15).

Once inside the mitochondria, β-hydroxybutyrate is converted to AcAc and then to AcAc-CoA by 3-oxoacid-CoA-transferase, also known as succinyl-CoA-AcAc-CoA-transferase. As the name implies, this conversion requires commensurate conversion of succinyl-CoA to succinate. This reaction lowers the succinyl-CoA concentration and relieves the product feedback inhibition of α-ketoglutarate dehydrogenase, the rate-limiting enzyme of the Krebs cycle. It is possible that reduced blood glucose and increased blood ketones may induce the activity of this enzyme (16).

SCIENTIFIC BASIS OF THE DIET

Scientific studies of the ketogenic diet have revealed important biochemical and metabolic observations. The animal model designed by Appleton and De Vivo permitted study of the effect of the ketogenic diet on cerebral metabolism (5). Adult male albino rats were placed on either (i) a high-fat diet containing (by weight) 38% corn oil, 38% lard, 11% vitamin-free casein, 6.8% glucose, 4% United States Pharmacopeia (USP) salt mixture, and 2.2% vitamin diet fortification mixture; or (ii) a high-carbohydrate diet containing (by weight) 50% glucose, 28.8% vitamin-free casein, 7.5% corn oil, 7.5% lard, 4% USP salt mixture, and 2.2% vitamin diet fortification mixture. Parallel studies were conducted to evaluate electroconvulsive shock responses and biochemical alterations. These studies revealed that the mean voltage necessary to produce a minimal convulsion remained constant for 12 days before the high-fat diet was started and approximately 10 days after beginning the feedings (69.75 ± 1.88 V). After 10 to 12 days on the high-fat diet, the intensity of the convulsive response to the established voltage decreased, necessitating an increase in voltage in order to re-establish a minimal convulsive response. Approximately 20 days after beginning the high-fat diet, a new convulsive threshold was achieved (81.25 ± 2.39 V; $P < 0.01$). When the high-fat diet was replaced by the high-carbohydrate diet, a rapid change in response to the voltage was observed. Within 48 hours, the animal exhibited a maximal convulsion to the electrical stimulus that previously had produced only a minimal convulsion, and the mean voltage to produce a minimal convulsion returned to the prestudy value (70.75 ± 1.37 V).

Blood concentrations of β-hydroxybutyrate, AcAc, chloride, esterified fatty acids, triglycerides, cholesterol, and total lipids increased in the rats fed on the high-fat diet. Brain levels of β-hydroxybutyrate and sodium were also significantly increased in the fat-fed rats.

Hori and associates studied the efficacy of the ketogenic diet in kindled animals—an appropriate model for partial seizures—and found the diet to have transient anticonvulsant properties (17). The investigators studied 32 male Sprague–Dawley rats, 20 of which were kindled and underwent behavioral testing; the 12 others underwent behavioral testing alone. Rats were kindled from P56 to 60 and then randomized (10 in each group) to treatment with either a ketogenic diet or regular rat chow. Afterdischarge threshold and seizure thresholds were tested at 1, 2, 4, and 5 weeks. Behavioral testing using both a water maze test and an open-field test was performed at week 3. During the period of administration of the ketogenic diet, statistically significant elevations of β-hydroxybutyrate were reported. Both the afterdischarge thresholds and seizure thresholds were raised for the first 2 weeks of the diet; however, this effect disappeared by weeks 4 and 5. There was no difference in behavioral performance between the ketogenic diet rats and the controls (17).

Stafstrom and coworkers reported on electrophysiologic observations using hippocampal slices from rats treated with the ketogenic diet (18). They found that the ketogenic diet did not alter baseline electrophysiologic parameters in normal rats (excitatory postsynaptic potential [EPSP] slope, input and output relationship, responses to evoked stimulation, and Mg(++)-free burst frequency), but that it was associated with fewer spontaneous seizures and reduced CA1 excitability in rats made chronically epileptic by administration of kainic acid. The researchers concluded that at least part of the ketogenic diet mechanism of action might involve long-term changes in network excitability. In another experiment, rats fed the ketogenic diet after kainic acid–induced status epilepticus had significantly fewer and briefer spontaneous seizures, and less supragranular mossy fiber sprouting, compared with animals on a normal diet (19). These results provide evidence that the ketogenic diet has an antiepileptogenic effect in an experimental model.

Bough and Eagles demonstrated that the ketogenic diet increases the resistance to pentylenetetrazole-induced seizures in the rat (20). In their experiment, seizures were induced by tail-vein infusion of pentylenetetrazole in rats fed either a ketogenic diet or a normal diet for 35 days. The rats fed a ketogenic diet had a significantly increased threshold for seizure induction ($P < 0.01$) compared with controls. These observations are particularly relevant because this model may mimic the condition of myoclonic seizure disorders in humans (20). In subsequent experiments, Bough and other collaborators performed recordings in the dentate gyrus of rats fed ketogenic calorie–restricted (KCR), normal calorie–restricted (NCR), or normal ad libitum (NAL) diets. In vivo extracellular field responses to angular bundle stimulation were recorded. Input and output curves and paired-pulse relations were used to assess network excitability, and a maximal dentate activation (MDA) protocol was used to measure electrographic seizure threshold and duration. The animals fed the KCR diet showed greater paired-pulse inhibition, elevated MDA threshold, and an absence of spreading depression-like events. Perhaps even more importantly, in the MDA model, the rate of increase in seizure duration after repeated stimuli was markedly reduced in the rats fed the KCR diet. These results agree with clinical observations made in the early 20th century that calorie restriction may be anticonvulsant, but they also show that the KCR diet has special properties and may, in fact, be antiepileptogenic (21).

De Vivo and colleagues reported on the change in cerebral metabolites in chronically ketotic rats (22), and found no changes in brain water content, electrolytes, and pH. As expected, fat-fed rats had significantly lower blood glucose concentrations and higher blood β-hydroxybutyrate and AcAc concentrations. More importantly, brain concentrations of adenosine triphosphate (ATP), glycogen, glucose-6-phosphate, pyruvate, lactate, β-hydroxybutyrate, citrate, α-ketoglutarate, and alanine were higher, and brain concentrations of fructose 1,6-diphosphate, aspartate, adenosine diphosphate (ADP), creatine, cyclic nucleotides, acid insoluble CoA, and total CoA were lower in the fat-fed group. Cerebral energy reserves were significantly higher in the fat-fed rats (26.4 ± 0.6) compared with controls (23.6 ± 0.2; $P < 0.005$). Many of these changes in metabolites could be explained by the higher energy state of the brain cells in the fat-fed group, specifically by the ratio of ATP to ADP. In addition, the normal oxaloacetate, elevated α-ketoglutarate, and decreased succinyl-CoA imply maximal tricarboxylic acid (TCA) cycle activity—quite contrary to the metabolite profile observed with anesthetic–sedative agents. Pan and associates used ^{31}P spectroscopic imaging at 4.1 T to demonstrate an elevated ratio of phosphocreatine to inorganic phosphorus in patients on the ketogenic diet and concluded that there was improvement in energy metabolism with use of the diet (23). Using a mouse model of succinic semialdehyde dehydrogenase deficiency, Nylen et al. found marked increases in the number of mitochondria and levels of ATP in animals treated with the ketogenic diet (24). The ketogenic diet also reversed the clinical phenotype.

Another possible mechanism of action may be suggested from these biochemical alterations. Elevated α-ketoglutarate may indicate increased flux through the α-aminobutyric acid

(GABA) shunt, which may, in turn, be expected to increase cerebral GABA levels. One study of adult male rats fed a ketogenic diet, however, failed to demonstrate elevated cerebral GABA levels (25).

GABA, β-hydroxybutyrate, and AcAc have very similar chemical structures raising the possibility that there might be some direct anticonvulsant action of the ketone bodies. This notion was advanced in the 1930s by Helmholz and Keith, and only recently has begun to attract some widespread attention (26,27). Likhodii and colleagues suggested that there may be a direct anticonvulsant action of acetone. Rats were administered acetone intraperitoneally and tested in four models: maximal electroshock, subcutaneous pentylenetetrazole, amygdala kindling, and the AY-9944 test—a model of chronic atypical absence seizures. Acetone suppressed seizures in all models (28). The therapeutic index of acetone was comparable or superior to VPA (29).

These observations demonstrate that the ketogenic diet has broad anticonvulsant properties and possibly antiepileptogenic activity. In addition, the available biochemical data suggest that the diet favorably influences cerebral energetics, and that increased cerebral energy reserves and increased GABA shunt activity may be important factors bestowing an increased resistance to seizures in ketotic brain tissue (30).

A variety of other plausible hypotheses have been advanced to explain the beneficial actions of the ketogenic diet including antioxidant properties (31,32), altered purine metabolism due to enhanced energy reserves (33), action of neuropeptides (34), and alteration of mitochondrial uncoupling protein (35). Like many anticonvulsant drugs, it is highly likely that the ketogenic diet has multiple mechanisms of action that summate and account for its rather unique therapeutic properties. Further basic science experiments will help to elucidate other novel effects of the ketogenic diet. In turn, these may lead to the development of new pharmaceutical agents. At the same time, a careful and systematic study of the clinical effects of the ketogenic diet in specific epilepsy syndromes with particular causes might provide useful clues regarding mechanisms of action (36).

ADMINISTRATION OF THE DIET

Implementation

Patients should be hospitalized for the initiation of the ketogenic diet. Close observation is important, because children with certain underlying inborn errors of metabolism, particularly ones that interfere with the utilization of ketone bodies, could quickly decompensate (37). The hospitalization also provides the opportunity for family members to be instructed on the maintenance of the diet and the monitoring of blood β-hydroxybutyrate concentrations. We strive for blood beta hydroxybutyrate (BOHB) concentrations of 4 to 5 mM. Urine ketones may be misleading and should not be monitored if blood measurements are available.

In the traditional approach, the first step is to promote ketosis with a fast. This can be done by the patient fasting after dinner (6:00 PM) on the evening of admission and continuing the fast until breakfast at 8:00 AM on the third day (38 hours). This allows metabolic adaptation to the state of ketosis and an opportunity to screen the child for any severe hypoglycemic predisposition. It is typical to see a transient hypoglycemia during the first few days, which does not require any treatment unless the child demonstrates symptoms. Treatment of asymptomatic hypoglycemia delays the metabolic adaptation of the child to the state of chronic ketosis. During the fast, the patient is offered water, sugar-free beverages, and unsweetened gelatin.

As an alternative, the diet can be offered without a period of fasting. This approach was compared to the traditional fasting implementation by Kim and colleagues. They found greater tolerability in the nonfasting group with no difference in time to ketosis or ultimate effectiveness of the diet at 3 months (38). In another study comparing fasting to nonfasting initiations, no difference was found in ultimate effectiveness of the diet, though the fasting group achieved ketosis more rapidly (39). If the child is fasted, then the urine usually reveals medium to large ketones after the 38-hour fast, and the diet is started. We never have children fast any longer than this, and a shorter period of fasting (24 hours) often suffices with infants and young children. Our current protocol at Children's Memorial Hospital in Chicago does not involve routine fasting. Instead, the diet is begun at a reduced concentration on the first day of admission.

The long-chain triglyceride (LCT) diet consists of three or four parts fat to one part nonfat (carbohydrate and protein), calculated based on weight. It is computed to provide 75 to 100 kcal/kg body weight and 1 to 2 g of dietary protein/kg body weight per day. Caloric requirements are adjusted to minimize weight gain and to maximize ketonemia. If a 3:1 (fat-to-nonfat) ratio is insufficient to produce the required ketosis, then a ratio of 4:1 is used.

The Conventional Ketogenic Diet or Long-Chain Triglyceride Diet

Prior to initiating the conventional ketogenic or LCT diet, a dietary prescription is made. Calculation of this prescription is straightforward. For example, if a 10-kg child is to be started on a 3:1 diet, one begins by estimating the calorie requirements of the child as follows:

$$10 \text{ kg} \times 100 \text{ kcal/day} = 1000 \text{ kcal/day}$$

Alternatively, consulting a table of recommended daily allowances (RDAs) may derive this figure. In either case, it may require adjustment based on the child's specific metabolic needs.

The 3:1 ratio of the diet stipulates that 4 g of food must contain 3 g of fat and 1 g of nonfat. The nonfat consists of both carbohydrate and protein. One gram of fat has the calorie equivalent of 9 calories, whereas 1 g of protein or carbohydrate has the calorie equivalent of approximately 4 calories. Four grams of food (arbitrarily referred to as 1 unit here) on a 3:1 diet is then equal to 31 calories:

$$1 \text{ g fat} = 9 \text{ calories} \times 3 = 27 \text{ calories}$$

$$1 \text{ g protein and carbohydrate} = 4 \text{ calories} \times 1 = 4 \text{ calories}$$

$$\text{Total calories} = 27 + 4 = 31 \text{ calories/unit}$$

To calculate the daily fat intake, one first divides the daily requirements of calories by this figure of 31 calories/unit, which generates the number of units required for the day:

$$\frac{1000 \text{ calories/day}}{31 \text{ calories/unit}} = 32.25 \text{ units/day}$$

Next, multiplying by 27 calories of fat/unit provides the daily fat requirement:

32.26 units/day × 27 calories of fat/unit
= 871 calories of fat/day, which is equivalent to 96 g.

The protein requirement is 10 kg × 2 g/kg, or 20 g/day (80 calories). Alternatively, one may consult the RDA table to determine the protein requirement.

Thus far, the combination of 871 calories of fat and 80 calories of protein leaves only 49 calories (1000 − 951) not accounted for in the daily allowance. The carbohydrate intake is then calculated to supply the necessary remaining calories (49 calories), which in this case is approximately 12 g.

The dietary prescription for this 10-kg patient on a 3:1 LCT diet is then:

Fat: 96 g/day or 32 g/meal

Protein: 20 g/day or 6.6 g/meal

Carbohydrate: 12 g/day or 4 g/meal

Although the calculation of the calorie requirements is straightforward, the generation of the actual food prescription requires more time and effort. The approach may vary from institution to institution. In ours, the nutrition support team does the calculation and generates the prescription, and in order to provide a successful regimen, the constituents are customized to fit the individual's preferences and special needs. In so doing, the various elements of the diet may be "juggled" to conform to the nutritional requirements. A food substitution approach may be used, which is analogous to that used for diabetic diets. This approach is simple to implement and increases the flexibility of the diet (40). A variety of computer programs are now available that facilitate calculation of the ketogenic diet, but we believe these calculations should be reviewed and accepted by qualified dieticians with special experience with the ketogenic diet.

Maintenance

After initiation of the diet, the patient remains in the hospital for another 2 to 3 days. This time is used to carefully instruct the parents or caretakers on the techniques of providing the diet, weighing the food, offering food substitutions, and monitoring ketosis. Patients on the ketogenic diet are often supplemented with calcium, iron, folate, and multivitamins, including vitamin D, to satisfy the RDA requirements. Protein requirements are carefully monitored and increased on an individual basis to account for weight gain and growth.

After discharge from the hospital, the child is initially seen on a monthly basis by the nutrition support team or registered dietitian. At each visit, the child's height, weight, and head circumference are charted. Electrolytes, liver function tests, serum lipids and proteins, and a complete blood count are periodically checked. On average, the calorie and nutritional needs are readjusted monthly for infants and every 6 to 12 months for children.

Termination of the Ketogenic Diet

The ketogenic diet should be stopped gradually. A sudden stop of the diet or sudden administration of glucose may aggravate seizures and precipitate status epilepticus (41). Livingston advocated maintaining the diet at a ratio 4:1 for 2 years and, if successful, weaning down to a 3:1 diet for 6 months, followed by 6 months of a 2:1 diet (42). At this point, a regular diet is given. We usually taper the diet more quickly, often making changes in the ratio by 0.5 increments on a monthly basis, liberalizing the diet when ketosis is consistently absent.

ADVERSE EVENTS

The ketogenic diet may be lethal in certain circumstances in which cerebral energy metabolism is deranged. An example of this is pyruvate carboxylase deficiency, in which patients may present early in life with refractory myoclonic seizures (37).

Mitochondrial disorders or diseases that involve the respiratory chain, such as myoclonic epilepsy and ragged-red fiber (MERRF+) disease; mitochondrial encephalopathy, lactic acidosis, and strokelike (MELAS) syndrome; and cytochrome oxidase deficiency might naturally raise some concerns because of the increased stress on respiratory chain and TCA cycle function. However, Kang and colleagues showed that the ketogenic diet may be used in selected circumstances, particularly in patients with respiratory chain defects (43). Patients with fatty acid oxidation problems would also be adversely affected by use of the ketogenic diet, but such patients do not, as a rule, present with seizures. The diet is contraindicated in patients with organic acidurias and porphyria (44).

Complications

Patients on the ketogenic diet exhibit a significantly reduced quantity of bone mass, which improves in response to vitamin D supplementation (5000 IU/day) (45). Renal calculi may develop but the occurrence is rare. Lipemia retinalis developed in two of Dr. Livingston's patients (42). Bilateral optic neuropathy has been reported in two children who were treated with a 4:1 "classic" ketogenic diet; these patients were not originally given vitamin B supplements. After administration of vitamin B supplements, vision was restored in both patients. Thinning of hair and, rarely, alopecia may occur. Cardiovascular complications have not been observed in those adults who were examined (42). In a prospective study, Ballaban-Gil and associates reported serious adverse events in 5 of 52 children: severe hypoproteinemia (two patients), with lipemia and hemolytic anemia developing in one of these patients; renal tubular acidosis (one patient), and marked increases in liver function tests (two patients). Four of these patients were comedicated with VPA (46).

Potential Adverse Drug Interactions

Carbonic anhydrase inhibitors, such as acetazolamide and topiramate, should be avoided, particularly in the early stages of treatment with the ketogenic diet. VPA is an inhibitor of fatty acid oxidation and a mitigator of hepatic ketogenesis.

At our institutions, we have encountered marked elevation of liver transaminases in two patients during coadministration of VPA and the diet, as have Ballaban-Gil and colleagues (46). When possible, therefore, we avoid the use of this agent.

Carnitine supplementation is complex. The agent is often used to supplement the diet of patients with various metabolic derangements whose defects allow a build-up of undesirable intermediates. It is also not uncommon that in patients who need the ketogenic diet, a metabolic disorder of this sort is either suspected or confirmed (another reason to avoid VPA is possible). Carnitine supplementation may be desirable for these patients; however, high doses of carnitine may interfere with ketogenesis. These factors must be weighed in each patient, and the decision to use the supplement should be individualized. This topic has been thoroughly reviewed (47).

CLINICAL INDICATIONS FOR USE AND EFFECTIVENESS

Primary Therapy

The ketogenic diet is first-line therapy for the treatment of seizures in association with glucose transporter type 1 (Glut1) deficiency and pyruvate dehydrogenase (E1) deficiency (48,49). The ketogenic diet provides fuel for brain metabolism and the degree of ketonemia must be monitored closely for maximal therapeutic benefit. We strive for blood BOHB concentrations of 4 to 5 mM. In both cases, the diet effectively treats seizures while providing essential fuel for brain metabolic activity. In patients with E1 deficiency, early initiation of the diet was associated with increased longevity and improved mental development.

Secondary Treatment

Multiple investigators have found the ketogenic diet to be effective in the treatment of patients with symptomatic or cryptogenic forms of generalized epilepsy. Prasad and coworkers have summarized the efficacy data (50) and a recent consensus panel issued a comprehensive report (44). It is clear from these compilations that the diet may be particularly helpful when the symptomatic epilepsy manifests with myoclonic and related seizures. Dr. Livingston found that the diet completely controlled seizures in 54% of his patients with myoclonic epilepsy (7). Freeman and colleagues performed a prospective evaluation of the ketogenic diet in 150 children with refractory epilepsy (51). At 1 year, 55% of the children remained on the diet and 27% had a greater than 90% reduction in seizure frequency. In 63 studies of 55 patients conducted by Schwartz and associates, a total of 51 studies (81%) showed a greater than 50% reduction in seizure frequency regardless of the type of diet used (52). The particular type of ketogenic diet used may not be critically important, although some investigators have found the medium-chain triglyceride (MCT) diet slightly less effective. In one study, 44% of patients treated with the MCT diet achieved a greater than 50% reduction in the number of seizures (53). A corn oil ketogenic diet was found to be equally beneficial to the MCT diet (54). Regardless of the type of diet used, seizure control may be inconsistently accompanied by electroencephalographic improvement (55).

The most definitive efficacy study of the ketogenic diet to date was reported by Neal et al. (8). They randomized 145 children with epilepsy refractory to two drugs to either immediate treatment with the ketogenic diet or a 3-month delay. Using intent-to-treat analysis, they found that the mean percentage reduction of baseline seizures at 3 months was 62% for the diet group and 136.9% for the control ($P < 0.001$). There was no difference in efficacy between those with symptomatic focal and symptomatic generalized syndromes. The most common side effects were constipation, vomiting, and lack of energy and hunger. They also found no efficacy differences between the classic and MCT diet (8).

Appropriate epilepsy syndromes in which to consider early treatment with the ketogenic diet include early myoclonic epilepsy, early infantile epileptic encephalopathy, and myoclonic absence epilepsy. Given the effectiveness of the diet in the treatment of myoclonic epilepsies, it could also be considered early for patients with severe epileptogenic myoclonic encephalopathies that are notoriously difficult to control, such as Lennox–Gastaut syndrome, myoclonic–astatic epilepsy, severe infantile myoclonic epilepsy, and early infantile epileptogenic encephalopathy. However, in our experience, most parents prefer the convenience of a medication, and it is unusual to try the ketogenic diet before at least one or two AEDs have failed. The ketogenic diet can be beneficial in infants with West syndrome who are refractory to corticosteroids and other medications (56). Based on Keith's data and our own experience, the ketogenic diet may also be useful in the treatment of children with refractory absence epilepsy without myoclonus (57). Since the brain's ability to extract ketone bodies diminishes with age, there has been concern about the use of the ketogenic diet in adolescents. However, Mady and associates have shown that the ketogenic diet can be well tolerated and effective for adolescents (58).

The Atkins diet, which also induces a ketotic state, may have a therapeutic role in patients with medically resistant epilepsy similar to the ketogenic diet.

Further Possible Indications

Focal Epilepsies

It is somewhat more difficult to precisely determine the efficacy of the ketogenic diet in the treatment of focal epilepsies. The recent data from Neal et al. suggest that it may be as effective in symptomatic localization-related as symptomatic generalized epilepsies (8). Livingston, however, did not find that the diet was not effective in treating patients with focal seizures (7). Our own experience has been mixed.

In the study by Schwartz and coworkers, 9 of the 55 children appeared to have partial seizures as their main seizure type (52). Overall, 81% of patients showed a greater than 50% reduction in seizures (52). Although the number of children in each group was small, seizure type did not seem to predict response to treatment. There have been reports of improvement in language, behavior, and seizure control in patients with acquired epileptic aphasia (59,60). Villeneuve and colleagues found the diet effective in a subgroup of children with focal epilepsy who had a history of recent deterioration (61). Results from the kindling animal model (17) could be used to predict efficacy in localization-related epilepsies, but such extrapolations from animal models to human are fraught with hazards. Taken together, these observations support the use of the ketogenic diet in this context, but there is no compelling clinical data to favor its use over newer medications or potentially curative surgery. Therefore, children with refractory focal seizures should be evaluated to determine whether they are candidates for focal resective surgery. If they are, then in our opinion, surgery need not be delayed to institute a trial of the ketogenic diet. On the other hand, if AEDs have failed and the patient is deemed to be a poor surgical candidate, then the diet should be tried. A more definitive statement would require further data comparing the efficacy of the diet in patients with localization-related epilepsy versus those with generalized forms of epilepsy.

CONCLUSIONS

It is remarkable that nearly 90 years and scores of drugs later, the ketogenic diet still retains a role in the modern treatment of children with refractory epilepsy. The diet is the treatment of choice for children with E1 deficiency and Glut1 deficiency. It is an effective and safe treatment for children with refractory generalized cryptogenic or symptomatic epilepsies. Recent work has suggested that it may be equally effective in those with refractory localization-related epilepsy, although this contrasts with older literature and our own clinical experience. The diet has clear anticonvulsant properties in a wide variety of animal models, including maximal electroshock, pentylenetetrazole, kindling, and kainic acid.

The ketogenic diet is generally safe but not risk-free. It may have devastating effects, particularly upon initiation, in children with inborn errors of metabolism. For this reason, we believe that it should be initiated in the hospital under the careful observation of professionals well versed in its use. Other side effects, including bone demineralization, growth failure, and kidney stones, may occur with continued administration and must be carefully followed.

Given its record of success, it is likely that the ketogenic diet will stay with us in the years to come. It deserves careful study, both by virtue of its clinical utility as well as the potential insights to be gleaned from analyzing its effective and nonsedating mechanisms of action.

References

1. Geyelin HR. Fasting as a method for treating epilepsy. *Med Rec.* 1921;99: 1037–1039.
2. Wilder RM. Effects of ketonuria on the course of epilepsy. *Mayo Clin Bull.* 1921;2:307–314.
3. Krebs HA. The physiological role of the ketone bodies. *Biochem J.* 1961; 80:225–233.
4. Owen OE, Morgan AP, Kemp HG, et al. Brain metabolism during fasting. *J Clin Invest.* 1967;46:1589–1595.
5. Appleton DB, DeVivo DC. An animal model for the ketogenic diet. *Epilepsia.* 1974;15:211–227.
6. Huttenlocher PR. Ketonemia and seizures: metabolic and anticonvulsant effects of two ketogenic diets in childhood epilepsy. *Pediatr Res.* 1976;10: 536–540.
7. Livingston S, Pauli LL, Pruce I. Ketogenic diet in the treatment of childhood epilepsy. *Dev Med Child Neurol.* 1977;19:833–834.
8. Neal EG, Chaffe H, Schwartz RH, et al. The ketogenic diet for the treatment of childhood epilepsy: a randomised controlled trial. *Lancet Neurol.* 2008;7(6):471–472.
9. Robinson AM, Williamson DH. Physiological roles of ketone bodies as substrates and signals in mammalian tissues. *Physiol Rev.* 1980;60: 143–187.
10. McGarry JD, Mannaerts GP, Foster DW. A possible role for malonyl CoA in the regulation of hepatic fatty acid oxidation and ketogenesis. *J Clin Invest.* 1977;60:265–270.
11. McGarry JD, Leatherman GF, Foster DW. Carnitine palmitoyltransferase I. The site of inhibition of hepatic fatty acid oxidation by malonyl-CoA. *J Biol Chem.* 1978;253:4128–4136.
12. Pan JW, Telang FW, Lee JH, et al. Measurement of beta-hydroxybutyrate in acute hyperketonemia in human brain. *J Neurochem.* 2001;79:539–544.
13. Cremer JE, Braun LD, Oldendorf WH. Changes during development in transport processes of the blood-brain barrier. *Biochim Biophys Acta.* 1976;448:633–637.
14. Bentourkia M, Tremblay S, Pifferi F, et al. PET study of 11C-acetoacetate kinetics in rat brain during dietary treatments affecting ketosis. *Am J Physiol Endocrinol Metab.* 2009;296(4):E796–E801.
15. Pan JW, de Graff RA, Rothman DL, et al. 13C-[2,4]-b-hydroxybutyrate metabolism in human brain. *J Neurochem.* 2002;81:45.
16. Fredericks M, Ramsey RB. 3-Oxo acid coenzyme A transferase activity in brain and tumors of the nervous system. *J Neurochem.* 1978;31:1529–1531.
17. Hori A, Tandon P, Holmes GL, et al. Ketogenic diet: effects on expression of kindled seizures and behavior in adult rats. *Epilepsia.* 1997;38:750–758.
18. Stafstrom CE, Wang C, Jensen FE. Electrophysiological observations in hippocampal slices from rats treated with the ketogenic diet. *Dev Neurosci.* 1999;21:393–399.
19. Muller-Schwarze AB, Tandon P, Liu Z, et al. Ketogenic diet reduces spontaneous seizures and mossy fiber sprouting in the kainic acid model. *Neuroreport.* 1999;10:1517–1522.
20. Bough KJ, Eagles DA. A ketogenic diet increases the resistance to pentylenetetrazole-induced seizures in the rat. *Epilepsia.* 1999;40:138–143.
21. Bough KJ, Schwartzkroin PA, Rho JM. Calorie restriction and ketogenic diet diminish neuronal excitability in rat dentate gyrus *in vivo. Epilepsia.* 2003;44:752–760.
22. DeVivo DC, Leckie MP, Ferrendelli JS, et al. Chronic ketosis and cerebral metabolism. *Ann Neurol.* 1978;3:331–337.
23. Pan JW, Bebin EM, Chu WJ, et al. Ketosis and epilepsy: 31P spectroscopic imaging at 4.1 T. *Epilepsia.* 1999;40:703–707.
24. Nylen K, Velazquez JL, Sayed V, et al. The effects of a ketogenic diet on ATP concentrations and the number of hippocampal mitochondria in Aldh5a1(-/-) mice. *Biochim Biophys Acta.* 2009;1790(3):208–212.
25. Al-Mudallal AS, LaManna JC, Lust WD, et al. Diet-induced ketosis does not cause cerebral acidosis. *Epilepsia.* 1996;37:258–261.
26. Helmholz HF, Keith HM. Eight years' experience with the ketogenic diet in the treatment of epilepsy. *JAMA.* 1930;95;707–709.
27. Keith HM. The effect of various factors on experimentally produced convulsions. *Am J Dis Child.* 1931;41:532–543.
28. Likhodii SS, Serbanescu I, Cortez MA, et al. Anticonvulsant properties of acetone, a brain ketone elevated by the ketogenic diet. *Ann Neurol.* 2003; 54:219–226.
29. Likhodii S, Nylen K, Burnham WM. Acetone as an anticonvulsant. *Epilepsia.* 2008;49(suppl 8):83–86.
30. Nordli DR, De Vivo DC. The ketogenic diet revisited: back to the future. *Epilepsia.* 1997;38:743–749.
31. Haces ML, Hernández-Fonseca K, Medina-Campos ON, et al. Antioxidant capacity contributes to protection of ketone bodies against oxidative damage induced during hypoglycemic conditions. *Exp Neurol.* 2008;211(1): 85–96.
32. Jarrett SG, Milder JB, Liang LP, et al. The ketogenic diet increases mitochondrial glutathione levels. *J Neurochem.* 2008;106(3):1044–1051.
33. Masino SA, Geiger JD. Are purines mediators of the anticonvulsant/neuroprotective effects of ketogenic diets? *Trends Neurosci.* 2008;31(6): 273–278.
34. Weinshenker D. The contribution of norepinephrine and orexigenic neuropeptides to the anticonvulsant effect of the ketogenic diet. *Epilepsia.* 2008;49(suppl 8):104–107.
35. Bough KJ, Rho JM. Anticonvulsant mechanisms of the ketogenic diet. *Epilepsia.* 2007;48(1):43–58.
36. Hartman AL. Does the effectiveness of the ketogenic diet in different epilepsies yield insights into its mechanisms? *Epilepsia.* 2008;49(suppl 8): 53–56.
37. DeVivo DC, Haymond MW, Leckie MP, et al. The clinical and biochemical implications of pyruvate carboxylase deficiency. *J Clin Endocrinol Metab.* 1977;45:1281–1296.
38. Kim DW, Kang HC, Park JC, et al. Benefits of the nonfasting ketogenic diet compared with the initial fasting ketogenic diet. *Pediatrics.* 2004;114(6): 1627–1630.

39. Kossoff EH, Laux LC, Blackford R, et al. When do seizures usually improve with the ketogenic diet? *Epilepsia.* 2008;49(2):329–333.

40. Carroll J, Koenigsberger D. The ketogenic diet: a practical guide for caregivers. *J Am Dietetic Assoc.* 1998;98:316–321.

41. Nordli DR, Koenigsberger D, Schroeder J, et al. Ketogenic diets. In: Resor S, Kutt H, eds. *The Medical Treatment of Epilepsy.* New York: Marcel Dekker, Inc.; 1992:455–472.

42. Livingston S. *Comprehensive Management of Epilepsy in Infancy, Childhood and Adolescence.* Springfield, IL: Charles C Thomas; 1972.

43. Kang HC, Lee YM, Kim HD, et al. Safe and effective use of the ketogenic diet in children with epilepsy and mitochondrial respiratory chain complex defects. *Epilepsia.* 2007;48(1):82–88.

44. Kossoff EH, Zupec-Kania BA, Amark PE, et al. Charlie Foundation, Practice Committee of the Child Neurology Society; Practice Committee of the Child Neurology Society; International Ketogenic Diet Study Group. Optimal clinical management of children receiving the ketogenic diet: recommendations of the International Ketogenic Diet Study Group. *Epilepsia.* 2009;50(2):304–317.

45. Hahn TJ, Halstead LR, De Vivo DC. Disordered mineral metabolism produced by ketogenic diet therapy. *Calcif Tissue Int.* 1979;28:17–22.

46. Ballaban-Gil K, Callahan C, O'Dell C, et al. Complications of the ketogenic diet. *Epilepsia.* 1998;39:744–748.

47. De Vivo DC, Bohan TP, Coulter DL, et al. L-carnitine supplementation in childhood epilepsy: current perspectives. *Epilepsia.* 1998;39:1216–1225.

48. De Vivo DC, Trifiletti RR, Jacobson RI, et al. Defective glucose transport across the blood-brain barrier as a cause of persistent hypoglycorrhachia, seizures, and developmental delay. *N Engl J Med.* 1991;325:713–721.

49. Wexler ID, Hemalatha SG, McConnell J, et al. Outcome of pyruvate dehydrogenase deficiency treated with ketogenic diets. Studies in patients with identical mutations. *Neurology.* 1997;49:1655–1661.

50. Prasad AN, Stafstrom CE, Holmes GL. Alternative epilepsy therapies: the ketogenic diet, immunoglobulins, and steroids. *Epilepsia.* 1996;37:S81–S95.

51. Freeman JM, Vining EP, Pillas DJ, et al. The efficacy of the ketogenic diet-1998: a prospective evaluation of intervention in 150 children. *Pediatrics.* 1998;102:1358–1363.

52. Schwartz RH, Eaton J, Bower BD, et al. Ketogenic diets in the treatment of epilepsy: short-term clinical effects. *Dev Med Child Neurol.* 1989;31:145–151.

53. Sills MA, Forsythe WI, Haidukewych D, et al. The medium chain triglyceride diet and intractable epilepsy. *Arch Dis Child.* 1986;61:1168–1172.

54. Woody RC, Brodie M, Hampton DK, et al. Corn oil ketogenic diet for children with intractable seizures. *J Child Neurol.* 1988;3:21–24.

55. Janaki S, Rashid MK, Gulati MS, et al. A clinical electroencephalographic correlation of seizures on a ketogenic diet. *Indian J Med Res.* 1976;64:1057–1063.

56. Nordli DR, Koenigsberger D, Carroll J, et al. Successful treatment of infants with the ketogenic diet [abstract]. *Ann Neurol.* 1995;38:523.

57. Keith HM. *Convulsive Disorders in Children. With Reference to Treatment with Ketogenic Diet.* Boston, Mass: Little, Brown, and Company; 1963.

58. Mady MA, Kossoff EH, McGregor AL, et al. The ketogenic diet: adolescents can do it, too. *Epilepsia.* 2003;44:847–851.

59. Bergquist AG, Chee CM, Lutchka LM, et al. Treatment of acquired epileptic aphasia with the ketogenic diet. *J Child Neurol.* 1999;14:696–701.

60. Kang HC, Kim HD, Lee YM, et al. Landau-Kleffner syndrome with mitochondrial respiratory chain-complex I deficiency. *Pediatr Neurol.* 2006;35(2):158–161.

61. Villeneuve N, Pinton F, Bahi-Buisson N, et al. The ketogenic diet improves recently worsened focal epilepsy. *Dev Med Child Neurol.* 2009;51(4):276–281.

CHAPTER 70 ■ VAGUS NERVE STIMULATION THERAPY

JAMES W. WHELESS

Epilepsy and seizures affect at least 2.3 million individuals in the United States. Although antiepileptic drugs (AEDs) are the primary form of treatment, recent outcome surveys reveal only mixed success even with the new AEDs that have become available over the past decade (1,2). Approximately one third of patients have seizures that are unresponsive to pharmacologic therapy (3–5). In addition, safety and tolerability issues associated with both the acute and chronic side effects and toxicity complications further diminish the effectiveness of AEDs (6–12). Nonadherence to AEDs, which is highly prevalent in the epilepsy population, also diminishes treatment effectiveness and further increases mortality as well as significantly increases health care utilization (13). Other treatment options are available for select subgroups of patients, including the ketogenic diet, which provides benefit to some children (14,15), and epilepsy surgery, which may manage or lessen poorly controlled seizures in 10% to 25% of patients (16). However, children and adults with uncontrolled seizures continue to carry a sad burden of higher mortality rates, higher rates of accidents and injuries, greater incidence of cognitive and psychiatric impairment, poor self-esteem, higher levels of anxiety and depression, and social stigmatization or isolation compared with the nonepileptic population (17,18). The shortcomings of AEDs, the ketogenic diet, and epilepsy surgery in improving overall outcome highlight the need for other treatments, one of which is vagus nerve stimulation therapy (VNS Therapy).

HISTORY

The effect of VNS on central nervous system (CNS) activity has been documented, with early attempts in the 1880s linking electrical vagal nerve and cervical sympathetic stimulation and carotid artery compression to the treatment of seizures (19). In the mid-1980s, Jacob Zabara, a biophysicist at Temple University, again suggested that electrical stimulation of the vagus nerve might prevent seizures. VNS therapy resulted from a hypothesis, formulated during his wife's Lamaze class, that the Lamaze method activated stretch receptors in the lungs, which in turn activated the vagus nerve (20). Vagus stimulation in the neck could quiet the abdominal muscle contractions that produce vomiting; Dr. Zabara likened these contractions to convulsions. Zabara believed that if VNS could alleviate vomiting and affect electroencephalographic (EEG) findings, it might ameliorate epilepsy. This theory was proved in his first canine studies (21), and a company—Cyberonics, Inc. (Houston, TX)—was founded in 1987 to develop VNS therapy, which would be delivered by a patented method using a generator device modeled after a cardiac pacemaker.

In 1988, the first patient to have a VNS therapy device implanted became seizure free (Table 70.1) (22). Five acute-phase clinical studies analyzing the safety and effectiveness of VNS therapy followed (Table 70.2). The first two single-blind trials showed improved control in adults with intractable partial seizures who were not candidates for epilepsy surgery (22–24). The subsequent two randomized, blinded, active-control trials (E03, E05) led to approval of VNS therapy by the U.S. Food and Drug Administration (FDA) in July 1997 for the adjunctive treatment of refractory partial-onset seizures among patients 12 years of age or older. VNS therapy is also approved for the treatment of epilepsy without age or seizure type restrictions (in most countries) and treatment-resistant depression in 68 countries around the world, including member nations of the European Union, Canada, Australia, and China. As of January 2009, more than 50,000 patients have received VNS therapy worldwide.

The VNS therapy system is made up of a pulse generator, a bipolar VNS lead, a programming wand with accompanying software for an IBM-compatible laptop or handheld computer, a tunneling tool, and handheld magnets (Fig. 70.1) (24,25). The generator transmits electrical signals to the vagus nerve through the lead. The software allows placement of the programming wand over the generator for reading and altering stimulation parameters (Fig. 70.2; Table 70.3; see VNS Therapy programming video). Each stimulation period is preceded by 2 seconds of ramp-up time and followed by 2 seconds of ramp-down time.

Two models of the VNS therapy generators are currently available: the Pulse Model 102 (single pin) and Pulse Duo Model 102R (dual pin) and the newer Demipulse Model 103

TABLE 70.1

HISTORY OF VNS THERAPY

1985	First animal studies
1988	First human implant
1992	First randomized active control study (E03) completed
1994	European community approval
1996	Second randomized active control study (E05) completed
1997	U.S. Food and Drug Administration commercial approval
February 2009	50,000+ implants worldwide for both epilepsy and depression

TABLE 70.2

EFFICACY OF VNS THERAPY IN CLINICAL STUDIES

Study	Design	Seizure type	No. of patients	Age of patients (years)	First implant	No. of patients with >50% response (%)	Mean reduction in seizures/day (%)
E01	Pilot, longitudinal	Partial	11	20–58	1998	30	24[a]
E02	Pilot, longitudinal	Partial	5	18–42	1990	50	40
E04	Open, longitudinal	All types	124	3–63	1990	29	7[a]
E03	Randomized, parallel, high/low	Partial	115	13–57	1991	31/14	24[a]/6
E05	Randomized, parallel, high/low	Partial	198	13–60	1995	23/16	28[b]/15[b]

[a]$P \leq 0.05$, by Student t test.
[b]$P < 0.0001$, by analysis of variance.

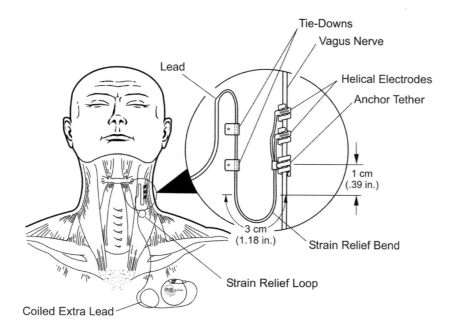

FIGURE 70.1 Implantable components of the VNS Therapy system.

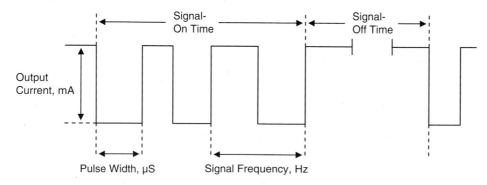

FIGURE 70.2 VNS Therapy stimulation parameters.

(single pin) and Demipulse Duo Model 104 (dual pin) (Fig. 70.3). The Demipulse generators, which are smaller and lighter than the Pulse generators, have improved diagnostics and faster communication with the programming system, but may have shorter battery life at higher duty cycles than the Pulse generators. Currently, three leads are available: the Model 302, Perennia Model 303, and PerenniaFLEX Model 304. All lead models are single pin and come in two sizes: 2.0 or 3.0 mm

(inner diameters of the helical coil) to account for various sizes of the vagus nerve. Dual-pin leads are no longer available. Therefore, the dual-pin generators (Model 102R and Model 104) are for replacement procedures only in patients with the previous dual-pin lead models. The Demipulse generators and Perennia model leads are not yet available in all countries. (See the Addendum for sources of information on the VNS therapy system.)

TABLE 70.3

VNS THERAPY PARAMETERS

	High	Low	Rapid cycling[a]
VNS current (mA)	Up to **3.5**	**1.2** (0.25–2.75)	Up to **3.5**
Frequency (Hz)	**30** (20–50)	**1** (to 2)	30
Pulse width (ms)	**500**	**130**	500
On time (s)	**30** (to 90)	**30**	7
Off time (min)	**5** (to 10)	**180** (60–180)	0.2
Magnet current (mA)	Same as VNS	0	Same as VNS
On time (s)	**30** (to 90)	**30**	30
Pulse width (μs)	**500**	**130**	500

Values in bold type are the most common settings from the E03 and E05 studies.
VNS, vagus nerve stimulation.
[a]From Refs. 27, 33, and 109.

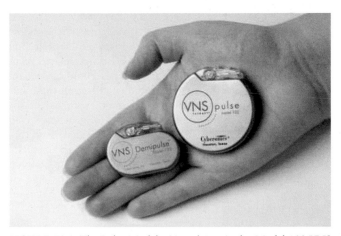

FIGURE 70.3 The Pulse Model 102 and Demipulse Model 103 VNS Therapy generators.

EFFICACY

The two pivotal studies—E03 and E05—were designed to demonstrate that high (therapeutic) and low (nontherapeutic) stimulation of the vagus nerve had different effects on the frequency of partial seizures (26,27). The effects of VNS therapy during the 12-week randomized phases of the studies, which began 2 weeks after implantation, were gauged against 12- to 16-week baseline periods. E03 acute-study patients (27) (N = 114 implanted) had epilepsy for an average of 22 years. Seizure frequency was reduced by at least half in 31% of patients in the high-stimulation group, compared with 14% in the low-stimulation group. No patients became seizure free during the acute phase, but some reported reduced seizure severity and improved postictal recovery periods. Patients in the high-stimulation group either aborted or decreased 59.8% of seizures with the magnet. No factors were identified that predicted response.

The similarly designed E05 study was the largest prospective, controlled trial of a device for epilepsy treatment ever conducted (26). Patients (N = 199) had a median of 0.51 to 0.58 seizures per day during baseline. One patient receiving high stimulation became seizure free, and 23.4% of patients had a 50% or more reduction in seizure frequency after 3 months of treatment. The presence or absence of aura did not predict efficacy. Of the implanted patients, 99% completed the study.

Long-Term Studies

All patients exiting Study E03 were offered indefinite open-label treatment at high (effective) stimulation; 100 (88%) of the 114 patients completed an additional 12 months of VNS therapy at therapeutic stimulation levels (14 patients discontinued because of lack of efficacy but were included in the analysis as intent to treat) (28). A median 20% reduction in seizure frequency occurred in the first 3 months of the extension study and improved over the ensuing months. In two thirds of patients, a minimum 50% reduction during the initial 3 months continued during months 10 through 12. Results among the 195 patients in the continuing long-term E05 study showed a 50% or more reduction in seizure frequency in 35% of patients and a 75% or more reduction in 20% of patients after an additional 12 months of VNS therapy at therapeutic stimulation levels (29). The median reduction in seizure frequency was 45%, with seizure frequency reductions sustained over time and only mild to moderate side effects reported.

Real-World Outcomes

In addition to the clinical trial data, real-world outcome studies show that VNS therapy is an effective treatment with increasing or sustained response rates over time. Response rates from the literature for studies reporting on at least 50 patients with a minimum of 3 months to more than 12 months of follow-up range from 50% to 59% (30–33). A retrospective study of 138 patients with at least 12 months of follow-up (mean of 44 months; range of 12 to 120 months) across multiple centers showed a 51% reduction in mean monthly seizure frequency (32). The overall responder rate was 59%, with an additional 13% of patients having a seizure frequency decrease between 30% and 50%. The seizure-free rate in this study was 9%. One study of 10 adults with intractable partial seizures revealed a 10-fold increase in the mean number of 14-day seizure-free periods after 50 months of VNS therapy with stable AED dosages (34). Seizure-free periods increased every year; one patient continued to be seizure free after 36.5 months. A prospective, open evaluation of 64 patients reported results for up to 5 years of follow-up (35). No change in AED dosages occurred during the first 6 months of VNS therapy, which lasted for an average of 20 months. Nineteen of 47 patients with partial seizures, 5 of 9 with idiopathic generalized seizures, and 5 of 8 with Lennox–Gastaut syndrome had a seizure reduction of greater than 50% or more. In this population with refractory seizures, 44% experienced a substantial reduction in severity and frequency over a long period. A report on long-term outcomes of 30 patients receiving VNS therapy (36) showed continued improvements over time, with 54% of patients at 1 year and 61% at 2 years exhibiting seizure frequency reductions of 50% or more compared with baseline. In a study of 269 patients on unchanged AEDs over 1 year, seizure frequency rates decreased over time from a median decrease of 45% at 3 months to a median of 58% at 12 months, indicating that response to VNS therapy over the long term is sustained and independent of AED changes (31). Small, prospective studies report similar results as well as additional benefits beyond seizure reduction such as reduced postictal periods and seizure duration (37,38). The mechanisms underlying the gradual improvements in response to VNS therapy seen over time in these long-term studies, however, have yet to be elucidated.

Pediatric, Elderly, and Special Populations

Studies indicate that response to VNS therapy is independent of age, seizure type, or epilepsy syndrome. The largest retrospective pediatric study to date showed the same median reduction in seizure frequency of 51% at 6 months among patients aged 12 to 18 years ($N = 56$) and among those less than 12 years of age ($N = 20$) (39). Longer-term retrospective studies among pediatric patients treated with VNS therapy showed increasing response rates over time similar to those seen in the real-world outcome data for adults with VNS (40–42). A retrospective study of 46 children implanted under the age of 18 (median age of 12.1 years) showed median seizure frequency reductions in the range of 60% over 3 years with VNS therapy, with response rates more favorable among patients less than 12 years of age (40). Particularly favorable results, including reduced seizure frequency and severity and improved quality of life (QoL), have been reported among patients in open studies of Lennox–Gastaut syndrome and other refractory childhood epilepsies, such as hypothalamic hamartomas, epileptic encephalopathies, Rett syndrome, and tuberous sclerosis complex (39,43–61). Verbal performance, alertness, motor and cognitive functions, and general behavior improved, sometimes dramatically (45,47,56,62,63). A retrospective study (63) showed that improved QoL (particularly in the area of alertness) was associated with VNS therapy in patients with autism ($N = 59$) or Landau–Kleffner syndrome (LKS; $N = 6$), with more than half of the patients in each group also experiencing a 50% or more reduction in seizure frequency at follow-up (12 months of follow-up for autism and 6 months for LKS patients). Studies have also shown both

seizure frequency reductions and improved QoL among both institutionalized and noninstitutionalized patients with mental retardation/developmental delay (MRDD) (64,65). VNS therapy also successfully stopped a case of refractory generalized convulsive status epilepticus in a patient 13 years of age (66). Another report among three children admitted to the intensive care unit (ICU) after developing status epilepticus showed that VNS therapy allowed early cessation of status and discharge from the ICU (57). Although the effectiveness of VNS therapy in the treatment of generalized seizures is not well documented, open studies indicate that VNS is a favorable treatment option among this patient population irregardless of age (67–72). Seizure frequency reductions among these studies ranged from 40% to >70% (67–69,71,72).

In a study of VNS therapy among patients 50 years of age or more, 21 of 31 patients experienced a 50% or greater decrease in seizure frequency at 1 year, accompanied by significant improvements in QoL from baseline over time (73). These studies indicate that age and seizure type or syndrome are not contraindications for the use of VNS therapy. A recent review (74) also indicated that VNS therapy is well tolerated among various patient populations, with rare withdrawals from treatment. A study of stimulation parameters among patients of different ages (75) recommended age-related stimulation adjustments based on age-related changes seen in vagus nerve characteristics. Early studies indicated that children might respond more rapidly than adults, with reductions in the interval between stimulations resulting in improved control (Table 70.3) (47,58,62). Additional pediatric studies reported that higher output currents might be required, particularly when lower pulse durations are used (76–78). Optimal stimulus parameter settings for patients of various ages or with specific seizure types or syndromes, however, have not yet been defined.

MECHANISM OF ACTION

The mechanisms by which VNS reduces seizure activity in humans were not known at the time VNS therapy was approved by the FDA. However, considerable progress in mechanistic VNS research has been made over the last 6 years. Electrical stimulation of the peripheral vagus nerve requires polysynaptic transmission to mediate the antiseizure effect. The anatomical distribution of vagal projections underlies the therapeutic actions of VNS therapy. Vagal visceral afferents have a diffuse CNS projection, with activation of these pathways broadly affecting neuronal excitability (25,79,80). Another review (79) examined the vagus nerve projections and CNS connections, as well as the current animal and human imaging studies, which indicate that VNS exerts both acute and long-term antiepileptic effects.

EXPERIMENTAL STUDIES

The first studies of the antiepileptic effects of VNS were conducted in 1937 (80). Subsequent experiments in cats showed that vagal stimulation produced EEG desynchronization (81) or synchronization, depending on the parameters used (82,83). Stimulation of the slow-conducting fibers most effectively resulted in EEG desynchronization. Hypersynchronized cortical and thalamocortical neuronal interactions characterize seizures; therefore, it was postulated that desynchronizing these activities would lead to antiseizure effects of VNS.

Initial work in cats and recent studies of strychnine-induced seizures in the dog, maximal electroshock and pentylenetetrazol-induced seizures in the rat, and the alumina-gel monkey model (21,81,84–87) showed that cervical vagal stimulation decreased interictal epileptiform discharges (IEDs) and shortened or aborted seizures; the antiepileptic effects outlasted the stimulus (21,84,87,88) and depended on its frequency and cumulative duration (84,84–86,88). These effects are now known to be mediated by activation of myelinated A and B fibers (89–91). Most central projections of the vagus nerve terminate in the nucleus of the solitary tract, with extensions to brain stem nuclei, thalamus, amygdala, and hypothalamus. Increased release of α-aminobutyric acid (GABA) and glycine by brain stem and subcortical nuclei was proposed as the antiepileptic mechanism of VNS therapy (85,86). Brain stem nuclei are known to influence seizure susceptibility (92–96); based on animal studies, the nucleus of the tractus solitarius is likely the key brain stem structure involved in transmitting and modulating VNS antiseizure effects.

Also unknown are the processes that mediate the sustained anticonvulsant effect of VNS therapy, but this effect, which outlasts the stimulation, suggests long-term changes in neural activity. Expression of *fos* immunoreactivity was induced by VNS in regions of the rat brain important in epileptogenesis (97); *fos* immunolabeling in the locus ceruleus suggested VNS modulation of norepinephrine release. Increased norepinephrine release by the locus ceruleus is antiepileptogenic. In rats with chronic or acute locus ceruleus lesions, VNS-induced seizure suppression was attenuated, supporting a noradrenergic mechanism (92). This first evidence of a structure mediating the anticonvulsant action of VNS may have pharmacologic implications for clinical practice. Drugs that activate the locus ceruleus or potentiate norepinephrine effects may enhance the efficacy of VNS. Pending the results of further animal testing, it is likely that the antiepileptic action of VNS is mediated through neuronal networks that project from brain stem to forebrain structures. Vagal projections to noradrenergic and serotonergic neuromodulatory systems of the brain may also explain the positive effects of VNS in improving mood disorders.

In summary, animal studies have established three distinct temporal patterns for the antiseizure effects of VNS: (i) acute abortive effects, in which an ongoing seizure is attenuated by VNS; (ii) acute prophylactic effects, in which seizure-inducing agents are less effective in provoking seizures when applied at the end of VNS; and (iii) chronic progressive prophylactic effects, in which total seizure counts are reduced more following chronic VNS stimulation. In addition, animal studies have shown that VNS can antagonize the development of epilepsy in the kindling model of epileptogenesis (98). Based on these studies, the mechanism of action of VNS therapy appears to be largely distinct from that of AED therapies (79).

CLINICAL STUDIES

Initial scalp recording performed in a small number of adults did not demonstrate a significant effect of VNS on EEG total power, median frequency, power in any of the conventional frequency bands (99), interictal epileptiform activity, or the waking or sleep background rhythms (22,99–101). At seizure onset, however, VNS has terminated both the clinical and the EEG seizure activity (101). Studies that are more recent have suggested that some patients may have a change in IEDs with VNS. Fifteen adults with refractory partial-onset seizure disorders showed a significant reduction in IEDs during stimulation and the interstimulation period immediately following stimulation, compared with baseline, with the reduction in IEDs greater among patients whose seizures decreased by more than 50% on VNS. Additionally, the patients who had a significant decrease in IEDs experienced the positive effect of magnetic extra stimulation in abolishing seizures (102). A single adult patient undergoing presurgical evaluation with intrahippocampal depth electrodes showed alteration of IEDs by VNS (increased spikes at 5 Hz, decreased at 30 Hz) (103). Chronic VNS in children was recently reported to reduce IEDs (104). However, this population was quite different from that in the earlier adult series. Included were patients with generalized and partial-onset seizures, greater frequency of IEDs, and younger age. During 12 months of VNS therapy, both generalized and focal spikes were diminished; however, this did not correlate well with seizure reduction. Pattern-reversal visual-evoked potentials, brain stem auditory-evoked potentials, and cognitive (P300) potentials were all unaffected by VNS (105).

Release of anticonvulsant neurotransmitters at the projection sites of vagus nerve afferent fibers was hypothesized as a mechanism of action (105,106). Cerebrospinal fluid samples assayed for amino acid and neurotransmitter metabolites in 16 patients before and after 3 months of VNS therapy showed a treatment-induced increase in GABA (an inhibitory amino acid), a decrease in aspartate (an excitatory amino acid), and an increase in ethanolamine (a membrane lipid precursor) (106).

Positron emission tomography (PET) $H_2^{15}O$ cerebral blood flow (CBF) imaging identifies the neuroanatomical structures recruited by VNS in humans. A pilot study of three adults showed activation of the right thalamus, right posterotemporal cortex, left putamen, and left inferior cerebellum (107). Localization to the thalamus may explain the therapeutic benefit of VNS and is consistent with the role of that structure as a generator and modulator of cerebral activity. Moreover, anatomic and physiologic evidence from both animal and human data further support the role of the thalamus in epilepsy (108), with stimulation of either the anterior thalamic nucleus or centromedian thalamic nucleus in animals being associated with antiepileptic effects (109). In a study of high and low stimulation (110), PET demonstrated CBF alterations at sites that receive vagal afferents and projections, including dorsal medulla, right postcentral gyrus, thalamus, cerebellum bilaterally, and limbic structures (bilateral hippocampus and amygdala). The high-stimulation group had more activation and deactivation sites, although the anatomical patterns during VNS were similar in both groups. Finally, acute CBF alterations were correlated with long-term therapeutic response, in an attempt to exclude those regions that show changes in VNS-induced synaptic activity but may not participate in VNS-related antiseizure actions (111). Decreased seizure frequency was associated with increased CBF only in the right and left thalami. Studies of chronic VNS therapy have shown the same anatomical distribution of CBF

(107,112). Demonstration of these acute regional alterations does not clarify the mechanism of action of long term, intermittent VNS, which may involve neurotransmitters or neurochemicals at those sites that outlast the stimulation.

Functional magnetic resonance imaging (fMRI) evaluating the time course of regional CBF alterations during VNS therapy can be performed safely in patients implanted with a vagal nerve stimulator (113). Preliminary fMRI studies have agreed with the PET studies, with the most robust activation observed in the thalami and insular cortices, with some activation also seen in ipsilateral basal ganglia, anterior parietal cortex, and other cortical areas (113,114).

SELECTION OF CANDIDATES

In the United States, VNS therapy is indicated as an adjunctive treatment for adults and adolescents 12 years of age or older with refractory partial-onset seizures (24). In the European Union, VNS therapy is indicated as an adjunctive treatment for patients with partial- or generalized-onset seizures without an age limitation. However, indications for VNS therapy were derived from the clinical trial experience, not from an understanding of its physiologic action. Age, sex, and frequency of seizures, secondarily generalized seizures, or interictal EEG spikes do not predict response to VNS therapy. The type or number of coadministered AEDs also do not predict response (67,115). Therefore, children may benefit considerably from VNS therapy, but randomized, controlled studies have not been completed. Patients with other seizure types or epilepsy syndromes also may benefit from VNS therapy.

Although optimal use parameters continue to be defined, candidates should meet the following criteria: (i) medically refractory seizures, (ii) adequate trials of at least two AEDs, (iii) exclusion of nonepileptic events, and (iv) ineligibility for epilepsy surgery (Fig. 70.4). Focal resective surgery (temporal lobectomy or lesional neocortical epilepsy) is preferred for appropriate patients because of its superior seizure-free rate (116–118). Recent open studies suggest that VNS therapy may be used among patients considered for corpus callosotomy, producing lower rates of morbidity (119–121), and among those who have previously undergone epilepsy surgery (39,122,123). Earlier use (within 2 years of seizure onset or after failure of two or three AEDs) of VNS therapy may also produce a higher response rate, as well as reduce the negative side effects associated with long-term epilepsy and AED therapy, which hinder development (30,124,125). Patients with a history of nonadherence to their AED regimens, particularly those on polypharmacy, may also be good candidates for VNS therapy because of the assured compliance and lack of further drug–drug interactions with VNS therapy.

Use of VNS therapy is contraindicated in patients with prior bilateral or left cervical vagotomy, and safety and efficacy have not been established for stimulation of the right vagus nerve. Patients with existing pulmonary or cardiac disease should be evaluated carefully before implantation; chronic obstructive pulmonary disease may increase the risk for dyspnea. Patients with cardiac conduction disorders were not studied in the controlled trials. A cardiologist's evaluation should precede implantation, with postprocedural Holter monitoring performed if clinically indicated. Patients with a history of obstructive sleep apnea should be treated with care, as an increase in apneic events during stimulation is possible (126,127). Lowering stimulation frequency (i.e., pulse width and signal frequency to 250 μsec and 20 Hz, respectively) may prevent exacerbation of this condition (126). However, most studies showing a decrease in airflow during sleep with VNS therapy reported this condition to be clinically insignificant (127). Moreover, beneficial effects on sleep and increases in slow wave sleep also have been reported with VNS therapy, which may play a role in the antiepileptic mechanisms of VNS (128,129).

Treatment Sequence for VNS Therapy

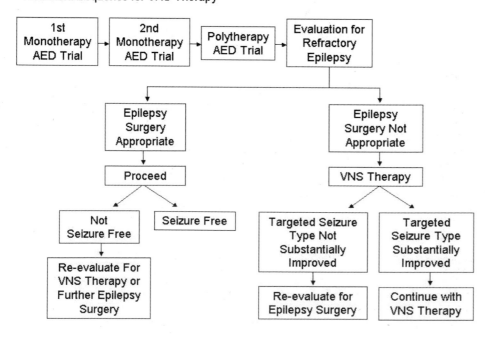

FIGURE 70.4 Treatment selection flow chart. AED, antiepileptic drug; VNS, vagus nerve stimulation therapy.

INITIATION AND MAINTENANCE

Hospitalization for implantation of the device is preceded by evaluations by a neurologist and by a surgeon with experience in the carotid sheath. With the patient typically under general anesthesia (although local or regional anesthesia has been used successfully as well) (130), the lead wires are placed on the left cervical vagus nerve and the generator is placed in a subcutaneous pocket in the left upper chest (131,132) (see VNS Therapy surgical implant video). Intraoperative electrical impedance testing ensures integrity of the system. Rare cases of bradycardia, asystole, or both mandate initial lead testing in the operating room (24,133,134); the anesthesiologist should be notified immediately before this test. Stimulation following intraoperative bradycardia has been shown to be safe, with no change in cardiac rhythm upon initiation of postoperative VNS, which was started under ECG monitoring (135). Reimplant of a second VNS therapy generator upon battery depletion in two patients also showed no occurrence of bradycardia (135). Correct placement of the lead electrodes around the vagus nerve is critical. Two methods have been developed to help confirm correct placement of the electrodes intraoperatively (136), depending on the type of anesthesia used for the procedure. For patients receiving general anesthesia, the larynx and vocal cords can be monitored by fiberoptic endoscopy for contraction of the left lateral larynx wall and vocal cord tightening. For patients being implanted under local and regional anesthesia, stimulation intensities can be increased until a voice alteration is noticed. Neither procedure is harmful to the patient nor greatly extends the length of the surgery.

Prophylactic antibiotics may be administered both in the operating room and postoperatively. The patient can be discharged after the procedure, which usually lasts for less than 1 hour, or can be observed overnight. Discharge education should include care of the incisions and use of the magnet. In clinical studies, the generator's output current was kept at 0 mA for the first 2 weeks; however, programmed stimulation is now being initiated at 0.25 mA in some operating rooms (39). Dosages of AEDs are generally kept stable for the first 3 months of stimulation unless an early response is noted.

A few weeks after implantation, the patient is examined to confirm wound healing and proper generator operation either to begin or to continue programming. Output current is increased in 0.25-mA increments until stimulation is comfortable (Table 70.1). The subsequent stimulation schedule is determined by patient response. Standard parameter settings range from 20 to 30 Hz at a pulse width of 250 to 500 μsec and an output current of 0.25 to 3.5 mA for 30 seconds "on" time and 5 minutes "off" time (78). At each visit, the generator and the battery are assessed for end of service; the battery's life expectancy of 7 to 10 years depends on the programmed stimulation parameters. If VNS therapy is to be continued, the generator can be replaced at the appropriate time in less than 20 minutes.

VNS may be continued indefinitely and without damage to the vagus nerve as long as the stimulation is less than 50 Hz and the on time remains less than the off time (24,137,138). Two safety features that protect patients from continuous stimulation or uncomfortable side effects are the magnet and the watchdog timer. The magnet can act as an "off" switch when held or taped over the generator. The watchdog timer is an internal monitor that limits the number of pulses to be delivered without an "off" time to prevent excess stimulation.

COMPLICATIONS AND ADVERSE EFFECTS

Surgical complications and difficulties are rare. Fracture of the electrode, related to fatigue at the junction between contact and the lead wire, was a common problem with early devices (23,139–142). Substitution of a quadrifilar wire and, later, a trifilar lead body coil improved electrode tolerance that had been compromised by repetitive neck motion. The two newest lead models (Perennia Model 303 and PerenniaFLEX Model 304) are designed to be even more resistant to fractures than previous models. The PerenniaFLEX is similar in design to the Model 302 but has a lead body designed with three high fatigue silicone tubes; the bifurcation is still caudal to the anchor tether, but designed with a smoother transition to facilitate a smooth strain relief bend. The Perennia is constructed with a trifilar lead body coil and a continuous bilumen lead body silicone tube with the bifurcation cephalad to the anchor tether; this design makes the handling characteristics of the Perennia lead feel stiffer during the implantation procedure compared with the Model 302 and 304 leads. The Perennia model leads are approved by the FDA but are not currently available in all countries.

Incisional infections are unusual and generally respond to antibiotic therapy. Fluid accumulation at the generator site with or without infection occurs in 1% to 2% of implantations and resolves with aspiration and antibiotics; the rare cases of refractory infection require removal of the generator. However, one case of deep wound infection associated with implantation of the generator was reported to be managed successfully with open wound treatment without removal of the device, an alternative option if removal of the device appears hazardous (143). Unilateral vocal cord paralysis, which accompanies approximately 1% of implants, may be caused by excess manipulation of the vagus nerve, and subsequent damage to the vagal artery and its reinforcing arterioles (144); in most cases, it remits completely over several weeks.

Common side effects, which occur primarily when the stimulator is actually delivering a pulse (Table 70.4), are dose dependent and usually mild or absent when VNS parameters are appropriately programmed (26,27,145); many patients become accustomed to them with time. Most patients experience hoarseness or a change in vocal quality and tingling over the left cervical region on delivery of the electrical pulse. Subjective dyspnea or a sensation of muscle tightening in the neck may occur, without changes on pulmonary function testing (26). Cough or throat pain during stimulus delivery sometimes necessitates a reduction in current or pulse width (146).

Despite the widespread visceral efferent projections of the vagus nerve, systemic effects are rare. Pulmonary function does not change significantly in patients without concomitant lung disease (26,147), but may deteriorate in the face of intense stimulation and obstructive lung disease (147).

TABLE 70.4

ADVERSE EVENTS WITH VAGUS NERVE STIMULATION[a]

	No. of patients (%)	
Adverse event	E03 and E05 patients (N = 314; 591 device years) > 3 months' follow-up	E03 and E05 patients with high stimulation (N = 152) > 3 months' follow-up
Voice alteration	156 (50)	91 (60)
Increased coughing	129 (41)	57 (38)
Paresthesia	87 (28)	32 (21)
Dyspnea	55 (18)	32 (21)
Dyspepsia	36 (12)	22 (15)
Laryngismus	10 (3.2)	9 (5.9)

[a]Number of patients reporting the adverse event at least once in the E03 and E05 randomized studies.

Inhalation of ipratropium bromide or lowering of the stimulus frequency or current is recommended. No substantial effects on cardiac function were reported during clinical studies (24,26, 27,145,148). An analysis of total mortality and sudden death in epileptic patients (to August 1996) revealed the expected rate in individuals with severe, intractable epilepsy (149,150). The clinical studies demonstrated no clinically relevant effects on the gastrointestinal system, serum chemistries, AED concentrations, vital signs, or weight.

Rare reported side effects associated with VNS therapy include diarrhea (151), sternocleidomastoid muscle spasm (152), phrenic nerve stimulation (153), tonsillar pain (154), emergent psychiatric disorders (155,156), and prominent drooling and vomiting (157). Of seven patients treated with VNS therapy who developed a major psychiatric disorder (155), all had a history of a dysphoric disorder and most had daily seizures before treatment with VNS. The severe dysphoric or psychotic conditions emerged once seizure frequency was reduced by 75% or more, but remitted or improved satisfactorily with psychotropic medication, with two patients also requiring a decrease or interruption of VNS therapy. Children with a history of dysphagia may experience swallowing difficulties during VNS therapy (157–159); using a magnet to turn off the stimulator during mealtime may help. The majority of side effects, including many of the rare incidents reported, are amenable to stimulus modifications, which could include changes in output current and/or pulse width.

ADVANTAGES AND DISADVANTAGES

Many patients maintained on VNS therapy can decrease their total AED burden, which typically results in a more alert patient who, while still receiving polytherapy, is without the cognitive or systemic side effects typically associated with multiple therapies. Therefore, use of AED monotherapy with VNS therapy may produce a better risk to benefit ratio than that with two AEDs. Even when AEDs cannot be substantially decreased or withdrawn, however, VNS therapy may allow amelioration of seizures with no risk of toxic organ reactions, drug interactions or failures, allergies, rashes, and other

systemic adverse effects or cognitive side effects (160,161); in some patients, memory, alertness, mood, and communication have been shown to improve (100,162–166). Improvements in QoL independent of treatment effect on seizure frequency, as well as increased daytime vigilance, have also been reported (167–169). In addition, because the beneficial results are maintained without active patient participation, VNS therapy may be an ideal treatment for the partially compliant. Teratogenesis is not expected with VNS therapy. Although no controlled studies of VNS therapy in pregnancy have been conducted, animal studies showed no harm to fertility or to the fetus (24). Cases also have been reported in the literature of patients who became pregnant while on VNS therapy and gave birth to healthy babies (35,170). Finally, VNS therapy can both prevent and abort seizures. The ability to trigger the device externally (with the magnet) and to interrupt the seizure or improve the postictal phase empowers the patient and provides a sense of control over epilepsy.

On the other hand, VNS is an empiric therapy, with no way to predict response except by trial. The initial cost (often between $15,000 and $25,000) can be prohibitive without coverage by a third-party payer. Over the life of the system, however, this cost approximates that of many of the new AEDs (171). Moreover, although weeks to months may elapse before seizure frequency decreases, cost-effectiveness studies indicate that VNS therapy provides a substantial cost-savings benefit to hospitals over the long-term course of treatment (172,173). These cost benefits are sustained over time and are sufficient to cover or exceed the cost of the device. Further savings can be seen in significant reductions in health care utilization and time spent on epilepsy-related matters with VNS therapy over time. A Kaiser study, which looked at health care utilization of 138 patients with refractory epilepsy comparing 1 year of baseline data followed by 4 years of quarterly follow-up data with VNS therapy, showed significant reductions in the numbers of emergency department visits (decreased by 99%), hospitalizations (70% decrease), and hospital lengths of stay (67% decrease) beginning with the first quarter after implantation with VNS Therapy (P < 0.05 for all postimplantation quarters) (174). A 91% decrease was also seen in outpatient visits post-VNS therapy, and significant decreases were seen for average number of days on which patients could not work because of health-related concerns ($P = 0.002$) and average time spent caring for health problems ($P < 0.001$), which further reflect positive changes in the QoL of both patients and their caregivers as a result of VNS therapy in addition to health care utilization savings.

According to the manufacturer of the device, a transmit-and-receive head coil MRI should be performed rather than a full-body MRI, with the generator programmed to 0 mA for the procedure and returned to the original settings thereafter (24). However, successful head coil MRIs have been performed among patients both with and without the device turned off (175). If the device does remain on during the MRI, the device should be interrogated postprocedure to ensure that the magnetic field did not deactivate the device or change the pre-MRI settings. Although not recommended by the manufacturer, successful body coil MRIs with the use of an ice pack over the area of the device leads have been reported among three patients (176). Diathermy, which could heat the system above safe levels and thereby cause either temporary or permanent tissue or nerve damage, should be avoided in patients receiving VNS therapy.

FUTURE DEVELOPMENTS

VNS therapy has raised interest in the role of neurostimulation as a treatment for refractory epilepsy. Since the first device implantation more than 20 years ago, the number of AEDs has increased, yet uncontrolled seizures continue. The question not answered in clinical studies is, when should VNS therapy be used? Currently, VNS is not used until multiple medications have failed and surgery is not an option. However, preliminary studies indicate that VNS therapy may be more effective when used earlier in the treatment process, particularly within 2 years of diagnosis after two or three AEDs have failed to control seizures (30).

Other research questions, if answered, have the potential to dramatically improve the overall treatment of all patients with epilepsy. Are there unique stimulation parameters for certain seizure types (e.g., partial vs. generalized), syndromes (e.g., Lennox–Gastaut), or age groups? Might some AEDs or other medications enhance the effectiveness of VNS therapy? What are the psychosocial effects of VNS therapy on the families of individuals with epilepsy? Answers to such questions and improvements in technology will expand the role of VNS therapy for uncontrolled epilepsy.

ADDENDUM

Videotapes and information on the VNS Therapy system are available free to patients, nurses, and physicians from Cyberonics, Inc.

References

1. Brodie MJ, Kwan P. Staged approach to epilepsy management. *Neurology.* 2002;58:S2–S8.
2. Schmidt D. The clinical impact of new antiepileptic drugs after a decade of use in epilepsy. *Epilepsy Res.* 2002;50:21–32.
3. Kwan P, Brodie MJ. Early identification of refractory epilepsy. *N Engl J Med.* 2000;342:314–319.
4. Mohanraj R, Brodie MJ. Diagnosing refractory epilepsy: response to sequential treatment schedules. *Eur J Neurol.* 2006;13:277–282.
5. Hitiris N, Mohanraj R, Norrie J, et al. Predictors of pharmacoresistant epilepsy. *Epilepsy Res.* 2007;75:192–196.
6. Jallon P. The problem of intractability: the continuing need for new medical therapies in epilepsy. *Epilepsia.* 1997;38(suppl 9):S37–S42.
7. Patsalos PN, Duncan JS. Antiepileptic drugs. A review of clinically significant drug interactions. *Drug Saf.* 1993;9:156–184.
8. Pellock JM, Pippenger CE. Adverse effects of antiepileptic drugs. In: Dodson WE, Pellock JM, eds. *Pediatric Epilepsy: Diagnosis and Therapy.* New York, NY: Demos; 1993:253–264.
9. Schmidt D. *Adverse Effects of Antiepileptic Drugs.* New York, NY: Raven Press; 1982.
10. Pellock JM. Antiepileptic drug therapy in the United States: a review of clinical studies and unmet needs. *Neurology.* 1995;45:S17–S24.
11. Kwan P, Brodie MJ. Effectiveness of first antiepileptic drug. *Epilepsia.* 2001;42:1255–1260.
12. Camfield P, Camfield C. Acute and chronic toxicity of antiepileptic medications: a selective review. *Can J Neurol Sci.* 1994;21:S7–S11.
13. Faught E, Duh MS, Weiner JR, et al. Nonadherence to antiepileptic drugs and increased mortality: findings from the RANSOM Study. *Neurology.* 2008;71:1572–1578.
14. Wheless JW, Ashwal S. The ketogenic diet. In: Swaiman KF, Ashwal S, eds. *Pediatric Neurology: Principles and Practice.* Philadelphia, PA: CV Mosby Co.; 1999:719–728.
15. Vining EP, Freeman JM, Ballaban-Gil K, et al. A multicenter study of the efficacy of the ketogenic diet. *Arch Neurol.* 1998;55:1433–1437.
16. Epilepsy Foundation of America. *Epilepsy: A Report to the Nation.* Landover, MD: Epilepsy Foundation of America; 1999.
17. Fisher RS, Parks-Trusz SL, Lehman C. Social issues in epilepsy. In: Shorvon S, Dreifus F, Fish D, et al., eds. *The Treatment of Epilepsy.* Cambridge, MA: Blackwell Science; 1996:357–369.
18. Wheless JW. Intractable epilepsy: a survey of patients and caregivers. *Epilepsy Behav.* 2006;8:756–764.
19. Lanska DJ. J.L. Corning and vagal nerve stimulation for seizures in the 1880s. *Neurology.* 2002;58:452–459.
20. Lesser RP. Unexpected places: how did vagus nerve stimulation become a treatment for epilepsy? *Neurology.* 1999;52:1117–1118.
21. Zabara J. Inhibition of experimental seizures in canines by repetitive vagal stimulation. *Epilepsia.* 1992;33:1005–1012.
22. Penry JK, Dean JC. Prevention of intractable partial seizures by intermittent vagal stimulation in humans: preliminary results. *Epilepsia.* 1990;31(suppl 2):S40–S43.
23. Uthman BM, Wilder BJ, Penry JK, et al. Treatment of epilepsy by stimulation of the vagus nerve. *Neurology.* 1993;43:1338–1345.
24. Cyberonics, Inc. *VNS Therapy Physician's Manual.* Houston, TX: Cyberonics, Inc.; 2006. Available at: http://www.vnstherapy.com/epilepsy/hcp/manuals/default.aspx
25. Schachter SC, Saper CB. Vagus nerve stimulation. *Epilepsia.* 1998;39:677–686.
26. Handforth A, DeGiorgio CM, Schachter SC, et al. Vagus nerve stimulation therapy for partial-onset seizures: a randomized active-control trial. *Neurology.* 1998;51:48–55.
27. A randomized controlled trial of chronic vagus nerve stimulation for treatment of medically intractable seizures: The Vagus Nerve Stimulation Study Group. *Neurology.* 1995;45:224–230.
28. Salinsky MC, Uthman BM, Ristanovic RK, et al. Vagus nerve stimulation for the treatment of medically intractable seizures. Results of a 1-year open-extension trial. Vagus Nerve Stimulation Study Group. *Arch Neurol.* 1996;53:1176–1180.
29. DeGiorgio CM, Schachter SC, Handforth A, et al. Prospective long-term study of vagus nerve stimulation for the treatment of refractory seizures. *Epilepsia.* 2000;41:1195–1200.
30. Renfroe JB, Wheless JW. Earlier use of adjunctive vagus nerve stimulation therapy for refractory epilepsy. *Neurology.* 2002;59:S26–S30.
31. Labar D. Vagus nerve stimulation for 1 year in 269 patients on unchanged antiepileptic drugs. *Seizure.* 2004;13:392–398.
32. De Herdt V, Boon P, Ceulemans B, et al. Vagus nerve stimulation for refractory epilepsy: a Belgian multicenter study. *Eur J Paediatr Neurol.* 2007;11:261–269.
33. Vonck K, Thadani V, Gilbert K, et al. Vagus nerve stimulation for refractory epilepsy: a transatlantic experience. *J Clin Neurophysiol.* 2004;21:283–289.
34. Clarke BM, Upton AR, Griffin H, et al. Seizure control after stimulation of the vagus nerve: clinical outcome measures. *Can J Neurol Sci.* 1997;24:222–225.
35. Ben-Menachem E, Hellstrom K, Waldton C, et al. Evaluation of refractory epilepsy treated with vagus nerve stimulation for up to 5 years. *Neurology.* 1999;52:1265–1267.
36. Chavel SM, Westereld M, Spencer S. Long-term outcome of vagus nerve stimulation for refractory partial epilepsy. *Epilepsy Behav.* 2003;4:302–309.
37. Ardesch JJ, Buschman HP, Wagener-Schimmel LJ, et al. Vagus nerve stimulation for medically refractory epilepsy: a long-term follow-up study. *Seizure.* 2007;16:579–585.

38. Abubakr A, Wambacq I. Long-term outcome of vagus nerve stimulation therapy in patients with refractory epilepsy. *J Clin Neurosci.* 2008;15: 127–129.

39. Helmers SL, Wheless JW, Frost M, et al. Vagus nerve stimulation therapy in pediatric patients with refractory epilepsy: retrospective study. *J Child Neurol.* 2001;16:843–848.

40. Alexopoulos AV, Kotagal P, Loddenkemper T, et al. Long-term results with vagus nerve stimulation in children with pharmacoresistant epilepsy. *Seizure.* 2006;15:491–503.

41. Benifla M, Rutka JT, Logan W, et al. Vagal nerve stimulation for refractory epilepsy in children: indications and experience at The Hospital for Sick Children. *Childs Nerv Syst.* 2006;22:1018–1026.

42. You SJ, Kang HC, Kim HD, et al. Vagus nerve stimulation in intractable childhood epilepsy: a Korean multicenter experience. *J Korean Med Sci.* 2007;22:442–445.

43. Frost M, Gates J, Helmers SL, et al. Vagus nerve stimulation in children with refractory seizures associated with Lennox–Gastaut syndrome. *Epilepsia.* 2001;42:1148–1152.

44. Murphy JV. Left vagal nerve stimulation in children with medically refractory epilepsy. The Pediatric VNS Study Group. *J Pediatr.* 1999;134: 563–566.

45. Parker AP, Polkey CE, Binnie CD, et al. Vagal nerve stimulation in epileptic encephalopathies. *Pediatrics.* 1999;103:778–782.

46. Lundgren J, Amark P, Blennow G, et al. Vagus nerve stimulation in 16 children with refractory epilepsy. *Epilepsia.* 1998;39:809–813.

47. Hornig GW, Murphy JV, Schallert G, et al. Left vagus nerve stimulation in children with refractory epilepsy: an update. *South Med J.* 1997;90: 484–488.

48. Parain D, Penniello MJ, Berquen P, et al. Vagal nerve stimulation in tuberous sclerosis complex patients. *Pediatr Neurol.* 2001;25:213–216.

49. Parker AP, Polkey CE, Robinson RO. Vagal nerve stimulation in the epileptic encephalopathies: 3-year follow-up. *Pediatrics.* 2001;108:221.

50. Murphy JV, Wheless JW, Schmoll CM. Left vagal nerve stimulation in six patients with hypothalamic hamartomas. *Pediatr Neurol.* 2000;23: 167–168.

51. Hosain S, Nikalov B, Harden C, et al. Vagus nerve stimulation treatment for Lennox-Gastaut syndrome. *J Child Neurol.* 2000;15:509–512.

52. Aicardi J. Vagal nerve stimulation in epileptic encephalopathies. *Pediatrics.* 1999;103:821–822.

53. Hornig G, Murphy JV. Vagal nerve stimulation: updated experience in 60 pediatric patients. *Epilepsia.* 1998;39:169.

54. Schallert G, Murphy J. Vagal nerve stimulation: experience in 60 children. *Neurology.* 1998;50:A14.

55. Aldenkamp AP, Majoie HJM, Berfelo MW, et al. Long-term effects of 24-month treatment with vagus nerve stimulation on behaviour in children with Lennox-Gastaut syndrome. *Epilepsy Behav.* 2002;3:475–479.

56. Wilfong AA, Schultz RJ. Vagus nerve stimulation for treatment of epilepsy in Rett syndrome. *Dev Med Child Neurol.* 2006;48:683–686.

57. Zamponi N, Rychlicki F, Corpaci L, et al. Vagus nerve stimulation (VNS) is effective in treating catastrophic 1 epilepsy in very young children. *Neurosurg Rev.* 2008;31:291–297.

58. Rossignol E, Lortie A, Thomas T, et al. Vagus nerve stimulation in pediatric epileptic syndromes. *Seizure.* 2009;18:34–37.

59. Major P, Thiele EA. Vagus nerve stimulation for intractable epilepsy in tuberous sclerosis complex. *Epilepsy Behav.* 2008;13:357–360.

60. Koenig SA, Longin E, Bell N, et al. Vagus nerve stimulation improves severely impaired heart rate variability in a patient with Lennox–Gastaut syndrome. *Seizure.* 2008;17:469–472.

61. You SJ, Kang HC, Ko TS, et al. Comparison of corpus callosotomy and vagus nerve stimulation in children with Lennox–Gastaut syndrome. *Brain Dev.* 2008;30:195–199.

62. Murphy JV, Hornig G, Schallert G. Left vagal nerve stimulation in children with refractory epilepsy. Preliminary observations. *Arch Neurol.* 1995;52: 886–889.

63. Park YD. The effects of vagus nerve stimulation therapy on patients with intractable seizures and either Landau–Kleffner syndrome or autism. *Epilepsy Behav.* 2003;4:286–290.

64. Gates J, Huf R, Frost M. Vagus nerve stimulation for patients in residential treatment facilities. *Epilepsy Behav.* 2001;2:563–567.

65. Andriola MR, Vitale SA. Vagus nerve stimulation in the developmentally disabled. *Epilepsy Behav.* 2001;2:129–134.

66. Winston KR, Levisohn P, Miller BR, et al. Vagal nerve stimulation for status epilepticus. *Pediatr Neurosurg.* 2001;34:190–192.

67. Labar D, Murphy J, Tecoma E. Vagus nerve stimulation for medication-resistant generalized epilepsy. E04 VNS Study Group. *Neurology.* 1999;52: 1510–1512.

68. Ng M, Devinsky O. Vagus nerve stimulation for refractory idiopathic generalized epilepsy. *Seizure.* 2004;13:176–178.

69. Holmes MD, Silbergeld DL, Drouhard D, et al. Effect of vagus nerve stimulation on adults with pharmacoresistant generalized epilepsy syndromes. *Seizure.* 2004;13:340–345.

70. Nei M, O'Connor M, Liporace J, et al. Refractory generalized seizures: response to corpus callosotomy and vagal nerve stimulation. *Epilepsia.* 2006;47:115–122.

71. Kostov H, Larsson PG, Roste GK. Is vagus nerve stimulation a treatment option for patients with drug-resistant idiopathic generalized epilepsy? *Acta Neurol Scand Suppl.* 2007;187:55–58.

72. Labar D, Nikolov B, Tarver B, et al. Vagus nerve stimulation for symptomatic generalized epilepsy: a pilot study. *Epilepsia.* 1998;39:201–205.

73. Sirven JI, Sperling M, Naritoku D, et al. Vagus nerve stimulation therapy for epilepsy in older adults. *Neurology.* 2000;54:1179–1182.

74. Privitera MD, Welty TE, Ficker DM, et al. Vagus nerve stimulation for partial seizures. *Cochrane Database Syst Rev.* 2002;(1):CD002896.

75. Koo B, Ham SD, Sood S, et al. Human vagus nerve electrophysiology: a guide to vagus nerve stimulation parameters. *J Clin Neurophysiol.* 2001; 18:429–433.

76. Majoie HJ, Berfelo MW, Aldenkamp AP, et al. Vagus nerve stimulation in children with therapy-resistant epilepsy diagnosed as Lennox–Gastaut syndrome: clinical results, neuropsychological effects, and cost-effectiveness. *J Clin Neurophysiol.* 2001;18:419–428.

77. Crumrine PK. Vagal nerve stimulation in children. *Semin Pediatr Neurol.* 2000;7:216–223.

78. Heck C, Helmers SL, DeGiorgio CM. Vagus nerve stimulation therapy, epilepsy, and device parameters: scientific basis and recommendations for use. *Neurology.* 2002;59:S31–S37.

79. Henry TR. Therapeutic mechanisms of vagus nerve stimulation. *Neurology.* 2002;59:S3–S14.

80. Rutecki P. Anatomical, physiological, and theoretical basis for the antiepileptic effect of vagus nerve stimulation. *Epilepsia.* 1990;31(suppl 2): S1–S6.

81. Zanchetti A, Wang SC, Moruzzi G. The effect of vagal afferent stimulation on the EEG pattern of the cat. *Electroencephalogr Clin Neurophysiol.* 1952;4:357–361.

82. Chase MH, Nakamura Y, Clemente CD, et al. Afferent vagal stimulation: neurographic correlates of induced EEG synchronization and desynchronization. *Brain Res.* 1967;5:236–249.

83. Chase MH, Sterman MB, Clemente CD. Cortical and subcortical patterns of response to afferent vagal stimulation. *Exp Neurol.* 1966;16:36–49.

84. Takaya M, Terry WJ, Naritoku DK. Vagus nerve stimulation induces a sustained anticonvulsant effect. *Epilepsia.* 1996;37:1111–1116.

85. Woodbury JW, Woodbury DM. Vagal stimulation reduces the severity of maximal electroshock seizures in intact rats: use of a cuff electrode for stimulating and recording. *Pacing Clin Electrophysiol.* 1991;14:94–107.

86. Woodbury DM, Woodbury JW. Effects of vagal stimulation on experimentally induced seizures in rats. *Epilepsia.* 1990;31(suppl 2):S7–S19.

87. Lockard JS, Congdon WC, DuCharme LL. Feasibility and safety of vagal stimulation in monkey model. *Epilepsia.* 1990;31(suppl 2):S20–S26.

88. McLachlan RS. Suppression of interictal spikes and seizures by stimulation of the vagus nerve. *Epilepsia.* 1993;34:918–923.

89. Krahl SE, Senanayake SS, Handforth A. Destruction of peripheral C-fibers does not alter subsequent vagus nerve stimulation-induced seizure suppression in rats. *Epilepsia.* 2001;42:586–589.

90. Zagon A, Kemeny AA. Slow hyperpolarization in cortical neurons: a possible mechanism behind vagus nerve simulation therapy for refractory epilepsy? *Epilepsia.* 2000;41:1382–1389.

91. Banzett RB, Guz A, Paydarfar D, et al. Cardiorespiratory variables and sensation during stimulation of the left vagus in patients with epilepsy. *Epilepsy Res.* 1999;35:1–11.

92. Krahl SE, Clark KB, Smith DC, et al. Locus coeruleus lesions suppress the seizure-attenuating effects of vagus nerve stimulation. *Epilepsia.* 1998;39: 709–714.

93. Walker BR, Easton A, Gale K. Regulation of limbic motor seizures by GABA and glutamate transmission in nucleus tractus solitarius. *Epilepsia.* 1999;40:1051–1057.

94. Depaulis A, Vergnes M, Liu Z, et al. Involvement of the nigral output pathways in the inhibitory control of the substantia nigra over generalized non-convulsive seizures in the rat. *Neuroscience.* 1990;39:339–349.

95. Miller JW. The role of mesencephalic and thalamic arousal systems in experimental seizures. *Prog Neurobiol.* 1992;39:155–178.

96. Magdaleno-Madrigal VM, Valdes-Cruz A, Martinez-Vargas D, et al. Effect of electrical stimulation of the nucleus of the solitary tract on the development of electrical amygdaloid kindling in the cat. *Epilepsia.* 2002;43:964–969.

97. Naritoku DK, Terry WJ, Helfert RH. Regional induction of fos immunoreactivity in the brain by anticonvulsant stimulation of the vagus nerve. *Epilepsy Res.* 1995;22:53–62.

98. Fernandez-Guardiola A, Martinez A, Valdes-Cruz A, et al. Vagus nerve prolonged stimulation in cats: effects on epileptogenesis (amygdala electrical kindling): behavioral and electrographic changes. *Epilepsia.* 1999;40: 822–829.

99. Salinsky MC, Burchiel KJ. Vagus nerve stimulation has no effect on awake EEG rhythms in humans. *Epilepsia.* 1993;34:299–304.

100. Hammond EJ, Uthman BM, Reid SA. Electrophysiological studies of cervical vagus nerve stimulation in humans: I. EEG effects. *Epilepsia.* 1992;33:1013–1020.

101. Hammond EJ, Uthman BM, Reid SA, et al. Vagus nerve stimulation in humans: neurophysiological studies and electrophysiological monitoring. *Epilepsia.* 1990;31(suppl 2):S51–S59.

102. Kuba R, Guzaninova M, Brazdil M, et al. Effect of vagal nerve stimulation on interictal epileptiform discharges: a scalp EEG study. *Epilepsia.* 2002;43:1181–1188.
103. Olejniczak PW, Fisch BJ, Carey M, et al. The effect of vagus nerve stimulation on epileptiform activity recorded from hippocampal depth electrodes. *Epilepsia.* 2001;42:423–429.
104. Koo B. EEG changes with vagus nerve stimulation. *J Clin Neurophysiol.* 2001;18:434–441.
105. Hammond EJ, Uthman BM, Wilder BJ, et al. Neurochemical effects of vagus nerve stimulation in humans. *Brain Res.* 1992;583:300–303.
106. Ben-Menachem E, Hamberger A, Hedner T, et al. Effects of vagus nerve stimulation on amino acids and other metabolites in the CSF of patients with partial seizures. *Epilepsy Res.* 1995;20:221–227.
107. Ko D, Heck C, Grafton S, et al. Vagus nerve stimulation activates central nervous system structures in epileptic patients during PET H2(15)O blood flow imaging. *Neurosurgery.* 1996;39:426–430; discussion 430–431.
108. Salanova V, Worth R. Neurostimulators in epilepsy. *Curr Neurol Neurosci Rep.* 2007;7:315–319.
109. Krauss GL, Koubeissi MZ. Cerebellar and thalamic stimulation treatment for epilepsy. *Acta Neurochir Suppl.* 2007; 97:347–356.
110. Henry TR, Bakay RA, Votaw JR, et al. Brain blood flow alterations induced by therapeutic vagus nerve stimulation in partial epilepsy: I. Acute effects at high and low levels of stimulation. *Epilepsia.* 1998;39:983–990.
111. Henry TR, Votaw JR, Pennell PB, et al. Acute blood flow changes and efficacy of vagus nerve stimulation in partial epilepsy. *Neurology.* 1999; 52:1166–1173.
112. Henry TR, Votaw JR, Bakay RAE, et al. Vagus nerve stimulation-induced cerebral blood flow changes differ in acute and chornic therapy of complex partial seizures. *Epilepsia.* 1998;39:92.
113. Sucholeiki R, Alsaadi TM, Morris GL 3rd, et al. fMRI in patients implanted with a vagal nerve stimulator. *Seizure.* 2002;11:157–162.
114. Narayanan JT, Watts R, Haddad N, et al. Cerebral activation during vagus nerve stimulation: a functional MR study. *Epilepsia.* 2002;43:1509–1514.
115. Labar DR. Antiepileptic drug use during the first 12 months of vagus nerve stimulation therapy: a registry study. *Neurology.* 2002;59(suppl 4): S38–S43.
116. Van Ness PC. Surgical outcome for neocortical (extrahippocampal) focal epilepsy. In: Luders HO, ed. *Epilepsy Surgery.* New York, NY: Raven Press; 1992:613–624.
117. Sperling MR, O'Connor MF, Saykin AJ, et al. Temporal lobectomy for refractory epilepsy. *JAMA.* 1996;276:470–475.
118. Fisher RS, Handforth A. Reassessment: vagus nerve stimulation for epilepsy: a report of the Therapeutics and Technology Assessment Subcommittee of the American Academy of Neurology. *Neurology.* 1999;53:666–669.
119. Baumgartner JE, Clifton GL, Wheless JW, et al. Corpus callosotomy. *Tech Neurosurg.* 1995;1:45–51.
120. Sorenson JM, Wheless JW, Baumgartner JE, et al. Corpus callosotomy for medically intractable seizures. *Pediatr Neurosurg.* 1997;27:260–267.
121. Camfield PR, Camfield CS. Vagal nerve stimulation for treatment of children with epilepsy. *J Pediatr.* 1999;134:532–533.
122. Schwartz TH, Spencer DD. Strategies for reoperation after comprehensive epilepsy surgery. *J Neurosurg.* 2001;95:615–623.
123. Amar AP, Apuzzo ML, Liu CY. Vagus nerve stimulation therapy after failed cranial surgery for intractable epilepsy: results from the vagus nerve stimulation therapy patient outcome registry. *Neurosurgery.* 2004;55: 1086–1093.
124. Scherrmann J, Hoppe C, Kral T, et al. Vagus nerve stimulation: clinical experience in a large patient series. *J Clin Neurophysiol.* 2001;18:408–414.
125. Helmers SL, Griesemer DA, Dean JC, et al. Observations on the use of vagus nerve stimulation earlier in the course of pharmacoresistant epilepsy: patients with seizures for six years or less. *Neurologist.* 2003;9:160–164.
126. Malow BA, Edwards J, Marzec M, et al. Effects of vagus nerve stimulation on respiration during sleep: a pilot study. *Neurology.* 2000;55:1450–1454.
127. Hsieh T, Chen M, McAfee A, et al. Sleep-related breathing disorder in children with vagal nerve stimulators. *Pediatr Neurol.* 2008;38:99–103.
128. Hallbook T, Lundgren J, Kohler S, et al. Beneficial effects on sleep of vagus nerve stimulation in children with therapy resistant epilepsy. *Eur J Paediatr Neurol.* 2005;9:399–407.
129. Kotagal P, Yardi N. The relationship between sleep and epilepsy. *Semin Pediatr Neurol.* 2008;15:42–49.
130. Bernard EJ, Passannante AN, Mann B, et al. Insertion of vagal nerve stimulator using local and regional anesthesia. *Surg Neurol.* 2002;57:94–98.
131. Reid SA. Surgical technique for implantation of the neurocybernetic prosthesis. *Epilepsia.* 1990;31(suppl 2):S38–S39.
132. Amar AP, Heck CN, Levy ML, et al. An institutional experience with cervical vagus nerve trunk stimulation for medically refractory epilepsy: rationale, technique, and outcome. *Neurosurgery.* 1998;43:1265–1276; discussion 1276–1280.
133. Tatum WO 4th, Moore DB, Stecker MM, et al. Ventricular asystole during vagus nerve stimulation for epilepsy in humans. *Neurology.* 1999;52: 1267–1269.
134. Asconape JJ, Moore DD, Zipes DP, et al. Early experience with vagus nerve stimulation for the treatment of epilepsy: cardiac complications. *Epilepsia.* 1998;39:193.
135. Ardesch JJ, Buschman HP, van der Burgh PH, et al. Cardiac responses of vagus nerve stimulation: intraoperative bradycardia and subsequent chronic stimulation. *Clin Neurol Neurosurg.* 2007;109:849–852.
136. Vaughn BV, Bernard E, Lannon S, et al. Intraoperative methods for confirmation of correct placement of the vagus nerve stimulator. *Epileptic Disord.* 2001;3:75–78.
137. Agnew WF, McCreery DB. Considerations for safety with chronically implanted nerve electrodes. *Epilepsia.* 1990;31(suppl 2):S27–S32.
138. Agnew WF, McCreery DB, Yuen TG, et al. Histologic and physiologic evaluation of electrically stimulated peripheral nerve: considerations for the selection of parameters. *Ann Biomed Eng.* 1989;17:39–60.
139. Murphy JV, Hornig GW, Schallert GS, et al. Adverse events in children receiving intermittent left vagal nerve stimulation. *Pediatr Neurol.* 1998; 19:42–44.
140. Landy HJ, Ramsay RE, Slater J, et al. Vagus nerve stimulation for complex partial seizures: surgical technique, safety, and efficacy. *J Neurosurg.* 1993;78:26–31.
141. Terry RS, Tarver WB, Zabara J. The implantable neurocybernetic prosthesis system. *Pacing Clin Electrophysiol.* 1991;14:86–93.
142. Terry R, Tarver WB, Zabara J. An implantable neurocybernetic prosthesis system. *Epilepsia.* 1990;31(suppl 2):S33–S37.
143. Ortler M, Luef G, Kofler A, et al. Deep wound infection after vagus nerve stimulator implantation: treatment without removal of the device. *Epilepsia.* 2001;42:133–135.
144. Fernando DA, Lord RS. The blood supply of vagus nerve in the human: its implication in carotid endarterectomy, thyroidectomy and carotid arch aneurectomy. *Anat Anz.* 1994;176:333–337.
145. Ramsay RE, Uthman BM, Augustinson LE, et al. Vagus nerve stimulation for treatment of partial seizures: 2. Safety, side effects, and tolerability. First International Vagus Nerve Stimulation Study Group. *Epilepsia.* 1994;35:627–636.
146. Liporace J, Hucko D, Morrow R, et al. Vagal nerve stimulation: adjustments to reduce painful side effects. *Neurology.* 2001;57:885–886.
147. Lotvall J, Lunde H, Augustinson LE, et al. Airway effects of direct left-sided cervical vagal stimulation in patients with complex partial seizures. *Epilepsy Res.* 1994;18:149–154.
148. Setty AB, Vaughn BV, Quint SR, et al. Heart period variability during vagal nerve stimulation. *Seizure.* 1998;7:213–217.
149. Annegers JF, Coan SP, Hauser WA, et al. Epilepsy, vagal nerve stimulation by the NCP system, all-cause mortality, and sudden, unexpected, unexplained death. *Epilepsia.* 2000;41:549–553.
150. Annegers JF, Coan SP, Hauser WA, et al. Epilepsy, vagal nerve stimulation by the NCP system, mortality, and sudden, unexpected, unexplained death. *Epilepsia.* 1998;39:206–212.
151. Sanossian N, Haut S. Chronic diarrhea associated with vagal nerve stimulation. *Neurology.* 2002;58:330.
152. Iriarte J, Artieda J, Alegre M, et al. Spasm of the sternocleidomastoid muscle induced by vagal nerve stimulation. *Neurology.* 2001;57: 2319–2320.
153. Leijten FS, Van Rijen PC. Stimulation of the phrenic nerve as a complication of vagus nerve pacing in a patient with epilepsy. *Neurology.* 1998; 51:1224–1225.
154. Duhaime AC, Melamed S, Clancy RR. Tonsillar pain mimicking glossopharyngeal neuralgia as a complication of vagus nerve stimulation: case report. *Epilepsia.* 2000;41:903–905.
155. Blumer D, Davies K, Alexander A, et al. Major psychiatric disorders subsequent to treating epilepsy by vagus nerve stimulation. *Epilepsy Behav.* 2001;2:466–472.
156. Klein P, Jean-Baptiste M, Thompson JL, et al. A case report of hypomania following vagus nerve stimulation for refractory epilepsy. *J Clin Psychiatry.* 2003;64:485.
157. Pearl PL, Conry JA, Yaun A, et al. Misidentification of vagus nerve stimulator for intravenous access and other major adverse events. *Pediatr Neurol.* 2008;38:248–251.
158. Schallert G, Foster J, Lindquist N, et al. Chronic stimulation of the left vagal nerve in children: effect on swallowing. *Epilepsia.* 1998;39: 1113–1114.
159. Lundgren J, Ekberg O, Olsson R. Aspiration: a potential complication to vagus nerve stimulation. *Epilepsia.* 1998;39:998–1000.
160. Ben-Menachem E. Vagus-nerve stimulation for the treatment of epilepsy. *Lancet Neurol.* 2002;1:477–482.
161. Hoppe C, Helmstaedter C, Scherrmann J, et al. No evidence for cognitive side effects after 6 months of vagus nerve stimulation in epilepsy patients. *Epilepsy Behav.* 2001;2:351–356.
162. Clarke BM, Upton AR, Griffin H, et al. Chronic stimulation of the left vagus nerve in epilepsy: balance effects. *Can J Neurol Sci.* 1997;24: 230–234.
163. Clarke BM, Upton AR, Griffin H, et al. Chronic stimulation of the left vagus nerve: cognitive motor effects. *Can J Neurol Sci.* 1997;24:226–229.
164. Harden CL. Mood changes in patients treated with vagus nerve stimulation. *Epilepsy Behav.* 2001;2:S17–S20.
165. Clark KB, Naritoku DK, Smith DC, et al. Enhanced recognition memory following vagus nerve stimulation in human subjects. *Nat Neurosci.* 1999;2:94–98.

166. Ghacibeh GA, Shenker JI, Shenal B, et al. The influence of vagus nerve stimulation on memory. *Cogn Behav Neurol.* 2006;19:119–122.

167. Cramer JA. Exploration of changes in health-related quality of life after 3 months of vagus nerve stimulation. *Epilepsy Behav.* 2001;2:460–465.

168. Malow BA, Edwards J, Marzec M, et al. Vagus nerve stimulation reduces daytime sleepiness in epilepsy patients. *Neurology.* 2001;57:879–884.

169. Galli R, Bonanni E, Pizzanelli C, et al. Daytime vigilance and quality of life in epileptic patients treated with vagus nerve stimulation. *Epilepsy Behav.* 2003;4:185–191.

170. Husain MM, Stegman D, Trevino K. Pregnancy and delivery while receiving vagus nerve stimulation for the treatment of major depression: a case report. *Ann Gen Psychiatry.* 2005;4:16.

171. Graves N. Anticonvulsants: choices and costs. *Am J Manag Care.* 1998; 49:S463–S474.

172. Boon P, D'Have M, Van Walleghem P, et al. Direct medical costs of refractory epilepsy incurred by three different treatment modalities: a prospective assessment. *Epilepsia.* 2002;43:96–102.

173. Ben-Menachem E, Hellstrom K, Verstappen D. Analysis of direct hospital costs before and 18 months after treatment with vagus nerve stimulation therapy in 43 patients. *Neurology.* 2002;59(6 suppl 4):S44–S47.

174. Bernstein AL, Barkan H, Hess T. Vagus nerve stimulation therapy for pharmacoresistant epilepsy: effect on health care utilization. *Epilepsy Behav.* 2007;10:134–137.

175. Benbadis SR, Nyhenhuis J, Tatum WO 4th, et al. MRI of the brain is safe in patients implanted with the vagus nerve stimulator. *Seizure.* 2001; 10:512–515.

176. Wilfong AA. Body MRI and vagus nerve stimulation. *Epilepsia.* 2002; 43(suppl 7):347.

CHAPTER 71 ■ ISSUES OF MEDICAL INTRACTABILITY FOR SURGICAL CANDIDACY

PATRICK KWAN AND MARTIN J. BRODIE

Although the concept of medically intractable (often used interchangeably with "medically refractory," "drug resistant," or "pharmacoresistant") epilepsy may appear self-explanatory and intuitive, a precise definition has remained elusive (1,2). This has resulted in diverse criteria used by different clinicians and researchers, or even a lack of explicit criteria in some cases, rendering it difficult to compare findings across studies and to make recommendation for clinical practice (3). Adopting a common definition of medical intractability is of particular relevance to selecting patients for epilepsy surgery because one of the prerequisites for epilepsy surgery is demonstrated "medical intractability" (4). This chapter explores the issues surrounding the definition of intractable epilepsy, with particular reference to its relevance to selection of surgical candidacy.

RULING OUT PSEUDORESISTANCE

The term "pseudoresistance" has been introduced to describe the condition in which seizures persist because the disorder has not been adequately or appropriately treated (1). It may arise in a number of situations, and must be excluded or corrected before antiepileptic drug (AED) treatment can be declared as having failed.

Incorrect Diagnosis

If a patient does not have epilepsy, AED therapy is unlikely to be helpful. A wide range of conditions can mimic epileptic seizures and must be considered in the differential diagnosis. Syncopal attacks, during which there may be clonic movements and incontinence, are commonly misdiagnosed as epileptic seizures (5). Pseudoseizures or nonepileptic psychogenic seizures are estimated to account for 10% to 45% of patients with apparently refractory epilepsy (6). Diagnosis can be challenging, as nonepileptic attacks often coexist with epilepsy or may develop as a substitute for seizures once the epilepsy is controlled (7). Mistaking other conditions for epilepsy can lead to unnecessary and potentially harmful treatments and delays in initiating appropriate therapy.

Incorrect Drug Choice or Inadequate Dosage

Incorrect classification of syndrome/seizure type is another common cause of drug failure. The profile of activity against different seizure types varies among the AEDs (8). AEDs may be inappropriately chosen for a particular seizure type, resulting in increase in seizure frequency and/or severity, presumably due to adverse pharmacodynamic interactions between the mode of action of the specific drug and the pathogenetic mechanisms underlying the specific seizure type. The idiopathic generalized epilepsies seem to be more vulnerable to aggravation by inappropriately chosen AEDs compared with focal epilepsies. For instance, phenytoin and carbamazepine are well documented to aggravate generalized seizures, including typical and atypical absence seizures, myoclonic and atonic seizures in a substantial proportion of patients (9). It is not uncommon at an initial clinic visit to be uncertain whether a young patient is reporting generalized absence or short-lived complex partial seizures, resulting in inappropriate drug choice.

In some circumstances, failure of an AED is not due to an incorrect drug choice for a particular seizure type(s), but rather because the agent is not prescribed at optimal dosage. Because of genetic and environmental factors, wide interindividual variability exists in the dosages at which beneficial and toxic effects are observed (10). Patients are often switched to an alternative treatment before the maximum tolerated dose of their current AED is reached, resulting in persistent seizures that could have been controlled at higher dosages. One of the reasons for failure to optimize the dose in an individual patient is injudicious reliance on monitoring serum drug concentration, including a "therapeutic range" that can be interpreted as dictating dosage adjustment without adequate clinical correlation. Although "therapeutic" or "target" ranges are often quoted for established AEDs in standard textbooks (11), these should only be used as an aid in dosage adjustment. The treating clinician must realize that some patients will do well below the lower limit of the range, whereas others will tolerate higher levels with benefits and without toxicity. In a study of 74 consecutive patients referred for epilepsy surgery for presumed drug resistance, a systematic protocol to titrate their AED to the maximally tolerated dose, regardless of serum levels, resulted in a greater than 80% reduction in seizure frequency and cancellation of planned surgery in seven patients (9.5%) (12). An individualized approach must, therefore, be adopted when titrating an AED to the maximally tolerated dose before being declared a failure.

Imperfect Medication Adherence or Inappropriate Lifestyle

As with other chronic medical conditions, imperfect adherence to the therapeutic regimen is one of the most common factors resulting in treatment failure. AED nonadherence is the most frequently identified etiology for status epilepticus in adults (13) and has been suggested to contribute to increased morbidity and mortality (14). The reasons for medication nonadherence are multifactorial, including socioeconomic, racial, and family factors (15). A survey of 232 adolescents identified support from the treating physician as the most powerful predictor of adherence with treatment regimens (16). Adherence to treatment may also be improved by simplifying the dosing regimen. Cramer and colleagues found that medication adherence rates in patients with epilepsy decreased as the frequency of drug administration increased, from 89% with once-daily dosing to 81% with twice-daily drug administration, 77% with 3-times-daily administration, dropping to only 39% with 4-times-daily administration (17).

Abuse of alcohol and recreational drugs can cause seizures and nonadherence to AED treatment. Similarly, sleep deprivation and stress are common precipitants. Social and lifestyle factors should, therefore, be considered when evaluating the efficacy of pharmacologic treatment.

INTENDED CONTEXT OF DEFINITION

Before the criteria for defining medical intractability are discussed, it should be emphasized that, by default, intractability is a relative concept rather than an absolute designation, which is influenced by the context in which it is intended to apply. This may include selection of patients for epilepsy surgery, recruitment in experimental drug trials, and identification for inclusion in epidemiologic studies. Because of these varying purposes, any core definition may need to be adapted in different settings. For instance, because industry-sponsored regulatory add-on trials of experimental agents are typically of relatively short duration, the definition of refractory epilepsy for enrollment purposes usually requires high baseline monthly seizure frequency in order to achieve adequate statistical power with minimum sample size (18). In epidemiologic studies, the definition of medical intractability should reflect the outcome of epilepsy in response to treatment—that is, the likelihood of success or failure with successive AED regimens. This requires an understanding of the natural history of treated and untreated epilepsy, which remains poorly documented (19).

The relativity of any definition of medical intractability is particularly poignant in the context of candidacy for potentially "curative" resective epilepsy surgery. Aided by technical advances in neuroimaging and video electroencephalographic (EEG) monitoring, improvements in technique, and a better understanding of the anatomic and pathophysiologic bases of the epilepsies, resective surgery has become a highly effective and safe treatment modality for certain remediable syndromes, the prototype of which is mesial temporal lobe epilepsy (20). With a reported postsurgery seizure-free rate of 60% to 70% from centers across the world, mortality close to zero, and permanent neurologic morbidity less than 5%, anterior temporal lobectomy has made mesial temporal lobe epilepsy, an often medically intractable condition, highly surgically treatable in appropriately selected patients (21). A clinically relevant, pragmatic definition of drug resistance for patients with this epilepsy syndrome must, therefore, take into account the potential success of surgical treatment. Indeed, since the effectiveness of surgery may vary for different types

of epilepsy, syndrome-specific predictive models may be required (22). Such definitions will have to be updated periodically, with the availability of new AEDs and improvement in surgical techniques and outcomes.

ELEMENTS OF THE DEFINITION

Bearing in mind the aforementioned considerations, a discussion of the criteria used to define medical intractability, with particular reference to epilepsy surgery, will follow. Although the definitions of medical intractability found in the medical literature seem to be highly variable (Table 71.1), three key elements are incorporated: number of AEDs failed, frequency of seizures, and duration of persisting seizures (23–34).

Number of Drugs Failed

An implicit assumption in any definition of medical intractability is that remission will not or is very unlikely to be attained with further manipulation of AED treatment. Therefore, the most important element in defining medical intractability is the number of AEDs failed at optimal dosage. Any definition must be based on an assessment of the probability of subsequent remission after each drug failure. Until recently, clinicians have had a relatively limited therapeutic armamentarium with which to treat epilepsy. With the global approval of at least 13 new AEDs in the past two decades, the choice has been substantially widened and the number of possible combinations is now almost limitless. No patient will be able to try all AED regimens. Therefore, to designate a patient's epilepsy as medically intractable, a number of questions need to be answered: How many trials of single AEDs should be used before a patient is treated with polytherapy? How many AEDs, either singly or in combination (and in how many combinations), have to fail before a seizure disorder can be recognized as medically refractory and surgery considered? At what stage does epilepsy become pharmacoresistant to AED treatment? Are there clinical features that will allow prediction of subsequent refractoriness? Answers to these questions depend on an understanding of the outcome of treated epilepsy, in particular its progress in response to treatment.

In a Veterans Affairs study, among the 82 patients who received polytherapy after failure of the first drug, only 9 (11%) became seizure free (35). In a relatively small cohort of 59 adult patients with chronic epilepsy poorly controlled on monotherapy, Schmidt and Richter (36) reported that substitution of another agent resulted in remission in only 12%.

The relationship between outcome and course of AED treatment has been specifically addressed in an ongoing, long-term study of patients with newly diagnosed epilepsy, conducted in Glasgow, Scotland, since 1982. In the first analysis reported in 2000, 525 unselected adolescent and adult patients (median age at onset, 26 years) were given a diagnosis of epilepsy, commenced on AED therapy, and followed for up to 16 years, with a median of 5 years (31). Among the 470 patients who had never before received AED treatment, 64% entered remission for at least 1 year. Forty-seven percent of patients became seizure free on their first drug, 13% on the second drug, but only 4% on the third drug or a combination of two drugs. Among those who became seizure free on their

TABLE 71.1

SELECTED DEFINITIONS OF MEDICALLY INTRACTABLE EPILEPSY FROM MEDICAL LITERATURE

Reference	Type of study	Definition
23	Epidemiology	One or more seizure per month for a period of at least 2 years, treated with at least three AEDs either singly or in combination
24	Epidemiology	Failure of two AEDs for seizure control or failure of one AED for seizure control and two others for intolerable side effects, with at least one seizure per month over an 18-month period
25	Surgery	20 complex partial seizures during the 24 months preceding surgical evaluation and a history of failure of two first-line AEDs
26	Epidemiology	One or more seizures every 2 months during the first 5 years of treatment or at least one seizure per year for longer treatment duration
27	Epidemiology	One or more seizures per month during the final 12 months of follow-up despite history of treatment with three or more AEDs
28	Phase 3 drug trial	At least 12 seizures within 12 weeks despite the use of at least two AEDs simultaneously or consecutively
29	Epidemiology (temporal lobe epilepsy)	Persistence of any seizures involving impairment of consciousness between 18 and 24 months after epilepsy onset despite at least two maximally tolerated AED trials
30	Epidemiology	One or more seizures per month for at least 2 years despite appropriate anticonvulsant agents at maximum tolerated blood levels
31	Epidemiology	Failure of two AEDs due to lack of efficacy, with one or more seizures over the past year
32	Epidemiology	At least one seizure per year during the last 10 years of observation
33	Phase 3 drug trial	An average of at least four seizures per month for 3 months prior to enrollment while taking one or two AEDs
34	Surgery	At least one seizure per month on average during the preceding year despite the use of two or more AEDs, one of which was phenytoin, carbamazepine, or valproic acid

AED, antiepileptic drug.

first drug, greater than 90% did so at moderate daily dosing (≤800 mg carbamazepine, ≤1500 mg sodium valproate, ≤300 mg lamotrigine) (37). Response to the first AED was the most powerful predictor of prognosis. Among the 248 patients in whom treatment with the first agent was unsuccessful, only 79 (32%) subsequently became seizure free, with worse prognosis for those failing due to lack of efficacy than those due to adverse effects.

Similar results were obtained in the analysis of the expanded cohort of 780 newly diagnosed patients, 47% of whom became seizure free with the first monotherapy. Another 10% responded to the second monotherapy. Only 2.3% became seizure free with the third monotherapy or with polytherapy (38,39). These observations suggest that when two appropriately chosen AEDs have failed, the chance of success with further agents becomes progressively less (Fig. 71.1) (40).

There is emerging evidence that the introduction of the newer AEDs have produced a modest improvement in the prognosis of adult epilepsy (41,42). Our ongoing analysis of outcomes in newly diagnosed epilepsy supports this observation. In our expanding population of patients starting treatment with their first AED at the Epilepsy Unit in Glasgow, outcomes have improved over the past 5 years with overall seizure-free rates increasing from 64% in 1997 ($N = 470$) (31), to 64.4% in 2005 ($N = 780$) (39), and most recently to 68.3% ($N = 1098$; unpublished data). More patients from the original cohorts are now seizure free with the introduction of a range of newer drugs (Fig. 71.2). Of these 1098 patients, epilepsy was controlled on more than one AED in only 70 with the vast majority ($N = 67$) receiving two AEDs. Only two patients remained seizure free on three AEDs, with just one person taking four drugs. Because of the broader range of pharmacologic

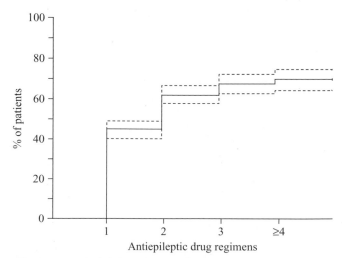

FIGURE 71.1 Probability of seizure freedom in patients with newly diagnosed epilepsy, according to the number of antiepileptic drug regimens. Dotted lines represent 95% confidence intervals. (From Brodie MJ, Kwan P. Staged approach to epilepsy management. *Neurology.* 2002;58(suppl 5):S2–S8, with permission).

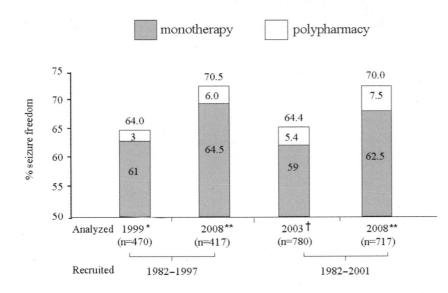

FIGURE 71.2 Percentage of patients with newly diagnosed epilepsy seizure free for at least the previous year in an expanding cohort analyzed at different time points. Numbers within bars represent percentage of patients seizure free on monotherapy (gray bars) or polypharmacy (open bars). Numbers on top of bars represent total percentage of patients seizure free. *Data from Ref. 31. †Data from Ref. 39. **Unpublished data.

options, a number of patients have been controlled with their third, fourth, and even fifth regimen (Table 71.2, unpublished data). Similar observations have also been made recently by Schiller and Najjar (43).

Existing data on pediatric epilepsy are encouraging and enable us to predict medical intractability early in the disease course. Camfield and colleagues (27) conducted an elegant population-based study that included 417 children (seizure onset between 1 month and 16 years), with an average follow-up of 8 years. Of the participants, 83% of the children received only one AED in the first year of treatment, which rendered 61% seizure free. These patients did not require AEDs at the end of their follow-up—that is, they achieved remission. Only 4% of the children receiving a single AED during the first year went on to develop intractable epilepsy. Of those patients (17%) who had inadequate seizure control with the first AED, only 42% achieved complete remission of their epilepsy, whereas 29% developed intractable epilepsy. However, the authors did not specify the number of successive AEDs tried in these children. In another retrospective analysis of 120 patients aged 1 to 18 years with recent-onset temporal lobe epilepsy, the only identified predictor of intractability at 2 years was failure of the first AED trial (29).

Seizure Frequency

There is no universal agreement as to how frequent and over what period of time seizures must be occurring to constitute intractability. Seizure frequency used by different authors in defining intractability ranges from one per month to one per year (see Table 71.1). However, studies including patients treated surgically (44–47) and medically (48) suggest that absolute seizure freedom is the only relevant outcome consistently associated with improvement in quality of life. In a community-based survey, patients with one or more seizures over the past 2 years had higher levels of anxiety and depression, greater perceived stigma and impact of epilepsy, and lower employment rates than did those in remission (49). In many countries, having even one seizure per year poses restrictions on driving (50,51). It may, therefore, be argued that in terms of the effect on psychosocial functioning, a patient's epilepsy may be considered intractable when one or more seizures per year are occurring (31). Because presurgical evaluation and surgery itself may entail risks, higher seizure frequency is often required for selection of surgical candidates (see Table 71.1). The impact of the seizures on a patient's

TABLE 71.2

RESPONDERSa (%) ACCORDING TO REGIMEN IN A POPULATION OF ADOLESCENT AND ADULT PATIENTS WITH NEWLY DIAGNOSED EPILEPSY

	Number of patients treated	Percentage responded to monotherapy	Percentage responded to polytherapy	Total percentage responded
First AED regimen	1098	49.5	0	49.5
Second AED regimen	398	25.4	11.3	36.7
Third AED regimen	168	15.5	8.9	24.4
Fourth AED regimen	68	8.8	7.4	16.2
Other AED regimens	46	6.5	10.8	17.3

AED, antiepileptic drug.
[a]Responders are seizure free for at least the previous year on the same antiepileptic drug regimen at unchanged dosage.

lifestyle and the likely outcome of surgical treatment must be taken into consideration.

Duration of Persistent Seizures and Time-Dependent Course

Even when the criteria for number of drugs failed and seizure frequency are fulfilled, it is unclear how long should recurrent seizures persist before the patient's epilepsy can be declared medically intractable and alternative therapies, such as surgery, considered. This question relates to the possibility of patients "switching" from one drug response status to the other over time, and in particular, whether a patient fulfilling the criteria of having medically intractable epilepsy will become drug responsive later with/without further drug manipulation. The critical issue would be how much longer such an individual should wait before surgery is considered.

Several recent studies have specifically addressed the outcome of patients with chronic epilepsy who have failed one or two AEDs. In an observational study of 155 adults who had previously failed one or more AEDs, 23% became seizure free for 12 months or more after further drug trials, although it took up to six trials for some (41). Observations from other cohorts of adult patients who had failed at least two AEDs previously suggest that subsequent seizure freedom occurs with further drug manipulation in approximately 4% to 5% per year (42,52), but with a probability of seizure relapse of 44% within 3 years (52). These data suggest that in patients who have failed two or more AEDs, seizure freedom may still be attained in a small proportion, but it may involve repeated drug manipulations over considerable time, and may often be temporary.

On the other hand, some patients become medically intractable after a period of seizure freedom. In the analysis of the Glasgow database including 780 adult patients with newly diagnosed epilepsy, 276 (35.4%) never obtained adequate control of seizures for any 1-year period during follow-up, suggesting a refractory course at the outset for such patients. However, among 504 patients who became seizure free initially for at least 1 year, seizures relapsed in 105 (21%), although seizure control was later regained in the majority (63 patients) (39).

Such a fluctuating or remitting–relapsing course might be particularly common in childhood onset epilepsy. In an observational study of 144 children with epilepsy onset in the 1960s and followed over an average of 37 years, delayed remission was observed in 50% of children and seizure relapse occurred after initial remission in 33% (53). Unfortunately the relationship with drug treatment was not detailed in the report. In a prospective cohort of 613 children, more than half with delayed intractability (defined as more than 3 years after initial diagnosis) had previously been in remission for at least 1 year, and of the 83 children with intractable epilepsy initially, 13% were in remission when last contacted (54). In an updated analysis of the 140 children who had failed trials of at least 2 different AEDs considered appropriate for their seizures and type of epilepsy, some experienced repeated remissions and relapses, and only a small proportion became seizure free for each of the additional drugs tried (55).

These observations imply that drug responsiveness in some patients can be regarded as a dynamic process rather than a permanent state. Instead of being constant, the course of epilepsy sometimes fluctuates, and apparent changes in responsiveness to AED treatment may merely represent shifts in the pathophysiology of the underlying disorder. Indeed, it is likely that treatment outcome is highly dependent upon the underlying epilepsy syndromes. A notable example is mesial temporal lobe epilepsy associated with hippocampal sclerosis, for which accumulating evidence suggests a progressive course in some patients (56) but not in others (57). In a retrospective survey of 333 patients who underwent resective surgery for medically refractory epilepsy (88% of whom had anterior temporal lobectomy), the average time to failure of two first-line AEDs was 9.1 years (median, 5 years). Of 284 patients from the cohort, 26% recalled a previous period of at least 1 year of seizure freedom since the onset of their epilepsy (25). This suggests that for some patients with temporal lobe epilepsy, medical intractability may not declare itself in the early stages of the disorder. Indeed, an initial apparently benign course seems to be one of the characteristics of this condition (58), but how often such a pattern is observed can only be accurately determined in a prospective study in which all patients with temporal lobe epilepsy are followed from the point of presentation with seizures. In the Glasgow cohort, newly diagnosed patients with underlying hippocampal sclerosis differed little in outcome from those with other localization-related epilepsies (38). Clearly, since epilepsy is not a single disease, syndrome and etiology-specific prospective prognostic studies are needed if individual patients are to be managed more appropriately.

Operational Definition

A pragmatic, unambiguous operational definition of medical intractability constituting the essential elements discussed above is needed in order to apply treatment rationally. Summarizing the available data, extensive evidence now exists that, once a patient has failed trials with two appropriate AEDs, the probability of achieving seizure freedom with subsequent AED treatments is low. After wrestling with the challenge of defining medical intractability a task force of the International League Against Epilepsy has recently proposed the following definition: "Failure of adequate trials of two tolerated and appropriately used AED regimens whether as monotherapy or in combination to achieve sustained seizure freedom" (59). The definition requires that the medication is failed despite being used at its clinically effective dose, that is, treatment failure is due to lack of efficacy instead of other reasons, such as an idiosyncratic reaction, and that the seizure-free period should be at least 1 year or 3 times the pre-treatment inter-seizure interval, whichever is longer. Fulfillment of the operational definition of medical intractability should prompt a comprehensive review of the diagnosis and management, preferably by an epilepsy center where epilepsy surgery may be offered as a therapeutic option.

Pediatric Issues

The timing of epilepsy surgery in children is further complicated by the need to consider the potential consequences of the insults from repeated seizures and from surgical intervention on the developing brain (60). This issue is particularly notable and sensitive when evaluating infants with catastrophic localization-related epilepsies, who may have many seizures per day. A large number of AEDs might have been tried and might have failed over a relatively short period. Although controlled studies are lacking, resumption of developmental progression after early surgery has been observed. For instance, Wyllie and colleagues (61) performed various forms of epilepsy surgery in 12 children with a variety of pathologies at a mean age of 15.3 months, with all but one becoming seizure free or having at least worthwhile improvement. In addition, "catch-up" developmental progress was noted in these infants. Therefore, the decision about the timing of surgery in children is strongly affected by the severity and natural history of the specific syndrome, taking into account the potential detrimental effects of continued seizures on neural plasticity, as well as on developmental and psychosocial outcomes. In some cases of catastrophic epilepsy, surgery should be considered even earlier than 2 years of onset following thorough, individualized evaluation (62,63).

FUTURE RESEARCH DIRECTIONS

Documentation of Natural History

The development of a valid, clinically relevant definition of medical intractability requires a better understanding of the natural history of each epilepsy syndrome. To this end, there is no substitution for population-based, long-term studies following patients from the point of presentation and diagnosis (64). With an ever-expanding list of AEDs, more well-designed prospective studies are needed to document the course of epilepsy in response to treatment and to provide data on the chance of remission with each successive drug regimen, so that a practical cutoff point of number of drugs failed may be applied when labeling the epilepsy pharmacoresistant. Complicating the matter is the use of AED polytherapy, which is often instituted when monotherapy fails. Whether this would be a more effective management strategy if used earlier and in what situations remain to be determined (40).

Outcome studies should also address the fundamental question of what constitutes drug failure. For example, should it be defined objectively by persistence of seizures despite attaining a target serum drug concentration, or dosage and duration of the AED regimen? Alternatively, should it be judged according to the individual circumstances of each drug trial? Whether drug withdrawal due to intolerability should be regarded as failure in defining drug resistance has not been thoroughly explored. In the Glasgow studies, withdrawal of the first AED due to intolerability was itself a predictive factor of poorer long-term outcome, compared with withdrawal due to idiosyncratic reactions or other factors unrelated to treatment (31). However, these studies and more recent data suggest that the eventual outcome is slightly more favorable if treatment failure is due to poor tolerability rather than to lack of efficacy.

Identification of Biomarkers of Drug Response

Coupled with improved epidemiologic documentation must be a better understanding of the biologic mechanisms underpinning drug resistance. This has been a challenging task because resistance to AEDs is generally thought to reflect a complex multifactorial phenomenon to which genetic and acquired factors may contribute. It is also likely that in many patients a combination of different mechanisms contribute to therapeutic failure, which may vary widely among individuals. Research during the last two decades has focused on two different major hypotheses. The "target hypothesis" postulates that changes in the AED target site(s) (e.g., neuronal voltage-gated sodium channels) may significantly alter affinity for or efficacy at the target, thereby reducing overall drug-sensitivity (65). In addition, the drug needs to reach the target site in sufficient concentrations, which may be restricted by the blood–brain barrier (BBB). Particularly, it has been suggested that enhanced BBB efflux transport due to overexpression of multidrug transporters (e.g., P-glycoprotein) at the epileptogenic focus may limit brain penetration of AEDs (the "transporter hypothesis") (66). Although a body of experimental data supporting both hypotheses has accumulated, much work needs to be done to determine their clinical relevance, if any.

The particular relevance of understanding the mechanisms of drug resistance to defining medical intractability is that biomarkers of drug response may be identified, which may have the potential to inform clinical decision making in terms of treatment approach and defining drug resistance in a more objective fashion. Genetic polymorphisms may represent one such marker (67). The influence of genetic variation in drug metabolizing genes, in particular those encoding the cytochrome P450 enzymes, on susceptibility to drug toxicity has long been recognized (68). Overwhelming evidence from recent studies shows that carriers of HLA-B*1502 allele across broad areas of Asia have greatly increased risk of developing severe cutaneous reactions after taking carbamazepine (69). Thus, the risk of this previously idiosyncratic response can now potentially be eliminated by avoiding carbamazepine in carriers of HLA-B*1502. However, reliable genetic markers for drug efficacy remain elusive. Evidence of association between drug resistance and genetic polymorphisms of candidate genes is either conflicting (e.g., polymorphisms of the efflux multidrug transporter *ABCB1* gene [70]) or preliminary and requires confirmation (e.g., polymorphisms of the neuronal sodium channel *SCN2A* gene [71]). In addition, given the likely multifactorial causes of AED resistance, it is perhaps only realistic that any individual genetic markers found would be expected to make a small clinical impact. Nonetheless, as the complexity of genetic influence on treatment responsiveness becomes better understood, pharmacogenetic profiling of a collection of markers may, in the future, be recognized as a practical determinant of medical intractability. Likewise, identification of biologic markers for surgical outcome could potentially avoid subjecting patients deemed to have poor outcome to the risks and complications of operation.

CONCLUSIONS

A consensus is being reached that, for operational purposes, medically intractable epilepsy may be defined when two appropriately chosen, well-tolerated, first-line AEDs (whether as monotherapies or in combination) have failed due to lack of efficacy (59). In practice, this minimum, core definition may be adapted for use in different contexts for example, surgical candidacy, experimental drug trials, or epidemiologic studies. There is a need to conduct syndrome-specific prognostic studies and to identify biomarkers of drug resistance.

In a patient with apparently medically intractable epilepsy, the decision to pursue epilepsy surgery and not continue pharmacologic manipulation must be made on a case-by-case basis, taking into consideration the patient's wishes, the likely prognosis with treatment modalities, the available medical and surgical expertise, and the potential risks and benefits of resective surgery. The challenge facing the clinician is to develop individualized protocols that maximize the likelihood of successful drug therapy but also efficiently identify patients suitable for curative resective surgery.

References

1. Perucca E. Pharmacoresistance in epilepsy: how should it be defined? *CNS Drugs.* 1998;10:171–179.
2. Regesta G, Tanganelli P. Clinical aspects and biological bases of drug-resistant epilepsies. *Epilepsy Res.* 1999;34:109–122.
3. Berg AT, Kelly MM. Defining intractability: comparisons among published definitions. *Epilepsia.* 2006;47:431–436.
4. Bourgeois BFD. General concepts of medical intractability. In: Lüders HO, Comair YG, eds. *Epilepsy Surgery.* Philadelphia, PA: Lippincott Williams & Wilkins; 2001:63–68.
5. Smith D, Defalla BA, Chadwick DW. The misdiagnosis of epilepsy and the management of refractory epilepsy in a specialist clinic. *QJM.* 1999;92:15–23.
6. Devinsky O. Patients with refractory seizures. *N Engl J Med.* 1999;340:1565–1570.
7. Kuyk J, Leijten F, Meinardi H, et al. The diagnosis of psychogenic non-epileptic seizures: a review. *Seizure.* 1997;6:243–253.
8. Kwan P, Brodie MJ. Emerging drugs for epilepsy. *Expert Opin Emerg Drugs.* 2007;12:407–422.
9. Genton P, Gelisse P, Thomas P, et al. Do carbamazepine and phenytoin aggravate juvenile myoclonic epilepsy? *Neurology.* 2000;55:1106–1109.
10. Perucca E, Dulac O, Shorvon S, et al. Harnessing the clinical potential of antiepileptic drug therapy: dosage optimisation. *CNS Drugs.* 2001;15:609–621.
11. Johannessen SI, Tomson T. Laboratory monitoring of antiepileptic drugs. In: Levy RH, Mattson RH, Meldrum BS, et al., eds. *Antiepileptic Drugs,* 4th ed. Philadelphia, PA, Lippincott Williams & Wilkins; 2002:103–111.
12. Hermanns G, Noachtar S, Tuxhorn I, et al. Systematic testing of medical intractability for carbamazepine, phenytoin, and phenobarbital or primidone in monotherapy for patients considered for epilepsy surgery. *Epilepsia.* 1996;37:675–679.
13. DeLorenzo RJ, Pellock JM, Towne AR, et al. Epidemiology of status epilepticus. *J Clin Neurophysiol.* 1995;12:316–325.
14. Faught E, Duh MS, Weiner JR, et al. Nonadherence to antiepileptic drugs and increased mortality. Findings from the RANSOM Study. *Neurology.* 2008;71:1572–1578.
15. Snodgrass SR, Vedanarayanan VV, Parker CC, et al. Pediatric patients with undetectable anticonvulsant blood levels: comparison with compliant patients. *J Child Neurol.* 2001;16:164–168.
16. Kyngas H. Predictors of good compliance in adolescents with epilepsy. *Seizure.* 2001;10:549–553.
17. Cramer JA, Mattson RH, Prevey ML, et al. How often is medication taken as prescribed? A novel assessment technique. *J Am Med Assoc.* 1989;261:3273–3277.
18. Committee for Proprietary Medicinal Products. The European Agency for the Evaluation of Medicinal Products. Note for guidance on clinical investigation of medicinal products in the treatment of epileptic disorders. London, November 16, 2000.
19. Kwan P, Sander JW. The natural history of epilepsy: an epidemiological view. *J Neurol Neuro Surg Psychiatry.* 2004;75:1376–1381.
20. Spencer S, Huh L. Outcomes of epilepsy surgery in adults and children. *Lancet Neurol.* 2008;7:525–537.
21. Engel J Jr, Wiebe S, French J, et al. Practice parameter: temporal lobe and localized neocortical resections for epilepsy: report of the Quality Standards Subcommittee of the American Academy of Neurology, in Association with the American Epilepsy Society and the American Association of Neurological Surgeons. *Neurology.* 2003;60:538–547.
22. Dlugos DJ. The early identification of candidates for epilepsy surgery. *Arch Neurol.* 2001;58:1543–1546.
23. Berg AT, Levy SR, Novotny EJ, et al. Predictors of intractable epilepsy in childhood: a case-control study. *Epilepsia.* 1996;37:24–30.
24. Berg AT, Shinnar S, Levy SR, et al. Defining early seizure outcomes in pediatric epilepsy: the good, the bad and the in-between. *Epilepsy Res.* 2001;43:75–84.
25. Berg AT, Langfitt J, Shinnar S, et al. How long does it take for partial epilepsy to become intractable? *Neurology.* 2003;60:186–190.
26. Camfield PR, Camfield CS. Antiepileptic drug therapy: when is epilepsy truly intractable? *Epilepsia.* 1996;37(suppl 1):S60–S65.
27. Camfield PR, Camfield CS, Gordon K, et al. If a first antiepileptic drug fails to control a child's epilepsy, what are the chances of success with the next drug? *J Pediatr.* 1997;131:821–824.
28. Cereghino JJ, Biton V, Abou-Khalil B, et al. Levetiracetam for partial seizures: results of a double-blind, randomized clinical trial. *Neurology.* 2000;55:236–242.
29. Dlugos DJ, Sammel MD, Strom BL, et al. Response to first drug trial predicts outcome in childhood temporal lobe epilepsy. *Neurology.* 2001;57:2259–2264.
30. Huttenlocher PR, Hapke RJ. A follow-up study of intractable seizures in childhood. *Ann Neurol.* 1990;28:699–705.
31. Kwan P, Brodie MJ. Early identification of refractory epilepsy. *N Engl J Med.* 2000;342:314–319.
32. Sillanpää M. Remission of seizures and predictors of intractability in long-term follow-up. *Epilepsia.* 1993;34:930–936.
33. US Gabapentin Study Group No. 5. Gabapentin as add-on therapy in refractory partial epilepsy: a double-blind, placebo-controlled, parallel-group study. *Neurology.* 1993;43:2292–2298.
34. Wiebe S, Blume WT, Girvin JP, et al. A randomized, controlled trial of surgery for temporal-lobe epilepsy. *N Engl J Med.* 2001;345:311–318.
35. Mattson RH, Cramer JA, Collins JF, et al. Comparison of carbamazepine, phenobarbital, phenytoin, and primidone in partial and secondarily generalized tonic-clonic seizures. *N Engl J Med.* 1985;313:145–151.
36. Schmidt D, Richter K. Alternative single anticonvulsant drug therapy for refractory epilepsy. *Ann Neurol.* 1986;19:85–87.
37. Kwan P, Brodie MJ. Effectiveness of first antiepileptic drug. *Epilepsia.* 2001;42:1255–1260.
38. Mohanraj R, Brodie MJ. Pharmacological outcomes in newly diagnosed epilepsy. *Epilepsy Behav.* 2005;6:382–387.
39. Mohanraj R, Brodie MJ. Diagnosing refractory epilepsy: response to sequential treatment schedules. *Eur J Neurol.* 2006;13:277–282.
40. Brodie MJ, Kwan P. Staged approach to epilepsy management. *Neurology.* 2002;58(suppl 5):S2–S8.
41. Luciano AL, Shorvon SD. Results of treatment changes in patients with apparently drug-resistant chronic epilepsy. *Ann Neurol.* 2007;62:375–381.
42. Callaghan BC, Anand K, Hesdorffer D, et al. Likelihood of seizure remission in an adult population with refractory epilepsy. *Ann Neurol.* 2007;62:382–389.
43. Schiller Y, Najjar Y. Quantifying the response to antiepileptic drugs: Effect of past treatment history. *Neurology.* 2008;70:54–65.
44. Vickrey BG, Hays RD, Engel J Jr, et al. Outcome assessment for epilepsy surgery: the impact of measuring health-related quality of life. *Ann Neurol.* 1995;37:158–166.
45. Wheelock I, Peterson C, Buchtel HA. Presurgery expectations, postsurgery satisfaction, and psychosocial adjustment after epilepsy surgery. *Epilepsia.* 1998;39:487–494.
46. Gilliam F, Kuzniecky R, Meador K, et al. Patient-oriented outcome assessment after temporal lobectomy for refractory epilepsy. *Neurology.* 1999;53:687–694.
47. Markand ON, Salanova V, Whelihan E, et al. Health-related quality of life outcome in medically refractory epilepsy treated with anterior temporal lobectomy. *Epilepsia.* 2000;41:749–759.
48. Birbeck GL, Hays RD, Cui X, et al. Seizure reduction and quality of life improvements in people with epilepsy. *Epilepsia.* 2002;43:535–538.
49. Jacoby A, Baker GA, Steen N, et al. The clinical course of epilepsy and its psychosocial correlates: findings from a U.K. Community study. *Epilepsia.* 1996;37:148–161.
50. Fisher RS, Parsonage M, Beaussart M, et al. Epilepsy and driving: an international perspective. *Epilepsia.* 1994;35:675–684.
51. Berg AT, Engel J Jr. Restricted driving for people with epilepsy. *Neurology.* 1999;52:1306–1307.
52. Choi H, Heiman G, Pandis D, et al. Seizure remission and relapse in adults with intractable epilepsy: a cohort study. *Epilepsia.* 2008;49:1440–1445.
53. Sillanpää M, Schmidt D. Natural history of treated childhood-onset epilepsy: prospective, long-term population-based study. *Brain.* 2006;129(pt 3):617–624.
54. Berg AT, Vickrey GB. Testa FM, et al. How long does it take for epilepsy to become intractable? A prospective investigation. *Ann Neurol.* 2006;60:73–79.
55. Berg AT, Levy SR, Testa FM, et al. Remission of epilepsy after 2 drug failures in children: a prospective study. *Ann Neurol.* 2009;65:510–519.
56. Fuerst D, Shah J, Shah A, et al. Hippocampal sclerosis is a progressive disorder: a longitudinal volumetric MRI study. *Ann Neurol.* 2003;53: 413–416.
57. Kobayashi E, Lopes-Cendes I, Guerreiro CA, et al. Seizure outcome and hippocampal atrophy in familial mesial temporal lobe epilepsy. *Neurology.* 2001;56:166–172.
58. Engel J Jr. Introduction to temporal lobe epilepsy. *Epilepsy Res.* 1996;26:141–150.
59. Kwan P, Arzimanoglou A, Berg AT, et al. Definition of drug resistant epilepsy. Consensus proposal by the *ad hoc* Task Force of the ILAE Commission on Therapeutic Strategies. *Epilepsia.* 2010;51:1069–77.

60. Cross JH, Jayakar P, Nordli D, et al. Proposed criteria for referral and evaluation of children for epilepsy surgery: recommendations of the subcommission for pediatric epilepsy surgery. *Epilepsia.* 2006;47:952–959.
61. Wyllie E, Comair YG, Kotagal P, et al. Epilepsy surgery in infants. *Epilepsia.* 1996;37:625–637.
62. Wyllie E. Surgical treatment of epilepsy in children. *Pediatr Neurol.* 1998;19:179–188.
63. Cross JH. Epilepsy surgery in childhood. *Epilepsia.* 2002;43(suppl 3): 65–70.
64. Baulac M, Pitkänen A. Research priorities in epilepsy for the next decade—a representative view of the European scientific community. *Epilepsia.* 2008 Sep 20. [Epub ahead of print]
65. Remy S, Beck H. Molecular and cellular mechanisms of pharmacoresistance in epilepsy. *Brain.* 2006;129:18–35.
66. Kwan P, Brodie MJ. Potential role of drug transporters in the pathogenesis of medically intractable epilepsy. *Epilepsia.* 2005;46:224–235.
67. Goldstein DB, Tate SK, Sisodiya SM. Pharmacogenetics goes genomic. *Nat Rev Genet.* 2003;4:937–947.
68. Szoeke CEI, Newton M, Wood JM, et al. Update on pharmacogenetics in epilepsy: a brief review. *Lancet Neurol.* 2006;5:189–196.
69. Man CBL, Kwan P, Baum L, et al. Association between HLA–B*1502 allele and antiepileptic drugs-induced cutaneous reactions in Han Chinese. *Epilepsia.* 2007;48:1015–1018.
70. Kwan P, Baum L, Wong V, et al. Association between *ABCB1* C3435T polymorphism and drug resistant epilepsy in Han Chinese. *Epilepsy Behav.* 2007;11:112–117.
71. Kwan P, Poon WS, Ng HK, et al. Multidrug resistance in epilepsy and polymorphisms in the voltage-gated sodium channel genes *SCN1A, SCN2A,* and *SCN3A:* correlation among phenotype, genotype and mRNA expression. *Pharmacogenet Genomics.* 2008;18:989–998.

CHAPTER 72 ■ THE EPILEPTOGENIC ZONE

ANITA DATTA AND TOBIAS LODDENKEMPER

Approximately 30% of patients with epilepsy have refractory seizures despite antiepileptic medications (1). In many of these patients epilepsy surgery leads to significant reduction in seizure frequency and frequently to seizure freedom. The concept of cortical zones, in particular the epileptogenic zone, is an important approach in the pursuit of determining the seizure focus in the presurgical workup of epilepsy patients. Careful delineation of these zones provides guidance in epilepsy surgery planning and may lead to better outcome after epilepsy surgery with only minimal or no functional deficits. A variety of clinical data and investigations are required to delineate different structural and functional abnormalities, leading to distinct, but often overlapping zones.

THE CONCEPT OF CORTICAL ZONES: HISTORICAL PERSPECTIVE AND TECHNIQUES

Techniques to estimate the epileptogenic zone can be traced back to ancient times. Seizure symptoms have been described for more than 3000 years and these help in the delineation of the symptomatogenic zone. One of the earliest description of detailed clinical seizure semiology stems from the Sakkiku (1050 BC) depicting observations of patients with seizures (2).

In the 19th century, John Hughlings Jackson localized and lateralized a seizure focus by confirmation of structural lesions in the cortex contralateral to the motor symptoms (3) and therefore introduced the concept of the functional deficit zone and its overlap with the epileptogenic zone. This was later corroborated by cortical stimulation studies performed in animals (4). A better understanding of the epileptogenic lesion and epileptogenic zone was possible when resection of lesions lead to seizure freedom in the 1870s to 1880s (5–7).

Another advance occurred with the introduction of the electroencephalogram (EEG) by Berger in the 1920s. The irritative and ictal onset zone could now be demarcated (8,9). In the 1940s, the symptomatogenic and ictal onset zones could be observed simultaneously with video EEG (10,11). Intracranial recordings were introduced in the 1950s and increased the armentarium of methods to determine the irritative and ictal onset zones (12). In the 1960s, magnetoencephalography (MEG) further helped to determine these zones as well as the functional deficit zone (13).

Advances in technology and availability of CT and MRI scans changed the presurgical work-up dramatically by enabling improved detection of the epileptogenic lesion (14,15). Closely linked in time to the development of anatomical imaging, functional neuroimaging techniques were developed. PET and SPECT scans permitted improved localization

of the functional deficit zone and eloquent cortex (16). Additionally, further determination of the functional deficit zone was possible with advances in neuropsychological testing and Wada testing (17–20).

As the scope of our knowledge of epilepsy and experience with newer techniques increases and newer technologies become available, there will continue to be better ways to define the epileptogenic zones. A historical outline defining a historical timeline and their relation to the concept of cortical zones is shown in Table 72.1.

CONCEPT OF ZONES AND DEFINITIONS

The Epileptogenic Zone

The epileptogenic zone is the "area of cortex that is indispensable for the generation of epileptic seizures" (Fig. 72.1) (31). This region needs to be resected or disconnected for successful epilepsy surgery. It cannot be measured directly. Because of overlap between the cortical zones, the location of the epileptogenic zone can be estimated based on concordant data from several investigations that delineate the other cortical zones, including ictal onset zone, irritative zone, epileptogenic lesion, ictal symptomatogenic zone, and functional deficit zone (31–34).

The epileptogenic zone includes two components, the *actual* seizure onset zone and the *potential* seizure onset zone. The *actual* seizure onset zone is cortex from where the recorded seizures arise. The *potential* seizure onset zone is adjacent or distant cortex that does not primarily generate seizures, but may lead to seizures once the actual seizure onset zone is resected. These two components comprise the epileptogenic zone.

When discrepancy between the different zones exists, additional tests can be useful, such as high-resolution MRI, ictal SPECT, PET, or invasive monitoring. It is unknown why a structural pathologic change turns into an epileptogenic region in one patient, but not in another. Changes in neighboring cortex, biochemical and genetic influences have been postulated (34).

The Irritative Zone

The irritative zone is the region that produces interictal epileptiform discharges. This may be delineated by scalp or invasive EEG recordings, MEG, and also functional MRI (fMRI). In selected cases, source analysis of EEG or MEG signals can assist with localization. Several factors influence the irritative zone, such as type of epilepsy syndrome, state of the patient,

TABLE 72.1

HISTORICAL EVOLUTION OF THE CONCEPT OF CORTICAL ZONES

Year and scientific advance	References	Epileptogenic zone	Irritative zone	Epileptic lesion	Symptomatogenic zone	Functional deficit zone	Ictal onset zone	Eloquent areas
1050 BC: Sakkiku	2				X			
400 BC: Hippocrates seizure classification	2				X			
1860s: J.H. Jackson: semiology and localization	3				X	X		
1870: Cortical stimulation	4				X			X
1870–1880s: Lesion resection leads to seizure freedom	5	X		X				
1912: Electrical stimulation to induce seizures	21				X		X	
1929: EEG	8		X				X	
1936: Interictal spikes	22,23		X					
1940: Video-EEG	10,11		X		X		X	
1950s: Intracranial electrodes	12		X				X	X
1950s: Neuropsychological testing	18–20					X		X
1959: Wada	17					X		X
1960s: MEG	13		X				X	
1960s: SPECT	16		X				X	X
1970: PET	24		X			X		
1970s: MRI	14,15,25,26			X				
Since 1980s: Functional MRI	27–30		X					X

medications, and even temperature (35). The irritative zone does not always necessarily overlap with the epileptogenic zone (34,36,37). An example would be a patient with a right mesial occipital tumor. This patient may have interictal left occipital discharges that disappear after tumor resection.

The Epileptic Lesion

The epileptic lesion is a lesion on neuroimaging or pathology that is considered to cause the seizures. Surgical outcome may be better with complete resection of the lesion (38,39). However, in some cases, more than just a simple "lesionectomy" is required. Tumors and vascular malformations often have a perilesional epileptogenic zone that is responsible for seizure generation. In other cases, even a partial lesion resection limited by eloquent cortex may render a patient seizure-free.

Lesions are best delineated with high-resolution MRI and this can be assisted by nuclear medicine techniques, such as PET. At times, lesions can be more extensive than visible on MRI alone. In particular, malformations of cortical develop-

ment can frequently not be fully identified on MRI but are responsible for seizures. Furthermore, not all lesions are related to the seizures. For example, a patient with tuberous sclerosis may have multiple tubers. However, history and other investigations may suggest that frequently only one tuber is the epileptic lesion. Alpha-C-methyl-L-tryptophan (AMT) PET has been found particularly useful in identifying an epileptogenic tuber in tuberous sclerosis (40–42).

The Symptomatogenic Zone

The symptomatogenic zone is the eloquent area that produces the clinical symptoms when activated during an epileptic seizure. Clinical features of seizures and video-EEG recording as well as knowledge of localization of cortical anatomy and functional imaging studies can be used to lateralize or localize the seizure focus. The seizure may start in a clinically silent area and then propagate into eloquent cortical areas. Therefore, the symptomatogenic zone is frequently close to the epileptogenic zone but there may be no direct overlap.

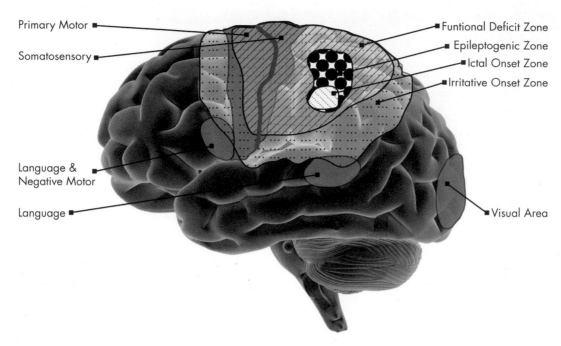

Primary Motor
Somatosensory
Language & Negative Motor
Language

Funtional Deficit Zone
Epileptogenic Zone
Ictal Onset Zone
Irritative Onset Zone
Visual Area

FIGURE 72.1 This diagram depicts an example of the cortical zones in a hypothetical epilepsy patient. The epileptogenic zone is "the area of cortex indispensable for the generation of clinical seizures" (31). Within the epileptogenic zone may be an epileptic lesion. The ictal-onset zone is a smaller region within the epileptogenic zone where seizures are generated. The irritative zone is the region that produces interictal epileptiform discharges. This is often larger than the epileptogenic zone. This is a lesion on neuroimaging or pathology that is considered to cause the seizures. The symptomatogenic zone is the eloquent area overlapping with the epileptogenic zone that produces the clinical symptoms when activated during an epileptic seizure. The functional deficit zone is the region that functions abnormally during the interictal period. The functional deficit may be related to interictal epileptiform discharges or to an underlying structural lesion. This can be large and encompass the other zones. Eloquent cortex is important for generating particular functions, including motor, sensory, language, memory, and other higher cortical functions. In this example, only some motor cortex, somatosensory cortex, visual cortex, and language areas are depicted. The goal of epilepsy surgery is to remove the epileptogenic zone, while at the same time preserving eloquent areas.

The Functional Deficit Zone

The functional deficit zone is the region that functions abnormally during the interictal period. The functional deficit may be related to interictal epileptiform discharges or to an underlying structural lesion. The functional deficit zone can be determined by neurologic exam, neuropsychological testing, EEG and MEG, evoked potentials, functional imaging, and other mapping techniques, such as fMRI, Wada testing, cortical stimulation, PET, and SPECT. It is useful if it corresponds to the other cortical zones. Sometimes, functional deficits exist distant to the epileptogenic zone as shown by areas of hypometabolism on FDG-PET distant to or beyond the epileptic lesion and epileptogenic zone (43).

The functional deficit zone may also be related to functional abnormalities, without structural abnormalities. It is known that there can be a momentary disruption of psychological function by subclinical EEG discharges that can contribute to the functional deficit zone (44,45). Janszky et al. demonstrated a relationship between the irritative zone, the functional deficit zone and eloquent cortex in patients with temporal lobe epilepsy. These authors concluded that interictal epileptiform discharges and seizure spread may influence speech reorganization (46). Binnie showed that frequent interictal spike discharges can lead to impairment during neu-

ropsychological testing (44). Patients improved after treatment with valproic acid, a spike suppressant (44).

The Ictal-Onset Zone

The ictal-onset zone is the region where seizures are generated and originate on ictal EEG. This can be estimated by scalp and invasive EEG as well as ictal SPECT and occasionally also MEG. A "secondary" ictal-onset zone is a different cortical region that is dependent on the primary ictal-onset zone. It is associated with a network of seizure propagation and has potential epileptogenic properties. However, this secondary epileptic focus may disappear after removal of the primary focus. At times, it may also be "independent," and present as a new epileptic focus (47,48). Patients with a prolonged history of seizures before epilepsy surgery have a poorer seizure outcome after resection of the primary focus when compared to individuals with a shorter history of seizures (49). This suggests that secondary epileptogenesis at sites located elsewhere in the brain may develop with persistence of uncontrolled seizures (49). Therefore, it is important to identify the ictal-onset zone as well as the associated "epileptic network." Additional tests, such as anatomical and functional studies, that is, PET, may be of help in this process (42). Ictal-onset zone and potential ictal-onset zone are part of the epileptogenic zone.

The Eloquent Cortex

Eloquent cortex encompasses regions of cortex that are responsible for particular functions, including motor, sensory, language, memory, and other higher cortical functions. Delineation of eloquent cortex in relationship to the epileptogenic zone is important in presurgical planning to prevent or predict postoperative deficits. Knowledge of eloquent areas may also help in the estimation of the functional deficit zone.

TECHNIQUES IN THE DELINEATION OF THE EPILEPTOGENIC ZONE

Presurgical planning requires a detailed evaluation of the cortical zones in order to estimate the epileptogenic zone. The process begins with a localization hypothesis using clinical history and ictal semiology. This information is then confirmed by other diagnostic modalities, including EEG recording, anatomical and functional neuroimaging and neuropsychological evaluations. When the data of the various tests are concordant, the localization hypothesis is corroborated leading to a higher likelihood for successful seizure reduction with minimal functional deficits.

History Taking

Taking a history may assist in the delineation of the symptomatogenic zone and functional deficit zone, and therefore provides additional information on the potentially adjacent epileptogenic zone. There are several ways to determine the symptomatogenic zone. The first step in developing a localization hypothesis is history taking. Detailed descriptions of the seizures by the patient and ideally also by a witness of the events are necessary. Clinical features, such as potential triggers, timing and diurnal patterns, warning including auras and prodromes, and sequence of clinical seizure presentation including motor features, loss of consciousness, secondary generalization, and lateralizing signs provide important clues to determine the symptomatogenic zone (Table 72.2).

Clues to etiology can also be provided by ante- and perinatal history, past medical history (including history of head trauma or infections and history of neonatal or febrile seizures), and developmental history. Family history can add important information, especially in the diagnosis of genetic forms of epilepsy or certain epilepsy syndromes. Video can be used to supplement the history in the determination of the symptomatogenic zone. Long-term video monitoring, routine EEG recordings, and patient materials such as home videos or photographs may also be helpful.

A detailed history is also useful for determination of the functional deficit zone. Patients with temporal lobe epilepsy may, for example, complain of memory difficulties or visual

TABLE 72.2

LOCALIZING AND LATERALIZING VALUE OF ICTAL AND POSTICTAL CLINICAL SYMPTOMS OR SIGNS AND RELATION TO EPILEPTOGENIC ZONE

Symptomatogenic zone: signs or symptoms	Epileptogenic zone estimation: lateralization	Epileptogenic zone estimation: location	References
AURA			
Olfactory auras		Medial TLE	50,51
Gustatory and olfactory auras		TLE	52
Vague general body sensation		FLE	53
Diffuse warm sensation		FLE	54
Pharyngeal dysesthesia		Medial TLE	55
Hemifield visual aura	Contralateral	OLE	56
Feeling of chills	Dominant	TLE (5 cases)	53
Experiential auras		TLE	54
Complex visual hallucinations		TLE, PLE	57
Simple visual hallucinations		OLE	58
Visual illusions		Close to geniculostriate radiation and visual cortex	57
Pallinopsia	Contralateral	OLE, OTLE, OPLE	59
Visual auras		OLE	56,60
Localized somatosensory auras	Contralateral	PLE	54
Ictal pain	Contralateral	PLE	58
Ictal pleasure and ecstasy	Left or right	Mesiobasal TLE	61
Ictal motor features and automatisms			
Hypermotor seizures		FLE	53
Upper extremity automatisms	Ipsilateral >80	TLE	62–64

(continued)

TABLE 72.2

LOCALIZING AND LATERALIZING VALUE OF ICTAL AND POSTICTAL CLINICAL SYMPTOMS OR SIGNS AND
RELATION TO EPILEPTOGENIC ZONE (*continued*)

Symptomatogenic zone: signs or symptoms	Epileptogenic zone estimation: lateralization	Epileptogenic zone estimation: location	References
Early motor involvement of contralateral upper extremity, experiential aura, auditory hallucinations and vertigo		Lateral TLE	57
Proximal automatisms (e.g., bicycling)		FLE	57
Unilateral ictal blinking	Ipsilateral 80%	FLE or TLE (dominant temporal in 1 case)	65
Early oral automatisms especially if accompanied by contralateral dystonic posturing, epigastric sensation		Medial TLE	66
Unilateral ictal dystonia	Contralateral 90%–100%	TLE, ETE	62,64,67,68
Forced head version less than 10 seconds before secondary generalization	Contralateral 90%	TLE, ETE	69
Focal clonic or tonic activity, unilateral spasms, nystagmus, and postictal hemiparesis in infants	Contralateral		70
Dystonic posturing of upper extremity or mouth deviation	Contralateral		63
Nonforced head turning within 30 seconds of seizure onset	Ipsilateral		71
Figure of four sign	Contralateral, often in secondarily generalized seizures		66,72
Lateral tongue biting[a]	Ipsilateral 71%		73
Affectionate kissing	Right	TLE (1 case)	74
Ictal smile	Right	Posterior quadrant of cortex	75,76
Ictal spitting		TLE	77
Ictal language and consciousness			
Ictal speech	Nondominant >80%	TLE	63,78
Ictal neologistic speech automatisms	Dominant	TLE (1 case)	79
Preserved consciousness during automotor seizures in TLE	Nondominant 100%		80,81
Preserved consciousness during versive movements	Contralateral 100%	FLE	82
Ictal autonomic features			
Ictal urinary urge	Nondominant	TLE	83
Ictal water drinking	Nondominant	TLE (20 cases)	84
Ictal piloerection	Ipsilateral		85
Ictal pallor	Left sided	TLE	76
Ictal vomiting	Nondominant >90% dominant (2 cases)		86,87
Postictal findings			
Postictal dysphasia	Dominant >80%	TLE	63,68,78,88
Postictal Todd's paralysis	Contralateral 93%		81
Postictal nose wiping	Ipsilateral 80%–90%	FLE 1 TLE	89,90

FLE, frontal lobe epilepsy; TLE, temporal lobe epilepsy; PLE, parietal lobe epilepsy; OLE, occipital lobe epilepsy; ETE, extratemporal lobe epilepsy.
[a]Lateralizing value of this finding has been debated.

spatial problems that can be used to lateralize the functional deficit zone.

Clinical Features

Localizing and lateralizing clinical features may provide additional evidence for the symptomatogenic and ultimately the epileptogenic zone. These can be observed when a seizure involves eloquent cortex. The first clinical features do not necessarily represent the ictal-onset zone, as the seizure may begin in clinically silent areas. For some lateralizing and localizing symptoms, frequency and reliability in prediction of the epileptogenic zone has been assessed (see Table 72.2). For example, 5% of patients with nondominant temporal lobe epilepsy may have ictal automatisms with preserved consciousness (45,46,80). Table 72.2 lists some clinical symptoms and signs that may be helpful in the determination of the symptomatogenic and subsequently the epileptogenic zone.

Examination

General and neurologic examination not only helps with localization and lateralization of focal neurologic findings, such as hemiparesis and hemianopia, but it may also provide further clues toward the etiology of seizures. Premature hand dominance, for example, may be suggestive of a functional or structural abnormality in the ipsilateral hemisphere. In pediatric patients, additional information may be obtained from a dilated eye examination, dysmorphic features, and neurocutaneous stigmata. A facial angioma in the V1 distribution in a patient with a history of seizures may indicate the possibility of ipsilateral Sturge–Weber syndrome. It can therefore help with lateralization of the epileptogenic zone and predict the functional deficit zone. In one study it was found that 69% of patients with Sturge–Weber syndrome have focal seizures contralateral to the facial lesion (91).

Studies

Electrophysiologic Studies

Scalp EEG. Interictal discharges from a scalp EEG can be used to determine the irritative zone. The irritative zone may be larger than the epileptogenic zone and may overlap with it. Long-term video-EEG, sleep recordings, and seizure-provocation techniques including sleep deprivation, hyperventilation, and photic stimulation can increase the yield of interictal discharges and occasionally seizures. Simultaneous video-EEG recordings are useful to correlate clinical and electrographic seizures. Seizures from a particular ictal onset zone strengthen the hypothesis for the epileptogenic zone due to at least partial overlap between both zones.

The localizing value of noninvasive ictal EEG depends on the location of the epileptogenic zone. Lateralized theta and alpha, fast activity at seizure onset, and postical slowing as criteria for localization correctly lateralized 47% to 65% of extratemporal seizures and 76% to 83% of temporal lobe seizures (92). There is limited data about yield of scalp EEG for seizures arising from different extratemporal areas. Source analysis is a supplemental technique that may complement surface EEG and determine the seizure-onset zone and estimation of the epileptogenic zone.

Invasive EEG Recordings. When noninvasive EEG recordings provide discordant information or when the suspected epileptogenic zone is near eloquent cortex, invasive EEG recordings may be used to estimate the epileptogenic zone better and tailor the extent of possible resective epilepsy surgery. Subdural and depth electrode EEG recordings are the current gold standard for epilepsy localization. Subdural electrodes with grids and strips as well as depth electrodes are used for cortical mapping of the seizure-onset zones, irritative zones, and eloquent cortex.

Intraoperative corticography can also be used to increase the precision of the presumed epileptogenic zone. For example, it can be useful in patients with tumors or focal cortical dysplasias without discrete margins on imaging or if they are located near eloquent cortex. A novel technique—laminar electrode recording—is mainly used for research purposes and may be able to record electrographic activity in different cortical layers (93).

Cortical Stimulation. Cortical stimulation can be performed intra- or extraoperatively to define the relationship between eloquent cortex and the epileptogenic zone. It can also rarely assist in the localization of the irritative zone based on after-discharge recordings. Cortical stimulation may help in the delineation and confirmation of eloquent cortical areas, including the motor area and sensory function, language areas, and auditory cortex as well as visual cortex. Symptoms experienced during stimulation allow mapping of eloquent cortex. Findings may include positive findings, such as movements, sensations, sounds or visual findings, or negative symptoms, such as loss of tone, and aphasia.

Evoked Potentials

Evoked potentials have high temporal and spatial resolution to localize eloquent cortical areas as well-functional deficit zones. In particular, somatosensory evoked potentials (SEPs) are used to identify the central sulcus, but have limited spatial resolution to localize to a lobe or gyrus (94–96). Subdural recording of evoked potentials can localize the primary sensory areas. Somatosensory, auditory, visual evoked potentials, and even event-related potential may also be helpful (97).

Evoked potentials are often used complementary to cortical stimulation and may also be useful if the origin of the seizures is uncertain. Giant SEPs can be used to identify the ictal-onset zone. In one report, electrical stimulation of the right median nerve revealed giant surface SEPs. Subdural recordings, performed to plan epilepsy surgery, demonstrated that the epileptogenic zone was in the left postcentral gyrus. The ictal-onset zone was confirmed to be in the hyperexcitable postcentral gyrus (98).

Magnetoencephalography (MEG)

MEG provides a new, noninvasive tool for localization of the irritative zone and occasionally of the ictal-onset zone allowing better estimation of the epileptogenic zone. In contrast to

EEG, the magnetic fields generated by electrical discharges are minimally affected by interposed tissue layers. MEG provides potentials oriented parallel to the scalp, unlike EEG which records potentials perpendicular to it. Therefore, both modalities may be complementary and each modality may detect spikes that are not detected by the other (99). However, at present, there are only a few comparisons of MEG to surface and invasive EEG, and evidence for the use of MEG in the presurgical workup is limited.

Structural Imaging

MRI provides additional noninvasive localization of the presumed source of seizures by demonstrating an epileptic lesion. Imaging can corroborate findings from history and physical exam. T1-weighted, T2-weighted, gadolinium contrast, fluid attenuated inversion recovery (FLAIR) coronal and axial images are usually obtained. Images with thin cuts of less than 5 mm and magnetization-prepared rapid gradient-echo (MPRAGE) sequences may assist in the documentation of cortical malformations.

Imaging may be nonlesional or demonstrate a variety of lesions, including tumors, cortical malformations, vascular malformations, tubers, and others. If a lesion is found, it may not necessarily reflect the epileptogenic zone and additional information is needed to support the hypothetical epileptogenic zone. For example, a patient with tuberous sclerosis may have multifocal tubers. However, history and other investigations may suggest that only one tuber is the epileptic lesion.

Several reformatting tools can be used to obtain more information on the epileptic lesion, especially if it is not clear on conventional MRI. To detect subtle abnormalities, curvilinear reformatting of 2D images is used to reconstruct the images into thin, curved slices where the distance from the surface of the hemispheric convexities is kept constant (100). Volumetric MRI is a tool to measure hippocampal volume and is particularly helpful in patients with mesial temporal sclerosis. Diffusion tensor imaging (DTI) is sensitive to the movement of water molecules, providing additional information on the microstructural arrangement of tissue and orientation of nerve fibers.

Functional Imaging

PET is helpful in localizing the epileptogenic zone and functional deficit zone, especially in patients with nonlesional epilepsy on MRI. PET scans are used to measure cerebral metabolic rate. At present, 2-deoxy-2-fluorodeoxyglucose (FDG) PET is most commonly used. Interical PET hypometabolism may be an indicator for the structural lesion that cannot easily be detected by MRI.

FDG accumulates in the intracellular compartment and reflects energy demand of cells (101). Decreased metabolism reflects decrease in glucose influx from reduced glucose transport across the blood–brain barrier and reduced phosphorylation (102). Decreased metabolism is thought to represent the functional deficit zone and may be related to various factors, such as underlying structural lesion, inhibitory mechanisms of seizures, atrophy, neuronal loss, decreased synaptic activity, and postictal depression of metabolism.

The sensitivity of FDG-PET varies with the location of the seizure focus and etiology (101). In patients with intractable seizures, PET was shown to detect cortical dysplasias that could not be identified with CT or MRI (103). It is also particularly helpful in infants with immature myelination in whom MRI studies are limited (104).

Recently, AMT-PET scans were found to be useful for the identification of an epileptic tuber in tuberous sclerosis and in the detection of cortical malformations (40–42). Benzodiazepine receptors ligands, such as flumazenil (FMZ) may be more sensitive than FDG-PET to identify the epileptogenic zone (105–107). Chugani et al. performed a study with 17 patients with various types of pathology, including cortical dysplasias, and found that FMZ-PET abnormality was larger than the structural lesion, but smaller than the findings on FDG-PET. The region delineated by FMZ-PET showed excellent concordance to intracortical cortical electrode recordings (108).

SPECT assists in the localization of the ictal-onset zone and serves as a surrogate for the localization of the epileptogenic zone (109). Blood flow is increased during a seizure and radiopharmaceuticals, like ^{99m}Technetium hexamethylpropylene amine oxime (^{99m}Tc-HMPAO) or ^{99m}Technetium ethyl cysteinate diethylester (^{99m}Tc-ECD), are used to measure this change. An interictal image is subtracted from the ictal image to derive the difference in cerebral blood flow related to focal seizures (110). Subtraction ictal SPECT coregistered to MRI (SISCOM) can give additional information of the epileptogenic zone and its relation with the anatomical structures. The presence of a localizing SISCOM alteration concordant with the epileptogenic zone was a favorable predictor of an excellent surgical outcome in patients with extratemporal lobe epilepsy (111).

ELOQUENT CORTEX

Eloquent cortex encompasses regions of cortex that are consistently important for generating particular functions, including motor, sensory, language, memory, and other higher cortical functions. The goal of epilepsy surgery is to remove the epileptogenic zone, while preventing functional deficits.

Neuropsychological testing is used to provide additional quantification and localizing information of cognitive deficits that hint at the functional deficit zone. Neuropsychological findings can also anticipate possible cognitive decline after epilepsy surgery. This is especially important if the epileptogenic zone or lesion is in close proximity or overlapping with eloquent areas. Besides defining eloquent cortex, it can be used to lateralize and localize the epileptogenic zone by showing regions of functional deficit.

The Wada test involves angiography and injection of a short-acting barbiturate into the internal carotid artery in order to temporarily simulate the effects of epilepsy surgery on language and memory. It is used to lateralize eloquent areas and functional deficit zone, in particular language and memory function (112–115). In patients with bilateral hypersynchrony on EEG, it has also rarely been used to localize the epileptogenic zone (116).

fMRI is based on increased cerebral blood flow during activation using blood oxygenation level dependent (BOLD) contrast. Blood flow increase exceeds the increase in local cerebral oxygen, and this leads to a localized increase in the ratio of oxyhemoglobin to deoxyhemoglobin (27,28). It can localize brain function and functional deficits, and may therefore serve as an estimate of the functional deficit zone. Additionally, EEG-triggered fMRI measures hemodynamics arising from spike discharge by using a combination of EEG and fMRI. This method can detect interictal spike-related changes and may be helpful in the localization of interictal epileptiform discharges. The superior spatial resolution of EEG-triggered fMRI may provide an additional noninvasive tool in the delineation of the irritative zone in patients with intractable focal seizures (29,30).

Other techniques may also provide additional information on eloquent cortex. MEG is a reliable tool for determining language localization when compared to Wada testing (117–119) and cortical stimulation results (120,121). Repetitive transcranial magnetic stimulation (rTMS) can be used for mapping of cortical motor representation and also be used to define eloquent cortex. Functional transcranial Doppler (fTCD) can also be used as in the presurgical work-up to assess eloquent cortex, especially lateralization of language, as well as interictal spiking (122–125).

RISKS AND BENEFIT OF EPILEPSY SURGERY

In pharmacologically intractable epilepsy patients, the risk of recurrent seizures, impairment of development and cognition as well as side effects of antiepileptic medications have to be weighed against the potential adverse effects of epilepsy surgery such as bleeding, infection, neurologic deficit, and continuing seizures. Dominant temporal lobe resections can lead to difficulties in learning or retaining verbal information (126–128). Deficit in nonverbal tasks after resection of the nondominant temporal lobe have also been described (129–131). Depending on the individuals' baseline functioning vocation and lifestyle, such deficits may lead to significant disability.

Effective epilepsy surgery can lead to a significant reduction of seizures or seizure freedom, leading to better quality of life, less injuries secondary to seizures, and possibly improvements in development and cognition. Successful surgery can only be performed after a detailed evaluation to define the epileptogenic zone pre- and perioperatively. The process begins with a localization hypothesis using clinical history of ictal semiology to delineate the symptomatogenic zone and possibly the functional deficit zone. Once medical intractability is confirmed, this hypothesis is corroborated by other diagnostic modalities. These confirm localization and prevent deficits, and add further information on ictal-onset zone and irritative zone as well as eloquent areas. Choice of studies depends on cost, availability, and experience at different institutions. Early surgical intervention is important, as hesitancy may lead to death as well as decreased development in the pediatric population (132,133). Brain plasticity in children secondary to neurogenesis and synapse formation may allow transfer of function and may lead to fewer deficits in patients undergoing with earlier surgery (134,135).

CONCLUSION

Definition and resection of the epileptogenic zone is critical to successful epilepsy surgery. New technologies will provide additional tools for the successful identification of this hypothetical region in the future. The preoperative evaluation relies strongly on history and seizure semiology, EEG, structural and functional imaging, and other testing methods described in this chapter. Main goal is development of a localization hypothesis on the basis of available information. The ultimate goal of preoperative planning is to provide patients with seizure reduction or freedom, improved quality of life, and minimal deficit. This can be achieved by an understanding and demarcation of the epileptogenic zone, which is unique to each epilepsy patient, and when completely resected renders the patient seizure-free.

References

1. Kwan P, Brodie MJ. Early identification of refractory epilepsy. *N Engl J Med.* 2000;342(5):314–319.
2. Temkin O. *The Falling Sickness: A History of Epilepsy from the Greeks to the Beginnings of Modern Neurology.* Baltimore, MD: Johns Hopkins University Press; 1971.
3. Jackson JH. Convulsive spasms of the right hand and arm preceding epileptic seizures. *Med Times Gazette.* 1863;1:110–111.
4. Hitzig E. John Hughlings Jackson and the cortical motor centres in the light of physiological research. *Brain.* 1900;23:545–581.
5. Macewen W. Tumor of the dura mater removed during life in a person affected with epilepsy. *Glasgow Med J.* 1879;12:210.
6. Bennet AH, Godlee RJ. Excision of a tumour from the brain. *Lancet.* 1984;1:1090–1091.
7. Green JR. The beginnings of cerebral localization and neurological surgery. *Barrow Neurol Inst.* 1985;1:12–28.
8. Berger H. Uber das electrenkephalogramm des Menschen. *Arch Psychiat Nervkrankh.* 1929;87:527–570.
9. Swartz BE, Goldensohn ES. Timeline of the history of EEG and associated fields. *Electroencephalogr Clin Neurophysiol.* 1998;106:173–176.
10. Hunter J, Jasper HH. A method of analysis of seizure patterns and electroencephalogram. *Electroencephalogr Clin Neurophysiol.* 1949;1:113–114.
11. Goldensohn ES. Simultaneous recording of EEG and clinical seizures using the kineoscope. *Electroencephalogr Clin Neurophysiol.* 1966;21:623.
12. Foerster O, Altnburger H. Elektrobiologische Vorgange an der menschlichen Hirnrinde. *Dt Z Nervheilk.* 1935;135:277–288.
13. Cohen D. Magnetoencephalography: evidence of magnetic fields produced by alpha-rhythm currents. *Science.* 1968;161:784–786.
14. Gadian DG. *Nuclear Magnetic Resonance and its Applications to Living Systems.* New York: Oxford University Press; 1982.
15. Kuznicky RI, Jackson GD. *Magnetic Resonance in Epilepsy.* New York: Raven Press;1995.
16. Kuhl DE, Engel J Jr, Phelps ME, et al. Epileptic patterns of local cerebral metabolism and perfusion in humans determined by emission computed tomography of 18FDG and 13NH3. *Ann Neurol.* 1980;8:348–360.
17. Wada J. A new method for the determination of the side of cerebral speech dominance. A preliminary report on the intracarotid injection of sodium amytal in man. *Igaku Seibutsugaku.* 1949;14:221–222.
18. Milner B, Penfield W. The effect of hippocampal lesions on recent memory. *Trans Am Neurol Assoc.* 1955;80:42–48.
19. Milner B. Psychological defects produced by temporal-lobe excision. *Res Publ Assoc Nerv Ment Dis.* 1958;36:244–257.
20. Milner B. Interhemispheric differences in the localization of psychological processes in man. *Br Med Bull.* 1971;27:272–277.
21. Kaufmann PY. Electrical phenomena in cerebral cortex. *Obz Psikhiatr Nev Eksper.* 1912;7–8:403.
22. Gibbs FA, Lennox WG, Gibbs EL. The electro-encephalogram in diagnosis and in localization of epileptic seizures. *Arch Neurol Psychiatry.* 1939;36: 1225–1235.
23. Jasper HH. Localized analyses of the function of the human brain by the electro-encephalogram. *Arch Neurol Psychiatry.* 1936;36:1131–1134.
24. Early PJ. Positron emission tomography (PET). In: Early PJ, Sodee DB, eds. *Principles and Practice of Nuclear Medicine.* St. Louis, MO: Mosby; 1995: 314–322.
25. Laster DW, Penry JK, Moody DM, et al. Chronic seizure disorders: contribution of MR imaging when CT is normal. *Am J Neuroradiol.* 1985;6: 177–180.
26. Latack JT, Abou-Khalil BW, Siegel GJ, et al. Patients with partial seizures: evaluation by MR, CT, and PET imaging. *Radiology.* 1986;159:159–163.
27. Pauling L. Magnetic properties and structure of oxyhemoglobin. *Proc Natl Acad Sci U S A.* 1977;74:2612–2613.
28. Thulborn KR, Waterton JC, Matthews PM, et al. Oxygenation dependence of the transverse relaxation time of water protons in whole blood at high field. *Biochem Biophys Acta.* 1982;714:265–270.
29. Krakow K, Lemieux L, Messina D, et al. Spatio-temporal imaging of focal interictal epileptiform activity using EEG-triggered functional MRI. *Epileptic Discord.* 2001;3(1):67–74.

30. Kikuchi K. Electroencephalogram-triggered functional magnetic resonance imaging in focal epilepsy. *Psychiatry Clin Neurosci.* 2004;58(3): 319–323.

31. Rosenow F, Luders HO. Presurgical evaluation of epilepsy. *Brain.* 2001; 124:1683–1700.

32. Luders H, Noachtar S, Burgess R. Semiologic classification of epileptic seizures. In: *Epileptic Seizures: Pathophysiology and Clinical Semiology.* Philadelphia: Churchill Livingstone; 2000:263–285.

33. Sperling MR, Shewmon DA. *Epilepsy, A Comprehensive Textbook.* Philadelphia, PA: Lippincott-Raven Publishers; 2007.

34. Klein KM, Rosenow F. *Textbook of Epilepsy Surgery.* London: Informa Healthcare; 2008.

35. Pedley TA, Traub RD. Physiological basis of the EEG. In: Daly DD, Pedley TA, eds. *Current Practice of Electroencephalography.* Philadelphia, PA: Lippincott-Raven; 1997.

36. Talairach J, Bancaud J. Lesions, "irriative" zone and epileptogenic focus. *Conf Neurol.* 1966;27:61–64.

37. Wyllie E, Luders HO, Morris HH IIII, et al. Clinical outcome after complete or partial cortical resection for intractable epilepsy. *Neurology.* 1987; 37:1634–1641.

38. Van Ness PC. *Textbook of Epilepsy Surgery.* New York: Raven Press.

39. Krsek P, Maton B, Jayakar P, et al. Incomplete resection of focal cortical dysplasia is the main predictor of poor postsurgical outcome. *Neurology.* 2009;72(3):217–223.

40. Chugani DC, Chugani HT, Muzik O, et al. Imaging epileptogenic tubers in children with tuberous sclerosis complex using alpha-11(C)methyl-L-tryptophan positron emission tomography. *Ann Neurol.* 1998;44:858–866.

41. Asano E, Chugani DC, Muzik O, et al. Multimodality imaging for improved detection of epileptogenic lesions in children with tuberous sclerosis complex. *Neurology.* 2000;54:1976–1984.

42. Sood S, Chugani HT. Functional neuroimaging in the preoperative evaluation of children with drug-resistant epilepsy. *Childs Nerv Syst.* 2006;22: 810–820.

43. Diehl B, LaPresto E, Najm I, et al. Neocortical temporal FDG-PET hypometabolism correlates with temporal lobe atrophy in hippocampal sclerosis associated with microscopic cortical dysplasia. *Epilepsia.* 2003; 44:559–564.

44. Binnie CD. Cognitive effects of subclinical EEG discharges. *Neurophysiol Clin.* 1996;26(3):138–142.

45. Janszky J, Jokeit H, Heinemann D, et al. Epileptic activity influences the speech organization in medial temporal lobe epilepsy. *Brain.* 2003;126(9): 2043–2051.

46. Janszky J, Balogh A, Hollo A, et al. Automatisms with preserved responsiveness and ictal aphasia: contradictory lateralising signs during a dominant temporal lobe seizure. *Seizure.* 2003;12(3):182–185.

47. Morrell F. Secondary epileptogenesis in man. *Arch Neurol.* 1985;42: 318–335.

48. Morrell F. Varieties of human secondary epileptogenesis. *J Clin Neurophysiol.* 1989;6:227–275.

49. Eliashiv SD, Dewar S, Wainwright I, et al. Long-term follow-up after temporal lobe resection for lesions associated with chronic seizures. *Neurology.* 1997;48:621–626.

50. Acharaya V, Acharya J, Luders H. Olfactory epileptic auras. *Neurology.* 1998;51:56–61.

51. Chen C, Shih YH, Yen DJ, et al. Olfactory auras inpatients with temporal lobe epilepsy. *Epilepsia.* 2003;44:257–260.

52. Ebner A, Kerdar M. Olfactory and gustatory auras. In: Luders H, Noachtar S, eds. *Epileptic Seizures: Pathophysiology and Clinical Semiology.* Philadelphia: Churchill Livingstone; 2000:313–319.

53. Kotagal P, Arunkumar G, Hammel J, et al. Complex partial seizures of frontal lobe onset statistical analysis of ictal semiology. *Seizure.* 2003;12: 268–281.

54. Palmini A, Gloor P. The localizing value of auras in partial seizures: a prospective and retrospective study. *Neurology.* 1992;42:801–808.

55. Carmant L, Carrazana E, Kramer U, et al. Pharyngeal dysesthesia as an aura in temporal lobe epilepsy. *Epilepsia.* 1996;37:911–913.

56. Salanova V, Andermann FR, Olivier A, et al. Occipital lobe epilepsy: electroclinical manifestations, electrocorticography, cortical stimulation and outcome in 42 patients treated between 1930 and 1991. Surgery or occipital lobe epilepsy. *Brain.* 1992;115:1655–1680.

57. Obeid M, Wyllie E, Rahi AC, et al. Approach to pediatric epilepsy surgery: state of the art, Part I: general principles and presurgical workup. *Eur J Paediatr Neurol.* 2008;13:1–13.

58. Anand I, Geller EB. Visual auras. In: Luders HO, Soachter S, eds. *Epileptic Seizures: Pathophysiology and Clinical Semiology.* Philadelphia, PA: Churchill Livingstone; 2000:298–303.

59. Mailard L, Vignal JP, Anxionnat R, et al. Semiologic value of ictal autoscopy. *Epilepsia.* 2004;45:391–394.

60. Williamson PD, Thadani VM, Darcey TM, et al. Occipital lobe epilepsy: clinical characteristics, seizure spread patterns, and results of surgery. *Ann Neurol.* 1992;31:3–13.

61. Stefan H, Schulze-Bonhage A, Pauli E, et al. Ictal pleasant sensations: cerebral localization and lateralization. *Epilepsia.* 2004;45:35–40.

62. Kotagal P, Luders H, Morris HH, et al. Dystonic posturing in complex partial seizures of temporal lobe onset: a new lateralizing sign. *Neurology.* 1989;39:196–201.

63. Chee MW, Kotagal P, Van Ness PC, et al. Lateralizing signs in intractable partial epilepsy: blinded multiple-observer analysis. *Neurology.* 1993;43: 2519–2525.

64. Marks WJ Jr, Laxer KD. Semiology of temporal lobe seizures: value in lateralizing the seizure focus. *Epilepsia.* 1998;39:721–726.

65. Benbadis SR. Tongue biting as a lateralizing sign in partial epilepsy. *Seizure.* 1996;5:175–176.

66. Kotagal P, Bleasel A, Geller E, et al. Lateralizing value of asymmetric tonic limb posturing observed in secondarily generalized tonic-clonic seizures. *Epilepsia.* 2000;41:457–462.

67. Bleasel A, Kotagal P, Kankirawatana P, et al. Lateralizing value and semiology of ictal limb posturing and version in temporal lobe and extratemporal epilepsy. *Epilepsia.* 1997;38:168–174.

68. Steinhoff BJ, Schindler M, Herrendorf G, et al. The lateralizing value of ictal clinical symptoms in uniregional temporal lobe epilepsy. *Eur Neurol.* 1998;39:72–79.

69. Wyllie E, Luders H, Morris HH, et al. The lateralizing significance of versive head and eye movements during epileptic seizures. *Neurology.* 1986; 36:606–611.

70. Loddenkemper T, Wyllie E, Neme S, et al. Lateralizing signs during seizures in infants. *J Neurol.* 2004;251:1075–1079.

71. Chee WM. Versive seizures. In: Luders H, Noachtar S, eds. *Epileptic Seizures: Pathophysiology and Clinical Semiology.* Philadelphia: Churchill Livingstone; 2000:433–438.

72. Kotagal P. Automotor seizures. In: Luders H, Noachtar S, eds. *Epileptic Seizures: Pathophysiology and Clinical Semiology.* Philadelphia: Churchill Livingstone; 2000:449–457.

73. Benbadis SR, Kotagal P, Klem GH. Unilateral blinking: a lateralizing sign in partial seizures. *Neurology.* 1996;46:45–48.

74. Mikati MA, Comair YG, Shamseddine AN. Pattern-induced partial seizures with repetitive affectionate kissing: an unusual manifestation of right temporal lobe epilepsy. *Epilepsy Behav.* 2005;6:447–451.

75. Molinuevo JL, Arroyo S. Ictal smile. *Epilepsia.* 1998;39:1357–1360.

76. Fogarasi A, Janszky J, Tuxhorn I. Ictal smile lateralizes to the right hemisphere in childhood epilepsy. *Epilepsy Res.* 2005;67:117–121.

77. Kellinghaus C, Loddenkemper T, Kotagal P. Ictal spitting: clinical and electroencephalographic features. *Epilepsia.* 2003;44:1064–1069.

78. Gabr M, Luders H, Dinner D, et al. Speech manifestations in lateralization of temporal lobe seizures. *Ann Neurol.* 1989;25:82–87.

79. Bell WL, Horner J, Logue P, et al. Neologistic speech automatism during complex partial seizures. *Neurology.* 1990;40:49–52.

80. Ebner A, Dinner DS, Noachtar S, et al. Automatisms with preserved responsiveness: a lateralizing sign in psychomotor seizures. *Neurology.* 1995;45(1):61–64.

81. Luders H, Noachtar S, Burgess R. Semiologic classification of epileptic seizures. In: Luders H, Noachtar S, eds. *Epileptic Seizures: Pathophysiology and Clinical Semiology.* Philadelphia: Churchill Livingstone; 2000: 458–471.

82. McLachlan RS. The significance of head and eye turning in seizures. *Neurology.* 1987;37:1617–1619.

83. Loddenkemper T, Foldvary N, Raja S, et al. Ictal urinary urge: further evidence for lateralization to the nondominant hemisphere. *Epilepsia.* 2003;44:124–126.

84. Remillard GM, Andermann F, Gloor P, et al. Water-drinking as ictal behavior in complex partial seizures. *Neurology.* 1981;31:117–124.

85. Loddenkemper T, Kellinghaus C, Gandjour J, et al. Localising and lateralising value of ictal piloerection. *J Neurol Neurosurg Psychiatry.* 2004;75: 879–883.

86. Kramer RE, Luders H, Goldstick LP, et al. Ictus emeticus: an electroclinical analysis. *Neurology.* 1988;38:1048–1052.

87. Koutroumanidis M. Ictal vomiting in association with left temporal lobe seizures in a left hemisphere language-dominant patient. *Epilepsia.* 2003;44:1259.

88. Fakhoury T, Abou-Khalil B, Peguero E. Differentiating clinical features or right and left temporal lobe seizures. *Epilepsia.* 1994;35:1038–1044.

89. Leutmezer F, Series W, Lehrner J, et al. Postictal nose wiping: a lateralizing sign in temporal lobe complex partial seizures. *Neurology.* 1998;51:1175–1177.

90. Geyer JD, Payne TA, Faught E, et al. Postictal nose-rubbing in the diagnosis, lateralization, and localization of seizures. *Neurology.* 1999;51:1175–1177.

91. Pascual-Castroviejo I, Pascual-Pascual SI, Velazquez-Fraqua R, et al. Sturge–Webe syndrome: study of 55 patients. *Can J Neurol Sci.* 2008; 35(3):301–307.

92. Walczak TS, Radtke RA, Lewis DV. Accuracy and interobserver reliability of scalp ictal EEG. *Neurology.* 1992;42:2279–2285.

93. Ulbert I, Magloczky Z, Czirjak S, et al. In vivo laminar electrophysiology co-registered with histology in the hippocampus of patients with temporal lobe epilepsy. *Exp Neurol.* 2004;187(2):310–318.

94. Allison T, McCarthy G, Wood CC, et al. Human cortical potentials evoked by stimulation of the median nerve I. Cytoarchitectonic areas generating short-latency activity. *J Neurophysiol.* 1989;62:694–710.

95. Allison T, Wood CC, McCarthy G, et al. Cortical somatosensory evoked potentials II. Effects of excision of somatosensory or motor cortex in humans and monkeys. *J Neurophysiol.* 1991;66:64–82.

96. Allison T, McCarthy G, Wood CC, et al. Human cortical potentials evoked by stimulation of the median nerve II. Cytoarchitectonic areas generating long-latency activity. *J Clin Neurophysiol.* 1989;62:711–722.

97. Luders H, Dinner DS, Lesser RP, et al. Evoked potentials in cortical localization. *J Clin Neurophysiol.* 1986;3:75–84.

98. Noachtar S, Holthausen H, Luders HO. Epileptic negative myoclonus. Subdural EEG recordings indicate a postcentral generator. *Neurology.* 1997;49(6):1534–1537.

99. Rodin E, Funke M, Berg P, et al. Magnetoencephalographic spikes not detected by conventional electroencephalography. *Clin Neurophys.* 2004;115:2041–2047.

100. Pfluger T, Vollmar C, Wismüller A, et al. Quantitative comparison of automatic and interactive methods for MRI-SPECT image registration of the brain based on 3-dimensional calculation of error. *J Nucl Med.* 2000; 41(11):1823–1829.

101. Chugani HT, Mazziotta JC, Phelps ME. Sturge–Weber syndrome: a study of cerebral glucose utilization with positron emission tomography. *J Pediatr.* 1989;114:244–253.

102. Rintahaka PJ, Chugani HT, Messa C, et al. Hemimegalencephaly: evaluation with positron emission tomography. *Pediatr Neurol.* 1993;9: 21–28.

103. Chugani HT, Shields WD, Shewmon, DA, et al. Infantile spasms: I. PET identifies focal cortical dysgenesis in cryptogenic cases for surgical treatment. *Ann Neurol.* 1990;27:406–413.

104. Chugani HT, Conti JR. Etiologic classification of infantile spasms in 140 cases: role of positron emission tomography. *J Child Neurol.* 1996;11: 44–48.

105. Henry TR, Frey KA, Sackellares JC, et al. In vivo cerebral metabolism and central benzodiazepine-receptor binding in temporal lobe epilepsy. *Neurology.* 1993;43:1998–2006.

106. DaSilva EA, Chugani DC, Muzik O, et al. Identification of frontal lobe epileptic foci in children using positron emission tomography. *Epilepsia.* 1997;38:1198–1208.

107. Hong KS, Lee SK, Kim JY, et al. Pre-surgical evaluation and surgical outcome of 41 patients with non-lesional neocortical epilepsy. *Seizure.* 2002;11:184–192.

108. Juhasz C, Chugani DC, Mizik O, et al. Electroclinical correlates of flumazenil and fluorodeoxyglucose PET abnormalities in lesional epilepsy. *Neurology.* 2000;55:825–834.

109. O'Brien TJ, So EL, Mullan BP, et al. Subtraction ictal SPECT coregistered to MRI improves clinical usefulness of SPECT in localizing the surgical seizure focus. *Neurology.* 1998;50:445–454.

110. Ho SS, Berkovic SF, Berlangieri SU, et al. Comparison of ictal SPECT and interictal PET in the presurgical evaluation of temporal lobe epilepsy. *Ann Neurol.* 1995;37:738–745.

111. O'Brien TJ, So EL, Mulan BP, et al. Subtraction peri-ictal SPECT is predictive of extratemporal epilepsy surgery outcome. *Neurology.* 2000;55: 1668–1677.

112. Hamer HM, Wylie E, Stanford L, et al. Risk factors for unsuccessful testing during the intracarotid amobarbital procedure in preadolescent children. *Epilepsia.* 2000;41:554–563.

113. Schevon C, Carlson C, Zaroff CM, et al. Pediatric language mapping. sensitivity of neurostimulation and Wada testing in epilepsy surgery. *Epilepsia.* 2007;48:539–545.

114. Milner B, Branch C, Rasmussen T. Study of short-term memory after intracarotid injection of sodium Amytal. *Trans Am Neurol Assoc.* 1962; 87:224–226.

115. Perrine K, Devinsky O, Pacia S, et al. Posterior cerebral artery amobarbital injections following anomalous intracarotid injections. *Epilepsia.* 1994;35(suppl 8):S123–S178.

116. Dinner DS, Loddenkemper T. Wada test and epileptogenic zone. In: Luders H, ed. *Textbook of Epilepsy Surgery.* London: Informa Healthcare; 2008:844–857.

117. Breier JI, Simos PG, Zouridakis G, et al. Relative timing of neuronal activity in distinct temporal lobe areas during a recognition memory task for words. *J Clin Exp Neuropsychol.* 1998;20:782–790.

118. Maestu F, Ortiz AT, Fernandez A, et al. Spanish language mapping using MEG: a validation study. *Neuroimage.* 2002;17:1579–1586.

119. Bowyer SM, Moran JE, Weiland BJ, et al. Language laterality determined by MEG mapping with MR-FOCUSS. *Epilepsy Behav.* 2005;6: 235–241.

120. Simos PG, Breier JI, Maggio WW, et al. Atypical temporal lobe language representation: MEG and intraoperative stimulation mapping correlation. *Neuroreport.* 1999;10:139–142.

121. Simos PG, Papanicolaou AC, Breier JI, et al. Localization of language-specific cortex by using magnetic source imaging and electrical stimulation mapping. *J Neurosurg.* 1999;91:787–796.

122. Knecht S, Deppe M, Ebner A, et al. Noninvasive determination of language lateralization by functional transcranial Doppler sonography: a comparison with the Wada test. *Stroke.* 1998;29:82–86.

123. Floel A, Knecht S, Lohmann H, et al. Language and spatial attention can lateralize to the same hemisphere in healthy humans. *Neurology.* 2001;57: 1018–1024.

124. Deppe M, Ringelstein EB, Knecht S. The investigation of functional brain lateralization by transcranial Doppler sonography. *Neuroimage.* 2004;21: 1124–1146.

125. Jansen A, Floel A, Deppe M, et al. Determining the hemispheric dominance of spatial attention: a comparison between fTCD and fMRI. *Hum Brain Mapp.* 2004;23:168–180.

126. Binder JR, Swanson SJ, Hammeke TA, et al. Determination of language dominance using functional MRI: a comparison with the Wada test. *Neurology.* 1996;46:978–984.

127. Golby AJ, Poldrack RA, Illes J, et al. Memory lateralization in medial temporal lobe epilepsy assessed by functional MRI. *Epilepsia.* 2002;43: 855–863.

128. Benke T, Koylu B, Visani P, et al. Language lateralization in temporal lobe epilepsy: a comparison between fMRI and the Wada test. *Epilepsia.* 2006; 47:1308–1319.

129. Milner B. Psychological aspects of focal epilepsy and its neurosurgical management. *Adv Neurol.* 1975;8:299–321.

130. Jones-Gotman, M. Right hippocampal excision impairs learning and recall of a list of abstract designs. *Neuropsychologia.* 1986;24: 659–670.

131. Seidenberg M, Hermann B, Wyler AR, et al. Neuropsychological outcome following anterior temporal lobectomy in patients with and without the syndrome of mesial temporal lobe epilepsy. *Neuropsychology.* 1998;12: 303–316.

132. Wiebe S, Blume WT, Girvin JP, et al. Effectiveness and Efficiency for Surgery for a Temporal Lobe Epilepsy Study Group. A randomized, controlled trial of surgery for temporal-lobe epilepsy. *N Engl J Med.* 2001; 345(5):311–318.

133. Loddenkemper T, Holland KD, Stanford LD, et al. Developmental outcome after epilepsy surgery in infancy. *Pediatrics.* 2007;119(5):930–935.

134. Peacock WJ. Hemispherectomy for the treatment of intractable seizures in childhood. *Neurosurg Clin N Am.* 1995;6:549–563.

135. Johnston MV. Clinical disorders of brain plasticity. *Brain Dev.* 2004;26: 73–80.

CHAPTER 73 ■ MRI IN EVALUATION FOR EPILEPSY SURGERY

AHSAN N.V. MOOSA AND PAUL M. RUGGIERI

Prior to the advent of modern neuroimaging, candidates for epilepsy surgery were selected based on seizure semiology, neurologic examination, and EEG features. Direct cortical EEG, intraoperatively or with implanted electrodes, was often critical to identify the epileptogenic zone. The epileptogenic lesions per se were identified only after histopathologic analysis of resected brain tissue. CT and then MRI provided powerful tools for identifying the epileptogenic lesions preoperatively thereby changing the approach of presurgical evaluation in patients with lesions. Invasive neurophysiologic techniques became unnecessary in many cases and the pool of surgical candidates widened with improved postsurgical outcome (1–3).

Brain MRI is currently the best available tool for identification of epileptogenic lesions. It provides two critical details of a lesion—the presumptive pathology and the precise anatomic location. The strong soft tissue contrast of MRI makes it particularly well suited to identify even the most subtle structural abnormalities such as cortical dysplasias that are often associated with refractory epilepsy. The multiplanar capabilities of MRI allow study of the precise anatomic location of these lesions in relation to eloquent cortices, which is a critical point for surgical planning. Newer MRI techniques, including 3 T magnets, functional MRI (fMRI), and diffusion tensor imaging (DTI), have further improved the detection of subtle abnormalities and provided information about brain function and network connectivity.

The intent of this chapter is to provide the reader with a working knowledge of major anatomical landmarks on brain MRI relevant to the eloquent cortex location, and a general understanding of various MRI pulse sequences and how these images are applied to the evaluation of patients with epilepsy. A mini-atlas of common epileptogenic lesions is displayed at the end of the chapter. Diffusion tensor imaging and functional MRI are addressed in Chapters 77 and 79.

MAJOR ANATOMICAL LANDMARKS OF BRAIN ON MRI

Epileptogenic lesions resulting in medically refractory epilepsy commonly include mesial temporal sclerosis (MTS), malformations of cortical development (MCD), encephalomalacia, slow growing benign tumors, hamartomas, and vascular malformations. In most cases, the anatomic location and extent of these otherwise benign lesions is more critical than the pathology itself. Anatomic location of the lesion is the chief determinant of the type of epilepsy syndrome. The extent of the lesion and its spatial relationship to eloquent areas of the brain has major implications for the surgical strategy. Hence a

three-dimensional working knowledge of MRI neuroanatomy is critical for optimal interpretation of the lesions. Extensive review of neuroanatomy is beyond the scope of this chapter. The main focus of this section will be to review the anatomy relevant for the location of eloquent cortex, and temporal lobe anatomy, as temporal lobe epilepsy remains the most common surgically remediable epilepsy syndrome in most epilepsy centers.

Eloquent cortex refers to areas of cerebral cortex that is indispensable for defined cortical function and whose damage leads to predictable pattern of neurologic deficits. The key eloquent areas relevant to epilepsy surgery are the primary motor cortex, Broca's area, Wernicke's area, and visual cortex. Although routine MRI provides information about the expected location of these regions, fMRI provides additional functional information, particularly important when the lesions occur in early life or the anatomy is distorted by lesions.

Broca's and Wernicke's areas

In most right-handed subjects and a significant number of left-handed subjects, the language areas reside in the left hemisphere. Broca's area refers to expressive language area and the Wernicke's area refers to receptive comprehension center. The location of Broca's area in the dominant inferior frontal gyrus is relatively consistent. On the contrary, the location of Wernicke's area is variable. Identification of the presumptive location of Broca's and Wernicke's areas begins with the knowledge of anatomy of sylvian fissure.

Sylvian fissure has three major components: an anterior ascending and anterior horizontal rami, a central stem with its minor rami, and a posterior terminal ascending ramus. Broca's area is located in relation to the anterior end of sylvian fissure and the Wernicke's area is located in relation to the posterior end of sylvian fissure in the dominant hemisphere. The central stem of the sylvian fissure is in relation to the inferior regions of motor and sensory cortex.

Sagittal sections of MRI provide excellent view of the sylvian fissure and the various gyri in relation to it (Fig. 73.1A and B). In far lateral sagittal sections, the V or Y shaped anterior horizontal (anterior arm of V or Y) and anterior ascending rami (posterior arm of V or Y) of sylvian fissure can be identified (Fig. 73.1A and B). The sulcus that is superior and perpendicular to these anterior rami is the inferior frontal sulcus and the sulcus posterior and parallel to the anterior ascending rami of sylvian fissure denotes inferior precentral sulcus. The "M" shaped region around the banks of the V or Y shaped anterior rami of sylvian fissure forms the inferior frontal gyrus which is limited superiorly by the inferior frontal

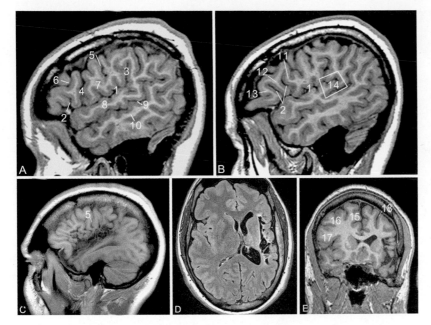

FIGURE 73.1 Broca'a and Wernicke's area: **A, B:** Major landmarks on sagittal images to identify Broca's and Wernicke's area. **C–E:** Left perisylvian encephalomalacia due to perinatally acquired ischemic injury displayed in sagittal, axial, and coronal planes. The lesion involves the region of potential Broca's and Wernicke's areas (Functional MRI in this subject confirmed language representation in the right hemisphere, likely a result of plasticity due to early brain injury.) 1, sylvian fissure; 2, "V" shaped anterior rami of sylvian fissure; 3, posterior ramus of sylvian fissure; 4, precentral sulcus—inferior part; 5, central sulcus; 6, inferior frontal sulcus; 7, precentral gyrus—inferior part; 8, superior temporal gyrus; 9, superior temporal sulcus; 10, middle temporal gyrus; 11, *pars* opercularis; 12, *pars* triangularis; 13, *pars* orbitalis; 14, usual location of Wernicke's area over the dominant hemisphere; 15, superior frontal gyrus; 16, middle frontal gyrus; 17, inferior frontal gyrus; 18, superior frontal sulcus.

sulcus (4,5). Inferior frontal gyrus consists of three regions, namely pars opercularis, pars triangularis, and pars orbitalis (Fig. 73.1B). In most normal subjects, pars opercularis, which lies between anterior ascending rami and the inferior precentral sulcus, and/or the region around the anterior ascending rami in pars triangularis harbors the Broca's area in the dominant hemisphere (4). On coronal sections, precise identification of location of Broca's area is difficult, but may be accomplished by tracing the inferior frontal sulcus posteriorly.

Wernicke's area is located in relation to the posterior end of sylvian fissure, which terminate in the temporoparietal region as the ascending posterior rami. Wernicke's area lies in the posterior part of superior temporal gyrus (4.5 cm posterior to tip of temporal pole) extending around the banks of the posterior terminal ascending ramus of sylvian fissure or around the superior temporal sulcus in the language dominant hemisphere (Fig. 73.1B). In a minority, the middle or inferior temporal gyrus harbors the Wernicke's area. Rarely, Wernicke's area may lie within the anterior part of superior temporal gyrus (6–8). On coronal sections, tracing the sylvian fissure and superior temporal sulcus posteriorly may assist to identify the region of Wernicke's area. Atypical locations of language area tend to occur when congenital or early acquired brain lesions are located in the vicinity of the presumptive language areas (Fig. 73.1C–E). These lesions may result in shift of the language areas to the perilesional regions or in extreme cases, to the contralateral homologous region of the brain. This can be confirmed by a Wada test or fMRI studies.

Primary Motor Area: The Precentral Gyrus

Surgery for epileptogenic lesions around the central sulcus pose special challenges due to the risk of motor deficits. A thorough knowledge of the anatomy of the central sulcus and precentral gyrus—the primary motor area, is crucial to localize the lesions around this region. Central sulcus and the precentral gyrus are best identified on the axial and sagittal images (Figs. 73.2 and 73.3). Precentral gyrus is outlined anteriorly

by the precentral sulcus and posteriorly by the central sulcus. Central sulcus begins near the interhemispheric fissure and descends in a slight forward angle toward the sylvian fissure. Central sulcus is longer than other adjacent sulci and is least intersected by other sulci. Precentral sulcus is frequently discontinuous and intersected by superior and inferior frontal sulci on its course toward the sylvian fissure.

On axial MR images (Fig. 73.2A and B), four features help to localize the central sulcus and precentral gyrus (9–11).

1. The sagittally oriented superior frontal sulcus at its posterior end meets the coronally oriented precentral sulcus; the adjacent gyrus posterior to the precentral sulcus is the precentral gyrus.
2. The right and left marginal sulci (the ascending terminal portion of the cingulate sulcus) on either side of the interhemispheric fissure produce an easily recognizable mustache-like image (Fig. 73.2A). Central sulcus is usually the first sulcus anterior to this marginal sulcus in most individuals.
3. Precentral gyrus is often 1.5- to 2-fold bigger (sagittal thickness) than the adjacent postcentral gyrus.
4. The hand motor area on precentral gyrus has an easily recognizable morphologic pattern in most individuals and can further aid in identification of precentral gyrus. The most common morphologic pattern described on axial image is the "inverted omega" or "knob" or "knuckle" like appearance, with its rounded knob abutting the central sulcus (12). Other morphologic patterns such as "horizontal epsilon" and "asymmetric horizontal epsilons" have been recognized (10,11).

On sagittal MR images, the central sulcus and precentral gyrus can be identified at three different levels—the far lateral surface, along the hand motor region, and over the medial surface (Figs. 73.1A and 73.2C and D).

1. As described earlier, in far lateral sagittal images, at the anterior end of sylvian fissure, the anterior ascending rami of sylvian fissure can be identified (Fig. 73.1A). The sulcus

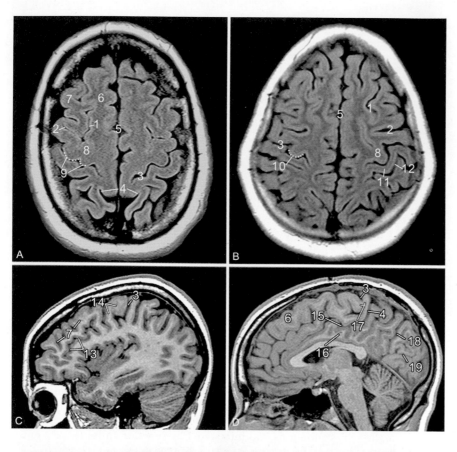

FIGURE 73.2 Primary motor area: Major landmarks on axial (**A** and **B**) and sagittal images (**C** and **D**) to identify the central sulcus and primary motor area (precentral gyrus). 1, superior frontal sulcus; 2, precentral sulcus; 3, central sulcus; 4, marginal sulcus (note mustache-like appearance); 5, interhemispheric fissure; 6, superior frontal gyrus; 7, middle frontal gyrus (note "zig-zag appearance" in sagittal image); 8, precentral gyrus; 9, "horizontal epsilon" shaped hand motor area; 10, "knob" shaped hand motor area in a different subject; 11, postcentral gyrus; 12, postcentral sulcus; 13, inferior frontal sulcus;14, posteriorly directed "hook" shaped hand motor area on sagittal plane; 15, cingulate sulcus; 16, cingulate gyrus; 17, paracentral lobule; 18, parieto-occipital sulcus; 19, calcarine fissure.

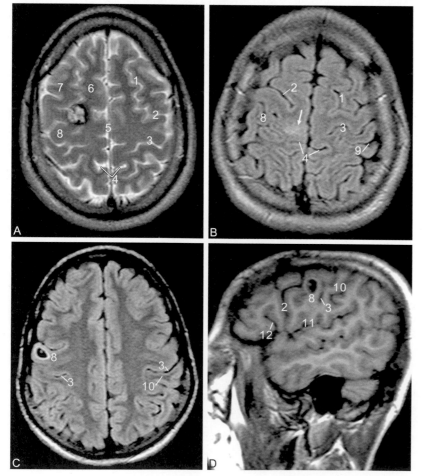

FIGURE 73.3 Lesions around the region of central sulcus and precentral gyrus. **A:** T2-weighted image shows a cavernoma at the junction of right superior frontal gyrus and precentral gyrus. **B:** FLAIR image shows an area of hyperintensity over the paramedian precentral and postcentral gyrus. **C, D:** A cystic lesion in the precentral gyrus over the lateral convexity displayed in axial and sagittal planes. 1, superior frontal sulcus; 2, precentral sulcus; 3, central sulcus; 4, marginal sulcus; 5, interhemispheric fissure; 6, superior frontal gyrus; 7, middle frontal gyrus; 8, precentral gyrus; 9, postcentral sulcus; 10, postcentral gyrus; 11, sylvian fissure; 12, anterior rami of sylvian fissure.

posterior and parallel to the anterior ascending rami denotes inferior precentral sulcus which descends inferiorly and often unites with the sylvian fissure. Central sulcus lies posterior and parallel to the precentral sulcus and it usually does not unite with the sylvian fissure unlike the precentral sulcus. Thus, the opercular (lower) ends of the precentral gyrus and postcentral gyrus (primary sensory cortex) unite to form the subcentral gyrus (4,5).

2. Further medially on sagittal sections (Fig. 73.2C), the hand motor area may be recognized as a posteriorly directed "hook" shaped appearance (the sagittal view of the "knob" described on axial), usually better visible if thin sagittal sections are obtained.

3. Further medially (Fig. 73.2D), in the medial aspect of the cerebral hemisphere, identification of cingulate sulcus and its ascending segment—the marginal sulcus, assist in delineation of central sulcus. Central sulcus makes a small dip in the medial surface and is often the first sulcus anterior to marginal sulcus. The region on either side of the central sulcus on the medial side forms the paracentral lobule which carries motor and sensory representation for contralateral lower extremity. Marginal sulcus marks the posterior margin of the paracentral lobule.

On coronal MR images, precise identification of central sulcus and precentral gyrus is difficult. On volume acquisition images, inferior precentral gyrus may be identified by tracing the inferior frontal sulcus posteriorly.

Visual Area: The Calcarine Cortex

Calcarine cortex, the primary visual area is located in the inferior and superior lips of the calcarine fissure in the occipital lobes. Calcarine fissure can be readily identified on the sagittal and coronal images (Figs. 73.4 and 73.5) (12). On sagittal images close to midline (Fig. 73.4A), in the medial surface of the occipital lobe, calcarine fissure extends from a point below the splenium of corpus callosum to the occipital pole. The

parieto-occipital sulcus extends from the anterior part of calcarine fissure and extends upwards in an oblique direction toward the dorsal surface of the brain. Between the parieto-occipital sulcus and the calcarine fissure lie the cuneus—a wedge-shaped region in medial occipital lobe. Precuneus lie anterior to this, between the parieto-occipital sulcus and the marginal sulcus. On axial images, parieto-occipital sulcus is more readily visualized on multiple slices because of the oblique orientation of the parieto-occipital sulcus (Fig. 73.4B).

On coronal MR images, both calcarine fissure and parieto-occipital sulcus are readily identified as the two major fissures in medial occipital lobes that diverge as they course posteriorly (Fig. 73.4C–E). Calcarine fissure becomes shallow as it courses posteriorly and does not quite extend to the occipital pole. The parieto-occipital sulcus is generally deeper and reaches dorsal surface, and can normally be somewhat asymmetric in depth and configuration (12).

Temporal Lobe

Temporal lobe epilepsy remains the most common surgically remediable medically refractory epilepsy syndrome. Broadly, temporal lobe epilepsy is categorized as mesial temporal epilepsy and lateral temporal epilepsy syndromes based on presumed anatomic origin of epileptogenicity. Temporal lobe on its outer surface is limited superiorly from the frontal lobe by sylvian fissure. The posterior limits of temporal lobe are poorly defined by an imaginary line from the preoccipital notch of the basal aspect of temporal lobe to the superior aspect of parieto-occipital sulcus. Lateral temporal region consists of three major gyri, namely the superior, middle, and inferior temporal gyri divided by the superior and inferior temporal sulci. There are two gyri on the basal aspect—the laterally located fusiform or occipito-temporal gyrus and the medially located parahippocampal gyrus (PHG). Fusiform gyrus is limited laterally from inferior temporal gyrus by lateral occipito-temporal sulcus and separated medially from

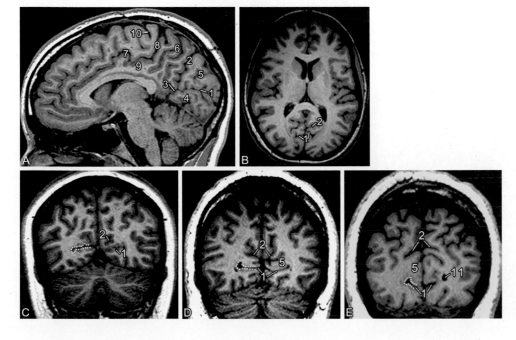

FIGURE 73.4 Visual cortex: Major landmarks on sagittal (**A**), axial (**B**), and coronal (**C–E**) planes to display calcarine fissure and parieto-occipital sulcus. 1, calcarine fissure; 2, parieto occipital sulcus; 3, anterior calcarine sulcus; 4, lingual gyrus; 5, cuneus; 6, precuneus; 7, cingulate sulcus; 8, marginal sulcus; 9, cingulate gyrus; 10, central sulcus; 11, occipital horn of lateral ventricle. Dotted lines on coronal images indicate region of visual cortex on the right side.

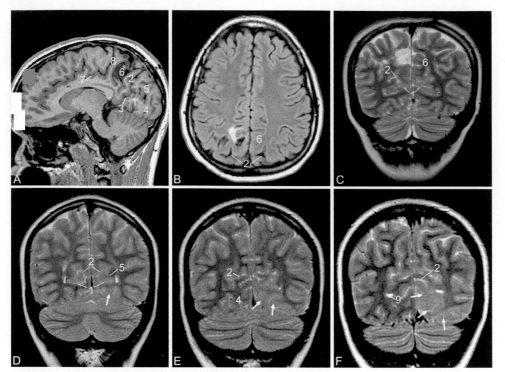

FIGURE 73.5 Lesions around the calcarine fissure and parieto-occipital sulcus. **A–C:** Residual tumor with postoperative changes noted in the right precuneus region displayed in sagittal, axial, and coronal planes. Note that the lesion is anterior to the parieto-occipital sulcus and posterior to the marginal sulcus. **D–F:** T2 weighted image shows hyperintensity *(arrows)* of the cortex and subcortical white matter in the left occipital lobe; lesion is inferior to calcarine fissure in anterior images (**D**) but involves calcarine fissure, cuneus and lateral occipital gyrus in posterior sections (**F**). 1, calcarine fissure; 2, parieto-occipital sulcus; 3, anterior calcarine sulcus; 4, lingual gyrus; 5, cuneus; 6, precuneus; 7, cingulate sulcus; 8, marginal sulcus; 9, occipital horn of lateral ventricle.

the PHG by collateral sulcus. Temporal structures medial to the collateral sulcus are referred to as mesial temporal structures (13–17).

Mesial temporal structures are best visualized on volumetric high-resolution coronal MR images (Fig. 73.6). Hippocampal formation, amygdala, and PHG are usually considered together as part of the mesial temporal epilepsy network. The term hippocampal formation is often used to denote the hippocampus proper along with dentate gyrus. Hippocampus derives its name from its morphologic resemblance to "seahorse," best

appreciated on sagittal images (Fig. 73.6A). It has three parts, namely head, body, and tail of hippocampus, from anterior to posterior. The head and body of hippocampus extend posteriorly along the inferomedial border of temporal horns of lateral ventricles (Fig. 73.6A and B). Head of hippocampus is the most voluminous part and occupies the anterior end of hippocampus (Fig. 73.6D). Head of hippocampus is further recognized by its typical undulating superior margin produced by the digitations on the ventricular surface of the structure, better visualized on coronal T2-weighted or inversion recovery images. Many

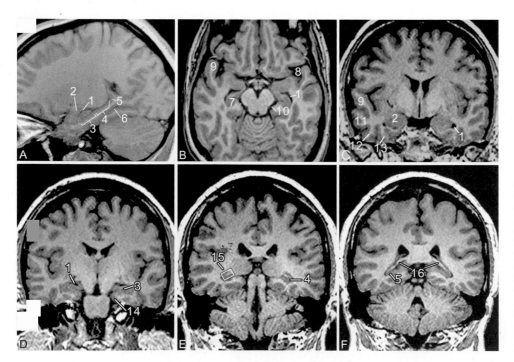

FIGURE 73.6 Temporal lobe structures displayed in sagittal (**A**), axial (**B**), and coronal (**C–F**) planes. 1, temporal horn of lateral ventricle; 2, amygdala; 3, head of hippocampus; 4, body of hippocampus; 5, tail of hippocampus; 6, collateral sulcus; 7, hippocampus; 8, sylvian fissure; 9, superior temporal gyrus; 10, ambiens cistern; 11, middle temporal gyrus; 12, inferior temporal gyrus; 13, occipito-temporal (fusiform) gyrus; 14, parahippocampal gyrus; 15, fimbriae—hyperintense structure within the box; 16, cruri of fornix.

landmarks have been used to identify body and tail of hippocampus, but the most useful would be internal landmarks such as fimbriae and crus fornix—the output tracts of hippocampus. On the coronal MR images, posterior to the head of hippocampus, the appearance of fimbriae signals the junction of head and body of hippocampus (Fig. 73.6E). Further posteriorly, the clear appearance of crus fornix signals the beginning of the tail of hippocampus (Fig. 73.6F). The tail of the hippocampus along with fornix course superiorly and medially along the medial margins of atria of lateral ventricles. The dentate gyrus is often indistinguishable from the hippocampus proper and forms a single unit. Dentate gyrus runs parallel to the hippocampus with its cuplike superior surface covering the CA4 region, forming the hilus of hippocampus. Dentate gyrus continues anteriorly as the band of Giacomini, also referred as tail of dentate gyrus and posteriorly curves around the callosum as indusium griseum. The amygdala, located on the roof of the temporal horn of the lateral ventricle is anterior and superior to the head of hippocampus (Fig. 73.6C). Amygdala fuses with the globus pallidus superiorly (13–18).

PHG is located inferolateral to the hippocampal formation and extends posteriorly along the margin of the tentorium cerebelli in contact with the ambiens cistern medially. Hippocampal sulcus separates the PHG from hippocampal formation superiorly, and collateral sulcus separates it from the fusiform gyrus laterally on the basal aspect (Fig. 73.6C and D). Anterior end of PHG is hooked backwards and medially, to form the uncus. PHG has two components, namely the subiculum and the entorhinal area. Subiculum, the superomedial part of PHG is continuous with the CA1 of hippocampus and forms the bed of hippocampal formation. Entorhinal area is a poorly demarcated area located in uncus and the anterior extension of PHG. In the posterior part, the anterior end of calcarine fissure divides the PHG into a superior and an inferior part. The superior part called isthmus curves up and continues with the cingulate gyrus, and the inferior part continues posteriorly with the lingual gyrus of occipital lobe (13–16).

MRI: TECHNICAL CONSIDERATIONS

Most centers use a 1.5 T MRI for routine imaging to evaluate for medically refractory partial epilepsy. 3 T MRI scanners are more expensive and are not widely available at present. 3 T MRI is likely to be used widely in the next few years and may potentially replace the 1.5 T MRI for imaging of potential epilepsy surgical candidates. Most MRI studies for evaluation of epilepsy incorporate a sagittal T1-weighted spin-echo acquisition as a scout image to position the slices of the subsequent pulse sequences. The other sequences and the imaging planes are tailored according to the referral information about presumptive epileptogenic zone. Broadly, two kinds of protocols are used in epilepsy imaging—temporal lobe protocol and extratemporal protocol. Different centers use different sets of sequences in these protocols. In general, high soft tissue contrast, thin sections, and imaging in all three planes, are critical to epilepsy protocols. A cost and time effective protocol, frequently employed at Cleveland Clinic is shown in Table 73.1.

In general, T1-weighted (short repetition time (TR), short echo time (TE)) images serve largely to define the anatomy

TABLE 73.1

EPILEPSY PROTOCOL MRI COMMONLY USED AT CLEVELAND CLINIC

Mandatory sequences[a]	Supplemental imaging that may be helpful
Temporal	
Sagittal T1 (4-mm slices)	Axial TSE T2
Coronal three-dimensional gradient-echo (1 mm slices) sequence (e.g., SPGR, MP-RAGE)	Axial TSE IR (4-mm slices)
Coronal TSE T2 (4-mm slices)	T2* gradient-echo—axial and coronal[c]
Coronal TSE FLAIR (4-mm slices)[b]	Contrast study as needed[d]
	DWI[e]
Extratemporal	
Sagittal T1 (4-mm slices)	Coronal TSE T2 (4-mm slices)[f]
Coronal three-dimensional gradient-echo sequence (e.g., SPGR, MP-RAGE) (1-mm slices)	Coronal TSE IR (4-mm slices)[f]
Axial TSE T2 (4-mm thick slices)	T2* gradient-echo—axial and coronal
Axial TSE FLAIR (4-mm slices)	Contrast study as needed[d]
	DWI[e]

TSE, Turbo spin echo; SPGR, spoiled gradient-recalled echo; MP-RAGE, magnetization prepared rapid acquisition gradient echo; IR, inversion recovery; FLAIR, fluid-attenuated inversion recovery; SWI, susceptibility weighted imaging; DWI, diffusion weighted imaging.
[a]3 T MRI is preferred.
[b]FLAIR is unhelpful and sometimes misleading in children below 18 to 24 months of age.
[c]Gradient-echo sequences or SWI—in cavernomas, arterio-venous malformations, remote hemorrhages, post-traumatic epilepsy, Sturge–Weber syndrome.
[d]Contrast study—for tumor-like lesions, vascular malformations, suspected Sturge–Weber syndrome, acute symptomatic seizures.
[e]DWI—acute symptomatic seizures, suspected strokes, cystic lesions (epidermoid cyst), tumors.
[f]Should ensure study of entire brain including frontal and occipital poles.

and T2-weighted (long TR and long TE) images are well suited for detecting most brain pathology. Fast spin-echo (FSE) or hybrid rapid acquisition relaxation enhancement sequences has replaced the earlier double echo T2-weighted imaging because of inherent advantages in signal-to-noise ratio, acquisition time, and reduction in motion artifacts (19,20). The heavily T2-weighted images provide strong contrast between CSF and brain parenchyma, and tissues with long T2 relaxation times. On the other hand, strong contrast produced by very long TRs and long echo trains can be detrimental and may obscure some parenchymal lesions and gray-white junction (19). The series of 180° pulses used in fast spin-echo T2 images reduces artifacts in plane with CSF motion as well as susceptibility artifacts at bone/CSF interfaces or adjacent to metallic foreign bodies. However, the same effect makes the visualization of some blood products

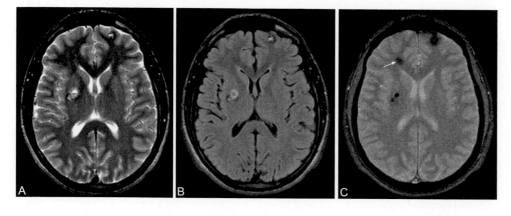

FIGURE 73.7 Axial T2-weighted (**A**), FLAIR (**B**), and gradient-echo images (**C**) show multiple cavernomas. Gradient-echo sequence reveals additional lesion in right frontal region (*arrow*) that is inconspicuous on T2 and FLAIR images.

less evident than on conventional spin-echo imaging. The absence of 180° rephasing pulse in the gradient-echo sequences accentuates the local susceptibility artifact related to blood by-products and compensates for this shortcoming of FSE sequences. Consequently, a gradient-echo sequence should be used in any patients in whom vascular malformations or prior trauma is the apparent etiology (Fig. 73.7).

FLAIR images improve the detection of lesions by suppressing the CSF signal, and accentuating the signal of lesions with relatively short T1 and long T2 relaxation times (21). Fast FLAIR incorporates a preparatory 180° pulse and inversion time before the long TR/long TE FSE sequence to nullify the signal intensity of CSF. Hence it has specific advantage over T2 for lesions in the brain–CSF interface, namely periventricular and subpial cortex location as the CSF signal appears dark. In MTS, the hyperintense signals in the hippocampus may be obscured by the hyperintense CSF in the temporal horns on T2 sequences (21–23). FLAIR, by suppressing the CSF signal accentuates the abnormality in the hippocampal region. Although FLAIR is often thought to be as "a heavily T2-weighted image with dark CSF," the nature of FLAIR sequence causes anything with relatively short T1 and long T2 relaxation times to be hyperintense on the FLAIR images. Some of these lesions may be overlooked on the T2-weighted study alone (Fig. 73.8). Direct comparison of T2 and FLAIR make it clear that the lesions that are evident on both sets of images are often more obvious on the fast FLAIR. Lesions that are better visualized by fast FLAIR

include subtle hyperintensity blurring the gray-white junction of MCD, subcortical foci of gliotic hyperintensity in areas of encephalomalacia, and the extent of infiltration of low-grade neoplasms.

FLAIR has its own limitations. (i) Motion artifacts due to CSF pulsations, often more striking in the basilar cisterns can blur the medial temporal regions. Fast T2 sequences are less susceptible to this and hence correlation with T2 makes this a relatively minor issue. (ii) Suppression of contrast between gray and white matter may obscure visualization of small foci of heterotopic gray matter without correlative pulse sequences. (iii) Detection of prior hemorrhages is limited with both fast FLAIR and fast T2 images because of the common sequence structure. (iv) Lastly, the contrast on fast FLAIR seems to be most limiting in young children (less than 2 years) with immature white matter. Normal children in this age group demonstrate patchy foci of hyperintensity in the subcortical and sometimes periventricular white matter that may be misinterpreted as abnormal. Conventional spin density images tend to be more helpful in this age group.

Volumetric High-Resolution Imaging

Conventional spin-echo imaging is generally sufficient to characterize a lesion when it is relatively large. In the case of smaller lesions, it may be difficult to interpret the nature of lesion or even identify the abnormality at all without high-resolution volumetric imaging. The best example of this would be the case of focal area of dysplastic cortex, which constitutes the major substrate in many patients with refractory extratemporal epilepsy. Diagnosis of these subtle malformations requires critical evaluation of the thickness and morphology of cortical mantle, delineation of the interface between gray and white matter, and detection of minor signal intensity changes in the subcortical white matter. The 4- to 5-mm thick slice of the routine T2 and FLAIR images frequently fail to detect such subtle abnormalities. Consequently, three-dimensional high-resolution volumetric imaging with T1-weighted gradient-echo protocols has become an integral and critical part of imaging for epileptogenic lesions.

Sequences such as fast spoiled gradient-recalled echo (SPGR), magnetization prepared rapid acquisition gradient echo (MP-RAGE), and fast spoiled gradient-recalled acquisition in a steady state (GRASS) can be performed rapidly with very short TRs and TEs that provide strong T1-like contrast between gray and white matter (24,25). The hypointensity of

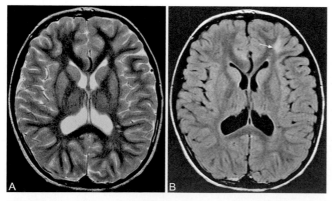

FIGURE 73.8 MR images to demonstrate superior visualization of subcortical hyperintensity associated with focal cortical dysplasia on FLAIR sequence. The dysplastic region in the left frontal region, nearly invisible on the T2-weighted image (**A**) is conspicuous (*arrow*) on the FLAIR image (**B**).

the gray matter is quite comparable to the adjacent CSF and hence signal abnormalities in the gray matter are generally quite subtle. Conversely, many lesions in the white matter are obvious, but the signal intensity characteristics are frequently nonspecific. Lesions such as gliosis, heterotopia, and neoplasm may have the same degree of hypointensity and may be indistinguishable based on volumetric sequence alone. Lesion morphology, correlation with other pulse sequences, and the clinical setting are necessary to distinguish the lesions. Images acquired through the volumetric study protocols do not have the true T1 contrast as they are gradient-echo sequences and not spin-echo sequences as in conventional T1 image. Hence lesions that are typically hyperintense on T1 images such as blood products, dystrophic calcification, and proteinaceous fluids may not be apparent on this high-resolution volumetric imaging using gradient-echo sequences.

These three-dimensional sequences are designed to cover the entire head with very thin 1 mm contiguous slices. These thin slices are especially sensitive to detection of subtle dysmorphism of the cortical mantle and can also highlight minimal mass effect by depicting effacement of adjacent sulcus in case of small tumors. Detection of subtle variations in configuration and volume of hippocampus are greatly improved by high-resolution volumetric imaging and has markedly reduced the need for invasive monitoring in patients with suspected MTS (26). Similarly, detection of concomitant malformation of cortical development in patients with MTS is critical in presurgical evaluation. Routine 4 to 5 mm FLAIR and T2 images are susceptible to volume averaging artifacts and thus misleading when one is trying to asses the morphology of hippocampus. Even minimal tilt of the head in the scanner may accentuate this problem. The thin, contiguous three-dimensional slices minimize the volume averaging errors and improve detection of selective atrophy, developmental dysplasia, and subtle masses such as gliomas in the hippocampal formation by visual inspections alone. Volume averaging errors are further minimized if the slices are taken perpendicular to the long axis of the hippocampal formation. Quantitative volumetric analysis of the hippocampal formation and T2 relaxometry—a technique to quantify the signal intensity, may potentially improve recognition of subtle variations in volume and signal abnormality respectively, than by visual inspection alone. But these techniques are time consuming with minimal additional advantage if any and are not routinely used in practice (27,28).

Other MRI Techniques and Their Utility in Epilepsy

In the last decade, newer MR imaging techniques have tremendously improved our understanding of the disorders of the brain. Careful selection of these sequences may provide useful information in selected causes of epilepsy such as cavernomas, posttraumatic epilepsy, epidermoid cyst, tuberous sclerosis, and acute symptomatic seizures. Some of the newer techniques provide information about the function and connections of the brain further assisting in surgical strategy.

Diffusion weighted imaging (DWI) has revolutionized the neuroimaging of acute stroke, but has limited role in epilepsy. In DWI, diffusion weighting is achieved by two strong diffusion-sensitizing gradients applied symmetrically around the 180° radiofrequency pulse of a spin-echo sequence. This leads to dephasing followed by rephasing of protons. Protons that have moved during and after the dephasing gradient move randomly which leads to incomplete rephasing and signal attenuation. Areas with restricted diffusion of water molecules retain the signal and appear bright on DWI. The degree of diffusion restriction can be quantified by apparent diffusion coefficient (ADC) value. Areas with restricted diffusion appear bright on DWI with low signal intensity (correspondingly low ADC values) on ADC maps (29,30). In focal epilepsies, peri-ictal changes with foci of hyperintensity on DWI with decreased ADC values presumably due to cytotoxic edema have been reported (31,32). Isolated low ADC values without overt hyperintensity on DWI are more common in the peri-ictal studies (33). On the other hand, interictal DWI has revealed increased ADC values which may reflect neuronal loss and increased extracellular space. Other disorders related to epilepsy that may show DWI abnormalities include the following: cortical and subcortical abnormalities in status epilepticus, tumors such as epidermoid cyst (Fig. 73.9), and transient lesions of splenium of corpus callosum related to seizures and antiepileptic drugs (34–36). A significant increase in ADC has been reported in epileptogenic tuber compared to other tubers in patients with tuberous sclerosis and may be helpful in surgical decisions (37).

Diffusion tensor imaging (DTI) is an emerging imaging modality that demonstrates the connections of different regions of the brain. Unlike conventional DWI, the diffusion-sensitizing gradients are applied in six different directions in DTI. As a result, the directionality of water diffusion is studied in addition to magnitude of diffusion. In general, the diffusivity

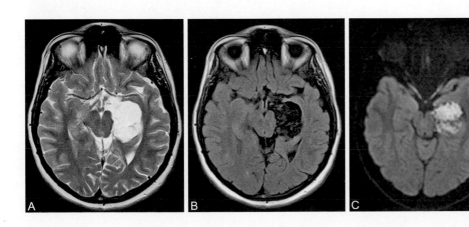

FIGURE 73.9 A cystic lesion in the left medial temporal region, with signal characteristics similar to CSF—hyperintense on T2-weighted image (**A**) and hypointense on FLAIR (**B**), shows diffusion restriction on DWI (**C**) consistent with epidermoid cyst. Histopathology confirmed the diagnosis.

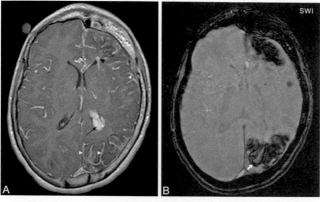

FIGURE 73.10 Contrast enhanced T1-weighted image (**A**), and susceptibility weighted image (SWI) (**B**) in a child with Sturge–Weber syndrome. Contrast study shows enlarged periventricular veins (*black arrow head*), abnormal leptomeningeal (*white arrow heads*), and choroid plexus enhancement (*black arrow*). SWI is superior to visualize the extent of cortical abnormality (*arrow*). Also note diffuse left hemispheric atrophy and thickening of ipsilateral calvarium. (Courtesy of Dr. Ingrid Tuxhorn, Cleveland, OH).

is greater parallel (i.e., along the long axis of the tracts) to than perpendicular to the fiber tracts and this can be quantified by DTI (38,39). DTI and its role in epilepsy evaluation are presented in greater detail in Chapter 77.

Susceptibility weighted imaging (SWI) techniques that exploit differences in magnetic susceptibility of tissue components may provide additional information in epileptogenic lesions containing blood products such as cavernomas, certain posttraumatic epilepsies, and Sturge–Weber syndrome. T2* gradient echo (GRE) is the most commonly used sequence for detecting remote blood products. However, SWI—now widely available commercially, is superior to T2* GRE in detection of remote hemorrhages. SWI is a high-resolution three-dimensional gradient-echo technique which exploits the small differences in magnetic susceptibility among different components of the tissue such as deoxygenated blood, iron, and calcium compared to the surrounding brain tissue. This also illustrates the smallest of veins (because veins contain higher deoxygenated blood) in the submillimeter caliber in great detail. Lesions such as cavernomas tend to be multiple, and some lesions not apparent on T2* GREs may be recognized with SWI (40). In Sturge–Weber syndrome, SWI improves detection of transmedullary and periventricular veins, and cortical gyral abnormalities compared to contrast enhanced T1 images (Fig. 73.10). The cortical gyral abnormalities on SWI seem to represent venous stasis related hypoxia and correspond to the hypometabolic areas detected on FDG PET. Thus SWI has the potential to show functional information in addition to anatomical details in Sturge–Weber syndrome (41,42).

STRATEGIES TO IMPROVE LESION DETECTION

Conventional epilepsy protocol imaging as outlined, using a 1.5 T MRI is sufficient for most cases of chronic epilepsy. However, the scenario of a patient with medically refractory epilepsy with no lesions detected on MRI is fairly common in epilepsy centers. Failure to diagnose a structural abnormality

reduces the likelihood of consideration for epilepsy surgery. Invasive monitoring with subdural grids and depth electrodes may be required in some of these patients. The success rates for epilepsy surgeries done on such patients with "unremarkable MRI" are substantially lower (43–45). The single most common epileptogenic substrate that evades detection in such situation is malformation of cortical development (MCD). Appropriate utilization of newer techniques in MRI may improve the detection of MCD and other subtle lesions missed by the routine epilepsy protocol. Reviewing the initial MRI with a more experienced reader familiar with characteristics of the subtle MCD is probably the first step to improve the detection. Localization data acquired from seizure semiology, EEG, and other imaging modalities such as PET and SPECT may guide to the area of interest and a more focused review of the images can be helpful in some cases. Some of the imaging strategies that may be employed to improve lesion detection are discussed in the following section.

3 T MRI

3 T MRI is being increasingly used in many epilepsy centers and is likely to replace 1.5 for refractory epilepsy imaging protocol. Increase in the magnetic field strength improves the signal-to-noise ratio and contrast-to-noise ratio thereby improving the detection of subtle lesions (46). The gray-white contrast is superior on the volumetric high-resolution imaging with 3 T MRI, despite the difference in T1 relaxation times

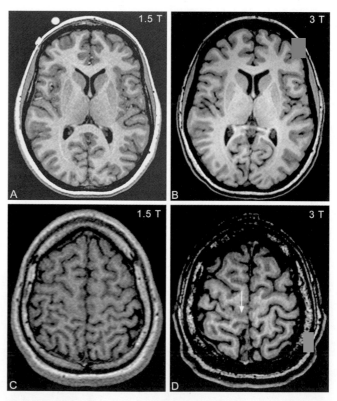

FIGURE 73.11 Comparison between 1.5 T and 3 T MRI (same patient). **A, B:** Axial MP-RAGE images with 1.5 T (**A**) and 3 T (**B**) MRIs show improved signal-to-noise ratio resulting in better gray-white contrast, on 3 T MRI. **C, D:** Subtle blurring of gray-white region on the banks of central sulcus (*arrow*), barely visible on the 1.5 T MRI (**C**) is better visualized on 3 T MRI (**D**).

of brain tissue at 3 T (Fig. 73.11). Subtle blurring at the gray-white junction without hyperintensity on T2 or FLAIR, a common and sometimes the only MRI finding of MCD is better visualized on these images. 3 T MRI is not without its disadvantages. One potential disadvantage with 3 T MRI is decreased gray-white contrast with T1 spin-echo imaging compared to 1.5 T MRI. Inversion recovery sequences can alleviate this effect but cannot be used when one attempts to compare with a contrast enhanced T1 image, as inversion recovery pulse interferes with visualization of contrast. Reducing the excitation flip angle improves gray-white contrast despite reduction in signal-to-noise ratio. Higher magnetic field strength also accentuates the susceptibility effects and this can cause artifacts. Conversely, studies that exploit the susceptibility effects, namely SWI and fMRI techniques such as BOLD (blood oxygenation level-dependent) are benefited by 3 T MRI. Other minor limitations of 3 T study include increased acoustic noise and increased device incompatibility (46–48).

Clinical experience with 3 T MRI in epilepsy suggests improved detection of lesions compared to 1.5 T imaging. Recent studies report a 20% to 48% increase in detection of new or additional information by 3 T study compared to 1 to 1.5 T MRI (46,49,50). Two of these three studies also used phased array coils and it is unclear whether the improved lesion detection rate was solely due to higher magnetic field strength. Higher detection rate of MCD is the main reason for improved yield of 3 T MRI in these studies. Anecdotal experience suggests that these lesions are often visible on 1.5 T studies but are diagnosed with more certainty by 3 T study.

Surface Coils and the Multichannel-Phased Array Coils

Surface coils instead of the routine head coils have been used in an attempt to improve imaging of selected regions of the brain and help to confirm or exclude suspicious abnormalities over the presumed epileptogenic zone. Surface coils improve the signal-to-noise ratio thereby improving the spatial resolution of the structures close the surface coils (Fig. 73.12). The structures away from the "view" of the surface coils are poorly visualized. As a result, poor imaging quality for deeper structures makes surface coils less desirable for evaluation of mesial temporal structures. In the past, limited coverage of brain by surface coils required careful planning with pre-imaging working hypothesis about the possible epileptogenic zone to guide the placement of surface coils. Localizing information from seizure semiology, EEG, video-EEG, prior MRI (in case of subtle questionable abnormalities) and other studies such as SPECT and PET should guide the placement of the coils (51). Limited coverage of cortex (and the resultant "tunnel vision"), overall increase in scan time, need for pre-imaging hypothesis, and decreased signal-to-noise ratio for the deeper structures were major limitations precluding routine use of surface coils.

Increased anatomical coverage by increase in the number of elements in the phased array coils has minimized the limitations of traditional surface coils. Using 3 T MRI with eight channel flexible phased array coils in 40 patients with focal epilepsy, a 65% increase in yield was reported in a subgroup of patients with previous unremarkable 1.5 T MRI (50). Though the differences appear robust, this study did not distinguish the effect of the higher field strength from the effect of surface coils. In another recent study of 25 patients with extratemporal epilepsy, 3 T MRI with two flexible surface coils was compared with 1 to 1.5 T MRI. Though additional abnormalities were seen in 20% of cases on 3 T MRI, authors concluded that there was no added benefit with the use of surface coils (49). Some centers use a 32-channel phased array coil in epilepsy imaging. More research on the use of such coils is required to guide routine use of this technique in clinical practice.

Three-Dimensional Reconstructions

Each of the pixels that constitute a two-dimensional MR image actually has a third dimension in anatomic imaging—the dimension of the thickness. As three-dimensional MRI produces slices without an interslice gap, it avoids the problem of lost data found with conventional two-dimensional imaging. If the imaging voxels in the three-dimensional acquisitions are designed to achieve an equivalent length in all three imaging planes (isotropic data), the images can be reconstructed in any alternate plane without compromising the spatial resolution or fidelity when compared to the original images. On the other hand, if the voxels were too anisotropic, the reconstructed images will be noticeably degraded compared with the original data. In practice, data can only be "nearly" isotropic as patients will not routinely tolerate the length of time required to acquire truly isotropic data.

With standard imaging planes, the complex interposition of gyrus and sulcus of normal brain's convolutional pattern

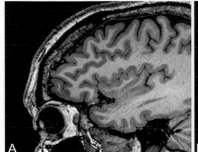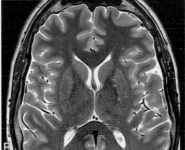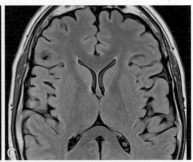

FIGURE 73.12 MRI with surface coils placed over the frontal regions yield high-resolution images of the frontal lobe. Deeper structures farther from the coil (temporal structures on sagittal image and basal ganglia on axial images) are poorly visualized due to decreased signal-to-noise ratio.

potentially lead to errors in interpretation of thickness in gray matter. Slices that cut through the in-plane cortex (along the gray matter) leads to apparent thickened cortex and potential misdiagnosis as malformed cortex. Conversely, cautious avoidance of such overcalls can potentially lead to underdiagnosis of truly thickened areas of malformed cortex as well. Subtle MCDs may be suspected on the original images but are difficult to confirm in the original plane, until after the images are reconstructed in other planes. Alternatively, the lesion may be clearly apparent on the original acquisition, yet there may be difficulty in delineating the spatial relationships of the lesion relative to adjacent eloquent cortex. Volumetric high-resolution images obtained in epilepsy protocols can be reconstructed in various planes. Reformatting the images in multiple planes may enable to view the images in a plane perpendicular to the gyri thereby reducing the spurious thickening of cortex seen in images in-plane with the gyri.

Image reconstruction in a curvilinear plane—a plane parallel to the cortical surface and perpendicular in relation to the gyri, is being performed in some centers. The resultant images show progressively deeper surfaces of the brain like "peeling an onion." In this technique, a surface is obtained initially by manually outlining the cortical surface in the coronal plane at selected intervals. This surface serves as a matrix to generate progressively deeper slices using a software. These curved slices will result in more uniform distribution of gray matter on both hemispheres assisting in comparison of homologous regions of the cortex (52–54). Apart from improving the detection of subtle MCDs, such surface reconstructions have the potential to assess the location of subdural grids and depth electrodes more precisely. However the clinical utility of these techniques in large patient population has not been studied.

Serial MRI in Infants and Young Children

Signal characteristics of immature myelin in infants and young children can pose significant challenges in interpretation of studies obtained in infancy. Lesions such as MCDs and cortical tubers have varying signal characteristics based on the developmental stage of the myelin of the lesions and the surrounding brain. For example, in infants, dysplastic cortex and adjacent subcortical regions may appear hypointense on T2-weighted images and hyperintense on T1 sequences, contrary to the reverse pattern seen in older children and adults (55–57). The lesions characteristics change to the more typical adult pattern over time with progressive myelination. In some patients, with progressive myelination these lesions tend to become less obvious or rarely "vanish" on follow-up imaging (58). Reviewing only the most recent images may fail to detect the lesions. Conversely, a "new lesion" of MCD may be detected on follow-up imaging in a child with previously "normal MRI" in early infancy. The poor visualization of the lesions on earlier MRI may be explained by the poor background contrast of the bright immature myelin on the T2 images (59). Follow-up MRI during second year of life or later allowing normal myelination to take place may unmask areas of MCD with decreased or absent subcortical myelin. Similarly, cortical tubers of tuberous sclerosis may be more evident on follow-up imaging (Fig. 73.13). Apart from changes in myelination, increased growth of tubers and dystrophic calcification may contribute to their better visibility on follow-up imaging. Serial MRIs are also helpful in other epileptic disorders such as Rasmussen's encephalitis and Sturge–Weber syndrome to demonstrate progressive regional or hemispheric cortical atrophy.

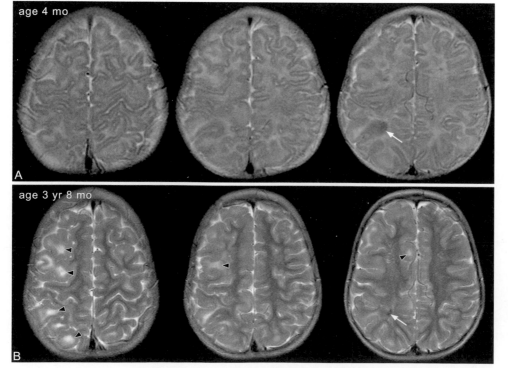

FIGURE 73.13 MRI in a child with tuberous sclerosis performed at 4 months of age (**A**), and at 3 years and 8 months of age (**B**). Cortical and subcortical tubers *(arrow heads)* were more evident on follow-up imaging because of myelination of white matter, improving the "background contrast." Increase in size of lesions with brain growth, calcification *(arrow)* and abnormal myelination around the lesions may also contribute to better visibility on follow-up MRI. (Courtesy of Dr. Ajay Gupta, Cleveland, OH).

MINI-ATLAS OF SOME TYPICAL EPILEPTOGENIC LESIONS

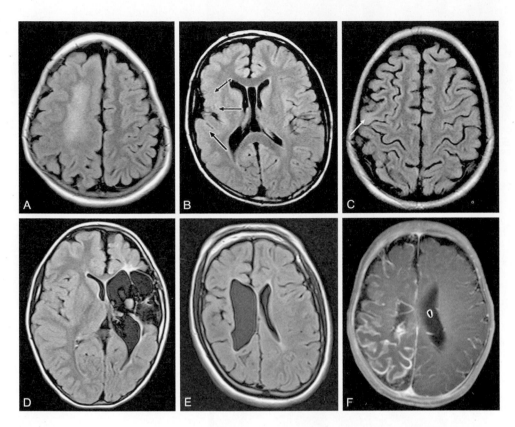

FIGURE 73.14 Hemispheric epileptogenic lesions. **A:** Right hemimegalencephaly; **B:** Right multilobar dysplasia with relative sparing of medial occipital region. **C:** A case of Rasmussen encephalitis with atrophy of right hemisphere and hyperintensity in the precentral gyrus *(arrow)*. **D:** Cystic encephalomalacia and gliosis on the left hemisphere due to remote ischemic stroke. **E:** Perinatal brain injury with right hemispheric atrophy—both cortical and subcortical. Note minimal involvement of the left hemisphere as well. **F:** A case of Sturge–Weber syndrome with right hemispheric atrophy with leptomeningeal enhancement and enlarged periventricular veins.

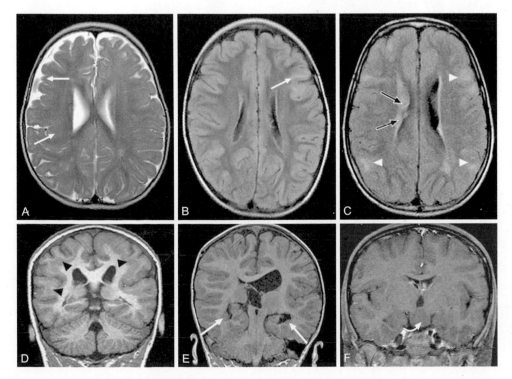

FIGURE 73.15 Focal malformations of cortical development and related disorders. **A:** Right frontal malformation with abnormal sulcal pattern and thickened cortex *(arrows)*. **B:** Left frontal dysplasia with subcortical hyperintensity. **C:** Cortical tubers *(white arrow heads)* and subependymal nodules *(arrows)* in tuberous sclerosis. **D:** Diffuse subcortical band heterotopia—"the double cortex." **E:** Multiple malformations including periventricular nodular heterotopia around temporal horns *(arrows)* and maloriented right hippocampus. **F:** Hypothalamic hamartoma—note signal intensity of the lesion similar to the gray matter.

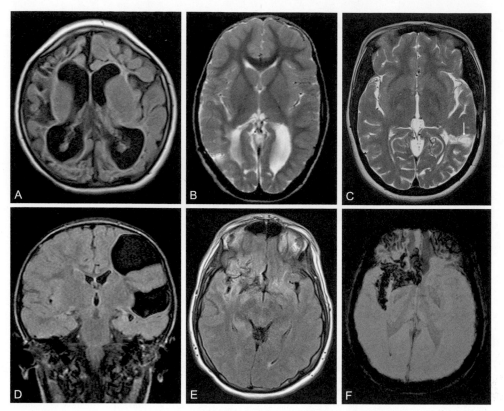

FIGURE 73.16 Porencephaly and encephalomalacia of various etiologies. **A:** Diffuse multicystic encephalomalacia and gliosis secondary to global hypoxic ischemic injury. **B:** Periventricular leukomalacia due to perinatal brain injury. **C:** Left posterior temporal encephalomalacia due to prior ischemic stroke in a patient with sickle cell anemia. **D:** Porencephalic cysts in left frontal and temporal lobes related to multiple hemorrhages in the neonatal period. Also note left mesial temporal sclerosis. **E, F:** Encephalomalacia due to remote herpes encephalitis on FLAIR images (**E**). Susceptibility weighted images (**F**) show marked hypointensity in the regions of prior petechial hemorrhages.

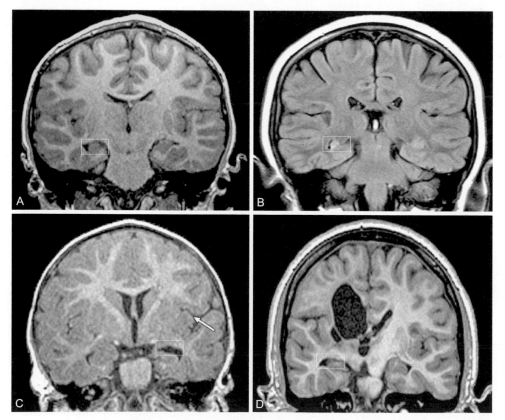

FIGURE 73.17 Mesial temporal sclerosis and dual pathology. **A, B:** Right mesial temporal sclerosis with prominent volume loss and hyperintense signal of hippocampus. **C:** Left hippocampal atrophy with atrophy of ipsilateral fronto-temporal cortex as evident from prominent left sylvian fissure (arrow). **D:** Right hippocampal atrophy associated with porencephaly right frontal subcortical region and basal ganglia.

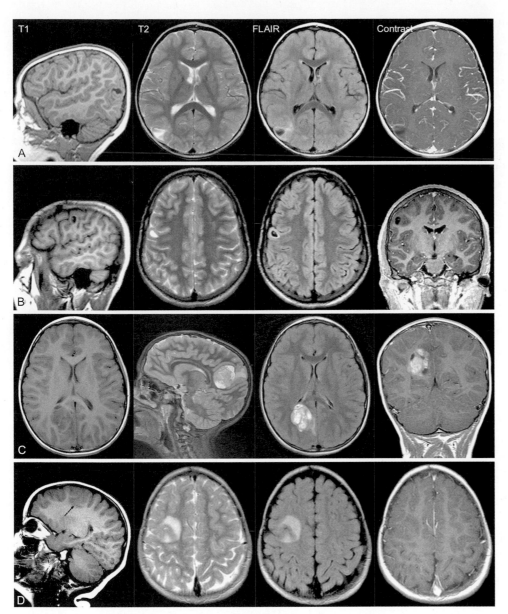

FIGURE 73.18 Tumors and hamartomas. **A:** A nonenhancing lesion with cystic and solid components in the right pareito-occipital junction without mass effect. Histopathology showed features of ganglioglioma. **B:** A predominantly cystic lesion in the right precentral gyrus without contrast enhancement or mass effect, similar to lesion on **A**. Histopathology confirmed dysembryoplastic neuroepithelial tumor. **C:** A predominantly solid tumor in the right precuneus and posterior cingulate region, with prominent heterogeneous contrast enhancement and mild mass effect. Histopathology showed evidence for pleomorphic xanthoastrocytoma. **D:** A nonenhancing lesion in the right posterior frontal region with evidence of vasogenic edema. A low-grade glioma was suspected. Histopathology showed features of meningioangiomatois, a hamartomatous lesion.

MAGNETIC RESONANCE SPECTROSCOPY

Magnetic resonance spectroscopy (MRS) offers the potential to noninvasively analyze the biochemical composition of an area of brain. Certain patterns of focal alterations in the biochemical structure may reflect altered neuronal or glial function providing localizing information. MRS can be acquired in any conventional high-field MRI system with appropriate software (60). Proton spectroscopy is the most widely accepted MRS technique in clinical settings, as it demands no additional hardware and has superior spatial resolution than alternative nuclei such as phosphorus. MRS generates a proton spectrum for a voxel or group of voxels that can be as small as 1 cm^3. Only limited areas of the brain can be studied in a time fashion that is acceptable for clinical practice. It is therefore necessary to have a preimaging hypothesis about the location of epileptogenic focus to decide on the placement of

spectroscopy voxels. The position of the voxel is chosen based on localizing information available from conventional MRI or other localizing information when MRI is normal. Restricted anatomic coverage with single-voxel techniques is a major limiting factor when the lesions are large or indistinct or absent on the MRI. Multivoxel technique provides the capability of greater anatomic coverage and is particularly appealing if the location of epileptogenic focus is uncertain.

The primary choice in parameters with conventional MRS is between short and long TEs. Long TE acquisition produce spectra that include N-acetylaspartate (NAA), choline, creatine/phosphocreatine, and possibly lactate. Short TE acquisitions include the same metabolites as well as myo-inositol, glutamate and glutamine, gamma aminobutyric acid (GABA), alanine, glucose, *scyllo*-inositol/taurine, and protein/lipids (61–63). Changes in relative quantities of these metabolites, in comparison with corresponding tissue on the presumably normal contralateral hemisphere or controls are used to characterize the tissue metabolically. NAA signal is the best studied and most sought after signal on MRS; NAA signal though signify neuronal loss or dysfunction, a linear correlation between the two has not been found. Mitochondrial dysfunction without actual neuronal loss has also been postulated as the mechanism for low NAA signal. Decreased regional NAA concentration in the epileptogenic zone is the most characteristic interictal abnormality described in intractable partial epilepsy. Abnormal lactate peaks in the epileptogenic zone may be identified when MRS study is performed within 6 hours of seizures.

Use of MRS in localization of epilepsy has been studied in both temporal and extratemporal epilepsies. In patients with bilateral mesial temporal abnormalities, the epilepsy may arise predominantly from one side. In such cases, studies using single-voxel technique comparing the two temporal lobes have provided additional concordant lateralizing information enabling surgical decisions (60,64,65). In a meta-analysis of MRS in temporal lobe epilepsy, presence of ipsilateral MRS abnormality and absence of bilateral abnormalities were associated with seizure good outcome. However, bilateral MRS abnormalities may be seen in as many as 35% of temporal lobe epilepsy patients with good outcome (66). In a study of nonlesional extratemporal epilepsy, widespread spectroscopic abnormality—greatest in the presumed epileptogenic zone has been reported (67,68). The true impact of MRS on surgical decision making for complex patients with poor localization information is unclear and has not been studied critically to provide meaningful integration of MRS in the presurgical epilepsy work up.

Ability to study tissue levels of glutamine and GABA by MRS offers lot of scope to study various epileptic disorders, as elevation of the excitatory glutamate and reduction of inhibitory GABA can result in seizures. Elevation of "glutamine plus glutamate" in frontal lobes has been reported in idiopathic generalized epilepsies as well (69,70). Despite the attractive concept of noninvasive biochemical sampling of the brain, MRS has not impacted epilepsy practice to earn a definitive role in routine presurgical work up. With the advent and wide availability of other tools such as PET and SPECT, the role of MRS has further diminished.

CONCLUSION

Anatomic visualization of substrates of epilepsy by MRI has tremendously advanced the field of epilepsy surgery. Various MRI techniques providing information on function and connections of the various areas of the brain has further helped the surgical strategy. Still, a significant number of patients with refractory partial epilepsy do not have an identifiable lesion on MRI. Epilepsy surgery in such cases, when performed often requires invasive intracranial monitoring with subdural grids and depth electrodes, despite which the outcome remains poor. Malformation of cortical development is the most common lesion that evades detection in these cases. Further improvements in MRI techniques and its integration with other modalities such as SPECT, PET, and MEG may help to improve the detection of these lesions and minimize the need for invasive monitoring. Development of newer MR techniques in future may also have the potential to improve the understanding of the cytoarchitectural and molecular abnormalities of brain with a greater impact in the field of epilepsy.

References

1. Penfield W, Jasper H. *Epilepsy and the Functional Anatomy of the Human Brain*. Boston, MA: Little Brown and Company; 1954.
2. Rosenow F, Luders H. Presurgical evaluation of epilepsy. *Brain*. 2001; 124(pt 9):1683–1700.
3. Wyllie E, Lachhwani DK, Gupta A, et al. Successful surgery for epilepsy due to early brain lesions despite generalized EEG findings. *Neurology*. 2007;69(4):389–397.
4. Ebeling U, Steinmetz H, Huang YX, et al. Topography and identification of the inferior precentral sulcus in MR imaging. *Am J Roentgenol*. 1989; 153(5):1051–1056.
5. Naidich TP, Valavanis AG, Kubik S. Anatomic relationships along the low-middle convexity: Part I—normal specimens and magnetic resonance imaging. *Neurosurgery*. 1995;36(3):517–532.
6. Ojemann G, Ojemann J, Lettich E, et al. Cortical language localization in left, dominant hemisphere—an electrical stimulation mapping investigation in 117 patients. *J Neurosurg*. 1989;71(3):316–326.
7. Devinsky O, Perrine K, Hirsch J, et al. Relation of cortical language distribution and cognitive function in surgical epilepsy patients. *Epilepsia*. 2000;41(4):400–404.
8. Pataraia E, Simos PG, Castillo EM, et al. Reorganization of language-specific cortex in patients with lesions or mesial temporal epilepsy. *Neurology*. 2004;63(10):1825–1832.
9. Kido DK, LeMay M, Levinson AW, et al. Computed tomographic localization of the precentral gyrus. *Radiology*. 1980;135(2):373–377.
10. Yousry TA, Schmid UD, Alkadhi H, et al. Localization of the motor hand area to a knob on the precentral gyrus. A new landmark. *Brain*. 1997; 120(pt 1):141–157.
11. Caulo M, Briganti C, Mattei PA, et al. New morphologic variants of the hand motor cortex as seen with MR imaging in a large study population. *Am J Neuroradiol*. 2007;28(8):1480–1485.
12. Tamraz JC, Outin-Tamraz C, Saban R. MR imaging anatomy of the optic pathways. *Radiol Clin North Am*. 1999;37(1):1–36.
13. DeFelipe J, Fernandez-Gil MA, Kastanauskaite A, et al. Macroanatomy and microanatomy of the temporal lobe. *Semin Ultrasound CT MR*. 2007; 28(6):404–415.
14. Naidich TP, Daniels DL, Haughton VM, et al. Hippocampal formation and related structures of the limbic lobe: anatomic-MR correlation. Part I. Surface features and coronal sections. *Radiology*. 1987;162(3):747–754.
15. Naidich TP, Daniels DL, Haughton VM, et al. Hippocampal formation and related structures of the limbic lobe: anatomic-MR correlation. Part II. Sagittal sections. *Radiology*. 1987;162(3):755–761.
16. Mark LP, Daniels DL, Naidich TP, et al. Limbic system anatomy: an overview. *Am J Neuroradiol*. 1993;14(2):349–352.
17. Hui F, Cavazos JE, Tien RD. Hippocampus. Normal magnetic resonance imaging anatomy with volumetric studies. *Neuroimaging Clin North Am*. 1997;7(1):11–30.
18. Bernasconi N, Bernasconi A, Caramanos Z, et al. Mesial temporal damage in temporal lobe epilepsy: a volumetric MRI study of the hippocampus, amygdala and parahippocampal region. *Brain*. 2003;126(pt 2):462–469.
19. Mulkern RV, Wong ST, Winalski C, et al. Contrast manipulation and artifact assessment of 2D and 3D RARE sequences. *Magn Reson Imaging*. 1990;8(5):557–566.
20. Jones KM, Mulkern RV, Schwartz RB, et al. Fast spin-echo MR imaging of the brain and spine: current concepts. *Am J Roentgenol*. 1992;158(6): 1313–1320.
21. De Coene B, Hajnal JV, Gatehouse P, et al. MR of the brain using fluid-attenuated inversion recovery (FLAIR) pulse sequences. *Am J Neuroradiol*. 1992;13:1555–1564.
22. Jack CR Jr, Rydberg CH, Krecke KN, et al. Mesial temporal sclerosis: diagnosis with fluid-attenuation inversion-recovery versus spin-echo imaging. *Radiology*. 1996;199:367–373.
23. Bergin PS, Fish DR, Shorvon SD, et al. Magnetic resonance imaging in partial epilepsy: additional abnormalities shown with the fluid attenuation inversion recovery (FLAIR) pulse sequence. *J Neurol Neurosurg Psychiatry*. 1995;58:439–443.
24. Mugler JP III, Spraggins TA, Brookeman JR. T2-weighted three-dimensional MP-RAGE MR imaging. *J Magn Reson Imaging*. 1991;1(6):731–737.
25. Barkovich AJ, Rowley HA, Andermann F. MR in partial epilepsy: value of high-resolution volumetric techniques. *Am J Neuroradiol*. 1995;16(2): 339–343.
26. Kilpatrick C, Cook M, Kaye A, et al. Non-invasive investigations successfully select patients for temporal lobe surgery. *J Neurol Neurosurg Psychiatry*. 1997;63:327–333.
27. Cheon JE, Chang KH, Kim HD, et al. MR of hippocampal sclerosis: comparison of qualitative and quantitative assessments. *Am J Neuroradiol*. 1998;19(3):465–468.
28. Jack CR Jr, Bentley MD, Twomey CK, et al. MR imaging-based volume measurements of the hippocampal formation and anterior temporal lobe: validation studies. *Radiology*. 1990;176(1):205–209.
29. Warach S, Chien D, Li W, et al. Fast magnetic resonance diffusion-weighted imaging of acute human stroke. *Neurology*. 1992;42(9):1717–1723.

30. Hossmann KA, Hoehn-Berlage M. Diffusion and perfusion MR imaging of cerebral ischemia. *Cerebrovasc Brain Metab Rev.* 1995;7(3):187–217.
31. Diehl B, Najm I, Ruggieri P, et al. Periictal diffusion-weighted imaging in a case of lesional epilepsy. *Epilepsia.* 1999;40(11):1667–1671.
32. Diehl B, Najm I, Ruggieri P, et al. Postictal diffusion-weighted imaging for the localization of focal epileptic areas in temporal lobe epilepsy. *Epilepsia.* 2001;42(1):21–28.
33. Oh JB, Lee SK, Kim KK, et al. Role of immediate postictal diffusion-weighted MRI in localizing epileptogenic foci of mesial temporal lobe epilepsy and non-lesional neocortical epilepsy. *Seizure.* 2004;13(7):509–516.
34. Milligan TA, Zamani A, Bromfield E. Frequency and patterns of MRI abnormalities due to status epilepticus. *Seizure.* 2009;18:104–108.
35. Nelles M, Bien CG, Kurthen M, et al. Transient splenium lesions in presurgical epilepsy patients: incidence and pathogenesis. *Neuroradiology.* 2006; 48(7):443–448.
36. Sirin S, Gonul E, Kahraman S, et al. Imaging of posterior fossa epidermoid tumors. *Clin Neurol Neurosurg.* 2005;107(6):461–467.
37. Jansen FE, Braun KP, van Nieuwenhuizen O, et al. Diffusion-weighted magnetic resonance imaging and identification of the epileptogenic tuber in patients with tuberous sclerosis. *Arch Neurol.* 2003;60(11):1580–1584.
38. Pierpaoli C, Jezzard P, Basser PJ, et al. Diffusion tensor MR imaging of the human brain. *Radiology.* 1996;201(3):637–648.
39. Basser PJ, Mattiello J, LeBihan D. Estimation of the effective self-diffusion tensor from the NMR spin echo. *J Magn Reson B.* 1994;103(3):247–254.
40. de Souza JM, Domingues RC, Cruz LC Jr, et al. Susceptibility-weighted imaging for the evaluation of patients with familial cerebral cavernous malformations: a comparison with t2-weighted fast spin-echo and gradient-echo sequences. *Am J Neuroradiol.* 2008;29(1):154–158.
41. Hu J, Yu Y, Juhasz C, et al. MR susceptibility weighted imaging (SWI) complements conventional contrast enhanced T1 weighted MRI in characterizing brain abnormalities of Sturge–Weber syndrome. *J Magn Reson Imaging.* 2008;28(2):300–307.
42. Juhasz C, Haacke EM, Hu J, et al. Multimodality imaging of cortical and white matter abnormalities in Sturge–Weber syndrome. *Am J Neuroradiol.* 2007;28(5):900–906.
43. Kuzniecky R, Burgard S, Faught E, et al. Predictive value of magnetic resonance imaging in temporal lobe epilepsy surgery. *Arch Neurol.* 1993; 50(1):65–69.
44. Mosewich RK, So EL, O'Brien TJ, et al. Factors predictive of the outcome of frontal lobe epilepsy surgery. *Epilepsia.* 2000;41(7):843–849.
45. Chapman K, Wyllie E, Najm I, et al. Seizure outcome after epilepsy surgery in patients with normal preoperative MRI. *J Neurol Neurosurg Psychiatry.* 2005;76(5):710–713.
46. Phal PM, Usmanov A, Nesbit GM, et al. Qualitative comparison of 3-T and 1.5-T MRI in the evaluation of epilepsy. *Am J Roentgenol.* 2008;191(3): 890–895.
47. Schmitz BL, Aschoff AJ, Hoffmann MH, et al. Advantages and pitfalls in 3T MR brain imaging: a pictorial review. *Am J Neuroradiol.* 2005;26(9): 2229–2237.
48. Schmitz BL, Gron G, Brausewetter F, et al. Enhancing gray-to-white matter contrast in 3T T1 spin-echo brain scans by optimizing flip angle. *Am J Neuroradiol.* 2005;26(8):2000–2004.
49. Strandberg M, Larsson EM, Backman S, et al. Pre-surgical epilepsy evaluation using 3T MRI. Do surface coils provide additional information? *Epileptic Disord.* 2008;10(2):83–92.
50. Knake S, Triantafyllou C, Wald LL, et al. 3T phased array MRI improves the presurgical evaluation in focal epilepsies: a prospective study. *Neurology.* 2005;65(7):1026–1031.
51. Grant PE, Barkovich AJ, Wald LL, et al. High-resolution surface-coil MR of cortical lesions in medically refractory epilepsy: a prospective study. *Am J Neuroradiol.* 1997;18(2):291–301.
52. Bastos AC, Korah IP, Cendes F, et al. Curvilinear reconstruction of 3D magnetic resonance imaging in patients with partial epilepsy: a pilot study. *Magn Reson Imaging.* 1995;13(8):1107–1112.
53. Bastos AC, Comeau RM, Andermann F, et al. Diagnosis of subtle focal dysplastic lesions: curvilinear reformatting from three-dimensional magnetic resonance imaging. *Ann Neurol.* 1999;46(1):88–94.
54. Montenegro MA, Li LM, Guerreiro MM, et al. Focal cortical dysplasia: improving diagnosis and localization with magnetic resonance imaging multiplanar and curvilinear reconstruction. *J Neuroimaging.* 2002;12(3): 224–230.
55. Tassi L, Colombo N, Garbelli R, et al. Focal cortical dysplasia: neuropathological subtypes, EEG, neuroimaging and surgical outcome. *Brain.* 2002; 125(pt 8):1719–1732.
56. Colombo N, Tassi L, Galli C, et al. Focal cortical dysplasias: MR imaging, histopathologic, and clinical correlations in surgically treated patients with epilepsy. *Am J Neuroradiol.* 2003;24(4):724–733.
57. Ruggieri PM, Najm I, Bronen R, et al. Neuroimaging of the cortical dysplasias. *Neurology.* 2004;62(6 suppl 3):S27–S29.
58. Sankar R, Curran JG, Kevill JW, et al. Microscopic cortical dysplasia in infantile spasms: evolution of white matter abnormalities. *Am J Neuroradiol.* 1995;16(6):1265–1272.
59. Eltze CM, Chong WK, Bhate S, et al. Taylor-type focal cortical dysplasia in infants: some MRI lesions almost disappear with maturation of myelination. *Epilepsia.* 2005;46(11):1988–1992.
60. Cross JH, Connelly A, Jackson GD, et al. Proton magnetic resonance spectroscopy in children with temporal lobe epilepsy. *Ann Neurol.* 1996;39(1): 107–113.
61. Birken DL, Oldendorf WH. N-acetyl-L-aspartic acid: a literature review of a compound prominent in 1H-NMR spectroscopic studies of brain. *Neurosci Biobehav Rev.* 1989;13(1):23–31.
62. Castillo M, Kwock L, Mukherji SK. Clinical applications of proton MR spectroscopy. *Am J Neuroradiol.* 1996;17(1):1–15.
63. Howe FA, Maxwell RJ, Saunders DE, et al. Proton spectroscopy in vivo. *Magn Reson Q.* 1993;9(1):31–59.
64. Achten E, Boon P, Van De Kerckhove T, et al. Value of single-voxel proton MR spectroscopy in temporal lobe epilepsy. *Am J Neuroradiol.* 1997; 18(6):1131–1139.
65. Achten E, Santens P, Boon P, et al. Single-voxel proton MR spectroscopy and positron emission tomography for lateralization of refractory temporal lobe epilepsy. *Am J Neuroradiol.* 1998;19(1):1–8.
66. Willmann O, Wennberg R, May T, et al. The role of 1H magnetic resonance spectroscopy in pre-operative evaluation for epilepsy surgery. A meta-analysis. *Epilepsy Res.* 2006;71(2–3):149–158.
67. Stanley JA, Cendes F, Dubeau F, et al. Proton magnetic resonance spectroscopic imaging in patients with extratemporal epilepsy. *Epilepsia.* 1998; 39(3):267–273.
68. Krsek P, Hajek M, Dezortova M, et al. (1)H MR spectroscopic imaging in patients with MRI-negative extratemporal epilepsy: correlation with ictal onset zone and histopathology. *Eur Radiol.* 2007;17(8):2126–2135.
69. Simister RJ, McLean MA, Barker GJ, et al. Proton MRS reveals frontal lobe metabolite abnormalities in idiopathic generalized epilepsy. *Neurology.* 2003;61(7):897–902.
70. Simister RJ, McLean MA, Barker GJ, et al. Proton magnetic resonance spectroscopy of malformations of cortical development causing epilepsy. *Epilepsy Res.* 2007;74(2–3):107–115.

CHAPTER 74 ■ VIDEO-EEG MONITORING IN THE PRESURGICAL EVALUATION

JEFFREY W. BRITTON

Surgery remains an important option in the treatment of intractable partial epilepsy (1). Thirty to 40% of patients with epilepsy will not respond to first or second-line medications (2). Such patients remain subject to the attendant psychosocial consequences and medical risks associated with inadequately controlled seizures. Surgery has been shown to be effective and safe for select patients with medically refractory temporal lobe and extratemporal partial epilepsy (3,4). Successful surgery requires the selection of appropriate candidates with surgically remediable syndromes and accurate localization of the epileptogenic zone. Video-EEG monitoring plays a crucial role in this process.

Video-EEG monitoring may provide the only localizing information in some patients, particularly in those without an underlying structural abnormality on neuroimaging. It also allows confirmation of the epileptogenic significance of structural lesions that may be present in a patient with intractable epilepsy. Video-EEG monitoring can also help verify the presence of a single seizure focus, and confirm the epileptic nature of a patient's clinical events prior to making final decisions about surgery. Finally, the video recordings can be shown to family and caretakers in order to verify that the patient's clinically disabling seizures have been recorded prior to making final decisions regarding surgical treatment.

This chapter will discuss the clinical applications, personnel, equipment, and environmental issues to consider in establishing an epilepsy monitoring unit. Safety factors and principles associated with video-EEG monitoring will also be discussed. The importance of ictal semiology and specific localizing signs are reviewed. Finally, the principles and limitations of ictal EEG are evaluated in detail, highlighting the findings most likely to be encountered in the evaluation of patients with surgically remediable partial epilepsy.

EQUIPMENT AND PERSONNEL

Guidelines for the technical and clinical aspects of video-EEG monitoring have been published (5,6). Important considerations pertaining to video-EEG monitoring safety and quality with respect to equipment, facilities, policies, and personnel are discussed below and summarized in Table 74.1.

Video-EEG Equipment

Most epilepsy centers use digital video-EEG acquisition systems for video-EEG monitoring. While analog video can be used to capture clinical seizure activity, navigating from one point in time to another on analog video is significantly less efficient than with digital. For any system used, care must be taken to ensure the video and EEG data time stamps are coordinated and integrated. If video and EEG data storage is parallel and separate, time correlation may be challenging and potentially inaccurate. Digital video allows viewing of recorded events remote from the video-EEG monitoring area, provided the hardware and network infrastructure available is

---

TABLE 74.1

SUMMARY OF IMPORTANT QUALITY AND SAFETY ATTRIBUTES OF A VIDEO-EEG MONITORING FACILITY

Video-EEG monitoring: equipment, safety, facilities and personnel
Video-EEG acquisition equipment
  Digital video-EEG acquisition systems with remote viewing capability, 20 channel minimum
  Redundant data storage in case of server and local hard drive failure
  Amplifiers with temporary local data storage capability
  Cameras (ceiling mounted) with remote control, auto-focus, low-light capabilities
Safety monitoring and intervention preparedness
  Continuous observation of patient by nurse or EEG technician
  Continuous monitoring of EEG by technologist preferred
  Continuous EKG monitoring
  Consider pulse oximetry
  IV access and maintenance
  Supplemental oxygen and airway availability
  Hand-off process for night coverage
  Standardized protocol and orders for acute seizure emergencies
  Standardized dismissal process
Facilities
  Inpatient preferred
  Single patient room for privacy
  Safe bathroom features
  Unobstructed path to patient
  Close proximity of EEG technicians and nursing staff to patient
Personnel
  EEG technician—24 hour coverage optimal
  Nursing—24 hour availability necessary
  Physician (primary and on-call)—24 hour availability necessary
  Rapid response team and Intensive Care availability

adequate to meet the high-volume data stream demands of digital video. Another advantage of digital video-EEG over analog relate to the costs of data storage space and data retrieval efficiency.

The video camera selected should have low-light recording capabilities in order to allow the capture of nocturnal events. Cameras selected should also have autofocus functionality and remote control capabilities for camera angle and zoom so as to enable technical staff to acquire optimum video during an event.

The advantages of digital EEG data over analog are significant. Digital EEG data lends itself to postacquisition filtering and montage reformatting which is not possible with analog EEG. The process of marking and retrieval of important portions of the EEG for data review purposes is far more efficient than with analog EEG. Spike and seizure detection algorithms can also be run on acquired digital EEG data which may increase the detection of abnormalities (7–9). Selection of amplifiers that allow local data storage with flash memory during disconnections from the primary network offers additional advantages, particularly in active patients such as young children, and those few patients who may require transport away from the central EEG recording area during evaluation.

Personnel

The presence of appropriately experienced EEG technologists is crucial in order to ensure quality recordings. Twenty-four hour technician coverage is optimal, as equipment issues can arise at any time potentially affecting several hours of data if not promptly addressed. Also, while spike and seizure detection hold promise for the future, the sensitivity and specificity of commercially available products are not currently sufficient to be considered an appropriate substitute for continuous EEG review by experienced technologists.

Nursing staff familiar with the identification and acute management of seizures are critical to epilepsy monitoring safety. Epilepsy monitoring patients are susceptible to falls, other seizure-related injuries and cardiorespiratory complications, which can be mitigated by prompt nursing intervention (10–12). Nursing and EEG technology personnel are also important in the performance of clinical testing during seizures for semiological analysis purposes.

Deaths and serious injury have occurred in association with video-EEG monitoring. In the few cases reported publicly, lapses in patient observation have been noted as contributing factors (10). It is essential to ensure continuous observation 24 hours a day when monitoring seizures in patients with intractable epilepsy by either nursing or technical staff. Back-up plans for busy times should also be developed to avoid gaps in patient observation.

Physician coverage needs to be available 24 hours a day for epilepsy monitoring patients. If continuous availability by the primary physician is not practical, appropriate cross-coverage by knowledgeable consulting or house staff needs to be established so that rapid evaluation and treatment of seizure-related emergencies can be provided. Twenty-four hour EEG interpretation should also be available in the event questions arise regarding the EEG or clinical status during off hours. Remote access to ongoing video-EEG monitoring data is very helpful for this purpose.

SEIZURE PROVOCATION, PATIENT MANAGEMENT, AND SAFETY CONSIDERATIONS

The goal of video-EEG monitoring in potential surgical patients is to record a complete sample of a patient's seizures in order to clarify the region or regions of seizure onset. The time needed to achieve this objective is often counterbalanced by cost constraints and other factors. Sleep deprivation, photic stimulation, hyperventilation, exercise, and supervised medication withdrawal are commonly used as seizure provocation modalities in order to increase the yield and efficiency of video-EEG monitoring. Most consider medication withdrawal to be the most effective method for seizure provocation but it is also the riskiest. Drug withdrawal should only be performed in an inpatient setting with appropriate personnel immediately available due to the attendant risks.

Supervised Medication Withdrawal

Medication withdrawal should be individualized for each patient, balancing the need to record a sufficient number of seizures and the risks based on the patient's individual seizure history. Medication withdrawal can result in status epilepticus, falls, postictal psychiatric complications, generalized convulsions in patients without a prior history, and seizure-related morbidity such as fractures, joint dislocations, aspiration, and cardiorespiratory arrest. Starting medication withdrawal prior to admission is not generally advisable given the risks. A common approach is to reduce the dose of one medication by 33% to 50% on the first monitoring day, then to continue reducing the dosages of one or more drugs at a similar rate on each successive day until a sufficient number of seizures have been recorded.

A few caveats should be kept in mind when withdrawing medications. Medication withdrawal may not be necessary in patients with a high seizure frequency on full medication therapy. Conversely, some patients with long seizure-free intervals may require a more abrupt withdrawal schedule in order to achieve the goals of monitoring within a realistic timeframe. Medication withdrawal may also predispose to secondary generalized seizures which can complicate ictal EEG localization and the yield of ictal SPECT imaging. Also, psychiatric difficulties may arise when withdrawing certain antiepileptic drugs with relatively favorable psychotropic properties such as valproate, topiramate, carbamazepine, and lamotrigine (13). Once a tapering plan is decided, it is important to clearly communicate the schedule and goals to the team so that medications are resumed as soon as the objectives have been met, even if this occurs after hours.

Patient Care, Monitoring, and Planning

A standardized rescue plan should be established in the monitoring unit in order to minimize treatment delay and potential for error in the treatment of an acute seizure emergency. This rescue plan should include objective criteria for treatment initiation, such as a number of seizures over a defined time period, or for seizures lasting beyond a defined maximal seizure duration. Other criteria for intervention may include the occurrence of a generalized seizure in a patient without a prior history, or the emergence of agitation in a patient with a history of postictal psychosis or violence. Any factor considered a threat to an individual patient's safety should be addressed in an adjunct to the standard rescue plan for that patient. Creation of an admission order set for the epilepsy monitoring unit containing the standard protocol is advised to ensure that rescue plan orders are put in place at admission. All health care team members need to be educated as to the unit's standard rescue plan. Immediate access to the patient's records is required and regular updates as to the goals of admission need to be documented clearly and communicated to the team and handed-off to cross-covering personnel so that once the goals of monitoring have been achieved, antiepileptic medication can be resumed.

Rescue plans typically entail use of intravenous (IV) medications as a component. It is therefore important that IV access be secured in all patients undergoing medication withdrawal upon admission, and that processes be in place to monitor IV viability so that it can be relied on in the event of an emergency. It is critical to inquire specifically about drug allergies and significant nonallergic idiosyncratic reactions to potential rescue medications at admission so that needs for deviation from the standard rescue plan can be identified early. IV lorazepam or diazepam at subanesthetic levels are typically used in epilepsy monitoring rescue plans. IV fosphenytoin can also be considered, but requires EKG and blood pressure monitoring for IV administration and should only be used in a setting where cardiac arrhythmia and hypotension can be effectively managed acutely if they arise.

Given the risk of cardiac arrhythmia associated with seizures (14–16), continuous EKG monitoring should be performed during video-EEG monitoring. Continuous pulse oximetry should also be considered as apnea can complicate seizures (12). Twenty-four hour physician availability is necessary to handle any acute situations that may arise during hospitalization. ICU and supportive services such as a rapid response team should be available in the event of the need for acute airway management and resuscitation.

Uniform policies for ambulation and activity should be established and made clear to patients upon admission due to the risk of seizure-related falls and injury. Sharp corners in the seizure-monitoring environment should be minimized. An unobstructed path to the patient bed needs to be ensured so that staff can attend to the patient in a timely manner. Bathroom fixtures pose safety risks and accommodations need to be considered to minimize the potential for injury in the event a seizure occurs there. Side rails with pads are reasonable to help prevent patients from falling out of bed during a seizure; however they can pose an unintended risk in some cases, particularly those with hypermotor semiologies.

Risks of Video-EEG Monitoring

Medication withdrawal can result in generalized tonic–clonic seizures in patients who never have them, which can be traumatic for the patient and family. Tongue bite wounds are not infrequent but rarely require treatment beyond conservative measures. Other injuries that can occur in association with video-EEG monitoring include vertebral compression fractures

and shoulder dislocations. Caution is required when reducing antiepileptic medications in patients with a previous history of shoulder dislocation and in patients with an established diagnosis of osteopenia. Seizure-related falls can lead to subdural hematoma and skull fractures. Exercise modalities that do not require an upright posture should also be considered. If treadmills and exercise bicycles are used, a nurse or aide need to be present to help prevent seizure-related falls.

Postictal psychosis can arise in the EEG monitoring setting (17–19). This typically occurs following a cluster of seizures. Postictal psychosis is more common in patients with a prior history of it, but can occur for the first time in the EEG monitoring setting. Postictal psychosis tends to occur in association with temporal lobe epilepsy, although it has also been reported in the setting of extratemporal seizures (20). Postictal psychosis may be associated with aggressiveness and combative behavior, posing a risk to the staff. An action plan needs to be anticipated in patients deemed at risk based on prior history. Monitoring and management options for postictal psychosis need to be discussed proactively with the health care team at admission.

Dismissal from the Video-EEG Monitoring Unit

Patient stability needs to be assured prior to dismissal. Patients undergoing EEG monitoring often have been subjected to significant changes in antiepileptic medication therapy over a short period of time which may predispose them to further seizures following discharge. Typically, the patient's usual medication regimen should be resumed 24 hours prior to dismissal. In some cases, it may be prudent to reload patients with parenteral or oral loading doses of their maintenance therapy in anticipation of dismissal. In particularly unstable patients, one should consider obtaining serum levels in order to ensure achievement of therapeutic drug concentrations prior to discharge. It is also ideal to ensure that patients being dismissed from epilepsy monitoring have appropriate supervision for the next 1 to 2 days by family or other appropriate caretakers given the potential for increased seizure activity.

VIDEO-EEG AND LOCALIZATION OF THE EPILEPTOGENIC ZONE

Clinical Localization: Ictal Semiology

Analysis of ictal semiology can provide valuable localizing information complementary to that provided by the ictal EEG (21,22). Concordance between the ictal semiology and EEG may help strengthen hypotheses regarding localization formed from the patient's ictal EEG, clinical data, and neuroimaging. Conversely, discordance between semiology and other data should raise concerns about the localization accuracy. Similarly, the presence of multiple semiologies should suggest the possibility of multiple seizure foci, which may influence the prospects for surgical success. Lateralizing and lobar localizing signs are not present in all seizures in all patients, however are specific when present. In one study, lateralizing signs

TABLE 74.2

LATERALIZING SIGNS IN ICTAL SEMIOLOGY: CONTRALATERAL AND IPSILATERAL SIGNS

Ictal semiology: lateralizing signs
Contralateral signs
Unilateral dystonic hand posturing
Unilateral forced head-turning at secondary generalization
Unilateral clonus
Eye deviation at secondary generalization
Ictal hemiparesis
Postictal (Todd's) paresis or visual field deficit
Figure of 4, fencing or M2E upper extremity limb posturing
Ipsilateral signs
Unilateral manual automatisms
Unilateral postictal nose wiping
Unforced early head-turning
Unilateral eye blinking
Unilateral piloerection
Dominant hemisphere
Postictal aphasia
Nondominant hemisphere
Ictal speech preservation
Ictal vomiting
Ictal spitting

TABLE 74.3

LOBAR LOCALIZING SIGNS IN ICTAL SEMIOLOGY

Ictal semiology: lobar localization
Temporal lobe localization
Aura characteristics
Epigastric rising; olfactory, dysgeusic, auditory hallucinations
Experiential—déjà/jamais-vu; dissociative symptoms
Oral and/or manual automatisms
Dystonic hand posturing
Ictal spitting, postictal nose wiping
Postictal confusion lasting several minutes
Postictal aphasia present (if dominant hemisphere involved)
Frontal lobe localization
Explosive onset
Hypermotor activity
Lower extremity automatisms (bicycling, kicking)
Nocturnal seizure clustering of several per night
Brief or absent postictal confusion
Postictal aphasia infrequent unless primary language cortex involved
Occipital lobe localization
Unilateral simple visual hallucinations (shapes and colors)
Eye deviation
Nausea/vomiting, migraine in children
Peri-Rolandic localization
Unilateral clonic activity as earliest seizure manifestation
Unilateral sensory disturbance as earliest seizure manifestation
Todd's paralysis

were present in 46% of recorded seizures and 78% of patients (23). Lateralization by ictal semiology was correct in 78% of a population with excellent surgery outcome in two studies (23,24). In terms of lobar localization, temporal versus frontal lobar localization could be correctly determined in 76% of patients by semiologic analysis of a cohort of patients with Engel Class 1 outcome (25). Lateralizing and localizing signs of significance in epilepsy surgery patients are summarized in Tables 74.2 and 74.3 and discussed further below.

A number of principles need to be kept in mind in ictal semiologic analysis. First, clinical seizure manifestations are influenced by the propagation of the discharge from one cortical region to another, which can lead to false localization (26,27). For example, aphasia may occur in patients with seizures of nondominant temporal origin if spread to the speech-dominant hemisphere occurs by the time language is tested during the seizure. Second, while the specificity of some of the semiologic signs approach 90%, the sensitivity is not as high (21). Indeed, localizing clinical signs may be completely absent in some patients (23,25). Third, seizures arising in functionally silent regions may not show clinical manifestations until spread to eloquent cortex has occurred, which might falsely suggest a seizure origin in the region of propagation. Finally, some regions of the brain lead primarily to subjective perceptual changes that are not appreciable on review of video data due to the absence of a motor or behavioral correlate. Despite these caveats, localization by analysis of ictal semiology is a useful and necessary part of the localizing process (21).

Lateralizing Signs

Some clinical signs are primarily of lateralizing value. These are summarized in Table 74.2 and are discussed in more detail in the following section. Select semiologic findings are illustrated in Figures 74.1 through 74.3.

Ictal Speech Preservation and Aphasia. Ictal speech preservation in temporal lobe seizures is highly suggestive of nondominant lateralization (28). Ictal aphasia may occur in nondominant temporal lobe seizures if contralateral propagation occurs (29). Measuring the time to speech recovery can help in such cases. In one prospective study, nearly all patients with nondominant temporal lobe seizures were able to read a test phrase within 1 minute of seizure onset, while no patient with dominant temporal lobe seizures were able to read until greater than 1 minute had passed (30). Ictal aphasia is less common in dominant hemisphere extratemporal seizures (31), except for those seizures arising in close proximity to the operculum. When assessing speech during seizure activity, it is important to make sure that any detected speech alteration is not primarily due to orolingual motor effects as opposed to language, as the localizing implications are different.

Unilateral Dystonic Hand Posturing. Unilateral dystonic hand posturing is associated with contralateral seizure onset (32). This sign is common in temporal lobe seizures, and thought to be due to seizure propagation to neighboring basal ganglia. This is depicted in Figure 74.1A showing a patient with unilateral dystonic hand posturing.

Ipsilateral Unilateral Manual Automatisms. Unilateral manual automatisms are of lateralizing significance primarily when seen in association with unilateral dystonic posturing affecting the contralateral hand (32). When present, unilateral automatisms usually involve the ipsilateral hand. Unilateral automatisms can be mistaken for unilateral upper extremity clonic activity. Distinguishing unilateral automatisms from clonus is important as the lateralizing implications are opposite.

Unilateral Forced Head-Turning at Secondary Generalization. Forced head-turning during transformation from a partial to a secondary generalized seizure typically occurs in the direction contralateral to the hemisphere of seizure onset (33). Figure 74.1B shows an example of forced head-turning. Conversely, early nonforced head-turning usually occurs ipsilateral to the seizure focus, but this is less reliable than late forced

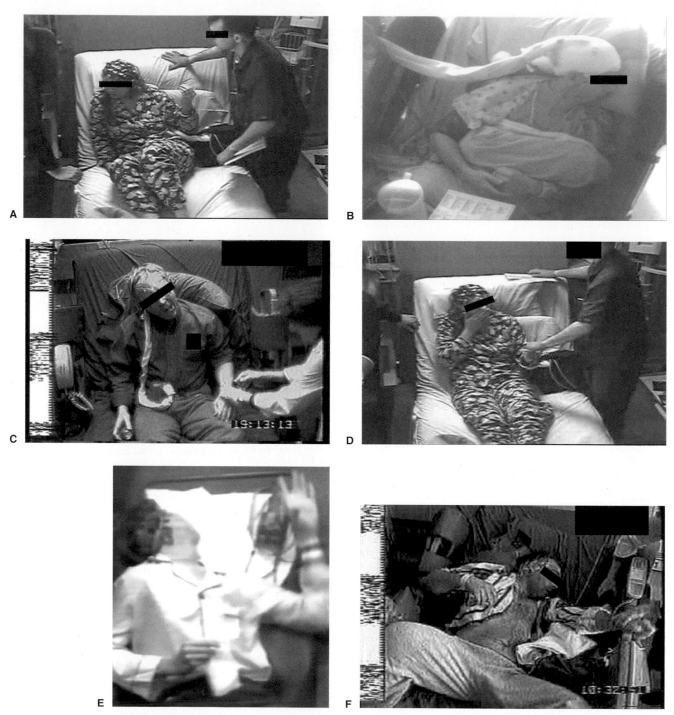

FIGURE 74.1 Lateralizing signs in patients with partial seizures. **A:** Unilateral dystonic hand posturing on the left and unforced head-turn to the right during a right temporal seizure in a patient with right mesial temporal sclerosis. **B:** Forced head-turning to the left during progression to a secondary generalized seizure in a seizure of right temporal origin secondary to mesial temporal sclerosis. **C:** Left facial contracture and clonus during a seizure of right frontocentral onset in a patient with a right peri-Rolandic cortical dysplasia. **D:** Unilateral postictal nose wiping involving the ipsilateral hand in a patient with right temporal seizures. **E:** "M2E" posturing in a patient with right temporal seizures of unknown etiology. **F:** "Fencing" posture in a patient with a secondary generalized seizure of right temporal neocortical onset.

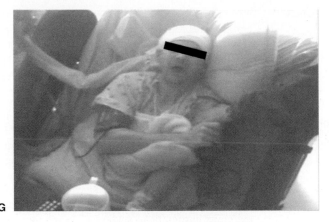

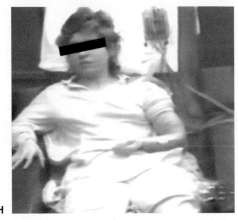

FIGURE 74.1 (*Continued*) **G:** "Figure of 4" posturing with left upper extremity extended during a secondary generalized seizure of right temporal origin. **H:** Ictal paresis involving the left upper extremity during a right parietal seizure of unknown etiology.

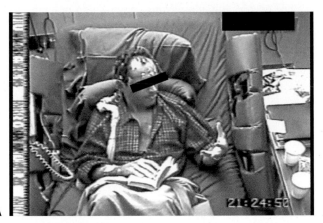

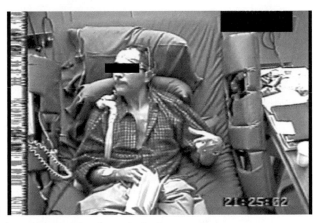

FIGURE 74.2 Semiologic signs of lobar localizing significance in partial epilepsy **A:** Oral automatisms and "regarding the hand" (left hand in this case) in a patient with temporal lobe epilepsy; (**B**) dystonic left hand posturing, continued oral automatisms and nonforced right head-turn during a right temporal lobe seizure.

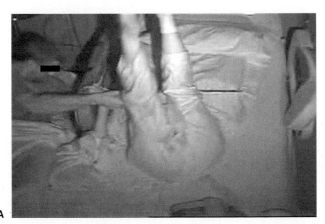

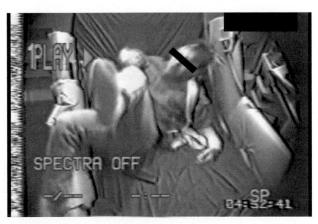

FIGURE 74.3 **A, B:** Complex lower extremity automatisms in two patients with frontal lobe epilepsy.

head-turning. Figure 74.1A shows ipsilateral nonforced head turning in addition to contralateral dystonic hand posturing.

Unilateral Facial or Limb Clonus. Unilateral clonus lateralizes to the contralateral hemisphere. Unilateral facial clonus can sometimes be appreciated on the scalp EEG in the form of asymmetric rhythmic muscle artifact involving the derivations overlying the affected facial and scalp muscles. Figure 74.1C

shows unilateral left facial contraction contralateral to a right frontocentral seizure focus secondary to a right precentral focal cortical dysplasia.

Ictal Vomiting. Ictal vomiting is an uncommon seizure manifestation that correlates with nondominant lateralization when present in the context of temporal lobe seizures (34). However, exceptions have been noted in the literature (35).

Ictal vomiting may also be seen in occipital seizures, in which case it is of less lateralizing significance (36).

Postictal Nose Wiping. Nose wiping with one hand following temporal lobe seizures typically involves the ipsilateral hand (37). Postictal nose wiping is more characteristic of temporal lobe than extratemporal seizures. Unilateral nose wiping is illustrated in a patient following a right temporal lobe seizure in Figure 74.1D.

Ictal Spitting. Ictal spitting is usually associated with nondominant temporal lobe seizures, however dominant lateralization has also been reported (38). It is thought to be due to hypersalivation secondary to stimulation of the central autonomic network.

Forced Eye Deviation. Similar to forced head-turning, this typically occurs contralateral to the seizure focus.

Unilateral Piloerection. This typically occurs ipsilateral to the seizure focus and is usually seen in temporal lobe seizures (39).

M2E, Fencing, Figure of 4 Posturing. "M2E" posturing refers to a posture consisting of contralateral shoulder abduction, elbow flexion, and head deviation toward the affected arm. This is depicted in Figure 74.1E in a patient with right frontal seizures. The "fencing" posture refers to a position assumed during secondary generalization where the contralateral upper extremity is extended, the ipsilateral arm flexed and abducted at the shoulder, and head rotated contralateral to the seizure focus. The hips may be abducted as well. An example is shown in Figure 74.1F. "Figure of 4" posturing refers to a position where the contralateral upper extremity is extended and the ipsilateral upper extremity flexed at the elbow so that it crosses the extended arm giving rise to the shape of the number "4". An example is shown in Figure 74.1G.

Todd's Paresis and Ictal Paresis. While relatively uncommon, unilateral postictal Todd's paralysis correlates with seizure lateralization to the contralateral hemisphere (40). Todd's paralysis is more commonly seen in extratemporal seizures. Similarly, "ictal paresis" is a rare semiologic manifestation typically occurring contralateral to the seizure focus in patients with extratemporal seizures. Ictal paresis can be mistaken for transient ischemic attacks. An example is shown in Figure 74.1H observed during a right parietal seizure.

Lobar Localization

Semiology can help with lobar localization as well, particularly in differentiating temporal and extratemporal seizures (25,41).

Temporal Localization. Temporal localization is suggested by the presence of an aura of experiential phenomena such as an out-of-body experience, epigastric rising sensation, and olfactory and dysgeusic hallucinosis. Manual and oral automatisms are commonly observed, and verbal and nonverbal vocalizations may be present. Cessation of activity at seizure onset is common. Upper extremity dystonic posturing may occur. Figure 74.2A and B show unilateral dystonic hand posturing and oral automatisms in a patient during a right temporal lobe seizure. Temporal lobe seizures typically last 1 to 3 minutes in duration. A postictal confusional period lasting a few to several minutes followed by a desire to sleep is typical in temporal lobe seizures; however nondominant temporal lobe seizures and those with limited bitemporal involvement may not be associated with a significant postictal period (25,41).

Frontal Lobe Seizures. The clinical presentations of extratemporal frontal lobe seizures are protean. A number of semiologic differences have been identified (25). In contrast to temporal lobe seizures, frontal lobe seizure auras, if present, are usually nondescript, consisting of vague light-headedness or fear. Frontal seizures are often brief, lasting 1 minute or less, and are sometimes characterized by an explosive onset, with prominent hypermotor activity and complex lower extremity automatisms such as bicycling movements and kicking (Fig. 74.3A and B). Vocalizations, such as the utterance of profanities and screaming, may also occur. Some patients with extratemporal seizures have them exclusively out of sleep. While nocturnal predominance may be seen in temporal lobe seizures as well, a seizure pattern of multiple brief clusters of seizures occurring exclusively during sleep is more characteristic of frontal lobe seizures. Nongeneralized seizures of frontal origin are often followed by a relatively brief postictal period in contrast to temporal lobe seizures. However, not all frontal lobe seizures behave in the same manner. Some frontal lobe seizures may evolve over prolonged periods of time, and postictal confusion may sometimes be seen. Semiology is particularly important in frontal lobe seizures as the ictal EEG is often nondiagnostic, particularly in seizures of supplementary motor or orbital frontal onset (21,42).

EEG Localization in Video-EEG Monitoring

Interictal and ictal EEG analysis are essential in the presurgical epilepsy patient. However, the EEG needs to be correlated with other localizing modalities, and can rarely be used alone in presurgical localization. An understanding of the localizing patterns seen in partial epilepsy and limitations of ictal EEG localization are essential in the evaluation of patients for epilepsy surgery.

A minimum of 20 scalp EEG channels should be used when performing prolonged video-EEG monitoring. Midline, right and left parasagittal and right and left temporal head electrodes should be utilized placed at standard interelectrode distances. Additional inferior temporal electrodes should be considered in patients where a temporal lobe focus is suspected. Nasopharyngeal, foramen ovale and transsphenoidal electrodes have been advocated by some to improve the sensitivity and specificity of ictal EEG localization, particularly in patients with mesial temporal seizures (43,44). The overall value of these electrodes has not been confirmed by all investigators, however, and are not routinely used (45,46).

Interictal Epileptiform Abnormalities

Although the ictal EEG receives the most scrutiny in video-EEG monitoring, the value of the interictal data acquired should not be overlooked. Correlating the interictal and ictal EEG provides a clearer picture of the complexity of the patient's seizure disorder. The interictal background may contain focal slowing or suppression, helping to localize areas of brain dysfunction. Also, the presence of interictal epileptiform abnormalities beyond the boundaries of the epileptogenic zone *or* contralateral to the suspected focus may influence surgical prognosis and the chances for eventual antiepileptic drug discontinuance. Generalized interictal activity may be seen in some cases which may suggest the presence of more than one epilepsy mechanism in a given patient. Finally, in some cases, the interictal EEG may contain abnormalities of greater localizing value than the ictal EEG, particularly in extratemporal partial epilepsy. Figure 74.4A–D show focal interictal epileptiform abnormalities in four patients undergoing epilepsy surgery evaluation. In the extratemporal cases (Fig. 74.4B–D), the interictal activity was more localizing than the ictal EEG.

The interictal record is of prognostic value in the epilepsy surgery patient. Concordance with other localizing data portends a more favorable prognosis than patients with discordant interictal EEG activity (47). In addition to the importance of localization concordance, the quantity of interictal abnormalities may be of prognostic value in certain epilepsy syndromes. In one study of temporal lobectomy patients, fewer (29%) patients with frequent spikes (>60 spikes per hour) experienced an excellent surgical outcome from a standard temporal lobectomy with amygdalohippocampectomy compared to 81% with infrequent spikes (<60 spikes per hour) (48). One explanation proposed for this observation was that frequent interictal abnormalities might be an indicator of neocortical rather than mesial temporal epilepsy.

The Ictal EEG

Analysis of the ictal EEG is essential in presurgical planning (49–52). However, limitations of the ictal EEG need to be recognized. In a retrospective study of patients with Engel Class 1 surgical outcomes, ictal EEG localization was possible in 57% of recorded seizures and 72% of patients, and false localization occurred in 6% (53). From this data, it is clear that the ictal EEG cannot be relied on in isolation in the selection of epilepsy surgery cases. The ictal EEG must be correlated with

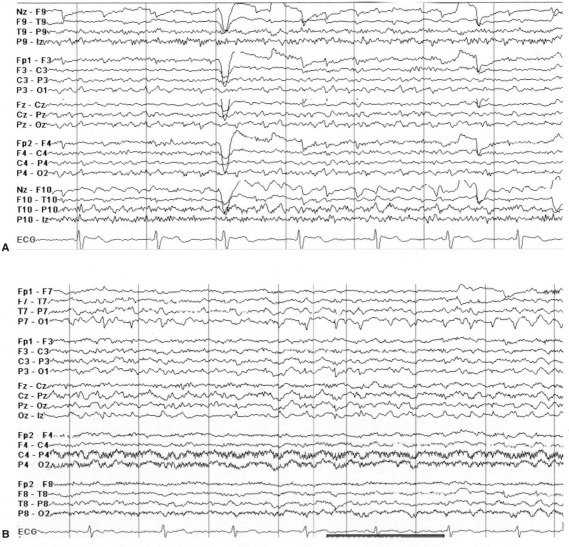

FIGURE 74.4 Localizing interictal abnormalities in epilepsy surgery patients with partial epilepsy. **A:** Right temporal sharp waves and temporal intermittent rhythmic delta activity in a patient with right temporal lobe epilepsy secondary to mesial temporal sclerosis. **B:** Left occipital-posterior temporal spikes in a patient with a left medial occipital cortical dysplasia.

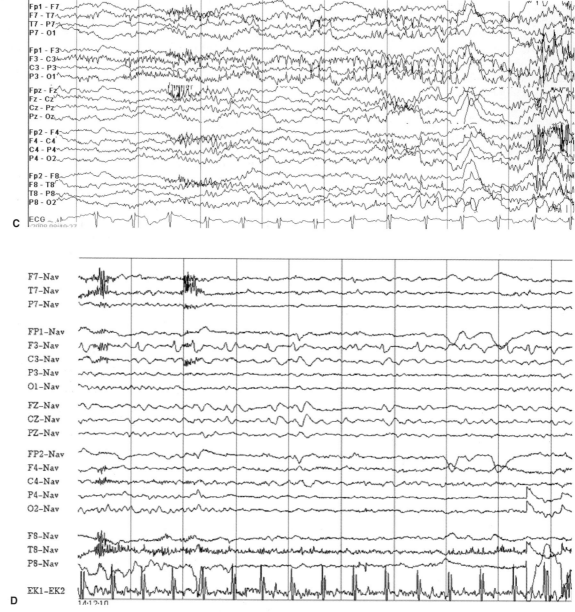

FIGURE 74.4 (*Continued*) **C:** Left centroparietotemporal spikes in a patient with a cortical dysplasia localized to the left inferolateral postcentral gyrus region. **D:** Repetitive left frontal spikes in a patient with nonlesional frontal lobe epilepsy localized to the left dorsolateral frontal region.

the interictal record, neuroimaging and semiology findings in making final decisions about surgical treatment (54,55).

Limitations of Ictal EEG. Acquisition of the ictal scalp EEG poses many technical challenges. In frontal lobe seizures, artifact secondary to hypermotor ictal behavior may obscure the recording. Oral automatisms during temporal lobe seizures may cause myogenic changes in the temporal derivations, shrouding the underlying ictal EEG discharge. While selective use of high- and low-pass filters may help in these situations, this often proves insufficient and filtering may alter or obscure features of the seizure discharge.

Other factors are important to consider when evaluating the ictal EEG. High-frequency discharges greater than 100 Hz are now recognized as important features of the epileptogenic zone on intracranial recordings using amplifiers with broad frequency

bandwidths (56). However, such high-frequency discharges are typically not appreciable with scalp EEG due to their low amplitude and the fact that their frequency lies outside the range of most routine EEG acquisition systems. The ictal EEG is also limited by the fact that the portion of the cortical surface amenable to scalp electrode acquisition is constrained by the discrepancy between the brain's convoluted surface and the relatively simple topography of the scalp surface (57,58). Because of this, certain regions of the brain such as the insula, interhemispheric regions, and inferior cortical surfaces do not lend themselves to scalp EEG recordings. Finally, it is recognized that two thirds of the cortical surface area lay in the cortical sulci as opposed to the gyral crests, giving rise to relatively distant dipoles oriented at an angle tangential to the electrode recording surface. These factors account for the observation that as few as 10% of spikes recorded with subdural electrodes are detectable on the scalp EEG (59,60).

The morphology and distribution of the ictal EEG depends on the localization, configuration, and size of the epileptogenic zone (58). The presence of cortical or cerebral pathology and anatomic changes secondary to previous surgeries may also affect the EEG. Lobar and sublobar EEG resolution is usually limited given the brain's complex anatomy and the relative limited electrode coverage accomplished with standard electrode placement (61). For example, while some investigators have identified ictal EEG features that distinguish mesial from neocortical temporal seizure onset (62–65), others have not been able to identify reliable features and intracranial monitoring is often necessary to resolve these situations (63,66). Also, seizures arising from some cortical regions may show their earliest expression on the ictal EEG in a brain region of propagation. For example, orbital frontal foci are often indistinguishable from temporal lobe foci based on EEG given the proximity of this area to the temporal head region. Occipital seizures are also known to propagate early to the temporal lobes, giving rise to the potential for false localization (25,27,57,58).

Another limitation to EEG localization arises in infants, children, and adolescents with refractory epilepsy due to congenital or early-acquired focal or hemispheric epileptogenic lesions. Such patients may have hypsarrhythmia, generalized slow spike wave complexes, or other generalized patterns on ictal and interictal EEG, with few or even no focal features. Selected children with such lesions may be favorable candidates for epilepsy surgery, despite the generalized manifestations on EEG (67). The mechanism for the diffuse EEG expression in such children is unknown, but a factor may be the earlier interaction between the focal lesion and the developing brain.

Features of Ictal EEG Recordings. The seizure pattern recorded in an individual patient with a single epileptogenic zone typically remains consistent from seizure to seizure in terms of the morphology and distribution of the discharge. Significant variability of the ictal EEG in a single patient should raise the possibility of a relatively large epileptogenic zone or multiple seizure foci. Conversely, seizures from the same brain region in different patients may show interindividual variability in the ictal EEG due to differences in anatomy and physiology.

A variety of ictal EEG discharges have been described in association with partial seizures in terms of discharge frequency and patterns seen (58,64,68,69). These include: (i) rhythmic theta, delta, or alpha activity; (ii) paroxysmal fast activity (rhythmic activity in the beta frequency range or beyond); (iii) suppression (focal, asymmetric, or diffuse); (iv) repetitive epileptiform abnormalities; and (v) arrhythmic mixed frequency activity (53,58,70). There is no clear association between pattern seen and surgical prognosis.

The distribution of the EEG discharge is also important. While focal, regional, or lateralized discharges are more typical in the partial epilepsy population, the presence of bisynchronous or diffuse activity at onset does not necessarily exclude the possibility of surgery if other localizing data are present. For example, bisynchronous and diffuse ictal EEG onset may be present in surgical candidates with supplementary motor area seizures (53). In such cases, intracranial monitoring may ultimately be required to resolve localization. Mesial temporal and lateral frontal seizure foci are the regions most amenable to localization with ictal scalp EEG (53,71). Conversely, mesial frontal, orbital frontal (72–74), parietal and occipital seizures (42,53,72–79) are difficult to localize with ictal EEG.

Determining the Ictal EEG Onset. The video and EEG should be reviewed in concert in order to determine whether the timing of the ictal EEG discharge correlates with the clinical onset. In general, the earlier the EEG onset, the more confident one can be that the discharge correlates with the epileptogenic zone. In general, the first 30–40 seconds of a seizure provide the most useful localizing information. Due to seizure propagation, later portions of the seizure discharge are of less value. The postictal record however can be useful, particularly in temporal lobe epilepsy where localized slowing can sometimes be seen in the ipsilateral temporal region (80).

Temporal lobe seizures: mesial versus neocortical temporal onset. Mesial temporal seizures typically are manifest as an evolving rhythmic theta discharge arising over the ipsilateral temporal derivations (50,58,70,81). A typical right mesial temporal seizure is shown in Figure 74.5A–D. The discharge morphology is often sinusoidal at onset, the individual waveforms showing a rounded contour rather than sharp in the

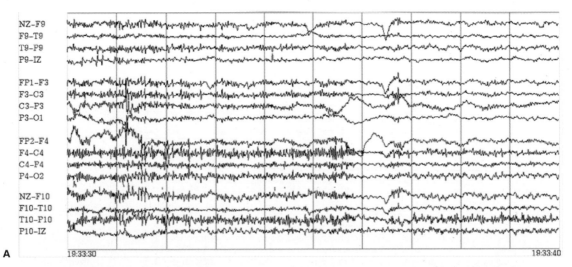

FIGURE 74.5 Ictal EEG evolution during a right temporal seizure in a patient with mesial temporal sclerosis. **A:** Ictal EEG onset consists of sinusoidal rhythmic theta over the right temporal derivations.

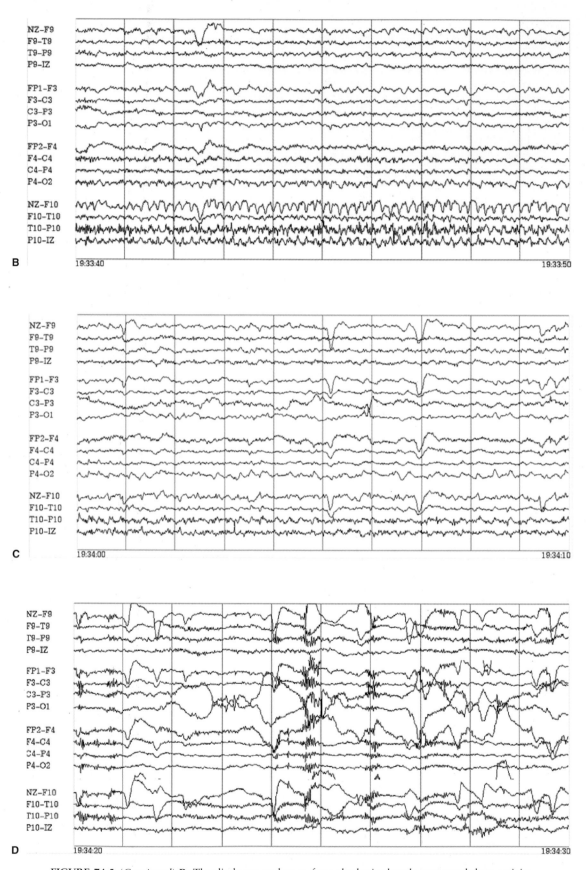

FIGURE 74.5 (*Continued*) **B:** The discharge evolves to form rhythmic sharply contoured theta activity with phase-reversal over the right anterior temporal derivations. **C:** The right temporal discharge frequency decreases toward the end of the seizure to the delta frequency range. **D:** Subtle lateralized postictal delta slowing and attenuation of the background is present over the right hemispheric derivations following seizure termination.

early portion of the seizure (Fig. 74.5A) (70). Sometimes temporal lobe seizures may be preceded by a transient suppression of the EEG background (70). This may be lateralized or diffuse and is more apparent in seizures arising out of sleep (82). Temporal lobe seizures may also begin with semirhythmic repetitive epileptiform potentials at onset rather than a sinusoidal morphology (58,70,83). While temporal seizures are typically focal or lateralized at onset, they may be bilateral or diffuse, evolving into a more lateralized discharge over the ipsilateral temporal region after the first several seconds of the seizure (43,70). As the seizure continues, the waveforms may become sharper in appearance and the frequency increases slightly (Fig. 74.5B) (58,70). Rhythmic activity then begins to appear in the parasagittal and midline regions, presumably secondary to propagation to the cingulum or due to formation of a vertical dipole in the mesial temporal region with the positive component oriented superiorly (84). Contralateral temporal spread often develops in the middle to latter portions of the seizure. At seizure termination, the discharge frequency typically decreases to the delta frequency range (Fig. 74.5C), and ipsilateral semirhythmic 1 to 2 Hz delta activity may be present in the postictal period (Fig. 74.5D) (80).

False ictal EEG lateralization is uncommon in temporal lobe epilepsy but can occur (85–87). This is typically seen in seizures which spread from one hippocampus to the other prior to propagation to the ipsilateral temporal neocortex. It can also occur when the seizure onset is such that the ictal EEG field is oriented tangential to the electrode recording surfaces. Sometimes a bitemporal discharge is seen at seizure onset, in which case ictal EEG lateralization may not be possible (43). Mesial temporal depth electrode recordings may be necessary to resolve seizure lateralization in such cases.

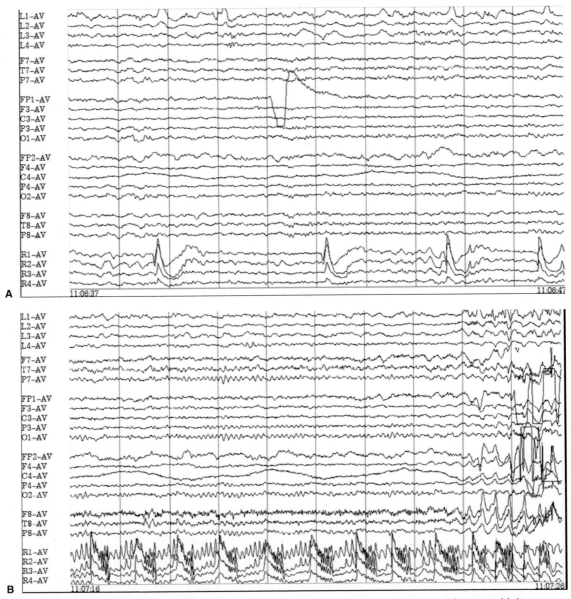

FIGURE 74.6 Simultaneous bitemporal depth and scalp EEG recording in a patient with temporal lobe epilepsy. **A:** Seizure onset in the right temporal depth (labeled R1-4-AV) without associated changes in the right temporal scalp derivations (labeled F8, T8, P8–AV). **B:** Right temporal scalp activation begins 48 seconds after right medial temporal depth onset, consisting of high amplitude rhythmic sharp activity involving F8, T8, P8—AV in the last two seconds of the Figure.

Figure 74.6A and B shows a recording in a patient undergoing simultaneous scalp and bitemporal depth electrode recordings demonstrating a relatively belated bitemporal scalp EEG discharge 48 seconds after right mesial temporal depth onset.

Neocortical temporal seizures cannot be reliably distinguished from medial temporal seizures on scalp EEG alone, however some features have been identified that may suggest neocortical localization. In one study, the mean discharge frequency at seizure onset in neocortical temporal seizures was 1 Hz less than mesial temporal seizures (65). In another study, mesial temporal seizures were characterized by an initial regular 5- to 9-Hz inferotemporal rhythm, and occasionally by a vertex/parasagittal positive rhythm of the same frequency. In contrast, neocortical temporal seizures were associated with an irregular polymorphic 2- to 5-Hz lateralized discharge, or by repetitive semiperiodic sharp waves at onset. Seizures without a clear lateralized EEG discharge were most commonly neocortical in this study (64). In another series, mesial temporal seizures were more likely to show fast rhythmic sharp waves (>4 Hz) at seizure onset than neocortical temporal seizures (mean 81% vs. 60%, $P = 0.05$) (66). Also, neocortical seizures were more often bilateral at onset (mean 55% vs. 26%, $P < 0.05$), and bilateral propagation occurred more rapidly (mean 23 vs. 74 second, $P < 0.005$) than did mesial temporal seizures (66). Sphenoidal electrodes can help delineate mesial and neocortical temporal seizures (44,62). However, intracranial monitoring is usually necessary when definitive electrophysiologic clarification is required (46).

Seizures from cortical regions other than the temporal lobe may show the earliest EEG activity over the temporal derivations, leading to false localization. This likely results from the fact that the temporal lobe receives connections from the extratemporal cortex via corticocortical pathways (27,43). In one study of 33 nonlesional patients with temporal lobe seizure activity on ictal scalp EEG, 11 were found to have an extratemporal seizure focus on intracranial monitoring with propagation to the temporal region (88). There is no EEG feature that can reliably distinguish a propagated temporal discharge from a temporal origin rhythm (89). In addition to propagation from other cortical regions, certain deep structures connected to the limbic system such as the hypothalamus may give show the earliest EEG discharge over the temporal regions, potentially leading to false localization (90). Dense array EEG acquisitions using multiple electrodes may hold promise in resolving sublobar localization and in distinguishing propagated versus temporal onset rhythms, but have not yet been validated extensively (91,92).

Frontal lobe seizures. The EEG is of less localizing value in frontal lobe seizures. There are several reasons for the limited ictal EEG localization in frontal lobe seizures, including artifact secondary to ictal behavior, the presence and extent of any underlying cortical pathology, prior surgical interventions, and the complex anatomy of the frontal lobe (57,93,94). While some ictal EEG features are relatively characteristic for frontal lobe seizures, ictal EEG localization was not found to be significant on multivariate analysis in one series of successful frontal lobe epilepsy surgery cases when compared to other factors (95).

The ictal EEG in *mesial frontal* seizures often does not show a discharge at clinical seizure onset (71,72). This, coupled with the unusual behavior that sometimes occurs in association with

this seizure type, may lead to a misdiagnosis of nonepileptic events. As the seizure progresses in mesial frontal seizures, rhythmic theta or delta activity may appear late over the midline and bilateral parasagittal regions. The EEG often remains obscured by artifact throughout seizures of mesial frontal origin, particularly in those with hypermotor semiology (72,96). Several other ictal patterns have been described in association with mesial frontal seizures including generalized spike and wave, a diffuse electrodecremental pattern, and rhythmic vertex alpha activity (72,96). It is often difficult to lateralize mesial frontal seizures on EEG or clinically. In the absence of a structural or functional imaging abnormality in such cases, intracranial monitoring is usually necessary (71,72,96,97).

Localizing ictal EEG abnormalities are more likely to be present in patients with *dorsolateral frontal* seizures due to the closer proximity of the area of seizure onset to the recording electrodes (53,71). The ictal onset in dorsolateral frontal seizures may manifest as a focal low-amplitude high-frequency discharge, an example of which is depicted in Figure 74.7 (98). The presence of a low-amplitude, high-frequency discharge at onset has been shown to be prognostically favorable (99,100). Recording multiple seizures may help increase the yield of the ictal scalp EEG in these patients.

Orbital frontal seizures often propagate to the ipsilateral temporal region (27,101). This can cause erroneous localization to the temporal lobe in such patients (102). Orbital frontal seizures can also spread to other regions of the frontal lobe (101). As a result, there is no diagnostic EEG pattern specific to seizures arising from this region.

Occipital lobe seizures. Occipital seizures are difficult to localize on ictal EEG even in lesional patients. Seizures arising from the calcarine cortex may give rise to bilateral or contralateral discharges due to the anatomic orientation of the medial occipital cortical surface relative to the scalp surface (53,103). A localizing ictal discharge may not be present in occipital epilepsy patients. In one large surgical series, a localizing discharge at onset was seen over the temporo-occipital region in only 46% of cases (75). Confounding matters further from an EEG standpoint is the fact that occipital seizures often spread to the temporal and frontal regions after onset which can result in false localization to these areas if other localizing data are lacking (73,79).

Parietal lobe seizures. The parietal lobe is the least common area of seizure onset in partial epilepsy. The ictal EEG is often not localizing in parietal seizures and other factors need to be taken into account (53,78). Like seizures from other extratemporal sites, parietal seizures often propagate to neighboring regions, leading to challenges in clinical and ictal EEG localization in the absence of a structural lesion on MRI (77,104,105). In one large surgical series, the sensitivity of ictal EEG in a seizure-free parietal lobe epilepsy cohort was 35.7%, compared to 64.3% for MRI, 50% for PET, and 45.5% for ictal SPECT (76).

CONCLUSION

Video-EEG monitoring is essential in the presurgical evaluation of patients with medically refractory epilepsy. There are some risks to video-EEG monitoring. Therefore, it is important to put in place appropriate policies and safety measures to minimize

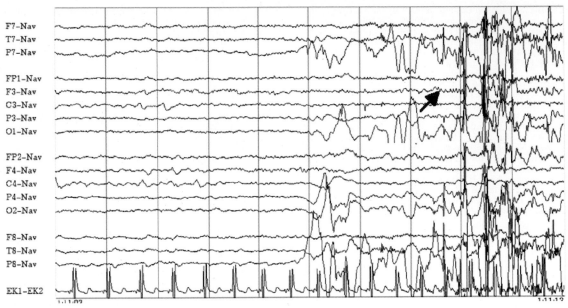

FIGURE 74.7 Ictal EEG during an extratemporal seizure of left lateral frontal onset. This patient's interictal EEG is shown in Figure 74.1D. At clinical onset, there is attenuation of the EEG background, and a high-frequency discharge ("beta buzz") present over the left frontal region *(arrow)*.

the potential for harm in these patients. Twenty-four hour patient observation by nursing or technical staff is essential to ensure prompt identification of seizure activity and associated complications in monitored patients. All data acquired during video-EEG monitoring, including ictal semiology, the interictal EEG, and the ictal EEG, should be analyzed in the process of seizure localization. Conclusions based on analysis of the video-EEG session then need to be correlated with neuroimaging and other localizing data prior to final surgical planning.

References

1. Engel J, Wieser HG, Spencer DD. Overview: surgical therapy. In: Engel J, Pedley TA, Aicardi J, et al., eds. *Epilepsy: A Comprehensive Textbook*. 2nd ed. Lippincott Williams & Wilkins: Philadelphia, PA; 2007: 1747–1749.
2. Kwan P, Brodie MJ. Early identification of refractory epilepsy. *N Engl J Med*. 2000;342:314–319.
3. Wiebe S, Blume WT, Girvin JP, et al. A randomized, controlled trial of surgery for temporal-lobe epilepsy [see comment]. *N Engl J Med*. 2001; 345:311–318.
4. Wetjen NM, Marsh WR, Meyer FB, et al. Intracranial electroencephalography seizure onset patterns and surgical outcomes in nonlesional extratemporal epilepsy. *J Neurosurg*. 2009;110:1147–1152.
5. Gumnit RJ, Walczak TS, National Association of Epilepsy C. Guidelines for essential services, personnel, and facilities in specialized epilepsy centers in the United States. *Epilepsia*. 2001;42:804–814.
6. Velis D, Plouin P, Gotman J, et al. Recommendations regarding the requirements and applications for long-term recordings in epilepsy. *Epilepsia*. 2007;48:379–384.
7. Flanagan D, Agarwal R, Wang YH, et al. Improvement in the performance of automated spike detection using dipole source features for artefact rejection. *Clin Neurophysiol*. 2003;114:38–49.
8. Gotman J, Wang LY. State-dependent spike detection: concepts and preliminary results. *Electroencephalogr Clin Neurophysiol*. 1991;79:11–19.
9. Gotman J, Wang LY. State dependent spike detection: validation. *Electroencephalogr Clin Neurophysiol*. 1992;83:12–18.
10. Phillips LA. Death in epilepsy monitoring unit raises questions about safety policies and practice standards. *Neurol Today*. 2008;8:1.
11. Ryvlin P, Tomson T, DuBois A, et al. MORTEMUS: mortality in epilepsy monitoring unit study, 2008 [cited 2009 Jan 27]. Central website for reporting deaths associated with EMU monitoring. Available at: http://mortemus.com/
12. So EL, Sam MC, Lagerlund TL. Postictal central apnea as a cause of SUDEP: evidence from near-SUDEP incident. *Epilepsia*. 2000;41:1494–1497.
13. Schmitz B. Effects of antiepileptic drugs on mood and behavior. *Epilepsia*. 2006;47(suppl 2):28–33.
14. Britton JW, Ghearing GR, Benarroch EE, et al. The ictal bradycardia syndrome: localization and lateralization. *Epilepsia*. 2006;47:737–744.
15. Schuele SU, Bermeo AC, Alexopoulos AV, et al. Video-electrographic and clinical features in patients with ictal asystole [see comment]. *Neurology*. 2007;69:434–441.
16. Tinuper P, Bisulli F, Cerullo A, et al. Ictal bradycardia in partial epileptic seizures: autonomic investigation in three cases and literature review [see comment]. *Brain*. 2001;124:2361–2371.
17. Kanner AM. Recognition of the various expressions of anxiety, psychosis, and aggression in epilepsy. *Epilepsia*. 2004;45(suppl 2):22–27.
18. Lancman M. Psychosis and peri-ictal confusional states. *Neurology*. 1999; 53:S33–S38.
19. Kanner AM, Dunn DW. Diagnosis and management of depression and psychosis in children and adolescents with epilepsy. *J Child Neurol*. 2004;19(suppl 1):S65–S72.
20. Adachi N, Onuma T, Nishiwaki S, et al. Inter-ictal and post-ictal psychoses in frontal lobe epilepsy: a retrospective comparison with psychoses in temporal lobe epilepsy. *Seizure*. 2000;9:328–335.
21. So EL. Value and limitations of seizure semiology in localizing seizure onset. *J Clin Neurophysiol*. 2006;23:353–357.
22. Luders H, Noachtar S. *Epileptic Seizures: Pathophysiology and Clinical Semiology*. New York, NY: Churchill Livingstone; 2000.
23. Serles W, Caramanos Z, Lindinger G, et al. Combining ictal surface-electroencephalography and seizure semiology improves patient lateralization in temporal lobe epilepsy. *Epilepsia*. 2000;41:1567–1573.
24. Chee MWL, Kotagal P, Van Ness PC, et al. Lateralizing signs in intractable partial epilepsy: blinded multiple-observer analysis. *Neurology*. 1993;43: 2519–2525.
25. O'Brien TJ, Mosewich RK, Britton JW, et al. History and seizure semiology in distinguishing frontal lobe seizures and temporal lobe seizures. *Epilepsy Res*. 2008;82:177–182.
26. Rusu V, Chassoux F, Landre E, et al. Dystonic posturing in seizures of mesial temporal origin: electroclinical and metabolic patterns. *Neurology*. 2005;65:1612–1619.
27. Lacruz ME, Garcia Seoane JJ, Valentin A, et al. Frontal and temporal functional connections of the living human brain. *Eur J Neurosci*. 2007;26:1357–1370.
28. Koerner M, Laxer KD. Ictal speech, postictal language dysfunction, and seizure lateralization. *Neurology*. 1988;38:634–636.
29. Ficker DM, Shukla R, Privitera MD. Postictal language dysfunction in complex partial seizures: effect of contralateral ictal spread. *Neurology*. 2001;56:1590–1592.
30. Privitera MD, Morris GL, Gilliam F. Postictal language assessment and lateralization of complex partial seizures. *Ann Neurol*. 1991;30: 391–396.

31. Goldberg-Stern H, Gadoth N, Cahill W, et al. Language dysfunction after frontal lobe partial seizures. *Neurology.* 2004;62:1637–1638.

32. Kotagal P, Luders H, Morris HH, et al. Dystonic posturing in complex partial seizures of temporal lobe onset: a new lateralizing sign [see comment]. *Neurology.* 1989;39:196–201.

33. Abou-Khalil B, Fakhoury T. Significance of head turn sequences in temporal lobe onset seizures. *Epilepsy Res.* 1996;23:245–250.

34. Kramer RE, Luders H, Goldstick LP, et al. Ictus emeticus: an electroclinical analysis. *Neurology.* 1988;38:1048–1052.

35. Schauble B, Britton JW, Mullan BP, et al. Ictal vomiting in association with left temporal lobe seizures in a left hemisphere language-dominant patient [see comment]. *Epilepsia.* 2002;43:1432–1435.

36. Panayiotopoulos CP. Vomiting as an ictal manifestation of epileptic seizures and syndromes. *J Neurol Neurosurg Psychiatry.* 1988;51:1448–1451.

37. Geyer JD, Payne TA, Faught E, et al. Postictal nose-rubbing in the diagnosis, lateralization, and localization of seizures. *Neurology.* 1999;52:743–745.

38. Kellinghaus C, Loddenkemper T, Kotagal P. Ictal spitting: clinical and electroencephalographic features. *Epilepsia.* 2003;44:1064–1069.

39. Loddenkemper T, Kellinghaus C, Gandjour J, et al. Localising and lateralising value of ictal piloerection. *J Neurol Neurosurg Psychiatry.* 2004;75:879–883.

40. Kellinghaus C, Kotagal P. Lateralizing value of Todd's palsy in patients with epilepsy [see comment]. *Neurology.* 2004;62:289–291.

41. Manford M, Fish DR, Shorvon SD. An analysis of clinical seizure patterns and their localizing value in frontal and temporal lobe epilepsies. *Brain.* 1996;119:17–40.

42. Quesney LF, Constain M, Rasmussen T, et al. Presurgical EEG investigation in frontal lobe epilepsy. *Epilepsy Res Suppl.* 1992;5:55–69.

43. Risinger MW, Engel J Jr, Van Ness PC, et al. Ictal localization of temporal lobe seizures with scalp/sphenoidal recordings. *Neurology.* 1989;39:1288–1293.

44. Velasco TR, Sakamoto AC, Alexandre V Jr, et al. Foramen ovale electrodes can identify a focal seizure onset when surface EEG fails in mesial temporal lobe epilepsy. *Epilepsia.* 2006;47:1300–1307.

45. Mintzer S, Nicholl JS, Stern JM, et al. Relative utility of sphenoidal and temporal surface electrodes for localization of ictal onset in temporal lobe epilepsy. *Clin Neurophysiol.* 2002;113:911–916.

46. Marks DA, Katz A, Booke J, et al. Comparison and correlation of surface and sphenoidal electrodes with simultaneous intracranial recording: an interictal study. *Electroencephalogr Clin Neurophysiol.* 1992;82:23–29.

47. Radhakrishnan K, So EL, Silbert PL, et al. Predictors of outcome of anterior temporal lobectomy for intractable epilepsy: a multivariate study. *Neurology.* 1998;51:465–471.

48. Krendl R, Lurger S, Baumgartner C. Absolute spike frequency predicts surgical outcome in TLE with unilateral hippocampal atrophy. *Neurology.* 2008;71:413–418.

49. Blume WT, Ganapathy GR, Munoz D, et al. Indices of resective surgery effectiveness for intractable nonlesional focal epilepsy. *Epilepsia.* 2004;45:46–53.

50. Blume WT, Holloway GM, Wiebe S. Temporal epileptogenesis: localizing value of scalp and subdural interictal and ictal EEG data. *Epilepsia.* 2001;42:508–514.

51. Blume WT, Ociepa D, Kander V. Frontal lobe seizure propagation: scalp and subdural EEG studies. *Epilepsia.* 2001;42:491–503.

52. Boon P, Michielsen G, Goossens L, et al. Interictal and ictal video-EEG monitoring. *Acta Neurol Belg.* 1999;99:247–255.

53. Foldvary N, Klem G, Hammel J, et al. The localizing value of ictal EEG in focal epilepsy. *Neurology.* 2001;57:2022–2028.

54. Spencer SS, Williamson PD, Bridgers SL, et al. Reliability and accuracy of localization by scalp ictal EEG. *Neurology.* 1985;35:1567–1575.

55. Swartz BE, Walsh GO, Delgado-Escueta AV, et al. Surface ictal electroencephalographic patterns in frontal vs. temporal lobe epilepsy. *Can J Neurol Sci.* 1991;18:649–662.

56. Gardner AB, Worrell GA, Marsh E, et al. Human and automated detection of high-frequency oscillations in clinical intracranial EEG recordings. *Clin Neurophysiol.* 2007;118:1134–1143.

57. Quesney LF. Extratemporal epilepsy: clinical presentation, pre-operative EEG localization and surgical outcome. *Acta Neurol Scand Suppl.* 1992;140:81–94.

58. Sharbrough FW. Scalp-recorded ictal patterns in focal epilepsy. *J Clin Neurophysiol.* 1993;10:262–267.

59. Devinsky O, Sato S, Kufta CV, et al. Electroencephalographic studies of simple partial seizures with subdural electrode recordings. *Neurology.* 1989;39:527–533.

60. Tao JX, Ray A, Hawes-Ebersole S, et al. Intracranial EEG substrates of scalp EEG interictal spikes. *Epilepsia.* 2005;46:669–676.

61. Tao JX, Baldwin M, Ray A, et al. The impact of cerebral source area and synchrony on recording scalp electroencephalography ictal patterns. *Epilepsia.* 2007;48:2167–2176.

62. Pfander M, Arnold S, Henkel A, et al. Clinical features and EEG findings differentiating mesial from neocortical temporal lobe epilepsy. *Epileptic Disord.* 2002;4:189–195.

63. Dantas FG, Yacubian EM, Jorge CL, et al. Clinical and EEG analysis of mesial and lateral temporal lobe seizures. *Arq Neuropsiquiatr.* 1998;56:341–349.

64. Ebersole JS, Pacia SV. Localization of temporal lobe foci by ictal EEG patterns. *Epilepsia.* 1996;37:386–399.

65. Foldvary N, Lee N, Thwaites G, et al. Clinical and electrographic manifestations of lesional neocortical temporal lobe epilepsy. *Neurology.* 1997;49:757–763.

66. O'Brien TJ, Kilpatrick C, Murrie V, et al. Temporal lobe epilepsy caused by mesial temporal sclerosis and temporal neocortical lesions. A clinical and electroencephalographic study of 46 pathologically proven cases. *Brain.* 1996;119:2133–2141.

67. Wyllie E, Lachhwani DK, Gupta A, et al. Successful surgery for epilepsy due to early brain lesions despite generalized EEG findings. *Neurology.* 2007;69:389–397.

68. Verma A, Radtke R. EEG of partial seizures. *J Clin Neurophysiol.* 2006;23:333–339.

69. Giagante B, Oddo S, Silva W, et al. Clinical-electroencephalogram patterns at seizure onset in patients with hippocampal sclerosis. *Clin Neurophysiol.* 2003;114:2286–2293.

70. Blume WT, Young GB, Lemieux JF. EEG morphology of partial epileptic seizures. *Electroencephalogr Clin Neurophysiol.* 1984;57:295–302.

71. Bautista RE, Spencer DD, Spencer SS. EEG findings in frontal lobe epilepsies. *Neurology.* 1998;50:1765–1771.

72. Toczek MT, Morrell MJ, Risinger MW, et al. Intracranial ictal recordings in mesial frontal lobe epilepsy. *J Clin Neurophysiol.* 1997;14:499–506.

73. Williamson PD, Spencer SS. Clinical and EEG features of complex partial seizures of extratemporal origin. *Epilepsia.* 1986;27(suppl 2):S46–S63.

74. Quesney LF. Preoperative electroencephalographic investigation in frontal lobe epilepsy: electroencephalographic and electrocorticographic recordings. *Can J Neurol Sci.* 1991;18:559–563.

75. Salanova V, Andermann F, Oliver A, et al. Occipital lobe epilepsy: electroclinical manifestations, electrocorticography, cortical stimulation and outcome in 42 patients treated between 1930 and 1991: surgery of occipital lobe epilepsy. *Brain.* 1992;115:1655–1680.

76. Kim DW, Lee SK, Yun C-H, et al. Parietal lobe epilepsy: the semiology, yield of diagnostic workup, and surgical outcome. *Epilepsia.* 2004;45:641–649.

77. Salanova V, Andermann F, Rasmussen T, et al. Parietal lobe epilepsy. Clinical manifestations and outcome in 82 patients treated surgically between 1929 and 1988. *Brain.* 1995;118:607–627.

78. Williamson PD, Boon P, Thadani VM, et al. Parietal lobe epilepsy: diagnostic considerations and results of surgery. *Ann Neurol.* 1992;31:193–201.

79. Williamson PD, Thadani VM, Darcey TM, et al. Occipital lobe epilepsy: clinical characteristics, seizure spread patterns, and results of surgery. *Ann Neurol.* 1992;31:3–13.

80. Blume WT, Ravindran J, Lowry NJ. Late lateralizing and localizing EEG features of scalp-recorded temporal lobe seizures. *J Clin Neurophysiol.* 1998;15:514–520.

81. Ebner A, Hoppe M. Noninvasive electroencephalography and mesial temporal sclerosis. *J Clin Neurophysiol.* 1995;12:23–31.

82. Buechler RD, Rodriguez AJ, Lahr BD, et al. Ictal scalp EEG recording during sleep and wakefulness: diagnostic implications for seizure localization and lateralization. *Epilepsia.* 2008;49:340–342.

83. Quesney LF. Clinical and EEG features of complex partial seizures of temporal lobe origin. *Epilepsia.* 1986;27(suppl 2):S27–S45.

84. Pacia SV, Ebersole JS. Intracranial EEG substrates of scalp ictal patterns from temporal lobe foci. *Epilepsia.* 1997;38:642–654.

85. Castro LH, Serpa MH, Valerio RM, et al. Good surgical outcome in discordant ictal EEG-MRI unilateral mesial temporal sclerosis patients. *Epilepsia.* 2008;49:1324–1332.

86. Chang V, Edwards J, Sagher O. False lateralization of electrographic onset in the setting of cerebral atrophy. *J Clin Neurophysiol.* 2007;24:438–443.

87. Fujimoto A, Masuda H, Homma J, et al. False lateralization of mesial temporal lobe epilepsy by noninvasive neurophysiological examinations. *Neurologia Medico-Chirurgica.* 2006;46:518–521.

88. Lee SK, Yun CH, Oh JB, et al. Intracranial ictal onset zone in nonlesional lateral temporal lobe epilepsy on scalp ictal EEG [see comment]. *Neurology.* 2003;61:757–764.

89. Barba C, Barbati G, Minotti L, et al. Ictal clinical and scalp-EEG findings differentiating temporal lobe epilepsies from temporal 'plus' epilepsies. *Brain.* 2007;130:1957–1967.

90. Cascino GD, Andermann F, Berkovic SF, et al. Gelastic seizures and hypothalamic hamartomas: evaluation of patients undergoing chronic intracranial EEG monitoring and outcome of surgical treatment. *Neurology.* 1993;43:747–750.

91. Holmes MD. Dense array EEG: methodology and new hypothesis on epilepsy syndromes. *Epilepsia.* 2008;49(suppl 3):3–14.

92. Morris HH III, Luders H, Lesser RP, et al. The value of closely spaced scalp electrodes in the localization of epileptiform foci: a study of 26 patients with complex partial seizures. *Electroencephalogr Clin Neurophysiol.* 1986;63:107–111.

93. Laskowitz DT, Sperling MR, French JA, et al. The syndrome of frontal lobe epilepsy: characteristics and surgical management. *Neurology.* 1995;45:780–787.

94. Walczak TS, Radtke RA, Lewis DV. Accuracy and interobserver reliability of scalp ictal EEG. *Neurology.* 1992;42:2279–2285.

95. Mosewich RK, So EL, O'Brien TJ, et al. Factors predictive of the outcome of frontal lobe epilepsy surgery. *Epilepsia.* 2000;41:843–849.
96. Morris HHIM, Dinner DS, Luders H, et al. Supplementary motor seizures: clinical and electroencephalographic findings. *Neurology.* 1988;38:1075–1082.
97. Jobst BC, Siegel AM, Thadani VM, et al. Intractable seizures of frontal lobe origin: clinical characteristics, localizing signs, and results of surgery. *Epilepsia.* 2000;41:1139–1152.
98. Allen PJ, Fish DR, Smith SJ. Very high-frequency rhythmic activity during SEEG suppression in frontal lobe epilepsy. *Electroencephalogr Clin Neurophysiol.* 1992;82:155–159.
99. Kazemi NJ, So EL, Mosewich RK, et al. Resection of frontal encephalomalacias for intractable epilepsy: outcome and prognostic factors [see comment]. *Epilepsia.* 1997;38:670–677.
100. Worrell GA, So EL, Kazemi J, et al. Focal ictal beta discharge on scalp EEG predicts excellent outcome of frontal lobe epilepsy surgery. *Epilepsia.* 2002;43:277–282.
101. Munari C, Bancaud J. Electroclinical symptomatology of partial seizures of orbital frontal origin. *Adv Neurol.* 1992;57:257–265.
102. Rougier A, Loiseau P. Orbital frontal epilepsy: a case report. *J Neurol Neurosurg Psychiatry.* 1988;51:146–147.
103. Blume WT, Wiebe S, Tapsell LM. Occipital epilepsy: lateral versus mesial. *Brain.* 2005;128:1209–1225.
104. Akimura T, Fujii M, Ideguchi M, et al. Ictal onset and spreading of seizures of parietal lobe origin. *Neurol Med Chir.* 2003;43:534–540.
105. Kasowski HJ, Stoffman MR, Spencer SS, et al. Surgical management of parietal lobe epilepsy. *Adv Neurol.* 2003;93:347–356.

CHAPTER 75 ■ NUCLEAR IMAGING (PET, SPECT)

WILLIAM DAVIS GAILLARD

Functional imaging studies using radiotracers, such as positron emission tomography (PET) and single photon emission computed tomography (SPECT), are performed primarily to identify or confirm the ictal focus in preparation for surgery and to investigate the pathophysiology of partial and generalized seizure disorders. Less commonly, PET is performed to identify eloquent cortical regions to be spared during epilepsy surgery.

PRINCIPLES: PET AND SPECT

Radiotracer studies using PET or SPECT allow for the in vivo assessment of physiologic function in humans. Such studies include glucose consumption ($[^{18}F]$fluoro-2-deoxyglucose, $[^{18}F]$FDG), cerebral blood flow ($[^{15}O]$water), and neurotransmitter synthesis (dopamine and serotonin) or receptor ligand binding (agonists or antagonists to benzodiazepine, opiate, serotonin, and N-methyl-D-aspartate [NMDA] receptors). A physiologic probe designed to assess a targeted function is labeled with a radioactive tag. The decay of the radioactive tag is associated with the emission of high-energy particles, or gamma rays, that are subsequently detected by the scanner; their origin is then computed. PET has a theoretical and practical resolution of 2 to 3 mm, which is superior to that of SPECT. Furthermore, unlike SPECT, PET studies can be quantitated. Use and application of PET ligands are in part determined by compound half-lives: ^{18}F-tagged compounds have a 110-minute half-life, ^{11}C a 20-minute half-life, and ^{15}O a 2-minute half-life. As a consequence of its longer half-life, $[^{18}F]$FDG cannot be used to assess short-lived physiologic phenomena such as ictal states, whereas the very short half-life of $[^{15}O]$water renders it suitable for capturing the brief activity of cognitive processes. Given the relatively short half-life of PET ligands, data acquisition must occur shortly or immediately after injection.

In contrast, SPECT ligands have a longer half-life. ^{99m}Tc-Hexamethyl-propyleneamine oxime (^{99m}Tc-HMPAO) or ^{99m}Tc-ethyl cysteinate dimer (^{99m}Tc-ECD) for cerebral perfusion has replaced ^{123}I-based ligands such as $[^{123}I]$iodoamphetamine and $[^{123}I]$trimethyl-hydroxymethyl-iodobenzylpropane diamine, so that data can be collected hours after injection. SPECT is less expensive and more readily available than PET, but the basic premises are similar. SPECT ligands used in epilepsy are primarily markers of perfusion, though some receptor ligands are also available, such as $[^{123}I]$iomazenil ($[^{123}I]$IMZ) for benzodiazepine receptor studies. The compounds that mark blood flow, HMPAO and ECD, have a distribution in the brain that is proportional to cerebral blood flow. Both ligands are lipophilic; they generally cross the blood–brain barrier on their first pass through brain tissue,

become trapped, and exhibit little subsequent redistribution. A potential limitation is that neither ligand has linear uptake at high cerebral blood flow rates, and thus cerebral blood flow is underestimated under certain circumstances (1). Although there are some individual differences in tracer distribution (1), the efficacy of HMPAO and ECD in epilepsy studies is comparable.

PET IN THE EVALUATION OF EPILEPSY

$[^{18}F]$FDG-PET and Temporal Lobe Epilepsy

The greatest clinical experience for evaluating patients with partial epilepsy has been gained with $[^{18}F]$FDG-PET. Several studies in patients with partial epilepsy have identified interictal regional decreases in glucose consumption that are invariably ipsilateral to the seizure focus—typically, but not always, most pronounced in the temporal lobe (Fig. 75.1) (2–4).

Sixty-five to 90% of patients with temporal lobe epilepsy (TLE) demonstrate regional hypometabolism; this figure is closer to 90% on recent generation scanners and to 60% for patients who show normal findings on MRI (5–8). The area of decreased glucose utilization is often more extensive than the epileptogenic zone, and it may extend into adjacent inferior frontal or parietal lobe neocortex (4,9) and occasionally into ipsilateral thalamus (10) and contralateral cerebellum (4). The regional abnormalities are invariably unilateral to the ictal focus; however, lobar localization is somewhat less reliable, about 80% to 90%. The few reports of false lateralization have occurred after surgery (3) was performed, when interpretation relied upon nonquantitative analysis, or occurred during subclinical seizures (3,11,12). Focal interictal regional hypometabolism also predicts a good surgical outcome (6,13–15). Different investigators using different methods and regional analyses have found several different regional hypometabolism patterns predictive of good outcome: inferior lateral temporal, anterior lateral, and uncus (6,13,15), and another study has found that extent of resection of PET abnormalities correlates with postoperative outcome (16). Bilateral temporal hypometabolism is associated with a less optimistic surgical outcome, and in half of patients reflects bilateral foci (17). Patients with focal temporal abnormalities have a 93% chance of good surgical outcome; those without have only a 63% chance (14,15). The ability to confirm the focus and predict surgical outcome is better when quantitative means are used, typically when asymmetry indexes (AIs; e.g., AI = 2[left − right]/[left + right]) are greater than two standard deviations from normative data, or about 10% to 15% (14).

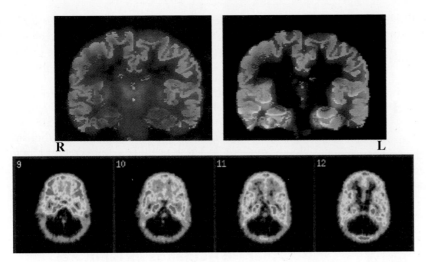

R   L

FIGURE 75.1 [^{18}F]FDG-PET (**upper row left**) showing normal glucose uptake. [^{18}F]FCWAY PET (**top row right**) shows decreased binding in left temporal lobe, most pronounced in amygdala and hippocampus. Lower row are axial views of [^{18}F]FCWAY PET in a normal volunteer. There is no ligand binding in cerebellum reflecting absence of 5HT1A receptors in cerebellar tissue. Raphe nucleus ligand binding can be seen. Left image is right brain. (Courtesy of Dr. William H. Theodore, National Institutes of Health, Bethesda, MD.) (Please see color insert.)

Lesser degrees of asymmetry, though visually apparent, may result in misleading information and erroneous conclusions (5,14). Voxel-based statistical methods performed in a standard anatomic atlas that allows comparison of individual patient images to normal control group data have been advocated as an alternative means of reliable analysis (18). Given that [^{18}F]FDG-PET is often performed to confirm the focus, focal abnormalities may reduce the need for, or extent of, invasive monitoring when laterality of the focus is in doubt (3,14,15). Issues of frontal versus temporal focus may not always reliably be resolved by interictal [^{18}F]FDG-PET studies, and invasive studies or other PET ligand studies may be needed. Conflicting, localizing, or lateralization data nearly always merit invasive monitoring.

Ictal [^{18}F]FDG-PET studies are uncommon because of technical constraints such as ligand availability and unpredictability of seizures. They may show profound focal increases in glucose consumption, but results may also be normal or show decreased consumption. The results depend on the delivery of ligand, time and duration of the seizure, and degree of offsetting postictal hypometabolism. Although of interest, they are of limited clinical use.

The reasons for regional hypometabolism are incompletely understood. Glucose consumption occurs primarily at the synapse. Regional hypometabolism appears to reflect a decrease in glucose influx from reduced glucose transport across the blood–brain barrier, which correlates with subsequent reduced phosphorylation. Cell loss with ensuing synaptic loss and altered remote projections, or degree of hippocampal atrophy in mesial temporal sclerosis (MTS), may account for a portion, but not all, of regional hypometabolism in TLE (19–21). Hypometabolism does not correlate with lifetime generalized tonic–clonic (GTC) seizures or complex partial seizures (CPS) frequency (22). Dysplastic tissue with aberrant synaptic connectivity can have either decreased or normal glucose consumption (23). The abnormalities in some circumstances appear to be functional, as some patients have profound decreases in glucose uptake and no discernible pathology; regional decreased glucose uptake may vary with relation to previous ictal events and clinical manifestations of the previous seizure (9). In patients with MTS, the predominant regions that may manifest decreased glucose consumption are the lateral neocortex and, to a lesser extent, the

frontal cortex. This may reflect the distant projection of functional loss in mesial structures. Frontal hypometabolism and contralateral hypometabolism appear to be reversible with successful temporal lobectomy (24).

Studies differ in the extent to which patients with mesial temporal seizures show pronounced lateral hypometabolism: mesial greater than lateral, lateral greater than mesial, and equal mesial and lateral temporal reductions in glucose uptake have been reported (4,5,25). Patients with neocortical temporal epilepsy may have greater lateral than mesial metabolic abnormalities (25). Patterns of hypometabolism may reflect seizure characteristics and seizure propagation. However, there is sufficient variability among patients that individual predictions of seizure focus within the temporal lobe based on [^{18}F]FDG-PET cannot be made.

[^{18}F]FDG-PET will be abnormal when MRI shows significant abnormalities, for example, in MTS, tumor, vascular malformation, infarct, and most instances of cortical dysplasia. In this setting, [^{18}F]FDG-PET provides little additional information beyond that of MRI. [^{18}F]FDG-PET may be more sensitive than MRI in TLE epilepsy under some circumstances. Current PET techniques are helpful in 85% to 90% of patients, volumetric MRI in 60% to 70%, and magnetic resonance spectroscopy (MRS) in 55%. Higher-resolution scanning techniques, including high-resolution fast spin echo, fluid-attenuated inversion recovery, T2 relaxometry, magnetization transfer, high-resolution thin-cut spoiled gradient recall anatomic sequences, and use of higher magnetic filed strength (3 T and now 7 T) have reduced the utility of [^{18}F]FDG-PET (7,26). Comparison studies report varying efficacy results with different imaging modalities, which generally reflect the particular research strengths of the investigators rather than the intrinsic advantages of the techniques studied.

Although glucose consumption in temporal cortex is decreased, perfusion is often maintained, especially in lateral neocortex (5,27). Interictal studies of cerebral blood flow using [^{15}O]water find a decrease in perfusion in only 50% of patients, but one fifth of these provide falsely localizing information (Fig. 75.1) (5). This experience is similar to that in interictal SPECT studies and quantitative perfusion ascertained by arterial spin labeled fMRI (6,28,29). These data suggest that vascular tone may be impaired in TLE and that the relationship between metabolism and perfusion is altered. For these reasons, interictal blood flow studies are unreliable markers of the epileptogenic zone and do not predict surgical outcome (5).

FDG-PET in Newly Diagnosed and Nonrefractory Localization Related Epilepsy

Metabolic abnormalities are less common in patients with recent-onset, nonrefractory, or well-controlled partial epilepsy. Thirty percent of adults with nonlesional epilepsy within less than 3 years of seizure onset have focal [18F]FDG-PET abnormalities (30). Forty to 50% of adults without refractory seizures of limited duration (<5 years) have focal abnormalities (30,31). Presence of focal abnormalities does not predict 2-year outcome. Other studies report 20% of adults with well-controlled partial seizures had regional metabolic abnormalities. In these adult populations, localization of seizures is less certain than in patients with refractory epilepsy—an important consideration because patients with extratemporal lobe epilepsy are less likely to have abnormal [18F]FDG-PET studies.

Chronic partial epilepsy typically begins during childhood. In a study of 40 children with recent-onset partial epilepsy (mean duration 1 year) and normal MRI (except for MTS), 20% demonstrated regional hypometabolism, all ipsilateral to the presumed focus. All the abnormalities were found among the 32 children with a suspected temporal lobe focus (32). Follow-up studies over 3 years did not show any change in extent or magnitude of regional hypometabolism; a combination of MRI and PET findings predicted outcome, those with

persistent abnormalities faired less well (33). In another study of 15 children, those with worsening seizures, regional hypometabolism changed in relation to seizure frequency (34). In contrast, 70% of children with chronic partial epilepsy (duration 10 years) have focal metabolic abnormalities. There is evidence that adult patients with a greater duration of epilepsy are more likely to have focal [18F]FDG-PET abnormalities (4,27,32). Partial seizures of greater duration are also associated with a greater dissociation between metabolism and blood flow (5,27). These [18F]FDG and cerebral blood flow studies, along with cross-sectional studies using volumetric MRI, may be taken as evidence that TLE in some patients is associated with chronic and continued neuronal injury (27,35).

Other PET Ligands in Temporal Lobe Epilepsy

In addition to widespread reduction in glucose utilization in cortical projection areas, with relatively preserved perfusion, ligand binding studies reveal additional functional abnormalities in patients with TLE (Table 75.1). These findings reflect hippocampal atrophy, loss of neuron populations, or a neuronal response to epilepsy.

GABA-A Receptor Studies

Unlike [18F]FDG-PET, which typically demonstrates hypometabolism that is more widespread than the epileptogenic zone, PET with [11C]flumazenil ([11C]FMZ), a benzodiazepine antagonist of the γ-aminobutyric acid-A (GABA-A) receptor, shows focal abnormalities confined to the hippocampal

---

TABLE 75.1

PET LIGANDS IN TEMPORAL AND NEOCORTICAL (NONLESIONAL) EPILEPSY

Ligand	Tracer	Action	TLE	Neocortical
FDG	18F	Glucose uptake and consumption	Decreased mesial, lateral	Decreased
FMZ	11C	GABA-A receptor benzodiazepine site antagonist	Decreased HF, amygdala	Mixed
FCWAY	18F	5HT1A receptor antagonist	Decreased HF, amygdala, insula	
MPPF	18F	5HT1A receptor antagonist	Decreased mesial temporal lobe	
AMT	11C	Precursor, 5HT/kynurenine synthesis	Increased in normal HF	Increased dysplasia; epileptogenic tubers
Carfentanil	11C	Opiate mu receptor agonist	Increased TL neocortex, decreased amygdala	
Cyclofoxy	18F	Opiate mu, kappa receptor antagonist	Increased ipsilateral TL	
Diprenorphine	11C	Opiate mu, kappa, delta receptor agonist	No change	
Methyl ketamine	11C	NMDA-receptor antagonist	Decreased	
Fallypride	18F	D2/D3-receptor	Decreased, ipsilateral temporal pole, lateral cortex	
SCH23390	11C	D1 receptor		ADNFLE, reduced in striatum
Fluoro-L-DOPA	18F	Dopamine precursor	Decreased, bilateral caudate, putamen and substantia nigra	
Doxepin	11C	H1 receptor agonist	Decreased	
Deprenyl	11C	MAO-B inhibitor (glial)	Increased	

ADNFLE, autosomal dominant nocturnal frontal lobe epilepsy; HF, hippocampal formation; TL, temporal lobe.

formation (8,36,37). Autoradiography of pathologic tissue indicates that most decreased [^{11}C]FMZ binding is proportional to cell loss (8,36). In contrast, some [^{11}C]FMZ binding studies performed in patients with MTS argue for an absence or downregulation of GABA receptors beyond that expected by atrophy alone. After accounting for partial volume effect, a 38% reduction in [^{11}C]FMZ binding is found in sclerotic hippocampus beyond reduction in hippocampal formation volume (37,38). In partial epilepsy, a greater degree and extent of decreased [^{11}C]FMZ binding are seen in patients with more frequent seizures, and decreased binding may extend to projection areas of the epileptogenic region (39). In MTS, there is decreased [^{11}C]FMZ binding in one third of patients in the contralateral hippocampal formation but to a lesser extent than in the epileptogenic hippocampus. This finding is similar to those in MRS studies (7). However, in patients with a temporal focus and normal MRI, [^{11}C]FMZ-PET is less useful (8). SPECT with [^{123}I]IMZ, a benzodiazepine ligand (40), shows results similar to those of the PET ligand.

Serotonin Receptor and Synthesis Studies

Serotonin (5HT)IA receptor binding is reduced, to a greater degree than reduced glucose uptake, in epileptogenic mesial temporal lobe and adjacent insula as deduced by the selective antagonists [^{18}F]trans-4-fluoro-N-2-[4-(2-methoxyphenyl) piperazin-1-yl]ethyl]-N-(2-pyridyl)cyclohexanecarboxamide ([^{18}F]FCWAY) and [^{18}F]2′-methoxyphenyl-(N-2′-pyridinyl)-p-18F-fluoro-benzamidoethylpiperazine ([^{18}F]MPPF) (Fig. 75.1) (41–44). Alpha-[^{11}C]methyl-L-tryptophan ([^{11}C]AMT) is increased in the hippocampus ipsilateral to mesial TLE in patients with normal hippocampal formation volumes, but not MTS (45). [^{11}C]AMT, designed as a serotonin precursor, may also be a marker for quinolinic or kynurenic acid, compounds implicated in excitatory neurotransmission (45–47). Decreased receptor binding in mesial temporal structures is more pronounced than reductions in cerebral metabolism. Decreased binding also correlates with severity of depression in epilepsy patients (48) comparable to patients with primary depression.

Opiate Receptor Binding Studies

Mu-opiate binding determined by [^{11}C]carfentanil, a selective mu agonist, is increased in temporal lobe neocortex ipsilateral to the seizure focus and decreased in amygdala, supporting either an increase in empty receptors or altered receptor affinity (49). [^{18}F]Cyclofoxy, a mu and kappa antagonist, has higher binding in the ipsilateral temporal lobe but shows no significant change in AI (50). Further studies using [^{11}C]diprenorphine, which labels mu-, kappa-, and delta-opiate receptors, do not show any significant changes.

NMDA, Histamine, and MAO-B Ligand Studies

In one study, (S)-[N-methyl-^{11}C]ketamine, an NMDA-receptor antagonist, showed a 9% to 34% decrease in the ipsilateral temporal lobe in eight patients with TLE (51). This observation may reflect either lowered NMDA-receptor density or neuronal cell loss. [^{11}C]Doxepin demonstrates an increase in H1-receptor binding in the epileptogenic zone that is hypometabolic, as shown with [^{18}F]FDG-PET. The ligand deuterium-L-[^{11}C]deprenyl measures the increased expression of monoamine oxidase B (MAO-B) and is thought to be a hallmark of gliosis. In patients with TLE, but not neocortical

epilepsy, there is a lower initial distribution in the ipsilateral temporal lobe but subsequent enhanced accumulation in the temporal lobe ipsilateral to the focus (52). This observation complements MRS employed to detect changes in choline signal, which also reflect gliosis (7). Similar results have been found in nine patients with TLE using the SPECT ligand and MAO-B inhibitor [^{123}I]Ro 43-0463 (53).

PET in Extratemporal Lobe Epilepsy

[^{18}F]FDG-PET is less efficacious in identifying the epileptogenic zone in extratemporal lobe epilepsy than in TLE (54). Most extratemporal lobe epilepsy series include patients with structural lesions that, not surprisingly, show concordant hypometabolism. When patients with abnormal MRI findings are excluded, 11% to 50% of the relatively small patient populations remaining show regional decreases in glucose consumption (8,55). Some investigators have found a good correlation between regional hypometabolism and the epileptogenic zone; others have found a reasonable correlation with side, but not site, of ictal origin. Coregistration of FDG-PET and high-resolution MRI may increase yield of identifying malformations of cortical development, the most common presumed cause of "nonlesional" epilepsy in children and adults (56).

[^{11}C]FMZ-PET studies yield mixed and inconsistent results (8,57). [^{11}C]FMZ binding may be reduced and is more restricted in cortical extent than [^{18}F]FDG-PET abnormalities, when present; appears to correlate with the site of ictal activity; and, if resected, associated with improved outcome (58,59). Patients with acquired lesions may have regional focal reductions in [^{11}C]FMZ binding concordant with the lesion, but most marked at the margins (57). In other studies, two thirds of patients with neocortical epilepsy and normal MRI had [^{11}C]FMZ abnormalities, either increased or decreased, which were bilateral in half of the subjects (57,60). Techniques that correct for gray matter volume averaging may be helpful in identifying abnormal [^{11}C]FMZ binding in cortical dysplasia, or ectopic neurons in white matter, as well as in avoiding false-positive interpretations (60,61). Given these mixed findings, the role of [^{11}C]FMZ in nonlesional epilepsy remains unclear. In patients with extratemporal lobe partial epilepsy, ictal SPECT may be a better identifier of epileptogenic cortex, which is discussed below.

PET in Generalized Epilepsy

PET has been used to explore generalized epilepsies, predominantly of the absence type. Glucose consumption and perfusion are globally increased (62). [^{15}O]Water studies performed during electroencephalographic (EEG) bursts of spike and wave demonstrate not only an increase in global perfusion but also a preferential increase in the thalamic regions, supporting the notion of the thalamus as the facilitator of absence events (63). There are no reported differences in [^{11}C]FMZ binding in the interictal or ictal state in absence epilepsy. However, valproate reduces [^{11}C]FMZ binding in patients with childhood or juvenile absence epilepsy. [^{11}C]Diprenorphine, the nonspecific opiate ligand, does not show any differences between patients with absence epilepsy and normal control subjects, especially in the thalamus.

PET in Children with Epilepsy

[¹⁸F]FDG-PET studies of normal development show increased glucose utilization in all brain areas, peaking around 5 to 8 years of age, that parallels synaptic density (64). Mature patterns of glucose uptake are established in primary motor and sensory cortex before they are consolidated in association cortex. [¹⁸F]FDG-PET studies of children with partial epilepsy show regional abnormalities similar to those seen in adults with temporal or extratemporal lobe epilepsy and are discussed above (Fig. 75.2). Although the primary generalized epilepsies are typically viewed as pediatric disorders, imaging studies in these populations have only been performed in adults (see above). Pediatric epilepsy syndromes that have been studied include infantile spasms, Lennox–Gastaut syndrome, Landau–Kleffner syndrome, Rasmussen encephalitis, and several of the cortical dysplasias, including tuberous sclerosis.

Though children with infantile spasms may show extensive hypometabolism, usually in posterior brain regions (23), these abnormalities often correspond to MRI abnormalities and may identify areas of dysgenesis not readily apparent with older MRI techniques. However, some children with a generalized EEG and normal MRI exhibit regional metabolic abnormalities (65). PET has been used in these cases to remove the epileptogenic zone in children with catastrophic epilepsy. In some children, however, the metabolic abnormalities seen at onset of infantile spasms may resolve with time and thus may represent a functional state that is potentially reversible with successful medical therapy (66). In children with Rasmussen encephalitis and hemimegalencephaly, widespread hemispheric hypometabolism is typically seen. PET has been advocated in some circumstances to assess the integrity of the good hemisphere before extensive cortical resection (23,67).

In tuberous sclerosis, tubers are often hypometabolic, whereas there is some evidence that the more epileptogenic tubers have increased serotonin or kynurenic acid synthesis, reflected by increased [¹¹C]AMT uptake (47,68). [¹¹C]AMT uptake is also increased in focal cortical dysplasia; MRI (especially in children less than 2 years) and [¹⁸F]FDG-PET may be normal (Fig. 75.3) (46,47,68).

PET studies in Lennox–Gastaut and Landau–Kleffner syndromes have yielded mixed results. Children with Lennox–Gastaut syndrome may have focal or multifocal abnormalities, diffuse cortical hypometabolism, or normal studies (69–71). Children with generalized EEG, nonfocal examinations, longer-duration seizures, and normal MRI have normal or diffusely hypometabolic studies. A minority of children exhibit regional metabolic abnormalities, either hypometabolic or hypermetabolic, but many of these children have focal neurologic examinations or partial seizures (69,71). In Landau–Kleffner syndrome and electrical status epilepticus of sleep, inconsistent results have been seen with [¹⁸F]FDG-PET, mostly involving temporal hypometabolism. However, other areas may be hypometabolic or hypermetabolic (72).

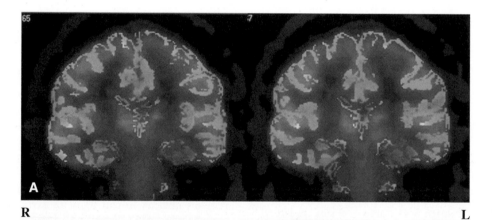

R   L

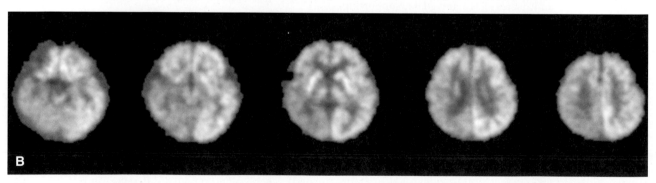

R   L

FIGURE 75.2 A: [¹⁸F]FDG-PET in adult with left temporal lobe epilepsy showing decreased glucose uptake in mesial temporal regions following partial volume correction. (Courtesy of Dr. William H. Theodore, National Institutes of Health, Bethesda, MD.) (Please see color insert.) **B:** [¹⁸F]FDG-PET scan in 14-month-old child with focal seizures (right posterior quadrant focus), and secondary generalization, and normal MRI. Figure shows right posterior quadrant hypometabolism. (National Institutes of Health, Bethesda, MD.)

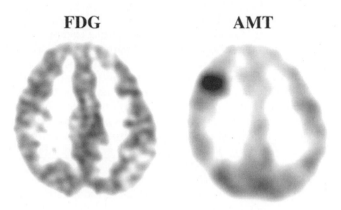

FIGURE 75.3 [^{18}F]FDG-PET (**left**) and [^{11}C] AMT-PET (**right**) in a 3.2-year-old child with frontal lobe epilepsy and normal MRI. [^{18}F]FDG-PET is normal. [^{11}C] AMT-PET shows marked increased ligand uptake in epileptogenic area; pathologic review of resected tissue demonstrated focal cortical dysplasia. (From Juhasz C, Chugani DC, Muzik O, et al. Alpha-methyl-L-tryptophan PET detects epileptogenic cortex in children with intractable epilepsy. *Neurology*. 2003; 60:960–968. Courtesy of Dr. Csaba Juhaz, Detroit Children's Hospital.)

PET and Antiepileptic Drugs

Several studies have examined the effect of antiepileptic drugs on glucose consumption and to a lesser extent on cerebral perfusion. The GABAergic receptor agonists, phenobarbital and benzodiazepine, reduce glucose consumption by 20% to 30%. In contrast, vigabatrin, an inhibitor of GABA degradation, which increases cerebrospinal fluid GABA, reduces glucose uptake by only 8.1% (73). The sodium channel blockers, carbamazepine and phenytoin, reduce glucose uptake by 9.5% and 11.5%, respectively. Valproate, when used in conjunction with carbamazepine in patients with epilepsy, results in a 22%

reduction; however, with monotherapy in normal volunteers, the reduction is only 9.5% with a decrease in perfusion of 14.9%. Although the effects of antiepileptic drugs appear to be global, there is some evidence with valproate of greater decreases in cerebral blood flow in the thalamus, which may reflect an effect of valproate in controlling the generalized epilepsies.

CEREBRAL BLOOD FLOW STUDIES USING SPECT

SPECT and Seizure Focus Identification

Interictal SPECT studies demonstrate regional hypoperfusion in 40% to 50% of patients with partial epilepsy of temporal lobe origin that is ipsilateral to a proven epileptogenic area. However, approximately 5% to 10% of studies are falsely lateralizing (5,6,8,28,74). These findings are similar to those of interictal perfusion studies performed with [^{15}O]water PET, discussed above. SPECT is more suitable for ictal studies than either [^{15}O]water or [^{18}F]FDG-PET and has provided both useful and reliable information. This is possible because both ^{99m}Tc-HMPAO and ^{99m}Tc-ECD have a rapid first-pass uptake but long half-life; the latter factor makes possible ligand availability for bedside injection at ictus as well as time to arrange for data acquisition scanning within 4 to 6 hours after injection. Ictal SPECT, when compared with an interictal study, demonstrates regional hyperperfusion in 67% to 90% of patients (Fig. 75.4). In a large majority of patients, this correlates with the ictal focus and has been validated with simultaneous invasive video-EEG. These findings hold true for temporal as well as extratemporal lobe epilepsy in both children and adults (6,28,75–77). The usefulness of ictal studies approaches that of [^{18}F]FDG-PET in patients with TLE, and ictal studies

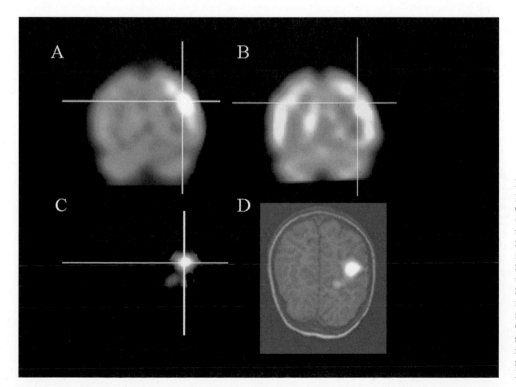

FIGURE 75.4 Ictal ^{99m}Tc-hexamethyl-propyleneamine oxime single photon emission computed tomography (SPECT) in a young adult with refractory partial seizures. **A:** Interictal SPECT. **B:** Ictal SPECT. **C:** Subtraction image of interictal from ictal SPECT. **D:** Subtraction SPECT coregistration with magnetic resonance image (SISCOM). Study demonstrates increased ictal perfusion in the parietal lobe. Here, the right side of the image is the left brain. Chronic invasive recording and surgery subsequently confirmed the ictal focus identified by subtraction SPECT techniques. (Courtesy Dr. Gregory Cascino, Mayo Clinic, Rochester, MN.)

are probably superior for extratemporal focus localization. Partial seizures often show more reliable results than generalized seizures. False localization is reported in 3% to 4% of studies, presumably because of seizure propagation, and is more likely to occur with later injection times (6). Subtraction techniques with MRI coregistration provide enhanced comparison and semiquantitation of perfusion changes between the interictal and ictal states compared with visual comparison alone (32% to 39% vs. 83% to 85%) (see Fig. 75.4) (78). Focal ictal SPECT also predicts whether surgical outcome will be good (79). Many SPECT studies have included patients with clear structural abnormalities such as tumor, MTS, and vascular malformations. As with [18F]FDG-PET, in this setting, it is unclear whether SPECT contributes to the patient evaluation. It is most useful in evaluating patients with nonlesional partial epilepsy, especially extratemporal partial epilepsy. Ictal subtraction SPECT is also useful in evaluating patients who have failed initial surgery: in a study of 58 patients, three quarters were abnormal—90% in the ipsilateral hemisphere, with 70% adjacent to the surgical margin, although only 20% were seizure free following second surgery (80).

Ictal SPECT findings are related to the timing of injection and the clinical manifestations of seizure propagation (81). For an ictal SPECT study to be useful, injection of the ligand must occur during the ictus and no later than 30 seconds after cessation of the seizure. The earlier the injection (<20 seconds from seizure onset), the more reliable are the study results, and better the surgical outcome (82). During the ictus, there is focal increase in cerebral blood flow to involved cortex, often with a surround of decreased perfusion. After the seizure, there is a postictal hypoperfusion, which may return to an interictal state rapidly (77). Postictal hypoperfusion abnormalities are more reliable than interictal hypoperfusion (60% to 70% vs. 40% to 50%, respectively). After ligand injection, lorazepam is sometimes administered to diminish the likelihood of subsequent seizures. The data from the scan can be acquired up to 6 hours after the injection. Furthermore, it is important to recall that if a patient has multiple seizure types, each type must be captured. Automated systems may be helpful to improve timing of ligand delivery; video-EEG monitoring is critical for interpretation of SPECT studies. Newer SPECT ligands (^{99m}Tc-HMPAO and ^{99m}Tc-ECD) have greater stability and offer a longer window of injectability (from 30 minutes to 4 hours after composition).

[15O]WATER PET AND BRAIN MAPPING OF CORTICAL FUNCTION

Although interictal [15O]water PET has not been useful in identifying the epileptogenic zone and the short half-life of [15O]water makes ictal studies impracticable, [15O]water PET have proved useful in identifying eloquent cortex to be spared during surgery. fMRI has supplanted most brain mapping with [15O]water PET (see Chapter 79 for more extensive discussion of brain mapping). The principles underlying brain evaluation with [15O]water PET and fMRI are similar. Both techniques rely on the observation that increased neuronal activity, primarily at the synapse, is associated with regional increases in cerebral blood flow (83–85). Detecting the location of changes in blood flow that occur during cognitive tasks (e.g., involving language) allows the mapping of neural networks involved in these tasks. PET is a direct measure of cerebral blood flow, has the advantage of measuring capillary rather than venous blood flow, and it is less sensitive to motion—thus allowing spoken and overt responses—and may be more suitable for patients who are less cooperative or who are cognitively impaired. PET can also be used to image patients with contraindications to MRI (e.g., implanted metallic devices).

Although [15O]water PET studies of language and cognition are typically analyzed and presented as group rather than individual data sets, advances in PET technology allow for repeated injections of [15O]water in individuals, resulting in less radiation exposure and making feasible reliable individual perfusion maps of cognitive processes (86). Such methods are reliable for lateralization and, unlike the intracarotid amobarbital procedure, localization of language function. Most of these studies rely on verbal fluency or naming tasks, similar to fMRI studies reviewed below, which readily identify anterior language areas.

Bookheimer et al. (87), using an auditory comprehension and naming task, compared individual activation patterns with PET and subdural grid stimulation and found excellent correlation between the disruption elicited by cortical stimulation and the cerebral blood flow activation elicited by task performance. Their study is the first to confirm the assumed reciprocal relationship between activation as defined by local increase in blood flow and the disruption of function elicited by cortical stimulation. Like other functional studies, these studies are valid only for specific aspects of language assessed by the experimental paradigm. Not all activated areas may be critical to language function. Furthermore, what is crucial may not exceed statistical threshold and may not be apparent. Other studies using PET to identify motor sensory cortex find good correlation (less than 5 mm) with corticography (88).

CLINICAL RECOMMENDATIONS FOR USE OF METABOLIC AND FUNCTIONAL IMAGING IN EVALUATION OF PATIENTS WITH PARTIAL EPILEPSY

MRI, MRS, PET, and SPECT provide complementary information. When a structural lesion is present, for example, with a tumor or MTS, then further imaging, though of interest, usually does not provide information relevant to clinical care. MRS and PET may add information in patients with TLE when routine MRI is normal. [18F]FDG-PET provides excellent lateralization of seizure focus but less reliable localization and a lower yield in patients with extratemporal epilepsy. Ictal SPECT is most useful in extratemporal lobe epilepsy, where other modalities are less helpful or unavailable; without EEG confirmation, invasive studies are usually indicated in these settings. The contribution of new PET ligands is not well established, but [11C]FMZ, [18F]FCWAY, and [11C]AMT may provide additional localizing information. [15O]water PET is a reliable technique for lateralization and localization of language and location of motor function.

References

1. Asenbaum S, Brücke T, Pirker W, et al. Imaging of cerebral blood flow with technetium-99m-HMPAO and technetium-99m-ECD: a comparison. *J Nucl Med.* 1998;39(4):613–618.

2. Engel J Jr, Brown WJ, Kuhl DE, et al. Pathological findings underlying focal temporal lobe hypometabolism in partial epilepsy. *Ann Neurol.* 1982; 12:518–529.

3. Engel J Jr, Henry TR, Risinger MW, et al. Presurgical evaluation for partial epilepsy: relative contributions of chronic depth-electrode recordings versus FDG-PET and scalp-sphenoidal ictal EEG. *Neurology.* 1990;40: 1670–1677.

4. Theodore WH, Fishbein D, Dubinsky R. Patterns of cerebral glucose metabolism in patients with partial seizures. *Neurology.* 1988;38: 1201–1206.

5. Gaillard WD, Fazilat S, White S, et al. Interictal metabolism and blood flow are uncoupled in temporal lobe cortex of patients with partial epilepsy. *Neurology.* 1995;45:1841–1848.

6. Ho SS, Berkovic SF, Berlangieri SU, et al. Comparison of ictal SPECT and interictal PET in the presurgical evaluation of temporal lobe epilepsy. *Ann Neurol.* 1995;37:738–745.

7. Knowlton, R.C., Laxer KD, Ende G, et al. Presurgical multimodality neuroimaging in electroencephalographic lateralized temporal lobe epilepsy. *Ann Neurol.* 1997;42:829–837.

8. Ryvlin P, Bouvard S, Le Bars D, et al. Clinical utility of flumazenil-PET versus [18F]fluorodeoxyglucose-PET and MRI in refractory partial epilepsy. A prospective study in 100 patients. *Brain.* 1998;121:2067–2081.

9. Savic I, Lindström P, Gulyás B, et al. Limbic reductions of 5-HT1A receptor binding in human temporal lobe epilepsy. *Neurology.* 2004;62(8). 1343–1351.

10. Khan N, Leenders KL, Hajek M, et al. Thalamic glucose metabolism in temporal love epilepsy measured with 18F-FDG positron emission tomography (PET). *Epilepsy Res.* 1997;28:233–243.

11. Nagarajan L, Schaul N, Eidelberg D, et al. Contralateral temporal hypometabolism on positron emission tomography in temporal lobe epilepsy. *Acta Neurol Scand.* 1996;93:81–84.

12. Sperling MR, Alavi A, Reivich M, et al. False lateralization of temporal lobe epilepsy with FDG positron emission tomography. *Epilepsia.* 1995; 36:722–727.

13. Manno EM, Sperling MR, Ding X, et al. Predictors of outcome after temporal lobectomy: positron emission tomography. *Neurology.* 1994;44: 2331–2336.

14. Theodore WH, Gaillard WD, Sato S, et al. PET measurement of cerebral blood flow and temporal lobectomy. *Ann Neurol.* 1994;36(2):241–244.

15. Theodore WH, Sato S, Kufta CV, et al. FDG-positron emission tomography and invasive EEG: seizure focus detection and surgical outcome. *Epilepsia.* 1997;38(1):81–86.

16. Vinton AB, Carne R, Hicks RJ, et al. The extent of resection of FDG-PET hypometabolism relates to outcome of temporal lobectomy. *Brain.* 2007; 130(pt 2):548–560.

17. Koutroumanidis M, Hennessy MJ, Seed PT, et al. Significance of interictal bilateral temporal hypometabolism in temporal lobe epilepsy. *Neurology.* 2000;54(9):1811–1821.

18. Lee SK, Lee DS, Yeo JS, et al. FDG-PET images quantified by probabilistic atlas of brain and surgical prognosis of temporal lobe epilepsy. *Epilepsia.* 2002;43(9):1032–1038.

19. Foldvary N, Lee N, Hanson MW, et al. Correlation of hippocampal neuronal density and FDG-PET in mesial temporal lobe epilepsy. *Epilepsia.* 1999;40:26–29.

20. Theodore WH, Gaillard WD, De Carli C, et al. Hippocampal volume and glucose metabolism in temporal lobe epileptic foci. *Epilepsia.* 2001;42(1): 130–132.

21. O'Brien TJ, Newton MR, Cook MJ, et al. Hippocampal atrophy is not a major determinant of regional hypometabolism in temporal lobe epilepsy. *Epilepsia.* 1997;38:74–80.

22. Spanaki MV, Kopylev L, Liow K, et al. Relationship of seizure frequency to hippocampus volume in temporal lobe epilepsy. *Epilepsia.* 2000;41: 1227–1229.

23. Chugani HT, Shields WD, Shewmon DA, et al. Infantile spasms: I. PET identifies focal cortical dysgenesis in cryptogenic cases for surgical treatment. *Ann Neurol.* 1990;27(4):406–413.

24. Spanaki MV, Kopylev L, DeCarli C, et al. Postoperative changes in cerebral metabolism in temporal lobe epilepsy. *Arch Neurol.* 2000;57(10): 1447–1452.

25. Hajek M, Antonini A, Leenders KL, et al. Mesiobasal versus lateral temporal lobe epilepsy: metabolic differences in the temporal lobe shown by interictal 18F-FDG positron emission tomography. *Neurology.* 1993;43: 79–86.

26. Gaillard WD, Bhatia S, Bookheimer SY, et al. FDG-PET and volumetric MRI in the evaluation of patients with partial epilepsy. *Neurology.* 1995; 45(1):123–126.

27. Breier JI, Mullani NA, Thomas AB, et al. Effects of duration of epilepsy on the uncoupling of metabolism and blood flow in the complex partial seizures. *Neurology.* 1997;48:1047–1053.

28. Rowe CC, Berkovic SF, Sia ST. Localization of epileptic foci with postictal single photon emission computed tomography. *Ann Neurol.* 1989;26: 660–668.

29. Ryvlin P, Philippon B, Cinotti L, et al. Functional neuroimaging strategy in temporal lobe epilepsy: a comparative study of 18FDG-PET and 99mTc-HMPAO-SPECT. *Ann Neurol.* 1992;31:650–656.

30. Matheja P, Kuwert T, Lüdemann P, et al. Temporal hypometabolism at the onset of cryptogenic temporal lobe epilepsy. *Eur J Nucl Med.* 2001;28(5): 625–632.

31. Weitemeyer L, Kellinghaus C, Weckesser M, et al. The prognostic value of [F]FDG-PET in nonrefractory partial epilepsy. *Epilepsia.* 2005;46(10): 1654–1660.

32. Gaillard WD, Kopylev L, Weinstein S, et al. Low incidence of abnormal 18FDG-PET in children with new onset partial epilepsy: a prospective study. *Neurology.* 2002;58:717–722.

33. Gaillard WD, Weinstein S, Conry J, et al. Prognosis of children with partial epilepsy: MRI and serial 18FDG-PET. *Neurology.* 2007;68(9):655–659.

34. Benedek K, Juhász C, Chugani DC, et al. Longitudinal changes in cortical glucose hypometabolism in children with intractable epilepsy. *J Child Neurol.* 2006;21(1):26–31.

35. Kalviainen R, Salmenperä T, Partanen K, et al. Recurrent seizures may cause hippocampal damage in temporal lobe epilepsy. *Neurology.* 1998; 50(5):1377–1382.

36. Henry TR, Frey KA, Sackellares JC, et al. In vivo cerebral metabolism and central benzodiazepine-receptor binding in temporal lobe epilepsy. *Neurology.* 1993;43:1998–2006.

37. Koepp MJ, Richardson MP, Brooks DJ, et al. Cerebral benzodiazepine receptors in hippocampal sclerosis. An objective in vivo analysis. *Brain.* 1996;119:1677–1687.

38. Koepp MJ, Hand KS, Labbé C, et al. In vivo [11C]flumazenil-PET correlates with ex vivo [3H]flumazenil autoradiography in hippocampal sclerosis. *Ann Neurol.* 1998;43:618–626.

39. Hammers A, Koepp MJ, Labbé C, et al. Neocortical abnormalities of [11C]-flumazenil PET in mesial temporal lobe epilepsy. *Neurology.* 2001;56(7):897–906.

40. Tanaka S, Yonekura Y, Ikeda A. Presurgical identification of epileptic foci with iodine-123 iomazenil SPECT: comparison with brain perfusion SPECT and FDG-PET. *Eur J Nucl Med.* 1997;24:27–34.

41. Toczek MT, Carson RE, Lang L, et al. PET imaging of 5-HT1A receptor binding in patients with temporal lobe epilepsy. *Neurology.* 2003;60(5): 749–756.

42. Giovacchini G, Toczek MT, Bonwetsch R, et al. 5-HT 1A receptors are reduced in temporal lobe epilepsy after partial-volume correction. *J Nucl Med.* 2005;46(7):1128–1135.

43. Didelot A, Ryvlin P, Lothe A, et al. PET imaging of brain 5-HT1A receptors in the preoperative evaluation of temporal lobe epilepsy. *Brain.* 2008;131(pt 10):2751–2764.

44. Merlet I, Ryvlin P, Costes N, et al. 5-HT1A receptor binding and intracerebral activity in temporal lobe epilepsy: an [18F]MPPF-PET study. *Brain.* 2004;127(pt 4):900–913.

45. Natsume J, Kumakura Y, Bernasconi N, et al. Alpha-[11C] methyl-L-tryptophan and glucose metabolism in patients with temporal lobe epilepsy. *Neurology.* 2003;60(5):756–761.

46. Juhasz C, Chugani DC, Muzik O, et al. Alpha-methyl-L-tryptophan PET detects epileptogenic cortex in children with intractable epilepsy. *Neurology.* 2003;60(6):960–968.

47. Fedi M, Reutens DC, Andermann F, et al. Alpha-[11C]-Methyl-L-tryptophan PET identifies the epileptogenic tuber and correlates with interictal spike frequency. *Epilepsy Res.* 2003;52(3):203–213.

48. Theodore WH, Hasler G, Giovacchini G, et al. Reduced hippocampal 5HT1A PET receptor binding and depression in temporal lobe epilepsy. *Epilepsia.* 2007;48(8):1526–1530.

49. Frost JJ, Mayberg HS, Fisher RS. Mu-opiate receptors measured by positron emission tomography are increased in temporal lobe epilepsy. *Ann Neurol.* 1988;23:231–237.

50. Theodore WH, Carson RE, Andreasen P, et al. PET imaging of opiate receptor binding in human epilepsy using [18F]cyclofoxy. *Epilepsy Res.* 1992;13:129–139.

51. Kumlien E, Hartvig P, Valind S, et al. NMDA-receptor activity visualized with (S)-[N-methyl-11C]ketamine and positron emission tomography in patients with medial temporal lobe epilepsy. *Epilepsia.* 1999;40:30–37.

52. Kumlien E, Nilsson A, Hagberg G, et al. PET with 11C-deuterium-deprenyl and 18F-FDG in focal epilepsy. *Acta Neurol Scand.* 2001;103(6): 360–366.

53. Buck A, Frey LD, Bläuenstein P, et al. Monoamine oxidase B single-photon emission tomography with [123I]Ro 43-0463: imaging in volunteers and patients with temporal lobe epilepsy. *Eur J Nucl Med.* 1998;25:464–470.

54. Lee JJ, Lee SK, Lee SY, et al. Frontal lobe epilepsy: clinical characteristics, surgical outcomes and diagnostic modalities. *Seizure.* 2008;17(6):514–523.

55. Kim YK, Lee DS, Lee SK, et al. (18)F-FDG PET in localization of frontal lobe epilepsy: comparison of visual and SPM analysis. *J Nucl Med.* 2002; 43(9):1167–1174.

56. Salamon N, Kung J, Shaw SJ, et al. FDG-PET/MRI coregistration improves detection of cortical dysplasia in patients with epilepsy. *Neurology.* 2008; 71(20):1594–1601.

57. Richardson MP, Koepp MJ, Brooks DJ. 11C-Flumazenil PET in neocortical epilepsy. *Neurology.* 1998;51:485–492.
58. Muzik O, da Silva EA, Juhasz C, et al. Intracranial EEG versus flumazenil and glucose PET in children with extratemporal lobe epilepsy. *Neurology.* 2000;54(1):171–179.
59. Juhasz C, Chugani DC, Muzik O, et al. Relationship of flumazenil and glucose PET abnormalities to neocortical epilepsy surgery outcome. *Neurology.* 2001;56(12):1650–1658.
60. Hammers A, Koepp MJ, Richardson MP, et al. Central benzodiazepine receptors in malformations of cortical development: a quantitative study. *Brain.* 2001;124(pt 8):1555–1565.
61. Hammers A, Koepp MJ, Richardson MP, et al. Abnormalities of grey and white matter [11C]flumazenil binding in temporal lobe epilepsy with normal MRI. *Brain.* 2002;125(pt 10):2257–2271.
62. Theodore WH, Brooks R, Margolin R, et al. Positron emission tomography in generalized seizures. *Neurology.* 1985;35:684–690.
63. Prevett MC, Duncan JS, Jones T, et al. Demonstration of thalamic activation during typical absence seizures using H2(15)O and PET. *Neurology.* 1995;45:1396–1402.
64. Chugani HT, Phelps ME, Mazziotta JC. Positron emission tomography study of human brain functional development. *Ann Neurol.* 1987;22(4):487–497.
65. Chugani HT, Conti JR. Etiologic classification of infantile spasms in 140 cases: role of positron emission tomography. *J Child Neurol.* 1996;11(1):44–48.
66. Metsahonkala L, Gaily E, Rantala H, et al. Focal and global cortical hypometabolism in patients with newly diagnosed infantile spasms. *Neurology.* 2002;58(11):1646–1651.
67. Chugani HT, Shewmon DA, Shields WD, et al. Surgery for intractable infantile spasms: neuroimaging perspectives. *Epilepsia.* 1993;34(4):764–771.
68. Chugani DC, Chugani HT, Muzik O, et al. Imaging epileptogenic tubers in children with tuberous sclerosis complex using alpha-[11C]methyl-L-tryptophan positron emission tomography. *Ann Neurol.* 1998;44:858–866.
69. Chugani HT, Mazziotta JC, Engel J Jr, et al. The Lennox-Gastaut syndrome: metabolic subtypes determined by 2-deoxy-2[18F]fluoro-D-glucose positron emission tomography. *Ann Neurol.* 1987;21(1):4–13.
70. Gaillard WD, Leiderman DB, White S. FDG-PET in children with seizures. *Epilepsia.* 1991;32(suppl 3):72.
71. Theodore W, Rose D, Patronas N, et al. Cerebral glucose metabolism in the Lennox–Gastaut syndrome. *Ann Neurol.* 1987;21(1):14–21.
72. Maquet P, Hirsch E, Metz-Lutz MN, et al. Regional cerebral glucose metabolism in children with deterioration of one or more cognitive functions and continuous spike-and-wave discharges during sleep. *Brain.* 1995;118:1497–1520.
73. Spanaki MV, Siegel H, Kopylev L, et al. The effect of vigabatrin on cerebral blood flow and metabolism. *Neurology.* 1999;53:1518–1522.
74. Markand ON, Salanova V, Worth R, et al. Comparative study of interictal PET and ictal SPECT in complex partial seizures. *Acta Neurol Scand.* 1997;95(3):129–136.
75. Harvey AS, Bowe JM, Hopkins IJ, et al. Ictal 99mTc-HMPAO single photon emission computed tomography in children with temporal lobe epilepsy. *Epilepsia.* 1993;34:869–877.
76. Harvey AS, Hopkins IJ, Bowe JM, et al. Frontal lobe epilepsy: clinical seizure characteristics and localization with ictal 99mTc HMPAO SPECT. *Neurology.* 1993;43:1966–1980.
77. Rowe CC, Berkovic SF, Austin MC, et al. Patterns of postictal cerebral blood flow in temporal lobe epilepsy: qualitative and quantitative analysis. *Neurology.* 1991;41(7):1096–1103.
78. Chang DJ, Zubal IG, Gottschalk C, et al. Comparison of statistical parametric mapping and SPECT difference imaging in patients with temporal lobe epilepsy. *Epilepsia.* 2002;43(1):68–74.
79. O'Brien TJ, So EL, Mullan BP, et al. Subtraction SPECT co-registered to MRI improves postictal SPECT localization of seizure foci. *Neurology.* 1999;52:137–146.
80. Wetjen NM, Cascino GD, Fessler AJ, et al. Subtraction ictal single-photon emission computed tomography coregistered to magnetic resonance imaging in evaluating the need for repeated epilepsy surgery. *J Neurosurg.* 2006;105(1):71–76.
81. Shin WC, Hong SB, Tae WS, et al. Ictal hyperperfusion patterns according to the progression of temporal lobe seizures. *Neurology.* 2002;58(3):373–380.
82. Lee SK, Lee SY, Yun CH, et al. Ictal SPECT in neocortical epilepsies: clinical usefulness and factors affecting the pattern of hyperperfusion. *Neuroradiology.* 2006;48(9):678–684.
83. Fox PT, Raichle ME. Focal physiological uncoupling of cerebral blood flow and oxidative metabolism during somatosensory stimulation of human subjects. *Proc Natl Acad Sci U S A.* 1986;323:806–809.
84. Roy CS, Sherrington CS. On the regulation of blood flow to the brain. *J Physiol.* 1980;11:85–108.
85. Logothetis NK. The underpinnings of the BOLD functional magnetic resonance imaging signal. *J Neurosci.* 2003;23(10):3963–3971.
86. Hunter KE, Blaxton TA, Bookheimer SY, et al. (15)O water positron emission tomography in language localization: a study comparing positron emission tomography visual and computerized region of interest analysis with the Wada test. *Ann Neurol.* 1999;45(5):662–665.
87. Bookheimer SY, Zeffiro TA, Blaxton T, et al. A direct comparison of PET activation and electrocortical stimulation mapping for language localization. *Neurology.* 1997;48:1056–1065.
88. Bittar RG, Olivier A, Sadikot AF, et al. Localization of somatosensory function by using positron emission tomography scanning: a comparison with intraoperative cortical stimulation. *J Neurosurg.* 1999;90:478–483.

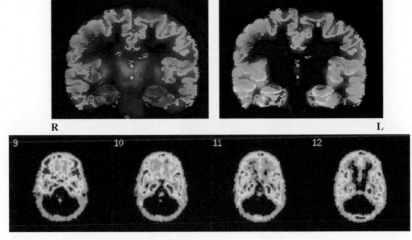

FIGURE 75.1 [^{18}F]FDG-PET (**upper row left**) showing normal glucose uptake. [^{18}F]FCWAY PET (**top row right**) shows decreased binding in left temporal lobe, most pronounced in amygdala and hippocampus. Lower row are axial views of [^{18}F]FCWAY PET in a normal volunteer. There is no ligand binding in cerebellum reflecting absence of 5HT1A receptors in cerebellar tissue. Raphe nucleus ligand binding can be seen. Left image is right brain. (Courtesy of Dr. William H. Theodore, National Institutes of Health, Bethesda, MD.)

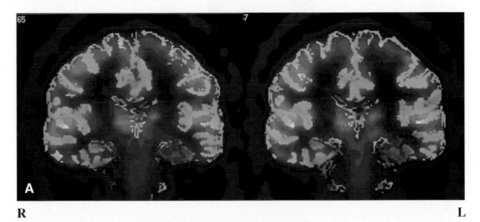

FIGURE 75.2 A: [^{18}F]FDG-PET in adult with left temporal lobe epilepsy showing decreased glucose uptake in mesial temporal regions following partial volume correction. (Courtesy of Dr. William H. Theodore, National Institutes of Health, Bethesda, MD.)

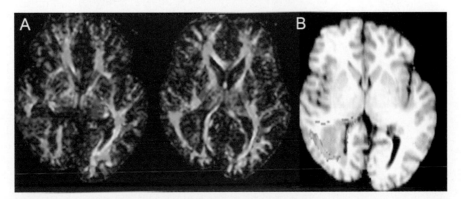

FIGURE 77.2 Malformations of cortical development and alterations of connectivity. Twenty-six-year-old with intractable focal epilepsy arising from the right temporo-occipital region. MRI showed right > left posterior quadrant polymicrogyria and heterotopic gray matter in the right posterior quadrant. **A:** Axial colorized fiber orientation maps showing displacement of the right superior fronto-occipital fasciculus and superior longitudinal fasciculus. **B:** Two-dimensional illustration of the tractography results overlaid onto the T1 image demonstrates the spatial relationship between the heterotopic gray matter and the white matter tracts.

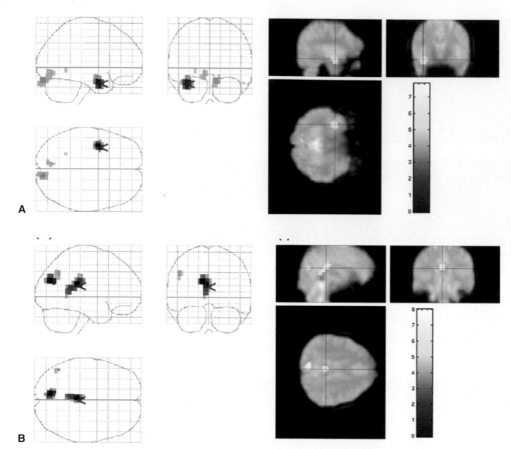

FIGURE 77.3 IED-related BOLD changes. Patient with left hippocampal sclerosis and left-temporal IEDs who underwent EEG–fMRI. **A:** BOLD increase in the left-temporal lobe with smaller clusters in the occipital region. The red arrow and cross-hair represent the location of the most significant BOLD change. The left of figure shows all statistically significant BOLD changes superimposed onto the SPM "glass-brain." The right of the figure shows parasagittal, coronal, and axial sections through the EPI data at the location of the statistical maximum. **B:** Retrosplenial BOLD decrease associated with the same IED. This effect, which is thought not to represent activity of the source of the spike seen on EEG, is commonly observed in relation to interictal activity in the temporal lobe. (Taken from Salek-Haddadi A, Diehl B, Hamandi K, et al. Hemodynamic correlates of epileptiform discharges: an EEG-fMRI study of 63 patients with focal epilepsy. *Brain Res.* 2006;1088(1): 148–166, with permission).

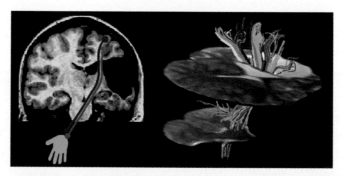

FIGURE 78.3 Diffusion tensor fiber tracking in a patient with corticosubcortical infarction. (From Staudt M, Erb M, Braun C, et al. Extensive peri-lesional connectivity in congenital hemiparesis. *Neurology.* 2006;66:771, with permission from Lippincott Williams & Wilkins, Copyright (2006).) Example of a patient with a pre- or perinatally acquired infarction in the territory of the middle cerebral artery, leaving only a small bridge of preserved white matter between the enlarged lateral ventricle and the large cystic lesion (**left:** T1-weighted coronal image). Nevertheless, TMS and MEG indicated preserved crossed corticospinal motor projections (red) and preserved crossed thalamocortical somatosensory projections (blue). Accordingly, MR diffusion tractography (**right;** in random colors) visualizes the extensive connectivity mediated by this small bridge of preserved white matter (= seed area for fiber tracking).

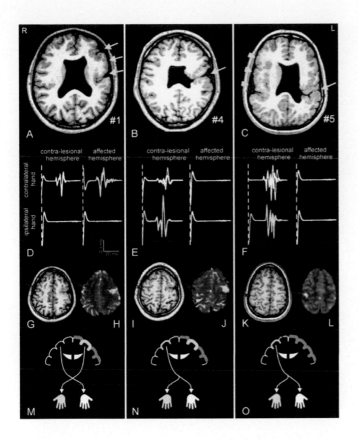

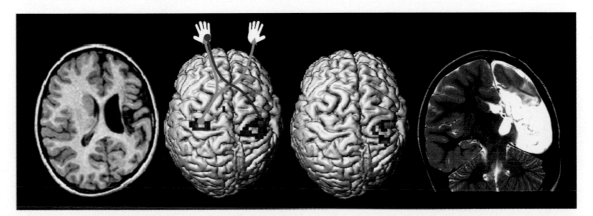

FIGURE 78.5 Function and reorganization in patients with malformations of cortical development. (From Staudt M, Krageloh-Mann I, Holthausen H, et al. Searching for motor functions in dysgenic cortex: a clinical transcranial magnetic stimulation and functional magnetic resonance imaging study. *J Neurosurg.* 2004;101:69–77, with permission from XX J Neurosurg XX, Copyright (2004)?) Structural MRI, TMS, and fMRI findings (paretic hand movement) are obtained in three patients with congenital hemiparesis due to malformations of cortical development, illustrating different possibilities of participation of the MCDs in hand motor functions. *Left column*: harboring the primary motor representation of the paretic hand (with crossed corticospinal projections originating in the dysgenic cortex); *middle column*: harboring the primary somatosensory (S1) representation of the paretic hand (MEG evidence not shown here)—with a reorganized primary motor representation (M1) of the paretic hand in the contralesional hemisphere; *right column*: showing no evidence of participation (with fMRI activation exclusively in the contralesional hemisphere). A–C: Axial reconstructions from the T1-weighted 3D data sets, depicting the frontoparietal polymicrogyria in Case 1 (arrows in A) and the schizencephalies in Cases 4 and 5 (*arrows* in B and C). D–F: Note the additional small area of polymicrogyria contralateral to the schizencephaly (*arrowheads* in C) after (*arrows* in B and C). Results of TMS for stimulation of the affected and contralesional hemispheres, with MEPs recorded simultaneously from target muscles of both the paretic hand (yellow MEPs) and the nonparetic hand (white MEP). G–L: fMRI activation patterns for movement of the paretic hand (yellow), superimposed on axial (functional) mean EPI sequences (H, J, and L). Red arrows indicate the central sulcus; corresponding slices from the 3D data sets are displayed in G, I, and K. M–O: Schematic illustration of the TMS and fMRI findings in the three patients. The thick gray cortical line represents the MCD; fMRI activation during movement of the paretic hand (yellow symbol) is also indicated.

FIGURE 78.10 Epilepsy surgery in a case of hemispheric dissociation between motor and sensory functions. An 8-year-old girl with pharmacorefractory seizures and congenital hemiparesis due to a pre- or perinatally acquired infarction in the territory of the middle cerebral artery. After hemispherectomy, the paretic hand could still be used for active grasping. **Left:** Axial T1-weighted image depicting the corticosubcortical lesion. **Middle left:** fMRI during active hand movement. Green arrows indicate TMS evidence of bilateral corticospinal projections from the contralesional hemisphere to the paretic hand; the blue arrow indicates preserved crossed spino-thalamo-cortical somatosensory projections to the central (Rolandic) region of the lesioned hemisphere. **Middle right:** fMRI during passive hand movement. **Right:** Coronal T2-weighted image after hemispherectomy.

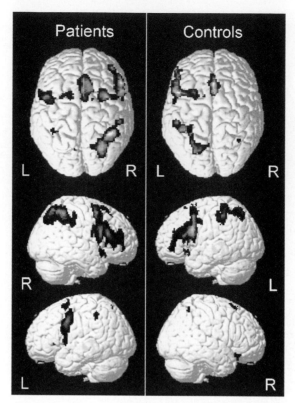

FIGURE 78.11 Architecture of lesion-induced right-hemispheric language organization. (From Staudt M, Lidzba K, Grodd W, et al. Right-hemispheric organization of language following early left-sided brain lesions: functional MRI topography. *Neuroimage.* 2002;16:954–967, with permission.) Functional MRI of speech production (silent generation of word chains) in five healthy right-handers (left) and five patients with predominantly right-hemispheric language representation due to left-sided periventricular brain lesions. SPM99, fixed-effect group analyses.

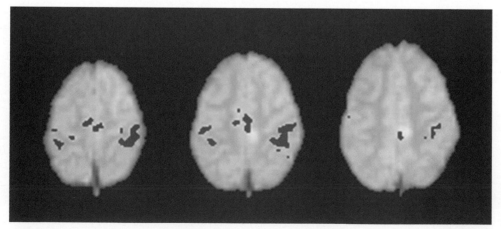

L　　　　　　　　　　　　　　　　　　　　**R**

FIGURE 79.1 A 10-year-old with a right mesial mass seen as increased signal. fMRI of motor tapping of left hand compared to rest yields activation (red), which identifies primary motor cortex, posterior to the lesion. Mirror activation ipsilateral to tapping hand is also seen. Supplementary motor cortex activation is seen adjacent to the lesion. This image is from raw fMRI data, rather than superimposed on high-resolution anatomic images (as seen in language/speech activation in Figure 79.3).

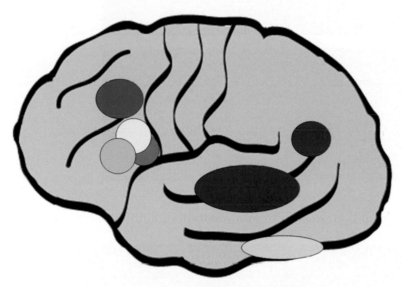

FIGURE 79.2 Schema showing areas activated with different paradigms advocated in individual studies. Areas adjacent to, and along, the superior temporal sulcus (blue) are activated by tasks that stress phrase or sentence comprehension such as listening to stories or reading stories or sentences. Supramarginal gyrus (and sometimes angular gyrus) (purple) may also be activated in auditory sentence processing tasks. Fusiform gyrus (light blue) is activated by tasks that require feature search or identification, such as identifying written characters or object naming. Middle frontal gyrus (red) is implicated in verbal working memory for reading, grammatical decipherment, or verbal recall. Inferior frontal gyrus subregions are activated by a variety of tasks, phonologic fluency (orange), syntactic/semantic decision (green), semantic fluency or recall (yellow).

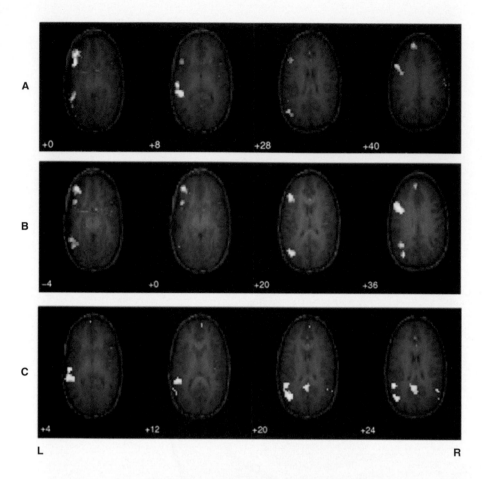

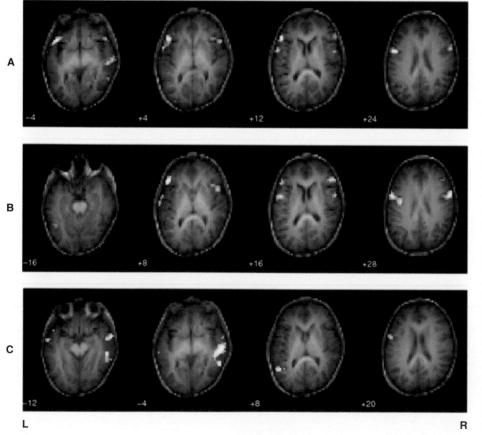

FIGURE 79.3 Functional magnetic resonance imaging (echo planar imaging, blood oxygenation level dependent) panel of tasks. I. Young adult with right temporal lobe focus; panel of tasks shows left frontal and left temporal activation demonstrating left-hemisphere dominance for language. II. A young adult with a left temporal lobe focus showing atypical language dominance. Activation predominantly occurs in right homologues of Broca's and Wernicke's Areas. The left side of the image is the left brain. "Activated" voxels representing brain regions involved in performing the task compared with a control condition (rest) are red. A. Auditory-based word definition task where patient decides whether a description of an object matches final answer (e.g., "a large pink bird is a flamingo"). Control conditions are the same clues in reverse speech and search for the presence of an after going tone; this controls for sound, pitch complexity, attention, and decision aspects of task. B. Auditory category decision task; the patient decides whether a presented word matches a given category (e.g., food: "pizza" "chair" "bean"); reverse speech tone control. C: Listening to stories; control reverse speech. For each paradigm there are five cycles, each consisting of a 30-second control condition and 30-second task condition.

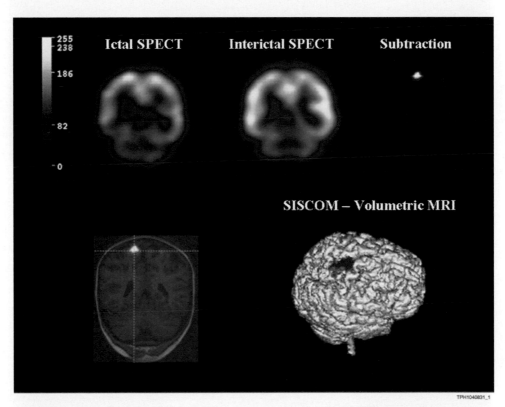

FIGURE 86.2 Steps to obtaining subtraction ictal SPECT (single photon emission computed tomography) coregistered to MRI (magnetic resonance imaging) (SISCOM) image. Ictal (**upper left**) and interictal (**upper middle**) SPECT images are obtained. After normalization of their mean intensities and coregistration with each other, subtraction is performed to obtain a "difference" image (**upper right**). The difference image is then coregistered with MRI images at specific planes (**lower left**) or on the surface of a three-dimensional MRI image (**lower right**). (From So E. Role of neuroimaging in the management of seizure disorders. *Mayo Clin Proc.* 2002;77:1251–1264, with permission.)

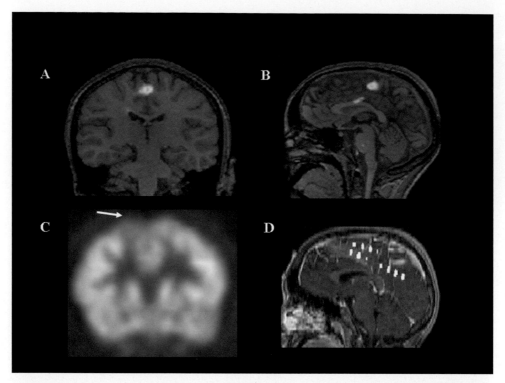

FIGURE 86.3 A: Coronal view of subtraction ictal SPECT (single photon emission computed tomography) coregistered to magnetic resonance imaging (MRI) (SISCOM) showing an apparently midline hyperperfusion focus in a 13-year-old male who had between 1 and 10 attacks per night of bilateral extremity movements and facial grimacing. Epilepsy-protocol MRI was normal and scalp ictal electroencephalogram was nonlocalizing. **B:** Sagittal view of SISCOM shows that the hyperperfusion focus was at the right posterior mesial frontal region. **C:** 2-[18F]fluoro-2-deoxy-D-glucose (FDG)–positron emission tomography (PET) shows a hypometabolic focus corresponding to the SISCOM hyperperfusion focus. **D:** MRI with coregistered CT (computed tomography)-derived images of subdural electrode contacts (white marks) on the SISCOM and PET abnormalities. The intracranial EEG recording confirmed ictal onset at the SISCOM and PET abnormalities. Surgical resection of the region rendered the patient free of seizures, with minimal weakness in the left toes. Pathologic examination of the specimen revealed cortical dysplasia.

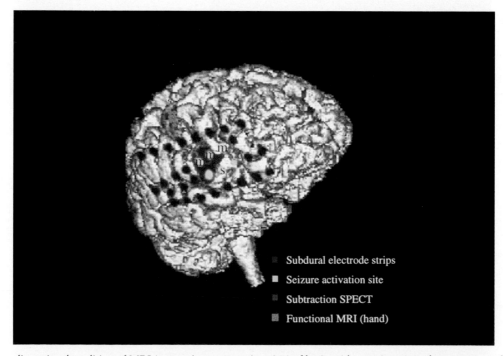

FIGURE 86.4 Three-dimensional rendition of MRI (magnetic resonance imaging) of brain with coregistration of sensory area of the hand identified with functional MRI (green), subtraction ictal SPECT (single photon emission computed tomography) coregistered to MRI (SISCOM) hyperperfusion focus (red), subdural electrodes (blue), and electrodes where electroencephalograph-detected seizures commenced (yellow). *m*, electrode sites where facial motor activity was elicited with electrocortical stimulation; *s*, electrode site where sensory function was elicited. (From So E. Role of neuroimaging in the management of seizure disorders. *Mayo Clin Proc.* 2002;77:1251–1264, with permission.)

CHAPTER 76 ■ MAGNETOENCEPHALOGRAPHY

THOMAS BAST

WHAT IS MAGNETOENCEPHALO-GRAPHY (MEG)?

Every electrical current produces an orthogonal magnetic flux and vice versa every magnetic flux produces an orthogonal current (Fig. 76.1). This also applies to biological intra- and extracellular currents generated by electrically active human body cells. Biomagnetism aims to measure and analyze these extracorporeal magnetic fields generated by somatic electric sources. In the 1960s, the first detection of magnetic fields generated by the heart gave way to magnetocardiography (1). Magnetoencephalography (MEG) is the completely noninvasive and contactless detection of tiny magnetic fields produced by neuronal activity in the cortex, pioneered by Cohen et al. (2) in 1968. Technical advances, that is, the development of shielded rooms and magnetometers based on supraconducting devices, became the basis for measurement of physiologic and pathologic brain activity (3). In 1982, Barth detected epileptic activity by MEG for the first time (4).

To date, MEG is mainly used by neurophysiologists in the analysis of complex and fast cortical activities, as it combines otherwise unreached high temporal resolution with satisfactory localization accuracy. Various event-related MEG activities, for example, triggered by somatosensory, acoustic, or visual stimuli, may provide information on the localization and (re-)organization of different eloquent cortical areas even in the clinical setting. However, this chapter focuses on the impact of MEG on the analysis of epileptic activities, which is the major clinical application. MEG has become an additional noninvasive diagnostic tool in the presurgical evaluation of children and adults with refractory epilepsy. Analysis of inter-ictal and ictal epileptic activity is usually based on algorithms for inverse electromagnetic source analysis. In 1997, MEG-based source localization in combination with structural imaging received Food and Drug Administration's approval for clinical use in the United States. In 2003, it was given Current Procedural Terminology (CPT) codes for epilepsy localization and presurgical brain mapping. Recent reviews valued MEG as useful in presurgical epilepsy workup (5–7).

TECHNICAL AND BIOLOGICAL BACKGROUND OF MEG

Amplitudes of magnetic fields measured by MEG are very small (typically 50 to 200 fT). Thus, patients are placed in a special room shielding recordings from environmental magnetic fields. Gradiometers detect magnetic field gradients based on direct-current superconducting quantum interference devices (SQUIDS) instead the actual field, which improves signal-to-noise ratio. Technical success in the 1970s allowed for direct detection of spontaneous neuronal activity, as well as evoked fields related to somatosensory, auditory, and visual stimuli. In 1993, whole-scalp MEG instruments were introduced and allowed for the application for clinical

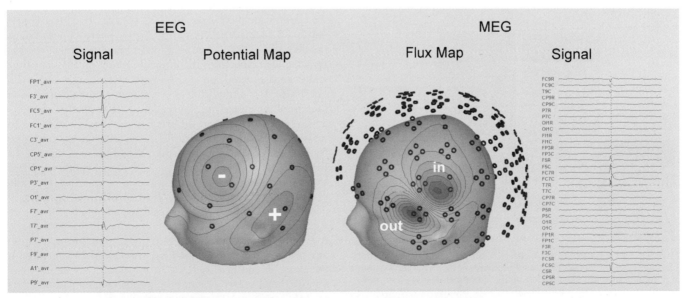

FIGURE 76.1 Simultaneous EEG and MEG in a child with benign epilepsy showing centrotemporal spikes. Principle morphology of an average of 45 interictal spikes is identical. Electric potential field and magnetic flux are orthogonal to each other.

studies in patients (8,9). The more common planar gradiometers detect changes of the magnetic field amplitudes between two very close localizations underlying one sensor. In other words, the largest signal is picked up above the strongest local current, where the field gradient reaches its peak allowing for an easier visual analysis. Signals detected by planar gradiometer systems are dominated by more superficial sources. This causes difficulties for detection of epileptic activity from deep regions like the hippocampus (i.e., in mesiotemporal epilepsy) (10,11). Axial gradiometers and magnetometers directly measure magnetic flux in a given location. Maxima and minima of the signals are located some centimeters from the center of an activated brain area. Magnetometers are more sensitive to deep brain sources than gradiometers. However, they are more sensitive to ambient noise, at least within the typical frequency spectrum used in analysis in clinical epileptology (12). To date, multichannel MEG systems with hundreds of sensors, some combining planar gradiometers and magnetometers, are increasingly implemented in epilepsy surgery programs.

EEG and MEG signals are generated by the same neurophysiologic processes, namely summated dipolar electric currents generated in the cerebral cortex. These dipolar currents are associated with dendritic excitatory and inhibitory postsynaptic potentials. Magnetic fields detectable outside the head are produced directly by intracellular current flow in the active neuron. In contrast, EEG signals are mainly determined by the distribution of the secondary extracellular volume currents (13). A considerable number of neurons functioning synchronously are necessary to generate electromagnetic fields measurable outside the head. Thus, the dendrites of pyramidal neurons aligned in parallel are considered the main contributors to MEG and EEG signals from the cerebral cortex.

EEG signals are dominated by activities from pyramidal neurons with an orientation radial to the head surface. Superficial pyramidal neurons in the gyral crowns contribute to the greatest extent. Activity from more tangentially oriented neurons, that is, pyramidal cells from fissural or basal cortex, also contributes to the EEG signal, but to a smaller extent (Fig. 76.2). Since the studies carried out by Cohen and

Cuffin in 1983, a higher MEG sensitivity to activity produced by tangential orientated neurons has been established (14–16). Magnetic fields due to intracellular currents of radial orientation are cancelled by those of the corresponding extracellular volume currents. The signal of neurons given this orientation will severely be attenuated below the noise level. Thus, MEG appears to be blind to pure radial sources (15,17,18). MEG detects only magnetic fields generated by currents tangential to the head surface, or by tangential components of sources with oblique orientation. The sources are localized in cortical sulci or in basal regions of the frontal or temporal lobe, comprising about two thirds of the cortex (see Fig. 76.2).

Table 76.1 summarizes the clinically relevant differences between MEG and surface EEG.

DETECTION OF EPILEPTIC ACTIVITY

A number of studies have compared spike detection rates in simultaneously recorded EEG and MEG in patients with epilepsy. Since there is no standardized definition of magnetic spikes (11), EEG criteria are usually applied. As a rule, MEG detects more spikes compared to EEG in neocortical epilepsies (11,19–23). Whereas detection rates of epileptic activity in anterotemporal epilepsies are comparable (11,20,24,25), EEG is superior in the detection of spikes in mesiotemporal epilepsies (10,24,25). Detecting epileptic activity in the mesial temporal cortex and deep orbitofrontal cortices directly by MEG is difficult, because gradiometers are relatively insensitive to deep sources (10,11). MEG seems to have a better sensitivity than EEG in posterior lateral sources (25). A recent review summarized the success rates of MEG regarding detection and analysis of epileptic activity from 25 studies (6). Success rates in the detection of epileptic activity by MEG measured to circa 75% in general; however, they dropped to 45% when temporal lobe epilepsy was specifically analyzed.

Not all epileptic MEG discharges are accompanied by simultaneous EEG spikes, and conversely not all EEG spikes are accompanied by MEG activity. This follows from the complementary sensitivities of the two techniques (11,20,22,23,25–30,53). In most research carried out to date, the detection of a spike population in one modality alone was principally attributed to the influence of characteristics of the spike source itself on MEG and EEG diagnostic yield (11,19,27,31). Amplitude, orientation, and localization (depth) of the underlying source influence appearance in EEG and/or MEG. However, differences in signal-to-noise ratio may also result from different background activities. Ramantani et al. compared spike detection in simultaneous EEG and MEG sleep recordings (22). They hypothesized that sleep changes, such as vertex waves and spindles, typically present with a radial potential field in EEG and may superpose low-amplitude spikes. Spikes detected only by MEG were significantly associated with simultaneous sleep changes. Averaging of pure MEG spikes reduced signal-to-noise ratio and resulted in clear epileptic discharges in the EEG in most of the cases. In contrast, spikes that appeared only in EEG had a more radial source orientation, and averaging had no effect on MEG visibility. Thus, appearance in MEG-only is mainly based on a better signal-to-noise ratio, whereas EEG-only spikes are usually generated by more radial-oriented sources.

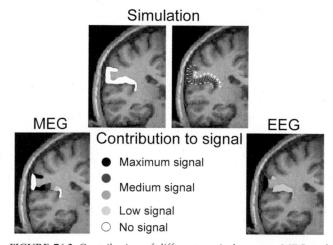

FIGURE 76.2 Contribution of different cortical areas to MEG and EEG signals. Top: Two-dimensional simulation of a cortical activation and dipolar currents. Bottom left: Only pyramidal neurons with tangential or oblique orientation relative to the head surface contribute to MEG signal. Bottom right: EEG signal is dominated by activities from radially oriented sources. Tangential sources contribute to the signal, but in a smaller extent.

TABLE 76.1

CLINICALLY RELEVANT DIFFERENCES BETWEEN SURFACE EEG AND MEG

EEG	MEG
Signals result from differences in surface potentials by secondary extracellular volume currents	**Signals** result from extracranial magnetic fields produced directly by intracellular neuronal currents
Dominated by radial sources	Exclusively generated by tangential sources
Predominantly pyramidal neurons in gyral crowns	Fissural and/or basal pyramidal neurons
Tangential sources contribute to the signal in a smaller extent	Discards any information in a radial direction
Marked influence of **volume conduction**	No relevant influence of **volume conduction**
Forward problem: Necessity of sophisticated head models for source analysis	Forward problem: Simple head models adequate. Higher accuracy
Widely available	Rare
Cheap	Expensive
Usually limited to 30 (max. 64) electrodes in clinical routine	High number of sensors (up to >300)
Long preparation time (h)	Short preparation time (min)
Fixed electrodes	Sensitive to head movements resulting a localization error
Suitable for use in children/handicapped	Cooperation required/sleep recording
Mobile	Shielded room
Suitable for long-term recordings	Recording time limited
Number of spikes "unlimited"	Number of spikes "limited"
Interictal and ictal recordings	Mainly interictal, ictal recordings rare

In general, more patients present with MEG-only spikes compared to patients with spikes only detected by EEG (20,23). Iwasaki et al. compared spike detection in simultaneous MEG and EEG (20). A median of 25.7% of total spikes was detectable by both modalities. A larger amount of spikes was detectable only in either EEG or MEG. Spike localization was similarly consistent with the epilepsy diagnosis in 85.2% (EEG) and 78.1% (MEG) of patients. Based on their findings, the authors concluded that independent spike identification in MEG provided clinical results comparable, but not superior, to EEG and underlined the importance of simultaneous EEG and MEG recordings.

An obvious cause of higher MEG spike detection rates is the higher number of sensors compared to surface EEG (32). The number of EEG channels considerably influences visual spike detection rates (31). Only few studies compared MEG with high-resolution EEG (23,24,33,34). Knake et al. studied 70 consecutive candidates for epilepsy surgery who underwent simultaneous 70-channel-EEG and 306-channel-MEG recordings (23). Massive artifacts did not allow for further analysis in three patients. Of the remaining 67 patients, interictal spikes were detected in 72% by 306-sensor MEG and in 61% by 70-channel EEG. Spikes were identified by both modalities in 55.7% of the cases. MEG-only spikes occurred in 13% and EEG-only spikes in 3% of the patients. Combined sensitivity of MEG and EEG was 75%. MEG recorded epileptiform activity in one third of the EEG-negative patients, particularly in patients with lateral neocortical epilepsy or focal cortical dysplasia. Thus, MEG added important information in a considerable number of cases.

It is of great importance to note that not all epileptic discharges in the cortex produce an external electromagnetic field detectable by either EEG or MEG. MEG positive spikes can be expected when the activated surface has an extent of at least 6 to 8 cm^2 in temporobasal (10,27,35), 3 cm^2 in temporolateral (36), and 3 to 4 cm^2 in frontolateral localization (35). In EEG, only a few spikes are recognizable when the activated anterior lateral cortex involves less than 10 cm^2. Most of the typical temporal anterior spikes reflect an activated area of 20 to 30 cm^2 (37). Lack of interictal spikes in either EEG or MEG is no proof for the absence of epileptic activity!

INTERICTAL VERSUS ICTAL MEG

Conditions for MEG acquisition do not usually allow for long-term recording. The fixed Dewar containing the SQUIDS surrounds the patient's head and this arrangement is sensitive to head movements (38). Algorithms for correction of head movements have recently been developed and will improve MEG accuracy in near future (39,40). Another limiting factor is that the patient has to stay in a shielded room and the acquisition unit is not mobile.

Due to limited acquisition time, ictal MEG recordings are rare and succeed in only about 5% of all recordings (41–45). A major shortcoming of MEG is that analysis of only interictal spikes may not reflect the actual localization of patients' epileptogenic, that is, seizure-generating, zone. This very true statement should, on the other hand, not disqualify MEG in epilepsy per se. Knowlton recently stated that spikes seen at the scalp by either EEG or MEG should not be confused with those recorded at the cortex, for which terms such as irritative zone are used (7). Spikes recognizable at the scalp are a strongly selected subset of robust, large amplitude discharges that contrast greatly with the far more numerous and scattered spikes recorded by electrocorticography (ECoG) (37,46). In lateral temporal or extratemporal neocortical epilepsies, frequent unifocal spikes that tightly cluster on source localization have a strong correlation with seizure onset recorded with intracranial EEG (47,48). There is few data from small patient series on the comparison of ictal and interictal epileptiform activity in MEG. Ictal MEG was superior in three out of six patients in one study (41) and sources of interictal spikes were found in the same area as the sources of ictal spikes in two further series (42,45).

ELECTROMAGNETIC SOURCE IMAGING OF EPILEPTIC ACTIVITY

MEG may not only detect interictal and ictal epileptic activity, but it additionally allows for a more accurate localization of the underlying source. The combination of MEG source localization with structural imaging by superposition is called magnetic source imaging (49). While MEG gained acceptance as a noninvasive tool for presurgical evaluation, there is still little research on the impact of EEG source analysis (50).

The "forward problem" is modeling an electromagnetic field on the surface for a three-dimensionally localized source with defined orientation and strength. The distribution of an EEG surface potential field is markedly influenced and distorted by the characteristics and conductivities of the surrounding tissues, that is, brain, CSF, meninges, skull, and skin (54). There is need for a multilayer and "realistic" head model to simulate a potential field on the surface that takes into account more of the complexities of the individual human head (51). All head models are limited, since conductivity values are rough estimations and age-depending effects are unknown at this time (52). Even the best individual "realistic" head model fails in case of skull breaches or large cystic brain lesions. One of the important advantages of MEG over EEG is the almost negligible influence of the surrounding volume conductor on the resulting external field distribution (53,54). Simple spherical head models are sufficient to face the forward problem in MEG analysis (51).

In the clinical setting, one searches for the localization of the generator, that is, source currents responsible for a given, actually measured extracranial electromagnetic field. This so-called "inverse problem" lacks a unique solution and remains unsolved for both, MEG and EEG analyses (Fig. 76.3).

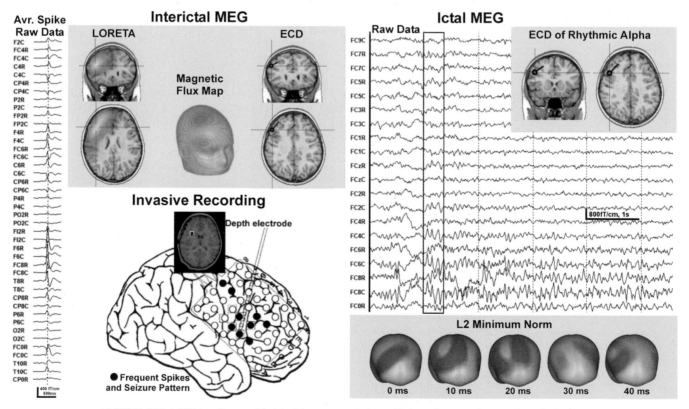

FIGURE 76.3 MEG in a 9-year-old girl with cryptogenic frontal lobe epilepsy. Left: Raw data of 35 averaged interictal spikes in a subset of the 122-channel whole-head gradiometer MEG. Top middle: Magnetic flux map of interictal spikes, Results from inverse source analysis (left: LORETA = distributed source model, right: single equivalent current dipole, filters 5-Hz forward and 45-Hz zero-phase). Top right: MEG raw data of a seizure pattern (clinically tonic seizure). Single equivalent current dipole of rhythmic alpha activity (filters 5- and 45-Hz zero-phase). Bottom right: L2-Minimum norm for alpha pattern. Note propagation from frontolateral to frontomesial region. Bottom middle: Results from an invasive recording with subdural grid and depth electrodes confirm preoperative findings (Prof. Schulze-Bonhage, Freiburg Epilepsy Center, Germany). The patient underwent a resection with outcome Engel 1A after 2 years. Histopathology: FCD 2A according to Palmini.

Consequently, a priori assumptions of the source structure are necessary in the interpretation of measured data. Source models, such as equivalent current dipoles, are needed. In MEG (and EEG) signal processing, the source location provides information about the approximate center of gravity of the activated area. The equivalent dipole model is the simplest, though nevertheless, mostly applied method. The forward model of an electric dipole is optimized regarding localization, orientation, and strength until it mathematically best fits the measured data. Usually the model with the highest goodness-of-fit (lowest residual variance) serves as the final solution. Usually, only dipole models fulfilling a cutoff criterion for residual variance are regarded as clinically relevant. However, goodness-of-fit may be markedly influenced by background activity, especially in low-amplitude spikes (55). Averaging of similar spikes may improve signal-to-noise ratio and allow for localization of dipoles modeling activity from smaller spikes (55,56). Cluster analysis of single spike dipoles and superposition with MRI is a typical procedure to generate a hypothesis about the location of the epileptogenic zone. However, single dipoles cannot discriminate activities from multiple, simultaneously active regions. Propagation of epileptic activity may result in such an overlap, and a single dipole will falsely localize the center in between these active regions. Thus, modeling of the spike onset is more important than localization of the peak source (18,32,55,57). Multiple source analysis is another discrete model that considers effects of spatiotemporal propagation and overlapping background activity (18,58–60).

In contrast to these discrete source models, distributed source models have the advantage that no a priori hypotheses regarding the number of activated regions are needed. However, modeling of hundreds or thousands of electromagnetic sources distributed throughout the solution space is based on the signals of only a limited number of sensors, which results in an underestimation bias. A number of mathematical and anatomical constraints are needed to obtain a reliable solution. Many different distributed and/or statistical inverse models have already been applied to the analysis of epileptic activity in clinical routine, that is, beamformer (61), dSPM (62), Loreta (63,64), "and others." or "and so on."

It is important to realize that all of the mentioned models aim to localize the center of an activated cortical area; however, to date none is able to give a trustful estimation of its extent. Impressive maps resulting from statistical and distributed source models are blurred due to the external constraints of minimum norm or maximum smoothness. The distributed models predominantly depict spatial smoothing and uncertainty of spatial resolution, and do not reflect extent!

Accuracy of dipole localization was 7 to 8 mm for EEG in phantom models and 2 to 4 mm for MEG (65,66). Many studies compared MEG source localization with data from ECoG and confirmed satisfactory accuracy and matches (35,67–71). Lower values of concordance were rarely described (72).

Knowlton et al. prospectively compared localization accuracy of noninvasive epilepsy workup, namely magnetic source imaging, ictal SPECT and PET, on a sublobar level with invasive recordings in 72 patients (73). Magnetic source imaging consistently showed sensitivity and specificity values greater than those of PET/SPECT. Depending on patient subgroup pairs, sensitivity of magnetic source imaging was 79% to 88% compared to 44% to 50% in SPECT and 53% to 63% in FDG-PET. In addition, localization concordance was greatest

with MEG. Direct clinical impact was demonstrated by high success of surgery in patients with nonlocalized intracranial EEG findings, where decision was based on a combination of MEG, SPECT, and PET.

A clinically relevant point is the risk of misinterpretation of MEG data when no simultaneous EEG is analyzed. Usually, EEG and MEG depict activities from the same regions and show no marked differences in localization (28,58,74). However, it was early stated by Cohen that MEG, because of its inability to detect radial sources, should be combined with EEG (14). MEG and EEG sources reflect the different anatomical aspects of the activated zone because of the different sensitivities of both modalities to the orientation of underlying neuronal currents. A lead of the MEG spike peak over the main EEG peak was reported for 7 out of 10 spike types in children suffering from different forms of epilepsy (16). The authors concluded that nonidentical neuronal currents underlie the MEG and EEG signals. Bast et al. compared MEG with EEG multiple source analysis in children with polymicrogyria. The loss of relevant fissures, that is, tangentially oriented sources, reduced MEG sensitivity in a number of cases (18). There is no doubt that MEG and EEG provide in parts complementary information and should be combined in the analysis of epileptic activity (18,21,28,58,68,75–77).

THE ROLE OF MEG IN THE PRESURGICAL EPILEPSY EVALUATION

MEG source localization is an auxiliary noninvasive method in the process of presurgical evaluation for epilepsy surgery (19,34,67,73,77–86). It can be readily applied in children with intractable epilepsy (58,70,87–92). MEG is helpful in the identification of epileptiform tubers in tuberous sclerosis (33,93,94), and revealed intrinsic epileptogenicity in focal cortical dysplasia (58,95–97) and polymicrogyria (18,98). MEG was applied to epileptic patients with cavernoma (99), arteriovenous malformations (100), and glioma (101).

In general, accuracy of MEG source localization is satisfactory compared to ECoG, and the impact in decision-making in the presurgical workup and prognosis, has been shown. Stefan et al. reported the largest series of 455 patients investigated by MEG for presurgical evaluation (86). Average sensitivity of MEG for specific epileptic activity has been found to be 70%. Crucial information for final decision-making was obtained in 10% of the patients. In a study by Knowlton et al., MEG sensitivity was 92% in extratemporal and 50% in temporal epilepsies, while overall sensitivity was measured to 73% (19). Pataraia et al. reported additional focus information obtained by MEG in 40% out of 82 patients (84). In this study, MEG was superior to noninvasive long-term video-EEG with 70% localizing in the resected area. Only 40% concordant results were obtained by EEG. Paulini et al. investigated the contribution of routinely used MEG in addition to long-term video-EEG monitoring (85). MEG localized to one anatomical lobe in 72%, comparable to ictal EEG (72%) and superior to interictal EEG (60%). MEG localized within the resection lobe in 11 out of 25 patients with noninformative EEG, resulting in an excellent to good postoperative outcome in 10 patients. Typical for most comparative studies, methods applied in analysis of MEG and EEG data were different. While MEG was analyzed by source localization, EEG was only analyzed by visual inspection and assessment of the field distribution based on channel activities.

Whether MEG is in general superior to EEG is still not clear, because fair comparisons are lacking. In fact, the simultaneous application of the two techniques seems to offer superior results in clinical application compared to either modality alone (18,20,22,28,58,75–77,84,90,102,103). MEG and EEG should particularly be combined in children with epileptic encephalopathies, in which rapidly generalizing spikes carry high risk for permanent intellectual development. Combined EEG and MEG can identify the source areas and their activation sequences, thereby helping to select children with a single pacemaker area and a prospect for good outcome after surgery (78,87,104,105).

Lau et al. concluded in their review that there is insufficient evidence in the current literature to support the relationship between the use of MEG in surgical planning and seizure-free outcome after epilepsy surgery (106). Lewine calculated positive and negative predictive values of MEG for the identical population, but asked the authors of the quoted original studies more detailed information and applied a more uniform and clinically relevant analysis (107). Based on the "modified" data, MEG offered a significant positive predictive value of 0.72 for seizure-free outcome whereas negative prediction was lower (0.39).

Knowlton et al. investigated the impact of magnetic source imaging on surgical outcome in 62 patients who underwent resection after evaluation by invasive EEG (82). When only patients with diagnostic MEG, that is, data containing spikes, were included, sensitivity for a conclusively localized study was 72%. Positive prediction value regarding seizure freedom was 78% and negative predictive value was 64% for these cases. MEG results were comparable to FDG-PET and ictal SPECT. MEG yield was greatest in extratemporal lobe epilepsy in contrast to PET, which was best in aiding localization of mesiotemporal lobe epilepsy. In this study, ictal SPECT had a high overall diagnostic value with the highest predictive value regarding Engel 1 outcome.

Papanocolaou et al. asked if MEG is already able to replace invasive EEG in presurgical evaluation (108). They found no statistical differences regarding overlap of epileptogenic regions identified by each of the both methods with the resection zone. However, some methodical limitations have to be considered, mainly the sampling bias of some invasive recordings performed with only few depth electrodes.

At time, there is no convincing evidence that MEG is able to replace invasive EEG monitoring. Reduction of both, the total number of invasive recordings and the number or insufficient invasive evaluations due to false electrode positions or incomplete coverage of the epileptogenic zone, seems a realistic goal. MEG source localization may guide the positioning of electrodes for invasive long-term monitoring or intraoperative ECoG (41,72). On the other hand, MEG results have to be handled with care, since there is an unknown risk of useless invasive EEG tests or too expanded implantation schemes to evaluate further potentially false MEG results. This risk needs to be considered in each case until there is more data available.

MEG seems particularly beneficial in the study of (i) patients with frontal lobe epilepsies (34), (ii) patients with nonlesional neocortical epilepsy (91), and (iii) patients who

are evaluated after a first craniotomy, for instance after unsuccessful epilepsy surgery (92,109).

Compared to EEG, signal-to-noise ratio in MEG is markedly better for sources in the frontal lobe (110). In addition, positioning of surface electrodes is limited and frontobasal areas are not adequately covered by EEG. Ossenblok et al. (34) investigated patients with frontal lobe epilepsies. Dipole cluster analysis was successful for MEG in twice the number of patients compared to EEG. MEG was more often localizable in general and particularly helpful in nonlesional cases.

Ramachandran Nair et al. investigated 22 children with normal or subtle and nonfocal MRI findings by MEG and 10-20 surface EEG (91). Good postsurgical outcome was correlated with the inclusion of MEG dipoles clusters to the resected area. Neither patients with a resection not including the MEG dipole cluster, nor patients with bilateral clusters or scattered dipoles became seizure-free. Seizure-free outcome after epilepsy surgery was most likely to occur when there was a concordance between EEG and MEG localization and least likely to occur when these results were divergent.

In addition to the direct impact to the decision for or against surgery in nonlesional cases, a hypothesis based on MEG may guide for high-resolution MRI. Even reviewing existing MRI data in the knowledge of the MEG sources may help to identify previously undetected anatomic cortical lesions (83).

MEG is useful in the analysis of epileptiform activity after incomplete removal of the epileptogenic zone by an unsuccessful epilepsy surgery and after craniotomy for any other reason. Surface EEG signals may be distorted by breach phenomena and dural adhesions may hamper the insertion of subdural electrode grids in these patients (111). Mohammed et al. applied MEG source localization to 17 children after failed epilepsy surgery (92). Out of these, 13 patients underwent further surgery with favorable outcome in 11. No additional intracranial EEG was necessary in cases with dipole clusters near the resection zone of the previous surgery.

SUMMARY

MEG is a noninvasive tool with the major advantage of a high temporal resolution in combination with satisfactory spatial accuracy. Electromagnetic source analysis adds information to the localization and organization of both, epileptogenic and normal cortical areas, which turns out to be clinically relevant in at least 10% of the cases. Further clinical research is necessary to better characterize candidates, in which MEG has a high chance to add new information. In addition, the impact of electromagnetic source analysis in the prediction of postsurgical seizure outcome has to be further investigated. Studies comparing the different MEG systems, on the one hand, and algorithms for inverse source analysis, on the other hand, are needed to optimize the use of MEG source analysis in presurgical evaluation of epilepsy patients.

References

1. Baule G, McFee R. Detections of the magnetic field of the heart. *Am Heart J.* 1963;66:95–96.
2. Cohen D. Magnetoencephalography: evidence of magnetic fields produced by alpha rhythm currents. *Science.* 1968;161:784–786.

3. Cohen D. Magnetoencephalography: detection of the brain's electrical activity with a superconducting magnetometer. *Science.* 1972;11:664–666.
4. Barth DS, Sutherling W, Engel Jr J., et al. Neuromagnetic localization of epileptiform spike activity in the human brain. *Science.* 1982;218:891–894.
5. Mäkelä JP, Forss N, Jääskeläinen J, et al. Magnetoencephalography in neurosurgery. *Neurosurgery.* 2006;59:493–510.
6. Leijten FSS, Huiskamp G. Interictal electromagnetic source imaging in focal epilepsy: practices, results and recommendations. *Curr Opin Neurol.* 2008;437–445.
7. Knowlton RC. Can magnetoencephalography aid epilepsy surgery? *Epilepsy Curr.* 2008;8:1–5.
8. Vrba J, Betts K, Burbank M, et al. Whole cortex 64 channel SQUID biomagneter system. *IEEE Trans Appl Supracond.* 1993;3:1878–1882.
9. Ahonen A, Hämäläinen M, Kajola M, et al. 122-channel SQUITD instrument for investigating the magnetic signals from human brain. *Physica Scripta T.* 1993;49:198–205.
10. Mikuni N, Nagamine T, Ikeda A, et al. Simultaneous recording of epileptiform discharges by MEG and subdural electrodes in temporal lobe epilepsy. *Neuroimage.* 1997;5:298–306.
11. Zijlmans M, Huiskamp GM, Leijten FS, et al. Modality-specific spike identification in simultaneous magnetoencephalography/electroencephalography: a methodological approach. *J Clin Neurophysiol.* 2002;19:183–191.
12. Hari R, Karhu J, Hämäläinen M, et al. Functional organization of the human first and second somatosensory cortices: a neuromagnetic study. *Eur J Neurosci.* 1993;5:724–734.
13. Hämäläinen M, Hari R, Ilmoniemi R, et al. Magnetoencephalography: theory, instrumentation and applications to noninvasive studies of the working human brain. *Rev Mod Phys.* 1993;65:413–497.
14. Cohen D, Cuffin BN. Demonstration of useful differences between magnetoencephalogram and electroencephalogram. *Electroencephalogr Clin Neurophysiol.* 1983;56:38–51.
15. Lopes da Silva F, Van Rotterdam A. Biophysical aspects of EEG and magnetoencephalogram generation. In: Niedermeyer E, ed. *EEG, Basic Principles, Clinical Applications and Related Fields.* 4th ed. Baltimore: Lippincott Williams & Wilkins; 1999;93–109.
16. Merlet I, Paetau R, Garcia-Larrea L, et al. Apparent asynchrony between interictal electric and magnetic fields. *Neuroreport.* 1997;8:1071–1076.
17. Malmivuo J, Suihko V, Eskola H. Sensitivity distributions of EEG and MEG measurements. *IEEE Trans Biomed Eng.* 1997;44:196–208.
18. Bast T, Ramantani G, Boppel T, et al. Source analysis of interictal spikes in polymicrogyria: loss of relevant cortical fissures requires simultaneous EEG to avoid MEG misinterpretation. *Neuroimage.* 2005;25:1232–1241.
19. Knowlton RC, Laxer KD, Aminoff MJ, et al. Magnetoencephalography in partial epilepsy: clinical yield and localization accuracy. *Ann Neurol.* 1997; 42:622–631.
20. Iwasaki M, Pestana E, Burgess RC, et al. Detection of epileptiform activity by human interpreters: blinded comparison between electroencephalography and magnetoencephalography. *Epilepsia.* 2005;46:59–68.
21. Barkley GL, Baumgartner C. MEG and EEG in epilepsy. *J Clin Neurophysiol.* 2003;20:163–178.
22. Ramantani G, Scherg G, Boor R, et al. MEG vs. EEG: influence of background activity on interictal spike detection. *J Clin Neurophysiol.* 2006; 23:498–508.
23. Knake S, Halgren E, Shiraishi H, et al. The value of multichannel MEG and EEG in the presurgical evaluation of 70 epilepsy patients. *Epilepsy Res.* 2006;69:80–86.
24. Leijten FSS, Huiskamp GJM, Hilgersom I, et al. High-resolution source imaging in mesiotemporal lobe epilepsy: a comparison between MEG and simultaneous EEG. *J Clin Neurophysiol.* 2003;20:227–238.
25. Lin YY, Shih YH, Chang KP, et al. MEG localization of rolandic spikes with respect to SI and SII cortices in benign rolandic epilepsy. *Neuroimage.* 2003;20:2051–2061.
26. Sutherling WW, Levesque MF, Crandall PH, et al. Localization of partial epilepsy using magnetic and electric measurements. *Epilepsia.* 1991; 32(Suppl 5):29–40.
27. Baumgartner C, Pataraia E, Lindinger G, et al. Neuromagnetic recordings in temporal lobe epilepsy. *J Clin Neurophysiol.* 2000;17:177–189.
28. Yoshinaga H, Nakahori T, Ohtsuka Y, et al. Benefit of simultaneous recording of EEG and MEG in dipole localization. *Epilepsia.* 2002;43: 924–928.
29. Huiskamp G, van der Meij W, van Huffelen A, et al. High resolution spatio-temporal EEG-MEG analysis of rolandic spikes. *J Clin Neurophysiol.* 2003;21:84–95.
30. Fernandes JM, da Silva AM, Huiskamp G, et al. What does an epileptiform spike look like in MEG? Comparison between coincident EEG and MEG spikes. *J Clin Neurophysiol.* 2005;22:68–73.
31. Rodin R, Funke M, Berg P, et al. Magnetoencephalographic spikes not detected by conventional electroencephalography. *Clin Neurophysiol.* 2004;115:2041–2047.
32. Michel CM, Lantz G, Spinelli L, et al. 128-channel EEG source imaging in epilepsy: clinical yield and localization precision. *J Clin Neurophysiol.* 2004;21:71–83.
33. Jansen FE, Huiskamp G, van Huffelen AC, et al. Identification of the epileptogenic tuber in patients with tuberous sclerosis: a comparison of high-resolution EEG and MEG. *Epilepsia.* 2006;47:108–114.
34. Ossenblok P, de Munck JC, Colon A, et al. Magnetoencephalography is more successful for screening and localizing frontal lobe epilepsy than electroencephalography. *Epilepsia.* 2007;48:2139–2149.
35. Oishi M, Otsubo H, Kameyama S, et al. Epileptic spikes: magnetoencephalography versus simultaneous electrocorticography. *Epilepsia.* 2002; 43:1390–1395.
36. Shigeto H, Morioka T, Hisada K, et al. Feasibility and limitations of magnetoencephalographic detection of epileptic discharges: simultaneous recordings of magnetic fields and electrocorticography. *Neurol Res.* 2002;24:531–536.
37. Tao JX, Ray A, Hawes-Ebersole S, et al. Intracranial EEG substrates of scalp EEG interictal spikes. *Epilepsia.* 2005;46:669–676.
38. Wehner DT, Hämäläinen MS, Mody M, et al. Head movements of children in MEG: quantification, effects on source estimation, and compensation. *Neuroimage.* 2008;40:541–550.
39. Wilson HS. Continuous head-localization and data correction in a whole-cortex MEG sensor. *Neurol Clin Neurophysiol.* 2004;30:56.
40. Medvedovsky M, Taulu S, Bikmullina R, et al. Artifact and head movement compensation in MEG. *Neurol Neurophysiol Neurosci.* 2007;29:4.
41. Eliashiv DS, Elsas SM, Squires K, et al. Ictal magnetic source imaging as a localizing tool in partial epilepsy. *Neurology.* 2002;59:1600–1610.
42. Tilz C, Hummel C, Kettenmann B, et al. Ictal onset localization of epileptic seizures by magnetoencephalography. *Acta Neurol Scand.* 2002;106:190–195.
43. Assaf BA, Karkar KM, Laxer KD, et al. Ictal magnetoencephalography in temporal and extratemporal lobe epilepsy. *Epilepsia.* 2003;44:1320–1327.
44. Yoshinaga H, Ohtsuka Y, Watanabe Y, et al. Ictal MEG in two children with partial seizures. *Brain Dev.* 2004;26:403–408.
45. Shiraishi H, Watanabe Y, Watanabe M, et al. Interictal and ictal magnetoencephalographic study in patients with medial frontal lobe epilepsy. *Epilepsia.* 2001;42:875–882.
46. Ray A, Tao JX, Hawes-Ebersole SM, et al. Localizing value of scalp EEG spikes: a simultaneous scalp and intracranial study. *Clin Neurophysiol.* 2007;118:69–79.
47. Oishi M, Kameyama S, Masuda H, et al. Single and multiple clusters of magnetoencephalographic dipoles in neocortical epilepsy: significance in characterizing the epileptogenic zone. *Epilepsia.* 2006;47:355–364.
48. Knowlton RC, Elgavish R, Howell J, et al. Magnetic source imaging versus intracranial electroencephalogram in epilepsy surgery: a prospective study. *Ann Neurol.* 2006;59:835–842.
49. Hämäläinen M. Anatomical correlates for magnetoencephalography: integration with magnetic resonance images. *Clin Phys Physiol Meas.* 1991;12(Suppl A):29–32.
50. Plummer C, Harvey AS, Cook M. EEG source localization in focal epilepsy: where are we now? *Epilepsia.* 2008;49:201–218.
51. Scheler G, Fischer MJ, Genow A, et al. Spatial relationship of source localizations in patients with focal epilepsy: comparison of MEG and EEG with a three spherical shells and a boundary element volume conductor model. *Hum Brain Mapp.* 2007;28:315–322.
52. Wolters CH, Anwander A, Tricoche X, et al. Influence of tissue conductivity anisotropy on EEG/MEG field and return current computation in a realistic head model: a simulation and visualization study using high-resolution finite element modeling. *Neuroimage.* 2006;30:813–826.
53. Ko DY, Kufta C, Scaffidi D, et al. Source localization determined by magnetoencephalography and electroencephalography in temporal lobe epilepsy: comparison with electrocorticography: technical case report. *Neurosurgery.* 1998;42:414–422.
54. Sato S, Balish M, Muratore R. Principles of magnetoencephalography. *J Clin Neurophysiol.* 1991;8:144–156.
55. Bast T, Boppel T, Rupp A, et al. Non-invasive source localization of interictal EEG spikes: effects of signal-to-noise ratio and averaging. *J ClinNeurophysiol.* 2006;23:487–497.
56. Thickbroom GW, Davies HD, Carroll WM, et al. Averaging, spatio-temporal mapping and dipole modeling of focal epileptic spikes. *Electroencephalogr Clin Neurophysiol.* 1986;64:274–277.
57. Huppertz HJ, Hof E, Klisch J, et al. Localization of interictal delta and epileptiform EEG activity associated with focal epileptogenic brain lesions. *Neuroimage.* 2001;13:15–28.
58. Bast T, Oezkan O, Rona S, et al. EEG and MEG source analysis of single and averaged interictal spikes reveals intrinsic epileptogenicity in focal cortical dysplasia. *Epilepsia.* 2004;45:621–631.
59. Scherg M, Bast T, Berg P. Multiple source analysis of interictal spikes: goals, requirements and clinical value. *J Clin Neurophysiol.* 1999;16:214–224.
60. Scherg M, Ille N, Bornfleth H, et al. Advanced tools for digital EEG review: virtual source montages, whole-head mapping, correlation and phase analysis. *J Clin Neurophysiol.* 2002;19:91–112.
61. Ward DM, Jones RD, Bones PJ, et al. Enhancement of deep epileptiform activity in the EEG via 3-D adaptive spatial filtering. *IEEE Trans Biomed Eng.* 1999;46:707–716.
62. Shiraishi H, Ahlfors SP, Stufflebeam SM, et al. Application of magnetoencephalography in epilepsy patients with widespread spike or slow-wave activity. *Epilepsia.* 2005;46:1264–1272.
63. Lantz G, Michel CM, Pascual-Marqui RD, et al. Extracranial localization of intracranial interictal epileptiform activity using LORETA (low resolution electromagnetic tomography). *Electroencephalogr Clin Neurophysiol.* 1997;102:414–422.

64. Zumsteg D, Friedman A, Wennberg RA, et al. Source localization of mesial temporal interictal epileptiform discharges: correlation with intracranial foramen ovale electrodes. *Clin Neurophysiol.* 2005;117:562–571.

65. Gharib S, Sutherling WW, Nakasato N, et al. MEG and ECoG localization accuracy test. *Electroencephalogr Clin Neurophysiol.* 1995;94:109–114.

66. Leahy RM, Mosher JC, Spencer ME, et al. A study of dipole localization accuracy for EEG and MEG using a human skull phantom. *Electroencephalogr Clin Neurophysiol.* 1998;107:159–173.

67. Nakasato N, Levesque MF, Barth DS, et al. Comparisons of MEG, EEG, and ECoG source localization in neocortical partial epilepsy in humans. *Electroencephalogr. Clin Neurophysiol.* 1994;91:171–178.

68. Cohen D, Cuffin BN, Yunokuchi K, et al. MEG versus EEG localization test using implanted sources in the human brain. *Ann Neurol.* 1990;28:811–817.

69. Lamusuo S, Forss N, Ruottinen HM, et al. [18F]FDG-PET and whole-scalp MEG localization of epileptogenic cortex. *Epilepsia.* 1999;40:921–930.

70. Otsubo H, Och A, Elliott I, et al. MEG predicts epileptic zone in lesional extrahippocampal epilepsy: 12 pediatric surgery cases. *Epilepsia.* 2001;42:1523–1530.

71. Krings T, Chiappa KH, Cuffin BN, et al. Accuracy of EEG dipole source localization using implanted sources in the human brain. *Clin Neurophysiol.* 1999;110:106–114.

72. Mamelak AN, Lopez N, Akhtari M, et al. Magnetoencephalography-directed surgery in patients with neocortical epilepsy. *J Neurosurg.* 2002;97:865–873.

73. Knowlton RC, Elgavish RA, Limdi N, et al. Functional imaging: I. Relative predictive value of intracranial electroencephalography. *Ann Neurol.* 2008;64:25–34.

74. Kirsch HE, Mantle M, Nagarajan SS. Concordance between routine interictal magnetoencephalography and simultaneous scalp electroencephalography in a sample of patients with epilepsy. *J Clin Neurophysiol.* 2007;24:215–231.

75. Barkley GL. Controversies in neurophysiology. MEG is superior to EEG in localization of interictal epileptiform activity: pro. *Clin Neurophysiol.* 2004;115:1001–1009.

76. Baumgartner C. Controversies in neurophysiology. MEG is superior to EEG in localization of interictal epileptiform activity: con. *Clin Neurophysiol.* 2004;115:1010–1020.

77. Fischer MJ, Scheler G, Stefan H. Utilization of magnetoencephalography results to obtain favourable outcomes in epilepsy surgery. *Brain.* 2005;128:153–157.

78. Baumgartner C, Pataraia E. Revising the role of magnetoencephalography in epilepsy. *Curr opin Neurol.* 2006;1:181–186.

79. Ebersole JS. Magnetoencephalography/magnetic source imaging in the assessment of patients with epilepsy. *Epilepsia.* 1997;38(Suppl 4):1–5.

80. Genow A, Hummel C, Scheler G, et al. Epilepsy surgery, resection volume and MSI localization in lesional frontal lobe epilepsy. *Neuroimage.* 2004;21:444–449.

81. Kirchberger K, Schmitt H, Hummel C, et al. Clonidine and methohexital-induced epileptic magnetoencephalographic discharge in patients with focal epilepsies. *Epilepsia.* 1998;39:841–849.

82. Knowlton RC, Elgavish RA, Bartolucci A, et al. Functional imaging: II. Prediction of epilepsy surgery outcome. *Ann Neurol.* 2008;64:35–41.

83. Moore KR, Funke ME, Constantino T, et al. Magnetoencephalographically directed review of high-spatial-resolution surface-coil MR images improves lesion detection in patients with extratemporal epilepsy. *Radiology.* 2002;225:880–887.

84. Pataraia E, Simos PG, Castillo EM, et al. Reorganization of language-specific cortex in patients with lesions or mesial temporal epilepsy. *Neurology.* 2004;63:1825–1832.

85. Paulini A, Fischer M, Rampp S, et al. Lobar localization information in epilepsy patients: MEG- a useful tool in routine presurgical diagnosis. *Epilepsy Res.* 2007;76:124–130.

86. Stefan H, Hummel C, Scheler A, et al. Magnetic brain source imaging of focal epileptic activity: a synopsis of 455 cases. *Brain.* 2003;126:2396–2405.

87. Lewine JD, Andrews R, Chez M, et al. Magnetoencephalographic patterns of epileptiform activity in children with regressive autism spectrum disorders. *Pediatrics.* 1999;104:405–418.

88. Minassian BA, Otsubo H, Weiss S, et al. Magnetoencephalographic localization in pediatric epilepsy surgery: comparison with invasive intracranial electroencephalography. *Ann Neurol.* 1999;46:627–633.

89. Paetau R, Hamalainen M, Hari R, et al. Magnetoencephalographic evaluation of children and adolescents with intractable epilepsy. *Epilepsia.* 1994;35:275–284.

90. Paetau R, Kajola M, Karhu J, et al. Magnetoencephalographic localization of epileptic cortex–impact on surgical treatment. *Ann Neurol.* 1992;32:106–109.

91. Ramachandran Nair R, Otsubo H, Shroff MM, et al. MEG predicts outcome following surgery for intractable epilepsy in children with normal or nonfocal MRI findings. *Epilepsia.* 2007;48:149–157.

92. Mohamed IS, Otsubo H, Ochi A, et al. Utility of magnetoencephalography in the evaluation of recurrent seizures after epilepsy surgery. *Epilepsia.* 2007;48:2150–2159.

93. Xiao Z, Xiang J, Holowka S, et al. Volumetric localization of epileptic activities in tuberous sclerosis using synthetic aperture magnetometry. *Pediatr Radiol.* 2006;36:16–21.

94. Kamimura T, Tohyama J, Oishi M, et al. Magnetoencephalography in patients with tuberous sclerosis and localization-related epilepsy. *Epilepsia.* 2006;47:991–997.

95. Morioka T, Nishio S, Ishibashi H, et al. Intrinsic epileptogenicity of focal cortical dysplasia as revealed by magnetoencephalography and electrocorticography. *Epilepsy Res.* 1999;33:177–187.

96. Widjaja E, Otsubo H, Raybaud C, et al. Characteristics of MEG and MRI between Taylor's focal cortical dysplasia (type II) and other cortical dysplasia: surgical outcome after complete resection of MEG spike source and MR lesion in pediatric cortical dysplasia. *Epilepsy Res.* 2008;82:147–155.

97. Ishii R, Canuet L, Ochi A, et al. Spatially filtered magnetoencephalography compared with electrocorticography to identify intrinsically epileptogenic focal cortical dysplasia. *Epilepsy Res.* 2008;81:228–232.

98. Burneo JG, Bebin M, Kuzniecky RI, et al. Electroclinical and magnetoencephalographic studies in epilepsy patients with polymicrogyria. *Epilepsy Res.* 2004;62:125–133.

99. Stefan H, Scheler G, Hummel C, et al. Magnetoencephalography (MEG) predicts focal epileptogenicity in cavernomas. *J Neurol Neurosurg Psychiatry.* 2004;75:1309–1313.

100. Morioka T, Nishio S, Hisada K, et al. Neuromagnetic assessment of epileptogenicity in cerebral arteriovenous malformation. *Neurosurg Rev.* 2000;23:206–212.

101. Patt S, Steenbeck J, Hochstetter A, et al. Source localization and possible causes of interictal epileptic activity in tumor-associated epilepsy. *Neurobiol Dis.* 2000;7:260–269.

102. Baillet S, Adam C, Schwartz D, et al. Combined MEG and EEG source imaging of interictal activity in partial epilepsy. In: Nowak H, Haueisen J, Gießler F, Huonker R, eds. *Proceedings in Biomagnetism.* Berlin, Offenbach:VDE; 2002:223–225.

103. Wheless JW, Willmore LJ, Breier JI, et al. A comparison of magnetoencephalography, MRI and V-EEG in patients evaluated for epilepsy surgery. *Epilepsia.* 1999;40:931–941.

104. Morrell F, Whisler WW, Smith MC, et al. Landau–Kleffner syndrome. Treatment with subpial intracortical transection. *Brain.* 1995;118:1529–1546.

105. Paetau R, Kajola M, Korkman M, et al. Landau–Kleffner syndrome: epileptic activity in the auditory cortex. *Neuroreport.* 1991;2:201–204.

106. Lau M, Yam D, Burneo JG. A systematic review on MEG and its use in the presurgical evaluation of localization-related epilepsy. *Epilepsy Res.* 2008;79:97–104.

107. Lewine JD. Commentary on Lau et al., 2008. A systematic review on MEG and its use in the presurgical evaluation of localization related epilepsy. *Epilepsy Res.* 2008;82:235–236.

108. Papanicolaou AC, Pataraia E, Billingsley-Marschall R, et al. Toward the substitution of invasive electroencephalography in epilepsy surgery. *J Clin Neurophysiol.* 2005;22:231–237.

109. Kirchberger K, Hummel C, Stefan H. Postoperative multichannel magnetoencephalography in patients with recurrent seizures after epilepsy surgery. *Acta Neurol Scand.* 1998;98:1–7.

110. de Jongh A, de Munck JC, Gonçalves SI, et al. Differences in MEG/EEG epileptic spike yields explained by regional differences in signal-to-noise ratios. *J Clin Neurophysiol.* 2005;22:153–158.

111. Kirchberger K, Schmitt H, Hummel C, et al. Clonidine- and methohexital-induced epileptiform discharges detected by magnetoencephalography (MEG) in patients with localization-related epilepsies. *Epilepsia* 1998;39:1104–1112.

CHAPTER 77 ■ DIFFUSION TENSOR IMAGING (DTI) AND EEG-CORRELATED FMRI

BEATE DIEHL AND LOUIS LEMIEUX

Magnetic resonance imaging (MRI) techniques have greatly improved our ability to investigate the structure and function of the epileptic brain (1). Detecting possible underlying structural abnormalities or causes of epilepsy is one important aspect of such advances, and currently pathologic lesions are identified in about 80% of all refractory focal epilepsies (2). In addition, novel imaging results are being explored to inform about cortical function or dysfunction in patients with epilepsy, as well as correlates of the ictal-onset zone and irritative zone (3).

The objective of epilepsy surgery in pharmacoresistant focal epilepsies is the complete resection or at least disconnection of the epileptogenic zone while preserving eloquent cortex (2,4). This chapter focuses on the contribution of two novel imaging technologies to optimize surgical results. Diffusion tensor imaging (DTI) is a novel MRI technology that allows measurement of water diffusion in the brain tissue, providing information of microstructural changes. In addition, white matter architecture and tract morphology can be interrogated allowing for the first time to reconstruct major tracts in vivo.

The simultaneous recording of EEG and functional MRI (fMRI) was first demonstrated in patients with epilepsy in the early 1990s, and has since become an important research tool in epilepsy and beyond (5). Simultaneous EEG–fMRI (or simply "EEG–fMRI") is uniquely capable of providing data to address the question: what patterns of hemodynamic change take place throughout the brain (5) in relation to epileptiform discharges seen on scalp EEG? For interictal pathological activity, simultaneous EEG is indispensable while ictal hemodynamic changes can be studied meaningfully without reference to concurrent EEG in some patients. Although EEG–fMRI has been primarily used as a localization technique, it can be combined with ever more advanced modeling methodologies to study the dynamics of networks. Together, both technologies may allow for novel insights in understanding the ictal-onset zone, irritative zone, and functional deficit zone.

DIFFUSION MR IMAGING

Principles of Diffusion Imaging

The MRI signal results from the RF excitation of water protons in tissue. In a medium without any boundaries, the random translational motion or Brownian motion of water molecules results from the thermal energy carried by these molecules. In the brain, however, such diffusion is restricted by intra- and extracellular boundaries. Various animal models have been used to assess the most important boundaries affecting

diffusion in the brain, revealing that myelin is the main barrier to water diffusion (6–9).

The principles of diffusion MRI were first developed in vivo in the mid-1980s (10,11). In diffusion-weighted imaging (DWI), images are sensitized to diffusion by using pulsed magnetic field gradients incorporated into a standard spin echo sequence (10,12). Taking measurements in at least three directions allows for characterization of the mean diffusion properties within a voxel in the image.

By applying diffusion gradients in six or more directions, the diffusion tensor, a mathematical construct, can be calculated. This allows assessing not only the amplitude of diffusional motion, but also the directionality (13–15). The fact that diffusion is not the same in the three main spatial directions, but is asymmetric in the brain and restricted in certain directions, gave rise to the concept of "anisotropy" (13,16). DTI has been developed to explore this directional information and to gain greater insights in the structural changes, possibly on a microscopic level. Fractional anisotropy (FA) is a scalar (unitless) index most commonly used to assess the overall degree of directionality; it ranges from 0 (full isotropy) to 1 (complete anisotropic diffusion). Diffusion in different directions, such as parallel (main direction of diffusion) and perpendicular to the main fiber tract orientation, can be studied. Together, these quantitative measures help to characterize the integrity of the underlying white matter and may allow understanding of the pathophysiologic mechanisms consistent with such diffusion abnormalities.

Exploring white matter changes in epilepsy, how they relate to epileptogenicity, and whether they may be a surrogate marker for cognitive difficulties is a matter of ongoing research. Furthermore, DTI in combination with tractography has become a powerful opportunity to subdivide compartments of white matter representing different tracts and study their diffusion properties selectively.

Experimental Insights into Tissue Structure Using DTI

Several animal models of tissue injury and degeneration have been used to measure serially diffusion changes and correlate them carefully with histology. Using an in vitro model of Wallerian degeneration in frog sciatic nerve, axonal and myelin degeneration causes a decrease in diffusion anisotropy due to reduced parallel and increased perpendicular diffusivity (9). Myelin has been shown to modulate perpendicular diffusivity (7,8), although it is not the only factor involved (17). In humans, reductions in the principal direction and increases in radial diffusivities have been shown in chronically degenerated white matter tracts (18). Serial DTI measurements in three patients who underwent corpus callosotomy to treat medically refractory seizures and drop attacks revealed interesting insights into the diffusion changes in the corpus callosum after the surgery (19). An initial decrease in parallel diffusivities evidencing the breakdown of the axons (19,20) is followed in the chronic stage (2 to 4 months later) by an increase of the radial diffusivities as myelin sheath degeneration is noted. Water molecules become more mobile perpendicular to the axons, resulting in an increase in radial diffusivities.

Tractography

Lastly, anisotropy information forms the basis of reconstructing tracts. Anisotropy in white matter results from the organization of tissue as bundles of axons and myelin sheaths run in parallel, and the diffusion of water is freer and quicker in the long axis of the fibers than in the perpendicular direction (17). By assuming that the largest principal axis of the diffusion tensor aligns with the predominant fiber orientation in an MRI voxel, we can obtain vector fields that represent the fiber orientation at each voxel. The three-dimensional reconstruction of tract trajectories, or tractography, is an extension of such vector fields (21). However, tractography only came into use in the late 1990s, due to the complexities to develop reliable computer algorithms to reconstruct the tracts. Some of the limitations and technical difficulties of tractography include the spatial resolution of DTI, which is in the order of several millimeters, as well as noise. Various acquisitions and postprocessing analysis techniques have been proposed (21), and methods continue to evolve. Voxel sizes are much larger than the resolution needed to image single axons. Hence, in vivo DTI studies can at present only display an approximation of the main tract direction, and do not have a resolution even close to a cellular level. White matter tractography is generally done in two different ways; either with a method known as "deterministic" tractography or with a "probabilistic" method. Using deterministic methods, seed points are placed and the tract grows in both directions along the dominant diffusion direction. This requires a preset threshold for angles and FA, and track is terminated when it reaches a voxel with subthreshold FA, or when the turning angle exceeds this threshold. As the main direction of water diffusion is used for tract reconstruction, crossing fibers will not be represented, and only the main tracts and its main direction will be displayed. The probabilistic methods probe fiber orientation distributions at each voxel and are computationally more intensive, but can more reliably reconstruct crossing fibers.

To date atlases have been published of anatomical correlation of the DTI based FA maps and tractography results (22–24), which are largely based on comparison to anatomical drawings and dissection maps.

There is no doubt that validation is of central importance for the development of tractography; how to validate and against what gold standard is a matter of debate.

Peri-Ictal DWI and DTI Changes in Humans

DWI has initially been introduced in clinical practice for the early detection of stroke. It has proven to be very sensitive to areas affected by ischemia (10). Subsequently, peri-ictal and postictal changes in diffusivity have been observed in animal

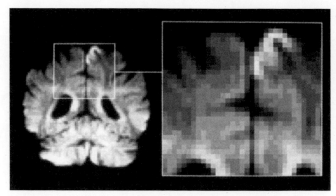

FIGURE 77.1 Area of restricted diffusion in the left superior frontal gyrus shown in a patient with right leg clonic status epilepticus. (From Wieshmann UC, Symms MR, Shorvon SD. Diffusion changes in status epilepticus. *Lancet.* 1997;350(9076):493–494, with permission.)

models of status epilepticus and in patients both after status epilepticus and after single short seizures. Systematic investigations of diffusion changes in rats following bicuculline-, kainic acid-, and pilocarpine-induced status epilepticus have highlighted changes closely correlated with the presumed area of seizure onset and the resulting histopathologic changes. Furthermore, such changes are dynamic, leading initially to restricted diffusion due to cytotoxic edema, and after several days, to normalization or facilitated diffusion (25–28). Diffusion imaging may, therefore, provide an opportunity to directly image the areas involved in seizure generation and possibly spread.

The first report of diffusion changes in a patient with focal status epilepticus was published in 1997 (29). Status consisted of clonic jerking of the right leg, which continued for 22 days and was followed by transient paresis. DWI during status showed decreased diffusion in the motor cortex of the right leg (Fig. 77.1) and an area of facilitated diffusion in the underlying white matter. This was explained by a shift of water into cortical neurons at the site of the seizure focus, that is, cytotoxic edema that is associated with restricted diffusion and vasogenic edema with a shift of water in the extracellular space in the underlying white matter (30).

Following this case report, multiple systematic investigations have explored peri-ictal DWI in an attempt to assess the usefulness of this novel technology to delineate the ictal-onset zone. Overall, the presence of dynamic diffusion changes has been documented in the majority of cases, but the correlation between the presumed epileptogenic zone and the diffusion changes is quite variable (31–35). Correlations seem closer in patients with longer seizures (or status) and short duration between seizure end and scan (31,33). A single case report in man confirms that restricted diffusion is a marker of the ictal-onset zone: An area of restricted diffusion adjacent to the lesion in the right frontal lobe in a patient with repetitive prolonged focal motor seizures corresponded to the region of focal electrocorticographic seizures that was mapped intraoperatively (36).

Studies using DTI to study peri-ictal changes allowed for comparison of the sensitivity of diffusivity changes versus anisotropy changes, and to assess whether DTI provides higher sensitivity to seizure-induced changes. The results remain rather disappointing, and it has become apparent that dynamic changes affected the diffusivity to a much higher degree than the directionality (32). Peri-ictal mean diffusivity reductions are seen in about half of the patients investigated, but only a relatively small proportion (20%) colocalized with the presumed ictal-onset zone, even when patients were scanned within 45 minutes after the seizure (35). In addition, whole-brain analysis using statistical parametric mapping (SPM) revealed distant areas of diffusivity change, possibly highlighting the network involved in ictal spread.

In order to minimize delays between seizure and scanning, flumazenil was used to induce seizures in patients assessed for epilepsy surgery (37). Even then diffusivity decreases were seen in the hippocampus on the seizure-onset side, as also some bilateral decreases in the parahippocampal gyrus.

Therefore, it seems possible that diffusion changes after single seizures appear more transient and require immediate access to scanning. If in the future such an environment can be provided, in combination with higher resolution scanning and possibly also higher field strengths of MR scanners, postictal studies may be of higher yield.

Interictal DTI and DWI Changes

Temporal Lobe Epilepsy

Patients with mesial temporal lobe epilepsy (TLE) due to hippocampal sclerosis reveal increased diffusivity in the ipsilateral hippocampus, indicative of structural disorganization and expansion of extracellular space, reflecting neuronal loss and other microstructural changes (38–43). These changes parallel the abnormalities noted on conventional MRI scans with atrophy and T2 signal increase. When assessing DWI compared to conventional MRI using volumetric T1 acquisitions and FLAIR, it was not more sensitive in detecting hippocampal sclerosis (40). In addition, in patients without lateralizing differences between the hippocampal formations, often both hippocampi showed increased apparent diffusion coefficient (ADC) compared to a control population, indicating bilaterality of the disease. Such bilateral abnormalities are present throughout the limbic system, including fornix and cingulum in both adults (44,45) and children (46).

When patients with TLE were evaluated using a region-of-interest approach, diffusion abnormalities extend into the ipsilateral hemisphere, and even into contralateral hemisphere (44,45,47–50). Such more widespread changes have been confirmed using voxel-based approaches, which compare one individual to a group of normal controls and thus do not have selection bias to a particular region of interest (50). These changes are not reversible after successful temporal lobectomy, which may suggest structural abnormalities as opposed to functional changes due to seizures (51).

DTI can also identify abnormal areas in temporal and extratemporal focal epilepsy with normal conventional MRI. Out of 30 patients, increases in diffusivity were found in eight patients (26%), six of the eight diffusivity alterations were in the presumed epileptogenic zone (52). In addition, group analysis of nonlesional left TLE patients revealed increased diffusivity and reduced anisotropy within the ipsilateral temporal lobe; the right TLE group displayed a trend in the same direction (52). Although such a group effect is not helpful in an individual patient, it suggests that given greater sensitivity and increased signal-to-noise ratios, an effect in individual patients may be demonstrated. Overall, such occult lesions are most likely caused by disruption of white matter architecture due to dysgenesis, or by seizure-related damage leading to atrophy, gliosis, and expansion of the extracellular space, resulting in increased diffusivity and potentially also decreased anisotropy.

Extratemporal Lobe Epilepsy

Extratemporal epilepsies represent a growing group being evaluated for epilepsy surgery, and often are challenging as precise localization of the epileptogenic zone in relation to cortical function is mandatory. Diffusion changes are seen in a variety of lesions associated with focal epilepsy and often localize outside the temporal lobe, such as cortical dysplasia.

Reductions in anisotropy and increase in diffusivity within the MRI visible lesion and also outside of it have been reported in a variety of cortical dysplasias (53,54). Reductions in FA in most patients in normal appearing white matter surrounding dysplastic lesions are likely due to gliosis, axonal loss, poor myelination, or increased cell bodies (e.g., ectopic or abnormal neurons, balloon cells). In addition, distant anisotropic changes can also be observed, possibly be due to Wallerian degeneration of tracts or gliosis resulting from chronic seizures. Investigations on the impact of cortical dysplasia on connectivity and adjacent tracts showed decreased tract size and displacement of tracts in larger dysplasias, as well as rarefaction of subcortical connections surrounding cortical dysplasia (55). Figure 77.2 shows altered connectivity in a patient with right temporo-occipital epilepsy, with polymicrogyria and heterotopic gray matter in the same region.

Probing Diffusion Changes: What Can It Tell Us in Human Epilepsy

Analyzing the pattern of diffusion changes with respect to diffusivities parallel and perpendicular (radial) to the main axonal direction provides in vivo insights into the underlying

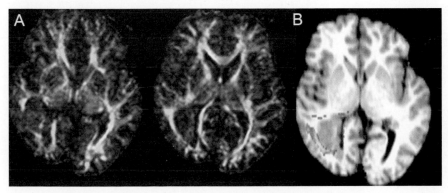

FIGURE 77.2 Malformations of cortical development and alterations of connectivity. Twenty-six-year-old with intractable focal epilepsy arising from the right temporo-occipital region. MRI showed right > left posterior quadrant polymicrogyria and heterotopic gray matter in the right posterior quadrant. **A:** Axial colorized fiber orientation maps showing displacement of the right superior fronto-occipital fasciculus and superior longitudinal fasciculus. **B:** Two-dimensional illustration of the tractography results overlaid onto the T1 image demonstrates the spatial relationship between the heterotopic gray matter and the white matter tracts. Please see color insert.

cause of diffusivity increase and decreased FA. Several studies revealed that the most commonly seen pattern of DTI changes associated with focal epilepsy was unchanged parallel diffusivity and increased perpendicular diffusivity (45,47,48,56,57). As detailed above, such a pattern of FA changes seen in most studies evaluating DTI in TLE is most consistent with chronic Wallerian degeneration, possibly due to cell loss in the temporal lobe secondary to seizure-induced cell death.

In order to evaluate potential mechanisms for such more widespread diffusion changes in TLE, it was investigated if different underlying pathologies as determined by preoperative MRI cause differential diffusion changes (45). Patients with TLE and hippocampal sclerosis were compared to nonlesional TLE: While some white matter bundles are affected equally in both forms of TLE, abnormalities of the bundles directly related to the mesial temporal structures (i.e., the fornix and cingulum) appear to be unique to TLE with hippocampal sclerosis.

It has been demonstrated that DTI can be used to delineate the neurocognitive correlates of localized white matter damage in TLE, such as memory and language dysfunction (57,58), and research into such structure function relationships is ongoing.

Interictal DTI and DWI Changes: Conclusion

Interictal DTI highlights areas of abnormal diffusion measures in temporal and extratemporal lobe epilepsies, both lesional and nonlesional. Specifically, mean diffusivity appears more sensitive to changes seen in patients with chronic refractory epilepsy compared to FA. The only exception may be cortical dysplasias. DTI abnormalities are seen in all areas, indicating pathology on conventional MRI. In addition, DTI changes may often be found outside the lesions, both contiguous and less frequently also noncontiguous to the lesion. Abnormalities mostly with increased diffusivity and reduced FA have also been found in patients with cryptogenic focal epilepsy. Analysis of water diffusivity changes reveals a pattern of increase in perpendicular diffusivity and not of parallel diffusivity. This may indicate Wallerian degeneration as one of the main mechanisms accounting for the structural changes underlying the DTI abnormalities remote from focus and lesion.

Such abnormal areas in patients with intractable epilepsy, therefore, probably represent structural disruption, possibly reflecting either an underlying pathology or gliosis due to secondary damage. This requires further study with MRI–histology correlation in more patients.

Interictal DTI and Irritative and Ictal-Onset Zone

Close correlations between the interictal abnormalities highlighted using DTI, pathology, and epileptogenicity are rare. Intracranial recordings in a patient with cryptogenic focal epilepsy showed seizure onset in the right orbitofrontal region, colocalizing with an area of abnormal diffusivity (59), and postresection pathology revealed gliosis. Of note, however, is that this patient is not completely seizure-free.

Few papers have evaluated in detail the concordance between diffusion abnormalities and irritative zone and ictal-onset zone as evaluated using invasive recordings. Two studies have used voxel-based statistical approaches to highlight areas

of abnormal diffusion in a small number of patients undergoing stereo-EEG evaluations (60,61). In one study (61), 13 of the 16 patients were found to have DTI abnormalities, consisting mainly of increases in mean diffusivity and concordant with the epileptogenic zone in 7. FA abnormalities added little in localization. The specificity of DTI abnormalities was better in extratemporal lobe epilepsy: 20% of TLE had congruent findings, whereas four of five extratemporal epilepsies concurred.

Another study investigated 14 patients with frontal lobe epilepsy (9 nonlesional), almost all patients showed areas of increased diffusivity (60). In this study, the sensitivity of diffusion imaging in defining regions that were the site of electrical abnormalities was about 57% for the area of seizure onset and 65% for the irritative zone, and the specificity was low. It is of note, however, that areas of diffusion abnormalities may not have been sampled, as coverage is necessarily limited with Stereo EEG. An interesting aspect in this study is that lesional epilepsies had very high sensitivity, as the lesion led to diffusion abnormalities, but very low specificity. In nonlesional epilepsies, cases in which epileptologists may particularly turn to novel imaging for additional support of a hypothesis for invasive recordings, three out of the nine patients had diffusion changes in the seizure-onset zone.

Overall, the limited data available lead to conclude that diffusion changes correlate better with areas of interictal spiking than the ictal onset. Furthermore, the presence of DTI abnormalities certainly does not mean that the seizures are arising in the vicinity. However, DTI changes may provide some additional information to guide placement of invasive electrodes. Correlating electroclinical abnormalities using invasive recordings with diffusion changes may allow for better insights in the future.

Tractography and Epilepsy Surgery

DTI is the first imaging modality that allows direct noninvasive visualization of white matter tracts. Several investigations have focused on retrospectively correlating DTI-based tractography with postoperative deficits, to assess if the technology could provide predictive information for a deficit, and maybe even could aid in preservation of function if such information were integrated in neuronavigation systems. Anterior temporal lobectomies can cause a contralateral superior quadrantanopsia in up to 10% of patients by disrupting Meyer's loop. The anterior extent of Meyer's loop has large interindividual variability and cannot be visualized using conventional imaging (62). Tractography has been used to demonstrate the optic radiation in normal subjects (63), and its use was subsequently explored for temporal lobectomies (64). Pre- and intraoperative DTI-based fiber tracking (65) showed significant correlation between the fiber tracking estimation and the outcome of visual field deficits after surgery.

These data provide evidence that tractography has the potential to inform about risks of epilepsy surgery procedures. Once successfully implemented into neuronavigation systems, this information may also be used intraoperatively to tailor resections (66). Aside from the technical issues of performing tractography in health and disease, the intraoperative brain shift after craniotomy is another significant impediment. The availability of intraoperative MRI may represent one method to correct for this movement and may improve the accuracy of the data to aid surgical planning.

Extratemporal surgeries will also benefit from visualizing of the tracts such as the pyramidal tract. Implementation of DTI-based tractography has already been shown to benefit in brain tumor surgeries and resections of vascular malformations (67–70), and will certainly be increasingly used in epilepsy surgery.

EEG–fMRI

Up to now, the localization of the generators of interictal epileptiform discharges has been mainly addressed through EEG and MEG, techniques with exquisite temporal resolution. fMRI offers good spatial resolution and localization of events that are accompanied by a blood oxygen level-dependent (BOLD) response (5). A question that must be addressed first when considering fMRI as an epilepsy localization tool is whether epileptiform paroxysmal events (interictal and ictal) are associated with detectable BOLD signal changes. In this regard, the evidence from sources as varied as visual observation of the cortex during surgery, or using tools such as PET, SPECT, and near infrared spectroscopy (NIRS), is conclusive: seizures are commonly accompanied by regional hemodynamic changes. In the case of interictal discharges, the above techniques are unsuitable; some due to their fundamentally limited temporal resolution (PET, SPECT), others due to limited spatial sensitivity profiles, such as NIRS. fMRI with its temporal resolution of the order of a few seconds and excellent mapping capability combined with the intrinsically sluggish nature of the hemodynamic changes may offer a way to map out hemodynamic changes throughout the brain linked to short events from individual interictal epileptiform discharges, to runs of spikes, and sharp waves to seizures. The EEG is used as an indicator of events of interest, such as spikes or ictal discharges, from which a model of the fMRI signal is derived a posteriori and used for analysis of the fMRI time series data.

fMRI of Spontaneous Brain Activity: Data Acquisition, Analysis, and Interpretation

In the following we discuss some of the main technical aspects, applications, and findings of fMRI used to map spontaneous hemodynamic changes in patients with epilepsy. In most studies, the patient is asked to lie in the scanner and whole-brain scanning is performed in the expectation of capturing events of interest, usually interictal discharges, although drugs have been used in a small number of studies to modulate epileptiform activity specifically for the purpose of fMRI (71,72). Because of the random nature and temporal characteristics of epileptic activity, the fMRI data thus acquired is commonly analyzed within the framework of event-related designs, in contrast to the more conventional block designs used in many cognitive studies. This is done using the EEG as a basis for modeling the variations in the BOLD signal related to epileptic activity. For this purpose, short epileptiform discharges such as single spikes have been likened to brief stimuli. As described in Chapter 79, the BOLD response to brief stimuli develops and resolves over a period of

roughly 25 seconds, generally peaking between 5 and 7 seconds, then undershoots the baseline slightly, roughly 15 seconds poststimulus, before returning to baseline, and is therefore essentially bi-phasic (i.e., it has positive and negative phases); this is the *hemodynamic response function* (HRF) (73). We note that a substantial amount of intersubject and interregional variability of the HRF in healthy subjects has been documented (74). The possibility of deviation of the shape of the HRF in patients with epilepsy due to the effects of pathology or other factors has implications for the technique's sensitivity and potential clinical usefulness. Furthermore, the choice of an accurate representation of the HRF is greater for the detection of regions of BOLD change in event-related designs than for block designs. Importantly, event-related designs are generally less efficient than block designs for the detection of BOLD changes.

Before embarking on a review of the application of EEG–fMRI in focal epilepsy, we discuss a small number of fMRI studies of seizures for which concurrent EEG was not used.

fMRI of Seizures (Without Concurrent EEG)

fMRI data acquired in the resting state has been used to map BOLD signal changes linked to ictal or peri-ictal events. The lack of concurrent EEG means that the analysis and interpretation of the fMRI is heavily reliant on clinical changes noted during events. Apparent BOLD changes were revealed by subtraction of scans acquired at baseline from scans acquired during motor seizures in a child (75). In one study (76), the authors identified patterns of signal change in the absence of any overt ictal activity that were consistent with invasive localization. In another case report, ictal signs identified in relation to scan acquisition times were used to plot T2* signal changes relative to a baseline value voxel by voxel, revealing regions of signal increase and decrease preceding and during the motor seizure (77). Federico et al. studied preictal fMRI changes based on visual observation without concurrent EEG in two cases (78). Regions of signal change were identified by comparing blocks of scans immediately preceding the seizures to blocks acquired 3 to 5 minutes before ictal onset. Inspection of the signal time course in those regions and "control" regions revealed patterns suggestive of specific preictal BOLD increases and decreases to a lesser extent taking place around 10 minutes before seizure onset in one of case, similarly to a case in which EEG was recorded during fMRI. Although interesting, this type of analysis of fMRI data is suboptimal in many respects such as potential subjectivity of the identification of the event onset (and the resulting model of the BOLD signal) and possible bias associated with physiological and scanner-related artifacts (5).

EEG-Correlated fMRI: The Technique

While the clinical manifestations may be used as event markers for seizures, this is not the case for subclinical events such as interictal epileptiform discharges (IED). Therefore, the study of the hemodynamic changes associated with IED necessitates the recording of EEG during fMRI. Concurrent EEG may also help in the interpretation of ictal events for the purpose of fMRI modeling. The technique that consists in the simultaneous acquisition of EEG and fMRI data is commonly referred to as EEG-correlated fMRI, or EEG–fMRI. Due to the various interactions between the two technologies, data quality and patient safety are serious concerns, and have been the subject of a large amount of work since the first ever EEG recording took place inside an MR scanner (79). The main problems are: pulse-related and image acquisition artifacts on EEG, image artifacts due to passive components (EEG leads and electrodes) and active components (EEG amplifier/digitizer) (80).

While many developments have led to the commercialization of EEG recording systems capable of providing the investigator with basic tools capable of producing good quality data for some applications, such as EEG–fMRI of visually identifiable IED, EEG and image data quality continue to preoccupy many users partly because some problems may never be completely solved (e.g., pulse-related artifact on EEG) and partly because the application boundaries continue to be pushed (increasing scanner field strength, study of ever more subtle EEG features, etc.). Therefore, EEG–fMRI data acquisition continues to be a field of development and investigators undertaking EEG–fMRI investigations in epilepsy are advised to obtain continuous technical support.

EEG–fMRI of Seizures

Although potentially most relevant for presurgical localization, the study of the hemodynamic changes during ictal patterns is problematic due to safety concerns, and the rarity and unpredictability of seizures in most patients mean that ictal EEG–fMRI studies are generally fortuitous. Once such data have been acquired, their analysis is made difficult due to the effects of head motion, the long duration of the events (same time scale as some fMRI artifacts), and the uncertain relationship between clinical and EEG manifestations on one hand and the pathological neurophysiological activity on the other. Nonetheless, based on simple fMRI modelling assumptions ictal EEG–fMRI has shown BOLD increases often of larger amplitude and extent than interictal patterns, and associated higher yield[1] than interictal EEG–fMRI. For example, using a flexible modeling strategy adapted to long events, a large, electroclinically concordant BOLD increase was revealed in relation to a single subclinical seizure (81). In a patient with multiple seizures, a similarly concordant pattern of BOLD increase was revealed with large contralateral areas of simultaneous BOLD decreases (82). In a series of eight selected cases with malformations of cortical development in whom seizures were studied using EEG–fMRI, the relationship between ictal and interictal BOLD patterns and MR-visible lesions seemed to reflect the specific pathology; for example, in cases with nodular heterotopia, there was a tendency for the ictal BOLD changes to involve the overlying cortex (83). As previously mentioned, patterns suggestive of preictal hemodynamic changes were observed with and without the assistance of synchronous EEG (78).

EEG–fMRI of Interictal Epileptiform Discharges

The overwhelming majority of cases studied using EEG–fMRI have focused on revealing BOLD changes linked to IED. The primary aim of early studies in patients with focal epilepsy has been the demonstration of IED-related changes to localize the generators of the discharges, with the focus gradually shifting to the study of the details of the BOLD map localization in relation to other tests (MRI, EEG, etc.) and other aspects of these patterns such as the sign of BOLD change.

Two variants of the technique have been used for this purpose: IED-triggered fMRI and the more flexible and now widely used continuous EEG–fMRI. In IED-triggered fMRI, the MR acquisition was started following the identification of a spike or sharp wave; a fixed delay of a few seconds between spike and scan was employed, calculated based on the assumption that IED-related BOLD change will follow the course of the normal HRF.[2] A set of images acquired following IED were compared to images acquired following periods of background EEG. Such studies revealed significant BOLD increases in a large proportion of cases mostly concordant with the presumed or suspected generator localization (71,72,84–88). We note that these studies largely ignored the possibility of IED-related BOLD decreases. The finding of BOLD increases in expected locations in the majority of cases in which IED were captured confers a degree of validity to the assumption that IED-related changes are roughly in line with the HRF derived from physiological stimuli in healthy subjects, peaking at around 6 seconds postspike.

Due to the appeal of having access to the entire EEG record during scanning, IED-triggered fMRI has now been superseded by continuous EEG–fMRI that was made possible by EEG scanning-related artifact correction algorithms (89,90). In continuous EEG–fMRI, scans are acquired without interruption resulting in a continuous time series of scan data. Importantly, the analysis of continuous EEG–fMRI data to reveal regions of increase or decrease BOLD signal related to events of interest (e.g., pathological EEG discharges) is based on building models (GLM) of the BOLD signal over the *entire scanning session* which can be challenging due to spontaneous changes in brain state at rest (91,92).

The analysis of EEG–fMRI is commonly based on conventional, visual EEG interpretation by expert observers, and therefore suffers from the same limitations, although the impact of this subjectivity has not been thoroughly investigated (see [5] for a review of the technique's principles and limitations; see [93] for a rare study on the impact of EEG interpretation on the fMRI results). Using this approach in selected case series in focal epilepsy, and assuming that the IED-related HRF does not deviate substantially from the norm, regions of statistically significant BOLD signal changes were revealed in around 70% of the cases in whom IED were captured during scanning sessions with durations of the order of 40 to 60 minutes (84,94). Overall, the pattern of BOLD increases and decreases is often complex, although the localization of the BOLD increases tends to match the presumed or

---

[1] Yield: proportion of cases in which significant event-related BOLD changes are revealed.

[2] The actual delay may have varied due to the manual nature of the process but an uncertainty of the order of +/−1 second would be of little consequence given the time scale of BOLD changes.

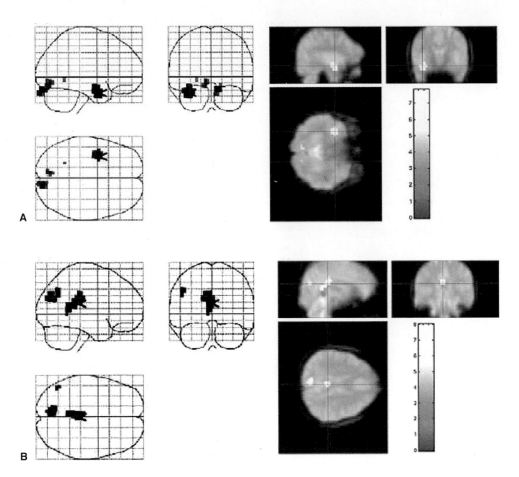

FIGURE 77.3 IED-related BOLD changes. Patient with left hippocampal sclerosis and left-temporal IEDs who underwent EEG–fMRI. **A:** BOLD increase in the left-temporal lobe with smaller clusters in the occipital region. The red arrow and cross-hair represent the location of the most significant BOLD change. The left of figure shows all statistically significant BOLD changes superimposed onto the SPM "glass-brain." The right of the figure shows parasagittal, coronal, and axial sections through the EPI data at the location of the statistical maximum. **B:** Retrosplenial BOLD decrease associated with the same IED. This effect, which is thought not to represent activity of the source of the spike seen on EEG, is commonly observed in relation to interictal activity in the temporal lobe. Please see color insert (94). (Taken from Salek-Haddadi A, Diehl B, Hamandi K, et al. Hemodynamic correlates of epileptiform discharges: an EEG-fMRI study of 63 patients with focal epilepsy. *Brain Res.* 2006;1088(1): 148–166, with permission).

confirmed IED- generator localization. BOLD decreases tend to be more remote and less representative of the IED field distribution (94,95). In TLE, a similar mix of BOLD increases and decreases involving the ipsilateral and contralateral (homologous) cortex was observed (94–96), with a consistent pattern of BOLD decrease in the precuneus (97), reminiscent of the so-called default-mode network (Fig. 77.3) (98).

One of the advantages of continuous EEG–fMRI over spike-triggered fMRI is that it allows one to estimate the shape of the IED-related HRF which is important if deviations from the norm are suspected with potential impact for analysis sensitivity. This can be done by using different sets of functions instead of the canonical HRF such as Fourier expansions or series of Gamma functions (99–101). The results of this type of study are somewhat conflicting and differences of opinion persist on the best approach for modeling IED-related BOLD changes in terms of sensitivity. For example, a study has revealed BOLD signal changes seemingly preceding IEDs mostly generalized in nature; these have been labeled "non causal" (101). However, the specificity of such deviations is uncertain. On the other hand, it has been shown that rare statistically significant deviations from the normal HRF, such as time course with a peak earlier than the normal 6 seconds postevent, are mostly remote from the presumed generators and suggestive of data-fitting artifacts (103), and perhaps most importantly, that no notable increase in yield results from the inclusion of causal noncanonical HRF in the GLM (94). Deviations from the causal relationship: EEG abnormality → time-locked BOLD change may be particularly relevant in studies of seizures (78) where it is known that scalp EEG often does not reflect the earliest electro-

physiological changes. No such evidence, from simultaneous scalp and intracerebral measurements for example, exists for interictal discharges to our knowledge.

There has been limited comparison of the localization of IED-related BOLD changes with either intracranial EEG or spike source analysis based on high-density EEG. Comparisons of fitted point dipoles or more sophisticated distributed source model with IED-related BOLD clusters from spike-triggered fMRI data showed a relatively coherent pattern of spatial concordance and the complementary and valuable nature of the information derived from the two techniques, although the agreement criteria, and fMRI modeling and source imaging procedures vary greatly between studies (102,104–107). When considered, the sign of IED-related BOLD change[3] did not significantly affect the degree of concordance with the presumed or confirmed generators (105,107). Comparison of IED fMRI and intracranial EEG in a small group showed that in cases where one electrode was located near BOLD clusters, at least one of the contacts of the electrode showed epileptiform activity (102).

EEG–fMRI has been used to study the characteristics of the IED-related BOLD changes in specific pathologies (108–110). In relation to gray matter heterotopia and malformations of cortical development (MCD), variability in the BOLD patterns was in line with previous findings, with a tendency for BOLD increases within the pathologically abnormal

---

[3] Taken in this context to be the sign of the first or dominant peak (or through) of the average IED-related BOLD time course relative to baseline.

regions and decreases generally but not exclusively more remote from the abnormality (109,110). The neurobiology of the observed patterns remains to be fully elucidated, but IED-related BOLD decreases in MCD have been attributed to either a loss of neuronal inhibition in the presence of normal neurovascular coupling in the regions surrounding the abnormality or abnormality of neurovascular coupling. Similar patterns of IED-related BOLD signal changes were revealed, involving the lesion and remote regions in patients with cavernomas (111) and tuberous sclerosis (in children) (112).

While the promising results of studies comparing localization based on EEG–fMRI to other forms of localization, the technique's role in presurgical evaluation remains unknown. To our knowledge no prospective randomized, controlled trial has been performed to assess the efficacy of imaging techniques for the purpose of presurgical evaluation to date, and this also applies to EEG–fMRI (113). In a group of 29 patients in whom surgery could not be offered based on the results of routine investigations, clusters of significant IED-correlated BOLD signal change concordant with presumed seizure focus were revealed in eight cases (93). In four patients, the BOLD maps consisted of multiple clusters, in line with the results of other tests. In the other four cases, the BOLD maps consisted of a single cluster, two of which were concordant with intracranial EEG, allowing surgery to be considered. Based on this evaluation as a second-line technique, the authors suggested that EEG–fMRI can play a significant role in presurgical evaluation. Further evaluation of the role of EEG–fMRI as part of the panoply of presurgical localization tests is required.

CONCLUSION

DTI and EEG–fMRI offer novel and complementary information to localize the epileptogenic zone. EEG–fMRI's unique characteristics among functional imaging techniques make it likely to make a strong contribution to the definition of the irritative zone, and of the ictal-onset zone in a smaller proportion of cases. However, its role in focus localization and contribution to the presurgical evaluation remains to be determined.

DTI may increase the sensitivity of MRI to lesions and improve our understanding of the local and remote impacts of the epileptogenic lesion on pathways and networks. In addition, it may help us better understand the often progressive cognitive changes seen in uncontrolled focal epilepsy and the functional deficit zone. Whether this information will be useful in predicting deficits following epilepsy surgery is unknown. MRI tractography will be increasingly used for neuronavigation during epilepsy surgery and may help limit surgical morbidity. Lastly, combining tractography and EEG–fMRI may provide novel insights in propagation of epileptic activity, and for identifying effective and functional connectivity between cerebral areas involved in the epileptic network and the structural basis of this. However, continued active research is required to translate these impressive advances in neuroimaging to improved outcomes.

References

1. Duncan J. The current status of neuroimaging for epilepsy: editorial review. *Curr Opin Neurol*. 2003;16(2):163–164.
2. Diehl B, Luders HO. Temporal lobe epilepsy: when are invasive recordings needed? *Epilepsia*. 2000;41(Suppl 3):S61–S74.
3. Koepp MJ, Woermann FG. Imaging structure and function in refractory focal epilepsy. *Lancet Neurol*. 2005;4(1):42–53.
4. Rosenow F, Luders H. Presurgical evaluation of epilepsy. *Brain*. 2001;124(Pt 9):1683–1700.
5. Salek-Haddadi A, Friston KJ, Lemieux L, et al. Studying spontaneous EEG activity with fMRI. *Brain Res Rev*. 2003;43(1):110–133.
6. Song SK, Sun SW, Ramsbottom MJ, et al. Dysmyelination revealed through MRI as increased radial (but unchanged axial) diffusion of water. *Neuroimage*. 2002;17(3):1429–1436.
7. Song SK, Sun SW, Ju WK, et al. Diffusion tensor imaging detects and differentiates axon and myelin degeneration in mouse optic nerve after retinal ischemia. *Neuroimage*. 2003;20(3):1714–1722.
8. Song SK, Yoshino J, Le TQ, et al. Demyelination increases radial diffusivity in corpus callosum of mouse brain. *Neuroimage*. 2005;26(1):132–140.
9. Beaulieu C, Does MD, Snyder RE, et al. Changes in water diffusion due to Wallerian degeneration in peripheral nerve. *Magn Reson Med*. 1996;36(4):627–631.
10. Le Bihan D, Mangin JF, Poupon C, et al. Diffusion tensor imaging: concepts and applications. *J Magn Reson Imaging*. 2001;13(4):534–546.
11. Le Bihan D, Van Zijl P. From the diffusion coefficient to the diffusion tensor. *NMR Biomed*. 2002;15(7–8):431–434.
12. Taylor DG, Bushell MC. The spatial mapping of translational diffusion coefficients by the NMR imaging technique. *Phys Med Biol*. 1985;30(4):345–349.
13. Basser PJ, Pierpaoli C. Microstructural and physiological features of tissues elucidated by quantitative-diffusion-tensor MRI. *J Magn Reson B*. 1996;111(3):209–219.
14. Basser PJ, Jones DK. Diffusion-tensor MRI: theory, experimental design and data analysis—a technical review. *NMR Biomed*. 2002;15(7–8):456–467.
15. Pierpaoli C, Jezzard P, Basser PJ, et al. Diffusion tensor MR imaging of the human brain. *Radiology*. 1996;201(3):637–648.
16. Basser PJ. Inferring microstructural features and the physiological state of tissues from diffusion-weighted images. *NMR Biomed*. 1995;8(7–8):333–344.
17. Beaulieu C, Allen PS. Determinants of anisotropic water diffusion in nerves. *Magn Reson Med*. 1994;31(4):394–400.
18. Pierpaoli C, Barnett A, Pajevic S, et al. Water diffusion changes in Wallerian degeneration and their dependence on white matter architecture. *Neuroimage*. 2001;13(6 Pt 1):1174–1185.
19. Concha L, Gross DW, Wheatley BM, et al. Diffusion tensor imaging of time-dependent axonal and myelin degradation after corpus callosotomy in epilepsy patients. *Neuroimage*. 2006;32(3):1090–1099.
20. Kerschensteiner M, Schwab ME, Lichtman JW, et al. In vivo imaging of axonal degeneration and regeneration in the injured spinal cord. *Nat Med*. 2005;11(5):572–577.
21. Mori S, van Zijl PC. Fiber tracking: principles and strategies—a technical review. *NMR Biomed*. 2002;15(7–8):468–480.
22. Wakana S, Jiang H, Nagae-Poetscher LM, et al. Fiber tract-based atlas of human white matter anatomy. *Radiology*. 2004;230(1):77–87.
23. Mori S, Wakana S, Nagae-Poetscher L, et al. *MRI Atlas of Human White Matter*. 1st ed. Amsterdam: Elsevier; 2005:61.
24. Jellison BJ, Field AS, Medow J, et al. Diffusion tensor imaging of cerebral white matter: a pictorial review of physics, fiber tract anatomy, and tumor imaging patterns. *Am J Neuroradiol*. 2004;25(3):356–369.
25. Nakasu Y, Nakasu S, Kizuki H, et al. Changes in water diffusion of rat limbic system during status epilepticus elicited by kainate. *Psychiatry Clin Neurosci*. 1995;49(3):S228–S230.
26. Nakasu Y, Nakasu S, Morikawa S, et al. Diffusion-weighted MR in experimental sustained seizures elicited with kainic acid. *Am J Neuroradiol*. 1995;16(6):1185–1192.
27. Righini A, Pierpaoli C, Alger JR, et al. Brain parenchyma apparent diffusion coefficient alterations associated with experimental complex partial status epilepticus. *Magn Reson Imaging*. 1994;12(6):865–871.
28. Wang Y, Majors A, Najm I, et al. Postictal alteration of sodium content and apparent diffusion coefficient in epileptic rat brain induced by kainic acid. *Epilepsia*. 1996;37(10):1000–1006.
29. Wieshmann UC, Symms MR, Shorvon SD. Diffusion changes in status epilepticus. *Lancet*. 1997;350(9076):493–494.
30. Lux HD, Heinemann U, Dietzel I. Ionic changes and alterations in the size of the extracellular space during epileptic activity. *Adv Neurol*. 1986;44:619–639.
31. Diehl B, Najm I, Ruggieri P, et al. Postictal diffusion-weighted imaging for the localization of focal epileptic areas in temporal lobe epilepsy. *Epilepsia*. 2001;42(1):21–28.
32. Diehl B, Symms MR, Boulby PA, et al. Postictal diffusion tensor imaging. *Epilepsy Res*. 2005;65(3):137–146.
33. Hufnagel A, Weber J, Marks S, et al. Brain diffusion after single seizures. *Epilepsia*. 2003;44(1):54–63.
34. Oh JB, Lee SK, Kim KK, et al. Role of immediate postictal diffusion-weighted MRI in localizing epileptogenic foci of mesial temporal lobe epilepsy and non-lesional neocortical epilepsy. *Seizure*. 2004;13(7):509–516.
35. Salmenpera TM, Symms MR, Boulby PA, et al. Postictal diffusion weighted imaging. *Epilepsy Res*. 2006;70(2–3):133–143.
36. Diehl B, Najm I, Ruggieri P, et al. Periictal diffusion-weighted imaging in a case of lesional epilepsy. *Epilepsia*. 1999;40(11):1667–1671.

37. Konermann S, Marks S, Ludwig T, et al. Presurgical evaluation of epilepsy by brain diffusion: MR-detected effects of flumazenil on the epileptogenic focus. *Epilepsia.* 2003;44(3):399–407.
38. Yoo SY, Chang KH, Song IC, et al. Apparent diffusion coefficient value of the hippocampus in patients with hippocampal sclerosis and in healthy volunteers. *Am J Neuroradiol.* 2002;23(5):809–812.
39. Wieshmann UC, Clark CA, Symms MR, et al. Water diffusion in the human hippocampus in epilepsy. *Magn Reson Imaging.* 1999;17(1):29–36.
40. Wehner T, LaPresto E, Tkach J, et al. The value of interictal diffusion-weighted imaging in lateralizing temporal lobe epilepsy. *Neurology.* 2007;68(2):122–127.
41. Hugg JW, Butterworth EJ, Kuzniecky RI. Diffusion mapping applied to mesial temporal lobe epilepsy: preliminary observations. *Neurology.* 1999;53(1):173–176.
42. Hakyemez B, Erdogan C, Yildiz H, et al. Apparent diffusion coefficient measurements in the hippocampus and amygdala of patients with temporal lobe seizures and in healthy volunteers. *Epilepsy Behav.* 2005;6(2):250–256.
43. Assaf BA, Mohamed FB, Abou-Khaled KJ, et al. Diffusion tensor imaging of the hippocampal formation in temporal lobe epilepsy. *Am J Neuroradiol.* 2003;24(9):1857–1862.
44. Concha L, Beaulieu C, Gross DW. Bilateral limbic diffusion abnormalities in unilateral temporal lobe epilepsy. *Ann Neurol.* 2005;57(2):188–196.
45. Concha L, Beaulieu C, Collins DL, et al. White matter diffusion abnormalities in temporal lobe epilepsy with and without mesial temporal sclerosis. *J Neurol Neurosurg Psychiatry.* 2009;80(3):312–9.
46. Nilsson D, Go C, Rutka JT, et al. Bilateral diffusion tensor abnormalities of temporal lobe and cingulate gyrus white matter in children with temporal lobe epilepsy. *Epilepsy Res.* 2008;81(2–3):128–135.
47. Gross DW, Concha L, Beaulieu C. Extratemporal white matter abnormalities in mesial temporal lobe epilepsy demonstrated with diffusion tensor imaging. *Epilepsia.* 2006;47(8):1360–1363.
48. Govindan RM, Makki MI, Sundaram SK, et al. Diffusion tensor analysis of temporal and extra-temporal lobe tracts in temporal lobe epilepsy. *Epilepsy Res.* 2008;80(1):30–41.
49. Arfanakis K, Hermann BP, Rogers BP, et al. Diffusion tensor MRI in temporal lobe epilepsy. *Magn Reson Imaging.* 2002;20(7):511–519.
50. Focke NK, Yogarajah M, Bonelli SB, et al. Voxel-based diffusion tensor imaging in patients with mesial temporal lobe epilepsy and hippocampal sclerosis. *Neuroimage.* 2008;40(2):728–737.
51. Concha L, Beaulieu C, Wheatley BM, et al. Bilateral white matter diffusion changes persist after epilepsy surgery. *Epilepsia.* 2007;48(5):931–940.
52. Rugg-Gunn FJ, Eriksson SH, Symms MR, et al. Diffusion tensor imaging of cryptogenic and acquired partial epilepsies. *Brain.* 2001;124(Pt 3):627–636.
53. Eriksson SH, Rugg-Gunn FJ, Symms MR, et al. Diffusion tensor imaging in patients with epilepsy and malformations of cortical development. *Brain.* 2001;124(Pt 3):617–626.
54. Dumas dlR, Oppenheim C, Chassoux F, et al. Diffusion tensor imaging of partial intractable epilepsy. *Eur Radiol.* 2005;15(2):279–285.
55. Widjaja E, Blaser S, Miller E, et al. Evaluation of subcortical white matter and deep white matter tracts in malformations of cortical development. *Epilepsia.* 2007;48(8):1460–1469.
56. Diehl B, Busch RM, Duncan JS, et al. Abnormalities in diffusion tensor imaging of the uncinate fasciculus relate to reduced memory in temporal lobe epilepsy. *Epilepsia.* 49(8):1409–18.
57. Kim H, Piao Z, Liu P, et al. Secondary white matter degeneration of the corpus callosum in patients with intractable temporal lobe epilepsy: a diffusion tensor imaging study. *Epilepsy Res.* 2008;81(2–3):136–142.
58. McDonald CR, Ahmadi ME, Hagler DJ, et al. Diffusion tensor imaging correlates of memory and language impairments in temporal lobe epilepsy. *Neurology.* 2008;71(23):1869–1876.
59. Rugg-Gunn FJ, Eriksson SH, Symms MR, et al. Diffusion tensor imaging in refractory epilepsy. *Lancet.* 2002;359(9319):1748–1751.
60. Guye M, Ranjeva JP, Bartolomei F, et al. What is the significance of interictal water diffusion changes in frontal lobe epilepsies? *Neuroimage.* 2007;35(1):28–37.
61. Thivard L, Adam C, Hasboun D, et al. Interictal diffusion MRI in partial epilepsies explored with intracerebral electrodes. *Brain.* 2006;129(Pt 2):375–385.
62. Ebeling U, Reulen HJ. Neurosurgical topography of the optic radiation in the temporal lobe. *Acta Neurochir (Wien).* 1988;92(1–4):29–36.
63. Yamamoto T, Yamada K, Nishimura T, et al. Tractography to depict three layers of visual field trajectories to the calcarine gyri. *Am J Ophthalmol.* 2005;140(5):781–785.
64. Powell HW, Parker GJ, Alexander DC, et al. MR tractography predicts visual field defects following temporal lobe resection. *Neurology.* 2005;65(4):596–599.
65. Chen X, Weigel D, Ganslandt O, et al. Prediction of visual field deficits by diffusion tensor imaging in temporal lobe epilepsy surgery. *Neuroimage.* 2009;45(2):286–97.
66. Nimsky C, Ganslandt O, Fahlbusch R. Implementation of fiber tract navigation. *Neurosurgery.* 2007;61(Suppl 1):306–317.
67. Wu JS, Zhou LF, Tang WJ, et al. Clinical evaluation and follow-up outcome of diffusion tensor imaging-based functional neuronavigation: a prospective, controlled study in patients with gliomas involving pyramidal tracts. *Neurosurgery.* 2007;61(5):935–948.
68. Nimsky C, Grummich P, Sorensen AG, et al. Visualization of the pyramidal tract in glioma surgery by integrating diffusion tensor imaging in functional neuronavigation. *Zentralbl Neurochir.* 2005;66(3):133–141.
69. Nimsky C, Ganslandt O, Hastreiter P, et al. Preoperative and intraoperative diffusion tensor imaging-based fiber tracking in glioma surgery. *Neurosurgery.* 2007;61(Suppl 1):178–185.
70. Chen X, Weigel D, Ganslandt O, et al. Diffusion tensor-based fiber tracking and intraoperative neuronavigation for the resection of a brainstem cavernous angioma. *Surg Neurol.* 2007;68(3):285–291.
71. Lazeyras F, Blanke O, Perrig S, et al. EEG-triggered functional MRI in patients with pharmacoresistant epilepsy. *J Magn Reson Imaging.* 2000;12:177–185.
72. Seeck M, Lazeyras F, Michel CM, et al. Non-invasive epileptic focus localization using EEG-triggered functional MRI and electromagnetic tomography. *Electroenceph Clin Neurophysiol.* 1998;106:508–512.
73. Friston KJ, Josephs O, Rees G, et al. Nonlinear event-related responses in fMRI. *Magn Reson Med.* 1998;39:41–52.
74. Aguirre GK, Zarahn E, D'Esposito M. The variability of human, BOLD hemodynamic responses. *Neuroimage.* 1998;8:360–369.
75. Jackson GD, Connelly A, Cross JH, et al. Functional magnetic resonance imaging of focal seizures. *Neurology.* 1994;44(5):850–856.
76. Detre JA, Alsop DC, Aguirre GK, et al. Coupling of cortical and thalamic ictal activity in human partial epilepsy: demonstration by functional magnetic resonance imaging. *Epilepsia.* 1996;37(7):657–661.
77. Krings T, Topper R, Reinges MHT, et al. Hemodynamic changes in simple partial epilepsy: a functional MRI study. *Neurology.* 2000;54(2):524–527.
78. Federico P, Abbott DF, Briellmann RS, et al. Functional MRI of the pre-ictal state. *Brain.* 2005;128(Pt 8):1811–1817.
79. Ives JR, Warach S, Schmitt F, et al. Monitoring the patient's EEG during echo planar MRI. *Electroenceph Clin Neurophysiol.* 1993;87(6):417–420.
80. Laufs H, Daunizeau J, Carmichael DW, et al. Recent advances in recording electrophysiological data simultaneously with magnetic resonance imaging. *Neuroimage.* 2008;40(2):515–528.
81. Salek-Haddadi A, Merschhemke M, Lemieux L, et al. Simultaneous EEG-correlated ictal fMRI. *Neuroimage.* 2002;16(1):32–40.
82. Kobayashi E, Hawco CS, Grova C, et al. Widespread and intense BOLD changes during brief focal electrographic seizures. *Neurology.* 2006;66(7):1049–1055.
83. Tyvaert L, Hawco C, Kobayashi E, et al. Different structures involved during ictal and interictal epileptic activity in malformations of cortical development: an EEG-fMRI study. *Brain.* 2008;131(Pt 8):2042–2060.
84. Al Asmi A, Benar CG, Gross DW, et al. fMRI Activation in continuous and spike-triggered EEG-fMRI studies of epileptic spikes. *Epilepsia.* 2003;44(10):1328–1339.
85. Jager L, Werhahn KJ, Hoffmann A, et al. Focal epileptiform activity in the brain: detection with spike-related functional MR imaging—preliminary results. *Radiology.* 2002;223:860–869.
86. Krakow K, Woermann FG, Symms MR, et al. EEG-triggered functional MRI of interictal epileptiform activity in patients with partial seizures. *Brain.* 1999;122(Pt 9):1679–1688.
87. Krakow K, Lemieux L, Messina D, et al. Spatio-temporal imaging of focal interictal epileptiform activity using EEG-triggered functional MRI. *Epileptic Disord.* 2001;3(2):67–74.
88. Patel MR, Blum A, Pearlman JD, et al. Echo-planar functional MR imaging of epilepsy with concurrent EEG monitoring. *Am J Neuroradiol.* 1999;20:1916–1919.
89. Allen PJ, Polizzi G, Krakow K, et al. Identification of EEG events in the MR scanner: the problem of pulse artifact and a method for its subtraction. *Neuroimage.* 1998;8(3):229–239.
90. Allen PJ, Josephs O, Turner R. A method for removing imaging artifact from continuous EEG recorded during functional MRI. *Neuroimage.* 2000;12(2):230–239.
91. Lemieux L, Salek-Haddadi A, Lund TE, et al. Modelling large motion events in fMRI studies of patients with epilepsy. *Magn Reson Imaging.* 2007;25(6):894–901.
92. Liston AD, Lund TE, Salek-Haddadi A, et al. Modelling cardiac signal as a confound in EEG-fMRI and its application in focal epilepsy studies. *Neuroimage.* 2006;30(3):827–834.
93. Zijlmans M, Huiskamp G, Hersevoort M, et al. EEG-fMRI in the preoperative work-up for epilepsy surgery. *Brain.* 2007;130(Pt 9):2343–2353.
94. Salek-Haddadi A, Diehl B, Hamandi K, et al. Hemodynamic correlates of epileptiform discharges: an EEG-fMRI study of 63 patients with focal epilepsy. *Brain Res.* 2006;1088(1):148–166.
95. Kobayashi E, Bagshaw AP, Grova C, et al. Negative BOLD responses to epileptic spikes. *Hum Brain Mapp.* 2005;27(6):488–497.
96. Kobayashi E, Bagshaw AP, Benar CG, et al. Temporal and extratemporal BOLD responses to temporal lobe interictal spikes. *Epilepsia.* 2006;47(2):343–354.
97. Laufs H, Hamandi K, Salek-Haddadi A, et al. Temporal lobe interictal epileptic discharges affect cerebral activity in "default mode" brain regions. *Hum Brain Mapp.* 28:1023–1032 (2007).
98. Raichle ME, MacLeod AM, Snyder AZ, et al. A default mode of brain function. *Proc Natl Acad Sci USA.* 2001;98(2):676–682.

99. Bagshaw AP, Aghakhani Y, Benar CG, et al. EEG-fMRI of focal epileptic spikes: analysis with multiple haemodynamic functions and comparison with gadolinium-enhanced MR angiograms. *Hum Brain Mapp.* 2004; 22(3):179–192.

100. Benar CG, Grova C, Kobayashi E, et al. EEG-fMRI of epileptic spikes: concordance with EEG source localization and intracranial EEG. *Neuroimage.* 2006;30(4):1161–1170.

101. Lemieux L, Salek-Haddadi A, Josephs O, et al. Event-related fMRI with simultaneous and continuous EEG: description of the method and initial case report. *Neuroimage.* 2001;14(3):780–787.

102. Hawco CS, Bagshaw AP, Lu Y, et al. BOLD changes occur prior to epileptic spikes seen on scalp EEG. *Neuroimage.* 2007;35(4):1450–1458.

103. Lemieux L, Laufs H, Carmichael D, et al. Noncanonical spike-related BOLD responses in focal epilepsy. *Hum Brain Mapp.* 2007;29:329–345.

104. Bagshaw AP, Kobayashi E, Dubeau F, et al. Correspondence between EEG-fMRI and EEG dipole localisation of interictal discharges in focal epilepsy. *Neuroimage.* 30(2006) 417–425.

105. Grova C, Daunizeau J, Kobayashi E, et al. Concordance between distributed EEG source localization and simultaneous EEG-fMRI studies of epileptic spikes. *Neuroimage.* 2008;39(2):755–774.

106. Lemieux L, Krakow K, Fish DR. Comparison of spike-triggered functional MRI BOLD activation and EEG dipole model localization. *Neuroimage.* 2001;14(5):1097–1104.

107. Vulliemoz S, Thornton R, Rodionov R, et al. The spatio-temporal mapping of epileptic networks: combination of EEG-fMRI and EEG source imaging. *Neuroimage.* 2009;46:834–843. .

108. Diehl B, Salek-Haddadi A, Fish DR, et al. Mapping of spikes, slow waves, and motor tasks in a patient with malformation of cortical development using simultaneous EEG and fMRI. *Magn Reson Imaging.* 2003;21(10): 1167–1173.

109. Federico P, Archer JS, Abbott DF, et al. Cortical/subcortical BOLD changes associated with epileptic discharges: an EEG-fMRI study at 3 T. *Neurology.* 2005;64(7):1125–1130.

110. Kobayashi E, Bagshaw AP, Jansen A, et al. Intrinsic epileptogenicity in polymicrogyric cortex suggested by EEG-fMRI BOLD responses. *Neurology.* 2005;64(7):1263–1266.

111. Kobayashi E, Bagshaw AP, Gotman J, et al. Metabolic correlates of epileptic spikes in cerebral cavernous angiomas. *Epilepsy Res.* 2007;73(1): 98–103.

112. Jacobs J, Rohr A, Moeller F, et al. Evaluation of epileptogenic networks in children with tuberous sclerosis complex using EEG-fMRI. *Epilepsia.* 2008;49(5):816–825.

113. Whiting P, Gupta R, Burch J, et al. A systematic review of the effectiveness and cost-effectiveness of neuroimaging assessments used to visualise the seizure focus in people with refractory epilepsy being considered for surgery. *Health Technol Assess.* 2006;10(4):1–4.

CHAPTER 78 ■ ELOQUENT CORTEX AND THE ROLE OF PLASTICITY

TOBIAS LODDENKEMPER AND MARTIN STAUDT

Epilepsy surgery aims at the resection of the epileptogenic zone with minimal or no damage to the surrounding brain tissue and eloquent cortex. Structural and functional lesions may lead to plasticity of eloquent cortex, making it impossible to predict location of function based on anatomy alone. Noninvasive mapping of eloquent cortex is, therefore, crucial in successful planning of epilepsy surgery. Mapping techniques vary in their sensitivity and specificity to predict postsurgical deficits, their temporal and spatial resolution, cost, and invasiveness (1). Test paradigms may be either activating or inhibiting function and thereby demonstrating different functional aspects.

In this chapter we will discuss plasticity of eloquent cortex in the setting of epilepsy, as assessed with various invasive and noninvasive mapping techniques.

METHODS TO ASSESS FUNCTIONAL (RE)ORGANIZATION

Functional reorganization following focal brain lesions can be assessed with several neurophysiological and imaging techniques, most of which are described in detail elsewhere in this book (Chapters 73, 74, 75, 76 and 77). This chapter briefly summarizes the particular roles of these techniques in the investigation of functional (re)organization after early brain lesions (Table 78.1).

Functional magnetic resonance imaging (fMRI) (see Chapter 79) can be used to map the cortical representations (and, thus, the reorganization) of various brain functions, such as motor, somatosensory, visual, or language functions. One major limitation of this technique is that it requires active patient cooperation for most paradigms, which makes it challenging and sometimes impossible to obtain reliable information in children. Consequently, child-friendly fMRI paradigms have been developed for motor, somatosensory, and also language studies (2–5). Only for passive stimulation paradigms (such as visual stimulation), fMRI studies are also possible in sedated or anesthetized patients (6,7).

Magnetoencephalography (MEG) (see Chapter 76), *evoked potentials (EP)*, *event-related potential (ERP)*, and EEG can be used to monitor cortical areas receiving input from peripheral sensory stimulation (e.g., tactile, auditory, visual, or electrical stimulation), with a superior temporal resolution (especially as compared with fMRI), but only a moderate spatial resolution is available, especially when 3D information is sought.

TABLE 78.1

OVERVIEW OF FUNCTIONAL BRAIN MAPPING TECHNIQUES

Technique	Spatial resolution	Temporal resolution	Invasiveness	Applications
PET	4 mm	s	++	Seizure focus identification
FMRI	2–5 mm	s	+	Seizure focus and eloquent area identification
DTI	<1 mm3	N/A	+	Localization and evaluation of WM tracts
MEG	Poor	ms	+	Seizure focus and eloquent area identification
IAP	Hemispheric	N/A	+++	Language and memory lateralization
Subdural electrodes recordings and stimulation	Excellent (on brain surface)	Instantaneous	++++	Eloquent area mapping and seizure focus identification
TMS	Medium	ms	++	Eloquent area mapping

Modified after Tharin S, Golby A. Functional brain mapping and its applications to neurosurgery. *Neurosurgery.* 2007;60:185–201, with permission.

Consequently, a combination of fMRI with these electrophysiological techniques will yield information with both a good spatial resolution in three dimensions (fMRI) and a good temporal resolution (MEG/EP/ERP), which allows a better understanding of reorganizational processes. Evoked potential (EP), such as visual, auditory, and somatosensory EP are useful tools in testing the integrity and localization of eloquent cortical areas prior to resection in epilepsy surgery candidates. Additionally, event-related potentials (ERP) have been implicated in memory, language, motor function, and other higher cortical functions (8). An example are well-circumscribed lesions of the medial temporal lobe that cause an amnestic syndrome and that have been shown to produce altered plasticity of the late positive P600 component, and usually spare P300 and N400 components (9). EEG spectral analysis has also been shown to vary based on development and intervention during development (10). Examples for the superiority of this combination will be given in this chapter.

Diffusion tensor imaging (DTI) and MR diffusion tractography (*"fiber tracking"*) (see Chapter 77) can visualize trajectories of fiber bundles in the cerebral white matter, and can thus be used to investigate reorganizational processes at the axonal level. The validity of this relatively new imaging technique still needs to be determined; therefore, a confirmation of its results by neurophysiological methods (see examples in this chapter) seems to be advisable whenever possible.

The *intracarotid amobarbital procedure (Wada test)* (see Chapter 80) is an inactivation technique that has been used for language and memory lateralization, and in selected cases for epilepsy lateralization and seizure outcome prediction after epilepsy surgery. Due to emergence of other mapping techniques, due to the relative invasiveness of the procedure and due to its low spatial resolution, Wada testing has decreased. However, it remains the gold standard when comparing mapping of language areas with other techniques, if cortical stimulation is not available.

Finally, for the investigation of corticospinal (re)organization following early brain lesions, the technique of *transcranial magnetic stimulation* (TMS) is extremely useful. This technique uses short magnetic pulses applied transcranially to induce electric currents in brain tissue. Thus, when TMS is applied over the primary motor cortex (M1), a volley of action potentials is generated, which travels down the corticospinal tract, reaches alpha-motor neurons in the spinal cord, and finally elicits a peripheral muscular response. This response can be recorded by surface EMG electrodes attached over the respective target muscle—the so-called motor evoked potential (MEP). Such MEPs are mostly recorded from hand muscles; when these MEPs in hand muscles have short latencies (around 20 ms or less), this finding can be regarded as evidence for the presence of direct, monosynaptic, fast-conducting corticospinal pathways from the stimulated area to hand muscles (11). Thus, when focal ("figure-eight-shaped") coils are used, TMS allows a topographic identification of the primary motor representation of a target muscle on the surface of the head, as well as an assessment of the integrity of corticospinal pathways in the case of brain lesions. This information cannot be obtained with the same degree of reliability by any other noninvasive technique. When combined with fMRI of active hand movements, TMS can thus test each of often multiple activation sites for the presence of corticospinal projections originating from the respective brain region. This is of particular importance in patients with early unilateral lesions, since these might have induced the

development of ipsilateral corticospinal projections from the contralesional hemisphere. Limitations of this technique (in the presurgical context) are:

- low spatial resolution and the lack of cortical reference points. This can be overcome either by combining TMS with other modalities (such as fMRI, see examples below) or by using neuronavigational systems.
- high stimulation intensities which are often needed in preschool children, and also in patients on antiepileptic medication, which sometimes makes reproducible elicitation of MEPs impossible. Therefore, under these circumstances, the inability to elicit MEPs from certain brain regions cannot be regarded as evidence for lack of corticospinal projections originating from these sites.

As opposed to the single-pulse TMS as described above, repetitive TMS (rTMS) is a new development that holds the potential to produce "virtual lesions" of a stimulated brain region. This methodology has, however, to our knowledge not yet been introduced into the field of routine preoperative functional diagnostic evaluations.

Functional transcranial Doppler ultrasound (fTCD) has been widely used to assess stenoses of intracranial vessels. As an extension of this technique, functional activation of brain areas has been introduced as functional TCD (fTCD). fTCD is—similar to fMRI—based on the assumption of increased vascular perfusion in corresponding brain areas during activity. Averaging of epochs during continuous measurement of cerebral blood flow velocity (CBFV) in homologous basal brain arteries may reveal hemispheric differences. Epochs are time-locked to a repeatedly performed cognitive paradigm. Blood flow in both hemispheres is compared during activation and compared to a resting period. A relative functional dominance is assumed for the hemisphere with greater increase in CBFV (12) (Fig. 78.1). Multiple cognitive functions have been demonstrated by fTCD including attention (13), visual and visuospatial functions (14,15), motor function (16), processing of music (17), math skills (18), and language (19,20). Language lateralization with fTCD had high concordance with Wada testing (21) and fMRI (22).

Positron emission tomography (PET) and single photon emission computed tomography (SPECT) are based on cerebral perfusion imaging. These techniques are capable of detecting areas of eloquent cortex or altered biochemical metabolism by means of radioactive compounds. Whereas PET tracers are attached to physiological molecules, SPECT radionucleotides are either not associated with biological molecules or may bind to specific receptors, that is, benzodiazepine receptors. PET and SPECT have both been used in the assessment of eloquent cortex (23).

Electrical cortical stimulation (ECS) was the first mapping technique establishing the concept of functional localization and eloquent areas. It remains the gold standard of functional mapping. Subdural grid electrode recordings and ECS may aid in the seizure focus determination as well as eloquent cortex mapping (Fig. 78.2). Responses to ECS may either be positive signs, such as motor movements, or negative findings that can only be detected when the patient is examined while performing specific tasks. Eloquent areas and plasticity defined by cortical stimulation include primary motor and sensory cortex, supplementary sensory motor area, secondary sensory area, language areas, visual and auditory cortices, as well as negative motor areas (24).

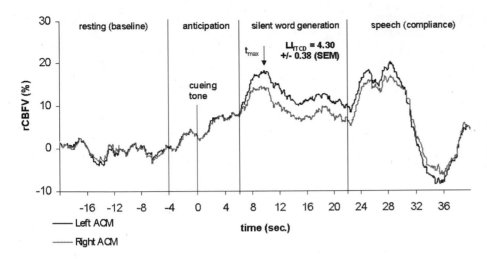

FIGURE 78.1 Language lateralization by fTCD. This figure displays averaged relative change in cerebral blood flow velocity (rCBFV) over 20 task repetitions compared to baseline CBFV during language assessment by fTCD. *Annotations:* MCA: Middle cerebral artery; t_{max}: time point of maximum difference in left-right rCBFV throughout word generation; LI: laterality index; SEM; standard error of the mean LI over task repetitions (from Loddenkemper & Haag, 2010 (12), with permission).

PLASTICITY IN SPECIALIZED ELOQUENT SYSTEMS

Motor System

During normal development of the motor system, corticospinal motor projections sprout from the motor cortex and grow in a corticofugal manner. By the 20th week of gestation, these descending corticospinal projections have reached the spinal cord (25) and enter a process of synaptogenesis with target cells, especially with alpha-motor neurons, at the spinal segmental level. During this phase, each hemisphere initially develops bilateral projections, that is, projections to both the contra- and the ipsilateral extremities, which results in a situation of "competition" between ipsi- and contralateral projections for motor neurons in the spinal cord. During ongoing normal development, a gradual withdrawal of ipsilateral projections can be observed, paralleled by strengthening of contralateral projections (26). During this process, neuronal

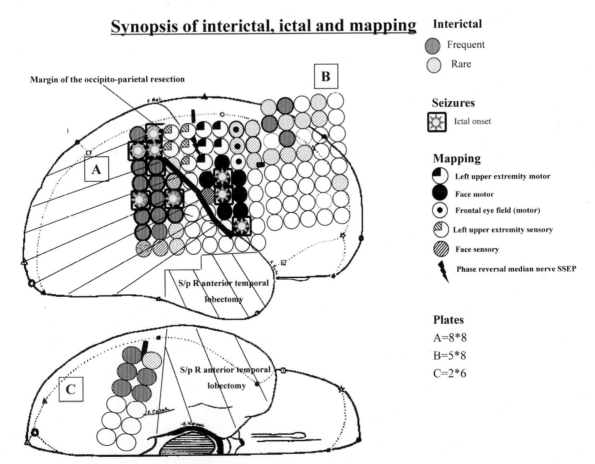

FIGURE 78.2 Synopsis of interictal, ictal, and subdural electrode mapping. This figure demonstrates a synopsis of cortical stimulation and EEG monitoring including seizure-onset and interictal EEG data. The patient underwent right temporal lobectomy in the past. Right posterior quadrant resection was tailored based on cortical stimulation mapping of primary sensory cortex areas in the postcentral gyrus.

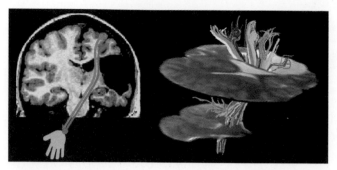

FIGURE 78.3 Diffusion tensor fiber tracking in a patient with corticosubcortical infarction. (From Staudt M, Erb M, Braun C, et al. Extensive peri-lesional connectivity in congenital hemiparesis. *Neurology.* 2006;66:771, with permission from Lippincott Williams & Wilkins, Copyright 2006.) Example of a patient with a pre- or peri-natally acquired infarction in the territory of the middle cerebral artery, leaving only a small bridge of preserved white matter between the enlarged lateral ventricle and the large cystic lesion (**left:** T1-weighted coronal image). Nevertheless, TMS and MEG indicated preserved crossed corticospinal motor projections (red) and preserved crossed thalamocortical somatosensory projections (blue). Accordingly, MR diffusion tractography (**right;** in random colors) visualizes the extensive connectivity mediated by this small bridge of preserved white matter (= seed area for fiber tracking). See color plate section.

activity seems to be a crucial factor in determining which projections are preserved and which are withdrawn.

This normally transient existence of ipsilateral corticospinal projections provides the basis for a peculiar type of motor (re)organization with ipsilateral corticospinal projections following early unilateral brain damage: When such unilateral brain damage occurs before or during the time of synaptogenesis of corticospinal motor projections with spinal alpha-motor neurons, this can put the crossing corticospinal projections from the affected hemisphere at a "disadvantage" with regards to the neuronal activity in these projections. Thus, the ipsilateral projections from the contralesional hemisphere can exceed the contralateral projections in their neuronal activity. Subsequently, the ipsilateral projections persist and are strengthened during further development, while the (now weaker) contralateral projections are withdrawn. Eventually, the contralesional hemisphere can become equipped with fast-conducting ipsilateral projections to the paretic extremities (26) (Fig. 78.3). This type of corticospinal (re)organization can occur throughout the pre- and perinatal period (27), during the first months of life (28), and in case reports even up to the age of 2 years (29). In children beyond this age and in adult stroke patients, such fast-conducting projections have, to date, never been reported. When ipsilateral projections are present in such patients, the MEPs have longer latencies and are therefore thought to be either oligosynaptic (11) or, alternatively, monosynaptic projections with slower conduction velocities (26). In adult stroke patients, these long-latency projections are associated with poor hand motor function outcome (30).

Corticospinal motor projections typically pass through the periventricular white matter on their way from the primary motor cortex (precentral gyrus/central sulcus) to the internal capsule. Thus, damage to these projections is frequent in patients with periventricular white matter lesions ("early third trimester lesions"; (31)), but more rare in patients with corticosubcortical "infarct-type" lesions ("late third trimester lesions"; (27)). Corticosubcortical "infarct-type" lesions often do not extend so far medially to also affect the periventricular

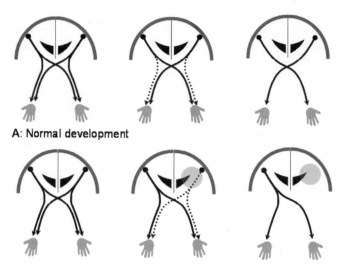

A: Normal development

B: Development after an early unilateral lesion

FIGURE 78.4 Normal and abnormal development of the corticospinal tract. Schematic illustration of corticospinal tract development under normal conditions (**A**) and in the case of an early unilateral brain lesion (**B**). At the beginning of the third trimester of pregnancy, descending corticospinal motor projections have already reached their spinal target zones, with initially bilateral projections from each hemisphere (**A** and **B**—*left*). During normal development (top row), the ipsilateral projections are gradually withdrawn, whereas the contralateral projections persist (**A**—*middle*). Thus, in the mature system, the hand is (nearly) completely controlled by the contralateral hemisphere (**A**—*right*). In the case of a unilateral lesion acquired during this phase (**B**—*middle*), both the ipsilateral and the contralateral projections from the lesioned hemisphere are weakened, so that ipsi- and contralateral projections from the contralesional hemisphere persist. Thus, in the mature system, the paretic hand can be controlled by the ipsilateral (contralesional) hemisphere (**B**—*right*).

white matter. Thus, crossed corticospinal projections from the lesioned hemisphere are often at least partially intact in such patients even with surprisingly large corticosubcortical lesions (Fig. 78.4).

Aside from these "defective" lesions, reorganization with ipsilateral corticospinal projections can also be induced by malformations of cortical development (MCD) involving the central region and/or the underlying white matter. On the other hand, MCDs can also harbor primary motor cortex, with "normal" fast-conducting monosynaptic corticospinal projections originating from these MCDs (32). Thus, when epileptogenic MCDs are located in the precentral region or in the central (Rolandic) white matter, individual assessment of motor system organization should be performed (Fig. 78.5).

Concerning the quality of hand functions which can be achieved by this motor (re)organization with ipsilateral corticospinal projections, many patients show a useful grasp function with their paretic hand, some even with preserved individual finger movements (31,32). A normal (or near to normal) function of the paretic hand has, however, never been reported. On the other hand, many patients cannot use their paretic hand for active grasping, although such fast-conducting pathways are present. This variability in the quality of paretic hand function can, at least partially, be explained by different stages of development at the time of the insult: The earlier during development a brain lesion occurs, the better the paretic hand function will be (32). Consequently, in many children with brain damage acquired around term birth or

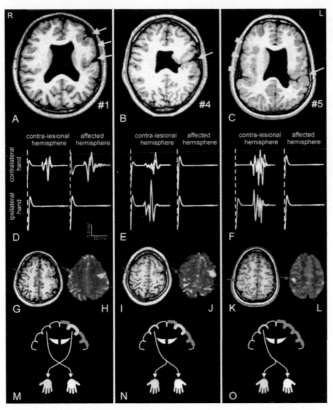

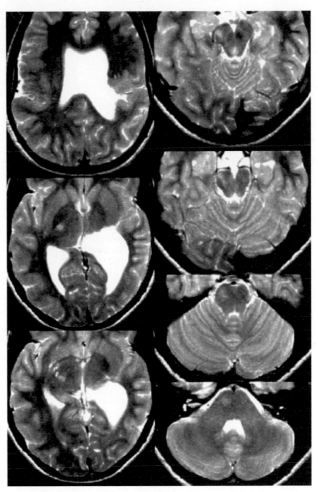

FIGURE 78.5 Function and reorganization in patients with malformations of cortical development. (From Staudt M, Krageloh-Mann I, Holthausen H, et al. Searching for motor functions in dysgenic cortex: a clinical transcranial magnetic stimulation and functional magnetic resonance imaging study. *J Neurosurg.* 2004;101:69–77, with permission from Journal of Neurosurgery, copyright 2004.) Structural MRI, TMS, and fMRI findings (paretic hand movement) are obtained in three patients with congenital hemiparesis due to malformations of cortical development, illustrating different possibilities of participation of the MCDs in hand motor functions. *Left column*: harboring the primary motor representation of the paretic hand (with crossed corticospinal projections originating in the dysgenic cortex); *middle column*: harboring the primary somatosensory (S1) representation of the paretic hand (MEG evidence not shown here)—with a reorganized primary motor representation (M1) of the paretic hand in the contralesional hemisphere; *right column*: showing no evidence of participation (with fMRI activation exclusively in the contralesional hemisphere). **A–C:** Axial reconstructions from the T1-weighted 3D data sets, depicting the frontoparietal polymicrogyria in Case 1 (arrows in A) and the schizencephalies in Cases 4 and 5 (*arrows* in B and C). **D–F:** Note the additional small area of polymicrogyria contralateral to the schizencephaly (*arrowheads* in C) after (*arrows* in B and C). Results of TMS for stimulation of the affected and contralesional hemispheres, with MEPs recorded simultaneously from target muscles of both the paretic hand (yellow MEPs) and the nonparetic hand (white MEP). **G–L:** fMRI activation patterns for movement of the paretic hand (yellow), superimposed on axial (functional) mean EPI sequences (H, J, and L). Red arrows indicate the central sulcus; corresponding slices from the 3D data sets are displayed in G, I, and K. **M–O:** Schematic illustration of the TMS and fMRI findings in the three patients. The thick gray cortical line represents the MCD; fMRI activation during movement of the paretic hand (yellow symbol) is also indicated. See color plate section.

postnatally, no useful hand function can be observed despite TMS evidence for ipsilateral tracts (28,32).

The existence of preserved crossed projections from the affected hemisphere and of ipsilateral projections from the contralesional hemisphere can easily be assessed using focal transcranial magnetic stimulation (TMS; see Methods

FIGURE 78.6 Evidence for ipsilateral corticospinal projections on conventional T2-weighted MRI. (From Staudt M, Krageloh-Mann I, Grodd W. Ipsilateral corticospinal pathways in congenital hemiparesis on routine magnetic resonance imaging. *Pediatr. Neurol.* 2005;32: 37–39; with permission from Elsevier, Copyright 2005.) A patient (= patient #5 in Fig. 78.5) with congenital hemiparesis due to unilateral schizencephaly (note the additional small area of polymicrogyria contralateral to the schizencephaly!), in whom conventional T2-weighted MRI shows hyperintense areas in the position of the pyramidal tract of the contralesional hemisphere as a potential correlate for the ipsilateral corticospinal projections originating in this hemisphere, as detected by TMS.

section). fMRI during active movements of the paretic hand demonstrates activation of the "hand knob" area of the contralesional hemisphere, thus depicting the cortical site from where these projections originate. Indirect evidence for the existence of ipsilateral corticospinal projections can also be observed on conventional MRI: Many of these patients show abnormal T2-hyperintensities in the course of the corticospinal tract of the contralesional hemisphere, especially in the pons. This sign was not observed in patients without ipsilateral projections (33) (Fig. 78.6).

All patients who depend on ipsilateral corticospinal projections to control their paretic hands by the contralesional hemisphere show a distinct clinical feature. During voluntary one-handed movements both with the paretic and with the nonparetic hand, the respective other hand shows involuntary cocontractions, the so-called "mirror movements." This phenomenon is also frequently observed in hemiparetic patients without ipsilateral corticospinal projections (such as in adult

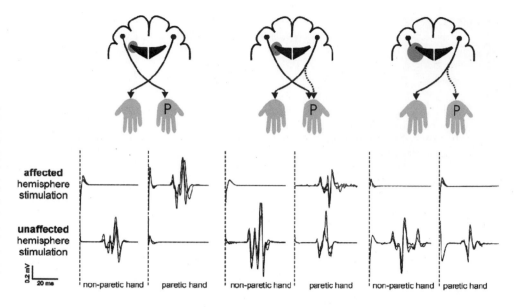

FIGURE 78.7 Types of corticospinal (re)organization in congenital hemiparesis. (Adapted from Staudt M, Grodd W, Gerloff C, et al. Two types of ipsilateral reorganization in congenital hemiparesis: a TMS and fMRI study. *Brain.* 2002;125:2222–2237, with permission from Brain, copyright 2002.) Schematic illustration of the three types of corticospinal (re)organization in patients with early unilateral brain lesions (P = paretic hand; gray circle = lesion) and TMS results from one representative patient from each type. Vertical dashed line = time of the TMS stimulus.

hemiparetic stroke), but only in the nonparetic hand (during voluntary movements of the paretic hand). Furthermore, some mirror movements can also be observed in healthy children up to the age of 10 years (34). Therefore, only mirror movements in patients after the age of 10 years and in the paretic hand during voluntary movements with the nonparetic hand can be regarded as a clinical sign for the presence of ipsilateral projections from the contralesional hemisphere to the paretic hand.

Several TMS studies demonstrated that, apart from patients with exclusively contralateral projections and patients with exclusively ipsilateral projections to the paretic hand, a third subgroup of patients can be identified who possess bilateral projections, that is, corticospinal projections to the paretic hand from both the contra- and the ipsilateral hemisphere. Concerning the quality of paretic hand functions, patients from this third subgroup seem to range "in-between" the other two groups (29,31,35) (Fig. 78.7). Little is known to date about the "differential" functional involvement of the contra- versus the ipsilateral hemisphere in such patients.

Aside from motor (re)organization with ipsilateral corticospinal tracts, a second type of (re)organization in the contralesional hemisphere can be observed: Hemiparetic patients with preserved crossed corticospinal projections can show an increased activation in a network of nonprimary motor areas such as the supplementary motor area or the ventral premotor cortex. This phenomenon has been reported in both patients with early unilateral periventricular brain lesions (31) and adult patients with hemiparetic stroke (36,37). In fact, due to the often widespread bilateral fMRI activation patterns of these patients during active movements with the nonparetic hand, fMRI alone can often not distinguish these patients from those with ipsilateral corticospinal pathways. This can only be accomplished by TMS (31) (Fig. 78.8).

Relevance to Epilepsy Surgery

Gardner and colleagues (38) were probably the first to report the phenomenon of a surprisingly good hand motor outcome post hemispherectomy in some patients with congenital hemiparesis contrasting with an almost completely plegic hand as

the typical result of hemispherectomy performed for brain tumors in previously healthy adults. The authors concluded that this observation could be explained by reorganizational processes that were induced by the early brain lesions in the children with congenital hemiparesis. Reorganization may have led to a take-over of motor control over the paretic hand by the contralesional hemisphere, which would then be spared after hemispherectomy.

One possible explanation for this potential of the developing brain is its ability to develop (or maintain) ipsilateral corticospinal projections from the contralesional hemisphere. And indeed, there is at least casuistic evidence that the preoperative TMS detection of such ipsilateral corticospinal pathways (and the failure to detect preserved crossed corticospinal projections from the affected hemisphere) correctly predicted preserved grasp function of the paretic hand post hemispherectomy (27,39). Therefore, even if the interpretation and

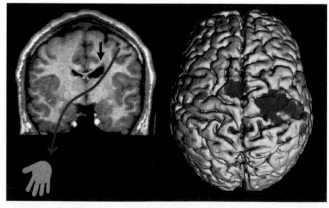

FIGURE 78.8 Ipsilateral reorganization in "nonprimary" motor areas. Example of a patient with a unilateral periventricular brain lesion (*short arrow*) and preserved contralateral corticospinal projections from the affected hemisphere to the paretic hand (*curved arrow*). fMRI during active movements of the paretic hand reveals activation in the (unchanged) primary sensorimotor cortex (M1S1) of the affected hemisphere and additional activation in a network of "nonprimary" sensorimotor regions especially in the contralesional hemisphere.

the predictive value of TMS in these situations is not yet entirely clear, it seems advisable to obtain this information by performing focal TMS when hemispherectomy is considered in a hemiparetic child with partially preserved paretic hand functions.

Unfortunately, this type of corticospinal reorganization seems to be functionally effective only following lesions acquired in the pre- or perinatal period. Hence, one cannot expect that such ipsilateral projections will "develop" after epilepsy surgery—in other words, when such ipsilateral projections are detected postoperatively, they very likely had already been present before the operation. Thus, the availability of this type of motor reorganization should not be used as an argument for early versus late operation.

Somatosensory System

In contrast to the motor system, the primary somatosensory hand representation (S1) apparently never shows an ipsilateral location, neither transiently during normal development nor as a consequence of an early unilateral lesion (40,41). In the somatosensory system, however, a different mechanism of postlesional reorganization can be observed:

During normal development, outgrowing thalamocortical afferent projections reach their cortical destination sites over a prolonged period of time, which starts at the beginning of the third trimester of pregnancy (42). This explains why developing thalamocortical somatosensory projections can still "bypass" even large periventricular brain lesions ("early third trimester lesions" (43)) acquired during this phase to reach their original cortical destination areas in the postcentral gyrus (44). Functionally, such patients typically show no or only little somatosensory deficits, which sometimes contrasts with marked motor dysfunctions (41,44) (Fig. 78.9).

Patients with corticosubcortical lesions ("late third trimester lesions" (43)) located in the vascular territory of the middle cerebral artery (MCA) often show a direct involvement of the postcentral gyrus. Even in these patients, no clear evidence has yet been found for reorganization of S1. During fMRI of passive hand movements, these patients typically activate the intact portions of the postcentral gyrus, with a somewhat more variable topography as determined in group analyses (41). Functionally, many of these patients show severe somatosensory deficits—which sometimes contrasts with relatively spared motor abilities (41).

Some of these corticosubcortical lesions extend deeply into the central white matter, leaving only a small bridge of preserved tissue between the lateral ventricle and the cystic lesion. Still, these patients can show preserved crossed corticospinal motor and somatosensory projections on TMS and MEG studies. Accordingly, diffusion tensor tractography can visualize extensive connectivity provided by such small bridges (45) (see Fig. 78.4).

The fact that only the motor system (but not the somatosensory system) has the capacity to develop an ipsilateral "alternative," and that the somatosensory system shows a protracted maturation of its cortical connections allowing the formation of "axonal bypasses" around defective brain areas, can lead to a situation of "hemispheric dissociation" between M1 and S1 in patients with early unilateral brain lesions: In these patients, M1 is organized in the ipsilateral (contralesional) hemisphere (with ipsilateral corticospinal projections), whereas S1 is still organized in the contralateral (lesioned) hemisphere). It is still unclear what the functional relevance of this dissociation might be. First studies suggest different mechanisms of cortical neuromodulation induced by functional therapy such as Constraint Induced Movement Therapy (CIMT) (46).

Relevance to Epilepsy Surgery

Patients with this peculiar "hemispheric M1–S1 dissociation" are particularly challenging in the interpretation of noninvasive functional mapping results.

When only *fMRI of passive hand movements* is used, such patients typically show activation only in the contralateral Rolandic area—representing the primary somatosensory representation of the paretic hand (S1). Therefore, the results of these studies are quite similar to findings in normal subjects

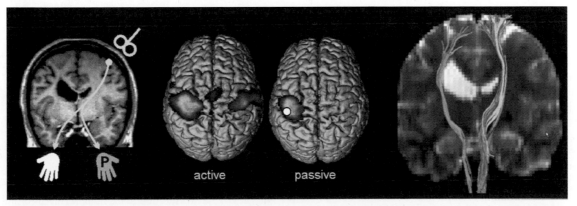

FIGURE 78.9 Axonal plasticity after early periventricular brain lesion. (Adapted from Staudt M, Braun C, Gerloff C, et al. Developing somatosensory projections bypass periventricular brain lesions. *Neurology.* 2006;67:522–525, with permission.) Example of a patient with a large unilateral periventricular brain lesion and ipsilateral corticospinal projections from the contralesional hemisphere to the paretic hand (left). fMRI during active movements of the paretic hand (P) reveals bilateral activation of the Rolandic (pericentral) cortices; during passive movement of the paretic hand, only the contralateral Rolandic area in the affected hemisphere is activated, indicating a contralaterally preserved primary somatosensory (S1) representation of the paretic hand in the affected hemisphere. Accordingly, the white dot represents the topography of the magnetoencephalographically determined S1 representation of the paretic hand. Finally, diffusion tensor tractography (right) visualized trajectories of somatosensory afferent fibers that bypass the lesion on their way to the Rolandic cortex of the affected hemisphere.

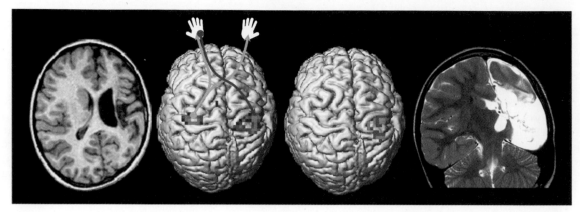

FIGURE 78.10 Epilepsy surgery in a case of hemispheric dissociation between motor and sensory functions. An 8-year-old girl with pharmacorefractory seizures and congenital hemiparesis due to a pre- or perinatally acquired infarction in the territory of the middle cerebral artery. After hemispherectomy, the paretic hand could still be used for active grasping. **Left:** Axial T1-weighted image depicting the corticosubcortical lesion. **Middle left:** fMRI during active hand movement. Green arrows indicate TMS evidence of bilateral corticospinal projections from the contralesional hemisphere to the paretic hand; the blue arrow indicates preserved crossed spino-thalamo-cortical somatosensory projections to the central (Rolandic) region of the lesioned hemisphere. **Middle right:** fMRI during passive hand movement. **Right:** Coronal T2-weighted image after hemispherectomy. See color plate section.

(both during active and passive hand movements): One could easily perceive a "normal" sensorimotor hand representation in these patients—and thus "miss" the ipsilateral M1 representation of the paretic hand in the contralesional hemisphere.

This information can be obtained either by fMRI of active hand movements or by TMS—or, ideally, by a combination of both techniques, since neither approach has a sensitivity of 100% (Fig. 78.10) (44). When hemispherectomy is performed, there is casuistic evidence that such patients retain an active grasp function with their paretic hand (despite the removal or disconnection of the contralaterally preserved S1 representation of the paretic hand) (H. Holthausen, personal communication).

Few studies investigated brain activation induced by somatosensory stimulation in hemispherectomized children, and observed activation in nonprimary somatosensory cortices (with variable, but mostly minimal residual somatosensory function) (47,48).

Language

In the majority of normal subjects, language develops predominantly in the left hemisphere. This is true for almost all right-handers, and also for most left-handers, although bilateral or right-hemispheric language organization occurs more frequently in these subjects (49).

Despite this clear "preference" of normal language development for the left hemisphere, even extensive damage to the left hemisphere can be fully or almost fully compensated when the insult occurs during the pre- or perinatal period. In these subjects, language functions develop in the right hemisphere (50,51), in areas homotopic to the classical language zones in the left hemisphere of healthy subjects (52) (Fig. 78.11).

Patients with such lesion-induced right-hemispheric language organization often have normal verbal IQs. However, their early phases of language development are typically slower (53), and there is preliminary evidence that, on more

detailed tests of language proficiency, these subjects score lower than IQ-matched controls (K. Lidzba, personal communication).

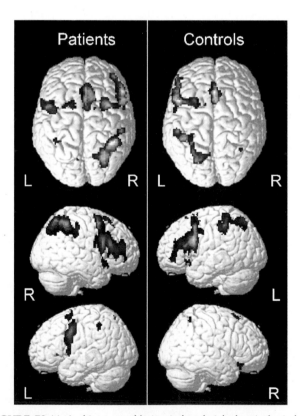

FIGURE 78.11 Architecture of lesion-induced right-hemispheric language organization. (From Staudt M, Lidzba K, Grodd W, et al. Right-hemispheric organization of language following early left-sided brain lesions: functional MRI topography. *Neuroimage.* 2002;16:954–967, with permission.) Functional MRI of speech production (silent generation of word chains) in five healthy right-handers (left) and five patients with predominantly right-hemispheric language representation due to left-sided periventricular brain lesions. SPM99, fixed-effect group analyses. See color plate section.

The efficacy of this compensation for structural damage to the left-hemispheric language areas decreases already during early childhood (54), and older children and adults with extensive left-hemisphere damage often remain aphasic. However, the type and onset of lesion may prolong the critical period in these patients (55). Prediction of language outcome after childhood lesions is, to date, quite vague, since data are scarce, mostly based on case reports and frequently "contaminated" by epilepsy as an additional relevant factor with often undetermined or imprecise "timing." Similarly, it is often difficult to predict the degree of left- and right-hemisphere involvement in language processing based on type, timing, and location of the lesion (56).

A right-hemispheric take-over of language functions shows noticeable effects on "originary" right-hemispheric functions: Patients with lesion-induced right-hemispheric language often show deficits, for example, in visuospatial functions, the severity of which correlates with the degree of right-hemispheric involvement in language (57) due to common use of right-hemispheric networks (the crowding effect) (58), which has been confirmed in fMRI studies (59).

Relevance for Epilepsy Surgery

Due to our still only marginal understanding of the mechanisms of language reorganization, their dependency on development, and their variable efficacy, a preoperative assessment of language dominance is often advisable when potentially language-relevant brain structures are targeted by surgical procedures. This is traditionally accomplished by the Wada test (see Chapter 81). However, due to the high degree of invasiveness and complications (60), this procedure may be supplemented or, ideally, replaced by noninvasive methods such as language fMRI and other noninvasive techniques as outlined above (61).

A second consequence for epilepsy surgery arises from the age dependency of language organization described above: The decreasing efficacy of right-hemispheric language reorganization during early childhood may justify calls for an early versus late operation when language-relevant structures have to be targeted (51).

Visual System

Still little is known to date about developmental plasticity in the human visual system. Several authors reported casuistic evidence for residual visual function in MCDs (62,63). But as opposed to the motor system, only case reports have, to our knowledge, yet been reported for an ipsilateral take-over of visual representations (64); that is, most early acquired lesions to the primary visual cortex will result in a corresponding visual field defect. Interestingly, a recent FDG-PET study in children with Sturge–Weber-syndrome demonstrated higher than normal metabolism (at rest) in the contralesional occipital lobe, which was interpreted as indicating reorganizational processes (65). The functional significance of this hypermetabolism is, however, still to be elucidated (66). Finally, lesions in the occipital white matter might be compensated by "axonal bypasses" of optic radiation pathways, similar to the somatosensory system (A. Guzzetta, personal communication). There is also increasing evidence that the temporal lobes play an important role in memory formation of more complex visual stimuli (67).

Memory

Severe anterograde amnesia, as seen in the case of H.M., lead to the introduction of the intracarotid amobarbital procedures (IAP) for memory assessment in epilepsy patients (68). Although H.M. lost both hippocampi after bilateral epilepsy surgery, it was noted that he was still able to learn certain visual spatial elements (68) suggesting a cortical memory and plasticity component even in adults. The IAP was introduced based on the notion that anesthesia of part of one hemisphere may transiently mimic the effects of the resection. This assumption is based on the models of functional adequacy (of the resected hippocampus) and functional reserve (of the remaining hippocampus) complementing each other (69). Recent studies also indicated that careful neuropsychological assessment, structural imaging, and possibly fMRI memory paradigms may replace Wada testing for memory assessment (70,71).

The degree of correlation between language and memory lateralization as assessed by IAP in patients with epilepsy differed depending on the presence and type of lesion (72). Laterality indices between language and memory correlated significantly higher in patients with congenital lesions, such as cortical dysplasia, as compared to nonlesional patients. Patients with later acquired lesions, such as hippocampal sclerosis, fell between these two groups (72).

Relevance for Epilepsy Surgery

Improvement and plasticity of memory function is possible after epilepsy surgery. Although up to a third of epilepsy patients experience memory decline following a temporal lobe resection, up to 20% may experience a postoperative improvement in function (73). A shorter duration of epilepsy and the cognitive capacity to develop compensatory strategies were positive predictors for improvements (73). It is unclear whether this is related to plasticity after surgery or relief from a structural or functional lesion.

COMMON PATHOPHYSIOLOGICAL MECHANISMS BETWEEN EPILEPSY AND PLASTICITY

Plasticity and increased ability to learn may be related to early developmental glutamate receptor changes and mechanisms associated with long-term potentiation.

AMPA Receptors and Epilepsy in the Immature Brain

Glutamatergic alpha-amino-3-hydroxy-5-methyl-4-isoxazole-propionic acid (AMPA) subunit expression has been shown to vary in the perinatal period (74). AMPA receptors without the GluR2 subunit are more frequently expressed in early life and may increase susceptibility to brain injury and subsequent seizures later in life (75,76). Additionally, early alterations of AMPA receptors reversibly mediate synaptic potentiation induced by neonatal seizures (77). Animal research has demonstrated that the expression of AMPA receptors after seizures and status epilepticus depends on the age of the animal, the timing of the first insult, and that this influences the formation of subsequent AMPA subunit compositions (78).

NMDA Receptors and Epilepsy in the Immature Brain

In the immature brain an obligate NR1 unit is paired with the NR2B subunit that leads to longer current decay time as compared to subunit in the mature brain, NR2A (79). NMDA receptors are also more excitable due to reduced magnesium sensitivity deriving from immature receptor subunits NR2C, NR2D, and NR3A (80,81). Due to the role of the NMDA receptor in memory, learning, and development, NMDA antagonist treatment strategies are limited (82,83). Seizures induced by GABA(A) antagonist in the developing brain actually lead to decreased expression of NMDA and AMPA receptors, possibly explaining cognitive deficits associated with seizures in the developing brain (84,85). Decreased expression may only occur after 5 days but then persists for at least 3 to 4 weeks. These effects were related to the number of seizures experienced, and were not observed when seizures were induced in adult mice (86).

Long-Term Potentiation (LTP) as a Model of Memory and Plasticity

LTP is most readily produced in the hippocampus and involves activation of glutamate receptors in many neuronal models. Depolarization of the postsynaptic neuron expels the blocking magnesium from the NMDA receptor. This leads to influx of calcium and sodium. Subsequently, calcium triggers an enzymatic cascade leading to the early and late phases of LTP (87). Although a detailed discussion of LTP is beyond the scope of this chapter, it is noteworthy that there is significant overlap in the mechanisms underlying memory formation and plasticity as well as epilepsy. Both, seizures and memory formation are induced by gamma–theta activity (87). Seizure may saturate synapses with long-term facilitation and decrease the capacity for plasticity (87), in particular, early in life when receptors are more excitable as outlined above. In this period infants may be also be more susceptible to changes related to seizures and epilepsy.

INFLUENCE OF THE TIMING AND TYPE OF LESION ON PLASTICITY

The type of lesion and in particular the timing of the pathological lesion may, therefore, determine the impact on development, plasticity, memory, and learning. We illustrate the impact of the timing of the lesion and the type of lesion based on plasticity in language development.

Previous studies have emphasized that language lateralization is related to handedness and to presence and localization of brain lesions (50).

Lesions causing plasticity may present as structural pathological lesions or as functional lesions with ongoing spiking. Patients with frequent spiking in the left hippocampus and mesial temporal sclerosis had more frequently left to right language shift (88).

In a series of epilepsy patients and IAP language lateralization, Moddel et al. found that right-handers with left-sided lesions did not differ from patients without lesions with regards to language lateralization. However, left-handers with early left lesions were most likely right-language dominant and left-handers with late neocortical left lesions had most likely bilateral language distribution. Right-hemispheric language development may be in part related to early insults and bilateral dominant language development may indicate defective maintenance of right-hemispheric language caused by a late left-hemispheric insult at a time when left dominance has already started to develop (51). Later lesions may lead to incomplete transfer of language (53,54) and aphasia when resected (89). However, later transfer may be related to the type of pathology. Language transfer in early teenage years was seen in patients with Rasmussen encephalitis (55).

The timing of the lesion may also result in different clinical epilepsy presentations. Recent patient series demonstrated that patients with early developmental lesions may present with generalized EEG features (90,91). These patients did well after epilepsy surgery and resection of the lesion. Findings may possibly indicate that early developmental lesions may trigger a different, more generalized EEG presentation, possibly due to epilepsy onset early in life during a critical period.

EPILEPSY SURGERY AND PLASTICITY

Basic Principles of Epilepsy Surgery

In preparation for epilepsy surgery, the epileptogenic zone is estimated based on history, clinical examination, video-EEG monitoring (sometimes complemented by MEG), and neuroimaging techniques. Simultaneously, eloquent cortex is localized, and developmental level is determined allowing an estimate of plasticity and developmental potential. This may include assessment of visual, motor, sensory, language, memory, and other higher cortical functions by neuropsychological assessment, by clinical examination, and by additional techniques as outlined above. In case of overlap of eloquent areas with the epileptogenic zone, or in case of a poorly localized epileptogenic zone based on noninvasive techniques, subdural grid and depth electrode implantation or intraoperative subdural recordings can be used for better localization of epileptogenic zone and eloquent cortex as well as detection of possible plasticity (see Fig. 78.2). Chances of seizure freedom are then weighed against possible complications, including morbidity and mortality from surgery, risks of ongoing seizures, and potential resection of eloquent areas such as vision, motor function, memory, language, and potential for neuronal plasticity. Consideration of potential developmental benefits and surgical timing are crucial.

Developmental Benefits and Plasticity after Epilepsy Surgery

Longer duration of seizures and higher percentage of lifetime with epilepsy leads to worse developmental outcome in pediatric epilepsy patients (92). Earlier epilepsy surgery and relief from seizures during a critical period improves developmental outcome in pediatric epilepsy patients (93). In a study in infants, at the time of epilepsy surgery the median developmental quotient (DQ) improved after surgery for the group overall and individual DQs improved for 71% of infants. Developmental status before surgery predicted developmental function after surgery. Mental age increased after surgery in every case. Many infants develop at a faster rate or pick up development, but remain abnormal. Meaningful changes may be seen in all infants that develop at a faster rate than their preoperative baseline (93,94). Patients operated at younger age and with epileptic spasms showed the largest increase in DQ after surgery (93,94). Other series also suggested that early epilepsy surgery in infants with catastrophic epilepsy may allow the resumption of developmental progression during critical stages of brain development and maturation (95,96). Mental development tends to progress in the majority of children after epilepsy surgery, in particular in those with initially no measurable development.

Another series also showed a statistically significant increase in developmental levels at an average age of 21 months after surgery as compared to presurgical results (94). These authors also compared the developmental outcome of their study with all other previously reported infants receiving medical treatment for infantile spasms and found that the developmental outcome in their surgical group was equal and sometimes superior to children treated with either ACTH or valproic acid (94). Early treatment and seizure control appear to be the key to improved developmental outcome. This has also been confirmed by a recent study on long-term cognitive outcomes of a cohort of children with infantile spasms of unknown etiology that were treated with high-dose ACTH (97).

CONCLUSION

Functional imaging and other novel techniques to map eloquent cortex play an increasingly important role in the presurgical workup of epilepsy patients. Consideration regarding the eloquent cortex involved and onset and type of lesion provide clues towards the necessary techniques for assessment of plasticity of function in the pediatric brain. Noninvasively presurgically obtained maps help guide further evaluation with subdural and depth electrodes, and may in the future even replace invasive monitoring in selected patients. Plasticity decreases as patients grow older. There is increasing evidence that earlier treatment of epileptic seizures leads to improved developmental outcome.

References

1. Tharin S, Golby A. Functional brain mapping and its applications to neurosurgery. *Neurosurgery.* 2007;60:185–201.
2. Staudt M, Pieper T, Grodd W, et al. Functional MRI in a 6-year-old boy with unilateral cortical malformation: concordant representation of both hands in the unaffected hemisphere. *Neuropediatrics.* 2001;32:159–161.
3. Wilke M, Holland SK, Myseros JS, et al. Functional magnetic resonance imaging in pediatrics. *Neuropediatrics.* 2003;34:225–233.
4. Wilke M, Lidzba K, Staudt M, et al. Comprehensive language mapping in children, using functional magnetic resonance imaging: what's missing counts. *Neuroreport.* 2005;16:915–919.
5. Wilke M, Lidzba K, Staudt M, et al. An fMRI task battery for assessing hemispheric language dominance in children. *Neuroimage.* 2006;32:400–410.
6. Gasser T, Sandalcioglu E, Schoch B, et al. Functional magnetic resonance imaging in anesthetized patients: a relevant step toward real-time intraoperative functional neuroimaging. *Neurosurgery.* 2005;57:94–99.
7. Souweidane MM, Kim KH, McDowall R, et al. Brain mapping in sedated infants and young children with passive-functional magnetic resonance imaging. *Pediatr Neurosurg.* 1999;30:86–92.
8. Usui K, Ikeda A. Event-related potentials in patients with epilepsy. In: Lüders H, ed. *Textbook of Epilepsy Surgery.* London: Informa Healthcare; 2008:858–867.
9. Taylor JR, Olichney JM. From amnesia to dementia: ERP studies of memory and language. *Clin EEG Neurosci.* 2007;38:8–17.
10. Marshall PJ, Reeb BC, Fox NA, Nelson CA III, Zeanah CH. Effects of early intervention on EEG power and coherence in previously institutionalized children in Romania. *Dev Psychopathol.* 2008;20:861–880.
11. Benecke R, Meyer BU, Freund HJ. Reorganisation of descending motor pathways in patients after hemispherectomy and severe hemispheric lesions demonstrated by magnetic brain stimulation. *Exp Brain Res.* 1991;83: 419–426.
12. Loddenkemper T, Haag A. The role of the Wada test, and functional transcranial Doppler sonography (fTCD), in the presurgical diagnosis of MTLE. In: Rosenow F, Lüders H, Ryvlin R, Kahane P, eds. *The mesial temporal lobe epilepsies.* London: John Libbey Eurotexts Editions, 2009: in press.
13. Floel A, Lohmann H, Breitenstein C, et al. Reproducibility of hemispheric blood flow increases during line bisectioning. *Clin Neurophysiol.* 2002; 113:917–924.
14. Sturzenegger M, Newell DW, Aaslid R. Visually evoked blood flow response assessed by simultaneous two-channel transcranial Doppler using flow velocity averaging. *Stroke.* 1996;27:2256–2261.
15. Floel A, Knecht S, Lohmann H, et al. Language and spatial attention can lateralize to the same hemisphere in healthy humans. *Neurology.* 2001; 57: 1018–1024.
16. Matteis M, Caltagirone C, Troisi E, et al. Changes in cerebral blood flow induced by passive and active elbow and hand movements. *J Neurol.* 2001;248:104–108.
17. Matteis M, Silvestrini M, Troisi E, et al. Transcranial doppler assessment of cerebral flow velocity during perception and recognition of melodies. *J Neurol Sci.* 1997;149:57–61.
18. Vingerhoets G, Stroobant N. Reliability and validity of day-to-day blood flow velocity reactivity in a single subject: an fTCD study. *Ultrasound Med Biol.* 2002;28:197–202.
19. Silvestrini M, Cupini LM, Matteis M, et al. Bilateral simultaneous assessment of cerebral flow velocity during mental activity. *J Cereb Blood Flow Metab.* 1994;14:643–648.
20. Knecht S, Henningsen H, Deppe M, et al. Successive activation of both cerebral hemispheres during cued word generation. *Neuroreport.* 1996;7: 820–824.
21. Rihs F, Sturzenegger M, Gutbrod K, et al. Determination of language dominance: Wada test confirms functional transcranial Doppler sonography. *Neurology.* 1999;52:1591–1596.
22. Deppe M, Knecht S, Papke K, et al. Assessment of hemispheric language lateralization: a comparison between fMRI and fTCD. *J Cereb Blood Flow Metab.* 2000;20:263–268.
23. Reis J, Rosenow F. Eloquent cortex and tracts: overview and noninvasive evaluation methods. In: Lüders H, ed. *Textbook of Epilepsy Surgery.* London, UK: Informa Healthcare; 2008:871–880.
24. Schüle S, McIntyre C, Lüders H. General principles of cortical mapping by electrical stimulation. In: Lüders H, ed. *Textbook of Epilepsy Surgery.* London, UK: Informa Healthcare; 2008:963–977.
25. Eyre JA, Miller S, Clowry GJ, et al. Functional corticospinal projections are established prenatally in the human foetus permitting involvement in the development of spinal motor centres. *Brain.* 2000;123(Pt 1):51–64.
26. Eyre JA, Taylor JP, Villagra F, et al. Evidence of activity-dependent withdrawal of corticospinal projections during human development. *Neurology.* 2001;57:1543–1554.
27. Staudt M, Gerloff C, Grodd W, et al. Reorganization in congenital hemiparesis acquired at different gestational ages. *Ann Neurol.* 2004;56:854–863.
28. Eyre JA, Smith M, Dabydeen L, et al. Is hemiplegic cerebral palsy equivalent to amblyopia of the corticospinal system? *Ann Neurol.* 2007;62: 493–503.
29. Maegaki Y, Maeoka Y, Ishii S, et al. Mechanisms of central motor reorganization in pediatric hemiplegic patients. *Neuropediatrics.* 1997;28:168–174.
30. Turton A, Wroe S, Trepte N, et al. Contralateral and ipsilateral EMG responses to transcranial magnetic stimulation during recovery of arm and hand function after stroke. *Electroencephalogr Clin Neurophysiol.* 1996; 101:316–328.
31. Staudt M, Grodd W, Gerloff C, et al. Two types of ipsilateral reorganization in congenital hemiparesis: a TMS and fMRI study. *Brain.* 2002;125: 2222–2237.
32. Staudt M, Krageloh-Mann I, Holthausen H, et al. Searching for motor functions in dysgenic cortex: a clinical transcranial magnetic stimulation and functional magnetic resonance imaging study. *J Neurosurg.* 2004; 101:69–77.
33. Staudt M, Krageloh-Mann I, Grodd, W. Ipsilateral corticospinal pathways in congenital hemiparesis on routine magnetic resonance imaging. *Pediatr Neurol.* 2005;32:37–39.
34. Muller K, Kass-Iliyya F, Reitz M. Ontogeny of ipsilateral corticospinal projections: a developmental study with transcranial magnetic stimulation. *Ann Neurol.* 1997;42:705–711.
35. Carr LJ, Harrison LM, Evans AL, et al. Patterns of central motor reorganization in hemiplegic cerebral palsy. *Brain.* 1993;116(Pt 5):1223–1247.

36. Weiller C, Chollet F, Friston KJ, et al. Functional reorganization of the brain in recovery from striatocapsular infarction in man. *Ann Neurol.* 1992;31:463–472.

37. Weiller C, Ramsay SC, Wise RJ, et al. Individual patterns of functional reorganization in the human cerebral cortex after capsular infarction. *Ann Neurol.* 1993;33:181–189.

38. Gardner WJ, Karnosh LJ, McClure JR, et al. Residual function following hemispherectomy for tumour and for infantile hemiplegia. *Brain.* 1995; 78:478–502.

39. Shimizu T, Nariai T, Maehara T, et al. Enhanced motor cortical excitability in the unaffected hemisphere after hemispherectomy. *Neuroreport.* 2000; 11:3077–3084.

40. Guzzetta A, Bonanni P, Biagi L, et al. Reorganisation of the somatosensory system after early brain damage. *Clin Neurophysiol.* 2007;118:1110–1121.

41. Wilke M, Staudt M, Juenger H, et al. Somatosensory system in two types of motor reorganization in congenital hemiparesis: topography and function. *Hum Brain Mapp.* 2009;30:776–788.

42. Kostovic I, Judas M. Correlation between the sequential ingrowth of afferents and transient patterns of cortical lamination in preterm infants. *Anat Rec.* 2002;267:1–6.

43. Krageloh-Mann I. Imaging of early brain injury and cortical plasticity. *Exp Neurol.* 2004;190(Suppl 1):S84–S90.

44. Staudt M, Braun C, Gerloff C, et al. Developing somatosensory projections bypass periventricular brain lesions. *Neurology.* 2006;67:522–525.

45. Staudt M, Erb M, Braun C, et al. Extensive peri-lesional connectivity in congenital hemiparesis. *Neurology.* 2006;66:771.

46. Kuhnke N, Juenger H, Walther M, et al. Do individuals with congenital hemiparesis and ipsilateral cortico-spinal projections to the paretic hand respond differently to constraint-induced Movement Therapy? *Dev Med Child Neurol.* 2008 Dec;50(12):898–903.

47. Bernasconi A, Bernasconi N, Lassonde M, et al. Sensorimotor organization in patients who have undergone hemispherectomy: a study with (15)O-water PET and somatosensory evoked potentials. *Neuroreport.* 2000;11:3085–3090.

48. Holloway V, Gadian DG, Vargha-Khadem F, et al. The reorganization of sensorimotor function in children after hemispherectomy. A functional MRI and somatosensory evoked potential study. *Brain.* 2000;123(Pt 12):2432–2444.

49. Pujol J, Deus J, Losilla JM, et al. Cerebral lateralization of language in normal left-handed people studied by functional MRI. *Neurology.* 1999;52: 1038–1043.

50. Rasmussen T, Milner B. The role of early left-brain injury in determining lateralization of cerebral speech functions. *Ann N Y Acad Sci.* 1977;299: 355–369.

51. Moddel G, Lineweaver T, Schuele SU, et al. Atypical language lateralization in epilepsy patients. *Epilepsia.* 2009;50(6):1505–1516.

52. Staudt M, Lidzba K, Grodd W, et al. Right-hemispheric organization of language following early left-sided brain lesions: functional MRI topography. *Neuroimage.* 2002;16:954–967.

53. Vargha-Khadem F, Isaacs E, Muter V. A review of cognitive outcome after unilateral lesions sustained during childhood. *J Child Neurol.* 1994; 9(Suppl 2):67–73.

54. Hertz-Pannier L, Chiron C, Jambaqué I, et al. Late plasticity for language in a child's non-dominant hemisphere: a pre- and post-surgery fMRI study. *Brain.* 2002;125:361–372.

55. Loddenkemper T, Wyllie E, Lardizabal D, et al. Late language transfer in patients with Rasmussen encephalitis. *Epilepsia.* 2003;44:870–871.

56. Liegeois F, Connelly A, Cross JH, et al. Language reorganization in children with early-onset lesions of the left hemisphere: an fMRI study. *Brain.* 2004;127:1229–1236.

57. Lidzba K, Staudt M, Wilke M, et al. Visuospatial deficits in patients with early left-hemispheric lesions and functional reorganization of language: consequence of lesion or reorganization? *Neuropsychologia.* 2006;44: 1088–1094.

58. Teuber HL. Why two brains? In: Schmitt FO, Worden FG, eds. *The Neurosciences: Third Study Program.* Cambridge: MIT Press; 1974:71–74.

59. Lidzba K, Staudt M, Wilke M, et al. Lesion-induced right-hemispheric language and organization of nonverbal functions. *Neuroreport.* 2006; 17:929–933.

60. Loddenkemper T, Morris HH, Moddel G. Complications during the Wada test. *Epilepsy Behav.* 2008;13:551–553.

61. Loddenkemper T. Quo vadis Wada? *Epilepsy Behav.* 2008;13:1–2.

62. Dumoulin SO, Jirsch JD, Bernasconi A. Functional organization of human visual cortex in occipital polymicrogyria. *Hum Brain Mapp.* 2007;28: 1302–1312.

63. Innocenti GM, Maeder P, Knyazeva MG, et al. Functional activation of microgyric visual cortex in a human. *Ann Neurol.* 2001;50:672–676.

64. Slotnick SD, Moo LR, Krauss G, et al. Large-scale cortical displacement of a human retinotopic map. *Neuroreport.* 2002;13:41–46.

65. Batista CE, Juhasz C, Muzik O, et al. Increased visual cortex glucose metabolism contralateral to angioma in children with Sturge–Weber syndrome. *Dev Med Child Neurol.* 2007;49:567–573.

66. Staudt M. Reorganization of the developing human brain after early lesions. *Dev Med Child Neurol.* 2007;49:564.

67. Kreiman G, Koch C, Fried I. Category-specific visual responses of single neurons in the human medial temporal lobe. *Nat Neurosci.* 2000;3:946–953.

68. Corkin S. What's new with the amnesic patient H.M.? *Nat Rev Neurosci.* 2002;3:153–160.

69. Chelune GJ. Hippocampal adequacy versus functional reserve: predicting memory functions following temporal lobectomy. *Arch Clin Neuropsychol.* 1995;10:413–432.

70. Baxendale S, Thompson P, Harkness W, et al. Predicting memory decline following epilepsy surgery: a multivariate approach. *Epilepsia.* 2006;47: 1887–1894.

71. Golby AJ, Poldrack RA, Illes J, et al. Memory lateralization in medial temporal lobe epilepsy assessed by functional MRI. *Epilepsia.* 2002;43: 855–863.

72. Kovac S, Möddel G, Reinholz J, et al. Memory performance is related to language dominance as determined by the intracarotid amobarbital procedure. *Epilepsy Behav.* 2009;16(1):145–149.

73. Baxendale S, Thompson PJ, Duncan JS. Improvements in memory function following anterior temporal lobe resection for epilepsy. *Neurology.* 2008; 71:1319–1325.

74. Jensen FE, Follett PL, Kinney HC, et al. Developmental expression of AMPA receptors in human telencephalic white matter. *Soc Neurosci Abs.* 2001;27:612.

75. Talos DM, Fishman RE, Park H, et al. Developmental regulation of alpha-amino-3-hydroxy-5-methyl-4-isoxazole-propionic acid receptor subunit expression in forebrain and relationship to regional susceptibility to hypoxic/ischemic injury. I. Rodent cerebral white matter and cortex. *J Comp Neurol.* 2006;497:42–60.

76. Talos DM, Follett PL, Folkerth RD, et al. Developmental regulation of alpha-amino-3-hydroxy-5-methyl-4-isoxazole-propionic acid receptor subunit expression in forebrain and relationship to regional susceptibility to hypoxic/ischemic injury. II. Human cerebral white matter and cortex. *J Comp Neurol.* 2006;497:61–77.

77. Rakhade SN, Zhou C, Aujla PK, et al. Early alterations of AMPA receptors mediate synaptic potentiation induced by neonatal seizures. *J Neurosci.* 2008;28:7979–7990.

78. Friedman LK, Avallone JM, Magrys B. Maturational effects of single and multiple early-life seizures on AMPA receptors in prepubescent hippocampus. *Dev Neurosci.* 2007;29:427–437.

79. Silverstein FS, Jensen FE. Neonatal seizures. *Ann Neurol.* 2007;62: 112–120.

80. Hollmann M, Heinemann S. Cloned glutamate receptors. *Annu Rev Neurosci.* 1994;17:31–108.

81. Wong HK, Liu XB, Matos MF, et al. Temporal and regional expression of NMDA receptor subunit NR3A in the mammalian brain. *J Comp Neurol.* 2002;450:303–317.

82. Johnston MV. Excitotoxicity in perinatal brain injury. *Brain Pathol.* 2005;15:234–240.

83. Jensen FE. Developmental factors regulating susceptibility to perinatal brain injury and seizures. *Curr Opin Pediatr.* 2006;18:628–633.

84. Swann JW. The impact of seizures on developing hippocampal networks. *Prog Brain Res.* 2005;147:347–354.

85. Swann JW, Le JT, Lam TT, et al. The impact of chronic network hyperexcitability on developing glutamatergic synapses. *Eur J Neurosci.* 2007; 26:975–991.

86. Swann JW, Le JT, Lee CL. Recurrent seizures and the molecular maturation of hippocampal and neocortical glutamatergic synapses. *Dev Neurosci.* 2007;29:168–178.

87. Meador KJ. The basic science of memory as it applies to epilepsy. *Epilepsia.* 2007;48(Suppl 9):23–25.

88. Janszky J, Mertens M, Janszky I, et al. Left-sided interictal epileptic activity induces shift of language lateralization in temporal lobe epilepsy: an fMRI study. *Epilepsia.* 2006;47:921–927.

89. Loddenkemper T, Dinner DS, Kubu C, et al. Aphasia after hemispherectomy in an adult with early onset epilepsy and hemiplegia. *J Neurol Neurosurg Psychiatry.* 2004;75:149–151.

90. Loddenkemper T, Cosmo G, Kotagal P, et al. Epilepsy surgery in children with electrical status epilepticus in sleep. *Neurosurgery.* 2009;64: 328–337.

91. Wyllie E, Lachhwani DK, Gupta A, et al. Successful surgery for epilepsy due to early brain lesions despite generalized EEG findings. *Neurology.* 2007;69:389–397.

92. Vendrame M, Alexopoulos AV, Boyer K, et al. Duration of epilepsy during infancy correlates with impaired cognitive development. *Neurology.* 2009;in print.

93. Loddenkemper T, Holland KD, Stanford LD, et al. Developmental outcome after epilepsy surgery in infancy. *Pediatrics.* 2007;119:930–935.

94. Asarnow RF, LoPresti C, Guthrie D, et al. Developmental outcomes in children receiving resection surgery for. *Dev Med Child Neurol.* 1997; 39:430–440.

95. Chugani HT, Shewmon DA, Shields WD, et al. Surgery for intractable infantile spasms: neuroimaging perspectives. *Epilepsia.* 1993;34: 764–771.

96. Wyllie E, Comair YG, Kotagal P, et al. Epilepsy surgery in infants. *Epilepsia.* 1996;37:625–637.

97. Kivity S, Lerman P, Ariel R, et al. Long-term cognitive outcomes of a cohort of children with cryptogenic infantile spasms treated with high-dose adrenocorticotropic hormone. *Epilepsia.* 2004;45:255–262.

CHAPTER 79 ■ FUNCTIONAL MRI FOR MAPPING ELOQUENT CORTEX

WILLIAM DAVIS GAILLARD

fMRI is a fast imaging technique that is used for mapping the location of neural function ("activation") based on detecting surrogates of blood flow, comparable to [^{15}O]water PET (see Chapter 77). fMRI is most often used to identify eloquent areas to be spared during epilepsy surgery: sensory cortex, motor cortex, language, and memory. fMRI is less commonly used to identify the epileptogenic zone for resection, primarily through interictal spike localization, and rarely ictal onset. Increasingly, fMRI is used to provide insights into the neurobiology of epilepsy, and effects of chronic epilepsy on higher-ordered brain function and development.

fMRI PRINCIPLES

The principles underlying brain evaluation with fMRI are similar to [^{15}O]water PET. Both rely on the observation that increased neuronal activity, primarily at the synapse, is associated with regional increases in cerebral blood flow (1–3). Detecting the location of changes in blood flow that occur during cognitive tasks (e.g., involving motor control, language, and memory) allows the mapping of neural networks involved in these tasks. PET has the advantage of imaging capillary rather than venous blood flow, but confers radiation and has less spatial resolution. fMRI does not confer radiation; thus, it is easier to do more tasks and conditions. It is also easier to collect normal data, especially in children, and fMRI can be more easily repeated.

fMRI relies primarily on blood oxygenation level–dependent (BOLD) contrast techniques, which take advantage of MRI signal changes that differ when hemoglobin is in a deoxygenated versus an oxygenated state. Increased neural activity is associated with tightly regulated increases in blood flow that often exceed local metabolic demand. This physiologic epiphenomenon of luxury hyperperfusion underlies BOLD fMRI; thus, unlike [^{15}O]water PET, which is a direct measure of capillary flow, BOLD fMRI is an indirect measure of cerebral blood flow. The phenomenon is most pronounced on the venous side of the capillary bed, where there is a relative increase in quantity, and hence ratio, of oxygenated to deoxygenated hemoglobin. The change in MRI signal is proportional to this effect. Because the signal change is small (0.5% to 5%), multiple observations are necessary to reliably detect it. Optical imaging studies show that the vascular response follows the stimulus onset by 2 seconds and reaches a peak effect in 5 to 7 seconds (3). The reasons for vascular response are unknown. It may be to ensure adequate oxygen and glucose to meet unanticipated demand, to drive oxygen

diffusion given increased cerebral blood flow, or it may be a means of removing metabolic and potentially toxic waste products (4).

The fMRI signal is nonquantitative; it measures a relative signal change between two conditions. Choice of task and control conditions is critical to an effective study. Stimuli must be of sufficient distinction to initiate a hemodynamic response, and the control tasks should not elicit blood flow changes in the brain regions studied. Also, the temporal resolution (4 seconds) is considerably slower than neuronal firing frequency but is superior to that of [^{15}O]water PET (60 seconds). Fast MRI techniques, such as echo planar or spiral imaging, detect signal change over time by obtaining whole-brain data every 2 to 5 seconds. Spatial resolution is typically 3 to 5 mm, but with proper coils may achieve whole-brain resolution of 1 mm.

Different statistical methods have been used to determine significance of signal change in a voxel between control and task conditions, identified as "activated." The results are similar using t maps, z maps, cross-correlation, linear regression, and nonparametric maps (4). Most methods involve overly rigorous thresholds, to mitigate spurious activation that may not identify brain areas truly involved in the experimental task. Many cognitive studies are performed with group analysis; however, for evaluation of epilepsy patients, individual rather than group studies are important. The practical statistical threshold appears to vary among individuals (5,6). As with PET, activated regions may not be critical to the task, and all critical areas may not be activated.

For any patient-oriented functional brain-mapping studies, neuropsychological testing is important to ensure the tasks are appropriate for the individual. Multiple tasks, multiple repetitions of a task, and well-characterized control conditions are important. Tasks that a subject cannot perform will not produce activation in brain regions of interest. Cognitive deficits, common among epilepsy populations, may affect fMRI. If activation maps are atypical, then repeat studies need to be performed to ensure replicability. Studies that cannot be rationally interpreted are not diagnostic and may require confirmation from invasive means such as the intracarotid amobarbital test or cortical stimulation. fMRI studies are sensitive to motion and require subject cooperation, which is problematic in cognitively impaired, claustrophobic, or very young patients (younger than 4 years). In scan monitoring of task, response may ensure task performance but may also change cognitive aspects of the paradigm and involve additional cognitive networks.

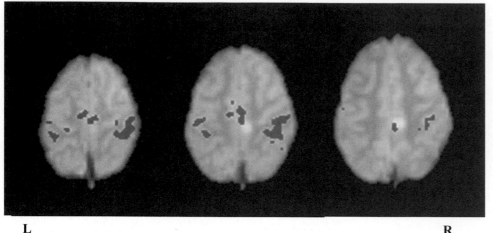

L   **R**

FIGURE 79.1 A 10-year-old with a right mesial mass seen as increased signal. fMRI of motor tapping of left hand compared to rest yields activation (red), which identifies primary motor cortex, posterior to the lesion. Mirror activation ipsilateral to tapping hand is also seen. Supplementary motor cortex activation is seen adjacent to the lesion. This image is from raw fMRI data, rather than superimposed on high-resolution anatomic images (as seen in language/speech activation in Figure 79.3). Please see color insert.

fMRI MOTOR AND SENSORY MAPPING

fMRI studies readily identify primary motor and sensory cortex (7–9), as signal changes in these brain areas are 5% on a 1.5-T scanner. In contrast, a 0.5% to 1.5% signal change is seen in cognitive studies in association cortex. Surgery in patients with parietal or frontal lobe epilepsy often requires identification of the sensory or motor cortex. Most reports of motor and sensory fMRI involve patients evaluated for surgical resection of lesions: tumor, vascular malformation, dysplasia, or encephalomalacia. Several series encompassing numerous patients demonstrate the capacity of fMRI to readily and reliably identify motor and sensory cortex (Fig. 79.1) (10). Motor cortex representing tongue, hand, finger, arm, and foot areas can be identified with tongue movement, finger tapping, and toe wiggling; analogous sensory areas are identified with brushing or an air puff. The supplementary motor area can be identified with complex finger movements (11). Correlation at the time of resection, confirmed with corticography or evoked potential mapping in these patients, is excellent. Cortical stimulation and fMRI activation typically lie within 3 to 5 mm of each other. Dysplastic tissue can also demonstrate activation. Primary and secondary visual cortices can also be easily identified with the use of visual stimuli, such as a reversing checkerboard pattern. Activation maps from these modalities may be used as seed regions to identify long white matter tracts essential to motor control and vision (12).

fMRI LANGUAGE LATERALIZATION AND LOCALIZATION

Numerous studies demonstrate that fMRI language paradigms reliably identify hemispheric dominance for language, including bilateral and right-hemisphere language representation in adults and in children 5 years and older. For language, and perhaps memory, fMRI may serve as a replacement of the intracarotid amobarbital test (IAT, Wada procedure). fMRI not only provides lateralization, but also localization of language (or speech) networks; this is important as chronic partial epilepsy is associated with altered cerebral representation of language functions. The cerebral location of language function is often difficult to predict and may involve transfer of language capacity partially or wholly to the typically nondominant hemisphere (13,14), or to intrahemispheric redistribution of language function (15).

Many fMRI studies typically rely on tests of verbal fluency: word generation to letters or generating a rhyming word, word stem completion (phonetic tasks), and word generation to categories or verb generation from nouns (both semantic tasks) (6,10,16). Verbal fluency paradigms reliably activate inferior cortex (Brodmann's areas 44 and 45) and midfrontal (MF) cortex (Brodmann's areas 9 and 46; dorsolateral prefrontal cortex). Fluency tasks can be semantically based—generate words that fall in categories ("food," "animals"), or generate a verb (or verbs) associated with a presented noun ("ball"; throw, pitch, kick)—or they may be phonologically based—generate words that begin with a presented letter (C, L, F; P, R, W) or that rhyme with a presented word ("bat", cat, bat, mat). Phonological emphasis generates more activation in posterior Broca's, semantic fluency greater activation inferior, superior Broca's. Semantic decision tasks (determining whether a word pair was abstract or concrete; or whether a presented word falls into a previously stated category) activate the same midfrontal and inferior frontal brain regions as well as Brodmann's area 47 (5,17). Verbal fluency and semantic decision tasks show marked activation in frontal cortex, most of which occurs in the dominant hemisphere (67% to 90%) (Fig. 79.2). A limitation, especially for evaluating patients with temporal lobe epilepsy, is the relatively limited ability to activate temporal language cortex (Fig. 79.3) (18).

Paradigms designed to identify receptive language fields in the temporal lobe in individual subjects use more linguistically complex auditory or visual language stimuli—sentences or phrases rather than single words (see Fig. 79.3). Reading paradigms using sentences and stories are potent identifiers of dominant superior and middle temporal cortex (18). As with fluency and semantic decision tasks, there is some bilateral activation, but the bulk of activation (70% to 90%) is found in the dominant hemisphere. These tasks may also engage dominant middle frontal and, to a lesser extent, inferior frontal lobes. Listening to sentences activates the left superior temporal sulcus, with minor activation in right regions, when control tasks involving unfamiliar languages or reverse speech are used to control for primary and secondary auditory processing (19,20). Reading and auditory language processing reliably

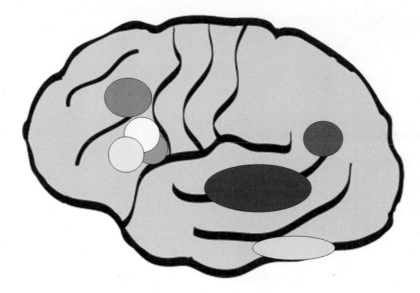

FIGURE 79.2 Schema showing areas activated with different paradigms advocated in individual studies. Areas adjacent to, and along, the superior temporal sulcus (blue) are activated by tasks that stress phrase or sentence comprehension such as listening to stories or reading stories or sentences. Supramarginal gyrus (and sometimes angular gyrus) (purple) may also be activated in auditory sentence processing tasks. Fusiform gyrus (light blue) is activated by tasks that require feature search or identification, such as identifying written characters or object naming. Middle frontal gyrus (red) is implicated in verbal working memory for reading, grammatical decipherment, or verbal recall. Inferior frontal gyrus subregions are activated by a variety of tasks, phonologic fluency (orange), syntactic/semantic decision (green), semantic fluency or recall (yellow). Please see color insert.

identify dominant language cortex in the temporal lobe, as well as the dorsolateral prefrontal cortex, in patients with refractory partial epilepsy confirmed by the IAT (18,21). Tasks may be designed to combine both language comprehension and expression: deciding whether a three-word sentence is syntactically and semantically correct (21) or deciding whether a description or a definition of an object is correct (18).

There is excellent agreement between IAT and fMRI using the above-mentioned tasks for identifying left-, bilateral, and right-language dominance (18,21). Most studies, however, report partial disparity in 10% to 15% of patients regardless of paradigm employed—in these instances, one method is unilateral while the other is bilateral (18,21). It is difficult to know which method, fMRI or IAT, is correct as both have defined limitations. Direct comparisons are imperfect as IAT relies heavily on object naming which has not proved useful in individual fMRI series. Partial disparity may be reduced to 5% to 8% by employing a panel of tasks (see Fig. 79.3) (18,22). This strategy may employ similar paradigms targeted at one process to increase reliability (16,23), or employ tasks

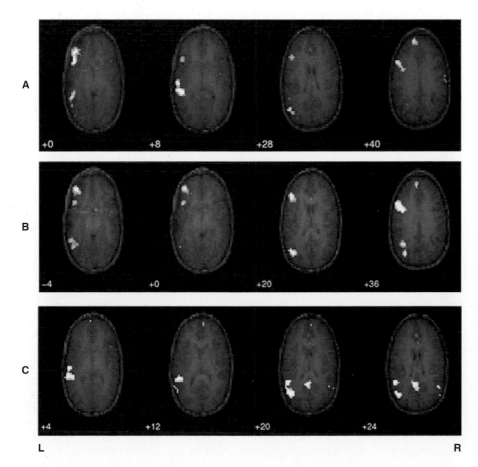

FIGURE 79.3 Functional magnetic resonance imaging (echo planar imaging, blood oxygenation level dependent) panel of tasks. I. Young adult with right temporal lobe focus; panel of tasks shows left frontal and left temporal activation demonstrating left-hemisphere dominance for language. II. A young adult with a left temporal lobe focus showing atypical language dominance. Activation predominantly occurs in right homologues of Broca's and Wernicke's Areas. The left side of the image is the left brain. "Activated" voxels representing brain regions involved in performing the task compared with a control condition (rest) are red. I. Auditory-based word definition task where patient decides whether a description of an object matches final answer (e.g., "a large pink bird is a flamingo"). Control conditions are the same clues in reverse speech and search for the presence of an after going tone; this controls for sound, pitch complexity, attention, and decision aspects of task.

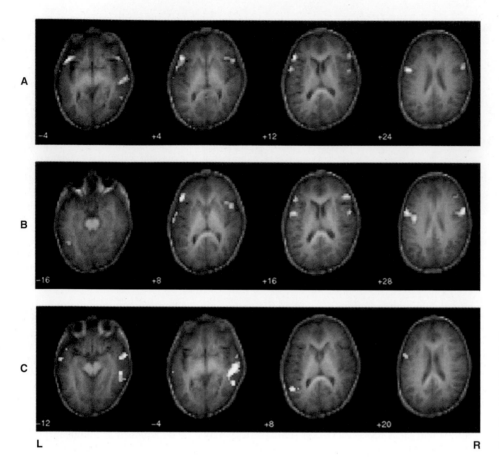

A −4 +4 +12 +24

B −16 +8 +16 +28

C −12 −4 +8 +20

L R

FIGURE 79.3 (*Continued*) II. Auditory category decision task; the patient decides whether a presented word matches a given category (e.g., food: "pizza" "chair" "bean"); reverse speech tone control. C: Listening to stories; control reverse speech. For each paradigm there are five cycles, each consisting of a 30-second control condition and 30-second task condition. Please see color insert.

used to assess varied aspects of language in frontal and temporal regions (18). Complete discordance is uncommon, but when described, either IAT or fMRI, depending on circumstances, has proved correct (24) (see below). Agreement with IAT using verbal fluency tasks may be less strong when MRI is normal or when atypical patterns are present (25–27). Asymmetry indices (AIs) are higher when region-of-interest (ROI) analysis targeted at language cortex is used, in comparison to hemispheric AIs (18,28), though visual and ROI analysis provide similar results (18,29). fMRI semantic decision tasks predict postoperative language measures, primarily in naming, in adults (30,31).

Although rare, there are circumstances where fMRI yields falsely lateralizing information, mostly derived from activation seen in homologous regions because "true" activation is obscured by physiologic factors that alter the BOLD response: large tumors with edema and mass effect; vascular malformations which induce a steal effect (32); and studies performed in a postictal state (33).

The evidence suggests there is good correspondence between cortical stimulation and fMRI activation, but results do not entirely overlap. fMRI–ECS comparison studies for language find 65% to 70% of activated areas to lie within 10 mm of positive ECS (closer to 5 mm for frontal lobe); fMRI negative sites in 90% of patients are never falsely negative (the other 10% were performed during circumstances where BOLD response may have been impaired) (10,23). Minor differences amount to millimeters (usually less than 5 mm) and may arise from coregistration program error, BOLD identification of draining veins rather than capillaries, or the loss of

true positives with overly stringent thresholds. Several language tasks during mapping are necessary because different aspects of language are variously expressed (23).

The temporal lobe appears primed to process elements of language. These systems appear to process sounds and language even when the sensorium is depressed, either by cerebral injury or by sedation. When sedation is light then activation of dominant temporal lobe may be achieved with presentation of sentences, and sensorimotor cortex can be identified by passive motion of joints and limbs (34,35).

Atypical language dominance may take many patterns: bilateral activation in both frontal and temporal regions, activation on one side in frontal and in contralateral temporal (crossed dominance), different laterality between tasks (e.g., reading showing left dominance, auditory comprehension left dominance), or one region bilateral and the other unilateral. Atypical patterns of language dominance are common in epilepsy populations (25% to 35%) and may vary depending on the location and extent of pathology or focus (25,36,37). All patients with left middle cerebral artery infarcts who retain speech have some degree of atypical speech representation. Damage to mesial temporal structures (MTS) implicated in verbal memory is associated with atypical language in 25% of patients (36,38). Small tumors and cortical dysplasia are associated with 15% to 30% atypical language representation depending on the extent and location of the lesion (36,39,40). Occasionally, extensive dysplasia can sustain activation for motor, sensory, and language tasks (41). Up to 30% of patients with left-hemisphere focus, with normal MRI, who are right-handed may exhibit atypical patterns (42). The age at insult, injury, or epilepsy onset appears to be more important than duration of epilepsy. Processes that affect the left hemisphere before the age of 7 years—such as meningitis, encephalitis, traumatic brain injury, stroke, developmental tumors, malformations of cortical development, and seizures—are more strongly associated with atypical language. Atypical language activation patterns may represent persistence of immature networks rather than reorganization as a shift from left to right homologs (36). When atypical language occurs, be it compensation or reorganization, activation occurs in right-hemisphere homologs or in regions immediately adjacent to areas that typically sustain language. Activation outside these areas is uncommon (43–46).

There is mounting evidence that imaging white matter tracts that connect temporal and frontal areas—the arcuate fasciculus, the extreme capsule fiber system, and the uncinate fasciculus (47–49)—may provide equivalent or complementary information to fMRI data. These methods measure the difference in size of white matter tracts either by using fMRI to establish seed regions (50,51) or by identifying white matter bundles (47). Other imaging methods that investigate the strength of functional connections between regions in epilepsy patients are in their infancy (52).

fMRI MEMORY STUDIES

From a practical perspective, the ability to assess the integrity of hippocampal function is desirable for planning mesial temporal tissue resection. Memory is difficult to study, however, because almost everything humans do requires memory, and presumably the hippocampus, in some capacity. Designing paradigms to achieve signal differences between task and control conditions is therefore difficult. Paradigms using encoding and retrieval of complex images demonstrate activation of posterior and bilateral hippocampus and parahippocampal gyrus, whereas retrieval using verbal identifiers of encoded memory for pictures appears to involve anterior subiculum bilaterally. Encoding of novel stimuli followed by recall is associated with activation of posterior parahippocampal.

Preferential activation of right and/or left mesial temporal structures reflects material specificity. Verbal encoding appears to preferentially activate left mesial temporal structures, whereas nonverbal stimuli such as patterns preferentially activate right mesial temporal. Viewing complex pictures, which likely involves verbal encoding as well as visual imagery, activates bilateral mesial temporal regions; face encoding is bilateral with a right bias; and mental navigation yields similar patterns as picture encoding (53–56). Most memory studies examine encoding rather than recall. Unlike language studies, where a number of paradigms have been successfully studied in normal and patient populations, an insufficient, but growing, number of normal volunteers have been studied to establish normative data for memory tasks. These techniques have not been extensively used for evaluating patients, and predictive paradigms have not yet been replicated and validated.

Bellgowan et al. (57) found activation of the middle left parahippocampal gyrus and hippocampus during the verbal encoding of the semantic decision task described previously (5) in patients with right temporal lobe epilepsy, but not left temporal lobe epilepsy. However, the analysis is reported as a group study, and individual variation may have been lost in the left temporal lobe epilepsy group. Jokeit et al. (56) found a mental navigation task predicted side of seizure onset but had insufficient data to correlate IAT on an individual basis. Temporal lobe epilepsy patients have substantially greater dorsolateral prefrontal cortex (DLPF) activation than hippocampal activation in MTS patients suggesting compensatory strategies and networks for verbal encoding (54,55).

An increasing number of small series studies have explored application of memory techniques in patients with epilepsy on an individual basis (50,51,54,58–60). One study found bilateral parahippocampal activation using a visual encoding paradigm based on encoding of scenes (58). It found a slightly greater activation in right posterior parahippocampal in normal subjects. Furthermore, an asymmetry index involving activation in posterior mesial temporal regions matched IAT lateralization in patients with temporal lobe epilepsy (58). Extensions of this study yielded good, but not excellent agreement with IAT. fMRI activation predicted postsurgical outcome for that specific encoding task (61), but not other measures of memory. A paradigm employing indoor and outdoor scene decisions compared to a scrambled image match decision control also found good, but incomplete, correlation with IAT (61). Two groups that examined the use of a panel of encoding tasks—combinations of verbal, face, scene, and pattern encoding—found encouraging preliminary findings (12,54). In the Roland hometown navigation task—walking, a covert recollection task—activation in right hippocampal formation was associated with memory performance on Rey visual design learning task for right ATL (62). Studies have not yet accounted for partial averaging effects of sclerotic hippocampus in their analysis.

Studies that employ verbal and face encoding paradigms as probes of left hippocampal integrity are based on models of material specificity. They find that there is greater activation in contralateral hippocampus from seizure focus, but that outcome depends on activation within the targeted HF. These data support the notion that hippocampal adequacy rather than hippocampal reserve are important for outcome, regardless of activation in contralateral hippocampus—and suggest that compensatory mechanisms are incomplete (50,51,59,62). Language appears to follow the hippocampus that supports verbal memory processing; resection on side of language dominance established by fMRI predicts verbal memory deficits (31).

Unlike language or sensory-motor paradigms, block designs work less well in memory studies. Signal is best identified using an event-related design. In this design, items are presented individually and the peak BOLD signal 5 seconds later is assessed. The versatility of this design is that one can examine BOLD signal for correctly encoded or recalled items (as the improperly encoded tasks will have a lesser or null BOLD signal). Approximately 25 to 30 encoded items are necessary for each condition; the analysis needs to be individualized based on behavior confirmation of properly encoded/recalled items.

To be efficacious, memory fMRI paradigms need to establish memory capacity of the side not targeted for resection as well as predict postoperative memory performance. As with language-mapping strategies, a panel of different memory probes will likely be required that include material specificity as well as encoding and recall.

fMRI: ICTAL AND INTERICTAL LOCALIZATION

In rare and serendipitous circumstances, fMRI can identify regional blood flow changes that accompany partial seizures (63). Several instances of ictal fMRI have involved patients with frequent seizures (epilepsia partialis continua in two patients), accompanied by minimal head movement and confirmed either by interictal and ictal SPECT studies or by cortical ictal recordings. It is possible to capture focal seizures in patients who have been removed from medications for video monitoring. Moreover, the time course analysis can demonstrate the anatomic distribution of seizure onset and propagation (63). In this instance, the superior temporal resolution of fMRI provides additional information beyond SPECT or PET cerebral blood flow–based studies. It may be possible to detect changes in BOLD signal that precedes ictal events (52).

fMRI of absence seizures shows increased thalamic signal and decreased cortical signal, thus providing supporting human evidence implicating thalamus in pathophysiology of absence seizures (64) and also "deactivations" in other cortical areas, and may be able to distinguish BOLD effects induced by spike in contrast to slow wave. Time-locked fMRI data acquisition of spikes detected by EEG can measure regional increases in MRI signal associated with interictal activity in mesial temporal structures, neocortex, and structural lesions (65). Such methods may ultimately prove to be reliable ways of localizing epileptogenic cortex and do not rely on the chance occurrence of seizures during scanning.

fMRI using arterial spin labeling provides a direct measure of blood flow—water is tagged with a magnetic signature in the carotid, and then traced through the brain. With these techniques, interictal blood flow can be assessed and quantitated, similar to [^{15}O]water PET, or unquantifiable SPECT. Interictal hypoperfusion, however, is not necessarily a reliable indicator of the epileptogenic zone (66,67).

fMRI ADVANTAGES AND LIMITATIONS

Unlike PET, fMRI technology is common and relatively inexpensive. Studies can be performed with little risk and no radiation. Most importantly, studies can be repeated to confirm findings, especially if no or unusual activation patterns are found. A number of different paradigms can be performed to map different aspects of language and speech—often more than can be performed in the operating room. Additionally, fMRI identifies language areas deep in sulci, areas that are often inaccessible to cortical stimulation. It can also be used to reliably study children over the age of 4 years.

fMRI is restricted to patients who will be medically safe in the scanner. To be studied successfully, patients must be awake and cooperative and must lie still. Motion artifact remains the principal cause of failed studies, a particular issue in very young, fidgety, or cognitively impaired patients (though older cognitively impaired patients may do quite well). Activation is task and control specific; a given task may not be optimal for identifying targeted cortex. Patients must be able to perform the task.

As a clinical tool, fMRI can be reliably used to lateralize language function and to identify motor or sensory strip in anticipation of surgery. It can also localize language function and, therefore, is a useful guide for sparing eloquent cortex. Activated areas are likely to be involved in task processing, although not all activated areas may be critical for language function. The statistical threshold used may underestimate the extent of area activated. Under certain clinical circumstances (tumor, vascular malformation, postictal state), fMRI may be unreliable. Memory paradigms are coming to be established. Application for seizure mapping is limited with current technology, is almost entirely fortuitous, and cannot be used reliably, except in rare circumstances.

CLINICAL RECOMMENDATIONS FOR USE OF FUNCTIONAL IMAGING IN EVALUATION OF PATIENTS WITH PARTIAL EPILEPSY

fMRI is a reliable technique for the location of sensory and motor function, and for the lateralization and localization of language functions, particularly when a panel of tasks is used and directed at regional activation in relation to the surgical target. Care should be taken to recall circumstances when the BOLD effect may be compromised and activation maps interpreted with caution. Null or peculiar activation maps should also be cautiously viewed, repeated, and when necessary resort made to invasive means. Memory assessment with fMRI is likely to ultimately prove reliable. As with language, different aspects of memory will likely be probed for best overall view. Information obtained by functional mapping can be used to direct surgery and cortical mapping necessary for anatomic confirmation and resection. Linking fMRI to DTI tractography may increase the impact on planning epilepsy surgery. Spike and seizure localization appears promising but may be problematic.

References

1. Fox PT, Raichle ME. Focal physiological uncoupling of cerebral blood flow and oxidative metabolism during somatosensory stimulation of human subjects. *Proc. Nat Acad Sci.* 1986;323:806–809.
2. Roy CS, Sherrington CS. On the regulation of blood flow to the brain. *J Physiol.* 1980;11:85–108.
3. Logothetis NK, The underpinnings of the BOLD functional magnetic resonance imaging signal. *J Neurosci.* 2003;23(10):3963–3971.
4. Moonen CTW, Bandettini PA. Functional MRI. In: Baert AL, Sartor K, Youker JE, eds. Heidelberg: Springer; 2000.
5. Binder JR, Swanson SJ, Hammeke TA, et al. Determination of language dominance using functional MRI: a comparison with the Wada test. *Neurology.* 1996;46:978–984.
6. Hertz-Pannier L, Gaillard WD, Mott SH, et al. Assessment of language hemispheric dominance in children with epilepsy using functional MRI. *Neurology.* 1997;48:1003–1012.
7. Kim SG, Ashe J, Georgopoulos AP, et al. Functional imaging of human motor cortex at high magnetic field. *J. Neurophysiol.* 1993;69:297–302.
8. Kwong K, Belliveau JW, Chesler DA, et al. Dynamic magnetic resonance imaging of human brain activity during primary sensory stimulation. *Proc Natl Acad Sci.* 1992;89:5675–5679.
9. Rao SM, Binder JR, Bandettini PA, et al. Functional magnetic resonance imaging of complex human movements. *Neurology.* 1993;43:2311–2318.
10. Fitzgerald DB, Cosgrove GR, Ronner S, et al. Location of language in the cortex: a comparison between functional MR imaging and electrocortical stimulation. *Am J Neuroradiol.* 1997;18:1529–1539.
11. Nelson L, Lapsiwala S, Haughton VM, et al. Preoperative mapping of the supplementary motor area in patients harboring tumors in the medial frontal lobe. *J Neurosurg.* 2002;97(5):1108–1114.
12. Powell HW, Parker GJ, Alexander DC, et al. MR tractography predicts visual field defects following temporal lobe resection. *Neurology.* 2005; 65(4):596–599.
13. Loring DW, Strauss E, Hermann BP, et al. Effects of anomalous language representation on neuropsychological performance in temporal lobe epilepsy. *Neurology.* 1999;53(2):260–264.

14. Rasmussen, T, Milner B. The role of early left-brain injury in determining lateralization of cerebral speech functions. *Ann N Y Acad Sci.* 1977;299: 355–369.

15. Ojemann G, Ojemann J, Lettich E, et al. Cortical language localization in left, dominant hemisphere. An electrical stimulation mapping investigation in 117 patients. *J Neurosurg.* 1989;71(3):316–326.

16. Ramsey NF, Sommer IE, Rutten GJ, et al. Combined analysis of language tasks in fMRI improves assessment of hemispheric dominance for language functions in individual subjects. *Neuroimage.* 2001;13:719–733.

17. Binder JR, Rao SM, Hammeke TA, et al. Functional magnetic resonance imaging of human auditory cortex. *Ann Neurol.* 1994;35:662–672.

18. Gaillard WD, Balsamo L, Xu B, et al. Language dominance in partial epilepsy patients identified with an fMRI reading task. *Neurology.* 2002; 59(2):256–265.

19. Schlosser MJ, Aoyagi N, Fulbright RK, et al. Functional MRI studies of auditory comprehension. *Hum Brain Mapp.* 1998;6:1–13.

20. Ahmad Z, Balsamo LM, Sachs BC, et al. Auditory comprehension of language in young children: neural networks identified with fMRI. *Neurology.* 2003;60(10):1598–1605.

21. Carpentier A, Pugh KR, Westerveld M, et al. Functional MRI of language processing: dependence on input modality and temporal lobe epilepsy. *Epilepsia.* 2001;42(10):1241–1254.

22. Gaillard W, Balsamo L, Xu B, et al. fMRI panel of verbal fluency, auditory, and reading comprehension identifies language dominance compared to the intracarotid amytal test. *Epilepsia.* 2002;43(Suppl 7):89.

23. Pouratian N, Bookheimer SY, Rex DE, et al. Utility of preoperative functional magnetic resonance imaging for identifying language cortices in patients with vascular malformations. *J Neurosurg.* 2002;97:21–32.

24. Hunter K, Blaxton TA, Bookheimer SY, et al. 15O water positron emission tomography in language localization: a study comparing positron emission tomography visual and computerized region of interest analysis with the Wada Test. *Ann Neurol.* 1999;45(5):662–665.

25. Woermann FG, Jokeit H, Luerding R, et al. Language lateralization by Wada test and fMRI in 100 patients with epilepsy. *Neurology.* 2003;61(5): 699–701.

26. Benke T, Köylü B, Visani P, et al. Language Lateralization in Temporal Lobe Epilepsy: a comparison between fMRI and the Wada Test. *Epilepsia.* 2006;47(8):1308–1319.

27. Brazdil M, Chlebus P, Mikl M, et al. Reorganization of language-related neuronal networks in patients with left temporal lobe epilepsy—an fMRI study. *Eur J Neurol.* 2005;12(4):268–275.

28. Spreer J, Arnold S, Quiske A, et al. Determination of hemisphere dominance for language: comparison of frontal and temporal fMRI activation with intracarotid amytal testing. *Neuroradiology.* 2002;44(6):467–474.

29. Fernandez G, de Greiff A, von Oertzen J, et al. Language mapping in less than 15 minutes: real-time functional MRI during routine clinical investigation. *Neuroimage.* 2001;14(3):585–594.

30. Sabsevitz DS, Swanson SJ, Hammeke TA, et al. Use of preoperative functional neuroimaging to predict language deficits from epilepsy surgery. *Neurology.* 2003;60(11):1788–1792.

31. Binder JR, Sabsevitz DS, Swanson SJ, et al. Use of preoperative functional MRI to predict verbal memory decline after temporal lobe epilepsy surgery. *Epilepsia.* 2008;49(8):1377–1394.

32. Lehericy S, Biondi A, Sourour N, et al. Arteriovenous brain malformations: Is functional MR imaging reliable for studying language reorganization in patients? Initial observations. *Radiology.* 2002;223(3):672–682.

33. Jayakar P, Bernal B, Santiago Medina L, et al. False lateralization of language cortex on functional MRI after a cluster of focal seizures. *Neurology.* 2002;58(3):490–492.

34. Souweidane MM, Kim KH, McDowall R, et al. Brain mapping in sedated infants and young children with passive-functional magnetic resonance imaging. *Pediatr Neurosurg.* 1999;30(2):86–92.

35. Altman NR, Bernal B. Brain activation in sedated children: auditory and visual functional MR imaging. *Radiology.* 2001;221(1):56–63.

36. Gaillard WD, Weinstein S, Conry J, et al. Prognosis of children with partial epilepsy: MRI and serial 18FDG-PET. *Neurology.* 2007;68(9):655–659.

37. Thivard L, Hombrouck J, du Montcel ST, et al. Productive and perceptive language reorganization in temporal lobe epilepsy. *Neuroimage.* 2005; 24(3):841–851.

38. Weber B, Wellmer J, Reuber M, et al. Left hippocampal pathology is associated with atypical language lateralization in patients with focal epilepsy. *Brain.* 2006;129(Pt 2):346–351.

39. Hadac J, Brozová K, Tintera J, et al. Language lateralization in children with pre- and postnatal epileptogenic lesions of the left hemisphere: an fMRI study. *Epileptic Disord.* 2007;9(1):S19–S27.

40. Briellmann RS, Labate A, Harvey AS, et al. Is language lateralization in temporal lobe epilepsy patients related to the nature of the epileptogenic lesion? *Epilepsia.* 2006;47(5):916–920.

41. Vitali P, Minati L, D'Incerti L, et al. Functional MRI in malformations of cortical development: activation of dysplastic tissue and functional reorganization. *Neuroimaging.* 2008;18(3):296–305.

42. Gaillard WD, Berl MM, Moore EN, et al. Atypical language in lesional and nonlesional complex partial epilepsy. *Neurology.* 2008;70(23):2266–2267.

43. Mbwana J, Berl MM, Ritzl EK, et al. Limitations to plasticity of language network reorganization in localization related epilepsy. *Brain.* 2009; 132(2):347–356.

44. Rosenberger LR, et al. fMRI evidence for inter and intra-hemispheric language re-organization in complex partial epilepsy. *Neurology.* In Press.

45. Voets NL, Adcock JE, Flitney DE, et al. Distinct right frontal lobe activation in language processing following left hemisphere injury. *Brain.* 2006;129(Pt 3):754–766.

46. Liegeois F, Connelly A, Baldeweg T, et al. Speaking with a single cerebral hemisphere: fMRI language organization after hemispherectomy in childhood. *Brain Lang.* 2008.

47. Catani M, Jones DK, Ffytche DH. Perisylvian language networks of the human brain. *Ann. Neurol.* 2005;57(1):8–16.

48. Catani M, Allin MP, Husain M, et al. Symmetries in human brain language pathways correlate with verbal recall. *Proc Natl Acad Sci USA.* 2007;104(43):163–168.

49. Frey S, Campbell JS, Pike GB, et al. Dissociating the human language pathways with high angular resolution diffusion fiber tractography. *J Neurosci.* 2008;28(45):11435.

50. Powell HW, Parker GJ, Alexander DC, et al. Abnormalities of language networks in temporal lobe epilepsy. *Neuroimage.* 2007;36(1):209–221.

51. Powell HW, Parker GJ, Alexander DC, et al. Imaging language pathways predicts postoperative naming deficits. *J Neurol Neurosurg Psychiatry.* 2008;79(3):327–330.

52. Federico P, Abbott DF, Briellmann RS, et al. Functional MRI of the pre-ictal state. *Brain.* 2005;128(Pt 8):1811–1817.

53. Kelley WM, Miezin FM, McDermott KB, et al. Hemispheric specialization in human dorsal frontal cortex and medial temporal lobe for verbal and nonverbal memory encoding. *Neuron.* 1998;20(5):927–936.

54. Golby AJ, Poldrack RA, Illes J, et al. Memory lateralization in medial temporal lobe epilepsy assessed by functional MRI. *Epilepsia.* 2002;43(8): 855–863.

55. Dupont S, Van de Moortele PF, Samson S, et al. Episodic memory in left temporal lobe epilepsy: a functional MRI study. *Brain.* 2000;123(Pt 8): 1722–1732.

56. Jokeit H, Okujava M, Woermann FG. Memory fMRI lateralizes temporal lobe epilepsy. *Neurology.* 2001;57(10):1786–1793.

57. Bellgowan PSF, Binder JR, Swanson SJ, et al. Side of seizure focus predicts left medial temporal lobe activation during verbal encoding. *Neurology.* 1998;51(2):479–484.

58. Detre JA, Maccotta L, King D, et al. Functional MRI lateralization of memory in temporal lobe epilepsy. *Neurology.* 1998;50:926–932.

59. Richardson MP, Strange BA, Thompson PJ, et al. Pre-operative verbal memory fMRI predicts post-operative memory decline after left temporal lobe resection. *Brain.* 2004;127(Pt 11):2419–2426.

60. Janszky J, Jokeit H, Kontopoulou K, et al. Functional MRI predicts memory performance after right mesiotemporal epilepsy surgery. *Epilepsia.* 2005;46(2):244–250.

61. Binder JR, Detre JA, Jones-Gotman M, et al. Functional MRI of episodic memory in temporal lobe epilepsy. *Epilepsia.* 2002;43(Suppl 7)(2).

62. Rabin ML, Narayan VM, Kimberg DY, et al. Functional MRI predicts post-surgical memory following temporal lobectomy. *Brain.* 2004;127 (Pt 10):2286–2298.

63. Jackson GD, Berkovic SF, Duncan JS, et al. Functional magnetic resonance imaging of focal seizures. *Neurology.* 1994;44:850–856.

64. Salek-Haddadi A, Lemieux L, Merschhemke M, et al. Functional magnetic resonance imaging of human absence seizures. *Ann Neurol.* 2003;53(5): 663–667.

65. Krakow K, Lemieux L, Messina D, et al. Spatio-temporal imaging of focal interictal epileptiform activity using EEG-triggered functional MRI. *Epileptic Disord.* 2001;3:67–74.

66. Wolf RL, Alsop DC, Levy-Reis I, et al. Detection of mesial temporal lobe hypoperfusion in patients with temporal lobe epilepsy by use of arterial spin labeled perfusion MR imaging. *Am J Neuroradiol.* 2001;22(7):1334–1341.

67. Lim YM, Cho YW, Shamim S, et al. Usefulness of pulsed arterial spin labeling MR imaging in mesial temporal lobe epilepsy. *Epilepsy Res.* 2008; 82:183–189.

CHAPTER 80 ■ THE INTRACAROTID AMOBARBITAL PROCEDURE

ROHIT DAS AND TOBIAS LODDENKEMPER

INTRODUCTION AND HISTORY

Juhn Wada pioneered the idea of unilateral hemispheric anesthesia as a presurgical test of eloquent areas, particularly language (1). The intracarotid amobarbital procedure (IAP) is therefore often called the Wada test. The devastating memory loss observed in patient H.M. led to the introduction of a memory component to the IAP by Brenda Milner (2). In the last decade, indications for performing the IAP decreased (Table 80.1) (3). New developments in noninvasive mapping procedures have since further limited its use, although some indications may remain.

PROCEDURE AND TESTING PARADIGMS

Numerous different protocols are used during the IAP at different centers. Paradigm variations primarily involve the procedure, stimulus presentation, and testing methodology (4). Here we discuss the Cleveland Clinic protocol for the IAP in adults.

Cleveland Clinic Adult IAP Protocol

At Cleveland Clinic, prior to the actual test, a "practice test" is performed in order to orient patients to the test as well as to assess the patients' baseline memory function. Some centers

TABLE 80.1

PREVIOUS INDICATIONS FOR THE IAP TEST IN 1997

Language	Left-handed subjects
	Patients with history or imaging suggestive of early life insult to left-sided speech areas
	Patients with a discordance between anatomic and neuropsychological lateralization
Memory	Significant deficits on verbal and nonverbal memory tests
	Discordance between EEG and imaging findings

From Jones-Gotman M, Smith M, Weiser H-G. Intraarterial amobarbital procedures. In: Engel J, Pedley T, eds. *Epilepsy: A Comprehensive Textbook.* Vol. II. Philadelphia: Lipincott Raven; 1997:1767–1776, with permission of the copyright holder.

may perform upper extremity strength testing or language testing. The anesthetic drug most commonly used is a barbiturate, either amobarbital or methohexital.

The initial step consists of completion of a cerebral angiogram via the transfemoral route to assess cerebral vasculature and cross-filling from one hemisphere to the other. Immediately after the angiogram, the catheter is moved into the internal carotid artery, and the location of the catheter is confirmed on fluoroscopy. Prior to barbiturate injection, the patient is instructed to lift both hands in the air and to start counting. The barbiturate is then injected, and after a few seconds, the patient's contralateral upper extremity drifts due to incipient hemiparesis. If the injected hemisphere is dominant for language, the patient may stop counting. Duration of muteness may last several minutes and slow recovery of speech may initially be associated with paraphasic errors. Once the injection is completed, the clinician assesses motor strength to determine if there is complete contralateral hemiparesis, which serves as a surrogate marker of hemispheric inactivation. The level of consciousness may be then assessed by utilizing a simple one-step command. Additionally, multiple areas of language are continuously assessed including spontaneous language production, repetition, reading, comprehension, and naming of objects. Injection of the nondominant hemisphere may lead to dysarthria but usually no speech arrest. Occasionally, a patient may be mute for a few seconds with nondominant hemisphere injection.

Benbadis et al. have suggested a laterality index with three components that include the absolute duration of speech arrest, the absolute difference of arrest times between both hemispheres, and a laterality index (the difference of the two arrest times divided by the sum of the two arrest times). These three measurements can each provide information on laterality, and frequently only the laterality index is used (5,6).

Memory testing is carried out by presentation of a variable number of objects that include real objects, object line drawings, photographs or pictures, and designs. At Cleveland Clinic, 12 to 16 memory items are presented immediately after the development of hemiparesis, following the first nonverbal response.

Alternative IAP Language Paradigms

There is considerable variability in language testing paradigms between centers. In a survey of epilepsy centers, Snyder et al. found that the vast majority used object naming as the primary language outcome measure (7). Some epilepsy centers may only use speech arrest and inability to respond following barbiturate injection, while others may test speech to evaluate paraphasic and other dysphasic errors (8).

Alternative IAP Memory Test Paradigms

Centers may present items before and after speech returns. Testing paradigms may be divided into two broad categories: presentation of discrete items and a stimulation–distraction–recognition format (4). Number and quality of items presented may vary as well. Some centers may exclusively present words, pictures, or real objects. Others may use a combination of these items. The recall of presented words, phrases, and commands may also be used to assess memory function (3).

Language and memory testing should be completed during the period of hemiparesis. An electroencephalogram (EEG) is performed at the same time, and slowing on the EEG is also monitored to assess return to baseline. Usually the hemisphere ipsilateral to the seizure focus is the first to be injected and tested.

IAP INDICATIONS

The IAP for Assessment of Language

The guiding principle behind the use of the IAP for language lateralization is that functional inactivation of the language-dominant hemisphere renders the subject mute while inactivation of the nondominant hemisphere allows the subject to continue to speak, albeit with some dysarthria but with no aphasia. The IAP, therefore, serves as a transient mimic of the effects of the proposed surgery (9). In their survey of epilepsy centers, Snyder et al. reported that nearly 90% of patients were found to be left-hemispheric language-dominant based on IAP results (7). Even in individuals with bilateral language, the representation of language subcomponents was left dominant (10). Bilateral language representation is noted if there is preservation of some language function with anesthesia of each hemisphere or if language is bilaterally impaired (11). There is considerable variability between centers in the determination of bilateral language and this may again be in part related to testing protocol heterogeneity (7). A major limitation of the IAP in bilaterally dominant individuals is that the test usually does not reliably identify specific aspects of language function (9).

The IAP for Assessment of Memory

Similar to language testing, the effect of the memory IAP is thought to transiently mimic the postsurgical outcome. If one hippocampus is unable to support memory, its removal may lead to minimal postoperative memory deficits. Two models have been suggested to explain memory function observed during the IAP: the *functional adequacy* and the *functional reserve* models. The functional reserve model hypothesizes that the contralateral temporal lobe has limited "reserve" to support memory secondary to structural abnormalities (12). The paradigm of functional adequacy suggests that postoperative memory decline, even in the setting of adequate contralateral functional reserve, is secondary to the residual memory

functions of the resected mesial temporal lobe structures (13). Surgical decision-making has been guided by IAP memory testing paradigms in the past. Patients with bilateral low scores or contralateral low scores were not offered surgery for fear of precipitating severe amnesia following surgery. This practice currently changes with the decline of the IAP and improved methods of memory testing (14).

IAP to Predict Global Amnesia

The term global amnesia has been poorly defined in the IAP literature (4). The hypothesis that the IAP may predict global amnesia following surgery is controversial and there are only a small number of cases reported of patients who failed the IAP, underwent surgery, and subsequently developed devastating memory loss (15). Authors have estimated a postoperative amnesia rate of only 1% or less if no temporal lobe resection was screened with an IAP (4). More recently, other test paradigms than the IAP have been suggested to identify patients at risk, including structural MRI review and neuropsychological evaluation (16).

IAP to Predict Material-Specific Memory Decline

In the past, the IAP had been used primarily to study global amnesia after surgery. More recent studies have attempted to correlate material-specific memory decline, in particular examining whether memory subtypes decline after surgery. These may be dichotomized into auditory and verbal memory decline following dominant temporal lobe surgery versus visual and spatial deficits after nondominant lobe surgery (4). It is thought that selective memory deficits are more common when IAP memory scores are symmetrical between the two hemispheres (17).

Verbal Memory Assessment

Baxendale et al. have shown that left-sided resections produce significant verbal memory decline as compared to right-sided resections. Multivariate analyses showed that good presurgical memory and asymmetric IAP memory scores were predictive of verbal memory decline with left-sided resection (16). However, left-hemispheric language dominance tends to bias memory scores with the recall of verbal stimuli appearing to be the hallmark of left-hemispheric function (16,18,19).

Visual-Spatial Memory

The IAP has been less robust in predicting visual-spatial memory decline after right temporal lobe surgery. This may be related to the facts that verbal memory loss confounds visual memory decline and that the construct validity of visual memory tests is not as strong as those for verbal memory (4,13).

IAP to Predict Postsurgical Seizure Outcome

Studies have examined the relationship between IAP memory scores and postresection seizure outcomes. Several studies have reported that asymmetrical recall on IAP was predictive of achieving Engel Grade I and II outcomes after surgery, with a higher degree of specificity than sensitivity. Positive predictive values ranged from 87% to 100% and negative predictive values ranged from 38% to 56% (20,21). While one study found that the magnitude of asymmetry was not predictive of seizure freedom, another study reported that those patients who had an asymmetry of greater than three recalled items had a higher degree of seizure freedom (22–24).

IAP and Lateralization of the Epileptogenic Zone

The use of the IAP for prediction of postoperative seizure outcome was based on the observation that injection of the hemisphere contralateral to the seizure focus was associated with poor memory scores (25,26). The IAP memory scores, therefore, serve as a proxy for identifying a dysfunctional medial temporal lobe and possibly also the epileptogenic zone (21,27). Recent surveys have found that the overwhelming majority of epilepsy centers do not utilize the IAP to lateralize the epileptogenic zone (28,29). IAP memory scores have been shown to reliably identify the seizure-onset hemisphere in three fourth of patients with lesional temporal lobe epilepsy. In patients with nonlesional MRI, the IAP identified the seizure onset in only one third of the cases (30). Unilateral memory deficits on IAP also indicated an additional medial temporal lobe ictal onset zone in selected patients with frontal and lateral temporal lobe epilepsy (31).

Other Potential Indications for the IAP

Primary versus Secondary Bilateral Synchrony

Secondary bilateral synchrony refers to focal seizures or inter-ictal epileptiform discharges that appear as bilaterally synchronous discharges on surface EEG (32). Lombroso et al. have used amobarbital in rabbits and sodium thiopental in humans to abolish secondary synchrony and to reveal the location of seizure onset (32,33). Today, the IAP is used only in very rare cases to differentiate between primary and secondary bilateral synchrony (28,29).

Lateralization of Mathematic Skills and Music

Mathematical ability lateralizes to the left in all patients with left-hemispheric language dominance, while the majority of those with bilateral or right-hemispheric language lateralize math ability to the right (34). Researchers have used IAP data to demonstrate right-sided dominance for music and singing (29).

FACTORS AFFECTING IAP RESULTS

Several factors may influence IAP and may confound results, including timing of the injection, side of initial injection, dosing of amobarbital, the timing of presentation of stimuli during the procedure, as well as the effect of anticonvulsants, other medications and additional patient- or situation-related factors. Finally, the IAP may provide nonconclusive results.

Timing of Injection

Grote et al. evaluated the effect of injection timing on IAP memory scores. Using univariate statistical analysis, the authors showed that patients who received their IAPs on succeeding days had significantly better memory scores than those who received the test the same day (35).

Side of Injection

The difference in memory scores was more significant for left- as compared to right-hemisphere injections when the left hemisphere was anesthetized first (35). An injection interval of less than 40 minutes was associated with prolonged electrographic slowing. Faster electrographic recovery was seen if the seizure focus hemisphere was injected first (36). The typical sequence is the injection of the hemisphere slated for surgery followed by the contralateral hemisphere. Bengner et al. demonstrated that memory scores of the epileptogenic hemisphere improved when the contralateral hemisphere was tested first (37).

Dose of Amobarbital

The dose effect of amobarbital has been evaluated by two studies with contradictory results. A dose of greater than 125 mg amobarbital was associated with worse object recognition, while a second study found no effect of amobarbital dosage on memory outcomes (38,39). However, lower doses of amobarbital may not induce adequate hemiparesis or amnesia.

Timing of presentation of stimuli during the procedure may also play a role. Loring et al. evaluated the effect of the timing of presentation of stimuli during the IAP on memory testing in two separate studies. In lesional temporal lobe epilepsy, recall of objects presented within 45 seconds of amobarbital injection was more strongly associated with lateralized temporal dysfunction (40). In nonlesional temporal lobe epilepsy, memory scores for objects presented in the first 50 seconds were predictive of the seizure-onset hemisphere (41). Memory outcomes did not change with presentation of stimuli either before or after return of speech (42).

Effect of Carbonic Anhydrase Inhibitors

A single center review of all cases of inadequate anesthetization during the IAP test found that all patients took carbonic anhydrase (CA) inhibitors (topiramate and zonisamide). Bookheimer et al. suggest that CA inhibition reduces amobarbital anesthetization by disabling the effect of amobarbital on GABA-A channels (43).

Reasons for Equivocal IAP Results

The IAP can occasionally provide equivocal results. If no inactivation of language occurs with right and left injections, the procedure may have been technically inadequate. Other reasons include vascular abnormalities causing shunting, reorganized language areas from pre-existing early cerebral insults and testing limitations imposed by behavior (9).

IAP VARIANTS

Posterior Circulation Amobarbital Injection

A drawback of the IAP is that the anterior circulation does not supply most of the hippocampus and temporal lobes, the very structures that frequently may be resected. The posterior circulation supplies most of the middle and posterior hippocampus and temporal lobe (44,45). Two major studies from the Mayo Clinic nearly 20 years ago pioneered the use of the posterior circulation amobarbital test. Disadvantages of this procedure include a procedural complication rate of 2% as well as a lengthier posterior circulation catherization and, therefore, greater manipulation of the intracranial vessels (46,47). The higher complication rate and replacement by newer techniques as well as continued anterior circulation IAP have prevented widespread use of this variant.

IAP in Children

The IAP test is less often used in children. In children and in patients with developmental delay and mental retardation, cooperation limits the testing paradigm. IAP testing in children may require modifications from the adult testing protocol. At Children's Hospital Boston, the child is asked to follow simple commands, name pictures, and point to stimuli on a card (to assess neglect) after development of hemiparesis. The child is also asked to repeat simple sentences and recite months of the year or days of the week forward and backward. At 2 minutes after injection, memory stimuli are presented, and this typically includes the presentation of two written words, two abstract designs that are not visually encoded, one mathematical calculation, and three pictured objects. An interference task is then performed and thereafter, at approximately 8 minutes after injection, memory recall testing is performed.

The majority of children who undergo the IAP are adolescents, though children as young as 3 years old have been tested (3,48). As compared to adults, children are rehearsed for the test. This helps to reduce anxiety and to improve cooperation with testing (3,48). Language testing protocols in children have been adapted from those created for adults (49). Memory testing is more difficult in children, in part due to anxiety, shorter attention span, and possibly less well-developed memory and learning strategies (3,50). Factors that are known to influence memory performance of IAPs in children include the side that is injected and the age of the child. Younger children are likely to have worse memory performance when the left hemisphere is injected. There is no definite relationship between IQ scores and memory performance (51). In a single center study, frequency of complications in children was similar to adults with comparable language lateralization data (48).

IAP asymmetry scores may predict postsurgical memory changes in children. Lee et al. evaluated whether these scores help predict memory after extratemporal surgery and found evidence suggesting that, while the epileptic focus does not directly affect the ipsilateral hippocampus, children with non-temporal lobe epilepsy, nevertheless, demonstrate worse memory ipsilateral to the seizure focus (52). IAP testing

methodology is also important. In younger children with left-hemispheric seizure focus, the use of real objects significantly improved memory scores as compared to mixed stimuli (53,54).

Intracarotid Propofol, Methohexital, and Etomidate (ESAM) Tests

Shortages of amobarbital lead to the use of methohexital, propofol, and etomidate during Wada testing. Methohexital has a shorter onset of action than amobarbital (within 1 minute) and shorter duration of action (less than 10 minutes). In a comparison of methohexital and amobarbital, Andelman et al. found that the methohexital group demonstrated better memory scores when the hemisphere ipsilateral to the epileptogenic zone was tested. There was no significant difference in scores when the contralateral hemisphere was tested (55). Two other studies have found no major difference between methohexital and amobarbital except for shorter speech arrest times with methohexital (56,57).

Takayama et al. examined the use of propofol as an alternative to amobarbital in a series of 14 subjects. Propofol testing was comparable to IAP results in a historical cohort. However, this pilot trial was limited by a small number of patients (58). Another study found that while multiple repeated doses of propofol were required to maintain sedation, propofol anesthetization was a safe and effective alternative to the IAP (59).

Jones-Gotman et al. described the use of etomidate as an amobarbital substitute and named this test the etomidate speech and memory test (eSAM). The authors suggest that the injection of etomidate, a short-acting anesthetic, provided investigators with the ability to control the degree of hemiparesis better. Because of the short half-life of this drug, the initial signs of clinical recovery appeared only when the etomidate infusion was discontinued (60).

ALTERNATIVE METHODS

Several noninvasive testing methods have been researched to evaluate memory and language lateralization. Alternative techniques include functional MRI (fMRI), functional transcranial Doppler ultrasound (fTCD), magnetoencephalography (MEG), positron emission tomography (PET), single photon emission CT (SPECT), near-infrared spectroscopy (NIRS), cortico-cortical evoked potentials, event-related brain potentials, and repetitive transcranial magnetic stimulation (rTMS) among others (11). fMRI is the most commonly used newer technique to evaluate speech and language.

Language lateralization by fMRI has been the focus of many studies. Numerous studies have compared fMRI and IAP. Word generation tasks appear to be the most reliable test paradigm for language. Language lateralization scores on fMRI correlate with IAP results (61). In one study the fMRI, verb generation paradigm demonstrated erroneous lateralization in 3% of left temporal lobe epilepsy but up to 25% in left-sided extratemporal lobe epilepsy (62). A reading and naming paradigm also adequately identified frontal and temporal speech areas and correlated well with IAP language lateralization (63).

fMRI memory localization is more controversial. In the past, fMRI complex image encoding and retrieval techniques have shown activation of the hippocampal and parahippocampal areas (64). An imaginative walk with a self-paced protocol to test long-term memory retrieval found that reduced activation of the ipsilateral medial temporal region was associated with better memory outcomes after right temporal lobectomy (65). Golby et al. found that fMRI memory lateralization (as defined by an asymmetry of activated voxels), using projected visual stimuli, was highly concordant with IAP in eight of nine cases (66).

DRAWBACKS OF THE IAP

Complications

In a study of more than 600 IAPs, roughly 11% of patients developed minor or major complications during or after the procedure. The most frequent complication was encephalopathy (7.2%), followed by seizures (1.1%), strokes (0.5%), catheter site hematomas (0.5%), and carotid artery dissection (0.4%). Uncommon complications included contrast-induced allergy, infection, and prolonged bleeding from the catheter insertion site. Almost all complications were detected immediately. However, carotid artery dissection was noted after several days in one patient (67). In 2% of patients, the procedure was terminated due to complications.

Variability of the Procedure

Validity

A test is valid if it accurately measures what it claims to measure. Validity in the IAP refers to how well the IAP actually predicts postsurgical language and memory decline after resection of eloquent areas. Given the variations of the IAP methodology between different centers, there are concerns regarding the validity and reliability of the IAP.

Simkins-Bullock categorized validity studies of the IAP prediction of global amnesia risk using standard epidemiological methodology into true positives, false positives, true negatives, and false negatives (4). True positives are those patients who fail the IAP and postsurgically demonstrate global amnesia. In a historical review, Baxendale estimated that there are approximately 20 of these cases (68). False positives are those patients

who fail the IAP for memory test but have postsurgical preservation of memory. Girvin et al. report three mentally challenged patients with bitemporal epilepsy and bihemispheric IAP failure who underwent left temporal lobe resection with little or no baseline decline in memory (69). False negatives are those patients who pass the memory test but have postoperative memory loss. Only one such case has been reported in the past (70). However, in a survey of epilepsy centers, several respondents noted that they were aware of at least one such patient (4). True negatives are those who pass the IAP and proceed to surgery. The vast majority of patients fall within this group and they are at very low risk of postoperative memory decline. Overall no definite information on validity is available due to lack of evidence in the false negative group.

Reliability is a measure of consistency of a test. There is evidence from studies involving repeat IAPs that the test is a reliable measure of language but not of memory (71). Loddenkemper et al. reviewed all cases with repeat IAPs at the Cleveland Clinic and found significant variability in memory testing but not language testing. Although this study was not specifically designed to test reliability, it may imply variability of results with repeated memory testing. Therefore, these results may also provide an estimate of the reliability of the memory IAP paradigm (71).

Content validity of the IAP is another concern. Testa et al. found that in patients with left temporal epilepsy and ipsilateral injection, the right hemisphere encoded and recalled faces and drawings but not verbal stimuli. In patients with right temporal epilepsy and ipsilateral injection, the left hemisphere performed well on memory encoding for both verbal and visual stimuli with one important exception: recall of faces was poor (17). In a multicenter trial, actual objects were recalled better than line diagrams in patients with left temporal epilepsy. Memory scores were not significantly different in patients with right temporal epilepsy (72).

CONCLUSION AND PERSPECTIVE

Decline of the IAP

In the early 1990s, most centers performed IAPs on almost all patients considered for epilepsy surgery (73). Today, Wada test frequency is declining. Currently, it is only used in selected patients to assess language and memory, and several epilepsy centers stopped performing Wada tests. Table 80.2 summarizes

TABLE 80.2

EPIDEMIOLOGY OF THE DECLINE OF THE IAP

Authors	Year	IAPs per year	Number of centers	Percentage of epilepsy surgery candidates who undergo IAP
Rausch et al. (74)	1992	1569	68	
Haag et al. (28)	2000	282	16	
	2005	210		
Loddenkemper (14)	2001	124	1	72%
	2007	76		20%
Helmstaedter (75)	1988–1995	—	1	50–70%
	2004–2008	—	1	<10%

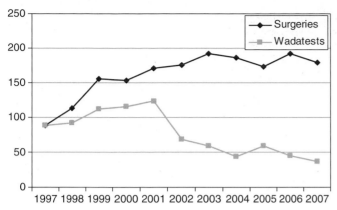

FIGURE 80.1 Frequency of IAP and epilepsy surgeries at the Cleveland Clinic. (From Loddenkemper T. Quo vadis Wada? *Epilepsy Behav.* 2008;13:1–2, with permission of copyright holder.)

the declining frequency of the IAP over the past decades and Figure 80.1 illustrates decreasing IAP frequency at Cleveland Clinic between over the last decade despite increasing epilepsy surgery numbers. In a multinational survey, Baxendale et al. found that more than half of all respondents would be comfortable to proceed to surgery in most or all cases without IAP data to predict risk of global and modality-specific postoperative memory loss (29). About two thirds of respondents were of the opinion that in most or all cases they would be confident of postsurgical outcome without IAP language data. In a European survey, Haag et al. found that respondents thought that the IAP was both reliable and valid in testing language but not memory (28).

Remaining Indications for IAP

In Figure 80.2, we present the previous algorithm that was clinically used to determine the indications for IAP testing. The IAP was used only if activation measures (fMRI or MEG) were inconclusive or if comprehensive memory testing was required. In Figure 80.3, we propose further limiting IAPs even in the aforementioned circumstances after consideration of risks, benefits, and the variety of alternative techniques available (14).

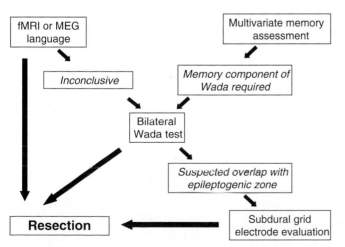

FIGURE 80.2 Algorithm for the indications of IAP testing. (From Loddenkemper T. Quo vadis Wada? *Epilepsy Behav.* 2008;13:1–2, with permission of copyright holder.)

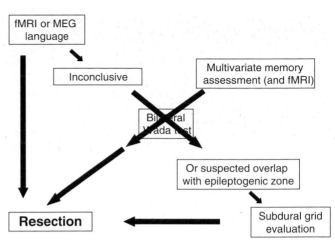

FIGURE 80.3 Revised algorithm for the indications of IAP testing. (From Loddenkemper T. Quo vadis Wada? *Epilepsy Behav.* 2008;13:1–2, with permission of copyright holder.)

TABLE 80.3

REMAINING "SOFT" INDICATIONS FOR INTRACAROTID AMOBARBITAL TESTS[a]

1. Inconclusive or bilateral lateralization on noninvasive testing for language and memory
2. Intracranial grids and strips in extratemporal epilepsy surgery demonstrating possible overlap of resection areas with language or eloquent areas
3. Dominant temporal lobe memory assessment prior to temporal lobe epilepsy surgery

[a]**Comment:** Some epileptologists argue that there may be no need for IAP at all as additional information may be obtained from invasive studies, and memory Wada testing may not be superior to estimation of memory loss risk with noninvasive techniques. Ultimately, the procedure may vanish depending on availability of alternative techniques and comfort level of epileptologists.

At this point, only a few "soft" indications for the IAP remain (Table 80.3) and the IAP may ultimately vanish.

Although the IAP has been a crucial component of epilepsy surgery, the attendant risks of this invasive procedure, the variability of the test, the poor reliability and the limited validity of the IAP, and the development of noninvasive functional testing has lead to a decline in the number of IAPs. IAP test numbers may decline further based on experience and comfort levels with new lateralization and mapping techniques.

ACKNOWLEDGMENT

We would like to acknowledge the assistance of Katrina Boyer, PhD, Children's Hospital Boston, for advising us on the Children's Hospital Boston IAP protocol.

References

1. Wada J, Rasmussen T. Intracarotid injection of sodium amytal for the lateralization of cerebral speech dominance. *J Neurosurg.* 1960;17:266–282.
2. Branch C, Milner B, Rasmussen T. Intracarotid sodium amytal for the lateralization of cerebral speech dominance; observations in 123 patients. *J Neurosurg.* 1964;21:399–405.

3. Jones-Gotman M, Smith M, Weiser H-G. Intraarterial amobarbital procedures. In: Engel J, Pedley T, eds. *Epilepsy: A Comprehensive Textbook.* Vol. II. Philadelphia: Lipincott Raven;1997:1767–1776.

4. Simkins-Bullock J. Beyond speech lateralization: a review of the variability, reliability, and validity of the intracarotid amobarbital procedure and its nonlanguage uses in epilepsy surgery candidates. *Neuropsychol Rev.* 2000; 10:41–74.

5. Moeddel G, Lineweaver T, Schuele S, et al. Atypical language lateralization in epilepsy patients. *Epilepsia.* 2009;50:1505–1516.

6. Benbadis SR, Dinner DS, Chelune GJ, et al. Objective criteria for reporting language dominance by intracarotid amobarbital procedure. *J Clin Exp Neuropsychol.* 1995;17:682–690.

7. Snyder PJ, Novelly RA, Harris LJ. Mixed speech dominance in the Intracarotid Sodium Amytal Procedure: validity and criteria issues. *J Clin Exp Neuropsychol.* 1990;12:629–643.

8. Ravdin LD, Perrine K, Haywood CS, et al. Serial recovery of language during the intracarotid amobarbital procedure. *Brain Cogn.* 1997;33: 151–160.

9. Meador KJ. Ambiguous language in Wada evaluations. *Epilepsia.* 2004; 45(Suppl 4):24–25.

10. Loring DW, Meador KJ, Lee GP, et al. Cerebral language lateralization: evidence from intracarotid amobarbital testing. *Neuropsychologia.* 1990;28: 831–838.

11. Abou-Khalil B. An update on determination of language dominance in screening for epilepsy surgery: the Wada test and newer noninvasive alternatives. *Epilepsia.* 2007;48:442–455.

12. Penfield W, Milner B. Memory deficit produced by bilateral lesions in the hippocampal zone. *AMA Arch Neurol Psychiatry.* 1958;79:475–497.

13. Kneebone AC, Chelune GJ, Dinner DS, et al. Intracarotid amobarbital procedure as a predictor of material-specific memory change after anterior temporal lobectomy. *Epilepsia.* 1995;36:857–865.

14. Loddenkemper T. Quo vadis Wada? *Epilepsy Behav.* 2008;13:1–2.

15. Trenerry MR, Loring DW. Intracarotid amobarbital procedure. The Wada test. *Neuroimaging Clin N Am.* 1995;5:721–728.

16. Baxendale S, Thompson P, Harkness W, et al. Predicting memory decline following epilepsy surgery: a multivariate approach. *Epilepsia.* 2006;47: 1887–1894.

17. Testa SM, Ward J, Crone NE, et al. Stimulus type affects Wada memory performance. *Epilepsy Behav.* 2008;13:458–462.

18. Vingerhoets G, Miatton M, Vonck K, et al. Clinical relevance of memory performance during Wada is stimulus type dependent. *J Neurol Neurosurg Psychiatry.* 2006;77:272–274.

19. Vingerhoets G, Miatton M, Vonck K, et al. Memory performance during the intracarotid amobarbital procedure and neuropsychological assessment in medial temporal lobe epilepsy: the limits of material specificity. *Epilepsy Behav.* 2006;8:422–428.

20. Lancman ME, Benbadis S, Geller E, et al. Sensitivity and specificity of asymmetric recall on WADA test to predict outcome after temporal lobectomy. *Neurology.* 1998;50:455–459.

21. Rausch R, Langfitt JT. Memory evaluation during intracarotid amobarbital procedures. In: Luders H, ed. *Epilepsy Surgery.* New York: Raven Press; 1991:507–514.

22. Sperling MR, Saykin AJ, Glosser G, et al. Predictors of outcome after anterior temporal lobectomy: the intracarotid amobarbital test. *Neurology.* 1994;44:2325–2330.

23. Loring DW, Meador KJ, Lee GP, et al. Wada memory performance predicts seizure outcome following anterior temporal lobectomy. *Neurology.* 1994;44:2322–2324.

24. Wieshmann UC, Larkin D, Varma T, et al. Predictors of outcome after temporal lobectomy for refractory temporal lobe epilepsy. *Acta Neurol Scand.* 2008;118:306–312.

25. Dinner D. Use of the intracarotid amobarbital procedure in the lateralization of the epileptogenic zone. In: Luders H, Comair Y, eds. *Epilepsy Surgery.* 2nd ed. Philadelphia: Lipincott, Williams and Wilkins; 2001.

26. Engel J, Jr., Rausch R, Lieb JP, et al. Correlation of criteria used for localizing epileptic foci in patients considered for surgical therapy of epilepsy. *Ann Neurol.* 1981;9:215–224.

27. Wyllie E, Naugle R, Awad I, et al. Intracarotid amobarbital procedure: I. Prediction of decreased modality-specific memory scores after temporal lobectomy. *Epilepsia.* 1991;32:857–864.

28. Haag A, Knake S, Hamer HM, et al. The Wada test in Austrian, Dutch, German, and Swiss epilepsy centers from 2000 to 2005: a review of 1421 procedures. *Epilepsy Behav.* 2008;13:83–89.

29. Baxendale S, Thompson PJ, Duncan JS. The role of the Wada test in the surgical treatment of temporal lobe epilepsy: an international survey. *Epilepsia.* 2008;49:715–720. Discussion 720–715.

30. Salanova V, Markand O, Worth R. Focal functional deficits in temporal lobe epilepsy on PET scans and the intracarotid amobarbital procedure: comparison of patients with unitemporal epilepsy with those requiring intracranial recordings. *Epilepsia.* 2001;42:198–203.

31. Spencer DC, Morrell MJ, Risinger MW. The role of the intracarotid amobarbital procedure in evaluation of patients for epilepsy surgery. *Epilepsia.* 2000;41:320–325.

32. Lombroso CT, Erba G. A test for separating secondary from primary bilateral synchrony in epileptic subjects. *Trans Am Neurol Assoc.* 1969;94:204–209.

33. Lombroso CT, Erba G. Primary and secondary bilateral synchrony in epilepsy; a clinical and electroencephalographic study. *Arch Neurol.* 1970; 22:321–334.

34. Delazer M, Karner E, Unterberger I, et al. Language and arithmetic–a study using the intracarotid amobarbital procedure. *Neuroreport.* 2005; 16:1403–1405.

35. Grote CL, Wierenga C, Smith MC, et al. Wada difference a day makes: interpretive cautions regarding same-day injections. *Neurology.* 1999;52: 1577–1582.

36. Selwa LM, Buchtel HA, Henry TR. Electrocerebral recovery during the intracarotid amobarbital procedure: influence of interval between injections. *Epilepsia.* 1997;38:1294–1299.

37. Bengner T, Haettig H, Merschhemke M, et al. Memory assessment during the intracarotid amobarbital procedure: influence of injection order. *Neurology.* 2003;61:1582–1587.

38. Loring DW, Meador KJ, Lee GP. Amobarbital dose effects on Wada Memory testing. *J Epilepsy.* 1992;5:171–174.

39. Baxendale S, Thompson P. Amobarbital dose effects on the intracarotid amobarbital procedure. *Epilepsia.* 1996;37:134.

40. Loring DW, Meador KJ, Lee GP, et al. Stimulus timing effects on Wada memory testing. *Arch Neurol.* 1994;51:806–810.

41. Loring DW, Meador KJ, Lee GP, et al. Wada memory and timing of stimulus presentation. *Epilepsy Res.* 1997;26:461–464.

42. Morris RG, Polkey CE, Cox T. Independent recovery of memory and language functioning during the intracarotid sodium amytal test. *J Clin Exp Neuropsychol.* 1998;20:433–444.

43. Bookheimer S, Schrader LM, Rausch R, et al. Reduced anesthetization during the intracarotid amobarbital (Wada) test in patients taking carbonic anhydrase-inhibiting medications. *Epilepsia.* 2005;46:236–243.

44. Muller J, Shaw L. Arterial vascularization of the human hippocampus. 1. extracerebral relationships. *Arch Neurol.* 1965;13:45–47.

45. Yasargil MG, Teddy PJ, Roth P. Selective amygdalo-hippocampectomy. Operative anatomy and surgical technique. *Adv Tech Stand Neurosurg.* 1985;12:93–123.

46. Jack CR Jr., Nichols DA, Sharbrough FW, et al. Selective posterior cerebral artery Amytal test for evaluating memory function before surgery for temporal lobe seizure. *Radiology.* 1988;168:787–793.

47. Jack CR Jr., Nichols DA, Sharbrough FW, et al. Selective posterior cerebral artery injection of amytal: new method of preoperative memory testing. *Mayo Clin Proc.* 1989;64:965–975.

48. Loddenkemper T, Moddel G, Pestana E, et al. Intracarotid amobarbital test in children. *Epilepsia.* 2005;46:308–309.

49. Hinz AC, Berger MS, Ojemann GA, et al. The utility of the intracarotid Amytal procedure in determining hemispheric speech lateralization in pediatric epilepsy patients undergoing surgery. *Childs Nerv Syst.* 1994;10: 239–243.

50. Szabo CA, Wyllie E. Intracarotid amobarbital testing for language and memory dominance in children. *Epilepsy Res.* 1993;15:239–246.

51. Williams J, Rausch R. Factors in children that predict performance on the intracarotid amobarbital procedure. *Epilepsia.* 1992;33:1036–1041.

52. Lee GP, Westerveld M, Blackburn LB, et al. Prediction of verbal memory decline after epilepsy surgery in children: effectiveness of Wada memory asymmetries. *Epilepsia.* 2005;46:97–103.

53. Mani J, Busch R, Kubu C, et al. Wada memory asymmetry scores and postoperative memory outcome in left temporal epilepsy. *Seizure.* 2008;17: 691–698.

54. Lee GP, Park YD, Westerveld M, et al. Effect of Wada methodology in predicting lateralized memory impairment in pediatric epilepsy surgery candidates. *Epilepsy Behav.* 2002;3:439–447.

55. Andelman F, Kipervasser S, Reider G II, et al. Hippocampal memory function as reflected by the intracarotid sodium methohexital Wada test. *Epilepsy Behav.* 2006;9:579–586.

56. Buchtel HA, Passaro EA, Selwa LM, et al. Sodium methohexital (brevital) as an anesthetic in the Wada test. *Epilepsia.* 2002;43:1056–1061.

57. Loddenkemper T, Moddel G, Dinner D, et al. Language assessment in Wada test: comparison of methohexital and amobarbital. *Seizure.* 2009; 18:656–659.

58. Takayama M, Miyamoto S, Ikeda A, et al. Intracarotid propofol test for speech and memory dominance in man. *Neurology.* 2004;63:510–515.

59. Mikati M, Naasan G, Tarabay H, et al. Intracarotid propofol testing: a comparative study with amobarbital. *Epilepsy and Behav.* 2009;14:503–507.

60. Jones-Gotman M, Sziklas V, Djordjevic J, et al. Etomidate speech and memory test (eSAM): a new drug and improved intracarotid procedure. *Neurology.* 2005;65:1723–1729.

61. Yetkin FZ, Swanson S, Fischer M, et al. Functional MR of frontal lobe activation: comparison with Wada language results. *Am J Neuroradiol.* 1998; 19:1095–1098.

62. Woermann FG, Jokeit H, Luerding R, et al. Language lateralization by Wada test and fMRI in 100 patients with epilepsy. *Neurology.* 2003;61:699–701.

63. Gaillard WD, Balsamo L, Xu B, et al. Language dominance in partial epilepsy patients identified with an fMRI reading task. *Neurology.* 2002; 59:256–265.

64. Stern CE, Sherman SJ, Kirchhoff BA, et al. Medial temporal and prefrontal contributions to working memory tasks with novel and familiar stimuli. *Hippocampus.* 2001;11:337–346.

65. Janszky J, Jokeit H, Kontopoulou K, et al. Functional MRI predicts memory performance after right mesiotemporal epilepsy surgery. *Epilepsia.* 2005;46:244–250.

66. Golby AJ, Poldrack RA, Illes J, et al. Memory lateralization in medial temporal lobe epilepsy assessed by functional MRI. *Epilepsia.* 2002;43: 855–863.

67. Loddenkemper T, Morris HH, Moddel G. Complications during the Wada test. *Epilepsy Behav.* 2008;13:551–553.

68. Baxendale S. Amnesia in temporal lobectomy patients: historical perspective and review. *Seizure.* 1998;7:15–24.

69. Girvin J, McGlone J, McLachlan R, et al. Validity of the sodium amobarbital test for memory in selected patients. *Epilepsia.* 1987;28:636.

70. Barr W, Schaul N, Decker R, et al. Post operative amnesia after "passing" memory testing during the intracarotid amobarbital procedure. *Epilepsia.* 1992;33:138.

71. Loddenkemper T, Morris HH, Lineweaver TT, et al. Repeated intracarotid amobarbital tests. *Epilepsia.* 2007;48:553–558.

72. Loring DW, Hermann BP, Perrine K, et al. Effect of Wada memory stimulus type in discriminating lateralized temporal lobe impairment. *Epilepsia.* 1997;38:219–224.

73. Baxendale SA, Thompson PJ, Duncan JS. Evidence-based practice: a reevaluation of the intracarotid amobarbital procedure (Wada test). *Arch Neurol.* 2008;65:841–845.

74. Rausch R, Silfenius H, Wieser H-G, et al. Intraarterial amobarbital procedures. In: Engel J, ed. *Surgical Treatment of the Epilepsies.* New York: Raven Press; 1993:341–358.

75. Helmstaedter C. The role of the Wada test in the surgical treatment of temporal lobe epilepsy: an international perspective–commentary on Baxendale, et al. *Epilepsia.* 2008;49:720–722.

CHAPTER 81 ■ INTRACRANIAL ELECTROENCEPHALOGRAPHY AND LOCALIZATION STUDIES

FERNANDO L. VALE AND SELIM R. BENBADIS

Recent advances in neuroimaging have improved the diagnosis and treatment of intractable epilepsy. Subtle epileptogenic lesions such as focal cortical dysplasias, heterotopias, and, even, hippocampal sclerosis are better identified with high-resolution magnetic resonance imaging (MRI). When concordant information is obtained among extracranial electroencephalogram (EEG), video recordings, and radiographic findings, success from surgical intervention remains high. Unfortunately, extracranial EEG has its limitations, and sometimes focal EEG findings are not well defined. In situations where discordant information is obtained, or poorly defined epileptogenic areas are found in noninvasive testing, or in cases of close proximity of the epileptogenic zone to eloquent cortex, the need from chronically implantable invasive electrodes becomes an acceptable alternative. Invasive electrodes should be part of the team's amentarium in the evaluation of intractable epilepsy. The success of epilepsy surgery depends on the identification of a focal epileptogenic zone and invasive recordings may offer in-depth evaluation for patients that may otherwise have no other option.

EXTRACRANIAL ELECTROENCEPHALOGRAPHY: THE STARTING POINT

The questions to be answered with intracranial electrodes are shaped by the results of the noninvasive evaluation, including extracranial EEG (1,2). Surface EEG provides a broad survey of EEG rhythms throughout both hemispheres and should be designed to yield the maximum localizing information about the epileptogenic zone (3). As an example, the combination of extracranial EEG and sphenoidal electrodes (Fig. 81.1) may be helpful when mesial temporal lobe epilepsy is suspected. More generally, surface EEG–video monitoring is the starting point for any patient whose seizures continue frequently despite medications, since some patients (20% to 30% of adults) will be shown to have nonepileptic (psychogenic) seizures.

The main limitation of extracranial EEG is decreased sensitivity to cortical generators (2,3). Intracranial electrodes overcome the sensitivity limitations of extracranial electrodes because they are closer to the cortical focus and free of the dampening effect of the skull and scalp. This increased sensitivity, however, is at the expense of more restricted sampling, or "vision," and involves an enhanced risk of complications.

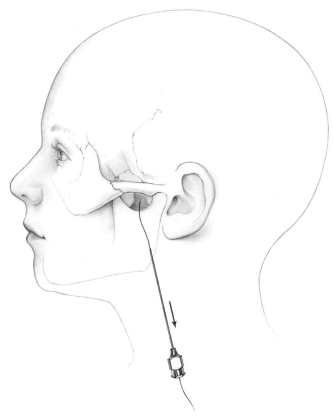

FIGURE 81.1 Placement of a sphenoidal electrode. A thin electrode wire is introduced into the subtemporal fossa within a 22-gauge lumbar puncture needle. After the needle is inserted to a depth of 3 to 5 cm, the cannula is withdrawn and the wire is left in place. The wire is looped and taped into place on the cheek, and the distal end soldered to connectors for use in the electrode jackbox.

Intracranial EEG may fail to define further the epileptogenic zone if problem areas are insufficiently covered, but the use of large numbers of electrodes is limited by the proportional increase in the rate of complications. For this reason, intracranial electrodes should be used only after noninvasive testing (i.e., EEG, video semiology, and imaging) has "narrowed down" the epileptogenic zone to a limited brain region that can be covered safely and adequately by the chosen invasive technique.

The strength of the hypothesis (based on the results of the noninvasive evaluation) is a key to successful use of invasive techniques. The clearer the question formulated for testing, the greater the chance of success with the invasive evaluation.

This chapter provides an overview of the invasive techniques available for these difficult cases, and reviews the major clinical situations and how they can be approached.

INTRACRANIAL ELECTRODES: AN OVERVIEW

Depth and subdural electrodes are the two types of intracranial electrodes used most commonly. Improvement in neuroradiology (high-resolution MRI) and neuronavigation (frame and frameless stereotaxis) allows for better surgical coverage (more accurate placement) and most likely a lower complication rate. The surgeon's clinical experience, in addition to the clinical findings, is also important for surgical planning.

DEPTH ELECTRODES

Surgical Aspects

Depth electrodes are multiple-contact "needles" of polyurethane or other material that typically are inserted into the brain by way of twist-drill skull holes under stereotactic guidance (4–9). Modern computer-assisted image-based stereotaxy has greatly improved the ease and precision of depth electrode placement. A target is chosen on the MRI or CT scan, and entry point, trajectory, and depth are calculated by the computer to result in precise placement of the electrode tip within 1 to 2 mm of the target. Framed or frameless stereotaxis allows for a more precise target placement.

A common approach for patients with suspected bitemporal epilepsy uses three electrodes placed under stereotaxis guidance, each with eight contacts that are advanced transversely through punctures in the middle or inferior temporal gyri into the amygdala and anterior and posterior hippocampus on each side (Fig. 81.2). These allow the survey of electrical activity from the mesial structures, from infolded gray matter of basal temporal gyri, and from the lateral temporal lobe.

An alternative trajectory for the evaluation of mesial temporal epilepsy is the longitudinal placement of depth electrodes by way of occipital burr holes (10,11). Usually placed with framed stereotaxis under local or general anesthesia, in this approach the electrode traverses the course of the hippocampus along its axis, sampling electrical activity throughout its length. Extratemporal foci are surveyed by carefully locating the electrodes according to structural lesions or particular gyri with suspected involvement in the epileptogenic zone (12).

Depth electrodes may be placed under local or general anesthesia (with the help of neuronavigation), with the latter preferred for lengthy procedures involving multiple insertions, and can be removed under local anesthesia. Previous insertion of depth electrodes does not significantly limit further options of epilepsy surgery, including the subsequent use of other electrode types.

Advantages

The main advantage is direct access to deep structures for EEG recording very close to potential generators (13–15). Electrodes can be left in place for days to weeks with minimal risk of infection, permitting extensive ictal recording. Ictal

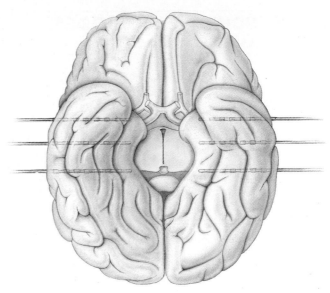

FIGURE 81.2 Bitemporal depth electrodes. In this array, three multi-contact electrodes are inserted on each side so that the contacts distal to the insertion site lie within the amygdale, anterior hippocampus, and posterior hippocampus. The contacts most proximal to the insertion site lie within the lateral cortex of the middle temporal gyrus. Other arrays place electrodes in an anterior–posterior or superior–inferior orientation.

EEG onset with depth electrodes often precedes onset with scalp and sphenoidal electrodes by 20 or 30 seconds, and in some cases, especially auras, the EEG seizure pattern may be seen only with depth recording. Depth electrodes may clearly locate seizure onset when extracranial localization is unclear. In addition to seizure onset, seizure termination may also have localizing and prognostic value, with unilateral termination (as opposed to simultaneous bilateral, contralateral, or mixed termination) predicting better outcome following temporal lobectomy (16).

Disadvantages

Depth electrodes sample only a relatively small brain region, providing a very detailed but also "very" focused EEG sample. This focus may be inadequate when the issue is localization of seizure onset within a relatively large region such as the frontal lobe. In addition, placement requires brain penetration. This raises theoretical concerns about damage to cortical areas outside the resection site and also makes depth electrodes inappropriate for the study of potential epileptogenic foci near vascular malformations. The examination of resected tissues has revealed gliosis, cystic degeneration, or microabscesses along the tracks of depth electrodes, but several studies (11) have failed to demonstrate any functional sequelae in the absence of clinically apparent bleeding or infection, and overall depth electrodes are safe (4,17).

The risk of bleeding or infection is only 0.5% to 5% (13,18). Routine imaging studies commonly reveal asymptomatic subdural collections of blood, but intraparenchymal hemorrhage is very rare (less than 1% in series (4,7,11) using modern stereotactic techniques). The risk of significant hemorrhage is decreased by careful attention to electrode trajectories on preoperative planning studies so as to avoid major vascular structures.

SUBDURAL ELECTRODES (GRIDS AND STRIPS)

Surgical Aspects

Probably the most commonly used invasive electrodes, subdural electrodes are embedded in strips or sheets of polyurethane or other material, and may be implanted subdurally over epileptogenic regions (Fig. 81.3) (19–24). These disks of stainless steel or platinum alloy, approximately 2 to 4 mm in diameter, are embedded in polyurethane at fixed interelectrode distances, typically 10 mm, in various arrays. The strips and grids include one or more cables with bundled insulated wires connecting to the individual electrodes. Cables can be connected by means of various interface blocks to conventional EEG equipment for recording and stimulation. Other subdural grids have been designed with electrode contacts on both sides of the polyurethane sheet for recording from both surfaces, as in interhemispheric locations.

Strips are usually inserted under frameless stereotaxis guidance through individual burr holes or trephines for bilateral placement when the side of seizure onset must be determined. Neuronavigation techniques allow for more accurate placement of the subdural electrodes. The cables exit through a stab wound separate from the main incision to assist with anchoring of the strip and to decrease cerebrospinal fluid leakage and infection. Subdural strips may be placed under local or general anesthesia, although general anesthesia is preferred for multiple burr holes and multiple strip insertions. The risk of infection and hemorrhage with insertion of subdural strips has been reported to be less than 1% (10). Because mobility of implanted subdural strips may change the position of electrodes in relation to the intended recording target, serial skull roentgenograms should be performed to verify stability of position.

Grids are inserted by way of open craniotomy (Fig. 81.4). Flap design allows coverage of all regions of suspected epileptogenicity and subsequent access to any possible resection to the region of interest. Subdural plates may be "slid" beyond the edges of the craniotomy to cover adjacent areas, including basal temporal, basal frontal, and interhemispheric regions. Subdural grids are sutured to the overlying dura mater to prevent movement. A water-tight dural closure around the electrode cables lessens the possibility of cerebrospinal fluid leakage. If possible, the overlying bone flap should be osteoplastic (attached to a vascularized muscle and periosteal pedicle) to prevent flap osteomyelitis. The electrode cable exits through a stab wound separate from the main incision, and water-tight sutures are used at the exit site to reduce cerebrospinal fluid leakage. Despite these precautions, minor leakage frequently occurs without serious complications.

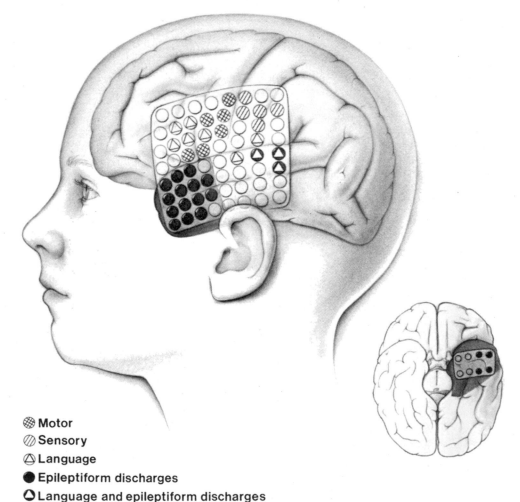

⊛ **Motor**
⦸ **Sensory**
△ **Language**
● **Epileptiform discharges**
◖ **Language and epileptiform discharges**

FIGURE 81.3 Results of electroencephalography (EEG) and cortical stimulation with subdural electrode grids. With scalp and sphenoidal EEG, this patient had epileptiform discharges from the anterior and posterior left temporal lobe. Extraoperative subdural EEG showed interictal sharp waves from anterolateral, posterolateral, and basal temporal areas. Seizures arose from anterior and basal temporal regions. The posterior temporal area with interictal sharp waves was within Wernicke language area, so this region was left untouched by the extensive left temporal lobectomy. Resection extended 7.5 cm posteriorly from the anterior temporal tip. Histopathologic examination of resected tissue showed cortical dysplasia; the magnetic resonance imaging techniques at that time were not adequate to reveal the subtle malformation. The patient remains seizure-free on medication 12 years after surgery but has had seizures when medications were withdrawn.

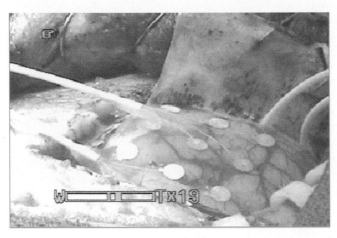

FIGURE 81.4 Temporal craniotomy with intraoperative placement of a subdural grid. Note the cable connecting the contacts to the EEG amplifier, and the retracted dura matter in the upper portion.

After completion of the evaluation with subdural electrodes, the patient is returned to the operating room for reopening of the craniotomy, removal of the subdural electrodes, and final resection of the mapped epileptogenic zone. This second operation typically is performed using general anesthesia, although local anesthesia is an option when further brain mapping is necessary. At reoperation, cultures are obtained from all layers of the wound, all electrode hardware, and the bone flap. If bacterial colonization of one or more wound layers is observed, the patient receives vigorous intravenous antibiotic therapy directed against the cultured organism(s) for 2 weeks following removal of the electrodes to reduce the risk of flap osteomyelitis.

Subdural grids have the greatest potential for complications, with an overall rate of 26% (25). These include infection (12%), transient neurologic deficit (11%), epidural hematoma (2.5%), increased intracranial pressure (2.5%), infarction (1.5%), and death (0.5%). Complication occurrence is associated with greater number of grids/electrodes (especially >60 electrodes), longer duration of monitoring (especially >10 days), older age of the patient, left-sided grid insertion, and burr holes in addition to the craniotomy. Improvements in grid technology, surgical technique, and postoperative care may reduce the complication rate (21,25–27).

OTHER TECHNIQUES

Foramen ovale and epidural peg electrodes are not commonly used due to limited sensitivity, but both techniques can be a useful adjunct to more invasive procedures (5). They are considered less accurate but safer when compared to subdural or depth electrode placement. Intraventricular electrode is another technique that involves endoscopically placed temporal horn electrodes. Frameless image guidance can be used to place a 10-contact depth electrode through a rigid neuroendoscope within the atrium of the lateral ventricle. Invasiveness is less than transcortical depth electrode placement, and complications may be fewer (28). Another less-known technique is cavernous sinus electrodes. This newer semi-invasive option may be useful for lateralization of temporal lobe epilepsy (29). Wire electrodes can be placed in the cavernous sinus (CS) and the superior petrosal sinus (SPS), via the jugular vein.

FUNCTIONAL LOCALIZATION STUDIES

Functional studies for mapping eloquent cortex (motor, sensory and language) are frequently used when the suspected seizure generator is in close proximity. Resection of the epileptogenic focus with preservation of function is the goal in this situation. Also, intra- or extraoperative electrocorticography is a helpful technique for better delineation of the epileptic zone.

Functional localization techniques with subdural electrodes include cortical stimulation and evoked potential studies. The addition of neuronavigation during surgical planning allows for accurate placement of contact electrodes along the suspected cortical surface. This is followed by cortical stimulation, which involves passage of a small electrical current through individual electrodes with close observation for symptoms or interference of cortical function. An alternating current is applied for 5 to 10 seconds with subsequent stepwise advancement from 1 mA to a maximum of 15 mA, until symptoms developed or afterdischarges are identified on EEG. Symptoms during stimulation may include positive motor phenomena (tonic or clonic contraction of a muscle group), negative motor phenomena (inhibition of voluntary movements of the tongue, fingers, or toes), somatosensory phenomena (tingling, tightness, or numbness of a part of the body), or language impairment (speech hesitation or arrest, anomia, or receptive difficulties). To screen for negative motor or language impairment during stimulation, the patient may be challenged to read or perform rapid alternating movements of the fingers, toes, or tongue. Signs or symptoms during stimulation of an electrode are interpreted to mean that the underlying cortex has importance for the affected function.

In another method of functional localization (30), median or posterior tibial evoked potentials may be recorded directly from the cortical surface by means of subdural electrodes, with maximum amplitudes over the postcentral gyrus. Results may confirm rolandic sensorimotor localization by cortical stimulation.

In addition to mapping eloquent cortex, stimulation may also be helpful in localizing epileptogenic cortex. Following single pulse stimulation, "early responses" (starting within 100 ms after the stimulus) are found in all areas of cortex, delayed responses (spikes or sharp waves occurring between 100 ms and 1 s after stimulation) appear to be significantly associated with the epileptogenic zone (31).

EXTRAOPERATIVE ELECTROCORTICOGRAPHY AND FUNCTIONAL MAPPING

Advantages

Extraoperative functional mapping requires placement of surface subdural electrodes (grids or strips) for seizure recordings and bedside mapping. This is a useful technique for patients in whom further localization studies are required or who are not able to tolerate intraoperative testing (anxious patients or patients who refused awake surgery).

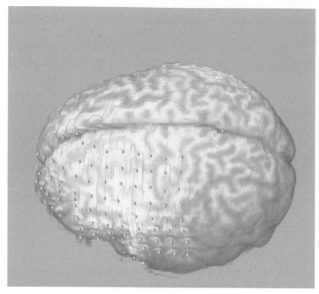
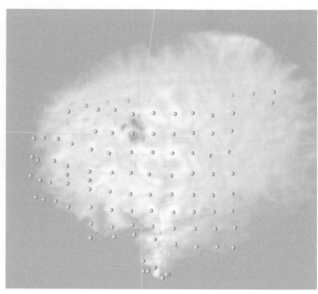

FIGURE 81.5 A 12-year-old female with 2-year history of left frontal lobe epilepsy underwent invasive evaluation with subdural grid electrodes. Preoperative MRI showed a hyperintense lesion on the FLAIR and T2 weighted images in the left superior frontal gyrus extending to the ependymal surface of the lateral ventricle. **A:** A volume-rendered brain image of the patient constructed from the postoperative three-dimensional T1-weighted MRI. Electrode location was identified by flow-void artifacts and coregistered on the image (dots). The lateral convexity of the frontal lobe is covered by an 8 by 8 array with 1 cm interelectrode spacing. **B:** The relationship of the lesion (shaded area) to the electrode. The FLAIR images were linearly overlaid on the same 3D MRI, and the hyperintense lesion was highlighted after making the T1 volume translucent. The lesion is located beneath the first two electrodes in the third column from the anterior superior edge. The EEG seizure onset of her habitual seizure (aura and right arm tonic seizure) was recorded from these electrodes as well as from the mesial frontal electrodes. The patient underwent resection of the superior and middle frontal gyri including the lesion. The pathological diagnosis was consistent with cortical dysplasia.

Subdural electrodes permit detailed definition of the epileptogenic zone in relation to eloquent cortex (Fig. 81.5). Epileptiform discharges may be recorded during wakefulness, sleep, and seizures and then mapped to define the safest, most complete resection of epileptogenic zones (23,24). Ictal EEG patterns are usually well defined if electrodes are over the epileptogenic zone. There is some evidence (at least for temporal lobe seizures) that the time from EEG onset to clinical onset has a prognostic value (32).

In infants and young children, cortical stimulation studies are more challenging. Sensory, negative motor, and language function cannot be assessed reliably during stimulation in infants. Special stimulation paradigms are required to elicit positive motor effects in children younger than 3 or 4 years (30,33). Evoked potential studies with subdural electrodes may help to identify the postcentral gyrus at any age.

Disadvantages

The risks of wound infection and flap osteomyelitis are the main disadvantages of chronically implanted subdural electrode grids. The incidence of 5% to 15% (21,23,24) about a decade ago has decreased in recent years, but occasional infections have occurred despite compulsive intraoperative culturing of all wound layers and vigorous prophylactic use of antibiotics. Infection may be less frequent with subdural strips (33) than with grids.

Other complications of subdural electrodes—acute meningitis, cerebral edema, and hemorrhage—are rare. Meningitis necessitates immediate electrode removal and vigorous antibiotic therapy. Brain edema can, rarely, be symptomatic, requiring early removal of electrodes, but usually it can be

successfully combated with judicious fluid and electrolyte management. Occurring in approximately 2% of patients, subdural or epidural hemorrhage may prompt premature removal of electrodes and evacuation of hemorrhage.

Concerns about intracranial pressure limit the number of subdural electrodes, so that only restricted unilateral cortical areas can be covered with grids. Strips can cover widespread areas through multiple burr holes, but mobility of the strips can be a problem and blind insertion of the strips may be impeded by subdural scarring or other structural lesions.

INTRAOPERATIVE ELECTROCORTICOGRAPHY AND FUNCTIONAL MAPPING

Surgical Aspects

Intraoperative electrocorticography (ECoG), the recording from electrodes placed directly over exposed cortex after craniotomy (34,35), can be performed with the patient under local anesthesia (fully awake) or under general anesthesia. General anesthetic agents may affect the ECoG, so the anesthesiologist needs to discontinue all inhalation agents approximately 30 minutes before the recording. Intravenous narcotics and nitrous oxide are continued to maintain a state of manageable general anesthesia without potential effects of inhalation agents.

Intraoperative ECoG may (occasionally) include the recording of evoked potentials to localize the rolandic fissure and orient the surgeon toward gyral anatomy so as to avoid resections in functional motor or sensory areas. Interictal epileptiform activity can be recorded for a stated period to define a zone of frequent interictal spiking. This may help the surgeon tailor the resection for maximal excision of areas with frequent interictal epileptiform activity. Surgical manipulation itself, however, may create some spike activity ("injury spikes"), and the practice of "chasing spikes" to maximize resection has not been shown convincingly to improve the outcome of resective epilepsy procedures. Most investigators have found that spikes on postresection ECoG do not reliably predict a less favorable outcome in temporal lobe resections (22,36–42). Preexcision spikes on three or more gyri that persist after resection, especially at a distance from the resection border, carry a poor prognosis, at least in nontumoral frontal lobe epilepsy (42).

Intraoperative cortical stimulation can delineate areas of primary motor, sensory, and speech function under local anesthesia. Even under light general anesthesia (without paralytic agents), this technique can reliably identify primary motor areas by allowing direct observation of clonic or tonic movement in respective muscle groups, assisting in tailored resections close to motor regions.

Advantages

Intraoperative techniques permit definition of functional cortex in relation to the epileptogenic zone while avoiding the potential complications of long-term invasive electrodes. The procedure lengthens the operating time but otherwise imparts no added risk to the patient. Detailed intraoperative cortical stimulation under local anesthesia is readily performed in cooperative adolescents and adults (39), but it is more difficult in young children or uncooperative adults. Even in young or difficult patients, however, it is usually possible to identify primary motor cortex intraoperatively with cortical stimulation and evoked potential studies using light general anesthesia (47).

Disadvantages

Because the total recording time of intraoperative techniques is limited to a few hours, recording during seizures is almost never obtained. Another limitation to intraoperative techniques is the stressful nature of the conditions for cortical stimulation while the patient is awake.

COMMON CLINICAL SCENARIOS

Suspected Bilateral Mesial Temporal Lobe Epilepsy

The need for invasive EEG in temporal lobe epilepsy has diminished as more powerful MRI has enhanced identification of hippocampal pathology. Nevertheless, bilateral mesial temporal lobe epilepsy is the most common indication for depth electrodes implanted into the amygdala and anterior and posterior hippocampus on both sides (15,43).

Bitemporal strips may also be used in this setting. Some authors (38) have found that subdural and depth electrodes are comparably sensitive for detection of interictal spikes in both mesial and neocortical temporal lobe epilepsy. Depth electrodes, however, are the only ones to lie within the mesial epileptogenic cortex, and thus may better allow detection of mesial-onset seizures than do subdural strips, which can reach only the parahippocampal gyrus (44,45). For example, studies that used both methods simultaneously reported cases in which bitemporal strips failed to provide adequate information to proceed with surgery (45–47), and occasionally subdural strips can even be falsely lateralizing (48). Only depth electrodes reliably record faster frequencies at onset (49,50), suggesting closer proximity to the generator. Although depth electrodes probably remain the gold standard for recording hippocampal onset, subdural strips are probably adequate when the issue is only lateralization of temporal lobe epilepsy (51). When extratemporal onset is a concern (e.g., in the setting of an extratemporal lesion of uncertain relevance), a combination of depth and subdural electrodes is appropriate (10,12,52).

Epileptogenic Zone Near Eloquent Cortex

Subdural electrodes are the method of choice whenever eloquent cortex must be clearly separated from the epileptogenic zone. For example, subdural electrodes may be used to define a frontal or parietal focus in relation to rolandic sensorimotor areas, a left lateral temporal focus in relation to Wernicke's language area, or a mesial frontal or parietal focus in relation to the supplementary motor area and primary motor cortex for the leg.

Although either extraoperative or intraoperative technique can be used to resolve such localization problems, the considerable variability in preferred methods depends largely on the familiarity of the surgery team with each approach. In general, intraoperative techniques may be preferable when the primary objective is localization of rolandic motor areas, for example, in preparation for anatomic frontal lobectomy or lesionectomy. In fact, intraoperative mapping is often used before resection in patients without seizures. Extraoperative techniques may be preferable if ictal recording is required to define the epileptogenic zone. The two techniques can also be combined, with extraoperative seizure recording followed by intraoperative mapping just before resection.

Poor Localization of Epileptogenic Zone

Hemisphere Known but Exact Localization Uncertain

A relatively common scenario is that the results of the noninvasive evaluation unequivocally point to a hemisphere, but the lobe cannot be confidently identified. In these patients, prognosis for surgical outcome is typically guarded, but an attempt to better define the epileptogenic zone with invasive techniques may be appropriate in some cases. Outcome sometimes can be excellent. Because this requires coverage of large areas on one side, grids can be combined with strips or depth electrodes. Depth EEG has been used, with good results, to resolve other discrete localization issues such as mesial temporal versus orbitofrontal or cingulate seizure onset. In these cases, depth and subdural electrodes may be used together (46,52), especially for a presumed extratemporal onset such as orbitofrontal (10) or occipital (12,53).

In the presence of a lesion apparent on MRI, even subtle lesions such as a suspected cortical dysplasia, invasive EEG may not be necessary (54). However, any lesion should not be assumed to be the source of the seizures ("dual pathology"), as some are often incidental (e.g., arachnoid cysts). If there is an extratemporal lesion but electroclinical data (EEG-video) suggest temporal onset, or there is MRI evidence for mesiotemporal sclerosis but electroclinical data suggest extratemporal onset, then invasive EEG (strips or grids) is needed.

Scenarios When Intracranial Localization May Be Limited

Although most cases of extratemporal onset involve difficult intrahemispheric localization, lateralization is occasionally at issue. This is particularly common in seizures arising from the supplementary sensorimotor area, where symptomatology and midline epileptiform discharges indicate mesial frontal onset, but lateralization is unclear in the absence of imaging abnormalities or clinical lateralizing signs (55). These cases are very challenging and may be difficult to clarify even with invasive EEG.

When the noninvasive presurgical evaluation does not sufficiently narrow the possibilities for localization, invasive studies may be of limited benefit.

CONCLUSIONS

With the advent of modern neuroimaging, the use of invasive electrodes has diminished. Presurgical evaluation strategies in patients with localization-related epilepsy remain variable and controversial. No universal scheme is accepted by all epilepsy surgery centers, and techniques continue to evolve (56). In each case, the decisions whether or not to use an invasive technique and, if so, which one should be based on results of an extensive noninvasive evaluation including extracranial EEG, video/seizure semiology analysis, structural and functional neuroimaging, and neuropsychological testing. Appreciating the brain coverage, strengths, and weaknesses of each invasive technique will help in this choice. In addition, the risk of invasive techniques varies among surgeons; as with other types of surgical procedures, experience and successful practice are important. Advancement in neuronavigation techniques allows for more accurate placement of the electrodes with less complication rate. Of course, the lowest complication rates can be expected from experienced epilepsy neurosurgeons at high-volume epilepsy surgery centers.

ACKNOWLEDGMENT

The drawings in this chapter are original art by Elaine Bammerlin.

References

1. Lüders H, Dinner DS, Morris HH, et al. EEG evaluation for epilepsy surgery in children. *Cleve Clin J Med.* 1989;56:S53–S61.
2. Jayakar P, Duchowny M, Resnick TJ. Localization of seizure foci: pitfalls and caveats. *J Clin Neurophysiol.* 1991;8:414–431.
3. Foldvary-Schaefer N. Noninvasive electroencephalography in the evaluation of the ictal onset zone. In: Luders HO, ed. *Textbook of Epilepsy Surgery.* 1st ed. London, UK: Informa Healthcare; 2008:603–613.
4. Afif A, Chabardes S, Minotti L, et al. Safety and usefulness of insular depth electrodes implanted via an oblique approach in patients with epilepsy. *Neurosurgery.* 2008;62(5 Suppl 2):ONS471–ONS479. Discussion 479–480.
5. Kim OJ, Ahn JY, Lee BI. Analysis of electrical discharges made with the foramen ovale electrode recording technique in mesial temporal lobe epilepsy patients. *J Clin Neurophysiol.* 2004;21(6):391–398.
6. Mehta AD, Labar D, Dean A, et al. Frameless stereotactic placement of depth electrodes in epilepsy surgery. *J Neurosurg.* 2005;102(6):1040–1045.
7. Pillay PK, Barnett GH, Awad IA, et al. MRI-guided placement of depth electrodes in temporal lobe epilepsy: a comparison of the CRW and BRW arc systems. *Br J Neurosurg.* 1992;6:47–53.
8. Shenai MB, Ross DA, Sagher O. The use of multiplanar trajectory planning in the stereotactic placement of depth electrodes. *Neurosurgery.* 2007;60(4 Suppl 2):272–276. Discussion 276.
9. Spire WJ, Jobst BC, Thadani VM, et al. Robotic image-guided depth electrode implantation in the evaluation of medically intractable epilepsy. *Neurosurg Focus.* 2008;25(3):E19.
10. Blatt DR, Roper SN, Friedman WA. Invasive monitoring of limbic epilepsy using stereotactic depth and subdural strip electrodes: surgical technique. *Surg Neurol.* 1997;48:74–79.
11. Spencer DD. Stereotactic methods in the management of epilepsy. In: Heilbrun MP, ed. *Stereotactic Neurosurgery.* Baltimore, MD: Williams & Wilkins; 1988:161–178.
12. Palmini A, Andermann F, Dubeau F, et al. Occipitotemporal epilepsies: evaluation of selected patients requiring depth electrode studies and rationale for surgical approaches. *Epilepsia.* 1993;34:84–96.
13. So NK, Gloor P, Quesney F, et al. Depth electrode investigations in patients with bitemporal epileptiform abnormalities. *Ann Neurol.* 1989;25:423–431.
14. Spencer SS. Depth electroencephalography in selection of refractory epilepsy for surgery. *Ann Neurol.* 1981;9:207–214.
15. Spencer SS, Spencer DD, Williamson PD, et al. The localizing value of depth electroencephalography in 32 patients with refractory epilepsy. *Ann Neurol.* 1982;12:248–253.
16. Verma A, Lewis D, VanLandingham KE, et al. Lateralized seizure termination: relationship to outcome following anterior temporal lobectomy. *Epilepsy Res.* 2001;47:9–15.
17. Fernandez G, Hufnagel A, Van Roost D, et al. Safety of intrahippocampal depth electrodes for presurgical evaluation of patients with intractable epilepsy. *Epilepsia.* 1997;38:922–929.
18. Spencer SS. Controversies in epileptology. Depth vs. subdural electrode studies for unlocalized epilepsy. *J Epilepsy.* 1989;2:123–127.
19. Nair DR, Burgess R, McIntyre CC, et al. Chronic subdural electrodes in the management of epilepsy. *Clin Neurophysiol.* 2008;119(1):11–28. Epub 2007 Nov 26. Review.
20. Steven DA, Andrade-Souza YM, Burneo JG, et al. Insertion of subdural strip electrodes for the investigation of temporal lobe epilepsy. Technical note. *J Neurosurg.* 2007;106(6):1102–1106.
21. Van Gompel JJ, Worrell GA, Bell ML, et al. Intracranial electroencephalography with subdural grid electrodes: techniques, complications, and outcomes. *Neurosurgery.* 2008;63(3):498–505. Discussion 505–506.
22. Wyler AR, Walker G, Somes G. The morbidity of long-term seizure monitoring using subdural strip electrodes. *J Neurosurg.* 1991;74:734–737.
23. Wyllie E, Lüders H, Morris HH, et al. Clinical outcome after complete or partial cortical resection for intractable epilepsy. *Neurology.* 1987;37:1634–1641.
24. Wyllie E, Lüders H, Morris HH, et al. Subdural electrodes in the evaluation for epilepsy surgery in children and adults. *Neuropediatrics.* 1988;19:80–86.
25. Hamer HM, Morris HH, Mascha EJ, et al. Complications of invasive video-EEG monitoring with subdural grid electrodes. *Neurology.* 2002;58:97–103.
26. Onal C, Otsubo H, Araki T, et al. Complications of invasive subdural grid monitoring in children with epilepsy. *J Neurosurg.* 2003;98:1017–1026.
27. Simon SL, Telfeian A, Duhaime AC. Complications of invasive monitoring used in intractable pediatric epilepsy. *Pediatr Neurosurg.* 2003;38:47–52.
28. Song JK, Abou-Khalil B, Konrad PE. Intraventricular monitoring for temporal lobe epilepsy: report on technique and initial results in eight patients. *J Neurol Neurosurg Psychiatry.* 2003;74:561–565.
29. Kunieda T, Ikeda A, Mikuni N, et al. Use of cavernous sinus EEG in the detection of seizure onset and spread in mesial temporal lobe epilepsy. *Epilepsia.* 2000;41:1411–1419.
30. Nespeca M, Wyllie E, Lüders H, et al. Subdural electrodes in infants and young children. *J Epilepsy.* 1990;3(Suppl 1):107–124.
31. Valentin A, Anderson M, Alarcon G, et al. Responses to single pulse electrical stimulation identify epileptogenesis in the human brain in vivo. *Brain.* 2002;125(Pt 8):1709–1718.
32. Weinand ME, Kester MM, Labiner DM, et al. Time from ictal subdural EEG seizure onset to clinical seizure onset: prognostic value for selecting temporal lobectomy candidates. *Neurol Res.* 2001;23:599–604.
33. Jayakar P, Alvarez LA, Duchowny MS, et al. A safe and effective paradigm to functionally map the cortex in childhood. *J Clin Neurophysiol.* 1992;9:288–293.

34. Ojemann GA, Sutherling WW, Lesser RP, et al. Cortical stimulation. In: Engel J Jr, ed. *Surgical Treatment of the Epilepsies.* 2nd ed. New York, NY: Raven Press; 1993:399–414.

35. Penfield W, Jasper H. *Epilepsy and the Functional Anatomy of the Human Brain.* Boston, MA: Little, Brown & Co;1954.

36. Cascino GD, Trenerry MR, Jack CR, et al. Electrocorticography and temporal lobe epilepsy: relationship to quantitative MRI and operative outcome. *Epilepsia.* 1995;36:692.

37. Kanazawa O, Blume WT, Girvin JP. Significance of spikes at temporal lobe electrocorticography. *Epilepsia.* 1996;37:50–55.

38. Schwartz TH, Bazil CW, Walczak TS, et al. The predictive value of intraoperative electrocorticography in resections for limbic epilepsy associated with mesial temporal sclerosis. *Neurosurgery.* 1997;40:302–309.

39. Tran TA, Spencer SS, Javidan M, et al. Significance of spikes recorded on intraoperative electrocorticography in patients with brain tumor and epilepsy. *Epilepsia.* 1997;38:1132–1139.

40. Tran TA, Spencer SS, Marks D, et al. Significance of spikes recorded on electrocorticography in nonlesional medial temporal lobe epilepsy. *Ann Neurol.* 1995;38:763–770.

41. Tuunainen A, Nousiainen U, Mervaala E, et al. Postoperative EEG and electrocorticography: relation to clinical outcome in patients with temporal lobe surgery. *Epilepsia.* 1994;35:1165–1173.

42. Wennberg R, Quesney F, Olivier A, et al. Electrocorticography and outcome in frontal lobe epilepsy. *Electroencephalogr Clin Neurophysiol.* 1998;106:357–368.

43. So NK, Olivier A, Andermann F, et al. Results of surgical treatment in patients with bitemporal epileptiform abnormalities. *Ann Neurol.* 1989; 25:432–439.

44. Spencer SS, Spencer DD, Williamson PD, et al. Combined depth and subdural electrode investigation in uncontrolled epilepsy. *Neurology.* 1990;40: 74–79.

45. Sperling MR, O'Connor MJ. Comparison of depth and subdural electrodes in recording temporal lobe seizures. *Neurology.* 1989;39:1497–1504.

46. Brekelmans GJ, van Emde Boas W, Velis DN, et al. Comparison of combined versus subdural or intracerebral electrodes alone in presurgical focus localization. *Epilepsia.* 1998;39:1290–1301.

47. Eisenschenk S, Gilmore RL, Cibula JE, et al. Lateralization of temporal lobe foci: depth versus subdural electrodes. *Clin Neurophysiol.* 2001;112: 836–844.

48. Alsaadi TM, Laxer KD, Barbaro NM, et al. False lateralization by subdural electrodes in two patients with temporal lobe epilepsy. *Neurology.* 2001;57:532–534.

49. Spencer SS, Guimaraes P, Katz A, et al. Morphological patterns of seizures recorded intracranially. *Epilepsia.* 1992;33:537–545.

50. van Veelen CW, Debets RM, van Huffelen AC, et al. Combined use of subdural and intracerebral electrodes in preoperative evaluation of epilepsy. *Neurosurgery.* 1990;26:93–101.

51. Risinger MW, Gumnit RJ. Intracranial electrophysiologic studies. *Neuroimag Clin North Am.* 1995;5:559–573.

52. Privitera MD, Quinlan JG, Yeh H. Interictal spike detection comparing subdural and depth electrodes during electrocorticography. *Electroencephalogr Clin Neurophysiol.* 1990;76:379–387.

53. Caicoya AG, Macarrón J, Albísua J, et al. Tailored resections in occipital lobe epilepsy surgery guided by monitoring with subdural electrodes: characteristics and outcome. *Epilepsy Res.* 2007;77(1):1–10. Epub 2007 Oct 17.

54. Mariottini A, Lombroso CT, DeGirolami U, et al. Operative results without invasive monitoring in patients with frontal lobe epileptogenic lesions. *Epilepsia.* 2001;42:1308–1315.

55. Laich E, Kuzniecky R, Mountz J, et al. Supplementary sensorimotor area epilepsy. Seizure localization, cortical propagation and subcortical activation pathways using ictal SPECT. *Brain.* 1997;120:855–864.

56. Benbadis SR, Tatum WO IV, Vale FL. When drugs don't work: an algorithmic approach to medically intractable epilepsy. *Neurology.* 2000;55: 1780–1784.

CHAPTER 82 ■ SURGICAL TREATMENT OF REFRACTORY TEMPORAL LOBE EPILEPSY

TONICARLO R. VELASCO AND GARY W. MATHERN

Temporal lobe epilepsy (TLE) is the most common epilepsy syndrome surgically treated in adolescents and adults, accounting for about 75% of operated patients (1,2). Of surgical patients, mesial TLE associated with hippocampal sclerosis (MTLE-HS) is the most frequent pharmacoresistant etiology (3). In this chapter, we will review the history of epilepsy neurosurgery for TLE, describe the clinical subtypes of TLE by location of the focus and etiology, denote the diagnostic accuracy of presurgery neuroimaging techniques, and outline expected outcomes after surgery. Our goal is to demonstrate that surgery for the treatment of refractory TLE has become the standard of care for this epilepsy syndrome.

HISTORY OF TLE SURGERY

The discovery of localized cortical language function by Paul Broca in 1861, the description of motor cortex using cortical stimulation by Fritsh and Hitzig and Daniel Ferrier in the 1870s, and the analysis of ictal motor symptoms by John Hughlings Jackson provided the intellectual foundations for the development of epilepsy neurosurgery. Based on a patient's typical motor seizures, Rickman Godlee localized and operated upon a brain tumor in 1884, with Jackson, Ferrier, and the neurosurgeon Victor Horsley present in the operating room. Two years later, Sir Victor Horsley performed his first epilepsy surgery. The patient was a 22-year-old man with focal motor seizures as a result of traumatic brain injury from a carriage accident. In the same year, Horsley resected a brain tumor and adjacent cerebral cortex guided by analysis of ictal semiology "in order to prevent, as far as possible, the recurrence of the epilepsy" (4).

After Horsley's report of successful epilepsy surgery, the field developed over the next several decades and included TLE surgery. Initially, most cases reported in the literature were resections in the frontal and parietal regions in close proximity to the motor and sensory cortices. Clinical observations made by Jackson associated "dreamy states" and psychical experience with lesions of the mesial temporal lobe. Penfield confirmed these ictal clinical features when he noticed that patients with complex auditory and visual hallucinations as part of their seizures could have their symptoms elicited by focal stimulation of the temporal neocortex and amygdale (5). The discovery of the electroencephalogram (EEG) (6) permitted better characterization of "psychomotor epilepsy" in the late 1940s (7). Consequently, by the 1950s successful surgical treatments of patients with TLE were reported by several groups (8,9).

Despite the macroscopic descriptions of HS by Bouchet and Cazauvieilh in 1825, and the microscopic studies of Sommer in 1880 and Bratz in 1899, the first temporal resections usually did not include the hippocampus (10–12). The predominant view at that time was that HS was most likely the consequence of repeated seizures and did not "cause" epilepsy. Many believed that HS was a coincidental finding, seen in the brains of persons without epilepsy, as illustrated by the words of Gowers (13):

It is more than doubtful whether any importance is to be ascribed to the induration of the cornu Ammonis . . . they cannot be regarded as significant, being found apart from epilepsy. All physiological and pathological consideration renders it improbable that the lesion has any direct relation with epilepsy.

By the 1950s and 1960s, however, this view changed as clinical studies pointed to the mesial and inferior temporal cortex as important in reproducing ictal phenomena in patients with TLE (5,14). More evidence that the mesial temporal region was important in the generation of TLE came from surgical studies. Penfield described successful control of seizures when he extended the resection to include the uncus and hippocampus in patients whose anterior and lateral resections did not initially eliminate seizures. In addition, during the 1957 International Colloquium of Epilepsy at Bethesda, Maryland, Paulo Niemeyer described a creative surgical technique to remove the amygdala and hippocampus by a transventricular approach, without resection of adjacent temporal cortex, and demonstrated that many TLE patients became seizure free (15). These results, added to clinicopathologic studies associating the presence of HS with TLE (16–18). Finally, the most convincing evidence came from intracranial depth electrode studies showing that EEG ictal onsets began in mesial temporal structures before the clinical ictal behavior (19,20). Since the 1970s, most of the advancements in treatment of TLE patients have been from improved neuroimaging and microsurgical techniques in the operating room.

TLE SYNDROMES AMENABLE TO SURGERY

Refractory TLE syndromes are typically classified by the anatomical location of the apparent seizure onsets and etiology. Based on ictal-onset zones, TLE is usually characterized as mesial TLE (MTLE), when the seizures begin from the hippocampus, uncus, and amygdala, or neocortical TLE (NTLE), if the seizures seem to originate from the lateral and inferior surfaces of the temporal lobe. Most experts use a classification that combines anatomical, clinical, and neuroimaging criteria into the following clinicopathologic categories:

1. Mesial temporal lobe epilepsy associated with hippocampal sclerosis (MTLE-HS). HS can be bilateral or there can be asymmetric hippocampal injury.
2. Temporal lobe epilepsy associated with other histopathologic lesions (brain tumors, CD, vascular lesions). Patients may have MTLE or NTLE depending on the lesion location.
3. Temporal lobe epilepsy without an identified epileptogenic lesion (termed cryptogenic, nonlesional, and paradoxical).
4. Dual pathology, which consists of HS plus extrahippocampal pathology.

Mesial Temporal Lobe Epilepsy Associated with Hippocampal Sclerosis (MTLE-HS)

In the modern neuroimaging era, HS is the most frequent etiology in surgically treated medically refractory TLE patients (21). In patients with MTLE-HS, there is a frequent association with an initial precipitating injury (IPI) that usually occurs during infancy and early childhood (22–24). Habitual seizures with limbic characteristics typically begin during the end of the first decade of life. Complex partial seizures (CPS) are the predominant seizure type. Most patients experience auras that probably arise from brain regions adjacent to the hippocampus. MTLE-HS auras usually consist of:

1. An unpleasant epigastric sensation that may rise to the throat.

2. A crude sensation of smell or taste, generally of an unpleasant nature.
3. Emotional phenomena, such as fear, anger, and occasionally pleasure.
4. Memory-related symptoms, ranging from a feeling of familiarity or strangeness, to elaborate hallucinations, when the patient may feel that he is taking part in a scene experienced before.

If the MTLE-HS seizure continues past the aura, patients lose consciousness. In its simplest form, the patient may stare quietly, or carry on simple automatic activities such as walking. When MTLE-HS seizures involve the dominant temporal lobe, the patient may not be able to speak or respond to a verbal command. Chewing, sucking, swallowing automatisms associated with tonic or dystonic postures of the contralateral arm are frequently observed. Secondarily generalized tonic–clonic (SGTC) seizures are usually infrequent, unless medications are discontinued (25,26). After the seizure is over, patients typically need to rest for a period. A proportion of MTLE patients are reported to have a family history of epilepsy (17,27,28).

Neurologic examination is generally normal. A mild central-type facial paresis has been reported contralateral to the side of HS (29). Interictal scalp EEG usually reveals focal slowing along with spikes and sharp-waves over the anterior, inferior, and mesial temporal regions. Ictal scalp EEG changes typically consist of lateralized buildup of rhythmic 5 to 7 Hz seizure activity (30,31). Neuropsychological testing may reveal material-specific memory loss (32). MRI typically depicts the classic signs of decreased volume and abnormal increased signal in T2 or fluid attenuated inversion recovery (FLAIR) sequences of the hippocampus (Fig. 82.1A; arrow) (33). This is generally associated with decreased FDG-PET hypometabolism in ipsilateral temporal lobe (34,35).

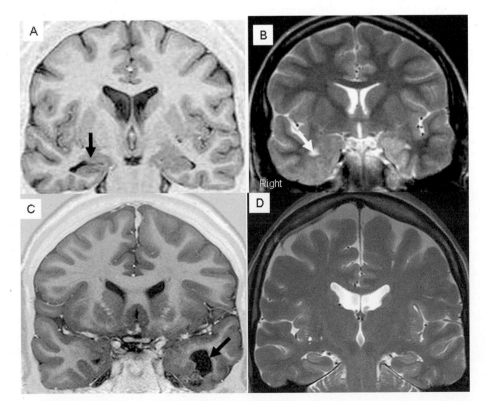

FIGURE 82.1 A: MRI showing atrophy of the right hippocampus *(arrow)* and ipsilateral temporal lobe in a patient with hippocampal sclerosis. **B:** An MRI reveals increased signal intensity and distortion of right mesial temporal structures *(arrow)* in a patient whose histopathologic diagnosis was cortical dysplasia. **C:** A T2 sequence showing a large cystic lesion in left temporal lobe with sharply defined borders and no surrounding edema in a patient with low-grade temporal lobe tumor. **D:** An MRI T2 sequence showing normal mesial structures in a patient with cryptogenic temporal lobe epilepsy.

CLINICAL VALUE OF ABDOMINAL AURAS, INTERICTAL TEMPORAL SPIKES, AND 5 TO 7 HZ ICTAL EEG PATTERN

The most common aura in patients with TLE is an epigastric sensation (25,36,37). One study evaluated the localizing value of abdominal auras in 491 consecutive patients with refractory epilepsy (38). They reported that abdominal auras were found in 52% of TLE patients, in comparison with 11% of patients with extratemporal epilepsy. Although the sensitivity was relatively low (52%), the specificity for abdominal aura as a diagnostic feature of TLE was high (90%; 95% CI = 84% to 94%, likelihood ratio = 4.56).

Interictal spikes (IS) are a marker of hyperexcitable cortex, arising in or near an area with high epileptogenic potential. In fact, interictal discharges that exhibit a consistent unilateral focal preponderance over a single region usually predict seizure origin (39). In TLE, temporal IS are found in 95% of studies, being unilateral in 70% to 80% of cases and bilateral in 20% to 30%. The laterality of temporal IS predicts lateralization of other diagnostic tests (40–42). For example, ictal EEG patterns at seizure onset and during its evolution are more often lateralized in patients with unilateral IS than in those with bilateral IS, which frequently exhibit bilateral independent, falsely lateralizing, and nonlateralizing ictal EEGs. The specificity of temporal IS for the diagnosis of TLE remains unclear, but it is well known that temporal spikes can be frequently found in patients with inferior lateral frontal lobe epilepsy and occipital epilepsy (43,44).

Unilateral temporal 5 to 7 Hz ictal EEG pattern correctly predicts seizure lateralization in 82% to 94% of cases of TLE (30). One study found 5 to 7 Hz ictal EEG pattern in 46% of seizures in patients with TLE, compared with 8% of seizures in patients with extratemporal epilepsy. With a 5 to 7 Hz ictal EEG pattern, the probability of the patient having TLE was 85% (likelihood ratio = 5.75) (45).

When Does Hippocampal Damage Occur in HS?

Investigations in animal models and clinical studies of TLE patients indicate that excessive neural activity, such as status epilepticus, is associated with seizure-induced neuronal loss, neurogenesis, abnormal collateral axonal sprouting and synaptic reorganization, gliosis, and molecular plasticity of glutamate and GABA receptors, transporters, and other signaling systems (46). This has led some authors to suggest that, after the development of epilepsy, continuous neural reorganization could contribute to progressive brain damage and HS. In patients with TLE, there is evidence for slowly progressive hippocampal damage that surpasses that which could be attributed to aging (24,47). The findings from pathologic studies have been confirmed by longitudinal neuroimaging studies showing that, in patients with refractory MTLE, progressive hippocampal and neocortical atrophy occur (48). However, at present, there is little clinical evidence that repeated seizures over many years "cause" HS. Instead, there is a strong association of HS with IPIs. Clinicopathologic

studies indicate that HS can be found in infants with refractory TLE (23,24). In addition, HS has been linked to developmental brain abnormalities. Neuroimaging studies have shown that HS can be associated with hippocampal anomalies, such as heterotopia and cortical dysplasia. This suggests that preexisting lesions might predispose an individual to developing febrile seizures, which in turn could produce HS and TLE (49).

Associated Extrahippocampal Abnormalities in Patients with MTLE-HS

Although the vast majority of MRI studies focus on the hippocampus, changes in other brain areas have also been documented in patients with MTLE-HS. In the temporal lobe, involvement of amygdala was described in 11 of 29 autopsy cases (16). Quantified neuroimaging studies have also shown amygdala damage in up to 55% of TLE patients, including 10% of isolated amygdala sclerosis (50). Extrahippocampal damage has also been described in the entorhinal cortex in 25% of patients with MTLE-HS (51), and in the fornix (52). Furthermore, quantitative MRI studies demonstrate that the temporal pole is frequently atrophic in drug-resistant TLE patients, and generally associated with increased T2-weighted signal in the white matter (53).

Studies have found involvement of the thalamus, extratemporal white matter, and cerebral hemispheres in patients with TLE. Thalamic damage suggests involvement of a thalamo-hippocampal network in MTLE-HS patients (54). White matter changes in patients with TLE were first described in the 19th century (11). In fact, Bouchet and Cazauvilh thought that "sclerosis" of white matter was more important than HS in the pathogenesis of epilepsy. Modern neuroimaging studies using voxel-based methods have reported diffuse white matter abnormalities in TLE patients (55). TLE is characterized by a relatively diffuse reduction in total gray and white matter cerebral volume, which appears to be associated with global neuropsychological deficits (56). A recent study suggested that left hippocampal atrophy was associated with extrahippocampal gray matter atrophy, which may explain the more pronounced cognitive impairments in patients with dominant lobe TLE (57). Widespread preoperative MRI changes and extratemporal hypometabolism on FDG-PET are associated with unsuccessful seizure control after temporal resections (58,59).

Bitemporal HS

By histopathology and neuroimaging, most patients with MTLE-HS have some degree of bilateral hippocampal atrophy (60). Approximately 20% of MTLE-HS patients will have bilateral hippocampal atrophy and sclerosis (17,47,60,61). The presence of bilateral hippocampal abnormalities on MRI increases the likelihood of bitemporal independent seizure onsets, but TLE surgery is still possible. If the presurgical evaluation can determine that most of the TLE seizures originate predominantly from one hippocampus and that resection will not induce an unacceptable postsurgical memory deficit, patients with bitemporal hippocampal atrophy may be surgical candidates. This usually requires intracranial EEG recording to confirm ictal onsets (62). Furthermore, one study indicated that even patients with intracranially recorded bilateral independent temporal seizures could have a seizure-free outcome after temporal lobectomy. The authors offered temporal lobectomy if at least 50% of seizures originated from one mesial temporal lobe, no focal extratemporal seizure or epileptogenic lesion was detected, and there was adequate contralateral memory function on Wada memory test. They found that two thirds of patients became seizure free, with a mean follow-up of 4 years (63).

TLE Associated with Other Histopathologic Lesions

After HS, the most common lesions identified in surgically treated TLE patients are tumors, cortical dysplasia, and vascular lesions. Of these, brain tumors are the next most common (Fig. 82.1C; arrow), consisting of low-grade astrocytomas (46%), ganglioglioma (21%), oligodendroglioma (18%), dyscmbryoplastic neuroepithelial tumor (6%), anaplastic astrocytoma (6%), and meningioma (3%) (64). The age at seizure onset is reported to be older in TLE patients with tumors than MTLE-HS cases, and febrile seizures and other IPIs occur rarely. The incidence of dual pathology is low in TLE patients with tumors. Confirming the concept that seizure semiology in TLE depends more on the location rather than type of lesion, auras consisting of déjà vu and epigastric sensations are reported to occur almost exclusively in mesial temporal tumors, while visual symptoms were exclusive of posterolateral temporal lesions (64).

Cortical dysplasia (CD) is the most common histopathologic finding in pediatric and the third most frequent abnormality in adult TLE patients (Fig. 82.1B; arrow) (21,65). The most common type of CD in TLE patients is termed mild or Type I CD, consisting of cortical dyslamination often with increased neurons in the subcortical white matter (66). TLE patients with CD are often associated with HS and dual pathology (67,68). The surgical treatment of refractory TLE associated with CD can be challenging because the area of dysplasia may not be completely visible on structural MRI scans. In addition, ictal propagation patterns in TLE patients with CD are often more complex, with patients exhibiting tonic seizures or even infantile spasms in infants. Moreover, patients with TLE from CD may have multilobar lesions involving nontemporal lobe structures making complete resection difficult.

Vascular lesions are identified in 5% of TLE patients (21). Cavernous malformations (CM) and arteriovenous malformations (AVM) were the most common types of vascular lesions associated with TLE. The temporal lobe was the most common site of AVMs associated with seizures (69). Similar to patients with brain tumors, the age of seizure onset has been reported as older in patients with vascular lesions compared with MTLE-HS cases, and IPIs are infrequent. In addition to seizures, patients with CM and AVM can present with acute bleeding, headache, and focal neurologic deficits. A longer epilepsy duration, a higher number of preoperative seizures, and female gender were reported as associated with pharmacoresistance in TLE patients with vascular lesions (70).

CRYPTOGENIC TEMPORAL LOBE EPILEPSY

In a subgroup of TLE patients, there is no lesion on neuroimaging and histopathology fails to show an abnormality that can explain the epilepsy (Fig. 82.1D). This group has been termed cryptogenic, nonlesional, and paradoxical temporal lobe epilepsy (PTLE) by different authors (71). Presurgical evaluation is more difficult in PTLE compared with MTLE-HS and lesional TLE. In one study, a group of 12 patients with PTLE evaluated with depth electrodes was compared with a randomly selected MTLE-HS group. In the PTLE group, febrile seizures were uncommon, their first seizure was at an older age, they had a higher incidence of generalized tonic–clonic seizures, and reduced rate of seizure freedom after surgery (50% compared with 76%). These features suggest a more extensive and complex epileptogenic region and network in patients with PTLE (71). When compared with patients with neocortical TLE, patients with PTLE are reported to have a higher proportion with contralateral hand dystonia, oral or manual automatisms, and abdominal auras. Nonspecific cephalic auras, early clonic activity, and a higher proportion of more diffuse EEG spikes (hemispheric or parasagittal) are more frequent in patients with neocortical TLE than PTLE (72). The absence of an IPI helps differentiate neocortical TLE from MTLE-HS (73), but not from PTLE.

Dual Pathology

Dual pathology is defined when an extrahippocampal epileptogenic lesion is found in association with HS. With better neuroimaging, dual pathology has been reported more frequently than previously appreciated in TLE patients. In a series of 178 patients with TLE, one study found evidence of dual pathology in 52% of patients, and it was more common in TLE patients with heterotopia than those with brain tumors (74). In a series from Montreal, hippocampal atrophy was present in 15% of patients with lesions involving other temporal structures. The authors found more intense hippocampal damage by MRI, indicating probable dual pathology in patients with CD and porencephalic cysts than in those with brain tumors (75). The clinical characteristics of TLE patients with dual pathology is similar to patients with MTLE-HS. In a series of 37 patients with dual pathology, the mean age of habitual seizure onset was 12.9 years, the aura consisted of epigastric sensation, fear, déja-vu, olfactory, and gustatory sensation, followed by loss of contact, automatisms, and dystonic posturing (76).

TYPES OF TEMPORAL RESECTIONS IN REFRACTORY TLE PATIENTS

For patient with TLE, typical resection can be tailored or anatomically standardized. In tailored operations, the findings from the clinical history, seizure semiology, neuroimaging, ictal EEG, and neuropsychological evaluations are used to

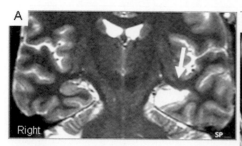
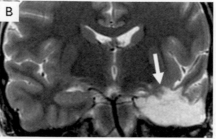

FIGURE 82.2 Postoperative MRIs showing selective amygdalohippocampectomy (SAH; **Panel A**) and standardized resection of the anterior temporal lobe (ATL; **Panel B**). (**Panel A**, courtesy of Dr. Eliseu Paglioli.)

guide the resection, and usually include intracranial electro-corticography and brain electrical stimulation. A tailored operation is frequently used in patients with cryptogenic TLE where the MRI is normal, patients with neocortical TLE associated with CD and tumors. Standardized resections are generally divided into two types: anterior temporal lobectomy (ATL) with hippocampectomy and selective amygdalohypocampectomy (SAH) (Fig. 82.2) (15,77). ATL is generally used to treat patients with MTLE-HS, TLE patients with dual pathology, and those with anterolateral neocortical lesions where the epileptic network appears to include the mesial temporal structures. For SAH, the presurgical workup usually indicates that the epileptogenic zone is exclusively localized to the mesial temporal lobe mostly involving the hippocampus and parahippocampal gyrus.

TIMING OF TLE SURGERY

Studies indicate that patients with refractory epilepsy are at risk for neuropsychological, psychiatric, and social impairments that limit employment and decrease quality of life (78). Moreover, refractory epilepsy is associated with higher mortality from sudden unexpected death than nonepileptic patients (79). Early control of epileptic seizures once a patient is considered drug refractory is crucial in preventing irreversible psychological disabilities and progressive cerebral dysfunction, as well as epilepsy-related death. If patients with

TLE do not respond to medical treatment after trials of two to three appropriate antiepilepsy drugs (AEDs), surgical candidacy should be considered and the patient offered referral for comprehensive evaluation. The time required to determine medical refractoriness and the number of AEDs used should not take 10 to 20 years. Epilepsy surgery is not the treatment of last resort. Early intervention can prevent epilepsy-induced disabilities, especially in children and adolescents (2).

Diagnostic Accuracy of Neuroimaging Techniques in TLE

The development of neuroimaging has had a substantial impact on the presurgical evaluation of refractory TLE patients. The diagnostic accuracy of tests in TLE patients is assessed in this section (Table 82.1; Fig. 82.3).

Qualitative Structural MRI

Structural MRI is the most accurate diagnostic tool in the presurgical evaluation of refractory TLE patients with HS and tumors (see Table 82.1). Structural MRI has reduced the need for intracranial EEG studies in patients with discrete lesions. For example, in patients with MTLE-HS by MRI, depth electrodes are used in less than 20% of patients in whom scalp EEG raised the question of bilateral mesial temporal epilepsy. By comparison, in TLE patients with CD, over 50% have normal structural MRI studies (Table 82.1). In fact, in TLE

TABLE 82.1

ACCURACY OF MRI IN IDENTIFYING EPILEPTOGENIC LESION IN TLE PATIENTS FROM DIFFERENT STUDIES

Study	Tumor	Hippocampal sclerosis	Cortical dysplasia/mMCD
Zentner, 1995	98.7% (76/77)		
Brooks, 1990	91.6% (11/12)	—	—
Hwang, 2001	100% (13/13)	—	46.4% (13/28)
Srikijvilaikul, 2003	—	—	46.4% (13/28)
Porter, 2003			14.3% (3/21)
Kuzniecky, 2001	—	—	70% (7/10)
Cendes, 1997	—	97% (97/100)	—
McBride, 1998	—	95.7 (44/46)	—
Kuzniecky, 1997	—	90% (36/40)	—
Jack, 1990	—	97.2% (35/36)	—
Pooled	98% (100/102)	95% (112/222)	41% (36/87)

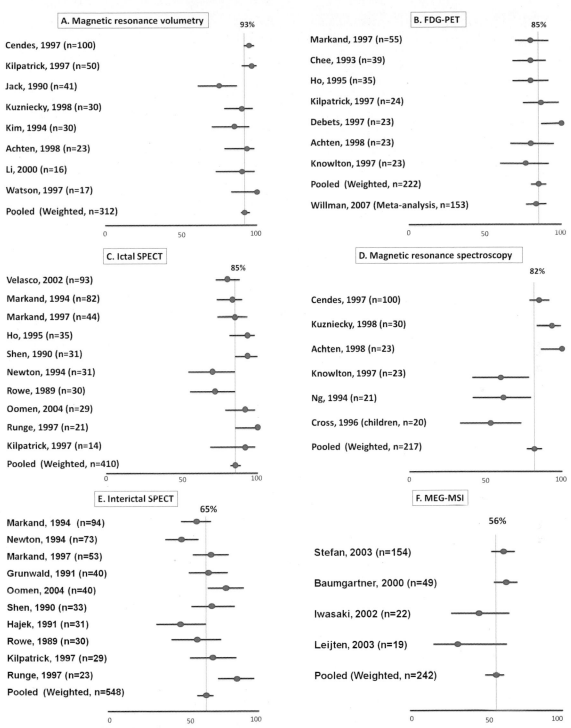

FIGURE 82.3 Panels depicting the diagnostic accuracy of neuroimaging tools used to identify the epileptogenic zone in patients with refractory TLE. Individual studies are depicted with their corresponding CI_{95} *(small horizontal bars)*. The pooled proportions weighted by number of patients are also represented by the large vertical bar. In MRI volumetry and MRS studies, only patients with nonlesional TLE were included.

patients with negative MRI scans, histopathologic evaluation of the resected temporal lobe will identify CD in about 25% of cases, but rarely HS or tumors (Table 82.2).

Quantified MRI Volumetric Studies

MRI volumetric analysis can provide quantified data of temporal lobe structures, including the temporal pole, hippocampus, amygdala, and entorhinal cortex. MRI volumetric studies

can accurately identify volume reduction of mesial structures in over 90% of patients with MTLE-HS (Fig. 82.3A). The severity of hippocampal histopathology correlates with MRI volume loss (80).

PET Studies

PET can evaluate in vivo biochemical and physiologic processes. Glucose metabolism reflecting interictal neural

TABLE 82.2

HISTOPATHOLOGIC DIAGNOSIS IN TLE PATIENTS WITH NEGATIVE MRI SCANS

Study	Gliosis/ nonspecific	Cortical dysplasia/ mMCD	Hippocampal sclerosis	Tumor	Total
Carne, 2004	45% (9)	50% (10)	5% (1)	—	20
Holmes, 2000	95% (19)	—	5% (1)	—	20
McGonigal, 2007	48% (11)	44% (10)	9% (2)	—	23
Siegel, 2001	67% (16)	25% (6)	5% (1)	4% (1)	24
Sylaya, 2004	65% (11)	—	35% (6)	—	17
Pooled	63%	25%	11%	1%	104

activity can be studied with FDG-PET. Also, neurotransmitter systems can be studied including homologs for GABA ([11C]FMZ-PET), opioid (mu opioid PET), and serotonin (5-HT1A-PET) receptors. Using FDG-PET, studies report that more than 85% of TLE cases correctly localized to the side of seizure onset (Fig. 82.3B). Many patients that are MRI negative are often FDG-PET positive, reducing the need for intracranial EEG evaluations in these patients. A study compared the diagnostic accuracy of FDG-PET with [11C]FMZ-PET in 100 patients with refractory epilepsy. The authors found a similar diagnostic accuracy, with both studies showing more than 90% correctly lateralization in patients with TLE (81).

Interictal and Ictal SPECT

Interictal and ictal SPECT can provide information about cerebral blood flow during the interictal state and during the initial portion of a seizure. Pooled studies indicate that interictal SPECT is accurate in about 65% of cases (Fig. 82.3E). By comparison, in TLE patients the accuracy of ictal SPECT is around 85% (Fig. 82.3C) (40).

Magnetic Resonance Spectroscopy (MRS)

Proton magnetic spectroscopy imaging (MRS) provides spatially encoded information about the chemical composition of brain structures. Studies reporting the diagnostic accuracy of MRS show variable results with an average accuracy of 81% (Fig. 82.3D). In studies of children with TLE, 55% of MRS studies correctly lateralized to the side of surgery. In studies of adult TLE patients MRS was reported to have 100% correct lateralization.

Magnetoencephalography–Magnetic Source Imaging (MEG-MSI)

MEG-MSI identifies magnetic fields generated by the brain and are less distorted by the resistive properties of the skull and scalp than EEG signals. Studies comparing source localizations of scalp EEG and MEG-MSI revealed that MEG results are more consistent and precise than scalp EEG (82). However, precision does not translate into accuracy. In pooled studies, the diagnostic yield of MEG-MSI in MTLE-HS is substantially lower than in neocortical epilepsy, with a sizable number of negative individual patient studies (Fig. 82.3F).

Seizure Outcome: Randomized Controlled Trial and Case-Control Series

One randomized controlled trial has reported the superiority of surgery over continued medical therapy in patients with refractory TLE. Eighty patients with mesial TLE were randomized to surgical or continued medical therapy after presurgical evaluation. The authors found that 58% of patients in the surgical group were seizure free at 1 year compared with 8% in the medical group (P < 0.001, Fig. 82.4) (83). The authors also found that compared to the medical group, patients in the surgery arm had better scores for quality of life, rates of employment, and school attendance. Finally, they reported an unexpected death for one patient in the medical group and no deaths in the surgical cohort.

A case-control study compared long-term seizure outcome and health-related quality of life (HRQL) for patients who underwent epilepsy surgery (mostly TLE patients) and matched medically treated nonsurgical controls with intractable epilepsy. After an average of more than 15 years of follow-up, the authors found that epilepsy surgery patients had fewer seizures, used less antiepileptic medication, and had better HRQL than controls (84). Another study has reported that a larger proportion of patients who had temporal resections were seizure free in comparison with medically treated patients (72% versus 23%) (85).

Seizure Outcome: Systematic Reviews and Meta-analysis

Four systematic reviews and meta-analysis published since 2003 have reported the postsurgical outcomes of patients with TLE (2,86–88). These studies included patients with variable pathologic substrates, and the time period covered by the authors and the number of incorporated papers were similar (Table 82.3). As might be expected, seizure outcomes reported by the different reviews were very similar, with seizure freedom after surgery averaging from 65% to 68% of patients. After reviewing the literature, the Quality Standards Subcommittee of the American Academy of Neurology stated that the results demonstrate that surgical outcome was consistent, differing little among stratifications, such as geographical region, longer follow-up, and surgery after the advent of MRI. The report recommended that "patients who meet established criteria for a temporal lobe resection and who accept the risks

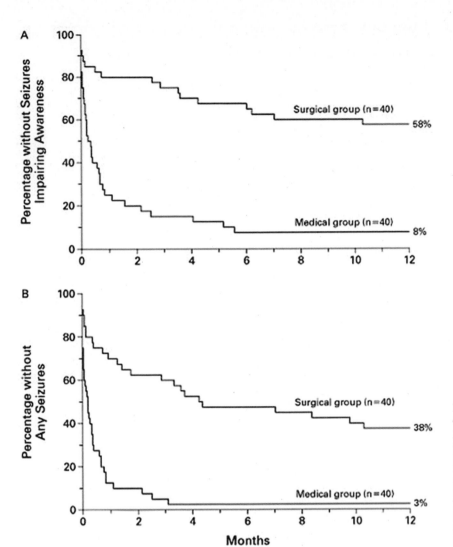

FIGURE 82.4 Kaplan–Meier event-free survival curves comparing the cumulative percentages of patients in groups which were free of disabling seizures (**Panel A**) and completely seizure-free (**Panel B**). More patients in the surgical group were free of seizures ($P < 0.001$) in both analysis. (From Wiebe S, Blume WT, Girvin JP, Eliasziw M, for the Effectiveness and Efficiency of Surgery for Temporal Lobe Epilepsy Study Group. A randomized, controlled trial of surgery for temporal lobe epilepsy. *N Engl J Med.* 2001;345(5):311–318, with permission.)

and benefits of this procedure, as opposed to continuing pharmacotherapy, should be offered surgical treatment" (2).

Seizure Outcome: Long-Term Outcome Studies

In addition to meta-analyses, recent studies have reported long-term outcomes after surgery for TLE patients (Table 82.4).

Most studies included multiple types of pathologic substrates, with an overall percentage of seizure freedom at 62% ranging from 41% to 74% at 10 years. All but one study reported more than 60% seizure freedom at 10 years follow-up. These studies strongly support the conclusion that temporal resections are an effective treatment, with approximately two

TABLE 82.3

SYSTEMATIC REVIEWS AND META-ANALYSIS OF SURGICAL OUTCOMES FOR PATIENTS WITH REFRACTORY TLE

Author, publication year	Time span	Number of studies	Number of patients	Seizure freedom	95% confidence interval
Engel et al., 2003	1990–1999	24	1952	67%	64–68%
Tonini et al., 2004	1984–2001	45	1769	65%	62–67%
Tellez-Zenteno et al., 2005	1991–2003	40	3895	66%	62–70%
Chapell et al., 2003[a]	1985–2003	73	3978	—	—
Seizure free without aura		20	734	55%	50–60%
Seizure free with aura		26	1396	68%	65–72%
Engel Class I		33	1549	67%	65–71%
Seizure-free undefined		16	977	61%	55–65%

[a]U.S. Department of Health and Human Services. Evidence Report/Technology Assessment on Management of Treatment-Resistant Epilepsy, 2003.

TABLE 82.4

SURGICAL OUTCOMES OF TEMPORAL RESECTIONS IN RECENT LONG-TERM OUTCOME STUDIES

Author, year	Age at surgery (years)	Follow-up (years)	Number of patients	Percent seizure freedom	Percent seizure freedom (HS patients)	Percent seizure freedom (non-MTLE-HS patients)
Luyken et al., 2003	2–54	8	170	81% at 10 years		82% (only TL tumors)
McIntosh et al., 2004	6.7–58.8	9.6 (0.7 to 23)	325	41% at 10 years	47% at 10 years	60%
Mittal et al., 2005	0.1–17	10.9	109	82% at 10 years	78.4 at 10 years	89.8%
Cohen-Gadol et al., 2006	3–69	6.2 (0.6–15.7)	372	74% at 10 years	79% at 10 years	62 (normal MRI) to 71% (gliosis)
Kelemen et al., 2006	15–60	2 to 17	94	61% at 10 years	—	—
Asztely et al., 2007	32–58	12.4 (8–16)	65	59% at 12 years	—	—
Elsharkawy et al., 2008	16 or older	16	434	69% at 16 years	75.5% at 16 years	33.3 (FCD) to 66.7 (Tu)
Pooled			1569	62%		

thirds of patients becoming free of disabling seizures after anterior temporal lobectomy, and this rate is maintained over time (21,88–93).

Predictors of Surgical Outcome: MRI and Histopathology

The probability of being seizure free after TLE surgery depends on the histopathology and MRI findings, with brain tumors and MTLE-HS showing the best outcomes. In two systematic reviews, the authors reported a higher proportion of long-term seizure freedom in patients with tumors when compared with other etiologies (86,87). In patients with temporal lobe tumors, two studies report that 65% of patients remain seizure free with follow-up of 9 years or more (21,64). In a series of 207 patients with brain tumors, of which 170 were in the temporal lobe, 82% patients were free of disabling seizures after 1 year, and 81% remained seizure free over a 10-year follow-up period (91). In another study, 86% of patients who had temporal lobe tumors were free of disabling seizures after surgery (94).

In the MTLE-HS patients, most studies report a high rate of becoming seizure free with surgery. A recent study reported 75% of patients as Engel Class I at 16 years after surgery (21). These results were similar to two other studies that reported a likelihood of remaining free of disabling seizures at 79% after 10 years of follow-up (88) and 78% in children (89). By comparison, other authors reported that the likelihood of remaining free of disabling seizures by 2-year postsurgery was 61%, and 41% at 10 years (90).

The likelihood of seizure freedom in patients with normal MRI scans and CD is lower than in patients with TLE associated with HS, tumors, and vascular lesions. In patients with normal MRI, 62% were reported as seizure free at 10 years in one study (88). These results were similar to another series that reported 56% of patients were seizure free after surgery in 39 patients with normal MRI followed for at least 2 years (95). In TLE associated with CD, long-term outcome studies have reported that the seizure-free rate decreases over time (68). Only 33.3% (95%CI 23% to 43%) of TLE patients with CD remained seizure free of disabling seizures after 16 years of follow-up in one study (21). Another series revealed similar

results, with only 38% of TLE patients with CD completely seizure free at 10 years of follow-up (96). A recent study reported surgical outcome in 166 patients with CD. In 52 patients, the CD was localized to the temporal lobe, with 46% of cases reported as seizure-free with a mean follow-up of 7.9 years (97). Finally, another study reported that 54% children with TLE from CD were Engel Class I at 5 years of follow-up (98).

In patients with dual pathology, 73% of patients are reported as free of disabling seizures when both the lesion and HS were removed. When only the lesion or the hippocampus were resected, the rate of seizure freedom decreased to 20% or less (99). Their results indicate that, in patients with dual pathology, removal of both the lesion and the atrophic hippocampus is the best surgical approach to optimize the chance of becoming seizure free after surgery (100). There are few studies reporting seizure outcome in TLE associated with CM and AVM. One study revealed that 78% of patients were seizure free in 14 patients with temporal lobe AVMs (70).

Clinical Predictors of Surgical Outcome

Multiple studies have attempted to identify clinical factors that would predict outcomes after epilepsy surgery; the results are often inconsistent (Table 82.5). In addition, many studies fail to control for clinical factors that are highly correlated. For example, a meta-analysis studying predictors of seizure outcome in patients with TLE concluded that a history of febrile seizures was associated to good postsurgical outcome (86). What that analysis did not consider was that most studies that reported this association pooled patients with MTLE-HS and patients with normal MRI. This could explain such association, because in patients with MTLE-HS, who have a better outcome than those with normal MRI, a history of febrile convulsion is more common than in patients with normal MRI. In fact, analyzing exclusively patients with MTLE-HS, several authors reported no association between febrile seizures and good postsurgical outcomes (21,101–103).

Looking at multiple published studies that included only one type of pathologic substrate, a clearer picture of possible

TABLE 82.5

CLINICAL PREDICTORS OF OUTCOME IN TLE PATIENTS

Predictor	Study (*n* of patients)	Pathologic substrate	*P* value or odds ratio
Age at surgery	Aull-Warschinger et al., 2008 (135)	MTLE-HS	NS
	Elsharkawy et al., 2008 (269)	MTLE-HS	NS
	Burneo et al., 2006 (252)	MTLE-HS	NS
	Janszky et al., 2005 (171)	MTLE-HS	OR = 0.93 (0.88–0.98)
	Kilpatrick et al., 1999 (56)	MTLE-HS	NS
	Hardy et al., 2003 (147)	MTLE-HS	NS
	Henessy et al., 2000 (116)	MTLE-HS	NS
	Tezer et al., 2008 (109)	MTLE-HS	NS
	Paglioli et al., 2004 (135)	MTLE-HS	NS
	Henessy et al., 2001 (80)	Tu/CD	0.006
	Zaatreh et al., 2003 (68)	Tumor	NS
Age at seizure onset	Aull-Warschinger et al., 2008 (135)	MTLE-HS	NS
	Elsharkawy et al., 2008 (269)	MTLE-HS	NS
	Janszky et al., 2005 (171)	MTLE-HS	NS
	Kilpatrick et al., 1999 (56)	MTLE-HS	NS
	Henessy et al., 2000 (116)	MTLE-HS	NS
	Hardy et al., 2003 (147)	MTLE-HS	NS
	Tezer et al., 2008 (109)	MTLE-HS	NS
	Paglioli et al., 2004 (135)	MTLE-HS	0.01
	Clusmann et al., 2004 (74)	Tu/CD	0.004
	Henessy et al., 2001 (80)	Tu/CD	NS
Epilepsy duration	Aull-Warschinger et al., 2008 (135)	MTLE-HS	NS
	Elsharkawy et al., 2008 (269)	MTLE-HS	NS
	Burneo et al., 2006 (252)	MTLE-HS	NS
	Janszky et al., 2005 (171)	MTLE-HS	OR = 0.92 (0.88–0.97)
	Kilpatrick et al., 1999 (56)	MTLE-HS	NS
	Henessy et al., 2000 (116)	MTLE-HS	0.02
	Tezer et al., 2008 (109)	MTLE-HS	NS
	Paglioli et al., 2004 (135)	MTLE-HS	NS
	Elsharkawy et al., 2008 (75)	Gliosis	0.021
	Elsharkawy et al., 2008 (30)	FCD	0.028
	Zaatreh et al., 2003 (68)	Tu	0.06
	Elsharkawy et al., 2008 (87)	Tu	0.006
History of febrile seizures	Aull-Warschinger et al., 2008 (135)	MTLE-HS	NS
	Elsharkawy et al., 2008 (269)	MTLE-HS	NS
	Burneo et al., 2006 (252)	MTLE-HS	NS
	Janszky et al., 2005 (171)	MTLE-HS	NS
	Kilpatrick et al., 1999 (56)	MTLE-HS	NS
	Hardy et al., 2003 (147)	MTLE-HS	NS
	Henessy et al., 2000 (116)	MTLE-HS	NS
	Tezer et al., 2008 (109)	MTLE-HS	NS
	Henessy et al., 2001 (80)	Tu/CD	NS
	Sylaja et al., 2004	Normal MRI	0.003
Family history of epilepsy	Elsharkawy et al., 2008 (269)	MTLE-HS	0.001
	Hardy et al., 2003 (147)	MTLE-HS	NS
	Tezer et al., 2008 (109)	MTLE-HS	NS
	Henessy et al., 2001 (80)	Tu/CD	NS

(continued)

TABLE 82.5

CLINICAL PREDICTORS OF OUTCOME IN TLE PATIENTS (*continued*)

Predictor	Study (*n* of patients)	Pathologic substrate	*P* value or odds ratio
History of SGS	Aull-Warschinger et al., 2008 (135)	MTLE-HS	NS
	Janszky et al., 2005 (171)	MTLE-HS	NS
	Kilpatrick et al., 1999 (56)	MTLE-HS	NS
	Henessy et al., 2000 (116)	MTLE-HS	0.01
	Tezer et al., 2008 (109)	MTLE-HS	NS
	Clusmann et al., 2004 (74)	Tu/CD	NS
	Zaatreh et al., 2003 (68)	Tu	NS
Preoperative seizure frequency	Aull-Warschinger et al., 2008 (135)	MTLE-HS	0.057
	Clusmann et al., 2004 (74)	Tu/CD	NS
Presence of dystonic posturing	Aull-Warschinger et al., 2008 (135)	MTLE-HS	NS
	Janszky et al., 2005 (171)	MTLE-HS	OR = 0.36 (0.14–0.97)
Versive seizure	Elsharkawy et al., 2008 (269)	MTLE-HS	0.022
Gender	Aull-Warschinger et al., 2008 (135)	MTLE-HS	0.007
	Elsharkawy et al., 2008 (269)	MTLE-HS	NS
	Burneo et al., 2006 (252)	MTLE-HS	OR = 0.5 (0.3–0.8)
	Janszky et al., 2005 (171)	MTLE-HS	NS
	Kilpatrick et al., 1999 (56)	MTLE-HS	NS
	Hardy et al., 2003 (147)	MTLE-HS	NS
	Tezer et al., 2008 (109)	MTLE-HS	NS
	Clusmann et al., 2004 (74)	Tu/CD	NS
	Zaatreh et al., 2003 (68)	Tumor	NS
Race/Ethnical group	Burneo et al., 2006 (252)	MTLE-HS	NS
Presence of unilateral HA	Elsharkawy et al., 2008 (269)	MTLE-HS	0.021
	Arruda et al., 1996 (74)	MTLE-HS	<0.001
Presence of HS at neuropathologic examination	Sylaja et al., 2004	Normal MRI	0.001
Side of surgery	Burneo et al., 2006 (68)	MTLE-HS	NS
	Tezer et al., 2008 (109)	MTLE-HS	NS
	Paglioli et al., 2004 (135)	MTLE-HS	NS
	Henessy et al., 2001 (80)	Tu/CD	NS
	Zaatreh et al., 2003 (68)	Tumor	NS
Total/Subtotal resection	Bonilha et al., 2004 (30)	MTLE-HS	NA[a]
	Zaatreh et al., 2003 (68)	Tumor	0.002
	Li et al., 1999 (38)	Dual pathology	<0.001
Spike frequency	Krendl et al., 2008 (55)	MTLE-HS	0.001
Focal ictal EEG	Tatum et al., 2008 (39)	Normal MRI	0.0005
	Holmes et al., 2000 (23)	Normal MRI	0.04
Presence unilateral IED	Aull-Warschinger et al., 2008 (135)	MTLE-HS	0.044
	Elsharkawy et al., 2008 (269)	MTLE-HS	0.004
	Janszky et al., 2005 (171)	MTLE-HS	NS
	Henessy et al., 2000 (116)	MTLE-HS	0.04
	Paglioli et al., 2004 (135)	MTLE-HS	NS
	Radhakrishnan et al., 1998 (175)	MTLE-HS	<0.01
	Henessy et al., 2001 (80)	Tu/CD	NS
	Radhakrishnan et al., 1998 (175)	Tu/CD	0.01
	Holmes et al., 2000 (23)	Normal MRI	0.04

[a]The *P*-value was not reported.

predictors of surgical outcomes in TLE patients emerges. These features include:

1. In patients with MTLE-HS, most studies did not report a relationship between age at surgery, age at seizure onset, epilepsy duration, history of febrile seizures, family history of epilepsy, history of secondary generalized seizures, and side of seizure with better seizure outcome. When an association was found, the effect size was small, or the association was weak.
2. In patients with MTLE-HS, two of seven studies showed an association between male gender and better postsurgical outcome. In both studies, the association was strong, but was not significant in other studies.
3. In patients with MTLE HS, three of five studies showed an association between ipsilateral interictal discharges and good postsurgical outcomes.
4. In lesions other that HS (tumors, CD, and vascular), there was an association between a longer epilepsy duration and poorer postsurgical seizure outcomes (four of four studies). This suggests that duration of epilepsy is important for TLE patients with tumors, CD, and vascular lesions.
5. In TLE patients with normal MRI, a history of febrile seizures and a focal temporal ictal EEG appears to be associated with better postsurgery seizure outcomes.

What Are the Chances that Antiepileptic Drugs Are Discontinued after Surgery?

Some consider that the ultimate goal of TLE surgery is to make patients seizure- and drug-free (cured). To address this question, Schmidt et al. reviewed studies reporting long-term seizure control of AEDs in 1658 patients following temporal lobe surgery. They found that 25% of adult patients (95% CI: 21% to 30%) and 33% of children and adolescents (95% CI: 20% to 41%) were seizure free for 5 years without AEDs (104). In another meta-analysis, using more stringent selection criteria, only 16% of patients with temporal lobe surgery patients were seizure free and not taking medications with more than 5 years of follow-up (104). Some studies have reported that patients who discontinued AEDs had a higher risk of seizure recurrence (105). These data contrast with others showing that the risk of seizure recurrence in people who stopped AEDs was similar to those remaining on AEDs (90).

Successful TLE Surgery Improves Quality of Life

Until the 1980s, few studies in patients with epilepsy included measurements of HRQL. The number of articles about HRQL in patients with epilepsy in the literature climbed from six articles published before 1980 to 467 articles published in the 1990s and 1041 articles between 2000 and 2009. These studies indicate that, compared with healthy controls, patients with TLE exhibit impairment in HRQL (106), and the impairments are related to having seizures (107). In patients with refractory seizures, the deleterious effects on individual health and quality of life are greater than in people with controlled seizures.

HRQL measures improve after epilepsy surgery, and the improvement is related to seizure control (108,109). In a prospective multicenter study, HRQL was evaluated using the Quality of Life in Epilepsy Inventory-89 (QOLIE-89) before surgery, within 6 months, and yearly intervals after surgery. They found that HRQL improved early after surgery, regardless of seizure outcome. However, a long-lasting improvement in HRQL was found in patients whose seizures remained controlled after surgery. In patients with recurrent seizures, the scores in QOLIE-89 returned to presurgical values 24 to 30 months after surgery (109). A systematic review of psychosocial outcome after epilepsy surgery concluded that all studies regarding psychosocial outcomes reported better outcomes after surgery (108).

HRQL measures can become worse after temporal resections. A study evaluated HRQL after temporal resection in patients with and without postoperative memory loss. They hypothesized that the "double losers," those who did not achieve seizure control and sustain a memory loss after surgery, would have the worst scores on QOLIE-89. They found that HRQL improved or remains stable in seizure-free patients despite memory decline. However, HRQL declined when persistent seizures were accompanied by memory loss (110).

Cognitive Outcome

Studies evaluating intelligence have consistently reported no long-term postsurgical worsening of full-scale IQ scores in TLE patients (108). However, unilateral resection of the mesial temporal structures can result in reduced memory function in 25% to 40% of patients with TLE (108,110). The presurgical evaluation team needs to discuss the risk of cognitive deficits and identify those patients at risk for memory loss. A study evaluating patients before and after temporal resections found that in subjects with dominant hemisphere surgery, MRI findings other than unilateral HS, intact preoperative delayed recall verbal memory, relatively poorer preoperative immediate recall verbal memory, and intact contralateral injection IAP memory were more likely to experience a significant decline in postoperative memory (111). Temporal lobe resections in the language-dominant hemisphere are also associated with declines in object naming. A study comparing naming scores reported that, in temporal resections in the nondominant hemisphere, the scores improved by two points after surgery whereas the dominant ATL group declined by an average of seven points ($P < 0.001$). Consistent with previous studies, they found that patients with later age at seizure onset (IPI or first seizure after age 5) experienced significantly greater naming declines than those with early age at seizure onset. They also found that words acquired later in life were more susceptible to being lost postoperatively than words learned earlier in life (112).

Psychiatric Outcome

Patients with epilepsy have an increased prevalence of mental health disorders compared with the general population (108). The prevalence is much higher in patients with refractory epilepsy, with up to 50% of patients reported as having affective disorders (depression, mania, and anxiety), psychosis, or personality disorders (1,108). Among 300 consecutive patients with refractory TLE, 47% had psychiatric comorbidity. An axis I diagnosis (DSM-III-R) was made in 29% and an axis II diagnosis (personality disorder) in another 18%. The most common axis I diagnosis were anxiety disorders (11%), schizophrenia-like psychosis (4%), and mood disorders (3%) (113).

Two prospective studies have reported less mood problems when patients underwent surgery and seizures became controlled. A study of 147 patients with TLE reported that the prevalence of depression in patients seizure free after surgery was 12%, compared to 44% in patients with continuing seizures (114). In addition, a prospective, multicenter study with 360 patients reported moderate to severe levels of depression symptoms in 18% of the patients experiencing seizures following surgery, but in only 8% of those with a seizure-free outcome (115). However, it has been reported that after TLE surgery, 4% to 30% of patients develop new affective disorders, and 1% to 5% develops new-onset psychosis (1).

Neurologic Outcome and Mortality After Temporal Resections

The prevalence of neurologic complications in patients after ATL is low and mostly mild or transient (2). The prevalence varies from 0.4% to 4% of patients, and generally consists of partial hemianopsia, aphasia, motor deficit, sensory deficit, or cranial nerve palsy (third and fourth cranial nerves). Permanent and severe deficits can occur and most often consist of occlusion of the anterior choroidal artery or remote cerebellar hemorrhage. The AHRQ meta-analysis found 40 articles totaling 2091 temporal lobe surgery patients, and 42 serious permanent complications were reported. This corresponds to 2% of the patients or 20 serious complications per 1000 surgery patients. Among the 2065 temporal lobe surgery patients, five deaths were reported (0.24% or 2.4 deaths per 1000 patients) (116).

Temporal Resections in Elderly

Until recently, few reports had described epilepsy surgery in older patients. A recent study reported surgical outcome and rate of complications in 52 patients older than 50 years for treatment of refractory TLE. They found that complete seizure relief was achieved in 71% of patients, plus 19% Class II outcomes, resulting in 90% "satisfactory" seizure control. However, complications occurred significantly more frequently in the older TLE patient group, compared with a younger control group. Permanent morbidity occurred in two patients who developed dysphasia, and one of whom had a moderate hemiparesis due to MCA infarction (3.8%), compared to 0.7% in younger patients (117). In addition, the authors also found that neuropsychological deterioration was more pronounced in the older subgroup, probably due to decreased cognitive reserve.

Radiosurgery

Stereotactic radiosurgery is an emerging treatment modality introduced as an alternative to temporal resections in patients with refractory TLE. It is based on multiple X-ray beams from a highly collimated radiation source oriented by stereotactic localization. About 1 year after radiation treatment, MRI signal changes characterized by heterogeneous T2 signal within a swollen hippocampus and diffusely increased T2 signal within the temporal lobe and adjacent white matter appear. These MRI changes are associated with a higher chance of eventual seizure control, but the clinical improvement can be slow, with persisting seizures up to 2 years after the procedure. The mechanisms underlying seizure control in patients submitted to radiosurgery are not fully understood.

Seizure outcome 2 to 3 years after radiosurgery has been reported to be similar to surgical resection at doses above 24 Gray (118,119). However, a small series of five patients submitted to nearly the same protocol showed disappointing results. Two patients died 1 month and 1 year after the radiosurgery and none of the three survivors had seizure reduction (120). More evidence from a randomized study comparing radiosurgery with resective procedures for patient with TLE is necessary.

CONCLUSIONS AND FUTURE DIRECTIONS

TLE is frequently refractory to pharmacologic treatment and has a significant impact in patient's quality of life. The most frequent pathologic substrates in TLE are HS, tumors, CD, vascular lesions, and gliosis. In selected cases, temporal resections can control seizures in 40% to 80% of cases and the most important predictor of surgical outcome is the pathologic substrate and MRI findings. In patients with tumors, the rate of seizure freedom in long-term studies is 60% to 80%, in HS 55% to 75%, in patients with normal MRI 50% to 60%, and in patients with CD is 35% to 60%. The prevalence of neurologic complications in patients after ATL is low and mostly mild or transient.

TLE surgery has a positive impact on quality of life if the patient is seizure free. Cure, seizure freedom without AEDs, is infrequent after temporal resection, occurring in less than 20% of cases. Finally, early recognition of surgical candidacy can help prevent future disability, especially in children and adolescents and in those with tumors, CD, and vascular lesions where longer durations of epilepsy are associated with worse outcomes.

Newer neuroimaging techniques and multimodality presurgical evaluations have increased accuracy in identifying TLE patients as surgical candidates, reduced the need for intracranial EEG studies, and improved the chance of becoming seizure-free postsurgery. However, not all patients are seizure free after TLE surgery. To further improve surgical treatment, our challenge in the near future will be to identify surgical candidates earlier in their epilepsy, further improve neuroimaging, and develop new treatment options for those who are not candidates for temporal lobe resections, such as brain stimulation and radiosurgery.

Another future challenge will be the ability to offer surgical treatment to more people of the world. A survey of regional advisers of the six WHO regions reported that epilepsy surgery was available in only 13% of low-income countries, compared with 66% of high-income countries. Thus, a treatment gap exists in the world and future efforts should reduce this gap so that more patients with refractory epilepsy have the opportunity to be evaluated and treated to reduce the global burden of epilepsy.

References

1. Spencer S, Huh L. Outcomes of epilepsy surgery in adults and children. *Lancet Neurol.* 2008;7(6):525–537.
2. Engel J, Jr, Wiebe S, French J, et al. Practice parameter: temporal lobe and localized neocortical resections for epilepsy: report of the Quality Standards Subcommittee of the American Academy of Neurology, in association with the American Epilepsy Society and the American Association of Neurological Surgeons. *Neurology.* 2003;60(4):538–547.

3. Semah F, Picot MC, Adam C, et al. Is the underlying cause of epilepsy a major prognostic factor for recurrence? *Neurology.* 1998;51(5):1256–1262.
4. Horsley V. Brain surgery. *Br Med J.* 1886;1:670–676.
5. Penfield W. Observations on the anatomy of memory. *Folia Psychiatr Neurol Neurochir Neerl.* 1950;53(2):349–351.
6. Berger H. Über das Elektroenkephalogramm des Menschen. *Archiv für Psychiatrie und Nervenkrankheiten.* 1929;87:527–570.
7. Gibbs EL, Gibbs FA, Fuster B. Psychomotor epilepsy. *Arch Neurol Psychiatry.* 1948;60(4):331–339.
8. Penfield W, Flanigin H. The surgical therapy of temporal lobe seizures. *Trans Am Neurol Assoc.* 1950;51:146–149.
9. Bailey P, Gibbs FA. The surgical treatment of psychomotor epilepsy. *J Am Med Assoc.* 1951;145(6):365–370.
10. Sommer W. Erkrankung des ammonshorns als aetiologiches moment der epilepsie. *Arch Psychiatr Nervenkr.* 1880;10:631–675.
11. Bouchet C, Cazauvielh Y. De l'épilepsie considérée dans ses rapports avec l'aliénation mentale. *Arch Gen Med Par.* 1825;9:510–542.
12. Bratz E. Ammonshornbefunde bei epileptikern. *Arch Psychiatr Nervenkr.* 1899;32:820–835.
13. Gowers W. Epilepsy and other convulsive diseases: their causes, symptoms, and treatment. In: Brinklow M, ed. *Pathology.* Philadelphia, PA: P. Blakiston's Son & Co; 1901:213–228.
14. Kaada BR. Somato-motor, autonomic and electrocorticographic responses to electrical stimulation of rhinencephalic and other structures in primates, cat, and dog; a study of responses from the limbic, subcallosal, orbito-insular, piriform and temporal cortex, hippocampus-fornix and amygdala. *Acta Physiol Scand Suppl.* 1951;24(83):1–262.
15. Niemeyer P. The transventricular amygdalo hipocampectomy in temporal lobe epilepsy. In: MBP B, ed. *Temporal Lobe Epilepsy.* Springfield, IL: Charles C. Thomas; 1958:461–482.
16. Sano K, Malamud N. Clinical significance of sclerosis of the cornu ammonis: ictal psychic phenomena. *AMA Arch Neurol Psychiatry.* 1953;70(1):40–53.
17. Margerison JH, Corsellis JA. Epilepsy and the temporal lobes. A clinical, electroencephalographic and neuropathological study of the brain in epilepsy, with particular reference to the temporal lobes. *Brain.* 1966;89(3):499–530.
18. Green JR, Duisberg RE, Mc GW. Focal epilepsy of psychomotor type: a preliminary report of observations on effect of surgical therapy. *J Neurosurg.* 1951;8(2):157–172.
19. Crandall PH, Walter RD, Rand RW. Clinical applications of studies on stereotactically implanted electrodes in temporal-lobe epilepsy. *J Neurosurg.* 1963;20:827–840.
20. Brown W. Structural substrates of seizure foci in the human temporal lobe. In: Brazier M, ed. *Epilepsy: Its Phenomena in Man.* New York: Academic Press; 1973:339–374.
21. Elsharkawy AE, Alabbasi AH, Pannek H, et al. Long-term outcome after temporal lobe epilepsy surgery in 434 consecutive adult patients. *J Neurosurg.* 2009;110(6):1135–1146.
22. Meyer A, Falconer MA, Beck E. Pathological findings in temporal lobe epilepsy. *J Neurol Neurosurg Psychiatry.* 1954;17(4):276–285.
23. Mathern GW, Babb TL, Vickrey BG, et al. The clinical-pathogenic mechanisms of hippocampal neuron loss and surgical outcomes in temporal lobe epilepsy. *Brain* 1995;118(Pt 1):105–118.
24. Mathern GW, Adelson PD, Cahan LD, et al. Hippocampal neuron damage in human epilepsy: Meyer's hypothesis revisited. *Prog Brain Res.* 2002;135:237–251.
25. Falconer MA. Clinical manifestations of temporal lobe epilepsy and their recognition in relation to surgical treatment. *Br Med J.* 1954;2(4894):939–944.
26. French JA, Williamson PD, Thadani VM, et al. Characteristics of medial temporal lobe epilepsy: I. Results of history and physical examination. *Ann Neurol.* 1993;34(6):774–780.
27. Berkovic SF, McIntosh A, Howell RA, et al. Familial temporal lobe epilepsy: a common disorder identified in twins. *Ann Neurol.* 1996;40(2):227–235.
28. Kobayashi E, Santos NF, Torres FR, et al. Magnetic resonance imaging abnormalities in familial temporal lobe epilepsy with auditory auras. *Arch Neurol.* 2003;60(11):1546 1551.
29. Lin K, Carrete H, Lin J, et al. Facial paresis in patients with mesial temporal sclerosis: clinical and quantitative MRI-based evidence of widespread disease. *Epilepsia.* 2007;48(8):1491–1499.
30. Risinger MW, Engel J, Jr., Van Ness PC, et al. Ictal localization of temporal lobe seizures with scalp/sphenoidal recordings. *Neurology.* 1989;39(10):1288–1293.
31. Williamson PD, French JA, Thadani VM, et al. Characteristics of medial temporal lobe epilepsy: II. Interictal and ictal scalp electroencephalography, neuropsychological testing, neuroimaging, surgical results, and pathology. *Ann Neurol.* 1993;34(6):781–787.
32. Hermann BP, Seidenberg M, Woodard AR. Memory and epilepsy: current perspectives. *Clin Nurs Pract Epilepsy.* 1996;3(4):4–8.
33. Jack CR, Jr., Bentley MD, Twomey CK, et al. MR imaging-based volume measurements of the hippocampal formation and anterior temporal lobe: validation studies. *Radiology.* 1990;176(1):205–209.
34. Stefan H, Pawlik G, Bocher-Schwarz HG, et al. Functional and morphological abnormalities in temporal lobe epilepsy: a comparison of interictal and ictal EEG, CT, MRI, SPECT and PET. *J Neurol.* 1987;234(6):377–384.
35. Engel J, Jr., Henry TR, Risinger MW, et al. Presurgical evaluation for partial epilepsy: relative contributions of chronic depth-electrode recordings versus FDG-PET and scalp-sphenoidal ictal EEG. *Neurology.* 1990;40(11):1670–1677.
36. Manford M, Fish DR, Shorvon SD. An analysis of clinical seizure patterns and their localizing value in frontal and temporal lobe epilepsies. *Brain.* 1996;119(Pt 1):17–40.
37. Fried I, Spencer DD, Spencer SS. The anatomy of epileptic auras: focal pathology and surgical outcome. *J Neurosurg.* 1995;83(1):60–66.
38. Henkel A, Noachtar S, Pfander M, et al. The localizing value of the abdominal aura and its evolution: a study in focal epilepsies. *Neurology.* 2002;58(2):271–276.
39. Holmes MD, Dodrill CB, Wilensky AJ, et al. Unilateral focal preponderance of interictal epileptiform discharges as a predictor of seizure origin. *Arch Neurol.* 1996;53(3):228–232.
40. Velasco TR, Wichert-Ana L, Leite JP, et al. Accuracy of ictal SPECT in mesial temporal lobe epilepsy with bilateral interictal spikes. *Neurology.* 2002;59(2):266–271.
41. Steinhoff BJ, So NK, Lim S, et al. Ictal scalp EEG in temporal lobe epilepsy with unitemporal versus bitemporal interictal epileptiform discharges. *Neurology.* 1995;45(5):889–896.
42. Serles W, Pataraia E, Bacher J, et al. Clinical seizure lateralization in mesial temporal lobe epilepsy: differences between patients with unitemporal and bitemporal interictal spikes. *Neurology.* 1998;50(3):742–747.
43. Jeha LE, Najm I, Bingaman W, et al. Surgical outcome and prognostic factors of frontal lobe epilepsy surgery. *Brain.* 2007;130(Pt 2):574–584.
44. Blume WT, Wiebe S, Tapsell LM. Occipital epilepsy: lateral versus mesial. *Brain.* 2005;128(Pt 5):1209–1225.
45. Foldvary N, Klem G, Hammel J, et al. The localizing value of ictal EEG in focal epilepsy. *Neurology.* 2001;57(11):2022–2028.
46. Mathern GW, Babb TL, Armstrong DL. Hippocampal sclerosis. In: Engel J, Jr., Pedley TA, eds. *Epilepsy: A Comprehensive Textbook.* 2nd ed. Philadelphia, PA: Lippincott-Raven Press; 1997:133–155.
47. Mouritzen-Dam A. Hippocampal neuron loss in epilepsy and after experimental seizures. *Acta Neurol Scand.* 1982;66(6):601–642.
48. Fuerst D, Shah J, Kupsky WJ, et al. Volumetric MRI, pathological, and neuropsychological progression in hippocampal sclerosis. *Neurology.* 2001;57(2):184–188.
49. VanLandingham KE, Heinz ER, Cavazos JE, et al. Magnetic resonance imaging evidence of hippocampal injury after prolonged focal febrile convulsions. *Ann Neurol.* 1998;43(4):413–426.
50. Miller LA, McLachlan RS, Bouwer MS, et al. Amygdalar sclerosis: preoperative indicators and outcome after temporal lobectomy. *J Neurol Neurosurg Psychiatry.* 1994;57(9):1099–1105.
51. Salmenpera T, Kalviainen R, Partanen K, et al. Quantitative MRI volumetry of the entorhinal cortex in temporal lobe epilepsy. *Seizure.* 2000;9(3):208–215.
52. Kuzniecky R, Bilir E, Gilliam F, et al. Quantitative MRI in temporal lobe epilepsy: evidence for fornix atrophy. *Neurology.* 1999;53(3):496–501.
53. Bonilha L, Kobayashi E, Rorden C, et al. Medial temporal lobe atrophy in patients with refractory temporal lobe epilepsy. *J Neurol Neurosurg Psychiatry.* 2003;74(12):1627–1630.
54. Bonilha L, Rorden C, Castellano G, et al. Voxel-based morphometry of the thalamus in patients with refractory medial temporal lobe epilepsy. *Neuroimage.* 2005;25(3):1016–1021.
55. Gross DW, Concha L, Beaulieu C. Extratemporal white matter abnormalities in mesial temporal lobe epilepsy demonstrated with diffusion tensor imaging. *Epilepsia.* 2006;47(8):1360–1363.
56. Hermann B, Seidenberg M, Bell B, et al. Extratemporal quantitative MR volumetrics and neuropsychological status in temporal lobe epilepsy. *J Int Neuropsychol Soc.* 2003;9(3):353–362.
57. Bonilha L, Rorden C, Castellano G, et al. Voxel-based morphometry reveals gray matter network atrophy in refractory medial temporal lobe epilepsy. *Arch Neurol.* 2004;61(9):1379–1384.
58. Sisodiya SM, Moran N, Free SL, et al. Correlation of widespread preoperative magnetic resonance imaging changes with unsuccessful surgery for hippocampal sclerosis. *Ann Neurol.* 1997;41(4):490–496.
59. Choi JY, Kim SJ, Hong SB, et al. Extratemporal hypometabolism on FDG PET in temporal lobe epilepsy as a predictor of seizure outcome after temporal lobectomy. *Eur J Nucl Med Mol Imaging.* 2003;30(4):581–587.
60. Araujo D, Santos AC, Velasco TR, et al. Volumetric evidence of bilateral damage in unilateral mesial temporal lobe epilepsy. *Epilepsia.* 2006;47(8):1354–1359.
61. Quigg M, Bertram EH, Jackson T, et al. Volumetric magnetic resonance imaging evidence of bilateral hippocampal atrophy in mesial temporal lobe epilepsy. *Epilepsia.* 1997;38(5):588–594.
62. Diehl B, Luders HO. Temporal lobe epilepsy: when are invasive recordings needed? *Epilepsia.* 2000;41(suppl 3):S61–S74.
63. Sirven JI, Malamut BL, Liporace JD, et al. Outcome after temporal lobectomy in bilateral temporal lobe epilepsy. *Ann Neurol.* 1997;42(6):873–878.

64. Zaatreh MM, Firlik KS, Spencer DD, et al. Temporal lobe tumoral epilepsy: characteristics and predictors of surgical outcome. *Neurology.* 2003;61(5):636–641.

65. Harvey AS, Cross JH, Shinnar S, et al. Defining the spectrum of international practice in pediatric epilepsy surgery patients. *Epilepsia.* 2008;49(1):146–155.

66. Palmini A, Najm I, Avanzini G, et al. Terminology and classification of the cortical dysplasias. *Neurology.* 2004;62(6 suppl 3):S2–S8.

67. Fauser S, Huppertz HJ, Bast T, et al. Clinical characteristics in focal cortical dysplasia: a retrospective evaluation in a series of 120 patients. *Brain.* 2006;129(Pt 7):1907–1916.

68. Fauser S, Schulze-Bonhage A, Honegger J, et al. Focal cortical dysplasias: surgical outcome in 67 patients in relation to histological subtypes and dual pathology. *Brain.* 2004;127(Pt 11):2406–2418.

69. Bronen RA, Fulbright RK, Spencer DD, et al. MR characteristics of neoplasms and vascular malformations associated with epilepsy. *Magn Reson Imaging.* 1995;13(8):1153–1162.

70. Cohen DS, Zubay GP, Goodman RR. Seizure outcome after lesionectomy for cavernous malformations. *J Neurosurg.* 1995;83(2):237–242.

71. Cohen-Gadol AA, Bradley CC, Williamson A, et al. Normal magnetic resonance imaging and medial temporal lobe epilepsy: the clinical syndrome of paradoxical temporal lobe epilepsy. *J Neurosurg.* 2005;102(5):902–909.

72. Foldvary N, Lee N, Thwaites G, et al. Clinical and electrographic manifestations of lesional neocortical temporal lobe epilepsy. *Neurology.* 1997;49(3):757–763.

73. Pacia SV, Devinsky O, Perrine K, et al. Clinical features of neocortical temporal lobe epilepsy. *Ann Neurol.* 1996;40(5):724–730.

74. Levesque MF, Nakasato N, Vinters HV, et al. Surgical treatment of limbic epilepsy associated with extrahippocampal lesions: the problem of dual pathology. *J Neurosurg.* 1991;75(3):364–370.

75. Cendes F, Cook MJ, Watson C, et al. Frequency and characteristics of dual pathology in patients with lesional epilepsy. *Neurology.* 1995;45(11):2058–2064.

76. Salanova V, Markand O, Worth R. Temporal lobe epilepsy: analysis of patients with dual pathology. *Acta Neurol Scand.* 2004;109(2):126–131.

77. Wieser HG, Yasargil MG. Selective amygdalohippocampectomy as a surgical treatment of mesiobasal limbic epilepsy. *Surg Neurol.* 1982;17(6):445–457.

78. Brodie MJ. Diagnosing and predicting refractory epilepsy. *Acta Neurol Scand Suppl.* 2005;181:36–39.

79. Cockerell OC, Johnson AL, Sander JW, et al. Mortality from epilepsy: results from a prospective population-based study. *Lancet.* 1994;344(8927):918–921.

80. Cascino GD, Jack CR, Jr., Parisi JE, et al. Magnetic resonance imaging-based volume studies in temporal lobe epilepsy: pathological correlations. *Ann Neurol.* 1991;30(1):31–36.

81. Ryvlin P, Bouvard S, Le Bars D, et al. Clinical utility of flumazenil-PET versus [18F]fluorodeoxyglucose-PET and MRI in refractory partial epilepsy. A prospective study in 100 patients. *Brain.* 1998;121(Pt 11):2067–2081.

82. Nakasato N, Levesque MF, Barth DS, et al. Comparisons of MEG, EEG, and ECoG source localization in neocortical partial epilepsy in humans. *Electroencephalogr Clin Neurophysiol.* 1994;91(3):171–178.

83. Wiebe S, Blume WT, Girvin JP, et al. A randomized, controlled trial of surgery for temporal-lobe epilepsy. *N Engl J Med.* 2001;345(5):311–318.

84. Stavem K, Bjornaes H, Langmoen IA. Long-term seizures and quality of life after epilepsy surgery compared with matched controls. *Neurosurgery.* 2008;62(2):326–334. Discussion 334–335.

85. Kumlien E, Doss RC, Gates JR. Treatment outcome in patients with mesial temporal sclerosis. *Seizure.* 2002;11(7):413–417.

86. Tonini C, Beghi E, Berg AT, et al. Predictors of epilepsy surgery outcome: a meta-analysis. *Epilepsy Res.* 2004;62(1):75–87.

87. Tellez-Zenteno JF, Dhar R, Wiebe S. Long-term seizure outcomes following epilepsy surgery: a systematic review and meta-analysis. *Brain.* 2005;128(Pt 5):1188–1198.

88. Cohen-Gadol AA, Wilhelmi BG, Collignon F, et al. Long-term outcome of epilepsy surgery among 399 patients with nonlesional seizure foci including mesial temporal lobe sclerosis. *J Neurosurg.* 2006;104(4):513–524.

89. Mittal S, Montes JL, Farmer JP, et al. Long-term outcome after surgical treatment of temporal lobe epilepsy in children. *J Neurosurg.* 2005;103(suppl 5):401–412.

90. McIntosh AM, Kalnins RM, Mitchell LA, et al. Temporal lobectomy: long-term seizure outcome, late recurrence and risks for seizure recurrence. *Brain.* 2004;127(Pt 9):2018–2030.

91. Luyken C, Blumcke I, Fimmers R, et al. The spectrum of long-term epilepsy-associated tumors: long-term seizure and tumor outcome and neurosurgical aspects. *Epilepsia.* 2003;44(6):822–830.

92. Kelemen A, Barsi P, Eross L, et al. Long-term outcome after temporal lobe surgery—prediction of late worsening of seizure control. *Seizure.* 2006;15(1):49–55.

93. Asztely F, Ekstedt G, Rydenhag B, et al. Long term follow-up of the first 70 operated adults in the Goteborg Epilepsy Surgery Series with respect to seizures, psychosocial outcome and use of antiepileptic drugs. *J Neurol Neurosurg Psychiatry.* 2007;78(6):605–609.

94. Bauer R, Dobesberger J, Unterhofer C, et al. Outcome of adult patients with temporal lobe tumours and medically refractory focal epilepsy. *Acta Neurochir (Wien).* 2007;149(12):1211–1216. Discussion 1216–1217.

95. Tatum WO, IV, Benbadis SR, Hussain A, et al. Ictal EEG remains the prominent predictor of seizure-free outcome after temporal lobectomy in epileptic patients with normal brain MRI. *Seizure.* 2008;17(7):631–636.

96. Hamiwka L, Jayakar P, Resnick T, et al. Surgery for epilepsy due to cortical malformations: ten-year follow-up. *Epilepsia.* 2005;46(4):556–560.

97. Kim DW, Lee SK, Chu K, et al. Predictors of surgical outcome and pathologic considerations in focal cortical dysplasia. *Neurology.* 2009;72(3):211–216.

98. Krsek P, Maton B, Jayakar P, et al. Incomplete resection of focal cortical dysplasia is the main predictor of poor postsurgical outcome. *Neurology.* 2009;72(3):217–223.

99. Li LM, Cendes F, Andermann F, et al. Surgical outcome in patients with epilepsy and dual pathology. *Brain.* 1999;122(Pt 5):799–805.

100. Nakasato N, Levesque MF, Babb TL. Seizure outcome following standard temporal lobectomy: correlation with hippocampal neuron loss and extrahippocampal pathology. *J Neurosurg.* 1992;77(2):194–200.

101. Tezer FI, Akalan N, Oguz KK, et al. Predictive factors for postoperative outcome in temporal lobe epilepsy according to two different classifications. *Seizure.* 2008;17(6):549–560.

102. Hennessy MJ, Elwes RD, Honavar M, et al. Predictors of outcome and pathological considerations in the surgical treatment of intractable epilepsy associated with temporal lobe lesions. *J Neurol Neurosurg Psychiatry.* 2001;70(4):450–458.

103. Burneo JG, Black L, Martin R, et al. Race/ethnicity, sex, and socioeconomic status as predictors of outcome after surgery for temporal lobe epilepsy. *Arch Neurol.* 2006;63(8):1106–1110.

104. Schmidt D, Baumgartner C, Loscher W. The chance of cure following surgery for drug-resistant temporal lobe epilepsy. What do we know and do we need to revise our expectations? *Epilepsy Res.* 2004;60(2–3):187–201.

105. Schiller Y, Cascino GD, So EL, et al. Discontinuation of antiepileptic drugs after successful epilepsy surgery. *Neurology.* 2000;54(2):346–349.

106. Hermann BP, Seidenberg M, Bell B, et al. Comorbid psychiatric symptoms in temporal lobe epilepsy: association with chronicity of epilepsy and impact on quality of life. *Epilepsy Behav.* 2000;1(3):184–190.

107. Birbeck GL, Hays RD, Cui X, et al. Seizure reduction and quality of life improvements in people with epilepsy. *Epilepsia.* 2002;43(5):535–538.

108. Tellez-Zenteno JF, Dhar R, Hernandez-Ronquillo L, et al. Long-term outcomes in epilepsy surgery: antiepileptic drugs, mortality, cognitive and psychosocial aspects. *Brain.* 2007;130(Pt 2):334–345.

109. Spencer SS, Berg AT, Vickrey BG, et al. Health-related quality of life over time since resective epilepsy surgery. *Ann Neurol.* 2007;62(4):327–334.

110. Langfitt JT, Westerveld M, Hamberger MJ, et al. Worsening of quality of life after epilepsy surgery: effect of seizures and memory decline. *Neurology.* 2007;68(23):1988–1994.

111. Stroup E, Langfitt J, Berg M, et al. Predicting verbal memory decline following anterior temporal lobectomy (ATL). *Neurology.* 2003;60(8):1266–1273.

112. Ruff IM, Swanson SJ, Hammeke TA, et al. Predictors of naming decline after dominant temporal lobectomy: age at onset of epilepsy and age of word acquisition. *Epilepsy Behav.* 2007;10(2):272–277.

113. Manchanda R, Schaefer B, McLachlan RS, et al. Psychiatric disorders in candidates for surgery for epilepsy. *J Neurol Neurosurg Psychiatry.* 1996;61(1):82–89.

114. Helmstaedter C, Kurthen M, Lux S, et al. Chronic epilepsy and cognition: a longitudinal study in temporal lobe epilepsy. *Ann Neurol.* 2003;54(4):425–432.

115. Devinsky O, Barr WB, Vickrey BG, et al. Changes in depression and anxiety after resective surgery for epilepsy. *Neurology.* 2005;65(11):1744–1749.

116. Chapell R, Reston J, Snyder D. *Management of Treatment-Resistant Epilepsy: Evidence Report/Technology Assessment No 77.* Rockville, MD: Agency for Healthcare Research and Quality; 2003.

117. Grivas A, Schramm J, Kral T, et al. Surgical treatment for refractory temporal lobe epilepsy in the elderly: seizure outcome and neuropsychological sequels compared with a younger cohort. *Epilepsia.* 2006;47(8):1364–1372.

118. Regis J, Rey M, Bartolomei F, et al. Gamma knife surgery in mesial temporal lobe epilepsy: a prospective multicenter study. *Epilepsia.* 2004;45(5):504–515.

119. Barbaro NM, Quigg M, Broshek DK, et al. A multicenter, prospective pilot study of gamma knife radiosurgery for mesial temporal lobe epilepsy: seizure response, adverse events, and verbal memory. *Ann Neurol.* 2009;65(2):167–175.

120. Srikijvilaikul T, Najm I, Foldvary-Schaefer N, et al. Failure of gamma knife radiosurgery for mesial temporal lobe epilepsy: report of five cases. *Neurosurgery.* 2004;54(6):1395–1402. Discussion 1402–1394.

CHAPTER 83 ■ FOCAL AND MULTILOBAR RESECTION

PAULA M. BRNA AND MICHAEL DUCHOWNY

It is well established that 25% to 30% of patients with epilepsy are medically resistant and that surgery offers the best chance of seizure freedom. After a single failed antiepileptic drug (AED), 11% of patients respond to a second drug but only 3% respond to two or more AEDs (1). There is, thus, little support for undertaking an exhaustive trial of AEDs before declaring a patient medically intractable and referring for surgical evaluation.

A high proportion of medically refractory epilepsies are focal in origin. While the majority arise in the temporal lobe, extratemporal foci are common particularly in childhood. The neocortical epilepsies are a diverse group with a broad spectrum of pathology, which present significant challenges to localizing the epileptogenic focus. The presurgical evaluation focuses on accurate and precise localization of the epileptogenic zone so that complete resection can be achieved. The compilation of clinical, electrographic, and neuroimaging data are directed toward this goal. Surgical procedures vary according to the location and extent of the epileptogenic zone and its proximity to eloquent cortex.

Epilepsy surgery should be advocated early in the course of medically intractable seizures (2). Early surgical management will prevent long-term disability, social maladjustment, and impaired quality of life. Timely surgical referral in childhood is particularly important to improve cognitive development and promote neuronal plasticity.

PRESURGICAL EVALUATION OF FOCAL EXTRATEMPORAL EPILEPSY

The goals of the presurgical evaluation are to identify the epileptogenic zone, define abnormal cortex, and determine the proximity of these regions to eloquent regions. Complete removal of the epileptogenic zone is the major prerequisite for postoperative seizure freedom (3,4). Patients generally fall into one of the three broad categories: (i) a discrete structural lesion and concordant electrophysiology, (ii) an identifiable developmental lesion with more diffuse abnormality and a less circumscribed epileptogenic zone, and (iii) no evidence of a lesion on MRI or functional imaging. MRI-negative patients are most challenging as the absence of a demonstrable lesion often mandates placement of intracranial electrodes.

Clinical Data

The preoperative evaluation begins with careful analysis of seizure semiology for essential clues to localization. The importance of documenting seizure history and ictal sequence of events cannot be overstated. For example, semiology helps distinguish frontal versus mesial temporal seizure origin. Motor symptomatology at seizure onset suggests frontal lobe involvement whereas oroalimentary automatisms and psychic symptoms indicate mesial temporal activation (5). Late motor symptoms in temporal lobe cases suggest secondary rather than primary activation of the frontal lobe.

The history provides important antecedent factors related to prenatal, perinatal, or postnatal etiologies. The family history will identify genetic syndromes that are not surgically amenable. Assessment of developmental status is important in pediatric patients as catastrophic epilepsies associated with developmental stagnation or regression mandate more urgent surgical referral. Neurologic deficits on examination such as hemiparesis or visual field defects raise suspicion of contralateral seizure origin.

Localizing Clinical Semiology

Frontal lobe epilepsy accounts for up to 30% of epilepsy surgeries, second only to temporal lobectomies (6,7). An anterior frontal wedge resection is illustrated in Figure 83.1. Frontal lobe seizures are typically brief, may occur in clusters, and manifest a nocturnal predisposition (8). Although motor manifestations and vocalization are the most common ictal features (9–11), frontal lobe functions are diverse and associated with a variety of ictal manifestations depending on the region involved.

Seizures involving the dominant inferior frontal lobe commonly produce aphasia, dysarthria, and contralateral facial motor deficits, whereas involvement of the nondominant inferior frontal gyrus induces speech arrest and tonic facial contractions. Salivation and swallowing are characteristic features of seizures arising in the frontal operculum, whereas contralateral head and eye, tonic elevation, and contralateral clonic movements of the arms and face occur with mesial frontal or dorsolateral frontal seizures (12). Classic supplementary motor area (SMA) seizures lead to speech arrest and a "fencing posture" with bilateral motor movements and contralateral head and eye version (13). However, callosal connections result in rapid activation of the contralateral hemisphere and may lead to difficulties lateralizing seizure onset (14). Resection of the SMA may result in transient weakness and contralateral apraxia.

The orbitofrontal region has extensive connections with the anterior temporal lobe, cingulum, and operculum. Orbitofrontal seizures commonly induce autonomic changes

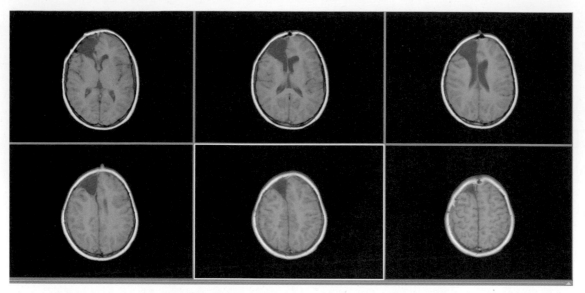

FIGURE 83.1 Postoperative MRI showing a right frontal anterior lobar wedge resection.

and heightened motor activity ("hypermotor seizures"), while behavioral arrest and automatisms indicate propagation to the temporal lobe or cingulate gyrus (15,16). The insula has extensive connections to the limbic system leading to visceral, gustatory, and somatosensory hallucinations (17,18).

Premotor seizures are associated with tonic versive upper extremity posturing (unilateral > bilateral) mimicking SMA semiology. Seizures originating from the precentral gyrus manifest as distal contralateral clonic movement. Although complete resection of primary motor cortex is rarely possible, localized resections may be beneficial in patients with an expectant motor deficit.

Parietal resections account for a modest proportion of epilepsy surgeries. Postcentral gyrus seizures often present with somatosensory auras, whereas seizure more posterior are often silent until they propagate to the frontal or temporal lobes (19). Parietal foci are often MRI-positive but scalp EEG rarely localizes the epileptogenic zone (19,20). Large posterior resections may be safely achieved in the nondominant parietal lobe.

Seizures of basal posterior temporal onset manifest with behavioral arrest followed by motor manifestations (mainly contralateral head version and contralateral arm tonic stiffening); clonic activity may occur late in the ictus (21). Late motor semiology is a clue to ictal onset outside of the frontal lobe.

Medically resistant occipital epilepsies are uncommon and present with elementary visual hallucinations, ictal amaurosis, rapid eye blinking and fluttering, sensations of eye movement, and variable spread to the temporal lobe (22). The majority of cases are MRI-positive with one surgical series reporting structural lesions in 96% of patients (23). A significant proportion of occipital lobe resections cause postoperative visual field deficits.

Seizure localization in infants presents special challenges. Seizures in children under age 3 years are often motor or hypomotor (24,25). Bilateral asymmetric motor and versive manifestations consistently demonstrate focal ictal EEG patterns, but even clinically generalized motor seizures in young children often show focal ictal EEG changes (26,27). Although infantile spasms, for example, are typically considered to represent

generalized epilepsy, focal abnormalities on EEG or neuroimaging are not uncommon (28).

Electrophysiology

Capturing habitual events ensures consistency and accuracy of localization, but multiple EEG studies may be required. Patients with frontal lobe epilepsy, for example, may exhibit either no interictal epileptiform discharges or patterns that are poorly localized, bifrontal, or generalized (12). While ictal capture is the most accurate noninvasive method to define the seizure focus, caution must be exercised for parietal and occipital foci where the ictal data may be falsely localizing (29,30). Consistent unifocal interictal epileptiform discharges are a strong predictor of good surgery outcome for both lesional and nonlesional epilepsies (31). In many cases, a large epileptogenic zone necessitates the placement of intracranial electrodes for accurate localization, though advances in neuroimaging have reduced the need for invasive monitoring.

Anatomic Neuroimaging

High-resolution MRI identifies a structural abnormality in up to 85% of partial epilepsy patients (32) and predicts favorable outcome (33–36). The MRI protocol for epilepsy patients includes T1 and T2 thin contiguous slices with three-dimensional volumetric acquisition, gadolinium enhancement, and fluid-attenuated inversion recovery (FLAIR) sequences to detect subtle cortical dysplasia (37). Despite modern imaging modalities and sequences, 25% of intractable epilepsies have a negative MRI (38). Frontal lobe epilepsies are especially problematic as up to 29% of pediatric cases reportedly demonstrate no anatomic abnormality (39).

Functional Neuroimaging

Diffusion tensor imaging (DTI) and functional MRI (fMRI) provide additional clues to abnormal function or aberrant pathways and a noninvasive means of examining critical functions. Functional MRI, for example, can assess language dominance without the need for invasive assessment (40,41). Functional neuroimaging offers greater sensitivity for detecting abnormalities but lacks the specificity of MRI (42). The techniques are often complimentary with each having distinct advantages and disadvantages. Unfortunately, there are no clear guidelines on which patients benefit from these studies and thus clinical practice varies widely among epilepsy surgery centers.

Interictal 2-deoxy-2-[18F] fluoro-D-glucose (FDG) positron emission tomography (PET) depicts cerebral metabolism by providing a topographic view of cerebral glucose uptake. Epileptogenic regions may show relative hypometabolism though the cause of this hypometabolism is poorly understood. Presumably it reflects cerebral dysfunction in the epileptogenic tissue. FDG-PET identifies regions of hypometabolism in 70% to 90% with temporal lobe epilepsy but has reduced sensitivity in extratemporal cases (42–46). For temporal cases, the surgical outcomes are better when a greater volume of the PET abnormality is resected, though complete removal is not required for success (47). The region of hypometabolism often extends beyond the epileptogenic zone and limits its specificity (48,49). PET rarely discloses a functional lesion in MRI-negative cases (28). Flumazenil-PET has shown increased sensitivity in detecting the area of ictal onset in children (48) and alpha[C]methyl-L-tryptophan (AMT) PET is useful in identifying the epileptogenic tuber in tuberous sclerosis complex (TSC) surgery candidates (50,51).

Interictal and ictal single photon emission computed tomography (SPECT) may provide additional localizing information in patients as young as 1 year of age (52,53). SPECT uses technetium-based radioisotopes that image ictal blood flow due to their ability to become trapped on first-pass through the cerebral vasculature following injection. Ictal SPECT reveals increased cerebral blood flow in the region affected by epileptic discharges (53), though the timing of radiopharmaceutical injection must be rapid for an accurate representation. SPECT injection should be performed within 20 seconds of seizure onset (54,55) as ictal regional blood flow may increase by 300% (56,57). Ictal hyperperfusion helps differentiate temporal and extratemporal epilepsy, confirms suspected epileptogenicity of a structural lesion, and guides placement of intracranial electrodes. It shows concordance with intracranial localization in 74% of cases (58) and identifies the ictal-onset zone rather than areas of propagation (59). This may be particularly useful for focal cortical dysplasia (FCD) where the epileptogenic zone frequently extends beyond the anatomic margins on MRI.

Ictal SPECT has shown good agreement with other noninvasive techniques (42) and clinical semiology for localization (52,60). The sensitivity of ictal SPECT is generally under 50% for extratemporal epilepsy but improves to 90% with subtraction techniques (61,62). Pediatric studies have shown sensitivities of 70% to 85% for frontal lobe localization but nocturnal and brief events pose logistical challenges (52,63). Rapid seizure propagation may provide confusing or conflicting results.

Magnetoencephalography (MEG)

MEG is an adjuvant technology to assist in localization of the interictal spike field on scalp EEG. MEG shows excellent concordance with intracranial ictal EEG studies in tumor and cortical malformation cases (64,65). In one pediatric study, 10/11 children with nonlesional, extratemporal focal epilepsy demonstrated MEG dipole localization concordant with ictal onset on intracranial EEG (66). MEG source localization may be coregistered to MRI to provide three-dimensional representation of the dipole.

Invasive Electrophysiology

Intrinsically epileptogenic lesions such as cortical malformations often exhibit near-continuous epileptiform activity on electrocorticography which can be used to guide the cortical resection (67,68). The application of intracranial EEG in adults has improved rates of seizure freedom for extratemporal epileptogenic lesions by 44% (69,70). Chronic intracranial recordings utilize a variety of electrodes including subdural grids, strips, and depth electrodes. Depth electrodes require strategic placement and have limited ability to sample widespread convexity and basal cortical surfaces. There are several indications for subdural electrode implantation (71). When epilepsy is nonlesional or poorly localized, subdural monitoring provides accurate localizing information. Even for widespread epileptogenic zones, implantation yields valuable information about its borders. Children with intractable epilepsy often have multifocal or multilesional epileptiform abnormalities necessitating implantation of subdural electrodes. This strategy is particularly important for children with TSC and intractable epilepsy where multiple tubers are the rule but a single lesion is epileptogenic.

Functional Mapping

Functional mapping is employed for resections of the central region, dominant inferior frontal cortex, dominant posterior temporal, parietal or occipital lobe, and can be employed in very young children using modified paradigms (72). Direct cortical stimulation also reveals aberrant regions of critical cortex owing to redistribution in regions of cortical dysplasia (73). Primary motor cortex may be mapped to define the boundaries of frontal lobectomy or paracentral corticectomy. Neocortical temporal and parietal resections may necessitate receptive language mapping depending on language lateralization and the posterior extent of the proposed resection.

Neuropsychological Evaluation

Formal neuropsychologic assessment serves as a baseline to identify specific deficits associated with the epileptogenic region, but often fails to lateralize dysfunction in pediatric cases. Older children and adults demonstrate discrepancies in verbal and performance intelligence quotients, memory deficits, or language lateralization.

SURGICAL CONTRAINDICATIONS

Contraindications to epilepsy surgery include underlying metabolic or neurodegenerative processes and benign epilepsy syndromes (benign rolandic epilepsy, benign occipital epilepsy).

Overlap of functional cortex and the epileptogenic zone may also preclude resection.

PATHOLOGIC SUBSTRATES

Major etiologies of the neocortical epilepsies are listed in Table 83.1. For extratemporal surgeries, the major pathologies at the Cleveland Clinic (74) were cortical dysplasia (38%), tumors (28%), remote infarct/ischemic lesions (18%), and vascular malformations (3%), while 17% had no pathological substrate and 26% of tumors had coexistent cortical dysplasia. Zentner et al. (35) reported a similar experience in 60 cases of extratemporal surgeries with pathology showing tumors in 28%, non-neoplastic focal lesions in 55%, and negative in 17%. The most common non-neoplastic focal lesions were glioneuronal and vascular malformations. The most common etiologies in the perirolandic region are neoplastic (50%), vascular (15%), cortical dysplasia (12%), and Rasmussen encephalitis (6%) (75).

Malformations of Cortical Development (MCDs)

MCDs are a frequent cause of intractable partial epilepsies in lesional and nonlesional MRI cases and constitute a spectrum from FCD to more extensive malformations including pachygyria, polymicrogyria, schizencephaly, and lissencephaly (73). FCD accounts for the majority of nonlesional surgical cases; 75% have medically refractory epilepsy (76) making surgical treatment important for this group (77). Patients with FCD are predisposed to early onset intractable seizures and status epilepticus, and are overrepresented in extratemporal cases (68,78). MCDs account for 20% to 30% of pediatric and adult resections (79). The most frequent locations FCD are frontal (68%), temporal (28%), and multilobar (4%) (78).

TABLE 83.1

LESIONAL EPILEPSY SUBSTRATES

Mesial temporal sclerosis
Neoplasms
Glial tumors
Ganglioglioma
Dysembryoplastic neuroepithelial tumors
Developmental lesions
Malformations of cortical development
Tuberous sclerosis complex
Hamartoma
Vascular malformations
Arteriovenous malformations
Cavernous angiomas
Inflammatory lesions
Rasmussen encephalitis
Postencephalitic lesions
Traumatic lesions
Gliosis
Focal encephalomalacia

FCD is also over-represented in the central and insular areas and 54% have epileptogenic zones within or in close proximity to critical cortex (78).

In severe FCD, cytomegalic neurons exhibit epileptogenic potential due to dendritic and axonal overgrowth; hyperexcitability is indicated by repetitive calcium spikes, but their absence in milder forms indicates that other factors must be involved (80).

FCD histopathology is categorized as: mild malformation of cortical development (mMCD), FCD type 1a (isolated architectural abnormalities) in which the MRI is often negative or shows focal gray-white blurring, type 1b (with additional immature or giant neurons), type 2a (with additional dysmorphic neurons), and type 2b (with additional balloon cells) (81). Taylor type 2 lesions are associated with focal thickening of cortex and blurring of the gray-white junction. Type 2b frequently shows increased signal intensity extending from the cortex to the ventricular surface.

Tuberous Sclerosis Complex (TSC)

TSC is a genetic disorder of neuronal differentiation and proliferation resulting in multiple hamartomatous central nervous system lesions (82). Up to 90% of TSC patients develop seizures in childhood, many of whom ultimately become medically refractory. Tubers are classically multiple and bilateral but partial seizures are often attributable to a single epileptogenic tuber (83,84). Excision of the epileptogenic tuber is associated with high rates of seizure freedom (83,85–87).

Tumors

Brain tumors account for 15% to 30% of patients undergoing epilepsy surgery for neocortical epilepsy (17,88). Approximately 50% of patients with supratentorial tumors will have seizures, though not all are medically intractable. Cerebral tumors may be of glial origin (astrocytomas, oligodendrogliomas, or mixed) or neuroglial (dysembryoplastic neuroepithelial tumors [DNET], ganglioglioma). Indolent benign tumors show a greater propensity towards intractable seizures. Seizures are often the first presentation of low-grade tumors and their presence is a favorable tumor prognosticator.

DNETs and gangliogliomas represent a small proportion of primary brain tumors but account for a disproportionate number of tumor-related intractable epilepsies (89,90). These tumors may have intrinsic epileptogenic activity because of their neuronal components. Gangliogliomas are composed of both neoplastic neural and neoplastic glial cells situated most frequently in the temporal lobe (91). These tumors appear hypointense on T1-weighted MRI and hyperintense on T2-weighted sequences. DNETs are cortically based tumors accounting for 10% to 20% of tumor-related intractable epilepsy (92). These lesions occur frequently in younger patients and most are located in the temporal or frontal lobe (93,94). These lesions may coexist with an area of FCD, a finding which has important implications for ensuring complete resection (95).

Low-grade glial tumors account for a substantial proportion of tumor-related epilepsies and most often occur in the temporal lobe (96). These include low-grade gliomas, pilocytic asytrocytomas, pleiomorphic xanthoastrocytomas, and oligo-dendrogliomas.

Prior Cerebral Injury (Trauma/Infarct/ Previous Cortical Resection)

Cranial injuries are frequently subdivided into penetrating or missile injuries and nonpenetrating head injuries. Penetrating injuries commonly produce focal tissue damage and hemorrhage. Approximately 50% to 75% of cortical contusions involve the frontal and temporal lobes, particularly the lateral convexity and basal frontal cortex (97). These lesions of the superficial gray matter are associated with acute hemorrhage. More severe trauma produces encephalomalacia with bilateral asymmetric frontal lesions. The frontal pole and orbitofrontal regions are particularly vulnerable to closed head trauma and post-traumatic epilepsy (98). Pathologic changes in post-traumatic epilepsy vary with the type of injury and vary significantly between affected regions (99,100). Encephalomalacia is nonspecific and results from perinatal insults, head injury, or previous surgical resections.

Vascular Malformations

The majority of vascular lesions associated with epilepsy are arteriovenous malformations (AVMs) and cavernous angiomas. Because these lesions consist of malformed blood vessels, they lack functioning neuronal tissue and their epileptogenic potential arises from hemorrhage, gliosis, and encephalomalacia in surrounding brain tissue. Surgical resection of vascular malformations has two primary treatment goals: seizure freedom and prevention of future hemorrhages, particularly for AVMs which have a 4% annual risk of hemorrhage (101).

AVMs are vascular abnormalities with direct communication between mature arteries and veins without an intervening capillary bed accompanied by gliosis of the adjacent brain tissue. AVMs are associated with focal epilepsy and are readily identified on MRI as a serpiginous cluster of signal void due to abnormally dilated vessels with slow blood flow.

Cavernous angiomas are clusters of fragile sinusoidal enlarged vessels which lack mature vessel walls and, therefore, are prone to repeated hemorrhages. These lesions account for 10% to 20% of intracranial vascular abnormalities with 30% to 40% resulting in seizures (102). They may be sporadic or familial. The cavernoma has a stereotyped appearance on MRI with a round area of mixed signal intensity surrounded by a ring of surround hypointensity on T2-weighted and gradient echo sequences caused by hemosiderin deposition from old hemorrhages (103). Their epileptogenic potential likely reflects pathologic changes in the surrounding tissue from chronic microhemorrhages (104,105), and there is experimental support for epileptogenicity of hemosiderin-induced damage (106). Resection of cavernous angiomas should include the hemosiderin-stained rim (107) as the vascular malformation itself is not epileptogenic. Cavernomas may be multiple and a careful search for other lesions is critical.

Venous angiomas rarely cause epilepsy but may be discovered incidentally on neuroimaging. Their importance lies in avoiding surgical resection as it can lead to venous infarction.

Inflammatory Lesions

Infectious

Though much less common in North America, neurocysticercosis is a major cause of seizures in Latin America, Asia, and Africa (108). Focal seizures occur in 70% of symptomatic patients and are a rare cause of intractable epilepsy due to calcifications or remote epileptogenesis (108,109). Postinfectious encephalitis is associated with multifocal abnormalities that may preclude focal resection.

Noninfectious

Rasmussen encephalitis is a chronic encephalopathy of unknown, though suspected autoimmune etiology resulting in progressive atrophy and inflammatory changes in one cerebral hemisphere. It is characterized by progressive hemiparesis, hemianopia, and intractable focal seizures (110). Seizures often include epilepsia partialis continua, and hemispherectomy remains the only known effective treatment (111). Focal resections or brain biopsies may be performed to confirm the diagnosis.

MULTILOBAR RESECTIONS

Multilobar resections are considered for management of intractable seizures in settings where epileptogenic zones affect more than one lobe of the brain while attempting to preserve visual, language, and motor integrity. Thus, these procedures are undertaken in cases of unilateral extensive or hemispheric pathology and epileptogenesis where minimal hemiparesis, visual field defect, and speech disturbance remain minimal or absent. Multilobar resections may involve any combination of lobar surgery. Surgical procedures vary from multiple lobectomies to multilobar corticectomies or lobar disconnection and may be staged with the initial resection targeting the most active region or most damaged lobe.

Etiologies of Multilobar Resections

Multilobar cases are a small proportion of epilepsy surgeries. In one series of 2000 epilepsy surgeries, multilobar resections accounted for only 1.6% of procedures (112). In a large pediatric series, the most commonly performed multilobar procedure was temporal–occipital–parietal (posterior quadrant) resection which accounted for 44% of multilobar cases (113). A typical posterior quadrant resection is illustrated in Figure 83.2. The most frequent etiology for multilobar resections is cortical dysplasia (55%). Indications for multilobar resections are similar to those for hemispherectomy including prenatal and neonatal insults, vascular insults leading to porencephalic cysts, tumors, trauma and gliosis, hemispheric cortical dysplasia, or other malformations of cortical development and Sturge–Weber syndrome (114).

Multilobar resections should only be performed when the etiology is static. Sturge–Weber syndrome, for example, is a neurocutaneous disorder with extensive unilateral leptomeningeal angiomatosis that often spares a portion of the hemisphere (115). If vascular compromise is nonprogressive, multilobar resection that spares sensorimotor cortex may be a reasonable goal. Similarly, in cases of extensive multilobar

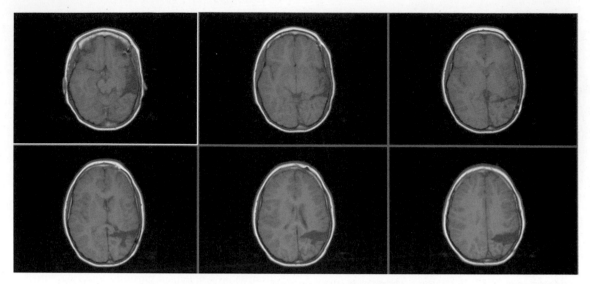

FIGURE 83.2 Postoperative MRI showing a typical left posterior quadrantectomy.

cortical dysplasia without hemiplegia, multilobar resection may help preserve sensorimotor function. In contrast, patients with Rasmussen encephalitis are unlikely to benefit from a multilobar resection given the relentlessly progressive nature of the disorder (111,116).

Posterior quadrantic surgery is the most commonly employed multilobar procedure and accounts for less than 5% of the surgical caseload (117). Most candidates have ischemic prenatal insults, cortical dysplasia, and Sturge–Weber syndrome (117). The posterior quadrant resection is a useful approach when the epileptogenic zone entails large portions of the temporal, parietal, and occipital lobes but spares the frontal and central areas. This large multilobar surgery may be completed as an excision or disconnection, but careful attention to preserving primary motor and sensory cortices is critical. A pre-existing visual field defect makes the decision for proceeding with this resection strategy more convincing. The early onset or congenitally acquired nature of many of these lesions frequently has led to transfer of language to the contralateral hemisphere, but this must be confirmed either invasively or noninvasively. Daniel et al. report five patients with left posterior quadrant surgeries with no postoperative language dysfunction (117).

Presurgical Evaluation for Multilobar Resections

The presurgical evaluation for multilobar resections applies the same principles as that for focal epilepsies. The more extensive electrographic and imaging abnormalities may require placement of intracranial electrodes to delineate eloquent cortical regions.

Clinical Data

The goal of multilobar surgery is generally to preserve motor, visual field, or language function in a hemisphere with extensive damage. In multilobar cases, the clinical details may be confusing or misleading as the seizure semiology may vary or localize to one affected region despite extensive abnormalities. Temporal lobe epilepsy, for example, may involve regional structures such

as the temporal–parietal–occipital junction, orbitofrontal cortex, insula, or the frontal or parietal operculum. The clinical semiology may suggest temporal lobe involvement while other affected regions remain clinically silent. However, more extensive epileptogenic zones are frequently associated with auditory illusions, piloerection, ipsilateral tonic motor or versive signs, and gustatory or vestibular auras (118).

Electrophysiology

Multilobar cases typically show widespread interictal abnormalities on EEG and the poorly circumscribed ictal-onset zones. Invasive electroencephalography may demonstrate focal ictal onset with independent electrographic sequences in adjacent cortex during the seizure. For example, anterior temporal lobe seizures may reveal extralobar intraictal activation of the frontal convexity (Fig. 83.3). Sites of intraictal activation are important markers of epileptogenicity. The illustrated example in Figure 83.4 prompted a multilobar resection of the left temporal and orbitofrontal regions. Under such circumstances, failure to resect the region of intraictal activation is associated with surgical failure (119).

Neuroimaging

Anatomic imaging localizes the lobes involved, but the epileptogenic zone often extends beyond the anatomic abnormality. PET may be a useful adjunct in better defining the epileptogenic zone. In Sturge–Weber syndrome, for example, PET can delineate functional involvement of regions beyond the angioma. Chugani et al. have demonstrated the benefit of combining PET with intraoperative electrocorticography to define the boundaries for multilobar resections (120). However, if there is hemiplegia with impaired hand function, a diffusely abnormal EEG and hemispheric pathology on MRI hemispherectomy are often preferred.

POSTSURGICAL OUTCOME

Seizure outcome according to the Engel classification system (121) reveals comparable adult and pediatric neocortical resection outcomes with seizure-free rates of 36% to 76% and

A

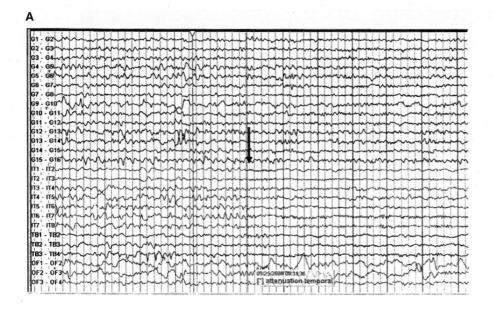

B

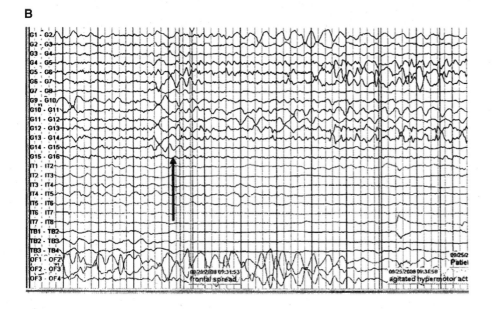

C

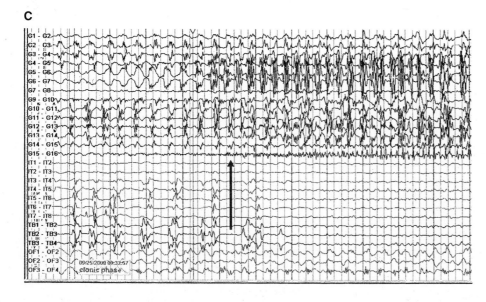

FIGURE 83.3 Intraictal activation of a secondary epileptogenic focus. **A:** Subdural EEG recordings over the left frontal and temporal lobes show a focal seizure onset over the temporal contacts IT 1-8 and TB1-4 *(arrow)*. **B:** An intraictal secondarily activated focus is evident over the frontal convexity grid at electrodes G 5/6 and G13 *(arrow)*. **C:** Persistent activity at this secondary focus is shown to outlast the temporal seizure activity *(arrow)*.

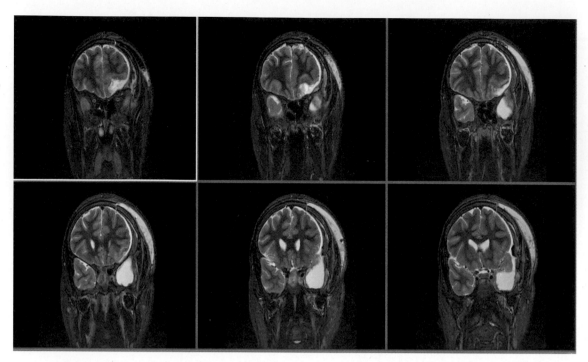

FIGURE 83.4 Postoperative MRI showing a multilobar resection involving left orbitofrontal and left temporal lobes.

54% to 66%, respectively (4,79,113,122–124). The single most consistent predictor of outcome is completeness of resection of the epileptogenic zone (4,24,70,125). Paolicchi et al. reported that the probability of poor outcome was 11 times greater for incomplete resections (4). Awad et al. reported 88% seizure freedom after complete resection of structural lesions (94).

Many studies report lower rates of seizure freedom in MRI-negative patients (31,126). In a large Mayo clinic nonlesional series, 72% had Engel Class I outcomes at 10-year follow-up (127). Patients remaining seizure-free in the first postoperative year had a high probability of long-term seizure freedom (127). In a smaller series of 24 patients with focal medically intractable, only 37% were seizure-free while 75% experienced at least 90% reduction in seizure frequency (126).

Several studies have analyzed the pathologic substrate for prognostic value. Typically, FCD has a less favorable surgical outcome than discrete lesions such as tumors or vascular malformations with an overall rate of seizure freedom of approximately 45% (128). Hader et al. reported that 72% of 39 pediatric patients with FCD had good outcome (129). Wyllie et al. reported seizure freedom in 52% of pediatric FCD cases (122). In a combined adult/pediatric study, 49% with FCD were seizure-free and independent of lesion location (130). Rates of seizure freedom declined with increasing age at surgery.

Recent retrospective studies have shown dramatically improved epilepsy surgery outcomes for FCD in patients with unilobar lesions and early surgery (70,79,131). The best outcomes are observed for mMCD and FCD type 1a (Engel Class I in 63% and 67%, respectively) and the poorest outcomes for FCD type 2a (Engel Class I in 57%) (132). Higher grade abnormalities are often more extensive which may contribute to less favorable outcomes, while the presence of balloon cells portend a better outcome (70,133,134). Tumors generally

show higher rates of seizure control (up to 96%) following surgical resection (135). The most favorable outcomes are seen with neoplastic lesions (80% seizure-free and 20% had no more than two seizures per year) compared to 52% seizure freedom in the non-neoplastic group (35).

While operative location appears to influence postoperative outcome, this may relate to underlying pathology and juxtaposition to eloquent cortex. In the pre-MRI era of pediatric epilepsy surgery between 1940 and 1980, the Montreal Neurological Institute performed 118 nontumoral frontal and temporal lobectomies and 47% had good outcome at minimum 2-year follow-up (136). Temporal resections had higher rates of favorable outcome but success in frontal lobe cases was influenced by the presence of a discrete, resectable structural abnormality. In a more recent Canadian pediatric epilepsy surgery study, 75% of frontal resections achieved Engel Class I outcomes whereas only 50% of parietal and occipital resections were seizure-free (123). Jeha et al. reviewed the outcome of 70 patients undergoing frontal lobectomy at Cleveland Clinic Foundation between 1995 and 2003 and reported 53% seizure freedom at 1 year but only 30% seizure freedom at 5 years (137). The most important prognosticator for seizure freedom was completeness. In contrast, rates of seizure freedom 10 years after temporal lobectomy are more favorable (124).

In the setting of FCD, temporal lobe dysplasia is more frequently mMCD or type 1a/1b while FCD type 2 is more commonly extratemporal (132) and contributes to lower rates of seizure freedom. Rates of postoperative seizure freedom are 31% to 44% in perirolandic cortex (75,138).

Despite one study reporting 92% Class I outcomes for posterior quadrant resections (117), patients with multilobar resections generally experience significantly lower rates of seizure freedom (4,113,130). Lower rates are not surprising given the extensive abnormalities seen electrographically, structurally, and pathologically in most patients. For patients with catastrophic epilepsies and multiple daily seizures, a substantial reduction in seizure frequency or elimination of the most disabling seizure semiology will improve quality of life.

The goal of epilepsy surgery is complete seizure freedom. However, in children experiencing multiple daily seizures and developmental regression, a significant reduction in the seizure frequency may positively impact cognitive development and quality of life. Under such circumstances, palliative surgery is a reasonable option if complete resection is not possible. Intractable epilepsy in childhood may cause major developmental ramifications, but the importance of early seizure control and early epilepsy surgery is only now being elucidated.

COMPLICATIONS

Mortality rates for pediatric epilepsy surgery are 0% to 2% (124) and overall mortality for epilepsy surgery is less than 0.5% (139). Permanent neurologic sequelae are reported in 2.3% of patients following epilepsy surgery (140). The majority of these deficits are anticipated based on the resection location and most commonly include hemiplegia, homonymous hemianopsia, quadrantanopsia, dysphasia, and reduced verbal memory. Subtle cognitive sequelae may be overlooked without detailed neuropsychological testing.

References

1. Kwan P, Brodie MJ. Early identification of refractory epilepsy. *N Engl J Med.* 2000;342(5):314–319.
2. Cross JH, Jayakar P, Nordli D, et al. Proposed criteria for referral and evaluation of children for epilepsy surgery: recommendations of the Subcommission for Pediatric Epilepsy Surgery. *Epilepsia.* 2006;47(6):952–959.
3. Duchowny M, Jayakar P, Koh S. Selection criteria and preoperative investigation of patients with focal epilepsy who lack a localized structural lesion. *Epileptic Disord.* 2000;2(4):219–226.
4. Paolicchi JM, Jayakar P, Dean P, et al. Predictors of outcome in pediatric epilepsy surgery. *Neurology.* 2000;54(3):642–647.
5. Manford M, Fish DR, Shorvon SD. An analysis of clinical seizure patterns and their localizing value in frontal and temporal lobe epilepsies. *Brain.* 1996;119(Pt 1):17–40.
6. Janszky J, Jokeit H, Schulz R, et al. EEG predicts surgical outcome in lesional frontal lobe epilepsy. *Neurology.* 2000;54(7):1470–1476.
7. Hosking PG. Surgery for frontal lobe epilepsy. *Seizure.* 2003;12(3):160–166.
8. Jobst BC, Williamson PD. Frontal lobe seizures. *Psychiatr Clin North Am.* 2005;28(3):635–651, 648–649.
9. Salanova V, Morris HH, Van Ness P, et al. Frontal lobe seizures: electroclinical syndromes. *Epilepsia.* 1995;36(1):16–24.
10. Lee JJ, Lee SK, Lee SY, et al. Frontal lobe epilepsy: clinical characteristics, surgical outcomes and diagnostic modalities. *Seizure.* 2008;17(6):514–523.
11. Laskowitz DT, Sperling MR, French JA, et al. The syndrome of frontal lobe epilepsy: characteristics and surgical management. *Neurology.* 1995;45(4):780–787.
12. Quesney LF, Constain M, Rasmussen T, et al. Presurgical EEG investigation in frontal lobe epilepsy. *Epilepsy Res Suppl.* 1992;5:55–69.
13. Bass N, Wyllie E, Comair Y, et al. Supplementary sensorimotor area seizures in children and adolescents. *J Pediatr.* 1995;126(4):537–544.
14. Tonini C, Beghi E, Berg AT, et al. Predictors of epilepsy surgery outcome: a meta-analysis. *Epilepsy Res.* 2004;62(1):75–87.
15. Bancaud J, Talairach J. Clinical semiology of frontal lobe seizures. *Adv Neurol.* 1992;57:3–58.
16. Munari C, Bancaud J. Electroclinical symptomatology of partial seizures of orbital frontal origin. *Adv Neurol.* 1992;57:257–265.
17. Cascino GD. Epilepsy and brain tumors: implications for treatment. *Epilepsia.* 1990;31(suppl 3):S37–S44.
18. Isnard J, Guenot M, Sindou M, et al. Clinical manifestations of insular lobe seizures: a stereo-electroencephalographic study. *Epilepsia.* 2004;45(9):1079–1090.
19. Cascino GD, Hulihan JF, Sharbrough FW, et al. Parietal lobe lesional epilepsy: electroclinical correlation and operative outcome. *Epilepsia.* 1993;34(3):522–527.
20. Williamson PD, Boon PA, Thadani VM, et al. Parietal lobe epilepsy: diagnostic considerations and results of surgery. *Ann Neurol.* 1992;31(2):193–201.
21. Duchowny M, Jayakar P, Resnick T, et al. Posterior temporal epilepsy: electroclinical features. *Ann Neurol.* 1994;35(4):427–431.
22. Williamson PD, Thadani VM, Darcey TM, et al. Occipital lobe epilepsy: clinical characteristics, seizure spread patterns, and results of surgery. *Ann Neurol.* 1992;31(1):3–13.
23. Binder DK, Von Lehe M, Kral T, et al. Surgical treatment of occipital lobe epilepsy. *J Neurosurg.* 2008;109(1):57–69.
24. Duchowny M, Jayakar P, Resnick T, et al. Epilepsy surgery in the first three years of life. *Epilepsia.* 1998;39(7):737–743.
25. Duchowny MS. Complex partial seizures of infancy. *Arch Neurol.* 1987;44(9):911–914.
26. Acharya JN, Wyllie E, Luders HO, et al. Seizure symptomatology in infants with localization-related epilepsy. *Neurology.* 1997;48(1):189–196.
27. Yamamoto N, Watanabe K, Negoro T, et al. Complex partial seizures in children: ictal manifestations and their relation to clinical course. *Neurology.* 1987;37(8):1379–1382.
28. Chugani HT, Shields WD, Shewmon DA, et al. Infantile spasms: I. PET identifies focal cortical dysgenesis in cryptogenic cases for surgical treatment. *Ann Neurol.* 1990;27(4):406–413.
29. Foldvary N, Klem G, Hammel J, et al. The localizing value of ictal EEG in focal epilepsy. *Neurology.* 2001;57(11):2022–2028.
30. Sharbrough FW. Scalp-recorded ictal patterns in focal epilepsy. *J Clin Neurophysiol.* 1993;10(3):262–267.
31. Radhakrishnan K, So EL, Silbert PL, et al. Predictors of outcome of anterior temporal lobectomy for intractable epilepsy: a multivariate study. *Neurology.* 1998;51(2):465–471.
32. Duncan JS. Neuroimaging for epilepsy: quality and not just quantity is important. *J Neurol Neurosurg Psychiatry.* 2002;73(6):612–613.
33. Cascino GD. Surgical treatment for extratemporal epilepsy. *Curr Treat Options Neurol.* 2004;6(3):257–262.
34. McIntosh AM, Wilson SJ, Berkovic SF. Seizure outcome after temporal lobectomy: current research practice and findings. *Epilepsia.* 2001;42(10):1288–1307.
35. Zentner J, Hufnagel A, Ostertun B, et al. Surgical treatment of extratemporal epilepsy: clinical, radiologic, and histopathologic findings in 60 patients. *Epilepsia.* 1996;37(11):1072–1080.
36. Zentner J, Hufnagel A, Wolf HK, et al. Surgical treatment of temporal lobe epilepsy: clinical, radiological, and histopathological findings in 178 patients. *J Neurol Neurosurg Psychiatry.* 1995;58(6):666–673.
37. Guidelines for neuroimaging evaluation of patients with uncontrolled epilepsy considered for surgery. Commission on Neuroimaging of the International League Against Epilepsy. *Epilepsia.* 1998;39(12):1375–1376.
38. Sisodiya SM. Surgery for malformations of cortical development causing epilepsy. *Brain.* 2000;123(Pt 6):1075–1091.
39. Lawson JA, Cook MJ, Vogrin S, et al. Clinical, EEG, and quantitative MRI differences in pediatric frontal and temporal lobe epilepsy. *Neurology.* 2002;58(5):723–729.
40. Hertz-Pannier L, Chiron C, Vera P, et al. Functional imaging in the work-up of childhood epilepsy. *Childs Nerv Syst.* 2001;17(4–5):223–228.
41. Hertz-Pannier L, Gaillard WD, Mott SH, et al. Noninvasive assessment of language dominance in children and adolescents with functional MRI: a preliminary study. *Neurology.* 1997;48(4):1003–1012.
42. Hwang SI, Kim JH, Park SW, et al. Comparative analysis of MR imaging, positron emission tomography, and ictal single-photon emission CT in patients with neocortical epilepsy. *Am J Neuroradiol.* 2001;22(5):937–946.
43. Spencer SS. The relative contributions of MRI, SPECT, and PET imaging in epilepsy. *Epilepsia.* 1994;35(suppl 6):S72–S89.
44. Gaillard WD, White S, Malow B, et al. FDG-PET in children and adolescents with partial seizures: role in epilepsy surgery evaluation. *Epilepsy Res.* 1995;20(1):77–84.
45. Ryvlin P, Philippon B, Cinotti L, et al. Functional neuroimaging strategy in temporal lobe epilepsy: a comparative study of 18FDG-PET and 99mTc-HMPAO-SPECT. *Ann Neurol.* 1992;31(6):650–656.
46. Swartz BE, Tomiyasu U, Delgado-Escueta AV, et al. Neuroimaging in temporal lobe epilepsy: test sensitivity and relationships to pathology and postoperative outcome. *Epilepsia.* 1992;33(4):624–634.
47. Vinton AB, Carne R, Hicks RJ, et al. The extent of resection of FDG-PET hypometabolism relates to outcome of temporal lobectomy. *Brain.* 2007;130(Pt 2):548–560.
48. Muzik O, da Silva EA, Juhasz C, et al. Intracranial EEG versus flumazenil and glucose PET in children with extratemporal lobe epilepsy. *Neurology.* 2000;54(1):171–179.
49. Juhasz C, Chugani DC, Muzik O, et al. Is epileptogenic cortex truly hypometabolic on interictal positron emission tomography? *Ann Neurol.* 2000;48(1):88–96.
50. Fedi M, Reutens DC, Andermann F, et al. Alpha-[11C]-Methyl-L-tryptophan PET identifies the epileptogenic tuber and correlates with interictal spike frequency. *Epilepsy Res.* 2003;52(3):203–213.
51. Fedi M, Reutens D, Okazawa H, et al. Localizing value of alpha-methyl-L-tryptophan PET in intractable epilepsy of neocortical origin. *Neurology.* 2001;57(9):1629–1636.

52. Harvey AS, Bowe JM, Hopkins IJ, et al. Ictal 99mTc-HMPAO single photon emission computed tomography in children with temporal lobe epilepsy. *Epilepsia.* 1993;34(5):869–877.

53. Newton MR, Berkovic SF, Austin MC, et al. SPECT in the localisation of extratemporal and temporal seizure foci. *J Neurol Neurosurg Psychiatry.* 1995;9(1):26–30.

54. Habert MO, Huberfeld G. Ictal single photon computed tomography and SISCOM: methods and utility. *Neurochirurgie.* 2008;54(3):226–230.

55. Hong SB, Joo EY, Tae WS, et al. Preictal versus ictal injection of radiotracer for SPECT study in partial epilepsy: SISCOM. *Seizure.* 2008;17(4):383–386.

56. Hougaard K, Oikawa T, Sveinsdottir E, et al. Regional cerebral blood flow in focal cortical epilepsy. *Arch Neurol.* 1976;33(8):527–535.

57. Engel J, Jr., Kuhl DE, Phelps ME, et al. Local cerebral metabolism during partial seizures. *Neurology.* 1983;33(4):400–413.

58. Thadani VM, Siegel AH, Lewis P, et al. SPECT in neocortical epilepsies. *Adv Neurol.* 2000;84:425–433.

59. Kaminska A, Chiron C, Ville D, et al. Ictal SPECT in children with epilepsy: comparison with intracranial EEG and relation to postsurgical outcome. *Brain.* 2003;126(Pt 1):248–260.

60. Ho SS, Berkovic SF, Newton MR, et al. Parietal lobe epilepsy: clinical features and seizure localization by ictal SPECT. *Neurology.* 1994;44(12):2277–2284.

61. O'Brien TJ, So EL, Cascino GD, et al. Subtraction SPECT coregistered to MRI in focal malformations of cortical development: localization of the epileptogenic zone in epilepsy surgery candidates. *Epilepsia.* 2004;45(4):367–376.

62. Widdess-Walsh P, Diehl B, Najm I. Neuroimaging of focal cortical dysplasia. *J Neuroimaging.* 2006;16(3):185–196.

63. Lawson JA, O'Brien TJ, Bleasel AF, et al. Evaluation of SPECT in the assessment and treatment of intractable childhood epilepsy. *Neurology.* 2000;55(9):1391–1393.

64. Morioka T, Nishio S, Ishibashi H, et al. Intrinsic epileptogenicity of focal cortical dysplasia as revealed by magnetoencephalography and electrocorticography. *Epilepsy Res.* 1999;33(2–3):177–187.

65. Knowlton RC, Laxer KD, Aminoff MJ, et al. Magnetoencephalography in partial epilepsy: clinical yield and localization accuracy. *Ann Neurol.* 1997;42(4):622–631.

66. Minassian BA, Otsubo H, Weiss S, et al. Magnetoencephalographic localization in pediatric epilepsy surgery: comparison with invasive intracranial electroencephalography. *Ann Neurol.* 1999;46(4):627–633.

67. Palmini A, Gambardella A, Andermann F, et al. Intrinsic epileptogenicity of human dysplastic cortex as suggested by corticography and surgical results. *Ann Neurol.* 1995;37(4):476–487.

68. Hirabayashi S, Binnie CD, Janota I, et al. Surgical treatment of epilepsy due to cortical dysplasia: clinical and EEG findings. *J Neurol Neurosurg Psychiatry.* 1993;56(7):765–770.

69. Palmini A, Andermann F, Olivier A, et al. Neuronal migration disorders: a contribution of modern neuroimaging to the etiologic diagnosis of epilepsy. *Can J Neurol Sci.* 1991;18(Suppl 4):580–587.

70. Chassoux F, Devaux B, Landre E, et al. Stereoelectroencephalography in focal cortical dysplasia: a 3D approach to delineating the dysplastic cortex. *Brain.* 2000;123(Pt 8):1733–1751.

71. Jayakar P. Invasive EEG monitoring in children: when, where, and what? *J Clin Neurophysiol.* 1999;16(5):408–418.

72. Jayakar P, Alvarez LA, Duchowny MS, et al. A safe and effective paradigm to functionally map the cortex in childhood. *J Clin Neurophysiol.* 1992;9(2):288–293.

73. Guerrini R, Dobyns WB, Barkovich AJ. Abnormal development of the human cerebral cortex: genetics, functional consequences and treatment options. *Trends Neurosci.* 2008;31(3):154–162.

74. Frater JL, Prayson RA, Morris IH, et al. Surgical pathologic findings of extratemporal-based intractable epilepsy: a study of 133 consecutive resections. *Arch Pathol Lab Med.* 2000;124(4):545–549.

75. Pondal-Sordo M, Diosy D, Tellez-Zenteno JF, et al. Epilepsy surgery involving the sensory-motor cortex. *Brain.* 2006;129(Pt 12):3307–3314.

76. Semah F, Picot MC, Adam C, et al. Is the underlying cause of epilepsy a major prognostic factor for recurrence? *Neurology.* 1998;51(5):1256–1262.

77. Lee SK, Lee SY, Kim KK, et al. Surgical outcome and prognostic factors of cryptogenic neocortical epilepsy. *Ann Neurol.* 2005;58(4):525–532.

78. Widdess-Walsh P, Jeha L, Nair D, et al. Subdural electrode analysis in focal cortical dysplasia: predictors of surgical outcome. *Neurology.* 2007;69(7):660–667.

79. Kral T, Clusmann H, Blumcke I, et al. Outcome of epilepsy surgery in focal cortical dysplasia. *J Neurol Neurosurg Psychiatry.* 2003;74(2):183–188.

80. Cepeda C, Andre VM, Vinters HV, et al. Are cytomegalic neurons and balloon cells generators of epileptic activity in pediatric cortical dysplasia? *Epilepsia.* 2005;46(suppl 5):82–88.

81. Palmini A, Najm I, Avanzini G, et al. Terminology and classification of the cortical dysplasias. *Neurology.* 2004;62(6 suppl 3):S2–S8.

82. Monaghan HP, Krafchik BR, MacGregor DL, et al. Tuberous sclerosis complex in children. *Am J Dis Child.* 1981;135(10):912–917.

83. Koh S, Jayakar P, Dunoyer C, et al. Epilepsy surgery in children with tuberous sclerosis complex: presurgical evaluation and outcome. *Epilepsia.* 2000;41(9):1206–1213.

84. Lachhwani DK, Pestana E, Gupta A, et al. Identification of candidates for epilepsy surgery in patients with tuberous sclerosis. *Neurology.* 2005;64(9):1651–1654.

85. Guerreiro MM, Andermann F, Andermann E, et al. Surgical treatment of epilepsy in tuberous sclerosis: strategies and results in 18 patients. *Neurology.* 1998;51(5):1263–1269.

86. Bye AM, Matheson JM, Tobias VH, et al. Selective epilepsy surgery in tuberous sclerosis. *Aust Paediatr J.* 1989;25(4):243–245.

87. Gillberg C, Uvebrant P, Carlsson G, et al. Autism and epilepsy (and tuberous sclerosis?) in two pre-adolescent boys: neuropsychiatric aspects before and after epilepsy surgery. *J Intellect Disabil Res.* 1996;40(Pt 1):75–81.

88. Spencer DD, Spencer SS, Mattson RH, et al. Intracerebral masses in patients with intractable partial epilepsy. *Neurology.* 1984;34(4):432–436.

89. Lee J, Lee BL, Joo EY, et al. Dysembryoplastic neuroepithelial tumors in pediatric patients. *Brain Dev.* 2009;31(9):671–81.

90. Luyken C, Blumcke I, Fimmers R, et al. The spectrum of long-term epilepsy-associated tumors: long-term seizure and tumor outcome and neurosurgical aspects. *Epilepsia.* 2003;44(6):822–830.

91. Blumcke I, Wiestler OD. Gangliogliomas: an intriguing tumor entity associated with focal epilepsies. *J Neuropathol Exp Neurol.* 2002;61(7):575–584.

92. Daumas-Duport C, Scheithauer BW, Chodkiewicz JP, et al. Dysembryoplastic neuroepithelial tumor: a surgically curable tumor of young patients with intractable partial seizures. Report of thirty-nine cases. *Neurosurgery.* 1988;23(5):545–556.

93. Daumas-Duport C, Dysembryoplastic neuroepithelial tumours. *Brain Pathol.* 1993;3(3):283–295.

94. Awad IA, Rosenfeld J, Ahl J, et al. Intractable epilepsy and structural lesions of the brain: mapping, resection strategies, and seizure outcome. *Epilepsia.* 1991;32(2):179–186.

95. Takahashi A, Hong SC, Seo DW, et al. Frequent association of cortical dysplasia in dysembryoplastic neuroepithelial tumor treated by epilepsy surgery. *Surg Neurol.* 2005;64(5):419–427.

96. Britton JW, Cascino GD, Sharbrough FW, et al. Low-grade glial neoplasms and intractable partial epilepsy: efficacy of surgical treatment. *Epilepsia.* 1994;35(6):1130–1135.

97. Hesselink JR, Dowd CF, Healy ME, et al. MR imaging of brain contusions: a comparative study with CT. *Am J Roentgenol.* 1988;150(5):1133–1142.

98. Salazar AM, Jabbari B, Vance SC, et al. Epilepsy after penetrating head injury. I. Clinical correlates: a report of the Vietnam Head Injury Study. *Neurology.* 1985;35(10):1406–1414.

99. Jabbari B, Prokhorenko O, Khajavi K, et al. Intractable epilepsy and mild brain injury: incidence, pathology and surgical outcome. *Brain Inj.* 2002;16(6):463–467.

100. Makarov A, Sadykov EA, Kiselev VN. Posttraumatic epilepsy: diagnosis and clinical variety. *Zh Nevrol Psikhiatr Im S S Korsakova.* 2001;101(6):7–11.

101. Brown RD, Jr., Wiebers DO, Forbes G, et al. The natural history of unruptured intracranial arteriovenous malformations. *J Neurosurg.* 1988;68(3):352–357.

102. Rigamonti D, Hadley MN, Drayer BP, et al. Cerebral cavernous malformations. Incidence and familial occurrence. *N Engl J Med.* 1988;319(6):343–347.

103. Kesava PP, Turski PA. Magnetic resonance angiography of vascular malformations. *Magn Reson Imaging Clin N Am.* 1998;6(4):811–833.

104. Awad I, Jabbour P. Cerebral cavernous malformations and epilepsy. *Neurosurg Focus.* 2006;21(1):e7.

105. Awad IA, Robinson JR, Jr., Mohanty S, et al. Mixed vascular malformations of the brain: clinical and pathogenetic considerations. *Neurosurgery.* 1993;33(2):179–188. Discussion 188.

106. Kraemer DL, Awad IA. Vascular malformations and epilepsy: clinical considerations and basic mechanisms. *Epilepsia.* 1994;35(suppl 6):S30–S43.

107. Baumann CR, Schuknecht B, Lo Russo G, et al. Seizure outcome after resection of cavernous malformations is better when surrounding hemosiderin-stained brain also is removed. *Epilepsia.* 2006;47(3):563–566.

108. Singh G, Singh P, Singh I, et al. Epidemiologic classification of seizures associated with neurocysticercosis: observations from a sample of seizure disorders in neurologic care in India. *Acta Neurol Scand.* 2006;113(4):233–240.

109. Del Brutto OH. Neurocysticercosis. *Semin Neurol.* 2005;25(3):243–251.

110. Rasmussen T, Olszewski J, Lloydsmith D. Focal seizures due to chronic localized encephalitis. *Neurology.* 1958;8(6):435–445.

111. Zupanc ML, Handler EG, Levine RL, et al. Rasmussen encephalitis: epilepsia partialis continua secondary to chronic encephalitis. *Pediatr Neurol.* 1990;6(6):397–401.

112. Engel J, Pedley T, eds. *Epilepsy: A Comprehensive Textbook.* 2nd ed. Vol. II. Philadelphia: Lippincott Williams & Wilkins; 2008:1885–1886.

113. Leiphart JW, Peacock WJ, Mathern GW. Lobar and multilobar resections for medically intractable pediatric epilepsy. *Pediatr Neurosurg.* 2001;34(6):311–318.

114. Farrell MA, DeRosa MJ, Curran JG, et al. Neuropathologic findings in cortical resections (including hemispherectomies) performed for the treatment of intractable childhood epilepsy. *Acta Neuropathol.* 1992;83(3):246–259.

115. Di Rocco C, Tamburrini G. Sturge–Weber syndrome. *Childs Nerv Syst.* 2006;22(8):909–921.
116. Bien CG, Widman G, Urbach H, et al. The natural history of Rasmussen's encephalitis. *Brain.* 2002;125(Pt 8):1751–1759.
117. Daniel RT, Meagher-Villemure K, Farmer JP, et al. Posterior quadrantic epilepsy surgery: technical variants, surgical anatomy, and case series. *Epilepsia.* 2007;48(8):1429–1437.
118. Barba C, Barbati G, Minotti L, et al. Ictal clinical and scalp-EEG findings differentiating temporal lobe epilepsies from temporal "plus" epilepsies. *Brain.* 2007;130(Pt 7):1957–1967.
119. Jayakar P, Duchowny M, Alvarez L, et al. Intraictal activation in the neocortex: a marker of the epileptogenic region. *Epilepsia.* 1994;35(3):489–494.
120. Chugani HT, Mazziotta JC, Phelps ME. Sturge-Weber syndrome: a study of cerebral glucose utilization with positron emission tomography. *J Pediatr.* 1989;114(2):244–253.
121. Engel J, Van Ness PC, Rasmussen TB, et al. Outcome with respect to epileptic seizures. In: Engel J Jr., ed. *Surgical Treatment of the Epilepsies.* New York, NY: Raven Press; 1993:609–621.
122. Wyllie E, Comair YG, Kotagal P, et al. Seizure outcome after epilepsy surgery in children and adolescents. *Ann Neurol.* 1998;44(5):740–748.
123. Sinclair DB, Aronyk K, Snyder T, et al. Extratemporal resection for childhood epilepsy. *Pediatr Neurol.* 2004;30(3):177–185.
124. Spencer S, Huh L. Outcomes of epilepsy surgery in adults and children. *Lancet Neurol.* 2008;7(6):525–537.
125. Krsek P, Maton B, Jayakar P, et al. Incomplete resection of focal cortical dysplasia is the main predictor of poor postsurgical outcome. *Neurology.* 2009;72(3):217–223.
126. Chapman K, Wyllie E, Najm I, et al. Seizure outcome after epilepsy surgery in patients with normal preoperative MRI. *J Neurol Neurosurg Psychiatry.* 2005;76(5):710–713.
127. Cohen-Gadol AA, Ozduman K, Bronen RA, et al. Long-term outcome after epilepsy surgery for focal cortical dysplasia. *J Neurosurg.* 2004;101(1):55–65.
128. Sisodiya SM. Surgery for focal cortical dysplasia. *Brain.* 2004;127(Pt 11):2383–2384.
129. Hader WJ, Mackay M, Otsubo H, et al. Cortical dysplastic lesions in children with intractable epilepsy: role of complete resection. *J Neurosurg.* 2004;100(2 suppl Pediatrics):110–117.
130. Edwards JC, Wyllie E, Ruggeri PM, et al. Seizure outcome after surgery for epilepsy due to malformation of cortical development. *Neurology.* 2000;55(8):1110–1114.
131. Tassi L, Colombo N, Garbelli R, et al. Focal cortical dysplasia: neuropathological subtypes, EEG, neuroimaging and surgical outcome. *Brain.* 2002;125(Pt 8):1719–1732.
132. Fauser S, Schulze-Bonhage A, Honegger J, et al. Focal cortical dysplasias: surgical outcome in 67 patients in relation to histological subtypes and dual pathology. *Brain.* 2004;127(Pt 11):2406–2418.
133. Urbach H, Scheffler B, Heinrichsmeier T, et al. Focal cortical dysplasia of Taylor's balloon cell type: a clinicopathological entity with characteristic neuroimaging and histopathological features, and favorable postsurgical outcome. *Epilepsia.* 2002;43(1):33–40.
134. Urbach H, Binder D, von Lehe M, et al. Correlation of MRI and histopathology in epileptogenic parietal and occipital lobe lesions. *Seizure.* 2007;16(7):608–614.
135. Packer RJ, Sutton LN, Patel KM, et al. Seizure control following tumor surgery for childhood cortical low-grade gliomas. *J Neurosurg.* 1994;80(6):998–1003.
136. Fish DR, Smith SJ, Quesney LF, et al. Surgical treatment of children with medically intractable frontal or temporal lobe epilepsy: results and highlights of 40 years' experience. *Epilepsia.* 1993;34(2):244–247.
137. Jeha LE, Najm I, Bingaman W, et al. Surgical outcome and prognostic factors of frontal lobe epilepsy surgery. *Brain.* 2007;130(Pt 2):574–584.
138. Malone SA, Brna P, Dunoyer C, et al. Sensorimotor cortex surgery for intractable epilepsy in a predominantly pediatric subgroup. *Epilepsia.* 2008;49(suppl 7):295.
139. Sperling MR, Harris A, Nei M, et al. Mortality after epilepsy surgery. *Epilepsia.* 2005;46(suppl 11):49–53.
140. Behrens E, Schramm J, Zentner J, et al. Surgical and neurological complications in a series of 708 epilepsy surgery procedures. *Neurosurgery.* 1997;41(1):1–9. Discussion 9–10.

CHAPTER 84 ■ HEMISPHERECTOMIES, HEMISPHEROTOMIES, AND OTHER HEMISPHERIC DISCONNECTIONS

JORGE A. GONZÁLEZ-MARTÍNEZ AND WILLIAM E. BINGAMAN

Hemispheric resections or disconnections are performed successfully to treat medically intractable hemispheric epilepsy in adolescents and older children, proving remarkable results in terms of seizure outcome and quality of life. New techniques are being constantly added to the surgical armamentarium, resulting in a diminished rate of complications and better seizure outcome in most recent surgical series. In this chapter, we will review the current different surgical methods related to hemispheric resections and disconnections, including a historical perspective, selection criteria, complications, and seizure outcome.

HISTORICAL PERSPECTIVE

The first neurosurgeon to describe hemispheric disconnection procedures was Walter Dandy in 1928, who performed in a patient with glioblastoma (1). It was only after 10 years that McKenzie first attempted to perform hemispherectomy in a patient with intractable epilepsy (2). Krynauw, in 1950, systematically performed hemispherectomies in patients with intractable seizures, infantile hemiplegia, and behavioral disorders (3). Only then, the technique gained acceptance in the management of handicapped patients with intractable epilepsy. According to Krynauw, predictors for good outcome depended on proper case selection.

Later in 1966, Oppenheimer and Griffith described a delayed complication, probably caused by a chronic intraventricular bleeding that was named superficial hemosiderosis (4). In order to prevent this complication, subtotal hemispherectomies were performed. These procedures were adequate to prevent the long-term complications; however, the results for seizure control were clearly less effective than those of anatomical hemispherectomy. In order to accomplish a better seizure control with minimal complications, Rasmussen developed the so-called functional hemispherectomy, where a complete functional disconnection is performed, leaving the disconnected hemisphere in place, avoiding previous complications (5–7). Other techniques included the Oxford variation (or Adam's modification), which included an anatomical hemispherectomy associated with tacking the dura to the falx and tentorium to collapse the subdural space at the expense of the epidural space (8). Hemidecortication and hemicorticectomy have also been used (9).

The term "hemispherotomy" was first defined by Delalande and colleagues in 1992 to describe a modified functional hemispherectomy, in which cortical resection is minimized and the rest of the hemisphere is functionally isolated by disconnecting the neuronal fibers (10). Other techniques include the peri-insular hemispherotomy of Villemure (11) and the transsylvian functional "keyhole approach" hemispherectomy of Schramm and colleagues (12). All variants of functional hemispherectomy represent attempts to perform a complete disconnection of the epileptic brain with minimal tissue removal.

SELECTION CRITERIA

Surgical candidates must satisfy the criteria common to all epilepsy surgery patients, which include the presence of intractable seizures, possible interference with neurodevelopmental milestones, and an epileptogenic focus located in one single hemisphere. Anatomical and electrophysiological investigations should indicate that the epileptogenic activity arises only from the hemisphere to be resected and that the side ipsilateral to the hemiparesis is essentially normal. In general, patients will also need to demonstrate the presence of hemiplegia or severe hemiparesis contralateral to the damaged hemisphere with loss of digital dexterity on the affected side, but the absence of these findings will not necessarily contraindicate the procedure. If the procedure is performed at younger age (before 6 years), clinically significant functional recovery is expected, even in cases in which speech appears to be localized to the abnormal side (13). Patient's age at the time of surgery is controversial. Surgical therapy for infants with medically intractable epilepsy is traditionally viewed as an extreme measure, but this view has being challenged in recent surgical series, which suggested a better seizure and cognitive outcome if patients are operated in younger ages. In a recent published study, the authors reviewed the seizure and cognitive outcome of 18 young children (less than 2 year olds) who underwent hemispheric disconnection or total removal. Seizure control was excellent (90% seizure-free) with an acceptable complication rate. No death occurred (14). In another study, Peacock et al. reported a pediatric series with 58 children (median: 2.8 years); 23 children were younger than 2 years. After 1 year of follow-up, 60% of the group was seizure-free and 28% had >90% reduction in seizure frequency. Two deaths occurred (13). Duchowny and colleagues reported a surgical series with 31 children younger than 3 years (mean age, 18.3 months). Fourteen hemispherectomies were performed in this series, with a favorable outcome in 76.9% (>90% seizure reduction). Nearly half of the patients were younger than 1 year, suggesting that extremely young age is not an absolute contraindication to this procedure (15). Based on literature, we concluded that hemispherectomy is a relatively safe procedure in younger ages (in appropriate settings regarding facilities and personal), providing dramatic results in terms of seizure outcome. The results support the concept that early surgery should be indicated in highly selected patients with catastrophic epilepsy.

The presence of bilateral electroencephalographic (EEG) abnormalities or bilateral lesions on the magnetic resonance imaging (MRI) should not be a contraindication for hemispheric surgery. Over the last few years, we observed seizure-free outcome in a number of older children and adolescents who underwent epilepsy surgery as a last resort despite various generalized or contralateral-maximum ictal and interictal EEG patterns. In the Cleveland Clinic, during the last 10 years, approximately 32 patients with bilateral EEG abnormalities underwent a hemispheric procedure, and 72% of these patients were seizure-free at the end of the follow-up (16).

PREOPERATIVE EVALUATION

Patients are selected based on the presence of medically intractable epilepsy arising from one hemisphere. In the preoperative period, a team of specialists, including adult and/or pediatric epileptologists, neurosurgeons, neuroradiologists, and neuropsychologists, evaluates these patients and the routine preoperative evaluation includes the following.

History and Physical Examination

A detailed history including prenatal events, birth and developmental history, and possible epilepsy risk factors are obtained. The neurological examination focuses on sensorimotor, language, visual, and cognitive functions. The ideal hemispherectomy candidate has a contralateral hemiparesis and hemianopsia with the absence of fine finger movements. The degree of motor impairment needs to be accurately documented to help counsel the parents on what to expect postoperatively. Similarly, the presence or absence of a hemianopsia should be assessed and parents need to be counseled about the presence of a contralateral hemianopsia postoperatively. This specific visual field deficit will preclude driving later in life. Any associated medical illness/syndrome such as epidermal nevus syndrome should be documented.

Clinical Semiology and Video Electroencephalography (VEEG)

All patients will have VEEG monitoring to document seizure semiology and interictal/ictal EEG data preoperatively. The seizure type(s) and location are documented and characterized. EEG findings can be variable with lateralization to the ipsilateral diseased hemisphere or in a bilateral/generalized pattern.

Magnetic Resonance Imaging (MRI)

Routine MRI including volumetric T1, T2, and FLAIR sequencing is performed in all patients. This is perhaps the most important preoperative data as the individual patient

anatomy influences the operative technique utilized. The MRI is also necessary to document the integrity of the unaffected hemisphere. Patients with bilateral imaging pathology are not necessarily excluded from consideration for hemispherectomy but appropriate caution should be taken in these circumstances. Specific anatomical details involving ventricular size, presence of heterotopic cortical dysplasia, the anatomy of the posterior basal frontal cortex, and location of the midline help to define the surgical plan.

Other Adjunctive Preoperative Tests

Single photon emission computed tomography (SPECT) and/or 18-fluorodeoxyglucose positron emission tomography (FDG-PET) scanning were infrequently performed to gain additional metabolic information, especially if bilateral disease was present on MRI. The intracarotid sodium amytal test was not routinely performed due to pediatric age considerations and poor baseline language function in some patients. It may be of use in the older patient where language transfer might not occur following dominant hemispherectomy. Finally, neuropsychological evaluation should be attempted to help gauge developmental delay and establish the preoperative baseline. Any associated behavioral problems should also be documented.

TIMING OF SURGERY

The appropriate timing for surgery is controversial. Many well-established epilepsy centers recommend early intervention to stop seizures and maximize chances for neurodevelopment (17–25). Despite this, there is little evidence supporting early surgery and the risks related to the surgical procedure, especially in infants, need to be considered. In general, for noncatastrophic epilepsy, we consider a body weight of 10 kg or above acceptable. All patients and/or families are asked to donate blood prior to the operative procedure. For catastrophic hemispheric epilepsy, surgery is performed earlier with appropriate informed consent on the risks of excessive blood loss and mortality (14).

ANATOMICAL REMARKS AND SURGICAL TECHNIQUES

Several techniques of hemispherectomy, hemispherotomy, and others hemispheric disconnections have been described. According to several authors (26,27), all of these variations have four common principles: (i) disruption of the descending and ascending fibers through the corona radiata and internal capsule; (ii) removal of the mesial temporal structures; (iii) complete callosotomy; (iv) disruption of the frontal horizontal fibers, including the occipitofrontalis fasciculus and uncinate fascicle. The main difference among these techniques lies in how the lateral ventricle is accessed, whether access starts from the temporal horn or from the body of the lateral temporal, and the extent of brain resection necessary to gain access to the ventricular system. Other differences include the removal or preservation of the insula and the preservation or ligation of branches of the middle cerebral artery. In the following paragraphs, we simplistically describe the differences in the several techniques.

Anatomical Hemispherectomy

Patient positioning is optimized to allow access to the lateral surface of the affected cerebral hemisphere and to minimize neck torsion. The head may be positioned in rigid point fixation or resting on a head support, depending on the patient's age. The head is turned 90° with ipsilateral shoulder support and the vertex slightly down to allow access to the mesial temporal lobe structures and interhemispheric fissure (Fig. 84.1).

The head is then shaved and a "T"-shaped incision planned to allow access from the floor of the middle fossa to the midline of the head. Superficial landmarks useful for incisional planning include anatomic midline from nasion to inion, the lateral edge of the anterior fontanelle, the transverse sinus location, the greater wing of the sphenoid bone, and the zygomatic arch (Fig. 84.2).

The T-incision is designed by a line at least 0.5 cm from midline and a perpendicular line from the zygomatic root just anterior to the tragus. The midline incision extends from the hairline to a point 4 to 5 cm above the inion. The incision is made with a surgical knife with care in the younger patient with an open anterior fontanelle to avoid inadvertent sagittal

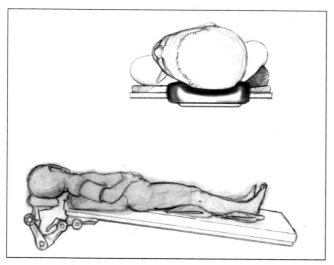

FIGURE 84.1 Patient's position for anatomical hemispherectomy.

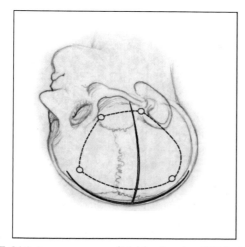

FIGURE 84.2 Important superficial landmarks, "T" incision and planned.

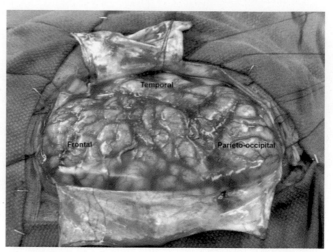

FIGURE 84.3 "H" dural opening and hemimegalencephalic brain.

sinus injury. The skin edges are then reflected, and periosteum and temporalis muscle fascia visualized. The muscle is mobilized off the underlying bone with a "T" incision, reflecting each muscle cuff inferiorly. Burr holes are done at the keyhole, the floor of the middle fossa just above the zygomatic arch, and lastly along the parasagittal areas just off the midline to avoid sagittal sinus injury (if anterior fontanelle is closed). The optimal craniotomy flap allows exposure to the midline, orbitofrontal base, floor of the middle fossa, and total length of the sylvian fissure. The craniotomy flap is carefully removed with a high-speed airdrill craniotome.

After the dura mater is opened in an H-fashion, the sylvian fissure is identified and venous drainage patterns inspected. The distance from the superior craniotomy edge to the interhemispheric fissure is verified. The locations of major draining veins to the sagittal sinus are noted and carefully protected until later in the procedure to avoid early and often devastating blood loss. The orbitofrontal region is inspected and the position of the olfactory tract visualized as an anatomic guide to the gyrus rectus and midline structures (Fig. 84.3).

The dissection of the sylvian fissure begins with early exposure and control of the middle cerebral artery trunk in the sylvian fissure just distal to the lenticulostriate branches. The sylvian fissure is split along its entire length using bipolar electrocautery, suction, and sharp microdissection (loupe magnification is preferred for this portion of the procedure). This should be done carefully to minimize bleeding, but cortex can be aspirated as necessary to aid in exposure. Once opened, the insular cortex including the inferior and superior circular sulci should be visualized along the length of the sylvian fissure.

The middle cerebral artery is then ligated with bipolar cautery and surgical hemostatic clips (Fig. 84.4).

The inferior circular sulcus is identified and the white matter of the temporal stem is localized just deep to the sulcus. Using suction aspiration, the white matter is removed along the temporal stem and the temporal horn of the lateral ventricle is entered. A cottonoid patty is placed here to protect the choroid plexus and prevent blood from entering the ventricular system. The pial dissection along the anterior (temporal) aspect of the sylvian fissure is carried below the main sylvian vein to the floor of the anterior aspect of the middle fossa. The anterior temporal pole is then aspirated to expose the edge of the

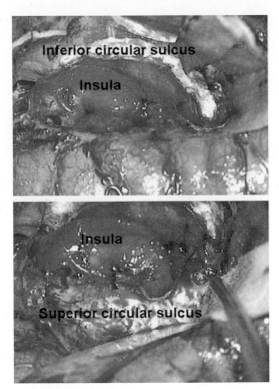

FIGURE 84.4 Exposure of superior and inferior circular sulcus surrounding insula.

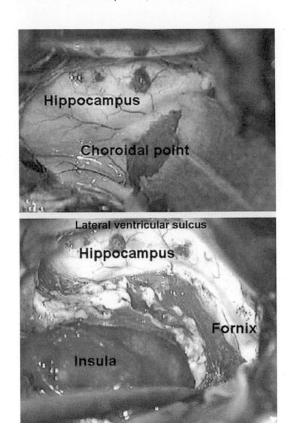

FIGURE 84.5 Temporal horn access through inferior circular sulcus and identification of important landmarks for mesial structures dissection.

tentorium. The white matter dissection of the temporal stem is then continued posteriorly to achieve exposure of the temporal horn from the anterior aspect to the trigonal region (Fig. 84.5). A long, thin cottonoid is then placed posteriorly into the ventricle passing from the trigone up into the lateral ventricle.

The posterior trigonal area is then plugged with a large cotton ball to prevent blood from entering the lateral ventricle. Exposure of the tentorial edge and basomesial temporal pia is then achieved by dissection of the lateral ventricular sulcus (collateral eminence) from within the temporal horn, just lateral to the hippocampus. This can be done with bipolar coagulation and suction or ultrasonic aspiration. In either case, the amygdala, hippocampus, and choroid plexus are protected from injury with cottonoid patties. Once the mesiobasal pia is identified just lateral to the parahippocampal gyrus, the dissection can be extended anteriorly to meet the prior pial dissection at the floor of the anterior middle fossa. The parahippocampus is then aspirated to identify the tentorial edge. The tentorial edge is then followed from anterior to posterior, curving back behind the mesencephalon. At this point, the posterior cerebral artery branches can be ligated as they pass from the perimesencephalic cistern over the tentorial edge to the temporo-occipital cortex. At the conclusion of this phase of the operation, the temporal lobe lateral to the parahippocampal gyrus has been disconnected and the posterior cerebral artery branches divided. The amygdala, hippocampus, and a remnant of the parahippocampal gyrus remain in place.

Supra-sylvian dissection through the superior limiting (circular) sulcus of the insula takes place to divide the coronal radiata and expose the lateral ventricle along its length. This can be done by careful dissection from above the insula or by following the previous trigonal ventricular opening around the posterior aspect of the insula to the lateral ventricle (Fig. 84.6).

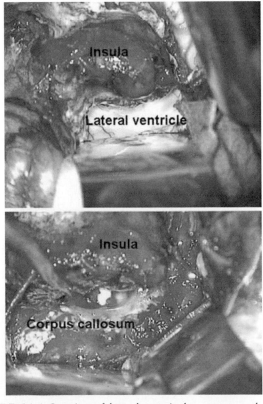

FIGURE 84.6 Opening of lateral ventricular system and corpus callosotomy. (Tip of the shunt from the opposite hemisphere is also seen.)

Dissection is facilitated by dividing the posterior branches of the MCA at the end of the sylvian fissure. Once the corona radiata is divided, the entire length of the lateral ventricle is opened and the foramen of Monro plugged with a small cotton ball to prevent blood from entering the dependent ventricular system. Care should be taken to protect the choroid plexus to avoid unnecessary bleeding. Similarly, basal ganglia disruption can be prone to bleed and is best controlled by the application of hemostatic agents to the exposed surfaces.

The corpus callosum is identified from within the ventricle at the junction of the septum pellucidum and the roof of the lateral ventricle. Aspiration of the roof of the lateral ventricle just above this area leads to the gray matter of the ipsilateral cingulate gyrus and falx cerebri. This is meticulously aspirated to prevent injury to the contralateral cingulum. Once this area is exposed, identification of the pericallosal arteries and corpus callosum proper is easily achieved. The corpus callosum and ipsilateral cingulate gyrus is then aspirated from the genu to the splenium. Complete sectioning is important to achieve and can be accomplished by following the pericallosal artery as it closely follows the characteristic course of the callosum. Special attention should be given to the genu and splenium to assure complete disruption of the horizontal fibers. Additional assistance is achieved by removal of the cingulate gyrus and identification of the inferior edge of the interhemispheric falx. Finally, the ipsilateral fornix is disrupted by aspiration at a point just anterior to the splenium. Next, the mesial dissection should continue anteriorly coagulating and dividing the pia of the ipsilateral mesial frontal lobe including the arterial branches from the anterior circulation. This mesial frontoparietal disconnection is followed anteriorly to the base of the frontal lobe just above the olfactory nerve (frontal pole). Posteriorly, the edge of the falx is followed as it transitions to the tentorium. This mesial parieto-occipital resection should connect with the basal temporal disconnection below the sylvian fissure, which was performed earlier. At this point, the callosum is disconnected and the pia along the mesial aspect of the entire hemisphere is coagulated and divided. The only remaining portion of the hemisphere in place is the basal–frontal lobe below the genu and the draining veins to the venous sinuses.

The last remaining pia to be divided extends from the anterior aspect of the sylvian fissure down along the posterior–basal–frontal lobe. This pia is coagulated and divided along with the MCA branches to the frontal cortex. The posterior–basal–frontal lobe is aspirated maintaining a plane just anterior to the anterosuperior insula (Fig. 84.7).

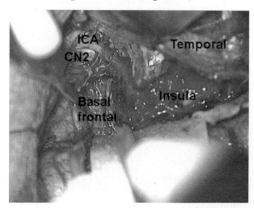

FIGURE 84.7 Important surgical landmarks of right fronto–basal disconnection.

The orbitofrontal pia is then coagulated and divided down to the olfactory nerve, and the pia overlying the gyrus rectus is identified and divided. The gyrus rectus is then aspirated to expose the contralateral gyrus rectus and a cottonoid patty placed to mark the midline. The pial dissection along the olfactory nerve is then carried anteriorly to avoid disruption of the nerve. The remaining gyrus rectus is then aspirated with the posterior removal limited by the internal carotid artery. The deep white matter and mesial frontal gyri are removed in subpial fashion by a dissection plane marked by the anterior aspect of the frontal horn starting below the prior dissection of the genu of the corpus callosum. This dissection is carried out through the caudate nucleus along the course of the anterior cerebral artery to where it joins the internal carotid artery. Special care should be taken after the hemisphere is removed to ensure complete removal of the basal–posterior–frontal lobe. Once all the pial surfaces and white matter tracts have been cut, the draining veins to the sinuses are circumferentially coagulated and divided and any bleeding points packed with hemostatic agent. At this point the entire hemisphere can be removed in one anatomic piece and sent for pathologic study. The remaining amygdala–hippocampus bloc is then removed as the last portion of the procedure.

The insular cortex can be removed if so desired by subpial aspiration using the ultrasonic aspirator or suction coagulation. As the middle cerebral artery has already been controlled, arterial injury is of less concern than in the functional hemispherectomy operation. Care must be taken to limit resection to the insular gyri to avoid injury to deeper thalamic/brainstem structures. Perhaps stereotactic imaging would be useful at this stage, although a practical approach is to stop the dissection when underlying white matter is reached.

Adam's Hemispherectomy Modification

Adam's modification is an attempt to avoid the complications of hemosiderosis and hydrocephalus. The classic anatomic hemispherectomy is supplemented by a muscle plug in the foramen of Monro on the resection side and by folding down the stripped dura of the convexity bone onto the falx, central block (composed by basal ganglia and thalamus and middle fossa cavity). The subdural space is occluded and outflow of cerebrospinal fluid (CSF) from the good side is prevented. Using this technique, there seems to be a higher rate of infection, but the rate of hydrocephalus seems to be reduced, compared to the classic anatomic resection (8).

Functional Hemispherectomy and Other Disconnection Techniques

Classic Functional Hemispherectomy

This technique was first described in Montreal by Rasmussen and colleagues in an effort to prevent the late hemorrhagic complications described after anatomical hemispherectomy, mainly hemosiderosis (5–7,28). It is unclear if late hemosiderosis was caused by chronic insidious bleeding into the remaining ventricular cavity or by chronic hydrocephalus, since the description of such complication was 40 to 50 years ago, before computerized tomography. In our anatomical hemispherectomy series, no signs of hemosiderosis were observed, even in patients with more than 20 years in follow-up. In the functional hemispherectomy procedure, the same T-shaped scalp incision is performed. The craniotomy is smaller than in the anatomical hemispherectomy, especially in the anterior–posterior orientation, and is mainly centered in the topographic location of the insula. The dura is open at the same matter as it has been described for the anatomical hemispherectomy. The overall goal of the functional hemispherectomy is to disconnect the frontal lobe from an incision that is placed just anterior to the genu of the corpus callosum and to disconnect the parietal and occipital lobe through a posterior incision, and then to remove the temporal lobe and its mesial structures. The fiber tracts projecting from the remaining parts of the frontal, parietal, and occipital lobes to the brainstem and spinal cord are then transected. The blood supply to the disconnected cortical regions is kept intact.

The first cortical incision is made along the upper margin of the sylvian fissure, by coagulating and incising the pia and its blood vessels, dissecting down into the frontal and parietal operculum, down to the plane of the insular cortex. From the anterior and posterior ends of this dissection, a central resection is performed, exposing the entire limitans sulcus of the insula and, consequently, the insula cortex. The incisions are extended to the medial surface to the level of the cingulate gyrus, which is preserved at this stage to protect the pericallosal artery, but removed later. By deepening the dissections in the superior limitans sulcus of the insula, the body of the lateral ventricle is entered and the central bloc of tissue removed.

The temporal lobe is removed by coagulating and dividing the pia and its vessels along the superior temporal gyrus, back to the posterior limb of the upper resection, and anteriorly around the temporal pole, down to the uncus. The roof of the temporal horn is entered and then the lateral portion of the temporal lobe is removed through the collateral sulcus. The hippocampus is dissected and removed through the coagulation of the hippocampus sulcus. The hippocampus is dissected free, and the amygdaloid nucleus is removed.

The deep white matter of the medial and inferior aspects of the frontal lobe is divided in the coronal plane, from the central resection area to the most basal and posterior area of the frontal lobe, just rostral to the anterior perforated substance and medial and lateral olfactory striae. The anterior portion of the corpus callosum is also divided, from its body to the knee and rostrum portions, stopping at the level of lamina terminalis. In the same way, the white matter of the parietal lobe is divided posterior to the splenium from the ventricular ependyma, from the body and atrium of the lateral ventricle to the pia overlying the falx and the floor of the middle fossa. Following subpial dissection, the cingulate gyrus is removed. In the same way as the anterior callosotomy, the posterior corpus callosum is also divided, from the topography of the central resection to the splenium. Just anterior to the splenium, the fimbrias and fornixes from both hippocampus formations join, forming the hippocampus comissure, which will need to be completely disconnected. After irrigation, the craniotomy is closed as previously described for anatomical hemispherectomy.

Hemidecortication

It is based on the principle that only the epileptogenic cortex needs to be removed in order to achieve seizure freedom. The concept was first delineated by Ignelzi and Bucy in 1968 (9). The integrity of the lateral ventricle is largely preserved, except

at the temporal lobe, where removal of the hippocampus requires opening of the temporal horn. There are several disadvantages with this technique as, although the main aim is to avoid opening the ventricular system, removal of the hippocampus makes opening of the temporal horn a necessary step. A large wound surface is created and, in cases of hemimegalencephaly (HME), where dysplastic ectopic gray matter is located in the white matter, orientation can be difficult.

Trans-Sylvian, Transventricular Functional Hemispherectomy

This approach was developed and refined by Schramm and colleagues (12). The key features of this approach are: (i) small craniotomy and trans-sylvian exposure of the insular cortex; (ii) anterior mesial temporal lobe resection, including amygdala and hippocampus; (iii) transcortical access to the ventricular system through the sulcus limitans of the insula, from the tip of the temporal horn to the tip of the frontal horn; (iv) frontal–basal disconnection anterior to the anterior cerebral artery; (v) mesial disconnection following the anterior cerebral artery through the anterior portions of the corpus callosum to the splenium; and (vi) posteromedial disconnection in the ventricular trigone following the outline of the falcotentorial border to the temporomesial resection cavity. This procedure is especially suited for cases with enlarged ventricles, porencephalic cysts, and marked atrophy of the insula–basal ganglia block or for cases with larger ventricle and cisterns.

The size of the craniotomy is chosen guided by the length of the corpus callosum, the anteroposterior diameter of the basal ganglia thalamus–insula block (limen insulae to pulvinar), and the degree of ventricular enlargement. The sylvian fissure is then opened, and the circular sulcus is exposed, taking advantage of the fact that the temporal operculum is overlying the inferior limb of the limitans sulcus only about 0.5 to 1 cm, whereas the frontal operculum can overlie the frontal limb of the circular sulcus up to 3 cm. Access to the temporal horn is gained through the inferior circular sulcus approach. The uncus and the lateral parts of the amygdala are removed, and the hippocampus also is taken out either by suction or en bloc. Sparing the major branches of the middle cerebral artery, the ventricular system is then opened all around the insular cortex. From inside the anterior horn of the lateral ventricle, a dissection line is now created by suction and bipolar coagulation from the frontal horn floor, just anterior from the foramen of Monro, down to the basal arachnoid, just anterior to the middle and anterior cerebral arteries. The mesial disconnection can now be continued around the corpus callosum following the anterior cerebral artery. Callosotomy is then performed within the ventricle, back to the area of the splenium. The fornix and the hippocampus tail are disconnected and resected, until the mesial temporal lobe resection cavity is reached.

According to Schramm and colleagues (12), the trans-sylvian–transventricular hemispherectomy with only a minimal mesial temporal lobe resection should not be used for HME cases, even if ventricles are enlarged, for two reasons: the insular cistern may be atypically configurated and the trans-sylviam approach can be more difficult even with enlarged hemisphere. In HME patients, the trans-sylvian–transventricular hemispherectomy should be combined with resection of the entire temporal lobe or with resection of the frontal operculum to the level of the insular cortex. This resection facilitates the transcortical access from the limitans sulcus of the insula to the lateral ventricle and creates room for postoperative swelling.

According to Bonn' series, possible disadvantages of this procedure include problems identifying anatomical landmarks due to the limited exposure. Hydrocephalus, possibly induced by the large wound surface and the transventricular approach, was not seen in the trans-sylvian "keyhole" hemispherectomies for all causes so far. No case of incomplete disconnection toward the midline was detected, but too anteriorly placed disconnections were seen. There was one death in the series, where a 5-year-old boy was found dead on the fifth postoperative day, with the cause remaining unknown.

Peri-insular Hemispherotomy

Peri-insular hemispherotomy was initially developed by Villemure and colleagues (11). The main features of this approach are: (i) medium-sized craniotomy exposing the frontal, parietal, and temporal operculum in the whole length of the sylvian fissure; (ii) resection of the frontal and parietal operculum and underlying white matter, opening the whole lateral ventricle through the anterior and superior limitans sulcus of the insula and disconnection of the frontobasal area through the intraventricular approach; (iii) resection of the temporal operculum (T1 gyrus and underlying white matter) and exposure of the temporal horn through the inferior limitans sulcus of the insula; (iv) mesial disconnection through the corpus callosum, from the rostrum and knee to the splenium; (v) temporomesial disconnection with only anterior resection of the amygdala, anterior aspect of the hippocampus and uncus.

Peri-insular hemispherotomy is best indicated in patients with enlarged ventricle and certain degree of atrophy, but because of the more extensive resection of the operculum and underlying white matter, it can be also applied for HME cases. Kestle and colleagues used this technique in 11 of their 16 cases. Estimated blood loss was 462 cc, compared to 1.3 L for decortication, 73% of their patients needed a transfusion, and there was no need for shunts (29).

Central Vertical Hemispherotomy

This approach was first decribed by Delalande and colleagues in 1992 (10) and, together with Schramm (trans-sylvian approach) and Villemure (peri-insular approach) techniques, consists in another variation of the classical functional hemispherectomy described by Rasmussen. It includes initially a small parasagittal craniotomy, complete callosotomy with opening of the roof of the lateral ventricle. Once the entire lateral ventricle is unroofed, posterior disconnection of the hippocampus is achieved by cutting the columns of the fornix at the level of the ventricular trigone. The vertical incision is performed lateral to the thalamus, choroid plexus, and choroidal fissure of the temporal horn, then following the temporal horn from the trigone to the most anterior part of the ventricle, keeping the incision in the white matter. The callosotomy is then completed by resecting the genu and the rostrum of the corpus callosum to the anterior comissure. The next step is the resection of the posterior part of the gyrus rectus, which will allow the visualization of the anterior cerebral artery and optic nerve and provide enough space for the last disconnection step, which is a straight incision anterolaterally through the caudate nucleus from the rectus gyrus to the anterior temporal horn.

The results in 53 cases, including 20 patients with focal cortical dysplasia (CD) or HME cases and six Sturge–Weber syndrome (SWS) cases, were recently reported. There was one death in the series. Ten patients (all HME cases) needed a shunt. In general, results were excellent, with 80% of patients seizure-free.

ANATOMICAL HEMISPHEREC-TOMY VERSUS FUNCTIONAL HEMISPHERECTOMY AND OTHER DISCONNECTION TECHNIQUES

The discussion about what would be the appropriate surgical technique for treatment of intractable hemispheric epilepsy is controversial. The literature is full of personal series, specifically reporting seizure outcome and complications related to one specific technique. In addition, most of the studies are retrospective in nature, reporting results in populations that differ in age, severity of seizure, and pathological substrate. There are no studies that directly compare functional versus anatomical hemispherectomy. In the largest series of patients treated with anatomical hemispherectomy, the surgical outcome is similar to that for functional disconnection (24,30–33). The group at John Hopkins reviewed their experience with anatomical hemispherectomy in infants and children (17). Of 21 patients with cortical dysplasia, 8 (38%) were seizure-free and an additional six (29%) had mild seizures after surgery. In contrast, surgical series after functional hemispherectomy for CD report 50% to 67% of seizure-free rate with an additional 11% to 33% having only rare seizures. Although number are small in all these studies and the radiological involvement of CD is not well outlined in some of these reports, these results suggest that functional hemispherectomy is at least as effective as anatomical hemispherectomy. The frequency of complications may also be lower after functional hemispherectomy. Nevertheless, of five patients with HME who continue to have seizures after functional hemispherectomy, three had seizures that arose from the operated hemisphere and two had seizures arising from the contralateral hemisphere. These results suggest that anatomic hemispherectomy may be more effective in patients with HME and that functional hemispherectomy may be better suited for patients with more restricted hemispheric CD. At the Cleveland Clinic, we believe that anatomical hemispherectomy provides a better seizure outcome in patients with CD and HME. In a series of patients with catastrophic epilepsy in young ages, incomplete disconnection was the only variable statiscally associated with persistent seizures after surgery (14). In a total of 18 patients, 6 patients had persistent seizures after surgery. Two patients had the diagnosis of HME and four the diagnosis of CD. From this group, four patients had incomplete disconnection, always located in the posterior basal frontal areas. All four patients underwent reoperation, converting the procedure to anatomical hemispherectomy. All four patients achieved seizure freedom. In our studied group, we found that for patients with HME, antomical hemispherectomy is the best option. In general, the lateral ventricle from patients with HME is characterized by an irregular shape, a relative hypoplasia of the temporal horn. Such anatomical peculiarities, together with irregular and abnormal thickness of the cerebral mantle, deep heterotopic gray matter, distorted trajectory of the anterior cerebral arteries, abnormal large veins at the level of the malformed sylvian fissure, and the possible interdigitation of the mesial aspect of the hemispheres make the functional hemispherectomy a technically difficult procedure in this group of patients. In our surgical series, all patients with HME who underwent functional hemispherectomy resulted in uncontrolled seizures after surgery; the conversion to anatomical hemispherectomy resulted in seizure freedom in all patients.

Although several authors reported higher complications rates in anatomical hemispherectomy (5,34–36), particularly hemosiderosis and secondary hydrocephalus, we did not find such findings in our patients. With specific regard to hemosiderosis associated with anatomic hemispherectomy, one could speculate whether late mortality from hemispherectomy was caused by the effects of chronic deposition of Fe^{2+} on the cerebral parenchyma, from repeated intracranial hemorrhages, or it was simply the outcome of hydrocephalus, which escaped detection before the introduction of CT. It is worth noting that reports concerning hemosiderosis have been practically absent in the literature since the 1970s; nevertheless, hemosiderosis is still quoted as a common reason for avoiding anatomic hemispherectomy.

SEIZURE OUTCOME AND COMPLICATIONS

Most studies reporting outcomes of hemispherectomies are in children, mainly because catastrophic epilepsy is more incident in the pediatric population. Additionally, children tolerate the procedure better than adults because of plasticity of the developing brain. Most studies reporting outcomes after hemispherectomy are related to children. Regarding hemispherectomies in adults, Cukiert et al. recently reported a retrospective outcome study of 14 adult patients with intractable epilepsy due to early middle cerebral artery infarct. Twelve out of 14 patients had Engel I outcome at the end of the follow-up period (64 months). The two remaining patients had at least 90% improvement in severity and seizure frequency. No mortality or major morbidity was reported (37).

There are different perspectives in assessing outcome after hemispherectomy. Seizure outcome is the primary concern, but the morbidity associated with the different procedures has to be considered. Outcomes will vary depending on the etiology of the refractory seizures. In large surgical series involving hemispherectomies and hemispherotomies, between 43% and 90% of patients have been described as seizure-free after surgery. In all the series in which outcomes were analyzed with respect to etiology, Rasmussen's encephalitis, SWS, and perinatal infarction had better outcome (70% to 90%) than those with CD and HME (60% to 80%) (38–42). Holthausen et al. included in a review 33 patients who underwent hemispherectomy at 13 centers. As previously mentioned, Rasmussen syndrome and SWS had a better prognosis than other etiologies (41). Different techniques had similar outcomes compared to the hemispherectomy group.

In terms of complications, hydrocephalus is, by far, the most prevalent complication across all surgical series, varying from 2% to 28%. Mortality was reported in almost all series, up to 7% reported in John Hopkins series (17).

Several publications discussed if hemispherectomy or hemispherotomy procedures can improve the postoperative development of children by decreasing the number of seizures. While some publications show no improvement (43), others show some improvement (23,24). The presurgical developmental level seems to be important not only for the capacity of the brain to improve but also for seizure outcome, favoring the concept that in young children with intractable hemispheric epilepsy, early surgical indication should be favored instead of more conservative measures. In infants with epilepsy, even with greater plasticity, recurrent seizures can be catastrophic for functional reorganization during a critical period in development, and therefore, if surgery is delayed, the outcome might not be as good as expected. Once again, patients with severe CD and HME tend to have the worst prognosis for cognitive recovery (22).

CONCLUSION

Hemispherectomy and other disconnection procedures for intractable epilepsy provide excellent and dramatic results with a satisfactory complication rate. A dramatic evolution in surgical technique, patient's selection criteria, and perioperatory care were observed in the last 60 years. Despite this, discrepancies related to complication rate and seizure outcome among different techniques are still unsolved. A large prospective multicenter study is necessary to indicate the better surgical technique for a specific pathology and population group. Nevertheless, early surgery in patients with catastrophic epilepsy seems to be associated with better seizure control and cognitive prognosis.

References

1. Dandy WE. Removal of right cerebral hemisphere for certain tumors. *J Am Med Assoc.* 1928;90:823–825.
2. McKenzie KG. The present status of a patient who had the right hemisphere removed. *J Am Med Assoc.* 1938;111:168–183.
3. Krynauw RA. Infantile hemiplegia treated by removing one cerebral hemisphere. *J Neurol Neurosurg Psychiatry.* 1950;13:243–267.
4. Oppenheimer DR, Griffith HB. Persistent intracranial bleeding as a complication of hemispherectomy. *J Neurol Neurosurg Psychiatry.* 1966;29:229–240.
5. Rasmussen T. Cerebral hemispherectomy: indications, methods, and results. In: Schmidek HH, Sweet WH, eds. *Operative Neurosurgical Techniques.* Orlando, FL: Grune & Stratton; 1988:1235–1241.
6. Rasmussen T. Hemispherectomy for seizures revisited. *Can J Neurol Sci.* 1983;10:71–80.
7. Rasmussen T, Villemure JG. Cerebral hemispherectomy for seizures with hemiplegia. *Cleve Clini J of Med.* 1989;56(suppl pt 1):S62–S68. Discussion S79–S83.
8. Adams CB. Hemispherectomy—a modification. *J Neurol Neurosurg Psychiatry.* 1983;46:617–619.
9. Ignelzi RJ, Bucy PC. Cerebral hemidecortication in the treatment of infantile cerebral hemiatrophy. *J Nerv Ment Dis.* 1968;147:14–30.
10. Delalande O, Pinard JM, Basdevant C, et al. Hemispherotomy: a new procedure for central disconnection. *Epilepsia.* 1992;33(suppl 3):99–100.
11. Villemure JG, Mascott CR. Peri-insular hemispherotomy: surgical principles and anatomy. *Neurosurgery.* 1995;37(5):975–981.
12. Schramm J, Behrens E, Entzian W. Hemispherical deafferentation: an alternative to functional hemispherectomy. *Neurosurgery.* 1995;36(3):509–515.
13. Peacock WJ, Wehby-Grant MC, Shields WD, et al. Hemispherectomy for intractable seizures in children: a report of 58 cases. *Childs Nerv Syst.* 1996;12(7):376–384.
14. Gonzalez-Martinez JA, Gupta A, Kotagal P, et al. Hemispherectomy for catastrophic epilepsy in children. *Epilepsia.* 2005;46(9):1518–1525.
15. Duchowny M, Jayakar P. Functional cortical mapping in children. *Adv Neurol.* 1993;40:31–38.
16. Wyllie E, Lachhwani D, Gupta A, et al. Successful surgery for epilepsy due to early brain lesions despite generalized EEG findings. *Neurology.* 2007;69:389–397.
17. Carson BS, Javedan SP, Freeman JM, et al. Hemispherectomy: a hemidecortication approach and review of 52 cases. *J Neurosurg.* 1996;84(6):903–911.

18. Cross JH. Epilepsy surgery in childhood. *Epilepsia*. 2002;43(suppl 3):65–70.
19. Daniel RT, Joseph TP, Gnanamuthu C, et al. Hemispherotomy for paediatric hemispheric epilepsy. *Stereotact Funct Neurosurg*. 2001;77(1–4):219–222.
20. Sugimoto T, Otsubo H, Hwang PA, et al. Outcome of epilepsy surgery in the first three years of life. *Epilepsia*. 1999;40(5):560–565.
21. Vining EP, Freeman JM, Pillas DJ, et al. Why would you remove half a brain? The outcome of 58 children after hemispherectomy—the Johns Hopkins experience: 1968 to 1996. *Pediatrics*. 1997;100(2 Pt 1):163–171.
22. Wyllie E. Surgery for catastrophic localization-related epilepsy in infants. *Epilepsia*. 1996;37(suppl 1):S22–S25.
23. Wyllie E. Surgical treatment of epilepsy in children. *Pediatr Neurol*. 1998; 19(3):179–188.
24. Wyllie E, Comair YG, Kotagal P, et al. Seizure outcome after epilepsy surgery in children and adolescents. *Ann Neurol*. 1998;44(5):740–748.
25. Wyllie E, Comair YG, Kotagal P, et al. Epilepsy surgery in infants. *Epilepsia*. 1996;37(7):625–637.
26. Morino M, Shimizu H, Ohata K, et al. Anatomical analysis of different hemispherotomy procedures based on dissection of cadaveric brains. *J Neurosurg*. 2002;97:423–431.
27. Wen HT, Rothon A, Marino R Jr. Anatomical landmarks for hemispherotomy and their clinical applications. *J Neurosurg*. 2004;101:747–755.
28. Kalkanis SN, Blumenfeld H, Sherman JC, et al. Delayed complications thirty-six years after hemispherectomy: a case report. *Epilepsia*. 1996;37:758–762.
29. Kestle J, Connolly M, Cochrane D. Pediatric peri-insular hemispherotomy. *Pediatr Neurosurg*. 2000;3244–3247.
30. Kossoff EH, Vining EP, Pillas DJ. Hemispherectomy for intractable unihemispheric epilepsy etiology vs. outcome. *Neurology*. 2003;18(3):228–232.
31. Di Rocco C, Iannelli A. Hemimegalencephaly and intractable epilepsy: complications of hemispherectomy and their correlations with the surgical technique: a report on 15 patients. *Pediatr Neurosurg*. 2000;33:198–207.

32. Duchowny M, Jayakar P, Resnick T, et al. Epilepsy surgery in the first three years of life. *Epilepsia*. 1998;39(7):737–743.
33. Tinuper P, Adermann F, Villemure JG, et al. Functional hemispherectomy for treatment of epilepsy associated with hemiplegia: rationale, indications, results, and comparisons with callosotomy. *Ann Neurol*. 1988;24:27–34.
34. Falconer MA, Wilson PJ. Complications related to delayed hemorrhage after hemispherectomy. *J Neurosurg*. 1969;30:413–426.
35. Villemure JG. Anatomical to functional hemispherectomy from Krynauw to Rasmussen. *Epilepsy Res Suppl*. 1992;5:209–215.
36. Wilson PJE. Cerebral hemispherectomy for infantile hemiplegia. A report of 50 cases. *Brain*. 1970;93:147–180.
37. Cukiert A, Cukiert CM, Argentoni M, et al. Outcome after hemispherectomy in hemiplegic adult patients with refractory epilepsy associated with middle cerebral artery infarcts. *Epilepsia*. 2009;50(6):1381–1384.
38. Engel JJ, VanNess PC, Rasmussen TB, et al. Outcome with respect to epilepsy seizures. In: Engel J, Jr, ed. *Surgical Treatment of The Epilepsies*. 2nd ed. New York, NY: Raven Press; 1993:609–621.
39. Hoffman HJ, Hendrick EB, Dennis M, et al. Hemispherectomy for Sturge–Weber syndrome. *Child's Brain*. 1979;5:233–248.
40. Holmes GL. Intractable epilepsy in children. *Epilepsia*. 1996;37(suppl 3): 14–27.
41. Holthausen H, May TW, Adams CTB, et al. Seizure post hemispherectomy. In: Tuxhorn I, Holthausen H, Boenigk H, eds. *Paediatric Epilepsy Syndromes and Their Surgical Treatment*. London: John Libbey; 1997: 749–773.
42. Palmini A, Gambardella A, Andermann F, et al. Operative strategies for patients with cortical dysplastic lesions and intractable epilepsy. *Epilepsia*. 1994;35(suppl 6):S57–S71.
43. Pulsifer MB, Brandt J, Salorio CF, et al. The cognitive outcome of hemispherectomy in 71 children. *Epilepsia*. 2004;45:243–254.

CHAPTER 85 ■ MULTIFOCAL RESECTIONS OR FOCAL RESECTIONS IN MULTIFOCAL EPILEPSY

HOWARD L. WEINER, JONATHAN ROTH, AND STEPHEN P. KALHORN

The concept of focal resections in multifocal medically refractory epilepsy directly contradicts the core philosophical basis of epilepsy surgery. Epilepsy surgery, as a concept, has traditionally relied on the precise localization and removal of a single seizure *focus* in the brain, the *epileptogenic zone*, for a successful outcome (1). The literature clearly demonstrates that if this zone can be targeted surgically, with accuracy, then the patient may be rendered seizure-free in the majority of cases. The emphasis in the field has been on methods of correctly identifying the focus noninvasively and invasively. Examples of the success of epilepsy surgery for focal epileptogenic disorders include temporal lobectomy for mesial temporal lobe epilepsy and focal resection for malformations of cortical development, tumors, and vascular lesions (2–12). With the increasingly widespread recognition of the benefits of epilepsy surgery in properly selected patients, as well as the emergence of new comprehensive epilepsy centers across the world, specialists in the field have been faced with managing patients who do not meet the strict classical selection criteria for seizure surgery. This is especially relevant in the pediatric population, in which seizures very often occur in the setting of a developmental brain disorder located outside the temporal lobe. After failing multiple antiepileptic drugs (AEDs), a risk–benefit analysis of other treatment options including epilepsy surgery is appropriate. Assuming that the preoperative evaluation localizes the ictal onset to more than one location in the brain, the epilepsy surgeon is faced with the possibility of a multifocal neurosurgical resection and an unlikely chance of achieving seizure freedom.

Before proceeding with a discussion of multifocal resections for epilepsy, it is important for us to better define this concept. Under the strictest definition, multifocal refers to three or more foci. This holds true whether referring to the ictal-onset zones, interictal discharge foci, or sites of resection. It seems logical that multifocal epilepsy begets a multifocal resection. However, that depends upon how one is defining epilepsy as multifocal. A patient with independent electrographic ictal onsets within three or more locations has multifocal epilepsy. This is in contrast to the presence of three or more distinct interictal epileptiform discharge populations, which represent multifocal cortical hyperexcitability, but may or may not represent multifocal epilepsy; whether one requires an observed ictal onset in a location, or just a demonstration of cortical hyperexcitability, to designate a new focus is ultimately a discussion outside of the scope of this chapter. The case of a patient with nonlocalizable and nonlateralizable seizure onsets (or generalized seizure onsets) with or without multiple interictal discharges, raises an interesting gray area in terms of defining multifocal epilepsy. In many cases, the term "multifocal epilepsy" is utilized to describe a difficult epilepsy case in which surgery is felt not to be an option. With these issues in mind, when and why does one pursue a multifocal resection? As noted above, one theory holds that multifocal resections for epilepsy are performed because of the presence multifocal ictal-onset zones and must be addressed individually. However, it is not clear whether this is always true. The attitude towards this definition is often not positive because it is felt that patients with seizures arising from multiple sites in the brain are usually not helped by surgery. Based on this thinking, one could easily make the argument that such patients are not candidates for surgery.

However, an alternative and compelling theory is that in multifocal epilepsy, seizures are actually spreading rapidly between brain regions such that the true ictal-onset zone eludes detection by current methods. Correlating the outcome and electrographic ictal patterns in 26 patients with neocortical epilepsy, Kutsy et al. found that patients with slow ictal spread had the best outcomes, whereas those with fast contiguous and noncontiguous spread did worse (13). Experience in specific patient populations, in particular those with tuberous sclerosis complex (TSC), suggests that surgery, in fact, may be quite effective if the site of seizure onset can be determined (14,15). Intriguingly, a critical review of the literature reveals several examples of successful epilepsy surgery in which a targeted, *focal*, surgical approach was utilized to treat apparent multifocal epilepsy, rather than resections in multiple areas of the brain. The challenge, therefore, is to utilize technological advances in anatomic imaging and functional studies to unmask the possibility of an occult seizure focus that may not yet be revealed in a seemingly multifocal seizure network.

The goal of treatment in patients with multifocal epilepsy is the elimination of seizures. Especially in children, one should strive to eliminate seizures as soon as possible, in order to optimize the neurologic setting for improved cognitive development, education, and quality of life (16). Of course, any decision one makes about multifocal resections should be made together with members of a comprehensive team and the family, weighing all the possible risks and potential benefits as they pertain to the individual patient. The potential risks of surgery, especially the possibility that it may be ineffective, must be considered against the risks of continued refractory epilepsy to the patient's neurologic function and life expectancy (17–20). The concept that successful epilepsy surgery may have a positive impact on development and quality of life has gained increasing support over time, and this applies to multifocal resections as well (21–28).

A review of the literature on multifocal resections for epilepsy does not provide a clear understanding of the indications and outcome of this approach. In fact, very few investigators have directly studied this group of patients as an independent entity. Moreover, the available outcome data on the likelihood of becoming seizure-free after resections in multifocal epilepsy are disappointing. For example, only 37% of patients with seizures secondary to viral encephalitis, a classic etiology for multifocal epilepsy, were seizure-free at long-term follow-up (29). With some exception, it is difficult to discern how many patients within individual series actually underwent resections for multifocal epilepsy. A recent international survey analyzing the spectrum of international practice in 543 pediatric epilepsy surgery patients reported that only 70 (13%) underwent multifocal resections for multifocal epilepsy (30). Two thirds of this group had resections involving two lobes, whereas the remaining one third underwent operations in three distinct lobes. They do not comment on how many patients had multifocal resections within a single lobe. An Italian group of investigators recently reported that 20 of 113 (18%) children they studied had multilobar resections (31). They found that a unifocal lesion on magnetic resonance imaging (MRI), temporal unilobar resection, and complete lesionectomy were all associated with a significantly lower risk of seizure recurrence. In contrast, 30% of those undergoing multifocal resections underwent a second operation because of persistent seizures (31). Our center reported 13 patients who underwent surgical treatment of multifocal epilepsy involving eloquent cortex (32). The multiple independent seizure foci documented in this group rendered these patients unconventional candidates for epilepsy surgery. Independent seizure foci were defined by subdural electrode recordings, when separate regions were identified as onsets for different seizures (32). Utilizing surgical resection when possible, plus multiple subpial transactions (MSTs) when eloquent cortex was found to be a seizure focus, Devinsky et al. reported a 31% modified Engel class I outcome and a 23% class IV outcome (32). This group concluded that "further studies are necessary to assess prospectively the indications for multilobar surgery and MST in patients with multifocal epilepsy involving eloquent cortex" (32).

Faced with increasing numbers of patients being referred to our center who did not meet the strict conventional selection criteria for epilepsy surgery, we developed a novel strategy with the goal of improving outcomes in this worst prognostic group, based on a rational treatment philosophy (33). We utilized multistage surgery, in which more than two operative stages were performed during the same hospital admission, with subdural electrodes, to treat a select group of patients, including those with multifocal seizure foci. The rationale was to identify which seizure foci were primarily epileptogenic, and therefore needed to be resected, in a multifocal setting. We noted seizure-free outcomes in 60% of all patients, with acceptable risk (33). We applied this strategy to a group of patients representing the paradigm for those with the worst prognosis for success with epilepsy surgery, those with TSC (15). This cohort of 25 TSC patients with multiple bilateral potentially epileptogenic cortical tubers included several patients who had been rejected elsewhere as surgical candidates because the preoperative evaluation indicated multifocal epileptogenicity (15). The surprising result that two thirds of these patients were free of seizures at long-term follow-up mandates that we attempt to understand the underlying difference between this population and those others that fare less well with multifocal resections (15). One

possible explanation for this better-than-predicted outcome might be that, in TSC, one can more easily detect the foci within the multifocal background. More specifically, multifocal surgery in TSC, in fact, entails *multilesional* resections. Surgery may be more successful because the lesions are more easily detected and dealt with surgically. Analogously, when multiple seizure "foci" are involved, and are confined to a single hemisphere of the brain, surgery can also be very effective (23,34–37).

One conceptual framework for understanding the way in which TSC may shed light on this challenging multifocal patient population involves the notion that epilepsy is a network (38–40). Multifocal epilepsy is likely one manifestation of this concept, with TSC being a good specific example (41). In TSC for instance, an ictal-onset zone may exist, initiating a secondary network; in some people (perhaps over time), other regions of that network become more active and can generate spikes and eventually can become independent foci to actually start the seizure; in this model one would expect a basically unified seizure semiology with variable onset zones. In other multifocal patients, independent onset zones may start truly independently with different semiologies (e.g., metastatic cancer, encephalitis). Can a strategic surgical intervention targeting an occult primary focus alter this network? The hypothesis that this question is based on is that multifocal epilepsy is the observed phenotype of a primary seizure focus driving a complex epileptic network. The multifocal EEG may, in fact, be masking a primary epileptogenic focus. A careful review of the literature indicates that this theme has been repeatedly observed over the history of epilepsy surgery. The successful surgical outcomes seen in several of these scenarios support the idea that if a primary focus can be identified, it can be strategically targeted with a resection that disrupts the network. Despite advances in anatomic and functional imaging as well as electrophysiologic studies, the challenge remains how to enhance the detection of a primary focus when it is not apparent.

Hirsch et al. showed that they were able to achieve excellent results following unilateral temporal lobectomy in selected patients with independent bilateral temporal ictal onsets documented with depth electrodes (42). They demonstrated that certain patients with temporal lobe epilepsy with bilateral independent seizures could be cured with a focal resection, a unilateral temporal lobectomy. These patients would have been rejected as surgical candidates by standard selection criteria at that time. They concluded that "having fewer than 80% of seizures originate in one temporal lobe should not be an absolute contraindication for temporal lobectomy" in bitemporal patients in whom most evidence implicates one temporal lobe (42). They posited three theories to explain their observation: the contralateral lobe is secondarily epileptogenic ("mirror focus") (43,44), surgery disconnects the pathway of ictal spread to involved extratemporal foci, or that it is a truly bilateral disease responsive to unilateral lobectomy (43,44).

Using positron emission tomography (PET), Chugani and colleagues developed the concept that previously unrecognized focal brain lesions could be the underlying etiology in certain cases of infantile spasm (45). These four patients, who were seizure-free after focal resection, all had normal computerized tomography (CT) scans, and would have all been rejected as potential surgery candidates based on the conventional work up at that time (45). Clearly, functional brain imaging was able to transform a seemingly nonsurgical case, with generalized multifocal EEG findings, into one amenable for cure with focal resection. Similarly, multifocal epileptiform activity observed in patients with hypothalamic hamartoma, responsive to focal therapy directed at the lesion, supports the hypothesis that patients with a more generalized epileptic phenotype may be harboring a focal, intrinsically epileptogenic pathology curable with lesionectomy (46–48). After resection of the hamartoma, 11 of 12 patients had resolution of generalized and gelastic seizures, with a significant reduction in multifocal EEG changes (47). Finally, Wyllie et al. advanced the understanding of this phenomenon by analyzing the role of resective epilepsy surgery in 50 children with generalized or bilateral EEG findings and congenital or perinatal abnormalities, and in 10 similar patients with focal brain lesions on MRI (49,50). They argue that selected children and adolescents with congenital or early acquired focal epileptogenic brain lesions may benefit from epilepsy surgery, despite a multifocal EEG (49,50). Their goal was to identify patients who had focal resection or hemispherectomy despite "abundant generalized or bilateral multifocal epileptiform discharges on preoperative EEG," given their experience that "infants and young children with a focal brain lesion may be favorable candidates for epilepsy surgery . . . despite generalized EEG seizures . . . with multifocal bilateral interictal epileptiform discharges" (49–52). The significant majority of these patients were either seizure-free or markedly improved, leading them to speculate that the timing of a lesion early in development may result in a more multifocal EEG pattern, due to either kindling or secondary epileptogenesis, masking this epileptogenic lesion (49,50).

We believe that our experience treating children with TSC also supports this hypothesis that multifocal epilepsy may be the observed phenotype when an occult ictal focus is driving a complex epileptic network (14,15). Many of the TSC children that we encountered in our practice did not meet traditional selection criteria for epilepsy surgery and, in fact, were rejected for consideration despite a progressive downward developmental course. Moreover, many of them were still deemed multifocal after having undergone extensive evaluations including MRI, MEG, PET, SPECT, and video-EEG monitoring. When we initiated this work, our treatment goal was not necessarily seizure freedom. We, and the patients' families, were willing to accept a partial benefit from surgery, given the poor prognosis with continued seizures despite multiple AEDs. In fact, we were surprised by many of the unexpected good outcomes, which challenged our group to pursue this therapeutic strategy even further. This philosophy is not unique to our group. Radhakrishnan et al. highlighted the role of palliative resection in an adolescent with multifocal epilepsy involving frontal and occipital lobes following radiation therapy for leukemia (53). Removal of a radiation-induced frontal lobe cavernous malformation resulted in amelioration of his disabling seizure type, illustrating how focal resection of the more deleterious focus may dramatically improve quality of life, despite the multifocal background (53).

Of 52 TSC patients who underwent epilepsy surgery by a surgeon during a 10-year period, 20 of them were in this worst prognostic category, with completely nonlateralizing work-ups (54). The hypothesis we began with was that, despite the multifocal findings on imaging and electrophysiology, an ictal

focus could be identified and resected in these patients. Our thinking was that, given the overall poor quality of life associated with refractory seizures and multiple AEDs, as well as the likelihood that these events were partial in nature, perhaps a bilateral electrode survey could identify a discrete focus that could be targeted. The multidisciplinary epilepsy team felt that the alternative path, a continued course of severe epilepsy despite multiple medications, entailed significant risk as well. Of the 20, 15 had a focus that was detected on bilateral intracranial EEG, whereas in the other five no respectable focus was found. Of the 14 who underwent resection, seven (50%) were seizure-free at follow-up. Interestingly, those children eventually found to have a resectable focus were younger at the time of diagnosis with both TSC and refractory seizures. Moreover, video-EEG, MRI, MEG, PET, or SPECT findings in this group did not predict those patients who went on to resection or success from surgery (54). Hidden within this group of TSC patients with apparent multifocal epilepsy is a cohort with a resectable focus.

The real challenge facing the treating team lies in not only identifying a potentially discrete resectable focus in patients with multifocal epilepsy, but in distinguishing whether this focus is primary, necessitating removal, or secondary. Ultimately, this is determined by whether the removal of a presumed primary ictal focus results in cessation of seizures. Therefore, the goal in multifocal epilepsy should be to identify a primary epileptogenic zone for strategic resection. However, in reality, this is often not possible, raising the need to consider multifocal resection, in which the aim is to remove all individual sites of presumed ictal onset. However, this too, is often not feasible in many cases, due to several factors, which include the presence of too many disparate epileptogenic zones to be handled surgically, bilaterally homologous foci, or their overlap with eloquent cortex (32). Indeed, it is often difficult to define the epileptogenic zone with precision when only a single seizure focus exists (14). Chassoux et al. utilized a depth electrode analysis in four patients with focal unilateral polymicrogyria, demonstrating an epileptic network much larger than the anatomic lesion (55). Their surgical approach for addressing this multifocal situation was to utilize extensive surgery, with resection of not only the polymicrgyria lesion, but also distal brain areas that were determined to be part of this large network (55). Their excellent outcomes allowed them to argue that this strategy was optimal, although they did not definitively prove that removing the extralesional sites was required for seizure freedom.

We have proposed multistage epilepsy surgery as one possible approach for rationally trying to distinguish which foci need to be resected in the patient with presumed multifocal epilepsy (14,33,56). Intracranial electrodes are reimplanted at the time of resection of the primary focus identified following the initial intracranial EEG monitoring session, for an additional phase on monitoring, in order to determine the importance of additional distal and/or adjacent seizure foci. Theoretically, this strategy should define those multifocal epilepsy settings in which one needs to carry out actual multifocal resections. We have found this technique to be useful, with acceptable risk, in a subset of pediatric patients with poorly localized medically refractory epilepsy (14,15,33). Disadvantages of this surgical strategy include the extra cost, hospital length-of-stay, and the theoretical risk associated with an additional operation. Second, the alternative strategy may be better: resecting the presumed primary focus only and "seeing how the patient does." According to this view, should surgery fail, additional surgery remains an option in the future. Our experience indicates that families seem more willing to undergo an additional surgical stage acutely rather than return to the operating room at a later date. Finally, we do not know definitively whether what is recorded between the second and third surgical stages is actually clinically significant. Perhaps seizures recorded after the initial resection would simply dissipate over time, obviating the need for further resection.

While we have been encouraged by the utility and safety of the multistage approach, it, nevertheless, clearly reflects the philosophy and referral bias of our institution. The limitations of this strategy point to the need for better noninvasive modalities for defining those specific situations that demand multifocal resection. Interestingly, Wyllie et al. used only clinical criteria, combined with developmental pathology on MRI scanning, to make surgical decisions (50). They did not rely on PET, SPECT, or invasive EEG to "prove that the generalized or contralateral epileptiform discharges represented spread from epileptogenic cortex near the MRI lesion, but instead accepted that the discharges were a manifestation of disturbed circuitry resulting from interaction between the early lesion and the developing brain" (50). But, lacking this experience, how can one transform an occult primary seizure focus within a multifocal background into a revealed one that can be targeted? Emerging technological advances indicate that continued progress in the field is being made. A review of the literature clearly shows that nonoperative methods for uncovering the symptomatic lesion show promise, including MEG, PET, and advanced MRI scanning techniques (57–65).

CASE EXAMPLE

The following case illustrates how a resective surgical strategy was utilized successfully for a case of apparent multifocal epilepsy in a young girl who, as a result of the nonlocalizing work up, was not felt to be a surgical candidate. Because the extensive preoperative evaluation did not precisely localize a seizure focus that could be targeted with epilepsy surgery, and in light of her severe medically refractory epilepsy and developmental regression, the patient initially was offered, and underwent, a bilateral electrode survey, which surprisingly revealed unilateral right hemisphere ictal onsets. She subsequently underwent multifocal resections (frontal, parietal, and temporal) of the epileptogenic zones within the involved right hemisphere. After 4 years of follow-up, she remains seizure-free (Engel class I).

A 3.5-year-old girl was diagnosed with TSC after presenting with a brief complex partial seizure (CPS) at 3 months of age and infantile spasms at 4 months. After brief seizure control on ACTH, she continued to have CPSs. She developed relatively well until age 2, when she experienced an episode of nonconvulsive status, resulting in the loss of language that had developed up to that point, and developmental regression in general. She also began experiencing secondarily generalized seizures. Despite multiple antiepileptic medications, she continued to have daily seizures, about four events per day on average. The seizures consisted of staring spells, eyes rolling up to the right, a smile appearing on her face with twitching of the left and

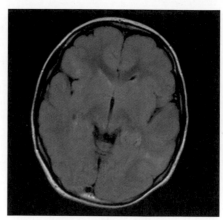

FIGURE 85.1 Preoperative FLAIR sequence MRI showing bilateral tubers.

occasionally the right corner of her mouth, followed by a series of head drops and upper extremity elevation. This was at times associated with grunting lasting 30 seconds to 2.5 minutes. Postictally, she was confused and ataxic. Occasionally, secondary generalization was seen. Other seizures were characterized by right arm clonic activity, right head deviation, and tongue thrusting lasting less than 1 minute.

On examination, she was nonverbal and had autistic features. When she presented to our Epilepsy Center, she was on four AEDs, had a vagal nerve stimulator in place, and had failed the ketogenic diet. Her MRI scan revealed multiple bilateral areas of ill-defined signal abnormality seen on the FLAIR images, consistent with cortical tubers (Fig. 85.1). All of these lesions were relatively small in size, and no lesion was calcified or enhanced with gadolinium contrast. Several video-EEG monitoring studies showed bilateral, multifocal ictal onsets. Interictally, very frequent spike-and-wave discharges were seen diffusely from multiple regions. Bilateral rhythmic synchronous delta bursts lasting over 20 seconds were also seen. Ictal events were characterized by staring, bilateral arm jerking, gaze deviation to the right, left facial "pulling," and behavioral arrest that were associated with diffuse polyspike and wave activity followed by attenuation. Both FDG-PET and AMT-PET were performed. The FDG-PET showed 11 areas of nodular hypometabolism, likely representing tubers, in multiple regions bilaterally. The AMT-PET suggested that the epileptic foci might be located in both hemispheres, in the temporal–parietal regions. EEG during PET scans showed very frequent generalized spike and wave, less frequent independent spike and wave in the left central–temporal–parietal region, and less frequent independent spike and wave in the right temporal–frontal–central–parietal regions. Seizure semiology and the EEG findings also suggested the diagnosis of multifocal epilepsy. Ictal SPECT demonstrated increased perfusion in the posterior right parietal lobe.

In brief, she was experiencing multiple daily seizures which were not responsive to several antiepilpetic medications. Her case was discussed in detail at the Multidisciplinary Presurgical Epilepsy Conference. Her data were suggestive of multifocal seizures, which could not be localized to a specific region of the brain. Weighing the risks and benefits in detail with her parents, and given her poor course and quality of life, the group recommended a bilateral electrode survey, targeting the tubers seen on MRI with subdural strip electrodes. The goal was to identify one or maybe two seizure foci which could then be approached for resection. The understanding was that bilateral epileptiform activity was likely to be detected and that a complete surgical cure was unlikely. The parents agreed to proceed with this plan, and the patient underwent bilateral subdural strip electrode placement at age 4. Interictally, during the 5 days of intracranial monitoring, very frequent spikes were seen in multiple bilateral strips. Twenty-one typical seizures were recorded: these showed diffuse attenuation with high frequency, low amplitude beta activity seen earliest in the right anterior and posterior frontal strips with fast spread to the right posterior temporal, midtemporal, temporooccipital, right parietal, and right anterior parasagittal strips.

After a multidisciplinary discussion and detailed conversations with the family, it was decided to proceed with a surgical resective strategy targeting this right frontal epileptogenic zone. She underwent a staged approach: at the first stage, the right inferior frontal tuber was resected and subdural electrodes were then placed primarily over the remaining frontal lobe, with additional coverage over the parietal and temporal tubers (Fig. 85.2A). During the 6 days of monitoring, seizure onsets were detected from the orbitofrontal area, along the margin of the prior frontal resection. Additionally, there was independent seizure activity arising from the right temporal lobe, in the region of a tuber. At the second stage, therefore,

these two active areas (frontal and temporal) were resected, and new electrodes were placed to determine if adjacent or distal areas would continue to be active (Fig. 85.2B). During the following week, monitoring showed residual seizures originating posterior and superior to the frontal resection cavity, beyond the margins of any apparent tubers. The frontal region was resected further based on the ictal map and the electrodes were removed (Fig. 85.2C–D).

Postoperatively, she was seizure-free for 3 months, during which time her parents noted developmental gains. However, her parents then began noting an occasional left-sided "grin" and facial twitching, which were suspicious for recurrent seizures. These worsened, and eventually she had a recurrence of her typical seizures despite maximal AEDs. Video-EEG monitoring confirmed right frontal–parietal seizure onsets.

Her case was discussed in detail with the parents, who were anxious to consider surgery once again because of seizure recurrence and their impression that the initial surgery helped her significantly. Weighing all the possible options, we considered reoperative surgery when her case was presented again at the Conference, because her evaluation suggested that seizures were arising from the same regions that were approached previously.

Approximately 1 year following her initial surgery, she underwent reoperation on the right hemisphere, with the initial stage consisting of placement of subdural grid, strip, and depth

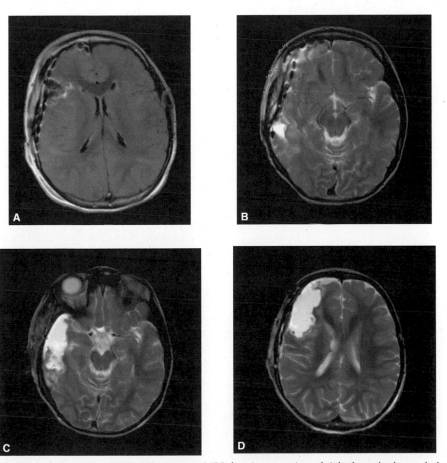

FIGURE 85.2 A: Postoperative FLAIR sequence MRI showing resection of right frontal tuber and placement of subdural electrodes (Stage 1). **B:** Postoperative T2-weighted MRI showing further resection of right frontal focus and new resection cavity within right temporal lobe, new subdural electrodes (Stage 2). **C–D:** Postoperative T2-weighted MRI showing further frontal and temporal lobe resection and removal of subdural electrodes (Stage 3).

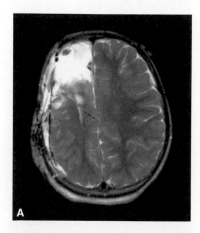

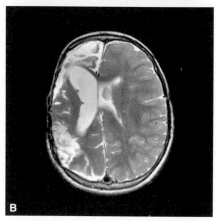

FIGURE 85.3 A: Postoperative T2-weighted MRI showing placement of subdural electrodes surrounding old resection bed as well as depth electrodes (Stage 1). **B:** Postoperative T2-weighted MRI showing final resection and removal of subdural electrodes (Stage 3).

electrodes via a right-sided craniotomy, targeting the frontal and parietal lobes (Fig. 85.3A). She was monitored for a week, during which time seizure onsets were recorded from the right posterior frontal and anterior parietal lobe regions, beyond the margins of any obvious tubers. At the second stage, these areas were resected, with intraoperative motor mapping, and electrodes were replaced for an additional phase of monitoring. Seizures persisted from the parietal lobe, beyond the margin of the prior resection, necessitating additional resection in this region. At the final stage, the residual parietal seizure focus was resected (Fig. 85.3B). The patient was discharged with a mild left hemiparesis, which resolved completely over the next 2 months, and was seizure-free.

At the most recent follow-up, surveillance EEGs have failed to show any seizure activity, and clinically this patient has remained seizure-free for over 4 years (Engel class I). She has also had significant gains in her language and cognitive development.

SUMMARY

Successful treatment of multifocal epilepsy remains an elusive goal, something like "chasing a ghost." Over the last few years, our treatment philosophy has evolved to include the multistage procedure when we feel it is indicated. The basic task is to find the hidden focus in the network. Initially,

patients undergo noninvasive testing, including video-EEG monitoring, MRI, MEG, PET, and SPECT scans, all trying to reveal the hidden focus. If at this stage no primary resectable focus is found, we proceed with intracranial EEG monitoring, using subdural grids, strips, and depth electrodes as needed. Invasive recordings are performed uni- or bilaterally according to the presurgical impression, and are used for seizure as well as functional mapping. We can then define the syndrome as either a focal or a multifocal one. For the truly multifocal syndrome, we consider nonresective treatments such as the ketogenic diet, additional medication trials, or the implantation of a vagal nerve stimulator (VNS) in addition to possible multifocal resections. If, however, a focus is determined, we resect it, possibly leaving grids, strips, and depth electrodes in place after resection to verify the cessation of the electrical network. Our goal is both clinical (no seizures) and electrical (no ictal activity). We acknowledge that, sometimes, persistent electrographic activity will have no clinical significance and may even regress spontaneously over time. As presented in the case above, sometimes reoperation is indicated and can be successful. The down side of this treatment regimen is a long hospitalization (up to 3 to 4 weeks), higher risk of infection, and surgical induced morbidity (including neurological insult). However, over the last few years, we have treated many children this way, and found the complication rate to be low and the epilepsy outcome to be worthwhile.

Multifocal epilepsy has traditionally been considered, in most situations, a contraindication for epilepsy surgery. However, with advances in surgical technique and functional and anatomic neuroimaging, a better understanding has emerged of the situations in which true multifocal resections are necessary. Several questions remain, however: how can we apply our experience in TSC to multifocal epilepsy in general? Is it possible to unmask a primary seizure focus in most cases of multifocal epilepsy? In what cases will a strategic approach to the presumed primary focus in multifocal epilepsy be sufficient? The lessons of the history of epilepsy surgery, combined with continued progress in technological modalities for defining the true epileptogenic zone, provide great optimism for patients who previously had no hope for a cure, but who now may find this elusive goal within reach. "Chasing the ghost" is sometimes successful, offering some of these children a meaningful solution to their incapacitating disease.

ACKNOWLEDGMENTS

We would like to acknowledge Dr. Chad Carlson of the NYU Comprehensive Epilepsy Center for his intellectual contributions that were key to preparing this chapter. We would also like to thank all of the other members of the NYU Comprehensive Epilepsy Center, under the direction of Dr. Orrin Devinsky and Dr. Ruben Kuzniecky, for their collaboration in all aspects of our work.

References

1. Luders HO, Najm I, Nair D, et al. The epileptogenic zone: general principles. *Epileptic Disord.* 2006;8(suppl 2):S1–S9.
2. Engel J, Jr., Wiebe S, French J, et al. Practice parameter: temporal lobe and localized neocortical resections for epilepsy. *Epilepsia.* 2003;44:741–751.
3. Cohen-Gadol AA, Ozduman K, Bronen RA, et al. Long-term outcome after epilepsy surgery for focal cortical dysplasia. *J Neurosurg.* 2004;101:55–65.

4. Park CK, Kim SK, Wang KC, et al. Surgical outcome and prognostic factors of pediatric epilepsy caused by cortical dysplasia. *Childs Nerv Syst.* 2006;22:586–592.

5. Siegel AM, Cascino GD, Meyer FB, et al. Surgical outcome and predictive factors in adult patients with intractable epilepsy and focal cortical dysplasia. *Acta Neurol Scand.* 2006;113:65–71.

6. Cataltepe O, Turanli G, Yalnizoglu D, et al. Surgical management of temporal lobe tumor-related epilepsy in children. *J Neurosurg.* 2005;102:280–287.

7. Giulioni M, Galassi E, Zucchelli M, et al. Seizure outcome of lesionectomy in glioneuronal tumors associated with epilepsy in children. *J Neurosurg.* 2005;102:288–293.

8. Luyken C, Blumcke I, Fimmers R, et al. The spectrum of long-term epilepsy-associated tumors: long-term seizure and tumor outcome and neurosurgical aspects. *Epilepsia.* 2003;44:822–830.

9. Schramm J, Aliashkevich AF. Surgery for temporal mediobasal tumors: experience based on a series of 235 patients. *Neurosurgery.* 2007;60: 285–294. Discussion 285–294.

10. Baumann CR, Schuknecht B, Lo Russo G, et al. Seizure outcome after resection of cavernous malformations is better when surrounding hemosiderin-stained brain also is removed. *Epilepsia.* 2006;47:563–566.

11. Hammen T, Romstock J, Dorfler A, et al. Prediction of postoperative outcome with special respect to removal of hemosiderin fringe: a study in patients with cavernous haemangiomas associated with symptomatic epilepsy. *Seizure.* 2007;16:248–253.

12. Wiebe S, Blume WT, Girvin JP, et al. A randomized, controlled trial of surgery for temporal-lobe epilepsy. *N Engl J Med.* 2001;345:311–318.

13. Kutsy RL, Farrell DF, Ojemann GA. Ictal patterns of neocortical seizures monitored with intracranial electrodes: correlation with surgical outcome. *Epilepsia.* 1999;40:257–266.

14. Bollo RJ, Kalhorn SP, Carlson C, et al. Epilepsy surgery and tuberous sclerosis complex: special considerations. *Neurosurg Focus.* 2008;25:E13.

15. Weiner HL, Carlson C, Ridgway EB, et al. Epilepsy surgery in young children with tuberous sclerosis: results of a novel approach. *Pediatrics.* 2006;117:1494–1502.

16. Cross JH, Jayakar P, Nordli D, et al. Proposed criteria for referral and evaluation of children for epilepsy surgery: recommendations of the Subcommission for Pediatric Epilepsy Surgery. *Epilepsia.* 2006;47:952–959.

17. Bourgeois BF, Prensky AL, Palkes HS, et al. Intelligence in epilepsy: a prospective study in children. *Ann Neurol.* 1983;14:438–444.

18. Nolan MA, Redoblado MA, Lah S, et al. Intelligence in childhood epilepsy syndromes. *Epilepsy Res.* 2003;53:139–150.

19. Racoosin JA, Feeney J, Burkhart G, et al. Mortality in antiepileptic drug development programs. *Neurology.* 2001;56:514–519.

20. Vasconcellos E, Wyllie E, Sullivan S, et al. Mental retardation in pediatric candidates for epilepsy surgery: the role of early seizure onset. *Epilepsia.* 2001;42:268–274.

21. Asarnow RF, LoPresti C, Guthrie D, et al. Developmental outcomes in children receiving resection surgery for medically intractable infantile spasms. *Dev Med Child Neurol.* 1997;39:430–440.

22. Battaglia D, Chieffo D, Lettori D, et al. Cognitive assessment in epilepsy surgery of children. *Childs Nerv Syst.* 2006;22:744–759.

23. Devlin AM, Cross JH, Harkness W, et al. Clinical outcomes of hemispherectomy for epilepsy in childhood and adolescence. *Brain.* 2003;126: 556–566.

24. Gleissner U, Clusmann H, Sassen R, et al. Postsurgical outcome in pediatric patients with epilepsy: a comparison of patients with intellectual disabilities, subaverage intelligence, and average-range intelligence. *Epilepsia.* 2006;47:406–414.

25. Jonas R, Asarnow RF, LoPresti C, et al. Surgery for symptomatic infant-onset epileptic encephalopathy with and without infantile spasms. *Neurology.* 2005;64:746–750.

26. Jonas R, Nguyen S, Hu B, et al. Cerebral hemispherectomy: hospital course, seizure, developmental, language, and motor outcomes. *Neurology.* 2004; 62:1712–1721.

27. Loddenkemper T, Holland KD, Stanford LD, et al. Developmental outcome after epilepsy surgery in infancy. *Pediatrics.* 2007;119:930–935.

28. Sabaz M, Lawson JA, Cairns DR, et al. The impact of epilepsy surgery on quality of life in children. *Neurology.* 2006;66:557–561.

29. Davies KG, Hermann BP, Wyler AR. Surgery for intractable epilepsy secondary to viral encephalitis. *Br J Neurosurg.* 1995;9:759–762.

30. Harvey AS, Cross JH, Shinnar S, et al. Defining the spectrum of international practice in pediatric epilepsy surgery patients. *Epilepsia.* 2008;49: 146–155.

31. Cossu M, Lo Russo G, Francione S, et al. Epilepsy surgery in children: results and predictors of outcome on seizures. *Epilepsia.* 2008;49:65–72.

32. Devinsky O, Romanelli P, Orbach D, et al. Surgical treatment of multifocal epilepsy involving eloquent cortex. *Epilepsia.* 2003;44:718–723.

33. Bauman JA, Feoli E, Romanelli P, et al. Multistage epilepsy surgery: safety, efficacy, and utility of a novel approach in pediatric extratemporal epilepsy. *Neurosurgery.* 2005;56:318–334.

34. Basheer SN, Connolly MB, Lautzenhiser A, et al. Hemispheric surgery in children with refractory epilepsy: seizure outcome, complications, and adaptive function. *Epilepsia.* 2007;48:133–140.

35. Kossoff EH, Buck C, Freeman JM. Outcomes of 32 hemispherectomies for Sturge–Weber syndrome worldwide. *Neurology.* 2002;59:1735–1738.

36. Kossoff EH, Vining EP, Pillas DJ, et al. Hemispherectomy for intractable unihemispheric epilepsy etiology vs outcome. *Neurology.* 2003;61:887–890.

37. Terra-Bustamante VC, Inuzuka LM, Fernandes RM, et al. Outcome of hemispheric surgeries for refractory epilepsy in pediatric patients. *Childs Nerv Syst.* 2007;23:321–326.

38. Blumenfeld H. From molecules to networks: cortical/subcortical interactions in the pathophysiology of idiopathic generalized epilepsy. *Epilepsia.* 2003;44(suppl 2):7–15.

39. Cavazos JE, Cross DJ. The role of synaptic reorganization in mesial temporal lobe epilepsy. *Epilepsy Behav.* 2006;8:483–493.

40. Spencer SS. Neural networks in human epilepsy: evidence of and implications for treatment. *Epilepsia.* 2002;43:219–227.

41. Jacobs J, Rohr A, Moeller F, et al. Evaluation of epileptogenic networks in children with tuberous sclerosis complex using EEG-fMRI. *Epilepsia.* 2008;49:816–825.

42. Hirsch LJ, Spencer SS, Spencer DD, et al. Temporal lobectomy in patients with bitemporal epilepsy defined by depth electroencephalography. *Ann Neurol.* 1991;30:347–356.

43. Morrell F. Secondary epileptogenesis in man. *Arch Neurol.* 1985;42: 318–335.

44. Morrell F. Varieties of human secondary epileptogenesis. *J Clin Neurophysiol.* 1989;6:227–275.

45. Chugani HT, Shields WD, Shewmon DA, et al. Infantile spasms: I. PET identifies focal cortical dysgenesis in cryptogenic cases for surgical treatment. *Ann Neurol.* 1990;27:406–413.

46. Fenoglio KA, Wu J, Kim do Y, et al. Hypothalamic hamartoma: basic mechanisms of intrinsic epileptogenesis. *Semin Pediatr Neurol.* 2007;14: 51–59.

47. Freeman JL, Harvey AS, Rosenfeld JV, et al. Generalized epilepsy in hypothalamic hamartoma: evolution and postoperative resolution. *Neurology.* 2003;60:762–767.

48. Harvey AS, Freeman JL. Epilepsy in hypothalamic hamartoma: clinical and EEG features. *Semin Pediatr Neurol.* 2007;14:60–64.

49. Gupta A, Chirla A, Wyllie E, et al. Pediatric epilepsy surgery in focal lesions and generalized electroencephalogram abnormalities. *Pediatr Neurol.* 2007;37:8–15.

50. Wyllie E, Lachhwani DK, Gupta A, et al. Successful surgery for epilepsy due to early brain lesions despite generalized EEG findings. *Neurology.* 2007;69:389–397.

51. Wyllie E, Comair Y, Ruggieri P, et al. Epilepsy surgery in the setting of periventricular leukomalacia and focal cortical dysplasia. *Neurology.* 1996;46:839–841.

52. Wyllie E, Comair YG, Kotagal P, et al. Epilepsy surgery in infants. *Epilepsia.* 1996;37:625–637.

53. Radhakrishnan A, Sithinamsuwan P, Simon Harvey A, et al. Multifocal epilepsy: the role of palliative resection—intractable frontal and occipital lobe epilepsy secondary to radiotherapy for acute lymphoblastic leukaemia. *Epileptic Disord.* 2008;10:362–370.

54. Carlson C, Teutonico F, Elliott R, et al. The utility of bilateral intracranial electroencephalographic monitoring in medically refractory epilepsy and tuberous sclerosis. Submitted for publication, 2009.

55. Chassoux F, Landre E, Rodrigo S, et al. Intralesional recordings and epileptogenic zone in focal polymicrogyria. *Epilepsia.* 2008;49:51–64.

56. Madhavan D, Weiner HL, Carlson C, et al. Local epileptogenic networks in tuberous sclerosis complex: a case review. *Epilepsy Behav.* 2007;11: 140–146.

57. Chandra PS, Salamon N, Huang J, et al. FDG-PET/MRI coregistration and diffusion-tensor imaging distinguish epileptogenic tubers and cortex in patients with tuberous sclerosis complex: a preliminary report. *Epilepsia.* 2006;47:1543–1549.

58. Chugani DC, Chugani HT, Muzik O, et al. Imaging epileptogenic tubers in children with tuberous sclerosis complex using alpha-[11C]methyl-L-tryptophan positron emission tomography. *Ann Neurol.* 1998;44:858–866.

59. Iida K, Otsubo H, Mohamed IS, et al. Characterizing magnetoencephalographic spike sources in children with tuberous sclerosis complex. *Epilepsia.* 2005;46:1510–1517.

60. Jansen FE, Huiskamp G, van Huffelen AC, et al. Identification of the epileptogenic tuber in patients with tuberous sclerosis: a comparison of high-resolution EEG and MEG. *Epilepsia.* 2006;47:108–114.

61. Kagawa K, Chugani DC, Asano E, et al. Epilepsy surgery outcome in children with tuberous sclerosis complex evaluated with alpha-[11C]methyl-L-tryptophan positron emission tomography (PET). *J Child Neurol.* 2005;20: 429–438.

62. Kamimura T, Tohyama J, Oishi M, et al. Magnetoencephalography in patients with tuberous sclerosis and localization-related epilepsy. *Epilepsia.* 2006;47:991–997.

63. Knowlton RC, Elgavish R, Howell J, et al. Magnetic source imaging versus intracranial electroencephalogram in epilepsy surgery: a prospective study. *Ann Neurol.* 2006;59:835–842.

64. RamachandranNair R, Otsubo H, Shroff MM, et al. MEG predicts outcome following surgery for intractable epilepsy in children with normal or nonfocal MRI findings. *Epilepsia.* 2007;48:149–157.

65. Wu JY, Sutherling WW, Koh S, et al. Magnetic source imaging localizes epileptogenic zone in children with tuberous sclerosis complex. *Neurology.* 2006;66:1270–1272.

CHAPTER 86 ■ NONLESIONAL CASES

ELSON L. SO

Nonlesional epilepsy refers to the *absence of a potentially epileptogenic lesion on magnetic resonance imaging (MRI)*, regardless of what the postsurgical histopathologic examination may eventually reveal. Before MRI is said to be "negative" and epilepsy is considered "nonlesional," it is necessary to verify that the MRI was performed with techniques that optimize the ability to detect potentially epileptogenic lesions. Standard MRI studies are insufficient for the evaluation of patients for epilepsy surgery. Sensitivity in detecting a lesion was only 50% with expert review of standard MRI studies, but it increased to 91% with expert review of epilepsy-protocol MRI studies of the same patients (1). Specific MRI imaging techniques and sequences must be used to minimize the risk of missing an epileptogenic lesion that would have facilitated presurgical localization and subsequent resection of the seizure focus. The requisite imaging techniques and sequences are described in the literature (2) and are affirmed by the Commission on Neuroimaging of the International League Against Epilepsy.

CHALLENGES IN NONLESIONAL CASES

Limitations in Noninvasive Evaluation

The concordance of interictal epileptiform discharges (IEDs), ictal discharges, and lesion in the temporal lobe is associated with 3.5 times greater probability of excellent postsurgical seizure control than when IEDs are absent or nonconcordant (3). Moreover, in patients with lesional epilepsy, exclusively concordant scalp-recorded IEDs improve the surgical prognosis beyond that conferred by the presence of an MRI lesion. The rate of excellent postsurgical outcome is 94% when exclusively concordant IEDs are present versus 60% when they are absent. In contrast, concordance between temporal lobe IEDs and ictal discharges is not associated with better prognosis for seizure control in patients undergoing nonlesional temporal lobe surgery. The probability of excellent postsurgical outcome is approximately 60% to 65%, regardless of the presence or absence of concordant IEDs in patients with nonlesional epilepsy.

As for frontal lobe epilepsy, IEDs are often absent or widespread. In one study, nearly 20% of patients with frontal lobe epilepsy do not have scalp-recorded IEDs and, when present, IEDs were discordant with the frontal epileptogenic zone in 45% of patients (4). The presence and location of scalp-recorded IEDs are not independently associated with the outcome of frontal lobe epilepsy surgery, which is the most common type of extratemporal epilepsy surgery (5).

Between 25% and 30% of all seizures recorded in patients with unilateral mesial temporal lobe epilepsy or MRI-detected hippocampal atrophy could not be lateralized to the diseased temporal lobe (6). Of temporal lobectomy candidates, 10% had extracranially recorded seizures with conflicting features and 18% had falsely localizing seizures (7). The situation is no better in patients with extratemporal epilepsy. Approximately 35% to 50% of seizures extracranially recorded in extratemporal epilepsy are nonlateralizing (8). In one study, 11 of 33 intractable epilepsy patients with negative MRIs had proven extratemporal seizure onset despite apparent onset of scalp-recorded EEG seizures at the temporal lobe region (9).

Complexity of Invasive Electroencephalogram (EEG) Recordings and Surgical Resection

In nonlesional cases, the adequacy of the extent of intracranial electrode implantation or surgical resection is not as apparent as when a lesion is present. The situation often calls for extensive intracranial electrode implantation over large regions in one or both hemispheres. Unfortunately, the risk for major complications is estimated to increase by 40% for every 20 additional subdural electrodes implanted (10).

In nonlesional epilepsy surgery, clinicians and surgeons are deprived of neuroanatomic landmarks to guide the extent of resection. In such cases, resection is then based on the extent of EEG abnormalities, but extensive resection based on abnormal EEG discharges raises the risk of perioperative morbidity. Conversely, restricted resection that spares electrophysiologically abnormal tissues may reduce the probability of postsurgical seizure control, especially in patients with extratemporal neocortical epilepsy.

Less Favorable Postsurgical Outcome

The probability of excellent postsurgical outcome following nonlesional surgery is uniformly lower than lesional surgery across many studies in the literature. In one series of 157 consecutive patients who underwent anterior temporal lobotomy, 62% of those with no MRI lesion versus 85% of those with an MRI lesion had an excellent (3). The outcome in patients undergoing nonlesional frontal lobe surgery is even less favorable (excellent outcome in only 40% vs. 72% in lesional cases (5)).

DIAGNOSTIC APPROACH IN NONLESIONAL EPILEPSY SURGERY

Despite their limitations, seizure semiology and extracranial EEG must still be fully explored for clues that help lateralize or localize seizure onset. Also, some types of extracranial IEDs and ictal discharges have value in determining the location of a seizure focus and in guiding intracranial electrode implantation. Exclusively unifocal IEDs are strong predictors of the site of the ictal-onset zone in both lesional and nonlesional temporal and extratemporal epilepsies (3,11). The presence of a fast discharge in the beta-frequency range at the onset of a frontal seizure is highly indicative of the location of the epileptogenic zone (12) (Fig. 86.1). Approximately 90% of patients with this focal ictal beta-discharge pattern at seizure onset became seizure-free following resection of the frontal lobe focus, even when the MRI was negative. In comparison, postsurgical seizure freedom occurred in only 16.7% of nonlesional frontal lobe epilepsy patients who did not have the focal ictal beta-discharge pattern.

In the absence of a structural lesion on MRI, functional imaging becomes important for guiding intracranial electrode implantation and for limiting the extent of the implantation. In some cases, functional imaging results can obviate the need for intracranial electrode implantation. More commonly utilized functional imaging tests in epilepsy surgery evaluation include positron emission tomography (PET), single photon emission computed tomography (SPECT), magnetic resonance spectroscopy (MRS), and magnetoencephalography (MEG) or magnetic source imaging (MSI).

Advanced MRI Techniques

Experienced reviews of 3 T phase array MRI studies have been reported to yield additional information in 48% of patients compared with routine reviews of their 1.5 T MRI studies (13). However, it is unclear whether the 1.5 T studies had been optimized for detecting epileptogenic lesions. Similarly, diffusion tensor imaging technique holds promise for increasing the yield of detecting MRI abnormalities. In a group of 16 predominantly nonlesional intractable epilepsy patients, diffusion tensor imaging specificity was found to be better in extratemporal than in temporal lobe epilepsy (14).

Ideally, three-dimensional rendition of the brain surface should be performed when needed, along with the capability for accurate coregistration of images from other diagnostic procedures. Finally, physicians who review the MRI images must be highly skilled in detecting and interpreting the structural alterations associated with epileptic seizure disorders.

Quantitative MRI has been assessed in a group of 44 temporal and 49 frontal lobe epilepsy patients whose conventional

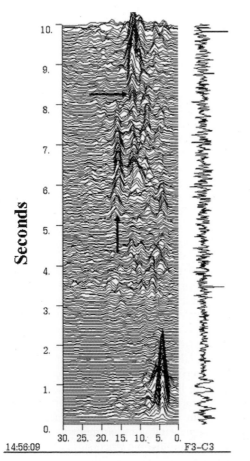
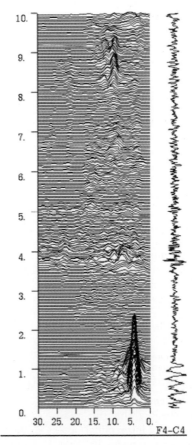

FIGURE 86.1 Time–frequency analysis of two channels: F_3–C_3 (**left**) and F_4–C_4 (**right**). The graph shows the spectral power (z axis [V^2/m^2]) as a function of time (y axis [seconds]) and frequency (x axis [Hertz]). At seizure onset, there is a 17-Hz discharge at the F_3–C_3 channel *(vertical arrow)*. The beta-frequency discharge precedes the build-up of lower-frequency and higher-amplitude activity *(horizontal arrow)*. (From Worrell G, So E, Kazemi J, et al. Focal ictal beta discharge on scalp EEG predicts excellent outcome of frontal lobe epilepsy surgery. *Epilepsia.* 2002;43:277–282, with permission.)

Frequency (Hz)

MRI showed no lesion. Techniques such as fast fluid attenuation inversion recovery-based T2 measurement, double inversion recovery, magnetization transfer ratio, and gray matter voxel-based morphometry were uniformly of low yield in revealing a focus that is concordant with the video-EEG localized focus (15).

Positron Emission Tomography (PET)

The most commonly used radioactive ligand in PET studies of patients with epilepsy is 2-[^{18}F]fluoro-2-deoxy-D-glucose (FDG). In nonlesional temporal lobe epilepsy patients with well-lateralized EEG abnormalities, FDG-PET lateralized hypometabolism to the same side in 90% (16). It was noted that PET abnormality is more extensive in nonlesional patients than in patients with MRI-detected hippocampal sclerosis. Analysis of the PET data using statistical parametric mapping demonstrated that the abnormality was mainly at the inferolateral temporal area in nonlesional patients and at the antero–inferomesial area in those with MRI-detected hippocampal sclerosis.

Quantitative measurement of FDG uptake improves the sensitivity of PET studies in patients with focal epilepsy. The interictal hypometabolic zone detected by quantitative measurement has very high concordance with the intracranial ictal EEG onset zone. In one study, 75% of patients who had reduced lateral temporal FDG uptake of 15% or more, as compared with the other side, became seizure-free after temporal lobectomy (17). About 67% of the patients in the study did not have a relevant MRI lesion. The finding of a hypometabolic temporal lobe is particularly useful when the extracranial ictal EEG is not localizing. Meta-analysis of the literature showed that ipsilateral PET hypometabolism has a predictive value of 80% for good postsurgical outcome in nonlesional patients and 72% in those with nonlocalized ictal scalp EEG (18).

PET is less useful in extratemporal lobe epilepsy than in temporal lobe epilepsy. Although 85% of nonlesional frontal lobe epilepsy patients reportedly had a unilateral frontal hypometabolic region, the location of the hypometabolic region observed did not correspond to the ictal EEG onset zone in 20% of the patients. Caution must be exercised when using FDG-PET for localizing the focus for either temporal or extratemporal epilepsy surgery. In temporal lobe epilepsy, the hypometabolic PET defect frequently involves the lateral or inferior neocortical region, even in patients with mesial temporal sclerosis or with mesial temporal ictal onset. Furthermore, the abnormal FDG-PET focus extends into the ipsilateral frontal lobe region in 30% of patients with proven mesial temporal lobe epilepsy. As for nonlesional frontal lobe epilepsy, the size of the hypometabolic region may exceed the ictal EEG onset zone in nearly 40% of patients (19).

Despite the low yield of FDG-PET in extratemporal epilepsy, its clinical application is not limited to patients with suspected temporal lobe epilepsy. PET can be considered as a means of detecting additional evidence for distinguishing between temporal and extratemporal epilepsies, or for lateralizing seizure onset to one hemisphere. The PET abnormality is then used to guide the location and extent of intracranial electrode implantation. A wide region of PET abnormality that affects both temporal and extratemporal areas can be still be implanted with intracranial electrodes to detect a more discrete focus of ictal EEG onset. PET abnormalities confined to one hemisphere can obviate the need for bilateral hemispheric implantation of intracranial electrodes.

PET using the radiotracer α-[^{11}C]methyl-L-tryptophan (AMT) to assess aberrant serotonin synthesis has also yielded encouraging results in patients with nonlesional partial epilepsy. A study compared AMT-PET with FDG-PET in 27 patients, 19 of whom had normal MRI (20). The sensitivity of AMT-PET in terms of agreement with intracranial ictal EEG onset was lower than that of FDG-PET (39% vs. 73%, respectively), but specificity of AMT-PET was better than that of FDG-PET (100% vs. 63%, respectively). Nine (47%) of the 19 MRI-negative patients had an abnormal AMT-PET.

Subtraction Ictal Single Photon Emission Computed Tomography Coregistered to Magnetic Resonance Imaging (SISCOM)

The conventional method of interpreting ictal SPECT studies is based on the subjective visual appreciation of differences in perfusion patterns between the ictal and the interictal images. The SISCOM technique was subsequently developed so that ictal images can be digitally subtracted from interictal images to derive images of the difference in perfusion intensity between the two studies (Fig. 86.2). The technique thresholds the difference image to display only pixels with intensities of perfusion that are more than two standard deviations from the mean. This peak intensity image is then registered on the MRI.

The SISCOM technique is superior to the conventional method in detecting a hyperperfusion focus (sensitivity rates of 88% vs. 39%, respectively) (21). Furthermore, the results of SISCOM studies are independently predictive of epilepsy surgery outcome, whereas the results of the conventional method of SPECT reviews are not. SISCOM is also useful in individuals with nonlesional epilepsy. In a group of 24 patients with either nonlesional temporal lobe or nonlesional extratemporal epilepsy, SISCOM revealed a hyperperfusion focus in 22 patients (91%). Furthermore, the predictive value of SISCOM for surgical outcome was independent of MRI, even when MRI-positive patients were included in the analysis. The rate of excellent postsurgical outcome was nearly 70% when the SISCOM focus was resected, but the rate was only 20% when the SISCOM focus was absent or excluded from the resection.

Despite the best efforts in attempting to inject the SPECT radioligand during seizure activity, the radioligand is often injected postictally instead, especially when seizures are brief in duration. When the seizure activity ends, the initially hyperperfused focus becomes progressively but transiently hypoperfused relative to the interictal state (i.e., postictal hypoperfusion). The dual SISCOM method of detecting hyperperfusion or hypoperfusion changes is specifically useful in the presurgical evaluation of nonlesional extratemporal epilepsy, revealing an abnormal focus in 77% of patients (22). When surgical resection involved the SISCOM focus, 55% of the patients had an excellent outcome. In contrast, none of the patients had an excellent outcome when surgical resection did not involve the SISCOM focus or when the SISCOM focus was absent. The modest rate of 55% excellent outcome

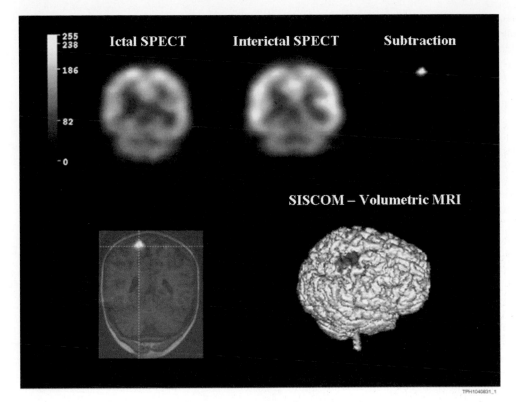

FIGURE 86.2 Steps to obtaining subtraction ictal SPECT (single photon emission computed tomography) coregistered to MRI (magnetic resonance imaging) (SISCOM) image. Ictal (**upper left**) and interictal (**upper middle**) SPECT images are obtained. After normalization of their mean intensities and coregistration with each other, subtraction is performed to obtain a "difference" image (**upper right**). The difference image is then coregistered with MRI images at specific planes (**lower left**) or on the surface of a three-dimensional MRI image (**lower right**). (From So E. Role of neuroimaging in the management of seizure disorders. *Mayo Clin Proc.* 2002;77:1251–1264, with permission.) Please see color insert.

in SISCOM-inclusive surgery must be viewed from the historical perspective of only 40% of nonlesional frontal lobe epilepsy patients at the same center having an excellent surgical outcome prior to development and use of the SISCOM technique. Of patients in the SISCOM series, 35% had no localized ictal EEG discharges. The intracranial ictal onset of patients in the series often involved the parietal or occipital regions, which harbored eloquent cortex that had restricted the extent of surgical resection. On the other hand, the majority of patients in the earlier non-SISCOM series had wide resection of the frontal lobe, largely unconstrained by the absence of eloquent cortex.

Magnetic Resonance Spectroscopy (MRS) in Patients with Nonlesional Epilepsy

In patients with MRI-detected loss of amygdala–hippocampal volume, the sensitivity of ^{1}H-MRS in revealing a lateralized abnormality is 85%, with nearly all agreeing with the MRI abnormality or the ictal EEG focus. However, the proportion of nonlesional temporal lobe epilepsy patients with an ^{1}H-MRS abnormality that lateralized to the ictal EEG focus ranged from 27% to 92% in several studies (23). Of 10 nonlesional temporal and extratemporal epilepsy patients, advanced MRS using statistical analysis techniques detected an abnormal focus that was concordant with localization by seizure semiology and EEG in 6 (24). There is still no evidence that a ^{1}H-MRS abnormality involving a nonlesional temporal lobe independently predicts seizure control after surgical resection of the lobe.

The usefulness of MRS in nonlesional extratemporal epilepsy surgery remains to be proven. Moreover, MRS abnor-

malities often extend well beyond the ictal EEG focus in patients with either temporal or extratemporal epilepsy. This occurred in 35% of patients in one series of temporal and extratemporal epilepsies (25).

As many as 60% of intractable epilepsy patients have been reported to have bilateral MRS abnormalities. Care must be exercised in treating these patients, in order to ascertain that the temporal lobe to be surgically resected is more severely abnormal than the contralateral temporal lobe. Prognosis for postsurgical seizure freedom is poor when the ^{1}H-MRS at the nonresected temporal lobe is more severely abnormal than the resected temporal lobe. Moreover, an abnormal ^{1}H-MRS in the language-dominant temporal lobe is associated with verbal memory deficits following contralateral temporal lobectomy (26). Therefore, a potential use of MRS is to assess the status of the temporal lobe contralateral to the side of contemplated temporal lobectomy, especially when the temporal lobes are normal in size or symmetrically atrophic.

Magnetic Source Imaging (MSI) in Patients with Nonlesional Epilepsy

Because of technical requirements and limitations, MSI recording sessions are typically a few hours in duration; consequently, this technique is limited to the detection and analysis of interictal spike discharges. The question of whether present MSI abnormalities could guide recognition of abnormalities in high-spatial-resolution MRI was assessed in a small number of patients (27). MSI abnormalities led to detection of MRI abnormalities upon repeat review of the MR images in three of eight patients. Thus far, data on the experience of MSI in nonlesional epilepsy surgery involve only a small number of patients in each reported series. The sensitivity of MSI in detecting interictal spikes was only 32% in nonlesional mesial temporal lobe epilepsy (28). The correlation between MSI and EEG localizations was only partial in these patients.

Spike discharges that are restricted to the mesial temporal regions are not as easily detected by MSI as are discharges occurring at the neocortical regions. Accordingly, MSI studies in extratemporal neocortical epilepsy have higher yields than do studies in patients with mesial temporal lobe epilepsy. The extent of the MSI focus resection is associated with surgical outcome in nonlesional extratemporal surgery. Smith and colleagues reported that 8 of 10 patients became seizure-free when their nonlesional extratemporal MSI focus was extensively resected, versus 1 of 10 when the focus was partially or totally unresected (29). Another study showed that the positive predictive value of MSI was 90% and the negative predictive value was 44% for successful short-term surgical outcome when MRI shows no lesion or ambiguous lesions (e.g., large, multiple, subtle, or questionable lesions) (30). A recent study in 22 children with normal MRI or nonlocalizing MRI abnormalities showed that multiple or scattered MSI spike clusters reduced the likelihood of postsurgical seizure freedom, and so did presence of multiple seizure-types and incomplete resection of the surgically intended region (31).

In patients with nonlesional epilepsy, MSI findings cannot be relied upon as the sole determinant of the location or the extent of surgical resection. MSI spikes indicate the probable location of the center of epileptiform activity, but they do not represent the entire extent of the irritative zone (32). Intracranial EEG recordings need to be considered to delineate the full extent of the irritative and the ictal-onset zones prior to surgery. MSI localization is useful in guiding the location and the extent of the intracranial electrode implantation in patients with nonlesional epilepsy. The complementary roles of MSI and EEG must be recognized. MSI records tangentially oriented magnetic fields generated by spike discharges, whereas EEG preferentially records radially oriented electrical fields of spike discharges. The superiority of MSI in spatial resolution complements the benefit of EEG in temporal resolution.

OPERATIVE STRATEGY IN NONLESIONAL EPILEPSY SURGERY

Intracranial Electrode Implantation

Intracranial electrode implantation and recording are required in most cases of nonlesional epilepsy surgery, especially when the suspected focus is in the extratemporal region. Intracranial electrode implantation can be obviated in some patients who possess sufficient noninvasive electroclinical and functional imaging abnormalities that are concordant in identifying an abnormal focus that is distant from the eloquent cortex. Such a situation is more obvious when a standard anterior temporal lobectomy is already the preferred surgical technique, especially in epilepsy involving the nondominant temporal lobe. Otherwise, to optimize postsurgical seizure control and to minimize perioperative complications, intracranial electrodes have to be implanted for tailoring the extent of surgical resection or transection.

False localization has occurred with each of the diagnostic modalities discussed in the previous sections. It has been difficult to determine which functional imaging modality is the most useful in evaluating patients with nonlesional epilepsy. Very few institutions routinely use all or most of the functional imaging modalities for evaluating intractable epilepsy patients for surgery. One exceptional study revealed that SISCOM had the best sensitivity, positive predictive value, and negative predictive value for postsurgical freedom from disabling seizures in patients whose MRI shows no lesion or ambiguous lesions (e.g., large, multiple, or questionable lesions) (33) (Table 86.1).

Concordance of the results from clinical, electrophysiologic, and functional imaging evaluation enhances confidence in selecting the site for intracranial electrode implantation or

---

TABLE 86.1

MAGNETIC SOURCE IMAGING, FDG-PET, SISCOM WITH RESPECT TO POSTSURGICAL FREEDOM FROM DISABLING SEIZURES

Diagnostic value	MSI (CI)	PET (CI)	SISCOM (CI)
Sensitivity	31%	54%	62%
	(12.0–46.9)	(31.6–66.3)	(38.8–74.0)
Specificity	79%	86%	86%
	(61.2–93.6)	(65.0–97.3)	(64.6–97.3)
PPV	57%	78%	80%
	(22.4–87.2)	(45.6–95.8)	(50.4–96.2)
NPV	55%	67%	70.6%
	(42.8–65.5)	(50.6–75.7)	(53.2–80.1)

FDG-PET, 2-[18F]fluro-2-deoxy-D-glucose positron emission tomography; MSI, magnetic source imaging; CI, confidence interval; SISCOM, subtraction ictal SPECT coregistered to magnetic resonance imaging; PPV, positive predictive value; NPV, negative predictive value.

Adapted from Knowlton RC, Elgavish RA, Bartolucci A, et al. Functional imaging: II. Prediction of epilepsy surgery outcome. *Ann Neurol.* 2008;64:35–41, with permission.

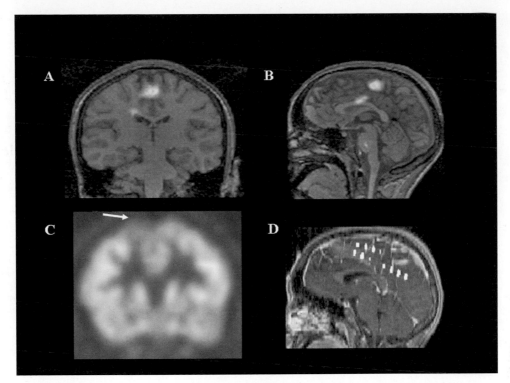

FIGURE 86.3 A: Coronal view of subtraction ictal SPECT (single photon emission computed tomography) coregistered to magnetic resonance imaging (MRI) (SISCOM) showing an apparently midline hyperperfusion focus in a 13-year-old male who had between 1 and 10 attacks per night of bilateral extremity movements and facial grimacing. Epilepsy-protocol MRI was normal and scalp ictal electroencephalogram was nonlocalizing. **B:** Sagittal view of SISCOM shows that the hyperperfusion focus was at the right posterior mesial frontal region. **C:** 2-[18F]fluoro-2-deoxy-D-glucose (FDG)–positron emission tomography (PET) shows a hypometabolic focus corresponding to the SISCOM hyperperfusion focus. **D:** MRI with coregistered CT (computed tomography)-derived images of subdural electrode contacts (white marks) on the SISCOM and PET abnormalities. The intracranial EEG recording confirmed ictal onset at the SISCOM and PET abnormalities. Surgical resection of the region rendered the patient free of seizures, with minimal weakness in the left toes. Pathologic examination of the specimen revealed cortical dysplasia. Please see color insert.

surgical treatment (Fig. 86.3). In nonlesional epilepsy surgery, concordance between two or more modalities has been shown to be associated with higher seizure-free rates than lack of concordance (34). If the modalities reveal conflicting findings or if only one modality has localizing features, more extensive implantation may have to be considered to ensure that ictal-onset and irritative zones are not overlooked.

There are patients whose electroclinical data and functional imaging studies are all devoid of clues as to the potential location of the seizure focus. These patients are generally considered to be very poor surgical candidates. Continued pursuit of seizure localization would require extensive bilateral hemisphere implantation with subdural electrodes, or selective implantation of both hemispheres with strip and depth electrodes. The risk-to-benefit ratio of these approaches should be carefully weighed in each patient. Every effort must be made to note any lateralizing feature in the diagnostic modalities, which, when present, may warrant the concentration of electrodes in one hemisphere or at one region.

Currently, no evidence in nonlesional epilepsy favors resection of the functional imaging abnormality over resection of the abnormal EEG focus, or vice versa. To date, the extent of resection has prognostic implications in three functional imaging modalities: SISCOM, MSI, and PET. Nonetheless, EEG abnormalities were not completely disregarded in the studies

that evaluated these three modalities. Therefore, the putative principle and practice in nonlesional epilepsy surgery is to resect both functional imaging and EEG abnormalities, whenever this can be safely accomplished. An FDG-PET abnormality can appear very diffuse, such that complete resection of the abnormality may be impractical or unsafe. In planning the extent of surgical resection in such a situation, the relationship between the diffuse functional imaging abnormality and the EEG abnormality must be fully elucidated in each patient. For this purpose, intracranial electrode coverage should encompass as much as possible the functional imaging abnormality and also extend beyond its dimensions. The extent of the coverage is also dictated by the proximity of the abnormalities to anatomical structures that serve critical cortical functions, such as cognitive, speech, or motor functions. For this purpose, the integration of images of functional imaging, EEG, and cortical functions into the patient's MRI is essential when planning electrode implantation and surgical resection or transection.

Integration of Multimodality Images for Surgical Planning

The spatial concordance of abnormalities of different diagnostic modalities can be assessed by coregistering the abnormalities

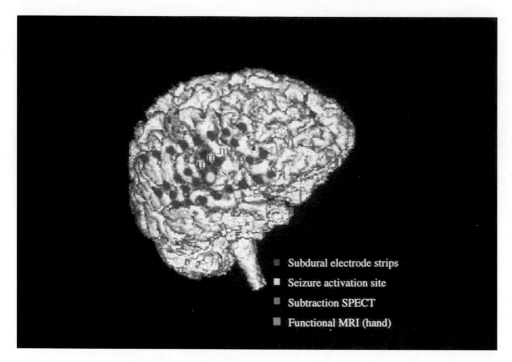

Subdural electrode strips
Seizure activation site
Subtraction SPECT
Functional MRI (hand)

FIGURE 86.4 Three-dimensional rendition of MRI (magnetic resonance imaging) of brain with coregistration of sensory area of the hand identified with functional MRI (green), subtraction ictal SPECT (single photon emission computed tomography) coregistered to MRI (SISCOM) hyperperfusion focus (red), subdural electrodes (blue), and electrodes where electroencephalograph-detected seizures commenced (yellow). *m*, electrode sites where facial motor activity was elicited with electrocortical stimulation; *s*, electrode site where sensory function was elicited. (From So E. Role of neuroimaging in the management of seizure disorders. *Mayo Clin Proc.* 2002;77:1251–1264, with permission.) Please see color insert.

on the background of the patient's brain MRI (Fig. 86.4). The coregistration makes it possible to study the spatial relationship of the abnormalities to each other, and also to appreciate their relationship to neuroanatomical structures. Computed tomography (CT)- or MRI-derived images of intracranial electrodes also can be registered on the patient's brain MRI. At the conclusion of the prolonged video-EEG monitoring session, the location of the ictal-onset and interictal discharges can be noted on the coregistered intracranial electrodes. Through this method, the irritative and the ictal-onset zones are related topographically to the functional imaging abnormalities. The risk of surgery in compromising eloquent functions of the brain can be inferred by recognizing the underlying and surrounding MRI anatomy, and then confirmed by using the implanted electrodes to electrically stimulate the cortical surface. Allowance must be made for a small, inherent degree of error when coregistering images on the MRI. Therefore, the coregistration technique used must be validated to determine the "worst case" degree of error.

Image-Guided Navigational Surgical Technique

During surgery for nonlesional epilepsy, the surgeon has to be able to determine how the images of different diagnostic modalities correspond to the surgically exposed brain surface. The Stealth Image Guided System can be used to relate the MRI graphic space to the physical space of the operative field (Fig. 86.5). The technology requires the presurgical performance of a frameless stereotactic MRI procedure that registers fiduciary scalp markers into an MRI matrix. After this procedure, the positions of these fiduciary scalp markers are manually registered by an infrared probe into a transformational matrix. With the use of the transformational matrix during surgery, the surgeon can see how a spot on the patient's

exposed brain relates to the location of the functional imaging abnormality on the MRI. This is accomplished by pointing the tip of a probe at the spot of interest on the exposed brain. The tip of the probe is represented by the crosshair cursor on the computer screen that illustrates the MRI containing the functional imaging abnormality. The cursor guides the surgeon's movement of the probe in locating the functional imaging abnormality on the exposed brain surface. This technology makes it possible to locate the functional imaging abnormality on a normal-appearing brain surface. The technology is especially useful when a discrete functional imaging abnormality, such as a SISCOM focus, is the target of electrode implantation. Furthermore, the technique makes it possible to identify the location of the electrode contacts that recorded abnormal EEG activity or critical cortical functions, even when the electrodes have been removed to allow surgical resection or transection of underlying brain tissue.

SUMMARY

Epilepsy surgery in the absence of an MRI lesion presents special challenges in the presurgical identification and the surgical treatment of the epileptogenic focus. Evidence of lateralizing or localizing abnormalities must be sought from noninvasive sources and tests, specifically from the results of clinical, electrophysiologic, neuropsychologic, and functional imaging studies. Careful presurgical evaluation in both intractable temporal and extratemporal nonlesional epilepsy patients can lead to favorable postsurgical outcome similar to that in lesional patients (35). However, the limitations and drawbacks of each noninvasive or minimally invasive modality must be considered. Concordance of the results serves as an important basis for further evaluation with invasive EEG recording, or, in some cases, for obviating the need for invasive recording. The absence of a visible abnormality on the

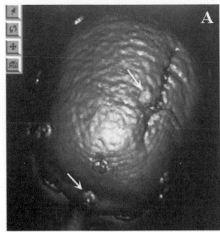

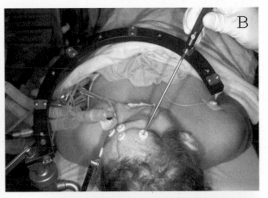

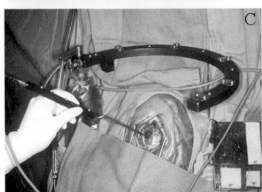

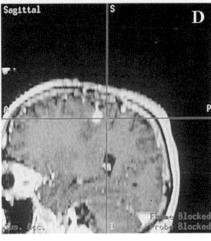

FIGURE 86.5 A: Three-dimensional reconstruction of the patient's head from frameless stereotactic MRI (magnetic resonance imaging) procedure showing scalp fiduciary markers *(lower arrow)* and the surface-rendered subtraction ictal SPECT (single photon emission computed tomography) coregistered to MRI (SISCOM) focus *(upper arrow)*. **B:** Scalp fiduciary markers are then registered into a computer to create a transformational matrix, so that the MRI image space can be related to the physical space of the patient's head. **C:** During surgery, the surgeon uses a probe to point at the location in the operative field. **D:** The surgeon views the computer screen where the crosshairs indicate how close the tip of the probe is to the SISCOM-detected abnormality. This observation is used to guide implantation of intracranial electrodes or surgical resection or transection of the abnormal focus. (Adapted from So E, O'Brien T, Brinkmann B, et al. The EEG evaluation of single photon emission computed tomography: abnormalities in epilepsy. *J Clin Neurophysiol.* 2000; 17:10–28; So E. Integration of EEG, MRI, and SPECT in the evaluation of patients for epilepsy surgery. *Epilepsia.* 2000;41(suppl 3):S48–S54, with permission.)

surgically exposed brain makes it essential to use the technology of image-guided navigational surgery. Patients should understand that the outcome of nonlesional epilepsy surgery is generally not as favorable as that of lesional surgery.

References

1. Von Oertzen J, Urbach H, Jungbluth S, et al. Standard magnetic resonance imaging is inadequate for patients with refractory focal epilepsy. *J Neurol Neurosurg Pyschiatry.* 2002;73:643–647.
2. Jack Jr C, Theodore W, Cook M, et al. MRI-based hippocampal volumetrics: data acquisition, normal ranges, and optimal protocol. *Magn Reson Imaging.* 1995;13:1057–1064.
3. Radhakrishnan K, So E, Silbert P, et al. Predictors of outcome of anterior temporal lobectomy for intractable epilepsy. A multivariate study. *Neurology.* 1998;51:465–471.
4. Vadlamudi L, So E, Worrell G, et al. Factors underlying extracranial interictal epileptiform discharges in intractable frontal lobe epilepsy. *Epileptic Disord.* 2004;6:89–95.
5. Mosewich R, So E, O'Brien T, et al. Factors predictive of the outcome of frontal lobe epilepsy surgery. *Epilepsia.* 2000;41:843–849.
6. Cambier D, Cascino G, So E, et al. Video-EEG monitoring in patients with hippocampal atrophy. *Acta Neurol Scand.* 2001;103:1–7.
7. Sirven J, Liporace J, French J, et al. Seizures in temporal epilepsy: I. Reliability of scalp/sphenoidal ictal reading. *Neurology.* 1997;48: 1041–1046.
8. Walczak T, Radtke R, Lewis D. Accuracy and interobserver reliability of scalp ictal EEG. *Neurology.* 1992;42:2279–2285.
9. Lee S, Yun C, Oh J, et al. Intracranial ictal onset zone in nonlesional lateral temporal lobe epilepsy on scalp ictal EEG. *Neurology.* 2003;61:757–764.
10. Hamer H, Morris H, Mascha E, et al. Complications of invasive video-EEG monitoring with subdural grids. *Neurology.* 2002;58:98–103.
11. Holmes M, Kutsky R, Ojemann G, et al. Interictal, unifocal spikes in refractory extratemporal epilepsy predict ictal origin and postsurgical outcome. *Epilepsy Res.* 2000;111:1802–1808.
12. Worrell G, So E, Kazemi J, et al. Focal ictal beta discharge on scalp EEG predicts excellent outcome of frontal lobe epilepsy surgery. *Epilepsia.* 2002;43:277–282.
13. Knake S, Triantafyllou C, Wald LL, et al. 3T phased array MRI improves the presurgical evaluation in focal epilepsies: a prospective study [see comment]. *Neurology.* 2005;65:1026–1031.
14. Thivard L, Adam C, Hasboun D, et al. Interictal diffusion MRI in partial epilepsies explored with intracerebral electrodes. *Brain.* 2006;129: 375–385.
15. Salmenpera TM, Symms MR, Rugg-Gunn FJ, et al. Evaluation of quantitative magnetic resonance imaging contrasts in MRI-negative refractory focal epilepsy. *Epilepsia.* 2007;48:229–237.
16. Carne RP, O'Brien TJ, Kilpatrick CJ, et al. MRI-negative PET-positive temporal lobe epilepsy: a distinct surgically remediable syndrome. *Brain.* 2004;127:2276–2285.
17. Theodore W, Sato S, Kufta C, et al. Temporal lobectomy for uncontrolled seizures: the role of positron emission tomography. *Ann Neurol.* 1992;32: 789–794.
18. Willmann O, Wennberg R, May T, et al. The contribution of 18F-FDG PET in preoperative epilepsy surgery evaluation for patients with temporal lobe epilepsy: a meta-analysis. *Seizure.* 2007;16:509–520.
19. da Silva E, Chugani D, Muzik O, et al. Identification of frontal lobe epileptic foci in children using positron emission tomography. *Epilepsia.* 1997; 38:1198–1208.
20. Juhasz C, Chugani DC, Muzik O, et al. Alpha-methyl-L-tryptophan PET detects epileptogenic cortex in children with intractable epilepsy. *Neurology.* 2003;60:960–968.
21. O'Brien T, So EL, Mullan BP, et al. Subtraction ictal SPECT co-registered to MRI improves clinical usefulness of SPECT in localizing the surgical seizure focus. *Neurology.* 1998;50:445–454.
22. O'Brien T, So E, Mullan P, et al. Subtraction peri-ictal SPECT is predictive of extratemporal epilepsy surgery outcome. *Neurology.* 2000;55: 1668–1676.
23. Connelly A, Van Paesschen W, Porter D, et al. Proton magnetic resonance spectroscopy in MRI-negative epilepsy. *Neurology.* 1998;51:61–66.
24. Mueller SG, D Laxer K, Barakos JA, et al. Identification of the epileptogenic lobe in neocortical epilepsy with proton MR spectroscopic imaging. *Epilepsia.* 2004;45:1580–1589.
25. Li L, Andermann F, Dubeau F, et al. Spatial extent of neuronal metabolic dysfunction measured by proton MR spectroscopic imaging in patients with localization-related epilepsy. *Epilepsia.* 2000;41:666–674.
26. Incisa della Rochetta A, Gadian D, Conelly A, et al. Verbal memory impairment after right temporal lobe surgery: the role of contralateral damage as revealed by ^{1}H magnetic resonance spectroscopy and T2 relaxometry. *Neurology.* 1995;45:797–802.

27. Moore K, Funke M, Constantino T, et al. Magnetoencephalography directed review of high-spatial resolution surface-coil MR images improves lesion detection in patients with extratemporal epilepsy. *Radiology.* 2002;225:880–887.

28. Leijten F, Huiskamp G.-J.M, Hilgerson I, et al. HIgh-resolution source imaging in mesiotemporal lobe epilepsy: a comparison between MEG and simultaneous EEG. *J Clin Neurophysiol.* 2003;20:227–238.

29. Smith JR, King DW, Park YD, et al. A 10-year experience with magnetic source imaging in the guidance of epilepsy surgery. *Stereotact Funct Neurosurg.* 2003;80:14–17.

30. Knowlton RC, Elgavish R, Howell J, et al. Magnetic source imaging versus intracranial electroencephalogram in epilepsy surgery: a prospective study [see comment]. *Ann Neurol.* 2006;59:835–842.

31. RamachandranNair R, Otsubo H, Shroff MM, et al. MEG predicts outcome following surgery for intractable epilepsy in children with normal or nonfocal MRI findings. *Epilepsia.* 2007;48:149–157.

32. Baumgartner C, Pataraia E, Lindinger G, et al. Neuromagnetic recordings in temporal lobe epilepsy. *J Clin Neurophysiol.* 2000;17:177–189.

33. Knowlton RC, Elgavish RA, Bartolucci A, et al. Functional imaging: II. Prediction of epilepsy surgery outcome. *Ann Neurol.* 2008;64:35–41.

34. Lee SK, Lee SY, Kim K-K, et al. Surgical outcome and prognostic factors of cryptogenic neocortical epilepsy [see comment]. *Ann Neurol.* 2005;58:525–532.

35. Alarcon G, Valentin A, Watt C, et al. Is it worth pursuing surgery for epilepsy in patients with normal neuroimaging? [see comment]. *J Neurol Neurosurg Psychiatry.* 2006;77:474–480.

CHAPTER 87 ■ HYPOTHALAMIC HAMARTOMA

JOHN F. KERRIGAN

Hypothalamic hamartomas (HH) result in a rare but distinctive epilepsy syndrome. Clinical research over the past two decades has led to improved understanding of the complex natural history of this disorder, including the recognition that HH are intrinsically epileptogenic. The last 10 years have also witnessed the emergence of several different therapeutic options, a revolutionary development for what was once considered an untreatable disease. Nevertheless, the availability of these therapies is still under-recognized in the United States and elsewhere around the world. HH is the best human model for subcortical epileptogenesis, and is an excellent clinical model for studying some of the fundamental questions associated with catastrophic epilepsy in children, such as secondary epileptogenesis and epileptic encephalopathy. This chapter will explore this unique form of epilepsy.

HISTORY

Pathological laughter, most likely representative of gelastic (or laughing) seizures, was first described by Trousseau in 1877 (1). In 1950, Martin drew attention to the floor of the third ventricle as a possible site of origin for gelastic seizures (2). List was the first to clearly identify the association between HH and epilepsy in 1958 (3). (An earlier publication in 1934 by Dott describes refractory epilepsy in a patient with what was likely an HH, although described in that autopsy report as an astrocytoma (4).) The syndrome of HH as we now know it, consisting of treatment-resistant gelastic seizures, cognitive impairment, and behavioral disturbance, accompanied by a natural history in which each of these clinical features may worsen, was described by Berkovic et al. in 1988 (5).

Since seizures generally arise from cerebral cortex (including the hippocampus), it was initially assumed that the HH was a marker for epileptogenic abnormalities elsewhere in the brain. However, in 1994, using implanted intracranial electrodes for seizure monitoring, Kahane et al. demonstrated that the ictal discharges associated with gelastic seizures arise within the HH lesion itself (6). A host of subsequent reports have confirmed that the HH is intrinsically epileptogenic, and therefore a suitable target for surgical treatment. However, early efforts with subfrontal or subtemporal surgical resection were disappointing for most patients. The current era of HH treatment was initiated with the innovation of using the transcallosal approach for open surgical resection by Rosenfeld and colleagues in Melbourne in 2001 (7).

CLINICOPATHOLOGIC SUBTYPES AND EPIDEMIOLOGY

HH lesions are associated with two distinct, though overlapping, clinicopathological syndromes (8–12). Pedunculated HH lesions, also referred to as parahypothalamic HH, are associated with central precocious puberty (CPP). These patients usually do not have epilepsy or developmental and behavioral problems. The second subtype, known as sessile (or intrahypothalamic) HH, is associated with gelastic seizures, cognitive impairment, and psychiatric problems. Approximately 40% of these patients will also have CPP.

There are no recognized differences in the histopathology of resected HH tissue between these two subtypes. Rather, the differences are more likely related to the anatomy of HH lesion attachment to the hypothalamus. HH lesions associated with CPP have an attachment to the tuber cinereum, usually with a narrow stalk and base of attachment, while those associated with epilepsy have a more posterior, and broader, base of attachment in the region of the mammillary bodies, or to the walls of the third ventricle. Patients with HH lesions that attach both to the tuber cinereum and the mammillary bodies can be expected to have both epilepsy and CPP. This is more likely to occur with larger HH lesions. This chapter will focus its discussion on HH lesions associated with epilepsy, unless otherwise stated.

HH lesions are rare, but a recent report from Sweden, where nationwide surveys are more readily conducted, showed the prevalence of HH with epilepsy to be 1 in 200,000 children and adolescents (13). There are no known racial or ethnic predilections for HH occurrence, although it may be slightly more common in males.

Most HH lesions are sporadic, and are not associated with other congenital malformations or a positive family history. However, approximately 5% of all HH cases are associated with a dysmorphic syndrome, and the vast majority of these patients have Pallister–Hall syndrome, which includes other malformations such as polydactaly, imperforate anus, and bifid epiglottis (14,15). Additional syndromes in which HH can occur include Waardenburg syndrome (16), oral–facial–digital syndrome (15,17), Bardet–Biedl syndrome (15), and, rarely, neurofibromatosis I (18).

NEUROPATHOLOGY

In comparison to other intrinsically epileptogenic tissues, such as mesial temporal sclerosis within the hippocampus or focal cortical dysplasia of neocortex, HH has a relatively simple histopathology. As a hamartoma, the individual constituent cells appear normal, but cellular relationships and spatial organization are disordered. HH tissue consists of intermixed neurons and glia, although the relative proportion of these differs significantly from case to case (19). A universal feature of all epileptic HH lesions appears to be the tendency of neurons to cluster, although the abundance, size, and cellular density of these clusters also varies significantly (20). The current mechanistic model for HH epileptogenicity hypothesizes that these clusters are the "functional unit" of HH tissue (21).

While the array of HH neuron phenotypes will undoubtedly become more diverse with further investigation, current studies have recognized two types, the small and the large HH neuron. Small HH neurons (generally 8 to 12 μm in diameter) have an interneuron-like phenotype, as they express glutamic acid decarboxylase (GAD), the synthetic enzyme responsible for the presynaptic production of gamma-aminobutyric acid (GABA) (22). These cells are abundant (accounting for approximately 90% of all HH neurons) and have a relatively simple, bipolar morphology (23). Functionally, these neurons also have intrinsic pacemaker-like firing activity with microelectrode recordings of perfused HH tissue slices or acutely dissociated single small HH neurons (22,24).

Large HH neurons (diameter 20 to 30 μm) are less abundant, have a pyramidal appearance more consistent with projection-type neurons, and do not show intrinsic pacemaker-like firing activity. However, they do have the interesting property of depolarizing and firing in response to pharmacological exposure to GABA$_A$-receptor agonists, such as muscimol, in slice preparations obtained from freshly resected HH tissue (25,26). A preliminary model for HH epileptogenesis is presented in Figure 87.1 (21).

ETIOLOGY

As noted above, most HH cases are sporadic, and the underlying cause is unknown. However, HH is a cardinal feature of Pallister–Hall syndrome, which is known to result from haploinsufficiency of *GLI3*, a zinc-finger transcription factor in the sonic hedgehog pathway. Two recent publications have reported that somatic mutations (mutations present in the tumor only) in *GLI3* are associated with HH in approximately 15% of sporadic cases, based upon current genotyping technology (27,28).

Accordingly, while somatic mutations in *GLI3* may be responsible for sporadic HH in some cases, other mutations are also likely to be discovered. At least two other susceptibility loci have been reported, specifically *SOX2* and 6p25.1-25.3, a locus which includes *FOXC1* (29,30). Like *GLI3*, *SOX2* and *FOXC1* are known to be transcription factors that are active during morphogenesis of the ventral forebrain. However, the specific molecular mechanisms controlling cellular proliferation that result in HH are unknown.

CLINICAL FEATURES

In patients with the intrahypothalamic subtype of HH, there is a great deal of variability with respect to the age of onset, severity, and evolution of the neurological symptoms (31). The tremendous clinical diversity from case to case must be kept in mind when evaluating patients with a possible diagnosis of HH. Additionally, these same clinical features, particularly the presence or absence of neurological deterioration and the pace

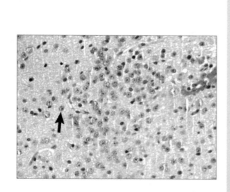
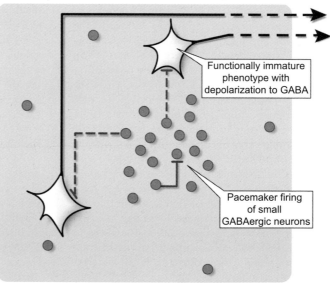

Functionally immature phenotype with depolarization to GABA

Pacemaker firing of small GABAergic neurons

FIGURE 87.1 Preliminary cellular model for HH epileptogenesis based upon laboratory findings derived from surgically resected HH tissue (Refs. 20 and 22–26; reviewed in Ref. 21). A photomicrograph of HH tissue is shown on the left side of the figure (hematoxylin and eosin stain). A small HH neuron (typically 8 to 12 μm in diameter) is indicated by the *arrow*, characterized by the well-defined nuclear membrane and densely staining nucleolus (20). A cluster of small neurons is seen immediately to the right of the *arrow*. The working model for epileptogenesis is shown on the right side of the figure. Small HH neurons tend to occur in clusters (20). They also express glutamic acid decarboxylase, and demonstrate intrinsic, spontaneous pacemaker-like firing activity in microelectrode recordings from freshly resected HH slice preparations (22). Their projections appear to be local, indicated by the solid line connecting two small HH neurons (23). Large HH neurons (typically 20 to 30 μm in diameter) have the morphology of projection neurons, and may express excitatory neurotransmitters (23). These large neurons *depolarize* to GABA agonist administration (25,26). The evidence for structural and functional connections between small and large HH neurons is incomplete, indicated by the use of a *dashed line*. The destination of the axonal projections of large HH neurons is unknown, also indicated by *dashed lines*. We hypothesize that clusters of small spontaneously firing HH neurons are linked in a functional network, resulting in the synchronized release of GABA, which has an excitatory effect on the larger projection neurons (21). (Copyright Barrow Neurological Institute 2009.)

at which it is occurring, affect the decision-making process for deciding the type and timing of therapeutic intervention.

Epilepsy: Gelastic Seizures

Gelastic seizures are the most specific symptom associated with HH. They are usually brief, typically just a few seconds in duration, and usually last less than 30 seconds. They can be very frequent, however, with multiple seizures per hour in more severely affected patients. Gelastic seizures can be associated with little or no change in consciousness, particularly early in the clinical course, although making this determination in infants and young children can be challenging. Superficially resembling laughter, the patients generally do not experience mirth, and most family members can readily distinguish the gelastic seizure from true laughter. Not uncommonly, patients may have clinical events that more closely resemble crying rather than laughing (ictal crying or dacrystic seizures). Gelastic seizures can also be quite subtle. A purely subjective sensation, described as a pressure to laugh, can be described by communicative patients (32). They are commonly mistaken for other conditions, particularly during early infancy, including colic and gastroesophageal reflux disease (GERD) (33).

Gelastic seizures associated with HH usually begin at an early age, and are usually the first seizure type (34). In our experience, the clinical diagnosis is almost always delayed by months or even years. In retrospect, the parents can identify the onset of peculiar laughing spells at a very early age. The mean age of onset for gelastic seizures in our series of HH patients with refractory epilepsy ($n > 130$) is 9 months, and 48% of all patients had onset before 1 month of age. Gelastic seizures become less frequent during the first decade, and may disappear entirely as other seizure types develop (35). Uncommonly, patients with HH may not develop gelastic seizures until early adulthood (36).

The EEG features associated with HH and gelastic seizures deserve emphasis, specifically because ictal recordings, obtained with the conventional placement of electrodes over the scalp, often show no change in the EEG from the ongoing background, which itself is often normal (37–39). Hence, clinicians need to be alert to this fact so as to not miss the correct diagnosis of epileptic seizures. Alternatively, nonlocalizing ictal changes may be observed, such as relative flattening of the EEG background, generalized paroxysmal fast activity, or an absence of interictal spikes (5,31,40).

As we shall see, gelastic seizures do not usually respond to antiepilepsy drugs (AEDs). Consequently, the timing of surgical intervention (here, this term includes gamma knife radiosurgery) is the major decision point facing the patient, family, and clinician. Brief, infrequent gelastic seizures are not disabling. If the child is making good developmental progress, a decision to withhold surgical intervention may be appropriate. However, under these circumstances, the clinical course needs to be observed carefully for any adverse changes in symptoms.

Epilepsy: Other Seizure Types

Over time, 75% of patients with gelastic seizures and HH will develop other types of seizures (34,35). The age at which other seizure types will appear varies, but is most likely to occur

between 4 and 10 years of age (5). Mullati and colleagues have reported two to five seizure types for each patient with childhood onset of epilepsy due to HH (35), and virtually all seizure types have been reported, including infantile spasms accompanied by hypsarrhythmia (41). A review of the published reports regarding lifetime prevalence of seizure types in patients with HH suggests that complex partial seizures occur in 50% to 60% of patients, tonic–clonic seizures in 40% to 60%, atypical absence in 40% to 50%, tonic seizures in 15% to 35%, and "drop attacks" in 30% to 50% (31,34,35,42–44). Seizures associated with HH are usually refractory to management with AEDs (45).

When they occur, complex partial seizures often suggest temporal lobe localization (most frequently) or frontal lobe localization based upon seizure semiology and the results from conventional video-EEG seizure monitoring utilizing scalp electrodes. However, surgical outcomes following temporal lobe or frontal lobe resections in HH patients are universally poor (46).

Freeman and colleagues have reported the presence of a symptomatic generalized epilepsy phenotype in 12 of 20 patients undergoing HH resection (47). Their cohort of patients demonstrated features of Lennox–Gastaut syndrome, including tonic seizures, and slow spike-wave and polyspike activities on interictal EEG. Seizure onset (gelastic seizures were the first seizure type in 92% of these patients) began between birth and 24 months of age (mean 0.3 years), while tonic seizures developed between 2 months and 9 years of age (mean 6 years) (47).

The interictal EEG is frequently normal early in the natural history of epilepsy associated with HH, particularly when gelastic seizures may be the only seizure type (31,34,35). However, the appearance and subsequent evolution of abnormal EEG findings parallels the worsening of the epilepsy with the emergence of multiple seizure types (5,34,35,47). In the review of Tassinari and colleagues, EEG studies in HH patients with multiple seizure types showed normal results in only 2%, generalized spike or spike-wave findings in 47%, multifocal independent spikes in 18%, and focal spikes (most frequently over the temporal regions) in 33% (34). Localization of the epileptic process in HH is complex, as seizures (simple partial, complex partial, or secondarily generalized) can originate within the HH and spread to cortical regions. These seizures may or may not have a clinically apparent gelastic component at the onset.

However, the observed changes in seizure type and the evolution of EEG findings also suggest a process of secondary epileptogenesis, in which distant cortical structures begin to generate seizure events that are independent of the original seizure focus (in this case, the HH lesion) (48–51). Initially, the new focus is dependent upon the presence of the original focus, such that removal of the HH will lead to a decrease in seizure frequency and eventually complete disappearance of seizures arising from the second focus (the "running-down phenomenon") (49). With time, however, usually over a period of years, the second focus becomes entirely independent of the original, inciting focus, such that its removal does not influence the independent epileptogenesis of the second focus. The original concept of secondary epileptogenesis was formulated in the context of temporal lobe epilepsy (52), but epilepsy associated with HH is also consistent with this conceptual model (44).

Indeed, video-EEG recordings with intracranial electrode implantation have demonstrated that seizure activity developing later in the course of the disease may not arise from the

HH lesion (6,47,48,53). Approximately 10% of patients undergoing resective surgery for HH experience the running-down phenomenon, in which seizures of neocortical origin decrease in frequency and eventually stop over a period of weeks or months (54). The running-down phenomenon is observed in 21% to 40% of those HH patients who are ultimately *seizure-free* following surgical resection (at least 1 year of postoperative follow-up) (54,55). Conversely, failure of surgical treatment in HH cases may be attributed to secondary epileptogenesis, as patients with 100% HH lesion resection may continue to have residual seizures in the absence of any other identifiable structural lesion (54).

Although the possibility that there are other cerebral abnormalities must be considered (56,57), most HH patients do not have observable neocortical or hippocampal structural abnormalities by high-resolution magnetic resonance imaging (MRI) (54,58–61). The cellular mechanisms for secondary epileptogenesis and the running-down phenomenon are unknown (51).

Cognition and Development

The clinical course of worsening epilepsy and increasingly abnormal EEG findings can also be accompanied by developmental regression and cognitive decline (5,31,62–65). There is a great deal of individual variability in this regard, but approximately 50% of HH patients with the onset of seizures during infancy will experience this deteriorating clinical course (45). Therefore, the degree of impairment demonstrated by any individual patient is a potentially moving target. There are no published series that document this natural history with longitudinal study of a large cohort of patients, but those detailed individual case reports that are available are compelling (62,66).

Cognitive impairment is common in HH patients, with or without the deterioration noted above, occurring in 80% or more of the patients with the intrahypothalamic subtype of HH (34,42,67). Cognitive problems correlate with the presence of epilepsy as a comorbid feature (patients with parahypothalamic HH lesions typically do not have epilepsy, and also have little or no cognitive impairment). The severity of cognitive impairment and developmental retardation correlates with an earlier age of seizure onset (45), and HH lesion size and subtype (67).

Behavior and Psychiatric Symptoms

Patients with epilepsy and intrahypothalamic HH lesions also show a very high likelihood for serious behavioral and psychiatric problems (5,42,68). These symptoms can be disabling, and often represent the most significant day-to-day problem for the family, in some instances leading to placement out of the home. Mood lability and rage attacks are the most frequent symptoms. Patients can have poor frustration tolerance, with acting-out behavior and excessive reactivity to relatively minor stimuli, sometimes with destructive and aggressive features (69).

There is a strong positive association between the incidence of refractory epilepsy, cognitive impairment, and behavioral disturbance in HH patients (45). There is abundant descriptive literature that worsening seizures, cognitive decline, and behavioral deterioration occur simultaneously (5,62,63,70,71).

HH appears to be an excellent clinical model for epileptic encephalopathy, although the basic mechanisms responsible for this are poorly understood.

TREATMENT

Rationale for the HH as the Therapeutic Target

There is now compelling evidence that gelastic seizures arise from HH tissue (64). This idea was slow to gain acceptance, since localization-related seizures were thought to arise exclusively from cortical structures (72,73). However, Kahane and colleagues reported in 1994 then if ictal video-EEG recordings included intracranial monitoring *with an electrode in the HH*, then the ictal EEG pattern associated with gelastic seizures was initially seen in the HH lesion (6,53). This has subsequently been confirmed by multiple additional reports (48,68,74–76). Electrical stimulation of the electrode contacts within the HH has also provoked the patient's habitual gelastic seizures (48,74,76). Functional imaging with single photon emission computed tomography (SPECT) has demonstrated increased perfusion in the HH with ictal SPECT imaging (74,77), and ictal imaging with flourodeoxyglucose positron emission tomography (FDG-PET) has also shown increased metabolism within the HH lesion (57,78). Perhaps the most important evidence for the intrinsic epileptogenesis of HH lesions are the outcomes observed with surgical resection, in which gelastic seizures can be immediately and completely controlled with surgical removal or disconnection.

Absence of Controlled Treatment Trials

There are no controlled trials investigating treatment issues for HH and epilepsy. Most clinical reports consist of a small number of cases due to the relative rarity of the disease at single centers. However, over the past decade, increasingly large uncontrolled treatment series have been published (54,55,59,61,79–81).

Antiepilepsy Drugs

There is broad consensus in the literature about the lack of efficacy of AEDs (45). It is likely that the number of medication-responsive patients is underestimated due to the ascertainment bias of epilepsy referral centers, and a small number of cases responsive to AEDs have been reported (9,32,78). However, probably <5% of patients with intrahypothalamic HH and epilepsy achieve complete and sustained seizure control with medications alone. AEDs are often reported to have little impact on the frequency of gelastic seizures, but may be valuable for patient management by reducing the frequency of secondary spread from seizures originating within the HH or by controlling seizures originating from cortical regions as a result of secondary epileptogenesis (64). At this time, no AED has emerged as demonstrating superior efficacy for treating epilepsy associated with HH. As a consequence, AEDs are probably best chosen based upon other factors, such as their side-effect profile and ease of administration.

Presurgical Evaluation

Video-EEG seizure monitoring is conventionally used as a component of the evaluation process for epilepsy surgery. However, as the HH lesion is deep in the brain, the results of seizure monitoring with electrode placement over the scalp have limited utility, and these results should be used with *extreme caution* when planning surgical interventions. In general, in HH cases seizure monitoring is more likely to identify patterns of ictal spread, rather than localizing seizure onset. Even for those patients with secondary epileptogenesis, seizure activity arising from the second focus is dependent (for an undetermined time) upon the presence of the HH (see the discussion of the running-down phenomenon). Accordingly, for almost all patients with HH and epilepsy, the HH lesion is the appropriate surgical target.

Invasive seizure monitoring, with electrodes implanted into the HH as well as multiple other brain regions, was necessary to "prove" seizure localization in HH cases. However, this type of implantation is technically challenging, has a low but definite risk of surgical complications, and rarely alters the decision-making process. Accordingly, intracranial monitoring is *not recommended* for most HH patients.

The timing of surgical intervention is influenced by the emergence of multiple seizures types, often accompanied by cognitive and behavioral regression. Neuropsychological testing is recommended at yearly intervals, if possible, to monitor for changes that may not be immediately apparent in the classroom or in the home.

MRI is the most important modality for diagnosis and surgical planning. For HH patients, MRI should include a coronal T2 fast-spin echo (FSE) sequence with thin cuts and no imaging gaps through the hypothalamus. Imaging for HH patients must also include a rigorous visual search to exclude abnormalities elsewhere in the brain.

Surgical Resection/Disconnection

Patients with the parahypothalamic (or pedunculated) subtype of HH usually do not have epilepsy or cognitive disturbance,

and are medically treated with gonadotropin-releasing hormone agonists (such as leuprolide acetate). Accordingly, surgical resection is usually not indicated for this subgroup of HH patients (9,82).

However, some of the early case reports of resective surgery for patients with CPP secondary to HH happened to include children with gelastic seizures, and improvement in seizure control was noted (83,84). Subsequent reports with HH resection specifically for epilepsy indicated encouraging results for seizure control in some patients, and suggested an improved outcome for cognitive and behavioral functioning (65,85,86).

The last decade has seen significant improvements in the operative techniques available for surgical resection and/or disconnection of HH lesions associated with epilepsy, and as well as the emergence of noninvasive measures for ablating HH lesions, such as gamma knife radiosurgery. The relative merits of one treatment approach over another are based upon the individual circumstances of each patient, including the surgical anatomy of the HH. The clinical course for each patient, particularly as it relates to any signs of regression or worsening, also influences the decision to use one treatment modality over another, as well as the timing of intervention.

HH Classification and Surgical Anatomy

When considering the surgical options, the classification of HH lesions must be refined beyond the binary model used thus far, specifically, intrahypothalamic and parahypothalamic HH subtypes. Several authors have proposed classification schemes for HH lesions, including Valdueza et al. (9), Regis et al. (60), and Delalande and Fohlen (79,87). Regardless of the classification system that is used, our experience suggests that there is a relatively smooth continuum between these subtypes. However, while the advantages of one classification scheme over another are debatable, each of these schemes addresses an important issue: the surgical anatomy of the HH lesion. Currently, our preference is to utilize the Delalande classification system (79,87) (Fig. 87.2).

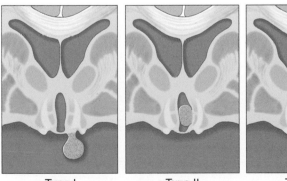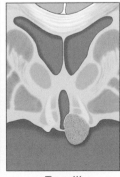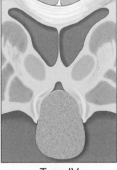

Type I   Type II   Type III   Type IV

FIGURE 87.2 Classification system for HH, proposed by Delalande and Fohlen (87). Type I lesions have a horizontal base of attachment, below the normal position of the floor of the third ventricle. If attached by a narrow stalk to the tuber cinereum, they result in central precocious puberty (CPP), whereas more posterior attachment to the region of the mammillary bodies may result in epilepsy. Larger Type I lesions can result in both CPP and epilepsy. Type II lesions have a vertical plane of attachment to the wall of the third ventricle, completely above the normal position of the floor of the third ventricle. Type III lesions may be unilateral or bilateral, and have a plane of attachment that extends both above and below the floor of the third ventricle. Consequently, these lesions have both vertical and horizontal planes of attachment when viewed on a coronal sequence. Type IV lesions are termed "giant," though features clearly distinguishing them from Type III lesions were not provided (87). We have used a measured volume of 10 cm^3 as our criteria for using the Type IV designation. (Copyright Barrow Neurological Institute 2009.)

Selecting the optimal surgical approach must take into account the location and size of the HH lesion, and most importantly, the anatomy of its base of attachment to the hypothalamus (79,87–90). Type I lesions in the Delalande system are attached to the inferior (horizontal) surface of the hypothalamus. This type includes those HH lesions with a thin peduncle or stalk, often attached to the tuber cinereum, and associated with only with CPP, but can also include HH lesions with a broader or more posterior base of attachment that are associated with epilepsy. These lesions are best resected or disconnected by an inferior or pterional approach. Conversely, Delalande Type II lesions have a vertical plane of attachment within the third ventricle, and are best suited to a superior approach with a transcallosal interforniceal or transventricular endoscopic resection/disconnection. Delalande Types III and IV have both vertical and horizontal planes of attachment (both above and below the normal position of the floor of the third ventricle). The superior approaches noted above may be adequate, but some of these cases may require a combined approach, with either simultaneous or staged resections.

Pterional Approach

Until relatively recently, resective surgery for HH was always performed with a surgical approach from below the lesion. As reported by Nishio et al. (86,91) and Machado et al. (65) in detailed case studies, resection of the HH via a pterional approach had the potential to control seizures and improve the patient's cognitive and behavioral level of functioning. Other surgical approaches for the HH lesion from below have also been reported, including orbitozygomatic (90), subfrontal (68), and lamina terminalis approaches (68). In those instances where a complete resection via a pterional approach is possible, seizure outcomes are good (66% seizure-free with complete resection of the lesion) (45).

However, the pterional approach is not suited to the surgical anatomy of most HH cases, where a substantial component of the HH has a vertical plane of attachment within the third ventricle (Delalande Types II to IV). Additionally, the complication rate, including stroke and cranial nerve injury, was substantial in earlier series (45,68). The advantage of approaching HH lesions from below includes a shorter distance. However, these approaches traverse territory with important vascular structures, including the internal carotid artery, anterior and posterior communicating arteries, and their associated perforating branches. The optic tracts and chiasm, and the third cranial nerve are also vulnerable (88).

Transcallosal Anterior Interforniceal (TAIF) Approach

Although utilized previously for other pathologies (92), Rosenfeld and colleagues in Melbourne, Australia were the first to utilize the transcallosal anterior interforniceal (TAIF) approach to the third ventricle to resect HH lesions in patients with refractory epilepsy (7,89). This approach, utilizing microsurgical technique and intracranial guidance systems, allows for excellent direct visualization of the HH and its base of attachment within the third ventricle. Rosenfeld's modification of the transcallosal approach to the third ventricle, with a more anterior, transseptal trajectory, minimizes retraction of the columns of the fornix, and also avoids injury to the internal cerebral veins, located more posteriorly (89).

The Melbourne group has published a series of 29 consecutive patients undergoing intrahypothalamic HH resection via the TAIF approach (55). Age at surgery ranged from 4 to 23 years (mean age 10 years). All patients had multiple seizure types, including gelastic seizures. Coexisting morbidities included a history of CPP in 13 (45%), intellectual disability in 21 (72%), and behavioral problems, most frequently rage and aggression, in 18 (62%).

At least 95% resection of HH lesion volume was achieved in 18 patients (62%). Postoperative follow-up for a minimum of 12 months showed 15 patients (52%) who were completely seizure-free and 7 patients (24%) with at least a 90% improvement in seizure frequency. Surgical resection was generally well tolerated. Small, unilateral ischemic strokes of the thalamus and internal capsule occurred in two cases (7%), both with complete recovery, and transient third cranial nerve injury was reported in one patient. The majority of patients (55%) developed mild, asymptomatic hypernatremia postoperatively, but no patients had persistent disturbances in fluid or electrolyte homeostasis. Five patients (17%) required thyroid hormone replacement therapy following surgery. Increased appetite with weight gain was reported in 45% of patients, but resolved in half of these with time.

Impairment of short-term memory was, however, a significant issue. The TAIF surgical approach, despite its more anterior trajectory, requires retraction of the columns of the fornix. Transient memory disturbance was noted in 14 patients (48%) during the immediate postoperative period, but residual difficulties were reported by only four (14%). Attention and behavior were noted to improve in many of the patients in this series, but further details were not available (55).

Remarkably similar results were subsequently reported by Rekate and colleagues at the Barrow Neurological Institute in Phoenix (54). In this series of 26 consecutive patients undergoing TAIF, 54% were completely seizure-free. The likelihood of complete seizure freedom (with at least 1 year of postoperative follow-up) had a positive correlation with the percentage of HH lesion volume that was successfully resected ($P < 0.05$). The risk and type of surgical complications were also similar. Notably, transient short-term memory impairment was noted in 58% of the patients, but persisted in only two patients (8%).

The impact on memory, cognition, and behavior resulting from TAIF HH resection/disconnection requires further study. Based upon postoperative interviews with the patients and their families 1 year after surgery, subjective improvement in cognition (65% of patients) and behavior (88%) were reported (54). However, neuropsychological studies comparing pre- and postoperative functioning have not yet been published.

Transventricular Endoscopic (TE) Approach

Transcortical transventricular endoscopic (TE) resection and/or disconnection has also been recently developed as a treatment option for HH patients with refractory epilepsy (59,68,79,87,93–97). Barrow has reported their series of 37 consecutive HH patients treated with endoscopic resection/disconnection for treatment-resistant seizures (59). All patients had at least 1 year of follow-up. The mean age at the time of surgery was 11.8 years (range 0.7 to 55 years). All patients had a history of gelastic seizures at some time point during their clinical course, and 29 (78%) had active gelastic seizures at the time of surgery. Twenty-eight patients (76%) had Type II HH lesions by the Delalande classification, and the median lesion volume was 1.0 cm^3. (In comparison, in the Barrow series of transcallosal resections noted above, 42% had a Type II lesion, and the median HH lesion volume was 2.4 cm^3, reflecting the different selection criteria for each approach (54).)

Median follow-up was at 21 months. Eighteen patients (49%) were completely seizure-free, while seizure frequency was reduced at least 90% in an additional eight patients (22%). Twelve patients were determined to have 100% of their HH lesions resected. Of these, eight (67%) were 100% seizure-free (59).

As observed with the TAIF approach, most patients tolerated endoscopic resection well. However, some differences from the TAIF approach were observed, with a significantly shorter total length of hospital stay in the endoscopic group (mean 4.1 days) versus the previously reported transcallosal group (mean 7.7 days, $P < 0.001$) (54,59). Only five patients (14%) experienced postoperative short-term memory loss, but this appeared to be a permanent residual problem (by history) in three (8%), which is comparable to the TAIF approach. No patients with endocrine disturbance, either transient or permanent, were observed. However, 11 patients (30%) showed small unilateral thalamic infarcts on diffusion-weighted MRI sequences. These were entirely asymptomatic in 9 of 11 cases, and the remaining two made a complete clinical recovery. These infarcts were attributed to disruption or injury to small thalamic perforators as a result of local brain movement with excursions of the endoscope.

For those HH patients who require surgical resection/disconnection from above, the factors that favor the endoscopic approach include smaller lesions with unilateral attachment to the wall of the third ventricle, adequate space within the third ventricle to manipulate the endoscope, and adequate size of the lateral ventricle and foramina of Monro for safe instrumentation. Factors which are more favorable for the TAIF approach include a younger age at the time of surgery (the columns of the fornix and leaves of the septum tend to fuse with age), larger lesions, and bilateral attachment.

Gamma Knife Radiosurgery

Gamma knife (GK) radiosurgery has also been investigated as an ablative or destructive therapy for HH lesions (53,80,93,98–104). GK is noninvasive, and can deliver a "killing" dose of radiation to a small volume of tissue via a large number of independent trajectories, with little or no injury to surrounding brain.

Regis et al. have described a series of 27 patients with intractable epilepsy and HH with at least three years of follow-up after GK therapy (105). GK delivers its maximal destructive energy to the interior of the targeted lesion, and the intensity of energy delivery falls off toward the periphery of the lesion. A dose of at least 17 Gy is ideally delivered to the entire lesion. The peripheral treatment margin (usually referred to as the 50% isodose margin) is matched to the outer edge of the HH lesion, but may need to be modified due to the proximity of the optic tracts or other radiosensitive structures.

A maximal threshold of 10 Gy to the optic tracts and 8 Gy to the optic chiasm and optic nerve were utilized for treatment planning for this prospective treatment study (105). In this series, the median HH diameter was 0.95 cm (range 0.5 to 2.6 cm) and the median volume of the marginal isodose was 0.65 cm^3 (range 0.13 to 2.67 cm^3). The median radiosurgery dose to the 50% isodose margin was 17 Gy (range 13 to 26 Gy, mean 16.9 Gy). Of the 27 patients reported, 10 (37%) were completely seizure-free and an additional 6 (22%) were substantially improved with only rare gelastic seizures (105).

Efficacy is delayed from the time of GK treatment. Changes in the frequency of seizures following GK can be anticipated, although variability from patient to patient should also be expected. Initially after treatment, seizure frequency may be improved, or patients may continue to have seizures at their preintervention baseline. Several months following therapy, an increase in seizure frequency, sometimes lasting for only a few days, may be observed. Subsequent to this, patients responding to treatment will experience progressively fewer seizures, with complete seizure control after a period of 6 to 24 months. Regis and colleagues recommend waiting 36 months from the time of treatment to assess final efficacy.

GK has an excellent adverse event profile. Most patients have no complications or side effects attributable to GK treatment. No patients among the 27 treated were reported to have a permanent complication (105). Three patients (11%) experienced transient poikilothermia. In contrast to side effects that may be seen with resective surgery, there were no patients in this series that experienced weight gain, endocrine disturbance, adverse changes in cognition or short-term memory complaints. The disadvantage of GK is the delayed onset of action for controlling seizures and the more limited anatomical spectrum of HH lesions to which it is suited.

GK is an important treatment option for many patients with HH and epilepsy, and should be the preferred treatment modality for smaller lesions, particularly for patients who are clinically stable and capable of tolerating the delay in efficacy to obtain improved seizure control. It is a less desirable approach for those patients who are progressively worsening with their epilepsy, or experiencing cognitive decline or behavioral deterioration with uncontrolled seizures. Additional study to define the optimal role of GK compared to other treatment modalities is required.

Stereotactic Thermoablation

Radiofrequency thermoablation has been described in a relatively small number of patients (36,74,76,106–109). This technique involves stereotactic placement of a depth wire into the HH target, then causing a destructive thermal lesion by physically heating the probe tip. Most of these publications are single case reports.

Kuzniecky reported a series of 12 patients treated with this modality, eight with stereotactic thermoablation alone and four with endoscopic resection followed by thermoablation (74). In the first group of eight, three (38%) were seizure-free and two (25%) were at least 90% improved with regard to seizure frequency. One patient developed transient third-nerve palsy. In the second group of four, two patients are seizure-free and one was improved at least 90% for seizure frequency. There was one death due to brainstem infarction, and one patient had transient difficulties with short-term memory.

Interstitial Radiosurgery

Interstitial radiosurgery with stereotactic implantation of ^{125}I radioactive seeds has also been proposed as an ablative therapy for HH associated with epilepsy (61,110). Schulze-Bonhage and colleagues in Freiburg, Germany, have reported a series of 24 patients (mean age 21.9 years), all of whom had

treatment-resistant gelastic seizures, in addition to other seizure types (110). Mean HH lesion volume was 1.2 cm³.

The treatment plan was designed to deliver a dose of 60 Gy at the outer margin of the HH, followed by radioisotope seed removal. Thirteen of 24 patients (54%) required at least one reimplantation for a second course of therapy if the response to the initial course was unsatisfactory. With follow-up of at least 2 years, 12.5% were seizure-free (Engel IA outcome) while 41.7% had at least a 90% improvement in seizure frequency (110). Treatment response is described as occurring within 8 weeks following treatment. No complications were noted, but follow-up MRI 3 months after treatment revealed local

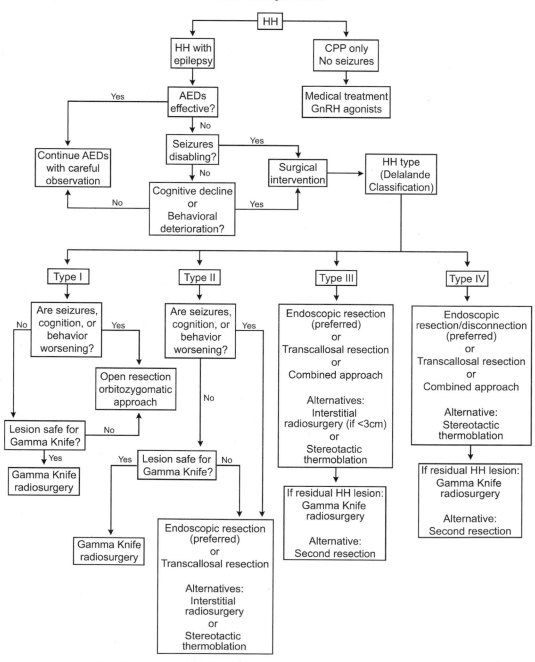

FIGURE 87.3 Suggested treatment algorithm for HH patients with treatment-resistant epilepsy. This approach is based upon the patient care experience at the Barrow Neurological Institute in Phoenix, Arizona (>130 treated HH patients since February 2003). This algorithm is meant to provide a frame of reference for the clinician and researcher. None of the options presented here are supported by randomized, controlled trials.

cerebral edema in five of 23 patients (22%), in some instances associated with headache and fatigue. Neuropsychological testing prior to implantation and at least 1 year following treatment showed no significant group differences with interstitial radiosurgery intervention (110).

Alternative Therapies

A limited number of HH patients were treated with alternative therapies such as the ketogenic diet (KD) (71), vagus nerve stimulation (VNS) (13,111), corpus callosotomy (46,66,112), and deep brain electrical stimulation (DBS) (48,66,113,114). With the possible exception of corpus callosotomy, the use of which should be discouraged in this patient population based upon universally unsatisfactory published reports, the other alternative therapies should be regarded as unproven therapeutic options (KD and VNS), or investigational treatment (DBS).

CONCLUSION

There has been tremendous progress in our understanding of HH over the past 15 years. Although uncommon, the intrahypothalamic subtype of HH can present with catastrophic epilepsy of early childhood. Many of these patients will experience a deteriorating course with worsening of seizures, cognitive functioning, and behavior. We now know that the HH itself is intrinsically epileptogenic and surgically treatable. A number of different therapeutic options are now available. While comparative trials have not been performed, it seems increasingly clear that no one treatment modality is appropriate for all HH patients. At our center, we utilize surgical resection/disconnection by TAIF, endoscopic and pterional approaches, and GK as treatments of first choice. The therapy selection is based upon the individual circumstances of each patient, and each option is discussed with the family. The most important factors for consideration include the stability of the patient (seizure severity and the presence or absence of clinical deterioration) and the surgical anatomy of the patient's HH lesion. A proposed treatment algorithm, based upon our experience over the past 6 years, is presented in Figure 87.3.

References

1. Trousseau A. De l'epilepsie. In: Michel Peter M, ed. *Clinique Medicale de l'Hotel-Dieu de Paris*. Paris: Librairie J. B. Bailliere; 1877.
2. Martin JP. Fits of laughter (sham mirth) in organic cerebral disease. *Brain*. 1950;73:453–464.
3. List CF, Dowman CE, Bagchi BK, et al. Posterior hypothalamic hamartomas and gangliogliomas causing precocious puberty. *Neurology*. 1958;8:164–174.
4. Dott NM. Surgical aspects of the hypothalamus. In: Le Gros Clark WE, Beattie J, Riddoch G, Dott NM, eds. *The Hypothalamus: Morphological, Functional, Clinical and Surgical Aspects*. Edinburgh: Oliver and Boyd; 1938:131–185.
5. Berkovic SF, Andermann F, Melanson D, et al. Hypothalamic hamartomas and ictal laughter: evolution of a characteristic epileptic syndrome and diagnostic value of magnetic resonance imaging. *Ann Neurol*. 1988;23:429–439.
6. Kahane P, Tassi L, Hoffmann D, et al. Crises dacrystiques et hamartome hypothalamique. A propos d'une observation video-stereo-EEG. *Epilepsia*. 1994;6:259–279.
7. Rosenfeld JV, Harvey AS, Wrennall J, et al. Transcallosal resection of hypothalamic hamartomas, with control of seizures, in children with gelastic epilepsy. *Neurosurgery*. 2001;48:108–118.
8. Boyko OB, Curnes JT, Oakes WJ, et al. Hamartomas of the tuber cinereum: CT, MR, and pathologic findings. *Am J Neuroradiol*. 1991;12:309–314.
9. Valdueza JM, Cristante L, Dammann O, et al. Hypothalamic hamartomas: with special reference to gelastic epilepsy and surgery. *Neurosurgery*. 1994;34:949–958.
10. Arita K, Ikawa F, Kurisu K, et al. The relationship between magnetic resonance imaging findings and clinical manifestations of hypothalamic hamartoma. *J Neurosurg*. 1999;91:212–220.
11. Debeneix C, Bourgeois M, Trivin C, et al. Hypothalamic hamartoma: comparison of clinical presentation and magnetic resonance images. *Horm Res*. 2001;56:12–18.
12. Jung H, Probst EN, Hauffa BP, et al. Association of morphological characteristics with precocious puberty and/or gelastic seizures in hypothalamic hamartoma. *J Clin Endocrinol Metab*. 2003;88:4590–4595.
13. Brandberg G, Raininko R, Eeg-Olofsson O. Hypothalamic hamartoma with gelastic seizures in Swedish children and adolescents. *Eur J Paediatr Neurol*. 2004;6:35–44.
14. Biesecker LG, Abbott M, Allen J, et al. Report from the workshop on Pallister–Hall syndrome and related phenotypes. *Am J Med Genet*. 1996;65:76–81.
15. Biesecker LG. Heritable syndromes with hypothalamic hamartoma and seizures: using rare syndromes to understand more common disorders. *Epileptic Disord*. 2003;5:235–238.
16. Sener RN. Cranial MR imaging findings in Waardenburg syndrome: anophthalmia, and hypothalamic hamartoma. *Comput Med Imaging Graph*. 1998;22:409–411.
17. Stephan MJ, Brooks KL, Moore DC, et al. Hypothalamic hamartoma in oral-facial-digital syndrome type VI (Varadi syndrome). *Am J Med Genet*. 1994;51:131–136.
18. Leal AJR, Passao V, Calado E, et al. Interictal spike EEG source analysis in hypothalamic hamartoma epilepsy. *Clin Neurophysiol*. 2002;113:1961–1969.
19. Amstutz DR, Coons SW, Kerrigan JF, et al. Hypothalamic hamartomas: correlation of MR imaging and spectroscopic findings with tumor glial content. *Am J Neuroradiol*. 2006;27:794–798.
20. Coons SW, Rekate HL, Prenger EC, et al. The histopathology of hypothalamic hamartomas: study of 57 cases. *J Neuropathol Exp Neurol*. 2007;66:131–141.
21. Fenoglio KA, Wu J, Kim DY, et al. Hypothalamic hamartoma: basic mechanisms of intrinsic epileptogenesis. *Semin Pediatr Neurol*. 2007;14:51–59.
22. Wu J, Xu L, Kim DY, et al. Electrophysiological properties of human hypothalamic hamartomas. *Ann Neurol*. 2005;58:371–382.
23. Beggs J, Nakada S, Fenoglio K, et al. Hypothalamic hamartomas associated with epilepsy: ultrastructural features. *J Neuropathol Exp Neurol*. 2008;67:657–668.
24. Wu J, Chang Y, Li G, et al. Electrophysiological properties and subunit composition of GABA$_A$ receptors in patients with gelastic seizures and hypothalamic hamartoma. *J Neurophysiol*. 2007;98:5–15.
25. Kim DY, Fenoglio KA, Simeone TA, et al. GABA$_A$ receptor-mediated activation of L-type calcium channels induces neuronal excitation in surgically resected human hypothalamic hamartomas. *Epilepsia*. 2008;49:861–871.
26. Wu J, DeChon J, Xue F, et al. GABA$_A$ receptor-mediated excitation in dissociated neurons from human hypothalamic hamartomas. *Exp Neurol*. 2008;213:397–404.
27. Craig DW, Itty A, Panganiban C, et al. Identification of somatic chromosomal abnormalities in hypothalamic hamartoma tissue at the GLI3 locus. *Am J Hum Genet*. 2008;82:366–374.
28. Wallace RH, Freeman JL, Shouri MR, et al. Somatic mutations in GLI3 can cause hypothalamic hamartoma and gelastic seizures. *Neurology*. 2008;70:653–655.
29. Kelberman D, Rizzoti K, Avilion A, et al. Mutations within *Sox2/SOX2* are associated with abnormalities in the hypothalamo-pituitary-gonadal axis in mice and humans. *J Clin Invest*. 2006;116:2442–2455.
30. Kerrigan JF, Kruer MC, Corneveaux J, et al. Chromosomal abnormality at 6p25.1-25.3 identifies a susceptibility locus for hypothalamic hamartoma associated with epilepsy. *Epilepsy Res*. 2007;55:70–73.
31. Arzimanoglou AA, Hirsch E, Aicardi J. Hypothalamic hamartoma and epilepsy in children: illustrative cases of possible evolutions. *Epileptic Disord*. 2003;5:187–199.
32. Sturm JW, Andermann F, Berkovic SF. "Pressure to laugh": an unusual epileptic syndrome associated with small hypothalamic hamartomas. *Neurology*. 2000;54:971–973.
33. Sweetman LL, Ng Y-t, Kerrigan JF. Gelastic seizures misdiagnosed as gastro esophageal reflux disease. *Clin Pediatr (Phila)*. 2007;46:325–328.
34. Tassinari CA, Riguzzi P, Rizzi R, et al. Gelastic seizures. In: Tuxhorn I, Holthausen H, Boenigk K, eds. *Paediatric Epilepsy Syndromes and Their Surgical Treatment*. London: John Libbey; 1997:429–446.
35. Mullati N, Selway R, Nashef L, et al. The clinical spectrum of epilepsy in children and adults with hypothalamic hamartoma. *Epilepsia*. 2003;44:1310–1319.
36. Mullatti N. Hypothalamic hamartoma in adults. *Epileptic Disord*. 2003;5:201–204.

37. Sher PK, Brown SB. Gelastic epilepsy: onset in neonatal period. *Am J Dis Child.* 1976;130:1126–1131.
38. Castro LH, Ferreira LK, Teles LR, et al. Epilepsy syndromes associated with hypothalamic hamartoma. *Seizure.* 2007;16:50–58.
39. Garcia-Morales I, Marinas A, del Barrio A, et al. Hypothalamic hamartoma: clinical characteristics. Electroencephalogram and brain magnetic resonance imaging in 10 patients. *Neurologia.* 2007;22:11–18.
40. Striano S, Striano P, Sarappa C, et al. The clinical spectrum and natural history of gelastic epilepsy-hypothalamic hamartoma syndrome. *Seizure.* 2005;14:232–239.
41. Kerrigan JF, Ng Y-t, Prenger E, et al. Hypothalamic hamartoma and infantile spasms. *Epilepsia.* 2007;48:89–95.
42. Frattali CM, Liow K, Craig GH, et al. Cognitive deficits in children with gelastic seizures and hypothalamic hamartoma. *Neurology.* 2001;57:43–46.
43. Leal AJR, Moreira A, Robalo C, et al. Different electroclinical manifestations of the epilepsy associated with hamartomas connecting to the middle or posterior hypothalamus. *Epilepsia.* 2003;44:1191–1195.
44. Kerrigan JF, Ng Y-t, Chung SS, et al. The hypothalamic hamartoma: a model of subcortical epileptogenesis and encephalopathy. *Semin Pediatr Neurol.* 2005;12(2):119–131.
45. Nguyen D, Singh S, Zaatreh M, et al. Hypothalamic hamartomas: seven cases and review of the literature. *Epilepsy Behav.* 2003;4:246–258.
46. Cascino GD, Andermann F, Berkovic SF, et al. Gelastic seizures and hypothalamic hamartomas: evaluation of patients undergoing chronic intracranial EEG monitoring and outcome of surgical treatment. *Neurology.* 1993;43:747–750.
47. Freeman JL, Harvey AS, Rosenfeld JV, et al. Generalized epilepsy in hypothalamic hamartoma: evolution and postoperative resolution. *Neurology.* 2003;60:762–767.
48. Kahane P, Ryvlin P, Hoffmann D, et al. From hypothalamic hamartoma to cortex: what can be learnt *(sic)* from depth recordings and stimulation. *Epileptic Disord.* 2003;5:205–217.
49. Morrell F. Secondary epileptogenesis in man. *Arch Neurol.* 1985;42:318–335.
50. Cibula JE, Gilmore RL. Secondary epileptogenesis in humans. *J Clin Neurophysiol.* 1997;14:111–127.
51. Dudek FE, Spitz M. Hypothetical mechanisms for the cellular and neurophysiologic basis of secondary epileptogenesis: proposed role of synaptic reorganization. *J Clin Neurophysiol.* 1997;14:90–101.
52. Wilder BJ. The mirror focus and secondary epileptogenesis. *Int Rev Neurobiol.* 2001;45:435–446.
53. Munari C, Kahane P, Francione S, et al. Role of the hypothalamic hamartoma in the genesis of gelastic fits (a video-stereo-EEG study). *Electroencephalogr Clin Neurophysiol.* 1995;95:154–160.
54. Ng Y-t, Rekate HL, Prenger EC, et al. Transcallosal resection of hypothalamic hamartoma for intractable epilepsy. *Epilepsia.* 2006;47:1192–1202.
55. Harvey AS, Freeman JL, Berkovic SF, et al. Transcallosal resection of hypothalamic hamartomas in patients with intractable epilepsy. *Epileptic Disord.* 2003;5:257–265.
56. Sisodiya SM, Free SL, Stevens JM, et al. Widespread cerebral structural changes in two patients with gelastic seizures and hypothalamic hamartomata. *Epilepsia.* 1997;38:1008–1010.
57. Palmini A, Van Paesschen W, Dupont P, et al. Status gelasticus after temporal lobectomy: ictal FDG-PET findings and the question of dual pathology involving hypothalamic hamartomas. *Epilepsia.* 2005;46:1313–1316.
58. Freeman JL, Coleman LT, Wellard RM, et al. MR imaging and spectroscopic study of epileptogenic hypothalamic hamartomas: analysis of 72 cases. *Am J Neuroradiol.* 2004;25:450–462.
59. Ng Y-t, Rekate HL, Prenger EC, et al. Endoscopic resection of hypothalamic hamartomas for refractory symptomatic epilepsy. *Neurology.* 2008;70:1543–1548.
60. Regis J, Hayashi M, Eupierre LP, et al. Gamma knife surgery for epilepsy related to hypothalamic hamartoma. *Acta Neurochir Suppl.* 2004;91:33–50.
61. Schulze-Bonhage A, Homberg V, Trippel M, et al. Interstitial radiosurgery in the treatment of gelastic epilepsy due to hypothalamic hamartomas. *Neurology.* 2004;62:644–647.
62. Deonna T, Ziegler A-L. Hypothalamic hamartoma, precocious puberty and gelastic seizures: a special model of "epileptic" developmental disorder. *Epileptic Disord.* 2000;2:33–37.
63. Berkovic SF, Kuzniecky RI, Andermann F. Human epileptogenesis and hypothalamic hamartomas: new lessons from an experiment of nature. *Epilepsia.* 1997;38:1–3.
64. Berkovic SF, Arzimanoglou A, Kuzniecky R, et al. Hypothalamic hamartoma and seizures: a treatable epileptic encephalopathy. *Epilepsia.* 2003;44:969–973.
65. Machado HR, Hoffman HJ, Hwang PA. Gelastic seizures treated by resection of a hypothalamic hamartoma. *Childs Nerv Syst.* 1991;7:462–465.
66. Savard G, Bhanji NH, Dubeau F, et al. Psychiatric aspects of patients with hypothalamic hamartoma and epilepsy. *Epileptic Disord.* 2003;5:229–234.
67. Prigatano GP, Wethe JV, Gray JA, et al. Intellectual functioning in presurgical patients with hypothalamic hamartoma and refractory epilepsy. *Epilepsy Behav.* 2008;13:149–155.
68. Palmini A, Chandler C, Andermann F, et al. Resection of the lesion in patients with hypothalamic hamartoma and catastrophic epilepsy. *Neurology.* 2002;58:1338–1347.
69. Weissenberger AA, Dell ML, Liow K, et al. Aggression and psychiatric comorbidity in children with hypothalamic hamartomas and their unaffected siblings. *J Am Acad Child Adolesc Psychiatry.* 2001;40:696–703.
70. Andermann F, Arzimanoglou A, Berkovic SF. Hypothalamic hamartoma and epilepsy: the pathway of discovery. *Epileptic Disord.* 2003;5:173–175.
71. Palmini A, Paglioli-Neto E, Montes J, et al. The treatment of patients with hypothalamic hamartomas, epilepsy and behavioural abnormalities: facts and hypotheses. *Epileptic Disord.* 2003;5:249–255.
72. Breningstall GN. Gelastic seizures, precocious puberty, and hypothalamic hamartoma. *Neurology.* 1985;35:1180–1183.
73. Breningstall GN. Gelastic seizures, precocious puberty, and hypothalamic hamartoma. Reply to Letter. *Neurology.* 1986;36:444.
74. Kuzniecky R, Guthrie B, Mountz J, et al. Intrinsic epileptogenesis of hypothalamic hamartomas in gelastic epilepsy. *Ann Neurol.* 1997;42:60–67.
75. Tasch E, Cendes F, Li LM, et al. Hypothalamic hamartomas and gelastic epilepsy: a spectroscopic study. *Neurology.* 1998;51:1046–1050.
76. Fukuda M, Kaeyama S, Wachi M, et al. Stereotaxy for hypothalamic hamartoma with intractable gelastic seizures. Technical case report. *Neurosurgery.* 1999;44:1347–1350.
77. Arroyo S, Santamaria J, Sanmarti F, et al. Ictal laughter associated with paroxysmal hypothalamopituitary dysfunction. *Epilepsia.* 1997;38:114–117.
78. Shahar E, Kramer U, Mahajnah M, et al. Pediatric-onset gelastic seizures: clinical data and outcome. *Pediatr Neurol.* 2007;37:29–34.
79. Fohlen M, Lellouch A, Delalande O. Hypothalamic hamartoma with refractory epilepsy: surgical procedures and results in 18 patients. *Epileptic Disord.* 2003;5:267–273.
80. Regis J, Bartolomei F, de Toffol B, et al. Gamma knife surgery for epilepsy related to hypothalamic hamartomas. *Neurosurgery.* 2000;47:1343–1352.
81. Kuzniecky RI, Guthrie BL. Stereotactic surgical approach to hypothalamic hamartomas. *Epileptic Disord.* 2003;5:275–280.
82. Mahachoklertwattana P, Kaplan SL, Grumbach MM. The luteinizing hormone-releasing hormone-secreting hypothalamic hamartoma is a congenital malformation: natural history. *J Clin Endocrinol Metab.* 1993;77:118–124.
83. Northfield DW, Russell DS. Pubertas praecox due to hypothalamic hamartoma: report of two cases surviving surgical removal of the tumour. *J Neurol Neurosurg Psychiatry.* 1967;30:166–173.
84. Takeuchi J, Handa H, Miki Y, et al. Precocious puberty due to a hypothalamic hamartoma. *Surg Neurol.* 1979;11:456–460.
85. Sato M, Ushio Y, Arita N, et al. Hypothalamic hamartoma: report of two cases. *Neurosurgery.* 1985;16:198–206.
86. Nishio S, Morioko T, Fukui M, et al. Surgical treatment of intractable seizures due to hypothalamic hamartoma. *Epilepsia.* 1994;35:514–519.
87. Delalande O, Fohlen M. Disconnecting surgical treatment of hypothalamic hamartoma in children and adults with refractory epilepsy and proposal of a new classification. *Neurol Med Chir (Tokyo).* 2003;43:61–68.
88. Polkey CE. Resective surgery for hypothalamic hamartoma. *Epileptic Disord.* 2003;5:281–286.
89. Rosenfeld JV, Freeman JL, Harvey AS. Operative technique: the anterior transcallosal transeptal interforniceal approach to the third ventricle and resection of hypothalamic hamartomas. *J Clin Neurosci.* 2004;11:738–744.
90. Feiz-Erfan I, Horn EM, Rekate HL, et al. Surgical strategies to approach hypothalamic hamartomas causing gelastic seizures in the pediatric population: transventricular versus skull base approaches. *J Neurosurg Pediatr.* 2005;103:325–332.
91. Nishio S, Fujiwara S, Aiko Y, et al. Hypothalamic hamartoma. Report of two cases. *J Neurosurg.* 1989;70:640–645.
92. Apuzzo ML, Chikovani OK, Gott PS, et al. Transcallosal, interfornicial approaches for lesions affecting the third ventricle: surgical considerations and consequences. *Neurosurgery.* 1982;10:547–554.
93. Akai T, Okamoto K, Iizuka H, et al. Treatments of hamartoma with neuroendoscopic surgery and stereotactic radiosurgery: a case report. *Minim Invasive Neurosurg.* 2002;45:235–239.
94. Choi JU, Yang KH, Kim TG, et al. Endoscopic disconnection for hypothalamic hamartoma with intractable seizure. Report of four cases. *J Neurosurg.* 2004;100(5 suppl Pediatrics):506–511.
95. Rekate HL, Feiz-Erfan I, Ng Y-t, et al. Endoscopic surgery for hypothalamic hamartomas causing medically refractory gelastic epilepsy. *Childs Nerv Syst.* 2006;22:874–880.
96. Procaccini E, Dorfmuller G, Fohlen M, et al. Surgical management of hypothalamic hamartomas with epilepsy: the stereoendoscopic approach. *Neurosurgery.* 2006;59(ONS Suppl 4):ONS336–ONS346.
97. Shim KW, Chang JH, Park YG, et al. Treatment modality for intractable epilepsy in hypothalamic hamartomatous lesions. *Neurosurg.* 2008;62:847–856.
98. Arita K, Kurisu K, Iida K, et al. Subsidence of seizure induced by stereotactic radiation in a patient with hypothalamic hamartoma. Case report. *J Neurosurg.* 1998;89:645–648.

99. Unger F, Schrottner O, Haselberger K, et al. Gamma knife radiosurgery for hypothalamic hamartomas in patients with medically intractable epilepsy and precocious puberty. Report of two cases. *J Neurosurg.* 2000;92:726–731.

100. Dunoyer C, Ragheb J, Resnick T, et al. The use of radiosurgery to treat intractable childhood partial epilepsy. *Epilepsia.* 2002;43:292–300.

101. Regis J, Scavarda D, Tamura M, et al. Gamma knife surgery for epilepsy related to hypothalamic hamartoma. *Semin Pediatr Neurol.* 2007;14: 73–79.

102. Barajas MA, Ramirez-Guzman MG, Rodriguez-Vazquez C, et al. Gamma knife surgery for hypothalamic hamartomas accompanied by medically intractable epilepsy and precocious puberty: experience in Mexico. *J Neurosurg.* 2005;102(suppl):53–55.

103. Mathieu D, Kondziolka D, Niranjan A, et al. Gamma knife radiosurgery for refractory epilepsy caused by hypothalamic hamartomas. *Stereotact Funct Neurosurg.* 2006;84:82–87.

104. Romanelli P, Muacevic A, Striano S. Radiosurgery for hypothalamic hamartomas. *Neurosurg Focus.* 2008;24:e9 (1–7).

105. Regis J, Scavarda D, Tamura M, et al. Epilepsy related to hypothalamic hamartomas: surgical management with special reference to gamma knife surgery. *Childs Nerv Syst.* 2006;22:881–895.

106. Parrent AG. Stereotactic radiofrequency ablation for the treatment of gelastic seizures associated with hypothalamic hamartoma. Case report. *J Neurosurg.* 1999;91:881–884.

107. Fujimoto Y, Kato A, Saitoh Y, et al. Stereotactic radiofrequency ablation for sessile hypothalamic hamartoma with an image fusion technique. *Acta Neurochir (Wien).* 2003;145:697–701.

108. Homma J, Kameyama S, Masuda H, et al. Stereotactic radiofrequency thermocoagulation for hypothalamic hamartoma with intractable gelastic seizures. *Epilepsy Res.* 2007;76:15–21.

109. de Almeida AN, Fonoff ET, Ballester G, et al. Stereotactic disconnection of hypothalamic hamartoma to control seizure and behavior disturbance: case report and literature review. *Neurosurg Rev.* 2008;31:343–349.

110. Schulze-Bonhage A, Trippel M, Wagner K, et al. Outcome and predictors of interstitial radiosurgery in the treatment of gelastic epilepsy. *Neurology.* 2008;71:277–282.

111. Murphy JV, Wheless JW, Schmoll CM. Left vagal nerve stimulation in six patients with hypothalamic hamartomas. *Pediatr Neurol.* 2000;23: 167–168.

112. Pallini R, Bozzini V, Colicchio G, et al. Callosotomy for generalized seizures associated with hypothalamic hamartoma. *Neurol Res.* 1993;15: 139–141.

113. van Rijckevorsel K, Serieh BA, de Tourtchaninoff M, et al. Deep EEG recordings of the mammillary body in epilepsy patients. *Epilepsia.* 2005; 46:781–785.

114. Khan S, Wright I, Javed S, et al. High frequency stimulation of the mamil-lothalamic tract for the treatment of resistant seizures associated with hypothalamic hamartoma. *Epilepsia.* 2009; [Epub ahead of print].

CHAPTER 88 ■ CORPUS CALLOSOTOMY AND MULTIPLE SUBPIAL TRANSECTION

MICHAEL C. SMITH, RICHARD BYRNE, AND ANDRES M. KANNER

Multiple subpial transection (MST) and corpus callosotomy share some common traits. Both are palliative surgical disconnection procedures that are effective in the treatment of medically intractable epilepsy in select patient populations. They both work by disrupting neuronal synchrony of epileptic activity in a critical population of neurons to stop the expression of seizures. MST breaks up the epileptic neuronal synchrony among cortical columns disrupting the epileptic focus itself by the transection of the horizontal fiber system disrupting the critical neuronal synchrony necessary to produce an epileptic spike. Corpus callosotomy disrupts the hemispheric synchrony that is critical in the expression of some generalized seizures such as atonic, tonic, and generalized tonic–clonic seizures. Both procedures are occasionally curative, but effectively treat epileptic seizures that cannot be helped by cortical resection.

CORPUS CALLOSOTOMY

Corpus callosotomy was first introduced as a surgical treatment for medically intractable epilepsy by Van Wagenen and Herren in 1939 (1). The ultimate goal of callosal section is to abolish the bilateral synchrony (or near-synchrony) of cortical epileptiform activity, which can result in seizures with bilateral motor manifestations, such as atonic, tonic, myoclonic, and tonic–clonic seizures. However, as cited by Blume, synchronous corticofugal epileptic discharges can also disrupt brainstem mechanisms affecting posture and tone of proximal limb and axial muscles, leading to atonic or akinetic seizures (2). In the following section, we briefly review some of the more relevant studies that have played an important role in the development and refinement of the techniques used in corpus callosotomy.

Neurophysiologic Basis

The corpus callosum is the most important interhemispheric commissural connection in the brain, with approximately 180 million axons in humans (3). These axons connect homotopic as well as heterotopic cortical regions (4) and exert inhibitory as well as excitatory effects (5). This latter property of the corpus callosum has been suggested as an explanation for the clinical reports of increased partial seizures after callosotomy in humans (6,7) and in animals (8). Studies in rhesus monkeys have shown that section of the two-third anterior corpus callosum resulted in the development of partial seizures five times faster than in nonbisected animals (9). In the amygdala kindling model of the cat, Wada and Sato (10)

reported that section of the corpus callosum accelerated the final stages of generalized convulsions.

The corpus callosum provides interhemispheric connection, unifying of certain motor functions and sensory perceptions of the axial or midline visual and somatosensory world. Axons connecting the frontal lobes occupy a rostral position, whereas those connecting parietal, temporal, and occipital cortices are positioned more caudally, in that order.

The role of the corpus callosum in epileptogenesis is evident from various studies in animals. In the feline model of generalized epilepsy, Musgrave and Gloor (11) demonstrated the loss of bilateral synchrony of spike and slow-wave discharges following the total section of the corpus callosum and anterior commissure. Callosal section in the photosensitive baboon, *Papio papio*, resulted in a decrement in the synchronization of epileptiform discharges and of seizures triggered by photic stimulation (12,13). In a study carried out on four monkeys by Kopeloff et al. (8) in 1950, seizures generated by unilateral application of aluminum oxide cream had a bilateral motor expression. Following callosal section, their clinical manifestations were restricted to a distribution contralateral to the seizure focus.

It must be remembered that although the corpus callosum may be the most important anatomic structure for the interhemispheric spread of epileptic activity, it is not the only one. Anterior and posterior commissures, thalamus, and brainstem structures may all play a role in the spread of discharge from one hemisphere to the other. Suppression of synchronized epileptic activity is routinely and repeatedly seen in acute models of generalized seizures. However, in most models of chronic epilepsy, after callosotomy, some synchronized epileptic activity returns over the ensuing months. This suggests that the epileptic activity utilizes alternate pathways over time. In patients who demonstrate lateralized epileptic activity postoperatively, there is a general tendency for these discharges to synchronize again over the first postoperative year.

Studies in Humans

The first series of 10 patients was published in 1940 by Van Wagenen and Herren (1). However, the real interest in this procedure developed almost 30 years later when Wilson reported on the Dartmouth series of callosotomies (14). In general, the clinical series have confirmed the animal studies, demonstrating the efficacy of callosotomy in treating seizures requiring bilateral synchrony for their clinical expression. In 1985, Spencer et al. (15) reported the abolition of a bilaterally synchronous ictal onset in 5 of 5 patients who underwent a complete section of the corpus callosum, but in only 5 of 10 patients who underwent a two-third anterior section. In contrast, interictal bisynchronous discharges persisted even after a complete section, albeit with a significantly lower frequency. A significant reduction in bisynchronous discharges has been reported in several other patient series (14,16–19). However, as with animal studies, there are a number of reports of an increase in partial seizures (2,20–24) and Spencer et al. described them as being more intense as well (25). Other authors report a conversion of generalized to partial seizures following callosotomy.

Indications

In 1985, Williamson suggested the use of corpus callosotomy to treat the following disorders: (i) infantile hemiplegia and its forme fruste; (ii) Rasmussen syndrome; (iii) Lennox–Gastaut syndrome; and (iv) frontal lobe epilepsy. However, its primary use has been in the treatment of patients with Lennox–Gastaut syndrome.

Efficacy

In general, the purpose of corpus callosotomy is to palliate the patient's intractable seizure condition by decreasing or abolishing the most incapacitating of the generalized seizures and improving the patient's quality of life. Overall, 50% to 77% of patients with Lennox–Gastaut syndrome have been reported to have a satisfactory outcome, defined as seizure reduction of 50% to 80% or more in the different series. The best response has been observed in patients with "drop attacks" presenting as tonic and atonic seizures. However, there is evidence that patients with atonic seizures derived a greater benefit from the procedure than those with tonic seizures (18,19,22,26–28). In 1996, Phillips and Sakas (29) reported the results of anterior callosotomy in 20 patients. They divided outcome into freedom from seizures and significant reduction (70%) of seizures. Using these criteria, 16 of 20 patients (80%) had significant improvement of at least a 70% decrease in seizure frequency. Patients with atonic seizures (11–13) had the best outcome, and favorable results were found in 14 of 18 patients with generalized tonic–clonic seizures. Gates et al. (30) reported that tonic seizures in the presence of an ictal electroencephalographic pattern consisting of an electrodecremental response were associated with a very good outcome in 92% of patients aged 10 years or older. However, this association of seizure type and ictal electroencephalographic pattern was not predictive of outcome in younger patients (16,30).

Corpus callosotomy has yielded a significant reduction of generalized tonic–clonic seizures in 50% to 80% in several patient series (6). Oguni et al. (28) and Spencer et al. (7) have suggested that patients with secondarily generalized tonic–clonic seizures in the presence of electroencephalographic evidence of secondary bilateral synchrony and clinical or neuroradiologic evidence of focality derive greater benefit than those with generalized tonic–clonic seizures without these characteristics. This view has not been universally accepted; Phillips and Sakas did not find neuroimaging or electroencephalographic findings to be predictive of outcome (29).

Patients with complex partial seizures are less likely to respond to this procedure; approximately 40% achieve a significant seizure reduction. Simple partial seizures are rarely affected by callosotomy. Corpus callosotomy had been used in patients with frontal lobe seizures in whom the seizure focus could not be lateralized because of very rapid spread of epileptiform activity. Clark in 2007 found that a planned palliative corpus callosotomy may help identify a resectable epileptic foci (31). However, Purves et al. (32) reported six such patients who underwent a two-third anterior callosotomy without favorable results.

Corpus callosotomy may be performed as a partial resection involving the anterior two third (in the majority of cases) or a complete section. The decision to use one technique rather than the other remains controversial. Studies by Cendes et al. (33), Harbaugh et al. (27), and Reutens et al. (34) showed no differences in seizure control between complete and partial sections. On the other hand, Spencer et al. (7) reported elimination of generalized tonic–clonic seizures in 77% of patients who underwent a complete section of the corpus callosum, compared with 35% of patients who underwent a two third anterior callosotomy. Rahimi in 2007 concurred that in patients with secondarily generalized intractable epilepsy complete callosotomy was superior to partial callosotomy (35). Following a reanalysis of 50 callosotomy patients, Spencer et al. (24) concluded that a two-third anterior section should be considered for patients with tonic, atonic, or myoclonic seizures, whereas a complete section should be reserved for patients with incomplete response to the two-third anterior section. Maehara and Shimizu advocate a complete callosotomy, especially in children and in adults with widespread epilepsy (36). In any event, when a complete section is considered, it should be carried out as a two-stage procedure to minimize neuropsychological complications.

Impact on Quality of Life

In 1997, Rougier et al. reviewed the literature on the efficacy of corpus callosotomy and its effect on quality of life (37). They found a favorable outcome, defined as a 50% reduction of seizures reported in 60% to 80% of all patients with atonic seizures and tonic seizures resulting in falls. Favorable outcome for tonic–clonic seizures varied from 40% to 80%. Complex and simple partial seizures were significantly improved less often. Improvements in quality-of-life indices and social adjustment did not always coincide with reduction in seizure frequency. The length of time for which the patient had had intractable epilepsy and its deleterious effect on his or her cognitive and social function were important variables in predicting quality-of-life improvements. In a study conducted at the Cleveland Clinic, 9 of 17 patients experienced a greater than 80% reduction in their targeted seizures and 15 of 17 reported satisfaction with the surgical outcome. However, improvement in alertness and responsiveness, not necessarily reduction in seizure frequency, was most closely associated with satisfaction with surgical outcome (38). Papo et al. (38) reviewed 36 patients with intractable seizures of mixed seizure types. Twenty-seven had had an anterior callosotomy; eight had a complete callosotomy in two stages, and one had a posterior callosotomy. Of the 36 patients, 30 had adequate follow-up to report meaningful results. Fourteen had excellent results (defined as more than 90% reduction in targeted seizure type), five had good results (more than 50% reduction), six had poor results (less than 50% reduction), and five showed no change. As reported above, global measures of quality of life did not always coincide with improvement of seizure frequency. In some patients with excellent seizure results, there was no clear change in quality of life. The authors suggest that this might be related to the long duration of uncontrolled seizures and their effect on cognitive function (38). Gilliam et al. (39) have also noted that overall clinical improvement did not always correlate with seizure reduction.

Asadi-Pooya, in a recent review, documents that corpus callosotomy's effectiveness and low permanent morbidity is demonstrated by over six decades of experience with this procedure. They note that besides seizure reduction, quality of life often improves (40).

VAGUS NERVE STIMULATION VERSUS CORPUS CALLOSOTOMY

While vagus nerve stimulation (VNS) has gained increasing use in the various seizure types in the Lennox–Gastaut syndrome, there have been a number of recent studies comparing VNS with corpus callosotomy. You et al. compared 14 patients with total callosotomy with 10 patients with VNS implantation and followed them for over 1 year. All patients had multiple seizure types of the Lennox–Gastaut syndrome, primarily atonic seizures and tonic seizures. Efficacy in seizure reduction was similar in the two groups. They reported that 64.3% in the callosotomy group versus 70% in the VNS group had a 50% reduction in targeted seizures (41). The authors concluded the efficacy and safety of VNS and corpus callosotomy were comparable. This differs somewhat from Nei's report that compared corpus callosotomy ($n = 53$) with VNS ($n = 25$) with refractory generalized seizures (generalized tonic–clonic, tonic, and atonic). They found 79.5% in the corpus callosotomy group had 50% or greater response versus 50% in the VNS group. However, morbidity in the corpus callosotomy group was higher (21% vs. 8%), although only 3.8% of the complications in the corpus callosotomy group were permanent. The authors concluded while both procedures were efficacious, corpus callosotomy had greater efficacy, though with transiently higher morbidity (42).

Surgical Technique

Under general anesthesia, the patient is placed in the supine position with pressure points padded. The head is placed in pin fixation in neutral position with the neck slightly flexed. The hair is clipped and the skin prepped. A lumbar drain may be placed to aid in retraction of the midline. A variety of skin incisions may be used for anterior callosal sectioning, all of which give access to the anterior midline. A coronally oriented skin incision 2 cm anterior to the coronal suture exposing both sides of midline will give the needed exposure. Usually, this incision should expose more right side than left because approach from the right allows retraction of the nondominant hemisphere. Hodaie et al. propose the use of image guidance in part to analyze the parasagittal veins in order to decide the side of entry (43). A craniotomy is performed just anterior to

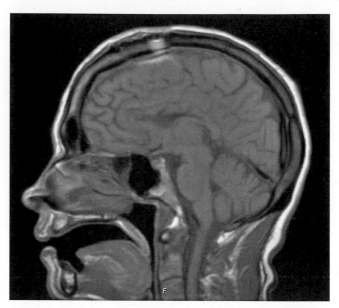

FIGURE 88.1 Sagittal T1 magnetic resonance image showing an anterior two-third callosotomy.

the coronal suture, crossing midline to expose the sagittal sinus. The procedure can be done without exposing the sinus, but retraction of the sinus is then not possible and sinus bleeding is more difficult to control if encountered. The dural flap is based on the sinus, and retraction of the dura allows retraction of the sinus. Although the exposure is anterior to the coronal suture, all but the most insignificant bridging veins should be spared. Planning the approach and exposure thus may be aided by examining preoperative magnetic resonance imaging (MRI) or magnetic resonance angiography (MRA) scans (Figs. 88.1 through 88.3). If a bridging vein complex does not allow retraction because of a far lateral entry of the vein into the sagittal sinus, a dural incision may be made in the

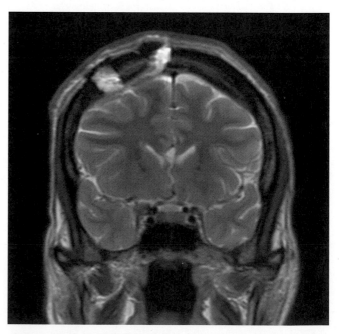

FIGURE 88.2 Coronal T2 magnetic resonance image showing the position of the craniotomy and the division of the genu into the midline cavum.

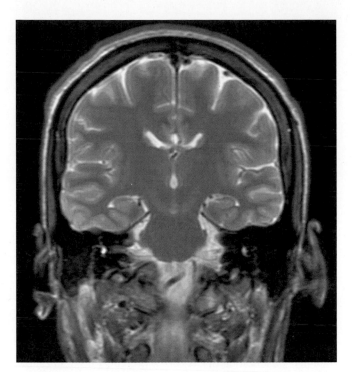

FIGURE 88.3 Coronal T2 magnetic resonance image showing division of the posterior body of the corpus callosum. Note the position of the fornices below the corpus callosum.

form of a triangle around the laterally entering vein to allow retraction of the dural flap without disturbing the vein.

Once an unencumbered view of the intrahemispheric fissure is obtained, the medial aspect of the exposed frontal lobe is covered with moist cottonoids, and self-retaining retractors are gently advanced. The falx is followed down the midline until the cingulated gyri are encountered. An error that is sometimes made is to mistake this view of the adherent cingulate gyri for the corpus callosum. The cingulated gyri are separated under magnification in the midline, exposing the corpus callosum and the pericallosal arteries. Once this view is obtained and the retractors are set, a final check of the anterior exposure confirms the exposure of the anterior corpus callosum if the genu is visible.

The actual division of the anterior corpus callosum is done with a microdissection instrument and gentle suction. This should begin in the midline of the callosum just posterior to the genu. Great care is taken to separate, but not disturb, the pericallosal arteries. At this level, certain landmarks, such as the cavum of the septum pellucidum, are visible beneath the corpus callosum, even if it is only a potential space in the individual patient. This midline landmark is valuable, if found, because it confirms the complete transection of the callosal fibers and it allows one to stay out of the lateral ventricles. If the lateral ventricle is entered, intraoperative or postoperative bleeding may cause hydrocephalus. The transection is then carried forward into the genu and the rostrum of the corpus callosum. The disconnection is carried out downwards following the A2 branches as they approach the anterior communicating artery complex. The extent of posterior callosal sectioning is decided preoperatively. Some surgeons advise a simple one-half callosal sectioning, which can be measured by comparing the intraoperative transection to the length of the callosum on the

preoperative sagittal MRI. This and other techniques, such as intraoperative plain films and stereotaxy, have been described to confirm the length of callosotomy (44). Other authors advocate a three-quarter sectioning, as there is some indication that seizure control may be more complete. If a complete corpus callosotomy is to be performed, the sectioning may be done with a microdissector or suction aspiration to the splenium. A complete posterior sectioning is confirmed by viewing the arachnoid covered vein of Galen in the posterior midline. If only an anterior transection is planned, an MRI-compatible marker should be placed at the posterior border of the anterior transection in order to see on imaging studies and to note on reoperation, if necessary, the extent of the first procedure. Hemostasis is obtained, and any entry into a lateral ventricle is covered with Gelfoam. A standard craniotomy closure is performed.

Over the past few years, there have been increasing reports in the use of radiosurgery or Gamma Knife to perform a corpus callosotomy, as reported by both Feichtinger et al. (45) and Eder et al. (46) in 2006. While the numbers in each series were small, efficacy was comparable to traditional surgical callosotomy (44–46).

Complications

Complications unique to corpus callosotomy as a surgical procedure are neuropsychological in nature. Well-described acute and chronic neuropsychological sequelae are possible after callosotomy (47,48). Varying degrees of the acute disconnection syndrome are commonly seen. This syndrome is characterized by a lethargic, apathetic mutism during the first few days after surgery. In our experience and in the experience of other investigators, this is always transient. The predictors of this transient state are related to the extent of callosal sectioning, baseline cognitive impairments, and the amount of traction necessary to gain access to the corpus callosum. Other early complications of the acute syndrome are incontinence, bilateral Babinski's sign, and apraxia.

The chronic disconnection syndrome was initially not well recognized when callosotomy was initially described (1). Detailed neuropsychological testing reveals deficits that are common after callosotomy, but are not usually clinically significant. The majority of the neuropsychological alterations, other than mutism, occur with posterior callosotomy. This is caused by disruption of communication between visual and tactile cortical sensory functions and verbal expression. Because of the disconnection between the hemispheres, an object placed only in the left visual field of a left-hemisphere-dominant patient will be seen by the right hemisphere, but the information will not be transferred to the left hemisphere for speech production. Thus, the patient recognizes the object but cannot name it. Similarly, an object placed in the left hand, but not seen, may be recognized by its shape and size but it will not be named. This is interesting but not clinically disabling to the patient because objects are normally seen by both hemispheres and can be felt with either hand. If a patient has bilateral speech representation, dysphasia may be a postoperative complication. This should be considered before complete callosotomy is undertaken on a patient with mixed speech dominance.

A disturbing complication known as alien hand syndrome has been reported (48). In this syndrome, poor cooperation or even antagonistic behavior between the left and right hand is noted. The verbal dominant hemisphere may express displeasure with the actions of the ipsilateral extremities. This phenomenon is usually short lived and is usually seen only in the immediate postoperative period; however, on rare occasions it may persist. Initially, performing only an anterior callosotomy can minimize the likelihood and the extent of these neuropsychological sequelae. If the anterior callosotomy is unsuccessful in controlling seizures, a completion of the callosotomy may be performed at a later time.

Other complications that have been observed are related to frontal lobe retraction: cingulate gyrus injury, injury to the pericallosal arteries, bridging veins or superior sagittal sinus, and hydrocephalus following entry into the lateral ventricle. Postoperative hydrocephalus secondary to entry into the ventricular system and a subsequent ventriculitis have been dramatically reduced by using an operative microscope and carefully respecting ventricle boundaries. Transient mutism may be reduced by minimizing the retraction of frontal cortex and retracting the nondominant frontal lobe, if possible. Despite this, mutism may occur transiently in up to 30% of patients.

Spencer and colleagues reported a meta-analysis of long-term neurologic sequelae of both anterior and complete corpus callosotomy (7). They found that motor sequelae were reported in 56% of complete and 8% of anterior callosotomy patients; language impairments in 14% and 8%, respectively; and both cognitive impairment and behavioral impairment in 11% and 8%, respectively.

Some authors have suggested certain contraindications to corpus callosotomy. Spencer et al. (7,15) found that patients with severe mental retardation (IQ lower than 45) did not derive any benefit from the procedure. Other studies, however, have not found any relationship between IQ and outcome (32,33,49–51). A relative contraindication has been proposed concerning patients whose hemisphere of language dominance is not that of hand dominance (52). Speech difficulties, with sparing of writing, have been identified in patients who are right-hemisphere-dominant for speech and are right handed, and dysgraphia with intact speech has been identified in left-handed patients with a left-dominant hemisphere.

In conclusion, corpus callosotomy is an effective surgical technique for the treatment of selected pharmacoresistant epileptic syndromes, particularly certain types of seizure (i.e., atonic seizures). Over the past 10 years, its use has decreased as a result of the introduction of new antiepileptic drugs, especially lamotrigine and topiramate, and a rekindling of interest in the ketogenic diet. The vagus nerve stimulator has clear benefit for atonic/tonic seizures and cortical stimulation may be beneficial for "drop" seizures, but no conclusive data are yet available. Certain epilepsy centers in the United States are routinely performing vagus nerve stimulation before considering corpus callosotomy. In general, anterior corpus callosotomy is still an underutilized procedure, especially for patients with intractable atonic seizures associated with recurrent falls and subsequent head injury. Radiosurgery has been proposed as an alternative to surgical callosotomy by Pendl et al. (53) and others. Although this is a promising approach, several questions about volume-dose analysis and long-term efficacy are yet to be fully answered (54,55).

MULTIPLE SUBPIAL TRANSECTION

Focal-onset medically intractable epilepsy has been surgically treated for 70 years by location of the seizure focus and resection of the involved cortex. A certain proportion of patients who undergo evaluation for possible surgical resection are found to have an epileptogenic zone originating in, or overlapping with, eloquent cortex. These patients traditionally have been denied surgery because resection of primary speech, motor, sensory, or visual cortex would result in unacceptable deficits. MST was developed specifically to address this problem. The purpose of this technique is to disrupt the intracortical horizontal fiber system while preserving the columnar organization of the cortex (i.e., its vertically oriented input and output systems and vascular supply) (56). The transection of horizontal fibers is aimed at preventing the propagation of epileptic discharges, thus averting the synchronous neuronal activation that ultimately results in the development of clinical seizures. The preservation of the columnar organization of the cortex prevents or minimizes the disruption of the functional state of the transected cortex.

The development of this technique was derived from three sets of experiments, each unrelated to the others or to the field of epilepsy surgery. The first set of experiments by Asanuma and Sakata (57), Hubel and Wiesel (58), and Mountcastle (59) demonstrated that the vertically oriented micro- and macrocolumns (with their vertically oriented input, output, and vascular supply) are the organizational unit of functional cortical architecture. The functional role of the intracortical horizontal fiber system is yet to be firmly established. However, this system is composed of fibers responsible for recurrent inhibition and excitation underlying neuronal plasticity. In the second set of experiments, Sperry (60) demonstrated that surgical disruption of the horizontal fiber system in the visual cortex of the cat, while sparing its columnar organization, does not affect its testable functional status. In the third set of experiments, Tharp related to the importance of the horizontal fiber system as a "critical component in cortical circuit necessary for generation and elaboration of paroxysmal discharges" (61). Epileptic activity in the form of spikes or sharp waves requires a synchronous neuronal activation of a contiguous cortical surface of at least 12 to 25 mm² (61,62). Tharp found that epileptic foci would synchronize their activity if the distance between them was 5 mm or less, and disrupting the neuropil between the foci would desynchronize the epileptic activity.

With this information, Morrell and colleagues hypothesized that sectioning of the intracortical horizontal fibers at 5-mm intervals, while preserving the columnar organization of the cortex, could abolish epileptic activity yet preserve the functional status of the transected cortex (56,63). Testing this hypothesis in the monkey, Morrell produced an epileptic focus with aluminum gel lesions in the left precentral motor cortex, which resulted in the development of focal motor seizures. Using a small wire, he disconnected the horizontal fibers at 5-mm intervals throughout the epileptogenic zone. This procedure, the first subpial transection for epilepsy, stopped the seizures, and the monkey suffered no motor deficits from the procedure. To confirm that what he had transected was motor cortex, 1 year later Morrell surgically removed the transected area, resulting in the expected hemiparesis. With this experimental evidence, Morrell and colleagues moved forward into the treatment of intractable human neocortical epilepsy arising in or overlapping eloquent cortex.

Indications for Multiple Subpial Transection

MST is indicated in any patient in whom the epileptic zone arises from or overlaps with eloquent cortex. The procedure is performed after a detailed presurgical evaluation, which includes closed-circuit television/electroencephalographic recording of habitual seizures using scalp and intracranial electrodes, mainly subdural grids. In addition, detailed functional mapping to identify eloquent cortex by electrical cortical stimulation and evoked potentials is performed. Neuropsychological testing and intracarotid amobarbital tests, as well as functional neuroimaging studies, all assist in defining the baseline function and risks of the procedure. Magnetoencephalography studies have also been very useful in the evaluation of children with an acquired epileptic aphasia of childhood or Landau–Kleffner syndrome (LKS) (64). It allows more accurate identification of the source of the dipole, especially its depth within a sulcus.

MST can be performed as the sole procedure or in conjunction with resection of noneloquent cortex, depending on the extent to which the epileptogenic zone involves eloquent cortex. Most cases of MST occur in conjunction with a cortical resection. Candidates are typically patients with dominant temporal neocortical epilepsy, dominant frontal lobe epilepsy, or primary sensory, motor, or visual cortex involvement. In patients undergoing resection/transection, resection of noneloquent cortex is performed to within 1.5 cm of the identified eloquent cortex. We recognize that this patient group is problematic for the evaluation of the clinical effectiveness of MST.

Cortical Surgical Anatomy

Human cortex is arranged in a gyral pattern, which is fairly constant between individuals. However, the microgyral patterns of individual gyri may be considerably variable. These cortical variations must be taken into account in a procedure where transections are being made perpendicular to the long axis of a gyrus. Thus, careful inspection of each gyrus prior to the procedure is important. Gray matter is, on average, 5-mm thick over the crown of a gyrus. However, the depth of each sulcus is variable.

These points are critical in subpial transection procedures because the objective is to divide the neuropil into 5-mm intervals perpendicular to the long axis of the gyrus while preserving the overlying pia with its blood vessels and the underlying white matter tracts and U fibers.

About a quarter of our patients have undergone MST as their primary procedure. These patients mainly had epilepsia partialis continua due to Rasmussen encephalitis or LKS. In the patients with Rasmussen syndrome, the epileptogenic zone arose from primary language and/or motor cortex, whereas in patients with LKS, it involved posterior language cortex.

Operative Procedure

Patients are given preoperative antibiotics and often steroids and are positioned so that the surgical site is at the highest point in the operative field. This makes intraoperative electrocorticography (ECoG), resection, and transection easier. The head is held in Mayfield head fixation and all pressure points are padded. If the operation is done with the patient awake, the patient's comfort is especially important.

Anesthesia is accomplished with intravenous methohexital and a generous amount of local anesthesia. Although methohexital has been shown to activate interictal epileptiform activity, such activation does not extend beyond the epileptogenic zone (65). Furthermore, the degree of activation of epileptiform activity can be minimized by lowering the infusion rate of methohexital. At our center, we perform intraoperative ECoG in all cases, even when mapping with subdural grids has been done, to ensure that the initial transections result in the desired abolition of epileptic activity.

Transections

Before performing the transections, careful inspection of the gyri, microgyral pattern, sulci, and vascular supply is carried out. Transections are first performed in the more dependent areas to avoid the problem of subarachnoid blood obscuring the other areas. At the edge of the visible gyrus, in an avascular area, a 20-gauge needle is used to open a hole in the pia. The tip of the subpial transection hook is introduced into the gray matter layer and advanced to the next sulcus in a direction perpendicular to the long axis of the gyrus. The tip of the hook is held upward and is visible immediately beneath the pia. It is important that the pia be left undisturbed to minimize vascular injury and scarring. The transection hook is designed with a handle, a malleable shaft, and a tip that is 4-mm long (paralleling the cortical width) and 1-mm wide. If the 4-mm tip is introduced just below the pia, it should remain in the gray matter layer, leaving the white matter undisturbed. The tip is angled at 105° and is blunt. These two features make snagging or injuring a vessel less likely. However, it is important to avoid crossing a sulcus where buried vessels are unprotected. While this procedure is simple in principle, we have found that to master it requires considerable experience.

After the first transection is completed, bleeding from the pial opening is controlled with small pieces of Gelfoam and a cottonoid. The 4-mm tip is then placed up against the cortex next to the transection so as to select the next transection site 5 mm from the first. This is repeated until the identified epileptogenic zone is transected. Over a few minutes, the lines take on a striped appearance from the petechial hemorrhages along the lines. Minimal bleeding is encountered if the transections are done properly. ECoG is repeated at the conclusion of the transections. The transected area displays a significant attenuation of the background activity with elimination of the spikes. In cases of persistent epileptiform activity, the possibility that activity is coming from the depth of a sulcus or from remote areas must be considered. On rare occasions, when persistent activity is clearly identified as originating in an area that has been transected, transecting down into the sulcus may be done. In order to perform this safely, the tip of the probe should be turned away from the sulcus as the instrument is advanced.

Favorable outcomes using alternative instruments and methods of transection have been described by neurosurgeons (66,67).

Seizure Outcome

Evaluation of seizure outcome should be carried out in patients who underwent MST without additional cortical resection. We have previously reported our series of patients with partial epilepsy with 37.5% of patients becoming seizure-free at 2-year follow-up with an additional 37.5% having a worthwhile outcome (Class II–III). However, as has been reported by other centers, there is a late reoccurrence rate in seizures following MST (68). Orbach reported a relapse rate of 18.6% over several years (69). Schramm reported on the efficacy of MST alone in 20 patients with drug-resistant epilepsy. One patient had a previous temporal resection; there were two cases each of LKS and electrical status epilepticus of sleep (ESES). In this series, 10% had a Class I outcome and 45% had a Class II–III outcome. They also noted the relapse in seizures over time (70). Zhao reported in 2005 on 80 patients treated with MST alone as part of his larger series. He reported 51.7% seizure freedom in patients with at least 1 year follow-up (71).

In a meta-analysis of MST with or without additional cortical resection, Spencer (2002) reviewed 211 patients who underwent MST for intractable epilepsy and found an excellent outcome (greater than 95% reduction in seizure frequency) in 87% of patients who had generalized seizures and 68% of patients with simple and complex partial seizures (72). Zhao et al., in 2005, in the largest series reported to date, reported on 200 patients (80 MST alone) treated with MST for intractable partial epilepsy involving eloquent cortex between 1991 and 2000. They reported complete control of seizures in 62.5% with another 20% of patients having a significant reduction (greater than 75%), with 160 patients having at least 1 year follow-up (71).

Pondal-Sordo, in 2006, reported the neurosurgical experience of London, Ontario, with perirolandic epileptic foci with cortical resection with or without additional MST. The most common etiology was neoplastic. Average follow-up was 4.2 years. At follow-up, 46% had worthwhile outcome (Engel Class I, 31%; Engel Class II, 15%). Residual deficits were seen in 50%, but were mild in half. Those patients whose postoperative ECoG showed infrequent or no epileptiform activity had better surgical outcomes (73).

In pediatric patients, Shimizu reported on 25 cases where MST was utilized with 10 out of 25 having an Engel Class I or II outcome (74). In 2006, Benifla et al. reviewed two studies of MST efficacy that included 60 patients (10 MST alone). They found that between 33% and 46% of patients in the respective series had Engel Class I or II outcomes (75).

MST had been used to treat hippocampal epilepsy and preserve verbal memory. Shimizu in 2006 reported 21 patients who underwent multiple transections of the pyramidal layer of the hippocampus under the alveus using a modification of the MST procedure. Of the 21 patients, 17 were followed for more than 1 year. Fourteen patients (82%) became seizure-free and two (12%) had rare seizures. Eight patients underwent a full postoperative battery of neuropsychological testing of verbal memory. Verbal memory was completely spared in seven, with one patient having a transient worsening that cleared over 6 months

(76). The authors were encouraged with the above results; however, a longer follow-up and greater numbers of patients are required before transection of hippocampus is confirmed to be efficacious and sparing of verbal memory function.

MST had been used to treat LKS for the past 15 years at our institution. Kanner et al. reviewed the outcome of 24 patients with classic LKS. Thirteen of the 24 had MST alone and 7 had resection and MST (77). All had continuous spike and wave in slow-wave sleep from a unilateral perisylvian source, and all had been mute for at least 2 years. After MST of the perisylvian epileptic abnormality, follow-up revealed that two third of the children speak in complex sentences at their last formal speech evaluation with significant improvement of language coming within the first 6 months postoperatively. Nine of these children had achieved complete recovery of language and were not requiring any speech therapy (77).

Irwin in 2001 reported five cases of classic LKS who underwent MST. All had ESES, clinical seizures, severe language dysfunction or no language, and a behavioral disorder. The frequency of seizures and behavioral disorders were significantly improved in all; however, improvement in language function was not dramatic. This might be related to the duration of the epileptic abnormality prior to surgery (78). The mean duration was 4.6 years and studies have suggested that duration over 3 years is a predictor of the severity of chronic language disturbance, even with treatment (78).

MST with cortical resection has also been used in patients with multifocal multilobar epilepsy with clinical seizures and developmental regression. In reports by Patel and the Devinsky groups, a moderate improvement in language, social and behavioral function with a significant improvement in seizure frequency was reported (79).

MST had been used in Rasmussen encephalitis in seven patients from Morrell's series. In four patients, the targeted seizures were eliminated but the progression of the disease continued. In three of seven, MST did not eliminate the epileptic process due to the fact that it arose from the depth of the sulcus (56). MST had also been used in patients with refractory status epilepticus that involved eloquent cortex. In both cases, MST successfully stopped the status epilepticus (80,81).

Surgical Morbidity

Acute Postoperative Morbidity

Cerebral edema is expected after MST, peaking on the third to fourth postoperative day. Consequently, patients are expected to experience transient dysfunction of transected cortex, with ensuing neurological deficits lasting for 2 to 3 weeks. Sometimes mild deficits may persist for several months. Similar observations have been made at the other centers where MST is performed (see the following section).

Chronic Morbidity

The incidence of chronic morbidity varies, in part, with the experience of the neurosurgeon performing the MST procedure. We have reported previously a neurological complication rate of 15% with 7% suffering a permanent deficit. These included foot drop in 2%, language deficit in 2%, and a parietal sensory loss in 1%. Mild, but clear, diminution in rapid skilled movements was seen in the majority of those undergoing MST of the parietal sensory cortex.

Spencer in the meta-analysis of 211 patients reported the highest morbidity with new neurologic deficits found in 19% of those with pure MST including 4 with memory decline, 5 with hemiparesis, and 1 with partial visual field defect. A total of 23% of the patients with resection and MST had persistent neurologic deficit (72). Schramm in the 20 cases of pure MST reported transient neurologic deficit in 29% but all deficits resolved to the point that they would not be noted on standard clinical exams (70). In Zhao's larger series of 200 patients, 80 MST alone, he reported transient neurologic deficits in just 3% (71). Likewise, in review of pediatric MST, Benifla reported no permanent language or motor disabilities after MST (75).

CONCLUSIONS

Corpus callosotomy and multiple subpial transection are different surgical techniques in which the basic modus operandi is a disconnection procedure. Both procedures offer therapeutic options in patients previously rejected for more traditional resective surgery. The efficacy of corpus callosotomy has now been demonstrated in multiple centers around the world. MST, while used with increasing frequency in epilepsy centers worldwide, has yet to gain universal acceptance. Additional experimental and clinical studies are needed before this surgical procedure is fully integrated into the therapeutic armamentarium at all major epilepsy centers. Much of the success of both procedures depends on the proper selection of patients and the experience of the neurologic and neurosurgical teams. A learning curve should be expected whenever these procedures are newly implemented at a center.

ACKNOWLEDGMENT

We thank Irene O'Connor for her editorial assistance and encouragement.

References

1. Van Wagenen WP, Herren RY. Surgical division of commissural pathways in the corpus callosum: relation to spread of an epileptic attack. *Arch Neurol Psychiatry.* 1940;44:740–759.
2. Blume WT. Corpus callosotomy: a critical review. In: Tuxhom I, Holthausen H, Boenigk H, eds. *Pediatric Epilepsy Syndromes and Their Surgical Treatment.* London: John Libbey; 1997:815–829.
3. Tomasch J. Size, distribution, and number of fibres in the human corpus callosum. *Anat Rec.* 1954;119:119–135.
4. Pandya DN, Seltzer B. The topography of commissural fibers. In: Lepore F, Ptito M, Jaspar HH, eds. *Two Hemispheres—One Brain: Functions of the Corpus Callosum.* New York, NY: Alan R. Liss; 1986:47–73.
5. Asanuma H, Okuda O. Effects of transcallosal volleys on pyramidal tract cell activity of cat. *J Neurophysiol.* 1962;25:198–208.
6. Gates JR, dePaola L. Corpus callosum section. In: Sliovon S, Dreifuss F, Fish D, et al., eds. *The Treatment of Epilepsy.* London: Blackwell Scientific; 1996:722–738.
7. Spencer SS, Spencer DD, Williamson PD, et al. Corpus callosotomy for epilepsy. I: seizure effects. *Neurology.* 1988;38:19–24.
8. Kopeloff N, Kennard MA, Pacalla BL, et al. Section of corpus callosum in experimental epilepsy in the monkey. *Arch Neurol Psychiatry.* 1950;63:719–727.
9. Shorvon S, Perucca E, Fish D et al. eds. The Treatment of Epilepsy. 2nd ed. Massachusetts: Blackwell Science Ltd., 2004;67:798–811.
10. Wada JA, Sata M. The generalized convulsive seizures induced by daily electrical stimulation of the amygdala in split brain cats. *Epilepsia.* 1975; 16:417–430.
11. Musgrave J, Gloor P. The role of the corpus callosum in bilateral interhemispheric synchrony of spike and wave discharge in feline generalized penicillin epilepsy. *Epilepsia.* 1980;21:369–378.
12. Naquet R, Wada JA. Role of the corpus callosum in photosensitive seizures of epileptic baboon *Papio papio. Adv Neurol.* 1992; 57:579–587.
13. Wada JA, Jomai S. Effect of anterior two-thirds callosal bisection upon bisymmetrical and bisynchronous generalized convulsions kindled from amygdala in epileptic baboon, *Papio papio.* In: Reeves AG, ed. *Epilepsy and the Corpus Callosum.* New York, NY: Plenum Press; 1985:75–97.
14. Wilson DH, Reeves AG, Gazzaniga MS, et al. Cerebral commissurotomy for control of intractable seizures. *Neurology.* 1977;27:708–715.
15. Spencer SS, Spencer DD, Williamson PD, et al. Effects of corpus callosum section on secondary bilaterally synchronous interictal EEG discharges. *Neurology.* 1985;35:1689–1694.
16. Courtney W, Gates JR, Ritter F, et al. Prediction of seizure outcome after corpus callosotomy in patients ten years or older. *Epilepsia.* 1993; 34(suppl):43.
17. Huck FR, Radvany J, Avila JO, et al. Anterior callosotomy in epileptics with multiform seizures and bilateral synchronous spike and wave EEG pattern. *Acta Neurochir Suppl (Wein).* 1980;30:127–135.
18. Nordgren RE, Reeves AG, Viguera AC, et al. Corpus callosotomy for intractable seizures in the pediatric age group. *Arch Neurol.* 1991;48: 364–372.
19. Wilson DH, Reeves A, Gazzaniga MS. "Central" commissurotomy for intractable generalized epilepsy: series two. *Neurology.* 1982;32:687–697.
20. Gates JR. Candidacy for corpus callosotomy. In: Luders H, ed. *Epilepsy Surgery.* New York, NY: Raven Press; 1991:140–150.
21. Gates JR. Presurgical evaluation for epileptic surgery in the era of long-term monitoring for epilepsy. In: Apuzzo MLJ, ed. *Neurosurgical Aspects of Epilepsy.* Chicago, IL: AANS Publications; 1991:59–72.
22. Gates JR, Maxwell R, Leppik IE, et al. Electroencephalographic and clinical effects of total corpus callosotomy. In: Reeves AG, ed. *Epilepsia and the Corpus Callosum.* New York, NY: Plenum Press; 1986:315–328.
23. Gates JR, Mireles R, Maxwell RE, et al. Magnetic resonance imaging, electroencephalogram and selected neuropsychological testing in staged corpus callosotomy. *Arch Neurol.* 1986;43:1188–1191.
24. Spencer SS, Katz A, Ebersole J, et al. Ictal EEG changes with corpus callosum section. *Epilepsia.* 1993;34:568–573.
25. Spencer SS, Spencer DD, Glaser GH, et al. More intense focal seizure types after callosal section; the role of inhibition. *Ann Neurol.* 1984;16:686–693.
26. Fuiks KS, Wylfer AR, Hermann BP, et al. Seizure outcome from anterior and complete corpus callosotomy. *J Neurosurg.* 1991;74:573–578.
27. Harbaugh RE, Wilson DH, Reeves AG, et al. Forebrain commissurotomy for epilepsy: review of 20 consecutive cases. *Acta Neurochir (Wien).* 1983;68:263–275.
28. Oguni H, Olivier A, Andermann F, et al. Anterior callosotomy in the treatment of medically intractable epilepsies: a study of 43 patients with a mean follow-up of 39 months. *Ann Neurol.* 1991;30:357–364.
29. Philips J, Sakas DE. Anterior callosotomy for intractable epilepsy: outcome in a series of twenty patients. *Br J Neurosurg.* 1996;10:351–356.
30. Gates JR, Courtney W, Ritter F, et al. Prediction of seizure outcome after corpus callosotomy among young children. *Epilepsia.* 1993;34(suppl): 111.
31. Clarke DF, Wheless JW, Chacon MM, et al. Corpus callosotomy: a palliative therapeutic technique may help identify respectable epileptogenic foci. *Seizure.* 2007;16(6):545–553.
32. Purves SJ, Wada JA, Woodhurst WB. Anterior callosotomy for complex partial seizures. Paper presented at the Second Dartmouth International Conference on Epilepsy and the Corpus Callosum; August 12, 1991; Hanover, New Hampshire.
33. Cendes F, Ragazzo PC, da Costa V, et al. Corpus callosotomy in treatment of medically resistant epilepsy: preliminary results in a pediatric population. *Epilepsia.* 1993;34:910–917.
34. Reutens DC, Bye AM, Hopkins IJ, et al. Corpus callosotomy for intractable epilepsy: seizure outcome and prognostic factors. *Epilepsia.* 1993;34:904–909.
35. Rahimi SY, Park YD, Witcher MR, et al. Corpus callosotomy for treatment of pediatric epilepsy in the modern era. *Pediatr Neurosurg.* 2007;43(3):202–208.
36. Machara T, Shimizu H. Surgical outcome of corpus callosotomy in patients with drop attacks. *Epilepsia.* 2001;42:67–71.
37. Rougier A, Claverie B, Pedespan JM, et al. Callosotomy for intractable epilepsy: overall outcome. *J Neurosurg Sci.* 1997;41:51–57.
38. Papo I, Quattrini A, Ortenzi A, et al. Predictive factors of callosotomy in drug-resistant epileptic patients with a long follow-up. *J Neurosurg Sci.* 1997;41:31–36.
39. Gilliam F, Wyllie E, Kotagal P, et al. Parental assessment of functional outcome after corpus callosotomy. *Epilepsia.* 1996;37:753–757.
40. Asadi-Pooya AA, Sharan A, Nei M, et al. Corpus callosotomy. *Epilepsy Behav.* 2008;13(2):271–278.
41. You SJ, Kang HC, Ko TS, et al. Comparison of corpus callosotomy and vagus nerve stimulation in children with Lennox–Gastaut syndrome. *Brain Dev.* 2008;30(3):195–199.
42. Nei M, O'Connor M, Liporace J, et al. Refractory generalized seizures: response to corpus callosotomy and vagal nerve stimulation. *Epilepsia.* 2006;47(1):115–122.

43. Hodaie M, Musharbash A, Otsubo H, et al. Image-guided, frameless stereotactic sectioning of the corpus callosum in children with intractable epilepsy. *Pediatr Neurosurg.* 2000;34:286–294.

44. Awad IA, Wyllie E, Luders H, et al. Intraoperative determination of the extent of the corpus callosotomy for epilepsy: two simple techniques. *Neurosurgery.* 1990;25:102–106.

45. Feichtinger M, Schrottner O, Eder H, et al. Efficacy and safety of radio-surgical callosotomy: a retrospective analysis. *Epilepsia.* 2006;47(7): 1184–1191.

46. Eder Hg, Feichtinger M, Pieper T, et al. Gamma knife radiosurgery for callosotomy in children with drug-resistant epilepsy. *Childs Nerv Syst.* 2006;22(8):1012–1017.

47. Black PM, Holmes G, Lombroso CT. Corpus callosum section for intractable epilepsy in children. *Pediatr Neurosurg.* 1992;18:298–304.

48. Ferguson SM, Rayport M, Corrie WS. Neuropsychiatric observations on behavioral consequences of corpus callosum section for seizure control. In: Reeves AG, ed. *Epilepsy and the Corpus Callosum.* New York, NY: Plenum Press; 1985:501–514.

49. Sass KJ, Spencer SS, Novelly RA, et al. Amnestic and attention impairments following corpus callosum section for epilepsy. *J Epilepsy.* 1988;1: 61–66.

50. Gates JR, Rosenfeld WE, Maxwell RE, et al. Response of multiple seizure types to corpus callosum section. *Epilepsia.* 1987;28:28–34.

51. Gates JR, Ritter FJ, Ragazzo PC, et al. Corpus callosum section in children: seizure response. *J Epilepsy.* 1990;3:271–278.

52. Spencer SS, Gates JR, Reeves AG, et al. Corpus callosum section. In: Engel J Jr, ed. *Surgical Treatment of the Epilepsies.* New York, NY: Raven Press; 1987:425–444.

53. Pendl G, Eder H, Schroettner O, et al. Corpus callosotomy with radio-surgery. *Neurosurgery.* 1999;45:303–308.

54. Smyth MD, Klein EE, Dodson WE, et al. Radiosurgical posterior corpus callosotomy in a child with Lennox–Gastaut syndrome. Case report. *J Neurosurg.* 2007;106(4 suppl):312–315.

55. Celis MA, Moreno-Jimenez S. Larraga-Gutierrez JM, et al. Corpus callosotomy using conformal stereotactic radiosurgery. *Childs Nerv Syst.* 2007;23(8):917–920.

56. Morrell F, Whisler WW, Bleck T. Multiple subpial transection: a new approach to the surgical treatment of focal epilepsy. *J Neurosurg.* 1989; 70:231–239.

57. Asanuma H, Sakata H. Functional organization of a cortical efferent system examined with focal depth stimulation in cats. *J Neurophysiol.* 1967; 30(suppl):35–54.

58. Hubel DH, Wiesel TN. Receptive fields, binocular interaction and functional architecture in the cat's visual cortex. *J Physiol.* 1962;160:106–154.

59. Mountcastle VB. Modality and topographic properties of single neurons of cat's somatic sensory cortex. *J Neurophysiol.* 1957;20:408–434.

60. Sperry RW. Physiological plasticity and brain circuit theory. In: Harlow HF, Woolsey CN, eds. *Biological and Biochemical Bases of Behavior.* Madison, WI: University of Wisconsin Press; 1958:401–418.

61. Tharp BR. The penicillin focus: a study of field characteristics using cross-correlation analysis. *Electroencephalogr Clin Neurophysiol.* 1971; 31:45–55.

62. Lueders H, Bustamante I, Zablow L, et al. The independence of closely spaced discrete experimental spike foci. *Neurology.* 1981;31:846–851.

63. Morrell F, Whisler W. Multiple subpial transection: technique, results and pitfalls. *Jpn J Neurosurg.* 1993;12:101–107.

64. Morrell F. Electrophysiology of CSWS in Landau–Kleffner syndrome. In: Majno E, ed. *Continuous Spikes and Waves During Slow Sleep. Electrical Status Epilepticus During Slow Sleep Acquired Epileptic Aphasia and Related Conditions.* Milan, Italy: Mraiani Foundation; 1995:77–90.

65. Kanner AM, Kaydanova Y, de Toledo-Morrell L, et al. Tailored anterior temporal lobectomy: relation between effect of resection of mesial structures and post-surgical seizure outcome. *Arch Neurol.* 1995;52:173–178.

66. Wyler AR, Wilkus RJ, Rotard SW, et al. Multiple subpial transection for partial seizures in sensorimotor cortex. *Neurosurgery.* 1995;37:1122–1128.

67. Engel J. Outcome with respect to epileptic seizures. In: Engel J Jr, ed. *Surgical Treatment of the Epilepsies.* New York, NY: Raven Press; 1987: 553–571.

68. Sawhney IMS, Robertson IJA, Polkey CE, et al. Multiple subpial transection: a review of 21 cases. *J Neurol Neurosurg Psychiatry.* 1995;58: 344–349.

69. Orbach D, Romanelli P, Devinsky O, et al. Late seizure recurrence after multiple subpial transections. *Epilepsia.* 2001;42:1316–1319.

70. Schramm J, Aliashkevich AF, Grunwald T. Multiple subpial transections: outcome and complications in 20 patients who did not undergo resection. *J Neurosurg.* 2002;97:39–47.

71. Zhao Q, Tian Z, Liu Z, et al. Evaluation of the combination of multiple subpial transection and other techniques for treatment of intractable epilepsy. *Chin Med J.* 2003;116(7):1004–1007.

72. Spencer SS, Schramm J, Wyler A, et al. Multiple subpial transection for intractable partial epilepsy: an international meta-analysis. *Epilepsia.* 2002;43(I2):141–145.

73. Pondal-Sordo M, Diosy D, Tellez-Zenteno JF, et al. Epilepsy surgery involving the sensory-motor cortex. *Brain.* 2006;129(pt 12):3307–3314.

74. Shimizu H, Maehara T. Neuronal disconnection for the surgical treatment of pediatric epilepsy. *Epilepsia.* 2000;41(suppl 9):28–30.

75. Benifla M, Otsubo H, Ochi A. Multple subpial transection in pediatric epilepsy: indications and outcomes. *Child's Nerv Syst.* 2006;22(8):992–998.

76. Shimizu H, Kawai K, Sunaga S, et al. Hippocampal transection for treatment of left temporal lobe epilepsy with preservation of verbal memory. *J Clin Neurosci.* 2006;13(3):322–328. [Epub 2006 Mar 6.]

77. Kanner AM, Byrne R, Van Slyke P, et al. Functional language recovery following a surgical treatment of Landau–Kleffner syndrome. *Neurology.* 2005;64:(suppl 1):A359.

78. Irwin K, Birch V, Lees J. Multiple subpial transection in Landau–Kleffner syndrome. *Dev Med and Child Neurol.* 2001;43:248–252.

79. Patel AA, Andrew RV, Torkelson R. Surgical treatment of intractable seizures with multilobar or bihemispheric seizure foci. *Surg Neurol.* 1997; 47:72–78.

80. D'Giano CH, Del CG, Pomata H, et al. Treatment of refractory partial status epilepticus with multiple subpial transection: case report. *Seizure.* 2001;10(5):382–385.

81. Ma X, Liporace J, O'Connor MJ, et al. Neurosurgical treatment of medically intractable status epilepticus. *Epilepsy Res.* 2001;46(1):33–38.

CHAPTER 89 ■ SPECIAL CONSIDERATIONS IN CHILDREN

AJAY GUPTA AND ELAINE WYLLIE

Surgery is a well-established treatment for children with medically intractable seizures (1–5). With education and training of pediatric neurology practitioners, broad acceptance of surgery as a promising option, and improved safety of pediatric anesthesia, neurosurgery and intensive care techniques, pediatric epilepsy surgery has truly emerged to be a mature discipline with growth of academic programs in most developed countries. Consequently, surgical experience and seizure outcome data after surgery in children have now been published from several centers around the world, and results are encouraging from pediatric series involving infants and young children (1,3,6–11) and adolescents (12–17). There have been collaborative efforts to study pediatric epilepsy surgery practices and outcomes gathering data from programs in the United States, Europe, and Australia (18). However, identification of appropriate pediatric surgical candidates, especially infants and children, remains a challenge because of complex interactions of several unique and age-related factors (4,19).

In this chapter, we focus our discussion on these unique and age-related differences that interplay in the management of children who are likely to benefit from the surgical treatment of epilepsy. The step critical to surgical strategy in children as well as adults is the identification of a focal, resectable epileptogenic zone. Clues to the epileptogenic zone are found in seizure symptomatology, electroencephalography (EEG), and neuroimaging results. Some aspects of these features are similar to those in adult candidates, whereas others are unique to infants and children.

Table 89.1 compares common findings during diagnostic evaluation of pediatric and adult patients for epilepsy surgery.

SEIZURE SEMIOLOGY DURING VIDEO-EEG IN INFANTS AND CHILDREN

Clinical features of focal seizures may differ in pediatric and adult surgical candidates. Independent studies (20–23) of videotaped seizures from patients at separate institutions indicated that the classification of epileptic seizures of the International League Against Epilepsy (23), originally reflecting experience in older patients, was not applicable to infants younger than 3 years of age. In one study by Acharya and colleagues (20), only 3 of 21 infants had unmistakable characteristics of localized seizure onset, including clonic jerking of one extremity. In the remaining patients, seizures consisted of a decrease in behavioral motor activity with indeterminate level of consciousness and minimal or no automatisms, arising

from temporal or temporoparietal regions, or bilateral tonic stiffening sometimes preceded by bilateral eyelid blinking, arising from frontal or frontoparietal regions. In another study of 77 children with temporal lobe epilepsy examining the relationships between etiology, age at onset and electroclinical findings, auras were typically clear after the age of 6 years, and initial ictal symptomatology consisted of staring with behavior arrest, lip cyanosis, and bland or subtle oral automatisms again reiterating the lack of clear lateralizing or localizing semiology (24). Other authors (21,25) have also noted bilateral motor phenomena during partial seizures in infants. The mechanism is unknown but may include ictal activation of subcortical regions or of the supplementary sensorimotor area. A localized EEG seizure pattern clarifies the focal nature of the epileptogenic process.

Seizure characteristics signaling localized onset in older patients may be absent or unidentifiable in infants. For example, an aura is an important clue to focal onset in older children and adults, but sensory phenomena are difficult to detect and are rarely observed during video-EEG studies in infants (20). Clinical seizure onset may be difficult to notice, especially in mentally impaired young children, and this may create a challenge during diagnostic evaluation like video-EEG and ictal single photon emission computed tomography (SPECT) (26,27). Complex gestural automatisms and altered awareness are hallmarks of many partial seizures in older patients, but assessment of the ictal level of consciousness in infants is fraught with problems, and automatisms, when present, tend to be simple, bland, and predominantly oral. In infants, distinguishing automatisms from normal background behavioral activity can be difficult (20,21).

SCALP EEG PATTERNS, INFANTILE SPASMS, AND FOCAL CORTICAL LESIONS

Within the first 2 years of life, focal cortical lesions may manifest as infantile spasms and hypsarrhythmia (7,28–30). The spasms may be intermixed with partial seizures (Fig. 89.1) or may replace a previous partial seizure type altogether, becoming the only active seizure type (Fig. 89.2). The mechanism is unknown, but a clue may be the relationship between age of onset of spasms and location of the lesion. Koo and Hwang (31) found that spasms began earliest in patients with occipital lesions (mean age, 3 months), appeared later in patients with centrotemporoparietal lesions (mean age, 6 months), and occurred latest in patients with frontal lesions (mean age,

TABLE 89.1

COMMONLY ENCOUNTERED DIFFERENCES DURING DIAGNOSTIC EVALUATION AND SURGICAL DECISION MAKING IN PEDIATRIC AND ADULT PATIENTS

Characteristic findings	Infants/young children	Adult patients
History, seizure semiology, and examination		
Specific auras	Rare (unable to communicate)	Common
Seizure semiology	Stereotypic (like "epileptic spasms" or "bland stare")	May indicate symptomatogenic zone
Clinical seizure onset, ictal examination, postseizure recall	Unable or difficult to confirm	Easier
Ictal lateralizing features	Uncommon or unreliable	Common and reliable
Neurologic deficit on examination	Difficult to elicit (mild hemiparesis, visual fields)	Easy to elicit
Neuropsychological testing for surgical risk	Less objective (due to age, severe cognitive and behavior difficulties)	Helpful in pointing to specific deficits
Scalp EEG patterns		
Confounding factor of developmental EEG evolution	Present	Absent
Stereotypic and nonlocalizing interictal and ictal patterns	Common (hypsarrhythmia, generalized discharges)	Absent or uncommon
Imaging and pathologic substrates		
Confounding factor of developmental brain MRI changes	Present	Absent
Ictal SPECT	Difficult (brief frequent seizures, clusters, difficult ictal onset)	Easier
Common location and extent of lesions	Extratemporal large lesions	Temporal, smaller lesions
Common etiologies	Congenital (cortical dysplasia, malformation, tumor, perinatal stroke)	Hippocampal sclerosis, focal cortical dysplasia
Surgical considerations		
Morbidity and mortality	Higher (due to age, weight, larger resections, coexisting disabilities)	Lower
Timing and best techniques for surgery	More controversial and require planning and experience	Less controversial
Invasive mapping (intracranial grids or depth electrodes)	Not practical in most infants and young children	Possible
Intraoperative neurophysiologic techniques	Limited utility, more challenging in infants	Very useful
Goals of surgery/successful seizure control	Cognitive improvement, schooling, behavior, productive adult life	Job, driving, independence

EEG, electroencephalographic; MRI, magnetic resonance imaging; SPECT, single photon emission computed tomography.

10 months). This timing coincides with maturation in those regions; rapid increases in synaptic density and sequential myelination that proceed from the back to the front of the brain. Infantile spasms appear to result from an age-related pathologic interaction between a focal cortical lesion and normal developmental processes.

Chugani and colleagues (8,32,33) first emphasized the role of positron emission tomography (PET) and magnetic resonance imaging (MRI) in identifying focal cortical lesions in children with infantile spasms and hypsarrhythmia, describing several patients with cessation or dramatic reduction of seizures after cortical resection or hemispherectomy. Their experience has been replicated elsewhere (3,30). In that 65% of affected children are free of seizures after surgery (7), infantile spasms are not predictive of poor outcome. However, the

identification of appropriate surgical candidates may be complicated by the absence of focal EEG seizure patterns in the setting of spasms with diffuse electrodecrements.

The goal of the presurgical evaluation in patients with infantile spasms is to identify a region of cortical abnormality. The most common finding for surgical planning in this setting is a unilateral lobar, multilobar, or a hemispheric epileptogenic lesion on MRI or PET, usually a malformation of cortical development or encephalomalacia following perinatal cerebral infarction or ischemia. Helpful EEG findings may include a predominance of interictal sharp waves over one region; localized slowing, decreased background activity, or absent sleep spindles over the affected region or hemisphere; unilateral electrodecremental events; asymmetric EEG seizures; or a history of partial seizures (4). Neurologic examination may show evidence of unilateral hemispheric dysfunction with decreased spontaneous movement of one arm (hemiparesis) or gaze preference to one side (homonymous hemianopia).

Generalized epileptiform discharges on scalp EEG in the presence of a congenital or early-acquired focal lesion are not limited to infants. Recently, two reports from Cleveland Clinic described older children and adolescents with a unilateral or strongly asymmetric focal or hemispheric epileptogenic lesion who presented with generalized interictal abnormalities and ictal scalp EEG patterns (34,35). Initially, many of these children were rejected for surgical treatment owing to the presence of generalized EEG findings and lack of localizing

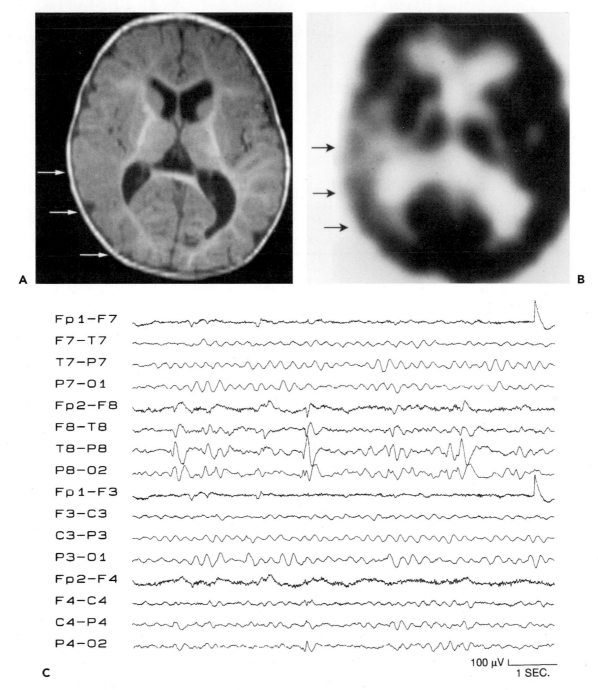

FIGURE 89.1 *Case 1.* (All images are of the same patient.) A: Axial magnetic resonance image from an 8-month-old boy, showing focal malformation of cortical development in the right temporo-occipital region *(arrows)*. Findings were subtle and included decreased arborization of the white matter and thickened, poorly sulcated cortex. Seizures began 14 hours after an unremarkable term birth and occurred 20 to 30 times per day. The boy was otherwise normal except for developmental delay. B: 2-[18F]fluoro-2-deoxy-D-glucose positron emission tomography scan at age 8 months, showing glucose hypometabolism in the right temporo-occipital region *(arrows)*. C: Interictal electroencephalogram at age 8 months, showing right posterior temporal sharp waves (maximum at the T8 and P8 electrodes), slowing, and decreased background activity.

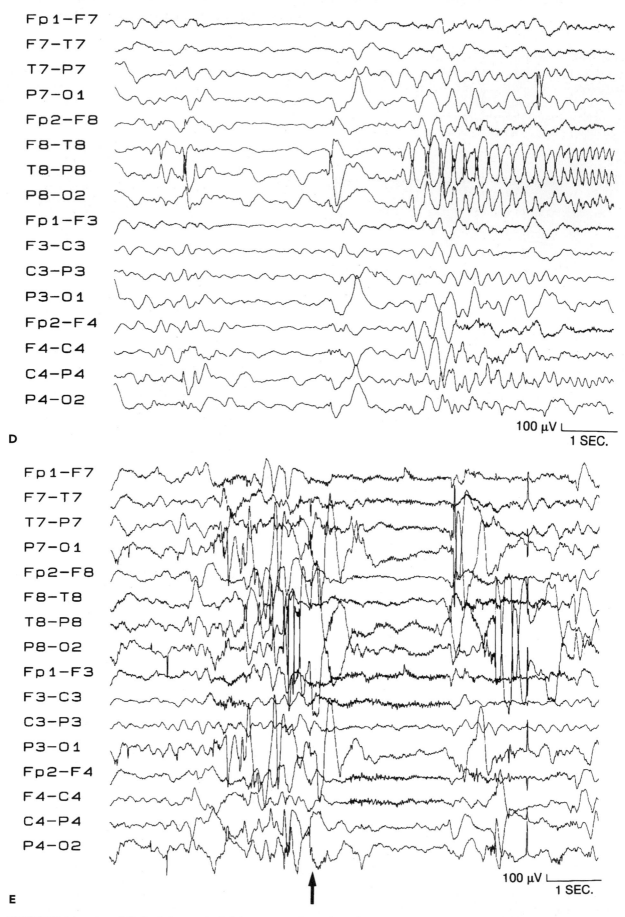

FIGURE 89.1 (*continued*) D: Ictal electroencephalogram at age 8 months with seizure pattern maximum in the right posterior temporal region (T8 electrode). Seizures involved bilateral clonic eyelid blinking, rhythmic interruption of crying, and bilateral clonic arm twitching. E: Ictal electroencephalogram at age 8 months, showing diffuse electrodecrement (*arrow*, preceded and followed by movement artifact) during an asymmetric spasm with extension and elevation of both arms (left more than right) and tonic closure of the left eyelid.

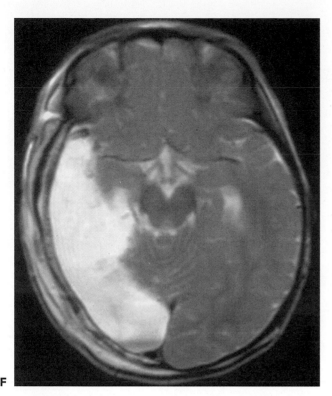

F

FIGURE 89.1 (*continued*) F: Magnetic resonance image showing the right temporo-occipital resection performed at age 22 months. Fourteen months later, the child still has developmental delay but remains free of seizures off all antiepileptic medication. (A and C–F are from Wyllie E. Surgical treatment of epilepsy in infants and children. *Can J Neurol Sci.* 2000;27:106–110, with permission.)

EEG data. Because of a high burden of seizures, failure of most treatment modalities, and minimal risk of new postoperative side effects, surgical treatment was generally offered as a last resort with resection of the brain MRI lesion or hemispherectomy in each case. Seizure-free outcome was obtained for 70% of these children with generalized or contralateral EEG abnormalities, and these results were similar to those in a comparison group of children with similar MRI lesions and localized EEG findings. On further analysis of the group with generalized video-EEG abnormalities, the rate of seizure freedom after resection of the lesion stood robust regardless of the presence or absence of focal ictal semiology, generalized slow spike and wave complexes, and proportion (30% to 100%) of the generalized or contralateral ictal and interictal epileptiform discharges (34). Postoperative EEG in seizure-free children typically showed resolution of the generalized or contralateral epileptiform discharges, which were often nearly continuous on preoperative EEG, especially during sleep.

A unifying feature in the Cleveland Clinic studies with generalized EEG was the early timing of the occurrence of the lesion seen on MRI, most commonly a malformation of cortical development or encephalomalacia following ischemia, infection, or trauma (34,35). Lesions were congenital or perinatal in 75% of patients, and acquired within the first 2 years of life or earlier in 90%. The latest timing of lesion acquisition in the series was 5 years. In contrast, the age at evaluation for

surgery ranged widely from infancy through young adulthood, with median at 8 years (34). Although mechanisms are unknown, the generalized epileptiform discharges seen later in childhood appear to result from complex early interactions between the epileptogenic lesion and the developing brain (34,35). These studies (34,35) highlight the limitations of scalp video-EEG in children, emphasize the importance of a brain MRI lesion, and show practical difficulties in establishing proof of focal epileptogenicity in some children before surgery. Therefore, in every child, the location of the focal epileptogenic zone must be preoperatively defined, whenever possible, by a convergence of results from clinical examination, video-EEG, anatomic, and functional neuroimaging, and other testing, while recognizing that in carefully selected cases with early MRI lesions, generalized EEG patterns may not contraindicate surgery (4).

ANATOMIC AND FUNCTIONAL NEUROIMAGING

Neuroimaging is a critical component of surgical strategy at every age. A focal epileptogenic lesion on the MRI seems to indicate a better prognosis for seizure-free outcome. In the Cleveland Clinic pediatric series from 1990 to 1996 (3), 54% of patients were seizure free and 19% had only rare seizures after extratemporal or multilobar resections. In contrast, in the Montreal Neurological Institute pediatric series (36) (excluding tumor cases) during the pre-MRI era between 1940 and 1980, only 27% had few or no seizures after frontal resection. The more favorable results from the Cleveland Clinic may be due to identification of a focal epileptogenic lesion on preoperative MRI in 85% of patients. Almost identical results were reported in an adult series of extratemporal resections performed in Bonn, Germany, from 1987 to 1993, with 54% of patients free of seizures after surgery (37). Seizure-free outcome in that series was significantly more common in lesional than nonlesional cases, with 82% of lesions identified preoperatively by MRI. The absence of MRI localization appears to be an unfavorable prognostic sign, although some patients may have good outcome after EEG-guided cortical resection. The yield of brain MRI, particularly in neocortical frontal and temporal lobe epilepsy, could be enhanced by use of high-resolution imaging with 3T magnets, specialized protocols with thin sections and surface coil MRI, and experience of the reader (38).

PET is also an important neuroimaging tool for pediatric epilepsy surgery. Chugani and colleagues found that a localized region of hypometabolism may identify focal cortical dysplasia even without abnormal features on MRI (7). This is especially helpful in infants because immature myelination challenges identification of subtle dysgenetic abnormalities of the gray-white junction on routine brain MRI protocols. PET scans using special tracers have been reported to be useful in some children with tuberous sclerosis (39). Ictal SPECT remains a challenging modality to use in children; however, it has been increasingly used in many centers in selected pediatric cases (26,40,41). Acquisition and interpretation of ictal SPECT in children are complicated as a result of several factors (26). First, interictal SPECT may be difficult to obtain owing to multiple daily seizures in this group of patients. Second, difficulty in promptly recognizing the clinical onset of

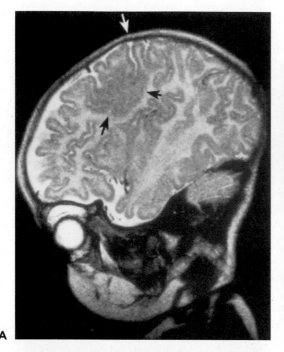

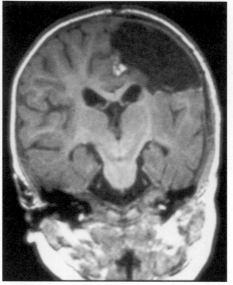

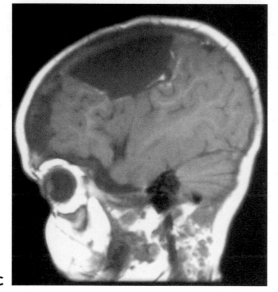

FIGURE 89.2 *Case 2.* **A:** Sagittal magnetic resonance image showing focal malformation of cortical development cerebral dysgenesis *(black arrow)* in the left posterior frontal lobe extending across the central sulcus *(white arrow)* into the anterior portion of the postcentral gyrus. The boy was 4 months old at the time of the magnetic resonance imaging, with intractable daily seizures since the first day of life after an uncomplicated full-term delivery. Seizures involved clonic jerking of the right arm and leg, with eye deviation toward the left, or opisthotonic posturing with stiffening and extension of all extremities. Ictal and interictal epileptiform discharges were localized to the left central region. Moderately severe right hemiparesis and mild developmental delay were also present. (From Wyllie E. Surgical treatment of epilepsy in children. *Pediatr Neurol.* 1998;19:179–188, with permission.) **B:** Coronal and (C) sagittal scans performed 2 days after cortical resection at age 9 months. Prior to resection, electroencephalographic seizure was recorded over the lesion with intraoperative electrocorticography, and primary hand motor cortex was identified in the same area by intraoperative cortical stimulation. Postoperatively, the hemiparesis was transiently minimally worse, returning to preoperative baseline within days. Twenty-two months later, the child is making developmental progress and has had no seizures on a reduced dose of antiepileptic medication.

ictal behavioral changes because of age and coexistent mental retardation may result in a late injection for an ictal SPECT. Third, some extratemporal seizures may be brief and spread rapidly. Fourth, children may require sedation on two occasions to obtain interictal and ictal scans. Newer noninvasive presurgical procedures, such as magnetoencephalography (MEG) and functional MRI (fMRI) are increasingly being used in children for source localization of interictal spikes (42–44) and mapping of language and motor function (fMRI) using standardized protocols (45). However, it remains to be seen if these techniques will independently expand the selection of pediatric surgical candidates, obviate the need for invasive video-EEG recordings, and improve the long-term surgical outcome in children.

ETIOLOGIES AND PATHOLOGIC SUBSTRATES OF EPILEPSY IN PEDIATRIC PATIENTS

Causes of epilepsy differ in children and adults. Figure 89.3 depicts the usual age of onset and common etiologies/pathologic substrates encountered in children with epilepsy. Hippocampal sclerosis, the most common etiologic factor in adult candidates for epilepsy surgery, is uncommon in children. In a multicenter, predominantly adult series (2), 73% of 5446 epilepsy surgeries (excluding corpus callosotomies) were performed for nonlesional temporal lobe epilepsy, including hippocampal sclerosis. In contrast, in a pediatric epilepsy surgery series

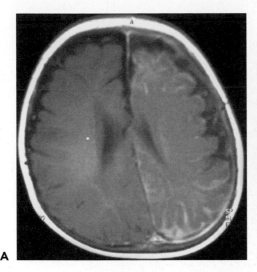 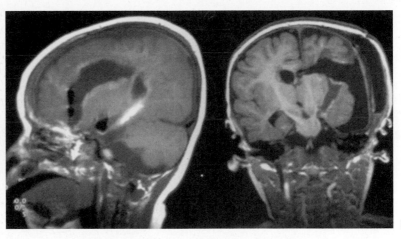

FIGURE 89.3 *Case 3.* **A:** Axial magnetic resonance image at age 12 months, showing Sturge–Weber malformation with left hemispheric atrophy and pial angiomatosis. Starting at age 2 months, seizures occurred once or twice per day characterized by jerking of the right arm or decreased behavioral activity with bilateral eye blinking and lip smacking. Physical examination revealed right hemiparesis, right hemianopia, and developmental delay. Ictal and interictal epileptiform abnormalities were seen in multiple areas of the left hemisphere. **B:** Sagittal (**left**) and coronal (**right**) magnetic resonance images showing the left hemispheric disconnection performed at age 12 months. No seizures occurred during the 8 months since surgery on a reduced dose of antiepileptic medications. Surgery did not worsen neurologic deficits, and the child has progressed developmentally.

from the Cleveland Clinic Foundation (3), hippocampal sclerosis was the cause in only 12% of 62 children (3 months to 12 years of age) and in 15% of 74 adolescents (13 to 20 years of age). Although hippocampal sclerosis may begin in childhood, the typical presentation for surgical evaluation is in early adulthood. When hippocampal sclerosis occurs in pediatric candidates for epilepsy surgery, the clinical and EEG features may be similar to those in adults (46). However, pediatric patients appear to have an especially high incidence of dual pathology with cortical dysplasia in addition to the hippocampal sclerosis (46).

In pediatric candidates, the predominant etiologic factors are focal, multilobar or extensive hemispheric malformation of cortical development (cortical dysplasia) (Figs. 89.1, 89.4, and 89.5), and low-grade tumor (3,47). These were the cause of the epilepsy in 57% of adolescents, 70% of children, 90% of infants younger than 3 years in the Cleveland Clinic series (3), and 90% of infants treated surgically in the series of Duchowny and colleagues (1). Less common causes are vascular malformation, arachnoid cyst, and localized injury due to infarction, trauma, or infection (1,3).

Hemispheric syndromes are also important etiologies in children undergoing epilepsy surgery in the form of hemispherectomy (47). Hemispheric malformations of cortical development like hemimegalencephaly (Fig. 89.5), Sturge–Weber syndrome (Fig. 89.6), and perinatal unilateral cerebral ischemic insults are the most common etiologic factors in children and adolescents who had hemispheric ablation procedures, with Rasmussen chronic focal encephalitis occurring less frequently (3,47,48).

The age-related differences in etiology result in an age-related spectrum of surgical procedures. Anteromesial temporal resections predominate in adults but not in children. In pediatric series, extratemporal or multilobar resections or hemispherectomies composed 44% of the surgeries in adolescents, 50% in children, and 90% in infants (1,3).

SURGICAL CONSIDERATIONS IN PEDIATRIC PATIENTS

Identification of Candidates: The Timing of Surgery

Critical features of surgical candidacy at any age include intractable epilepsy interfering with quality of life or development, clear identification of a localized epileptogenic zone, and low risk for new postoperative neurologic deficits. However, for each of these factors, age-related issues must be considered in light of results from an extensive presurgical evaluation. The risk of proceeding with surgery must be weighed against the risk of continuing with uncontrolled seizures treated medically. If careful analysis yields a favorable risk/benefit ratio for surgery, then the available data suggest that it is appropriate to proceed regardless of age.

The usual delay from onset of seizure intractability to surgery is still in the range of 12 to 15 years at most centers, reflecting a reluctance to consider surgery during childhood. Results from pediatric series do not justify this reluctance but instead suggest that children should be referred for surgical evaluation at whatever age they present with severe focal epilepsy. Complicated cases warrant referral to specialized centers with extensive pediatric experience.

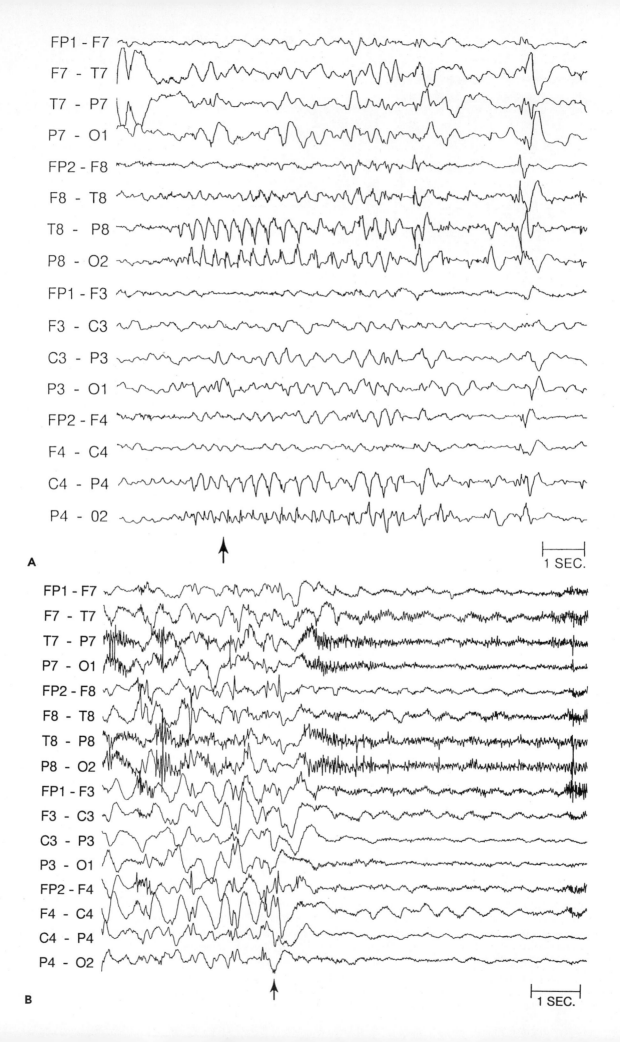

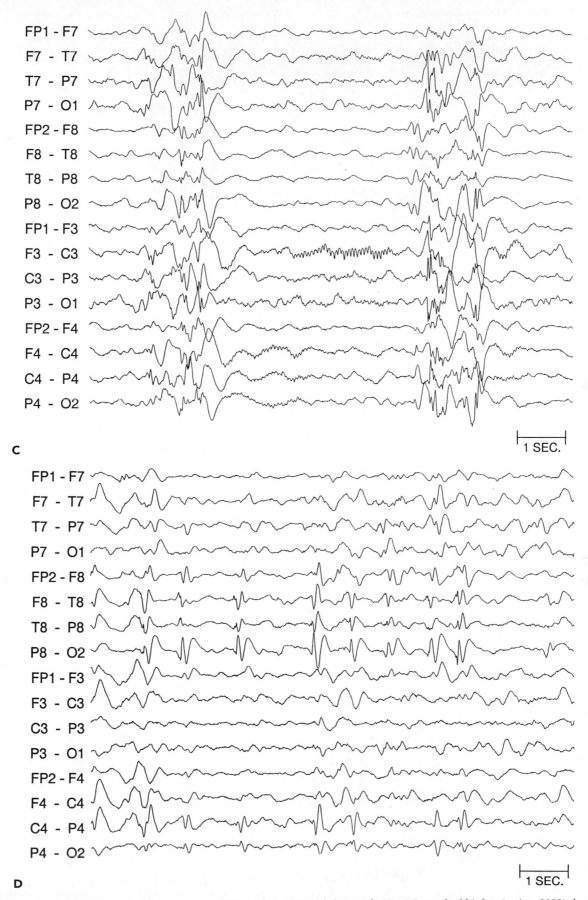

C

1 SEC.

D

1 SEC.

FIGURE 89.4 *Case 4.* (All images are of the same patient.) **A:** Ictal electroencephalogram from a 4.5-month-old infant (patient 2089) showing right parietal onset of a partial seizure *(arrow)*. Seizures began at age 2 months and occurred several times a day. **B:** Ictal electroencephalogram at age 13 months, showing hypsarrhythmia with diffuse electrodecrement at the onset of an infantile spasm *(arrow)*. Evolution from partial seizures to infantile spasms occurred at age 7 months. The infant had delayed cognitive development and reduced visual attentiveness but no motor deficits. **C:** Sleep spindles were consistently reduced over the right hemisphere, providing further evidence of right hemisphere dysfunction. **D:** This carefully selected segment of the interictal electroencephalogram shows that spikes were sometimes predominant over the right parietal region, despite the diffuse hypsarrhythmic pattern during most of the recording. Normal faster frequencies were reduced in that area.

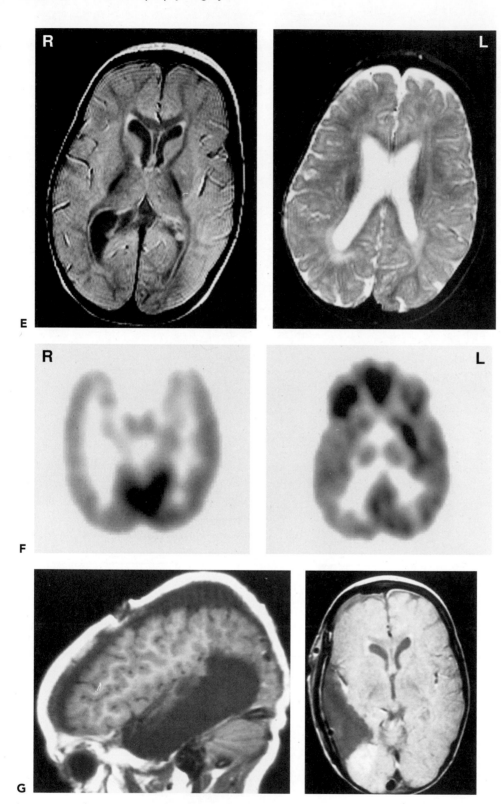

FIGURE 89.4 (*continued*) **E:** Magnetic resonance imaging (MRI) at 13 months showed bilateral periventricular leukomalacia, worse in the right parietal region. The findings could have resulted from intrauterine right germinal matrix hemorrhage several weeks before the uneventful term birth. No cortical dysplasia or gyral abnormality was evident on MRI. **F:** Interictal 2-[^{18}F]fluoro-2-deoxy-D-glucose positron emission tomography at 13 months showing right parieto-occipitotemporal hypometabolism. **G:** Postoperative MRI showing the right parieto-occipitotemporal resection performed at age 15 months. Histopathologic analysis of resected tissue revealed microscopic cortical dysplasia, possibly as a result of disturbance of late neuronal migration at the time of the intrauterine intraventricular hemorrhage. The infant remains free of seizures 17 months after operation and has made "catch-up" developmental progress. (**A, B, E,** and **F** are from Wyllie E, Comair Y, Ruggieri P, et al. Epilepsy surgery in the setting of periventricular leukomalacia and focal cortical dysplasia. *Neurology.* 1996;46:839–841, with permission; **A** and **G** are from Wyllie E, Comair YG, Kotagal P, et al. Epilepsy surgery in infants. *Epilepsia.* 1996;37: 625–637, with permission.)

Goals of Epilepsy Surgery in Children and Adolescents

The goals of epilepsy surgery may vary according to age. In adolescents and adults, the main goals are usually related to driving, independence, and employment, and their achievement requires complete postoperative freedom from seizures.

For infants and children, the goals often center on relief of catastrophic epilepsy, resumption of developmental progression, and improvement in behavior. These goals may sometimes be reached even in the absence of complete freedom from seizures. For infants and young children with many daily seizures and developmental stagnation or regression, a postoperative outcome with rare or infrequent seizures and resumption of developmental progression may be gratifying.

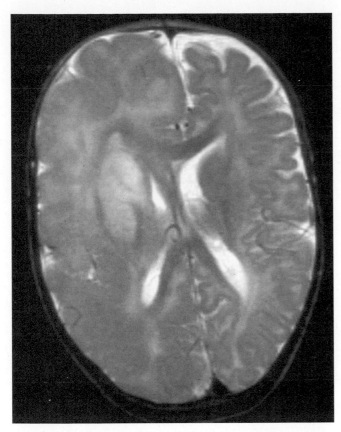

FIGURE 89.5 T2-weighted sagittal image of "typical" hemimegalencephaly showing diffuse right hemispheric enlargement and dysplasia. Midline shift with bulging of anterior falx to the left and compression of the right lateral ventricle suggest a mass effect as a result of increased volume of the brain parenchyma. Dysplastic changes are diffuse, with thick and disorganized cortex, poor gray-white matter differentiation, and abnormal signal in the white matter. Note that the basal ganglia are also dysplastic with abnormal increased signal.

Even in the less-favorable-outcome group with malformation of cortical development, 68% of patients in the Cleveland Clinic series had few or no seizures after surgery (3).

In pediatric practice, developmental outcome is of paramount importance. Developmental delay is common in pediatric epilepsy surgery candidates, especially infants. Duchowny and associates noted normal preoperative development in only 20% of infant candidates for epilepsy surgery, whereas the remainder had moderate (52%) or severe (28%) delay (1). Postoperatively, the developmentally normal infants remained normal after surgery, whereas the severely delayed infants remained severely delayed. Parents reported cognitive and social gains in children with seizure-free outcome, although these were difficult to appreciate on examination (1). Other researchers have made similar observations (7,28).

In a series of infants who had epilepsy surgery at the Cleveland Clinic (49), the developmental quotient indicated modest postoperative improvement in mental age. Developmental status before surgery predicted developmental function after surgery, and patients who were operated on at younger age and with epileptic spasms showed the largest increase in developmental quotient after surgery (49). These results suggest that early surgery for refractory epilepsy may offer an opportunity for improved developmental outcome.

Seizures that begin in the first few years of life, regardless of etiology, constitute a risk factor for mental retardation (50–52). Early surgical intervention may reduce this risk, but quantitative and prospectively collected data are scant. Asarnow and colleagues studied results of the Vineland assessment in 24 patients with infantile spasms who underwent focal cortical resection or hemispherectomy at a mean age of 21 months (53). Raw scores 2 years after surgery increased significantly compared with preoperative levels, although only four children had a normal rate of development. The Adjusted Behavioral Composite scores were significantly higher for

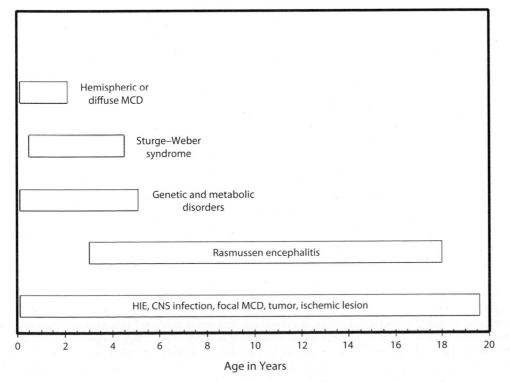

Hemispheric or diffuse MCD

Sturge–Weber syndrome

Genetic and metabolic disorders

Rasmussen encephalitis

HIE, CNS infection, focal MCD, tumor, ischemic lesion

0   2   4   6   8   10   12   14   16   18   20

Age in Years

FIGURE 89.6 Usual age of seizure onset and common etiologies/pathologic substrates often encountered in children with epilepsy. (Modified from Gupta A, Wyllie E. Presurgical evaluation in children with catastrophic epilepsy. In: Luders H, Rosenow F, eds. *Presurgical Assessment of the Epilepsies With Clinical Neurophysiology and Functional Imaging.* Amsterdam: Elsevier; 2004:451–459.)

children who had higher preoperative scores or earlier surgery. Surgery within the first year of life may therefore maximize developmental outcome by allowing resumption of developmental progression during critical stages of brain maturation (53). A more recent study (54) on cognitive outcome of hemispherectomy in 53 children who underwent presurgical and postsurgical testing reported moderate cognitive and behavioral improvement in most patients. The most significant predictor of cognitive skills after surgery was etiology, with dysplasia patients scoring lowest in intelligence and language but not in visual-motor skills (54). Other studies have also reported similar improvements in the cognitive and behavior spheres after hemispherectomy (55–57).

Psychosocial outcome may also be better after earlier surgery. At the advent of epilepsy surgery, Falconer urged that adolescents be considered for operative treatment before the end of secondary school so that they could pass more normally through the maturational stages of early adulthood (13). In patients who had temporal resection for childhood-onset epilepsy and were studied after a mean interval of 15 years, Mizrahi and colleagues noted that later surgery was associated with greater permanent psychosocial, behavioral, and educational problems (58). Delaying surgery for childhood-onset epilepsy may have disadvantages.

Age-Related Risks of Epilepsy Surgery

The extensive multilobar and hemispheric surgeries performed in children and adolescents may carry some risk. In the Cleveland Clinic series (3), 2 of 149 patients (1.3%) died immediately after surgery, and Paolicchi and colleagues (11) reported 1 postoperative death among 83 patients (1.2%) in a pediatric series from Miami Children's Hospital. Mortality may be slightly higher for infants, in part because of their small blood volumes. One or two infant deaths were reported in surgery series from UCLA (33), Johns Hopkins Medical Center (59,60), and Miami Children's Hospital (1,11). These results emphasize the need to reserve surgery for infants with severe epilepsy. Risk may be reduced by a dedicated team of pediatric anesthesiologists, intensivists, and surgeons.

At any age, the mortality from epilepsy surgery must be weighed against the mortality from uncontrolled seizures treated medically. Nashef and associates (61) found this risk to be 1:295 per year in children and adolescents with severe epilepsy and learning disabilities. In a population-based cohort study in children (62) (1 to 16 years of age) who developed epilepsy between 1977 and 1985, 26 (3.8%) of 692 children died by the year 1999. The majority (13/26) who died had secondarily generalized seizures. Neurologic deficit was the only independent factor that determined mortality. In this study, mortality in children with comorbid neurologic deficits (15/1000 person-years) was higher than in those without any deficits (0.7/1000 person-years). Mortality in the children with seizures and no neurologic deficits was no different from that in the reference nonepileptic population. A Dutch study has reported similar results (63,64). These epidemiologic data reinforce consideration for early surgical intervention, as children with catastrophic partial epilepsy who are candidates for surgery often have neurologic deficits and secondarily generalized seizures. The increased long-term mortality from epilepsy in children can also be seen in outcome studies of epilepsy

surgery. During long-term follow-up, late death occurred in 2% of the Cleveland Clinic series (3) and in 11% of a series from Guldvog and associates involving patients with persistent seizures (14).

Other risks of epilepsy surgery, including new postoperative neurologic deficits (e.g., hemiparesis or language impairment), may be reduced in pediatric patients as a result of developmental plasticity. Language may transfer to the right hemisphere during the course of destructive processes such as Rasmussen chronic focal encephalitis or may develop in an unusual region of the left hemisphere in a congenital left frontal or posterotemporal tumor (65,66). In these cases, the epileptogenic lesion may be resected or disconnected without producing new language deficits. Motor function may also partially develop outside a damaged or malformed rolandic region, so that resection of a perirolandic lesion results in little or no additional postoperative motor deficit (see Fig. 89.4). Factors favoring developmental plasticity include early onset of the lesion (e.g., perinatal infarction or congenital malformation) and surgery performed within the first few years of life.

Decrements in postoperative verbal memory scores may follow left mesial temporal resection in adults, especially in individuals with high preoperative scores (67,68). Little is known about this potential complication in children, although similar risk factors were identified in a small pediatric series examining cognitive outcome after temporal lobe resection (69). It is not known whether the intracarotid amobarbital procedure can accurately predict this complication in children. Low memory retention scores may occur during this testing in a significant proportion of children (70), and withholding mesial temporal resection from otherwise favorable candidates on the basis of this finding alone may not be appropriate.

Seizure Outcome after Epilepsy Surgery

Published studies on surgical outcome are reliable but difficult to compare owing to the inclusion of patients with diverse pathologic conditions, use of different evaluation and surgical techniques, and variable definitions of postoperative outcome and follow-up. Good postoperative outcomes with rare or no seizures occur with similar frequencies at all ages, according to recent series in infants, children, adolescents, and adults, despite age-related differences in causes and surgery types (1,3,11,28,71,72). The likelihood of a favorable seizure outcome postoperatively does not diminish significantly, even in infancy. These results compare favorably with those achieved during controlled trials of new antiepileptic drugs, in which the rate of "responders" (at least 50% improvement in seizure frequency) was 20% to 40% and seizure freedom was fairly rare (73). More recent studies show only modest chances of seizure freedom (<5%) after failure of two antiepileptic medications and report no difference between established and newer antiepileptic drugs used as initial monotherapy (74).

Certain subgroups appear especially likely to be free of seizures after surgery. In the Cleveland Clinic pediatric series (3), this outcome was significantly more common in patients who had temporal resection (78%) than in those who had extratemporal or multilobar resection (54%). However, this difference based on surgery type disappeared when results were analyzed by etiologic factors. Significantly more patients with low-grade tumor (82%) than patients with malformation of cortical development (52%) were seizure free, regardless of whether the surgery was temporal (86% for tumor vs. 56% for dysplasia) or extratemporal/multilobar (75% for tumor vs. 50% for dysplasia). Duchowny and colleagues (1) noted that it is relatively meaningless to consider pediatric patients treated with temporal resection as a special-outcome subgroup because of the varied etiologic factors in younger patients. In children, surgically managed temporal lobe epilepsy is not synonymous with hippocampal sclerosis. However, in the pediatric patients who have hippocampal sclerosis, postoperative seizure outcome appears similar to that in adults. In a series of 34 children and adolescents with hippocampal sclerosis who had anteromesial temporal resection at the Cleveland Clinic for intractable temporal lobe epilepsy, 78% of patients were free of seizures after surgery (46).

Published series (48,55,56) in children who underwent hemispherectomy for any indication report seizure freedom rates in the range of 50% to 65% after a postoperative follow-up of 3 months to 22 years. Rates of seizure freedom were consistently lower in children who underwent hemispherectomy for congenital malformations than in children who had the procedure for acquired diseases like Rasmussen encephalitis and ischemic stroke (47). From 30% to 50% of children with hemispheric malformations of cortical development and 55% to 80% of those with acquired causes were seizure free after hemispherectomy. Few reports that analyzed seizure outcome in subgroups of patients with hemispheric malformations of cortical development showed higher rates (68% to 80%) of seizure freedom in partial (sparing anterior or posterior brain regions) or nonhemimegalencephalic (without excessive growth of the affected hemisphere) types compared with classic hemimegalencephaly (47).

CONCLUSIONS

All children with catastrophic epilepsy, regardless of age, must be promptly evaluated for diagnosis and surgical candidacy. The risk/benefit ratio should then be cautiously weighed for every child in light of several complex age-related issues discussed in this chapter. Young age entails special challenges for presurgical evaluation, but it also provides a great opportunity to attain early freedom from daily seizures and to achieve the maximum cognitive potential. Even in some older children, it is now evident that surgically treatable epilepsy due to focal congenital or early-acquired lesion may manifest with a "generalized EEG phenotype" and global epileptic encephalopathy posing challenges for surgical selection. Evaluation and treatment of complex cases are best done at specialized centers with extensive experience in pediatric epilepsy surgery.

References

1. Duchowny M, Jayakar P, Resnick T, et al. Epilepsy surgery in the first three years of life. *Epilepsia.* 1998;39:737–743.
2. Engel J Jr. Surgery for seizures. *N Engl J Med.* 1996;334:647–652.
3. Wyllie E, Comair YG, Kotagal P, et al. Seizure outcome after epilepsy surgery in children and adolescents. *Ann Neurol.* 1998;44:740–748.
4. Gupta A, Wyllie E. Presurgical evaluation in children with catastrophic epilepsy. In: Luders H, Rosenow F, eds. *Presurgical Assessment of the Epilepsies with Clinical Neurophysiology and Functional Imaging.* Amsterdam: Elsevier; 2004:451–459.
5. Wiebe S, Blume WT, Girvin JP, et al. A randomized, controlled trial of surgery for temporal-lobe epilepsy. *N Engl J Med.* 2001;345:311–318.
6. Adelson PD, Peacock WJ, Chugani HT, et al. Temporal and extended temporal resections for the treatment of intractable seizures in early childhood. *Pediatr Neurosurg.* 1992;18:169–178.
7. Chugani HT, Shewmon DA, Shields WD, et al. Surgery for intractable infantile spasms: neuroimaging perspectives. *Epilepsia.* 1993;34:764–771.
8. Chugani HT, Shields WD, Shewmon DA, et al. Infantile spasms: I. PET identifies focal cortical dysgenesis in cryptogenic cases for surgical treatment. *Ann Neurol.* 1990;27:406–413.
9. Duchowny MS, Resnick TJ, Alvarez LA, et al. Focal resection for malignant partial seizures in infancy. *Neurology.* 1990;40:980–984.
10. Peacock WJ, Wehby-Grant MC, Shields WD, et al. Hemispherectomy for intractable seizures in children: a report of 58 cases. *Childs Nerv Syst.* 1996;12:376–384.
11. Paolicchi JM, Jayakar P, Dean P, et al. Predictors of outcome in pediatric epilepsy surgery. *Neurology.* 2000;54:642–647.
12. Davidson S, Falconer MA. Outcome of surgery in 40 children with temporal-lobe epilepsy. *Lancet.* 1975;1:1260–1263.
13. Falconer MA. Significance of surgery for temporal lobe epilepsy in childhood and adolescence. *J Neurosurg.* 1970;33:233–252.
14. Guldvog B, Loyning Y, Hauglie-Hanssen E, et al. Surgical treatment for partial epilepsy among norwegian children and adolescents. *Epilepsia.* 1994;35:554–565.
15. Meyer FB, Marsh WR, Laws ER Jr, et al. Temporal lobectomy in children with epilepsy. *J Neurosurg.* 1986;64:371–376.
16. Polkey CE. Selection of patients with intractable epilepsy for resective surgery. *Arch Dis Child.* 1980;55:841–844.
17. Whittle IR, Ellis HJ, Simpson DA. The surgical treatment of intractable childhood and adolescent epilepsy. *Aust N Z J Surg.* 1981;51:190–196.
18. Harvey AS, Cross JH, Shinnar S, et al. Defining the spectrum of international practice in pediatric epilepsy surgery patients. *Epilepsia.* 2008;49:146–155.
19. Wyllie E. Surgical treatment of epilepsy in children. *Pediatr Neurol.* 1998;19:179–188.
20. Acharya JN, Wyllie E, Luders HO, et al. Seizure symptomatology in infants with localization-related epilepsy. *Neurology.* 1997;48:189–196.
21. Nordli DR Jr, Bazil CW, Scheuer ML, et al. Recognition and classification of seizures in infants. *Epilepsia.* 1997;38:553–560.
22. Hamer HM, Wyllie E, Luders HO, et al. Symptomatology of epileptic seizures in the first three years of life. *Epilepsia.* 1999;40:837–844.
23. Proposal for revised clinical and electroencephalographic classification of epileptic seizures. from the commission on classification and terminology of the international league against epilepsy. *Epilepsia.* 1981;22:489–501.
24. Fontana E, Negrini F, Francione S, et al. Temporal lobe epilepsy in children: electroclinical study of 77 cases. *Epilepsia.* 2006;47(suppl 5):26–30.
25. Dravet C, Catani C, Bureau M, et al. Partial epilepsies in infancy: a study of 40 cases. *Epilepsia.* 1989;30:807–812.
26. Gupta A, Raja S, Kotagal P, et al. Ictal SPECT in children with partial epilepsy due to focal cortical dysplasia. *Pediatr Neurol.* 2004;31:89–95.
27. Lawson JA, O'Brien TJ, Bleasel AF, et al. Evaluation of SPECT in the assessment and treatment of intractable childhood epilepsy. *Neurology.* 2000;55:1391–1393.
28. Wyllie E, Comair YG, Kotagal P, et al. Epilepsy surgery in infants. *Epilepsia.* 1996;37:625–637.
29. Asanuma H, Wakai S, Tanaka T, et al. Brain tumors associated with infantile spasms. *Pediatr Neurol.* 1995;12:361–364.
30. Brockhaus A, Elger CE. Complex partial seizures of temporal lobe origin in children of different age groups. *Epilepsia.* 1995;36:1173–1181.
31. Koo B, Hwang P. Localization of focal cortical lesions influences age of onset of infantile spasms. *Epilepsia.* 1996;37:1068–1071.
32. Chugani HT, Shewmon DA, Sankar R, et al. Infantile spasms: II. Lenticular nuclei and brain stem activation on positron emission tomography. *Ann Neurol.* 1992;31:212–219.
33. Chugani HT, Shewmon DA, Peacock WJ, et al. Surgical treatment of intractable neonatal-onset seizures: the role of positron emission tomography. *Neurology.* 1988;38:1178–1188.
34. Wyllie E, Lachhwani DK, Gupta A, et al. Successful surgery for epilepsy due to early brain lesions despite generalized EEG findings. *Neurology.* 2007;69:389–397.
35. Gupta A, Chirla A, Wyllie E, et al. Pediatric epilepsy surgery in focal lesions and generalized electroencephalogram abnormalities. *Pediatr Neurol.* 2007;37:8–15.
36. Fish DR, Smith SJ, Quesney LF, et al. Surgical treatment of children with medically intractable frontal or temporal lobe epilepsy: results and highlights of 40 years' experience. *Epilepsia.* 1993;34:244–247.
37. Zentner J, Hufnagel A, Ostertun B, et al. Surgical treatment of extratemporal epilepsy: clinical, radiologic, and histopathologic findings in 60 patients. *Epilepsia.* 1996;37:1072–1080.
38. Grant PE, Barkovich AJ, Wald LL, et al. High-resolution surface-coil MR of cortical lesions in medically refractory epilepsy: a prospective study. *Am J Neuroradiol.* 1997;18:291–301.
39. Chugani DC, Chugani HT, Muzik O, et al. Imaging epileptogenic tubers in children with tuberous sclerosis complex using alpha-[11C]methyl-L-tryptophan positron emission tomography. *Ann Neurol.* 1998;44:858–866.
40. Koh S, Jayakar P, Resnick T, et al. The localizing value of ictal SPECT in children with tuberous sclerosis complex and refractory partial epilepsy. *Epileptic Disord.* 1999;1:41–46.

41. Vera P, Kaminska A, Cieuta C, et al. Use of subtraction ictal SPECT co-registered to MRI for optimizing the localization of seizure foci in children. *J Nucl Med.* 1999;40:786–792.

42. RamachandranNair R, Otsubo H, Shroff MM, et al. MEG predicts outcome following surgery for intractable epilepsy in children with normal or nonfocal MRI findings. *Epilepsia.* 2007;48:149–157.

43. Otsubo H, Ochi A, Elliott I, et al. MEG predicts epileptic zone in lesional extrahippocampal epilepsy: 12 pediatric surgery cases. *Epilepsia.* 2001;42: 1523–1530.

44. Ochi A, Otsubo H, Iida K, et al. Identifying the primary epileptogenic hemisphere from electroencephalographic (EEG) and magnetoencephalographic dipole lateralizations in children with intractable epilepsy. *J Child Neurol.* 2005;20:885–892.

45. Gaillard WD, Berl MM, Moore EN, et al. Atypical language in lesional and nonlesional complex partial epilepsy. *Neurology.* 2007;69:1761–1771.

46. Mohamed A, Wyllie E, Ruggieri P, et al. Temporal lobe epilepsy due to hippocampal sclerosis in pediatric candidates for epilepsy surgery. *Neurology.* 2001;56:1643–1649.

47. Gupta A, Carreno M, Wyllie E, et al. Hemispheric malformations of cortical development. *Neurology.* 2004;62:S20–S26.

48. Gonzalez-Martinez JA, Gupta A, Kotagal P, et al. Hemispherectomy for catastrophic epilepsy in infants. *Epilepsia.* 2005;46:1518–1525.

49. Loddenkemper T, Holland KD, Stanford LD, et al. Developmental outcome after epilepsy surgery in infancy. *Pediatrics.* 2007;119:930–935.

50. Dikmen S, Matthews CG, Harley JP. Effect of early versus late onset of major motor epilepsy on cognitive-intellectual performance: further considerations. *Epilepsia.* 1977;18:31–36.

51. Klove H, Matthews CG. Neuropsychological evaluation of the epileptic patient. *Wis Med J.* 1969;68:296–301.

52. Huttenlocher PR, Hapke RJ. A follow-up study of intractable seizures in childhood. *Ann Neurol.* 1990;28:699–705.

53. Asarnow RF, LoPresti C, Guthrie D, et al. Developmental outcomes in children receiving resection surgery for medically intractable infantile spasms. *Dev Med Child Neurol.* 1997;39:430–440.

54. Pulsifer MB, Brandt J, Salorio CF, et al. The cognitive outcome of hemispherectomy in 71 children. *Epilepsia.* 2004;45:243–254.

55. Taha JM, Crone KR, Berger TS. The role of hemispherectomy in the treatment of holohemispheric hemimegaloencephaly. *J Neurosurg.* 1994;81: 37–42.

56. Kossoff EH, Vining EP, Pillas DJ, et al. Hemispherectomy for intractable unihemispheric epilepsy etiology vs outcome. *Neurology.* 2003;61: 887–890.

57. Maehara T, Shimizu H, Kawai K, et al. Postoperative development of children after hemispherotomy. *Brain Dev.* 2002;24:155–160.

58. Mizrahi EM, Kellaway P, Grossman RG, et al. Anterior temporal lobectomy and medically refractory temporal lobe epilepsy of childhood. *Epilepsia.* 1990;31:302–312.

59. Vining EP, Freeman JM, Pillas DJ, et al. Why would you remove half a brain? The outcome of 58 children after hemispherectomy—the Johns Hopkins experience: 1968 to 1996. *Pediatrics.* 1997;100:163–171.

60. Kossoff EH, Vining EP, Pyzik PL, et al. The postoperative course and management of 106 hemidecortications. *Pediatr Neurosurg.* 2002;37:298–303.

61. Nashef L, Fish DR, Garner S, et al. Sudden death in epilepsy: a study of incidence in a young cohort with epilepsy and learning difficulty. *Epilepsia.* 1995;36:1187–1194.

62. Camfield CS, Camfield PR, Veugelers PJ. Death in children with epilepsy: a population-based study. *Lancet.* 2002;359:1891–1895.

63. Appleton RE. Mortality in paediatric epilepsy. *Arch Dis Child.* 2003;88: 1091–1094.

64. Callenbach PM, Westendorp RG, Geerts AT, et al. Mortality risk in children with epilepsy: the Dutch study of epilepsy in childhood. *Pediatrics.* 2001;107:1259–1263.

65. Janszky J, Ebner A, Kruse B, et al. Functional organization of the brain with malformations of cortical development. *Ann Neurol.* 2003;53: 759–767.

66. DeVos KJ, Wyllie E, Geckler C, et al. Language dominance in patients with early childhood tumors near left hemisphere language areas. *Neurology.* 1995;45:349–356.

67. Chelune GJ, Naugle RI, Luders H, et al. Prediction of cognitive change as a function of preoperative ability status among temporal lobectomy patients seen at 6-month follow-up. *Neurology.* 1991;41:399–404.

68. Seidenberg M, Hermann B, Wyler AR, et al. Neuropsychological outcome following anterior temporal lobectomy in patients with and without the syndrome of mesial temporal lobe epilepsy. *Neuropsychology.* 1998;12: 303–316.

69. Szabo CA, Wyllie E, Stanford LD, et al. Neuropsychological effect of temporal lobe resection in preadolescent children with epilepsy. *Epilepsia.* 1998;39:814–819.

70. Hamer HM, Wyllie E, Stanford L, et al. Risk factors for unsuccessful testing during the intracarotid amobarbital procedure in preadolescent children. *Epilepsia.* 2000;41:554–563.

71. Duchowny M, Levin B, Jayakar P, et al. Temporal lobectomy in early childhood. *Epilepsia.* 1992;33:298–303.

72. Wyllie E, Comair Y, Ruggieri P, et al. Epilepsy surgery in the setting of periventricular leukomalacia and focal cortical dysplasia. *Neurology.* 1996;46:839–841.

73. Marson AG, Kadir ZA, Chadwick DW. New antiepileptic drugs: a systematic review of their efficacy and tolerability. *BMJ.* 1996;313:1169–1174.

74. Kwan P, Brodie MJ. Early identification of refractory epilepsy. *N Engl J Med.* 2000;342:314–319.

75. Gupta A. Special characteristics of surgically remediable epilepsy in infants. In: Luders HO, ed. *Textbook of Epilepsy Surgery.* London, UK: Informa Healthcare; 2008:400–406.

CHAPTER 90 ■ OUTCOME AND COMPLICATIONS OF EPILEPSY SURGERY

LARA JEHI, JORGE MARTINEZ-GONZALEZ, AND WILLIAM BINGAMAN

The effectiveness of epilepsy surgery in the treatment of intractable focal epilepsy is currently widely accepted. With Engel Class I evidence showing obvious therapeutic superiority of temporal lobectomy (TL) over medical treatment with comparable complications (1), and multiple series since then replicating similar results with up to 50% to 55% of patients remaining seizure free as late as a decade after surgery (2–8), little doubt remains that once the determination of medical intractability has been made, a patient with temporal lobe epilepsy (TLE) should undergo an evaluation for surgical candidacy (9). Several studies have also shown encouraging, albeit less dramatic, results following extratemporal epilepsy surgery with chances of seizure freedom at 5 postoperative years ranging from 30% to 50% (10–15).

Our understanding of "favorable" surgical outcomes has, however, evolved significantly over time. We know now that postoperative seizure outcome is a dynamic state with chances of ongoing seizure freedom dropping steadily after surgery (4,6,8,10,11,16). Conversely, up to 20% to 30% of TL patients have intermittent seizures within the few months following surgery only to become seizure free later (5,17–19). So, assessing the "success" of surgery few months postoperatively represents a simplistic approach of limited long-term usefulness. Furthermore, while seizure outcome is indeed the most important determinant of quality of life (QOL) after surgery (20), it is not the only one, such that a comprehensive view of a surgical outcome should include consideration of neurocognitive, social, psychiatric, and functional implications of surgery, as well as its potential complications.

This chapter will provide an overview of the currently available information on surgical outcomes following the most commonly performed types of epilepsy surgery.

AVAILABLE OUTCOME MEASURES AND PITFALLS OF OUTCOME STUDIES

Definitions of "seizure free" vary. Two major seizure outcome classification systems are currently available. Traditionally, most studies have used Engel's classification (Table 90.1), reporting favorable seizure outcomes as being either "excellent," reflecting freedom from disabling seizures (Engel Class I), or "good" with the additional inclusion of patients having rare seizures (Engel Classes I and II). Disadvantages of this system include the following: (i) certain outcome criteria, such as "worthwhile improvement," are very ambiguous, leading to variation in interpretation among different centers; (ii) comparison to antiepileptic drug (AED) trials is virtually impossible

TABLE 90.1

ENGEL'S CLASSIFICATION OF POSTOPERATIVE OUTCOME

Class I: Free of disabling seizures[a]
  A: Completely seizure free since surgery
  B: Nondisabling simple partial seizures only since surgery
  C: Some disabling seizures after surgery, but free of disabling seizures for at least 2 years
  D: Generalized convulsions with AED discontinuation only

Class II: Rare disabling seizures ("almost seizure free")
  A: Initially free of disabling seizures but has rare seizures now
  B: Rare disabling seizures since surgery
  C: More than rare disabling seizures since surgery, but rare seizures for the last 2 years
  D: Nocturnal seizures only

Class III: Worthwhile improvement[b]
  A: Worthwhile seizure reduction
  B: Prolonged seizure-free intervals amounting to greater than half the followed-up period, but not <2 years

Class IV: No worthwhile improvement
  A: Significant seizure reduction
  B: No appreciable change
  C: Seizures worse

[a]Excludes early postoperative seizures (first few weeks).
[b]Determination of "worthwhile improvement" will require quantitative analysis of additional data such as percentage seizure reduction, cognitive function, and quality of life.

as those typically use "≥50% seizure reduction" as their outcome measure; (iii) the "seizure-free" category (Engel Class I) is not restricted to patients who are truly completely seizure free after surgery (Engel Class IA); it also includes those with persistent auras, simple partial seizures, and generalized convulsions upon AED withdrawal (Engel Classes IB to ID). Since studies do not usually report outcome using Engel's classification subcategories, the independent evaluation of truly seizure-free patients is not always possible.

To address the above issues, the International League Against Epilepsy (ILAE) issued a commission report proposing a new outcome classification scheme (Table 90.2). Completely seizure-free patients are classified separately; seizures are quantified in each category and compared to a well-defined baseline frequency, and results can be easily compared to AED trials. To date, only one study (19) compared both systems in its outcome assessment, and found similar results at the last available follow-up.

TABLE 90.2

PROPOSAL FOR A NEW CLASSIFICATION OF OUTCOME WITH RESPECT TO EPILEPTIC SEIZURES

Outcome classification	Definition
1	Completely seizure free[a]; no auras
2	Only auras[b]; no other seizures
3	1 to 3 seizure days per year; ± auras
4	4 seizure days[c] per year to 50% reduction of baseline seizure days[d]; ± auras
5	Less than 50% reduction of baseline seizure days to 100% increase of baseline seizure days; ± auras
6	More than 100% increase of baseline seizure days; ± auras

[a]"Neighborhood seizures" in the first postoperative month are not counted.
[b]Auras are only counted if they are short in duration, and similar or identical to the preoperative ones.
[c]A "seizure day" is a 24-hour period with one or more seizures. This may include an episode of status epilepticus.
[d]"Baseline seizure days" are calculated by determining the seizure-day frequency during the 12 months before surgery, with correction for the effects of AED reduction during diagnostic evaluation.

Some centers reported their outcomes using internally validated scoring systems (17,21,22). Others chose a prespecified period of seizure freedom—usually 12 to 24 months—as reflecting a favorable outcome (8,23,24).

This wide variation in outcome measures is only one of many pitfalls complicating the interpretation and comparison of the results among different surgical series. Other issues comprise: (i) including patients with heterogeneous disease pathologies and even surgeries in the same study limiting the validity of the results for any one group; (ii) using cross-sectional methods of analysis which, by definition, are inaccurate in analyzing longitudinal dynamic time-dependent outcomes like postoperative seizure freedom; and (iii) the limited number of studies with long-term follow-ups, especially in extratemporal lobe surgeries and hemispherectomies.

TEMPORAL LOBE SURGERY

Rate and Stability of Postoperative Seizure Freedom

TL is the most common type of resective epilepsy surgery performed. One randomized controlled trial (1) showed that only two intractable epilepsy patients need to be treated surgically for one patient to become free of disabling seizures. Table 90.3 summarizes the seizure outcomes of most major centers, showing relatively comparable results with about two thirds of the patients becoming seizure-free postoperatively, compared to 5% to 8% with medical therapy. More than 50% of patients remain seizure free beyond 10 years after Anterior temporal lobectomy (ATL) reflecting a sustained benefit (6,7,28,29,31).

If a patient is seizure free at 1 year postoperatively, the likelihood of remaining seizure free is 87% to 90% at 2 years,

74% to 82% at 5 years, and 67% to 71% at 10 years (6,28,31,32). If a patient is seizure free for 2 years postoperatively, chances of seizure freedom increase up to 95% at 5 years, 82% at 10 years, and 68% at 15 years (6,33). So, seizure freedom for 2 years might be a better predictor of long-term outcome, although both the 1-year and the 2-year conditions correlate fairly well with subsequent seizure-free status.

In surgical failures, more than half of seizure recurrences start within 6 postoperative months, and more than 95% recur within 2 to 5 postoperative years (4,34). There is therefore an initial phase of steep recurrence, followed by a relapse rate of 2% to 5% per year for 5 years with subsequent more stable seizure freedom (4,6,28). Recent data suggest that prognostic factors affecting those two phases of recurrence are distinct (4,23,35), possibly reflecting different mechanisms for early versus late relapses. "Early recurrences" occurring within 1 to 2 years of surgery may be due to incomplete removal of the initial epileptogenic zone, whereas later relapses may reflect an underlying diffuse epileptogenicity or progression of an "age-dependent" etiology such as mesial temporal sclerosis (2,8,28,36).

The counterpart of late seizure relapses also exists. In the "running-down" phenomenon, defined as the late remission of postsurgical seizures and occurring in 3.2% to 20% of TLE surgery cases, the frequency of seizures during the running-down interval may be up to several per month, but a seizure-free state is usually achieved within 2 years (36,37). The most accepted explanation for this phenomenon is a dekindling effect, an opposite process to secondary epileptogenesis, where the induced synaptic dysfunction gradually declines in the surrounding epileptogenic cortex after pace-maker resection, and eventually "runs itself down" (37).

Predictors of Recurrence

Clinical Variables and Seizure Outcome

Age at Onset of Epilepsy. Patients with an earlier age at onset of epilepsy (usually <5 years) or at the time of the initial neurologic insult may be up to three times more likely to have a favorable postoperative outcome (7,29). However, some investigators proposed that this variable actually predicts hippocampal sclerosis (HS) which is the actual good prognostic indicator (24,38). This hypothesis is supported by the observation that those patients were more likely to have features typical of HS such as unilateral hippocampal atrophy on MRI (39), focal ictal electroencephalogram (EEG) with predominantly partial seizures (29), and by the fact that age at onset per se was of no prognostic value in studies evaluating pure cohorts of HS (24,38) or controlling for pathology (4,6,8).

Duration of Epilepsy. A long history of seizures correlated with worse outcome in multiple studies on univariate analysis (17,34,36). In some of those same cohorts, this influence disappeared when multivariate analysis was performed adjusting for other more solid indicators of outcome (5,6). Furthermore, many more recent studies found no correlation of epilepsy duration with outcome (6–8,24,30,38). Various hypotheses have been proposed to explain those findings, including secondary epileptogenesis occurring with a long seizure history, varying degrees of maturation of different epileptogenic foci,

TABLE 90.3

SURGICAL OUTCOME IN MAJOR STUDIES EVALUATING PURE COHORTS OF PATIENTS WITH HIPPOCAMPAL SCLEROSIS

Author[a]	Study period	Years of follow-up: mean (range)	N	Surgery	Outcome measure used	Percentage of favorable outcome at				
						1 year[a]	2 year	5 year	>5 year	Date of last follow-up
Paglioli et al. (25)		6.7 (2–11)	80	ATL	Engel I					72%
		4.5 (2–11)	81	SAH	Engel I					71%
Jeba et al. (4)	1990–2000	5.5 (1–14.1)	371 (219 with MTS)	ATL or SAH	ILAE 1 — All		78%	66%	53% at 10 years	63%
					ILAE 1 — MTS		71%	64%	55% at 10 years	70%
Jeong et al. (5)	1994–2000	4.6 (1–n/a)	227	ATL	Engel I	81%		75%		
Spencer et al. (8)	1996–2001	4.6 (2–7.3)	339 (297 with MTS)	ATL	2-year remission from seizures ± auras		46%	69%		MTS 68% / Neocortical 50%
Janszky et al. (2)	1993–2002	n/a (0.5–n/a)	171	ATL	Complete seizure freedom to last follow-up or for "≥2 years at time of outcome assessment"		71%	58%		
Salanova et al. (26)	1984–2002	n/a	262	ATL	Engel I					65%
Paglioli et al. (7)	1992–2000	5.47 (2–11)	135	ATL or SAH	Engel IA	85%	77%	74%	66% at 10 years	
Urbach et al. (27)	1999–2000	2	209	n/a	Engel IA	73%				
McIntosh et al. (6)	1978–1998	9.6 (0.7–23)	325	ATL	Engel I (a, b, d) — All	61%	55%	48%	41% at 10 years, 37% at 15 years	
					HS	68%	62%	54%	47% at 10 years, 43% at 15 years	
Yoon et al. (28)	1972–1992	8.4 (3.1–20)	175	n/a	"Continuous 1 year seizure free"	51%				
Jutila et al. (29)	1988–1999	5.4 (3 months–10.5 years)	140	ATL or SAH	ILAE 1	64%	58%	50%	50% at 9 years	58%
Wieser et al. (19,30)	1975–1999	7.2 (1–24)	369 (with MTLE, 151 with HS)	SAH	Engel I	71%	70%	65%	62%	66.9%
Hennessy et al. (24)	1975–1995	5.2 (n/a)	116	ATL	ILAE Class 1a	56%	50%	38%	34% at 10 years	57.1%
					12 consecutive months of absolute seizure freedom ± auras			67%		

[a]Bold: Prospective studies; italic: all TLE (not distinguishing MTLE from neocortical).

and the increased development of generalized seizures with longer epilepsy duration (36).

Age at Surgery. Most studies found no correlation between age at surgery and seizure outcome (4,6,7,24), although one longitudinal study in HS patients found that cases who were ≤24 years old at surgery were about four times more likely to be seizure free at 5 postoperative years when compared to the older surgical group (36 years or older) (5). Few other studies found similar results (34,36).

One should note here that successful and safe ATLs have been performed in the elderly (>50 years old), with few reports suggesting slightly lower chances of seizure freedom albeit without increased risks of neuropsychological deficits (36). Therefore, older age by itself should not be a deterrent from surgery.

Absence of Secondarily Generalized Tonic–Clonic Seizures (SGTCS). Only 57% of mesial TLE patients with SGTCS achieved a 1-year remission compared to 80% remission rate in those who had only partial seizures in one study (24). Patients who had no GTCS were 2.2 times more likely to be seizure free 5 years after surgery in another study (5). This effect may be most significant when GTCS are frequent (more than two per year) and occurring within 3 years of surgery (6). The prognostic significance of SGTCS was confirmed in a recent prospective multicenter trial (8).

The occurrence of SGTCS in TLE correlates with more extensive HS, multifocal irritative areas, and extended positron emission tomography (PET) hypometabolism suggesting a diffuse potential epileptogenic zone with worse expected surgical outcome (36).

Other. Clinical variables where some studies suggested a favorable prognostic significance include low baseline seizure frequency and a history of febrile seizures. This, however, was not consistently confirmed. No correlation between occurrence of auras and outcome was proven (4).

Imaging Variables and Seizure Outcome

Magnetic Resonance Imaging. A consistently identified favorable outcome predictor has been the presence of a unilateral temporal lobe abnormality on MRI (8,36,38). Patients with MRI evidence of unilateral HS had a 54% chance of seizure freedom at 10 years after ATL compared to 18% if MRIs were normal in a recent longitudinal study (6). However, recent data suggest that such a favorable prognostic significance is actually conferred by ANY unilateral temporal MRI lesion, and not necessarily by HS, especially with concordant ictal and interictal EEG findings (6,26,36).

Although a normal MRI was traditionally considered as an automatic correlate to surgical failure (40,41), recent data have actually shown seizure freedom rates of up to 41% to 48% as far as 8 years after ATL (4,42,43). While some data suggest that these patients may actually have "MRI-negative" or undetected HS (36), one study concluded that most cases of normal appearing hippocampi on high-resolution MRI have neocortical TLE since they had less febrile seizures, more delta rhythms at ictal onset, and more extensive lateral neocortical changes on PET with surgical outcomes still comparable to those of MRI obvious HS (43). It should be emphasized, though, that surgery was successful in nonlesional patients only when

performed in context of concordant EEG and PET data (4,43). "Normal" MRIs correlating with bad outcomes in older studies using lower quality imaging may have included patients with extratemporal or contralateral pathology, findings that would currently exclude viable surgical options (4,43).

Bilateral MRI lesions, including grossly bilateral HS, reflect multiple potentially epileptogenic foci and correlate with a worse surgical outcome: 58% seizure free at 2 years compared to 78% when compared to unilateral lesions or even normal MRI (4,36). Subtle hippocampal asymmetries only detected using volumetric analyses were less predictive of outcome (36).

Nuclear Imaging. Unilateral temporal hypometabolism on FDG-PET is a good predictor of seizure freedom in patients with mesial TLE, independent of pathologic findings and regardless of whether MRI is normal or not. In a recent review of the literature, Casse (44) found that 86% of patients with unilateral temporal hypometabolism ipsilateral to the side of surgery had a good outcome as defined by more than 90% reduction in seizure frequency or Engel Class I or II, with those chances slightly reduced to 82% if the MRI was normal. This number significantly dropped to 62% when PET was normal and to 50% when it showed bitemporal hypometabolism (44). With extratemporal hypopmetabolism, chances of seizure freedom are even worse: complete seizure freedom at last follow-up (mean 6.1 years) was seen in 45% of patients with extratemporal cortical hypometabolism confined to the ipsilateral hemisphere, and only 22% with contralateral cortical hypometabolism (45).

Abundant data support the usefulness of ictal SPECT in localizing the epileptogenic zone in TLE, with 70% to 100% of ictal SPECTs being correctly localizing and only 0% to 7% incorrectly localizing (36). However, while the prognostic value of such localized SPECT findings is clear in extratemporal or poorly localized nonlesional epilepsy (46), its role in clear lesional TLE cases is less defined. In a recent analysis of patients with unilateral HS visible on MRI, surgical outcome was not influenced by contralateral increased flow on ictal SPECT (47). One hypothesis is that due to their low temporal resolution, ictal SPECT hyperperfusion patterns often contain both the ictal-onset zone and propagation pathways. These patterns often have a multilobulated "hourglass" appearance with the largest and most intense hyperperfusion cluster often representing ictal propagation and not necessarily requiring resection to render a patient seizure free (48). Results for interictal SPECT suggest that it is relatively poor at localizing the seizure focus (36).

Electrophysiologic Variables and Seizure Outcome

Noninvasive EEG. Focal interictal EEG predicts a favorable outcome when lateralized to the side of surgery, or when highly localized to the resected temporal lobe. Patients whose interictal EEGs showed ≥90% predominance on the operated-on side had an 80% chance of complete seizure freedom after a mean 5.5 years of follow-up versus 54% in those with lesser degrees of lateralization in a recent prospective study (7). In general, interictal evidence of a diffuse irritative zone predicts a worse outcome: postoperative seizure freedom is worse when interictal spiking was posterior temporal, extratemporal, or bitemporal (36). Posterior temporal and extratemporal spiking in patients with pathologically confirmed HS may reflect diffuse epileptogenicity or "dual pathology" with associated neocortical epileptogenic zones, thereby explaining the associated worse prognosis (24,40). However, prognostic implications of bitemporal interictal spiking on surface EEG deserve more careful consideration, as it does not automatically preclude postoperative seizure freedom. One study found that if ≥90% of surface interictal bitemporal spikes arise from one temporal lobe, excellent outcome is possible (92% seizure free in the second postoperative year vs. 50% if <90% lateralization), and further evaluation with depth EEG electrodes may not even be indicated (49). With a unilateral MRI temporal lesion, and with lateralizing WADA or neuropsychiatric testing, up to 64% of patients with bilateral interictal spikes achieved complete seizure freedom at ≥1 year postoperatively when seizure onset was strictly unilateral on invasive evaluation (50). Other findings consistent with unilateral HS, such as a history of febrile seizures or early onset of epilepsy (prior to age 3 to 6 years), also correlated with favorable outcome in patients with bitemporal interictal spikes suggesting that contralateral spiking may simply be spread from a surgically treatable hippocampus (36). However, if the MRI is normal or shows widespread abnormalities, then seizure recurrence is the rule as either an extratemporal focus spreading to both temporal lobes or bitemporal epilepsy becomes more likely (50).

Similar concepts apply to the prognostic value of ictal EEG. Again, focal or anterior ictal EEG correlate with a more favorable outcome, and patients who had bitemporal ictal onsets on surface EEG still achieved seizure freedom rates of up to 64% at 1 postoperative year if seizures were exclusively unilateral with depth recordings and imaging or neuropsychological testing were also consistent with unilateral temporal dysfunction (36,50).

Invasive EEG. Depth electrode evaluations have traditionally been used to clarify lateralization of the epileptogenic zone in patients with suspected bitemporal or falsely lateralized TLE, whereas subdural recordings are useful in neocortical epilepsy for extraoperative functional mapping and definition of the extent of the epileptogenic zone. A combination of the two is often used to clarify whether a patient has mesial versus neocortical TLE. Those modalities are therefore reserved for patients with a poorly defined epileptogenic zone, which may explain poorer outcomes seen in cases that required invasive recordings preoperatively compared to those that did not (4,26,31). Yet, specific findings obtained with such invasive evaluations may provide useful prognostic information. During depth recordings, more favorable outcomes are seen with exclusively unilateral seizure onset and ictal spiking as opposed to low-voltage fast activity, electrodecrement, or any other rhythmic sustained activity at seizure onset, whereas evolution into distinct contralateral electrographic seizures lowered seizure freedom from 84% to 47% at 1 postoperative year (36). Short interhemispheric propagation times ranging from <1 second to <8 second, a short duration between EEG and clinical seizure onset, and diffuse or posterior temporal onset as opposed to anterior and/or middle basal temporal ictal onset have all been also identified as predictors of seizure recurrence after surgery (36).

Surgical Technique and Seizure Outcome

Similar seizure freedom rates have been observed with selective amygdalohippocampectomy and anterior TL (4,7). Many studies failed to correlate the extent of temporal resection (29), the extent of hippocampal resection (31), or having a mesial versus neocortical resection (4,8) to outcome. Those studies, however, did not evaluate patients with mesial TLE separately. In the presence of unilateral mesial TLE with HS, the extent of mesial resection becomes a more significant predictor of postoperative seizure freedom (36). In a prospective, randomized, blinded clinical trial, Wyler et al. found that only 38% of patients in whom the hippocampal resection was limited posteriorly by the anterior edge of the cerebral peduncle (partial hippocampectomy) were seizure free at 1 year, compared to 69% of those in whom the hippocampus was removed further, to the level of the superior colliculus (complete resection) (51). The amount of amygdala that must be resected to achieve seizure freedom is unclear, although one study found no correlation between residual amygdalar tissue and surgical outcome (52). The ideal extent of lateral temporal resection also remains to be defined with conflicting data currently available (36).

In the presence of a well-circumscribed lesion, such as a tumor or a vascular malformation, a lesionectomy might suffice unless there is associated hippocampal atrophy. In such cases of dual pathology, complete seizure freedom after a mean follow-up of 37 months was lowered from 73% with lesionectomy plus mesial temporal resection to 20% with mesial temporal resection alone and 12.5% with lesionectomy alone (36).

Etiology, Pathology, and Seizure Outcome

When pathologic findings in the resected temporal lobe were restricted to nonspecific gliosis, worse short- and long-term outcomes have consistently been observed (36). In a recent longitudinal study of 371 ATL patients, 44% of cases who only had gliosis were seizure free 8 years after surgery, compared to 64% if a specific pathologic diagnosis was identified (4). However, once a specific pathologic abnormality is identified, it is not entirely clear that its nature is relevant for seizure outcomes. While the older literature has suggested more favorable outcomes with HS, seizure-freedom rates were similar between HS and other types of lesions in many recent (4,6) or prospective studies (8,16,27). One hypothesis is that outcome depends not only on the presence of HS, but also on its severity: worse disease may predict better outcome. One group found that 84% of patients with classical HS, as defined by neuronal loss and sclerosis in CA1, CA4, and the granule cells of the dentate gyrus, achieved at least 95% seizure reduction at last follow-up, compared to only 29% of those where cell loss was restricted to the dentate gyrus and/or CA4 (53). Another group also found that rates of Engel Class I outcomes at last follow-up increased from 60% to 76% to 89% as the pathologic severity of HS ranged from mild to moderate to severe (19).

FRONTAL LOBE SURGERY

Rate and Stability of Postoperative Seizure Freedom

Frontal lobectomy (FL) accounts for 6% to 30% of all epilepsy surgeries and represents the second most common procedure performed to treat intractable focal epilepsy after

TL. However, reported seizure-freedom rates with frontal resections have varied from 13% to 80% (10,15,54–59), suggesting, in general, significantly lower success rates than those observed with temporal resections. Only few studies evaluated seizure freedom after FL longitudinally, and can therefore provide useful information related to rate and stability of seizure outcome over time (10,56). In a retrospective study evaluating 97 adults who underwent resective FL surgery between 1991 and 2005, Elsharkawy et al. found that the probability of an Engel Class I outcome was 54.6% at 6 months, 49.5% at 2 years, 47% at 5 years, and 41.9% at 10 years (56). In a study reviewing patients operated at Cleveland Clinic between 1995 and 2003, and using a stricter "favorable outcome" definition (complete seizure freedom since surgery), we had previously identified a seizure-freedom rate of 55.7% at 1 postoperative year, 45.1% at 3 years, and 30.1% at 5 years and beyond (10). Eighty percent of seizure recurrences occur within the first 6 postoperative months, and although late remissions and relapses may occur, those are usually rare (10). One study showed that although a postoperative reduction in seizure frequency often occurred in patients who failed to become completely seizure free after surgery, this improvement was sustained until the last follow-up in only 35%, with seizure frequencies eventually returning to preoperative levels in the remainder (10). The running-down phenomenon previously described may occur following FL, but at a rate of <15%, also significantly less than that seen after TL (56).

Similar to TL, however, seizure freedom at 6 months to 2 postoperative years seems to be a very good predictor of a long-term seizure-free state. If a patient is seizure free at 2-year follow-up, the probability of remaining seizure free up to 10 years may increase up to 86% (56).

Predictors of Seizure Recurrence

Mechanistically, proposed hypotheses to explain the generally lower rates of seizure freedom following FL include (i) difficulty localizing the epileptogenic zone with EEG data secondary to rapid ictal spread through the frontal lobe, (ii) difficulty achieving a complete surgical resection secondary to proximity of functional/eloquent cortex, and (iii) a preponderance of cortical dysplasia, often invisible on MRI, as the epilepsy etiology in the frontal lobe as opposed to clearly localized HS in the temporal lobe (13,46,58). Practically, identified predictors of postoperative seizure recurrence have included incomplete resection of the epileptic lesion (10,56,60,61), the need to perform an invasive subdural grid evaluation (10,56), the occurrence of acute postoperative seizures (10), the persistence of auras postoperatively (10,56), a history of febrile seizures (62), predominantly generalized or poorly localized ictal EEG patterns on surface EEG prior to surgery—especially in the adult population (10,12,15,56)—and the lack of a distinct single MRI lesion (10,12,56,60). Of all the above prognostic indicators, the two most consistently reported and strongly predictive of postoperative seizure freedom are the presence of an MRI lesion and completeness of resection (Figs. 90.1 and 90.2).

MRI and Seizure Outcome

A normal MRI in a patient undergoing FL has consistently been found to predict a worse outcome. Twenty-five percent of the patients with negative MRI studies and 67% of those

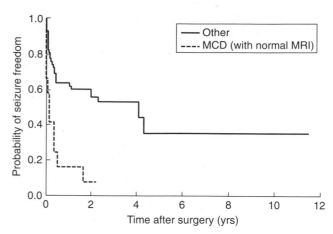

FIGURE 90.1 Survival curve illustrating lower long-term rates of seizure freedom in patients with normal MRI as opposed to lesional cases following frontal lobe resection. (Adapted from Jeha LE, Najm I, Bingaman W, et al. Surgical outcome and prognostic factors of frontal lobe epilepsy surgery. *Brain.* 2007;130(pt 2):574–584, with permission.)

with neuroimaging abnormalities restricted to the frontal lobe were seizure free at a minimum duration of follow-up of 1 year in one study (63). A focal MRI abnormality was the only variable significantly associated with a favorable surgical outcome in another report (64). Only 41% of nonlesional FLE patients had an excellent outcome versus 72% when MRI abnormality was present in yet another retrospective analysis (58). Most such "nonlesional" FLE cases are thought to have an underlying malformation of cortical development (MCD) (12,60). In a more recent longitudinal outcome analysis, all patients with normal MRI and pathologically proven MCD had recurrent seizures by 3 postoperative years (10). Knowing that milder forms of MCD such as microdysgenesis, cortical dyslamination, or focal MCD are often missed, even on high-resolution MRI may explain why one cannot "see" the extent of the epileptogenic tissue in those MRI-negative MCD cases making adequate surgical treatment harder.

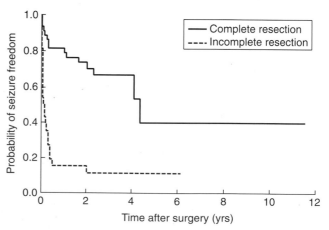

FIGURE 90.2 Survival curve illustrating lower long-term rates of seizure freedom in patients with incomplete resection as opposed to complete resections following frontal lobe resection. (Adapted from Jeha LE, Najm I, Bingaman W, et al. Surgical outcome and prognostic factors of frontal lobe epilepsy surgery. *Brain.* 2007;130(pt 2): 574–584, with permission.)

Techniques such as ictal SPECT imaging, FDG-PET, and subdural grid or stereo-EEG monitoring are often used to better localize the epileptogenic zone in nonlesional FLE cases. A study reporting on 193 patients with neocortical focal epilepsy (including 61 with FLE) showed that correct localization by FDG-PET was an independent predictor of a good outcome (12), and other case reports highlighted the usefulness of ictal SPECT in identifying a potential epileptogenic zone in nonlesional FLE (46). A recent analysis, however, found that while MRI, PET, and ictal SPECT all had good positive predictive values with correspondingly acceptable negative predictive values in correlating with the ictal-onset zone as later defined by invasive EEG recording, there was no significant relationship between the diagnostic accuracy of any of these modalities and surgical outcome, with the exception of MRI ($P = 0.029$) (54). So, the translation of "accurate" and "correct localization" of epileptic foci using either PET or SPECT into actual improvements in seizure outcome for nonlesional FLE has not always been consistently reproducible. The interpretation of the role of intracranial EEG monitoring is another delicate issue. In a cross-sectional study of 51 nonlesional, mostly FLE, cases operated on between 1992 and 2002, Wejten et al. found that 35.7% of the 28 patients who eventually underwent a focal resection after intracranial EEG recording became seizure free with high-frequency oscillations at ictal onset being predictive of seizure freedom (55). Since this study's patient population included cases operated on prior to the advent of FLAIR imaging and other high-resolution neuroimaging techniques, an unknown proportion of its cases may have had subtle structural abnormalities which potentially could have been detected using current imaging modalities. A longitudinal study of FLE patients imaged and operated on more recently found that for nonlesional cases, and despite the use of invasive EEG recordings, only 30% were seizure free at 1 year after surgery and 15% were seizure free at 3 years (10). In summary, while nonlesional FLE cases seem to be as a whole less than ideal surgical candidates for resective epilepsy surgery, efforts to identify the specific subgroup who might benefit from surgery while pursuing nonsurgical treatment options for the rest are still required.

Any extra frontal MRI abnormality also confers a poor prognosis. Favorable outcomes occurred in either none of the patients with multilobar MRI abnormalities (63) or at best in 10% to 14% (10,65). Tumors, well-circumscribed pathologies, usually have the best outcome with up to 62% seizure free at last follow-up in one report (10), and 65% Engel Class I or II at last follow-up in another series (13).

Extent of Resection and Seizure Outcome

Complete resection of the epileptogenic lesion has consistently been found to predict seizure freedom. In one report, of patients who had complete removal of their epileptogenic lesions, 81% were seizure free at 1 year and 66% at 3 years, compared to 13% and 11%, respectively, of those who did not (10). Complete removal of neuroimaging abnormalities (15,55,60), and abolition of residual ECoG spiking (66) or seizures (67) have also been linked with the most favorable outcomes following FLE surgery. Major challenges that hinder a complete resection in all cases include frequent proximity or overlap with eloquent cortex and difficulties identifying the true edges of the "abnormal" tissue in MCD cases where

the MRI-visible portion of the dysplasia may be surrounded by microscopically abnormal tissue that seems normal on imaging (10).

In summary, while the rates of seizure freedom are low, in general, following frontal resections, very successful seizure outcomes are possible in a selected group of patients, mainly those with a clear MRI lesion that is completely resectable.

POSTERIOR CORTEX SURGERY

Rate and Stability of Postoperative Seizure Freedom

Resections in the posterior cortex represent less than 10% of all epilepsy surgeries, with reported postoperative seizure-freedom rates varying from 25% to 90% (11,68–72). In a longitudinal analysis of a cohort of posterior cortex resections, the estimated chance of seizure freedom was 73.1% at 6 postoperative months, 68.5% at 1 year, 65.8% between 2 and 5 years, and 54.8% at 6 years and beyond. The median timing of recurrence was 2.0 months with 75% of the seizure recurrences occurring by 6.4 months, and late recurrences were rare with the latest being at 74 months (11). Similar rates of seizure freedom have been reported in another longitudinal analysis of 154 adult patients who underwent various types of extratemporal resections (about 40% frontal and the remaining being posterior cortex surgeries), with an Engel Class I at 2 postoperative years being correlated with an 88% chance of remaining seizure free 14 years after surgery (73). These findings suggest that in posterior cortex resections, we can expect an initial rate of seizure recurrence that is as fast as following FL, allowing a relatively early identification of surgical failures, but with a more optimistic long-term outlook with late seizure-free rates comparable to those following temporal resections. Figure 90.3 illustrates the longitudinal rates of seizure freedom in posterior quadrant resections in a cohort evaluated at Cleveland Clinic recently.

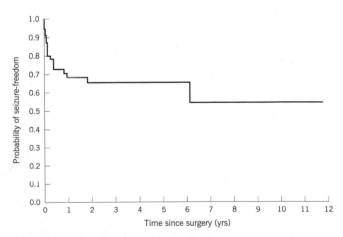

FIGURE 90.3 Survival curve illustrating long-term rates of seizure freedom following posterior quadrant surgery. (Adapted from Jeha et al. Longitudinal outcome and prognostic factors of posterior quadrant epilepsy surgery. *Epilepsia.* 2009, in print, with permission.)

Predictors of Seizure Recurrence

Patients with well-circumscribed focal lesions (tumors or MRI-visible MCD), who have more extensive resections (lobectomies or multilobar resections as opposed to lesionectomies), and no preoperative evidence of extralobar epileptogenicity extending to the ipsilateral temporal lobe (temporal spiking or auditory auras), and no postoperative evidence of residual epileptogenicity (spiking on 6 months postoperative EEG) had the most favorable outlook in most series of posterior cortex resections (11,68–73). Other less consistently reported predictors of seizure freedom include lateralizing seizure semiology (74), focal ictal EEG (75), and longer epilepsy duration (76).

In a series of 57 patients with posterior cortex resections, only a quarter of patients with either a tumor or lesional MCD had postoperative seizure recurrence, as opposed to more than half of the patients who had other pathologies after a mean follow-up of 3.3 years (11). Completeness of resection of such epileptogenic lesions was identified, among others, by Barba et al. in 2005 to be the strongest predictor of postoperative seizure freedom (75). The challenge though is that while it is easily understood that larger resections have a better chance of achieving seizure freedom, this may not always be possible secondary to risks of injury to eloquent cortex, especially in the dominant hemisphere. We found that a lesionectomy achieved seizure freedom in 67% of cases in tumor or MCD but in only 20% of other etiologies, suggesting that attempting a "smaller surgery" to avoid injuring eloquent cortex may be appropriate in selected cases of tumor/MCD but is rather ill-advised with other "unfavorable etiologies" (11). Invasive EEG recordings with subdural grids, depths, or the use of stereo-EEG are more extensively used for better delineation of the epileptogenic zone and for extraoperative functional mapping optimizing resections with multiple reports showing very promising seizure outcome data. Caicoya et al. found that five of seven occipital lobe epilepsy patients who underwent tailored resections guided by subdural EEG data were seizure free after a mean follow-up of 24.3 months (77). Cukiert et al. (78) reported on 16 patients with intractable extratemporal epilepsy who either had normal or "nonlocalizing" MRI finding that 13/14 were rendered seizure free with resections that used subdural EEG information (79). The use of preoperative invasive monitoring has even been shown in one report to actually correlate with a more favorable outcome in a large cohort of extratemporal resections, consisting mostly of posterior cortex surgeries (73).

PSYCHIATRIC OUTCOMES AFTER EPILEPSY SURGERY

Epilepsy surgery, especially when successful, appears to reduce the prevalence of commonly observed psychiatric comorbidities of epilepsy, including depression and anxiety. Kanner et al. reported a total remission rate off psychotropic medication in 45% of patients who underwent epilepsy surgery (79). The impact on psychotic disorders, however, is less clearly defined: it varied from unchanged in most cases to improved psychotic status/and or level of functioning (79). Conversely, patients may undergo an exacerbation of an underlying psychopathology or develop de-novo psychopathology after surgery. In a study by Wrench et al. comparing the psychiatric outcomes following temporal versus extratemporal resections over a 3-month period, it was found that although both groups had similar baseline rates of depression and anxiety, and more patients were seizure free after a temporal than after an extratemporal resection, the psychiatric outcome was significantly worse in the temporal resections group: at 1 month after surgery, 66% of TL versus 19% of ETL patients reported symptoms of anxiety or depression, which persisted until the 3-month follow-up in 30% of TL and 17% of ETL. In addition, by the 3-month follow-up, 13% of ATL patients had developed a de-novo depression as opposed to none in the ETL group. More notably, the occurrence of any of those psychiatric comorbidities was not related to seizure freedom (80). This reinforces the need to carefully evaluate and consider psychiatric outcomes after epilepsy surgery as an independent—albeit intimately connected—entity to the seizure outcomes.

PSYCHOSOCIAL OUTCOMES AFTER EPILEPSY SURGERY

The goals of surgery, as identified by epilepsy patients, extend beyond seizure control, to include driving, regaining or improving employment, and overall independence (80). Intimately linked to these goals is the absence of any "functional" worsening due to surgery, as might occur with a new neurologic deficit, memory loss, or language disturbance. A "successful" surgery is one where seizures are controlled, and where the patients' psychosocial goals materialize into an improved QOL. Several studies have found that for optimal improvement in QOL measurements, complete seizure freedom (even from auras) is required (34,81). Other possible predictors of an improved QOL include a higher presurgical IQ score, younger age at surgery, and a more stable mood at baseline (81). Studies evaluating the psychosocial and educational impacts of surgery in the pediatric population are very limited, but do suggest meaningful improvements in educational attainments and later employment (81).

SURGICAL COMPLICATIONS AFTER FOCAL EPILEPSY SURGERY

The main goal of the pre- and intraoperative evaluation for epilepsy surgery is to identify possible candidates in whom surgical intervention will totally or partially control seizures without increasing neurologic deficits or general morbidity.

In general, we can divide complications in focal neocortical epilepsy surgery based on physiopathologic mechanisms into: *Surgical Complications:*

- Infection
- Hematoma
- Brain swelling
- Hydrocephalus
- Vascular compromise (arterial or venous).

Injury to Eloquent Areas of the Brain Causing Neurologic Impairment:

- Hemiparesis
- Hemiplegia

- Visual field defect
- Aphasia
- Alexia
- Neuropsychological impairment (deficits in cognition, memory, language, attention and concentration)

Psychosocial Impairment:

- Family and interpersonal relationships
- Self-esteem
- Vocational/educational

Psychiatric Impairment:

- Depression
- Anxiety
- Psychosis

In regard to surgical procedures related to neocortical focal epilepsy, we can classify complications due to focal neocortical resections as follows:

Diagnostic Procedures:

- Complications associated with subdural grid and strip electrodes, depth electrode, and stereoelectroencephalograph (SEEG) complications.

Therapeutic Procedures—Resective Surgery:

- Complications associated with frontal (mesial and lateral) resections.
- Complications associated with temporal lobe resections.
- Complications associated with parietal and occipital resections.

Diagnostic Procedures

Subdural Grids/Strip Electrodes, Depth Electrode, and SEEG Complications

When noninvasive studies remain nonconcordant or inconclusive regarding the localization and the extent of the seizure-onset zone and/or the eloquent cortex, invasive studies using subdural grids, strips, or depth electrode may be needed (82,83). Jayakar and colleagues proposed the following relative indications for the evaluation with invasive monitoring: normal structural imaging, extratemporal location, divergent noninvasive data, and encroachment on eloquent cortex, tuberous sclerosis, and cortical dysplasia (82). Rosenow and Lüders (84) recommended the use of invasive monitoring only in patients with focal epilepsy (single focus) in whom there is a clear hypothesis regarding the location of the epileptogenic zone (derived from noninvasive studies).

The intracranial placement of subdural grid electrodes via craniotomy has received increasing acceptance over the past decade. Invasive EEG monitoring by subdural grid electrodes facilitates prolonged electrographic assessment as well as extraoperative functional brain mapping. Also, it is particular important in pediatric cases in which awake surgery and intraoperative functional mapping are often difficult.

The principal complications of grid electrode implantation include infection and subdural hematoma formation, which may be associated with neurologic deficits, elevations of intracranial pressure (ICP), and even death (85–87).

Other complications may include brain swelling, arterial or venous infarctions (Fig. 90.4). In a recent series, of the 228 cases from 9 centers, the reported complications included

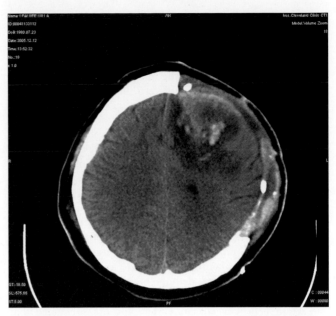

FIGURE 90.4 Complication of subdural grid placement: Venous infarction located in the left frontal lobe region after subdural grid placement. Postoperative CT after subdural grid removal and bone decompression.

infection, hemorrhage with transient deficit, increased preexisting hemiparesis, aseptic necrosis of the bone flap, and transient elevations in ICP (88). In an individual series from the Cleveland Clinic, an initial infection rate of 22% declined to 7% when subcutaneous tunneling of electrode cables was instituted (89). More recently, routine use of perioperative antibiotics and water-tight dural closure with sutures at cable exit sites has been advocated in our group (Awad, personal communication, 1992). Since these modifications were introduced, the infection rate has declined markedly.

In the absence of a multicenter, prospective complications survey, anecdotal reports of subdural hematoma formation, increased ICP, and death following grid placement have been documented in the literature (90). Some centers recommend routine, perioperative dexamethasone, and mannitol administration over 2 to 3 days after surgery, dural grafting, or leaving out the bone flap during the period of monitoring as responses to the threat of increased ICP. Circumferential dural incision, lining of the outer grid surface with hemostatic agents, and tapering of valproic acid are also recommended to reduce hematoma formation (90). There is no data with respect to the relative value of any of these practices in preventing individual complications.

Regarding subdural strip, epilepsy surgery literature suggests that subdural strip electrode insertion may be safer than depth electrode placement (86,91,92). No examples of significant hemorrhagic complications associated with prolonged neurologic deficit or death have been reported so far. Localized infections occur at a slightly lower frequency when compared with depth recordings and usually respond to antibiotic therapy alone. In a recent series of 350 patients, 2 cases of meningitis, 1 brain abscess associated with hemiparesis, and 3 superficial wound infections were reported (93). In two additional reports studying 122 patients, no hemorrhagic, neurologic, or infectious complications occurred following strip electrode placement (94).

Different techniques of invasive monitoring exist, and each has its advantages and disadvantages. Chronically implanted subdural electrodes allow recording from large superficial cortical areas, but they provide limited coverage of deeper structures, such as the hippocampus, the interhemispheric region, or cortex within sulci. Intracerebral electrodes have the advantage of excellent sampling from mesial structures and from deep cortical areas, with the disadvantage of providing information from a limited volume of tissue. Combined use of subdural and intracerebral electrodes also has been advocated. In a recent publication, Cossu et al. presented a retrospective study of a large series of patients (211 patients) who underwent SEEG evaluation. SEEG provided additional guidance towards epileptic focus resection in 183 patients (87%), resulting in seizure-free outcome in 44% of the cases, and an overall significant improvement in 82%. Major complications occurred in less than 1% of the patients, with an overall hemorrhagic event risk of 4.2%. Other complications included one brain abscess, not resulting in permanent deficit; one episode of focal cortical edema; and one retained broken electrode. The authors concluded that SEEG is a useful and relatively safe tool in the presurgical evaluation of focal epilepsy (95).

As highlighted by others, important issues relating to depth electrode placement and associated complications include (i) the relative safety of lateral, parasagittal, and tangential methods of insertion; (ii) the relative safety of flexible versus rigid electrodes; (iii) the role of computer-assisted work stations in the improvement of stereotactic accuracy and the reduction of vessel injury; (iv) the effect upon infectious complications of length of monitoring, antibiotics prophylaxis, tunneling of electrode leads, and methods of electrode removal (90).

Therapeutic Procedures

Complications of Temporal Neocortical Focal Resections

In general, there are at least four different surgical approaches to treat mesial TLE. These approaches include (i) en bloc temporal resection or standard TL; (ii) awake TL with tailored resection; (iii) amygdalohippocampectomy; and (d) radical hippocampectomy. Each technique represents a different approach to the identification and resection of the epileptogenic zone. Because this chapter is focused on complications in neocortical epilepsy surgery, complications related to amygdalohippocampal resections will not be discussed.

In an extensive review of the literature performed by Pilcher and Ojemann regarding complications of anterior TL, mortality occurred in less than 1%, mainly caused by hemorrhage, infarction, pulmonary complications, and sudden death. Other complications included hemiparesis (transient or permanent) in 2% to 4%, minimal visual field defects in more than 50%, and severe field defects (hemianopsia) in 2% to 4%. Infections (meningitis, abscess), epidural hematoma, and III nerve palsy (transient) occurred in less than 2%. Neurobehavioral complications included transitory anomia (less than 1 week) in 20% of the patients, persistent dysphasia in 1% to 3%, and transitory psychosis/depression in 2% to 20% (90).

Penfield reported a 2.5% *hemiplegia* in an early Montreal Neurological Institute (MNI) series. He attributed this complication to excessive manipulation of branches of the middle cerebral artery (MCA) during the trans-sylvian resection of insular cortex (96). Alternative explanations included direct capsular injury with insular resection as well as compromise of the lenticulostriate vessels and the anterior choroidal artery.

Visual field deficits occur following temporal lobe resections in approximately 50% of operated patients. These deficits are often incongruous or worse in the ipsilateral eye, due to the anterolateral location of ipsilateral fibers overlying the anterior portion of the temporal horn (Meyer's loop). Severe visual field deficits considered disabling by patients are less frequent and were reported in 8% in our previous series (89). Rasmussen et al. suggested that by limiting the extent of the superolateral ventricular opening to 1 cm, quadrantic deficits could be avoided entirely (97). Other studies also suggested that the magnitude of the visual field deficit was entirely related to the extension of the ventricular opening, mainly in the ventricular roof in the temporal horn. Alternatively, direct surgical injury to the optic tract, lateral geniculate nucleus, or optic radiation in the posterior temporal lobe white matter can also cause visual field deficits.

Postoperative *anomia* or *dysphasia* is not uncommon following dominant TL. These aphasias are largely resolved after 1 week. Transitory dysphasias are reported in up to 30% of operated patients in the setting of awake surgery with intraoperative language mapping. Removal of the anterior temporal or inferior-basal language sites may explain this phenomenon (98). Other explanations include resection of cortex within 1 to 2 cm from essential language areas, brain retraction, and disruption of white matter pathways connecting language areas. According to Crandall and colleagues, persistent language disorders were found in three of 53 patients undergoing temporal lobe resection (99). In another series, 5 of 25 patients were aphasic at the time of discharge (100). In the MNI series, using intraoperative language mapping, 2 of 250 patients were reported to have long-lasting aphasia after surgery (97). In both cases, aggressive resection near essential speech areas was performed. In the Seattle series, removal of brain within 1 to 2 cm of essential sites established by intraoperative mapping was associated with mild language deficits (101,102).

The "tailored operation" is designed to use language-mapping techniques to identify and protect neocortical language sites. In a comparison of "standard" versus tailored TLs performed by a single surgeon, a slight increase in postoperative dysnomia was identified 6 months after surgery following a "standard" operation (103).

Complications of Extratemporal Neocortical Focal Resections

The extratemporal epilepsies considered for resective therapy are less frequent, more variable in their presentation, and the epileptogenic zone is more likely to involve eloquent cortex and intraoperative or extraoperative brain mapping is often necessary. All of these facts have a direct impact upon the complications of extratemporal neocortical focal resections, most important of which are the functional consequences of adequate removal of the epileptogenic zone in a particular brain area. In a systematic fashion, we can divide extratemporal focal resections in frontal, central, parietal, and occipital resections.

Frontal Resections. Anatomically, Broca's area is located in the inferior frontal gyrus at *pars triangularis* and *pars opercularis* of the dominant frontal lobe, and this region is generally avoided when dominant frontal resections are performed under general anesthesia. The pattern of frontal language localization may be quite variable and many centers rely upon brain-mapping techniques to tailor frontal resections and avoid language complications. These investigations may identify zones of language cortex quite separate from Broca's area within middle, superior, and even parasagittal frontal cortex in the region of the supplementary motor area (SMA).

Transitory aphasic syndromes are often caused when resections are carried within 1 to 1.5 cm of these essential language areas (101). Long-lasting expressive aphasia can follow resection of language sites in the posterior inferior frontal gyrus or vascular compromise with postoperative ischemic injury to the region. Resections involving frontal cortex (superior frontal gyrus) may cause compromise of draining frontal veins with associated postoperative edema, venous infarction, as well as potential language and motor deficits.

The SMA is located in the mesial superior frontal cortex of the lower extremity and superior to the cingulate gyrus. Functional studies have shown that this area is activated during initiation of movement and vocalization. Stimulation of this area leads to a fencing posture with bilateral motor movement. Unilateral responses are rare. The SMA is extensively and somatotopically connected through the corpus callosum, resulting in fast spread of the ictal discharges to the contralateral side, making lateralization of the ictal-onset zone difficult (104). Resection of the SMA located in the mesial frontal lobe may produce supplementary motor cortex syndrome characterized by mutism, contralateral neglection or hemiparesis, and diminished spontaneous movement which gradually resolves over several weeks (105,106). On long-term follow-up, gross motor deficits are rare.

The orbitofrontal area is limited laterally by the orbitofrontal sulcus, medially by the olfactory sulcus, anteriorly and superiorly by the frontomarginal sulcus, and posteriorly by the anterior perforated area. The orbitofrontal cortex is extensively connected with the anterior and mesial temporal lobes, cingulum and opercular area, and for this reason, frequently misdiagnosed as anterior temporal seizures (107). Adequate sampling of these structures using invasive electrodes is recommended. On the nondominant side, extensive resection of the orbitofrontal cortex can be performed without deficits. The intersection of the optic nerve and the olfactory nerve and the anterior face of the M1 segment of the MCA are used as the posterior anatomical landmarks of the resection. On the dominant side, mapping of the Broca's area should be performed.

The cognitive effects of extensive nondominant frontal resections are thought to be of minimal consequences in daily life activities (108). Furthermore, provided that a careful subpial technique is employed, with preservation of the vascular supply to motor cortex, frontal excisions may be safely carried up to the pial bank of the precentral gyrus. Care must be taken, however, not to undermine the motor cortex if the resections are extended into the white matter.

Central Resections. Central type epilepsy or seizures arising from the primary motor and sensory area are infrequent. Patients with preserved motor function present considerable challenges. A more aggressive approach to the peri-Rolandic epilepsies is gaining acceptance in which extraoperative functional mapping of central cortex is supplemented by intraoperative remapping of this area by direct cortical stimulation, often under awake conditions.

Resection of the face motor cortex. The partial resection of the nondominant face motor cortex may be safely performed, resulting in a transitory contralateral facial asymmetry. Complete removal may be associated with perioral weakness in some patients. The superior resection margin should extend no higher than 2 to 3 mm below the lowest elicited thumb response. In the dominant hemisphere, some surgeons report postoperative dysarthrias and dysphasias following face motor cortex excision. Nevertheless, Rasmussen et al. reported that complete removal of dominant face motor and sensory cortex may be safely performed, provided that manipulation of underlying white matter or ascending vascular supply is avoided (97).

Resection of the hand/leg motor cortex. The resection of the primary hand motor cortex produces a permanent deficit of fine motor control and should be avoided if useful hand function is present preoperatively. Resection of the primary leg motor cortex will elicit an immediate flaccid leg paralysis followed by gradual partial recovery of ambulatory capacity over months (97). Proximal limb function is likely to recover; however, distal ankle and foot permanent weakness are often present, requiring use of orthoses for safe ambulation.

Resection of the sensory cortex. The resections of leg or face sensory cortex cause permanent but clinically insignificant deficit of proprioception in the leg or two-point discrimination in the lower face (109). In contrast, resection of hand sensory cortex is followed by important functional impairment, with the majority of patients showing deficits of pressure sensitivity, two-point discrimination, point localization, position sense, and tactual object recognition, which makes functional use of the involved hand difficult (109).

Parietal Resections. Very few articles reporting complications in parietal resections are available in the literature. Salanova et al. reported the MNI experience of 79 patients with nontumoral parietal lobe epilepsy (71). Of these, 45.5% were seizure free, 19% had rare seizures, and 21.5% had worthwhile improvement. Persistent dysphasia was noted in two patients, Gerstmann syndrome in one patient, and contralateral weakness in three patients.

Large parietal resections may be undertaken posterior to the central cortex in the nondominant hemisphere without causing a sensorimotor deficit and with a rate of hemiparesis of approximately 0.5% (97). A nondominant parietal syndrome may follow these resections in some individuals. In the dominant hemisphere, language mapping must be used to avoid postoperative language deficits. When resections are extended into the parietal operculum, contralateral lower quadrantic or hemianopic visual field deficits (rare) may occur as resections are performed beyond the depths of the sulci into the white matter (88,97).

Occipital Resections. In patients with hemianopsia, resective occipital surgery carries minimal risk. On the dominant hemisphere, the speech-related cortex should be identified and spared. The management of patients with intact vision is challenging. When a circumscribed lesion is found, lesionectomy can yield satisfactory results. In nonlesional cases, the ictal-onset area should be precisely localized using invasive electrodes (110). These are used in addition to mapping of the calcarine cortex and speech-related cortex. With this strategy, visual deficits can be minimized. Resections of the dominant basal temporal lobe should be carefully planned as this can yield to an alexia without agraphia deficit (98).

Contralateral homonymous hemianopsia may follow resections in this area. If vision is intact preoperatively, calcarine cortex and optic radiations must be spared as much as possible. The use of intraoperative visual-evoked potential (VEP), intraoperative direct stimulation, and radiologic techniques as diffuse tensor images (DTI) are still under investigation.

If adequate data from invasive monitoring are available to suggest that the superior calcarine gyrus may be spared, an inferior calcarine gyrus resection with or without an aggressive resection of mesial temporal lobe structures will result only in a superior quadrantic deficit associated with minimal disability. Excision to within 2 cm of Wernicke's area in the dominant hemisphere may elicit persistent dyslexia (97). Therefore, exposure at craniotomy should be adequate to provide access to the postcentral gyrus and parietotemporal language areas, which will serve as the anterior limits of resection.

CONCLUSIONS

A valid appreciation of the complications of epilepsy surgery is fundamental to balance the risks and benefits of diagnostic and therapeutic procedures. Unfortunately, the actual literature available in this topic does not reflect contemporary surgical practice. Available data are derived from the surgical experience of a few highly experienced surgeons who worked in a few well-established comprehensive epilepsy centers and used patient selection criteria and operative approaches which have since been modified or radically changed. A prospective multicenter study is necessary to determine the contemporary risks for invasive monitoring, the role of awake craniotomy with intraoperative mapping for speech mapping, and the complications rate in the epilepsy population.

References

1. Wiebe S, Blume WT, Girvin JP, et al. Effectiveness and Efficiency of Surgery for Temporal Lobe Epilepsy Study Group. A randomized, controlled trial of surgery for temporal-lobe epilepsy. *N Engl J Med.* 2001; 345(5):311–318.
2. Janszky J, Janszky I, Schulz R, et al. Temporal lobe epilepsy with hippocampal sclerosis: predictors for long-term surgical outcome. *Brain.* 2005;128(pt 2):395–404.
3. Tellez-Zenteno JF, Dhar R, Wiebe S. Long-term seizure outcomes following epilepsy surgery: a systematic review and meta-analysis. *Brain.* 2005; 128(pt 5):1188–1198.
4. Jeha LE, Najm IM, Bingaman WE, et al. Predictors of outcome after temporal lobectomy for the treatment of intractable epilepsy. *Neurology.* 2006;66(12):1938–1940.
5. Jeong SW, Lee SK, Hong KS, et al. Prognostic factors for the surgery for mesial temporal lobe epilepsy: longitudinal analysis. *Epilepsia.* 2005; 46(8):1273–1279.
6. McIntosh AM, Kalnins RM, Mitchell LA, et al. Temporal lobectomy: long-term seizure outcome, late recurrence and risks for seizure recurrence. *Brain.* 2004;127(pt 9):2018–2030.
7. Paglioli E, Palmini A, Paglioli E, et al. Survival analysis of the surgical outcome of temporal lobe epilepsy due to hippocampal sclerosis. *Epilepsia.* 2004;45(11):1383–1391.
8. Spencer SS, Berg AT, Vickrey BG, et al. Predicting long-term seizure outcome after resective epilepsy surgery: the multicenter study. *Neurology.* 2005 27;65(6):912–918.
9. Engel J, Jr., Wiebe S, French J, et al. Practice parameter: temporal lobe and localized neocortical resections for epilepsy. *Epilepsia.* 2003;44(6): 741–751.
10. Jeha LE, Najm I, Bingaman W, et al. Surgical outcome and prognostic factors of frontal lobe epilepsy surgery. *Brain.* 2007;130(pt 2):574–584.
11. Jehi LE, O'Dwyer R, Najm I, Alexopoulos A, Bingaman W. A longitudinal study of surgical outcome and its determinants following posterior cortex epilepsy surgery. *J Epilepsia.* 2009 Sep;50(9):2040–52. Epub 2009 Mar 23.
12. Yun CH, Lee SK, Lee SY, et al. Prognostic factors in neocortical epilepsy surgery: multivariate analysis. *Epilepsia.* 2006;47(3):574–579.
13. Zaatreh MM, Spencer DD, Thompson JL, et al. Frontal lobe tumoral epilepsy: clinical, neurophysiologic features and predictors of surgical outcome. *Epilepsia.* 2002;43(7):727–733.
14. Lee SK, Lee SY, Kim KK, et al. Surgical outcome and prognostic factors of cryptogenic neocortical epilepsy. *Ann Neurol.* 2005;58(4):525–532.
15. Janszky J, Jokeit H, Schulz R, et al. EEG predicts surgical outcome in lesional frontal lobe epilepsy. *Neurology.* 2000;54(7):1470–1476.
16. Spencer DC, Szumowski J, Kraemer DF, et al. Temporal lobe magnetic resonance spectroscopic imaging following selective amygdalohippocampectomy for treatment-resistant epilepsy. *Acta Neurol Scand.* 2005;112(1): 6–12.
17. Ficker DM, So EL, Mosewich RK, et al. Improvement and deterioration of seizure control during the postsurgical course of epilepsy surgery patients. *Epilepsia.* 1999;40(1):62–67.
18. Rasmussen T. Modern problems of pharmacopsychiatry. In: Niedermeyer E, ed. *The Neurosurgical Treatment of Focal Epilepsy.* 1st ed. New York, NY: Krager; 1970:306–325.
19. Wieser HG, Ortega M, Friedman A, et al. Long-term seizure outcomes following amygdalohippocampectomy. *J Neurosurg.* 2003;98(4): 751–763.
20. Cascino GD. Improving quality of life with epilepsy surgery: the seizure outcome is the key to success. *Neurology.* 2007;68(23):1967–1968.
21. Cascino GD, Trenerry MR, So EL, et al. Routine EEG and temporal lobe epilepsy: relation to long-term EEG monitoring, quantitative MRI, and operative outcome. *Epilepsia.* 1996;37(7):651–656.
22. Cascino GD, Trenerry MR, Jack CR, Jr, et al. Electrocorticography and temporal lobe epilepsy: relationship to quantitative MRI and operative outcome. *Epilepsia.* 1995;36(7):692–696.
23. Janszky J, Pannek HW, Janszky I, et al. Failed surgery for temporal lobe epilepsy: predictors of long-term seizure-free course. *Epilepsy Res.* 2005; 64(1–2):35–44.
24. Hennessy MJ, Elwes RD, Rabe-Hesketh S, et al. Prognostic factors in the surgical treatment of medically intractable epilepsy associated with mesial temporal sclerosis. *Acta Neurol Scand.* 2001;103(6):344–350.
25. Paglioli E, Palmini A, Portuguez M, et al. Seizure and memory outcome following temporal lobe surgery: selective compared with nonselective approaches for hippocampal sclerosis. *J Neurosurg.* 2006;104(1):70–78.
26. Salanova V, Markand O, Worth R. Temporal lobe epilepsy: analysis of failures and the role of reoperation. *Acta Neurol Scand.* 2005;111(2): 126–133.
27. Urbach H, Hattingen J, von Oertzen J, et al. MR imaging in the presurgical workup of patients with drug-resistant epilepsy. *Am J Neuroradiol.* 2004;25(6):919–926.
28. Yoon HH, Kwon HL, Mattson RH, et al. Long-term seizure outcome in patients initially seizure-free after resective epilepsy surgery. *Neurology.* 2003;61(4):445–450.
29. Jutila L, Immonen A, Mervaala E, et al. Long term outcome of temporal lobe epilepsy surgery: analyses of 140 consecutive patients. *J Neurol Neurosurg Psychiatr.* 2002;73(5):486–494.
30. Wieser HG, Blume WT, Fish D, et al. ILAE Commission Report. Proposal for a new classification of outcome with respect to epileptic seizures following epilepsy surgery. *Epilepsia.* 2001;42(2):282–286.
31. Kelley K, Theodore WH. Prognosis 30 years after temporal lobectomy. *Neurology,* 2005;64(11):1974–1976.
32. Schwartz TH, Jeha L, Tanner A, et al. Late seizures in patients initially seizure free after epilepsy surgery. *Epilepsia* 2006;47(3):567–573.
33. Sperling MR, Feldman H, Kinman J, et al. Seizure control and mortality in epilepsy. *Ann Neurol.* 1999;46(1):45–50.
34. Sperling MR, O'Connor MJ, Saykin AJ, et al. Temporal lobectomy for refractory epilepsy. *J Am Med Assoc.* 1996;276(6):470–475.
35. Kelemen A, Barsi P, Eross L, et al. Long-term outcome after temporal lobe surgery—prediction of late worsening of seizure control. *Seizure.* 2006; 15(1):49–55.
36. Jehi LE. Mesial temporal lobectomy: post-surgical seizure frequency. In: Lüders HO, ed. *Textbook of Epilepsy Surgery.* 1st ed. United Kingdom: Informa; 2008:1223–1235.
37. Salanova V, Andermann F, Rasmussen T, et al. The running down phenomenon in temporal lobe epilepsy. *Brain.* 1996;119 (pt 3):989–996.
38. Kilpatrick C, Cook M, Matkovic Z, et al. Seizure frequency and duration of epilepsy are not risk factors for postoperative seizure outcome in patients with hippocampal sclerosis. *Epilepsia.* 1999;40(7):899–903.
39. Mathern GW, Pretorius JK, Babb TL. Influence of the type of initial precipitating injury and at what age it occurs on course and outcome in patients with temporal lobe seizures. *J Neurosurg.* 1995;82(2):220–227.
40. Radhakrishnan K, So EL, Silbert PL, et al. Predictors of outcome of anterior temporal lobectomy for intractable epilepsy: a multivariate study. *Neurology.* 1998;51(2):465–471.

41. Berkovic SF, McIntosh AM, Kalnins RM, et al. Preoperative MRI predicts outcome of temporal lobectomy: an actuarial analysis. *Neurology.* 1995;45(7):1358–1363.
42. Sylaja PN, Radhakrishnan K, Kesavadas C, et al. Seizure outcome after anterior temporal lobectomy and its predictors in patients with apparent temporal lobe epilepsy and normal MRI. *Epilepsia.* 2004;45(7):803–808.
43. Carne RP, O'Brien TJ, Kilpatrick CJ, et al. MRI-negative PET-positive temporal lobe epilepsy: a distinct surgically remediable syndrome. *Brain.* 2004;127(pt 10):2276–2285.
44. Casse R, Rowe CC, Newton M, et al. Positron emission tomography and epilepsy. *Mol Imaging Biol.* 2002;4(5):338–351.
45. Choi JY, Kim SJ, Hong SB, et al. Extratemporal hypometabolism on FDG PET in temporal lobe epilepsy as a predictor of seizure outcome after temporal lobectomy. *Eur J Nucl Med Mol Imaging.* 2003;30(4):581–587.
46. Cascino GD. Surgical treatment for extratemporal epilepsy. *Curr Treat Options Neurol.* 2004;6(3):257–262.
47. Castro LH, Serpa MH, Valerio RM, et al. Good surgical outcome in discordant ictal EEG-MRI unilateral mesial temporal sclerosis patients. *Epilepsia.* 2008;49(8):1324–1332.
48. Van Paesschen W, Dupont P, Sunaert S, et al. The use of SPECT and PET in routine clinical practice in epilepsy. *Curr Opin Neurol.* 2007;20(2):194–202.
49. Chung MY, Walczak TS, Lewis DV, et al. Temporal lobectomy and independent bitemporal interictal activity: what degree of lateralization is sufficient? *Epilepsia* 1991;32(2):195–201.
50. Holmes MD, Miles AN, Dodrill CB, et al. Identifying potential surgical candidates in patients with evidence of bitemporal epilepsy. *Epilepsia.* 2003;44(8):1075–1079.
51. Wyler AR, Hermann BP, Somes G. Extent of medial temporal resection on outcome from anterior temporal lobectomy: a randomized prospective study. *Neurosurgery.* 1995;37(5):982–990. Discussion 990–991.
52. Bonilha L, Kobayashi E, Mattos JP, et al. Value of extent of hippocampal resection in the surgical treatment of temporal lobe epilepsy. *Arq Neuropsiquiatr.* 2004;62(1):15–20.
53. York MK, Rettig GM, Grossman RG, et al. Seizure control and cognitive outcome after temporal lobectomy: a comparison of classic Ammon's horn sclerosis, atypical mesial temporal sclerosis, and tumoral pathologies. *Epilepsia.* 2003;44(3):387–398.
54. Lee JJ, Lee SK, Lee SY, et al. Frontal lobe epilepsy: clinical characteristics, surgical outcomes and diagnostic modalities. *Seizure.* 2008;17(6):514–523.
55. Wetjen NM, Marsh WR, Meyer FB, et al. Intracranial electroencephalography seizure onset patterns and surgical outcomes in nonlesional extratemporal epilepsy. *J Neurosurg.* 2008.
56. Elsharkawy AE, Alabbasi AH, Pannek H, et al. Outcome of frontal lobe epilepsy surgery in adults. *Epilepsy Res.* 2008;81(2–3):97–106.
57. Tigaran S, Cascino GD, McClelland RL, . Acute postoperative seizures after frontal lobe cortical resection for intractable partial epilepsy. *Epilepsia.* 2003;44(6):831–835.
58. Mosewich RK, So EL, O'Brien TJ, et al. Factors predictive of the outcome of frontal lobe epilepsy surgery. *Epilepsia.* 2000;41(7):843–849.
59. Wyllie E, Comair YG, Kotagal P, et al. Seizure outcome after epilepsy surgery in children and adolescents. *Ann Neurol.* 1998;44(5):740–748.
60. Chung CK, Lee SK, Kim KJ. Surgical outcome of epilepsy caused by cortical dysplasia. *Epilepsia.* 2005;46(suppl 1):25–29.
61. Urbach H, Scheffler B, Heinrichsmeier T, et al. Focal cortical dysplasia of Taylor's balloon cell type: a clinicopathological entity with characteristic neuroimaging and histopathological features, and favorable postsurgical outcome. *Epilepsia.* 2002;43(1):33–40.
62. Mosewich RK, So EL, O'Brien TJ, et al. Factors predictive of the outcome of frontal lobe epilepsy surgery. *Epilepsia.* 2000;41(7):843–849.
63. Cascino GD, Jack CR, Jr, Parisi JE, et al. MRI in the presurgical evaluation of patients with frontal lobe epilepsy and children with temporal lobe epilepsy: pathologic correlation and prognostic importance. *Epilepsy Res.* 1992;11(1):51–59.
64. Ferrier CH, Engelsman J, Alarcon G, et al. Prognostic factors in presurgical assessment of frontal lobe epilepsy. *J Neurol Neurosurg Psychiatr.* 1999;66(3):350–356.
65. Schramm J, Kral T, Kurthen M, et al. Surgery to treat focal frontal lobe epilepsy in adults. *Neurosurgery.* 2002;51(3):644–654. Discussion 654–655.
66. Salanova V, Quesney LF, Rasmussen T, et al. Reevaluation of surgical failures and the role of reoperation in 39 patients with frontal lobe epilepsy. *Epilepsia.* 1994;35(1):70–80.
67. Ferrier CH, Alarcon G, Engelsman J, et al. Relevance of residual histologic and electrocorticographic abnormalities for surgical outcome in frontal lobe epilepsy. *Epilepsia.* 2001;42(3):363–371.
68. Boesebeck F, Schulz R, May T, et al. Lateralizing semiology predicts the seizure outcome after epilepsy surgery in the posterior cortex. *Brain.* 2002;125(pt 10):2320–2331.
69. Chung CK, Lee SK, Kim KJ. Surgical outcome of epilepsy caused by cortical dysplasia. *Epilepsia.* 2005;46(suppl 1):25–29.
70. Kim CH, Chung CK, Lee SK, et al. Parietal lobe epilepsy: surgical treatment and outcome. *Stereotact Funct Neurosurg.* 2004;82(4):175–185.
71. Salanova V, Andermann F, Rasmussen T, et al. Parietal lobe epilepsy. Clinical manifestations and outcome in 82 patients treated surgically between 1929 and 1988. *Brain.* 1995;118(pt 3):607–627.
72. Sinclair DB, Wheatley M, Snyder T, et al. Posterior resection for childhood epilepsy. *Pediatr Neurol.* 2005;32(4):257–263.
73. Elsharkawy AE, Behne F, Oppel F, et al. Long-term outcome of extratemporal epilepsy surgery among 154 adult patients. *J Neurosurg.* 2008;108(4):676–686.
74. Boesebeck F, Schulz R, May T, et al. Lateralizing semiology predicts the seizure outcome after epilepsy surgery in the posterior cortex. *Brain.* 2002;125(pt 10):2320–2331.
75. Barba C, Doglietto F, De Luca L, et al. Retrospective analysis of variables favouring good surgical outcome in posterior epilepsies. *J Neurol.* 2005;252(4):465–472.
76. Dalmagro CL, Bianchin MM, Velasco TR, et al. Clinical features of patients with posterior cortex epilepsies and predictors of surgical outcome. *Epilepsia.* 2005;46(9):1442–1449.
77. Caicoya AG, Macarron J, Albisua J, et al. Tailored resections in occipital lobe epilepsy surgery guided by monitoring with subdural electrodes: characteristics and outcome. *Epilepsy Res.* 2007;77(1):1–10.
78. Cukiert A, Buratini JA, Machado E, et al. Results of surgery in patients with refractory extratemporal epilepsy with normal or nonlocalizing magnetic resonance findings investigated with subdural grids. *Epilepsia.* 2001;42(7):889–894.
79. Kanner AM, Balabanov AJ. Psychiatric outcome of epilepsy surgery. In: Lüders HO, ed. *Textbook of Epilepsy Surgery.* United Kingdom: Informa; 2008:1254–1261.
80. Wrench J, Wilson SJ, Bladin PF. Mood disturbance before and after seizure surgery: a comparison of temporal and extratemporal resections. *Epilepsia.* 2004;45(5):534–543.
81. So N, Dodrill CB. Psychosocial outcome and quality of life outcome. In: Lüders HO, ed. *Textbook of Epilepsy Surgery.* United Kingdom: Informa; 2008:1269–1276.
82. Jayakar P. Invasive EEG monitoring in children: when, where and what? *J Clin Neurophysiol.* 1999;16:404–418.
83. Lüders H, Lesser R, Dinner D, et al. Commentary: chronic intracranial recording and stimulation with subdural electrodes. In: Engel JJ, ed. *Surgical Treatment of the Epilepsies.* New York, NY: Raven Press; 1987:297–321.
84. Rosenow F, Luders H. Presurgical evaluation of epilepsy [in process citation]. *Brain.* 2001;124:1683–1700.
85. Cahan L, Sutherling W, McCullough M, et al. Review of the 20 year UCLA experience with surgery for epilepsy. *Cleve Clin Q.* 1984;51:313–318.
86. Spencer DD. Depth electrode implantation at Yale University. In: Engel J, ed. *Surgical Treatment of the Epilepsies.* New York, NY: Raven Press; 1987:603–607.
87. King D, Flanigan H, Gallagher B, et al. Temporal lobectomy for partial complex seizures: evaluation, results and 1 year follow up. *Neurology.* 1986;334–339.
88. Van Buren JM. Complications of surgical procedures in the diagnosis and treatment of epilepsy. In: Engel J, ed. *Surgical Treatment of the Epilepsies.* New York, NY: Raven Press; 1987:465–475.
89. Wyllie E, Luders H, Morris H, et al. Clinical outcome after complete or partial cortical resection for intractable epilepsy. *Neurology.* 1987;37:1634–1641.
90. Pilcher WH, Ojemann GA. Surgical evaluation and treatment of epilepsy. In: Apuzzo MLJ, ed. *Brain Surgery: Complication, Avoidance and Management.* New York: Churchill Livingston, 1993.
91. Spencer SS. Depth versus subdural electrode studies for unlocalized epilepsy. *J Epilepsy.* 1989;2:123–127.
92. Sperling M, O'Connor M. Comparison of depth and subdural electrodes in recording temporal lobe seizures. *Neurology.* 1989;39:1497–1504.
93. Wyler AR, Walker G, Somes G. The morbidity of long-term seizure monitoring using subdural grid electrodes. *J Neurosurg.* 1991;74:734–737.
94. Rosenbaum TJ, Laxer KD. Subdural electrode recordings for seizure focus localization. *J Epilepsy.* 1989;2:129–135.
95. Cossu M, Cardinale F, Castana L, et al. Stereoelectroencephalography in the presurgical evaluation of focal epilepsy: a retrospective analysis of 215 procedures. *Neurosurgery.* 2005;57(4):706–718.
96. Silfvenius H, Gloor P, Rasmussen T. Evaluation of insular ablationin surgical treatment of temporal lobe epilepsy. *Epilepsia.* 1964;5:307–320.
97. Rasmussen T. Surgical treatment of patients with complex partial seizures. In: Penry JK, Daly DD, eds. *Advances in Neurology.* Vol. 8. New York, NY: Raven Press; 1975:197–205.
98. Lüders H, Lesser R, Dinner D, et al. Language deficits elicited by electrical stimulation of the fusiform gyrus. In: Engel J Jr, ed. *Fundamental Mechanisms of Human Brain Function.* New York, NY: Raven Press;1987;83–90.
99. Crandall PH. Postoperative management and criteria for evaluation. In: Purpura DP, Penry JK, Walter RD, eds. *Neurosurgical Management of the Epilepsies. Advances in Neurology.* Vol. 8. New York, NY: Raven Press; 1975:265–279.
100. Katz A, Awad I, Kong A, et al. Extent of resection in temporal lobectomy for epilepsy: II. Memory changes and neurological complications. *Epilepsia.* 1989;30:763–771.

101. Ojemann GA, Dodrill CB. Intraoperative techniques for reducing language and memory deficits with left temporal lobectomy. *Advances in Epileptology.* Vol 16. New York, NY: Raven Press; 1987;327–330.

102. Ojemann GA, Ojemann J, Lettich E, et al. Cortical language localization in left, dominant hemisphere. *J Neurosurg.* 1989;71:316–326.

103. Hermann BP, Wyler AR. Comparative results of temporal lobectomy under local or general anesthesia: language outcome. *J Epilepsy.* 1988;1: 127–134.

104. Tuxhorn I, Van Ness PC, Luders HO. Supplementary motor area seizures: EEG patterns with interhemispheric subdural plate electrodes. *Neurology.* 1992; 42(suppl 3):158.

105. Olivier A, Awad IA. Extratemporal resections. In: Engel J Jr, ed. *Surgical Treatment of the Epilepsies.* 2nd ed. New York, NY: Raven Press; 1993: 489–500.

106. Rostomily R, Berger M, Ojemann G, et al. Postoperative deficits and functional recovery following removal of tumors involving the dominant hemisphere supplementary motor area. *J Neurosurg.* 1991;75(1):62–68.

107. Tharp BR. Orbital frontal seizures. An unique electroencephalographic and clinical syndrome. *Epilepsia.* 1972;13:627–642.

108. Milner B. Visually-guided maze learning in man: effects of bilateral hippocampal, bilateral frontal and unilateral cerebral lesions. *Neuropsychologia.* 1965;3:317–338.

109. Corkin S, Milner B, Rasmussen T. Somatosensory thresholds: contrasting effects of postcentral gyrus and posterior parietal lobe excisions. *Arch Neurol.* 1970;23:41–58.

110. Comair Y, Choi HY, Van Ness P. Neocortical resections. In: Engel J Jr, ed. *Epilepsy: A Comprehensive Textbook.* Philadelphia, PA: Lippincott-Raven Publishers; 1997.

CHAPTER 91 ■ ELECTRICAL STIMULATION FOR THE TREATMENT OF EPILEPSY

S. MATTHEW STEAD AND GREGORY A. WORRELL

Electrical stimulation has a long history as a diagnostic and therapeutic modality for epilepsy (1,2). The application of electrical stimulation for mapping cortical function in animals was first reported by Fritsch and Hitzig in 1870 (3), and the first report in humans by Bartholow (4) followed in 1874. Krause and Foerster extended the clinical application of electrical stimulation for localization of brain function in patients undergoing surgery for epilepsy (5). These studies culminated in the seminal work of Penfield and Jasper (6) who established the routine clinical use of electrical stimulation for localization of cortical function in epilepsy surgery.

THERAPEUTIC STIMULATION FOR THE TREATMENT OF EPILEPSY

Cooper first began implanting cerebellar stimulators in patients with intractable epilepsy in the 1970s (8,9), but the idea of electrical stimulation as a treatment for epilepsy is much older (2,10). Cooper reported significant reductions in the number of seizures with chronic cerebellar stimulation (8,9). However, later controlled trials did not confirm a dramatic therapeutic effect (11). The failure of a controlled trial to confirm the efficacy reported in uncontrolled trials was later repeated for centromedian nucleus (CMN) of thalamus stimulation (12). These examples underscore the need for well-designed clinical trials to establish the efficacy of electrical stimulation before they can be recommended in routine clinical practice. Recent reviews have summarized the research in humans and animal models, and have laid the framework for future research and clinical trials of brain stimulation for treatment of epilepsy (2,13).

Advances in neural engineering are now poised to deliver new treatments for a range of neurological diseases. In epilepsy, active areas of research include the development of devices that modulate epileptogenic brain to prevent seizures, devices that directly detect seizures and deliver electrical stimulation to abort seizures, and devices that identify periods of increased probability of seizure occurrence (2,7). Two first-generation devices using electrical stimulation for treatment of epilepsy are currently in multicenter trials (Fig. 91.1), and are discussed below in detail.

Clinical Trial Design

Determining the efficacy of an epilepsy therapy is challenging. Epilepsy is characterized by unprovoked paroxysmal seizures that leave no lasting objective evidence of their occurrence. Clinical trials investigating treatment efficacy, for example, medications or brain stimulation, typically use reduction in seizure frequency as the primary outcome measure. Well-designed clinical trials have control and active

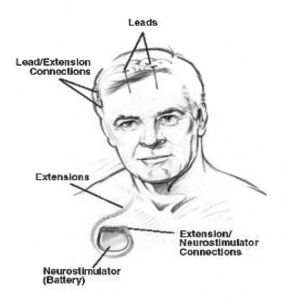

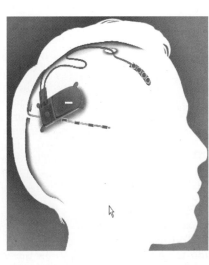

FIGURE 91.1 Brain stimulation devices. The Medtronic DBS device (**left**) and NeuroPace RNS device (**right**) panels are currently undergoing multicenter pivotal trials. Preliminary results for these devices are encouraging.

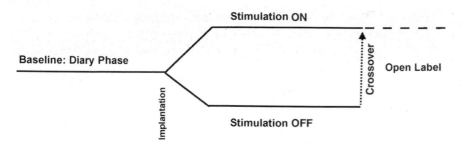

FIGURE 91.2 Study design. Baseline phase to determine frequency of seizures prior to therapeutic intervention. Note all phases of the study require patient diary entry to track seizure frequency. Implantation is followed by a period to minimize the confound of an acute implantation effect (e.g., 1 month). The patient is then randomized to therapy ON or OFF. After the evaluation phase (double-blind control phase) all patients are entered into an open-label phase during which the blinding is removed and all patients receive stimulation.

therapy arms (Fig. 91.2) with patients randomized to therapy ON or OFF. The patient and treating physicians are blinded to this information in order to limit bias. Nonetheless, because seizures occur sporadically without lasting objective evidence of their occurrence, the measure of treatment success depends on the seizure diary. Of course, many patients are amnesic for their seizures, and the limitations of seizure diaries are well known (14). This can be contrasted with investigation of a disease or disorder associated with a measurable signal, for example, the use of MRI to follow tumor size during a cancer drug trial.

To determine the efficacy of a particular brain stimulation paradigm (target of stimulation, timing of stimulation, stimulation parameters, etc.) for treatment of epilepsy requires an appropriate study design. Pilot studies in a small number of patients are often used to initially investigate the safety, feasibility, and evidence of possible efficacy. Pilot and feasibility studies are not adequately powered to prove efficacy, but should use an appropriate design with controls and blinding. Figure 91.2 is a schematic for a double-blind, placebo- controlled trial that has been adopted for two recent multicenter brain stimulation trials (Stimulation of the anterior nucleus of the thalamus for epilepsy [SANTE] trial by Medtronic, and the responsive neurostimulator system [RNS] trial by NeuroPace). As discussed in the following sections, a number of studies that reported positive results have not held up in better designed, more rigorous studies with a placebo-controlled arm.

Baseline

The baseline seizure frequency is determined from the patient diary in a defined period prior to the intervention under investigation. Studies of epilepsy, whether they are drug studies or brain stimulation, typically rely on the patient diary for determining seizure frequency. The reliability of patient reporting is a recognized weakness, but there are currently no reliable tools for counting seizures in the outpatient setting.

Implantation

The device is implanted in patients who have met the enrollment criteria of the study. For example, in the 3-month baseline seizure frequency phase, the patient had the required number of seizures. In order to minimize the acute effect of implantation, there is typically a period of time (~1 month) prior to randomization to stimulation ON/OFF and commencing the blinded treatment phase.

Randomization and Placebo Control

In order to rigorously differentiate the effect of electrode implantation, placebo, and stimulation, a sham surgery arm would be required. In most cases, it is not ethically possible to include sham surgery. The placebo response and efficacy of stimulation are determined by randomization of patients to therapy ON or OFF. In effect, a coin toss (heads/tails) determines whether stimulation is activated or remains inactivated after surgery. In this way, approximately half the patients in the trial are randomized to therapy ON or OFF.

Double-Blind Design

The placebo response is well established in clinical trials and can have a powerful impact on patient's and physician's perception of treatment efficacy. By blinding the patient and physician to the treatment information, that is, is stimulation ON or OFF, the placebo response can be determined. The efficacy of stimulation can be evaluated by directly comparing seizure frequency with stimulation ON versus OFF. A statistically significant reduction in seizures in the stimulation arm versus placebo (i.e., control) can be attributed to the therapy. Any seizure reduction occurring in the control arm is attributed to placebo response, chance, or possibly implantation effect. As mentioned in the two device trials currently under way (Medtronic SANTE and NeuroPace RNS), the implantation of the electrodes could conceivably create a therapeutic lesion.

Crossover

A crossover design allows patients who were initially randomized to therapy OFF to receive stimulation after completion of the double-blind study phase. The multicenter trials discussed in the following sections have utilized this single crossover design. In a *double* crossover study design, patients receiving therapy (ON) are crossed over to no therapy (OFF). In an attractive study design, the possible carryover effects of brain stimulation could confound the interpretation of the results. The "washout" period for anticonvulsant medications can be easily obtained, but the time required for "washout" of the effect of months of brain stimulation is not known.

Open-Label Extension

In the open-label portion of the trial, all patients receive stimulation without blinding. Often in the open-label phase medications are adjusted or added, so interpretation of results requires caution. In addition, the patients and physician are no longer blinded to the therapy. Interestingly, the three large-scale multicenter clinical trials (see vagus nerve stimulation [VNS], SANTE, and RNS studies discussed below) have all shown evidence for increasing efficacy of brain stimulation with duration of time of receiving stimulation. These results must be interpreted with caution since they come from the open-label portion of the trial, but raise the possibility that brain stimulation has a cumulative therapeutic benefit.

Measures of Efficacy

Commonly reported outcome measures are (i) responder rate (RR), defined as the percentage of patients with a 50% or greater reduction in seizures; (ii) mean reduction in seizures from all patients; (iii) number of seizure-free patients (defined over a specific duration of the trial, e.g., the most recent 3 months of the open-label phase of the trial). In addition, quality of life measures are often assessed, for example, Quality of Life in Epilepsy (QOLIE)-89 scale (15).

Measures of Safety

Side effects are categorized as serious or minor, and anticipated or unanticipated. For example, an intracranial hemorrhage associated with electrode placement would be a serious, but anticipated complication.

ELECTRICAL STIMULATION PARADIGMS

The parameter space defining the range of stimulation variables is large and includes the type of stimulation (constant current vs. constant voltage), amplitude, stimulation waveform, frequency, duration, etc. The paradigms of stimulation can be broadly categorized as follows.

Open-Loop Stimulation (Duty Cycle Stimulation)

To date, the majority of stimulation systems utilize duty cycle stimulation. The stimulation is given regardless of the occurrence of seizures or brain activity. For example, VNS for epilepsy, deep brain stimulation for tremor, and open-loop stimulation protocols for the SANTE trial.

Closed-Loop Stimulation (Intelligent, Automated, or Responsive Stimulation)

Recently developed systems utilizing implantable microprocessors make it possible for programmable stimulation to be delivered in response to seizures or other electrophysiological signals. The NeuroPace RNS system is a closed-loop device capable of recording continuous intracranial EEG and delivering therapeutic stimulation based on automated detection of seizures.

Control Law Stimulation (Feedback Control Stimulation)

Based on the hypothesis that seizures occur out of a particular brain state that can be characterized by some observable (e.g., iEEG), it may be possible to actually prevent seizures by continuously adjusting a therapy (such as stimulation) that is determined by the measured observable. This approach is commonly used in a wide range of engineering applications and has been applied to animal models of epilepsy (16–18).

STIMULATION TARGETS IN THE HUMAN NERVOUS SYSTEM

Vagus Nerve Stimulation

VNS is an adjunctive treatment for patients with medically refractory partial epilepsy (19–21). The device was approved by the U.S. Food and Drug Administration (FDA) for partial epilepsy in patients 12 years of age or older in 1997 (22). It delivers duty cycle electrical stimulation to the left vagus nerve. The implanted programmable pulse generator uses a helical electrode wrapped around the left vagus nerve in the neck. This is primarily seen as a palliative therapeutic modality with a response rate similar to antiepileptic drug (AED) therapy (23,24), with 50% reduction in seizure activity in approximately one third to one half of individuals. In medically refractory patients, it is uncommon for patients to achieve a seizure remission with this device (19,21,23–25).

Since patients can detect stimulation of the vagus nerve, VNS trials have utilized "low" versus "high" stimulation study designs. Unfortunately, in these study designs the placebo effect cannot be determined, since the patient is aware of the stimulation. Nonetheless, two well-designed controlled trials have demonstrated the efficacy of VNS for treatment of epilepsy (26,27). The trials have demonstrated that "high"-level stimulation (0.25 to 3.50 mA, 500 μsec pulse width, 30 Hz for 30 sec delivered every 5 min) is more effective than "low" stimulation (0.25 to 3.50 mA, 130 μsec pulse width, 1 Hz for 30 sec delivered every 180 min). The studies have shown that the reduction in seizure frequency was 25% to 30% for the "high" stimulation group and 6% to 15% for the "low" stimulation group. The responder rate (i.e., 50% reduction in seizures) was approximately 40% for the "high" stimulation group and 20% for the "low" stimulation group.

In the open-label extension of the E05 VNS trials (27), the median reduction in seizures was 45% versus 28% found at the end of the crossover, double phase. At 12 months, 35% of 195 subjects had a >50% reduction in seizures, and 20% had a >75% reduction in seizures (28).

Intracranial Stimulation

The idea of using electrical stimulation to treat epilepsy has a long history (1,2,10). Here some of the earlier studies will be reviewed, but particular focus is given to studies with control data and good clinical design.

The ability to accurately and safely implant electrodes into human brain has led to dramatically successful therapies for some neurological disorders, for example, tremor (1). Less successful has been the application of deep brain stimulation, hippocampus stimulation, and neocortical stimulation for treatment of epilepsy. Nonetheless, the field has moved steadily forward. Fortunately, the field of brain stimulation for epilepsy will soon have the results of two well-designed multicenter clinical trials (Medtronic SANTE and NeuroPace RNS), investigating the feasibility, safety, and efficacy of brain stimulation for treatment of medically resistant partial epilepsy. Preliminary results from both of these multicenter trials have recently been reported and are discussed below.

Cerebellar Stimulation

The cerebellum provides inhibitory outflow, and for this reason was an early candidate target for electrical stimulation to treat epilepsy (8,29). In early uncontrolled studies, cerebellar stimulation was reported to yield significant reductions seizures. An early uncontrolled trial of 115 patients reported 31 patients became seizure-free and 56 improved significantly (30). This was a remarkable result and generated considerable interest.

However, in a later controlled, double-blind study of 12 patients, only two patients showed improvement (11). The small number of patients studied in the trial limits the ability to draw conclusions, and the use of cerebellar stimulation is not currently pursued.

Caudate Nucleus Stimulation

Chkhenkeli and Chkhenkeli (31) reported a decrease in "interparoxysmal activity" in neocortical and mesial temporal epileptic foci in patients with partial epilepsy, but clinical seizures were not investigated.

Mammillary Nuclei

Mirski and Fisher (32) reported an increase in the seizure threshold for pentylenetetrazol treated rats. However, trials have not been performed in humans.

Centromedian Nucleus of the Thalamus

The CMN is implicated as part of the circuit involved in the generation of spike-and-wave discharges in generalized epilepsy (33). Early reports from Velasco et al. reported significant reductions in seizures for patients with generalized convulsive seizures and atypical absence seizures, but no benefit in patients with complex partial seizures (33,34).

Fisher (12) reported the first randomized, controlled trial of CMN stimulation in seven patients. The trial did not show a statistically significant difference between the stimulation ON versus OFF (although one patient showed marked improvement). The trial was a rigorous double-blind, placebo-controlled, crossover design. One patient experienced dramatic benefit, which prevented his crossover to the OFF arm. In addition, in this double crossover design, the possible "carryover" benefit from 3 months of stimulation may have confounded the results. Unfortunately, it is not known if there

is a carryover effect from stimulation and if there is the "washout" time required for its elimination.

Subthalamic Nucleus

Stimulation of the subthalamic nucleus (STN) for treatment of essential tremor and Parkinson disease is safe and effective (35). The use of stimulation of STN for epilepsy is based on evidence for a subcortical control network that influences cortical excitability (35).

Loddenkemper et al. (36) reviewed the studies supporting the existence of the nigral control of epilepsy system and preliminary results of STN stimulation in animals and humans. There are no controlled trials.

Anterior Nucleus of the Thalamus Stimulation

The antiepileptic effect of stimulation of the anterior nucleus of the thalamus is thought to be mediated by its integral role in the circuit of Papez (2). Sectioning the connection between the mammillary bodies and the anterior thalamus markedly increased the threshold for pentylentrazol-induced seizures in guinea pigs (37). Later studies showed that high-frequency electrical stimulation of the anterior thalamus in rat also significantly increased the threshold for pentylentrazol-induced seizures (32).

Upton and Cooper reported an antiepileptic effect associated with stimulation of the anterior nucleus of thalamus (38). Hodaie et al. (39) reported on five patients who underwent bilateral anterior thalamus stimulation. The patients experienced a 54% mean reduction in seizure frequency, with two patients having >75% reduction. Interestingly, however, there was not a significant difference between the stimulation ON and OFF arms of the trial, perhaps indicating a strong placebo component, carryover confound, or therapeutic lesion from implantation.

Medtronic SANTE Trial

The preliminary results from a large multicenter, randomized, controlled trial for SANTE using the Medtronic Deep Brain Stimulation stimulator have recently been reported by R.S. Fisher. The SANTE trial recently reported by Fisher et al. (Fisher R, et al. *Epilepsia* 51:899–908, 2010). new reference was a multi-center, double-blind, randomized trial of bilateral stimulation of the anterior nuclei of thalamus for partial epilepsy. In this study from 17 epilepsy centers, 110 participants were implanted with the Medtronic DBS device, and half randomized to sham stimulation and half to duty cycle stimulation. Baseline monthly median seizure frequency was 19.5. In the last month of the blinded phase the stimulated group had a 29% greater reduction in seizures compared with the control group as estimated by a generalized estimating equations (GEE) model (p = 0.002). Unadjusted median declines at the end of the blinded phase were 14.5% in the sham stimulation (control group) and 40.4% in the group receiving stimulation. After the blinded phase all patients received stimulation, and after two years 54% of patients had a seizure reduction of at least 50%.

The SANTE trial showed evidence of efficacy and modest complication rates. During the course of the trial five deaths occurred, but none were believed to be related to implantation or stimulation.

Hippocampus Stimulation

Velasco et al. (40) reported on nine patients with a 3-month-baseline-seizure count, after which they underwent bilateral hippocampus diagnostic electrode implantation to establish laterality and location of seizure onset. The patients were not surgical candidates, and were offered therapeutic stimulation. Three patients had bilateral, and six had unilateral seizure onset foci. Duty cycle stimulation was delivered using the Medtronic DBS system. Follow-up ranged from 18 months to 7 years. Patients were divided into groups: patients with normal MRI and patients with MRI consistent with mesial hippocampus sclerosis. Patients with normal MRIs had seizure reductions of >95%, while the four patients with hippocampus sclerosis had seizure reductions of 50% to 70% (40).

Vonck et al. reported on 10 patients with temporal lobe epilepsy and normal MRIs who received duty cycle stimulation to unilateral amygdalohippocampal stimulation. All patients had a >50% reduction in seizures at 5 months (41).

Tellez-Zenteno et al. (42), however, reported on a well-designed controlled trial of four patients who had a median reduction in seizures of only 15% using duty cycle hippocampus stimulation with the Medtronic DBS device. All but one patient's seizures improved; however, the results did not reach significance. The authors concluded that there are beneficial trends, some long-term benefits, and absence of adverse effects of hippocampus electrical stimulation in mesial temporal lobe epilepsy. However, the effect sizes observed were much smaller than those reported in nonrandomized, unblinded studies. Again, these results are from small groups of patients. More recently, the preliminary results from the safety and feasibility trial for the NeuroPace RNS device were reported at the 2008 AES meeting by Morrell (43) (see the following section).

NeuroPace Responsive Neurostimulation Trial

The responsive neurostimulator system (RNS NeuroPace) is an investigational device being tested in adults with medically resistant partial epilepsy. The RNS includes a cranially implanted programmable and depth or subdural leads, a physician programmer, a patient data transmitter, and a web-based interactive data repository. A 2-year multicenter safety and feasibility trial collected safety and efficacy data after implantation. These preliminary results were not powered to prove efficacy. However, because of the good safety data and encouraging results, a multicenter pivotal trial is now completed.

The RNS trial was a multi-center, double-blind, randomized trial of responsive neural stimulation applied to the region of brain generating seizures. In this study from 32 epilepsy centers, 191 participants were implanted with the Neuropace RNS system. In the pivotal trial phase 93 patients randomized to sham stimulation and 96 patients received responsive stimulation delivered on detection of epileptiform activity. Unadjusted median declines at the end of the blinded

phase were 41% reduction in seizures in the group receiving stimulation compared to a 9% reduction in the sham stimulation group. Using a generalized estimating equation there was a 21% greater reduction (p = 0.012) in the group receiving stimulation compared to the control (sham) group not receiving stimulation After the blinded phase all patients received stimulation, and over the most recent 3 months period 51% of patients had a seizure reduction of at least 50%.

The RNS trial showed evidence of efficacy and modest complication rates. During the course of the trial five deaths occurred, but none were believed to be related to implantation or stimulation.

CONCLUSIONS

Despite the development of numerous new anticonvulsant medications, the number of patients that remain refractory to best medical therapy is significant. The potential for therapeutic brain stimulation has attracted considerable attention over the past decades, and the technology is now matured to the point were devices are possible. There are two well-designed multicenter trials under way, investigating electrical stimulation for the treatment of epilepsy. The preliminary results from both trials, SANTE (Medtronic) and RNS (NeuroPace), show promise as viable therapies for medically resistant epilepsy.

The SANTE trial results are not yet published, but the results presented at the 2008 American Epilepsy Society 2008 are from a pivotal trial that demonstrated efficacy. The NeuroPace RNS trial results, also presented at AES 2008, are from a safety and feasibility trial, and while not powered to prove efficacy, the results are encouraging. A pivotal trial with the RNS device is now under way and should conclude within the next year. The safety record from both these device trials of long-term brain stimulation is very encouraging.

The next decade will hopefully see the emergence of viable therapeutic devices for patients with epilepsy.

References

1. Kringelbach ML, Jenkinson N, Owen SLF, et al. Translational principles of deep brain stimulation. *Nat Rev Neurosci.* 2007;8(8):623–635.
2. Theodore WH, Fisher RS. Brain stimulation for epilepsy. *Lancet Neurol.* 2004;3(2):111–118.
3. Fritsch G, Hitzig E. Über die elektrische Erregbarkeit des Grosshirns. *Arch Anat Physiol.* 1870;37:300–332.
4. Bartholow R. Experimental investigations into the functions of the human brain. *Am J Med Sci.* 1874;67:305–313.
5. Luders HO, Luders JC. Contributions of Fedor Krause and Otfrid Foerster to epilepsy surgery. In: Luders H, Comair Y, eds. *Epilepsy Surgery.* Philadelphia: Lippincott Williams & Wilkins; 2001.
6. Jasper H, Penfield W. *Epilepsy and the Functional Anatomy of the Human Brain.* Boston, MA: Little, Brown and Co.; 1954.
7. Stacey WC, Litt B. Technology insight: neuroengineering and epilepsy-designing devices for seizure control. *Nat Clin Pract Neurol.* 2008;4(4):190–201.
8. Cooper I. *Cerebellar Stimulation in Man.* New York: Raven Press; 1978.
9. Cooper I, Amin I, Gilman S. The effect of chronic cerebellar stimulation upon epilepsy in man. *Trans Am Neurol Assoc.* 1973;98:192–196.
10. Kellaway P. The part played by electric fish in the early history of bioelectricity and electrotherapy. *Bull Hist Med.* 1946;20:112–137.
11. Wright G, McLellan D, Brice J. A double-blind trial of chronic cerebellar stimulation in 12 patients with severe epilepsy. *J Neurol Neurosurg Psychiatr.* 1984;47:769–774.
12. Fisher RS, Uematsu S, Kraus GL, et al. Placebo-controlled pilot study of centromedian thalamic stimulation in treatment of intractable seizures. *Epilepsia.* 1992;33(5):841–851.
13. Morrell M. Brain stimulation for epilepsy: can scheduled or responsive neurostimulation stop seizures? *Curr Opin Neurol.* 2006;19(2):164–168.

14. Hoppe C, Poepel A, Elger CE. Epilepsy: accuracy of patient seizure counts. *Arch Neurol.* 2007;64(11):1595–1599.

15. Vickrey BG, Perrine KR, Hays RD, et al. Quality of Life in Epilepsy (QOLIE)-89: scoring manual and patient inventory. Santa Monica, CA: RAND; 1993.

16. Gluckman BJ, Neel EJ, Netoff TI, et al. Electric field suppression of epileptiform activity in hippocampal slices. *J Neurophysiol.* 1996;76(6): 4202–4205.

17. Richardson KA, Gluckman BJ, Weinstein SL, et al. In vivo modulation of hippocampal epileptiform activity with radial electric fields. *Epilepsia.* 2003;44(6):768–777.

18. Sunderam S, Chernyy N, Mason J, et al. Seizure modulation with applied electric fields in chronically implanted animals. *Conf Proc IEEE Eng Med Biol Soc.* 2006;1:1612–1615.

19. Ben-Menachem E, Hellström K, Waldton C, et al. Evaluation of refractory epilepsy treated with vagus nerve stimulation for up to 5 years. *Neurology.* 1999;52(6):1265–1267.

20. Schachter SC, Saper CB. Vagus nerve stimulation. *Epilepsia.* 1998;39(7): 677–686.

21. Ben-Menachem E. Vagus-nerve stimulation for the treatment of epilepsy. *Lancet Neurol.* 2002;1(8):477–482.

22. The Vagus Nerve Stimulation Study Group. A randomized controlled trial of chronic vagus nerve stimulation for treatment of medically intractable seizures. *Neurology.* 1995;45(2):224–230.

23. Cramer JA. Exploration of changes in health-related quality of life after 3 months of vagus nerve stimulation. *Epilepsy Behav.* 2001;2(5):460–465.

24. Cramer JA, Ben Menachem E, French J. Review of treatment options for refractory epilepsy: new medications and vagal nerve stimulation. *Epilepsy Res.* 2001;47(1–2):17–25.

25. Schachter SC. Vagus nerve stimulation therapy summary: five years after FDA approval. *Neurology.* 2002;59(6 suppl 4):S15–S20.

26. Ben-Menachem E, Mañon-Espaillat R, Ristanovic R, et al., First International Vagus Nerve Stimulation Study Group. Vagus nerve stimulation for treatment of partial seizures: 1. A controlled study of effect on seizures. *Epilepsia.* 1994;35(3):616–626.

27. Handforth A, DeGiorgio CM, Schachter SC, et al. Vagus nerve stimulation therapy for partial-onset seizures: a randomized active-control trial. *Neurology.* 1998;51(1): 48–55.

28. DeGiorgio CM, Schachter SC, Handforth A, et al. Prospective long-term study of vagus nerve stimulation for the treatment of refractory seizures. *Epilepsia.* 2000;41(9):1195–1200.

29. Cooper IS, Amin I, Riklan M, et al. Chronic cerebellar stimulation in epilepsy. Clinical and anatomical studies. *Arch Neurol.* 1976;33(8):559–570.

30. Davis R, Emmonds SE. Cerebellar stimulation for seizure control: 17-year study. *Stereotact Funct Neurosurg.* 1992;58(1–4):200–208.

31. Chkhenkeli SA, Chkhenkeli IS. Effects of therapeutic stimulation of nucleus caudatus on epileptic electrical activity of brain in patients with intractable epilepsy. *Stereotact Funct Neurosurg.* 1997;69(1–4 Pt 2):221–224.

32. Mirski MA, Fisher RS. Electrical stimulation of the mammillary nuclei increases seizure threshold to pentylenetetrazol in rats. *Epilepsia.* 1994; 35(6):1309–1316.

33. Velasco M, Velasco F, Velasco AL, et al. Effect of chronic electrical stimulation of the centromedian thalamic nuclei on various intractable seizure patterns: II. Psychological performance and background EEG activity. *Epilepsia.* 1993;34(6):1065–1074.

34. Velasco F, Velasco M, Velasco AL, et al. Electrical stimulation of the centromedian thalamic nucleus in control of seizures: long-term studies. *Epilepsia.* 1995;36(1):63–71.

35. Benabid AL, Wallace B, Mitrofanis J, et al. Therapeutic electrical stimulation of the central nervous system. *C R Biol.* 2005;328(2):177–186.

36. Loddenkemper T, Pan A, Neme S, et al. Deep brain stimulation in epilepsy. *J Clin Neurophysiol.* 2001;18(6):514–532.

37. Mirski MA, Ferrendelli JA. Interruption of the mammillothalamic tract prevents seizures in guinea pigs. *Science.* 1984;226(4670):72–74.

38. Upton AR, Cooper IS, Springman M, et al. Suppression of seizures and psychosis of limbic system origin by chronic stimulation of anterior nucleus of the thalamus. *Int J Neurol.* 1985;19–20:223–230.

39. Hodaie M, Wennberg RA, Dostrovsky JO, et al. Chronic anterior thalamus stimulation for intractable epilepsy. *Epilepsia.* 2002;43(6):603–608.

40. Velasco AL, Velasco F, Velasco M, et al. Electrical stimulation of the hippocampal epileptic foci for seizure control: a double-blind, long-term follow-up study. *Epilepsia.* 2007;48(10):1895–1903.

41. Vonck K, Boon P, Achten E, et al. Long-term amygdalohippocampal stimulation for refractory temporal lobe epilepsy. *Ann Neurol.* 2002;52(5): 556–565.

42. Tellez-Zenteno JF, McLachlan RS, Parrent A, et al. Hippocampal electrical stimulation in mesial temporal lobe epilepsy. *Neurology.* 2006;66(10): 1490–1494.

43. Martha J Morrell, Lawrence J Hirsch, G Bergey, et al. Long-term safety and efficacy of the RNS™ system in adults with medically intractable partial onset seizures. *Abstract Epilepsia.* 2008;0 suppl.

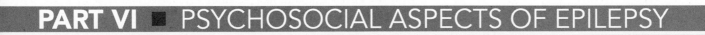

PART VI ■ PSYCHOSOCIAL ASPECTS OF EPILEPSY

CHAPTER 92 ■ COGNITIVE EFFECTS OF EPILEPSY AND ANTIEPILEPTIC MEDICATIONS

KIMFORD J. MEADOR

COGNITIVE DEFICITS IN EPILEPSY

As a group, individuals with epilepsy have impaired cognitive performance in comparison to healthy subjects matched for age and education (1); however, considerable intersubject variability exists. Most persons with epilepsy have intelligence in the normal range, and some have superior cognitive abilities. Various factors can have a detrimental effect on cognition in epilepsy patients, including (i) etiology of seizures; (ii) cerebral lesions acquired prior to onset of seizures; (iii) seizure type; (iv) age at onset of epilepsy; (v) seizure frequency; (vi) duration and severity of seizures; (vii) physiologic dysfunction (intraictal, interictal, or postictal) resulting from seizures; (viii) structural cerebral damage as a consequence of repetitive or prolonged seizures; (ix) hereditary factors; (x) psychosocial factors; (xi) sequelae of epilepsy surgery; and (xii) untoward effects of antiepileptic drugs (AEDs) (2,3).

Patients with new onset epilepsy have been shown to have impaired cognition (1,4). The etiology of seizures may be one of the strongest factors influencing cognitive abilities (5). Patients with seizures attributable to progressive cerebral degeneration usually exhibit dementia, those with mental retardation have an increased incidence of epilepsy, and those with seizures caused by a focal brain lesion may exhibit a specific neuropsychological pattern of deficits. In contrast, patients with idiopathic epilepsy are more likely to have normal intelligence (5). Seizure type may be strongly associated with cognition (6). Patients with juvenile myoclonic epilepsy usually have normal intelligence, but children with infantile spasms have a poor prognosis. In general, the earlier the age of seizure onset, the more likely it is that a patient will have cognitive impairment. Additionally, patients with mental retardation are more likely to have refractory epilepsy (6,7).

Seizure frequency, duration, and severity may affect cognition in several ways (3,8). Obviously, cognition is impaired interictally when consciousness is altered during generalized or complex partial seizures. Epileptiform discharges and postictal suppression may impair cognition interictally (9,10). Recent temporal lobe seizures impair consolidation of memory (11). Classic postictal Todd paralysis lasts less than 24 hours, but postictal cognitive dysfunction, such as dysphasia, may persist for several days. Chronic physiologic dysfunction may also exist beyond the area of epileptogenesis. For example, positron emission tomography (PET) scans reveal interictal hypometabolism extending to the lateral temporal cortex in patients with epilepsy caused by mesial temporal lobe sclerosis (12). Repetitive or prolonged seizures may permanently damage the cerebral substrate via anoxia, lactic acidosis, or excessive excitatory neurotransmitters. Even temporal lobe seizures of relatively modest frequency over several decades can increase the severity of hippocampal atrophy and reduce cognitive abilities (13,14). Memory problems are common in patients with epilepsy. Although many factors contribute to these problems, it is interesting that the molecular mechanisms of animal models for epilepsy (i.e., kindling) and memory formation (i.e., long-term potentiation) are very similar (15).

Factors indirectly related to epilepsy may also affect cognition. Hereditary factors strongly influence intelligence. In fact, maternal intelligence quotient (IQ) is the most influential factor overall in predicting a child's intelligence (16). Psychosocial factors may adversely affect cognition through such mechanisms as depression or restriction of environmental influences (17). Finally, surgical or pharmacological treatment of seizures may produce adverse cognitive effects.

EPILEPSY SURGERY

Epilepsy surgery usually does not cause a general cognitive decline because dysfunctional tissue is primarily removed (18). Surgery may even result in improved cognition because of the reduction in seizures and AEDs. However, clinically significant postoperative cognitive deficits may occur (19). For example, left temporal lobectomy may lead to declines in naming and in verbal memory. However, the risks are largely predictable (19–22). Risks are greater if age of epilepsy onset is later or if hippocampal gliosis/atrophy is not present. Verbal memory is at greater risk following left temporal lobectomy if baseline verbal memory is high in a patient with left cerebral language dominance or if functional assessments (e.g., functional magnetic resonance imaging [fMRI], PET, Wada) suggest greater residual preoperative function of the left temporal lobe. Thus, a patient undergoing left temporal lobectomy is at particular risk if the patient has high baseline verbal memory with left cerebral language dominance and lack of evidence of left temporal lobe dysfunction. High memory performance with right intracarotid amobarbital injection and low with left injection on the Wada test, absence of left temporal lobe PET hypometabolism, or robust left temporal lobe activation on fMRI memory task all suggest increased risk. In contrast, a decline in visuospatial memory is inconsistent following right temporal lobectomy. Rarely, unilateral temporal lobectomy has resulted in a severe global anterograde memory disorder. Fortunately, modern advances in preoperative evaluation techniques have minimized this risk. In addition, selective resections (e.g., amygdalohippocampectomy) may reduce the risk for memory loss compared with standard anterior two-thirds temporal lobectomy, but the effect of selective approaches may be affected by collateral white matter damage (23,24). Patients who become seizure-free from epilepsy surgery have a significant improvement in their emotional well being and perceived quality of life (QOL) (25), but those who fail epilepsy surgery are at risk for depression and poor QOL (26).

Vagus Nerve Stimulation

Some studies have reported mild cognitive or behavioral improvement following vagus nerve stimulation (VNS) (27,28), but this may be the result of reduced seizures. Other studies have shown no positive or negative effects of VNS on cognition or behavior in patients with epilepsy (29,30).

ANTIEPILEPTIC DRUGS

AEDs reduce neuronal irritability and thus may reduce neuronal excitability and impair cognition. Because AEDs are the major therapeutic intervention in epilepsy, their cognitive effects are of particular concern to physicians, who must consider the risk-to-benefit ratio of any treatment. Therefore, differentiating the cognitive effects of AEDs and placing them in the proper perspective are important.

Although all AEDs may impair cognition, such side effects are usually modest, as assessed by neuropsychological tests in patients on monotherapy in whom anticonvulsant blood levels are within standard therapeutic ranges (31). Furthermore, the cognitive effects may be partially offset by the reduction in seizures. It is clear that the risk of cognitive side effects rises with polypharmacy and with increasing AED dosages and anticonvulsant blood levels (32). Decreasing the number of AEDs frequently improves cognition and may reduce the number of seizures (33). However, the best drug regimen for an individual patient is the one that best controls seizures with the fewest side effects, and for some patients this regimen may involve polytherapy. Despite the modest cognitive effects of AEDs on formal neuropsychological testing, these effects can be clinically pertinent, as evidenced by the highly significant inverse correlation of neurotoxicity symptoms and QOL scores (34). Despite the absence of overt toxicity on examination, patients who exhibit more symptoms of neurotoxicity have lower perceived QOL. Further evidence of the clinical impact is the fact that certain AEDs can impair verbal paragraph memory by 15% to 20% (35–39) and withdrawal of AEDs (primarily carbamazepine and valproate) can produce an 11% to 28% improvement on neuropsychological tests (40).

Cognitive effects of AEDs differ across AEDs. For the older AEDs, the most consistent and marked adverse effects are observed with barbiturates and benzodiazepines, but adverse effects of carbamazepine, phenytoin, and valproate have been demonstrated (31,32). Several of the newer AEDs appear to have fewer cognitive side effects than the older AEDs, but the effects of the newer AEDs relative to each other and to older AEDs are not yet fully determined.

Historical Perspective

AED-induced cognitive deficits actually led to the discovery of the first effective AED. In 1850, Huette (41) noted that bromide produces general sedation, mental slowing, and depression of sexuality. The anticonvulsant effects of bromide were discovered in 1857 after Locock (42) suggested that the agent might be efficacious for patients with hysterical epilepsy, which was believed to result from excessive masturbation. The first systematic investigation of the cognitive effects of AEDs was conducted in 1940. Somerfeld-Ziskind and Ziskind (43) randomized 100 patients with epilepsy to phenobarbital or ketogenic diet. Phenobarbital controlled seizures better, but no differences were reported on limited neuropsychological testing. Numerous studies (31,32,44) have subsequently examined the cognitive side effects of AEDs.

Methodological Issues

The literature examining the cognitive effects of AEDs must be viewed critically, because flaws in experimental design, analysis, and interpretation occur frequently (32,44,45). Errors in experimental design include subject selection bias, nonequivalence of clinical variables, and nonequivalence of dependent variables. Selection bias is a problem when subjects are not randomly assigned to a treatment group or inadequately matched, or if the sample size is inadequate for a parallel-group design. Examples of nonequivalence of clinical variables include the failure to control for anticonvulsant blood levels or seizure frequency. Nonequivalence of dependent measures may occur when there is no assurance that treatment groups performed similarly on dependent measures prior to treatment. Additional design issues include sample size, test–retest effects, characteristics of behavioral tests, and effects of changes in seizures. Issues related to statistical analysis and interpretation include type I error, use of inappropriate statistics, nonorthogonal contrasts, and comparison of studies with nonequivalent designs/statistics. Even when statistically significant findings are apparent, the magnitude and impact of the findings have to be interpreted in terms of clinical significance, taking into account the overall risk-to-benefit ratio of the AED and the severity of the seizure disorder in question. The magnitude of AED effects on standard neuropsychological measures is generally modest and may be missed if appropriate study designs are not used (45).

Review of Selected Studies of Older Antiepileptic Drugs

Dodrill and Troupin (46) compared the cognitive effects of carbamazepine and phenytoin in patients with epilepsy using a double-blind, randomized, crossover, monotherapy design. When they reanalyzed controlling for anticonvulsant blood levels, no differences were observed (47). Meador and associates (48) also found no cognitive differences between carbamazepine and phenytoin in patients with epilepsy, but evidence of worse performance with phenobarbital.

Meador and colleagues examined the effects of several AEDs using randomized, double-blind, crossover designs in healthy volunteers, which controls for the confounding effects of seizures and preexisting brain abnormalities. The investigators found no overall difference between carbamazepine and phenytoin (35,36), but 52% of the variables were significantly worse with AEDs than with nondrug. In another study (49), 32% of the variables were significantly worse with phenobarbital than with phenytoin or valproate, with the latter two agents being similar to each other, and about half of all variables significantly worse than nondrug condition. Overall, phenobarbital has greater untoward cognitive effects versus other older AEDs, while carbamazepine, phenytoin, and valproate have similar cognitive effects.

The original Veterans Administration (VA) Cooperative Study (50), comparing the cognitive effects of carbamazepine, phenobarbital, phenytoin, and primidone in patients with new-onset epilepsy, found "no consistent pattern" across AEDs, but the study design was not optimal. In addition, the second VA Cooperative Study (51) found no cognitive differences between carbamazepine and valproate. Other studies comparing carbamazepine and phenytoin have described modest negative effects on cognition with both agents, but few differential effects (52–54).

A possible criticism of some of the crossover studies described above might be the relatively short duration of treatment. Dodrill and Wilensky (55) addressed this issue in a study that examined neuropsychological performance over 5 years in patients with epilepsy. The patients were on stable regimens consisting of phenytoin alone, phenytoin with other AEDs, or AED regimens exclusive of phenytoin. No differences in cognitive performance were observed over the 5-year follow-up.

Newer Antiepileptic Drugs

Although many questions remain unanswered, several studies offer insight into the cognitive/behavioral effects on the newer AEDs. Available published data are reviewed.

Felbamate

Given the restrictions imposed by the systemic toxic effects of felbamate, there are no systematic investigations of cognition, but anecdotally, it is reported to be alerting and can even produce insomnia. This effect can be beneficial or detrimental.

Gabapentin

Studies of add-on gabapentin in patients with epilepsy report subjective improvements in well being (56). When comparing gabapentin with placebo in patients with partial epilepsy, using a double-blind, dose-ranging (1200 to 2400 mg/day), add-on, crossover design, Leach and coworkers (57) found one positive effect and no negative effects, except for more subjective drowsiness. A double-blind, randomized, crossover study of healthy volunteers (37) compared gabapentin and carbamazepine during two 5-week treatment periods. Significantly better performance was seen with gabapentin versus carbamazepine on 26% of the variables, carbamazepine was worse than nondrug on 48% of the variables, and gabapentin was worse than nondrug on 19% of the variables. Although both agents produced some effects, significantly fewer untoward cognitive effects were seen with gabapentin compared with carbamazepine. These results have

been supported by two subsequent double-blind studies in healthy volunteers comparing treatment with carbamazepine and gabapentin. Greater electroencephalographic slowing and more frequent cognitive complaints were reported with carbamazepine in adults (58), and better overall tolerability was seen with gabapentin in healthy elderly adults (59). In contrast, gabapentin can produce irritability, hyperactivity, and agitation in children (60,61).

Lamotrigine

An adjunctive therapy study in patients with epilepsy found no cognitive effects with lamotrigine versus placebo on a limited neuropsychological battery (62). A double-blind, randomized, crossover design, with two 10-week treatment periods, in healthy adults revealed significantly better performance for lamotrigine versus carbamazepine on more than half of the variables (e.g., cognitive speed, memory, mood factors, sedation, perception of cognitive performance, and other QOL perceptions) (38). Other studies with healthy adults demonstrated fewer cognitive side effects with lamotrigine compared with carbamazepine, diazepam, phenytoin, placebo, and valproate (63–65). In clinical trials, lamotrigine was better tolerated than carbamazepine and phenytoin (66–69). See section "Topiramate" for additional studies. Several studies (62,66,70) using QOL measures demonstrated beneficial effects with lamotrigine compared with placebo or carbamazepine. Lamotrigine has positive psychotropic properties as evidenced in bipolar disorder patients and epilepsy patients with severe cognitive impairment (71–73). Significantly more improvements in mood occurred with lamotrigine compared to levetiracetam in a double-blind, randomized, parallel, adjunctive therapy study in epilepsy patients (74).

Levetiracetam

A double-blind, randomized, crossover healthy volunteer study with eight treatments arms found significantly less neuropsychological effects of levetiracetam versus carbamazepine on 44% of variables (75). An acute reversible adverse behavioral syndrome has been reported in children treated with levetiracetam (76); although the incidence of behavioral events in adult patients is reported to be low (77), it appears higher than some AEDs but lower than others (78).

Oxcarbazepine

No differences in cognitive effects were found between oxcarbazepine (OXC) and phenytoin in a small randomized, monotherapy, double-blind, parallel-group study (79) of patients with new-onset epilepsy. Mixed results were reported in a randomized, double-blind, placebo-controlled, crossover study (80) in 12 healthy volunteers treated for 2 weeks with low-dose (150 or 300 mg twice daily) OXC; reaction time slowed, but participants had slightly better subjective alertness and improved on a cancellation task. Only one significant neuropsychological difference was found for OXC versus phenytoin using a double-blind, randomized, parallel-group, healthy volunteer, 12-week treatment study (81); the Vigor scale from the Profile of Mood States favored OXC.

Rufinamide

A double-blind, randomized, parallel, placebo-controlled, multidose study found no statistically significant cognitive changes for any of the doses of rufinamide (82).

Tiagabine

Tiagabine inhibits the reuptake of the inhibitory neurotransmitter γ-aminobutyric acid (GABA). No significant cognitive effects were reported in a small, low-dose, add-on study (83) and in a large, randomized, double-blind, add-on, placebo-controlled, parallel-group, dose–response study in patients with epilepsy (84).

Topiramate

In clinical trials, topiramate produced somnolence, psychomotor slowing, memory difficulties, and language problems (e.g., difficulty with word-finding and fluency). Factors affecting these adverse effects include titration rate, maintenance time, dose, polytherapy, and individual susceptibility. In a single-blind, randomized, parallel-group study in healthy volunteers (85), topiramate was associated with more adverse cognitive effects than gabapentin and lamotrigine at 1 month, but the topiramate titration rate was faster than recommended. In a study of 38 patients with epilepsy tested on/off or off/on topiramate, declines in verbal fluency, attention, processing speed, and working memory, but not retention, were associated with topiramate use (86). Two randomized, multicenter, double-blind studies of topiramate versus valproate as adjunctive therapy in patients with epilepsy found less-profound neuropsychological effects after slow titration and 8 weeks' maintenance. Only 1/17 variables (i.e., verbal memory) in one study (87) and 2/30 variables (i.e., verbal fluency and a graphomotor task) in another study (88) were worse with topiramate compared with valproate. A double-blind, randomized, placebo-controlled, 12-week treatment, parallel-group study in healthy adults found that gabapentin had less adverse effects on 50% of the variables compared to topiramate (89). A double-blind, randomized, crossover study in healthy adults with 12-week treatment arms noted worse effects for topiramate on 88% of variables compared to lamotrigine (39). Similarly, a multicenter, double-blind, randomized, adjunctive therapy reported more adverse neuropsychological effects for topiramate versus lamotrigine (90).

Vigabatrin

In four double-blind, randomized, add-on studies of patients with epilepsy (91–95), vigabatrin had few adverse effects on cognition or QOL compared with placebo, despite elevated brain levels of GABA. A single-dose study in healthy volunteers showed less impairment than lorazepam (95), and vigabatrin produced fewer adverse effects than carbamazepine in a small, open-label, randomized, parallel-group study of patients with epilepsy (96). Abnormal behaviors, including depression and psychosis, have been reported in 3.4% of adults in controlled clinical trials, but vigabatrin has not been shown to be associated with a greater risk for these effects than other AEDs (97).

Zonisamide

Zonisamide appears to have a wide therapeutic index, but can cause sedation. The agent was reported to impair cognition (e.g., learning), but some tolerance appeared to develop over 24 weeks in a small, preliminary add-on study in patients (98). Long-term cognitive and mood effects of zonisamide were investigated in a randomized, monotherapy, multidose (100, 200, or 400 mg/day), open-label, 1-year investigation (99);

after 1 year, 47% complained of cognitive deficits; dose-related negative effects were seen on delayed word recall, Trail Making Test, and verbal fluency.

Effects of Antiepileptic Drugs at Age Extremes

Elderly

Fewer AED studies have been conducted at the extremes of the age spectrum. The increased susceptibility of the elderly to the cognitive effects of a variety of agents is attributable to both pharmacokinetic and pharmacodynamic factors. For example, it is well established that the elderly are at increased risk for untoward cognitive effects from benzodiazepines (100). Similar to studies in younger adults, one study (101) reported comparable cognitive effects of phenytoin and valproate in elderly patients. Reanalysis of the original VA Cooperative Study comparing carbamazepine, phenobarbital, phenytoin, and primidone revealed that elderly patients were easier to control but had greater cognitive side effects (102). The results from a VA Cooperative Study in elderly patients with new-onset epilepsy revealed that patients are more likely to remain on gabapentin or lamotrigine compared to carbamazepine (103). This finding was predominately a result of side effects that were least likely with lamotrigine, intermediate with gabapentin, and worse with carbamazepine.

Children

Because the modest effects of AEDs on attention and memory might be additive over the long-term during neurodevelopment, children may be at higher risk for developing cognitive side effects from AEDs. Further, the detrimental effects of AEDs might interact with seizures and underlying cerebral abnormalities to produce even greater impairments in neurodevelopment (104). Unfortunately, investigations in children are inadequate (105). A double-blind, randomized, crossover, monotherapy study (106) conducted in children with epilepsy, found performance on phenobarbital was worse than valproate. Adverse cognitive effects of phenobarbital have also been found in placebo-controlled, parallel-group studies of children with febrile convulsions (107,108). Similar to the outcomes of adult studies, comparisons of carbamazepine, phenytoin, and valproate in children have yielded few differences (109–112). No statistically significant differences in cognition were observed between OXC, carbamazepine, and valproate in an open-label, randomized, parallel-group study in children and adolescents with newly diagnosed partial seizures (113).

NEURODEVELOPMENTAL EFFECTS OF IN UTERO AED EXPOSURE

A variety of factors may contribute to the observed neurodevelopmental deficits in children of mothers with epilepsy, including AEDs, seizures during pregnancy, seizure type, heredity, maternal age/parity, and socioeconomic status (114,115). Data from animals and humans suggest that AEDs have an important role in this regard, but many issues remain unresolved.

Animal Studies

AED-induced malformations (i.e., anatomical teratogenesis) have been observed in animals (116–118). Further, cognitive/behavioral deficits (i.e., behavioral teratogenesis) have been observed in animals at dosages lower than those associated with somatic malformations (119).

Phenobarbital produces neuronal deficits, reduces brain weight, and impairs development of reflexes, open-field activity, schedule-controlled behavior, and brain levels of catecholamines in mice (120–124). Prenatal phenytoin produces dose-dependent, long-lasting impaired coordination and learning in rats (125–132). Significant, but less striking, neurobehavioral effects are seen with trimethadione and valproate (127,131,133,134). Phenytoin and valproate alter neuronal membranes in the hippocampus (135,136).

Human Studies

Although the risks for birth defects and neurodevelopmental deficits are increased in children of women with epilepsy (117,118,137–140), the role of AEDs and differential risks of AEDs have been unclear and remain only partially delineated (141). Disparities across studies are partly a result of differences in methodology and patient populations. Formal assessments of mental performance were made in most studies, but in many it is unclear whether investigators were blind as to AED exposure when assessments were made. In many prospective studies, follow-up began postnatally rather than during pregnancy. In many studies, the influences of possible confounding factors have not been addressed in an empirical fashion (e.g., parental IQ and education, seizure type and frequency, AED dose/blood levels, maternal age/parity, socioeconomic status, and home environment).

The majority of investigations report an increased risk for developmental delay in children of mothers with epilepsy (2,139–152), although a few studies (153–155) found no delays. The incidence of mental retardation is increased in children of mothers with epilepsy versus children of mothers without epilepsy, but not in children of fathers with epilepsy versus controls (148,156). A retrospective population-based study found that 19% of children exposed in utero to AEDs had developmental delay versus 3% of unexposed children (157). Animal studies suggest that AEDs play at least a partial role. Few data are available for AED effects in children of nonepileptic women, but one study suggests that the risk for somatic malformations is similar in children of mothers without epilepsy who take AEDs (158). The risk for mental impairment in children of mothers with epilepsy has been related to intrauterine growth retardation, reduced head circumferences, major malformations, numerous (nine or more) minor malformations, and in utero AED exposure (144,145,152,156,159–161), although contradictory findings have been reported (148,154,162–164). Fujioka and associates (142) suggested complex interrelationships, finding an increased risk with increased dose and numbers of AEDs, decreased maternal education, impaired maternal–child relationship, and maternal partial seizure disorder. Gaily and coworkers (143) related risk for cognitive dysfunction to seizures during pregnancy, maternal partial seizure disorder, and low paternal education, but not to AED exposure. Hattig

and colleagues (165) reported greater cognitive impairment with polytherapy compared with monotherapy and with valproate as monotherapy.

Two retrospective studies from Denmark (166) examined the effects of in utero phenobarbital exposure on intelligence in adult men of mothers without epilepsy. Men exposed prenatally to phenobarbital had significantly lower verbal IQ scores (about seven points) than predicted in both studies. Lower socioeconomic status and being the offspring of an "unwanted" pregnancy markedly increased the magnitude of negative effects (about 20 IQ points).

A retrospective study of 594 school-age children exposed in utero to AEDs suggested that valproate has greater detrimental effects on neurodevelopment than other AEDs or no drug (167). Special education was required in 30% of children exposed to valproate monotherapy, compared with 3% to 6% for other monotherapies, and 11% with no drug. A prospective study (168) found no effect of carbamazepine; however, the mean IQ of children exposed in utero to valproate was 83, compared to 96 for children exposed to carbamazepine, which did not differ from no drug exposure (IQ = 95), but the monotherapy valproate group was small and maternal IQ was not measured. A recent prospective study, which controlled for multiple possible confounding factors including maternal IQ, has confirmed the increased risk for impaired cognition from in utero valproate exposure (169); the IQ of children exposed to valproate was reduced six to nine points compared to children exposed to carbamazepine, lamotrigine, and phenytoin. Valproate's effect in this and other studies was dose-dependent. Two retrospective and one prospective study have also reported an increased risk for autistic spectrum disorder or behavioral abnormalities in children exposed to valproate (170–172). Although it is clear that in utero valproate exposure poses a greater risk for both anatomical and behavioral teratogenesis, the risks for other AEDs remains to be fully delineated.

Possible Mechanisms of Antiepileptic Drug Effects on Neurodevelopment

A teratogen operates on a susceptible genotype, and this process may involve the interaction of multiple-liability genes (173). For example, discordant outcomes have been observed for dizygotic twin fetuses exposed to phenytoin (174). It is unclear whether similar mechanisms may be involved in both functional and anatomical defects since anatomical risks are related to first trimester exposure, but functional deficits may be related primarily to third trimester exposure. Proposed possible mechanisms underlying functional teratogenicity of AEDs include folate, reactive intermediates (e.g., epoxides or free radicals), ischemia, apoptosis-related mechanisms, and neuronal suppression.

Reactive Intermediates

The fetotoxicity of some AEDs may be mediated not by the parent compound, but by toxic intermediary metabolites (175). AEDs may be bioactivated to free-radical reactive intermediates by means of embryonic prostaglandin H synthetase or lipoxygenases (176–178). Once generated, these reactive oxygen species may bind to DNA, protein, or lipids, resulting in teratogenesis.

Ischemia/Hypoxia

Ischemia-induced embryopathy in animals resembles phenytoin-induced defects, and hyperoxic chamber treatment reduces malformations caused by phenytoin (179). However, the resemblance to AED defects may be due to free-radical–induced ischemia.

Folate

During pregnancy, folate demand is increased because of its involvement in DNA and RNA synthesis. Phenobarbital, phenytoin, and primidone, but not carbamazepine, deplete folate (180–183), and valproate affects folate-dependent one-carbon metabolism (184). Blood folate concentrations are significantly lower in women with epilepsy who have abnormal pregnancy outcomes (185). In addition, Bialc and Lewenthal (186) found that infants of mothers with epilepsy who received no folate supplementation had a 15% rate of malformation, but no congenital abnormalities were identified in 33 folate-supplemented children.

Neuronal Suppression

AEDs suppress neuronal irritability and, as a consequence, impair neuronal excitation. Reduction of neuronal excitation in utero might alter synaptic growth and connectivity during these early stages of neurodevelopment, resulting in long-term deficits in cognition and behavior.

Apoptosis-Related Mechanisms

In utero ethanol exposure can result in widespread apoptotic neurodegeneration, reduced brain mass, and neurobehavioral deficits (187). The effect is primarily due to third trimester exposure and has been attributed to N-methyl-D-aspartic acid (NMDA) glutamate-receptor blockade and $GABA_A$ receptor activation (187). Studies in neonatal rats reveal widespread apoptosis in the developing brain as a result of exposure to clonazepam, diazepam, phenobarbital, phenytoin, vigabatrin, or valproate (188–190). The effect is dose-dependent, occurs at therapeutically relevant blood levels, and requires only relatively brief exposure. Valproate's increased risk may be because apoptosis occurs at relatively lower therapeutic concentrations compared to other AEDs. The effect appeared to be caused by reduced expression of neurotrophins and levels of protein kinases that promote neuronal growth and survival. Of note, the adverse effects were ameliorated by β-estradiol, which has neurotrophic effects. Many AEDs have not been tested in this model, but similar apoptotic effects were not seen at therapeutic dosages for carbamazepine, lamotrigine, levetiracetam, or topiramate monotherapy (191–194). The observations that many AEDs cause apoptosis in the immature brain of animals raise serious concern that certain AEDs, which are commonly used in women of childbearing potential, could produce similar adverse effects in children exposed in utero or in the neonatal period. Additional studies are needed to examine effects of other AEDs in this animal model and determine if a similar mechanism occurs in humans.

CONCLUSIONS

Patients with epilepsy are at increased risk for cognitive impairment, and a variety of factors may adversely affect cognition in this population. As the major therapeutic modality for epilepsy, AEDs are of special concern. All AEDs can produce some cognitive side effects, which are increased with polypharmacy and higher dosage/anticonvulsant blood levels. With polypharmacy, the effects are additive and can occur even when all anticonvulsant blood levels are within "standard therapeutic ranges." AEDs may also produce positive or negative behavioral alterations (e.g., mood stabilization, irritability/agitation, psychosis). Carbamazepine, lamotrigine, and valproate have positive psychotropic effects. However, the treatment goal in each patient is to achieve the best control of seizures while producing the fewest side effects. For an individual patient, the best risk-to-benefit ratio may be obtained with judicious use of polypharmacy or with anticonvulsant blood level above "standard therapeutic ranges." However, physicians should be alert to increased risk for cognitive side effects in these circumstances.

The magnitude of AED effect on cognition is commonly smaller than other epilepsy-related factors. When AEDs are used in monotherapy with anticonvulsant blood levels within standard therapeutic ranges, their cognitive effects on formal neuropsychological tests of cognition are modest. However, AED effects can be clinically significant, as evidenced by the adverse effects of subtle neurotoxic symptoms on patient's QOL. The major cognitive effects of AEDs are on psychomotor processing speed, sustained attention, memory, and dual processing. Cognitive impairments induced by AEDs may be of particular concern for adults with jobs requiring speed or sustained vigilance and for children in whom the additive effects during neurodevelopment may have long-lasting consequences.

Although data are incomplete, clinically significant differential adverse cognitive effects exist for patients taking AEDs and for children exposed in utero. Further studies are needed to examine more thoroughly the relative cognitive effects of the new AEDs and to delineate the cognitive effects of all AEDs at age extremes, especially in the fetus and in children.

References

1. Smith DB, Craft BR, Collins J, et al. VA Cooperative Study Group 118. Behavioral characteristics of epilepsy patients compared with normal controls. *Epilepsia*. 1986;27:760–768.
2. Lennox WG. Brain injury, drugs and environment as causes of mental decay in epilepsy. *Am J Psychiatry*. 1942;99:174–180.
3. Lesser RP, Lüders H, Wyllie E, et al. Mental deterioration in epilepsy. *Epilepsia*. 1986;27(suppl 2):S105–S123.
4. Hermann B, Jones J, Sheth R, et al. Children with new-onset epilepsy: neuropsychological status and brain structure. *Brain*. 2006;129: 2609–2619.
5. Perrine K, Gershengorm J, Brown ER. Interictal neuropsychological function in epilepsy. In: Devinsky O, Theodore WH, eds. *Epilepsy Behavior*. New York: Wiley-Liss; 1991:181–193.
6. Huttenlocher PR, Hapke RJ. A follow-up study of intractable seizures in childhood. *Ann Neurol*. 1990;28:699–705.
7. Dodrill CB. Neuropsychological aspects of epilepsy. *Psychiatr Clin North Am*. 1992;15:383–394.
8. Dikmen S, Matthews CG. Effect of major motor seizure frequency upon cognitive-intellectual functions in adults. *Epilepsia*. 1977;18:21–29.
9. Kasteleijn-Nolst Trenite DGA, Riemersma JBJ, Binnie CD, et al. The influence of subclinical epileptiform EEG discharges on driving behaviour. *Electroencephalogr Clin Neurophysiol*. 1987;67:167–170.
10. Shewmon DA, Erwin RJ. The effect of focal interictal spikes on perception and reaction time. I. General considerations. *Electroencephalogr Clin Neurophysiol*. 1988;69:319–337.
11. Jokeit H, Daamen M, Zang H, et al. Seizures accelerate forgetting in patients with left-sided temporal lobe epilepsy. *Neurology*. 2001;57: 125–126.
12. Henry TR, Chugani HT, Abou-Khalil BW, et al. Positron emission tomography. In: Engel J, ed. *Surgical Treatment of the Epilepsies*. New York: Raven Press; 1991:211–232.

13. Theodore WH, Bhatia S, Hatta J, et al. Hippocampal atrophy, epilepsy duration, and febrile seizures in patients with partial seizures. *Neurology.* 1999;52:132–136.
14. Jokeit H, Ebner A. Long term effects of refractory temporal lobe epilepsy on cognitive abilities: a cross sectional study. *J Neurol Neurosurg Psychiatry.* 1999;67:44–50.
15. Meador KJ. The basic science of memory as it applies to epilepsy. *Epilepsia.* 2007;48(suppl 9):1–3.
16. Sattler JM. *Assessment of Children.* 3rd ed. San Diego: Jerome M Sattler; 1992.
17. Hermann BP. Quality of life in epilepsy. *J Epilepsy.* 1992;5:153–165.
18. Loring DW, Meador KJ. Neuropsychological aspects of epilepsy surgery. In: Feinberg TE, Farah MJ, eds. *Behavioral Neurology and Neuropsychology.* New York: McGraw-Hill; 1997:657–666.
19. Téllez--Zenteno JF, Dhar R, Hernandez-Ronquillo L, Wiebe S. Long-term outcomes in epilepsy surgery: antiepileptic drugs, mortality, cognitive and psychosocial aspects. *Brain* 2007;130(Pt 2):334-45.
20. Clusman H, Schramm J, Kral T, et al. Prognostic factors and outcome after different types of resection for temporal lobe epilepsy. *J Neurosurg.* 2002;97:1131–1141.
21. Hamberger MJ, Drake EB. Cognitive functioning following epilepsy surgery. *Curr Neurol Neurosci Rep.* 2006;6(4):319–326.
22. Hoppe C, Elger CE, Helmstaedter C. Long-term memory impairment in patients with focal epilepsy. *Epilepsia.* 2007;48(suppl 9):26–29.
23. Helmstaedter C, Reuber M, Elger CC. Interaction of cognitive aging and memory deficits related to epilepsy surgery. *Ann Neurol.* 2002;52:89–94.
24. Helmstaedter C, Richter S, Röske S, et al. Differential effects of temporal pole resection with amygdalohippocampectomy versus selective amygdalohippocampectomy on material-specific memory in patients with mesial temporal lobe epilepsy. *Epilepsia.* 2008;49(1):88–97.
25. Markand ON, Salanova V, Whelihan E, et al. Health-related quality of life outcome in medically refractory epilepsy treated with anterior temporal lobectomy. *Epilepsia.* 2000;41:749–759.
26. Téllez-Zenteno JF, Wiebe S. Long-term seizure and psychosocial outcomes of epilepsy surgery. *Curr Treat Options Neurol.* 2008;10(4):253–259.
27. Hoppe C, Helmstaedter C, Scherrmann J, et al. Self-reported mood changes following 6 months of vagus nerve stimulation in epilepsy patients. *Epilepsy Behav.* 2001;2:335–342.
28. Majoie HJ, Berfelo MW, Aldenkamp AP, et al. Vagus nerve stimulation in children with therapy-resistant epilepsy diagnosed as Lennox-Gastaut syndrome: clinical results, neuropsychological effects, and cost-effectiveness. *J Clin Neurophysiol.* 2001;18:419–428.
29. Hoppe C, Helmstaedter C, Scherrmann J, et al. No evidence for cognitive side effects after 6 months of vagus nerve stimulation in epilepsy patients. *Epilepsy Behav.* 2001;2:351–356.
30. Aldenkamp AP, Majoie HJ, Berfelo MW, et al. Long-term effects of 24-month treatment with vagus nerve stimulation on behaviour in children with Lennox-Gastaut syndrome. *Epilepsy Behav.* 2002;3:475–479.
31. Meador KJ. Cognitive side effects of antiepileptic drugs. *Can J Neurol Sci.* 1994;21(suppl 3):S12–S16.
32. Meador KJ, Loring DW. Cognitive effects of antiepileptic drugs. In: Devinsky O, Theodore WH, eds. *Epilepsy and Behavior.* New York: Wiley-Liss; 1991:151–170.
33. Shorvon SD, Reynolds EH. Reduction in polypharmacy for epilepsy. *Br Med J.* 1979;2:1023–1025.
34. Gilliam F, Kuzniecky R, Faught E, et al. Impact of adverse antiepileptic drug effects on quality of life in refractory epilepsy. *Epilepsia.* 1999;40 (suppl):64–65.
35. Meador KJ, Loring DW, Abney OL, et al. Effects of carbamazepine and phenytoin on EEG and memory in healthy adults. *Epilepsia.* 1993;34:153–157.
36. Meador KJ, Loring DW, Allen ME, et al. Comparative cognitive effects of carbamazepine and phenytoin in healthy adults. *Neurology.* 1991;41:1537–1540.
37. Meador KJ, Loring DW, Ray PG, et al. Differential cognitive effects of carbamazepine and gabapentin. *Epilepsia.* 1999;40:1279–1285.
38. Meador KJ, Loring DW, Ray PG, et al. Differential cognitive and behavioral effects of carbamazepine and lamotrigine. *Neurology.* 2001;56:1177–1182.
39. Meador KJ, Loring DW, Vahle VJ, et al. Cognitive and behavioral effects of lamotrigine and topiramate in healthy volunteers. *Neurology.* 2005;64(12):2108–2114.
40. Lossius MI, Hessen E, Mowinckel P, et al. Consequences of antiepileptic drug withdrawal: a randomized, double-blind study (Akershus Study). *Epilepsia.* 2008;49(3):455–463.
41. Huette C. Recherches sur les proprietes physiologiques et thérapeutiques de bromure de potassium. *Memoirs de la Societe de Biologie.* 1850;2:19.
42. Locock C. Discussion of paper by EH Seiveking. Analysis of 52 cases of epilepsy observed by the author. *Lancet.* 1857;1:527–528.
43. Somerfeld-Ziskind E, Ziskind E. Effect of phenobarbital on the mentality of epileptic patients. *Arch Neurol Psychiatry.* 1940;43:70–79.
44. Vermeulen J, Aldenkamp AP. Cognitive side-effects of chronic antiepileptic drug treatment: a review of 25 years of research. *Epilepsy Res.* 1995;22:65–95.
45. Meador KJ. Cognitive and behavioral assessments in antiepileptic drug trials. In: French J, Dichter M, Leppik I, eds. *Antiepileptic Drug*
46. Dodrill CB, Troupin AS. Psychotropic effects of carbamazepine in epilepsy: a double-blind comparison with phenytoin. *Neurology.* 1977;27:1023–1028.
47. Dodrill CB, Troupin AS. Neuropsychological effects of carbamazepine and phenytoin: a reanalysis. *Neurology.* 1991;41:141–143.
48. Meador KJ, Loring DW, Huh K, et al. Comparative cognitive effects of anticonvulsants. *Neurology.* 1990;40:391–394.
49. Meador KJ, Loring DW, Moore EE, et al. Comparative cognitive effects of phenobarbital, phenytoin and valproate in healthy subjects. *Neurology.* 1995;45:1494–1499.
50. Smith DB, Mattson RH, Cramer JA, et al. Results of a nationwide Veterans Administration Cooperative Study comparing the efficacy and toxicity of carbamazepine, phenobarbital, phenytoin, and primidone. *Epilepsia.* 1987;28(suppl 3):S50–S58.
51. Prevey ML, Delaney RC, Cramer JA, et al., The Department of Veterans Affairs Epilepsy Cooperative Study 264 Group. Effect of valproate on cognitive functioning. Comparison with carbamazepine. *Arch Neurol.* 1996;53:1008–1016.
52. Pullianen V, Jokelainen M. Effects of phenytoin and carbamazepine on cognitive functions in newly diagnosed epileptic patients. *Acta Neurol Scand.* 1994;89:81–86.
53. Smith KR, Goulding PM, Wilderman D, et al. Neurobehavioral effects of phenytoin and carbamazepine in patients recovering from brain trauma: a comparative study. *Arch Neurol.* 1994;51:653–660.
54. Hessen E, Lossius MI, Reinvang I, et al. Influence of major antiepileptic drugs on neuropsychological function: results from a randomized, double-blind, placebo-controlled withdrawal study of seizure-free epilepsy patients on monotherapy. *J Int Neuropsychol Soc.* 2007;13(3):393–400.
55. Dodrill CB, Wilensky AJ. Neuropsychological abilities before and after 5 years of stable antiepileptic drug therapy. *Epilepsia.* 1992;33:327–334.
56. Dimond KR, Pande AC, Lamoreaux L, et al. Effect of gabapentin (Neurontin) [corrected] on mood and well-being in patients with epilepsy. *Prog Neuropsychopharmacol Biol Psychiatry.* 1996;20:407–417.
57. Leach JP, Girvan J, Paul A, et al. Gabapentin and cognition: a double-blind, dose-ranging, placebo-controlled study in refractory epilepsy. *J Neurol Neurosurg Psychiatry.* 1997;62:372–376.
58. Salinsky MC, Binder LM, Oken BS, et al. Effects of gabapentin and carbamazepine on the EEG and cognition in healthy volunteers. *Epilepsia.* 2002;43:482–490.
59. Martin R, Meador K, Turrentine L, et al. Comparative cognitive effects of carbamazepine and gabapentin in healthy senior adults. *Epilepsia.* 2001;42:764–771.
60. Lee DO, Steingard RJ, Cesena M, et al. Behavioral side effects of gabapentin in children. *Epilepsia.* 1996;37:87–90.
61. Wolf SM, Shinnar S, Kang H, et al. Gabapentin toxicity in children manifesting as behavioral changes. *Epilepsia.* 1995;36:1203–1205.
62. Smith D, Baker G, Davies G, et al. Outcomes of add-on treatment with lamotrigine in partial epilepsy. *Epilepsia.* 1993;34:312–322.
63. Aldenkamp AP, Arends J, Bootsma HP, et al. Randomized double-blind parallel-group study comparing cognitive effects of a low-dose lamotrigine with valproate and placebo in healthy volunteers. *Epilepsia.* 2002;43:19–26.
64. Cohen AF, Ashby L, Crowley D, et al. Lamotrigine (BW430C), a potential anticonvulsant. Effects on the central nervous system in comparison with phenytoin and diazepam. *Br J Clin Pharmacol.* 1985;20:619–629.
65. Hamilton MJ, Cohen AF, Yuen AW, et al. Carbamazepine and lamotrigine in healthy volunteers: relevance to early tolerance and clinical trial dosage. *Epilepsia.* 1993;34:166–173.
66. Gillham R, Baker G, Thompson P, et al. Standardization of self-report questionnaire for use in evaluating cognitive, affective and behavioural side-effects of anti-epileptic drug treatments. *Epilepsy Res.* 1996;24:47–55.
67. Brodie MJ, Overstall PW, Giorgi L, for the UK Lamotrigine Elderly Study Group. Multicentre, double-blind, randomised comparison between lamotrigine and carbamazepine in elderly patients with newly diagnosed epilepsy. *Epilepsy Res.* 1999;37:81–87.
69. Steiner TJ, Dellaportas CI, Findley LJ, et al. Lamotrigine monotherapy in newly diagnosed untreated epilepsy: a double-blind comparison with phenytoin. *Epilepsia.* 1999;40:601–607.
70. Brodie M, Richens A, Yuen AWC; for the UK Lamotrigine/Carbamazepine Monotherapy Trial Group. Double-blind comparison of lamotrigine and carbamazepine in newly diagnosed epilepsy. *Lancet.* 1995;345:476–479.
71. Buchanan N. The efficacy of lamotrigine on seizure control in 34 children, adolescents and young adults with intellectual and physical disability. *Seizure.* 1995;4:233–236.
72. Meador KJ, Baker GA. Behavioral and cognitive effects of lamotrigine. *J Child Neurol.* 1997;12(suppl 1):S44–S47.
73. Uvebrant P, Bauziene R. Intractable epilepsy in children. The efficacy of lamotrigine treatment, including non-seizure-related benefits. *Neuropediatrics.* 1994;25:284–289.
74. Labiner DM, Ettinger AB, Fakhoury TA, et al. Effects of lamotrigine compared with levetiracetam on anger, hostility, and total mood in patients with partial epilepsy. *Epilepsia.* 2009;50(3):434–42.

Development. Advances in Neurology Series. Vol 76. Philadelphia, PA: Lippincott-Raven Publishers; 1998:231–238.

75. Meador KJ, Gevins A, Loring DW, et al. Neuropsychological and neurophysiological effects of carbamazepine and levetiracetam. *Neurology.* 2007;69:2076–2084.

76. Kossoff EH, Bergey GK, Freeman JM, et al. Levetiracetam psychosis in children with epilepsy. *Epilepsia.* 2001;42:1611–1613.

77. Cramer JA, De Rue K, Devinsky O, et al. A systematic review of the behavioral effects of levetiracetam in adults with epilepsy, cognitive disorders, or an anxiety disorder during clinical trials. *Epilepsy Behav.* 2003;4:124–132.

78. Mula M, Sander JW. Negative effects of antiepileptic drugs on mood in patients with epilepsy. *Drug Saf.* 2007;30(7):555–567.

79. Aikia M, Kalviainen R, Sivenius J, et al. Cognitive effects of oxcarbazepine and phenytoin monotherapy in newly diagnosed epilepsy: one year follow-up. *Epilepsy Res.* 1992;11:199–203.

80. Curran HV, Java R. Memory and psychomotor effects of oxcarbazepine in healthy human volunteers. *Eur J Clin Pharmacol.* 1993;44:529–533.

81. Salinsky MC, Spencer DC, Oken BS, et al. Effects of oxcarbazepine and phenytoin on the EEG and cognition in healthy volunteers. *Epilepsy Behav.* 2004;5(6):894–902.

82. Aldenkamp AP, Alpherts WC. The effect of the new antiepileptic drug rufinamide on cognitive functions. *Epilepsia.* 2006;47(7):1153–1159.

83. Sveinbjornsdottir S, Sander JW, Patsalos PN, et al. Neuropsychological effects of tiagabine, a potential new antiepileptic drug. *Seizure.* 1994;3:29–35.

84. Dodrill CB, Arnett JL, Sommerville K, et al. Cognitive and quality of life effects of differing dosages of tiagabine in epilepsy. *Neurology.* 1997;48:1025–1031.

85. Martin R, Kuzniecky R, Ho S, et al. Cognitive effects of topiramate, gabapentin, and lamotrigine in healthy young adults. *Neurology.* 1999;52:321–326.

86. Lee S, Sziklas V, Andermann F, et al. The effects of adjunctive topiramate on cognitive function in patients with epilepsy. *Epilepsia.* 2003;44:339–347.

87. Aldenkamp AP, Baker G, Mulder OG, et al. A multicenter, randomized clinical study to evaluate the effect on cognitive function of topiramate compared with valproate as add-on therapy to carbamazepine in patients with partial-onset seizures. *Epilepsia.* 2000;41:1167–1178.

88. Meador KJ, Loring DW, Hulihan JF, et al. Differential cognitive and behavioral effects of topiramate and valproate. *Neurology.* 2003;60:1483–1488.

89. Salinsky MC, Storzbach D, Spencer DC, et al. Effects of topiramate and gabapentin on cognitive abilities in healthy volunteers. *Neurology.* 2005;64(5):792–798.

90. Blum D, Meador KJ, Biton V, et al. Cognitive effects of lamotrigine compared with topiramate in patients with epilepsy. *Neurology.* 2006;67:400–406.

91. Dodrill CB, Arnett JL, Sommerville KW, et al. Evaluation of the effects of vigabatrin on cognitive abilities and quality of life in epilepsy. *Neurology.* 1993;43:2501–2507.

92. Dodrill CB, Arnett JL, Sommerville KW, et al. Effects of differing dosages of vigabatrin (Sabril) on cognitive abilities and quality of life in epilepsy. *Epilepsy.* 1995;36:164–173.

93. Gillham RA, Blacklaw J, McKee PJW, et al. Effect of vigabatrin on sedation and cognitive function in patients with refractory epilepsy. *J Neurol Neurosurg Psychiatry.* 1993;56:1271–1275.

94. Grunewald RA, Thompson PJ, Corcoran R, et al. Effects of vigabatrin on partial seizures and cognitive function. *Neurol Neurosurg Psychiatry.* 1994;57:1057–1063.

95. Saletu B, Grunberger J, Linzmayer L, et al. Psychophysiological and psychometric studies after manipulating the GABA system by vigabatrin, a GABA-transaminase inhibitor. *Int J Psychophysiol.* 1986;4:63–80.

96. Kalviainen R, Aikia M, Saukkonen AM, et al. Vigabatrin versus carbamazepine monotherapy in patients with newly diagnosed epilepsy: a randomized controlled study. *Arch Neurol.* 1995;52:989–996.

97. Ferrie CD, Robinson RO, Panayiotopoulos CP. Psychotic and severe behavioural reactions with vigabatrin: a review. *Acta Neurol Scand.* 1996;93:1–8.

98. Berent S, Sackellares JC, Giordani B, et al. Zonisamide (CI-912) and cognition: results from preliminary study. *Epilepsia.* 1987;28:61–67.

99. Park SP, Hwang YH, Lee HW, et al. Long-term cognitive and mood effects of zonisamide monotherapy in epilepsy patients. *Epilepsy Behav.* 2008;12(1):102–108.

100. Taylor JL, Tinklenberg JR. Cognitive impairment and benzodiazepines. In: Meltzer HY, ed. *Psychopharmacology: The Third Generation of Progress.* New York: Raven Press; 1987:1449–1454.

101. Craig I, Tallis R. The impact of sodium valproate and phenytoin on cognitive function in elderly patients: results of a single-blind randomized comparative study. *Epilepsia.* 1994;35:381–390.

102. Ramsey RE, Pryor F. Epilepsy in the elderly. *Neurology.* 2000;55(suppl 1):S9–S14.

103. Rowan AJ, Ramsay RE, Collins JF, et al. New onset geriatric epilepsy: a randomized study of gabapentin, lamotrigine, and carbamazepine. *Neurology.* 2005;64:1868–1873.

104. Mikati MA, Holmes GL, Chronopoulos A, et al. Phenobarbital modifies seizure-related brain injury in the developing brain. *Ann Neurol.* 1994;36:425–433.

105. Loring DW, Meador KJ. Cognitive side effects of antiepileptic drugs in children. [Review]. *Neurology.* 2004;62:872–877.

106. Vining EPG, Mellitis ED, Dorsen MM, et al. Psychologic and behavioral effects of antiepileptic drugs in children: a double-blind comparison between phenobarbital and valproic acid. *Pediatrics.* 1987;80:165–174.

107. Camfield CS, Chaplin S, Doyle AB, et al. Side effects of phenobarbital in toddlers: behavioral and cognitive aspects. *J Pediatr.* 1979;95:361–365.

108. Farwell JR, Lee YJ, Hirtz DG, et al. Phenobarbital for febrile seizures—effects on intelligence and on seizure recurrence. *N Engl J Med.* 1990;322:364–369.

109. Aldenkamp AP, Alpherts WCJ, Blennow G, et al. Withdrawal of antiepileptic medication in children—effects on cognitive function: the multicenter Holmfrid study. *Neurology.* 1993;43:41–50.

110. Forsythe I, Butler R, Berg I, et al. Cognitive impairment in new cases of epilepsy randomly assigned to carbamazepine, phenytoin, and sodium valproate. *Dev Med Child Neurol.* 1991;33:524–534.

111. Forsythe WI, Sills MA. One drug for childhood grand mal: medical audit for three-year remissions. *Dev Med Child Neurol.* 1984;26:742–748.

112. Tonnby B, Nilsson HL, Aldenkamp AP, et al. Withdrawal of antiepileptic medication in children. Correlation of cognitive function and plasma concentration—the multicentre "Holmfrid" study. *Epilepsy Res.* 1994;19:141–152.

113. Donati F, Gobbi G, Campistol J, et al. The cognitive effects of oxcarbazepine versus carbamazepine or valproate in newly diagnosed children with partial seizures. *Seizure.* 2007;16(8):670–679.

114. Leavitt AM, Yerby MS, Robinson N, et al. Epilepsy in pregnancy: developmental outcome of offspring at 12 months. *Neurology.* 1992;42(suppl 5):141–143.

115. Yerby MS. Pregnancy and epilepsy. *Epilepsia.* 1991;32(suppl 6):S51–S59.

116. Dansky LV, Finnell RH. Parental epilepsy, anticonvulsant drugs, and reproductive outcome: epidemiologic and experimental findings spanning three decades; 2: human studies. *Reprod Toxicol.* 1991;5:301–335.

117. Finnell RH, Dansky LV. Parental epilepsy, anticonvulsant drugs, and reproductive outcome: epidemiologic and experimental findings spanning three decades; 1: animal studies. *Reprod Toxicol Rev.* 1991;5:281–299.

118. Fisher JE, Vorhees C. Developmental toxicity of antiepileptic drugs: relationship to postnatal dysfunction. *Pharm Res.* 1992;26:207–221.

119. Adams J, Vorhees CV, Middaugh LD. Developmental neurotoxicity of anticonvulsants: human and animal evidence on phenytoin. *Neurotoxicol Teratol.* 1990;12:203–214.

120. Fishman RHB, Gaathon A, Yanai J. Early barbiturate treatment eliminates peak serum thyroxine levels in neonatal mice and produces ultrastructural damage in brain of adults. *Dev Brain Res.* 1982;5:202–205.

121. Yanai J, Rosselli-Austin L, Tabakoff B. Neuronal deficits in mice following prenatal exposure to phenobarbital. *Exp Neurol.* 1979;64:237–244.

122. Middaugh LD, Santos CA III, Zemp JW. Effects of phenobarbital given to pregnant mice on behavior of mature offspring. *Dev Psychobiol.* 1975;8:305–313.

123. Middaugh LD, Santos CA III, Zemp JW. Phenobarbital during pregnancy alters operant behavior of offspring in C57BL/6J mice. *Pharmacol Biochem Behav.* 1975;3:1137–1139.

124. Middaugh LD, Thomas TN, Simpson LW, et al. Effects of prenatal maternal injections of phenobarbital on brain neurotransmitters and behavior of young C57 mice. *Neurobehav Toxicol Teratol.* 1981;3:271–275.

125. Elmazar MMA, Sullivan FM. Effect of prenatal phenytoin administration on postnatal development of the rat: a behavioral teratology study. *Teratology.* 1981;24:115–124.

126. Mullenix P, Tassinari MS, Keith DA. Behavioral outcome after prenatal exposure to phenytoin in rats. *Teratology.* 1983;27:149–157.

127. Vorhees CV. Fetal anticonvulsant syndrome in rats: dose- and period-response relationships of prenatal diphenylhydantoin, trimethadione, and phenobarbital exposure on the structural and functional development of the offspring. *J Pharmacol Exp Ther.* 1983;227:274–287.

128. Vorhees CV. Fetal anticonvulsant syndrome in rats: effects on postnatal behavior and brain amino acid content. *Neurobehav Toxicol Teratol.* 1985;7:471–482.

129. Vorhees CV. Fetal anticonvulsant exposure: effects of behavioral and physical development. *Ann N Y Acad Sci.* 1986;477:49–62.

130. Vorhees CV. Fetal hydantoin syndrome in rats: dose-effect relationships of prenatal phenytoin on postnatal development and behavior. *Teratology.* 1987;35:287–303.

131. Vorhees CV, Minck DR. Long-term effects of prenatal phenytoin exposure on offspring behavior in rats. *Neurotoxicol Teratol.* 1989;11:295–305.

132. Vorhees CV, Rindler JM, Minck DR. Effects of exposure period and nutrition on the developmental neurotoxicity of anticonvulsants in rats: short and long-term effects. *Neurotoxicology.* 1990;11:273–283.

133. Vorhees CV. Behavioral teratogenicity of valproic acid: selective effects on behavior after prenatal exposure to rats. *Psychopharmacology.* 1987;92:173–179.

134. Vorhees CV. Teratogenicity and developmental toxicity of valproic acid. *Teratology.* 1987;35:195–202.

135. Vorhees CV, Rauch SL, Hitzemann RJ. Prenatal phenytoin exposure decreases neuronal membrane order in rat offspring hippocampus. *Int J Dev Neurosci.* 1990;8:283–288.

136. Vorhees CV, Rauch SL, Hitzemann RJ. Prenatal valproic acid exposure decreases neuronal membrane order in rat offspring hippocampus and cortex. *Neurotoxicol Teratol.* 1991;13:471–474.

137. Delgado-Escueta AV, Janz D. Consensus guidelines: preconception counseling, management, and care of the pregnant woman with epilepsy. *Neurology.* 1992;42(suppl 5):149–160.

138. Dressens AB, Boer K, Koppe JG, et al. Studies on long-lasting consequences of prenatal exposure to anticonvulsant drugs. *Acta Paediatr.* 1994;83(suppl 404):54–64.

139. Granström ML, Gaily E. Psychomotor development in children of mothers with epilepsy. *Neurology.* 1992;42:144–148.

140. Janz D. On major malformations and minor anomalies in the offspring of parents with epilepsy: review of the literature. In: Janz D, Dam M, Richens A, et al., eds. *Epilepsy, Pregnancy, and the Child.* New York: Raven Press; 1982:211–222.

141. Meador KJ, Baker G, Cohen MJ, et al. Cognitive/behavioral teratogenetic effects of antiepileptic drugs. *Epilepsy Behav.* 2007;11:292–302.

142. Fujioka K, Kaneko S, Hirano T, et al. A study of the psychomotor development of the offspring of epileptic mothers. In: Sato T, Shinagawa S, eds. *Antiepileptic Drugs and Pregnancy.* Amsterdam: Excerpta Medica; 1984: 415–424.

143. Gaily E, Kantola-Sorsa E, Granström ML. Specific cognitive dysfunction in children with epileptic mothers. *Dev Med Child Neurol.* 1990;32: 403–414.

144. Hanson JW, Myrianthopoulos NC, Harvey MAS, et al. Risks to the offspring of women treated with hydantoin anticonvulsants, with emphasis on the fetal hydantoin syndrome. *J Pediatrics.* 1976;89:662–668.

145. Hill RM, Tennyson LM. Maternal drug therapy: effect on fetal and neonatal growth and neurobehavior. *Neurotoxicology.* 1986;7:121–140.

146. Jones KL, Lacro RV, Johnson KA, et al. Pattern of malformations in the children of women treated with carbamazepine during pregnancy. *N Engl J Med.* 1989;320:1661–1666.

147. Losche G, Steinhausen HC, Koch S, et al. The psychological development of children of epileptic parents. II. The differential impact of intrauterine exposure to anticonvulsant drugs and further influential factors. *Acta Paediatr.* 1994;83:961–966.

148. Nelson KB, Ellenberg DH. Maternal seizure disorder, outcome of pregnancy, and neurologic abnormalities in the children. *Neurology.* 1982;32: 1247–1254.

149. Speidel BD, Meadow SR. Maternal epilepsy and abnormalities of the fetus and newborn. *Lancet.* 1972;2:839–843.

150. Steinhausen HC, Losche G, Koch S, et al. The psychological development of children of epileptic parents. I. Study design and comparative findings. *Acta Paediatr.* 1994;83:955–960.

151. Vanoverloop D, Schnell RR, Harvey EA, et al. The effects of prenatal exposure to phenytoin and other anticonvulsants on intellectual function at 4 to 8 years of age. *Neurotoxicol Teratol.* 1992;14:329–335.

152. Vert P, Deblay MF, Andre M. Follow-up study on growth and neurological development of children born to epileptic mothers. In: Janz D, Dam M, Richens A, et al., eds. *Epilepsy, Pregnancy, and the Child.* New York: Raven Press; 1982:433–436.

153. Andermann E. Development in offspring of epileptic parents. In: Akimoto H, Kazamatsuri H, Seino M, et al., eds. *Advances in Epileptology: XIIIth Epilepsy International Symposium.* New York: Raven Press; 1982: 415–424.

154. Dieterich E, Steveling A, Lukas A, et al. Congenital anomalies in children of epileptic mothers and fathers. *Neuropediatrics.* 1980;11:274–283.

155. Granström ML, Hiilesmaa VK. Physical growth of the children of epileptic mothers: preliminary results from the prospective Helsinki study. In: Janz D, Dam M, Richens A, et al., eds. *Epilepsy, Pregnancy, and the Child.* New York: Raven Press; 1982:397–401.

156. Majewski F, Steger M, Richter B, et al. The teratogenicity of hydantoins and barbiturates in humans, with considerations on the etiology of malformations and cerebral disturbances in the children of epileptic parents. *Int J Biol Res Pregnancy.* 1981;2:37–45.

157. Dean JC, Hailey H, Moore SJ, et al. Long-term health and neurodevelopment in children exposed to antiepileptic drugs before birth. *J Med Genet.* 2002;39:251–259.

158. Holmes LB, Harvey EA, Coull BA, et al. The teratogenicity of anticonvulsant drugs. *N Engl J Med.* 2001;344:1132–1138.

159. Bertollini R, Kallen B, Mastroiacova P, et al. Anticonvulsant drugs in monotherapy. Effect on the fetus. *Eur J Epidemiol.* 1987;3:164–171.

160. Jäger-Roman E, Rating D, Koch S, et al. Somatic parameters, diseases and psychomotor development in the offspring of epileptic parents. In: Janz D, Dam M, Richens A, et al., eds. *Epilepsy, Pregnancy, and the Child.* New York: Raven Press; 1982:425–432.

161. Majewski F, Steger M. Fetal head growth retardation associated with maternal phenobarbitone/primidone and/or phenytoin therapy [letter]. *Eur J Pediatr.* 1984;141:188–189.

162. Dieterich E. Antiepileptika embryopathien. *Ergeb Inn Med Kinderheilkd.* 1980;43:93–107.

163. Gaily EK, Granström ML, Hiilesmaa VK, et al. Head circumference in children of epileptic mothers: contributions of drug exposure and genetic background. *Epilepsy Res.* 1990;5:217–222.

164. Kelly TE, Edwards P, Rein M, et al. Teratogenicity of anticonvulsant drugs, II: a prospective study. *Am J Med Genet.* 1984;19:435–443.

165. Hattig H, Helge H, Steinhausen HC. Infants of epileptic mothers: developmental scores at 18 months. In: Wolf P, Dam M, Janz D, et al., eds. *Advances in Epileptology: XVIth Epilepsy International Symposium.* New York: Raven Press; 1987:579–582.

166. Reinisch JM, Sanders SA, Mortensen EL, et al. In utero exposure to phenobarbital and intelligence deficits in adult men. *J Am Med Assoc.* 1995;274:1518–1525.

167. Adab N, Jacoby A, Smith D, et al. Additional educational needs in children born to mothers with epilepsy. *J Neurol Neurosurg Psychiatry.* 2001; 70:15–21.

168. Gailey E, Kantola-Sorsa E, Hiilesmaa V, et al. Intelligence in children of mothers with epilepsy [abstract]. *Epilepsia.* 2002;43(suppl 8):56.

169. Meador KJ, Baker GA, Browning N, et al. Fetal antiepileptic drug exposure and cognitive function at age 3. *New Engl J Med.* 2009;360(16):1597–605.

170. Rasalam AD, Hailey H, Williams JH, et al. Characteristics of fetal anticonvulsant syndrome associated autistic disorder. *Dev Med Child Neurol.* 2005;47(8):551–555.

171. Vinten J, Bromley RL, Taylor J, et al. The behavioral consequences of exposure to antiepileptic drugs in utero. *Epilepsy Behav.* 2009;14(1): 197–201.

172. Bromley RL, Mawer G, Clayton-Smith J, et al. Autism spectrum disorders following in utero exposure to antiepileptic drugs. *Neurology.* 2008; 71(23):1923–1924.

173. Finnell RH, Chernoff GF. Gene-teratogen interactions. An approach to understanding the metabolic basis of birth defects. In: Nau H, Scott WJ, eds. *Pharmacokinetics in Teratogenesis.* Boca Raton, FL: CRC Press; 1987:97–109.

174. Phelan MC, Pellock JM, Nance WE. Discordant expression of fetal hydantoin syndrome in heteropaternal dizygotic twins. *N Engl J Med.* 1982;307:99–101.

175. Buehler BA, Delimont D, Waes MV, et al. Prenatal prediction of risk of the fetal hydantoin syndrome. *N Engl J Med.* 1990;322:1567–1572.

176. Wells PG, Zubovits JT, Wong ST, et al. Modulation of phenytoin teratogenicity and embryonic covalent binding by acetylsalicylic acid, caffeic acid, and alpha-phenyl-N-t-butylnitrone: implications for bioactivation by prostaglandin synthetase. *Toxicol Appl Pharmacol.* 1989;97:192–202.

177. Wells PG, Kim PM, Laposa RR, et al. Oxidative damage in chemical teratogenesis. *Mutat Res.* 1997;396:65–78.

178. Wong M, Wells PG. Modulation of embryonic glutathione reductase and phenytoin teratogenicity by 1,3-bis(2-chloroethyl)-1-nitrosourea (BCNU). *J Pharmacol Exp Ther.* 1989;250:336–342.

179. Danielsson B, Skold AC, Azarbayjani F, et al. Pharmacokinetic data support pharmacologically induced embryonic dysrhythmia as explanation to fetal hydantoin syndrome in rats. *Toxicol Appl Pharmacol.* 2000;163: 164–175.

180. Carl GF, Smith DB. Interaction of phenytoin and folate in the rat. *Epilepsia.* 1983;24:494–501.

181. Carl GF, Smith DB. Effect of chronic phenobarbital treatment on folates and one-carbon enzymes in the rat. *Biochem Pharm.* 1984;21:3457–3463.

182. Carl GF, Smith ML. Chronic primidone treatment in the rat: an animal model of primidone therapy. *Res Commun Chem Path Pharmacol.* 1988; 61:365–376.

183. Carl GF, Smith ML. Chronic carbamazepine treatment in the rat: efficacy, toxicity, and effect on plasma and tissue folate concentrations. *Epilepsia.* 1989;30:217–224.

184. Carl GF, DeLoach C, Patterson J. Chronic sodium valproate treatment in the rat: toxicity versus protection against seizures induced by Indoklon. *Neurochem Int.* 1986;8:41–45.

185. Danksy LV, Andermann E, Rosenblatt D, et al. Anticonvulsants, folate levels and pregnancy outcome: a prospective study. *Ann Neurol.* 1987;21: 176–182.

186. Biale Y, Lewenthal H. Effect of folic acid supplementation on congenital malformations due to anticonvulsant drugs. *Eur J Obstet Gynecol Reprod Biol.* 1984;18:211–216.

187. Ikonomidou C, Bittigau P, Ishimaru MJ, et al. Ethanol-induced apoptotic neurodegeneration in fetal alcohol syndrome. *Science.* 2000;287:1056–1060.

188. Bittigau P, Sifringer M, Genz K, et al. Antiepileptic drugs and apoptotic neurodegeneration in the developing brain. *Proc Natl Acad Sci U S A.* 2002;99(23):15089–15094.

189. Bittigau P, Sifringer M, Ikonomidou C. Antiepileptic drugs and apoptosis in the developing brain. *Ann NY Acad Sci.* 2003;993:103–114.

190. Stefovska VG, Uckermann O, Czuczwar M, et al. Sedative and Anticonvulsant Drugs Suppress Postnatal Neurogenesis. *Ann Neurol.* 2008;64:434–445.

191. Glier C, Dzietko M, Bittigau P, et al. Therapeutic doses of topiramate are not toxic to the developing rat brain. *Exp Neurology.* 2004;187:403–409.

192. Manthey D, Asimiadou S, Stefovska V, et al. Sulthiame but not levetiracetam exerts neurotoxic effect in the developing rat brain. *Exp Neurol.* 2005;193(2):497–503.

193. Katz I, Kim J, Gale K, et al. Effects of lamotrigine alone and in combination with MK-801, phenobarbital or phenytoin on cell death in the neonatal rat brain. *J Pharmacol Exp Ther.* 2007;322(2):494–500.

194. Kim J, Kondratyev A, Gale K. Antiepileptic drug-induced neuronal cell death in the immature brain: Effects of carbamazepine, topiramate, and levetiracetam as monotherapy versus polytherapy. *J Pharmacol Exp Ther.* 2007;323:165–173.

CHAPTER 93 ■ PSYCHIATRIC COMORBIDITY OF EPILEPSY

BETH LEEMAN AND STEVEN C. SCHACHTER

Epilepsy is a model for brain–behavior relationships. Seizures affect behavior and behavior affects seizures. Psychiatric comorbidity is common among patients with epilepsy, the clinical presentation is frequently atypical, and there is often a temporal relationship with seizures. This chapter reviews four of the most commonly encountered psychiatric illnesses in patients with epilepsy: depression, anxiety, psychosis, and personality disorders.

DEPRESSION

Epidemiology

Depression is the most frequently occurring comorbid psychiatric disorder in patients with epilepsy, with a prevalence of 10% to 20% among patients with controlled seizures and 20% to 60% among those with refractory epilepsy (1,2). These rates are significantly higher than that of controls, with major depressive disorder (MDD) diagnosed in 4.9% to 17% of the general population. The relationship between seizures and depression is bidirectional, in that the presence of one predicts the other (3). Those with depression have a 1.7- to 6-fold higher risk of developing seizures than controls (4,5).

Depression is a better predictor of quality of life in patients with epilepsy than are verbal memory, psychomotor function, cognitive processing speed, mental flexibility, seizure frequency, and seizure severity (6,7). Depression has a negative effect and is associated with more disability, greater social difficulties, more drug side effects, lower employment rates, cognitive dysfunction and subjective memory complaints, and greater use of the medical system (8,9). In patients with epilepsy, morbidity, mortality, and overall prognosis are poorer in those with comorbid depression. Those with psychiatric disease are less likely to attain seizure freedom with antiepileptic drugs (AEDs) or anterior temporal lobectomy (10,11).

Potential risk factors for depression in patients with epilepsy include frequent seizures (>1 per month), symptomatic focal epilepsy, younger age, psychosocial difficulties with learned helplessness, and polypharmacy (12). Depression ratings negatively correlate with the presence of idiopathic generalized epilepsy (IGE) as opposed to other types of seizures (12). Mesial temporal structure (MTS) is a better predictor of the presence of depression compared to other forms of temporal lobe epilepsy (TLE). The effect in focal epilepsies appears to be independent of lateralization of the seizure focus, although studies are conflicting with some indicating left predominance (13). Frontal dysfunction may have etiologic significance as well. Unlike idiopathic depression, female predominance is not a consistent finding.

Clinical Features

Depression is categorized into MDD, dysthymia, or depressive disorder not otherwise specified (NOS). Criteria for major depression include low mood, feelings of worthlessness, guilt, loss of energy and interest, insomnia or hypersomnia, changes in appetite, loss of libido, psychomotor retardation or agitation, decreased concentration, and suicidal ideation (SI). Approximately 17% to 30% of depressed patients with epilepsy will meet formal criteria for MDD. In dysthymia, symptoms are more chronic but less severe. Depressive disorder NOS is diagnosed when the presentation does not meet full *Diagnostic and Statistical Manual of Mental Disorders* (DSM) criteria for MDD or dysthymia.

The clinical presentation in 25% to 71% of depressed patients with epilepsy does not meet any of the DSM Axis I category criteria (14). Atypical presentations are particularly common in children. The concept of an atypical depression in epilepsy, first noted by Kraepelin and later formalized by Blumer, has been termed "interictal dysphoric disorder" (IDD) (15) or "dysthymic-like disorder of epilepsy" (16). Symptoms resemble those of dysthymia, but occur intermittently, precluding the formal diagnosis of dysthymia. Patients may have intermittent irritability, depressed or euphoric moods, anergia, insomnia, atypical pains, anxiety, and fears in the setting of clear consciousness. Episodes begin and end abruptly. They may recur every few days to every few months and last from a few hours to upto 2 days or more. Onset generally occurs 2 years after the diagnosis of epilepsy. Data suggest an association with mesial TLE. A similar presentation in the setting of limbic lesions, but without overt seizures, has been termed "subictal dysphoric disorder." Depression in epilepsy may represent a continuum, perhaps with chronic dysthymia, intermittent episodes of IDD, and occasional worsening of symptoms meeting criteria for MDD (17). While IDD may be evident preictally, postictally, premenstrually, or in the setting of forced normalization, symptoms are typically independent of seizure occurrence. Many patients experience an increase in dysphoria over the 12 to 18 months following temporal lobectomy, after which symptoms resolve.

The Seizure Questionnaire (15) may be used to screen for IDD; presence of at least three of the key symptoms warrants the diagnosis. Ongoing treatment is often necessary. Patients with IDD tend to be sensitive to antidepressants, in that drugs are rapidly effective for their broad array of symptoms at low doses.

Major depressive symptoms vary according to the temporal relation to seizure activity. Symptoms may arise prior to seizure onset (preictal), as an expression of the seizure (ictal), following seizures (postictal), or, most commonly, unrelated to seizure occurrence (interictal). Preictal depression is characterized by a dysphoric mood that precedes a seizure by hours or days (18) and usually ends with the seizure. Ictal depression may manifest as a simple partial seizure (SPS) in which depression is the sole symptom, or as an aura leading to a complex partial seizure (CPS). Psychiatric symptoms occur in 25% of auras, 15% of which involve affective changes (19). Ictal depression is the second most common, after ictal anxiety or fear, and consists of anhedonia, guilt, and SI. In dacrystic seizures, auras consist of unprovoked and inappropriate crying. The mood alterations with ictal depression are stereotypical and occur out of context. Postictal depression has long been recognized but its frequency is unknown. In one series, postictal depression was evident in 43% of patients with partial seizures. Postictal symptoms often persist for hours to several days and may be severe, including SI (20).

Major depression may also develop paradoxically as seizure control or EEG abnormalities improve through medication or surgery, a sequence of events termed "forced normalization." Although many of those with depression will have resolution of their symptoms after epilepsy surgery (21), depression may also worsen or occur de novo posttemporal lobectomy (22). Postoperative depression often begins acutely within the first month after surgery. In 80% of patients, symptoms will begin within the first year. Risk factors include those with fear auras, especially those rendered seizure-free by surgery. Quigg et al. (23) also suggest higher risk with right-sided resections.

Treatment

Depression is both under-recognized and undertreated in patients with epilepsy. An estimated 80% of neurologists (24) do not screen for depression in patients with seizure disorders, perhaps due to unease with its management. Difficulty in recognition of symptoms may also play a role, as many patients present atypically or have confounding side effects of medications. A further limiting factor is the lack of controlled trials for depression in patients with epilepsy. Wiegartz et al. (25) found that 38% of patients with a lifetime history of MDD had never received treatment, and Kanner and Palac (14) observed that treatment was delayed by more than 6 months in 66% of patients with epilepsy and concomitant mood disorders of greater than 1-year duration.

When screening for depression, an initial, simple step is to inquire about anhedonia, which is the inability to experience pleasure. This is an excellent indicator of depression and generally unaffected by drug side effects or underlying medical issues. Referral to a psychiatrist, especially one who is knowledgeable about epilepsy, is advisable for diagnosis and initiation of treatment.

Before initiating treatment, iatrogenic factors should be considered, such as the recent discontinuation of an AED with mood-stabilizing properties (e.g., carbamazepine [CBZ], lamotrigine [LTG], valproate [VPA], and vagus nerve stimulation [VNS]); the recent introduction or dosage increase of an AED with potential negative psychotropic properties (e.g., primidone, phenobarbital [PB], topiramate [TPM], vigabatrin, tiagabine, felbamate, gabapentin, levetiracetam [LEV], or zonisamide [ZNS]); or the recent remission of seizures (i.e., "forced normalization"). Phenobarbital exerts particularly negative effects on mood, with 40% of those treated developing depression (26). Risk factors for AED-induced depressive episodes include a personal or family history of mood disorders, anxiety, or alcoholism; severe epilepsy; polytherapy; rapid titration; and high doses. Addition of an enzyme-inducing AED may also increase clearance of concurrently administered antidepressants, leading to breakthrough depressive symptoms (Table 93.1). If iatrogenic issues are a factor, their correction should be the first step in treatment. If it is not possible to alter the AED regimen, an antidepressant may be added. In addition, prior to initiation of therapy, patients should be screened for evidence of bipolar disorder to avoid precipitating a manic episode.

For those with peri-ictal depression, improved seizure control may be a sufficient treatment. For patients with resistant peri-ictal depression, or interictal MDD, dysthymia, or IDD, antidepressant treatment is indicated. In the absence of controlled trials, the choice of antidepressant should be based upon safety, tolerability, and ease of use (e.g., frequency of dosage, likelihood of drug–drug interactions). If a particular antidepressant was successful in the past for the patient or family member, another trial of this agent should be considered.

A common misconception is that all antidepressants significantly lower seizure threshold and should be avoided. These fears are largely based upon seizures associated with overdoses, which have little predictive value when levels are within therapeutic range (27,28). Lower doses of antidepressants may in fact have anticonvulsant properties (29). Rate of escalation and duration of treatment may also play a role. Patients with primary generalized epilepsy may have a greater propensity for seizure exacerbation secondary to antidepressants; depression in such patients appears to respond well to low doses of these agents (15).

The medications with substantial risk are few; however, it is prudent to avoid bupropion, maprotiline, clomipramine, and amoxapine because of their potential for exacerbating seizures (29). Seizures due to bupropion are classically generalized tonic–clonic convulsions (GTC), as may be seen particularly in patients with bulimia. The immediate-release preparation presents a particular concern, with a seizure incidence of 0.36% to 5.8%. The seizure-inducing potential is dose-related and the therapeutic index is low. Maprotiline induces seizures in 12.2% to 15.6% of patients; higher serum levels and longer durations of treatment are the risk factors. The epileptogenicity of clomipramine varies by dose, with seizures in up to 3% of patients taking >250 mg/day. Risk also increases with concomitant VPA, with status epilepticus occurring in some cases. Although the propensity for seizures is lower (0.5%) with doses <250 mg/day, this medication is best avoided. Likewise, seizure risk with amoxapine is 36.4%, with reports of status epilepticus.

In contrast, selective serotonin reuptake inhibitors (SSRIs; citalopram, escitalopram, fluoxetine, fluvoxamine, paroxetine, sertraline) are unlikely to worsen seizure frequency or severity and are generally effective for dysthymic disorders, symptoms of irritability, and poor frustration tolerance. Furthermore, an overdose of an SSRI is unlikely to be fatal,

TABLE 93.1

ANTIDEPRESSANTS COMMONLY USED IN PATIENTS WITH EPILEPSY

Medication	Initial monotherapy	Hepatic enzyme effects	Interactions with AEDs/Antidepressants	Seizure risk (percent incidence in general population)	Notes
SSRI					
Citalopram	Depression Adults Children	Little effect	Levels decreased by: DPH CBZ PB Primidone	0.1–0.3 18.0 at 600–1900 mg	
Escitalopram	Depression Adults Children	Little effect		0–0.04%	Myoclonus reported with concurrent LMT
Fluoxetine	Depression— children[a]	Inhibitor	↑DPH levels ↑CBZ levels ↑TCA levels ↑VPA levels (rare)	0–0.3	Possible anticonvulsant effects Serotonin syndrome; isolated case of Parkinsonian syndrome with concurrent CBZ Long half-life, less withdrawal
Fluvoxamine	Depression— children	Inhibitor	↑DPH levels Levels decreased by: DPH CBZ PB Primidon	0.05–0.2	
Paroxetine	Depression— children	Little effect		0.07–0.1	Increased risk of weight gain Short half-life, withdrawal syndrome
Sertraline	Depression— children[b]	Little effect	↑TCA levels Levels decreased by: DPH CBZ PB Primidone OXC (minimal) TPX (minimal)	0–0.3	Increased risk of weight gain
SNRI					
Venlafaxine	Depression— adults			0.1–0.3% 0 with XR formulation 5.0 with overdose	Not for use in young children; may use in older adolescents and those with resistant depression Higher remission rates than SSRI Faster onset of action For somatic symptoms; wide spectrum of action More complicated titration Significant withdrawal Use extended release May cause lethargy, irritability, hypertension Use at half starting dose in elderly
Tetracyclic					
Mirtazapine	Depression— adults			0.04	Not for use in young children; may use in older adolescents and those with resistant depression For melancholic features May cause sedation, weight gain Lacks SE of nausea, sexual dysfunction May cause agranulocytosis; do not use with CBZ

[a]FDA approved for age >8 years.
[b]FDA approved.
TCA, tricyclic antidepressant; SSRI, selective serotonin reuptake inhibitor; SNRI, selective serotonin norepinephrine reuptake inhibitor; DPH, phenytoin; CBZ, carbamazepine; PB, phenobarbital; OXC, oxcarbazepine; TPX, topiramate; VPA, valproic acid; LMT, lamotrigine; SE, side effects; AED, antiepileptic drug.

interactions with AEDs are minimal, and side effects are manageable. For these reasons, SSRIs are first-line treatments in adults and children with depressive disorders. Women tend to be more responsive than men, however, and sexual dysfunction and weight gain are common adverse reactions. Sexual dysfunction may occur in 70% of those treated with SSRIs. Weight gain is of particular concern when SSRIs are used in combination with AEDs that cause the same effect, including gabapentin, VPA, CBZ, and pregabalin.

Among the SSRIs, sertraline has been best studied. Kanner and associates used sertraline to treat depression in 100 patients with epilepsy. Depressive symptoms improved in the majority of subjects, with seizures definitely worsening in only one patient (16). Clinicians favor the use of the newer SSRIs, citalopram and escitalopram, due to their lack of hepatic enzyme effects. Starting with the lowest dose is recommended, with a gradual dose increase at 1- to 2-week intervals. If a more rapid increase is necessary due to severe symptoms, closer observation is required.

The tricyclic antidepressants (TCAs; amitriptyline, amoxapine, clomipramine, desipramine, doxepin, imipramine, nortriptyline, protriptyline, trimipramine) are not recommended as first-line agents in patients with epilepsy because of a greater likelihood of side effects and drug–drug interactions. Weight gain and sexual dysfunction are common. Also of concern are the potential for cardiac conduction abnormalities and the greater tendency to induce mania. The anticholinergic effects may exacerbate memory dysfunction in patients with Alzheimer disease as well. Finally, these medications have been shown to increase the risk of seizures in the general population in up to 0.1% to 4% at therapeutic levels and 8.4% to 22% in the setting of overdose (levels >1000 mg/mL). This class of medications is contraindicated in children with epilepsy due to the seizure risk. Imipramine and amitriptyline at dosages ≤200 mg/day, however, do not generally provoke seizures in adults. Imipramine, amitriptyline, and trimipramine may cause epileptiform EEG changes at high doses, although this is not generally accompanied by clinical seizures.

For these reasons, monitoring TCA levels may be helpful, particularly in the setting of polypharmacy or to identify slow metabolizers. Enzyme-inducing AEDs (e.g., phenytoin [DPH], PB, primidone, CBZ) may cause low TCA levels, while enzyme inhibitors (i.e., VPA) may increase TCA levels. Conversely, imipramine and nortriptyline may increase concentrations of DPH, CBZ, and PB, and amitriptyline may increase the volume of distribution of VPA. Drug–drug interactions may be quite complex, at times with increased formation of toxic metabolites but decreased activity of parent compounds. The common recommendation to start at a low dose and increase slowly applies.

The monoamine oxidase inhibitors (MAOIs; rasagiline, selegiline, isocarboxazid, phenelzine, tranylcypromine) are generally safe in patients with epilepsy. They are not often prescribed due to their side effect profile, however, which includes hypertensive crises due to interactions with tyramine-containing foods. The potentially fatal serotonin syndrome may also occur when an MAOI is combined with an SSRI or a TCA, with symptoms including restlessness, myoclonus, diaphoresis, tremor, hyperthermia, and seizures. Although useful for atypical features of depression, these are third-line agents and should be prescribed only by psychiatrists.

Of the selective norepinephrine reuptake inhibitors (SNRIs; duloxetine, venlafaxine), venlafaxine is a first-line agent in adults with depression, particularly for those with melancholic features. Dosages as high as 225 mg/day have been demonstrated to be safe in depressed patients with epilepsy. Lethargy, irritability, and hypertension are the main side effects. Blood pressure elevations are typically seen at higher doses, above 300 mg/day.

The goal of treatment for depression is symptom remission; those with any residual symptoms have a greater likelihood for relapse. A full response should be evident in 6 to 12 weeks. Continuation of medication is generally indicated for 4 to 9 months. If a patient has three or more episodes of depression, residual symptoms, suicidality, psychosis, or an otherwise severe episode, long-term prophylaxis is indicated. Children tend to have high relapse rates, with continuation of symptoms into adulthood (30).

In the elderly, SSRIs and venlafaxine may be used, but dosages should begin at one-half the usual starting dose, and treatment should be continued for at least 2 years in those with frequent or severe episodes (19).

In addition to pharmacotherapy, evidence supports use of cognitive-behavioral therapy (CBT) and interpersonal therapy in those with mild to moderate symptoms, and additional benefit may be attained from combined approaches with therapy plus medication. Psychotherapy can help patients cope with limitations imposed by epilepsy and may result in significant improvements in rating scales of depression and anxiety, as well as seizure frequency (31). Psychoeducation and therapy (e.g., CBT, interpersonal psychotherapy, or supportive therapy) is strongly recommended for children (32).

For refractory depression, alternative regimens may include dopamine agonists and electroconvulsive therapy (ECT), which is particularly useful for refractory depression or acute, severe episodes (e.g., including suicidality, psychosis). ECT is not contraindicated in epilepsy. Dose reduction of AEDs may be required during a course of ECT, and AEDs should be withheld the morning of a treatment unless there is concern for status epilepticus.

The Epilepsy Foundation's Mood Disorders Initiative has made the following recommendations regarding treatment of depression in adults with epilepsy (19):

Stage 1: Monotherapy with an SSRI (citalopram, escitalopram), venlafaxine or mirtazepine, and/or CBT is first-line treatment. If there is an incomplete response, proceed to Stage 2.

Stage 2: Monotherapy with a different agent is recommended (another SSRI, a TCA, venlafaxine, or mirtazapine). If there is an incomplete response, proceed to Stage 3.

Stage 3: Monotherapy with an SSRI, a TCA, venlafaxine, mirtazapine, or an MAOI is recommended. A medication from a different class than that used in Stages 1 or 2 should be administered. Alternatively, combination therapy may be used (TCA with SSRI, TCA with venlafaxine, TCA with mirtazepine, venlafaxine with mirtazepine). If there is an incomplete response, proceed to Stage 4.

Stage 4: Combination therapy is recommended (TCA with SSRI, TCA with venlafaxine, TCA with mirtazepine, venlafaxine with mirtazepine). If there is an incomplete response, proceed to Stage 5.

Stage 5: ECT.

When transitioning between drugs, an overlap and taper strategy should be used to avoid withdrawal symptoms.

Suicidality

Though estimates vary, the lifetime prevalence of SI in patients with epilepsy is approximately twice that of the general population, occurring at a rate of about 12%. Suicide attempts occur in 4.6% to 30% of patients with epilepsy, compared to 1.1% to 7% of controls. Patients with seizures are also at greater risk of completing suicide compared to controls: 2.32% to 14% and 0.74% to 1.4%, respectively (33). Elevated risk occurs in children and adolescents with epilepsy as well, with 20% of such children experiencing SI (34).

The prevalence of suicide in epilepsy increases with comorbid psychiatric diagnoses, including depression, psychosis, anxiety, personality disorders, and bipolar disorder (33). Ictal and postictal depression, mania, postictal psychosis, and command hallucinations present particular risks. In 90% to 95% of patients who commit suicide, prior psychiatric diagnoses were present (33).

Other risk factors include psychosocial stressors, poor physical health, young age in men (25 to 49 years), early age of seizure onset (<18 years, particularly during adolescence), presence of brain lesions, inadequate follow-up or treatment of seizures, access to firearms or other methods of self-harm, and interictal behavioral disorders (i.e., viscosity) (33,35). In TLE, the suicide rate is 25 times higher than in the general population, and a history of epilepsy surgery presents a risk five times of that presented by medical management. Furthermore, cognitive impairment carries a 10 to 25 times greater risk than normal cognition. The degree to which these factors are predictive, however, may differ between men and women (36).

Time periods for particular concern are in the first 6 months after the diagnosis of seizures (37) and within a few months to years of attaining good seizure control after a long history of refractory epilepsy (38). SI may also occur with a temporal relationship to seizure activity. Among patients with refractory seizures, 13% experience postictal SI, lasting 24 hours on average.

Of concern is suicidality associated with AEDs, especially PB (26,36), which carries a risk of SI in 47% of those treated with PB compared to 4% of those treated with CBZ (26). The relationship may be related to dose (36). Those taking PB should be specifically monitored for the development of SI, and use of the drug should be avoided in those with depression or cognitive dysfunction.

In early 2008, the FDA issued an alert regarding suicidality and use of AEDs (39). Based upon a meta-analysis of 199 placebo-controlled trials including 11 AEDs, they found approximately twice the risk of suicidal thoughts or behavior in those taking AEDs compared to placebo (0.43% vs. 0.22%, respectively). The FDA interpreted the findings as likely representing a class effect, generally consistent across medications. Rates differed, however, between the studied AEDs, and older AEDs were not included in the analysis. The risk began as early as 1 week, and continued to at least 24 weeks, at which time most trials ended. Demographic factors (i.e., age) did not clearly influence risk, although those using the drugs for seizure control had the highest relative risk of suicidality (3.6)

when compared to groups taking these agents for other indications. These findings are prompting labeling changes. Physicians are encouraged to discuss this issue with their patients and closely monitor those receiving AEDs for onset or worsening of depression.

Assessment should include direct questioning regarding risk factors. Risk for suicide may also be assessed by the suicidality modules of the Mini International Neuropsychiatric Interview (MINI), the Beck Depression Inventory-II (BDI-II), and the Children's Depression Inventory (CDI) (19,33). Physicians need to document the level of risk, interventions, and plans for monitoring. The patient must be kept safe, including the removal of firearms from the home, or should be provided potential hospitalization until the SI resolves. The clinician should also consider the patient's access to AEDs and the potential for overdose. The availability of PB, for example, poses great safety concerns. Antidepressants and psychotherapy are helpful, and referral to a psychiatrist is indicated.

ANXIETY DISORDERS

Anxiety disorders include generalized anxiety disorder (GAD), panic disorder (PD), obsessive–compulsive disorder (OCD), phobias, and posttraumatic stress disorder (PTSD). Studies suggest an increased prevalence of GAD, PD, OCD, and phobias in patients with either partial or primary generalized epilepsy, with prevalence estimates of 3% to 66% in patients with seizures and up to 29% in the general population (2). Patients may also have symptom complexes that overlap these defined categories. Anxiety may lead to significant distress, and the presence of anxiety in a depressed patient with epilepsy increases the risk of suicide (33).

Generalized Anxiety Disorder

GAD is characterized by excessive anxiety and worry about many issues, occurring almost daily. Patients with GAD may also experience restlessness, fatigue, poor concentration, irritability, muscle tension, and sleep dysfunction. Anxiety in epilepsy most commonly presents as GAD, seen in an estimated 21% of patients with refractory TLE (40).

Anxiety may occur prior to (preictal), during (ictal), or after (postictal) seizure onset. Preictal anxiety may precede the seizure by hours to days. Ictal anxiety is often described as "fear," occurring as part of the aura in approximately 15% of patients with partial seizures and 33% of patients with TLE. Ictal fear is more common with medial foci than with lateral regions of onset. It has been suggested that ictal fear may signify well-localized anterior TLE and predict a favorable surgical outcome compared to those without ictal fear. Ictal anxiety may also be present, however, with frontal, cingulate, or other limbic-onset seizures. While some authors suggest that fear lateralizes to the nondominant hemisphere (41), this is not entirely clear. Postictal anxiety occurs in an estimated 45% of those with refractory partial seizures. Symptoms last an average of 24 hours, and have been likened to a "psychiatric Todd's phenomenon." Those at greatest risk for postictal anxiety include patients with a psychiatric history (20).

Up to 66% of patients with epilepsy report interictal anxiety. While data are conflicting, interictal anxiety does not

TABLE 93.2

TREATMENT OF ANXIETY DISORDERS

T	GAD	PD	OCD	PTSD	Social anxiety
Antidepressants	SSRI Paroxetine	SSRI Sertraline Paroxetine	SSRI Sertraline Paroxetine Fluoxetine	SSRI Sertraline	SSRI Paroxetine
	Venlafaxine	Imipramine Phenelzine	Clomipramine		
Benzodiazepines	Clonazepam **Alprazolam**	**Clonazepam** **Alprazolam**			
Other Anticonvulsants		Valproic acid Gabapentin Oxcarbazepine	Carbamazepine		
Additional Agents	Propranolol				

Medications in bold are FDA approved for that indication.

necessarily correlate with seizure frequency (42,43), and symptoms may develop paradoxically with seizure freedom or reduction (i.e., postoperatively). A shorter duration (<2 years) of epilepsy may correlate with increased anxiety.

Contributing factors include the unpredictability of seizures, psychosocial difficulties, and iatrogenic effects. More specifically, the use of felbamate, vigabatrin, LTG, or TPM may predispose to anxiety, particularly with rapid titration. The withdrawal of AEDs, such as benzodiazepines or PB, may also precipitate GAD, particularly in those with ictal anxiety. Increased anxiety can occur as a paradoxical reaction to SSRIs as well.

GAD may affect quality of life even more than seizure frequency. Anxiety prior to epilepsy surgery is a marker of poorer postresection psychosocial adjustment, perceived memory function, and health-related quality of life. Hence, the importance of screening should be emphasized to aid in appropriate treatment and presurgical counseling. A number of assessment tools are available, including the State-Trait Anxiety Scale (STAI, revised scale Form Y), Goldberg's Depression and Anxiety Scales, the Beck Anxiety Inventory (BAI), the Symptoms Check List (SCL-90-R), the Hospital Anxiety and Depression Scale, and the Hamilton Anxiety Rating Scale (HAM-A or HARS) (44).

Treatment in patients with epilepsy currently varies little from that of the general population, although no controlled studies have been conducted to date. SSRIs, specifically paroxetine and escitalopram, are first-line agents (Table 93.2). Data also demonstrate efficacy of venlafaxine. Benzodiazepines may be used for insomnia and acute, severe distress, although continuous use should probably be limited due to their addictive properties. Pharmacologic treatments used empirically also include TCAs (i.e., imipramine), trazodone, propranolol, and AEDs. AEDs with anxiolytic effects include VPA, tiagabine, barbiturates, gabapentin, pregabalin, and oxcarbazepine (OXC). While buspirone is effective in the general population, this agent should be avoided in patients with epilepsy due to the risk of exacerbating seizures.

Nonpharmacologic treatment may be helpful in individual cases, including family counseling, supportive psychotherapy, psychoeducational programs, and self-help groups. CBT is often useful, either adjunctive to anxiolytics or alone, in patients with mild to moderate symptoms. CBT addresses the negative thought patterns that lead to anxiety, followed by desensitization to anxiety-provoking stimuli. In severe cases, anxiety may also be treated by ECT.

Panic Disorder

Panic attacks consist of episodic symptoms including light-headedness, tremor, fear of loss of control or death, paresthesias, shortness of breath, chest pain, palpitations, perspiration, chills, abdominal upset, sensation of choking, derealization, and persistent worry about future attacks. Clinicians must distinguish between seizures manifesting as panic ("ictal panic"), a primary panic disorder (PD), and comorbid epilepsy and PD. Factors favoring the diagnosis of PD include a gradual onset of symptoms, duration from minutes to hours, and lack of postepisode confusion (Table 93.3). Making the distinction, however, may be difficult. Sazgar et al. (45) identified 4.5% of patients with intractable TLE as having been initially misdiagnosed as PD. Mintzer et al. (46) have adapted the MINI with an "Epilepsy Addendum" that attempts to aid in the distinction between PD and ictal fear. Anecdotally, patients often report that they sense the difference between the two types of spells. Still, seizures may be diagnosed only after a long delay, when progression to more clear complex partial events occurs.

An estimated 21% of patients with epilepsy have comorbid PD (47), in contrast to a prevalence of PD in 1% to 3.5% of the U.S. general population. The comorbidity may occur in up to 33% of patients with ictal fear (46). PD may emerge or worsen after epilepsy surgery, particularly in those with ictal fear. The incidence of PD in epilepsy appears to increase with age.

Seizures manifesting as panic are uncommon. When present, ictal panic is most often associated with right midanterior temporal lobe onset. One study suggested that ictal panic is particularly rare in patients with extratemporal lobe seizures, with no cases observed in a series of 72 such patients

TABLE 93.3

DIFFERENTIATION OF PANIC ATTACKS AND PARTIAL SEIZURES

	Panic attacks	Partial seizures
Duration of episode	Longer duration, last at least 5–15 minutes up to several hours	Brief, typically lasting 30 seconds to 2 minutes
Variability of symptoms	Variable symptoms and sequence	More stereotyped
Consciousness	Preserved	May progress to alteration/loss of awareness
Postevent symptoms	No confusion/amnesia	May have confusion/amnesia
Symptom onset	Slow building of symptoms	Rapid shifts of symptoms
Déjà vu, olfactory or gustatory hallucinations	Rare	>5%
	Hallucinations in psychiatric disease perceived as internal to self, often with associated paranoia	Hallucinations perceived as external to self, without paranoia
Smothering or choking sensation, tachypnea	Common	Rare
Anticipatory anxiety	Common	Uncommon
Associated symptoms (aphasia, gustatory hallucinations, behavioral arrest, automatisms)	Uncommon	May be associated as progress to CPS
Treatment	Response to benzodiazepines, antidepressants; other AEDs occasionally helpful	Response to AEDs, resection. May rarely worsen with certain antidepressants (i.e., tricyclics)
Recurrence	More associated with periods of emotional upset; occur in wakefulness	Sporadic; may occur during sleep
Agoraphobia	50%	No association
Family History	25.1% first-degree relatives with panic disorder	Uncommon
Palpitations	Tachycardia	Brady or tachycardia
Paresthesias	Perioral, distal extremities associated with hyperventilation	May be generalized although bilaterality rare; often focal, unilateral
EEG	Usually normal	Often abnormal
MRI	Usually normal	Lesions common
Age of Onset	Most often 20–30 years	Any age

(45). Isolated case reports, however, suggest that ictal panic may occur with left parieto-occipital (48), right parietal (41), and left temporal lobe–onset seizures (49).

Panic attacks may also present as a postictal phenomenon. Like other forms of postictal anxiety, symptoms last 24 hours on average, and are predicted by psychiatric history and relatively low seizure frequency.

PD can cause significant distress and proper treatment should be initiated upon diagnosis. Serotonergic medications and benzodiazepines are the agents of choice (50). FDA-approved medications for the treatment of panic include sertraline, paroxetine, clonazepam, and alprazolam. The role for other anticonvulsants in the treatment of PD is unclear, although VPA, gabapentin, and OXC may be helpful.

Obsessive–Compulsive Disorder

OCD manifests as obsessive thoughts or repetitive, ritualistic behaviors, typically carried out in order to neutralize anxieties or prevent imagined negative events. The prevalence of OCD in the general population is estimated at 1% to 3%. Limited data suggest an increased frequency of OCD in patients with seizures, with studies demonstrating prevalence between 14.5% and 22% in patients with TLE (51). Several case reports also document the co-occurrence of OCD and epilepsy in patients with temporal lobe (52,53), anterior cingulate (54), frontorolandic (55), and primary generalized (56) seizures. Interictal personality characteristics associated with TLE, such as attention to detail or hyperreligiosity, may be viewed as a mild form of obsessions or compulsions.

OCD in the setting of epilepsy, however, remains under-recognized. In a series of nine patients with TLE meeting criteria for OCD, only one had been previously diagnosed (51). Barbieri et al. (52) described a patient who experienced symptoms of OCD for 17 years and never informed her physicians. These cases underscore the importance of screening and the involvement of neuropsychiatrists in epilepsy clinics.

No controlled trials have evaluated the treatment of OCD in patients with epilepsy, and no consensus regarding management exists. Idiopathic OCD may be treated with psychotherapy and antidepressants, with SSRIs as first-line agents. Although one case report documented a 50% improvement in symptoms, many attempts at nonpharmacologic, behavioral treatments have met with limited success in patients with comorbid seizures (53). Successful treatment with CBZ or OXC has been reported (56). Koopowitz and Berk (56) suggested that comorbid epilepsy may predict better response of OCD symptoms to AEDs than antidepressants, although many other case reports document a lack of effect.

Phobias

Phobias occur in 20% of patients with epilepsy. An estimated 8% to 9% of patients with refractory TLE have agoraphobia and 29% have social phobia (40). Underlying cognitive deficits, low self-esteem, depression, family psychiatric history, and lack of social support may predispose to phobias.

Rare, and perhaps unique to epilepsy, is a "seizure phobia" in which patients fear future seizures. Patients may specifically fear resultant death or brain damage, and relive prior seizures. Patients may develop agoraphobia or social phobia, stemming from fear that others would observe their seizures if they were to occur in public. While phobias are typically an interictal phenomenon, some patients experience postictal agoraphobia. The degree of anxiety may parallel the perceived severity of seizures.

Such phobias may be successfully treated by CBT in addition to other forms of counseling and seizure education (57). Caution should be used in the prescription of benzodiazepines, given concerns that they may lead to dependence and avoidance of the deeper cognitive-behavioral issues.

PSYCHOSIS

Epidemiology

The risk of psychosis varies with epilepsy syndrome, seizure severity, and seizure frequency. Psychosis is reported in 0.6% to 7% of patients with epilepsy in the community, and in 19% to 27% of hospital-derived populations (58). The overall frequency of psychosis among patients with epilepsy is approximately 7% to 14%. Most studies indicate a predilection for those with TLE (15.8%), particularly those with left MTS (59). Reports of an association with other localization-related epilepsies indicate, less commonly, a relationship with left frontal lobe–onset seizures (60). In addition, a prevalence of 3% has been documented in patients with IGE.

Preictal or ictal psychosis is rare. Shukla et al. described a series of patients with intractable right temporal or frontotemporal seizures and preictal psychosis (61). Symptoms consisted of hallucinations, delusions, affective changes, heightened religiosity, and abusive behavior lasting from 12 hours to 15 days prior to habitual seizures. The psychotic features resolved after each seizure.

Diagnosis

During seizures, patients may experience visual or auditory illusions and hallucinations, paranoia, depersonalization, derealization, autoscopy, or a sense of someone lurking behind them. As with most partial seizures, symptoms typically last less than 3 minutes duration. Prolonged ictal psychosis is rare, but may be evident in the setting of nonconvulsive partial or absence status. Often such patients have a corresponding central nervous system (CNS) lesion (i.e., tumor) (62).

The most common form of psychosis occurs between seizures (interictal). Interictal psychosis is present in up to 9.4% of patients with MTS. Features resemble that of schizophrenia, with persistent or recurrent positive symptoms, such as delusions and visual or auditory hallucinations, in the setting of otherwise clear consciousness (63,64). Themes are often persecutory or religious, and may have strong affective components. Common associated affective changes include irritability, depression, and aggressive behavior. As in schizophrenia, symptoms may be insidious in onset.

Many key differences to schizophrenia, however, have prompted the term "schizophrenia-like psychosis" of epilepsy (64). Compared with the psychosis of schizophrenia, patients with interictal psychosis typically have an absence of negative symptoms or formal thought disorder, better premorbid states, and less deterioration of personality (65). Patients with psychosis related to epilepsy also have an older age of onset compared to those with schizophrenia, with symptoms beginning in the late 20s to mid 30s (65,66). Those with epilepsy-related psychosis are more likely to be male, as opposed to patients with schizophrenia (65). Patients with interictal psychosis may also have a better prognosis, with a tendency for remissions and positive responses to treatment (65).

In some patients, a positive correlation exists between overall seizure frequency and psychotic symptoms. A notable exception to this pattern, however, is the concept of "forced normalization" or "alternative psychosis" introduced by Landolt in 1953 (63). Although evident with other psychiatric disorders as noted above, forced normalization is classically associated with psychotic behavior. The patient may have periods of psychosis coinciding with improved seizure control or reduced epileptiform discharges on EEG, often seen with the addition of a new AED. Such periods may alternate with epochs of improved psychiatric function in the setting of a paradoxical increase in seizure frequency or abnormalities on EEG. The underlying pathophysiology is unclear. As Nadkarni et al. note (62), the psychosis may also be a reaction to the new drug, with improved EEG patterns representing an epiphenomenon. Forced normalization has been documented with other treatments, however, including VNS (67).

De novo psychosis after epilepsy surgery has also been reported, with rates varying from <1% to 28.5%. Symptoms most often occur transiently after surgery, and the diagnosis may be easily missed. The time period of greatest concern is the first 6 months after resection. Risk factors include a family history of psychosis, surgery after 30 years of age, and preoperative psychosis. Some authors suggest an increased incidence in those undergoing nondominant temporal resections, although this is not a consistent finding. Etiology of epilepsy does not appear to affect risk assessment (62).

Postictal psychosis is less common, occurring in 6.4% of patients with MTS (59). It typically presents after a cluster of seizures or status epilepticus, oftentimes in someone whose seizures were otherwise well controlled. Postictal psychosis after a single seizure is rare. Symptoms often begin after 24 to 48 hours of normal baseline behavior, a period termed the "lucid interval." Episodes may last a few days to several weeks, terminating within 1 to 2 weeks on average. Approximately 95% of episodes will resolve within 1 month. A history of interictal psychosis, a family history of psychosis, and low intellectual functioning predict a longer duration of symptoms (68). Symptoms may include visual or auditory hallucinations, paranoia, delusions, confusion, affective changes, violence (i.e., suicidal acts), and amnesia (58,69). Religious or grandiose themes among hallucinations and delusions are common, while thought insertion, commenting/command

TABLE 93.4

COMPARISON OF POSTICTAL MANIA AND PSYCHOSIS (70)

Features of postictal mania versus psychosis		
	Postictal mania	**Postictal psychosis**
Duration of episode	Longer; mean 16.1 days	Shorter; mean 6 days
Recurrence	More likely	Less likely
Age of onset	Older; mean onset 18.4 years	Younger; mean onset 9.1 years
Localization	Frontal, temporal	Temporal
Lateralization	Dominant hemisphere	Less well lateralized
Symptoms	Elated/expansive/euphoric mood	Delusions (often persecutory, delusions of reference)
	Distractibility	Hallucinations (often auditory)
	Hyperactivity	Insomnia
	Pressured speech	Emotional lability (transient)
	Decreased need for sleep	Elated/euphoric mood (transient)
	Flight of ideas	
	Grandiosity	
	Hyperreligiosity	
Congruency	Mood congruent symptoms	Mood incongruent symptoms
Psychotic features	Rarely	Always

hallucinations, and negative symptoms are rare. Most religious conversions occur during this period.

It is important to distinguish between postictal psychosis and postictal mania, as treatment options differ (Table 93.4). The two entities may be easily confused, as both may involve manic features and exhibit a similar lucid period. Logsdail and Toone (69) suggested the following diagnostic criteria for postictal psychosis:

1. An episode of psychosis developing within 1 week of a seizure or cluster of seizures
2. Lasting ≥24 hours and ≤3 months
3. Characterized by disorientation, delirium, delusions, or hallucinations in clear or clouded consciousness
4. Without AED toxicity, nonconvulsive status on EEG, prior interictal psychosis, recent head trauma, or alcohol/drug intoxication.

Possible risk factors for postictal psychosis include age >30 years; male gender; focal-onset seizures; bilateral onset (often bitemporal) or spread of seizures (i.e., secondary generalization); history of status epilepticus; prior encephalitis or other widespread CNS injury; borderline intelligence; EEG slowing; psychiatric illness; clusters of seizure activity; and family history of mood disorders, alcohol use, or epilepsy (71–73). Age at seizure onset and seizure frequency are not predictive. These patients tend to have complex presentations, in that, bitemporal dysfunction on neuropsychological testing may be greater than that expected based upon structural imaging, and seizure onsets on video-EEG monitoring are often nonlateralizing (73). Postictal psychoses typically develop after at least 10 years of epilepsy and occur almost exclusively in adults, with the mean age of onset 32 to 35 years. Recurrent episodes have been documented in 12% to 50% of cases. As the frequency of psychotic episodes increases, the risk for developing chronic interictal psychosis becomes greater (62). In a series of 18 patients with postictal psychosis, 39% also experienced interictal psychosis (74).

Treatment

The first step in treatment is identification of the problem. Patients may not report their symptoms, hence direct questioning is necessary. As "psychotic episodes may beget psychotic episodes," once identified, symptoms should be treated immediately (62). For those with peri-ictal psychosis, optimal seizure control is advised. Symptoms may resolve with treatment of the seizures (i.e., with resection) (60). Antipsychotic medications are the mainstay of management for both acute episodes and prevention, as long-term treatment may be necessary for patients with interictal or frequent peri-ictal episodes (Table 93.5). Some patients require psychotherapy, day-treatment programs, case managers, or assisted living facilities (62). ECT may be helpful in refractory cases. Patients with psychosis are best referred to epilepsy centers with teams that include psychiatrists and social workers.

The "positive symptoms," such as delusions, hallucinations, and disordered thinking, respond best to medications. The "negative symptoms," such as apathy, social withdrawal, and catatonia, are notoriously difficult to treat, but may respond to the newer, atypical antipsychotics. In general, patients with psychosis associated with epilepsy have better response rates than patients with schizophrenia, with lower initial and maximum doses. These findings were likely due in large part, however, to better compliance (65).

The older, typical antipsychotics carry a greater risk of seizure exacerbation, with seizure induction rates of 0.5% to 1.2% in the general population. Risk is increased by a history of seizures or abnormal EEGs, CNS disorders, rapid titration, high doses and the concomitant use of other drugs that lower the seizure threshold (75). Hence, the atypical antipsychotics, with lower epileptogenic potential, are preferred. Due in part to a lack of controlled studies, specific treatment decisions are individualized and based upon side effect profiles. Of note, all of the atypical antipsychotics carry some risk of weight gain, hyperlipidemia, and type 2 diabetes mellitus. New data also

TABLE 93.5

ATYPICAL ANTIPSYCHOTICS

Atypical antipsychotics				
Drug	Levels decreased by	Levels increased by	Seizure risk	Notes
Clozapine	DPH CBZ PB Primidone OXC[a] TPX[a]	VPA	Avoid use; black box warning for higher seizure risk 4.4% at >600 mg/day[b] <1% at <300 mg/day[b] Patients with epilepsy had increased seizure frequency on <300 mg/day	Concomitant CBZ increases risk of leukopenia and neuroleptic malignant syndrome
Olanzapine	DPH CBZ PB Primidone	VPA	Higher seizure risk 0.9	
Ziprasidone	DPH CBZ PB Primidone OXC[a] TPX[a]		0.4–0.5	Affective and anxiolytic properties May cause akathisia
Risperidone	DPH CBZ PB Primidone OXC[a] TPX[a]		Lower seizure risk 0.3	More likely to cause extrapyramidal side effects
Quetiapine	DPH CBZ PB Primidone OXC[a] TPX[a]		0.8	Affective and anxiolytic properties Only neuroleptic that did not cause EEG changes
Aripiprazole	CBZ	Fluoxetine[c] Paroxetine[c]	0.4	May cause akathisia

[a]Moderate, dose-dependent effects.
[b]Studies in patients without epilepsy.
[c]May be minimal effects.
DPH, phenytoin; CBZ, carbamazepine; PB, phenobarbital; OXC, oxcarbazepine; TPX, topiramate; VPA, valproic acid.

suggest an increased risk of sudden cardiac death (76). Blood glucose and lipid profiles must be followed, particularly in those taking AEDs that are associated with weight gain (e.g., VPA, gabapentin, pregabalin, and CBZ). One may also consider checking pre- and post-treatment EKGs for evidence of prolonged QT intervals (77).

Ziprasidone is the most common agent used to treat postictal and interictal psychosis, followed by quetiapine and aripiprazole (62). Other options with relatively low rates of seizure induction include risperidone (78) and olanzapine. Among the typical antipsychotics, haloperidol appears to be the safest. Other typical agents with lower seizure-inducing potential include molindone, fluphenazine, perphenazine, and trifluoperazine (75). Lorazepam may also be used in conjunction with an antipsychotic for acute exacerbations and reinforcement of sleep schedules.

Clearly, psychotropic agents that are associated with a high incidence of seizures in nonepileptic patients should be avoided. These include the antipsychotics clozapine, chlorpromazine, and loxapine. Many antipsychotics can cause slowing of the EEG waveforms, particularly at higher doses. Clozapine, however, can cause frank epileptiform discharges. While these spikes and sharp waves are not predictive of seizure occurrence, severe disorganization of the EEG background may be a harbinger of seizures. Whether concurrent use of AEDs will protect against seizure-inducing potential is unknown. The adage "start low, go slow" applies to all antipsychotics.

Forced normalization is a unique entity, in that a breakthrough seizure may resolve the psychotic symptoms. In such patients, the goal of seizure freedom must be balanced by the risk of potentially disabling psychiatric disease. Seizure freedom may not be ideal for such patients. As Landolt stated, "there would seem to be epileptics who must have a pathological EEG in order to be mentally sane." For those with forced normalization due to VNS, decreasing the pulse intensity can improve symptoms (67). Gradual withdrawal of medications may be necessary, and antipsychotics, antidepressants, and anxiolytics may be used.

PERSONALITY DISORDERS

The association between epilepsy and certain personality characteristics dates back to Hippocrates in 400 BC. Reports suggest that up to 69% of patients with TLE and 72% of patients with generalized epilepsy suffer from personality disorders (PSD) (79). In a series of patients with juvenile myoclonic epilepsy (JME) (80), 14% had PSD, including borderline (6%), dependent (3%), histrionic (1%), and obsessive–compulsive (0.6%) personality disorders, as well as 3% with PSD NOS.

Perhaps more controversial is the notion of a specific personality type in the setting of TLE, thought to occur in 7% of TLE patients (81,82). In 1975, Waxman and Geschwind formalized the concept of an "interictal behavioral syndrome," alternatively termed "Geschwind syndrome" or "Gastaut–Geschwind syndrome," which consisted of deepened emotions, circumstantiality, hyper-religiosity, hyposexuality, and hypergraphia. Gastaut suggested that this cluster of personality traits was the opposite of that exhibited by patients with Kluver–Bucy syndrome. Bear and Fedio later expanded the cluster of traits to include the 18 items listed in Table 93.6. The most significant differences in patients with TLE compared to non-neurologic controls were in humorlessness, circumstantiality, dependence, and sense of personal destiny. These are not necessarily negative, pathological, or maladaptive

TABLE 93.6

CHARACTERISTICS OF THE "INTERICTAL BEHAVIORAL SYNDROME"

Characteristics of the interictal personality in temporal lobe epilepsy (83)
Emotionality
Elation/Euphoria
Sadness
Anger
Aggression
Altered sexual interest
Guilt
Hypermoralism
Obsessionalism
Circumstantiality
Viscosity
Sense of personal destiny
Hypergraphia
Religiosity
Philosophical interest
Dependence/Passivity
Humorlessness/Sobriety
Paranoia

traits, but rather a constellation of often subtle behavioral changes. The alterations in personality tend to develop gradually, after at least 2 years of seizures (82).

Overall, these behavioral characteristics may correlate with mild intellectual impairment and AED levels. The effect of laterality in TLE is likely minor, with mixed results. An observed trend is for those with right temporal foci to report more emotional traits and minimize their difficulties, while those with left temporal foci endorse more aberrant behaviors thereby "tarnishing their image" (81).

While much of this discussion focuses on patients with TLE, those with other localization-related epilepsies or IGE may have personality changes as well (81). Patients with anterior cingulate seizures can demonstrate aggressive, sociopathic, irritable, obsessive–compulsive, or impulsive traits (81). Orbitofrontal epilepsy may be characterized by abnormal emotionality, aggression, disinhibition, and confabulation. Patients with typical absence epilepsy may have poor social relationships, particularly in the setting of ongoing seizures. Patients with JME may exhibit irresponsibility, poor impulse control, self-interest, emotional instability, exaggeration, denial, inconsiderate behaviors, and distractibility (81,83). Although scores on PSD inventories are often higher in TLE than in generalized epilepsy, this is not a consistent finding.

A number of instruments are available for the evaluation of personality disorders. Administered most commonly is the Minnesota Multiphasic Personality Inventory-2 (MMPI-2). The Bear–Fedio Inventory (BFI), evaluating the characteristics outlined in Table 93.6, has been used less often in recent years. Other self-report batteries include the Questionnaire on Personality Traits, Neurobehavioral Inventory (NBI, a revised version of the BFI), Neurobehavioral Rating Scale (NBHRS), Overt Aggression Scale, Freiburg Personality Inventory/Form A (FPI-A), Index of Personality Characteristics (IPC), and Millon Behavioral Health Inventory (MBHI) (81).

Treatment options for PSD are limited. Patients may be referred for psychotherapy, although there is little data to formally support its use in epilepsy patients (81).

It is important, though difficult, to distinguish those behavioral components due to psychological comorbidities of the epileptic disorder from effects of underlying lesions, medications, or other behavioral issues. It may also be challenging to differentiate between the ictal, preictal, interictal, and postictal states, as boundaries may be indistinct. Studies are further confounded by difficulties in identifying the focus of onset and degree of spread of abnormal activity, particularly when using routine scalp recordings. Differing criteria for the diagnosis of a behavioral disorder, varying definitions of the epilepsy or control populations, and small sample sizes make studies complicated to interpret or compare. Furthermore, none of the symptoms above are pathognomonic for any one seizure subtype, or even to epilepsy as a whole. For these reasons, identification of a personality syndrome specific to TLE has met with criticism (85).

Aggression

Aggression and hostility have been documented in approximately 5% of patients with epilepsy (81,86). In more selected groups and prisoners with TLE, interictal aggressive behavior is present in up to 56% of patients. Nevertheless, violent behavior is likely underdiagnosed due to underreporting and a lack of appreciation that the behavior may constitute a treatable disorder.

Although classically associated with TLE and lesions of the amygdala, patients with JME, anterior cingulate seizures, and orbitofrontal epilepsy may also demonstrate interictal aggression. Such behavior is more likely in men and children. Onset of epilepsy before 10 years of age, traumatic brain injury, psychosis, cognitive deficits, fewer years of formal education, lower IQ, and lower socioeconomic status are possible risk factors (87,88).

The association between aggression and epilepsy may relate to common limbic pathways or psychosocial factors. Seizure treatments are also important contributors. Because AEDs may indirectly cause aggressive behavior as a consequence of forced normalization (89) or disinhibiting, anxiogenic side effects, iatrogenic causes should first be considered. Agents causing irritability or aggression include PB, LTG, and gabapentin, particularly in children and patients with learning disabilities. Aggressive behavior has also been noted after resection for refractory TLE (90).

Interictal aggression may be evident as a symptom of depression, or the more controversial IDD in which patients have "paroxysmal affects" ranging from mild irritability to rage. Violent behavior may also occur with a temporal relationship to seizures. Some patients exhibit irritability and aggression in the minutes, hours, or days leading up to a seizure (preictal) (18). Directed, purposeful, aggressive behavior during seizures (ictal), however, is rare (86,91,92). Postictal aggression is the best recognized entity.

Postictal violent behavior may result from attempts at physical restraint, termed "resistive violence" (93). The behavior is typically associated with impaired consciousness or confusion, and is most frequently seen in those with CNS pathology (e.g., prior head injury or CNS infection), mental retardation (MR), and psychiatric illness. Self-injury is more often evident in patients with developmental disabilities. Violent behavior may also occur in association with postictal psychosis (94). In the setting of psychosis, aggression may be more directed in response to hallucinations or delusions.

Subacute postical aggression (SPA) consists of stereotyped, directed violent or verbally abusive behavior beginning several minutes to hours after a seizure (95). Episodes may occur after waking from postictal sleep and are unrelated to ictal discharges or postictal confusion. The episodes are brief, lasting 5 to 30 minutes. Curious features include at least partially retained awareness and remorse after the episode. SPA tends to occur many years after the onset of epilepsy, in patients with long-standing refractory partial seizures and extensive neural dysfunction. These episodes are more common in men, and in patients with TLE and secondary generalized seizures. SPA is not a well-recognized clinical entity, and must be differentiated from the more common postictal psychosis (PIP).

Treatment depends upon the severity of the behavior and the temporal relationship to seizures. Ictal aggression should respond to AEDs. Postictal resistive violence is best treated by avoiding or limiting physical restraint during the postictal period (93). The treatment of interictal aggression is less certain, as it does not necessarily improve with seizure freedom and controlled studies are lacking. AEDs (particularly CBZ and VPA), antidepressants, and atypical neuroleptics (e.g., olanzapine, risperidone, quetiapine, and ziprasidone) have

been used empirically. Valproic acid, however, may also cause paradoxical irritability. Beta-adrenergic receptor blockers, including propranolol, nadolol, and pindolol, provide alternative treatment options. Drug–drug interactions are of concern, however, as beta blockade may be increased by SSRIs and decreased by CBZ. Amphetamines may be effective for the treatment of impulsivity and aggression, and are generally safe for use in epilepsy, although methylphenidate has been reported to increase seizure frequency in isolated cases. Lithium may be used for treatment of aggression and agitation, although patients with brain injuries are particularly sensitive to its neurotoxic side effects. Encephalopathy has also been noted with concomitant use of CBZ. While lithium has been used safely in patients with epilepsy and BPD, it is not generally recommended as initial therapy because of its potential for seizure exacerbation and induction. Similarly, while buspirone is effective for aggression in the general population, its use is discouraged in patients with epilepsy. Removal of anxiogenic agents and treatment of coexisting mood disorders should be pursued. Behavioral therapy may also be helpful, and psychiatric hospitalization should be considered for patients at risk for impulsive, potentially self-injurious behavior (93).

SUMMARY

Psychiatric disease is common and significantly impacts quality of life in patients with seizures. Physicians must actively screen for these disorders, and proper treatment is essential.

Depression, the most common comorbid psychiatric disorder in epilepsy, negatively affects quality of life and increases the risk for suicide. Unfortunately, depression in epilepsy remains under-recognized and undertreated. Many patients present with atypical symptoms and establishing a diagnosis may be challenging. The importance of screening and treatment for depression in this population, however, should be emphasized. The myth that all antidepressants significantly lower seizure threshold and should be avoided must be dispelled.

Anxiety disorders also occur more commonly in patients with seizures than in the general population. Symptoms typically manifest as GAD, and may occur inter- or peri-ictally.

Comorbid PD may be present in the setting of epilepsy, and must be distinguished from seizures manifesting as panic attacks. Anxiety may also present as OCD or phobias. Common phobias in patients with epilepsy include agoraphobia, social phobia, and a fear of having seizures. Anxiety disorders can be a source of significant distress, and proper treatment is essential.

Patients with epilepsy may also experience comorbid psychosis. Psychotic symptoms generally occur during the interictal state with features similar to that of schizophrenia (e.g., delusions and hallucinations). In contrast to schizophrenia, however, patients with epilepsy and psychosis often lack negative symptoms and deterioration of personality. Psychosis may also occur as a peri-ictal phenomenon. As an increased frequency of postictal psychotic episodes may evolve to chronic interictal psychosis, immediate treatment is indicated. Atypical antipsychotics and psychiatric consultation are the cornerstones of management.

Finally, clinicians should note the frequent presence of comorbid personality disorders in this patient population. Perhaps more controversial is the notion of a specific "interictal behavioral syndrome" in patients with TLE, including such traits as viscosity, hyper-religiosity, and hyposexuality. Aggression may also be evident in patients with seizures, and should be recognized as a treatable disorder.

References

1. Mendez MF, Cummings JL, Benson DF. Depression in epilepsy. Significance and phenomenology. *Arch Neurol.* 1986;43:766–770.
2. Tellez-Zenteno JF, Patten SB, Jette N, et al. Psychiatric comorbidity in epilepsy: a population-based analysis. *Epilepsia.* 2007;48:2336–2344.
3. Kanner AM. Depression in epilepsy: a complex relation with unexpected consequences. *Curr Opin Neurol.* 2008;21:190–194.
4. Hesdorffer DC, Hauser WA, Annegers JF, et al. Major depression is a risk factor for seizures in older adults. *Ann Neurol.* 2000;47:246–249.
5. Hesdorffer DC, Hauser WA, Olafsson E, et al. Depression and suicide attempt as risk factors for incident unprovoked seizures. *Ann Neurol.* 2006;59:35–41.
6. Perrine K, Hermann BP, Meador KJ, et al. The relationship of neuropsychological functioning to quality of life in epilepsy. *Arch Neurol.* 1995;52:997–1003.
7. Lehrner J, Kalchmayr R, Serles W, et al. Health-related quality of life (HRQOL), activity of daily living (ADL) and depressive mood disorder in temporal lobe epilepsy patients. *Seizure.* 1999;8:88–92.
8. Cramer JA, Blum D, Reed M, et al. The influence of comorbid depression on quality of life for people with epilepsy. *Epilepsy Behav.* 2003;4:515–521.
9. Kanner AM, Barry J, Gilliam FG, et al. Differential impact of mood and anxiety disorders on the quality of life and perception of adverse events to antiepileptic drugs in patients with epilepsy. *Epilepsia.* 2007;48(suppl 6):103.
10. Hitiris N, Mohanraj R, Norrie J, et al. Predictors of pharmacoresistant epilepsy. *Epilepsy Res.* 2007;75:192–196.
11. Anhoury S, Brown RJ, Krishnamoorthy ES, et al. Psychiatric outcome after temporal lobectomy: a predictive study. *Epilepsia.* 2000;41:1608–1615.
12. Kimiskidis VK, Triantafyllou NI, Kararizou E, et al. Depression and anxiety in epilepsy: the association with demographic and seizure-related variables. *Ann Gen Psychiatry.* 2007;6:28.
13. Quiske A, Helmstaedter C, Lux S, et al. Depression in patients with temporal lobe epilepsy is related to mesial temporal sclerosis. *Epilepsy Res.* 2000;39:121–125.
14. Kanner AM, Palac S. Depression in epilepsy: a common but often unrecognized comorbid malady. *Epilepsy Behav.* 2000;1:37–51.
15. Blumer D, Montouris G, Davies K. The interictal dysphoric disorder: recognition, pathogenesis, and treatment of the major psychiatric disorder of epilepsy. *Epilepsy Behav.* 2004;5:826–840.
16. Kanner AM, Kozak AM, Frey M. The use of sertraline in patients with epilepsy: is it safe? *Epilepsy Behav.* 2000;1:100–105.
17. Barry JJ, Lembke A, Gisbert PA, et al. Affective disorders in epilepsy. In: Ettinger AB, Kanner AM, eds. *Psychiatric Issues in Epilepsy: A Practical Guide to Diagnosis and Treatment.* 2nd ed. Philadelphia, PA: Lippincott Williams & Wilkins; 2006:203–247.
18. Blanchet P, Frommer GP. Mood change preceding epileptic seizures. *J Nerv Ment Dis.* 1986;174:471–476.
19. Barry JJ, Ettinger AB, Friel P, et al. Consensus statement: the evaluation and treatment of people with epilepsy and affective disorders. *Epilepsy Behav.* 2008;13(suppl 1):S1–S29.
20. Kanner AM, Soto A, Gross-Kanner H. Prevalence and clinical characteristics of postictal psychiatric symptoms in partial epilepsy. *Neurology.* 2004;62:708–713.
21. Glosser G, Zwil AS, Glosser DS, et al. Psychiatric aspects of temporal lobe epilepsy before and after anterior temporal lobectomy. *J Neurol Neurosurg Psychiatry.* 2000;68:53–58.
22. Blumer D, Wakhlu S, Davies K, et al. Psychiatric outcome of temporal lobectomy for epilepsy: incidence and treatment of psychiatric complications. *Epilepsia.* 1998;39:478–486.
23. Quigg M, Broshek DK, Heidal-Schiltz S, et al. Depression in intractable partial epilepsy varies by laterality of focus and surgery. *Epilepsia.* 2003;44:419–424.
24. Gilliam FG, Santos J, Vahle V, et al. Depression in epilepsy: ignoring clinical expression of neuronal network dysfunction? *Epilepsia.* 2004;45(suppl 2):28–33.
25. Wiegartz P, Seidenberg M, Woodard A, et al. Co-morbid psychiatric disorder in chronic epilepsy: recognition and etiology of depression. *Neurology.* 1999;53:S3–S8.
26. Brent DA, Crumrine PK, Varma RR, et al. Phenobarbital treatment and major depressive disorder in children with epilepsy. *Pediatrics.* 1987;80:909–917.
27. Balit CR, Lynch CN, Isbister GK. Bupropion poisoning: a case series. *Med J Aust.* 2003;178:61–63.
28. Cuenca PJ, Holt KR, Hoefle JD. Seizure secondary to citalopram overdose. *J Emerg Med.* 2004;26:177–181.
29. Pisani F, Spina E, Oteri G. Antidepressant drugs and seizure susceptibility: from in vitro data to clinical practice. *Epilepsia.* 1999;40(suppl 10):S48–S56.
30. Birmaher B, Arbelaez C, Brent D. Course and outcome of child and adolescent major depressive disorder. *Child Adolesc Psychiatr Clin N Am.* 2002;11:619–637.
31. Gillham RA. Refractory epilepsy: an evaluation of psychological methods in outpatient management. *Epilepsia.* 1990;31:427–432.
32. Birmaher B, Brent D, AACAP Work Group on Quality Issues, et al. Practice parameter for the assessment and treatment of children and adolescents with depressive disorders. *J Am Acad Child Adolesc Psychiatry.* 2007;46:1503–1526.
33. Jones JE, Hermann BP, Barry JJ, et al. Rates and risk factors for suicide, suicidal ideation, and suicide attempts in chronic epilepsy. *Epilepsy Behav.* 2003;4(suppl 3):S31–S38.
34. Caplan R, Siddarth P, Gurbani S, et al. Depression and anxiety disorders in pediatric epilepsy. *Epilepsia.* 2005;46:720–730.
35. Nilsson L, Ahlbom A, Farahmand BY, et al. Risk factors for suicide in epilepsy: a case control study. *Epilepsia.* 2002;43:644–651.
36. Kalinin VV, Polyanskiy DA. Gender differences in risk factors of suicidal behavior in epilepsy. *Epilepsy Behav.* 2005;6:424–429.
37. Christensen J, Vestergaard M, Mortensen PB, et al. Epilepsy and risk of suicide: a population-based case-control study. *Lancet Neurol.* 2007;6:693–698.
38. Blumer D, Montouris G, Davies K, et al. Suicide in epilepsy: psychopathology, pathogenesis, and prevention. *Epilepsy Behav.* 2002;3:232–241.
39. U.S. Food and Drug Administration. Information for healthcare professionals: suicidality and antiepileptic drugs. Available at: http://www.fda.gov/ Cder/Drug/InfoSheets/HCP/antiepilepticsHCP.htm; 2008. Accessed May 31, 2010.
40. Devinsky O, Barr WB, Vickrey BG, et al. Changes in depression and anxiety after resective surgery for epilepsy. *Neurology.* 2005;65:1744–1749.
41. Alemayehu S, Bergey GK, Barry E, et al. Panic attacks as ictal manifestations of parietal lobe seizures. *Epilepsia.* 1995;36:824–830.
42. Mattsson P, Tibblin B, Kihlgren M, et al. A prospective study of anxiety with respect to seizure outcome after epilepsy surgery. *Seizure.* 2005;14:40–45.
43. Goldstein MA, Harden CL. Epilepsy and Anxiety. *Epilepsy Behav.* 2000;1:228–234.
44. Harden CL, Goldstein MA, Ettinger AB. Anxiety disorders in epilepsy. In: Ettinger AB, Kanner AM, eds. *Psychiatric Issues in Epilepsy: A Practical Guide to Diagnosis and Treatment.* 2nd ed. Philadelphia, PA: Lippincott Williams & Wilkins; 2006:248–263.
45. Sazgar M, Carlen PL, Wennberg R. Panic attack semiology in right temporal lobe epilepsy. *Epileptic Disord.* 2003;5:93–100.
46. Mintzer S, Lopez F. Comorbidity of ictal fear and panic disorder. *Epilepsy Behav.* 2002;3:330–337.
47. Pariente PD, Lepine JP, Lellouch J. Lifetime history of panic attacks and epilepsy: an association from a general population survey. *J Clin Psychiatry.* 1991;52:88–89.
48. Paparrigopoulos T, Tzavellas E, Karaiskos D, et al. Left parieto-occipital lesion with epilepsy mimicking panic disorder. *Prog Neuropsychopharmacol Biol Psychiatry.* 2008;32:1606–1608.
49. Young GB, Chandarana PC, Blume WT, et al. Mesial temporal lobe seizures presenting as anxiety disorders. *J Neuropsychiatry Clin Neurosci.* 1995;7:352–357.
50. Scicutella A, B Ettinger A. Treatment of anxiety in epilepsy. *Epilepsy Behav.* 2002;3:10–12.
51. Monaco F, Cavanna A, Magli E, et al. Obsessionality, obsessive-compulsive disorder, and temporal lobe epilepsy. *Epilepsy Behav.* 2005;7:491–496.
52. Barbieri V, Lo Russo G, Francione S, et al. Association of temporal lobe epilepsy and obsessive-compulsive disorder in a patient successfully treated with right temporal lobectomy. *Epilepsy Behav.* 2005;6:617–619.
53. Kettl PA, Marks IM. Neurological factors in obsessive compulsive disorder. Two case reports and a review of the literature. *Br J Psychiatry: J Ment Sci.* 1986;149:315–319.
54. Levin B, Duchowny M. Childhood obsessive-compulsive disorder and cingulate epilepsy. *Biol Psychiatry.* 1991;30:1049–1055.
55. Guarnieri R, Araujo D, Carlotti CG, et al. Suppression of obsessive-compulsive symptoms after epilepsy surgery. *Epilepsy Behav.* 2005;7:316–319.
56. Koopowitz LF, Berk M. Response of obsessive compulsive disorder to carbamazepine in two patients with comorbid epilepsy. *Ann Clin Psychiatry.* 1997;9:171–173.
57. Newsom-Davis I, Goldstein LH, Fitzpatrick D. Fear of seizures: an investigation and treatment. *Seizure.* 1998;7:101–106.
58. Torta R, Keller R. Behavioral, psychotic, and anxiety disorders in epilepsy: etiology, clinical features, and therapeutic implications. *Epilepsia.* 1999;40(suppl 10):S2–S20.
59. Filho GM, Rosa VP, Lin K, et al. Psychiatric comorbidity in epilepsy: a study comparing patients with mesial temporal sclerosis and juvenile myoclonic epilepsy. *Epilepsy Behav.* 2008;13:196–201.
60. Luat AF, Asano E, Rothermel R, et al. Psychosis as a manifestation of frontal lobe epilepsy. *Epilepsy Behav.* 2008;12:200–204.
61. Shukla G, Singh S, Goyal V, et al. Prolonged preictal psychosis in refractory seizures: a report of three cases. *Epilepsy Behav.* 2008;13:252–255.

62. Nadkarni S, Arnedo V, Devinsky O. Psychosis in epilepsy patients. *Epilepsia.* 2007;48(suppl 9):17–19.

63. Krishnamoorthy ES, Trimble MR, Blumer D. The classification of neuropsychiatric disorders in epilepsy: a proposal by the ILAE Commission on Psychobiology of Epilepsy. *Epilepsy Behav.* 2007;10:349–353.

64. Slater E, Beard AW, Glithero E. The schizophrenia-like psychoses of epilepsy. *Br J Psychiatry: J Ment Sci.* 1963;109:95–150.

65. Tadokoro Y, Oshima T, Kanemoto K. Interictal psychoses in comparison with schizophrenia—a prospective study. *Epilepsia.* 2007;48:2345–2351.

66. Adachi N, Hara T, Oana Y, et al. Difference in age of onset of psychosis between epilepsy and schizophrenia. *Epilepsy Res.* 2008;78:201–206.

67. Keller S, Lichtenberg P. Psychotic exacerbation in a patient with seizure disorder treated with vagus nerve stimulation. *Isr Med Assoc J.* 2008;10:550–551.

68. Adachi N, Ito M, Kanemoto K, et al. Duration of postictal psychotic episodes. *Epilepsia.* 2007;48:1531–1537.

69. Logsdail SJ, Toone BK. Post-ictal psychoses. A clinical and phenomenological description. *Br J Psychiatry: J Ment Sci.* 1988;152:246–252.

70. Nishida T, Kudo T, Inoue Y, et al. Postictal mania versus postictal psychosis: differences in clinical features, epileptogenic zone, and brain functional changes during postictal period. *Epilepsia.* 2006;47:2104–2114.

71. Alper K, Kuzniecky R, Carlson C, et al. Postictal psychosis in partial epilepsy: a case-control study. *Ann Neurol.* 2008;63:602–610.

72. Devinsky O. Postictal psychosis: common, dangerous, and treatable. *Epilepsy Curr.* 2008;8:31–34.

73. Falip M, Carreño M, Donaire A, et al. Postictal psychosis: A retrospective study in patients with refractory temporal lobe epilepsy. *Seizure.* 2009; 18:145–149.

74. Kanner AM, Ostrovskaya A. Long-term significance of postictal psychotic episodes II. Are they predictive of interictal psychotic episodes? *Epilepsy Behav.* 2008;12:154–156.

75. Kanner AM. The use of psychotropic drugs in epilepsy: what every neurologist should know. *Semin Neurol.* 2008;28:379–388.

76. Ray WA, Chung CP, Murray KT, et al. Atypical antipsychotic drugs and the risk of sudden cardiac death. *N Engl J Med.* 2009;360:225–235.

77. Schneeweiss S, Avorn J. Antipsychotic agents and sudden cardiac death—how should we manage the risk? *N Engl J Med.* 2009;360:294–296.

78. Mahgoub NA. A report of successful treatment of psychosis in epilepsy with risperidone. *J Neuropsychiatry Clin Neurosci.* 2007;19:347–348.

79. Guerrant J, Anderson WW, Fischer A, et al. *Personality in Epilepsy.* Springfield, IL: Thomas; 1962.

80. Gelisse P, Genton P, Samuelian JC, et al. Psychiatric disorders in juvenile myoclonic epilepsy. *Rev Neurol.* 2001;157:297–302.

81. Devinsky O, Vorkas CK, Barr W. Personality disorders in epilepsy. In: Ettinger AB, Kanner AM, eds. *Psychiatric Issues in Epilepsy: A Practical Guide to Diagnosis and Treatment.* 2nd ed. Philadelphia, PA: Lippincott Williams & Wilkins; 2006:286–305.

82. Blumer D. Evidence supporting the temporal lobe epilepsy personality syndrome. *Neurology.* 1999;53:S9–S12.

83. Bear DM, Fedio P. Quantitative analysis of interictal behavior in temporal lobe epilepsy. *Arch Neurol.* 1977;34:454–467.

84. Plattner B, Pahs G, Kindler J, et al. Juvenile myoclonic epilepsy: a benign disorder? Personality traits and psychiatric symptoms. *Epilepsy Behav.* 2007;10:560–564.

85. Devinsky O, Najjar S. Evidence against the existence of a temporal lobe epilepsy personality syndrome. *Neurology.* 1999;53:S13–S25.

86. Rodin EA. Psychomotor epilepsy and aggressive behavior. *Arch Gen Psych.* 1973;28:210–213.

87. Herzberg JL, Fenwick PB. The aetiology of aggression in temporal-lobe epilepsy. *Br J Psychiatry: J Ment Sci.* 1988;153:50–55.

88. Mendez MF, Doss RC, Taylor JL. Interictal violence in epilepsy. Relationship to behavior and seizure variables. *J Nerv Ment Dis.* 1993; 181:566–569.

89. Pakalnis A, Drake ME Jr, John K, et al. Forced normalization. Acute psychosis after seizure control in seven patients. *Arch Neurol.* 1987;44: 289–292.

90. Hillemacher T, Kraus T, Stefan H, et al. Suicidal attempts and aggressive behaviours after temporal lobectomy in epilepsy. *Eur J Neurol.* 2007; 14:e10.

91. Delgado-Escueta AV, Mattson RH, King L, et al. Special report. The nature of aggression during epileptic seizures. *N Engl J Med.* 1981;305: 711–716.

92. King DW, Marsan CA. Clinical features and ictal patterns in epileptic patients with EEG temporal lobe foci. *Ann Neurol.* 1977;2:138–147.

93. Alper KR, Barry JJ, Balabanov AJ. Treatment of psychosis, aggression, and irritability in patients with epilepsy. *Epilepsy Behav.* 2002;3:13–18.

94. Kanemoto K, Kawasaki J, Mori E. Violence and epilepsy: a close relation between violence and postictal psychosis. *Epilepsia.* 1999;40: 107–109.

95. Ito M, Okazaki M, Takahashi S, et al. Subacute postictal aggression in patients with epilepsy. *Epilepsy Behav.* 2007;10:611–614.

CHAPTER 94 ■ DRIVING AND SOCIAL ISSUES IN EPILEPSY

JOSEPH F. DRAZKOWSKI AND JOSEPH I. SIRVEN

A person with epilepsy faces many social concerns that are taken for granted by those without the disorder (1,2). A recent quality-of-life (QOL) survey identified driving a motor vehicle as the number one concern for a person with epilepsy (1). In addition to driving, other important social issues for a person with epilepsy include obtaining and maintaining employment, and participating in athletic and recreational activities (2). This chapter explores important social issues that can influence the QOL of a person with epilepsy.

EVALUATION OF THE RISK OF ENGAGING IN A DESIRED ACTIVITY

Although on some level everyone must balance the risks of engaging in a desired activity against the potential benefits derived from that activity, this cost-to-benefit analysis assumes added significance for the person with epilepsy. A person with epilepsy must conduct the analysis in the context of a specific situation, with the consideration that a seizure-related injury might occur during the specific activity. To determine potential risk, a person with epilepsy needs to understand all aspects of the specific activity and must try to predict the potential exposure to injury should a seizure occur during participation. The risk of seizure recurrence will determine, at least in part, how safe it is to participate in a desired activity. Factors that influence seizure recurrence have been reported (3) and may provide important insight into determining the risks associated with a desired activity. These factors include the presence of an abnormal electroencephalogram (EEG), initial seizure type, and etiology of the seizure. Symptomatic seizures are twice as likely as idiopathic seizures to recur (4–6). Partial seizures are also more likely to recur compared with an initial major motor seizure (4,7). If the etiology of a seizure disorder is head injury, the risk for recurrence may be higher. In patients with severe head injury, the recurrence rates for seizures are 7.1% and 11.5% at 1 and 5 years, respectively (8), with severe head injury defined as amnesia and/or loss of consciousness for more than 24 hours, or the presence of an intracranial hematoma. Structural lesions, such as brain tumors, stroke, abscesses, and penetrating head wounds, all carry an increased risk for recurrent seizures. Seizures caused by alcohol use, on the other hand, are unlikely to recur if abstinence is maintained. After a new-onset major motor seizure in a patient with a normal examination and work-up, including magnetic resonance imaging (MRI), electroencephalography, and blood tests, seizure recurrence is estimated to range between 25% (5) and approximately 70% (9) at 3 years. Another review suggested a recurrence risk of 50%, also at 3 years (7). If one remains in remission (i.e., seizure free) for 2 years or longer, a good prognosis is possible (10).

The danger period for a particular activity should also be considered when evaluating potential risk. The person with epilepsy is exposed to less risk when the danger period for an activity is brief. For example, target shooting with a lethal weapon likely poses little risk to the shooter or people in close proximity except for that very short period of time when squeezing the trigger. In contrast, such activities as motorbike riding or hang gliding might present a relatively high risk for the person with epilepsy as danger periods encompass the entire time they are involved in the activity. Activities with inherent danger must also be factored into the decision of whether to participate. For example, table tennis is certainly less dangerous than bullfighting. Finally, other factors, such as medication compliance, medication side effects, age, concomitant medical problems, use of safety equipment, and a prolonged and consistent aura, can all influence the risks faced by a person with epilepsy when engaging in a specific activity.

DRIVING AND THE PERSON WITH EPILEPSY

The Risks

A person with epilepsy faces a risk of injury and a risk of causing injury if a seizure should occur while operating a motor vehicle. Driving is a privilege, not a right. This privilege is governed by individual country, state, or territorial governments (11). There are approximately 225 million registered vehicles in the United States. In 2002, an estimated 6.7 million motor vehicle crashes occurred in the United States (12). These crashes resulted in approximately 3 million injuries and more than 42,000 deaths (12). It is estimated that approximately 0.5% to 1.0% of the U.S. population has epilepsy (3), potentially placing more than 2.5 million drivers with epilepsy on the roads of the United States. However, the actual number of persons with epilepsy who drive with or without a valid license is unknown. Applicants for a motor vehicle license must answer questions about their medical status and affirm that they are healthy and fit to drive before they are allowed to operate a motor vehicle. One study suggested that only 14% of individuals had answered truthfully on their driving application when asked about the presence of epilepsy (13). In a prospective survey of 367 patients with localization-related epilepsy pooled from a consortium of comprehensive epilepsy programs, approximately 30% of the respondents had operated a motor vehicle in the previous 12 months (14). The paucity of available data makes it difficult to definitively establish the number of automobile crashes caused by persons with epilepsy who have a seizure while driving. Reports suggest that persons with epilepsy account for approximately 0.02% to 0.04% of all reported automobile car crashes (15,16). In contrast, alcohol-related crashes comprise approximately 7% of car crashes but account for approximately 40% of all fatalities nationwide (17).

Seizures are unpredictable, and the presumption is that longer seizure-free intervals translate into a decreased likelihood of seizure-related crashes. Verifying this is difficult, however, as individual driving records are generally not available for review. A recent retrospective survey of patients in several Maryland outpatient epilepsy clinics suggested that the risk of motor vehicle crashes was reduced by 85% and 93% if the patient did not have a seizure at 6 months and 12 months, respectively (18). This survey relied on self-reported crashes.

It has been suggested that self-reporting of crashes by respondents in surveys is unreliable (19,20). Drazkowski and colleagues (16) reviewed actual accident reports in Arizona from crashes caused by seizures before and after the seizure-free interval was reduced from 12 to 3 months (Table 94.1). Although no significant increases in seizure-related crashes were reported, the retrospective study provided some objective data on these crashes. To date, no controlled prospective data are available to guide regulating authorities as to the optimum seizure-free interval for the protection of both the person with epilepsy and the public.

The Regulatory Requirements

The first seizure-related car crash was reported near the turn of the 19th century. Since then, regulatory authorities have placed restrictions on driving for a person with epilepsy. Almost a decade ago, the American Academy of Neurology, the American Epilepsy Society, and the Epilepsy Foundation of America convened a conference of thought leaders to issue guidelines on the topic of driving and the person with epilepsy (21). Recommendations from the conference included (i) a seizure-free interval of 3 months, (ii) allowances for purely nocturnal seizures, and (iii) a provision allowing driving when there is an established pattern of a prolonged and consistent aura (21).

Determining the risk of a crash caused by the driver with epilepsy is difficult. Traditionally, the duration of seizure freedom is used by authorities to determine when it is safe for a person with epilepsy to drive. Seizure-free intervals adopted by jurisdictions vary widely and have many unique exceptions (22). State regulatory agencies and the Epilepsy Foundation of America website (www.efa.org) can be contacted for current laws governing driving and epilepsy, which has been recently updated (23). In an editorial, Krumholz suggested that it is time to consider uniform laws governing epilepsy and driving throughout the United States (24). International rules on driving have been reviewed, and because of the high variability among individual countries, it has been suggested that the appropriate national authority be consulted to determine current local laws regarding driving before traveling to these nations (25).

TABLE 94.1

CHANGES IN THE INCIDENCE RATES OF CRASHES (/10^9 MILES DRIVEN) AFTER REDUCING THE RESTRICTION ON DRIVERS WITH EPILEPSY FROM 12 TO 3 MONTHS, 3 YEARS BEFORE AND AFTER LAW CHANGE

Type/Cause	Before	After	Incidence[a] rate	95% CI	95% CI	RR[b]
Total						
Seizure	1.1	1.1	−0.028	−0.30–0.24	0.98	0.77–1.24
Other medical	2.6	2.6	−0.092	−0.51–0.33	0.97	0.82–1.13
Not seizure (103)	2.6	2.8	0.20	0.19–0.22	1.08	1.07–1.08
Injury						
Seizure	0.58	0.76	0.18	−0.03–0.39	1.31	0.95–1.80
Other medical	1.6	1.3	−0.21	−0.52–0.10	0.87	0.70–1.07
Not seizure (103)	1.0	1.1	0.045	0.037–0.053	1.04	1.04–1.05
Fatal[c]						
Seizure	0.046	0.016	−0.029	−0.076–0.017	0.36	0.07–1.85
Other medical	0.055	0.099	0.043	−0.027–0.11	1.79	0.67–4.8
Not seizure	20	21	1.6	0.39–2.7	1.08	1.02–1.14

CI, confidence interval; RR, relative risk.
[a]Incidence rate difference (before vs. after).
[b]Relative risk (before vs. after).
[c]Fatal crashes are a subset of the injury category and are segregated for separate analysis.
Modified from Drazkowski JF, Fisher RS, Sirven JI, et al. Seizure-related motor vehicle crashes in Arizona before and after reducing the driving restriction from 12 to 3 months. *Mayo Clin Proc.* 2003;78:819–825, with permission.

Six states currently have laws that require health care providers to report persons with epilepsy to the appropriate state driving authorities. The rationale behind the reporting requirement is that a person with epilepsy will not reliably self-report the presence of active or recurrent seizures to the proper authority. Laws that require a health care provider to report a person with epilepsy to authorities are criticized as impairing the physician–patient relationship and thus compromising optimal medical care. The premise is that when physicians are required to report epilepsy to driving authorities, persons with epilepsy may conceal information about their seizures to avoid being reported and potentially losing their license (19). Of persons with epilepsy who had been counseled about driving laws, only 27% reported their condition to the appropriate authorities (20). This is assuming that the health care professional knows the proper laws; in a recent review of ER visits requiring self-reporting to the driving authorities, less than 10% were counseled in a major metropolitan city in the southwest (26); in another survey, only 13% of providers knew the appropriate requirements in any event (27). In California, which is the most populous state requiring physician reporting, a survey again suggested that the physician reporting requirement impaired medical care and the doctor–patient relationship (28). There are no available studies showing that physician reporting reduces seizure-related automobile crashes. In Canada, a conference of invited experts concluded that the laws requiring health care professionals to report persons with epilepsy to authorities should be abolished and suggested that driving laws be uniform across Canada (29). McLachlan et al. reported on the impact of mandatory reporting to driving authorities in one province requiring reporting compared to a province that does not. Their conclusion was that mandatory reporting of Person with epilepsy (PWE) to the driving authorities by physicians did not reduce accident risk. They go on to suggest that the reporting requirements may be excessive compared to other medical conditions or nonmedical risk factors (30). An editorial by emergency department physicians suggested that mandatory reporting of seizures be abolished in the United States (31). This editorial highlighted several other medical conditions and situations that are associated with a similar or higher relative risk of a car crash compared with epilepsy, such as sleep, apnea, diabetes, dementia, and cell phone use (distraction) (29).

EMPLOYMENT AND THE PERSON WITH EPILEPSY

QOL surveys have identified employment issues and concerns of persons with epilepsy as significant (1,2). The economic impact that epilepsy has on society is huge (more than $10.8 billion/year) and is largely attributable to indirect employment-related costs, which account for 85% of all epilepsy costs (32). Persons with epilepsy are reported to have lower household incomes, which are estimated to be 93% of the U.S. median income (33), compared with the general population.

In the United States, the rate of unemployment for persons with epilepsy is reported to be between 25% and 69% (33,34). The overall nationwide rate of graduation from high school is approximately 82%; for persons with epilepsy, this rate is approximately 64% (33). Although many factors are likely to contribute to the high rate of unemployment among persons with epilepsy, poorly controlled epilepsy is associated with a high level of unemployment (34). Age of epilepsy onset also impacts employment status, with an earlier age of onset correlating with work difficulties later in life (35). In patients with adult-onset epilepsy, initial seizure control or lack of control does affect work status. Newly diagnosed, unprovoked seizures in adults do not seem to negatively impact employment rates. The same study associated the development of refractory seizures in adults with reduced income (36).

Many persons with epilepsy have to deal with the reality of employment discrimination. A survey of young persons with epilepsy enrolled in a job-training program in Ireland indicated that 50% of the participants believed they were being actively discriminated against when seeking employment (37).

The Americans with Disabilities Act (ADA) was enacted in 1990 to combat job discrimination against individuals with illnesses. The law was intended to help persons with epilepsy and persons with other disabilities obtain and retain employment. A prominent feature of the ADA is that a person with a covered malady cannot be discriminated against if "reasonable accommodations" can be made that would allow the covered individual to obtain or remain in a specific job. But the ADA exempts employers with 15 or fewer employees, thereby eliminating many small businesses. Furthermore, what constitutes a reasonable accommodation was left open to interpretation. The standard may be based on the actual cost of any modifications required that allow a person to keep a specific job. Finally, the employee must be able to perform the "essential" tasks of the job. Administrative and court rulings have made it clear that the protection sought has not been achieved (38). In a unanimous U.S. Supreme Court opinion, Justice O'Connor wrote that for an individual to be considered disabled, the person's disability must be "permanent or long-term," and the impairment must "prevent or severely restrict the individual from doing activities that are of central importance to most people's daily lives" (39). The following statement summarizes the court's opinion: "Merely having an impairment does not make one disabled for the purposes of the ADA." This ruling and others like it have changed the thinking on what defines disability for many patients. These uncertainties and restrictive rulings by the court have prompted a reevaluation of the issue by the United States Legislature which resulted in the passage of the "ADA Restoration Act of 2008." The law took effect on January 1, 2009. The law was passed in an effort to clarify and be more inclusive on what constitutes disability under the law. It still covers business and governmental agencies of 15 or more employees. The United States Equal Employment Opportunity Commission (EEOC) has reviewed and published guidelines for PWE and employers regarding employment and epilepsy issues (http://www.eeoc.gov/facts/epilepsy.html). Major life activities specifically covered in the law are highlighted in Table 94.2. The major life limitations due to epilepsy can result from seizures or the complications and side effects of medications used to treat the seizures. Specific examples of hiring practices' do's and don'ts for the PWE determinations about disability are fraught with complexities and should be considered on a case-by-case basis, taking into account the unique facts involved. Individual cases may require specialized legal advice. All the possible accommodations that may affect the PWE would be lengthy. A potentially helpful website, the Job accommodation network (JAN), with common examples of accommodation is http://www.jan.wvu.edu/media/epilepsy.html.

TABLE 94.2

LIFE ACTIVITIES THAT MUST BE IMPAIRED TO BE CONSIDERED DISABLED BY SEIZURE AS DEFINED BY THE AMERICANS WITH DISABILITIES ACT AMENDMENTS ACT OF 2008

Walking
Seeing
Speaking
Breathing
Thinking
Performing manual tasks
Concentrating
Learning
Social interaction
Reproduction
Sleeping

Limitations on one or more of the above life activities due to seizures or side effects of medications used to treat epilepsy must be present to be considered disabled.

TABLE 94.3

FACTORS REQUIRED FOR CONSIDERATION OF SOCIAL SECURITY ADMINISTRATION DISABILITY BENEFITS

- Four partial seizures per month
- One major motor seizure per month
- Continued seizures despite adequate use of medication for 3 months
- Electroencephalogram results
- Detailed description of the events documented in the medical record

code that covers conversion disorder/somatoform disorders. Although NES is not epilepsy, many of the patients evaluated in epilepsy centers around the country are ultimately diagnosed with this condition, which can be as debilitating as epilepsy.

SPORTS AND RECREATIONAL ACTIVITIES

Persons with epilepsy are often excluded or discouraged from participation in sports and recreational activities because of fear of what might occur during the activity. When making decisions about participating in any activity, a person with epilepsy must consider the consequences of a seizure that may occur at any moment during that particular activity.

Epilepsy and Recreational Vehicles

Motorized vehicles can potentially cause serious injury or death even in persons without epilepsy. The unpredictability of uncontrolled seizures might pose a serious threat should a seizure occur at the wrong time. Operating motorized vehicles is associated with a prolonged danger period.

A seizure that occurs while a person is piloting a private plane is likely to have disastrous consequences. Noncommercial aviation is at least partially regulated by the FAA. A third-class pilot's license is required for all general noncommercial aviation (40). If an individual has experienced a single unprovoked seizure with no EEG abnormalities, normal brain imaging, and no additional risk factors, that person can be considered for a third-class license if he or she has not taken an AED for 4 consecutive years. Uncomplicated childhood febrile seizures may not disqualify a person from obtaining a third-class license. The FAA uses certified examiners to assist in the decision-making process for granting licenses when there is a potential medical problem. Piloting ultralight aircraft, hang gliders, and other small aircraft may not require a license, but these are unlikely to be any safer than a private plane should a mishap occur.

Other motorized vehicles, such as motorcycles, personal watercraft, all terrain vehicle (four wheel), and boats may pose less of a threat to a person with epilepsy than does flying. If the person with epilepsy operating the vehicle has a prolonged and consistent aura, it may allow that person the opportunity to stop and protect ones self. However, other factors should be considered by a person with epilepsy when contemplating engaging in some of these activities. For example, drowning is a common accident among persons with epilepsy (42). The use

Certain jobs may be perfectly safe for many persons with epilepsy but other jobs may impose unacceptable risk. A person with epilepsy must carefully evaluate jobs involving dangerous machinery, or equipment heights, or situations in which there is a possibility for injury or death because of potentially dangerous conditions in the event of a seizure. Persons with epilepsy also face regulatory-imposed restrictions for some jobs. For example, a person with epilepsy's pursuit of a commercial pilot's license is severely limited by the Federal Aviation Administration (FAA) (40). Similarly, a person with epilepsy wishing to obtain a commercial driver's license (CDL) to operate a truck in interstate commerce must overcome significant hurdles imposed by the Federal Department of Transportation. The diagnosis of epilepsy and the use of antiepileptic drugs (AEDs) generally disqualify an applicant or current driver from obtaining a CDL. A CDL is required to operate a truck with a gross weight greater than 24,000 pounds. Although many states have mirrored the federal regulations with regard to state commercial driving laws, individual state regulations should be reviewed for accuracy. Commercial and military scuba diving is similarly restricted for the person with epilepsy (39). Tailoring the specific job to the person with epilepsy, based on the person's unique, individual situation, should be emphasized.

Under Social Security Administration (SSA) regulations, epilepsy is covered by specific listings (41). These listings, which define what constitutes a disability for the person with epilepsy, are used in determining who is eligible to receive disability payments. Persons with epilepsy are required to provide specific evidence, through medical records documenting that they "meet the listing," as featured in Table 94.3. Other factors, such as postictal effects of seizures and side effects of prescribed medications, may be considered in determining disability, especially during a hearing or an appeals process for a denied claim. The specific listings for epilepsy are sections 11.03 and 11.02 for minor motor and major motor seizures, respectively (41). The diagnosis of pseudoseizure or nonepileptic seizure (NES) may also be covered by SSA regulations under section 12.07. This listing is in the psychiatry section of the of a personal flotation device at all times when operating or riding in any watercraft should be considered. When operating off-road vehicles, safety equipment should also be considered, especially the use of boots, shoulder pads, protective clothing, and helmets. Although a person operating such a vehicle does not require a license, specific training courses are available and are highly recommended.

In contrast, organized motor sports generally require some form of medical clearance before participation (39). The different motor sport sanctioning bodies, such as the Sports Car Club of America (SCCA), the National Association of Stock Car Racers, and the IndyCar Series, all have specific requirements for a person to be allowed to drive in sanctioned events. Each series requires approval from a qualified health care professional before driving, and therefore specific rules should be reviewed.

The Person with Epilepsy and Athletics

The decision to participate in individual (i.e., one-on-one) and team sports should follow those principles outlined above in order to ensure maximum benefits (and thus satisfaction) and safety. The extent to which a person with epilepsy wishes to pursue athletics is an individual decision that should be based on individual circumstances. Each team or individual sport presents different challenges that may affect a person with epilepsy in different ways. Many one-on-one sports are less likely to pose a threat to a person with epilepsy. For example, the potential injury a person with epilepsy might sustain during golf, tennis, or running track is likely to be low, whereas a seizure sustained during boxing, hang gliding, ski flying, or waterskiing would pose a much higher risk. Table 94.4 classifies risks to the person with epilepsy according to the sport.

Participation in team sports should also be determined on an individual basis. Football could be dangerous if a player is unable to protect him- or herself during a play, whereas basketball is less likely to be dangerous. Noncommercial scuba diving is also not regulated from a medical standpoint, but good judgment is required on the part of the participant. Hyperventilation techniques and the high concentration of inspired oxygen used during scuba diving have the potential to provoke seizures. The person with epilepsy should also inform his or her dive buddy, instructor, and dive master of the potential risk should a seizure occur during diving. Water sports and drowning pose a likely threat to the person with epilepsy. A review of drowning deaths found that 40% of seizure-related drownings occurred during recreational activities (42). Among persons with epilepsy, 83% of deaths during drowning occurred in those with subtherapeutic levels of AEDs, with the remainder of such drownings occurring where bathing was unsupervised. A study by Gotze found no increase in seizure occurrence during strenuous swimming (43).

Exercise-provoked seizures are a controversial issue. The available data on such seizures are limited, suggesting that sports participation does not provoke seizure recurrence (44), and in some cases may even reduce seizure occurrence (43). Recent opinion has encouraged sports participation for the person with epilepsy despite the potential risks (45,46). The decision regarding person with epilepsy participation in sporting activities must be made on an individual basis.

TABLE 94.4

SPORTING ACTIVITIES CLASSIFIED ACCORDING TO POSSIBLE RISK FOR THE PERSON WITH EPILEPSY

Low risk
  Track
  Cross-country skiing
  Golf
  Bowling
  Ping-Pong
  Baseball
  Weight training (machines)
Moderate risk
  Football
  Biking
  Soccer
  Gymnastics
  Horseback riding
  Basketball
  Boating/sailing
High risk
  Scuba diving
  Hang gliding
  Motor sports
  Boxing
  Downhill skiing/ski flying
  Long-distance swimming
  Hockey
  Boxing

Modified from Mesad SM, Devinsky O. Epilepsy and the athlete. In: Jordan BD, Tsairis P, Warren PF, eds. *Sport Neurology*. 2nd ed. Philadelphia, PA: Lippincott Raven Publishers; 1998:285, with permission.

Often overlooked are the possible AED-associated side effects that may interfere with participation in sports. For example, zonisamide reduces sweating in children and could potentially lead to heat-related injury in hot climates. Tremor associated with the use of valproic acid could be dangerous when shooting target pistols. Phenytoin-induced ataxia could potentially be deadly while riding a motorbike (47). Many more potential examples could be conceived and listing all the potential combinations is beyond the scope of this chapter, thus the health care professional should be knowledgeable of the person with epilepsy's history, desires, and a basic understanding of the recreational activity considered. Individualizing the specific drug side-effect profile, patient characteristics, and particular recreational activity generally should all be considered when advising the person with epilepsy about participation in recreational and sporting activities.

CONCLUSIONS

The patient with epilepsy poses many challenges to the health care professional. In addition to the usual concerns persons with epilepsy have about seizure control and medication effects, social issues play an important role in their everyday lives. An understanding of the unique difficulties with respect to driving, employment, and recreational/sporting activities that confront the person with epilepsy can be used to improve the QOL of many of these patients. It must be emphasized that each patient has individual characteristics requiring knowledge of the specific activity in which the person with epilepsy wishes to participate. Recent changes to the U.S. laws governing disability and employment may prove helpful for the person with epilepsy.

References

1. Gilliam F, Kuzniecky R, Faught E, et al. Patient-validated content of epilepsy-specific quality-of-life measurement. *Epilepsia.* 1997;38:233–236.
2. Fisher RS, Vickrey BG, Gibson P, et al. The impact of epilepsy from the patient's perspective I. Descriptions and subjective perceptions. *Epilepsy Res.* 2000;41:39–51.
3. Hauser WA, Hesdorffer DC, eds. *Epilepsy: Frequency, Causes, and Consequences.* New York, NY: Demos; 1990.
4. Camfield PR, Camfield CS, Dooley JM, et al. Epilepsy after a first unprovoked seizure in childhood. *Neurology.* 1985;35:1657–1660.
5. Hauser WA, Anderson VE, Loewenson RB, et al. Seizure recurrence after a first unprovoked seizure. *N Engl J Med.* 1982;307:522–528.
6. Annegers JF, Shirts SB, Hauser WA. Risk of recurrence after an initial unprovoked seizure. *Epilepsia.* 1986;27:43–50.
7. Hopkins A, Garman A, Clarke C. The first seizure in adult life: value of clinical features, electroencephalography, and computerised tomographic scanning in prediction of seizure recurrence. *Lancet.* 1988;1:721–684.
8. Annegers JF, Grabow JD, Groover RV, et al. Seizures after head trauma: a population study. *Neurology.* 1980;30(7 pt 1):683–689.
9. Elwes RD, Johnson AL, Shorvon SD, et al. The prognosis for seizure control in newly diagnosed epilepsy. *N Engl J Med.* 1984;311:944–947.
10. Sander JWAS, Shorvon SD. Remission periods in epilepsy and their relations to long-term prognosis. In: Wolf P, Dam M, Janz D, et al., eds. *Advances in Epileptology: XVIth Epilepsy International Symposium.* New York, NY: Raven Press; 1987:353–356.
11. Fisher RS, Parsonage M, Beaussart, M, Joint Commission on Drivers' Licensing of the International Bureau for Epilepsy and the International League Against Epilepsy. Epilepsy and driving: an international perspective. *Epilepsia.* 1994;35:675–684.
12. National Highway Traffic Safety Administration, National Center for Statistics and Analysis. Available at: http://www-nrd.nhtsa. dot.gov/pdf/ nrd-30/NCSA/Rpts/2003/2002EARelease.pdf. Last accessed on June 28, 2003.
13. van der Lugt PJ. Is an application form useful to select patients with epilepsy who may drive? *Epilepsia.* 1975;16:743–746.
14. Berg AT, Vickrey BG, Sperling MR, et al. Driving in adults with refractory localization-related epilepsy. *Neurology.* 2000;54:625–630.
15. Millengen KS. Epilepsy and driving. *Proc Aust Assoc Neurol.* 1976;13:67–72.
16. Drazkowski JF, Fisher RS, Sirven JI, et al. Seizure-related motor vehicle crashes in Arizona before and after reducing the driving restriction from 12 to 3 months. *Mayo Clin Proc.* 2003;78:819–825.
17. *Arizona Motor Vehicle Crash Facts 1997.* Available at: http://www.dot. state.az.us/roads/crash/index.htm. Last accessed on March 24, 2003.
18. Krauss GL, Krumholz A, Carter RC, et al. Risk factors for seizure-related motor vehicle crashes in patients with epilepsy. *Neurology.* 1999;52: 1324–1329.
19. Salinsky MC, Wegener K, Sinnema F. Epilepsy, driving laws, and patient disclosure to physicians. *Epilepsia.* 1992;33:469–472.
20. Taylor J, Chadwick DW, Johnson T. Accident experience and notification rates in people with recent seizures, epilepsy or undiagnosed episodes of loss of consciousness. *Q J Med.* 1995;88:730–740.
21. Consensus conference on driver licensing and epilepsy: American Academy of Neurology, American Epilepsy Society, and Epilepsy Foundation of America. Washington, DC, May 31–June 2, 1991. Proceedings. *Epilepsia.* 1994;35:662–705.
22. Krauss GL, Ampaw L, Krumholz A. Individual state driving restrictions for people with epilepsy in the US. *Neurology.* 2001;57:1780–1785.
23. Epilepsy Foundation of America website: www.efa.org. Last accessed on Jan 29, 2009.
24. Krumholz A. To drive or not to drive: the 3-month seizure-free interval for people with epilepsy [editorial]. *Mayo Clin Proc.* 2003;78:817–818.
25. Ooi WW, Gutrecht JA. International regulations for automobile driving and epilepsy. *J Travel Med.* 2000;7:1–4.
26. Long L, Reeves AL, Moore JL, et al. An assessment of epilepsy patients' knowledge of their disorder. *Epilepsia.* 2000;41:727–731.
27. Shareef, Y, McKinnon, J, Gauthier SM, et al. Counselling for driving restrictions in epilepsy and other causes of temporary impairment of consciousness: how are we doing? *Epilepsy and Behavior.* 2009;14(3):550–552.
28. Rodrigues KM, Callanan MA, Risinger MW, et al. *Should Physicians be Responsible for Reporting Their Patients to the DMV?* Available at: http://www.cma.org. Last accessed on June 26, 2003.
29. Remillard GM, Zifkin BG, Andermann F. Epilepsy and motor vehicle driving—a symposium held in Quebec City, November 1998. *Can J Neurol Sci.* 2002;29:315–325.
30. McLachlan, R., Starreveld, E. Impact of mandatory physician reporting on accident risk in epilepsy. *Epilepsia.* 2007;48(8):1500–1505.
31. Lee W, Wolfe T, Shreeve S. Reporting epileptic drivers to licensing authorities is unnecessary and counterproductive. *Ann Emerg Med.* 2002;39:656–659.
32. Begley CE, Annegers JF, Lairson DR, et al. Methodological issues in estimating the cost of epilepsy. *Epilepsy Res.* 1999;33:39–55.
33. Fisher RS, Vickrey BG, Gibson P, et al. The impact of epilepsy from the patient's perspective II. Views about therapy and health care. *Epilepsy Res.* 2000;41:53–61.
34. Salgado PC, Souza EA. Impact of epilepsy at work: evaluation of quality of life. *Arq Neuropsiquiatr.* 2002;60:442–445.
35. Chaplin JE, Wester A, Tomson T. Factors associated with the employment problems of people with established epilepsy. *Seizure.* 1998;7:299–303.
36. Lindsten H, Stenlund H, Edlund C, et al. Socioeconomic prognosis after a newly diagnosed unprovoked epileptic seizure in adults: a population-based case-control study. *Epilepsia.* 2002;43:1239–1250.
37. Carroll D. Employment among young people with epilepsy. *Seizure.* 1992;1:127–131.
38. Epilepsy Foundation of America. *Civil Rights.* Available at: http://www. epilepsyfoundation.org/Advocacy/rights/rights.html. Last accessed on August 22, 2002.
39. Drazkowski JF. Management of the social consequences of seizures. *Mayo Clin Proc.* 2003;78:641–649.
40. Federal Aviation Administration Regulations Title 14 parts 67.109, 67.09, and 67.309. Available at: http://www.faa.gov. Last accessed on January 29, 2009.
41. Social Security Administration. *Disability Evaluation Under Social Security.* Publication 64-039. Baltimore, MD: Author; 1999. Available at: http://www.ssa.gov/disability/professionals/bluebook /11.00-neurological-adult.htm. Last accessed on January 29, 2009.
42. Ryan CA, Dowling G. Drowning deaths in people with epilepsy. *Can Med Assoc J* 1993;148:781–784.
43. Gotze W, Kubicki S, Munter M, et al. Effect of physical exercise on seizure threshold (investigated by electroencephalographic telemetry). *Dis Nerv Syst.* 1967;28:664–667.
44. Committee on the Medical Aspects of Sports. *Medical Evaluation of the Athlete: A Guide.* Chicago, IL: American Medical Association; 1979.
45. Livingston S, Berman W. Participation of epileptic patients in sports. *J Am Med Assoc.* 1973;224:236–238.
46. van Linschoten R, Backx FJ, Mulder OG, et al. Epilepsy and sports. *Sports Med.* 1990;10:9–19.
47. Mesad SM, Devinsky O. Epilepsy and the athlete. In: Jordan BD, Tsairis P, Warren PF, eds. *Sport Neurology.* 2nd ed. Philadelphia, PA: Lippincott-Raven Publishers; 1998.

CHAPTER 95 ■ ACHIEVING HEALTH IN EPILEPSY: STRATEGIES FOR OPTIMAL EVALUATION AND TREATMENT

FRANK G. GILLIAM

The many clinical manifestations, etiologies, and health effects of epilepsy can present formidable diagnostic and treatment challenges. Physicians traditionally are trained to evaluate seizure semiology, and look for electrophysiologic and structural brain abnormalities to support a diagnosis of epilepsy. If the diagnosis is confirmed, then an antiepileptic drug (AED) is selected based on a balance of efficacy and risk of negative side effects. New AEDs and neuroimaging techniques have allowed advances in the diagnosis and treatment of epilepsy in recent decades, but many challenges remain. For example, a recent study found that the average neurology outpatient visit for epilepsy in the community setting lasted 12 minutes (1). Such a short clinical interaction requires exquisite organization to render optimal care. Other studies indicate that side effects of antiepileptic medications and common comorbid psychiatric disorders severely limit quality of life (QOL) for many patients (2–5), and that easily accomplished health assessments such as screening for depression and adverse medication effects are infrequently performed by clinicians (6,7). Health outcomes research such as this provides information that offers opportunities to improve epilepsy care (8–10). This chapter reviews available data from clinical outcomes studies that support specific strategies to improve the results of outpatient care for epilepsy.

The initial steps toward optimal outpatient epilepsy care require that five questions be answered, which will be explored in the following sections:

1. Is the diagnosis and classification correct?
2. Is the reported seizure rate accurate?
3. Are adverse medication effects detectable?
4. Are comorbid depression and/or anxiety present?
5. Is a surgically correctable region identified by high-resolution MRI or EEG?

IS THE DIAGNOSIS AND CLASSIFICATION CORRECT?

Although few studies have addressed the accuracy of the clinical diagnosis of epilepsy, the studies that have utilized specific EEG criteria suggest surprisingly high error rates. For example, juvenile myoclonic epilepsy is estimated to be 10% of all epilepsy cases, but is frequently misdiagnosed for years after initial presentation. Benbadis et al. (11) described a consecutive series of 58 patients with idiopathic generalized epilepsy to determine appropriateness of diagnosis and subsequent treatment. About 70% of the group were on medications for partial seizures, and only 17 (29%) were on an appropriate regimen of broad-spectrum AEDs. An earlier study found that only a small minority of patients with juvenile myoclonic epilepsy (JME) were diagnosed and treated appropriately despite prior evaluations by neurologists, and the delay to accurate diagnosis averaged 14.5 years (12).

Nonepileptic, psychogenic seizures are estimated to be up to 10% of all cases of epilepsy and 20% to 30% of pharmacoresistant cases (13,14). Although limited research has specifically addressed the problem of misdiagnosis, the average delay in accurate classification of the seizures by video-EEG appears to be about 7 years (15). The magnitude of the health-related QOL effects and the unnecessary health care utilization and expenditures is immense. However, video-EEG monitoring for definitive diagnosis and classification has been shown to markedly reduce health care costs for nonepileptic psychogenic seizures. Martin et al. found an 84% reduction in seizure-related medical care costs in the 6 months following video-EEG diagnosis of psychogenic seizures compared to a similar period prior to evaluation (15). This reduction equated to $6850 per patient for the 6-month period.

Some clinicians assume that video-EEG monitoring is an inefficient means of evaluating and diagnosing epilepsy, but this view is not supported by substantial published data. Eisenman et al. (16) evaluated 150 consecutive admissions to the video-EEG monitoring unit and found that the mean time to record a diagnostic clinical event was 2.2 days for patients with nonepileptic, psychogenic seizures. Interestingly, time to first seizure did not correlate with self-reported seizure rate in the most recent outpatient clinic visit. The survival curve in Figure 95.1 demonstrates that patients with very low self-reported seizure rates of <1 seizure per month had a diagnostic event recorded by the third day and 90% by the sixth day. There was no significant difference in time to diagnostic event between the very low seizure rate patients and those with more frequent self-reported seizures. Although the reasons for this finding are not clear, inaccuracy of self-reported rates may be a major factor. These data support that low seizure rates reported in the outpatient setting should not influence decisions for definitive evaluation for accurate diagnosis by video-EEG. A very large majority of patients with self-reported seizure rates of <1 per month will have a diagnostic event recorded within 6 days. Based on the personal risks and substantial QOL effects, as well as health care expenditures, the argument can be reasonably made that video-EEG monitoring should be performed for accurate classification of the seizure disorder after the first or second AED has not completely controlled all seizures.

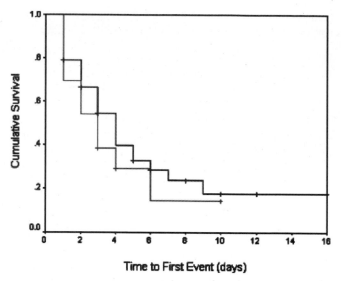

FIGURE 95.1 Kaplan–Meier curves for time to first seizure in very low (<1 per month; gray) and low (>1 but <2 per month; black) self-reported seizures rate groups.

IS THE REPORTED SEIZURE RATE ACCURATE?

Self-reported seizure rate, with supplemental input from family and friends, is the standard outcome measure for both clinical care and research. However, available data that have been replicated in adults and children indicate that patient or family reporting is highly inaccurate. Blum et al. (17) used the video-EEG monitoring unit to evaluate reliability of patients' ability to identify their own seizures. Only 26% of the cohort was able to identify every seizure recorded by video-EEG, and 30% did not correctly identify any of their recorded seizures. More than 60% of complex partial seizures were not identified by patients. A particularly problematic finding was that the patients with the lowest seizures rates reported in outpatient visits had the greatest proportion of seizures that were not identified by them in monitoring unit.

After more than 10 years of absence of publications on this important aspect of epilepsy care, Hoppe et al. (18) replicated the earlier study, finding that patients in the video-EEG

monitoring unit were unable to report 73.2% of recorded complex partial seizures and 41.7% of secondarily generalized tonic–clonic seizures, as summarized in Table 95.1. Of seizures occurring while asleep, 85.8% were not reported. Only 25% of patients identified every complex partial seizure, and only 50% identified every generalized tonic–clonic seizure. A left-sided seizure onset, but not temporal or frontal lobe localization, was associated with documentation failure. Based on this innovative study, the authors concluded that "patient seizure counts do not provide valid information."

Akman et al. (19) recently completed a similar study of parental accuracy for seizure identification in their children. The parents were asked to stay with the child throughout the video-EEG recording, and press the event button for every definite seizure that they identified. Only 38% of the 1095 seizures recorded were correctly identified by parents.

ARE ADVERSE MEDICATION EFFECTS DETECTABLE?

Toxic effects of pharmacologic treatment of epilepsy have been recognized since early experiences with bromides, and several studies have quantified the severity or frequency of adverse events with common AEDs using reliable and valid measures. The VA Cooperative Studies (20,21) utilized a combination of subjective self-report with clinicians' physical examination findings to create a composite score in combination with seizure control. At the final 36-month outcome assessment in the VA Cooperative I trial, the composite scores were closer to the poor than the good outcome category for each of the study drugs (22). The authors concluded that "the outcome of this project underscores the unsatisfactory status of antiepileptic therapy with the medications currently available. Most patients whose epilepsy is reasonably controlled must tolerate some side effects. These observations emphasize the need for new AEDs and other approaches to treatment" (20). Furthermore, most studies that have included medication use in the predictors of health-related quality of life (HRQOL) have found an association of poorer QOL with seizure-free patients taking AEDs compared to seizure-free patients not taking AEDs (23). A large prospective study of immediate versus delayed treatment for epilepsy (MESS Trial) demonstrated

TABLE 95.1

DOCUMENTATION ACCURACY OF SEIZURES BY PATIENTS

Type of seizure	Total no. of seizures (video-EEG)	No. (%) undocumented by patient	SFPM video-EEG	SFPM patient report
CPS	347	254 (73.2)	22.0	0
Awake	150	79 (52.7)	15.9	6.5
Asleep	197	175 (88.8)	16.8	0
sGTCS	48	20 (41.7)	10.4	6.3
Awake	28	9 (32.1)	7.3	6.2
Asleep	20	11 (55.0)	9.4	4.0

CPS, complex partial seizure; sGTCS, secondarily generalized tonic–clonic seizure; SFPM, estimated seizure frequency per month.

that medication toxicity was significantly worse in the group with recurrent seizures while taking AEDs compared to all other groups (24).

The Commission on Outcome Measurement in Epilepsy (COME) reviewed available reliable and valid instruments, and specifically mentions the Adverse Events Profile (AEP) as a simple and accurate assessment (6). The items in the AEP were selected based on the results of small group interviews of patients taking AEDs. It contains 19 items that are brief descriptions of a subjective experience of a toxic medication effect. The instructions ask the person to rank the frequency of each adverse effect on a 1 to 4 Likert-like scale during the past 4 weeks. The psychometric properties of reliability and validity of the AEP are robust (25). In a European study including 15 countries and over 5000 participants, the AEP demonstrated that 40% to 50% of patients on the most common AEDs reported excessive tiredness, poor concentration, sleepiness, and/or memory problems (5). In another study, the AEP strongly correlated with HRQOL (partial $r = 0.61$; $P < 0.001$), independent of seizure rate (2). This observation was replicated in a multicenter study (partial $r = 0.60$; $P < 0.0001$) after controlling for depression symptoms (Fig. 95.2) (26).

To demonstrate the clinical utility of the AEP to improve outcomes in the outpatient treatment of epilepsy, a randomized trial compared the use of the AEP by clinicians to usual care without the AEP (3). In this 4-month trial, the group for which the treating neurologists had access to the AEP at each visit had a 24% reduction in AEP scores and was nearly threefold more likely to have a medication change or dosage adjustment. Improvement in the AEP was significantly associated with improvement in quality of life in epilepsy inventory (QOLIE-89) scores. This study demonstrated the importance of systematic screening in clinical

epilepsy care, and also of value of the quantification of medication toxicity in health outcomes research in epilepsy.

ARE COMORBID DEPRESSION AND/OR ANXIETY PRESENT?

The final report of the COME (6), a remarkable document that elucidated the need for more comprehensive, patient-oriented assessments of the results of epilepsy interventions. Interestingly, a major portion of the paper focused on the interictal state.

Although by definition, epilepsy is a condition characterized by brief paroxysmal disturbances of brain function, the supposition that between seizures every person with epilepsy reverts to a condition without epilepsy is obviously too optimistic. The mere need for uninterrupted AED therapy implies a risk of treatment-emergent adverse events (AEs). Symptomatic epilepsies are a comorbidity, with disorders affecting the brain and, as indicated by the label cryptogenic, probably many more epilepsies than those diagnosed as symptomatic fall into that category. The primary brain disorder itself may determine to a great extent the condition of the person with epilepsy in the interictal period. Accurate recording of the effects of comorbidity should not be limited to routine neurologic, psychological, and psychiatric examination, but should include a measure of quantification (6).

The COME final report deserves careful consideration of its recommendations to support both improved outcomes research and clinical care in epilepsy.

Similar to epilepsy, depression may be a term used for a variety of disorders with differing etiologies and complex interactions with social, vocational, and neuropsychological functioning. Depression is recognized as a common comorbid condition in persons with epilepsy, especially in tertiary care samples (27,28) and more recently in population (29,30) and community-based studies (31). Although interpretation of the literature on depression in epilepsy is complicated by varying ascertainment methods, definitions of depression, and sample characteristics, available estimates indicate that the prevalence of clinically relevant depression is 30% to 50% in persons with refractory epilepsy and 10% to 30% in controlled epilepsy. Additional support for the significance of depression in epilepsy includes the observation that suicide rates are significantly higher than the general population (32,33).

The etiology of depression in epilepsy is not fully understood and is very likely multifactorial, even on an individual level (7,34). However, specific psychological and neurologic factors have been associated with depression in epilepsy. Hermann et al. (35) performed a study based on the learned helplessness theory and found that a pessimistic attributional style was significantly associated with increased self-reported depression and remained significant when the effects of several confounding variables were controlled (age, age at epilepsy onset, laterality of temporal lobe epilepsy [TLE], sex, and method variance). Other investigators have found association of depression with brain abnormalities based on structural and functional imaging (7,22,36–40). For example, extent of abnormal creatine/N-acetyl aspartate (NAA) MR spectroscopic maps in the hippocampi of a sample of patients with refractory TLE strongly correlated with severity of depression symptoms (39). Less information is available regarding the neurobiology of anxiety symptoms and epilepsy (41,42).

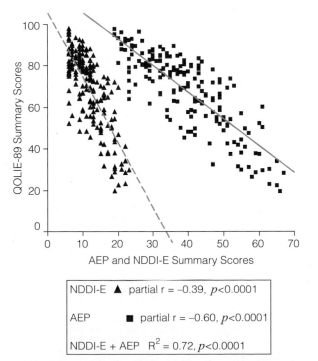

NDDI-E	▲	partial $r = -0.39$, $p < 0.0001$
AEP	■	partial $r = -0.60$, $p < 0.0001$
NDDI-E + AEP	$R^2 = 0.72$, $p < 0.0001$	

FIGURE 95.2 Comparison of severity of adverse medication effects and depression symptoms to quality of life in a large cohort of persons with epilepsy.

The importance of depression and anxiety in epilepsy is supported by their strong and consistent correlation with HRQOL, independent of seizure rates, in multiple clinical studies (2,4,41). A recent study of 200 epilepsy patients from five academic centers in the United States found that 72% of the variance in HRQOL was explained by reliable and valid measures of depression and adverse medication effects, shown in Figure 95.2 (26). Furthermore, depression is associated with increased health care utilization and costs in persons with epilepsy (25).

The optimal approaches to treatment of depression and anxiety in epilepsy have received relatively little attention compared to its impact on the epilepsy community. Several important issues must be considered, such as efficacy of antidepressant medications in the setting of epileptic brain dysfunction, additional adverse effects of antidepressants, and the unique social and vocational disabilities in epilepsy that may make cognitive and behavioral therapies particularly valuable (7). In 1985, Robertson and Trimble described the results of a randomized, double-blind comparison of amitriptyline, nomifesine, and placebo in 42 patients with depression and epilepsy (43). Although the mean scores of the Hamilton Depression Rating Scale and the Beck Depression Inventory scores improved by 50% after treatment, similar improvement in the placebo group resulted in no significant difference in outcome between any group at 6 weeks. A second 6-week treatment phase without placebo control compared higher doses of each drug (150 mg), and found that the nomifesine group had significantly better Hamilton Depression Rating Scale but not Beck Depression Inventory scores. The authors concluded "our results suggest that, in patients with depression and epilepsy, immediate prescription with antidepressants may not be indicated" (43). A more recent study compared the efficacy of citalopram, mirtazapine, and roboxetine in 75 subjects with TLE and major depression (44). Although each of the drugs was associated with significant reduction in depression symptoms at the 24- to 30-week assessment, mirtazapine had a higher dropout rate due to unacceptable side effects. Although the results indicate efficacy and differential tolerability of the antidepressants in TLE, only a small minority of the subjects achieved an improvement consistent with complete remission of depression. Similar to another study using sertraline (45), no significant increase in seizure was observed (44). Nonpharmacologic treatments for depression have not received adequate systematic evaluations to draw conclusions about efficacy in persons with epilepsy. Additional research is needed to provide the necessary evidence to guide optimal care of persons with epilepsy and comorbid depression and anxiety.

IS A SURGICALLY CORRECTABLE REGION IDENTIFIED BY HIGH-RESOLUTION MRI OR EEG?

The practice parameter on epilepsy surgery from the Quality Standards Subcommittee of the American Academy of Neurology (AAN) succinctly states that "a class I study and 24 class IV studies indicate that the benefits of anteromesial temporal lobe resection for disabling complex partial seizures is greater than continued treatment with AEDs, and the risks are at least comparable. For patients who are compromised by

such seizures, referral to an epilepsy surgery center should be strongly considered" (46). A recent publication in the *Journal of the American Medical Association* using decision-analysis methodology for temporal resection compared to continued medical therapy in persons who had failed at least two medications concluded that life expectancy is increased by 5 years (95% CI: 2.1 to 9.2 years) (47). The subset of patients with concordant lateralized interictal anterior temporal lobe sharp waves and mesial temporal sclerosis on MRI have a particularly favorable outcome, estimated to be between 75% and 89% in several large studies (48–50). The decision to perform surgery in neocortical epilepsy is less clear, especially in cases without a focal lesion on MRI. However, recent studies indicate that concordance of results of two or more of interictal EEG, ictal EEG, FDG-PET, or ictal SPECT predict a better than 60% chance for seizure freedom after epilepsy surgery in patients with a normal MRI (51).

The risk of recurrent seizures for life, injury, and QOL makes epilepsy surgery a treatment of choice for many persons for whom at least two medications have failed to fully control seizures. It is remarkable that the delay between onset of pharmacoresistant epilepsy and evaluation for potential surgery is >20 years in most studies, and does not appear to have decreased in the 5 years, since the AAN practice parameter was published (52). Identification of surgical candidates early in the course of their pharmacoresistance seems mandatory for optimal care. Therefore, high-resolution MRI with adequate fidelity to accurately identify mesial temporal sclerosis and video-EEG monitoring to evaluate interictal and ictal abnormalities should be considered as soon as pharmacoresistance is identified, because candidates with the best chance for long-term seizure freedom may not want to delay surgery or wait for a third, fourth, or fifth drug to fail. It is noteworthy that community-based MRI may not adequately assess for hippocampal sclerosis, with false negative rates >50% in some series (53).

SUMMARY

Epilepsy is a complex disorder with many different potential influences on an individual's health. This complexity creates challenges for the clinician in the outpatient clinic setting, especially considering common time and resource constraints. Organizing epilepsy care to efficiently confirm the diagnosis and syndromic classification, estimate as accurately as possible the actual seizure rate, systematically screen for adverse medication effects and comorbid depression, and identify pharmacoresistant epilepsy as early as possible can help ensure the best QOL for persons with epilepsy. Utilization of available reliable and valid screening tools and implementation of existing practice guidelines can support delivery of the most effective care for persons suffering the multifactorial disability of epilepsy.

References

1. Gilliam F, Penovich PE, Eagan CA, et al. Conversations between community-based neurologists and patients with epilepsy: results of an observational linguistic study *Epilepsy Behav.* 2009;16:315–320.
2. Gilliam F. Optimizing health outcomes in active epilepsy. *Neurology.* 2002;58:S9–S19.
3. Gilliam FG, Fessler AJ, Baker G, et al. Systematic screening allows reduction of adverse antiepileptic drug effects: a randomized trial. *Neurology.* 2004;62:23–27.

4. Boylan LS, Flint LA, Labovitz DL, et al. Depression but not seizure frequency predicts quality of life in treatment-resistant epilepsy. *Neurology.* 2004;62:258–261.
5. Baker GA, Jacoby A, Buck D, et al. Quality of life of people with epilepsy: a European study. *Epilepsia.* 1997;38:353–362.
6. Baker GA, Camfield C, Camfield P, et al. Commission on outcome measurement in epilepsy, 1994–1997: final report. *Epilepsia.* 1998;39: 213–231.
7. Gilliam FG, Santos J, Vahle V, et al. Depression in epilepsy: ignoring clinical expression of neuronal network dysfunction? *Epilepsia.* 2004; 45:28–33.
8. Vickrey BG. Getting oriented to patient-oriented outcomes [editorial; comment]. *Neurology.* 1999;53:662–663.
9. Vickrey BG, Hays RD, Rausch R, et al. Quality of life of epilepsy surgery patients as compared with outpatients with hypertension, diabetes, heart disease, and/or depressive symptoms. *Epilepsia.* 1994;35:597–607.
10. Baker GA. Quality of life and epilepsy: the liverpool experience. *Clin Ther.* 1998;20 (suppl A):A2–A12.
11. Benbadis SR, Tatum WO IV, Gieron M. Idiopathic generalized epilepsy and choice of antiepileptic drugs. *Neurology.* 2003;61:1793–1795.
12. Grunewald RA, Chroni E. Panayiotopoulos CP. Delayed diagnosis of juvenile myoclonic epilepsy. *J Neurol Neurosurg Psychiatry.* 1992;55:497–499.
13. LaFrance WC Jr. Psychogenic nonepileptic seizures. *Curr Opin Neurol.* 2008;21:195–201.
14. Krumholz A, Hopp J. Psychogenic (nonepileptic) seizures. *Semin Neurol.* 2006;26:341–350.
15. Martin RC, Gilliam FG, Kilgore M, et al. Improved health care resource utilization following video-EEG-confirmed diagnosis of nonepileptic psychogenic seizures. *Seizure.* 1998;7:385–390.
16. Eisenman LN, Attarian H, Fessler AJ, et al. Self-reported seizure frequency and time to first event in the seizure monitoring unit. *Epilepsia.* 2005;46:664–668.
17. Blum DE, Eskola J, Bortz JJ, et al. Patient awareness of seizures. *Neurology.* 1996;47:260–264.
18. Hoppe C, Poepel A, Elger CE. Epilepsy: Accuracy of patient seizure counts. *Arch Neurol.* 2007;64:1595–1599.
19. Akman CI, Montenegro MA, Jacob S, et al. Seizure frequency in children with epilepsy: factors influencing accuracy and parental awareness. *Seizure.* 2009;18:524–529.
20. Mattson RH, Cramer JA, Collins JF, et al. Comparison of carbamazepine, phenobarbital, phenytoin, and primidone in partial and secondarily generalized tonic–clonic seizures. *N Engl J Med.* 1985;313:145–151.
21. Mattson RH, Cramer JA, Collins JF, The Department of Veterans Affairs Epilepsy Cooperative Study No. 264 Group. A comparison of valproate with carbamazepine for the treatment of complex partial seizures and secondarily generalized tonic–clonic seizures in adults. *N Engl J Med.* 1992;327:765–771.
22. Theodore WH, Hasler G, Giovacchini G, et al. Reduced hippocampal 5HT1A PET receptor binding and depression in temporal lobe epilepsy. *Epilepsia.* 2007;48:1526–1530.
23. O'Donoghue MF, Goodridge DM, Redhead K, et al. Assessing the psychosocial consequences of epilepsy: a community-based study. *Br J Gen Pract.* 1999;49:211–214.
24. Jacoby A, Gamble C, Doughty J, et al. Medical Research Council MESS Study Group. Quality of life outcomes of immediate or delayed treatment of early epilepsy and single seizures. *Neurology.* 2007;68:1188–1196.
25. Cramer JA, Blum D, Fanning K, et al. The impact of comorbid depression on health resource utilization in a community sample of people with epilepsy. *Epilepsy Behav.* 2004;5:337–342.
26. Gilliam FG, Barry JJ, Hermann BP, et al. Rapid detection of major depression in epilepsy: a multicentre study. *Lancet Neurol.* 2006;5:399–405.
27. Mendez MF, Cummings JL, Benson DF. Depression in epilepsy: significance and phenomenology. *Arch Neurol.* 1986;43:766–770.
28. Jones JE, Hermann BP, Barry JJ, et al. Clinical assessment of axis I psychiatric morbidity in chronic epilepsy: a multicenter investigation. *J Neuropsychiatry Clin Neurosci.* 2005;17:172–179.
29. Gaitatzis A, Carroll K, Majeed A, et al. The epidemiology of the comorbidity of epilepsy in the general population. *Epilepsia.* 2004;45: 1613–1622.
30. Tellez-Zenteno JF, Patten SB, Jette N, et al. Psychiatric comorbidity in epilepsy: a population-based analysis. *Epilepsia.* 2007;48:2336–2344.
31. Ettinger A, Reed M, Cramer J. Depression and comorbidity in community-based patients with epilepsy or asthma. *Neurology.* 2004;63:1008–1014.
32. Jones JE, Hermann BP, Barry JJ, et al. Rates and risk factors for suicide, suicidal ideation, and suicide attempts in chronic epilepsy. *Epilepsy Behav.* 2003;(4 suppl 3):S31–S38.
33. Christensen J, Vestergaard M, Mortensen PB, et al. Epilepsy and risk of suicide: a population-based case-control study. *Lancet Neurol.* 2007;6:693–698.
34. Kanner AM. Depression in epilepsy: prevalence, clinical semiology, pathogenic mechanisms, and treatment. *Biol Psychiatry.* 2003;54:388–398.
35. Hermann BP, Trenerry MR, Colligan RC. Learned helplessness, attributional style, and depression in epilepsy. Bozeman epilepsy surgery consortium. *Epilepsia.* 1996;37:680–686.
36. Salzberg M, Taher T, Davie M, et al. Depression in temporal lobe epilepsy surgery patients: an FDG-PET study. *Epilepsia.* 2006;47:2125–2130.
37. Shamim S, Hasler G, Liew C, et al. Temporal lobe epilepsy, depression, and hippocampal volume. *Epilepsia.* 2009;50:1067–1071.
38. Lothe A, Didelot A, Hammers A, et al. Comorbidity between temporal lobe epilepsy and depression: a [18F]MPPF PET study. *Brain.* 2008;131: 2765–2782.
39. Gilliam FG, Maton BM, Martin RC, et al. Hippocampal 1H-MRSI correlates with severity of depression symptoms in temporal lobe epilepsy. *Neurology.* 2007;68:364–368.
40. Quiske A, Helmstaedter C, Lux S, et al. Depression in patients with temporal lobe epilepsy is related to mesial temporal sclerosis. *Epilepsy Res.* 2000;39:121–125.
41. Johnson EK, Jones JE, Seidenberg M, et al. The relative impact of anxiety, depression, and clinical seizure features on health-related quality of life in epilepsy. *Epilepsia.* 2004;45:544–550.
42. Kanner AM. Psychiatric issues in epilepsy: the complex relation of mood, anxiety disorders, and epilepsy. *Epilepsy Behav.* 2009;15:83–87.
43. Robertson MM, Trimble MR. The treatment of depression in patients with epilepsy. A double-blind trial. *J Affect Disord.* 1985;9:127–136.
44. Kuhn KU, Quednow BB, Thiel M, et al. Antidepressive treatment in patients with temporal lobe epilepsy and major depression: a prospective study with three different antidepressants. *Epilepsy Behav.* 2003;4:674–679.
45. Kanner AM, Kozak AM, Frey M. The use of sertraline in patients with epilepsy: is it safe? *Epilepsy Behav.* 2000;1:100–105.
46. Engel J Jr, Wiebe S, French J, et al. Practice parameter: temporal lobe and localized neocortical resections for epilepsy: report of the quality standards subcommittee of the American Academy of Neurology, in association with the American Epilepsy Society and the American Association of Neurological Surgeons. *Neurology.* 2003;60:538–547.
47. Choi H, Sell RL, Lenert L, et al. Epilepsy surgery for pharmacoresistant temporal lobe epilepsy: a decision analysis. *J Am Med Assoc.* 2008;300:2497–2505.
48. Gilliam F, Bowling S, Bilir E, et al. Association of combined MRI, interictal EEG, and ictal EEG results with outcome and pathology after temporal lobectomy. *Epilepsia.* 1997;38:1315–1320.
49. Radhakrishnan K, So EL, Silbert PL, et al. Predictors of outcome of anterior temporal lobectomy for intractable epilepsy: a multivariate study. *Neurology.* 1998;51:465–471.
50. Spencer SS, Berg AT, Vickrey BG, et al. Predicting long term seizure outcome after resective epilepsy surgery: the multicenter study. *Neurology.* 2005;65:912–918.
51. Lee SK, Lee SY, Kim KK, et al. Surgical outcome and prognostic factors of cryptogenic neocortical epilepsy. *Ann Neurol.* 2005;58:525–532.
52. Choi H, Carlino R, Heiman G, et al. Evaluation of duration of epilepsy prior to temporal lobe epilepsy surgery during the past two decades. *Epilepsy Res.* 2009;86:224–227.
53. McBride MC, Bronstein KS, Bennett B, et al. Failure of standard magnetic resonance imaging in patients with refractory temporal lobe epilepsy. *Arch Neurol.* 1998;55:346–348.

APPENDIX ■ INDICATIONS FOR ANTIEPILEPTIC DRUGS SANCTIONED BY THE UNITED STATES FOOD AND DRUG ADMINISTRATION

KAY C. KYLLONEN

Authors in this text have described uses of antiepileptic drugs based on clinical experience and results of clinical trials. In some cases, these clinical indications are broader than those sanctioned by the U.S. Food and Drug Administration (FDA) for product labeling.

To obtain specific FDA-approved indications, pharmaceutical companies present efficacy data from controlled clinical trials. If the data are judged scientifically sound, then the FDA may approve use of the drug for the specific types of patients and seizures studied in the trials. The approved indications are based only on the data presented by the pharmaceutical manufacturer and may not reflect all of the available research information. Once the indications are authorized by the FDA, the pharmaceutical manufacturers may not promote use of the drug for indications other than those specifically delineated in the labeling. However, this does not preclude the "off-label" use of these medications for other indications, including those discussed in this clinical text. By necessity, certain patient populations—most notably, children—are often treated outside of the labeled indications, because prior to recent FDA regulations, they were infrequently included in controlled clinical trials.

Antiepileptic medications mentioned in this text are listed in the following table with their FDA-approved epilepsy-related indications from the 2009 online editions of the *Pediatric Lexi-Drugs Online* (1), *MicroMedex* (2), or *Drug Facts and Comparisons* (3), all standard references for pharmacists. Some of the listed indications use outdated terminology because they were designated prior to the adoption of international standards for seizure and epilepsy classification. Some drugs not included in *Pediatric Lexi-Drugs Online*, *MicroMedex*, or *Drug Facts and Comparisons* are listed as investigational in the United States on the website *Inteleos* (4), which lists all currently investigational or recently approved drug applications filed by indication. Others are not yet in any part of the U.S. federal approval process and have been marked as "not listed" in the table.

Only four antiepileptics had specific FDA-approved pediatric indications listed in the 1999 *Physicians' Desk Reference* (5) or *Drug Facts and Comparisons* (6). At this writing, 20 medications carry specific FDA approval for pediatric indications. For many other antiepileptic drugs, use in children is implied in the approved product information by mentioning use in specific pediatric syndromes (e.g., infantile spasms or febrile seizures), by listing pediatric formulations (chewable tablets or elixirs), or by describing dosage schedules based on pediatric ages or body weights. The table also notes whether pediatric doses are listed in the any of the following: *DrugDex System*, *The Pediatric Lexi-Drugs Online*, or *Drug Facts and Comparisons*, regardless of whether or not the drug carries a specific FDA-approved pediatric indication. Dosing schedules are further discussed in "Part IV: Antiepileptic Medications" of this textbook; however, it is advisable to consult full prescribing information before clinical use.

References

1. Pediatric Drugs Online [database online], 2009. Available from: Lexicomp, Inc., accessed each anticonvulsant drug's monograph listed in table below. Last accessed on January 30, 2009.
2. Epilepsy treatment. In: MICROMEDEX [database online], 2009. Available from: Thomson MICROMEDEX. Last accessed on January 27, 2009.
3. CNS agents: anticonvulsants, and investigational drugs. In: *Drug Facts and Comparisons*, eFacts [database online], 2009. Available from Elsevier, Inc. Last accessed on January 27, 2009.
4. Epilepsy treatment. In: Inteleos [database online], 2009. Available from Wolters Kluwer Health, Inc. Last accessed on January 30, 2009.
5. Arky R (consultant). *Physicians' Desk Reference*. 53rd ed. Montvale, NJ: Medical Economics; 1999.
6. Olin BR, Hagemann RC, eds. *Drug Facts and Comparisons, 1999*. June update. St. Louis, MO: Facts and Comparisons; 1999.

Drug	Listed indications: seizure or epilepsy type	Pediatric dose	Pediatric labeling indication
Acetazolamide	Centrencephalic epilepsies (petit mal, unlocalized seizures)	Yes	
Brivaracetam	Adjunctive treatment of generalized epileptic syndrome in children of 1 month to 16 years of age; adjunctive treatment of partial onset seizures in adults; investigational in the United States		
Carbisamate	Adjunctive therapy for complex partial seizures, pending approval (1/09)		
Carbamazepine	Epilepsy—partial seizures with complex symptomatology (psychomotor, temporal lobe), generalized tonic–clonic seizures (grand mal), mixed seizures	Yes	Yes

(continued)

Drug	Listed indications: seizure or epilepsy type	Pediatric dose	Pediatric labeling indication
Clobazam	Investigational in the United States	Yes	
Clonazepam	Lennox–Gastaut syndrome (petit mal variant), akinetic and myoclonic seizures		
Clorazepate	Adjunctive therapy; management of partial seizures	Yes	≤9 years
Corticotropin	Infantile spasms, pending approval in the United States	Yes	
Diazepam	Status epilepticus, severe recurrent convulsive disorders	Yes	Yes (age >30 days parenteral)
Eslicarbazepine	Partial epilepsy, pending approval		
Ethosuximide	Absence (petit mal) epilepsy	Yes	Yes
Ethotoin	Tonic–clonic (grand mal) and complex partial seizures	Yes	Yes
Felbamate	Adjunctive therapy in Lennox–Gastaut syndrome, monotherapy for partial seizures in adults with epilepsy	Yes	Yes (age >2 years)
Fosphenytoin	Short-term treatment of acute seizures, including status epilepticus; prevention of seizures during and after neurosurgery; substitute for oral phenytoin	Yes	
Gabapentin	Adjunctive treatment of partial seizures with or without generalization	Yes	Yes (age >3 years)
IVIG—intravenous immunoglobulin	Intractable epilepsy (possible due to IgG2 subclass deficiency)	Yes	
Lamotrigine	Adjunctive treatment of partial seizures and Lennox–Gastaut syndrome	Yes	Yes (≥2 yrs)
Lacosamide	Partial onset seizures		
Levetiracetam	Treatment of partial seizures and primary generalized epilepsy	Yes	Yes (≥4 yrs)
Lorazepam	Status epilepticus	Yes	
Loreclezole	Not listed	Yes	
Mephenytoin	Withdrawn from market		
Mephobarbital	Grand mal and petit mal epilepsy	Yes	Yes
Metharbital	Not listed		
Methsuximide	Absence seizures refractory to other drugs	Yes	Yes
Midazolam	No FDA indication for seizure disorders		
Nitrazepam	Not available in the United States		
Oxcarbamazepine	Partial seizures	Yes	Yes (age ≥4 years)
Paraldehyde	Withdrawn from human use		
Paramethadione	Withdrawn from market	Yes	
Perampanel	Refractory seizures; partial onset seizure; investigational		
Phenacemide	Severe epilepsy, mixed forms of complex partial (psychomotor) seizures refractory to other drugs	Yes	Yes
Phenobarbital	Generalized and partial seizures, febrile seizures, status epilepticus	Yes	Yes
Phenytoin	Generalized tonic–clonic (grand mal) and complex partial (psychomotor, temporal lobe) seizures; prevention and treatment of seizures occurring during or following neurosurgery; status epilepticus	Yes	Yes
Pregabalin	Partial onset seizures in adults		
Primidone	Grand mal, psychomotor, and focal epileptic seizures	Yes	Yes (age >8 years)
Pyridoxine	Pyridoxine-dependent seizures	Yes	
Remacemide	Investigational in the United States		
Rufinamide	Lennox—Gastaut, complex partial onset seizures	Yes	
Seletracetam	Partial onset seizures, investigational in the United States		
Stiripentol	Adjunctive therapy for partial and generalized epilepsy, investigational in the United States	Yes	
Tiagabine	Adjunctive therapy for partial seizures	Yes	Yes (age ≥12 years)
Topiramate	Adjunctive therapy for partial seizures	Yes	Yes (age >2 years)
Trimethadione	Withdrawn from U.S. market		
Valproate	Simple and complex absence seizures; adjunctive therapy in multiple seizure types, including absence and complex partial seizures	Yes	
Vigabatrin	Adjunctive therapy for complex partial seizures	Yes	
Zonisamide	Adjunctive therapy for partial seizures	Yes	

INDEX

Page numbers followed by f indicate a figure; t following a page number indicates tabular material.